The Clinician's Guide to Dermatologic Differential Diagnosis

Paul I. Schneiderman · Marc E. Grossman

The Clinician's Guide to Dermatologic Differential Diagnosis

Second Edition

Volume II

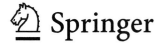

Springer

Paul I. Schneiderman
Clinical Professor of Dermatology
Columbia University
New York, NY
USA

Marc E. Grossman
Associate Clinical Professor of Dermatology
Department of Dermatology
Yale University School of Medicine
New Haven, CT
USA

Adjunct Clinical Professor of Dermatology
Department of Dermatology
Hofstra/Northwell Donald and
Barbara Zucker School of Medicine
New Hyde Park, NY
USA

ISBN 978-3-030-63526-8   ISBN 978-3-030-63527-5   (eBook)
https://doi.org/10.1007/978-3-030-63527-5

This Springer imprint is published by the registered company Springer Nature Switzerland AG
The registered company address is: Gewerbestrasse 11, 6330 Cham, Switzerland

There are a great number of people who made significant contributions to my personal and professional development, provided me with nurturing love and guidance, the opportunity to succeed, mentorship and encouragement, and valuable professional support which has enabled me to make a difference for my patients and my specialty. I am deeply grateful and indebted to them all. It is to these members of my life family that this book is lovingly dedicated.

Miriam and Morris Schneiderman
Steven and Arthur Schneiderman
Judy Schneiderman
Hyman Karmen
Arthur and Marcia Karmen
Etta and Louis Biblowitz
Iris and Jerry Schwartzbaum
Kenneth Barnett, PhD
Eric Tash
Bette Schneiderman
Andy and Scott Schneiderman
Judy and Morty Eydenberg
John J. Gullo, MD
Robert O. Knapp, MD
Frank Call, MD
Edward W. Hook, MD

Dwight Wooster, MD
David Stone, MD
Kenneth E. Greer, MD
Richard L. Edelson, MD
Barry S. Coller, MD
Edward P. Cawley, MD
Louis E. Harman, MD
Peyton E. Weary, MD
Larry Legum, MD
Steven R, Kohn, MD
Larry Bilsky, MD
Lindy Peta Fox, MD
Kristin Magnuson Nord, MD
Nicole LeBoeuf, MD
My co-author
Marc E. Grossman, MD, FACP

Paul I. Schneiderman

To Alexander and Natalie
For bringing pure joy to my life

Marc E. Grossman

Preface to the Second Edition

More than a decade has passed since the publication of the first edition of this textbook, *A Clinician's Guide to Dermatologic Differential Diagnosis*. In that period of time, the medical literature has expanded exponentially in print and online. We have updated, edited, and incorporated new material into all of the "old chapters" of the Text.

Almost a hundred additional new chapters have been added to the text. The expansion of topics was mostly the cutaneous manifestations of systemic disorders of the subspecialties of medicine and surgery for the adult and pediatric patient.

The atlas has been improved and expanded. All the new images are 20% larger, making them easier to visualize, with more emphasis on morphologic detail to increase diagnostic acumen. The fine points of the physical examination enable the pictures to do the teaching. This second edition atlas contains 6000 completely new and different images from the 4000 original non-digital photographs of the first edition. Some of the new illustrations are different views or perspectives of the diagnostic images, different time periods in the evolution of skin disease, or more complete images of the entire patient providing high-power and low-power or scanning views of the clinical disorder represented.

On a personal note, the atlas contains the only published photograph of the first case of cutaneous anthrax as a weapon of bioterrorism in New York City in 2001 (diagnosed, photographed, and treated by the author MG). Our collection of photographs of Nazi concentration camp serial identification number tattoos on the left forearms of survivors will outlive our patients and memorialize the Holocaust for the six million.

The original concepts, expectations, and usefulness of our textbook have been confirmed by its continued value as a reference in the hospital, in the classroom, and in the office by the seasoned practitioner, the resident, and medical student. The first edition passed the "use test."

The correct dermatologic diagnosis is essential for the treatment to be effective. Starting with a symptom, sign, or organ system dysfunction from the table of contents, a perusal of the differential diagnosis lists has successfully led us to a diagnosis we had not considered beforehand. The text provides the essential comprehensive differential diagnosis to avoid diagnostic traps and errors of dermatologic heuristics (cognitive shortcuts). The atlas augments visual observational skills by providing focused photographs of characteristic findings in common and exotic diseases. Common findings in rare diseases and rare or unusual findings in common diseases are illustrated as well as atypical locations for both. For the patient that defies diagnosis, going systematically through check lists of diseases ensures that none is missed before concluding that the patient has a new or undescribed disorder, or that the rash has not yet evolved into its recognizable form.

Writing and editing the "Red Books" have been as much self-education for us as teaching has been for us over the past 40 years. Education is a lifelong process augmented by historical perspective, remarkable one-case experiences, and gestalt/gut feeling/intuition.

Most of our dermatology resident and medical student teaching has been in the Washington Heights section of Manhattan at Columbia Presbyterian Medical Center; in New Haven, Connecticut, at Yale University School of Medicine; and in New Hyde Park, New York, at Hofstra/Northwell Donald and Barbara Zucker School of Medicine.

We expect that these companion volumes will be helpful in all clinical settings and used by all healthcare providers on the academic campus or in the community environment, anywhere in the world.

New York, NY, USA
New Haven, CT, USA

Paul I. Schneiderman
Marc E. Grossman

Contents

The Text

Volume I

Abdominal Pain, Cutaneous Manifestations 1

Abscess (Sterile and Non-sterile) 4

Acanthosis Nigricans-Like Lesions 11

Acidosis and Rash in the Newborn 15

Acneiform Eruptions 15

Acral Cyanosis 22

Acral Erythema and Scale With or Without Linear Cutoff 27

Acral Erythema 28

Acral Papules and Nodules; Knuckle Papules; Papules,
    Digital 32

Acrochordons (Skin Tags) 43

Acromegalic Features 43

Acro-Osteolysis 44

Adrenal Disease, Cutaneous Manifestations 45

Ainhum 45

Alopecia and Structural Abnormalities of the Nose and
    Hands 47

Alopecia, Eyebrows 48

Alopecia in Neonates, Infants, and Toddlers 52

Alopecia 54

Alveolar Hemorrhage 73

Angioedema 75

Angiokeratoma Corporis Diffusum 76

Annular Lesions of Penis with Surface Changes 77

Annular Lesions with Surface Changes 77

Annular Lesions Without Surface Changes 83

Annular Scars 90

Aortic Disease in the Young 91

Aphthous Stomatitis 92

Arthritis and Rash (Polyarthritis and Monoarthritis) 94

Aseptic Meningitis, Cutaneous Manifestations 107

Atrichia and Nail Abnormalities 107

Atrophic Glossitis 108

Atrophic Lesions 109

Autoinflammatory Diseases 126

Bariatric Surgery, Cutaneous Signs of Nutrient Deficiency ... 128

Basal Cell Carcinomas: Syndromes with Basal Cell
    Carcinomas 129

Bioweapons 129

"Black" Dermatologic Entities 130

Black Oral Lesions 134

Blaschko-esque Entities 134

Blindness, Cutaneous Manifestations 139

Blue Lunulae/Blue Nails 142

Blue Sclerae 143

Blue Spots 143

Blueberry Muffin Lesions, Neonate 153

Breast Asymmetry 154

Breast Cancer, Cutaneous Manifestations 154

Breast Hypertrophy (Gynecomastia) and Breast Masses 155

Breast Lesions 158

Buffalo Hump (Cervicodorsal Lipodystrophy) 161

Bullae and/or Vesicles 162

Bullae, Hemorrhagic 176

Bullae, Hemorrhagic, Septic 180

Bullae in Newborn 181

Bullae in Infants and Children 183

Bullae of the Fingers or Toes 187

Bullae, Transient, in Infants 190

Burning Tongue 190

Butterfly Rash 190

Café au lait macules (CALMs), Associations 195

Cardiac and/or Cardiovascular Disease and Skin Lesions 197

CDKN2A with p14 Loss 205

Cellulitis in the Immunocompromised Host 205

Cellulitis, INFECTIOUS, in the Immunocompetent Host 207

Cellulitis (Pseudocellulitis), Non-infectious Etiologies 207

Cerebriform Lesions 208

Chalky Material Extruded from Lesions 211

Cheilitis (Crusted Lips) 211

Chemotherapy, Cutaneous Manifestations 216

Chest Wall Tumors 219

Cleft Lip and/or Palate (Associated SKIN Disorders) 219

Coarse facies and Coarse Facial Skin 221

Cobblestone Appearance of Skin 222

Cobblestone Appearance of the Oral Mucosa 227

Cocaine Use, Cutaneous Manifestations 230

Concentric Lesions 230

Conjunctival Lesions, Pigmented 231

Craniosynostosis 231

Cutaneous Horns 231

Cutis Laxa-Like Appearance... 233
Cutis Verticis Gyrata 236
Cysts with or Without Drainage 238
Deafness or Hearing Impairment, Cutaneous Manifestations 243
Dermatitis (Spongiotic Dermatitis), Differential Diagnosis 248
Dermatitis, Facial, Pediatric.. 258
Dermatitis, Periorbital 261
Dermatitis, Periorificial 263
Dermatographism... 267
Desmoplakin Mutations.. 268
Diabetes Mellitus, Cutaneous Manifestations..................... 268
Diarrhea, Cutaneous Manifestations 269
Dimples.. 274
Doughy Skin 275
Drug Abuse, Cutaneous Manifestations 276
Dyschromatosis (Hypopigmentation and
   Hyperpigmentation)... 278
Dyshidrosis 282
Ear, Hard (Petrified Auricles) 284
Ear Lesions 285
Ears, Red, with or Without Nodules.............................. 296
Edema 299
Edema, Hands.. 307
Edema, Head 311
Edema, Legs 312
Erosions (Superficial Ulcers) 317
Erythrodermas (Exfoliative Erythroderma) 323
Erythrodermic Infant 329
Eschars... 332
Esophageal and Cutaneous Disease 334
Exanthem 336
Exfoliation (Desquamation) 347
Eyelid Lesions 350
Eyes, Red and Rash... 363
Facial Asymmetry 375
Facial Dermatitis, Scaly 375
FACIAL EDEMA... 378
Facial Papules and Plaques.. 382
Facial Papules 385
Facial Plaques, Scarring and Non-scarring 395
Facial Scars.. 400
Facial Ulcers 402
Facies 405
Fetal Akinesia Deformation Sequence 420
Fever and Rash, Noninfectious 421
Fever, Arthritis, and Exanthem 423
Fibromatoses in Children.. 427
Fibrous Tumors, Differential Diagnosis........................... 428
Figurate Erythemas 428
Fingertip Lesions 429
Fingertip Necrosis 432
Fingertip Ulcers 434
Flushing Disorders.. 436

Follicular Plugging 441
Foot Ulcers 442
Freckling of Hands... 444
Gastrointestinal Cancer and Skin Lesions...................... 445
Gastrointestinal Hemorrhage and Skin Lesions 445
Gastrointestinal Polyposis and Skin 446
Gingival Hyperplasia... 446
Gingivitis 450
Glomerulonephritis, Cutaneous Manifestations................. 454
Granulomas 455
Granulomatosis with Polyangiitis, Cutaneous Manifestations 456
Green Pigmentation.. 456
Hair Abnormalities 458
Hair Breakage.. 459
Hair Shaft Nodules or Nits (Particulate Matter) 461
Hair, Premature Graying.. 461
Heart Block and Rash... 463
Heart Failure, Cutaneous Manifestations 464
Heliotrope 465
Hematologic Malignancies, Cutaneous Signs 466
Hemihypertrophy (Asymmetric Overgrowth Syndromes)...... 467
Herpetiform Lesions 469
Heterochromia Iridum (IRIDIS)....................................... 471
Hoarseness, Cutaneous Manifestations........................... 471
Human Papilloma Virus-Associated Immunodeficiency
   Syndromes 473
Hyperhidrosis... 474
Hyperkeratotic Lesions 479
Hyperkeratotic Lesions of Feet...................................... 489
Hyperkeratotic Lesions of the Hands.............................. 493
Hyperkeratotic Papules of the Nipple 497
Hyperpigmentation in Blaschko's Lines........................... 498
Hyperpigmentation, Diffuse 499
Hyperpigmentation, Flagellate.. 503
Hyperpigmentation, Paronychial...................................... 503
Hyperpigmentation, Patchy 504
Hyperpigmentation, Segmental or Zosteriform.................. 513
Hyperpigmented Lesions, Discrete Annular 514
Hypertrichosis, Generalized 519
Hypertrichosis, Localized... 522
Hypohidrosis (Anhidrosis).. 531
Hypopigmented Patches or Plaques 537
Hypoplasia of Distal Phalanges..................................... 544
Hypotrichosis with Growth and Mental Retardation........... 545
Ichthyosiform Eruptions 546
Immune Deficiency Syndromes with Bacterial Infections...... 555
Inguinal Lymphadenitis and Rash 558
Intertrigo, Including Diaper Dermatitis 560
Iris Lesions, Pigmented 566
Islands of Sparing.. 566
Kaposi's Sarcoma, Differential Diagnosis......................... 568
Kinky Hair 569
Knuckle Papules... 569

Knuckles, Pebbly, with Scarring 572

Lacrimal Gland, Enlarged 573

Lentigines 573

Leonine Facies 576

Leukoderma, Guttate 578

Leukonychia 578

Leukoplakia 580

Linear Erythronychia.. 583

Linear Hypopigmentation.. 583

Linear Lesions 584

Linear Lesions Following Veins 596

Lip Lesions, Pigmented 599

Lip Papules.. 600

Lip Pits... 603

Lipoma Syndromes... 604

Lips, Swollen 605

Lithium, Cutaneous Side Effects 610

Livedo Reticularis with or Without Necrosis 610

Liver Disease, Cutaneous Manifestations and Hepatic
     Abnormalities of Skin Disease 617

Lymphadenopathy for the Dermatologist.............................. 622

Macrocephaly 627

Macrodactyly (Enlarged Digit) 628

Malodorous Skin Conditions... 633

Marfanoid Features 634

Masses of the Head and Neck 635

Melanoma, Clinical Simulators 639

Melanonychia 640

Microcephaly 642

Micronychia and Anonychia.. 646

Midline Facial Nodules of Children 648

Midline Nasal Mass 648

Milia or Milia-Like Lesions (Fine White Papules).................. 649

Monoclonal Gammopathy, Cutaneous Manifestations 652

Mucinoses 653

Mucocutaneous Candidiasis Syndromes 654

Muscle Weakness and Rash 654

Myocarditis, Cutaneous Manifestations................................ 657

Volume II

Nail Abnormalities.. 659

Nasal Infiltration or Enlargement.. 666

Nasal Septal Ulcerations/Perforations
     (Rhinophagic Ulceration) 670

Neck Lesions... 673

Neck Papules 682

Necrosis... 686

Neural Tube Dysraphism.. 699

Nevi, Associated Syndromes.. 699

Nipple Dermatitis 702

Nipple Lesions, Including Areola with Multiple Papules......... 703

No Fingerprint Syndromes (Adermatoglyphia, Absent
     Dermatoglyphics) 708

Nodules, Congenital 708

Nodules, Foot... 710

Nodules, Juxta-Articular 713

Nodules, Knee 716

Nodules, Multilobulated 717

Nodules, Multiple, Subcutaneous... 723

Nodules, Red, Extremities.. 727

Nodules, Red, Face.. 740

Nodules, Red, Hand 744

Nodules, Red or Violaceous, Vascular Appearance 746

Nodules, Skin Colored 756

Nodules, Ulcerated 769

Nodules, Unspecified Location 775

Normal Skin (Barely Perceptible Plaque) 779

Obesity Syndromes/Protuberant Abdomen 781

Onycholysis.. 781

Oral Mucosal Hyperpigmentation 784

Oral Mucosa, Blue Pigmentation 787

Oral Mucosa, Cysts 788

Oral Mucosa, Nodules 789

Oral Mucosa, Ulceration 794

Oral Mucosa, Verrucous and Vegetating Lesions................. 803

Osteoma Cutis.. 804

Overgrowth Syndromes.. 805

P63-Associated Disorders 807

Painful Tumors... 807

Palatal Necrosis (Necrotic Ulcers of the Palate)................... 808

Palmar and/or Plantar Erythema 809

Palmar and/or Plantar Nodules 813

Palmar Pits and Punctate Keratoses/Dyshidrosis-Like
     Lesions... 814

Palmoplantar Keratodermas 818

Palmoplantar Keratoderma with Atrichia or Hypotrichosis..... 831

Papules, Crusted 831

Papules, Digital.. 836

Papules, Dirty Brown 841

Papules, Distal Digital, White 842

Papules, Solitary Facial 842

Papules, Flat-Topped.. 844

Papules, Follicular (Folliculocentric, Including Folliculitis)..... 848

Papules, Hyperkeratotic 857

Papules, Hyperpigmented with Hypertrichosis (Hyperpigmented
     Hairy Papules) 864

Papules and Nodules, Hyperpigmented (with or Without
     Hyperkeratosis).. 865

Papules, Periorbital 870

Papules, Red 872

Papules, Skin Colored 884

Papulosquamous Eruptions.. 887

Paraneoplastic Dermatoses 889

Paraproteinemias, Cutaneous Manifestations...................... 892

Parathyroid Disease, Cutaneous Manifestations.................. 893

Paronychia... 894

Parotid Gland Enlargement 898

Particulate Matter/Exfoliation............................... 901

Pedunculated (Polypoid) Lesions.......................... 902

Penile Edema, Acute and Chronic......................... 907

Penile Lesions 908

Penile Ulcers 916

Perianal Dermatitis and Hypertrophic Plaques...... 918

Perianal Ulcers, Single or Multiple....................... 922

Periorbital Edema/Erythema (Dermatitis)............. 925

Periorbital Congenital Nodules, Pediatric............. 933

Periostitis... 933

Peripheral Eosinophilia....................................... 934

Peripheral Neuropathy, Cutaneous Manifestations ... 936

Phakomatoses.. 939

Pharyngitis... 948

Photoeruption and Seborrheic Dermatitis-Like Eruption ... 951

Pigmentary Retinopathy or Cone-Rod Dystrophy with
    Dermatologic Manifestations........................... 965

Pituitary Disease, Cutaneous Manifestations 966

Pityriasis Rosea-Like Eruptions........................... 967

Exogenous Agents.. 968

Infections and Infestations.................................. 968

Plantar Erythema 969

Pneumonia and Pneumonia-Associated Disease, Cutaneous
    Manifestations... 971

Poikilodermas of Adulthood................................. 978

Poikilodermas of Childhood................................. 979

Poliosis, Localized or Generalized (Canities)......... 980

Polydactyly (PPD, PAP, and Complex Types) 982

Pore.. 983

Port Wine Stain.. 984

Preauricular Sinuses (Ear Pits) 985

Pregnancy, Cutaneous Manifestations 986

Premature Aging Syndromes (Progeroid Syndromes) 987

Primary Immunodeficiencies with Granuloma Formation 989

Proptosis... 989

Pruritic Tumors 990

Pruritus, Anal 991

Pruritus, Erythematous Papules 992

Pruritus, Generalized, Without Primary Skin Lesions........... 994

Pruritus, Vulvar 998

Pseudoxanthoma Elasticum-Like Changes........... 999

Psoriasiform Dermatitis 1000

Psoriasiform Plaque, Focal or Solitary 1006

Pterygium (Webbing)... 1008

Pterygium of the Nail 1008

Puberty, Delayed (Hypogonadism)........................ 1010

Puberty, Premature... 1013

Pulmonary Disease Associated with Skin Disease... 1015

Pulsatile Papules 1021

Punctate and Reticulate Hyperpigmentation 1021

Purpura... 1023

Purpura, Neonatal 1040

Purpuric Rash and Fever..................................... 1041

Pustular and Vesicopustular Eruptions in the Newborn......... 1046

Pustules and Pustular Eruptions of the Palms and Soles 1048

Pustules and Pustular Eruptions 1049

Red Chest.. 1061

Red Elbow 1062

Red Face 1063

Red Feet.. 1068

Red Nose... 1071

Red Patch.. 1074

Red Plaque.. 1085

Red Scrotum.. 1100

Redundant Skin 1101

Renal Failure, Cutaneous Manifestations.............. 1104

Renal Tumor, Cutaneous Manifestations............... 1109

Reticulated Eruptions 1110

Reticulated Hyperpigmentation 1116

Rhinophymatous Eruptions 1119

Rippling of Skin.. 1119

Rosette Lesions 1119

Saddle Nose Deformity.. 1121

Scalp Cysts.. 1121

Scalp Dermatitis 1123

Scalp Nodules 1126

Scalp Poliosis 1135

Scalp, Red Plaques... 1135

Scarring of Neck 1136

Scars, Lesions in Scars....................................... 1137

Sclerodermoid Changes 1140

Scrotal Nodules with Erosions............................. 1147

Scrotal Papules and Nodules 1148

Scrotal Ulcerations... 1150

Serpiginous Lesions 1152

Short Stature 1158

Sickle Cell Disease, Cutaneous Manifestations 1169

Sinus Tracts... 1170

Spiky Skin.. 1173

Spinal Dysraphism (Cutaneous Stigmata)............. 1173

Splinter Hemorrhages.. 1174

Sporotrichoid Lesions 1174

Spotty Pigmentation of the Face 1176

Striae Distensae (Stretch Marks).......................... 1176

Stroke Syndromes, Cutaneous Manifestations 1177

Swollen Calf... 1178

Syndactyly 1179

Synophrys.. 1183

Tails 1184

Tall Stature Syndromes 1184

Target Lesions 1184

Tattoo, Palpable/Lesions in a Tattoo...................... 1189

Teeth... 1191

Telangiectasias 1199

Testicular Enlargement.. 1206

Thumbs.. 1207

Thyroid Disease, Cutaneous Manifestations.......... 1207

Tongue, Enlarged (Macroglossia)........................ 1209
Tongue, Hyperpigmentation............................... 1213
Tongue, Multilobulated..................................... 1214
Tongue Necrosis (Lingual Necrosis).................... 1216
Tongue Nodules, Solitary.................................. 1216
Tongue, Red... 1217
Tongue, Scrotal (Plicated Tongue, Fissured Tongue)........... 1219
Tongue, Ulcers.. 1220
Trichomegaly... 1222
Tropical Fever And Rash.................................. 1224
Tumors, Giant.. 1227
Ulcers, Leg... 1233
Ulcers, Leg, in a Young Patient.......................... 1239
Ulcers.. 1242
Umbilical Lesions.. 1255
Umbilical Nodules.. 1259
Umbilicated Lesions....................................... 1261
Unilateral Foot Edema..................................... 1265
Urticaria and Urticaria-Like Lesions..................... 1265
Uveitis, Cutaneous Manifestations....................... 1273
Uvula, Enlarged.. 1275
Valvular Heart Disease, Cutaneous Manifestations......... 1277
Vasculitis, Granulomatous................................ 1278
Vasculitis, Leukocytoclastic.............................. 1278
Vasculitis, Thrombotic.................................... 1280
Vasculitis, Types.. 1281
Vegetating Lesions.. 1282
Verrucous Lesions of the Legs............................ 1284
Verrucous Lesions, Periungual............................ 1285
Verrucous Plaques... 1286
Vulva, Hypertrophic, and/or Edematous Lesions.......... 1293
Vulvar Edema.. 1296
Vulvar Erythema With or Without Pruritus................ 1297
Vulvar Papules and Nodules.............................. 1299
Vulvar Ulcers.. 1303
White Feet... 1307
White Macules... 1307
White Papules, Nodules, and Plaques.................... 1314
Woolly Hair.. 1318
Xanthomatous Lesions.................................... 1320
Xerosis, Associations and Causes........................ 1320
Yellow Nails... 1325
Yellow or Skin-Colored Papules of the Neck............. 1325
Yellow Papules and Plaques.............................. 1327
Yellow Plaque... 1332
Yellow Skin (Xanthoderma)............................... 1334
Zebra Stripes.. 1337
Zosteriform Lesions/Segmental Disorders................ 1340

The Atlas

Volume III

Abscess.. 1346
Acanthosis Nigricans-Like Lesions....................... 1353

Acneiform Lesions... 1355
Acral Bullae... 1368
Acral Cyanosis.. 1369
Acral Erythema.. 1374
Acral Erythema and Scale................................ 1377
Acral Necrosis.. 1379
Acral Nodules... 1380
Acral Papules... 1383
Acral Papules and Nodules............................... 1396
Acral Pits... 1397
Acromegalic Features..................................... 1397
Ainhum.. 1398
Alopecia... 1400
Alopecia of the Eyebrows................................. 1410
Angioedema... 1411
Annular Lesions of the Penis............................. 1411
Annular Lesions with Scars............................... 1412
Annular Lesions with Surface Change..................... 1412
Annular Lesions Without Surface Change.................. 1423
Aphthae... 1431
Arthritis and Rash.. 1433
Atrophic Glossitis... 1440
Atrophy... 1442
Black Lesions... 1452
Blaschko-Esque Entities.................................. 1458
Blue Spots.. 1465
Blueberry Muffin Lesions, Neonate....................... 1477
Breast Asymmetry... 1477
Breast Lesions.. 1478
Bullae... 1485
Bullae in Children... 1498
Bullae in Children, Acral................................. 1498
Bullae, Fingers and Toes.................................. 1499
Bullae, Giant.. 1502
Bullae, Hemorrhagic...................................... 1508
Bullae, Hemorrhagic Septic............................... 1514
Bullae, Neonatal.. 1518
Butterfly Rash... 1518
Cafe au lait macules, Associations....................... 1530
Cellulitis-Like Lesions.................................... 1530
Cerebriform Lesions....................................... 1532
Cheilitis, Including Swollen Lips......................... 1534
Clitoromegaly... 1544
Clubbing.. 1545
Cobblestoned Oral Mucosa................................ 1546
Cobblestoned Skin.. 1548
Cocaine Abuse.. 1561
Columbia Presbyterian Medical Center................... 1563
Concentric Lesions.. 1563
Conjunctivae, Hyperpigmented............................ 1564
Conjunctivae, Red... 1565
Covid-19 Rashes.. 1567
Crix Belly... 1569
Cushingoid Appearance................................... 1569

Cutaneous Horn 1571

Cutis Laxa-Like Appearance 1573

Cysts 1575

Dermatitis 1579

Dermatitis of Hands or Feet 1587

Dermatitis of the Palms 1590

Dermatitis, Facial, Adult 1592

Dermatitis, Facial, Pediatric 1601

Dermatitis, Fingertips 1605

Dermatitis, Perianal 1606

Dermatitis, Periorificial, Adult 1606

Dermatitis, Periorificial, Pediatric 1610

Desquamatian (Exfoliation) 1611

Dimples 1616

Dyschromatosis 1618

Dyshidrosiform Lesions 1621

Ear Lesions 1626

Ear, Hard 1634

Ear, Red 1636

Ear, Swollen 1638

Edema 1639

Edema of Fingers or Toes 1642

Edema of the Foot 1645

Edema of the Hands 1648

Edema of the Legs 1653

Elbow Plaques 1656

Enanthem 1657

Erosions 1658

Erythroderma 1669

Erythroderma in Infancy 1680

Eschar 1682

Exanthem 1684

Exophthalmos 1700

Eyelid Lesions 1701

Eyes, Red 1711

Facial Asymmetry 1718

Facial Edema 1723

Facial Papules 1735

Facial Papules and Plaques 1744

Facial Plaques 1748

Facial Scars 1756

Facial Ulcer 1759

Facies 1765

Fever and Rash 1785

Filiform Lesions 1786

Fingertip Lesions 1786

Fingertip or Toetip Necrosis 1791

Fingertip or Toetip Ulcer 1796

Fissures 1798

Flagellate 1798

Flushing 1799

Foot Ulcers 1804

Gingival Hyperplasia 1806

Gingivitis 1807

Green Skin 1809

Hair Nodules (Particulate Matter) 1812

Hair, Unruly 1812

Hemihypertrophy 1814

Herpetiform Lesions 1815

Hyperelastic Skin 1818

Hyperkeratotic Lesions 1819

Hyperkeratotic Lesions of Feet 1828

Hyperkeratotic Lesions of Hands 1831

Hyperpigmentation, Discrete Annular 1833

Hyperpigmentation, Generalized 1839

Hyperpigmentation, Patchy 1845

Hyperpigmented Plaques 1849

Hypertrichosis, Generalized 1851

Hypertrichosis, Localized 1851

Hypopigmented Papules 1855

Hypopigmented Patches 1856

Ichthyosiform Eruptions 1860

Intertrigo 1871

Iris lesions, Pigmented 1881

Islands of Sparing 1882

Knee Lesions 1885

Knuckle Papules 1885

Koilonychia 1891

Lacrimal Gland Enlargement 1892

Lentigines 1893

Leonine Facies 1896

Leukonychia 1898

Leukoplakia 1900

Linear Lesions 1904

Linear Lesions Over Veins or Lymphatics 1914

Lip Lesions 1919

Lip Papules 1920

Lip Pigmentation 1922

Lip Ulcer 1923

Livedo Reticularis With or Without Necrosis 1924

Lymphadenopathy 1933

Volume IV

Macrocephaly 1936

Macrodactyly 1937

Macromano 1939

Marfanoid Features 1940

Melanoma Mimickers 1943

Melanonychia 1943

Micronychia and Anonychia 1944

Milia 1947

Mountain Range Lesions 1949

Nails 1956

Nails, Hyperkeratotic 1964

Nasal Destruction, Septal Perforation, or Ulcerations . 1967

Nasal Infiltration and/or Enlargement 1968

Neck Lesions 1970
Neck Papules 1979
Necrosis 1981
Nevi 1999
Nipple Dermatitis 1999
Nipple Lesions 2000
Nodules of the Elbows 2004
Nodules of the Foot 2004
Nodules of the Hands 2006
Nodules of the Knee 2007
Nodules, Juxtaarticular 2007
Nodules, Multilobulated 2010
Nodules, Multiple Subcutaneous 2017
Nodules, Purple Plum 2018
Nodules, Red 2020
Nodules, Red, of the Extremities 2021
Nodules, Red, of the Face 2032
Nodules, Red, of the Hand 2037
Nodules, Skin Colored 2038
Nodules, Ulcerated 2044
Nodules, Vascular Appearance 2052
Normal Skin (Barely Perceptible Lesions) 2058
Onycholysis 2060
Oral Mucosa, Red Plaques 2061
Oral Mucosa, Ulceration 2062
Oral Mucosal Pigmentation 2065
Oral Nodules 2066
Oral Vegetative Lesions 2068
Palmar and/or Plantar Pits and Punctate Keratoses 2069
Palmar Erythema 2071
Palmoplantar Keratoderma 2074
Papules and Nodules, Hyperpigmented 2081
Papules, Crusted 2085
Papules, Dirty Brown 2089
Papules, Flat-Topped 2089
Papules, Follicular 2092
Papules, Hyperkeratotic 2101
Papules, Red 2104
Papulosquamous Eruptions 2114
Papulovesicles 2119
Paraneoplastic Disorders 2119
Paronychia 2120
Parotid Gland Enlargement 2123
Particulate Matter 2124
Peau d'orange 2125
Pebbly Skin 2128
Pedunculated Lesions 2128
Penile Lesions 2130
Penile Ulcers 2137
Perianal Ulcers, Single or Multiple 2138
Perianal Dermatitis 2140
Perianal Nodules 2144
Periarticular Erythema 2144

Perifollicular Erythema 2145
Periorbital Edema, Erythema 2145
Periorbital Papules 2151
Photodermatitis – Seborrheic Dermatitis 2152
Pityriasis Rosea-Like 2167
Plantar Nodules 2171
Poikilodermas, Childhood and Adulthood 2172
Pore 2173
Pruritus Without Rash 2174
Pseudoxanthoma Elasticum-Like Changes 2177
Psoriasiform Dermatitis 2179
Psoriasiform Plaque, Solitary or Localized 2190
Pterygium of the Nails 2194
Pterygium Unguis Inversum 2195
Purpura 2195
Purpura in the Neonate 2209
Purpura of the Face 2210
Purpura with Fever 2211
Pustular Eruptions 2216
Pustular Eruptions of Infancy 2225
Pustular Eruptions of the Face 2226
Pustular Eruptions of the Neonate 2228
Pustular Eruptions of the Palms and Soles 2229
Red Elbow 2232
Red Face 2234
Red Feet 2255
Red Hand 2259
Red Knee 2260
Red Leg 2260
Red Lunula 2261
Red Nose 2261
Red Patch 2263
Red Plaque 2269
Red scrotum 2281
Redundant Skin 2283
Reticulated 2284
Reticulated Hyperpigmentation 2288
Rosette Lesions 2290
Scalp Dermatitis 2292
Scalp Nodules 2297
Scalp Ulcers 2302
Scalp, Red Plaques 2305
Scars, Lesions in Scars 2306
Sclerodermoid Changes 2315
Scrotal Edema 2320
Scrotal Papules and Nodules 2321
Scrotal Ulcers 2323
Serpiginous Lesions 2325
Short Stature 2334
Sinus Tracts 2335
Sporotrichoid Pattern 2338
Stellate Lesions 2340
Strange But True 2341

Striae 2342

Syndactyly 2343

Targetoid Lesions 2345

Tattoos 2350

Tattoos, Concentration Camp 2354

Teeth, Abnormalities 2355

Telangiectasias 2358

Tongue Hyperpigmentation........................... 2362

Tongue Lesions 2362

Tongue Papules 2363

Tongue Ulcers.. 2365

Tongue, Enlarged (Macroglossia) 2370

Tongue, Multilobulated................................. 2371

Tongue, Red 2372

Trichomegaly 2374

Tumors, Giant 2374

Ulcers 2381

Ulcers of the foot 2386

Ulcers of the hand 2390

Ulcers of the Leg 2391

Umbilical lesions.. 2399

Umbilicated lesions... 2402

Urticaria and Urticarial-Like Lesions................... 2408

Uvula 2414

Vegetative Plaques 2415

Verrucous Plaques 2417

Vulvar Edema 2424

Vulvar Erythema 2425

Vulvar Hyperpigmentation 2426

Vulvar Hypertrophic Lesions............................... 2426

Vulvar Hypertrophic Plaques 2426

Vulvar Papules and Nodules 2428

Vulvar Ulcers 2428

Wallace's Line.. 2432

White Macules or Patches................................... 2433

White Papules, Nodules, or Plaques 2440

Xerosis.. 2449

Yellow Papules and Nodules 2452

Yellow Skin 2456

Zebra Stripes... 2459

Zosteriform Eruptions 2465

Index... 2475

NAIL ABNORMALITIES

BJD 173:922–979, 2015

AUTOIMMUNE DISEASES AND DISORDERS OF IMMUNE DYSREGULATION

APECED syndrome *BJD 178:335–349, 2018*

Chronic mucocutaneous candidiasis – crusted plaques, cicatricial alopecia, leukoplakia, dystrophic nails *Ped Derm 34:609–611, 2017*

Dectin-1 deficiency – candidiasis of nails *BJD 178:335–349, 2018*

Epidermolysis bullosa acquisita – nail dystrophy *BJD 171:1022–1030, 2014*

Gain of function *STAT1* mutations – chronic mucocutaneous candidiasis; onychodystrophy, generalized dermatophytosis; disseminated coccidioidomycosis, histoplasmosis, sinopulmonary infections, herpes simplex infections; endocrine, dental, gastrointestinal disease; diabetes mellitus, hypothyroidism, autoimmune hepatitis, cerebral aneurysms, oral and esophageal squamous cell carcinomas; increased levels of interferon results in decreased IL-17A and IL-22 *JAAD 73:255–264, 2015*

Graft vs host disease – pterygium unguis inversum *J Eur Acad DV 33:637–642, 2019*

Hyper IgE syndrome – candida of nails; retained primary teeth leading to double rows of teeth; lack of eruption of secondary teeth, delayed resorption of roots of primary teeth *BJD 178:335–349, 2018; JAAD 60:289–298, 2009; JAAD 54:855–865, 2006*

Lupus erythematosus, systemic – pterygium; pterygium unguis inversum *J Drugs Dermatol 12:344–346, 2013;* melanonychia *JAAD 47:S187–188, 2002;* pincer nails *Lupus 26:1562–1563, 2017*

Rheumatoid arthritis – red lunulae

Sclerederma – trachyonychia, scleronychia, thickened nails, brachyonychia, parrot beaking, pterygium unguis inversum, splinter hemorrhages *JAAD 76:1115–1123, 2017*

STAT1 gain of function mutation – most common cause of chronic mucocutaneous candidiasis; demodicidosis with facial papulopustular eruptions, blepharitis, chalazion, dermatitis of the neck, nail dystrophy, congenital candidiasis *Ped Derm 37:159–161, 2020*

STING-associated vasculopathy with onset in infancy (SAVI) (type 1 interferonopathy) – red plaques of face and hands; chilblain-like lesions; atrophic plaques of hands, telangiectasias of cheeks, nose, chin, lips, acral violaceous plaques and acral cyanosis (livedo reticularis of feet, cheeks, and knees), distal ulcerative lesions with infarcts (necrosis of cheeks and ears), gangrene of fingers or toes with ainhum, nasal septal perforation, nail dystrophy; small for gestational age; paratracheal adenopathy, abnormal pulmonary function tests; interstitial lung disease with fibrosis with ground glass and reticulate opacities; gain of function mutation in *TMEM173* (stimulator of interferon genes); mimics granulomatosis with polyangiitis *Ped Derm 33:602–614, 2016; JAMADerm 151:872–877, 2015; NEJM 371:507–518, 2014*

T-cell immunodeficiency, congenital alopecia, and nail dystrophy *Clin in Dermatol 23:47–55, 2005*

CONGENITAL DISORDERS

Congenital malalignment of the great toenail – thickened nails *J Cut Med Surg 13:276–279, 2009*

Congenital malalignment of the great toenails *Dermatol Surg 45:1211–1213, 2019; Clin Exp Dermatol 8:619–623, 1983; Clin Exp Dermatol 4:309–313, 1979*

Congenital onychodysplasia of the index finger *Genetic Skin Disorders, Second Edition, 2010, pp.244*

Congenital paramedian canaliform dystrophy – personal observation

DRUG REACTIONS

Acitretin – trachyonychia *Cureus 12:e6703, 2020*

Actinomycin D – brown nails

Amiodarone pigmentation – personal observation

Anthralin – brown or orange nails

Antimalarials – blue nails

AZT (zidovudine) – blue lunulae, blue nails *JAAD 46:284–293, 2002*

Bleomycin – blue nails; brown nails

Chloroquine – black nail beds *AD 88:419–426, 1963*

Combination chemotherapy – cyclophosphamide, vincristine, doxorubicin, dacarbazine; blue lunulae *JAAD 32:296, 1995;* cisplatin, ifosfamide, temozolomide, and vincristine – blue lunulae *J Drugs Dermatol 12:223–226, 2013*

Cyclophosphamide – black nails

Daunorubicin – black nails

Docetaxel/paclitaxel – nail changes *JAAD 71:203–214, 2014*

Pegylated liposomal doxorubicin – red hands and feet (acral erythrodysesthesia); follicular exanthem, intertrigo, alopecia, nail changes, stomatitis *BJD 176:507–509, 2017*

Doxycycline – brown nails

Gefitinib – nail hyperpigmentation *JAAD 77:902–910, 2017*

Gold salts – black nails

Ibrutinib – diarrhea, brittle fingernails and toenails with onychorrhexis *JAMADerm 152:698–701, 2016*

Imatinib – nail hyperpigmentation *JAAD 77:902–910, 2017*

Ketoconazole – brown nails

Mepacrine – blue nails *BJD 130:794–795, 1994*

Minocycline – blue nails

Nitrogen mustard – brown nails

Penicillin allergy – onychomadesis (shedding of nail)

Phenolphthalein (X-Lax) – blue lunulae

Psoralen – brown nails

Sulfonamides – brown nails

Tetracycline – teeth; brown nails

Zidovudine – black nails

EXOGENOUS AGENTS

Argyria - blue lunulae and blue nails

Coal tar – black nails

Copper stains, swimming pool – personal observation

Ebony workers – black nails

Formaldehyde nail hardeners – blue discoloration of nails; gray nails

Gentian violet – purple nails; gray nails

Iodine – brown nails

Mercury-containing cosmetics – black nails

Nail polish, nail hardeners – brown or orange hyperpigmentation

Photographic developing (methyl or p-methyl aminophenyl sulfate hydroquinone) – black nails

Shoe polish – black nails

Silver nitrate – gray or black nails

Synthetic opioid MT-45 – hair depigmentation, hair loss, Mees' lines *BJD 176:1021–1027, 2017*

Wine – black nails

INFECTIONS AND INFESTATIONS

Aspergillus flavus – deep superficial white onychomycosis *JAAD 66:494–502, 2012*

Aspergillus niger – proximal subungual white onychomycosis *JAAD 66:494–502, 2012*

Bacterial subungual infections – *Pseudomonas aeruginosa, Klebsiella spp., Proteus spp.* – longitudinal melanonychia *Dermatol Surg 27:580–584, 2001*

Candidiasis – of skin; of nails in congenital candidiasis *Textbook of Neonatal Dermatology, p.513, 2001*

Chronic mucocutaneous candidiasis *Ped Inf Dis J 20:197–206, 2001; JAAD 31(PT 2)514–517, 1994*

Dermatophytoma – linear white or yellow nail band *JAAD 66:1014–1016; J Drugs Dermatol 14:524–526, 2015; JAAD 66:1014–1016, 2012; BJD 138:189–190, 1998*

Epidermophyton floccosum – green nails

Fusarium – superficial white onychomycosis *JAAD 66:494–502, 2012; JAAD 65:1219–1227, 2011*

Lymphogranuloma venereum – red nails, red lunulae

Onychomycosis – hypertrophic nail plates *JAAD 80:835–851, 2019; JAMA 316:1915–1916, 2016; AD 147:1277–1282, 2011;* distal subungual onychomycosis *JAAD 73:62–69, 2015;* onychomycosis in CARD9 deficiency; autosomal recessive *JAMADerm 151:192–194, 2015; Dermatol Clin 33:175–183, 2015;* superficial white onychomycosis – zebra stripes *JAAD 57:879–882, 2007*

Pseudomonas – green nails

Scabies – nail dystrophy *Ped Derm 35:829–830, 2018*

Scopulariopsis brevicaulis – opaque thick nails *JAAD 66:494–502, 2012*

Syphilis – brown nails; secondary – "onychia sicca syphilitica" – well demarcated purplish opaque rough vertically ridged plaque-like lesions of proximal portions of fingernails *SAGE Open Med Case Rep March 28, 2018; BJD 23:368–377, 1911*

Trichophyton rubrum – proximal white onychomycosis *JAAD 65:1219–1227, 2011*

Warts – wart over nail matrix – longitudinal nail groove

INFILTRATIVE DISORDERS

Amyloidosis – primary systemic amyloidosis – longitudinal ridging, onychorrhexis, zebra stripes; linear striations of nails *JAMADerm 152:1395–1396, 2016;* nail dystrophy *JAAD 54:712–714, 2006;* trachyonychia *JAMADerm 150:1357–1358, 2014;* brittleness, longitudinal ridging, subungual thickening, onycholysis, anonychia *Dermatology 228:97–102, 2014; Dermatologica 183:44–46, 1991;* primary systemic amyloidosis – atrophic nail dystrophy *JAAD 54:712–714, 2006*

Langerhans cell histiocytosis – pterygium of the nails *JAAD 78:1035–1044, 2018;* purpuric nail striae with paronychia *Ped Derm 37:182–183, 2020;* onycholysis and subungual hyperkeratosis *Ped Derm 34:732–734, 2017*

INFLAMMATORY DISORDERS

Erythema multiforme – atrophic nails

Sarcoidosis – pterygium, nail dystrophy *Skeletal Radiol 45:717–721, 2016; Clin Exp Dermatol 38:119–124, 2003*

Stevens-Johnson syndrome – hypertrophic nails; atrophic nails *Dermatol Clin 33:207–241, 2015;* Beau's lines or transverse lines; onychomadesis or shedding; anonychia *AD 113:970, 1977*

Toxic epidermal necrolysis *Pediatr 109:74–78, 2002*

METABOLIC DISORDERS

Acrodermatitis enteropathica – shedding and onychomadesis *Atlas of Clinical Syndromes A Visual Aid to Diagnosis, 1992, pp.462–463*

Acromegaly – onychauxis (hypertrophy of nail)

Beau's lines

Congenital erythropoietic porphyria *Genetic Skin Disorders, Second Edition, 2010,pp.608–612*

Congestive heart failure – red nails, lunulae

Hemochromatosis – thin nails *Genetic Skin Disorders, Second Edition, 2010,pp.308–311*

Hemoglobin M disease – blue lunulae

Hyperparathyroidism, acquired racket nails *J Eur Acad DV 28:257–259, 2014*

Koilonychia (spoon shaped nails) – iron deficiency anemia (Plummer-Vinson syndrome); repeated occupational trauma *NEJM 379:e13 2018; J Eur Acad DV 30:1985–1992, 2016*

Lindsay's nails – half and half nail of chronic renal failure

Melanonychia striata in regression – "dots and lines" *Ped Derm 34:e321–323, 2017*

Muehrcke's lines – zebra stripes; hypoalbuminemia, paired transverse hypopigmented bands *BMJ 1:1327–1328, 1956; AD 143:815–816, 2007*

Necrolytic migratory erythema (glucagonoma syndrome) – brittle nails *JAMADerm 155:1180, 2019; Int J Dermatol 49:24–29, 2010; J Eur Acad Dermatol 18:591–595, 2004*

Neapolitan nails – age related changes of nails in otherwise healthy individuals similar to Terry's, Lindsay's, or Muehrcke's nails

Ochronosis – blue-gray nails

Pernicious anemia, congenital – blue nails

Polycythemia vera – red lunulae

Porphyria cutanea tarda – photoonycholysis; discoloration of nails and onycholysis *Photodermatol Photoimmunol Photomed 18:202–207, 2002; Genetic Skin Disorders, Second Edition, 2010,pp.618–620*

Pregnancy – brown nails

Renal disease – hypopigmented hair; transverse white nail bands; half and half nails (Lindsay's nails)

Selenium deficiency – xerosis, alopecia, leukotrichia, leukonychia; pancytopenia, muscle weakness, muscle pain, cardiac arrhythmia, unsteady gait, distal paresthesias *JAAD 80:1215–1231, 2019; Nutrition 23:782–787, 2007; Nutrition 12:40–43, 1996*

Terry's nails – personal observation

Thyroid disease – white lunulae

NEOPLASMS

Atrial myxoma – emboli with nail degloving *JAAD 58:232–237, 2008*

Atypical melanocytic hyperplasia – longitudinal melanonychia *Dermatol Surg 27:580–584, 2001*

Bowen's disease – linear longitudinal melanonychia *JAAD 39: 490–493, 1998;* periungual erythematous squamous or eroded plaque; in lateral groove; a recalcitrant hyperkeratotic or papillomatous lesion

Chondroma – subungual soft tissue chondroma *Ped Derm 32:132–134, 2015*

Chondrosarcoma of distal phalanx *Acta DV 95:1026–1027, 2015*

Digital myxoid cyst – linear nail groove

Enchondromas – red nails

Fibrokeratoma – longitudinal linear groove *Dermatol Clin 33:243–255, 2015*

Glomus tumor – longitudinal erythronychia *JAMADerm 152:1271–1272, 2016*

Leiomyoma – subungual leiomyoma; erythronychia and nail dystrophy *J Drugs Dermatol 18:465–467, 2019*

Lentigo simplex – longitudinal melanonychia *Dermatol Surg 27:580–584, 2001*

Lymphoma – Sezary syndrome; onychauxis, anonychia, distal notching, onychoschizia *J Cut Med Surg 23:380–387, 2019; JAAD 79:972–973, 2018*

Melanoma of nail apparatus *JAAD 73:213–220, 2015;* subungual in situ melanoma – totally black nail *BJD 174:935, 2016;* melanoma in situ *J Drugs Dermatol 16:268–270, 2017;* subungual amelanotic melanoma – ulcerated nodule of nail bed *JAMA 319:713–714, 2018;* hemorrhagic nail bed with rim of hyperpigmentation *NEJM 381:1853, 2019;* amelanotic subungual melanoma; linear fissure of nail *AD 148:947–952, 2012*

Mucoepithelial dysplasia *Genetic Skin Disorders, Second Edition, 2010,pp.698–700*

Myxoid cyst (over nail matrix) – longitudinal nail groove often with Heberden's nodes

Onychomatricoma – parallel white and yellow nail bands with thickening of the nail plate; multiple subungual perforations *JAAD 76:S19–21, 2017;* localized yellow thickening with transverse overcurvature and splinter hemorrhages *BJD 173:1305–1307, 2015; Dermatol Clin 33:197–205, 2015;* hyperkeratotic nail with black dots *AD 147:1117–1118, 2011;* severe subungual hyperkeratosis *Society of Pediatric Dermatology Annual Meeting, July, 2015;* banded or diffuse thickening of nail with yellowish discoloration, splinter hemorrhages, and transverse overcurvature (thick yellow nail) *Cutis 96:121–124, 2015;*onycholysis with linear yellow band *JAAD 70:395–397, 2014*

    Differential diagnosis of onychomatricoma

        Acquired digital fibrokeratoma of nail matrix

        Aggressive angiomyxoma

        Angiokeratoma

        Basal cell carcinoma of nail unit

        Bowen's disease

        Nail fibroma

        Glomus tumor

        Juvenile xanthogranuloma of proximal nail fold

        Langerhans cell histiocytosis

        Longitudinal melanonychia

        Malignant proliferating onycholemmal cyst

        Melanocytic nevus

        Nail psoriasis

        Neurofibroma

        Onychodystrophy

        Onychogenic Bowen's disease

        Onychogryphosis

        Onycholemmal horn

        Onychomycosis

        Pachyonychia congenital

        Periungual and subungual warts

        Pyogenic granuloma

        Longitudinal melanonychia

        Nail bed fibrosarcoma

        Squamous cell carcinoma

        Subungual exostosis

        Subungual keratoacanthoma

        Subungual melanoma

        Subungual metastasis

        Subungual osteochondroma

        Subungual porocarcinoma

        Subungual eccrine syringofibroadenoma

        Subungual squamous cell carcinoma

        Superficial acral fibromyxoma

        Verruca vulgaris

        Yellow nail syndrome

Onychopapilloma – V-shaped distal split of nail, longitudinal erythronychia, longitudinal leukonychia, onycholysis, longitudinal melanonychia, splinter hemorrhages, distal subungual hyperkeratotic mass *JAAD 74:521–526, 2016; JAAD 63:541–542, 2010;* linear red streak with distal central fissure *Dermatol Clin 33:197–205, 2015;* onychopapilloma of nailbed and Bowen's disease – longitudinal erythronychia *BJD 143:132–135, 2000;* longitudinal leukonychia *JAAD 63:541–542, 2010;*

Osteochondroma – subungual osteochondroma; linear longitudinal nail ridge *Ped Derm 11:39–41, 1994*

Porokeratosis, linear – nail dystrophy *J Dermatol 43:286–287, 2016*

Squamous cell carcinoma – HPV and squamous cell carcinoma *JAAD 81:1358–1370, 2019;* dystrophic thumb nail *NEJM 373:2357, 2015*

Subungual elastoma *Dermatol Online J Sept 15, 2017*

Subungual exostosis – hyperkeratotic subungual papule of fingertip *Cutis 98:128–129, 2016*

Subungual onycholemmal cyst – pressure-induced onycholysis overlying blue discoloration *Cutis 98:107–110, 2016*

PARANEOPLASTIC DISORDERS

Glucagonoma syndrome – brittle crumbling nails; periorbital and perioral erythema; alpha cell tumor in the tail of the pancreas; 50% of cases have metastasized by the time of diagnosis; skin rash, angular stomatitis, cheilosis, beefy red glossitis, blepharitis, conjunctivitis, alopecia; rarely, associated with MEN I or IIA syndromes *BJD 174:1092–1095, 2016; JAMADerm 345–347, 2016; JAAD 54:745–762, 2006; JAAD 12:1032–1039, 1985; Int J Derm 43:12–18, 2004; AD 133:909, 912, 1997; JAAD 12:1032–1039, 1985; Ann Int Med 91:213–215, 1979; AD 45:1069–1080, 1942*

PRIMARY CUTANEOUS DISEASES

Acrodermatitis continua *JAMADerm 153:336–337, 2017; JAMADerm 153:331–332, 2017*

Acrokeratosis verruciformis – thin friable nails *Genetic Skin Disorders, Second Edition, 2010,pp.54–57*

Alopecia areata – red lunulae

Alpha6-beta4 epidermolysis bullosa – onychogryphosis; yellow-brown discoloration of teeth with enamel defects *BJD 169:115–124, 2013;* with alopecia totalis *BMJ Case Rep Nov 8, 2017*

Anonychia – autosomal recessive congenital anonychia – mutation in *RSPO4 BJD 173:922–979, 2015; Ped Derm 30:139–141, 2013;* congenital totalis *Int J Dermatol 41:397–399, 2002*

Anonychia of the thumbnails *Genetic Skin Disorders, Second Edition, 2010, pp.244–245*

Anonychia with flexural pigmentation *Genetic Skin Disorders, Second Edition, 2010, pp.244*

Autosomal recessive nail dysplasia – mutation in *FZD6* encoding Wnt receptor frizzled 6 *BJD 178:556–558, 2018; BJD 168:422–425, 2013; BJD 166:1088–1094, 2012*

Blue lunulae
   Amorolfine
   Antimalarials – quinacrine, chloroquine, camoquine
   Argyria
   AZT infection
   Bichloride of mercury (topical)
   Combination chemotherapy – cyclophosphamide, vinblastine, vincristine, doxorubicin, dacarbazine, 5-fluorouracil, cyclophosphamide, dactinomycin, bleomycin, busulfan
   Cupric acid
   Cyanotic disease
   Enchondromas
   Galvanizers (silver or cyanide)
   Glomus tumor
   Hemochromatosis
   Hemoglobin M disease
   Hereditary acrolabial telangiectasias
   HIV infection
   Minocycline
   Ochronosis
   Oxalic acid (in radiators)
   Phenolphthalein purgative
   Pseudomonas paronychia
   PUVA
   Quinacrine
   Thallium
   Zidovudine

Atrophic nails, congenital

Brachydactyly type B1 *Clin in Dermatol 23:47–55, 2005*

Brittle nails *Dermatol Clin 33:175–183, 2015*

Claw-shaped nails – onychauxis, hyponychia, onycholysis *BJD 173:922–979, 2015*

Darier's disease – red-white streaks; distal notching; thickening *SKINmed 13:313–315, 2015; Dermatol Clin 33:197–205, 2015; Clin in Dermatol 23:47–55, 2005;* red lunulae; Darier's disease – onychomadesis (shedding of nail); linear red, white, and pigmented streaks of nails *JAAD 27:40–50, 1992*

Epidermolysis bullosa – onychomadesis (shedding of nail)

Epidermolysis bullosa, all types

Epidermolysis bullosa – autosomal dominant epidermolysis bullosa – acral blisters of palms and soles and wrists; nail thickening progresses to anonychia; mutation in *ITGB4 JAMADerm 152:558–562, 2016*

Epidermolysis bullosa pruriginosa – anonychia *BJD 172:778–781, 2015*

Erythronychia *J Drugs Dermatol 18:465–467, 2019; SKINmed 9:327–329, 2011; Am J Clin Dermatol 12:217–231, 2011; JAAD 37:74–79, 2011; J Eur Acad Dermatol Venereol 15:85–86, 2001;* longitudinal erythronychia *BJD 155:219–221, 2006*
   Acantholytic dyskeratotic epidermal nevus

Acantholytic epidermolysis bullosa
Acrokeratosis verruciformis of Hopf
Amyloid
Darier's disease
Glomus tumor
Graft vs. host disease
Hemiplegia
Idiopathic
Leiomyoma
Lichen planus
Melanoma, amelanotic
Onychopapilloma
Post-surgical scar
Pseudo-bulbar syndrome
Squamous cell carcinoma
Verruca
Warty dyskeratoma

Familial dystrophic shedding of the nails *Genetic Skin Disorders, Second Edition, 2010,pp.236–238; Cutis 25:622–625, 1980; BJD 88:497–498, 1973; BJD 39:297, 1927*

Hereditary palmoplantar keratoderma with deafness *Genetic Skin Disorders, Second Edition, 2010,pp.58–60*

Hoof nail deformity *BJD 169:946–948, 2013*

Ichthyosis, gastric hyperplasia, subungual hyperkeratosis, immunologic dysfunction; *TTC7A* mutations *BJD 175:1061, 2016*

Ichthyosis en confetti – large lunulae with elongated nails *JAMADerm 151:64–69, 2015*

Isolated congenital nail dysplasia – autosomal dominant *Clin in Dermatol 23:47–55, 2005*

Junctional epidermolysis bullosa of late onset (skin fragility in childhood) – speckled hyperpigmentation of elbows; hemorrhagic bullae, teeth and nail abnormalities, oral blisters, disappearance of dermatoglyphics, palmoplantar keratoderma, small vesicles, atrophy of skin of hands *BJD 169:714–716, 2013*

Keratosis follicularis spinulosa decalvans – elevated cuticles *Genetic Skin Disorders, Second Edition, 2010,pp.104–107*

Keratosis punctata palmaris et plantaris – onychomadesis (shedding of nail)

Leukonychia *BJD 173:922–979, 2015; AD 90:392–399, 1964*

Leukonychia striata

Lichen planus – pterygium *JAAD 79:789–804, 2018;* atrophy of nail plate; including hemorrhagic nails in bullous lichen planus *Ped Derm 34:193–194, 2017; JAMADerm 151:674–675, 2015;* onychomadesis (shedding of nail)

Lichen striatus – linear nail striations *Ped Derm 36:859–863, 2019;* subungual hyperkeratosis *Ped Derm 33:95–96, 2016; Int J Dermatol 54:1255–1260, 2015*

Linear nail bands *JAAD 34:943–953, 1996*
   Black
      Longitudinal melanonychia striata
   Brown
      Antineoplastic agents
      Cyclophosphamide
      Doxorubicin
      Hydroxyurea
      Subungual keratosis of nail bed *BJD 140:730–733, 1999*
      Antiviral agents
      Zidovudine
   Red (longitudinal erythronychia) *AD 140:1253–1257, 2004*
      Cirsoid aneurysm
      Darier's disease
      Lichen planus
      Glomus tumor

Onychopapilloma
Squamous cell carcinoma, in situ
Ionizing radiation-induced keratosis
White
Darier's disease
Yellow
Onychomatricoma – longitudinal bands of yellow thickening of nail plate with transverse overcurvature and splinter hemorrhages; funnel-shaped nail *AD 145:1461–1462, 2009; BJD 126:510–515, 1992*

Longitudinal melanonychia *J Dermatol 46:e89–90, 2019*

Median canaliform dystrophy of the nails *Dermatol Clin 33:243–255, 2015; Hautarzt 25:629, 1974; Dermat Atschr 51:416–419, 1928;* familial *Cutis 75:161–165, 2005;* following cryosurgery of warts on proximal nail folds *Ped Derm 34:726–727, 2017*

Nagashima type palmoplantar keratoderma – autosomal recessive; transgredient; acral erythema of palms and soles; hyperkeratosis of elbows and knees and ears; toenail dystrophy; mutation in *SERPINB7 BJD 171:847–853, 2014; AD 144:375–379, 2008*

Onychogryphosis – acquired; inherited forms – autosomal dominant, congenital forms *SKINMed 13:355–359, 2015;*

Onycholysis *BJD 173:922–979, 2015; Dermatol Clin 33:175–183, 2015*

Onychomadesis *Dermatol Clin 33:243–255, 2015; BJD 172:592–596, 2015; AD 148:769–770, 2012*
Anti-epileptic medications
Cancer chemotherapy
Hand, foot, and mouth disease
Idiopathic
Major medical illness
Pemphigus vulgaris

Palmoplantar pustulosis – subungual postulation, nail destruction *Int J Dermatol 56:e28–29, 2017; BJD 134:1079, 1082, 1996*

Periodic nail shedding – thin or atrophic nails

Phylloid hypermelanosis – cicatricial alopecia, onychodystrophy, deafness, malformed ear, mental retardation, umbilicated nipples *JAAD 19:1037–1044, 1988; Rev Neurol (Paris)95:48–54, 1956*

Pincer nails *Clin Orthoped Surg 10:285–288, 2018*

Pitting *Int J Dermatol 56:3–17, 2017*

Pityriasis rubra pilaris *Genetic Skin Disorders, Second Edition, 2010,pp.46–49*

Proximal nail fold pterygium – longitudinal nail groove

Psoriasis *Ped Derm 34:58–63, 2017; Dermatol Clin 33:175–183, 2015*

Punctate palmoplantar keratoderma *Genetic Skin Disorders, Second Edition, 2010,pp.68–71*

Pure hair and nail ectodermal dysplasia (PHNED) *BMC Med Gen April 12, 2017*

Pterygium unguis inversum *Dermatol Clin 33:257–263, 2015*

Normal racial linear brown pigmented bands of nails

Racket nails – personal observation

Red nail matrix – personal observation

Retronychia *JAAD 73:849–855, 2015*

Trachyonychia *Dermatol Clin 33:243–255, 2015*

Transient bullous dermolysis of the newborn *Genetic Skin Disorders, Second Edition, 2010,pp.173–175*

Transient yellow discoloration of nails *Orphanet J Rare Dis 12:159, 2017*

Twenty nail dystrophy *Ped Derm 5:117–119, 1988; JAAD 7:349–352, 1982*

Universal melanosis – thin nails *Genetic Skin Disorders, Second Edition, 2010,pp.342–345*

Vitiligo – longitudinal ridging, leukonychia, absent lunula, onycholysis, nail bed pallor, onychomadesis, splinter hemorrhages, nail plate thinning *An Bras Dermatol 91:442–445, 2016*

Vohwinkel's palmoplantar keratoderma *Genetic Skin Disorders, Second Edition, 2010,pp.77–79*

PSYCHOCUTANEOUS DISEASES

Onychotillomania – total melanonychia; nail dystrophy *Am J Clin Dermatol 18:763–770, 2017; JAAD 75:1245–1250, 2016*

SYNDROMES

Acro-dermato-ungual-lacrimal-tooth syndrome (ADULT syndrome) – ectrodactyly or syndactyly, freckling and dry skin, dysplastic nails, superficial blisters and desquamation of hands and feet; lacrimal duct atresia, primary hypodontia, conical teeth, and early loss of permanent teeth; small ears hooked nose, sparse thin blond hair, frontal alopecia, hypohidrosis, lacrimal duct atresia, hypoplastic breasts and nipples, urinary tract anomalies; mutation in *TP63* gene (encodes transcription factor p63); p63 mutations also responsible for EEC, AEC, limb mammary, and Rapp-Hodgkin syndromes *Ped Derm 33:e322–326, 2016; BJD 172:276–278, 2015; Ped Derm 27:643–645, 2010; Hum Mol Genet 11:799–804, 2002; Am J Med Genet 45:642–648, 1993*

Activated STING in Vascular and Pulmonary syndrome – autoinflammatory disease; butterfly telangiectatic facies; acral violaceous psoriasiform, papulosquamous, and atrophic vasculitis of hands; nodules of face, nose, and ears; fingertip ulcers with necrosis; nail dystrophy; nasal septal perforation; interstitial lung disease with fibrosis; polyarthritis; myositis *NEJM 371:507–518, 2014*

Ankyloblepharon-ectodermal defects-clefting (AEC) syndrome – autosomal dominant; flat face, prominent nose, periorbital wrinkling, hypodontia, sparse hair, alopecia, sparse eyebrows and eyelashes; nail dystrophy; mutation in p63 *BJD 166:134–144, 2012*

Anonychia-lymphedema syndrome *BMJ Case Rep Nov 8, 2017*

ANOTHER syndrome – alopecia, nail dystrophy, ophthalmic complications, thyroid dysfunction, hypohidrosis, ephelides and enteropathy, respiratory tract infections *Clin Genet 35:237–242, 1989; J Pediatr 108:109–111, 1986*

Aplasia cutis congenita with limb defects *Genetic Skin Disorders, Second Edition, 2010,pp.455–460*

Aplasia cutis congenita associated with fetus papyraceus – cutaneous ulcers, linear atrophic scars, atrophic scars of scalp, dystrophic nails *Ped Derm 32:858–861, 2015*

Asymmetric gait nail unit syndrome (AGNUS) – clinical changes of toenails identical to onychomycosis *SKINmed 12:217–223, 2014*

Bart-Pumphrey syndrome – palmoplantar keratoderma, knuckle pads, deafness, and leukonychia

Cardiofaciocutaneous syndrome – shares findings of Costello syndrome such as cutis laxa, thin nails, curly hair, increased nevi, pruritus, hyperhidrosis *Ped Derm 30:665–673, 2013*

Cartilage-hair hypoplasia *Atlas of Clinical Syndromes A Visual Aid to Diagnosis, 1992, pp.264–265*

Cerebro-oculo-facial-skeletal syndrome (in aboriginal families) – onychogryphosis, microcephaly, facies – micrognathia, small eyes, enlarged ears, bulbous nose, prominent nasal bridge, microphthalmia with poor vision, cataracts, blepharophimosis, short palpebral fissures, photosensitivity, mental retardation, hyperkinesis, failure to thrive, developmental delay, hypotonia, orthopedic anomalies (kyphoscoliosis), joint contractures; overhanging upper lip, small jaw *JAAD 75:873–882, 2016; Ped Derm 26:97–99, 2009; JAMA Derm 149:1414–1418, 2013*

CHAND syndrome – autosomal recessive; curly hair, ankyloblepharon, nail dysplasia; *RIPK4* mutation *Am J Med Genet A 173:3114–3117, 2017; Genetic Skin Disorders, Second Edition, 2010, pp216–219*

Chevron nails (herring bone nails) – congenital nail dystrophy with V-shaped abnormalities *Society of Pediatric Dermatology Annual Meeting, July, 2015*

CHILD syndrome *Genetic Skin Disorders, Second Edition, 2010,pp.116–119*

Chondrodysplasia punctate, X-linked (Conradi-Hunermann-Happle syndrome) *Atlas of Clinical Syndromes A Visual Aid to Diagnosis, 1992, pp.226–227*

Cleidocranial dysplasia *Atlas of Clinical Syndromes A Visual Aid to Diagnosis, 1992, pp.3–33*

Clouston's syndrome (hidrotic ectodermal dysplasia) – pterygium, thinning of nails *J Dermatol 48:329–330, 2019;* may mimic nail changes of pachyonychia congenita *JID*

Cockayne's syndrome (cachectic dwarfism) – autosomal recessive; thin skin, dry hair, anhidrosis, short stature, facial erythema in butterfly distribution leading to mottled pigmentation and atrophic scars, premature aged appearance with loss of subcutaneous fat and sunken eyes (enophthalmos with loss of periorbital fat), lipoatrophy of temples; canities, nail dystrophy, hair loss, mental deficiency, photosensitivity, disproportionately large hands, feet, and ears, ocular defects, demyelination *JAAD 75:873–882, 2016; Ped Derm 20:538–540, 2003; J Med Genet 18:288–293, 1981*

Coffin-Siris syndrome – mutation in *ARID1B*; extreme obesity, macrocephaly, hepatomegaly, hyperinsulinemia, polycystic ovarian syndrome, hypertrichosis, hypoplastic or absent fifth distal phalanx or nail *Eur J Hum Genet 22:1327–1329, 2014; Am J Med Genet A176:1764–1767, 2018*

Costello syndrome – warty papules around nose and mouth, legs, perianal skin; loose thick skin of neck, hands, and feet, thick, redundant palmoplantar surfaces, hypoplastic nails, short stature, craniofacial abnormalities; linear papillomatous papules of upper lip *Ped Derm 30:665–673, 2013; BJD 168:903–904, 2013; Am J Med Genet 117:42–48, 2003; Eur J Dermatol 11:453–457, 2001; Am J Med Genet 82:187–193, 1999; JAAD 32:904–907, 1995; Am J Med Genet 47:176–183, 1993; Aust Paediat J 13:114–118, 1977* Cutis laxa (dermatochalasis connata) – autosomal dominant; mild disease of late onset *Ped Derm 21:167–170, 2004;* bloodhound appearance of premature aging *Ped Derm 19:412–414, 2002; JAAD 29:846–848, 1993; Clin Genet 39:321–329, 1991; Ped Derm 2:282–288, 1985*

Craniofrontal dysplasia – longitudinal ridges *Genetic Skin Disorders, Second Edition, 2010*

Cronkhite-Canada syndrome – diarrhea, protein-losing enteropathy, and peripheral edema; atrophic fingernails *NEJM 366:463–468, 2012*

Curry-Hall syndrome – polydactyly

Desmoplakin mutations – syndrome of dilated cardiomyopathy with severe left ventricular dysfunction, congenital alopecia, striate palmoplantar keratoderma, nail dystrophy, follicular hyperkeratosis with hyperpigmented plaques of elbows *Ped Derm 32:102–108, 2015*

DOOR syndrome (deafness and onychoosteodystrophy with mental retardation) *Int J Ped Otorhinolaryngol 117:57–60, 2019*

Dyskeratosis congenita (Zinsser-Engman-Cole syndrome) – Xq28; oral leukoplakia, bullae and erosions; distal ridging, splitting,

pterygia *BJD 178:335–349, 2018; JAAD 77:1194–1198, 2017; J Blood Med 5:157–167, 2014; Br J Haematol 145:164–172, 2009; Semin Cut Med Surg 16:72–80, 1997; Ped Derm 14:411–413, 1997; J Med Genet 33:993–995, 1996; Dermatol Clin 13:33–39, 1995; BJD 105:321–325, 1981*

Autosomal recessive – hypotrichosis, dystrophic nails; HOXC13 *Ped Derm 34:172–175, 2017*

Ectodermal dysplasia – X-linked anhidrotic ectodermal dysplasia; thin or atrophic nails

EEC syndrome *Genetic Skin Disorders, Second Edition, 2010,pp.279–282*

Ellis-van Creveld syndrome (achondroplastic dwarfism with defective teeth and nails, and polydactyly) (chondroectodermal dysplasia) – autosomal recessive; very short stature; chondrodysplasia, ectodermal dysplasia with ulnar polydactyly, cone- and peg-shaped teeth or hypodontia, enamel hypoplasia, fused incisors, molars with extra cusps, dental fissures and pits, neonatal teeth, malocclusion; short upper lip bound down by multiple labiogingival frenula; gingival hypertrophy, nail dystrophy, hair may be normal or sparse and brittle; cardiac defects; ichthyosis, palmoplantar keratoderma; asymmetric distal limb shortening; short distal phalanges with small dystrophic fingernails; congenital heart disease; hypospadias, cryptorchidism; mutations in EVC and EVC2 *Cutis 83:303–305, 2009; Ped Derm 18:485–489, 2001; J Med Genet 17:349–356, 1980; Arch Dis Child 15:65–84, 1940*

Erythrokeratoderma-cardiomyopathy syndrome – recurrent infections, wiry or absent hair, dental enamel defects, nail dystrophy, sudden onset congestive heart failure; early death; dominant mutation in desmoplakin *Cases of the Year, Pre-AAD Pediatric Dermatology Meeting*

Finlay-Marks syndrome (scalp-ear-nipple syndrome) – nipple or breast hypoplasia or aplasia, aplasia cutis congenita of scalp, abnormal ears and teeth, nail dystrophy, syndactyly, reduced apocrine secretion

Fried syndrome – autosomal recessive; thin sparse hair and eyebrows; everted lower lip

GAPO syndrome *Am J Med Genet A 146A:1523–1529, 2008; Genetic Skin Disorders, Second Edition, 2010,pp.284–286*

Goltz's syndrome (focal dermal hypoplasia) – atrophic nails; V-nicking; longitudinal ridging, micronychia; asymmetric linear and reticulated streaks of atrophy and telangiectasia; yellow-red nodules; raspberry-like papillomas of lips, perineum, acrally, at perineum, buccal mucosa; xerosis; hypopigmented atrophic macules, Blaschko-esque hyperpigmentation, yellow nodules of hand, oligodontia, wide-spaced teeth, cleft hand, syndactyly, mammary hypoplasia, scalp and pubic hair sparse and brittle; short stature; asymmetric face; syndactyly, polydactyly; ocular, dental, and skeletal abnormalities with osteopathia striata of long bones; thin or atrophic nails *JAMADerm 152:713–714, 2016; AD 148:85–88, 2012; AD 143:109–114, 2007; JAAD 25:879–881, 1991; AD 86:708–717, 1962;* aplasia cutis congenita *AD 145:218–219, 2009;* male mosaic Goltz's syndrome; blaschko-linear white atrophic depigmented lines, hyperpigmented linear streaks, linear alopecia, syndactyly, hydronephrosis *Ped Derm 28:550–554, 2011;* unilateral focal dermal hypoplasia, unilateral – PORCN gene mutation; PORCN encodes O-acyltransferase involved in palmitoylation and secretion of Wnt signaling proteins important in embryonic tissue development, fibroblast proliferation and osteogenesis *Am J Med Genet C Semin Med Genet 172C:44–51, 2016; AD 148:85–88, 2012; AD 145:218–219, 2009*

Hair-nail-skin-teeth dysplasias (dermo-odonto-dysplasia, pilo-dento-ungular dysplasia, odonto-onycho-dermal dysplasia, odonto-onychial dysplasia, tricho-dermo-dysplasia with dental alterations) *Am J Med Genet 14:335–346, 1983*

Huriez syndrome *Clin in Dermatol 23:47–55, 2005*

Hutchinson-Gilford syndrome – thin nails *Genetic Skin Disorders, Second Edition, 2010,pp.649–653*

Hypertrichosis, coarse face, brachydactyly, obesity, mental retardation, broad proximal phalanges, small dysmorphic nails *Clin Dysmorphol 5:223–229, 1996*

Hypohidrotic ectodermal dysplasia *Atlas of Clinical Syndromes A Visual Aid to Diagnosis, 1992, pp.456–457*

Hydantoin-barbiturate embryopathy *Atlas of Clinical Syndromes A Visual Aid to Diagnosis, 1992, pp.450–451*

Incontinentia pigmenti *Genetic Skin Disorders, Second Edition, 2010,pp.311–316*

IPEX syndrome – immune dysregulation (neonatal autoimmune enteropathy, food allergies), polyendocrinopathy (diabetes mellitus, thyroiditis), enteropathy (neonatal diarrhea), X-linked, rash (atopic dermatitis-like with exfoliative erythroderma and periorificial dermatitis; psoriasiform dermatitis, pemphigoid nodularis, painful fissured cheilitis, edema of lips and perioral area, urticaria secondary to foods); penile rash; thyroid dysfunction, diabetes mellitus, hepatitis, nephritis, onychodystrophy, alopecia universalis; mutations in *FOXP3* (forkhead box protein 3) gene – master control gene of T regulatory cells (Tregs); hyper IgE, eosinophilia *JAAD 73:355–364, 2015; BJD 160:645–651, 2009;* ichthyosiform eruptions *Blood 109:383–385, 2007; BJD 152:409–417, 2005; NEJM 344:1758–1762, 2001;* alopecia areata *AD 140:466–472, 2004*

Iso-Kikuchi syndrome – congenital onychodysplasia of the index finger *Actas Dermosifiliogr 109:e33–36, 2018*

Kindler's syndrome – thin nails *Genetic Skin Disorders, Second Edition, 2010,pp.636–666*

Laband syndrome *Genetic Skin Disorders, Second Edition, 2010,pp.190*

Laryngo-onycho-cutaneous syndrome – autosomal recessive type of junctional epidermolysis bullosa; skin ulceration with prominent granulation tissue, early hoarseness and laryngeal stenosis; scarred nares; chronic erosion of corners of mouth (giant perleche); paronychia with periungual inflammation and erosions; onycholysis with subungual granulation tissue and loss of nails with granulation tissue of nail bed, conjunctival inflammation with polypoid granulation tissue, and dental enamel hypoplasia and hypodontia; only in Punjabi families; mutation in laminin alpha-3 (*LAMA3A*) *BJD 169:1353–1356, 2013; Ped Derm 23:75–77, 2006; Biomedica 2:15–25, 1986*

Lelis syndrome – acanthosis nigricans with hypohidrosis, hypotrichosis, hypodontia, furrowed tongue, nail dystrophy, palmoplantar keratoderma *Genetic Skin Disorders, Second Edition, 2010, pp.94–97*

LOGIC syndrome *Genetic Skin Disorders, Second Edition, 2010,pp.161,163*

Multicentric reticulohistiocytosis – onychomadesis (shedding of nail)

Naegeli-Franceschetti-Jadassohn syndrome – autosomal dominant; abnormally shaped teeth, polydontia, yellow spotted enamel, caries, early total loss; reticulate gray to brown pigmentation of neck, upper trunk and flexures, punctate or diffuse palmoplantar keratoderma, hypohidrosis with heat intolerance, onycholysis, subungual hyperkeratosis *JAAD 60: 289–298, 2009; Ped Derm 22:122–126, 2005; Semin Cutan Med Surg 16:72–80, 1997; JAAD 28:942–950, 1993; Genetic Skin Disorders, Second Edition, 2010,pp.327–329*

Nail patella syndrome – triangular lunulae *J Drugs Dermatol 14:85–86, 2015; Indian J Dermatol Venereol Leprol 73:355–357, 2007; Clin in Dermatol 23:47–55, 2005*

Odonto-onycho-dermal dysplasia – oligodontia with small widely spaced conical peg-shaped teeth, hypodontia, absence of secondary teeth; palmoplantar keratoderma, hyperhidrosis, dystrophic

nails, erythematous telangiectatic, reticulated atrophic malar and ala nasal patches with vermiculate scarring *JAAD 57:732–733, 2007; Am J Med Genet 14:335–346, 1983*

Olmsted syndrome *Orphanet J Rare Dis March 17, 2015; Genetic Skin Disorders, Second Edition, 2010,pp.65–68*

Onychodystrophy with deafness *Genetic Skin Disorders, Second Edition, 2010,pp.246–248*

Onychomatricoma – parallel white and yellow nail bands with thickening of the nail plate; multiple subungual perforations *JAAD 76:S19–21, 2017*

Onychotrichodysplasia and neutropenia – thin nails *Clin Genet 15:147–152, 1979*

Otopalatal syndrome, type 1 – X-linked dominant *Clin in Dermatol 23:47–55, 2005*

Pachyonychia congenita – overcurvature of nails; subungual hyperkeratosis; facial steatocystoma multiplex and palmoplantar keratoderma; mutation in keratin 17 *Ped Derm 36:149–151, 2019; BJD 171:1565–1567, 2014; BJD 171:343–355, 2014; JAMADerm 150:146–153, 2014; Clin in Dermatol 23:6–14, 2005*

Pallister-Hall syndrome – autosomal dominant *Clin in Dermatol 23:47–55, 2005*

Papillon-Lefevre syndrome – splits, grooves, and pits *Genetic Skin Disorders, Second Edition, 2010,pp.83–86*

Peutz-Jeghers syndrome – brown pigmented bands of nails

PGM3 deficiency – autosomal recessive; dermatitis, conductive hearing loss, ataxia, myoclonus, narrow palpebral fissures; increased IgE; herpes simplex, molluscum contagiosum viral infections, sinopulmonary infections, chronic mucocutaneous candidiasis, developmental delay *JAAD 73:355–364, 2015*

POEMS syndrome – white nails *Int J Dermatol 52:1349–1356, 2013*

Pseudoglucagonoma syndrome – periorificial erythema, crusted migratory plaques, hair loss, brittle nails, diarrhea, poor weight gain, onycholysis; associated with cirrhosis, celiac disease inflammatory bowel disease, small cell lung cancers *Am J Med 126:387–389, 2013*

Psoriasis, pediatric *Ped Derm 35:202–207, 2018*

Pure hair and nail ectodermal dysplasia – autosomal dominant or autosomal recessive; alopecia of scalp; may be generalized; nail dystrophy; mutation in *HOXC13 BJD 169:478–480, 2013*

Pycnodysostosis – autosomal recessive *Clin in Dermatol 23:47–55, 2005*

Rabson-Mendenhall syndrome *Genetic Skin Disorders, Second Edition, 2010, pp.197*

Retronychia (disappearing nail bed) – hyperpigmentation of proximal nail fold *Ped Derm 34:717–718, 2017*

Revesz syndrome *Genetic Skin Disorders, Second Edition, 2010, pp.303*

Rothmund-Thomson syndrome *Genetic Skin Disorders, Second Edition, 2010, pp.669–673*

Rubinstein-Taybi syndrome – autosomal dominant *Clin in Dermatol 23:47–55, 2005*

Santos syndrome – ungula hypoplasia/anonychia *J Hum Genetics 62:1073–1078, 2017*

SASH1 related lentigines, hyper- and hypopigmentation, alopecia, nail dystrophy, palmoplantar keratoderma, skin cancer *BJD 177:945–959, 2017*

Schopf-Schulz-Passarge syndrome (hypotrichosis, palmoplantar hyperkeratosis, apocrine hidrocystomas of eyelid margins, nail dystrophy) – oligodontia; red palms and soles with focal dryness; maceration with hyperhidrosis; finger and toenail dystrophy; mutation in *WNT10A BJD 171:1211–1214, 2014; Ped Derm*

30:491–492, 2013; JAAD 65:1066–1069, 2011; AD 140:231–236, 2004; Acta DV 88:607–612, 2008; JAAD 10:922–925, 1984

Scleroatrophic and keratotic dermatosis of the limbs *Genetic Skin Disorders, Second Edition, 2010,pp.87–89*

Sclerosteosis – autosomal recessive *Clin in Dermatol 23:47–55, 2005*

Simpson–Golabi–Behmel syndrome – generalized somatic overgrowth; coarse facial features, hypertelorism, downslanting palpebral fissures, epicanthal folds, short nose with broad nasal bridge, macrostomia, macroglossia, central groove of lower lip and/or tongue; short broad hands, fingernail hypoplasia of index finger, supernumerary nipples *Cutis 83:255–261, 2009*

Temple-Baraitser syndrome – absent or hypoplastic first thumbnails and/or toenails *Clin Dysmorphol 24:55–60, 2015; Am J Med Genet A 146A:450–452, 2008*

Tooth and nail syndrome – thin nails *Genetic Skin Disorders, Second Edition, 2010,pp.291–292*

Trichorhinophalangeal syndromes types I and II – thin nails *BJD 171:1581–1573, 2014; Genetic Skin Disorders, Second Edition, 2010,pp.225–228*

Trichothiodystrophy *Genetic Skin Disorders, Second Edition, 2010,pp.229–233*

Turner's syndrome *Atlas of Clinical Syndromes A Visual Aid to Diagnosis, 1992, pp.192–193*

Weaver syndrome – generalized somatic overgrowth; macrocephaly, broad forehead, flattened occiput, large low set ears, hypertelorism; soft loose skin, redundant nuchal skin folds; umbilical hernia; thin deep set nails *J Ped Genet 4:136–143, 2015; Cutis 83:255–261, 2009*

Williams' syndrome *Atlas of Clinical Syndromes A Visual Aid to Diagnosis, 1992, pp.484–485*

Witkop tooth-nail syndrome – autosomal dominant; hypodontia with nail dysgenesis; teeth widely spaced; narrow crowns; hypoplastic spoon shaped nails, slow growing, prone to fracture; normal facies; mutation in *MSX1 Ped Derm 28:281–285, 2011; Clin in Dermatol 23:47–55, 2005; J Clin Pediatr Dent 28:107–112, 2004; Oral Surg 37:576–582, 1974*

Yellow nail syndrome *BJD 156:1230–1234, 2007; Clin in Dermatol 23:47–55, 2005; without a syndrome SKINMed 17:73–74, 2019*

TOXINS

Carbon monoxide – red lunulae

Mee's lines – arsenic poisoning; zebra stripes *JAAD 50:258–261, 2004*

Selenium toxicity – transverse white nail bands *JAAD 63:168–169, 2010*

Thallium poisoning – generalized hyperpigmentation; anagen effluvium, gastrointestinal upset, visual impairment, Mees' lines, perioral dermatitis, scaling of palms and soles, acneiform eruptions; treat with Prussian blue *JAMADerm 152:724–726, 2016*

TRAUMA

Beau's lines *Dermatol Clin 33:243–255, 2015; Arch Gen Med 11:447–458, 1846*

Habit tic deformity *Dermatol Clin 33:243–255, 2015* zebra stripes

Hyperpigmentation – physical trauma, habit tic deformity, radiation

Physical trauma – atrophic nails

Ski jump toenails – primary lymphedema *Vasc Med 20:268, 2015*

Traumatic nail damage

VASCULAR LESIONS

Arteriovenous malformation, subungual – red lunulae

Atherosclerosis and other vascular disorders – atrophic nails

Blue rubber bleb nevus syndrome – personal observation

Cholesterol emboli, splinter hemorrhages – personal observation

Clubbing *BJD 173:922–979, 2015*

Dissecting aortic aneurysm – transverse white nail bands

Glomus tumors – red nails, lunula

Hemangioma, proliferating – including red nails

Peripheral arterial disease – onychodystrophy *J Vasc Nurs 34:24–26, 2016*

Raynaud's phenomenon – atrophic nails

NASAL INFILTRATION OR ENLARGEMENT

AUTOIMMUNE DISEASES AND DISEASES OF IMMUNE DYSFUNCTION

Allergic rhinitis

Pemphigus vegetans

Pemphigus vulgaris *Cutis 34:394–395, 1984*

Relapsing polychondritis – personal observation

Rheumatoid nodule – nasal nodule *JAAD 53:191–209, 2005; JAAD 8:439–457, 1983*

CONGENITAL ANOMALIES

Anterior cephalocele – intranasal polypoid lesion with broad nasal bridge *Ped Derm 32:161–170, 2015*

Dermoid cyst *Ped Derm 36:745–746, 2019; AD 135:463–468, 1999*

Dermoid sinus – broad nasal root *Ped Derm 32:161–170, 2015; Dermatol Therapy 18:104–116, 2005*

Embryonal rhabdomyosarcoma – orbit, nasopharynx, nose

Encephalocele

Epidermoid cyst – congenital midline mass *Soc Ped Derm Annual Meeting, Poster Session, July 2005*

Hemangioma congenital midline mass *Soc Ped Derm Annual Meeting, Poster Session, July 2005*

Heterotopic brain tissue

Lacrimal duct cyst

Lymphoma – congenital midline mass *Soc Ped Derm Annual Meeting, Poster Session, July 2005*

Meningocele

Meningoencephalocele

Meningioma – extracranial meningioma

Metastatic tumor – congenital midline mass *Soc Ped Derm Annual Meeting, Poster Session, July 2005*

Nasal glioma (nasal glial heterotopia) – red or bluish nodules; resemble hemangiomas, nasal encephalocele, meningoencephalocele, extracranial meningioma, dermoid cyst, lacrimal duct cyst, neuroblastoma, rhabdomyosarcoma *Ped Derm 25:573–574, 2008; Ear Nose Throat J 80:410–411, 2001*

Nasal midline masses *Dermatol Therapy 18:104–116, 2005; AD 127:362–366, 1991*

Neuroblastoma – olfactory neuroblastoma *Soc Ped Derm Annual Meeting, Poster Session, July 2005*

Neurofibroma – congenital midline mass *Soc Ped Derm Annual Meeting, Poster Session, July 2005*

Olfactory neuroblastoma

Rhabdomyosarcoma – congenital midline mass *Soc Ped Derm Annual Meeting, Poster Session, July 2005; J Cut Med Surg 13:276–279, 2009*

Subcutaneous abscess – congenital midline mass *Soc Ped Derm Annual Meeting, Poster Session, July 2005*

Teratoma of nasal tip *Ann Plast Surg 35:522–524, 1995*

Trauma, facial congenital midline mass *Soc Ped Derm Annual Meeting, Poster Session, July 2005*

DRUGS

Methotrexate-associated lymphoproliferative disorder – red papules and plaques of nose, cheeks, eyelids *JAAD 56:686–690, 2007*

EXOGENOUS AGENTS

Silicone granulomas – nasal enlargement *JAAD 52:S53–56, 2005*

Smoking-induced nasopharyngeal lymphoid hyperplasia *Laryngoscope 107:1635–1642, 1997*

INFECTIONS AND INFESTATIONS

Abscess – nasal septal abscess – collection of pus between cartilaginous or bony septum and mucoperichondrium or periosteum; due to trauma; bilateral nasal obstruction, foreign body sensation, nasal pain, swelling and erythema of overlying skin, rhinorrhea, swollen upper lip, fever, headache, malaise *J Emerg Med 46:e81, 2014; Pediatr and Neonatology 53:213–215, 2012; Ear, Nose, and Throat J 90:144–145, 2011; J Laryngol and Otol 124:1014–1016, 2010; Rhinology 47:476–477, 2009*

Actinomycosis – indurated red nose *JAAD 38:310–313, 1998*

Aspergillosis *Oral Surg Oral Med Oral Pathol 59:499–504, 1985*

Bacillary angiomatosis *Cutaneous Manifestations of Infection in the Immunocompromised Host, second Ed, Grossman, et al*

Balamuthiasis (*Balamuthia mandrillaris*) – amoebic infection of soft tissues and central nervous system; edematous erythematous infiltrated plaque of face, abdomen, extremities; nasal enlargement *Clin Dermatol 32:744–751, 2014; JAAD 60:897–925, 2009; Advances Dermatol 23:335–350, 2007*

Basidiobolus ranarum

Candidiasis – chronic mucocutaneous candidiasis

Chromomycosis *JAAD 53:931–951, 2005*

Conidiobolus coronatus (rhinoentomophthoromycosis) *Med Mycol 48:870–879, 2010*

Cryptococcosis – indurated red nose *JAAD 38:310–313, 1998*

Erysipelas

Fusarium – of sinuses; nasal erythema with conjunctivitis *JAAD 47:659–666, 2002*

Herpes simplex virus

Herpes zoster

Histoplasmosis – indurated red nose *JAAD 38:310–313, 1998; Mycopathologia 115:13–18, 1991*

Leishmaniasis – mucocutaneous leishmaniasis – infiltrated nasal plaque *JAMA 312:1250–1251, 2014;*; lupoid leishmaniasis – verrucous plaque of nose *JAAD 73:911–926, 2015; JAAD 73:897–908, 2015;*indurated red nose (tapir face) *JAAD 60:897–925, 2009; JAAD 38:310–313, 1998; Am J Trop Med Hyg 59:49–52, 1998; L. tropica –* enlarged nose with crusted plaque *JAAD 71:271–277, 2014; L. aethiopica –* nasal infiltration with edema but no destruction *Trans R Soc Trop Med Hyg 63:708–737, 1969;* mucocutaneous leishmaniasis with destruction of the nose and midface *JAAD 34:257, 1996*

Leprosy – indurated red nose *JAAD 38:310–313, 1998*

Mycobacterium avium-intracellulare – nasal papules *JAAD 33:528–531, 1995*

Mycobacterium marinum Medicine 95:e3131, 2016

Mycobacterium tuberculosis – lupus vulgaris *Clin Dermatol 32:817–826, 2014;* indurated red nose *Dermatol Clin 26:285–294, 2008; JAAD 38:310–313, 1998;* starts as red-brown plaque; vegetating forms – ulcerate, areas of necrosis, invasion of mucous membranes with destruction of cartilage (lupus vorax); tumor-like forms – deeply infiltrative; soft smooth nodules or red-yellow hypertrophic plaque; nasal papules; *Int J Dermatol 26:578–581, 1987; Acta Tuberc Scand 39(Suppl 49):1–137, 1960;*

North American blastomycosis – pustulonodular infiltration of nose *JAMA 312:2564–2565, 2014;* indurated red nose *JAAD 38:310–313, 1998; Laryngoscope 103:53–58, 1993*

Paracoccidioidomycosis – indurated red nose *Dermatol Clin 26:257–269, 2008; JAAD 38:310–313, 1998*

Pinta – *Treponema carateum*

Rhinoscleroma – *Klebsiella rhinoscleromatis* (Frisch bacillus) exudative stage with rhinorrhea; then proliferative stage with exuberant friable granulation tissue of nose (Hebra nose), pharynx, larynx; progresses to nodules; then fibrotic stage*; Acta Otolaryngol 105:494–499, 1988; Cutis 40:101–103, 1987;* indurated red nose *JAAD 38:310–313, 1998*

Rhinosporidiosis (*Rhinosporidium seeberi*) – soft polyps with minute white spots; Indian sand dredgers; intranasal and conjunctival red polypoid lesions*; NEJM 380:1359, 2019;*

JAAD 53:931–951, 2005

Sinusitis, acute

Sporotrichosis – indurated red nose *JAAD 38:310–313, 1998;* fixed cutaneous

Staphylococcus aureus – nasal carriage with intranasal folliculitis or vestibulitis

Subcutaneous zygomycosis (*Conidiobolus*) – very disfiguring *JAAD 30:904–908, 1994*

Syphilis, tertiary

Verruga peruana – *Bartonella bacilliformis*

Yaws – tertiary yaws – hypertrophic proliferative periostitis of maxilla and nasal bridge (osseous form) (goundou); only in African children *Ped Derm 27:364–367, 2010*

Zygomycosis (*Basidiobolus coronatus*) *AD 141:1211–1213, 2005*

INFILTRATIVE DISEASES

Amyloid – rhinophyma-like *Aesthetic Plast Surg 28:98–99, 2004;* primary cutaneous nodular amyloid *Cutis 91:271,283–284, 2014;*

Juvenile hyaline fibromatosis (infantile systemic hyalinosis) *Ped Derm 23:458–464, 2006*

Juvenile xanthogranuloma

Langerhans cell histiocytosis

Lichen myxedematosus

Pseudolymphoma – personal observation

INFLAMMATORY DISEASES

Crohn's disease *J Otolaryngol 14:399–400, 1985*

Lymphocytoma cutis – idiopathic or due to Lyme borreliosis *JAAD 38:877–905, 1998*

Lymphoid hyperplasia of the nasal cavity in AIDS *Ann Otolaryngol Chir Cervicofac 105:543–547, 1988*

Pseudolymphomatous folliculitis – infiltration of columella *JAAD 60:994–1000, 2009; Am J Surg Pathol 23:1313–1319, 1999; AD 124:1272–1273, 1276, 1988*

Pyoderma vegetans (pseudoepithelioma of Azua; hyperinflammatory proliferative pyoderma; blastomycosis-like pyoderma) – ulcerated vegetative plaques and rhinophymatous changes of nose *JAMADerm 150: 773–774, 2014; Arch Dermatol Syphilol 43:289–306, 1898*

Pyostomatitis vegetans – pustular lips and nose; erosive plaques of lips with yellow crusts; association with ulcerative colitis and Crohn's disease *JAMADerm 156:335, 2020*

Rosai-Dorfman disease (sinus histiocytosis with massive lymphadenopathy) *J Cutan Pathol 25:563–567, 1998; BJD 134:749–753, 1996*

Sarcoid – rhinophymatous sarcoid *J Drugs Dermatol 3:333–334, 2003;* lupus pernio *JAAD 66:699–716, 2012; JAAD 39:835–838, 1998; Lupus 1:129–131, 1992; JAAD 22:439–443, 1990*

METABOLIC DISEASES

Acromegaly *Pituitary 20:22–32, 2017*

NEOPLASTIC DISEASES

Aggressive intranasal carcinoma – edema and erythema of nose *Cutis 42:288–293, 1988*

Angiosarcoma – indurated red nose *JAAD 54:883–885, 2006; Cutis 76:313–317, 2005; JAAD 38:310–313, 1998;JAAD 38:837–840, 1998; BJD 76:21–39, 1964;* resembling rhinophyma *JAAD 49:530–531, 2003*

Basal cell carcinoma mimicking rhinophyma – indurated red nose *JAAD 38:310–313, 1998*

Carcinoma of the nasal columella *Am J Surg 170:453–456, 1995*

Carcinoma of the nasal vestibule *Int J Radiat Oncol Biol Phys 10:627–637, 1984*

Cellular neurothekeoma – papule *Ped Derm 12:191–194, 1995*

Chondroid syringoma – infiltrated nodule of ala nasi *Dermatol Online J Nov 15, 2016; Ped Derm 24:505–507, 2007*

Cylindromatosis, familial *J Med Genet 35:841–845, 1988*

Epidermoid cyst

Folliculosebaceous cystic hamartoma – nasal nodule *JAAD 34:77–81, 1996*

Kaposi's sarcoma – enlargement of tip of nose in AIDS mimicking pyogenic granuloma of the nasal mucosa *J Laryngol Otol 112:280–282, 1998*

Keratoacanthoma, giant *Am J Dermatopathol 36:252–257, 2014; Clin Exp Dermatol 36:369–371, 2011*

Lacrimal duct cyst

Leukemia *J Laryngol Otol 106:261–263, 1992;* chronic lymphocytic leukemia – red infiltrated nose with necrosis *Cutis 80:208–210, 2007;* chronic lymphocytic leukemic infiltrates – rosacea-like appearance *BJD 150:1129–1135, 2004; Am J Surg Pathol 20:1000–1010, 1996;* CLL appearing as rhinophymatous rosacea *BJD 163:443, 2010;* angioimmunoblastic lymphoma – personal observation; HTLV-1 leukemia/lymphoma – personal observation

Lymphoma; *JAAD 38:310–313, 1998; Br J Haematol 97:821–829, 1997;* primary cutaneous B-cell lymphoma – rhinophyma-like enlargement of nose *AD 140:751–756, 2004;* midline malignant B-cell lymphoma *Cancer 70:2958–2962, 1992;* angiocentric T-cell lymphoma *JAAD 26:31–38, 1992;* primary cutaneous peripheral T-cell lymphoma – nasal enlargement – rhinophyma-like *AD 148:824–831, 2012; Ad 140:751–756, 2004; BJD 164:677–679, 2011;* hydroa vacciniforme-like cutaneous T-cell lymphoma, Epstein-Barr virus-related – edema, blisters, vesicles, ulcers, scarring, facial scars, swollen nose, lips, and periorbital edema, crusts with central hemorrhagic necrosis, facial dermatitis, photodermatitis, facial edema, facial papules and plaques, crusting of ears, fever *JAAD 69:112–119, 2013;* nasal type CD56 + natural killer cell/T-cell lymphoma *BJD 142:1021–1025, 2000;* primary cutaneous follicular center cell lymphoma *JAAD 52:S73–75, 2005;* cutaneous Richter syndrome (CLL rapidly developing into large cell lymphoma) *BJD 153:833–837, 2005;* primary cutaneous follicular center lymphoma *JAAD 65:887–889, 2011;* B-cell lymphomas (primary marginal zone lymphoma, chronic lymphocytic leukemia) mimicking rosacea or rhinophyma *AD 148:824–831, 2012*

Malignant eccrine spiradenoma *Dermatol Surg 27:417–420, 2001*

Malignant fibrous histiocytoma, myxoid *Ear Nose Throat J 91:e3–5, 2012*

Malignant histiocytosis *J Clin Pathol 35:599–605, 1982*

Melanocytic nevus, congenital

Melanoma – rhinophymatous amelanotic melanoma *Cutis 79:383–386, 2007*

Meningioma

Merkel cell carcinoma – reddish-blue nodules; legs, lip, eyelid, scalp, nose *Histopathology 7:229–249, 1983*

Metastasis – rhinophyma-like metastatic carcinoma *Cutis 57:33–36, 1996*

Microcystic adnexal carcinoma – rhinophyma-like *Laryngorhinootologie 83:113–116, 2004*

Nasal polyps

Nasal septal carcinoma – mimicking rosacea *J Derm Surg 13:1021–1024, 1987*

Nasopharyngeal carcinoma *Laryngoscope 111:645–649, 2001*

Neuroblastoma *Minim Invasive Neurosurg 44:79–84, 2001*

Neurofibroma

Neurothekeoma, atypical cellular – pink papule of the nasal tip *AD 147:1342–1343, 2011*

Osteosarcoma of the orbit *Ophthal Plast Reconstr Surg 14:62–66, 1998*

Plasmacytosis, mucocutaneous *Med Cutan Ibero Lat Am 16:339–342, 1988*

Polyps *Allergy 54 Suppl 53:7–11, 1999*

Post-transplant lymphoproliferative disorder *Ear Nose Throat Jan7, 2020*

Proliferating trichilemmal tumor *An Bras Dermatol 87:914–916, 2012*

Rhabdomyomatous mesenchymal hamartoma – sessile mass of nostril *Ped Derm 32:256–262, 2015*

Rhabdomyosarcoma

Schwannoma *No Shinkei Geka 20:1189–1194, 1992. Japanese*

Sebaceous adenoma

Sebaceous carcinoma – rhinophyma-like *BJD 124:283–284, 1991*

Sebaceous hyperplasia

Septal hamartoma *Int J Ped Otorhinolaryngol 67:669–672, 2003*

Spindle cell lipoma – facial asymmetry with deviated nasal tip *JAMADerm 156:210–211, 2020*

Striated muscle hamartoma of the nostril *J Dermatol 22:504–507, 1995*

Squamous cell carcinoma – personal observation

Trichoepitheliomas, multiple *BJD 95:225–232, 1976*

PARANEOPLASTIC DISEASES

Acrokeratosis paraneoplastica (Bazex syndrome) *Cutis 55:233–236, 1995; Medicine 70:269–280, 1991*

PRIMARY CUTANEOUS DISEASES

Acne necrotica varioliformis

Acne rosacea, granulomatous rosacea

Actinic rhinophyma – personal observation

Alopecia mucinosa

Darier's disease

Granuloma faciale *BJD 153:851–853, 2005; Am J Otolaryngol 4:184–186, 1983;* diffuse enlargement of entire nasal surface *Cutis 88:77–82, 2011; Dermatologica 105:85–99, 1952; Proc R Soc Med 38:125–126, 1945;* rhinophyma-like granuloma faciale *BJD 170:474–475, 2014;* eosinophilic angiocentric fibrosis – infiltration of mucosal surface of nose; thought to be mucosal variant of granuloma faciale

Granulosis rubra nasi *G Ital DV 125:275–276, 1990*

Malignant pyoderma *AD 122:295–302, 1986*

Rhinophyma – acne rosacea *JAAD 74:1276–1278, 2016; JAAD 72:49–58, 2015; NEJM 367:1838, 2012; BJD 161:814–818, 2009; JAAD 57:551–554, 2007;* nodular rhinophyma
    Mimickers of rhinophyma
        Amyloid *Aesthetic Plast Surg 28:98–99, 2004*
        Angiosarcoma *JAAD 49:530–531, 2003*
        Microcystic adnexal carcinoma *Laryngorhinootologie 83:113–116, 2004*
        Sebaceous carcinoma *BJD 124:283–284, 1991*
        Metastases *Cutis 57:33–36, 1996*
        Sarcoid *J Drugs Dermatol 2:333–334, 2003*

SYNDROMES

Bonnet-Dechaume-Blanc syndrome – midfacial arteriovenous malformation

Branchio-oculo-facial syndrome – bulbous nose *Ped Derm 12:24–27, 1995*

Costello's syndrome – nasal papillomas *Ped Derm 30:665–673, 2013; Ped Derm 11:277–279, 1994*

Cutaneous segmental heterotopic meningeal tissue with multifocal neural and mesenchymal hamartomas – skin colored pedunculated papules of forehead, eyelids, scalp, ala nasi; hypertrichotic heterotopic meningeal nodule *BJD 156:1047–1050, 2007*

Fibropapule multiplex of the nose – a possible variant of Cowden's disease *Dermatology 192:379–381, 1996*

Fibrous dysplasia

Hereditary progressive mucinous histiocytosis *JAAD 35:298–303, 1996*

Juvenile hyaline fibromatosis – bulbous nose *Ped Derm 6:68–75, 1989; Am J Med Genet 26:123–131, 1987;* infiltration and multi-nodularity of nose; mutation of capillary morphogenesis protein 2 gene *BJD 157:1037–1039, 2007*

Lipoid proteinosis – papules *Ped Derm 9:264–267, 1992*

Mucopolysaccharidoses

Muir-Torre syndrome

Multicentric reticulohistiocytosis *Hautarzt 46:118–120, 1995*

Proteus syndrome *J Craniofac Surg 6:151–160, 1995*

Pseudohypoparathyroidism – depressed nasal bridge *Ped Derm 9:11–18, 1993*

Steatocystoma multiplex, congenital linear *Ped Derm 17:136–138, 2000*

Tetrasomy 13q – facies with long forehead, thick eyebrows, hypertelorism, broad nasal bridge, malposition of teeth, prominent central incisors with diastema, bilateral clinodactyly of fifth fingers *Ped Derm 32:263–266, 2015*

Treacher Collins-Franceschetti syndrome (mandibulofacial dysostosis) – autosomal dominant; prominent nose, sunken cheeks, stretching of skin to side of neck, recessed chin, large down-turned mouth, wide-spaced eyes with antimongoloid slants, lateral coloboma of lower eyelids, absent eyelashes of lower lids, hairline extended to cheeks, small and crumpled pinnae, with skin tags or blind pits between tragus and angle of the mouth; hypoplastic or deformed teeth in older children *Ped Derm 23:511–513, 2006*

Trichorhinophalangeal syndrome type I – autosomal dominant; slow growing scalp hair; receding frontotemporal hairline with high bossed forehead; facial pallor, pear-shaped bulbous nose, elongated philtrum, thin upper lip, receding chin, tubercle of normal skin below the lower lip, distension, and deviation with fusiform swelling of the PIP joints; brachydactyly of thumbs and great toes, clinodactyly; hip malformation, brachydactyly, prognathism, fine brittle slow growing sparse hair, eyebrows sparse laterally, dense medially, short stature; mutation in zinc finger nuclear transcription factor (*TRPS1* gene) *BJD 163:416–419, 2010; BJD 157:1021–1024, 2007; AD 137:1429–1434, 2001; JAAD 31:331–336, 1994; Ped Derm 10:385–387, 1993; Hum Genet 74:188–189, 1986; Helv Paediatr Acta 21:475–485, 1966*

Trichorhinophalangeal syndrome type II – microcephaly with mental retardation, deep set eyes, exotropia, broad nasal bridge, thick ala nasi, cartilaginous exostoses, foot deformities, joint laxity; *EXT* gene *BJD 157:1021–1024, 2007*

Tuberous sclerosis – giant angiofibromas *JAAD 67:1319–1326, 2012*

Zimmermann-Laband syndrome *J Oral Pathol Med 19:385–387, 1990*

TRAUMA

Trauma – nasal fracture

VASCULAR DISEASES

Agminated eruptive pyogenic granuloma-like lesions over congenital vascular stains (capillary malformations) *Ped Derm 29:186–190, 2012*

Angioendotheliosarcoma *Acta DV 64:88–90, 1984*

Angiofibromas (tuberous sclerosis)

Angiomatous nevus

Arteriovenous malformation

Granulomatosis with polyangiitis

Hemangioma – infantile hemangioma *Sem Cut Med Surg 35:108–116, 2016; BJD 168:837–843, 2013; Ped Derm 26:399–404, 2009; Ped Derm 25:193–195, 2008;* diffuse hemangioma *AD 139:869–875, 2003*

NASAL SEPTAL ULCERATIONS/ PERFORATIONS (RHINOPHAGIC ULCERATION)

NEJM 352:609–615, 2005; Cutis 65:73–76, 2000

AUTOIMMUNE DISORDERS AND DISEASES OF IMMUNE DYSFUNCTION

Bullous pemphigoid *Clin Dermatol 32:817–826, 2014*

Dermatomyositis *J Rheum 13:231–232, 1986;* anti-MDA5 *J Eur Dermatol 26:315–316, 2016*

Hyper-IgE syndrome *Clin Dermatol 32:817–826, 2014; J Invest Allergol Clin Immunol 3:217–220, 1993*

IgG4 disease *Ann Rheum Dis 73:1434–1436, 2014*

Lupus erythematosus, systemic – acute exacerbation of SLE; discoid lupus erythematosus *Clin Dermatol 32:817–826, 2014; Arch Otolaryngol 99:456–457, 1974*

Mixed connective tissue disease

Pemphigus vulgaris *Clin Dermatol 32:817–826, 2014*

PLAID (*PLCG2*-associated antibody deficiency and immune dysregulation) – evaporative cold urticaria; neonatal ulcers in cold sensitive areas; granulomatous lesions sparing flexures; blotchy pruritic red rash, spontaneous ulceration of nasal tip with eschar of nose; erosion of nasal cartilage, neonatal small papules and erosions of fingers and toes; brown granulomatous plaques with telangiectasia and skin atrophy of cheeks, forehead, ears, chin; atopy; recurrent sinopulmonary infections *JAMADerm 151:627–634, 2015*

Relapsing polychondritis – saddle nose deformity, red ears, and airway collapse *NEJM 378:1715, 2018; NEJM 352:609–615, 2005; Chest 91:268–270, 1987; Medicine 55:193–216, 1976*

Rheumatoid arthritis *Int Med 58:3167–3171, 2019; Arthr Rheum 19:119–121, 1976;* methotrexate-associated lymphoproliferative disorder

Sclerederma *Arthr Rheum 19:119–121, 1976*

STING-associated vasculopathy with onset in infancy (SAVI) (type 1 interferonopathy) ((activated STING in Vascular and Pulmonary syndrome – autoinflammatory disease; red plaques of face and hands; chilblain-like lesions; atrophic plaques of hands, butterfly telangiectasias of cheeks, nose, chin, lips, acral violaceous psoriasiform, papulosquamous, and atrophic plaques of vasculitis and acral cyanosis (livedo reticularis of feet, cheeks, and knees), nodules of face, nose, and ears; distal ulcerative lesions with infarcts (necrosis of cheeks and ears), nasal septal perforation; gangrene of fingers or toes with ainhum, nasal septal perforation, nail dystrophy; polyarthritis; myositis small for gestational age; paratracheal adenopathy, abnormal pulmonary function tests; interstitial lung disease with fibrosis with ground glass and reticulate opacities; gain of function mutation in *TMEM173* (stimulator of interferon genes); mimics granulomatosis with polyangiitis *JAAD 74:186–189, 2016; Ped Derm 33:602–614, 2016; JAMADerm 151:872–877, 2015; NEJM 371:507–518, 2014*

CONGENITAL DISEASES

Nasal aplasia, heminasal aplasia with or without proboscis *Syndromes of the Head and Neck, p. 585–586, 1990*

Noma neonatorum – deep ulcers with bone loss, mutilation of nose, lips, intraorally, anus, genitalia; *Pseudomonas*, malnutrition, immunodeficiency

DEGENERATIVE DISEASES

Trigeminal trophic syndrome (Wallenberg's syndrome) *JAAD 67:325–327, 2012; AD 148:641–646, 2012; Cephalalgia 28:980–985, 2008; J Eur Acad Dermatol Venereol 21:725–731, 2007; JAAD 55:359–361, 2006; JAAD 50:549–552, 2004; BJD 141:758–759, 1999; Clin Exp Dermatol 21:299–301, 1996; AD 115:1118, 1979*

    Acoustic neuroma

    Alcohol or glycerol injection of Gasserian ganglion

    Astrocytoma

    Cortical and brainstem infarctions

    Herpes zoster ophthalmicus

    Intracranial meningioma

    Mycobacterium leprae neuritis

    Postencephalitic parkinsonism

    Posterior, inferior cerebellar artery insufficiency

    Spinal cord degeneration

    Syringobulbia

    Trauma

    Trigeminal rhizotomy

    Vertebrobasilar insufficiency

DRUGS

Aflibercept *Asia Pac J Clin Oncol 13:e179–180, 2017*

Bevacizumab *Am J Otolaryngol 38:354–355, 2017*

Corticosteroids, topical *Rhinology 36:128–132, 1998; J Pediatr 105:840–841, 1984;* intranasal steroid (nasal sprays) *Clin Dermatol 32:817–826, 2014; JAMA 253:2046, 1985*

Ketamine *ENT J 95:256, 2016*

Methotrexate *SKINMed 14:139–140, 2016; Ear Nose Throat J 88:e12–14, 2009*

Nicorandil – ulcer of forehead and nasal columella *BJD 171:662–663, 2014*

Sweet's syndrome, drug-induced – red plaques, nasal ulcers, perianal ulcers – celecoxib *JAAD 45:300–302, 2001*

Vasoconstrictors (rhinitis medicamentosa)

EXOGENOUS AGENTS

Agricultural aerosolized dust

Arsenic

Bromines

Button batteries – foreign body in the nose *J Otolaryngol 21:458–460, 1992*

Cement

Chemical and industrial dusts

Chlorines

Cocaine abuse – ulceronecrotic nasoparanasal lesions; cocaine sniffing ulcer *Clin Inf Dis 61:1840–1849, 2015; JAAD 69:135–142, 2013; AD 143:653–658, 2007; NEJM 352:609–615, 2005; Br Dent J 198:333–334, 2005; Cutis 65:73–76, 2000;* mimicking midline granuloma *JAAD 59:483–487, 2008; Eur Arch Otorhinolaryngol 255:446–447, 1998; JAAD 32:286–287, 1995; J Rheumatol 17:838–840, 1990*

Cyanides

Glass

Heavy metal

Hydrochloric acid

Lime

Methamphetamine *Iran J Otorhinolaryngol 25:53–56, 2013*

Rice and grain elevator dust

Salt

Sulfuric acid

INFECTIONS

Alternariosis

Amebiasis (*Entamoeba histolytica*) – nasal destruction with malodorous ulcer with gray-white necrotic base *Cutis 90:310–314, 2012*

Anthrax *JAAD 50:549–552, 2004*

Aspergillosis *JAAD 50:549–552, 2004*

Balamuthia mandrillaris (granulomatous amebic infection) – central facial destruction *JAAD 50:S38–41, 2004; J Trop Med Hyg 70:666–669, 2004*

Cancrum oris (noma) – nasopharyngeal mutilation *J Craniofac Surg 12:273–283, 2001*

Coccidioidomycosis

Cryptococcosis

Cytomegalovirus

Diphtheria *Clin Dermatol 32:817–826, 2014*

Fusarium falciforme – saddle nose deformity; immunosuppression *Clin Inf Dis 68:705,707–709, 2019*

Glanders – *Pseudomonas mallei* – cellulitis which ulcerates with purulent foul-smelling discharge, regional lymphatics become abscesses; nasal and palatal necrosis and destruction and mutilation; metastatic papules, pustules, bullae over joints and face, then ulcerate; deep abscesses with sinus tracts occur; polyarthritis, meningitis, pneumonia *Clin Dermatol 32:817–826, 2014*

Herpes simplex virus

Histoplasmosis *NEJM 352:609–615, 2005; Mycopathologia 176:145–150, 2013; Mycopathologia 115:13–18, 1991*

HIV/AIDS *Rhinology 37:93–95, 1999*

Leishmaniasis – *L. panamensis* – ulcera de Bejuco *JAAD 75:19–30, 2016; JAAD 73:897–908, 2015;* espundia (mucocutaneous leishmaniasis) – nasopharyngeal ulceration and/or mutilation *Clin Dermatol 32:744–751, 2014; JAAD 60:897–925, 2009; NEJM 352:609–615, 2005; Am J Trop Med Hyg 59:49–52, 1998;* post-kala azar dermal leishmanoid *Clin Dermatol 32:817–826, 2014;* masquerading as granulomatosis with polyangiitis *J Clin Rheumatol 16:125–128, 2010*

Leprosy – lepromatous leprosy – misshapen nose with collapse of nose and saddle nose deformity; nosebleeds *Ped Derm 32:863–864, 2015; NEJM 352:609–615, 2005;* primary diffuse lepromatous leprosy (la lepra bonita) *JAAD 51:416–426, 2004;* leprous trigeminal neuritis – nasopharyngeal mutilation

Mucormycosis (rhino-orbito-cerebral mucormycosis) – central facial destruction, hematoma, and ecchymosis *JAAD 65:241–243, 2011; JAAD 50:549–552, 2004;* unilateral localized facial edema with slight erythema; within days goes on to necrosis *JAAD 66:975–984,*

2012; slowly progressive cutaneous rhinofacial and pulmonary mucormycosis due to *Mucor irregularis Clin Inf Dis 56:993–995, 2013*

Mycobacterium africanum Clin Inf Dis 21:653–655, 1995

Mycobacterium kansasii J Laryngol Otol 117:992–994, 2003

Mycobacterium marinum Medicine 95:e3131, 2016

Mycobacterium tuberculosis – tuberculosis cutis orificialis *Dermatol Clin 33:541–562, 2015;* lupus vulgaris of external nose with nasal septal perforation *Indian J Tuberc 57:157–159, 2010;* vegetating forms – ulcerate, areas of necrosis, invasion of mucous membranes with destruction of cartilage (lupus vorax); saddle nose deformity; nasal involvement with friable nodules which ulcerate *J Lab Physic 159:26–30, 2017; J Formos Med Assoc 106:953–955, 2007; NEJM 352:609–615, 2005; Int J Dermatol 26:578–581, 1987; Acta Tuberc Scand 39(Suppl 49):1–137, 1960*

Myiasis *J Dermatol 22:348–350, 1995*

North American blastomycosis – nasopharyngeal mutilation *Laryngoscope 103:53–58, 1993*

Paracoccidioidomycosis – nasopharyngeal ulceration and/or mutilation *NEJM 352:609–615, 2005; JAAD 50:549–552, 2004*

Phagedenic ulcer – due to *Klebsiella Ped Derm 30:367–369, 2013*

Purpureocillium lilacinum Indian J Otolaryngol Head Neck Surg 65:184–185, 2013

Rhinoentomophthoromycosis *JAAD 50:S38–41, 2004*

Rhinoscleroma – nasopharyngeal mutilation *NEJM 352:609–615, 2005; Ped Derm 21:134–138, 2004; Acta Otolaryngol 105:494–499, 1988; Cutis 40:101–103, 1987; Wien Med Wochenschr 20:1–5, 1870*

Rhinosporidiosis – nasopharyngeal mutilation *NEJM 352:609–615, 2005*

Sporotrichosis *JAAD 50:549–552, 2004*

Staphylococcus aureus Clin Dermatol 32:817–826, 2014

Subcutaneous phaeohyphomycosis – *Corynespora cassiicola (*plant pathogen of leaf spotting disease) in CARD9 deficiency *BJD 174:176–179, 2016*

Syphilis – congenital – destruction of nasal septum; tertiary (gumma) *Arch Otolaryngol Rhinol 2:13–15, 2016; Dermatol Clin 24:497–507, 2006; NEJM 352:609–615, 2005;;* tertiary nasal syphilis; endemic (bejel) – nasopharyngeal mutilation

Typhoid *Clin Dermatol 32:817–826, 2014*

Yaws – nasopharyngeal mutilation (rhinopharyngitis mutilans) (gangosa) *JAAD 54:559–578, 2006; AD 142:12–13, 2006;*

INFLAMMATORY DISEASES

Crohn's disease *Ear Nose Throat J 79:520–523, 2000*

Lethal midline granuloma – nasopharyngeal mutilation

Malignant pyoderma – papulopustules, skin ulcers, violaceous nodules with central necrosis, tongue, pharyngeal, and nasal ulcers *AD 146:102–104, 2010; AD 98:561–576, 1968*

Pyoderma gangrenosum *Allergy Rhinol (Providence)6:122–124, 2015; Clin Dermatol 32:817–826, 2014; BJD 141:1133–1135, 1999*

Sarcoid, ulcerative – nasopharyngeal mutilation *Clin Dermatol 32:817–826, 2014; NEJM 352:609–615, 2005; Dermatology 199:265–267, 1999; JAAD 39:835–838, 1998; BJD 99(Suppl.16):54–55, 1978*

Ulcerative colitis *Inflamm Bowel Dis 18:e397–398, 2012*

METABOLIC DISORDERS

Cryoglobulinemia *J Laryngol Otol 110:668–669, 1996*

Porphyria – congenital erythropoietic porphyria – mutilation of the nose due to photosensitivity *Semin Liver Dis 2:154–63, 1982*

Prolidase deficiency – autosomal recessive; peptidase D mutation (PEPD); increased urinary imidopeptides; leg ulcers, anogenital ulcers, short stature (mild), telangiectasias, recurrent infections (sinusitis, otitis); mental retardation; splenomegaly with enlarged abdomen, atrophic scarring, spongy fragile skin with annular pitting and scarring; dermatitis, hyperkeratosis of elbows and knees, lymphedema, purpura, low hairline, poliosis, canities, lymphedema, photosensitivity, hypertelorism, saddle nose deformity, frontal bossing, dull expression, mild ptosis, micrognathia, mandibular protrusion, exophthalmos, joint laxity, deafness, osteoporosis, high arched palate *JAAD 62:1031, 1034, 2010; Ped Derm 13:58–60, 1996; JAAD 29:819–821, 1993; AD 127:124–125, 1991; AD 123:493–497, 1987*

NEOPLASTIC

Adenocarcinoma *Clin Dermatol 32:817–826, 2014*

Basal cell carcinoma *BJD 158:1386–1388, 2008; NEJM 352:609–615, 2005; Acta Pathol Microbiol Scand 88A:5–9, 1980*

Chondrosarcoma *Clin Dermatol 32:817–826, 2014*

Leukemia *Clin Dermatol 32:817–826, 2014*

Lymphoma, including extranodal nasal NK T-cell lymphoma (nasal lymphoma, polymorphic reticulosis, lymphomatoid granulomatosis, and malignant (lethal) midline granuloma) *JAAD 54:S192–197, 2006; JAAD 52:708–709, 2005; AD 133:1156–1157, 1997; Am J Surg Pathol 20: 103–111, 1996;* angiocentric lymphoma *Cancer 66:2407–2413, 1990;* B-cell lymphoma *Clin Dermatol 32:817–826, 2014*

Malignant epithelial and mesenchymal tumors (sarcomas) – nasopharyngeal mutilation *Clin Dermatol 32:817–826, 2014*

Malignant histiocytosis – mimicking lethal midline granuloma *Pathol Res Pract 171:314–324, 1981*

Melanoma

Multiple myeloma

Nasal polyps – nasopharyngeal mutilation

Squamous cell carcinoma *AD 143:889–892, 2007; NEJM 352:609–615, 2005;* associated with HPV-5 in epidermodysplasia verruciformis *J Laryngol Otol 102:834–835, 1988*

PHOTODERMATOSES

Hydroa vacciniforme – *Clin Dermatol 32:817–826, 2014*

PRIMARY CUTANEOUS DISEASES

Eosinophilic angiocentric fibrosis (variant of granuloma faciale) – red facial plaque with saddle nose deformity *Clin Dermatol 32:817–826, 2014; BJD 152:574–576, 2005; Histopathology 9:1217–1225, 1985*

Hydroa vacciniforme – saddle nose deformity *Ped Derm 21:555–557, 2004*

Neurodermatitis – personal observation

PSYCHOCUTANEOUS DISEASES

Factitial dermatitis *Clin Dermatol 32:817–826, 2014; JAAD 50:549–552, 2004*

SYNDROMES

Albright's hereditary osteodystrophy (pseudohypoparathyroidism) – osteoma cutis – periarticular calcified or ossified nodules (ectopic ossification); short stocky build; round face; low flat nasal bridge; short neck, brachymetaphalangism and brachydactyly; developmental delay, cataracts, hearing loss, seizures, poor dentition, basal ganglia calcification, osteomalacia, rickets, osteoporosis *JAMA Derm 149:975–976, 2013; JAAD 15:353–356, 1986; AD 104:636–642, 1971; Medicine 37:317–352, 1958*

Anhidrotic ectodermal dysplasia – saddle-nose deformity *Clin Dermatol 32:817–826, 2014*

Anti-phospholipid antibody syndrome – nasal tip necrosis *BJD 142:1199–1203, 2000*

Behcet's disease *Clin Dermatol 32:817–826, 2014*

CANDLE syndrome (chronic atypical neutrophilic dermatosis with lipodystrophy and elevated temperature) – annular erythematous edematous plaques of face and trunk which become purpuric and result in residual annular hyperpigmentation; limitation of range of motion with plaques over interphalangeal joints; periorbital edema with violaceous swollen eyelids, edema of lips (thick lips), lipoatrophy of cheeks, nose, and arms, chondritis with progressive ear and saddle nose deformities, hypertrichosis of lateral forehead, gynecomastia, wide spaced nipples, nodular episcleritis and conjunctivitis, epididymitis, myositis, aseptic meningitis; short stature, anemia, abnormal liver functions, splenomegaly, protuberant abdomen *Ped Derm 28:538–541, 2011; JAAD 62:487–495, 2010*

Hurler's syndrome – saddle-nose deformity *Clin Dermatol 32:817–826, 2014*

Laryngo-onycho-cutaneous syndrome – autosomal recessive type of junctional epidermolysis bullosa; skin ulceration with prominent granulation tissue, early hoarseness and laryngeal stenosis; scarred nares; chronic erosion of corners of mouth (giant perleche); paronychia with periungual inflammation and erosions; onycholysis with subungual granulation tissue and loss of nails with granulation tissue of nail bed, conjunctival inflammation with polypoid granulation tissue, and dental enamel hypoplasia and hypodontia; only in Punjabi families; mutation in laminin alpha-3 (*LAMA3A*) *BJD 169:1353–1356, 2013; Ped Derm 23:75–77, 2006; Biomedica 2:15–25, 1986*

Pseudohypoparathyroidism type IA (Albright's hereditary osteodystrophy) – subcutaneous nodule (osteoma cutis); short stature, round face, obesity, subcutaneous ossifications, bilateral brachydactyly, mental retardation, hypothyroidism, saddle nose deformity *Ped Derm 33:675–676, 2016; Atlas of Clinical Syndromes A Visual Aid to Diagnosis, 1992, pp188–189*

TOXINS

Alkaline dusts (soap powders)

Anhydrous sodium carbonate (soda ash)

Arsenic

Bromoderma – nasopharyngeal mutilation

Capsaicin (active agent in capsicum)

Chromium inhalation – chrome ulcers *Am J Ind Med 26:221–228, 1994;* chrome plating *Occup Med (Lond) 48:135–137, 1998* Copper salts

Dimethyl sulfate

Fluorides

Industrial irritants (nickel, chromium, copper, arsenic)

Iododerma – nasopharyngeal mutilation

Lime

Mercury organic compounds

Snuff

Soda ash *Br J Ind Med 11:31–37, 1954*

TRAUMA

Digital trauma

Nose picking with impacted foreign bodies *Clin Dermatol 32:817–826, 2014;* rhinotillexomania *AJNR 18:1949–1950, 1997*

Recurrent cautery

Surgery – postnasal surgery (rhinoplasty) *Plas Reconstr Surg Dec 2019;* external trauma *Clin Dermatol 32:817–826, 2014;* trophic ulcer following surgery – nasopharyngeal mutilation

VASCULAR DISEASES

Eosinophilic granulomatosis with polyangiitis *Clin Dermatol 32:817–826, 2014; Otolaryngol Head Neck Surg 88:85–89, 1980*

Hemangioma, infantile *Clin Dermatol 32:817–826, 2014*

Lymphomatoid granulomatosis – destruction of midline nasal structures; necrotic plaque of nose; crateriform nodule of cheek *JAMADerm 155:113–114, 2019*

Vasculitis

Vascular neoplasm

Granulomatosis with polyangiitis *Clin Dermatol 32:817–826, 2014; Laryngoscope 119:757–761, 2009; NEJM 352:609–615, 2005; NEJM 352:392, 2005AD 130:861–867, 1993; Ann Int Med 98:76–85, 1983*

Takayasu's arteritis *Intern Med 48:48:1551–1554, 2009;*

Arthr Rheum 19:119–121, 1976

Trigeminal trophic syndrome (posterior inferior cerebellar artery syndrome) (Wallenberg's syndrome) – nasal ulcers, facial ulcers *JAAD 74:215–228, 2016; Dt X Nervenheilk 19:227–231, 1901*

NECK LESIONS

AUTOIMMUNE DISEASES AND DISEASES OF IMMUNE DYSFUNCTION

Allergic contact dermatitis – cosmetics, nail polish *Contact Dermatitis 34:140–141, 1996;* fragrances, necklaces Compositae dermatitis – lichenified dermatitis along posterior hairline airborne allergic contact dermatitis *JAAD 15:1–10, 1986;* airborne omeprazole *Acta DV Croat 27:188–189, 2019*

Atopic dermatitis – poikiloderma-like lesions of the neck *J Dermatol 17:85–91, 1990*

Autoimmune progesterone dermatitis *S Afr Med J 17:48–50, 2016*

Brunsting-Perry cicatricial pemphigoid – herpetiform plaques with scarring *Lancet 381:320–332, 2013; J Dermatol 38:887–892, 2011; AD 75:489–501, 1957*

Bullous pemphigoid

Dermatitis herpetiformis – - personal observation

Dermatomyositis – erythema of neck

Epidermolysis bullosa acquisita

Folliculitis – pustules covering neck *J Drugs in Dermatol 12:369–374, 2013*

Graft vs. host disease, acute – papules *Taiwan I Hsueh Hui Tsa Chih 88:657–672, 1989;* pediatric – red macules or folliculocentric papules of face, ears, palms and soles, periungual areas, upper back and neck *AD 143:67–71, 2007*

Hyper IgE syndrome – papular, pustular, excoriated dermatitis of scalp, buttocks, neck, axillae, groin; furunculosis; growth failure *Clin Exp Dermatol 11:403–408, 1986; Medicine 62:195–208, 1983*

IgG4 related disease *J Dermatol 44:288–296, 2017*

Linear IgA disease (chronic bullous disease of childhood) *JAAD 54:652–656, 2006*

Lupus erythematosus – systemic LE; tumid lupus *Medicine 97:e0375, 2018; JAAD 41:250–253, 1999; Am J Dermatopathol 21:356–360, 1999;* bullous dermatosis of SLE (annular bullae) – face, neck, upper trunk, oral bullae *Semin Arthr Rheum 48:83–89, 2018; JAAD 27:389–394, 1992; Ann Int Med 97:165–170, 1982; Arthritis Rheum 21:58–61, 1978;* discoid lupus, subacute cutaneous lupus erythematosus – annular and polycyclic lesions *Med Clin North Am 73:1073–1090, 1989; JAAD 19:1957–1062, 1988;* neonatal *SKINMed 17:76–78, 2019*

Morphea

Pemphigus foliaceus of children – arcuate, circinate, polycyclic lesions *JAAD 46:419–422, 2002; Ped Derm 3:459–463, 1986*

Pemphigus vegetans – *Rom J Morph Embryol 56:563–568, 2015*

Pemphigus vulgaris – - personal observation

Rheumatoid neutrophilic dermatitis *AD 133:757–760, 1997*

Sclerederma

Sjogren's syndrome – enlarged submandibular glands *A Clinician's Pearls and Myths in Rheumatology pp.107–130; ed John Stone; Springer 2009;* annular erythema of forehead, temples, neck, and thigh *Clin Exp Rheumatol 22:55–62, 2004*

STAT1 gain of function mutation – most common cause of chronic mucocutaneous candidiasis; demodicidosis with facial papulopustular eruptions, blepharitis, chalazion, dermatitis of the neck, nail dystrophy, congenital candidiasis *Ped Derm 37:159–161, 2020*

Still's disease

Urticaria

CONGENITAL ANOMALIES

Dermatol Therapy 18:104–116, 2005

Branchial cleft cyst, sinus and/or fistula; overlying anterior border of the sternocleidomastoid muscle *Int J Oral Maxillofac Surg 25:449–452, 1996; Int J Dermatol 19:479–486, 1980;* confused with malignant or tuberculous lymphadenopathy, parotid or thyroid tumor, thymopharyngeal cyst, thyroglossal cyst, dermoid cyst, teratoma, carotid body tumor, hemangioma, neurofibroma *Plastic Reconstruct Surg 100:32–39, 1997; Arch Otolaryngol Head Neck Surg 123:438–441, 1997; J Pediatr Surg 24:966–969, 1989;* Melnick-Fraser syndrome – preauricular pits, hearing loss, and renal anomalies

Branchial cleft sinus – pit in lower third of the neck along anterior border of sternocleidomastoid muscle; skin tag at opening *Clin Otolaryngol 3:77–92, 1978*

Branchial vestige (wattles) (cervical chondrocutaneous branchial remnants) (cartilaginous rest of the neck (wattle)) – neck nodule in children – remnants include cysts (deep to middle or lower thirds of sternocleidomastoid muscles), sinus tracts, and cartilaginous remnants (overlying anterior border of sternocleidomastoid muscles); pinpoint firm masses or ear-like projections; (accessory tragus) (wattle or cervical auricle) *AD 134:499–504, 1998; Ped Clin North Amer 6:1151–1160, 1993; Cutis 58:293–294, 1996; Int J Derm 25:186–187, 1986; AD 127:404–409, 1985; JDSO 7:39–41, 1981*

Bronchogenic cyst – keratotic papule, sinus tract or cyst at the suprasternal notch; neck, shoulders, back and chest *AD 136:925–930, 2000; Ped Derm 15:277–281, 1998; Ped Derm 12:304–306, 1995; J Cutan Pathol 12:404–409, 1985*

Cervical braid *Br J Plastic Surg 43:369–370, 1990*

Cervical chondrocutaneous branchial remnants – rare benign congenital choristomas *Head Neck Pathol 12:244–246, 2018*

Cervical tab

Cervico-thymic cyst – resembles branchial cleft cyst

Congenital rhabdomyomatous mesenchymal hamartoma (striated muscle hamartoma) – skin colored pedunculated (polypoid) nodule of neck, midline of chin, upper lip *Ped Derm 16:65–67, 1999; Ped Derm 7:199–204, 1990; Ped Derm 3:153–157, 1986*

Cystic hygromas

Cystic hygroma (lymphatic malformation) *Ped Clin North Amer 6:1151–1160, 1993; NEJM 309:822–825, 1983*

Cystic teratoma – large neck mass

Dermoid cyst – lower neck *Ped Derm 36:999–1001, 2019;* neck, midline *Ped Clin NA 6:1151, 1993;* midline of nose, lateral eyebrow, scrotum, sternum, perineal raphe, and sacral areas *Curr Prob in Derm 8:137–188, 1996; Acta Neurochir (Wien) 128:115–121, 1994;* submental mass *BJD 158:415–417, 2008*

Ectopic thyroid gland *NEJM 363:1351, 2010*

Ectopic respiratory epithelium – red plaque of the neck *BJD 136:933–934, 1997*

Ectopic or christomatous salivary gland (heterotopic salivary gland tissue) – skin colored nodule along lower surface of the sternocleidomastoid muscle *JAAD 58:251–256, 2008*

Ectopic thyroid tissue *Ped Clin North Amer 6:1151–1160, 1993;* large midline subcutaneous nodule *NEJM 363:1351, 2010*

Esophageal diverticulum

Fibrous hamartoma of infancy – blue plaque of neck *AD 144:547–552, 2008*

Fourth branchial sinus causing recurrent cervical abscess *Aust N Z J Surg 67:119–122, 1997*

Laryngocele

Midline cervical clefts – vertically oriented atrophic area of lower anterior neck, associated skin tags or sinus tracts, fibrous bands connect to platysma muscle *Ped Derm 17:118–122, 2000; Int J Derm 19:479–486, 1980*

Myelomeningocele *Ped Derm 26:688–695, 2009*

Nevus simplex (capillary ectasias) – glabella, eyelids, nose, upper lip, nape of neck

Occult spinal dysraphism – papule *Ped Derm 12:256–259, 1995*

Pterygium colli medianum

Rhabdomyomatous mesenchymal hamartoma – pedunculated papule associated with a midline cervical cleft *AD 141:1161–1166, 2005*

Teratoma – bulky tumors of newborn *Ped Clin North Amer 6:1151–1160, 1993*

Thymopharyngeal cyst

Thyroglossal duct cyst and/or sinus – midline cervical mass *Ped Clin North Amer 6:1151–1160, 1993; J Pediatr Surg 24:966–969, 1989;* cleft with sinus tract *JAAD 26:885–902, 1992; J Pediatr Surg 19:437–439, 1984*

Thyroid gland – enlarged pyramidal lobe of the thyroid gland *Ped Clin North Amer 6:1151, 1993*

Wattle (cervical accessory auricle) – - personal observation

DEGENERATIVE LESIONS

Cervical trophic syndrome *JAAD 63:724–725, 2010*

DRUG REACTIONS

Bleomycin – pruritic hyperpigmented patches of neck, back, chest, thighs; not flagellate *BMJ Case Rep Sept 29, 2016*

Bortezomib (proteasome inhibitor for treatment of myeloma) – red nodules of trunk, face, neck, and extremities *JAAD 55:897–900, 2006*

Cetuximab – personal observation

Corticosteroid – topical steroid acne – - personal observation

Cyclosporine – acne keloidalis nuchae *BJD 143:465–466, 2000*

Efavirenz – HIV and HAART; bullfrog neck (HIV lipodystrophy) *AD 146:1279–1282, 2010*

Erlotinib – pustules of neck *JAAD 147:735–740, 2011*

Infliximab – symmetrical drug related intertriginous and flexural exanthems (baboon syndrome) *J Dermatol Case Rep 31:12–14, 2015*

Penicillamine – elastosis perforans serpiginosa *AD 138:169–171, 2002*

Protease inhibitor (saquinavir, nelfinavir, indinavir) – buffalo hump *JAAD 46:284–293, 2002*

Proton pump inhibitors – airborne contact dermatitis; red face and neck *Dermatitis 26:287–290, 2015*

Sirolimus (Rapamune) – acneiform eruptions of face, neck, and trunk *JAAD 55:139–142, 2006*

Thalidomide embryopathy *Atlas of Clinical Syndromes A Visual Aid to Diagnosis, 1992, pp.370–371*

Vancomycin – linear IgA disease – - personal observation

Vemurafenib – erythema and edema of face and neck *BJD 169:934–938, 2013*

EXOGENOUS AGENTS

Chrysiasis – papules *BJD 133:671–678, 1995*

Fiberglass dermatitis *Kao Hsiung I Hseveh Ko Hseueh Tsa Chih 12:491–494, 1996*

Filler (PDMS) (liquid silicone) migration – erythema and edema over cheeks and neck following lip augmentation *J Cosmet Dermatol 17:996–999, 2018*

Impaled tree branch *NEJM 373:366, 2015*

Iodide mumps – iodine contrast agent; giant acute inflammatory swelling of submandibular, sublingual, or parotid glands *Ann Int Med 145:155–156, 2006; Circulation 104:2384, 2001; Acta Radiol 36:82–84, 1995; Am J Roentgenol 159:1099–1100, 1992; JAMA 213:2271–2272, 1970; NEJM 255:433–434, 1956*

Iododerma *Australas J Dermatol 29:179–180, 1988*

Methylene blue phototoxicity – erythema of anterior neck *BJD 166:907–908, 2012*

Mudi-chood – due to oils applied to hair; papulosquamous eruption of nape of neck and upper back; begin as follicular pustules then brown-black papules with keratinous rim *Int J Dermatol 31:396–397, 1992*

Percutaneous long line – extravascular location; neck ulcer in infant *AD 147:512–514, 2011*

INFECTIONS AND INFESTATIONS

Abscess of neck – Salmonella *Head Neck 13:153–155, 1991*

Actinomycosis, cervicofacial – - midline cervical cleft with sinus tract *Laryngoscope 94:1198–1217, 1984*

AIDS – photosensitivity

Anthrax – eschar of neck *NEJM 372:954–962, 2015; Cutis 67:488–492, 2001; J Appl Microbiol 87:303, 1999; Clin Inf Dis 19:1009–1014, 1994; Cutis 48:113–114, 1991; Cutis 40:117–118, 1987*

Bacterial lymphadenitis

Beetle (*Paederus* dermatitis) – severe vesicating dermatitis *Mil Med 180:e1293–1295, 2015*

Brucellosis

Candidiasis – personal observation

Carbuncle

Cat scratch disease *Ped Clin NA 6:1151–1160, 1993*

Chromomycosis *AD 113:1027–1032, 1997; BJD 96:454–458, 1977; AD 104:476–485, 1971*

Coccidioidomycosis *AD 1345:365–370, 1998*

Corynebacterium diphtheriae – respiratory diphtheria; pharyngeal erythema with purulent exudate; swollen neck *NEJM 369:1544, 2013*

Cryptococcosis – supraclavicular mass *Head and Neck 21:239–246, 1999;* crusted plaque of neck *AD 142:921–926, 2006*

Cutaneous larva migrans *Mikrobiyol Bul 50:165–169, 2016*

Demodicidosis (demodex folliculitis) – erythema of face and neck mimicking acute graft vs. host reaction *JAMA Derm 149:1407–1409, 2013; Bone Marrow Transplant 37:711–712, 2006;* papular eruption in HIV patients of head and neck *J Med Assoc Thai 74:116–119, 1991; JAAD 20:197–201, 1989*

Dental sinus – midline cervical cleft with sinus tract *J Derm Surg Oncol 7:981–984, 1981; JAAD 2:521–524, 1980*

Diphtheria – swollen neck, fever, throat pain, difficulty swallowing, oral gray-white membrane, myocarditis *NEJM 381:1267, 2019*

Eikenella corrodens – neck wound *Clin Inf Dis 33:70–75, 2001*

Emergomyces pasteruianus Mycopathologia 185:193–200, 2020

Herpes simplex; eczema herpeticum (Kaposi's varicelliform eruption) *Clin Inf Dis 32:1480, 1500–1501, 2001;; Arch Dis Child 60:338–343, 1985;* herpes simplex folliculitis – - personal observation

Herpes zoster

Histoplasmosis

Horse fly bites *J Travel Med Sept, 2017*

Impetigo

Infectious eczematoid dermatitis

Infectious mononucleosis *Ped Clin NA 6:1151–1160, 1993*

Kaposi's varicelliform eruption

Leishmaniasis – red plaque – mucocutaneous leishmaniasis *JAMA 312:1250–1251, 2014;* nodule, crusting, ulceration, scarring *Trans R Soc Trop Med Hyg 81:606, 1987; Cutis 38:198–199, 1986; L. donovani J Trop Med May 27, 2019*

Lemierre's syndrome (human necrobacillosis) – *Fusobacterium necrophorum*; suppurative thrombophlebitis of tonsillar and peritonsillar veins and internal jugular vein; oropharyngeal pain, neck swelling, pulmonary symptoms, arthralgias *Clin Inf Dis 31:524–532, 2000*

Lobomycosis *Emerging Infect Dis 25:654–660, 2019*

Ludwig's angina – submandibular, submental swelling and edema of floor of mouth *NEJM 381:163, 2019*

Lymphadenitis *Ped Clin North Amer 6:1151, 1993*

Lymphadenopathy, reactive – supraclavicular mass *Head and Neck 21:239–246, 1999*

Mucormycosis – red plaque of neck *Cutis 89:167–168, 2012*

Molluscum contagiosum – giant ulceroproliferative neck lesion *Diagn Cytopathol 46:794–796, 2018*

Mycobacterium avium – intracellulare Ped Clin North Amer 6:1151–1160, 1993

Mycobacterium bovis – scrofuloderma *JAMADerm 155:610, 2019*

Mycobacterium fortuitum – following neck liposuction *Dermatol Surg 26:588–590, 2000;* red plaque mimicking lupus vulgaris *BJD 147:170–173, 2002*

Mycobacterium scrofulaceum Ped Clin NA 6:1151–1160, 1993

Mycobacterium tuberculosis – scrofuloderma – infected lymph node, bone, joint, lacrimal gland with overlying red-blue nodule which breaks down, ulcerates, forms fistulae, scarring with adherent fibrous masses which may be fluctuant and draining *Cutis 85:85–89, 2010; Dermatol Therapy 21:154–161, 2008; JAAD 54:559–578, 2006; BJD 134:350–352, 1996; Ped Clin North Amer 6:1151–1160, 1993;* scrofuloderma after BCG vaccination *Ped Derm 19:323–325, 2002; J Dermatol 21:106–110, 1924;* tuberculous cervical adenitis *Ped Derm 37:29–39, 2020;* tuberculous cold abscess of the neck *JAMADerm 150:909–910, 2014; BJD 142:387–388, 2000;* massive tuberculous lymphadenopathy (red nodule) of lower neck in paradoxical response to anti-tuberculous therapy associated with infliximab treatment *Clin Inf Dis 40:756–759, 2005;* lupus vulgaris – vegetative linear serpiginous lesion of neck *Ped Derm 36:955–957, 2019*

Myiasis – *Dermatobia hominis;* abscess of posterior neck *JAAD 57:716–718, 2007*

Necrotizing fasciitis of neck *Int J Surg Case Rep 59:220–223, 2019*

Nocardiosis *Cutis 104:226–229, 2019*

North American blastomycosis

Orf *Acta DV Croat 27:280–281, 2019*

Paracoccidioidomycosis – massive cervical adenopathy *JAAD 53:931–951, 2005; Br J Radiol 72:717–722, 1999;* cutaneous nodules *Annual Meeting AAD 2000*

Pasteurella multocida

Pediculosis

Phaeoacremonium inflatipes – fungemia in child with aplastic anemia; swelling and necrosis of lips, periorbital edema, neck swelling *Clin Inf Dis 40:1067–1068, 2005*

Pityrosporum folliculitis *Mycoses 40(suppl 1):29–32, 1997*

Plague

Rat-bite fever

Roseola infantum *(*human herpesvirus 6*)* – rose-pink macules start on neck and trunk, then spread to face and extremities

Scabies, nodular *Ped Derm 11:264–266, 1994;* crusted scabies; *Iran J Public Health 48:1169–1173, 2019*

Sporotrichosis – cutaneous lesions with or without cervical lymphadenopathy; head and neck most frequent in children *J Chiliena Infectol 33:315–321, 2016; JAAD 53:931–951, 2005*

Staphylococcus aureus – folliculitis; furunculosis; staphylococcal lymphadenitis *Head and Neck 21:239–246, 1999*

Subcutaneous phaeohyphomycosis – *Cladosporium cladosporioides*; cysts and nodules of the face and neck for 5 years; *Mycopathologia 181:567–573, 2016*

Sycosis barbae

Syphilis – primary chancre; secondary *AD 133:1027, 1030, 1997;* leukoderma syphiliticum *JAAD 55:187–189, 2006;* secondary – most commonly involved body site was the neck *Int J STD AIDS 29:1454–1456, 2018*

Tinea corporis

Tinea versicolor *Indian J Pathol Microbiol 59:159–165, 2016*

Toxoplasmosis

Trichophytosis barbae *Indian J Med Microbiol 33:444–447, 2015*

Tularemia

Verruca vulgaris

Verruga peruana *Am J Trop Med and Hygiene 50:143, 1994*

INFILTRATIVE DISEASES

Amyloidosis – nodular amyloidosis *AD 139:1157–1159, 2003*

Colloid milium *Clin Exp Dermatol 18:347–350, 1993; BJD 125:80–81, 1991*

Mastocytosis – - personal observation

Juvenile xanthogranuloma (generalized lichenoid juvenile xanthogranuloma) – face, neck, scalp, upper trunk *Child Nerv Syst 34:765–770, 2018; BJD 126:66–70, 1992;* multiple *BMJ Case Rep July 1, 2019*

Langerhans cell histiocytosis – in adults *SKINMed 14:147–149, 2016*

Scleredema, diabetes-associated – swollen neck *JAMA 315:1159–1160, 2016*

Xanthoma disseminatum *Iran J Otorhinolaryngol 29:365–368, 2019*

INFLAMMATORY DISEASES

Eosinophilic pustular folliculitis *J Dermatol 25:178–184, 1998*

Folliculitis nuchae scleroticans *Hautarzt 39:739–742, 1988*

Hidradenitis suppurativa – nodulocystic lesions of posterior neck and post-auricular areas *AD 147:1343–1344, 2011*

Malignant pyoderma

Pseudofolliculitis barbae

Rosai-Dorfman disease – sinus histiocytosis with massive lymphadenopathy

Sarcoid – mask-like hypopigmented plaque of posterior neck *The Dermatologist; February 2015; p.47–50; Laryngoscope 87:2038–2048, 1977;* subcutaneous sarcoid *World J Clin Cases 7:2505–2512, 2019*

Toxic epidermal necrolysis

METABOLIC DISEASES

Acrodermatitis enteropathica – - personal observation

Chronic alcoholism – telangiectatic mats – - personal observation

Alpha-1 anti-trypsin panniculitis

Congenital disorders of glycosylation (CDG-Ix) – nuchal skin folds, facial dysmorphism, inverted nipples, hypoplastic nails, petechiae and ecchymoses, edema; neurologic, gastrointestinal and genitourinary abnormalities, pericardial effusion, ascites, oligohydramnios *Ped Derm 22:457–460, 2005*

Congenital dyserythropoietic anemia type I – small or absent nails; partial absence or shortening of fingers and toes, mesoaxial polydactyly, syndactyly of hands and feet; short stature, vertebral abnormalities and Madelung deformity; mutation in *CDAN1 Clin Exp Dermatol 515–517, 2020*

Cryoglobulinemia – papules *JAAD 25:21–27, 1991*

Essential fatty acid deficiency

Fabry's disease – telangiectasias of the neck *J Dermatol 33:652–654, 2006*

Goiter

Pellagra (niacin deficiency) – Casal's necklace; red pigmented sharply marginated photodistributed rash, including drug-induced pellagra-like dermatitis – 6-mercaptopurine, 5-fluorouracil,INH (all of the above – also seborrheic dermatitis-like); resembles Hartnup disease *NEJM 371:2218–2223, 2014; Cutis 68:31–34, 2001; Ped Derm 16:95–102, 1999; BJD 125:71–72, 1991*

Porphyria – porphyria cutanea tarda with calcinosis; congenital erythropoietic porphyria *BJD 148:160–164, 2003;* bullae, erosions and crusts of neck and hands *Dermatol Ther 32:e13014, 2019*

Pregnancy – hyperpigmentation of neck, nipples, anogenital skin

Pretibial myxedema *JAAD 46:723–726, 2002*

Pruritic urticarial papules and plaques of pregnancy *Z Hautkr 65:831–832, 1990*

Xanthomas, including plane xanthomatosis *BJD 133:961–966, 1995;* eruptive *Acta Med Port 31:219–222, 2018*

Acquired zinc deficiency – - personal observation

NEOPLASTIC DISEASES

Acrochordon (skin tags)

Actinic keratosis

Adenoid cystic carcinoma *JAAD 17:113–118, 1987*

Angiomatoid fibrous histiocytoma *Dermatol Surg 26:491–492, 2000*

Apocrine carcinoma *Cancer 71:375–381, 1993;* carcinoma erysipelatoides (red plaque of head and neck) *AD 147:1335–1337, 2011*

Atypical fibroxanthoma *Auris Nasus Larynx 42:469–471, 2015*

Basal cell carcinoma *Cancer 92:354–358, 2001;* following radiotherapy *AD 108:523–527, 1973*

Basosquamous carcinoma *Otolaryngol Head Neck Surg 87:420–427, 1979*

Blastic plasmacytoid dendritic cell neoplasm *Rev Med Chil 145:1208–1212, 2017*

Bowenoid papulosis – neck papules *JAAD 41:867–870, 1999*

Carotid body tumor

Cephalic histiocytomas *Am J Dermatopathol 15:581–586, 1993*

Chondroid syringoma *Ear Nose Throat J 75:104–108, 1996*

Collagenoma – linear *Ped Derm 26:626–628, 2009;* Pacinian collagenoma (form of sclerotic fibroma) *J Cut Pathol 47:291–2020*

Cylindromas – scalp, face, nose, around ears, and neck

Cysts on neck
    Branchial cleft anomaly (cyst, sinus, and/or fistula)
        Bronchogenic cyst
    Dermoid cyst
        Epidermoid cyst
    Eruptive vellus hair cysts
    Heterotopic salivary gland tissue
    Milia
    Pilar cyst
    Steatocystoma multiplex/simplex
        Thyroglossal duct cyst
    Teratomas

Deep penetrating nevus *JAAD 71:1234–1240, 2014*

Dermatofibrosarcoma protuberans *Oncol Lett 10:3765–3768, 2015*

Dermatosis papulosa nigra *Int J Derm 56:975–980, 2017*

Desmoplastic trichoepithelioma *Acta DV Croat 27:282–284, 2019*

Epidermal nevus

Epidermoid inclusion cyst

Eruptive fibromas *J Cut Pathol 25(2):122–125, 1998*

Eruptive histiocytoma *J Dermatol 20:105–108, 1993*

Eruptive syringomas

Eruptive vellus hair cysts *Ped Derm 5:94–96, 1988*

Fibroblastic connective tissue nevus *J Cut Pathol 44:827–834, 2017*

Ganglioneuroma of cervical sympathetic chain *Ped Clin North Amer 6:1151–1160, 1993*

Giant cell fibroblastoma of soft tissue – neck and trunk *Ped Derm 18:255–257, 2001*

Heterotopic submandibular salivary glands – submental mass *Ped Clin North Amer 6:1151–1160, 1993*

Hibernoma – neck, axilla, central back; vascular dilatation overlying lesion *NEJM 367:1636, 2012; AD 73:149–157, 1956*

Benign cephalic histiocytosis – neck papules *AD 135:1267–1272, 1999*

Inflammatory linear verrucous epidermal nevus (ILVEN)

Infantile myofibromatosis – red to skin-colored nodules *AD 134:625–630, 1998*

Inverted follicular keratosis *J Clin Pathol 28:465–471, 1975*

Kaposi's sarcoma *Int J Dermatol 58:1388–1397, 2019; Otolaryngol Head Neck Surg 111:618–624, 1994; Ann Int Med 103:744–750, 1985*

Keloids – personal observation

Keratoacanthoma, including Ferguson-Smith tumors *Ann Dermatol Venereol 104:206–216, 1977;* solitary giant keratoacanthoma *Dermatol Surg 43:810–816, 2017*

Leukemia cutis *Laryngoscope 86:1856–1863, 1976;* cervical adenopathy *Ped Clin North Amer 6:1151–1160, 1993*

Lipofibromata, eruptive *AD 119:612–614, 1983*

Lipoma supraclavicular mass *Head and Neck 21:239–246, 1999;* spindle cell lipomas *JAAD 48:82–85, 2003;* large neck mass in infancy

Liposarcoma – swollen neck *NEJM 363:864, 2010*

Lymphadenoma, cutaneous – papules or nodules of head and neck *BJD 128:339–341, 1993;* adamantoid variant of trichoblastoma *J Cut Pathol 44:954–957, 2017*

Lymphadenopathy, malignant

Lymphoma – cutaneous T-cell lymphoma; folliculotropic CTCL – red plaque of face (periauricular), head, neck; comedo-like lesions, acneiform, cystic, follicular keratotic papules *JAAD 62:418–426, 2010;* and Ki-1+ lymphoma; anaplastic large cell B-cell lymphoma; cutaneous B-cell lymphomas *Am J Surg Pathol 10:454–463, 1986;* diffuse large cell B-cell lymphoma – acute violaceous indurated plaque of neck *Ped Derm 34:703–705, 2017;* angiocentric lymphoma – edema of face and neck *Indian J Pathol Microbiol 34:293–295, 1991;* Hodgkin's disease – ulcerated papules and nodules *AD 133:1454–1455, 1457–1458, 1997;* Hodgkin's disease mimicking scrofuloderma *Dermatology 199:268–270, 1999;* granulomatous slack skin syndrome (CTCL) *BJD 142:353–357, 2000; Ped Derm 14:204–208, 1997; AD 121:250–252, 1985;* lymphomatous lymphadenopathy – neck masses *Ped Clin North Amer 6:1151–1160, 1993;* Burkitt's lymphoma CD4+ small,/medium pleomorphic T-cell lymphoma – skin colored nodule of face, red nodule of scalp, red plaque of neck *JAAD 65:739–748, 2011;* primary cutaneous follicle center cell lymphoma – multilobulated nodules, red plaques of scalp, nodules of head and neck, papules of head and neck *JAAD 70:1010–1020, 2014;* subcutaneous panniculitis-like T-cell lymphoma – nodules of head and neck, legs, trunk, cheeks, lips *Ped Derm 32:526–532, 2015* angioimmunoblastic T-cell lymphoma – red plaque of neck *Cutis 102:179–182, 2018;* CD4/CD8

dual positive cutaneous peripheral C-cell lymphoma *Am J Dermatopathol 40:836–840, 2018*

Lymphoplasmacytoid immunocytoma *Hautarzt 44:172–175, 1993*

Malignant proliferating trichilemmal tumor *BJD 150:156–157, 2004*

Medallion-like dermal dendrocyte hamartoma – blue-brown oval depression of back of neonate; thin hair on surface *AD 142:921–926, 2006;* of neck *JAAD 51:359–363, 2004;* wrinkled pliable pink-yellow atrophic patch with plucked chicken appearance of lateral neck *Ped Derm 27:638–642, 2010*

Melanoma *Dermatology Nov 8, 2019; Acta Oncol 38:1069–1074, 1999; Am J Trop Med and Hygiene 50(2):143, 1994*

Merkel cell carcinoma *Arch Plast Surg 46:441–448, 2019*

Metastases – supraclavicular masses; breast, uterine, cervical, lung, stomach, oropharyngeal carcinomas *Head and Neck 21:239–246, 1999;* carcinoma erysipelatoides – violaceous plaques of neck and upper chest *AD 147:345–350, 2011;* carcinoma en cuirasse (gastric) *BMJ Case Rep April 30, 2019*

Mucoepidermoid carcinoma *Laryngoscope 93:464–467, 1983*

Neurilemmoma

Neuroblastoma of cervical sympathetic chain – neck mass *Ped Clin North Amer 6:1151–1160, 1993*

Neurofibroma – plexiform neurofibromas of brachial plexus *Ped Clin North Amer 6:1151–1160, 1993*

Neuroma – hypercellular encapsulated neuroma *Am J Dermatopathol 41:358–260, 2019*

Neurothekeoma *Am J Surg Pathol 14:113–120, 1990*

Nevi, melanocytic, including eruptive melanocytic nevi (papules) *JAAD 37:337–339, 1997; J Dermatol 22:292–297, 1995*

Nevus comedonicus *Dermatol Online J Sept 15, 2016*

Nevus sebaceous

Nevus spilus *Dermatol Ther July 30, 2014*

Nuchal fibroma – solitary subcutaneous mass of back of neck; multiple lesions associated with Gardner's syndrome *JAAD 66:959–965, 2012*

Paraganglioma – neck mass *Ped Clin NA 6:1151–1160, 1993;*

Pilomatrixoma *Am J Dermatopathol 41:293–295, 2019; Clin Exp Dermatol 42:400–402, 2017; Otolaryngol Head Neck Surg 125:510–515, 2001; J Cutan Pathol 18:20–27, 1991*

Porokeratosis – personal observation

Post-transplantation lymphoproliferative disorder – lymphadenopathy of head and neck *JAAD 54:657–663, 2006*

Primary histiocytic sarcoma *Ann Diag Pathol 32:56–62, 2018*

Rhabdomyosarcoma – neck nodule in children *JAAD 31:871–876, 1994; Ped Clin North Amer 6:1151–1160, 1993*

Schwannoma – supraclavicular mass *Head and Neck 21:239–246, 1999;* lateral neck nodule *Ped Derm 353–354, 2016*

Spinal cord tumor – excoriations – personal observation

Spindle cell lipoma – subcutaneous nodule of posterior neck *AD 142:921–926, 2006*

Squamous cell carcinoma *J Laryngol Otol 110:694–695, 1996;* metastatic squamous cell carcinoma – red nodule of submandibular region *J Drugs Dermatol 13:1277–1279, 2014;* Marjolin's ulcer *Exp Ther Med 17:3403–3410, 2019*

Syringocystadenoma papilliferum *AD 121:1198–1201, 1985;* linear vascular appearing nodules of neck *AD 144:1509–1514, 2008*

Syringoma – generalized eruptive *Dermatol Online J Sept 15, 2017*

Syringomatous carcinoma – neck plaque *Cutis 77:19–24, 2006*

Thymus gland rests – mass of lower neck or suprasternal notch *Ped Clin NA 6:1151–1160, 1993*

Thyroid adenoma, carcinoma, colloid cysts – neck nodules *Ped Clin NA 6:1151–1160, 1993*

Trichilemmal carcinoma *Saudi Med J 39:213–216, 2018*

Trichoblastic carcinoma *Arch Craniofac Surg 19:275–278, 2018*

Trichoepithelioma *Acta DV Croat 26:162–165, 2018;* unilateral trichoepitheliomas of neck *Dermatol Online J Nov 18, 2015*

Tumor of follicular infundibulum – facial and neck hypopigmented macules and patches (multiple) *JAMADerm 152:1155–1156, 2016*

Verrucous carcinoma

Warthin's tumor, extraparotid – skin colored neck nodule *JAAD 40:468–470, 1999*

Warty dyskeratoma

PARANEOPLASTIC DISORDERS

Acrokeratosis paraneoplastica (Bazex syndrome) *J Laryg Otol 110:899–900, 1996*

Necrobiotic xanthogranuloma with paraproteinemia *Case Rep Dermatol 8:350–353, 2016; Int J Clin Exp Pathol 8:3304–3307, 2015*

Normolipemic plane xanthomatosis *BJD 135:460–462, 1996*

PHOTODERMATOSES

Actinic granuloma *AD 122:43–47, 1986*

Berloque dermatitis

Cutis rhomboidalis nuchae

Photoallergic contact dermatitis – personal observation

Phytophotodermatitis – personal observation

Poikiloderma of Civatte *Ann Dermatol Syphilol 9:381–420, 1938*

Riehl's melanosis

PRIMARY CUTANEOUS DISORDERS

Acanthosis nigricans/pseudoacanthosis nigricans

Acne keloidalis nuchae *Plast Reconstr Surg Glob Open 7:e2215, 2019*

Acne vulgaris *AD 131:341–344, 1995*

Alopecia mucinosa (follicular mucinosis) – neck plaque *JAAD 38:622–624, 1998; Dermatology 197:178–180, 1998; JAAD 10:760–768, 1984; AD 76:419–426, 1957*

Atopic dermatitis

Anetoderma of Jadassohn *AD 120:1032–1039, 1984*

Annular lichenoid dermatitis of youth *Dermatol Ther 27:e13285, 2020*

Blaschkitis – personal observation

Bullous prurigo pigmentosa – pruritic reticulated bullous eruption of neck and trunk *JAMADerm 150:1005–1006, 2014; Dermatologica sinica 27:103–110, 2009*

Centrifugal lipodystrophy *Dermatology 188:142–144, 1994*

Confluent and reticulated papillomatosis *Actas Dermatosifiliogr 109:e7–911, 2018*

Cutis laxa

Darier's disease *Dermatology 188:157–159, 1994*

Diaper dermatitis with rapid dissemination – expanding nummular dermatitis of trunk, and red scaly plaques of neck and axillae ("psoriasiform id") *BJD 78:289–296, 1966*

Disseminate and recurrent infundibulofolliculitis – skin-colored papules and pustules of neck and upper chest *Indian J Dermatol 64:404–406, 2019*

Dowling-Degos disease

Elastoderma *JAAD 53:S147–149, 2005*

Elastosis perforans serpiginosa *J Dermatol 24:458–465, 1997; Hautarzt 43:640–644, 1992; AD 97:381–393, 1968*

Epidermodysplasia verruciformis – personal observation

Epidermolysis bullosa – epidermolysis bullosa simplex – neck bullae *BJD 162:980–989, 2010;* recessive inverse dystrophic – groin, axillae, neck, lower back, nail dystrophy, oral erosions (dermolytic dystrophic) *AD 124:544–547, 1988*

Epidermolytic hyperkeratosis

Erythema annulare centrifugum

Erythromelanosis follicularis of face and neck (faciei et colli) – red-brown pigmentation with telangiectasias, follicular papules involving preauricular and maxillary regions and extending to mandible and neck *Cutis 79:459–461, 2007; Ped Derm 23:31–34, 2006; JAAD 32:863–866, 1995; Hautarzt 9:391–393, 1960*

Fibroelastolytic papulosis of the neck *BJD 173:461–466, 1997*

Granular parakeratosis – red neck *Ped Derm 33:665–666, 2016*

Granuloma annulare *Citos 55:158–160, 1995*

Granuloma gluteal infantum – personal observation

Grover's disease (benign papular acantholytic dermatosis) *AD 112:814–821, 1976*

Hailey-Hailey disease *Open Acesi Maced J Med Sci 7:3070–3072, 2019; BJD 126:275–282, 1992; Arch Dermatol Syphilol 39:679–685, 1939*

Neonatal ichthyosiform erythroderma, hyperpigmented verrucous and cerebriform plaques of heels and neck *BJD 176:249–251, 2017*

Ichthyosis vulgaris – personal observation

Idiopathic eruptive macular hyperpigmentation – light brown non-confluent macules 3–25 mm of neck or extremities (distinguished from erythema dyschromicum perstans) *BJD 157:840-, 2007; JAAD 49:S280–282, 2003; JAAD 44: 351–353, 2001; Ped Derm 13:274–277, 1996; JAAD 11:159, 1984; Ann DV 105:177–182, 1978*

Impetigo herpetiformis

Juxtaclavicular beaded lines *J Cutan Pathol 18:464–468, 1991*

Kimura's disease *Exp Ther Med 16:1087–1093, 2018; Am J Kid Dis 11:353–356, 1988*

Lichen nitidus

Lichen planus including lichen planus pigmentosus *Clin Exp Dermatol 44:190–193, 2019*

Lichen sclerosus et atrophicus, guttate

Lichen simplex chronicus

Lichen spinulosus *JAAD 22:261–264, 1990*

Lupus miliaris disseminate faciei *Am J Dermatopathol 40:819–823, 2018*

Miliaria rubra in infants *BJD 99:117–137, 1978*

Napkin psoriasis

Nevoid hypertrichosis

Pityriasis rosea

Pityriasis rubra pilaris – personal observation

Prurigo nodularis

Prurigo pigmentosa – red papules with vesiculation and crusting arranged in reticulated pattern or reticulate plaques of back, neck, and chest; heals with reticulated hyperpigmentation; urticarial red pruritic papules, papulovesicles, vesicles, and plaques with reticulated hyperpigmentation *Ped Derm 24:277–279, 2007; JAAD 55:131–136, 2006; Cutis 63:99–102, 1999; JAAD 34:509–11, 1996; AD 130:507–12, 1994; BJD 120:705–708, 1989; AD 125:1551–1554, 1989; JAAD 12:165–169, 1985; J Dermatol 5:61–67, 1978; Jpn J Dermatol 81:78–91, 1971*

Pseudofolliculitis barbae

Psoriasis

Scleredema of Buschke (pseudoscleroderma) *JAAD 11:128–134, 1984*

Seborrhiasis

Syringolymphoid hyperplasia *JAAD 49:1177–1180, 2003*

Terra firme (Diogenes syndrome) (terra firme-forme dermatosis) – hyperpigmented hyperkeratotic plaques of neck of teenagers and pre-teens (teenage scruff neck) *Ped Derm 36:501–504, 2019; Ped Derm 29:297–300, 2012;* self-neglect *Lancet i:366–368, 1975*

Upper dermal elastolysis *J Cutan Pathol 21:533–540, 1994*

Vitiligo

White fibrous papulosis of the neck *Int J Derm 35:720–722, 1996; BJD 127:295–296, 1992*

X-linked ichthyosis

PSYCHOCUTANEOUS DISEASES

Factitial dermatitis *Ann DV 143:210–214, 2016; Ped Derm 32:604–608, 2015*

SYNDROMES

Acrogeria *Dermatology 192:264–268, 1996*

Aicardi syndrome *Atlas of Clinical Syndromes A Visual Aid to Diagnosis, 1992, pp.292–293*

Albright's hereditary osteodystrophy – pseudohypoparathyroidism, round face, short neck, osteomas of skin with overlying hyperpigmentation, short stature, hypogonadism, macrocephaly, psychomotor retardation, endocrinologic abnormalities; mutation in *GNAS1 JAMA Derm 149:975–976, 2013; Ped Derm 28:135–137, 2011; Endocrinology 30:922–932, 1942*

Barber-Say syndrome – generalized hypertrichosis, dysmorphic facies (bilateral ectropion, hypertelorism, macrostomia, abnormal ears, bulbous nose, sparse eyebrows and eyelashes, hypoplasia of nipples with absence of mammary glands, transposition of scrotum, club feet, short neck, lax skin, premature aged appearance, cleft palate, conductive hearing loss *Ped Derm 23:183–184, 2006; Syndrome Ident 8:6–9, 1982*

Baverstedt syndrome – linear horny excrescences of face and neck; mental retardation, seizures *Acta DV 22:207–212, 1941*

Becker's syndrome – discrete or confluent brown macules of neck, forearms *AD Syphilol 40:987–998, 1939*

Behcet's syndrome – superior vena cava syndrome – superior and inferior vena cava obstruction; dilated and tortuous veins of chest wall, facial edema, thickening of neck with neck vein distension, upper body edema and edema of arms and legs, proptosis; superficial and deep thrombophlebitis *BJD 159:555–560, 2008*

Birt-Hogg-Dube syndrome *AD 133:1163–1166, 1997;* comedonal or cystic fibrofolliculomas *JAMADerm 151:770–774, 2015*

Branchiooculofacial syndrome – autosomal dominant; congenital bilateral cervical ulcerations (bilateral ectopic thymus glands); congenital ulcerated neck mass (ectopic thymus), flattened nasal tip, pseudo-cleft lip, posterior rotated ears, pre-auricular pit, cleft lip, microphthalmia, coloboma, nasolacrimal duct stenosis or atresia, dolichocephaly; mutation in *TFAP2A* (retinoic acid responsive gene) *Ped Derm 29:759–761, 2012; Mol Vis 16:813–818, 2010; Arch Otolaryngol Head Neck Surg 128:714–717, 2002;* (pseudocleft of upper lip, cleft-lip-palate, and hemangiomatous branchial cleft) – atrophic neck lesions *Ped Derm 29:383–384, 2012; Am J Med Genet 27:943–951, 1987*

Branchio-oto-renal syndrome (Melnick-Fraser syndrome) – autosomal dominant, chromosome 8q – abnormal pinna, prehelical pits, renal anomalies, branchial cleft fistulae and/or cysts pre-auricular sinus tract or cyst *Am J Nephrol2:144–146, 1982; Am J Med Genet 2:241–252, 1978; Clin Genet 9:23–34, 1976*

Brooke-Spiegler syndrome – eccrine spiradenomas, cylindromas, trichoepitheliomas *Int J Surg Case Rep 51:277–281, 2018*

Buschke-Ollendorff syndrome *Eur J Dermatol 11:576–579, 2001*

Cleidocranial dysplasia *Atlas of Clinical Syndromes A Visual Aid to Diagnosis, 1992, pp.32–33*

Coffin-Siris syndrome – webbed neck, bifid scrotum, umbilical and inguinal hernias *JAAD 46:161–183, 2002*

Cornelia de Lange (Brachmann-de Lange) syndrome – generalized hypertrichosis, and hypertrichosis of posterior neck, confluent eyebrows, low hairline, hairy forehead and ears, hair whorls of trunk, single palmar crease, cutis marmorata, psychomotor and growth retardation with short stature, specific facies, hypertrichosis of forehead, face, back, shoulders, and extremities, bushy arched eyebrows with synophrys; long delicate eyelashes, skin around eyes and nose with bluish tinge, small nose with depressed root, prominent philtrum, thin upper lip with crescent shaped mouth, widely spaced, sparse teeth, hypertrichosis of forehead, and arms, low set ears, arched palate, antimongoloid palpebrae; congenital eyelashes *Ped Derm 24:421–423, 2007; JAAD 37:295–297, 1997; Am J Med Genet 47:959–964, 1993*

Costello syndrome – warty papules around nose and mouth, legs, perianal skin; loose skin of neck, hands, and feet, thick, redundant palmoplantar surfaces, hypoplastic nails, short stature, craniofacial abnormalities *Am J Med Genet 117:42–48, 2003; Eur J Dermatol 11:453–457, 2001; Am J Med Genet 82:187–193, 1999; JAAD 32:904–907, 1995; Am J Med Genet 47:176–183, 1993; Aust Paediat J 13:114–118, 1977*

Cowden's syndrome – skin tags *OSOMOPOR 125:209–214, 2018*

Craniocarpotarsal dysplasia (whistling face syndrome) – webbed neck *Birth Defects 11:161–168, 1975*

Delleman syndrome (oculocerebrocutaneous syndrome) – pedunculated facial papules and atrophic patches of neck; accessory tragi and aplasia cutis congenita *AD 147:345–350, 2011; J Med Genet 25:773–778, 1988*

Diffuse infiltrative lymphocytosis syndrome (DILS) – autoimmune syndrome with oligoclonal expansion of CD8+ T lymphocytes in response to HIV antigens; lymphocytic infiltration of salivary glands (parotid glands) and viscera *Clin Lab Haem 27:278–282, 2005*

Diffuse pigmentation of trunk and neck with subsequent white macules *Proc R Soc Med 48:179–180, 1955*

Diffuse pigmentation with macular depigmentation of trunk with reticulate pigmentation of neck *Hautarzt 6:458–460, 1955*

Distichiasis and lymphedema – webbed neck

Dowling-Degos disease *Indian J DV Leprol 84:70–72, 2018*

Down's syndrome – webbed neck

Dyskeratosis congenita (Zinsser-Engman-Cole syndrome) – Xq28 *J Med Genet 33:993–995, 1996; Dermatol Clin 13:33–39, 1995; BJD 105:321–325, 1981*

Ekbom's syndrome (myoclonic epilepsy and ragged muscle fibers) (mitochondrial syndrome) – cervical lipomas *JAAD 39:819–823, 1998*

Encephalocraniocutaneous lipomatosis *Ped Derm 10:164–168, 1993*

Epidermodysplasia verruciformis

Franceschetti-Jadassohn-Naegeli syndrome – generalized reticulated hyperpigmentation, accentuated in neck and axillae *JAAD 10:1–16, 1984*

Gardner's syndrome – nuchal-type fibroma *Am J Surg Pathol 24:1563–1567, 2000*

Goldenhar syndrome (oculoauriculovertebral syndrome) – epibulbar dermoid cysts, vertebral defects, accessory tragi *Int J Derm 19:479–486, 1980*

Hermansky-Pudlak syndrome – actinic keratoses *J Dermatol 44:219–220, 2017*

Hidrotic ectodermal dysplasia *Hautarzt 42:645–647, 1991*

Hunter's syndrome – skin colored to white papules of nape of neck *AD 113:602–605, 1977*

Infantile cortical hyperostosis *Atlas of Clinical Syndromes A Visual Aid to Diagnosis, 1992, pp.102–103*

Infantile myofibromatosis *Int J Pediatr Otorhinolaryngol 51:181–186, 1999; Ped Derm 8:306–309, 1991; Ped Derm 5:37–46, 1988*

Job's syndrome (hyper IgE syndrome) – autosomal dominant or sporadic; cold abscesses of neck and trunk; atrophoderma vermiculatum; coarse facial features with broad nose, rough thickened skin with prominent follicular ostia; papular and papulopustular folliculitis-like eruptions; oral candidiasis; chronic paronychia; otitis media common; mutation in *STAT3* (transcription 3 gene activator and signal transducer) *JAAD 65:1167–1172, 2011*

Juvenile hyaline fibromatosis (systemic hyalinosis) – translucent papules or nodules of scalp, face, neck, trunk, gingival hypertrophy, flexion contractures of large and small joints *JAAD 16:881–883, 1987*

Kawasaki's disease – cervical adenopathy *Ped Clin North Amer 6:1151–1160, 1993*

Klippel-Feil anomaly – webbed neck *J Bone Jt Surg 56:1246–1253, 1974;* neckless or short neck *Atlas of Clinical Syndromes A Visual Aid to Diagnosis, 1992, pp.296–297*

LEOPARD (Moynahan) syndrome – CALMs, granular cell myoblastomas, steatocystoma multiplex, small penis, hyperelastic skin, low set ears, short webbed neck, short stature, syndactyly *JAAD 46:161–183, 2002; Am J Med 60:447–456, 1976; JAAD 40:877–890, 1999; J Dermatol 25:341–343, 1998; Am J Med 60:447–456, 1976; AD 107:259–261, 1973*

Lymphedema-distichiasis syndrome – periorbital edema, vertebral abnormalities, spinal arachnoid cysts, congenital heart disease, thoracic duct abnormalities, hemangiomas, cleft palate, microphthalmia, strabismus, ptosis, short stature, webbed neck *Ped Derm 19:139–141, 2002; Atlas of Clinical Syndromes A Visual Aid to Diagnosis, 1992, pp.460–461*

Madelung's deformity

McCune-Albright syndrome – café au lait macule *Ped Derm 8:35–39, 1991*

Menkes' kinky hair syndrome – silvery hair, generalized hypopigmentation, lax skin of brows, neck, and thighs *Ped Derm 15:137–139, 1998*

Microphthalmia with linear skin defects syndrome (MLS syndrome) (microphthalmia, dermal aplasia, and sclerocornea (MIDAS) syndrome) – X-linked dominant; atrophic Blaschko linear scars of face and neck; linear red atrophic skin (resembles aplasia cutis) *Ped Derm 37:217–218, 2020; Am J Med Genet 49:229–234, 1994*

Mobius sequence *Atlas of Clinical Syndromes A Visual Aid to Diagnosis, 1992, pp.492–493*

Morquio syndrome (mucopolysaccharidosis type IV) – autosomal recessive; short neck, skeletal abnormalities, corneal clouding, cardiac valvulopathies, odontoid hypoplasia, hypermobile joints *Ped Derm 33:594–601, 2016*

Mottled pigmentation of neck and elbows *Z Haut-u Geschl Krankh 32:33–44, 1962*

Multiple endocrine neoplasia syndrome type II – medullary carcinoma of the thyroid *Ped Clin North Amer 6:1151–1160, 1993*

Multiple pterygium syndrome – webbed neck *J Med Genet 24:733–749, 1987*

Neu-Laxova syndrome – short neck; mild scaling to harlequin ichthyosis appearance; ichthyosiform scaling, increased subcutaneous fat and atrophic musculature, generalized edema and mildly edematous feet and hands, absent nails; microcephaly, intrauterine growth retardation, limb contractures, low set ears, sloping forehead; small genitalia, eyelid and lip closures, syndactyly, cleft lip and palate, micrognathia; autosomal recessive; uniformly fatal *Ped Derm 20:25–27,78–80, 2003; Curr Prob Derm 14:71–116, 2002; Clin Dysmorphol 6:323–328, 1997; Am J Med Genet 35:55–59, 1990*

Neurofibromatosis – type I; segmental neurofibromatosis *J La State Med Soc 146:183–186, 1994;* plexiform neurofibroma *NEJM 382:1430–1442, 2020*

Noonan's syndrome – malformed ears, nevi, keloids, transient lymphedema, ulerythema ophryogenes, keratosis follicularis spinulosa decalvans, joint hyperextensibility, hypertelorism, webbed neck, down slanting of palpebral fissures, keratosis pilaris atrophicans, short stature, chest deformity (pectus carinatum and pectus excavatum), cubitus valgus, radioulnar synostosis, clinobrachydactyly, congenital heart disease; PTPN 11 gene on chromosome 12; SOS1, RAF1, gain of function of non-receptor protein tyrosine phosphate SHP-2 or KRAS gene *Ped Derm 24:417–418, 2007; JAAD 46:161–183, 2002; J Med Genet 24:9–13, 1987; J Pediatr 63:468–470, 1963*

Occipital horn syndrome (Ehlers-Danlos syndrome, type IX) – long neck *Am J Hum Genet 41:A49, 1987*

Oculo-auricular vertebral syndrome – short neck, epibulbar dermoid tumors, abnormal hair *Ped Derm 20:182–184, 2003*

Pallister-Killian syndrome – short neck; streaks of hypo- and hyperpigmentation, mental retardation, coarse facies with prominent forehead with abnormally high anterior hairline, sparse temporal hair and sparse anterior scalp hair, hypertelorism, short nose with anteverted nostrils, flat nasal bridge, flat occiput, sparse eyelashes, long philtrum with thin upper lip, horizontal palpebral fissure, supernumerary nipples, Blaschko linear hypopigmented bands of face and shoulder; i(12p) (tetrasomy 12p); tissue mosaicism; pigmentary mosaicism and localized alopecia *Ped Derm 24:426–428, 2007; Ped Derm 23:382–385, 2006; Ped Derm 22:270–275, 2005*

PAPA (pyogenic arthritis, pyoderma gangrenosum, acne vulgaris) syndrome – autosomal dominant; mutation in proline serine threonine phosphatase-interacting protein 1 (PSTPIP1) *BJD 161:1199–1201, 2009; Mayo Clin Proc 72:611–615, 1997*

Patau's syndrome (trisomy 13) – loose skin of posterior neck, parieto-occipital scalp defects, abnormal helices, low set ears, simian crease of hand, hyperconvex narrow nails, polydactyly *Ped Derm 22:270–275, 2005*

Phakomatosis pigmentovascularis *J Dermatol 46:843–848, 2019*

Poland anomaly *Atlas of Clinical Syndromes A Visual Aid to Diagnosis, 1992, pp.390–391*

Proteus syndrome *Atlas of Clinical Syndromes A Visual Aid to Diagnosis, 1992, pp.352–355*

Pseudoxanthoma elasticum – linear and reticulated cobblestoned yellow papules and plaques *AD 124:1559, 1988; JAAD 42:324–328, 2000; Dermatology 199:3–7, 1999*; PXE and acrosclerosis *Proc Roy Soc Med 70:567–570, 1977*

Pterygium colli medianum *Atlas of Clinical Syndromes A Visual Aid to Diagnosis, 1992, pp.58–59*

Rigid spine syndrome *Atlas of Clinical Syndromes A Visual Aid to Diagnosis, 1992, pp.446*

SAPPHO syndrome *Oral Radiol Aug 14, 2019*

Short stature, mental retardation, facial dysmorphism, short webbed neck, skin changes, congenital heart disease – xerosis, dermatitis, low set ears, umbilical hernia *Clin Dysmorphol 5:321–327, 1996*

Sjogren-Larsson syndrome – verrucous hyperkeratosis of flexures, neck, and periumbilical folds; mental retardation, spastic diplegia, short stature, kyphoscoliosis, retinal changes, yellow pigmentation, intertrigo – deficiency of fatty aldehyde dehydrogenase *Chem Biol Interact 130–132:297–307, 2001; Am J Hum Genet 65:1547–1560, 1999; JAAD 35:678–684, 1996*

Spondylocostal dysostosis *Atlas of Clinical Syndromes A Visual Aid to Diagnosis, 1992, pp.294–295*

Steatocystoma multiplex

Sweet's syndrome – red plaque with or without bullae or pustules red plaque *NEJM 382:1543, 2020; JAAD 69:557–564, 2013; JAAD 40:838–841, 1999; AD 134:625–630, 1998; Eur J Gastro Heptl 9:715–720, 1997; JAAD 31:535–536, 1994; BJD 76:349–356, 1964*

Thrombocytopenia-absent radius syndrome (TAR syndrome) – cutis laxa of neck; congenital thrombocytopenia, bilateral absent or hypoplastic radii, port wine stain of head and neck *AD 126:1520–1521, 1990; Am J Pediatr Hematol Oncol 10:51–64, 1988*

Trisomy 13 (Patau syndrome) – redundant skin of neck *J Genet Hum 23:83–109, 1975*

Trisomy 18 syndrome – redundant skin of neck *J Med Genet 15:48–60, 1978*

Tuberous sclerosis – fibrous cephalic plaque of neck *JAAD 78:717–724, 2018; Head Neck Pathol 542–546, 2016*

Turner's syndrome (XO in 50%) – webbed neck, lymphedema of neck; low posterior hairline, low misshapen ears, peripheral edema at birth which resolves by age 2; redundant neck skin in newborn; small stature, broad shield-shaped chest with widely spaced nipples, arms show wide carrying angle, high arched palate, cutis laxa of neck and buttocks, short fourth and fifth metacarpals and metatarsals, hypoplastic nails, keloid formation, increased numbers of nevi; skeletal, cardiovascular, ocular abnormalities; increased pituitary gonadotropins with low estrogen levels *JAAD 50:767–776, 2004; JAAD 46:161–183, 2002; JAAD 40:877–890, 1999; NEJM 335:1749–1754, 1996;* halo nevi of the neck *JAAD 51:354–358, 2004*

Weaver-Williams syndrome (cleft palate, microcephaly, mental retardation, musculoskeletal mass deficiency) – long neck *Birth Defects 13:69–84, 1977*

Wildervanck syndrome *Atlas of Clinical Syndromes A Visual Aid to Diagnosis, 1992, pp.298–299*

49,XXXXY syndrome – webbed neck *Syndromes of the Head and Neck, p. 59–60, 1990*

TRAUMA

Chemical leukoderma – from dimethyl sulfate *An Bras Dermatol 91(suppl 1)26–28, 2016*

Dental treatment – soft tissue cervicofacial emphysema after dental treatment *AD 141:1437–1440, 2005*

Fiddler's neck – lichenification with erythema, hyperpigmentation, papules, pustules, and cysts *BJD 98:669–674, 1978*

Frostbite – bullous frostbite in a snowmobiler (Polaris vulgaris) *Cutis 63:21–23, 1999*

Hickey (passion mark)

Neck impalement with tree branch *NEJM 373:366, 2015*

Strangulation purpura

Subcutaneous emphysema *AD 134:557–559, 1998*

Thermal burn

VASCULAR DISORDERS

Acquired elastotic hemangioma – red plaque with vascular appearance *JAAD 47:371–376, 2002*

Acquired port wine stain – red patches of neck, upper back, lower leg, posterior thigh *Ped Derm 37:93–97, 2020*

Aneurysmal dilatation of the internal jugular vein – soft blue neck mass *Ped Clin North Amer 6:1151–1160, 1993*

Angiolymphoid hyperplasia with eosinophilia *Actas Dermosifiliogr 110:303–307, 2019; Dermatol Online J Dec 16, 2015*

Angiosarcoma *BJD 138:692–694, 1998; Australas Radiol 39:277–281, 1995; Cancer 44:1106–1113, 1979*

Angioma serpiginosum

Arteriovenous fistulae – congenital or acquired; red pulsating nodules with overlying telangiectasia – extremities, head, neck, trunk

Blue rubber bleb nevus syndrome *World J Gastroenterol 20:17254–17259, 2014*

CLAPO syndrome – capillary malformation of lower lip; lymphatic malformation of face and neck; swollen lip, prominent veins of neck, jaw and scalp, asymmetry of face and limbs, partial or generalized overgrowth reticulate erythema of neck; *PIK3CA* mutation *Ped Derm 35:681–682, 2018*

Dabska tumor (malignant endovascular papillary endothelioma) – head and neck of infants *JAAD 49:887–896, 2003*

Granulomatosis with polyangiitis – ulcer of posterior neck *JAMADerm 152:1375–1376, 2016;* pyoderma gangrenosum-like ulcers of neck in teenage boy *Tidsskr Nor Laegeforen April 8, 2019*

Hemangioma – symptomatic hemangiomas of the airway with airway obstruction and cutaneous hemangiomas in a "beard" distribution *J Pediatr 131:643–646, 1997;* large neck mass; hemangioma beyond proliferative stage – hypertrophy of lip, chin, and neck *Ped Derm 28:94–98, 2011*

Non-involuting congenital hemangioma *JAAD 53:185–186, 2005*

Kaposiform hemangioendothelioma *Ann Diagn Pathol 44:151434, 2020*

Lymphatic malformation

Port wine stain *JAAD 80:779–781, 2019*

Pseudo-Kaposi's sarcoma

Pyogenic granuloma – head and neck most common affected sites *Tokol J Exp Clin Med 20:110–114, 2015*

Salmon patch (nevus simplex) ("stork bite") – pink macules with fine telangiectasias of the nape of the neck, glabella, forehead, upper eyelids, tip of nose, upper lip, midline lumbosacral area *Ped Derm 73:31–33, 1983*

Thoracic duct obstruction – non-inflammatory swelling of supraclavicular fossa – obstruction of cervical portion of thoracic duct *AD 147:1337–1338, 2011; Vasc Med 9:141–143, 2004; Lymphology 28:118–125, 1995*

Tufted angioma – dull red, purple, or red-brown *JAAD 49:887–896, 2003; Ped Derm 19:388–393, 2002;* vascular nodule *Ped Derm 29:778, 2012*

Unilateral nevoid telangiectasia

Venous lakes

NECK PAPULES

AUTOIMMUNE DISEASES OR DISEASES OF IMMUNE DYSFUNCTION

Dermatitis herpetiformis AD 147:1313–1316, 2011

DOCK8 deficiency syndrome (dedicator of cytokinesis 8 gene) (aka autosomal recessive hyper-IgE syndrome) DOCK8 – involved in T cell polarization and activation; atypical guanine exchange factor; interacts with Rho GTPases (CDC42 AND RAC) which mediate actin cytoskeletal reorganization; hematologic stem cell homing and mobilization – immunodeficiency; resembles Job's syndrome; decrease T and B cells; increased IgE, decreased IgM, increased eosinophilia; recurrent sinopulmonary infections, severe cutaneous viral infections and lymphopenia; red papules of neck – molluscum contagiosum; warts, widespread dermatitis (atopic dermatitis-like) (24% at birth; Job's 81% dermatitis at birth), asthma, cutaneous staphylococcal abscesses; malignancies – aggressive T-cell lymphoma vulvar squamous cell carcinoma, diffuse large B-cell lymphoma; Job's syndrome may be differentiated by presence of pneumatoceles and bronchiectasis, rash at birth, osteoporosis, scoliosis, craniosynostosis, minimal trauma fractures, joint hyperextensibility; dominant negative STAT3 mutation *AD 148:79–84, 2012*

Graft vs. host reaction, acute *Taiwan I Hsueh Hui Tsa Chih 88:657–662, 1989*

IgG4-related disease *Mod Rheumatol 23:986–993, 2013*

Lupus erythematosus – papulonodular mucinosis; papules of neck *JAAD 32:199–205, 1995; AD 114:432–435, 1978*

Still's disease *Semin Arthr Rheum 42:317–326, 2012*

Urticaria

CONGENITAL DISORDERS

Accessory tragus – facial, glabellar papule – isolated, Treacher Collins syndrome (mandibulofacial dysostosis; autosomal dominant), Goldenhaar syndrome ((oculo-auriculo-vertebral syndrome) – macroglossia, preauricular tags, abnormal pinnae, facial asymmetry, macrostomia, epibulbar dermoids, facial weakness, central nervous system, renal, and skeletal anomalies), Nager syndrome, Wolf-Hirschhorn syndrome (chromosome 4 deletion syndrome), oculocerebrocutaneous syndrome *Ped Derm 17:391–394, 2000;* Townes-Brocks syndrome *Am J Med Genet 18:147–152, 1984;* VACTERL syndrome *J Pediatr 93:270–273, 1978*

Branchial remnants – branchial cleft cyst/sinus *Cutis 99:327–328, 2017; Plastic and Reconstructive Surgery 100:32–39, 1997*

Cervical braid *Brit J Plast Surg 43:369–370, 1990*

Congenital malalignment of the great toenails *Dermatol Surg 45:1211–1213, 2019; Clin Exp Dermatol 8:619–623, 1983; Clin Exp Dermatol 4:309–313, 1979*

Congenital onychodysplasia of the index finger *Genetic Skin Disorders, Second Edition, 2010, pp.244*

Congenital paramedian canaliform dystrophy – personal observation

Cutaneous cartilaginous rest (cervical accessory auricle (wattle)) *AD 121:22–23, 1985;* in oculo-auricular-vertebral spectrum

Syndromes of the Head and Neck; Oxford Monographs on Medical Genetics No. 19; Oxford University Press; Oxford/New York; 1990

Ectopic or christomatous salivary gland (heterotopic salivary gland tissue) – skin colored nodule along lower surface of the sternocleidomastoid muscle *JAAD 58:251–256, 2008*

Glandular congenital lymphadenoma *Ped Derm 24:547–550, 2007*

Midline cervical cleft *Int J Pediatr 2015:209418, 2015*

Occult spinal dysraphism *Ped Derm 12:256–259, 1995*

Rhabdomyomatous mesenchymal hamartoma – pedunculated papule associated with a midline cervical cleft *AD 141:1161–1166, 2005*

Supernumerary nipples *Cutis 71:344–346, 2003*

Thyroglossal duct cyst *Semin Pediatr Surg 15:70–75, 2006*

DRUG REACTIONS

Atorvastatin-induced dermatomyositis *Rheumatol Int 37:1217–1219, 2017*

Cyclosporine – pseudofolliculitis barbae-like lesions *Dermatologica 172:24–30, 1986*

EXOGENOUS AGENTS

Chrysiasis *BJD 133:671–678, 1995*

Fiberglass dermatitis *Kao Hsiung J Med Sci 12:491–494, 1996*

Silica granulomas from mine explosion – red nodules of face, neck, chest *JAMADerm 154:953–954, 2018*

INFECTIONS AND INFESTATIONS

Bed bug bites *Ped Derm 22:183–187, 2005*

Botryomycosis *Cutis 80:45–47, 2007*

Candidiasis – *Candida tropicalis* sepsis, papillary muscle rupture – personal observation

Cattle itch mite (*Sarcoptes scabiei var. bovis*) *Hautarzt 30:423–426, 1979*

Chromomycosis – feet, legs, arms, face, and neck *AD 113:1027–1032, 1997; BJD 96:454–458, 1977; AD 104:476–485, 1971*

Coccidioidomycosis *Acta Cytologica 38:422–426, 1994*

Cryptococcosis *AD 142:25–27, 2006*

Demodicidosis – erythema and papules of neck (demodex folliculitis) *Cutis 90:62,65–66, 2012; J Med Assoc Thai 74:116–119, 1991*

Dental sinus – neck nodule *Ped Derm 29:421–425, 2012; Am Fam Physician 40:113–116, 1989*

Histoplasmosis – disseminated histoplasmosis in AIDS; red papules of neck *AD 143:255–260, 2007*

HTLV III *JAAD 13:563–566, 1985*

Leishmania *ID Cases 18:60–62, 2014*

Molluscum contagiosum *Ann Dermatol 25:398–399, 2013*

Mucormycosis – red nodule of neck *Clin Inf dis 63:959,991–992, 2016*

Mycobacterium tuberculosis – after BCG vaccination *J Derm 21:106–110, 1924*

Myiasis – cuterebrid myiasis; neck nodules *Ped Derm 21:515–516, 2004*

Nematode larvae *JAAD 58:668–670, 2008*

Pediculosis – head lice – pruritic papules of nape of neck; generalized pruritic eruption *NEJM 234:665–666, 1946*

Pityrosporum folliculitis *Mycoses 40(supp 1)29–32, 1997; Med Cut Ibero Lat Am 13:357–361, 1985*

Prototheosis *Mycopathologia 179:163–166, 2015*

Rickettsialpox – personal observation

Scabies *JAAD 82:533–548, 2020; Ped Derm 11:264–266, 1994;* neonatal scabies *Am J Dis Child 133:1031–1034, 1979*

Sporotrichosis – lateral neck nodules *BJD 173:291–293, 2015*

Staphylococcus aureus – folliculitis

Sycosis barbae

Tinea barbae – *Trichophyton rubra,* Majocchi's granuloma *Mycopathologia 182:549–554, 2017*

Verruca vulgaris

Verruga peruana *Am J Trop Med and Hygiene 50:143, 1994*

INFILTRATIVE DISORDERS

Angioplasmocellular hyperplasia – red nodule with red rim, ulcerated nodule, vascular nodule of face, scalp, neck, trunk, and leg *JAAD 64:542–547, 2011*

Benign cephalic histiocytosis – cheeks, forehead, earlobes, neck *JAAD 47:908–913, 2002; Ped Derm 11:265–267, 1994; Ped Derm 6:198–201, 1989; AD 122:1038–43, 1986; JAAD 13:383–404, 1985*

Congenital self-healing reticulohistiocytosis (Hashimoto-Pritzker disease) *Ped Derm 23:273–275, 2006; JAAD 48:S75–77, 2003*

Primary and secondary intralymphatic histiocytosis – red papule or nodule of neck *J Dermatol 35:691–693, 2008;; red patch of back; livedo reticularis JAAD 70:927–933, 2014*

Follicular mucinosis *Indian Dermatol Online J 4:333–335, 2013*

Indeterminate cell histiocytosis *Am J Dermatopathol 19:276–283, 1997*

Juvenile xanthogranuloma *Ped Derm 26:238–240, 2009; Ped Derm 15:65–67, 1998*

Lichen myxedematosus (scleromyxedema) *JAAD 33:37–43, 1995;* discrete papular lichen myxedematosus *Cutis 75:105–112, 2005; Indian J DV Leprol 52:340–342, 1986*

Plane xanthomatosis *BJD 133:961–966, 1995*

Papular mucinosis – localized papular mucinosis associated with IgA nephropathy; cobblestoned shiny grouped follicular papules of the neck *AD 147:599–602, 2011*

Rosai-Dorfman disease *Chin Med (Engl) 124:793–794, 2011*

Self-healing (papular) juvenile cutaneous mucinosis – yellow papules and plaques; arthralgias *Ped Derm 32:e255–258, 2015; Ped Derm 20:35–39, 2003; JAAD 44:273–281, 2001; Ped Derm 14:460–462, 1997; AD 131:459–461, 1995; JAAD 11:327–332, 1984; Ann DV 107:51–57, 1980;* of adult *JAAD 50:121–123, 2004; BJD 143:650–651, 2000; Dermatology 192:268–270, 1996*

Urticaria pigmentosa *Pediatr Ann 43:e13–15, 2014*

Xanthoma disseminatum *J Postgrad Med 60:69–71, 2014*

INFLAMMATORY DISORDERS

Eosinophilic pustular folliculitis *J Dermatol 25:178–184*

Erythema nodosum

Folliculitis decalvans *J Dermatol 28:329–331, 2001*

Folliculitis nuchae scleroticans (acne keloidalis nuchae) *Hautarzt 39:739–742, 1988*

Kimura's disease *Am J Kidney disease 11:353–356, 1988*

Necrotizing infundibular crystalline folliculitis – red umbilicated papules of face, neck, and back *JAMA Derm 149:1233–1234, 2013; BJD 145:165–168, 2001; BJD 143:310–314, 1999*

Neutrophilic eccrine hidradenitis *SkinMed 15:297–299, 2017*

Sarcoid *JAAD 68:765–773, 2013; J Spec Oper Med 13:105–108, 2013; AD 133:882–888, 1997; NEJM 336:1224–1234, 1997; Clinics in Chest Medicine 18:663–679, 1997*

METABOLIC DISEASES

Cryoglobulinemia *JAAD 25:21–27, 1991*

Pruritic urticarial papules and plaques of pregnancy (PUPPP) *Z Hautkr 65:831–832, 1990*

Xanthomas, eruptive *Acta Med Port 30:219–222, 2018*

NEOPLASTIC DISORDERS

Acrochordon (skin tag)

Adenoid cystic carcinoma *JAAD 17:113–118, 1987*

Adenosquamous carcinoma of the skin – red keratotic papule or plaque of head, neck or shoulder; extensive local invasion *AD 145:1152–1158, 2009*

Angiosarcoma *BJD 138:692–694, 1998*

Apocrine adenoma – personal observation

Apocrine carcinoma *Cancer 71:375–381, 1993*

Apocrine hidrocystoma *Stat Pearls Dec 23, 2019*

Atypical fibroxanthoma *Semin Cut Med Surg 38:E65–66, 2019; Dermatol Surg 37:146–147, 2011; AD 146:1399–1404, 2010; Sem Cut Med Surg 21:159–165, 2002; Cutis 51:47–48, 1993; Cancer 31:1541–1552, 1973;* crusted pink papule of neck *Ped Derm 24:450–452, 2007*

Basal cell carcinoma *AD 126:102,104–105, 1990; Acta Pathol Microbiol Scand 88A:5–9, 1980*

Benign cephalic histiocytomas *Ped Derm 31:547–550, 2014; JAAD 47:908–913, 2002; Am J Dermatopathol 15:581–586, 1993*

Eruptive blue nevi *Cutis 102:E24–26, 2018;* rare, often a triggering event is present

Bowenoid papulosis – HPV 18 *JAAD 40:633–634, 1999*

Cardiac myxoma emboli *J Dermatol 22:600–605, 1995*

Cutaneous lymphadenoma – papules or nodules of head and neck *BJD 128:339–341, 1993*

Eruptive collagenoma *J Dermatol 29:79–85, 2002;* familial collagenoma *Ann Dermatol 23:S119–122, 2011*

Cylindromas *BJD 151:1084–1086, 2004*

Deep penetrating nevus – black or darkly pigmented nevus of head, neck, and scalp *JAAD 71:1234–1240, 2014*

Dermal duct tumor – red nodule of neck *AD 140:609–614, 2004*

Dermatomyofibroma – oval nodule or firm plaque *Ped Derm 34:347–351, 2017; Clin Exp Dermatol 21:307–309, 1996*

Dermatosis papulosa nigra *Stat Pearls April 30, 2020*

Desmoplastic trichoepithelioma *AD 138:1091–1096, 2002; AD 132:1239–1240, 1996; Cancer 40:2979–2986, 1977*

Encephalocraniocutaneous lipomatosis *Ped Derm 10:164–168, 1993*

Eruptive fibromas *J Cutan Pathol 25:122–125*

Eruptive histiocytoma *J Dermatol 20:105–108, 1993*

Eruptive lipofibromas *AD 119:612–614, 1983*

Eruptive vellus hair cysts

Fibrosarcoma, neonatal *JAAD 50:S23–25, 2004*

Fibrous hamartoma of infancy – neck nodule *Ped Dev Pathol 2:236–243, 1999*

Hamartoma moniliformis – linear array of skin-colored papules of face and neck *AD 101:191–205, 1970*

Infantile myofibromatosis – single or multiple; head, neck, trunk *JAAD 41:508, 1999; AD 134:625–630, 1998*

Inverted follicular keratosis *J Clin Pathol 28:465–471, 1975*

Kaposi's sarcoma *Ann Int Med 103:744–750, 1985*

Keratoacanthomas of Ferguson-Smith – multiple self-healing keratoacanthomas *JAAD 49:741–746, 2003; Ann DV 104:206–216, 1977; BJD 46:267–272, 1934;* generalized eruptive keratoacanthomas *Int J Dermatol 54:160–167, 2015*

Leiomyomas – grouped, linear or dermatomal (Reed syndrome) *The Dermatologist, July 2016, pp.47–49;JAAD 52:410–416, 2005; JAAD 46:477–490, 2002;* piloleiomyomas *Eur J Dermatol 9:309–310,1999*

Leiomyosarcoma – blue-black; also red, brown, yellow or hypopigmented *JAAD 46:477–490, 2002*

Leukemia – chronic lymphocytic leukemia *Laryngoscope 86:1856–1863, 1976*

Leukemid – personal observation

Lymphoepithelioma-like carcinoma *Mod Pathol 1:359–365, 1988*

Lymphoma – CTCL; Ki-1+ lymphoma; Hodgkin's disease *AD 133:1454–1455, 1457–1458, 1997;* B-cell lymphoma *JAAD 53:479–484, 2005;* xanthomatous infiltration of the neck *Eur J Derm 10:481–483, 2000;;* miliary and agminated primary follicle center lymphoma – multiple grouped papules of face, neck, trunk, and extremities *JAAD 65:749–755, 2011;* lymphoblastic lymphoma – red neck nodule *JAAD 70:318–325, 2014;* primary cutaneous follicle center cell lymphoma – multilobulated nodules, red plaques of scalp, nodules of head and neck, papules of head and neck *JAAD 70:1010–1020, 2014;* diffuse large cell B-cell lymphoma – multiple red subcutaneous nodules of neck *BJD 173:134–145, 2015;* post-transplant lymphoma *JAAD 81:600–602, 2019*

Lymphomatoid papulosis *Acta DV Croat 26:264–266, 2018*

Lymphoplasmocytoid immunocytoma *Hautarzt 44:172–175, 1995*

Melanocytic nevus – eruptive melanocytic nevi *JAAD 37:337–339, 1997; J Dermatol 22:292–297, 1995*

Melanoma, including metastatic melanoma – 2 mm brown papules of face and neck *Ped Derm 27:201–203, 2010*

Merkel cell carcinoma – pink to violaceous nodule *Sem Cut Med Surg 21:159–165, 2002*

Metastases – NUT (nuclear protein in testis) midline carcinoma *JAAD 67:323–324, 2012;* metastatic squamous cell carcinoma of the tongue *NEJM 370:558, 2014;* submandibular gland adenocarcinoma – personal observation; basaloid carcinoma of lung *JAAD 49:523–526, 2003;* renal cell carcinoma *SkinMed 17:65–66, 2019; Australas J Dermatol 46:158–160, 2005;* gastric adenocarcinoma *Dermatol Reports 8:6819, 2017;* salivary gland carcinoma *Cutis 93:E16–18, 2014*

Milia *Acta Derm Venereol 71:334–336, 1991*

Mucinous carcinoma *JAAD 52:S76–80, 2005*

Multiple myeloma *AD 139:475–486, 2003*

Myofibroma *J Cutan Pathol 23:445–457, 1996; Histopathol 22:335–341, 1993*

Neurilemmoma (schwannoma) – pink-gray or yellowish nodules of head and neck

Neurofibroma

Neuroma – palisaded encapsulated neuroma *AD 140:1003–1008, 2004*

Neurothekeoma *An Bras Dermatol 90:156–159, 2015; J Drugs Dermatol 11:252–255, 2012; Am J Surg Pathol 14:113–120, 1990*

Nevus sebaceous *Int J Dermatol 44:142–150, 2005*

Nuchal fibroma – solitary subcutaneous mass of back of neck; multiple lesions associated with Gardner's syndrome *JAAD 66:959–965, 2012*

Palisaded encapsulated neuroma – benign nerve sheath proliferation; skin colored solitary papules of the head and neck in adults *Am J Dermatopathol 41:358–360, 2019*

Pilomatrixoma *J Cutan Pathol 18:20–27, 1991*

Pilomatrix carcinoma – multiple of head and neck *Otolaryngol Head Neck Surg 109:543–547, 1993*

Plasmacytoid dendritic cell neoplasm – purple macules, violaceous papules, nodules, tumefactions; highly pigmented dark red, purpuric, necrotic lesions of face, neck *JAAD 66:278–291, 2012*

Porokeratotic eccrine ostial and dermal duct nevus (linear eccrine nevus with comedones) *AD 138:1309–1314, 2002*

Primary cutaneous adenoid cystic carcinoma – violaceous nodules of face and neck *JAAD 58:636–641, 2008*

Cutaneous pseudolymphoma *J Dermatol 32:594–601, 2005*

Rhabdomyomatous mesenchymal hamartoma – ventral midline skin colored polypoid papule of neck *Ped Derm 37:64–68, 2020; Ped Derm 33:449–450, 2016*

Rhabdomyosarcoma *JAAD 31:871–876, 1994*

Sebaceous hyperplasias – linear neck papules; prepubescent sebaceous hyperplasias *Ped Derm 28:198–200, 2011*

Solitary fibrous tumor of the skin – facial, scalp, posterior neck nodule *JAAD 46:S37–40, 2002*

Squamous cell carcinoma

Syringocystadenoma papilliferum *AD 144:1509–1514, 2008; AD 138: 1091–1096, 2002; AD 121:1198–1201, 1985;* linear verrucous papules *AD 138:1091–1096, 2002*

Syringomas, eruptive *Dermatol Online J 2016 Aug 15; 22(8)13030qt4mm751qr; Cureus Nov 21, 2018*

Tick bite – persistent atypical lymphocytic hyperplasia *Ped Derm 18:481–484, 2001*

Warty dyskeratoma – face, neck, scalp, axillae *Iran J Public Health 43:1145–1147, 2014*

PARANEOPLASTIC DISORDERS

Acrokeratosis paraneoplastica (Bazex syndrome) *J Laryng Otol 110:899–900, 1996*

Granulomatous rosacea-like leukemid in acute myelogenous leukemia *Vojnosanit Pregl 65:565–568, 2008*

Sweet's syndrome *Ear Nose Throat J 94:282–284, 2015; Clin Exp Rheumatol 27:588–590, 2009*

PHOTODERMATOSES

Actinic granuloma (annular elastolytic giant cell granuloma) *Dermatol Online J 18:23, 2012; AD 122:43–47, 1986*

PRIMARY CUTANEOUS DISORDERS

Acantholytic dermatosis *Nippon Hifuka Gakkai Zasshi 10:453–460, 1991*

Acne keloidalis *JAAD 56:699–701, 2007; J Dermatol Surg Oncol 15:642–647, 1989*

Acne rosacea *J Dermatol Case Rep 31:68–72, 2016*

Acne vulgaris *AD 131:341–344, 1995*

Alopecia mucinosa (follicular mucinosis) – neck papules *JAAD 38:622–624, 1998; Dermatology 197:178–180, 1998; JAAD 10:760–768, 1984; AD 76:419–426, 1957*

Anetoderma of Jadassohn *AD 120:1032–1039, 1984*

Angiolymphoid hyperplasia with eosinophilia *Stat Pearls April 23, 2020; Int J Dermatol 56:1373–1378, 2017; BJD 134:744–748, 1996*

Atopic dermatitis *Allergy Asthma Proc 40:433–436,2019*

Benign papular acantholytic dermatosis *AD 112:814–821, 1976*

Confluent and reticulated papillomatosis of Gougerot and Carteaud *Stat Pearls April 29, 2020; Ann DV 93:493–494, 2013*

Darier's disease *Case Rep Dermatol 11:327–333, 2019; J Oral Maxillofac Pathol 21:321, 2017; AD 143:535–540, 2007; Dermatology 188:157–159, 1994*

Degos' disease, benign cutaneous *J Dermatol 31:666–670, 2004*

Disseminated and recurrent infundibulofolliculitis – neck, trunk, extremities *Indian J Dermatol 64:404–406, 2019; J Derm 25:51–53, 1998; Dermatol Clin 6:353–362, 1988; AD 105:580–583, 1972*

Elastosis perforans serpiginosa *Acta DV 98:822–823, 2018; J Dermatol 24:458–465, 1997*

Erythromelanosis follicularis faciei *Case Rep Dermatol 27:335–339, 2015*

Erythromelanosis follicularis faciei et colli *An Bras Dermatol 85:923–925, 2010*

Fibroelastolytic papulosis of the neck – skin colored papules with cobblestoning of face and neck; possibly same as white fibrous papulosis of neck or PXE-like papillary dermal elastolysis *AD 148:849–854, 2012; BJD 173:461–466, 1997; post-menopausal and elderly white women Am J Dermatopathol 41:640, 2019; J Cutan Pathol 43:142–147, 2016; JAAD 67:128–135, 2012*

Focal dermal elastosis, late onset *J Cutan Pathol 39:957–961, 2012*

Granuloma annulare *Cutis 55:158–160, 1995*

Granuloma faciale, extrafacial *SkinMed 6:150–151, 2007; BJD 145:360–362, 2001*

Granulomatous perioral dermatitis *AD 128:1396–1397,1399, 1992*

Hailey-Hailey disease *JAMA Derm 150:97–99, 2014*

Juxtaclavicular beaded lines *J Cutan Pathol 18:464–468, 1991*

Lichen sclerosus et atrophicus, guttate *Indian J Dermatol 60:105, 2015*

Lichen spinulosus *JAAD 22:261–264, 1990*

Lichen striatus *An Bras Dermatol 86:142–145, 2011*

Lupus miliaris disseminate faciei *Ann Saudi Med 34:351–353, 2014*

Prurigo pigmentosa *Ann DV 146:219–222, 2019*

Psoriasis

Scruff (terra firme) – teenage neck – personal observation

Trichodysplasia spinulosa – follicular crusted papules with keratotic spines; lesions of face, neck with eyebrow alopecia; trichodysplasia spinulosa-associated polyoma virus *JAAD 76:suppl 1 AB269, June 1, 2017; AD 147:1215–1220, 2011*

Upper dermal elastolysis *J Cutan Pathol 21:533–540, 1994*

PXE-like papillary dermal elastolysis – side of neck, axilla; post-menopausal and elderly women *JAAD 67:128–135, 2012*

White fibrous papulosis (fibroelastotic papulosis) – cobblestoning with 2–4 mm skin colored papules, back or sides of neck *An Bras Dermatol 95:102–104, 2020; JAAD 67:128–135, 2012; Cut Ocul Toxicol*

30:69–71, 2011; JAAD 51:958–964, 2004; Int J Derm 35:720–722, 1996; Ann DV 119:925–926, 1992; JAAD 20:1073–1077, 1989

SYNDROMES

Acrogeria *Dermatol 192:264–268, 1996*

Atrichia with keratin cysts – face, neck, scalp; then trunk and extremities *Ann DV 121:802–804, 1994*

Basaloid follicular hamartoma syndrome (generalized basaloid follicular hamartoma syndrome) – multiple skin-colored, red, and hyperpigmented papules of the face, neck chest, back, proximal extremities, and eyelids; syndrome includes milia-like cysts, comedones, sparse scalp hair, palmar pits, and parallel bands of papules of the neck (zebra stripes) *JAAD 49:698–705, 2003; BJD 146:1068–1070, 2002; JAAD 43:189–206, 2000*

Bazex-Christol-Dupre syndrome – neck papules, trichoepitheliomas *Eur J Med Genet 52:250–255, 2009*

Behcet's syndrome – acneiform lesions; erythema nodosum; nodule *AD 138:467–471, 2002*

Birt-Hogg –Dube syndrome – autosomal dominant; fibrofolliculomas, trichodiscomas, acrochordon; lung cysts, pneumothorax, renal cancer; mutation in *FLCN (*folliculin) *Am J Clin Dermatol 19:87–101, 2018; AD 133:1163–1166, 1997*

Brooke-Spiegler syndrome – multiple familial trichoepitheliomas, bilateral symmetric skin colored papules of face, neck, or chest *Dermatol Online J 18:16, 2012*

Down's syndrome – deep folliculitis of posterior neck; elastosis perforans serpiginosa

Fibroblastic rheumatism – symmetrical polyarthritis, nodules over joints and on palms, elbows, knees, ears, neck, Raynaud's phenomenon, sclerodactyly; skin lesions resolve spontaneously *AD 131:710–712, 1995*

Hunter's syndrome – reticulated 2–10 mm skin colored papules over scapulae, chest, neck, arms; X-linked recessive; MPS type II; iduronate-2 sulfatase deficiency; lysosomal accumulation of heparin sulfate and dermatan sulfate; short stature, full lips, coarse facies, macroglossia, clear corneas (unlike Hurler's syndrome), progressive neurodegeneration, communicating hydrocephalus, valvular and ischemic heart disease, lower respiratory tract infections, adenotonsillar hypertrophy, otitis media, obstructive sleep apnea, diarrhea, hepatosplenomegaly, skeletal deformities (dysostosis multiplex), widely spaced teeth, dolichocephaly, deafness, retinal degeneration, inguinal and umbilical hernias *Ped Derm 21:679–681, 2004; AD 113:602–605, 1977*

Hypohidrotic ectodermal dysplasia *Hautarzt 42:645–647, 1991*

Juvenile hyaline fibromatosis (systemic hyalinosis) – translucent papules or nodules of scalp, face, neck, trunk, gingival hypertrophy, flexion contractures of large and small joints *Indian J DV Leprol 71:115–118, 2005; J Cutan Pathol 32:438–440, 2005; Ped Derm 21:154–159, 2004; JAAD 16:881–883, 1987*

Lipoid proteinosis *BJD 151:413–423, 2004; JID 120:345–350, 2003; Hum Molec Genet 11:833–840, 2002*

Neurofibromatosis type 1

Nevoid basal cell carcinoma syndrome *JAAD 42:939–969, 2000; basal cell carcinomas – skin tag-like lesions in children with nevoid basal cell carcinoma syndrome Clin in Dermatol 23:68–77, 2005; JAAD 44:789–794, 2001*

Nevus comedonicus syndrome *Yonajo Acta Med 56:59–61, 2013*

Phakomatosis pigmentokeratotica – 3 mm pigmented papules of neck (melanocytic nevi); Blaschko epidermal nevus; *HRAS* mosaic mutation; tendency for squamous cell carcinoma *NEJM 381:1458, 2019*

Pseudoxanthoma elasticum – linear and reticulated cobblestoned yellow papules and plaques *JAAD 42:324–328, 2000; Dermatology 199:3–7, 1999; AD 124:1559, 1988;* PXE and acrosclerosis *Proc Roy Soc Med 70:567–570, 1977;* agminated papules *Cutis 102:E5–7, 2018;* perforating PXE *Indian J DV Leprol 82:464–466, 2016*

PXE-like papillary dermal elastolysis *An Bras Dermatol 95:247–249, 2020; Int J Dermatol 58:93–97, 2019; J Cutan Pathol 21:252–255, 1994*

Reed syndrome – leiomyomatosis *The Dermatologist July, 2016, pp47–49*

Steatocystoma multiplex – autosomal dominant *BMJ Case Rep Sept 26, 2011:bcr0420114165.doi* https://doi.org/10.1136/bcr.4.2011.4165; *J Cut Aesthet Surg 2:107–109, 2009*

Sweet's syndrome – red papules and plaques of neck; *JAAD 69:557–564, 2013; Eur J Gastro Hepatol 9:715–720, 1997*

Tuberous sclerosis – angiofibromas; fibrous cephalic plaques *JAAD 78:717–724, 2018; Mymensingh Med J 13:82–85, 2004*

TRAUMA

Fiddler's neck *BJD 98:669–674, 1978*

Pseudofolliculitis barbae *BJD 172:878–884, 2015; Dermatol Clin 6:387–395, 1988*

Pseudofolliculitis barbae – razor bumps

VASCULAR LESIONS

Glomus tumor

Pseudo-Kaposi's sarcoma overlying arteriovenous anastomosis following carotid endarterectomy

Tufted angioma – deep red papule, plaque, or nodule of back or neck *JAAD 52:616–622, 2005*

Venous lakes

NECROSIS

AUTOIMMUNE DISEASES AND DISEASES OF IMMUNE DYSFUNCTION

Allergic contact dermatitis – poison ivy or oak *NEJM 352:700–707, 2005*

Anti-centromere antibodies – ulcers and gangrene of the extremities *Br J Rheumatol 36:889–893, 1997*

Antiphospholipid syndrome – ear necrosis *JAMA 316:450–451, 2016;* acral necrosis of toes *Cutis 100:206,209–210, 2017;* catastrophic anti-phospholipid antibody syndrome *Int J Dermatol 58:e130–132, 2019*

Arthus reaction – necrosis of skin over deltoid muscle due to hepatitis B virus vaccine *Clin Inf Dis 33:906–908, 2001;* erythema, edema, hemorrhage, occasional necrosis

Bowel arthritis dermatitis syndrome – necrotic papules *AD 135:1409–1414, 1999; Cutis 63:17–20, 1999; JAAD 14:792–796, 1986; Mayo Clin Proc 59:43–46, 1984; AD 115:837–839, 1979*

Chronic granulomatous disease – necrotic ulcers; bacterial abscesses, perianal abscesses *JAAD 36:899–907, 1997; AD 130:105–110, 1994; NEJM 317:687–694, 1987; AD 103:351–357, 1971*

Congenital deficiency of leucocyte-adherence glycoproteins (CD11a (LFA-1), CD11b, CD11c, CD18) (leukocyte adhesion deficiency syndrome) – necrotic cutaneous abscesses, psoriasiform dermatitis, gingivitis, periodontitis, septicemia, ulcerative stomatitis, pharyngitis, otitis, pneumonia, peritonitis *BJD 123:395–401, 1990*

Connective tissue disease – eosinophilic vasculitis in connective tissue diseases; digital microinfarcts *JAAD 35:173–182, 1996*

Dermatomyositis – epidermal necrosis associated with internal malignancy *Cutis 61:190–194, 1998*

Graft vs. host disease, acute – epidermal necrosis *AD 134:602–612, 1998*

Heparin necrosis *Thromb Haemost 91:196–197, 2004; Br J Haematol 111:992, 2000; Ann R Coll Surg Engl 81:266–269, 1999; JAAD 37:854–858, 1997; NEJM 336:588–589, 1997; Nephron 68:133–137, 1994;* low molecular weight heparin *Ann Haematol 77:127–130, 1998;* at injection site *Dermatology 196:264–265, 1998; Thromb Haemost 78:785–790, 1997; Australas J Dermatol 36:201–203, 1995;* eschar and ulceration *JAAD 47:766–769, 2002;* heparin induced thrombocytopenia (HITT) – blisters with surrounding erythema followed by necrosis; acute arterial or venous occlusion; skin necrosis; livedo racemosa; thrombocytopenia; heparin-PF4 antibodies *Curr Opinion Hematol 23:462–470, 2016; JAAD 61:325–332, 2009*

Hypersensitivity angiitis *AD 138:1296–1298, 2002*

Intrauterine blood transfusion – Rh incompatibility

Linear IgA disease (TEN) *JAAD 31:797–799, 1994*

Lupus erythematosus – systemic – necrosis of the proximal nail fold; epidermal necrosis mimicking toxic epidermal necrosis *Clin Rheum Dis 8:207, 1982;* vasculitis; gangrene of extremity due to vasculitis or thrombosis (anti-phospholipid antibodies) *J Rheumatol 13:740–747, 1986;* infarcts of fingertips *JAAD 48:311–340, 2003;* digital gangrene *Cureus 12:e6667, 2020;* toxic epidermal necrolysis *JAAD 48:525–529, 2003*

Mixed connective tissue disease; *J Cut Med Surg 21:425–451, 2017; Am J Med 52:148–159, 1972*

Myeloperoxidase deficiency – lip infection and necrosis *Ped Derm 20:519–523, 2003*

Pemphigus vegetans *NEJM 352:700–707, 2005*

PLAID (*PLCG2*-associated antibody deficiency and immune dysregulation) – autosomal dominant; evaporative cold urticaria; neonatal ulcers in cold sensitive areas; granulomatous lesions sparing flexures; blotchy pruritic red rash, spontaneous ulceration of nasal tip with eschar of nose; erosion of nasal cartilage, neonatal small papules and erosions of fingers and toes; brown granulomatous plaques with telangiectasia and skin atrophy of cheeks, forehead, ears, chin; crusted, ulcerated eroded plaque of nasal tip, ears, tips of fingers and toes (acral necrosis); atopy; recurrent sinopulmonary infections; autoimmune diseases *Ped Derm 37:147–149, 2020; JAMADerm 151:627–634, 2015*

Rheumatoid vasculitis – purpuric infarcts of paronychial areas (Bywater's lesions) *JAAD 53:191–209, 2005; BJD 77:207–210, 1965;* bullae of fingertips and toe-tips with purpura; *BJD 77:207–210, 1965;* large hemorrhagic lesions, gangrene with necrotizing arteritis; peripheral gangrene *JAAD 53:191–209, 2005;* mononeuritis multiplex; papulonecrotic lesions *JAAD 48:311–340, 2003*

SAVI – STING-associated vasculopathy with onset in infancy syndrome (type 1 interferonopathy) – autosomal dominant; gain of function mutation in transmembrane protein 173 (STING) leading to chronic activation of Type I interferon pathway; red plaques of face and hands; chilblain-like lesions; atrophic plaques of hands, telangiectasias of cheeks, nose, chin, lips, acral violaceous scaling plaques and acral cyanosis (livedo reticularis of feet, cheeks, ears, and knees), of fingers, toes, nose, ears, cheeks distal ulcerative lesions with infarcts (erythema then necrosis of cheeks and ears), gangrene of fingers or toes with ainhum, nasal septal perforation, nail dystrophy and nail loss, small for gestational age; paratracheal adenopathy, abnormal pulmonary function tests; severe interstitial lung disease with fibrosis with ground glass and reticulate opacities; gain of function mutation in *TMEM173* (stimulator of interferon genes); mimics granulomatosis with polyangiitis *Ped Derm 33:602–614, 2016; JAMADerm 151:872–877, 2015; NEJM 371:507–518, 2014*

Severe combined immunodeficiency – necrotic bacterial skin infections resembling ecthyma gangrenosum

CONGENITAL LESIONS

Anti-phospholipid antibody syndrome, neonatal – arterial thrombotic gangrene of lower leg *Ped Derm 28:343–345, 2011*

Gangrene of abdominal wall – due to intrauterine red-cell transfusion *Am J Dis Child 117:593–596, 1969*

Intrauterine epidermal necrosis *JAAD 38:712–715, 1998*

Subcutaneous fat necrosis of the newborn – necrotic bulla *Ped Derm 20:257–261, 2003*

Umbilical artery catheterization – legs, lumbar, buttocks (perinatal gangrene of the buttock); gangrene of legs *AD 113:61–63, 1977;* unilateral necrosis of buttock *Arch Dis Child 55:815–817, 1980; JAAD 3:596–598, 1980*

DRUG-INDUCED

Acetaminophen rectal suppositories – perianal necrosis (ergotism) *BJD 170:212–218, 2014*

Actinomycin D extravasation

Adriamycin – IV *J Surg Res 75:61–65, 1998; Cancer Treat Rep 63:1003–1004, 1979; Cancer 38:1087–1094, 1976*

Alendronate – osteonecrosis of mandible; halitosis, hypesthesia of lower lip, submental sinus; necrosis of mandible underlying gingiva *NEJM 367:551, 2012*

All-trans retinoic acid induction chemotherapy in acute promyelocytic leukemia – fever, scrotal, vulvar, or perineal necrotic ulcers *JAMADerm 153:1181–1182, 2017*

Amiodarone

Amitriptyline *Burns 25:768–770, 1999*

Arsenic – endothelial damage

Beta blockers *BJD 143:1356–1358, 2000*

Bevacizumab (VEGF inhibitor) and irinotecan – steroid-induced striae undergo necrosis *AD 147:1226–1227, 2011*

Bleomycin – gangrene *Eur J Dermatol 8:221, 1998; AD 107:553–555, 1973*

Buprenorphine – intra-arterial injection *AD 138:1296–1298, 2002*

Calcium gluconate infusion – IV *JAAD 6:392–395, 1982*

Capecitabine – personal observation

Chemotherapy injection site *BJD 143:1356–1358, 2000*

Cisplatin *Cancer Treat Rep 67:199, 1983*

IV cocaine *JAAD 16:462–468, 1987*

Crack cocaine – necrosis of ears and legs *JAAD 64:1004–1006, 2011;* necrotizing vasculitis *JAAD 59:483–487, 2008; Neurol Clin 15:945–957, 1997*

Compazine – intramuscular with infarction

Coumarin necrosis – eschar and ulceration; associations include acquired protein C deficiency in chronic liver disease, chronic renal failure and dialysis, acute leukemia, systemic lupus erythematosus, anti-phospholipid antibody syndrome, Epstein-Barr virus infection, acute respiratory distress syndrome, acute intravascular coagulation, plasmapheresis *JAAD 61:325–332, 2009; BJD 151:502–504, 2004; JAAD 47:766–769, 2002; Br J Surg 87:266–272, 2000; Thromb Haemost 78:785–790, 1997; Hematol Oncol Clin North Am 7:1291–1300, 1993; AD 128:105, 108, 1992; AD 123:1701a-1706a, 1987;* with mutation of prothrombin gene *NEJM 340:735, 1999;* with familial type II protein C deficiency *Am J Hematol 29:226–229, 1988;* with acquired protein C deficiency *Intensive Care Med 27:1555, 2001;* with protein S deficiency *Haemostasis 28:25–30, 1998;* with Factor V Leiden and protein S deficiency *Clin Lab Haematol 23:261–264, 2001;* intravascular coagulation necrosis *JAAD 25:882–888, 1991;* late onset coumarin warfarin necrosis *Am J Hematol 57:233–237, 1998;* other associations include bleeding, priapism, hepatitis, alopecia, morbilliform eruptions *JAAD 61:325–332, 2009;* massive necrosis mimicking calciphylaxis *J Drugs in Dermatol 9:859–863, 2010*

Cyclophosphamide *BJD 143:1356–1358, 2000*

Dactinomycin – flexural cutaneous necrosis with post-inflammatory hyperpigmentation *AD 142:1660–1661, 2006*

Daunorubicin extravasation *Oncol Nurs Forum 25:67–70, 1998*

Depo-Provera – intramuscular *BJD 143:1356–1358, 2000*

Dextran injections – intramuscular *AD 124:1722–1723, 1988*

Doxorubicin hydrochloride – epidermal necrosis *Pharmazie 48:772–775, 1993*

DPT vaccination site – embolia cutis medicamentosa (Nicolau syndrome) *Actas Dermosifiliogr 95:133–134, 2004*

Calcium salts – IV

Dextrose – IV

Dopamine – IV

Ergot poisoning

Enoxaparin *Ann Int Med 125:521–522, 1996*

Epidural blockade – necrosis of lower extremities *Can J Anaesth 35:628–630, 1988*

Epinephrine-containing cream *Br J Clin Pract 38:191, 1984*

Fluorescein extravasation *Retina 7:89–93, 1987*

5-fluorouracil – epidermal necrosis of psoriatic plaques following intravenous 5-FU *BJD 147:824–825, 2002*

Flunitrazepam abuse *Acta DV 79:171, 1999*

G-CSF – necrotizing vasculitis *Ped Derm 17:205–207, 2000*

Gemcitabine *SAGE Open Med Case Rep Oct 30, 2018; K Drugs Dermatol 17:582–585, 2018*

Heparin-induced skin necrosis – black necrotic bullae of abdomen *JAAD 71:1033–1035, 2014*

Hydantoin (Dilantin) extravasation

Hypertonic saline extravasation *J Derm Surg Oncol 19:641–646, 1993*

Infusion leakage in the newborn *Br J Plast Surg 54:396–399, 2001*

Interferon alpha injection site *JAAD 37:118–120, 1997;* pegylated interferon alpha *JAAD 53:62–66, 2005*

Interferon beta *J Cosmetic Dermatol Aug 22, 2019; JAAD 37:553–558, 1997; Dermatology 195:52–53, 1997*

Interleukin-2 *JAAD 29:66–70, 1993*

Interleukin-3 *BJD 143:1356–1358, 2000*

Intra-articular anesthesia *BJD 143:1356–1358, 2000*

Levophed ischemic necrosis – personal observation

Mannitol – IV

Methadone *BJD 143:1356–1358, 2000*

Methotrexate necrosis – necrosis of psoriatic plaques *JAAD 77:247–255, 2017; JAAD 73:484–490, 2015; Cutis 92:148–150, 2013; Cutis 81:413–416, 2008; BMJ 299:980–981, 1989; S Afr Med J 72:888, 1987*

Mitomycin C – spillage; penile necrosis *JAAD 55:328–331, 2006*

Nafcillin – IV

Nivolumab – ulcer of scalp; scalp necrosis; giant cell arteritis due to nivolumab *JAMADerm 155:1086–1087, 2019*

Norepinephrine – IV *BJD 143:1356–1358, 2000*

Oxymetazoline – intra-arterial injection *AD 138:1296–1298, 2002*

Paracetamol – fixed drug eruption with eyelid skin necrosis *Indian J Ophthalmol 66:1627–1629, 2018*

Parenteral nutrition formulation extravasation *J Miss State Med Assoc 40:307–311, 1999*

Phenergan injection

Phenylephrine-induced microvascular occlusion syndrome – livedo racemosa, acral cyanosis and necrosis with hemorrhagic bullae *AD 143:1314–1317, 2007*

Phenytoin – IV *JAAD 28:360–363, 1993;* hydantoin (Dilantin) extravasation

Photodynamic therapy *Photochem Photobiol 68:575–583, 1998*

Potassium salts – IV

Propylthiouracil vasculitis – blue necrotic ear lesions; fever, arthralgias, and myalgias *JAMADerm 151:551–552, 2015*

Quinine sulfate – acral necrosis *Hautarzt 51:332–335, 2000*

Radiation recall – capecitabine, doxorubicin, taxanes, gemcitabine; erythema and desquamation; edema; vesicles and papules; ulceration and skin necrosis *The Oncologist 15:1227–1237, 2010*

Radioopaque dye – IV

Sertraline – giant bulla with necrosis *BJD 150:164–166, 2004*

Sodium bicarbonate – IV

Sodium tetradecyl sulfate extravasation *J Derm Surg Oncol 19:641–646, 1993*

Streptokinase – IV *BMJ 309:378, 1994*

Toxic epidermal necrolysis *SKINmed 10:373–383, 2012; JAAD 40:458–461, 1999; JAAD 23:870–875, 1990*

Tumor necrosis factor *J Inflamm 47:180–189, 1995*

Ustekinumab – leukocytoclastic vasculitis – purpuric necrotic targetoid bullae *J Drugs Dermatol 15:358–361, 2016*

Vaccination – DPT – livedoid skin necrosis (Nicolau syndrome) *BJD 137:1030–1031, 1997*

Vasoconstricting agents

Vasopressin *BJD 143:1356–1358, 2000; Dermatology 195:271–273, 1997; Cutis 57:330–332, 1996; JAAD 15:393–398, 1986;* scrotal and abdominal skin necrosis *Dig Dis Sci 30:46–464, 1985*

Vasopressive agents – peripheral ischemia *NEJM 369:1047–1054, 2013*

Vinorelbine extravasation *Tumori 86:289–292, 2000*

Voriconazole – in graft vs. host disease – giant bullae of hands, feet, and legs which progress to necrosis *JAAD 58:484–487, 2008*

Warfarin-associated nonuremic calciphylaxis *JAMADerm 153–309–314, 2017*

EXOGENOUS AGENTS

Acids and alkali

Alcohol – percutaneous absorption and necrosis in a preterm infant *Arch Dis Child 57:477–479, 1982*

Anabolic steroids – acne fulminans with necrotic ulcers *AD 148:1210–1212, 2012*

Antiseptics (isopropyl alcohol) – in newborn *Pediatrics 68:587–588, 1981*

Buprenorphine, surreptitious intra-arterial administration – livedo racemosa (necrotic livedo reticularis) *AD 146:208–209, 2010;* high dose buprenorphine injections – livedo with necrosis *BJD 172:1412–1414, 2015*

Calcium – percutaneous calcium salts (calcium chloride-containing EEG paste on abraded scalp skin) *Ped Derm 15:27–30, 1998; Dermatologica 181:324–326, 1990*

Collagen implant (bovine) – Zyderm or Zyplast *JAAD 25:319–326, 1991;* sterile abscesses with local necrosis *JAAD 25:319–326, 1991*

Crack hands – free base cocaine crack pipe; black burns of fingertips *Curr Drug Abuse Rev 5:64–83, 2012; Chest 121:289–291, 2002; Cutis 50:193–194, 1992*

Dequalinium (quaternary ammonium antibacterial agent) – necrotizing ulcers of the penis *Trans St John's Hosp Dermatol Soc 51:46–48, 1965*

Drug abuse *NEJM 277:473–475, 1967*

Emmonsia pasteurina – verrucous and black necrotic nodule *JAMADerm 151:1263–1264, 2015*

Injectable filler necrosis of the face (glabella) *JAAD 73:15–24, 2015;* nasal ala *J Oral Maxillofac Surg 78:133–140, 2020; JAMA Facial Plast Surg 20:207–214, 2018; Plast Reconstr Surg 12:127e-12e, 2008*

Orthopedic braces *Am J Orthop 27:371–372, 1998*

Hepatitis B virus vaccine – Arthus reaction *Clin Inf Dis 33:906–908, 2001*

Hydrofluoric acid *Ann DV 122:512–513, 1995*

Intra-arterial injections

Irritant contact dermatitis

Krokodil (desomorphine) – intravenous drug abuse contaminated with paint thinner, lighter fluid, gasoline, lead, zinc, hydrochloric acid green scaly skin; gangrene down to bone leading to amputation *Clin Inf Dis 61:1840–1849, 2015*

Levamisole-adulterated cocaine – cutaneous necrosis (livedo racemosa) associated with cocaine abuse (cocaine cut with levamisole); retiform purpura with neutropenia and vasculitis; necrosis and purpura of face, ears, nose, and cheeks, trunk; thrombotic vasculopathy; perinuclear ANCA positivity *Cutis 102:169–170,175–176, 2018; Clin Inf Dis 61:1840–1849, 2015; J Drugs in Dermatol 10:1204–1207, 2011; Cutis 91:21–24, 2013; JAAD 69:135–142, 2013; Cutis 91:21–24, 2013; JAAD 65:722–725, 2011; AD 146:1320–1321, 2010; Ann Int Med 152:758–759, 2010;* paronychial necrosis *BJD 140:948–951, 1999;* ear necrosis *Pediatr Nephrol 14:1057–1058, 2000*

Marijuana – cannabis arteritis – peripheral necrosis over legs *JAAD 69:135–142, 2013;* toe tip ulcers *JAAD 58:S65–67, 2008*

Naphtha (charcoal lighter fluid), subcutaneous injection *Am J Emerg Med 16:508–511, 1998*

Parenteral nutrition – extravasation of parenteral nutrition in pre-term or low birth weight infants; edema and compartment syndromes; necrosis, acral necrosis, anonychia *Ped Derm 32:830–835, 2015*

Phosphoric acid

Potassium hydroxide, topically, as therapy for molluscum contagiosum *Ped Derm 37:224–225, 2020*

PPD *NEJM 295:1263, 1976*

Sclerotherapy – high-concentration sclerotherapy for varicose veins *Dermatol Surg 26:535–542, 2000*

Silicone, injected *AD 141:13–15, 2005; Derm Surg 27:198–200, 2001*

Tibial cement extrusion *J Arthroplasty 13:826–829, 1998*

Tongue ring – mucosal necrosis

INFECTIONS AND INFESTATIONS

Acanthamoeba *J Clin Inf Dis 20:1207–1216, 1995;* perianal gangrene *Trop Doct 12:162–163, 1982; Proc R Soc Med 66:677–678, 1973;* tender red nodules of trunk and extremities with necrosis and eschars *AD 147:857–862, 2011*

Acinetobacter baumannii – cellulitis with overlying vesicles progress to necrotizing fasciitis with bullae *JAAD 75:1–16, 2016; Surg Infect (Larchmt)11:49–57, 2010*

Acremonium – target-like lesions with central necrosis

Actinomycosis – necrotic oral plaques *Ped Derm 29:519–520, 2012*

Aeromonas hydrophilia sepsis – gangrene *JAAD 61:733–750, 2009*

African tick bite fever (*Rickettsia africae*) – crusted eschar *AD 142:1312–1314, 2006; BJD 143:1109–1110, 2000;* hemorrhagic pustule, purpuric papules; transmitted by *Amblyomma* ticks – high fever, regional adenopathy, arthralgia, myalgia, fatigue, rash in 2–3 days, with eschar, maculopapules, vesicles, and pustules *JAAD 48:S18–19, 2003*

Alternariosis – necrosis of large section of arm *Ped Derm 24:257–262, 2007*

Amebiasis (*Entamoeba histolytica*) – nasal destruction with malodorous ulcer with gray-white necrotic base; penile ulcers, genital and perianal ulcers *Cutis 90: 2012*

Angioinvasive fungal infections *JAAD 80:869–880, 2019; JAAD 80:883, 898, 2019*

Anthrax – eschar of the fingers, face, or neck *NEJM 372:954–962, 2015; Cutis 69:23–24, 2002; Cutis 67:488–492, 2001; Clin Inf Dis 19:1009–1014, 1994; Cutis 48:113–114, 1991; Cutis 40:117–118, 1987;* eschar and ulceration *NEJM 352:700–707, 2005; JAAD 47:766–769, 2002;* necrotic papulopustule *Ped Derm 24:330–331, 2007;* papule develops central vesicle with surrounding brawny edema becomes hemorrhagic, necrotic with satellite vesicles; black eschar, painless ulcer *JAAD 65; 1213–1218, 2011;* intravenous drug abuse – edema, necrosis, bullae, compartment syndrome, necrotizing fasciitis *Clin Inf Dis 61:1840–1849, 2015*

Arthropod bite *NEJM 352:700–707, 2005;* hypersensitivity to mosquito bites with intense erythema, edema and necrosis *AD 139:1601–1607*

Aspergillosis – necrotic papulonodules *JAAD 80:869–880, 2019; AD 125:952–956, 1989;* large (2–3 cm) eschar with thin erythematous halo *SKINmed 13:329–330, 2015; BJD 157:407–409, 2007; NEJM 352:700–707, 2005; AD 141:633–638, 2005; Clin Inf Dis 22:1102–1104, 1996; Ped Inf Dis 12:673–682, 1993;* A. flavus, primary cutaneous – necrotic ulcer *AD 141:1035–1040, 2005;* violaceous and necrotic plaque – primary cutaneous aspergillosis at site of cyanoacrylate skin adhesive *Ped Derm 35:494–497, 2018;* primary cutaneous aspergillosis in premature infant – necrotic eschar blanketing entire back *Ped Derm 36:709–710, 2019;* necrotizing dermal plaque *BJD 85(suppl 17):95–97, 1971;* primary cutaneous aspergillosis *JAAD 38:797–798, 1998; Infect Control Hosp Epidemiol 17:365–366, 1996;* primary cutaneous aspergillosis in premature infants *Ped Derm 19:439–444, 2002;* A. flavus *JAAD 46:945–947, 2002;* zosteriform A. flavus – black eschar *JAAD*

38:488–490, 1998; eschar and ulceration *JAAD 53:213–219, 2005; JAAD 47:766–769, 2002; Aspergillus fumigatus –* necrotic purpura with ulcers; verrucous crusted black giant plaque of back *Ped Derm 27:403–404, 2010; Aspergillus fumigatus –* painful, purpuric necrotic papules and pustules in tattoo *BJD 170:1373–1375, 2014*

Bacteroides – non-clostridial gas gangrene in diabetics *JAMA 233:958–963, 1975*

Balamuthia mandrillaris – red plaque with central necrosis; transmitted by organ transplant *Clin Inf Dis 63:878–888, 2016*

BCG lymphadenopathy with eschar *Ped Derm 21:646–651, 2004*

Beetle bite *J Cutan Med Surg 4:219–222, 2000*

Bejel

Bilophila wadsworthia and *Escherichia coli* – necrotizing fasciitis

Boutonneuse fever

Brown recluse spider bite – necrotic arachnidism – (*L. reclusa*) *Lancet 378:2039–2047, 2011; J Toxicol Clin Toxicol 21:451–472, 1983–1984;* ecchymosis, cyanotic pale hemorrhagic bulla progresses to eschar; sunken bluish patch; *Loxosceles rufescens;* eschar, necrosis, targetoid: 6 eyes *JAMADerm 156:203, 2020; JAMADerm 150:1205–1208, 2014; JAAD 67:347–354, 2012; NEJM 352:700–707, 2005;* dermonecrotic lesion with periorbital edema *Turk J Pediatr 53:87–90, 2011*

Brucellosis – necrotizing vasculitis

Burkholderia pseudomallei (melioidosis) – disseminated; ecthyma-like lesions *Clin Inf Dis 40:988–989, 1053–1054, 2005*

especially found in Thailand; ecthyma gangrenosum-like lesions *AD 135:311–322, 1999;* ecthymatous eschar *Clin Inf Dis 40:988–989,1053–1054, 2005*

Buruli ulcer – diffuse erythema, edema, and necrosis of dorsal hand *JAMADerm 130:669–671, 2014*

Calymmatobacterium granulomatis (Donovanosis) – penile necrosis *J Clin Inf Dis 25:24–32, 1997*

Cancrum oris (noma) – labial and buccal necrosis *J Dent Child 48:138–141, 1981*

Candida tropicalis – targetoid lesions with central necrosis *JAAD 80:869–880, 2019; J Hosp Infect 50:316–319, 2002; Rev Iberoam Micol 16:235–237, 1999; Mycoses 40:17–20, 1997; AD 115:234–235, 1979*

Candidiasis, disseminated – necrotic eschar and pustules; ecthyma gangrenosum-like lesion

Capnocytophaga canimorsus sepsis – dog and cat bites; necrosis with eschar *Cutis 60:95–97, 1997; JAAD 33:1019–1029, 1995*

Carbuncle

Caterpillars, poisonous *Toxicon 153:39–52, 2018; Ann DV 125:489–491, 1998*

Cellulitis, erysipelas

Cheyletiella mites – dogs, cats; papulovesicles, pustules, necrosis *JAAD 50:819–842, 2004; AD 116:435–437, 1980*

Chikungunya fever (Chikungunya virus) – Africa, Middle East, Europe, India, Southeast Asia; fever, arthralgias, morbilliform eruption; polyarthritis and tenosynovitis; hepatitis, myocarditis, hemorrhage, meningitis, encephalitis; palpebral edema; purpuric butterfly eruption of face; necrosis of skin of nose *Clin Inf Dis 62:78–81, 2016*

Chromobacterium violaceum NEJM 352:700–707, 2005; distal gangrene *JAAD 54:S224–228, 2006*

Clostridium botulinum – wound botulism in drug addicts *Clin Inf Dis 31:1018–1024, 2000*

Clostridial cellulitis of the newborn *AD 113:683–684, 1977*

Clostridium perfringens (gas gangrene) – most common cause of necrotizing anorectal and perianal infection *Surgery 86:655–662, 1979*

Clostridium septicum – gas gangrene and myonecrosis

Clostridium welchii

Coccidioidomycosis – primary cutaneous coccidioidomycosis; necrotic papule *JAAD 49:944–949, 2003*

Colletotrichum gloeosporioides (plant pathogen) – necrotic ulcers *JAMADerm 1511383–1384, 2015*

Corynebacterium urealyticum Clin Inf Dis 22:853–855, 1996

Covid-19 – coronavirus; hypercoagulability with acral necrosis – personal observation

Cowpox (feline orthopoxvirus) – eschar; necrotic papule; tongue ulcer, targetoid and umbilicated indurated papules, vesicles, pustules with central necrosis; exposure to pet rat *Clin Inf Dis 68:1063–1064, 2019; BJD 173:535–539, 2015; JAAD 49:513–518, 2003; BJD 145:146–150, 2001*

Cryptococcosis *NEJM 352:700–707, 2005;* umbilicated papules with central necrosis *AD 142:921–926, 2006*

Diphtheria, cutaneous (*Corynebacterium diphtheria*) – black n necrotic ulcers of penis and scrotum *Cutis 79:371–377, 2007*

Cytomegalovirus infection – necrotic ulcers of the scalp *Ped Derm 31:729–731, 2014*

Ecthyma – eschar and ulceration *JAAD 47:766–769, 2002*

Ecthyma gangrenosum – *Pseudomonas aeruginosa NEJM 352:700–707, 2005; JAAD 11:781–787, 1984; Pseudomonas cepacia AD 113:199–202, 1977;* gram-negative bacteria *Postgrad Med 106:249–250, 1999; AD 121:873–876, 1985; JAAD 11:781–787, 1984; Escherichia coli J Clin Gastroenterol 4:145–148, 1982; Rev Inf Dis 2:854–865, 1980; Aeromonas hydrophila NY State J Med 82:1461–1464, 1982; J Pediatr 83:100–101, 1973; Klebsiella pneumoniae Int J Dermatol 34:216–217, 1995; South Med J 84:790–793, 1991; Xanthomonas maltophilia Ann Int Med 121:969–973, 1994; Morganella morganii Mil Med 153:400–401, 1988; Serratia marcescens Rev Inf Dis 2:854–865, 1980; Citrobacter freundii JAAD 50:S114–117, 2004; Corynebacterium diphtheria JAAD 50:s114–117, 2004; Neisseria gonorrhoeae; Yersinia pestis; Citrobacter freundii; Staphylococcus aureus; Streptococcus pyogenes; Aspergillus fumigatus; Aspergillus niger Am J Clin Pathol 72:230–232, 1979; Candida albicans Am J Med 70:1133–1135, 1982; Exserohilum species Ped Derm 20:495–497, 2003; Vibrio, Rhizopus, Fusarium solani; Scytalidium dimidiatum J Clin Microbiol Infect Dis 12:118–121, 1993; Pseudallescheria boydii, Curvularia sp. Bone Marrow Transplant 27:1311–1313, 2001; herpes simplex Clin Infect Dis 29:454–455, 1999*

Endocarditis, bacterial – necrosis in children *AD 133:1500–1501, 1997;* subacute bacterial endocarditis with vasculitis; subacute bacterial endocarditis – *Streptococcus viridans* with cutaneous vasculitis; Osler's nodes (painful hemorrhagic bulla of thumb tip); extensive distal purpura with necrosis of legs; Janeway lesion – purpuric macule of sole; conjunctival hemorrhage *JAMADerm 150:494–500, 2014;* extensive cutaneous necrosis *Eur Heart J Dec 23, 2019*

Acute bacterial endocarditis – personal observation

Enteroviral infections – leukocytoclastic vasculitis – personal observation

Epidemic typhus (*Rickettsia prowazekii*) – pink macules on sides of trunk, spreads centrifugally; flushed face with injected conjunctivae; then rash becomes deeper red, then purpuric; gangrene of finger, toes, genitalia, nose *JAAD 2:359–373, 1980*

Chronic active Epstein-Barr virus – vulvitis, hemorrhagic cheilitis, necrotic ulcers, periorbital erythema and edema, maxillary sinusitis, hepatosplenomegaly *BJD 173:1266–1270, 2015*

Erysipelothrix rhusiopathiae – rare systemic form with localized swellings with central necrosis

Escherichia coli – non-clostridial gas gangrene in diabetics *JAMA 233:958–963, 1975*

Fire coral (*Millepora spp*) – scuba divers; dermatitis, bullae, hemorrhagic bullae, necrosis, ulceration, urticaria; late lichenoid and granulomatous reactions *JAAD 61:733–750, 2009*

Flavobacterium odoratum – necrotizing fasciitis *J Clin Inf Dis 21:1337–1338, 1995*

Fournier's gangrene *NEJM 376:1158: AD 142:797–798, 2006; Clin Inf Dis 40:990–996, 2005*

Fusarium – sepsis; red-gray macules or papules with central eschar *JAAD 47:659–666, 2002; Ped Derm 9:62–65, 1992; Fusarium solani –* target-like lesions with central necrosis; violaceous nodules with central necrosis *AD 146:1037–1042, 2010; Clin Inf Dis 32:1237–1240, 2001; Eur J Clin Microbiol Infect Dis 13:152–161, 1994;* purpuric eschar *AD 147:1317–1322, 2011;* cellulitis with necrosis *Am J Clin Pathol 75:304–311,1981;* necrotic nodule of temple *AD 146:439–444, 2010; J Pediatr 84:561–564, 1974; F. falciforme –* starts as red nodule then evolves into red plaques, vesicles, pustules, with or without central necrosis *BJD 157:407–409, 2007*

Fusobacterium – abscesses with necrosis

Gangrenous and crepitant cellulitis
 Clostridium perfringens
 Infected vascular gangrene
 Nonclostridial crepitant cellulitis (anaerobes)
 Phycomycotic gangrenous cellulitis
 Progressive bacterial synergistic gangrene
 Vibrio vulnificus

Gemella morbillorum – necrotizing fasciitis *JAAD 52:704–705, 2005*

Glanders – eschar and ulceration *JAAD 47:766–769, 2002*

Gonococcemia *NEJM 352:700–707, 2005;* periarticular lesions appear in crops with red macules, papules, vesicles with red halo, pustules, bullae becoming hemorrhagic and necrotic; suppurative arthritis and tenosynovitis *Ann Int Med 102:229–243, 1985; NEJM 282:793–794, 1970;* in children *AD 133:1500–1501, 1997*

Gypsy moth caterpillar reaction *JAAD 62:1–10,13–28, 2010*

Hepatitis C – with cryoglobulins; thrombotic vasculitis *AD 131:1185–1193, 1995*

Herpes simplex virus – necrotizing balanitis *JAMA 248:215–216, 1982; Br J Vener Dis 55:48–51, 1979;* necrotic digits in chronic herpes simplex *JAAD 60:484–486, 2009;* neonatal herpes simplex – necrotic plaque of scalp at site of fetal monitor electrode placement

Herpes zoster – cutaneous necrosis in AIDS *Clin Dermatol 38:160–175, 2020;* jaw necrosis *Oral Surg 56:39–46, 1983;* purpuric, umbilicated, necrotic bullae of leg *AD 147:235–240, 2011;* red plaque of face with necrosis *Cutis 96:364–390, 2015*

HHV6 and protein S deficiency (anti-protein S antibodies) – disseminated intravascular coagulation *BJD 161:181–183, 2009*

Histoplasmosis – necrotic papules and ulcers *BJD 113:345–348, 1985*

HIV disease – polyarteritis-like vasculitis with acral necrosis *J Clin Inf Dis 23:659–661, 1996*

Hyalohyphomycosis – necrotic papulonodules *JAAD 80:869–880, 2019; Clin Inf Dis 35:909–920, 2002; Rev Inst Trop Sao Paulo 39:227–230, 1997*

Insect bite – especially in Hodgkin's disease; eschar and ulceration *JAAD 47:766–769, 2002;* necrosis due to hypersensitivity to mosquito bites in patients with Epstein-Barr virus infection *JAAD 72:1–19, 2015;* mosquito bite hypersensitivity syndrome in EBV-associated natural killer cell leukemia/lymphoma – clear or hemorrhagic bullae with necrosis, ulceration and scar formation *JAAD 45:569–578, 2001*

Klebsiella sepsis – including non-clostridial gas gangrene in diabetics *JAMA 233:958–963, 1975*

Leclaria adecarboxylata – cellulitis with necrotic pustules in acute lymphoblastic leukemia *Ped Derm 28:162–164, 2011*

Leishmaniasis – eschar and ulceration *NEJM 352:700–707, 2005; JAAD 47:766–769, 2002;* large necrotic ulcer of dorsum of hand in AIDS *BJD 160:311–318, 2009;* necrosis of lips *Mycoses 41 Suppl2:78–80, 1998(German); JAAD 28:495–496, 1993; Dermatologica 150:292–294, 1975; L. aethiopica* – lip edema *Trans R Soc Trop Med Hyg 63:708–737, 1969;* espundia (mucocutaneous leishmaniasis) – nasopharyngeal mutilation with protuberant lips *Am J Trop Med Hyg 59:49–52, 1998;* erythema nodosum leprosum – targetoid red nodules with central necrosis *AD 144:821–822, 2008*

Leprosy – plantar necrotic blister; Lucio's phenomenon – bullae and necrosis leaving deep painful ulcers; necrotic ulcerated plaques of face and extremities *JAMADerm 152:333–334, 2016; Int J Lepr 47:161–166, 1979;* stellate necrosis due to hemorrhagic infarcts of legs, forearms, buttocks with lymphadenopathy, splenomegaly in Lucio's phenomenon; fever, anemia, hepatosplenomegaly *JAAD 83:17–30, 2020; JAAD 71:795–803, 2014; JAAD 51:416–426, 2004;* lepromatous leprosy including erythema nodosum leprosum (vasculitis) *JAAD 51:416–426, 2004; AD 111:1575–1580, 1975;* eschar and ulceration *JAAD 47:766–769, 2002;* erythema nodosum leprosum *Rheum (Oxford) 58:85, 2019;* Lucio's phenomenon – serpiginous polycyclic necrotic ulcers *J Clin Aesthet Dermatol 12:35–38, 2019*

Lyme disease – vesicular variant with secondary necrosis *NEJM 352:700–707, 2005; JAAD 49:363–392, 2003*

Malaria

Mediterranean spotted fever *AD 139:1545–1552, 2003*

Meningococcemia *Ann Plast Surg 46:199–200, 2001;* purpura fulminans *Burns 24:272–274, 1998;* chronic meningococcemia – necrotic papule *AD 144:770–773, 2008; Ped Derm 13:483–487, 1996*

Milker's nodule – eschar and ulceration *JAAD 47:766–769, 2002*

Millipede burns – necrosis of toes *Cutis 103:195–196, 2019*

Moths – *Podalia, Megalopyge, or Saturniidae* moths; necrosis due to envenomation with larval forms of moths (erucism) *JAAD 67:331–344, 2012*

Mucormycosis – necrotic papulonodules *JAAD 80:869–880, 2019; Rhizopus oryzae* (accounts for 70% of all mucormycosis), *Absidia corymbifera, Cunninghamella bertholletiae, Rhizomucor pusillus Clin Derm 37:447 = 467, 2019; BJD 150:1212–1213, 2004; Mucor circinelloides, Apophysomyces elegans, Saksenaea vasiformis;* face, scalp, extremities – necrotic ulcer *Ped Derm 20:411–415, 2003; AD 136:1165–1170, 2000; AD 133:249–251, 1997; J Clin Inf Dis 19:67–76, 1994;* necrotizing cutaneous mucormycosis *NEJM 367:2214–2225, 2012;* ptosis with upper eyelid edema and necrosis *JAMA 309:2382–2383, 2013;* rhino-orbital-cerebral mucormycosis – black necrotic plaque of medial eyelids *Cutis 94:168, 195–196, 2014;* palatal ulcer, necrosis *JAMADerm 155:109–110, 2019; Clin Inf Dis 40:990–996, 2005; Oral Surg 68:624–627, 1989;* unilateral localized facial edema with slight erythema; within days goes on to necrosis *JAAD 66:975–984, 2012;* eschar and ulceration *JAAD 47:766–769, 2002;* rhino-orbital mucormycosis – palatal and nasal mucosal necrosis *NEJM 341:265–273, 1999;* slowly progressive cutaneous rhinofacial and pulmonary mucormycosis due to *Mucor irregularis Clin Inf Dis 56:993–995, 2013; Rhizopus AD 125:952–956, 1989; Rhizopus azygosporus BJD 153:428–430, 2005*

Mycetoma *JAAD 32: 897–900, 1995*

Mycobacterium chelonei var. abscessus

Mycobacterium haemophilum – necrotic ulcer *J Infection 23:303–306, 1991*

Mycobacterium kansasii – papulonecrotic tuberculid *JAAD 40:359–363, 1999; JAAD 36:497–499, 1997*

Mycobacterium marinum

Mycobacterium tuberculosis NEJM 352:700–707, 2005; primary inoculation; miliary tuberculosis – large crops of blue papules, vesicles, pustules, hemorrhagic papules; red nodules; vesicles become necrotic to form ulcers *JAAD 50:S110–113, 2004; Practitioner 222:390–393, 1979; Am J Med 56:459–505, 1974; AD 99:64–69, 1969;* lupus vulgaris; starts as red-brown plaque, enlarges with serpiginous margin or as discoid plaques; vegetating forms – ulcerate, areas of necrosis, invasion of mucous membranes with destruction of cartilage (lupus vorax); head, neck, around nose, extremities, trunk *Int J Dermatol 26:578–581, 1987; Acta Tuberc Scand 39(Suppl 49):1–137, 1960;* lupus vulgaris, miliary, papulonecrotic tuberculid *Am J Clin Dermatol 3:319–328, 2002; Dermatologica 173:189–195, 1986; BJD 91:263–270, 1974;* congenital tuberculosis – red papule with central necrosis *AD 117:460–464, 1981;* penile gangrene; eschar and ulceration *JAAD 47:766–769, 2002*

Mycobacterium ulcerans (Buruli ulcer) – necrotic leg ulcer *JAMADerm 151:1137–1139, 2015; NEJM 352:700–707, 2005*

Mycoplasma pneumoniae – purpura and necrosis *Clin Exp Immunol 14:531–539, 1973*

Necrolytic acral erythema – hepatitis C infection *Int J Dermatol 35:252–256, 1996*

Necrotizing fasciitis – necrotic ulcer *Ped Derm 29:264–269, 2012; Streptococcus pyogenes Curr Prob in Dermatol 14:183–220, 2002; Ann DV 128:376–381, 2001;* methicillin-resistant *Staphylococcus aureus NEJM 352:1445–1453, 2005; Streptococcus pneumoniae* – due to intramuscular injection *Clin Inf Dis 33:740–744, 2001; Serratia marcescens Clin Inf Dis 23:648–649, 1996; JAAD 20:774–778, 1989; Bacteroides spp.* in penile necrotizing fasciitis *JAAD 37:1–24, 1997;* neonatal *Pediatrics 103:53, 1999;* in infancy *Ped Derm 2:55–63, 1984;* Clostridial cellulitis (gangrene); progressive synergistic gangrene; gangrenous cellulitis (*Pseudomonas*); Fournier's gangrene; periorbital *AD 140:664–666, 2004; Klebsiella pneumonia* – massive edema, erythema, necrosis of thigh *Clin Inf Dis 56:1457,1505–1506, 2013*

> Most common organisms of necrotizing soft tissue infections are: *Infection 47:677–679, 2019; Clin Infect Dis 41:1373–1406, 2005*
> *Streptococcus pyogenes*
> *Staphylococcus aureus*
> *Vibrio vulnificus*
> Anaerobic streptococci
> *Klebsiella pneumoniae*

New Jersey novel polyoma virus sepsis *JAAD 1:538–540, 2015*

Niquim toadfish envenomation *Am J Trop Med Hyg 101:476–477, 2019*

Nocardia asteroides AD 121:898–900, 1985; J Inf Dis 134:286–289, 1976

Noma (cancrum oris) (necrotizing gingivitis) – *Fusobacterium necrophorum, Prevotella intermedia, alpha-hemolytic streptococci, Actinomyces spp. Oral Dis 5:144–149,156–162, 1999;* associated with malnutrition, unsafe drinking water, poor sanitation, poor oral health *Am J Trop Med Hyg 60:150–156, 1999; Cutis 39:501–502, 1987; J Maxillofac Surg 7:293–298, 1979*

Noma neonatorum – *Pseudomonas* infection *Ped Inf Dis 21:83–84, 2002*

Non-clostridial gas gangrene – cellulitis with necrosis; *Streptococcus anginosus, Strep faecalis, aerobic strep, E. coli, Proteus, Bacteroides, Klebsiella spp. JAAD 40:347–349, 1999; Diabetalogia 13:373–376, 1977*

North American blastomycosis

North Asian tick typhus

Orf – eschar and ulceration *JAAD 47:766–769, 2002*

Orthopoxvirus – facial necrosis; on prednisone for Crohn's disease *Hautarzt 70:715–722, 2019*

Osteomyelitis-associated vasculitis – personal observation

Paecilomyces lilacinus – red nodules with necrotic centers *Ann Int Med 125:799–806, 1996;* ecthyma gangrenosum-like *JAAD 39:401–409, 1998*

Phaeoacremonium inflatipes – fungemia in child with aplastic anemia; swelling and necrosis of lips, periorbital edema, neck swelling *Clin Inf Dis 40:1067–1068, 2005*

Phaeohyphomycosis, subcutaneous *Ped Inf Dis 5:380–382, 1986;* phaeomycotic cyst of the hand – *Phialophora, Cladosporium, Alternaria JAAD 8:1–16, 1983*

Phagedenic balanitis

Phlegmon – necrotic cutaneous phlegmon

Plague (*Yersinia pestis*) – ecthyma gangrenosum-like lesions at site of initial flea bite; eschars *AD 135:311–322, 1999; Clin Inf Dis 19:655–663, 1994;* eschar and ulceration *JAAD 47:766–769, 2002*

Portuguese man-of-war stings *J Emerg Med 10:71–77, 1992*

Pseudallescheria boydii – mycetoma – bulla with central necrosis *AD 132:382–384, 1996*

Pseudomonas – ecthyma gangrenosum in Pseudomonas sepsis; *Pseudomonas aeruginosa* – ecthyma gangrenosum with severe facial edema *AD 142:1663–1664, 2006;* eschar and ulceration *JAAD 47:766–769, 2002; JAAD 11:781–787, 1984; Arch Int Med 128:591–595, 1971;* noma neonatorum – gangrenous changes in oronasal and perineal areas, scrotum, and eyelids (Pseudomonas in infants) *Lancet 2:289–291, 1978; Pseudomonas* sepsis – penile gangrene *J Urol 124:431–432, 1980;* non-clostridial gas gangrene in diabetics *JAMA 233:958–963, 1975;* abscess – personal observation

Pythium insidiosum (pythiosis) (alga) (aquatic oocyte) – necrotizing hemorrhagic plaque; ascending gangrene of legs; Thailand; painful subcutaneous nodules, eyelid swelling and periorbital cellulitis, facial swelling, ulcer of arm or leg, pustules evolving into ulcers *BJD 175:394–397, 2016; J Infect Dis 159:274–280, 1989;* cellulitis, infarcts, ulcers *JAAD 52:1062–1068, 2005*

Differential diagnosis includes:
   Aeromonas hydrophilia
   Aspergillus
   Fusarium
   Mucor, Rhizopus
   Vibrio vulnificus

Queensland tick typhus *AD 139:1545–1552, 2003*

Rat bite fever (Sodoku) – *Spirillum minor* – eschar (acrally); macular and petechial rash on palms and soles; palmar papules and pustules with necrosis; acral hemorrhagic pustules; acral morbilliform eruption with petechiae, vesicles, and pustules; headache, migratory polyarthralgias *AD 148:1411–1416, 2012; Clin Inf Dis 43:1585–1586, 1616–1617, 2006; JAAD 38:330–332, 1998; Ann Emerg Med 14:1116–1118, 1985;* eschar and ulceration *JAAD 47:766–769, 2002*

Rickettsia parkeri rickettsiosis – Southeastern United States; Gulf coast tick (*Amblyomma maculatum*); eschar with surrounding petechiae, fever, lethargy, fatigue, headache, myalgia, arthralgia, morbilliform or vesiculopapular or papulopustular rash of trunk and extremities, palms and soles, and occasionally the face 0.5 to 4 days after fever; some lesions with small vesicle or pustule; morbilliform eruptions, discrete round macules and papules *AD 146:641–648, 2010; Clin Inf Dis 47:1188–1196, 2008*

Rickettsialpox (*Rickettsia akari*) (Kew Gardens spotted fever) - house mouse mite bite (*Liponyssus (Allodermanyssus) sanguineus*) *Ped Derm 29:767–768, 2012; NY Med 2:27–28, 1946;* eschars in rickettsialpox, *R. conorii, R. sibirica, R. australis, R. japonicum AD 139:1545–1552, 2003; Clin Inf Dis 18:624–626, 1994;* eschar and ulceration *JAAD 47:766–769, 2002*

Rocky Mountain spotted fever *JAAD 49:363–392, 2003; Clin Inf Dis 16:629–634, 1993;* eschar at bite site; DIC *J Clin Inf Dis 21:429, 1995;* massive skin necrosis *South Med J 71:1337–1340, 1978*

Scedosporium apiospermum – septic hemorrhagic necrotic bullae *Cutis 84:275–278, 2009*

Scopulariopsis

Scorpion sting – pain, necrosis, hemorrhagic bullae; pulmonary edema, shock, death *JAAD 67:347–354, 2012*

Scrub typhus (*Orientia (Rickettsia) tsutsugamushi*) (larval stage of trombiculid mites (chiggers)) – headache and conjunctivitis; eschar with black crust; generalized macular or morbilliform rash *Clin Inf Dis 39:1329–1335, 2004; AD 139:1545–1552, 2003; JAAD 2:359–373, 1980;* eschar and ulceration *JAAD 47:766–769, 2002*

Sea anemone sting

Serratia marcescens – including necrotizing fasciitis *J Clin Inf Dis 23:648–649, 1996*

Siberian tick typhus *AD 139:1545–1552, 2003*

Smallpox vaccination *Clin Inf Dis 37:241–250, 2003;* progressive vaccinia *Clin Inf Dis 37:251–271, 2003*

Snake bites – edema, erythema, pain, and necrosis *NEJM 347:347–356, 2002;* green pit viper *Am J Trop Med 58:22–25, 1998;* spitting cobra (*Naja nigricollis*) *Toxicon 25:665–672, 1987;*

Spider bites *Trans R Soc Trop Med Hyg 92:546–548, 1998; South Med J 69:887–891, 1976;* brown recluse spider bite *JAAD 44:561–573, 2001;* eschar and ulceration *JAAD 47:766–769, 2002*

Sporotrichosis *NEJM 352:700–707, 2005;* necrotic plaques *Cutis 78:253–256, 2006;;* eschar of forehead – fixed cutaneous neonatal sporotrichosis *Ped Derm 26:563–565, 2009;* necrotic facial mass *Dermatol Online J July 15, 2017*

Staphylococcus aureus NEJM 352:700–707, 2005; Staphylococcus aureus purpura fulminans and toxic shock syndrome *Clin Inf Dis 40:941–947, 2005;* MRSA abscess – necrotic papule *AD 144:952–954, 2008;* methicillin-resistant *Staphylococcus aureus* – ecthyma gangrenosum (hemorrhagic necrotic bulla) *Cutis 90:67–69, 2012;* ecthyma gangrenosum lesion *Ped Derm 29:320–323, 2012*

Staphylococcal scalded skin syndrome

Stenotrophomonas maltophilia (formerly *Pseudomonas maltophilia*) (*Xanthomonas maltophilia*) – cellulitis, nodules, ecthyma gangrenosum lesions *Eur J Clin Microbiol Infect Dis 28:719–730, 2009lJ Eur Acad Dermatol Venereol 21:1298–1300, 2007; Ann Pharmacother 36:63–66, 2002; JAAD 37:836–838, 1997; Can J Infect Dis 7:383–385, 1996*

Stingray bite *Cutis 78:93–94, 2006; BJD 143:1074–1077, 2000*

Streptococcus pyogenes – necrotizing fasciitis with toxic shock syndrome *Clin Infect Dis 51:58–65, 2010;* acute necrotizing infection following bites or scratches of dogs or cats *NEJM 352:700–707, 2005; Ann DV 123:804–806, 1996;* ecthyma gangrenosum-like lesion (erythematous plaque with central black necrosis) in disseminated streptococcal disease *JAMA 311:957–958, 2014*

Streptococcus pneumoniae Clin Inf Dis 21:697–698, 1995; penile gangrene

Subcutaneous phaeohyphomycosis – *Corynespora cassiicola (*plant pathogen of leaf spotting disease) in CARD9 deficiency *BJD 174:176–179, 2016*

Synergistic necrotizing gangrene (Meleney's synergistic gangrene); *Surgery 86:655–662, 1979; Arch Surg 9:317–364, 1924*

Syphilis – malignant lues – necrotic papules and nodules *JAMA Derm 149:1429–1430, 2013; NEJM 352:700–707, 2005; JAAD 22:1061–1067, 1990;* penile gangrene

Talaromyces marneffei – necrotic papules and/or nodules *JAAD 54:730–732, 2006; JAAD 37:450–472, 1997; Clin Inf Dis 23: 125–130, 1996; Lancet 344:110–113, 1994; Mycoses 34: 245–249, 1991*

Tanapox – umbilicated papule progressing to necrosis *JAAD 44:1–14, 2001*

Tick bites – especially soft ticks *JAAD 49:363–392, 2003*

Tick typhus (Boutonneuse fever, Kenya tick typhus, African and Indian tick typhus) (ixodid ticks) – small ulcer at site of tick bite (tache noire) – black necrotic center with red halo; pink morbilliform eruption of forearms, then generalizes, involving face, palms, and soles; may be hemorrhagic; recovery uneventful *JAAD 2:359–373, 1980;* eschar and ulceration *JAAD 47:766–769, 2002*

Toxoplasmosis, congenital – necrotic papules *JAAD 60:897–925, 2009*

Trichosporon beigelii AD 129:1020–1023, 1993

Tropical ulcer – eschar and ulceration *JAAD 47:766–769, 2002*

Trypanosoma brucei rhodesiense – necrotic chancre *J Clin Inf Dis 23:847–848, 1996*

Tsutsugamushi fever *Dtsch Med Wochenschr 123:562–566, 1998*

Tularemia – necrotic papule *Cutis 54:279–286, 1994;* eschar and ulceration *NEJM 352:700–707, 2005; JAAD 47:766–769, 2002;* skin slough from hamster bite *MMWR 53:1202–1203, 2005*

Tungiasis – black eschar in paronychial fold

Vaccinia – progressive vaccinia *J Clin Inf Dis 25:911–914, 1997*

Varicella – varicella gangrenosa *Arch Dis Child 30:177–179, 1955;* chronic varicella zoster virus in AIDS *AD 124:1011–1012, 1988;* penile gangrene in infancy; atypical recurrent varicella with vesiculopapular lesions with central necrosis *JAAD 48:448–452, 2003;* varicella with anti-protein S antibodies, protein S deficiency and DIC *J Thromb Haemost 3: 1243–1249, 2005*

Venoms

Vibrio vulnificus sepsis *JAAD 46:S144–145, 2002; Ann DV 128:653–655, 2001; JAAD 24:397–403, 1991*

Yaws

Zygomycosis *AD 140:877–882, 2004; JAAD 32:346–351, 1995; Rhizopus arrhizus;* bull's eye infarct *JAAD 51:996–1001, 2004; JAMA 2254:737–738, 1973; Apophysomyces elegans, Saksenaea vasiformis J Clin Inf Dis 24:580–583, 1997; J Clin Inf Dis 19:67–76, 1994; Rhizopus* – necrotic purpuric plaque of arm *Ped Derm 31:249–250, 2014; Rhizopus azygosporus BJ Inf Dis 3:428–430, 2005*

INFILTRATIVE LESIONS

Langerhans cell histiocytosis *NEJM 352:700–707, 2005;* self-regressive Langerhans cell histiocytosis (Hashimoto-Pritzker disease) – hypopigmented macules of trunk, solitary papules with necrosis, erosive and ulcerated papules, keratotic plantar papules *AD 146:149–156, 2010*

Langerhans cell histiocytosis in the adult – scrotal ulcer; solitary pink papule; red papules of trunk; ulceronecrotic plaque of scalp; perianal plaque; perianal dermatitis *BJD 167:1287–1294, 2012*

Reactive intravascular histiocytosis – black necrotic eschar of scrotum and gluteal cleft; associated with tonsillitis; possibly related to reactive angioendotheliomatosis *BJD 154:560–563, 2006*

Waldenstrom's macroglobulinemia – necrotic papules and psoriasiform plaques of knees *Annual AAD Meeting 2000*

INFLAMMATORY DISORDERS

Chondrodermatitis nodularis chronica helicis – necrotic ear *Cutis 98:293,301–302, 2016*

Dermatitis gangrenosum infantum – multiple necrotic ulcers complicating varicella, seborrheic dermatitis *BJD 75:206–211, 1963*

Erythema multiforme *Medicine 68:133–140, 1989; JAAD 8:763–765, 1983;* Stevens-Johnson syndrome

Malignant pyoderma – papulopustules, skin ulcers, violaceous nodules with central necrosis, tongue, pharyngeal, and nasal ulcers *AD 146:102–103, 2010; AD 98:561–576, 1968*

Nodular panniculitis, idiopathic – overlying necrosis with drainage of oily brown serous fluid *Medicine 64:181–191, 1985*

Pyoderma gangrenosum *BJD 157:1235–1239, 2007; NEJM 352:700–707, 2005; Br J Plast Surg 53:441–443, 2000; JAAD 18:559–568, 1988*

Pyoderma gangrenosum-like lesions, polyarthritis, and lung cysts with ANCA to azurocidin – umbilicated necrotic lesions *Clin Exp Immunol 103:397–402, 1996*

Sarcoid – resembling papulonecrotic tuberculid *AD Syphilol 13:675–676, 1926*

Stevens-Johnson syndrome – personal observation

METABOLIC DISEASES

Acrodermatitis enteropathica – black necrotic lesions

Calcific uremic arteriolopathy *NEJM 352:700–707, 2005*

Calcific vasculopathy of chronic renal failure – personal observation

Calcinosis cutis – metastatic calcification *AD 106:398–402, 1972*

Calciphylaxis (vascular calcification cutaneous necrosis syndrome) (cutaneous calcinosis in end stage renal disease) – necrotic cutaneous ulcers, livedo racemosa (livedoid necrosis), hemorrhagic patches, indurated plaques, hemorrhagic bullae *NEJM 379:397–400, 2018; NEJM 378:1704–1714, 2018; JAAD 77:241–246, 2017; JAMA Derm 149:946–949, 2013; JAMA Derm 149:163–167, 2013;; Am J Dermatopathol 33:796–802, 2011; JAAD 58:458–471, 2008; CIASN 3:1139–1143, 2008; JAAD 56:569–579, 2007; Ped Derm 23:266–272, 2006; JAAD 58:458–471, 2008; AD 143:791–796, 2007; AD 140:1045–1048, 2004; J Dermatol 28:27–31, 2001; Br J Plast Surg 53:253–255, 2000; J Cutan Med Surg 2:245–248, 1998; JAAD 40:979–987, 1999; JAAD 33:53–58, 1995; JAAD 33:954–962, 1995; JAAD 33:954–962, 1995; AD 127:225–230, 1991;* stellate necrosis *JAMADerm 130:671–673, 2014;* stellate necrosis with calciphylaxis associated with pancreatic carcinoma *BJD 171:1247–1248, 2014;* penile necrosis *JAAD 54:736–737, 2006;* penile necrosis *JAAD 82:799–816, 2020;* calciphylaxis with stellate necrosis and retiform purpura unassociated with renal disease (non-uremic calciphylaxis) – stellate necrosis beginning as mottled purpuric reticulated patches; associated with hyperparathyroidism, malignancy, alcoholic liver disease, connective tissue disease, diabetes mellitus, chemotherapy-induced protein C or S deficiency *JAMA 310:1281–1282, 2013;* associated with hypoalbuminemia, malignancy, systemic corticosteroid therapy, coumarin, chemotherapy, systemic inflammation, cirrhosis, protein C or S deficiency, obesity, rapid weight loss, infection *AD 145:451–458, 2009;* warfarin associate *JAMADerm 153:309–314, 2017*

Catastrophic anti-phospholipid antibody syndrome – personal observation

Cold agglutinins *BJD 139:1068–1072, 1998; JAAD 19:356–357, 1988;* at site of transfusion *JAAD 19:356–357, 1988;* intravascular coagulation necrosis *JAAD 25:882–888, 1991;* digital necrosis *Ann DV 145:761–764, 2018*

Cryofibrinogenemia *AD 144:405–410, 2008; Am J Med 116:332–337, 2004; Clin Exp Dermatol 25:621–623, 2000; Am J Kidney Dis 32:494–498, 1998; AD 133:1500–1501, 1997; JAAD 24:342–345, 1991;* intravascular coagulation necrosis *JAAD 25:882–888, 1991*

Cryoglobulinemia – mixed cryoglobulinemia – hemorrhagic necrosis, urticaria, ulcers with necrosis, livedo reticularis; intravascular coagulation necrosis *JAAD 61:325–332, 2009; NEJM 352:700–707, 2005; JAAD 25:882–888, 1991;* necrotic ears *BJD 143:1330–1331, 2000;* type 1 cryoglobulinemia in multiple myeloma – acral cyanosis, Raynaud's phenomenon; livedoid necrosis of arms, ears *JAMADerm 151:659–660, 2015;* type 1 cryoglobulinemia in Waldenstrom's macroglobulinemia or myeloma *Medicine (Balt) 92:61–68, 2013; Am J Med 57:775–788, 1974;* monoclonal cryoglobulinemia; cutaneous necrosis *JAAD 48:311–340, 2003; JAAD Case Rep 5:736–738, 2019*

Diabetes – microangiopathy, neuropathy *NEJM 352:700–707, 2005;* dry or wet gangrene; arteriosclerotic peripheral vascular disease; penile gangrene *J Urol 132:560–562, 1984*

Disseminated intravascular coagulation – personal observation

Homocystinuria – cystathionine-beta synthase deficiency; distal cutaneous necrosis *Ann DV 126:822–825, 1999*

Hyperparathyroidism

Hyperphosphatemia *J Parent Enteral Nutr 21:50–52, 1997*

Hyperviscosity – cryos, paraproteinemia, dehydration

Kwashiorkor – personal observation

Methylenetetrahydrofolate reductase deficiency – nonuremic calciphylaxis; livedoid necrosis *JAAD 69:324–326, 2013; AD 147:450–453, 2011*

Oxalosis – acral necrosis with livedo; (primary oxalosis (hyperoxalosis) – type 1 – alanine glyoxylate aminotransferase (transaminase) deficiency; chromosome 2q36–37; type 2 (rare) – D-glyceric acid dehydrogenase deficiency *AD 137:957–962, 2001; JAAD 22:952–956, 1990; AD 131:821–823, 1995;* primary hyperoxalosis; necrosis with limb gangrene *JAAD 49:725–728, 2003;* livedo reticularis, ulcers, and peripheral gangrene *AD 136:1272–1274, 2000;* autosomal recessive; livedo reticularis, acrocyanosis, peripheral gangrene, ulcerations, sclerodermoid changes (woody induration of extremities), eschar of hand (calcium oxalate); acral and/or facial papules or nodules; end stage renal disease; primary hyperoxalosis – deficiency of alanine:glyoxylate aminotransferase; primary hyperoxalosis – deficiency of D-glycerate dehydrogenase/glyoxylate reductase *AD 147:1277–1282, 2011*

Paroxysmal nocturnal hemoglobinuria – petechiae, ecchymoses, hemorrhagic bullae; ulcers; red plaques which become hemorrhagic bullae with necrosis; lesions occur on legs, abdomen, chest, nose, and ears; fever; deficiency of enzymes – decay-accelerating factor (DAF) and membrane inhibitor of reactive lysis (MIRL) *AD 148:660–662, 2012; AD 138:831–836, 2002; AD 122:1325–1330, 1986; AD 114:560–563, 1978*

Protein C deficiency *Blood Coagul Fibrinolysis 9:351–354, 1998; AD 133:1500–1501, 1997; Semin Thromb Hemost 16:299–309, 1990; Blood Coagul Fibrinolysis 1:319–330, 1990; AD 123:1701a-1706a, 1987*

Protein S deficiency *JAAD 29:853–857, 1993; Semin Thromb Hemost 16:299–309, 1990;* Crohn's disease *J Med Vasc 44:291–294, 2019*

Prothrombin G20210A – mutation (heterozygous) *Pediatr Hematol Oncol 16:561–564, 1999*

Purpura fulminans, neonatal – purpura or cellulitis-like areas evolving into necrotic bullae or ulcers pneumococcal sepsis – personal observation

Short bowel syndrome – superficial skin necrosis *Harefuah 136:855–857, 915, 1999*

Sickle-cell anemia – stellate necrosis – personal observation

Thrombocythemia – livedo reticularis, acrocyanosis, erythromelalgia, gangrene, pyoderma gangrenosum *Leuk Lymphoma 22 Suppl 1:47–56, 1996; Br J Haematol 36:553–564, 1977; AD 87:302–305, 1963;* essential thrombocythemia with or without necrotizing vasculitis *JAAD 24:59–63, 1991*

NEOPLASTIC

Atrial myxoma *Am J Med 62:792–794, 1977*

Basal cell carcinoma *NEJM 352:700–707, 2005*

CD 30+ lymphoproliferative disorders – red tumors, red plaques with or without necrosis, giant tumor *JAAD 72:508–515, 2015*

Cutaneous lymphoproliferative disease associated with Epstein-Barr virus – necrotic leg nodule *JAAD 57:S69–71, 2007*

Eosinophilic histiocytosis *JAAD 13:952–958, 1985*

Fibrosarcoma/spindle cell sarcoma – necrotic red or violaceous nodule

Histiocytic lymphoma (true histiocytic lymphoma) *JAAD 50:S9–10, 2004*

Infantile myofibromatosis – brown plaque with central necrosis *JAAD 71:264–270, 2014*

Kaposi's sarcoma – gangrene and ulcerations of legs *JAMA Derm 149:1319–1322, 2013*

Keloids – suppurative necrosis

Leukemia cutis *NEJM 352:700–707, 2005; BJD 143:773–779, 2000;;* acute promyelocytic leukemia – necrotic red plaques *AD 143:1220–1221, 2007;* chronic lymphocytic leukemia – red infiltrated nose with necrosis *Cutis 80:208–210, 2007;* natural killer cell CD 56- large granular lymphocytic leukemia – necrotic papules and nodules, hydroa vacciniforme-like lesions *JAAD 62:496–501, 2010*

Lymphoma – cutaneous T-cell lymphoma *NEJM 352:700–707, 2005; JAAD 47:914–918, 2002;* tumor necrosis in CTCL *JAAD 58:S88–91, 2008;* hydroa vacciniforme-like primary CD8+ angiocentric T-cell lymphoma – necrotic facial ulcers *Cutis 77:310–312, 2006;* primary cutaneous epidermotropic CD8+ T-cell lymphoma – mixture of patches, plaques, papulonodules with central ulceration, necrosis, and hemorrhage *JAAD 62:300–307, 2010;* hydroa vacciniforme-like cutaneous T-cell lymphoma, Epstein-Barr virus-related – edema, blisters, vesicles, ulcers, scarring, facial scars, swollen nose, lips, and periorbital edema, crusts with central hemorrhagic necrosis, facial dermatitis, photodermatitis, facial edema, facial papules and plaques, crusting of ears, fever *JAAD 81:23–41, 2019; JAAD 69:112–119, 2013;* primary cutaneous aggressive epidermotropic cytotoxic CD8+ T-cell lymphoma – necrotic plaques and nodules *JAMADerm 156:155–156, 2020;* variant of extranodal NK/T cell lymphoma, nasal type/ CD8+ cytotoxic T cells – recurrent papulovesicles, necrosis, ulceration, facial edema, atrophic scars, lip ulcers, edema of hands, subcutaneous nodules; systemic manifestations; occurs on both sun-exposed and non-sun-exposed skin; necrotic ulcer of hard palate *NEJM 371:1629, 2014; Ped Derm 27:463–469, 2010; AD 142:587–595, 2006; BJD 151:372–380, 2004; JAAD 38:574–579, 1998* (angiocentric lymphoma associated with Epstein-Barr virus *BJD 147:587–591,*

2002; JAAD 38:574–579, 1998; AD 133:1156–1157, 1997); NK T-cell lymphoma – necrotic plaque *JAAD 67:328–330, 2012;* subcutaneous panniculitis-like T-cell lymphoma with necrotic nodules of legs *AD 141:1035–1040, 2005; Am J Surg Pathol 15:17–27, 1991;* primary cutaneous CD30+ lymphoproliferative disorder (CD8+/CD4+) – necrotic nodule *JAAD 51:304–308, 2004;* primary B-cell lymphoma – necrotic ulcer of lower back *JAAD 55:S24–27, 2006;* primary cutaneous epidermotropic aggressive CD8+ T-cell lymphoma – red plaques and nodules with central necrosis (targetoid); ulcerated nodule *BJD 173:869–871, 2015; JAAD 67:748–759, 2012*

Lymphomatoid papulosis – papules or nodules with central necrosis *BJD 172:372–379, 2015; JAAD 70:724–735, 2014; BJD 169:1157–1159, 2013; JAAD 55:903–906, 2006; NEJM 352:700–707, 2005; JAAD 49:1049–1058, 2003; Am J Dermatopathol 18:221–235, 1996; JAAD 17:632–636, 1987; JAAD 13:736–743, 1985*

Melanoma *NEJM 352:700–707, 2005*

Metastatic carcinoma – metastatic telangiectatic breast carcinoma – violaceous swelling with telangiectasia and necrosis *JAMADerm 155:615–616, 2019*

Cutaneous blastic plasmacytoid dendritic cell neoplasm – purple macules, violaceous papules, nodules, tumefactions; highly pigmented dark red, purpuric, necrotic lesions of face, neck *JAAD 66:278–291, 2012;* ulceronecrotic lesions of scalp; red nodules of back *BJD 172:298–300, 2015*

Polycythemia vera – ischemic digital necrosis *Acta Chir Scand 144:129–132, 1978*

Squamous cell carcinoma *NEJM 352:700–707, 2005*

Thrombocythemia *SKINMed 17:204–205, 2019; Am J Dermatopathol 39:637–662, 2017*

PARANEOPLASTIC DISORDERS

Choriocarcinoma – acne fulminans in prepubertal boy – personal observation

Type 1 cryoglobulinemia – with myeloma; livedo racemosa (necrotizing livedo reticularis) *J Drugs Dermatol 13:498–499, 2014*

Hypersensitivity to mosquito bites – associated with lymphoma/leukemia *BJD 153:210–212, 2005; JAAD 45:569–578, 2001; BJD 138:905–906, 1998*

Necrolytic migratory erythema (glucagonoma syndrome) – necrotic crusted plaques of legs *Int J Dermatol 57:642–645, 2018; BJD 174:1092–1095, 2016*

Paraneoplastic acral vascular syndrome – acral cyanosis and gangrene *JAAD 47:47–52, 2002; AD 138:1296–1298, 2002*

Paraneoplastic pemphigus – necrosis of eyelids and oral mucosa

Paraneoplastic vasculitis with myelodysplasia – personal observation

Paraneoplastic venous thrombosis

Pyoderma gangrenosum, atypical (bullous) – associated with myeloproliferative disease

Sweet's syndrome with myelodysplasia – necrotic bullae *BJD 178:595–602, 2018*

Venous thrombosis

PHOTODERMATITIS

Hydroa vacciniforme – vesiculopapular eruption of face; crusted papules, necrosis, facial ulcers *BJD 173:801–805, 2015;*

necrotic lip lesions with edema *AD 142:651, 2006; BJD 144:874–877, 2001; AD 118:588–591, 1982*

Ultraviolet recall manifested as edema, erythema, bullae, hemorrhagic crusting, macules, papules, ulceration, necrosis *JAAD 56:494–499, 2007*

PRIMARY CUTANEOUS DISEASE

Acne fulminans *JAAD 77:109–117, 2017*

Acne necrotica varioliformis

Acute parapsoriasis (pityriasis lichenoides et varioliformis acuta) (Mucha-Habermann disease) *NEJM 361:1787–1796, 2009; JAAD 51:606–624, 2004; JAAD 55:557–572, 2006; AD 123:1335–1339, 1987; AD 118:478, 1982; Dermatol Z 45:42–48, 1925; Arch Dermatol Syph (Wien) 123:586–592, 1916; Veth Dtsch Dermatol Ges 4:495–499, 1894;* febrile ulceronecrotic variant of Mucha-Habermann disease – papules and plaques with painful ulceration and necrosis *Acta DV 94:603–604, 2014; Ped Derm 90:93, 2013; Ped Derm 29:53–58, 2012; Dermatology 225:344–348, 2012; Ped Derm 27:290–293, 2010; JAAD 55:557–572, 2006; NJAAD 54:1113–1114, 2006; Ped Derm 22:360–365, 2005;BJD 152:794–799, 2005; JAAD 49:1142–1148, 2003; BJD 147:1249–1253, 2002; Ped Derm 8:51–57, 1991; Ann DV 93:481–496, 1966;* criteria *Int J Dermatol 55:729–738, 2016*

Degos' disease – personal observation

Erythema elevatum diutinum *BJD 67:121–145, 1955*

Necrolytic acral erythema - hepatitis C-related

Pityriasis rosea – vesicular variant

Pustular psoriasis

Pyoderma faciale

Subcutaneous fat necrosis of newborn

PSYCHOCUTANEOUS DISORDERS

Factitial dermatitis – linear lesions *Ped Derm 21:205–211, 2004; JAAD 1:391–407, 1979;* penile gangrene (Munchhausen syndrome) – ulcerated nodules; necrosis of legs; injection of paint thinner *JAAD 71:376–381, 2014; Lancet 1:339–341, 1951;* patchy areas of necrosis *Ped Derm 32:604–608, 2015;*

SYNDROMES

Anterior tibial syndrome (compartment syndrome) *Surg Clin NA 63:539–565, 1983*

Antiphospholipid antibody syndrome – eschar and ulceration *NEJM 352:700–707, 2005; JAAD 47:766–769, 2002; NEJM 346:752–763, 2002; Semin Arthritis Rheum 31:127–132, 2001; JAAD 36:149–168, 1997; JAAD 36:970–982, 1997; Clin Rheumatol 15:394–398, 1996; South Med J 88:786–788, 1995; BJD 120:419–429, 1989;* nasal tip necrosis *BJD 142:1199–1203, 2000;* neonatal digital gangrene *AD 143:121–122, 2007;* acral livedo and necrosis *AD 147:164–167, 2011;* lupus anticoagulant

Behcet's disease (bullous necrotizing vasculitis) *JAAD 21:327–330, 1989;* pyoderma gangrenosum-like lesions *JAAD 40:1–18, 1999*

Familial chilblain lupus – paronychia, acral erythema, acral papules, necrotic ulcers, facial ulcers, mutilation of fingers, ear lesions; mutation of exonuclease III domain of 3′ repair exonuclease 1 (*TREX1*) *JAMADerm 151:426–431, 2015*

Flood syndrome – sudden rush of ascitic fluid with spontaneous rupture of umbilical hernia in longstanding ascites and end stage liver disease *JAAD Case Reports 2015:1:5–6*

Hypereosinophilic syndrome – cutaneous necrotizing eosinophilic vasculitis with Raynaud's phenomenon *BJD 143:641–644, 2000;* hypereosinophilic syndrome associated with T-cell lymphoma *JAAD 46:S133–136, 2002;* fingertip necrosis with vasculitis *AD 132:535–541, 1996;* digital necrosis without vasculitis *BJD 144:1087–1090, 2001;* cutaneous infarction *BJD 148:817–820, 2003; JAAD 5:1041–1044, 2019*

IgG4-related disease – cutaneous plasmacytosis (papulonodules); pseudolymphoma; angiolymphoid hyperplasia with eosinophilia; Mikulicz's disease; psoriasiform dermatitis; morbilliform eruption; hypergammaglobulinemic purpura; urticarial vasculitis; ischemic digits; Raynaud's disease and digital gangrene *BJD 171:929,959–967, 2014*

Infantile myofibromatosis *Ped Derm 5:37–46, 1988*

Kawasaki's disease – erythema, crusting, or necrosis of BCG inoculation sites *JAAD 69:501–510, 2013;* peripheral gangrene *JAAD 69:501–510, 2013*

Neurofibromatosis type I – vasculopathy with acral necrosis, livedoid painful ulcerations *BJD 172:253–256, 2015; Pediatrics 100:395–397, 1997*

POEMS syndrome – vasculitis with necrosis *Clin Rheumatol 26:1989–1992, 2007;* calciphylaxis *Orphanet J Rare Dis April 12, 2016*

RACAND syndrome – acral or digital necrosis; Raynaud's phenomenon, anticentromere antibodies and necrosis of digits without sclerodactyly and sclerosis of internal organs *JAAD 43:621, 2001*

Rowell's syndrome – lupus erythematosus and erythema multi-forme-like syndrome – papules, annular targetoid lesions, vesicles, bullae, necrosis, ulceration, oral ulcers; perniotic lesions *JAAD 21:374–377, 1989*

SAPHO syndrome – palmoplantar pustulosis with sternoclavicular hyperostosis; non-palmoplantar pustulosis, acne fulminans, acne conglobata, hidradenitis suppurativa, psoriasis, multifocal osteitis *Cutis 71:63–67, 2003; Cutis 62:75–76, 1998; Rev Rheum Mol Osteoarthritic 54:187–196, 1987; Ann Rev Rheum Dis 40:547–553, 1981;* with neutrophilic dermatosis (ulceronecrotic bullous Sweet's syndrome) *AD 143:275–276, 2007*

Sjogren's syndrome – nail-fold infarcts, gangrene of fingers

Sweet's syndrome – necrotizing Sweet's syndrome presenting as necrotizing fasciitis *JAMADerm 155:79–84, 2019; Int J Rheum Dis 20:2197–2199, 2017*

Thoracic outlet obstruction *AD 138:1296–1298, 2002*

Werner's syndrome – acral necrosis *Medicine 45:177–221, 1966*

Wiskott-Aldrich syndrome

TOXINS

Carbon monoxide poisoning – endothelial cell damage; compartment syndrome, pressure necrosis, rhabdomyolysis *Pediatr 68:215–224, 1981*

TRAUMA

Blunt trauma – repetitive blunt trauma *AD 138:1296–1298, 2002*

Carpal tunnel syndrome

Chemical burns
  Acids and alkalis
    Cement (calcium hydroxide) *BJD 102:487–489, 1980; Br Med J i:1250, 1978*
  Chromic acid

Hydrofluoric acid
  Lime dust – necrosis with ulcers *Contact Dermatitis 1:59, 1981*
  Phenol
  Phosphorus

Chilblains – fingertips and toetips; with necrosis on fingers, toes, nose, and ears in patients with monocytic leukemia *AD 121:1048, 1052, 1985*

Cold – central facial necrosis after application of cold pack during cardiac surgery – personal observation

Coma bullae – sweat gland necrosis *Am J Dermatopathol 35:381–384, 2013; Ann DV 122:780–782, 1995*

Compartmental syndrome (crush injury of thorax) – skin necrosis

Condom catheter – gangrene of glans or shaft of penis *JAMA 244:1238, 1980*

Crush injury of fingertip *AD 138:1296–1298, 2002*

Cryosurgery *JAAD 8:513–519, 1983*

Electric shock – fingertip necrosis *AD 138:1296–1298, 2002*

External compression of arterial supply (popliteal entrapment, cervical rib)

Frostbite – vesicles, bullae, ischemic necrosis; calcification; congenital frostbite – acral necrosis *Ped Derm 26:625–626, 2009*

Gentian violet *Acta DV 52:55–60, 1972*

Heel sticks of neonate – gangrene of heel

Hypothenar hammer syndrome *AD 138:1296–1298, 2002*

Intravenous drug addiction – dorsal vein of penis; necrosis *BJD 150:1–10, 2004; Cutis 29:62–72, 1981*

"Krokodil" – injectable opiate; cooking cocaine with caustic chemicals; described in Russia since 2002; flesh-eating necrosis; possible first cases in Arizona in 2013 *Clin Inf Dis 57:ii, 2013*

Laser burns

Microwave radiation burns

Nerve injury, traumatic – small areas of acral necrosis

Negative pressure device for erectile impotence *J Urol 146:1618–1619, 1991;* penile ring; hair tourniquet; Fournier's gangrene

Nicolau syndrome – livedoid aseptic necrosis after injections; iatrogenic cutaneous necrosis; "embolia cutis medicamentosa" *Am J Dermatopathol 40:212–215, 2018; JAAD 54:S241–242, 2006*

Orthopedic braces *Injury 25:323–324, 1994*

Oxygen face mask with continuous positive pressure *Anaesthesia 48:147–148, 1993*

Penile gangrene – post-surgical; calciphylaxis *Clin Exp Dermatol 43:645–647, 2018*

Physical trauma- rock drillers, lumberjacks, riveters, grinders, pneumatic hammer operators

Post-surgical – penile gangrene

Pressure necrosis *NEJM 352:700–707, 2005;* due to continuous positive pressure ventilation *Ped Derm 29:45–48, 2012*

Pulse oximetry – acral necrosis *Cutis 48:235–237, 1991; Anesth Analg 67:712–713, 1988*

Radial or ulnar artery cannulation *AD 138:1296–1298, 2002; N Y State J Med 90:375–376, 1990*

Radiation dermatitis, acute or chronic – necrosis *JAAD 54:28–46, 2006; NEJM 352:700–707, 2005; J Laryngol Otol 112:1142–1146, 1998;* necrosis after fluoroscopy during coronary angioplasty *AD 139:140–142, 2003*

Skin popping *Clin Nucl Med 22:865–866, 1997*

Surgery – pressure necrosis of scalp, hips, occipital scalp

Surgical embolization – occipital scalp necrosis and scarring *Surg Neurol 25:357–366, 1988*

Thoracic outlet obstruction – cervical rib, external compression of arterial supply *AD 138:1296–1298, 2002*

Tourniquet injury (hair) – penile gangrene

Traumatic disruption of arterial wall

Trench foot, immersion foot – superficial gangrene *Clin Exp Dermatol 45:10–14, 2020*

VASCULAR

Acral necrotic livedo reticularis – surgical acrylic cement embolus following vertebroplasty *BJD 156:382–383, 2007*

Acute hemorrhagic edema of infancy – purpura in cockade pattern of face, cheeks, eyelids, and ears; may form reticulate pattern; edema of penis and scrotum *JAAD 23:347–350, 1990;* necrotic lesions of the ears, urticarial lesions; oral petechiae *JAAD 23:347–350, 1990; Ann Pediatr 22:599–606, 1975;* edema of limbs and face *Cutis 68:127–129, 2001; AD 133:1500–1501, 1997*

ANCA-associated vasculitis with acquired protein S deficiency *Throm Haemost 84:929–930, 2000*

Aneurysm – dissecting aneurysm, thrombosed aneurysm

Angiopericytomatosis (angiomatosis with cryoproteins) – painful red papules and ulcerated plaques acrally; necrotic plaques *JAAD 49:887–896, 2003*

Arterial fibromuscular dysplasia – fingertip necrosis *AD 138:1296–1298, 2002*

Arteriovenous fistulae – vascular steal syndrome in hemodialysis patients (dialysis-associated steal syndrome) with arteriovenous fistulae *JAAD 58:888–891, 2008; AD 138:1296–1298, 2002*

Atherosclerosis – ischemic necrosis, gangrene; leg ulcers with small areas of necrosis along margin *NEJM 363:2651, 2010 AD 138:1296–1298, 2002*

Atrophie blanche (livedoid vasculopathy) *JAAD 69:1033–1042, 2013; AD 119:963–969, 1983*

Benign (reactive) angioendotheliomatosis – red-brown or violaceous nodules or plaques with small areas of necrosis *JAAD 38:143–175, 1998*

Brachiocephalic thrombosis – breast necrosis – personal observation

Eosinophilic granulomatosis with polyangiitis *Autoimmunol Rev 14:341–348, 2015; AD 139:715–718, 2003; JAAD 48:311–340, 2003; JAAD 47:209–216, 2002; JAAD 37:199–203, 1997; JAAD 27:821–824, 1992; JID 17:349–359, 1951; Am J Pathol 25:817, 1949;* necrotic purpura of scalp *Ann DV 122:94–96, 1995;* umbilicated nodules with central necrosis of elbows and knees (papulonecrotic lesions) *JAAD 48:311–340, 2003; BJD 127:199–204, 1992;* skin infarcts *BJD 150:598–600, 2004; Mayo Clinic Proc 52:477–484, 1977;* presenting as purpura fulminans *Clin Exp Dermatol 29:390–392, 2004;* cutaneous infarcts *Autoimmun Rev 14:341–348, 2015; Dermatopathol 37:214–221, 2015; JAAD 37:199–203, 1997; JAAD 47:209–216, 2002; JID 17:349–359, 1951; Am J Pathol 25:817, 1949*

Cholesterol emboli *JAMADerm 150:903–905, 2014; J Dermatol Case Rep 24:27–29, 2009*

Cutaneous polyarteritis nodosa – atrophie blanche lesions, acrocyanosis, Raynaud's phenomenon, peripheral gangrene, red plaques and peripheral nodules, myalgias; macular lymphocytic arteritis – red or hyperpigmented reticulated patches of legs *JAAD 73:1013–1020, 2015*

Degos' disease (malignant atrophic papulosis) *BJD 100:21–36, 1979; Ann DV 79:410–417, 1954*

Dialysis shunt-associated steal syndrome *Ann Dermatol Venereol 133:264–267, 2006; Curr Surg 63:130–136, 2006; AD 138:1296–1298, 2002*

Diffuse dermal angiomatosis of the breast *Clin Exp Dermatol 45:107–109, 2020; Int J Dermatol 53:445–449, 2014*

Disseminated intravascular coagulation (DIC) – intravascular coagulation necrosis; associated with sepsis, snake envenomation, amniotic fluid embolization, fat emboli, abruption placentae, severe head injury, Kasabach-Merritt syndrome *JAAD 61:325–332, 2009; JAAD 25:882–888, 1991;* peripheral symmetric gangrene *AD 137:139–140, 2001*

Emboli – tumor; intravascular coagulation necrosis; cholesterol emboli – peripheral gangrene *JAAD 55:786–793, 2006; BJD 146:511–517, 2002; Medicine 74:350–358, 1995; JAAD 25:882–888, 1991; Angiology 38:769–784, 1987; AD 122:1194–1198, 1986; Angiology 37:471–476, 1986;* septic *NEJM 352:700–707, 2005*

Erythromelalgia – associated with thrombocythemia – may affect one finger or toe; ischemic necrosis *JAAD 22:107–111, 1990*

Glomeruloid angioendotheliomatosis – red purpuric patches and acral necrosis – associated with cold agglutinins *JAAD 49:887–896, 2003*

Granulomatosis with polyangiitis – acneiform facial and truncal lesions with crusted necrotic papules, ulcers; palpable purpura *JAAD 72:859–867, 2015;* cutaneous necrosis *NEJM 352:700–707, 2005;* papulonecrotic lesions *JAAD 48:311–340, 2003; Cutis 64:183–186, 1999; JAAD 31:615–622, 1994;* necrotic penile ulcers *Clin Rheumatol 17:239–241, 1998; JAAD 31:605–612, 1994; AD 130:1311–1316, 1994;* genital and perineal necrosis *Am J Med 108:680–681, 2000;* necrotic lesion of forehead *Ped Derm 16:277–280, 1999;* herpetiform necrotic purpuric papules over joints (ankles, elbows) *AD 148:849–854, 2012*

Granulomatous vasculitis, cutaneous – necrosis with ulcers *JAAD 58:S93–95, 2008;* breast necrosis, livedo reticularis, arthralgias *Rev Med Brux 33:112–115, 2012*

Hemangioma (proliferating hemangioma) – focal necrosis

Henoch-Schonlein purpura *Ped Derm 15:357–359, 1998; Ped Derm 12:314–317, 1995; Am J Dis Child 99:833–854, 1960;* in the adult *AD 125:53–56, 1989*

Heterozygous factor V Leiden deficiency *BJD 143:1302–1305, 2000*

Hypertensive ulcer (Martorell's ulcer) – starts as area of cyanosis with progression to ulcer of lower lateral leg with livedo at edges *Phlebology 3:139–142, 1988*

Hypotension

Intravascular thrombosis – DIC (meningococcemia, Rocky Mountain spotted fever, fungal, parasitic (Strongyloides)), atheroemboli, fat emboli, calciphylaxis, coumarin necrosis, protein C or S deficiency, antithrombin III deficiency, purpura fulminans, antiphospholipid antibody syndrome, thrombotic vasculitis (LE), cryoglobulins, cryofibrinogens, oxalosis

Ischemic limb gangrene with pulses *NEJM 373:642–655, 2015*
   Antiphospholipid antibody syndrome
   Cardiogenic shock
   Congenital hypercoagulability
   Disseminated intravascular coagulation
   Deep vein thrombosis in an ischemic limb
   Heparin-induced thrombocytopenia (HIT)
   Metastatic adenocarcinoma
   Septic shock (meningococcemia)
   Venous limb gangrene

Ischemic venous thrombosis (phlegmasia cerulae dolens) (venous gangrene) *JAAD 28:831–835, 1993; AD 123:933–936, 1987*

Juvenile gangrenous vasculitis of the scrotum

Kasabach-Merritt syndrome – personal observation

Livedoid vasculopathy *NEJM 352:700–707, 2005;* livedoid vasculopathy associated with anti-phosphatidylserine-prothrombin complex antibody – acral gangrene, foot ulcers *AD 147:621–623, 2011*

Lymphomatoid granulomatosis – destruction of midline nasal structures; necrotic plaque of nose; crateriform nodule of cheek *JAMADerm 155:113–114, 2019*

Neonatal gangrene – secondary to umbilical arterial catheterizations, polycythemia, prematurity *BJD 150:357–363, 2004*

Perinatal gangrene of the buttock, scrotum, and prepuce *AD 121:23–24, 1985*

Peripheral vascular disease – personal observation

Polyarteritis nodosa – livedoid necrosis *NEJM 352:700–707, 2005;* peripheral embolization of thrombi with necrosis of fingers or toes cutaneous – peripheral gangrene *Ped Derm 15:103–107, 1998; Ann Rheum Dis 54:134–136, 1995; JAAD 31:54–56, 1994;* palpable purpura, livedo, nodules, urticaria, skin necrosis with ulcers *BJD 159:615–620, 2008; JAAD 48:311–340, 2003;* petechiae or gross hemorrhage *JAAD 31:561–566, 1994;* cutaneous infarcts presenting as purpuric plaques; microscopic polyarteritis nodosa – arthralgias, leg ulcers, fever, livedo, nodules, urticaria, palpable purpura, petechiae, ecchymoses, acral bullae, plantar red plaque *JAAD 73:1013–1020, 2015; BJD 159:615–620, 2008; JAAD 57:840–848, 2007; Eur J Dermatol 14:255–258, 2004;* microscopic polyarteritis nodosa – hemorrhagic papules (palpable purpura) *JAAD 48:311–340, 2003; AD 128:1223–1228, 1992;* oral purpura *Oral Surg 56:597–601, 1983;* cutaneous (livedo with nodules) – purpura; painful or asymptomatic red or skin colored multiple nodules with livedo reticularis of feet, legs, forearms face, scalp, shoulders, trunk *BJD 146:694–699, 2002;* splinter hemorrhages; childhood cutaneous polyarteritis nodosa – acral extremity necrosis; fever, muscle weakness and myalgia, and livedo with necrosis (livedo racemosa) *BJD 171:201–202, 2014; Ped Derm 29:473–478, 2012*

Porcelain aorta – chest necrosis – personal observation

Purpura fulminans *JAAD 57:944–956, 2007; Semin Thromb Hemost 16:333–340, 1990; Br Med J 2:8–9, 1891;* neonatal *AD 123:1701a-1706a, 1987;* neonatal purpura fulminans – ecchymoses of limbs at sites of pressure in first day of life; enlarge rapidly, hemorrhagic bullae with central necrosis; homozygous protein C or protein S deficiency *Semin Thromb Hemost 16:299–309, 1990*

Pustular vasculitis – annular pustular plaques with central necrosis

Radial artery removal for coronary bypass grafting *AD 138:1296–1298, 2002*

Raynaud's phenomenon

Reactive angioendotheliomatosis – red purple-purpuric patches and plaques with necrotic ulcers; includes acroangiomatosis, diffuse dermal angiomatosis, intravascular histiocytosis, glomeruloid angioendotheliomatosis, angiopericytomatosis (angiomatosis with luminal cryoprotein deposition), reactive angiomatosis-like reactive angioendotheliomatosis; associated with subacute bacterial endocarditis, hepatitis, cholesterol emboli, cryoglobulinemia, arteriovenous shunt, anti-phospholipid antibody syndrome, chronic lymphocytic leukemia, monoclonal gammopathy, chronic renal failure, rheumatoid arthritis, severe peripheral vascular disease, arterio-venous fistulae *JAAD 49:887–896, 2003; BJD 147:137–140, 2002; JAAD 42:903–906, 2000*

Recurrent cutaneous eosinophilic necrotizing vasculitis – papules, purpura, necrosis *Acta DV 80:394–395, 2000*

Sickle-cell infarct – thrombotic vasculitis

Small vessel occlusive arterial disease – diabetes *NEJM 352:700–707, 2005*

Symmetric peripheral gangrene *Cutis 46:53–55, 1990*
   Primary arterial disease – polyarteritis nodosa, SLE, rheumatoid arthritis, arteriosclerosis obliterans, thromboangiitis obliterans
   Congestive heart failure
   Overwhelming infection – meningococcemia, pneumococcal, rickettsial, viral, fungal, other
   Miscellaneous – carbon monoxide poisoning, fibrin thrombi, cold injury, crutch pressure arteritis
   Mitral stenosis with or without left atrial wall thrombus
   Embolization – cholesterol, infectious, tumor, thromboembolic
   Myocardial infarction
   Pulmonary embolus
   Vasospastic – ergotism, Raynaud's
   Primary venous disease – venous gangrene

Syphilitic aortic aneurysm eroding through the sternum *Dur M Cardiothorac Surg 10:922–924, 1996*

Takayasu's arteritis – cutaneous necrotizing vasculitis *NEJM 352:700–707, 2005; Dermatology 200:139–143, 2000*

Temporal arteritis (giant cell arteritis) – headache, loss of vision, tender temporal artery, muscle or joint pain, malaise, weight loss, loss of appetite, jaw claudication, tongue necrosis, absent temporal pulses *JAAD 61:701–706, 2009; Arthritis Rheum 42:1296, 1999;* bilateral forehead necrosis with linear eschars *JAAD 63:343–344, 2010;* with scalp necrosis *JAAD 61:701–706, 2009; AD 143:1079–1080, 2007; Clin Rheumatol 26:1169, 2007; BJD 120:843–846, 1989; Q J Med 15:47–75, 1946;* gangrene of leg, tongue necrosis *BJD 151:721–722, 2004; BJD 76:299–308, 1964;* ulcer of scalp; scalp necrosis; giant cell arteritis due to nivolumab *JAMADerm 155:1086–1087, 2019;* lip necrosis *J Oral Maxillofac Surg 51:581–583, 1993;* scalp necrosis *J Neuro Ophthalmol Oct 15, 2019*

Thromboangiitis obliterans (Buerger's disease) *Am J Med Sci 136:567–580, 1908*

Thromboembolic phenomena – fingertip necrosis; cardiac source, arterial source, aneurysm (subclavian or axillary arteries), infection, hypercoagulable state *AD 138:1296–1298, 2002*

Thrombotic thrombocytopenic purpura

Thrombotic vasculitis – personal observation

Thrombosis of large vessels

Urticarial vasculitis *Clin Rev Allergy Immunol 23:201–216, 2002*

Vasculitis – large and/or small vessel – leukocytoclastic vasculitis *NEJM 352:700–707, 2005; AD 134:309–315, 1998;* urticarial vasculitis *AD 134:231–236, 1998;* Cutaneous small vessel vasculitis – ulcerated purpuric necrotic plaques *AD 148:887–888, 2012*

Vasoconstriction

Venous stasis ulceration (chronic venous insufficiency) – medial lower leg and medial malleolus *NEJM 352:700–707, 2005; AD 133:1231–1234, 1997; Semin Dermatol 12:66–71, 1993;* with subcutaneous calcification *J Derm Surg Oncol 16:450–452, 1990*

Venous limb gangrene (phlegmasia cerulea dolens) – during warfarin treatment of cancer-associated deep venous thrombosis; due to severe depletion of protein C and failure to reduce thrombin generation *Ann Int Med 135:589–593, 2001;* massive proximal venous thrombosis resulting in arterial insufficiency; triad of asymmetric leg edema, hemorrhagic bullae, cyanosis, acral necrosis, pain *NEJM 370:1742–1748, 2014*

Congenital Volkmann ischemic contracture (neonatal compartment syndrome) – upper extremity circumferential contracture from wrist to elbow; necrosis, cyanosis, edema, eschar, bullae, purpura; irregular border with central white ischemic tissue with formation of bullae, edema, or spotted bluish color with necrosis, a reticulated eschar or whorled pattern with contracture of arm; differentiate from necrotizing fasciitis, congenital varicella, neonatal gangrene, aplasia cutis congenital, amniotic band syndrome, subcutaneous fat necrosis, epidermolysis bullosa or protein C or S deficiency with disseminated intravascular coagulation; asymmetric, well-demarcated, stellate ulcers of arms with neuromuscular defects; in newborn; serpiginous border; muscle necrosis and nerve palsy due to increased intracompartmental pressure from amniotic band, oligohydramnios, or abnormal fetal position; begins as large bulla *Ped Derm 37:207–208, 2020; JAMADerm 150:978–980, 2014; Ped Derm 25:352–354, 2008; BJD 150:357–363, 2004*

NEURAL TUBE DYSRAPHISM

Ped Derm 32:161–170, 2015

Acrochordon, pseudotail, or true tail

Aplasia cutis and congenital

Anterior cephalocele – intranasal polypoid lesion, broad nasal root, soft compressible nodule of nose

Cephaloceles – overlying hypertrichosis, capillary malformation, or hair collar

Dermoid cysts and sinuses – broad nasal root; yellow plaque; skin colored nodule; pits

Lipoma

Lumbosacral stigmata – lipoma, acrochordon, pseudotail, true tail, aplasia cutis congenital and scars, dermoid cyst or sinus, infantile hemangioma >2.5 cm, atypical dimple, infantile hemangioma <2.5 cm, faun tail, dimple, hyper- or hypopigmentation, nevus, teratomas, port wine stain

Meningeal heterotopia (ectopic rests of meningeal tissue that have lost central nervous system connection) and rudimentary or atretic meningoceles – exophytic nodular or cystic mass of occipital or parietal scalp – normal skin; glistening or bullous appearance, alopecia, hair collar

Neuroglial heterotopia (encephaloceles that lost intracranial connection) – red nodule of nasal root; skin colored nodule; red blue firm non-compressible nodule (nasal glioma); intranasal polypoid masses; and rudimentary or atretic encephaloceles

NEVI, ASSOCIATED SYNDROMES

JAAD 29:374–388, 1993

CONGENITAL NEVI

CLOVES syndrome – with epidermal nevi *Cureus 11:e5772, 2019; PIK3CA* mutation *Human Genome Var June 24, 2019*

Congenital perifollicular nevus *Indian J Otorhinolaryngol Head Neck Surg 71(suppl 3):1705–1707, 2019*

Congenital pigmented nevus with cartilaginous differentiation – congenital pigmented nevus with giant pedunculated pink tumor *Ped Derm 30:501–502, 2013;* congenital melanocytic nevus *JAAD 67:495–511, 2012*

Epidermal nevus syndrome *Ped Derm 6:316–320, 1989;* Spitz nevi *Ped Derm 35:21–29, 2018*

Familial atypical mole syndrome *JAAD 74:395–407, 2016; Bull Cancer 85:627–630, 1998*

Halo nevi around congenital nevi *Ped Derm 26:755–756, 2009*

Limb hypoplasia *J Pediatr 120:906–911, 1992*

Linear nevus sebaceous syndrome

Malformations associated with congenital nevi – spinal cord, vascular, neurocutaneous melanosis

Melanocytic nevi along Blaschko's lines *Acta DV 78:378–380, 1998*

Mills syndrome – giant congenital nevus and chronic progressive ascending hemiparesis *Ital J Neurol Sci 13:259–263, 1992*

Multiple hamartoma syndrome with congenital melanocytic nevus, epidermal nevi, vascular malformations, aplasia cutis congenita of the scalp, cartilage hamartoma, lipodermoid fibroma of the conjunctiva, and intracranial malformation *Ped Derm 3:219–225, 1986*

NAME/LAMB (Carney) syndrome *Curr Prob in Derm VII:143–198, 1995*

Neurocutaneous melanosis *JAAD 35:529–538,1996; JAAD 24:747–755. 1991;* in association with large congenital nevi with satellite nevi *Ped Derm 26:79–82, 2009*

Neurofibromatosis Type I *Neurology 35(suppl 1):194, 1985*

Nevus psiloliparus – marker for encephalocraniocutaneous lipomatosis, neurocutaneous syndrome with ocular and CNS anomalies, irregularly shaped congenital scalp alopecia *J Cut Pathol Feb 7, 2020*

Nevi spili along Blaschko's lines *Acta DV 78:378–380, 1998*

Nevus comedonicus syndrome *Am J Med Genet A Jan 21, 2020*

Nevus spilus *Ped Derm 30:281–293, 2013*

Nevus spilus syndrome – ipsilateral hyperhidrosis, muscular weakness, dysesthesia *Eur J Dermatol 12:133–135, 2002*

Nevus spilus with torsion dystonia *Ped Derm 27:654–656, 2010*

Noonan syndrome *JAAD 46:161–183, 2002; Curr Prob in Derm VII:143–198, 1995*

Occult spinal dysraphism/tethered cord *Semin Perinatol 7:253–256, 1983*

Phakomatosis pigmentovascularis – pigmented nevus, vascular nevus, nevus spilus *JAAD 53:536–539, 2005;* nevus flammeus; blaschko-esque non-epidermolytic epidermal nevus, speckled lentiginous nevus with contralateral organoid nevus *Clin Exp Dermatol 25:51–54, 2000; Ped Derm 16:25–30, 1999; Ped Derm 15:321–323, 1998; Ped Derm 13:33–35, 1996;* type IIIB nevus spilus *AD 125:1284–1285, 1989;* nevus spilus in phakomatosis pigmentovascularis type IIIb *AD 125:1284–1285, 1989*

Phakomatosis pigmentokeratotica – coexistence of an organoid nevus and a checkerboard papular speckled lentiginous nevus; organoid nevus associated with hypophosphatemic vitamin D-resistant rickets *Ped Derm 28:715–719, 2011; JAAD 55:S16–20, 2006; Eur J Dermatol 10:190–194, 2000; Ped Derm 15:321–323, 1998; AD 134:333–337, 1998;* speckled lentiginous nevus in checkerboard pattern *AD 134:333–337, 1998*

Proliferative nodules in giant congenital melanocytic nevi *JAMADerm 152:1147–1151, 2016*

Mulvihill-Smith progeria-like syndrome (premature aging syndrome) – multiple congenital melanocytic nevi, freckles, blue nevi, short stature, unusual birdlike facies, lack of facial subcutaneous tissue, xerosis, telangiectasias, thin skin, fine silky hair, premature aging, low birth weight,, hypodontia, high-pitched voice, mental retardation, sensorineural hearing loss, hepatomegaly, microcephaly, immunodeficiency with chronic infections, progeroid, conjunctivitis, delayed puberty *Am J Med Genet A 149A:496–500, 2009; Am J*

Med Genet 69:56–64, 1997; J Med Genet 31:707–711, 1994; Am J Med Genet 45:597–600, 1993

Noonan's syndrome – webbed neck, short stature, malformed ears, nevi, keloids, transient lymphedema, ulerythema ophryogenes, keratosis follicularis spinulosa decalvans JAAD 46:161–183, 2002; J Med Genet 24:9–13, 1987

Ring chromosome 7 syndrome – multiple congenital melanocytic nevi; CALMs

Schimmelpenning syndrome, Feuerstein-Mims syndrome – neurocutaneous syndrome with organoid epidermal nevus J Pediatr Neurosci 12:288–290, 2017

ACQUIRED NEVI

Addison's disease – eruptive nevi Clin Exp Dermatol 38:927–929, 2013; JAAD 37:321–325, 1997

Alopecia areata – surrounding a nevus – personal observation

Alpha MSH – eruption of benign and atypical nevi AD 145:441–444, 2009

Asthma melanodermica – prior to attack, diffuse darkening of skin and increase in size and number of nevi AD 78:210–213, 1958

Ataxia telangiectasia – autosomal recessive; telangiectasias of face, ocular telangiectasia, extensor surfaces of arms and bulbar conjunctiva; café au lait macules, hypopigmented macules, melanocytic nevi, facial papulosquamous rash, hypertrichosis, bird-like facies; immunodeficiency, increased risk of leukemia, lymphoma; cerebellar ataxia with eye movement signs, mental retardation, and other neurologic defects; cafe au lait macules JAAD 68:932–936, 2013; Ann Int Med 99:367–379, 1983

Atypical mole syndrome (dysplastic nevus syndrome) (familial atypical multiple mole melanoma syndrome) – melanoma; pancreatic cancer JAAD 74:395–407, 2016; Methods Mol Biol 1102:381–393, 2014; Genes Dev 28:1–7, 2014; Cancer J 18:485–491, 2012; JAAD 29:373–388, 1993; Recent Results Cancer Res 128:101–118, 1993; Cancer 46:1787–1794, 1980; J Med Genet 15:352–356, 1978

Azathioprine – eruptive nevi Cutis 99:268–270, 2017

Cardiofaciocutaneous syndrome (NS) – autosomal dominant, xerosis/ichthyosis, eczematous dermatitis, alopecia, growth failure, hyperkeratotic papules, ulerythema ophryogenes (decreased or absent eyebrows), seborrheic dermatitis, CALMs, multiple melanocytic nevi (over 50), hemangiomas, keratosis pilaris, patchy or widespread ichthyosiform eruption, sparse curly scalp hair and sparse eyebrows and lashes, congenital lymphedema of the hands, redundant skin of the hands, short stature, abnormal facies with macrocephaly, broad forehead, bitemporal narrowing, hypoplasia of supraorbital ridges, short nose with depressed nasal bridge, high arched palate, low set posteriorly rotated ears with prominent helices, cardiac defects; gain of function sporadic missense mutations in BRAF, KRAS, MEK1, or MEK2, MAP2K1/MAP2K2 BJD 180:172–180, 2019; Ped Derm 30:665–673, 2013; BJD 164:521–529, 2011; BJD 163:881–884, 2010; Ped Derm 27:274–278, 2010; Ped Derm 17:231–234, 2000; JAAD 28:815–819, 1993; AD 129:46–47, 1993; JAAD 22:920–922, 1990; port wine stain Clin Genet 42:206–209, 1992

Cheetah phenotype JAAD 48:707–713, 2003

Costello syndrome – verrucous papillomas of nose and arms; growth and mental retardation, sociable, depressed nasal bridge, low set ears with thick earlobes, short neck, limited joint mobility, cardiac abnormalities, malignancies (rhabdomyosarcoma, ganglioneuroblastoma, neuroblastoma, bladder carcinoma), loose redundant skin of neck, hands and feet with deep creases of palms

and soles, acanthosis nigricans, increased numbers of pigmented acral nevi, vascular birthmarks, hyperkeratosis, hyperpigmentation of skin, thin nails, thick eyebrows, sparse curly scalp hair; mutation in HRAS gene Ped Derm 30:665–673, 2013; Am J Med Genet 117:42–48, 2003 JAAD 32:904–907, 1995

Craniofacial anomalies, ocular findings, pigmented nevi, camptodactyly, skeletal changes – autosomal recessive Clin Dysmorphol 9:61–62, 2000

Crouzon syndrome with acanthosis nigricans (CAN) – onset of acanthosis nigricans during childhood, melanocytic nevi, craniosynostosis, ocular proptosis, midface hypoplasia, choanal atresia, hypertelorism, anti-Mongoloid slant, posteriorly placed ears, hydrocephalus; mutation in FGFR3 JAMA Derm 149:737–741, 2013; Ped Derm 27:43–47, 2010; Am J Med Genet 84:74, 1999

Drug-induced – immunosuppressive therapy in transplant recipients associated with increased number of nevi; 6-mercaptopurine BJD 163:1095–1098, 2010; eruptive nevi AD 145:441–444, 2009; JAAD 28:51–53, 2001; JAAD 44:932–939, 2001; Dermatology 194:17–19, 1997; of the palms and soles JAAD 52:S96–100, 2005; cyclosporine – eruptive nevi AD 146:802–804, 2010; melanotan II (melanotropic peptide) BJD 161:707–708, 2009

Ectrodactyly, ectodermal dysplasia, and cleft palate syndrome (EEC syndrome) – increased numbers of nevi JAAD 29:374–388, 1993

Epidermolysis bullosa – nevi associated with EB ("EB nevi") AD 143:1164–1167, 2007; Ped Derm 22:338–343, 2005; atypical nevi JAAD 44:577–584, 2001; BJD 153:97–102, 2005; generalized atrophic benign EB (GABEB) (mitis) – non-lethal junctional – generalized blistering beginning in infancy; nevi or acquired macular pigmented lesions with irregular borders AD 122:704–710, 1986; GABEB – giant nevi at sites of blistering AD 132:145–150, 1996

Eruptive melanocytic nevi without associations JAAD Case Rep 6:128–130, 2020; JAMADerm 150:1209–1212, 2014

Eruptive melanocytic nevi with associations: Am J Clin Dermatol 20:669–682, 2019; JAAD 75:1045–1052, 2016
   Severe blistering disease – often TEN Acta DV Croat 26:183–185, 2018; after TEN-like cutaneous lupus Lupus 27:1220–1222, 2018
   Renal transplant
   Malignancy
   AIDS Dermatol Online J June 15, 2018; AD 135:397–401, 1989
   Medications: JAAD 75:1045–1052, 2016
      Adalimumab Ann Dermatol 28:777–779, 2016
      Azathioprine Clin Exp Dermatol 43:106–107, 2018; Cutis 99:268–1270, 2017
      6-mercaptopurine J Drugs Dermatol 16:516–518, 2017
      Carbidopa-levodopa JAAD Case Rep 5:21–23, 2018
      Cyclosporine
      Methotrexate
      Etanercept Ann DV 146:640–645, 2019
      Infliximab
      Rituximab
      Combination chemotherapy
      BRAF inhibitors (vemurafenib, encorafenib)
      Ponatinib JAAD Case Rep 4:1052–1054, 2018
      Sorafenib AD 144:821–822, 2008
      Sunitinib JAMADerm 149:624–626, 2013
      Encorafenib – In Vivo 34:441–445, 2020
      Erlotinib Cutis 104:e19–21, 2019
      Regorafenib
      Melanotan I and II
      Corticotropin
      Vemurafenib JAAD 67:1265–1272, 2012
      Voriconazole AD 146:300–304, 2010

Inflammatory disorders
Stevens-Johnson syndrome *BJD 177:924–935, 2017*

Eruptive atypical nevi – widespread dermatitis with underlying eruptive atypical nevi *An Bras Dermatol 95:71–74, 2020; JAMADerm 152:1021–1024, 2016*

Erythema multiforme – eruptive nevi following erythema multiforme *JAAD 37:337–339, 1997; JAAD 1:503–505, 1979*

Facial nevi, anomalous cerebral venous return, and hydrocephalus *Ann Neurol 3:316–318, 1978; J Neurosurg 45:20–25, 1976*

Harlequin ichthyosis – increased numbers of nevi and lentigines *Ped Derm 37:192–195, 2020*

Hypoplastic anemia with triphalangeal thumbs syndrome (Aase-Smith syndrome)

Idiopathic scoliosis – related to number of acquired melanocytic nevi *JAAD 45:35–43, 2001*

Langer-Giedion syndrome (trichorhinophalangeal syndrome Type II) *JAAD 29:373–388, 1993*

Langerhans cell histiocytosis – flexural agminated eruptive nevi *JAMA Derm 149:635–636, 2013*

Lichen sclerosus et atrophicus *AD 138:77–87, 2002*

Lymphoma – multiple nevi developing in cutaneous T-cell lymphoma *Ped Derm 36:232–235, 2019*

Melanocortin receptor agonists (melanotan I and II) – eruptive nevi *BJD 161:707–708, 2009*

Multiple deep penetrating nevi *AD 139:1608–1610, 2003*

Multiple melanocytic nevi and mental retardation *Dermatology 220:169–172, 2010*

Multiple schwannomas, multiple nevi, and multiple vaginal leiomyomas – autosomal dominant *Am J Med Genet 78:76–81, 1998*

Mustard gas – eruptive nevi *JAAD 40:646–647, 1999*

Neonatal blue light phototherapy *BJD 169:243–249, 2013*

Neurologic syndromes – eruptive nevi after loss of consciousness or seizures *BJD 92:207–211, 1975*

Post-transplant eruptive nevi (renal transplantation) – eruptive atypical nevi in renal transplantation *JAAD 54:338–340, 2006, JAAD 49:1020–1022, 2003; Clin Exp Dermatol 16:131–132, 1991*

Pyoderma gangrenosum *Ped Derm 28:32–34, 2011*

RAF inhibitors (MAPK pathway) – vemurafenib and dabrafenib – exanthema warts and other hyperkeratotic lesions, keratoacanthomas, squamous cell carcinoma, melanocytic nevi, keratosis pilaris, seborrheic dermatitis, hyperkeratotic hand-foot reactions, photosensitivity, panniculitis with arthralgias, alopecia *JAAD 72:221–236, 2015*

Signature nevi *JAAD 60:508–514, 2009*

Spitz nevi – multiple Spitz nevi *Eur J Dermatol 27:59–62, 2017; Ped Derm 32:e181–183, 2015; Int J Dermatol 51:1270–1271, 2012; AD 147:227–231, 2011*

Stevens- Johnson syndrome – eruptive nevi *AD 143:1555–1557, 2007; JAAD 37:337–339, 1997*

Sunburn, blistering – eruptive nevi

Telangiectasia macularis eruptiva perstans – mastocytosis – nevus-like appearance

Toxic epidermal necrolysis – eruptive nevi *Clin Exp Dermatol 3:323–326, 1978*

Tricho-odonto-onychodysplasia syndrome – multiple melanocytic nevi, freckles, generalized hypotrichosis, parietal alopecia, brittle nails, xerosis, supernumerary nipples, palmoplantar hyperkeratosis, enamel hypoplasia, deficient frontoparietal bone *JAAD 29:373–388, 1993; Am J Med Genet 15:67–70, 1983*

Turner's syndrome (XO in 80%) – multiple nevi; peripheral edema at birth which resolves by age 2; redundant neck skin in newborn; small stature, broad shield-shaped chest with widely spaced nipples, arms show wide carrying angle, webbed neck, low posterior hairline, low misshapen ears, high arched palate, cutis laxa of neck and buttocks, short fourth and fifth metacarpals and metatarsals, hypoplastic nails, keloid formation, increased numbers of nevi; skeletal, cardiovascular, ocular abnormalities; increased pituitary gonadotropins with low estrogen levels *JAAD 50:767–776, 2004; JAAD 46:161–183, 2002; JAAD 40:877–890, 1999*

UVB therapy – change in color and size of nevi *BJD 168:815–819, 2013*

Xanthoma disseminatum – nevi-like appearance of xanthoma disseminatum *AD 138:1207–1212, 1992*

Vulvar pemphigoid *Dermatology 213:159–162, 2006*

CONGENITAL AND/OR ACQUIRED NEVI

Baraitser syndrome – premature aging with short stature and pigmented nevi *J Med Genet 25:53–56, 1988*

Crouzon syndrome *Ped Derm 13:18–21, 1996*

Ectrodactyly-ectodermal dysplasia-cleft lip/palate (EEC) syndrome

Epidermolysis bullosa – generalized atrophic benign; EB (GABEB) (mitis) – non-lethal junctional – generalized blistering beginning in infancy; atrophic scarring; alopecia of scalp, eyebrows, eyelashes *Dermatologica 152:72–86, 1976;* nevi or acquired macular pigmented lesions with irregular borders *AD 122:704–710, 1986;* GABEB – giant nevi at sites of blistering *AD 132:145–150, 1996*

Familial multiple blue nevi *JAAD 39(pt 2):322–325, 1998*

Goeminne syndrome – X-linked incompletely dominant, multiple melanocytic nevi, multiple spontaneous keloids, basal cell carcinomas, varicose veins, muscular torticollis, renal dysplasia, cryptorchidism, urethral meatal stenosis, facial asymmetry, clinodactyly, scoliosis, dental caries *JAAD 29:373–388, 1993; Curr Prob in Derm VII:143–198, 1995*

Ichthyosis – increased number of atypical nevi lamellar ichthyosis and non-bullous congenital ichthyosiform erythroderma *Ped Derm 27:453–458, 2010*

Jaffe-Campanacci syndrome *Curr Prob in Derm VII:143–198, 1995*

Kuskokwim syndrome – autosomal recessive, multiple melanocytic nevi, joint contractures, muscle atrophy, decreased corneal reflexes, skeletal abnormalities *Curr Prob in Derm VII:143–198, 1995*

LEOPARD syndrome *The Dermatologist April 2015:46–48, 2015;*

Leukemia – eruptive nevi with chronic myelogenous leukemia *JAAD 35:326–329, 1996*

Moynahan syndrome *Proc R Soc Med 55:959–960, 1962*

Mulvihill-Smith syndrome (premature aging, microcephaly, unusual facies, multiple nevi, mental retardation) *Birth Defects 11:368–371, 1975*

Neurofibroma resembling congenital melanocytic nevus *JAAD 20:358–362, 1989*

Nevoid basal cell carcinoma syndrome

Nevus sebaceous syndrome *Syndromes of the Head and Neck, p.362, 1990*

Non-selective antiangiogenic multikinase inhibitors – sorafenib, sunitinib, pazopanib – hyperkeratotic hand foot skin reactions with knuckle papules, inflammatory reactions, alopecia, kinking of hair, depigmentation of hair; chloracne-like eruptions, erythema multiforme, toxic epidermal necrolysis, drug hypersensitivity, red scrotum with erosions, yellow skin, eruptive nevi, pyoderma gangrenosum-like lesions *JAAD 72:203–218, 2015*

Noonan's syndrome – short stature, webbed neck, shield chest, lymphedema, dystrophic nails, keloids, and increased numbers of nevi *Ped Derm 11:120–124, 1994*

Progeroid short stature with pigmented nevi *J Med Genet 25:53–56, 1988*

Proteus syndrome – partial gigantism of the hands and/or feet, nevi, hemihypertrophy, subcutaneous tumors, macrocephaly, other skull anomalies, accelerated growth *Eur J Pediatr 140:5–12, 1983*

SCALP syndrome – aplasia cutis congenita, pigmented nevus, nevus sebaceous; limbal dermoid, CNS malformations *JAAD 63:1–22, 2010*

Short stature, premature aging, pigmented nevi *J Med Genet 25:53–56, 1988*

Tricho-odonto-onychial dysplasia *JAAD 29:374–388, 1993; Am J Med Genet 15:67–70, 1983*

Tricho-onychodysplasia syndrome

Trisomy 22 – Turner-like changes

Turner's syndrome – webbed neck, hypoplastic nails, keloids and hypertrophic scars, xerosis, seborrheic dermatitis, abnormal dermatoglyphics, increased numbers of nevi, sexual infantilism, short stature, cubitus valgus *JAAD 74:231–244, 2016; Ped Derm 11:120–124, 1994; JAAD 36:1002–1004, 1996; NEJM 335:1749–1754, 1996; Curr Prob in Derm VII:143–198, 1995*

Vemurafenib (BRAF inhibitor) – cystic lesions of face, hidradenitis suppurativa, keratosis pilaris-like eruptions, eruptive melanocytic nevi; hyperkeratotic plantar papules, squamous cell carcinoma; multiple nodules of cheeks; follicular plugging; exuberant seborrheic dermatitis-like hyperkeratosis of face; hand and foot reaction; diffuse spiny follicular hyperkeratosis; cobblestoning of forehead *AD 1428:-1429, 2012; JAAD 67:1375–1379, 2012; AD 148:357–361, 2012*

NIPPLE DERMATITIS

JAAD 43:733–751, 2000

AUTOIMMUNE DISEASES AND DISEASES OF IMMUNE DYSREGULATION

Allergic contact dermatitis *Contact Dermatitis 45:44–45, 2001; Contact Dermatitis 33:440–441, 1995; Contact Dermatitis 24:139–140, 1991;* para-tertiary butylphenol formaldehyde resin in a padded bra *Ped Derm 29:540–541, 2012;* nipple piercing, nipple tattoos (including after radical mastectomy); lanolin, aloe vera, chlorhexidine, topical Vitamin E, fragrances *JAAD 80:1483–1494, 2019*

Bullous pemphigoid

Chronic granulomatous disease

DiGeorge's syndrome *Cutis 45:455–459, 1990*

Graft vs. host disease *AD 147:509–510, 2011*

Pemphigus foliaceus

Pemphigus vulgaris

Severe combined immunodeficiency *Ped Derm 9:49–51, 1992*

DRUG-INDUCED

Drug reaction with eosinophilia and systemic symptoms (DRESS) – morbilliform eruption, cheilitis (crusted hemorrhagic lips), diffuse desquamation, areolar erosion, periorbital dermatitis, vesicles, bullae, targetoid plaques, purpura, pustules, exfoliative erythro-derma, facial edema, lymphadenopathy *JAAD 68:693–705, 2013*

Heparin *JAAD 20:1130–1132, 1989*

Linear IgA disease – annular blisters of nipples *Acta DV Croat 16:21–217, 2008*

Sorafenib – hyperkeratotic dermatitis of nipple and areola *Eur J Dermatol 20:854–856, 2010*

EXOGENOUS AGENTS

Irritant contact dermatitis

Hair sinus

Silicone breast implant leakage – inflammatory changes of nipple *J Plast Reconstr Aesthet Surg 67:423–425, 2014*

INFECTIONS AND INFESTATIONS

Bejel – endemic syphilis

Candidiasis – candidal mastitis – areolar erythema and fissuring *JAAD 80:1483–1494, 2019*

Coxsackie A4 *Infez Med 25:274–276, 2017*

Herpes simplex virus – eczema herpeticum

Histoplasmosis *JAAD 25:418–422, 1991*

HIV infection in children *JAAD 22:1223–1231, 1990*

Lyme disease – Borrelial lymphocytoma *Med Mal Infect 37:540–547, 2007*

Molluscum contagiosum

Mycobacterium tuberculosis – tuberculous mastitis, lupus vulgaris *Pathologee 18:67–70, 1997*

Non-tuberculous mastitis *Eur J Surg 166:687–690, 2000*

Scabies

Syphilis – secondary; primary chancre – unilateral crusted plaque; bilateral nipple-areolar dermatitis lesions *Acta DV 94:617–618, 2014; JAMA 308:403–404, 2012;* unilateral nipple erosion *AD 146:81–86, 2010*

Staphylococcal infection of the nipple (inflammatory plaques) *JAAD 20:932–934,1989*

Subareolar abscess

Tinea corporis

Tinea versicolor

Verruca vulgaris

INFILTRATIVE

Mucopolysaccharidosis

INFLAMMATORY

Hidradenitis suppurativa

Idiopathic granulomatous mastitis *Ann DV 146:571, 2019;* with erythema nodosum *J Eur Acad DV 31:e391–393, 2017;* arthritis *Rheumatol Int 31:1093–1095, 2011*

Neutrophilic eccrine hidradenitis

Periductal mastitis – nipple discharge

Pyoderma gangrenosum *JAAD 55:317–320, 2006*

Superficial granulomatous pyoderma

METABOLIC DISEASES

Prolidase deficiency *JAAD 29:819–821, 1993*

NEOPLASTIC DISEASES

Adenocarcinoma

Basal cell carcinoma – crusted dermatitis *JAAD 22:207–210, 1990*

Blue nevus

Bowen's disease *Derm Surg 27:971–974, 2001*

Breast carcinoma – direct spread from underlying breast carcinoma; primary inflammatory breast carcinoma; nipple discharge; male breast carcinoma *Cutis 83:79–82, 2009; AD 134:517–518, 1998*

Clear cell acanthoma – psoriasiform plaque *JAAD 80:749–755, 2019; BJD 141:950–951, 1999*

Epidermal nevus

Keratoacanthoma

Lentigo maligna *Cutis 40:357–359, 1987*

Lymphoma – cutaneous T-cell lymphoma; cutaneous T cell lymphoma presenting as hyperkeratosis areolae mammae *JAAD 41:274–276, 1999*

Melanoma

Metastases – carcinoma erysipelatoides

Nevus, melanocytic

Paget's disease of the breast (nipple) *Cutis 83:240, 253–254, 2009; Breast J 12:83, 2006; Br J Clin Pract 41:694–696, 1987; Dermatologica 170:170–179, 1985; Surg Gynecol Obstet 123:1010–1014, 1966; in male J Cut Surg Med 4:208–212, 2000; St Barholomew Hosp Research London 10:87–89, 1874;* pigmented Paget's disease of the nipple in men; mimics melanoma of the breast *JAAD 55:S62–63, 2006; Melanoma Research 14:S13–15, 2004; Dermatology 202:134–137, 2001; Ann DV 128:649–652, 2001; Hautarzt 43:28–31, 1992; Histopathology 19:470–472, 1991; JAAD 23:338–341, 1990*

Sebaceous hyperplasia *Cutis 58:63–64, 1996*

Seborrheic keratoses

Verrucous acanthoma

Wart

PRIMARY CUTANEOUS DISEASES

Acanthosis of nipple

Acanthosis nigricans/pseudoacanthosis nigricans

Apocrine chromhidrosis – black dot of nipple *Ped Derm 12:48–50, 1995*

Atopic dermatitis *Ped Derm 22:64–66, 2005; Trans St John's Hosp Dermatol Soc 58:98–99, 1972;* unilateral *Ped Derm 32:718–722, 2015*

Confluent and reticulated papillomatosis *J Eur Acad Dermatol 27:e119–123, 2013*

Darier's disease – erosions *JAAD 23:893–897, 1990*

Erosive adenomatosis of the nipple – blood-stained or serous discharge; enlarged nipple; eroded, crusted, dermatitis; papule on nipple *AD 144:933–938, 2008; JAAD 40:834–837, 1999; Cutis 59:91–92, 1997; JAAD 12:707–715, 1985; Cancer 8:315–319, 1955;* papillary adenoma of the nipple *Plast Reconstr Surg 90:1077–1078, 1992* Erythema craquele

Florid papillomatosis of the nipple

Fox-Fordyce disease *J Eur Acad DV 29:7–13, 2015;*

JAAD 48:453–455, 2003; J Eur Acad DV 17:244–245, 2003

Hailey-Hailey disease

Hidradenitis suppurativa *JAAD 60:539–561, 2009*

Hyperkeratosis of the nipple (hyperkeratosis areolae mammae) *JAAD 80:1483–1494, 2019; NEJM 366:158–164, 2012; JAAD 41:274–276, 1999; Australas J Dermatol 40:220–222, 1999; JAAD 13:596–598, 1985;*

Idiopathic dermatitis of the nipple *Trans St John's Hosp Dermatol Soc 58:98–99, 1972*

Lichen sclerosus et atrophicus *BJD 129:748–749, 1993*

Lichen simplex chronicus

Mamillary fissure

Mammary duct ectasia *JAAD 40:834–837, 1999*

Milium

Nummular dermatitis

Psoriasiform dermatitis

Psoriasis

Seborrheic dermatitis

Subareolar duct papillomatosis

PSYCHOCUTANEOUS

Factitial dermatitis

SYNDROMES

Netherton's syndrome

Neurofibromatosis

TRAUMA

Breast feeding (lactation mastitis) – edema, erythema, and tenderness *JAMA 289:1609–1612, 2003*

Friction, exercise, breast feeding

Guitar nipple *Eur J Dermatol 25:375–383, 2015; BMC Dermatol 5:3, 2004; JAAD 22:657–663, 1990*

Jogger's nipple *Am J Ind Med 8:403–413, 1985; NEJM 297:1127, 1977*

Nipple ring

Radiation dermatitis, acute or chronic *Breast Cancer 9:313–323, 2017*

Surf rider's dermatitis *Contact Dermatitis 32:247, 1995*

VASCULAR

Granulomatosis with polyangiitis

Superficial thrombophlebitis of the breast (Mondor's disease)

NIPPLE LESIONS, INCLUDING AREOLA WITH MULTIPLE PAPULES

AUTOIMMUNE DISEASES AND DISEASES OF IMMUNE DYSFUNCTION

Acute graft vs host reaction – nipple erosions *BJD 168:906–908, 2013*

Allergic contact dermatitis *Cutis 92:253–257, 2013*

Pemphigus foliaceus

CONGENITAL ANOMALIES

Absent or rudimentary nipples with lumpy scalp and unusual pinnae (Finlay syndrome) – autosomal dominant *Genet Couns 2:233–236, 1991; BJD 99:423–430, 1978*

Adnexal polyp of neonatal skin *BJD 92:659–662, 1975*

Carbohydrate-deficient glycoprotein syndrome – inverted nipples; emaciated appearance; lipoatrophy over buttocks; lipoatrophic streaks extend down legs; high nasal bridge, prominent jaw, large ears, fat over suprapubic area and labia majora, fat pads over buttocks; hypotonia

Circumareolar telangiectasia *AD 126:1656, 1990*

Galactorrhea of newborn – witches' milk

Mamillary fistula

Pearls (milia) in newborn of areolae, scrotum, and labia majora of newborn

Rudimentary nipples *Humangenetik 15:268–269, 1972*

Supernumerary nipples (accessory nipple or nipple nevus) *Cutis 62:235–237, 1998;* accessory supernumerary axillary breast and nipple with breast carcinoma *Cutis 87:300–304, 2011*

DRUG-INDUCED

Diethylstilbestrol – florid papillomatosis after diethylstilbestrol therapy in males

Fixed drug eruption – personal observation

Nipple priapism *JAMA 258:3122, 1987*

Paroxetine – galactorrhea *JAAD 56:848–853, 2007; Mayo Clin Proc 76:215–216, 2001; Br J Clin Pharmacol 44:277–281, 1997*

Sorafenib – hyperkeratosis of nipple *JAAD 71:217–227, 2014*

EXOGENOUS AGENTS

Curcumin supplements – nipple hyperpigmentation – personal observation

Nipple rings

INFECTIONS AND INFESTATIONS

Subareolar abscess – personal observation

Candida albicans – lactation *Aust NZ J Obstet Gynaecol 31:378–380, 1991*

Cellulitis – personal observation

Herpes simplex

Lyme disease (*Borrelia burgdorferi*) – lymphocytoma cutis; bluish-red plaque of nipple or areola *JAAD 49:363–392, 2003; JAAD 47:530–534, 2002; Cutis 66:243–246, 2000; JAAD 38:877–905, 1998*

Molluscum contagiosum *Breast J 22:120–121, 2016; Dermatol Online J 19:18965, 2013*

Mycobacterium abscessus – subareolar abscess due to nipple piercing *Clin Inf Dis 33:131–134, 2001*

Mycobacterium tuberculosis – lupus vulgaris *Cutis 53:246–248, 1994*

Scabies

Syphilis – primary chancre bilateral nipple erosions *JAMADerm 154:719–720, 2018;* nipple ulcer *Cutis 102:26, 31–32, 2018;* unilateral crusted plaque *JAMA 308:403–404, 2012;* unilateral nipple erosion *AD 146:81–86, 2010;* secondary

INFILTRATIVE LESIONS

Mucinosis of the areolae – manifestation of CTCL *Clin Exp Dermatol 21:374–376, 1996*

Mucopolysaccharidoses

INFLAMMATORY LESIONS

Lactation mastitis *JAMA 289:1609–1612, 2003*

METABOLIC DISEASES

Addison's disease – hyperpigmentation of nipples

Androgen excess – hyperpigmentation of areolae, axillae, external genitalia, perineum

Congenital disorders of glycosylation (CDG-Ix) – nuchal skin folds, facial dysmorphism, inverted nipples, hypoplastic nails, petechiae and ecchymoses, edema; neurologic, gastrointestinal and genitourinary abnormalities, pericardial effusion, ascites, oligohydramnios *Ped Derm 22:457–460, 2005*

CDG-Ie – eyelid telangiectasia, hemangiomas, inverted nipples, microcephaly; neurologic abnormalities; dolichol-phosphate-mannose synthase *Ped Derm 22:457–460, 2005*

Congenital disorders of glycosylation (CDG-IIa) – N-acetylglucosaminyltransferase II; midfrontal capillary hemangioma, wide spaced nipples; facial dysmorphism, neurologic and gastrointestinal abnormalities *Ped Derm 22:457–460, 2005*

Persistent galactorrhea – familial hyperprolactinemia due to a mutant prolactin receptor (*PRLR*) *NEJM 369:2012–2020, 2013*

Nipple retraction of menopause *Br Med J 309:797–800, 1994*

Pregnancy – hyperkeratosis of the nipple *JAMA Derm 149:722–726, 2013;*

hyperpigmentation of nipples

NEOPLASTIC DISEASES

Acrochordon (adnexal polyp) *Ped Derm 26:618–620, 2009; Acta DV 78:391–392, 1998; BJD 92:659–662, 1975*

Adenoma of the nipple *Br J Hosp Med 50:639–642, 1994*

Basal cell carcinoma – red plaque *Derm Surg 27:971–974, 2001; Cutis 54:85–92, 1994;* including pigmented basal cell carcinoma (black nipple) *J Drugs Dermatol 13:767–768, 2014; AD 125:536–539, 1989;* red plaque in nevoid basal cell carcinoma syndrome *BJD 168:901–903, 2013;* pigmented nipple *Cutis 92:253–257, 2013*

Becker's nevus with supernumerary nipples *Am J Med Genet 77:76–77, 1998*

Blue nevus

Bowen's disease *Cutis 92:253–257, 2013*

Breast cancer – female or male; puckered nipple; primary breast cancer with epidermotropism *Cutis 92:253–257, 2013;* carcinoma erysipelatoides – personal observation

Carcinoma of the breast (primary), metastatic to nipple – cellulitis-like appearance of primary inflammatory breast carcinoma *JAAD 43:733–751, 2000;* female or male breast carcinoma – puckered nipple; ductal adenocarcinoma of male breast – translucent papule *JAMADerm 156:337–338, 2020*

Clear cell acanthoma – red nodule of nipple *AD 148:641–646, 2012;* psoriasiform plaque *JAAD 80:749–755, 2019*

Dermatofibroma – atypical polypoid dermatofibroma *JAAD 24:561–565, 1991*

Ductal papilloma *Cutis 92:253–257, 2013*

Epidermal nevus *Paris Med 28:63–66, 1938;* mimicking supernumerary nipple – personal observation

Epidermoid cyst

Folliculosebaceous cystic hamartoma *Am J Dermatopathol 28:205–207, 2006*

Fox-Fordyce disease

Granular cell myoblastoma – nipple-like lesion *AD 121:927–932, 1985*

Hidradenoma papilliferum *Hautarzt 19:101–109, 1968*

Hidradenoma

Hidrocystoma – personal observation

Keratoacanthoma *J Cutan Pathol 3:195–198, 1976*

Leiomyomas *Am J Clin Dermatol 16:35–46, 2015; AD 127:571–576, 1991*

Leiomyosarcoma – blue-black; also red, brown, yellow or hypopigmented *JAAD 46:477–490, 2002*

Lymphoma – cutaneous T-cell lymphoma mimicking hyperkeratosis of the nipple (hyperkeratosis areolae mammae) *JAAD 41:274–276, 1999*

Lymphocytoma cutis

Melanocytic nevus – personal observation

Melanoma – primary, metastatic, amelanotic *Cutis 92:253–257, 2013*

Melanosis of the areola and nipple *JAAD 59:S33–34, 2008; AD 126:542–543, 1990*

Metastases – vascular red papule (renal cell carcinoma) *Cutis 86:69, 73–74, 2010;* pigmented epidermotropic metastasis *Cutis 92:253–257, 2013;* prostatic carcinoma metastases *JAAD 18:391–393, 1988*

Milium *Ped Derm 26:485–486, 2009*

Neurofibromas

Nevi, melanocytic

Nevoid hyperkeratosis of the nipple *JAAD 46:414–418, 2002; BJD 142:382–384, 2000; JAAD 41:325–326, 1999*

Paget's disease of the breast (nipple) *Dermatologica 170:170–179, 1985; Surg Gynecol Obstet 123:1010–1014, 1966;* pigmented Paget's disease of the nipple in men; mimics melanoma of the breast; *JAAD 55:S62–63, 2006; Melanoma Research 14:S13–15, 2004; Dermatology 202:134–137, 2001; Ann DV 128:649–652, 2001; Hautarzt 43:28–31, 1992; Histopathology 19:470–472, 1991; JAAD 23:338–341, 1990;* pigmented macule of nipple *JAAD 65:247–249, 2011;* erosion of nipple *BJD 165:440–441, 2011* Papillomatosis *Cutis 92:253–257, 2013*

Sebaceous hyperplasia of areola *JAAD 13:867–868, 1985*

Seborrheic keratoses *Cutis 92:253–257, 2013*

Squamous cell carcinoma *Cutis 92:253–257, 2013*

Steatocystoma multiplex

Syringocystadenoma papilliferum

Syringomas

Syringomatous adenomas of the nipple – subareolar nodule of the nipple *JAMADerm 151:227–228, 2015; Cutis 92:253–257, 2013*

Verrucous acanthoma – personal observation

NORMAL

Montgomery's tubercles – ectopic sebaceous glands – 2 mm papules of areola *The Dermatologist Dec 2015;pp.47–50;* areolar sebaceous hyperplasia *BMJ Case Rep April 23, 2014 JAAD 10:929–940, 1984; BJD 86:126–133, 1972*

PRIMARY CUTANEOUS DISEASES

Acanthosis nigricans *JAAD 52:529–530, 2005; JAAD 31:1–19, 1994*

Acanthosis nigricans-like "neglected nipples"(poor cleansing) *Dermatol Pract Concept 31:81–84, 2014*

Atopic dermatitis *Cutis 92:253–257, 2013*

Epidermolytic hyperkeratosis – verrucous plaques of nipples

Erosive adenomatosis (papillary adenomatosis) (nipple adenoma) of the nipple – blood-stained or serous discharge; enlarged nipple; eroded nipple; erythema, ulcer, crusted dermatitis, granular appearance, papule or nodule on nipple *Ped Derm 27:399–401, 2010; JAAD 47:578–580, 2002; JAAD 43:733–751, 2000;* superficial papillary adenomatosis of the nipple *JAAD 33:871–875, 1995; JAAD 12:707–715, 1985*

Florid papillomatosis of the nipple

Fox-Fordyce disease

Hyperkeratosis of the nipple and areola (hyperkeratosis areolae mammae) *AD 137:1327–1328, 2001; JAAD 41:274–276, 1999; Eur J Dermatol 8:131–132, 1998; AD 126:687, 1990; JAAD 13:596–598, 1985;* estrogen-induced *Cutis 26:95–96, 1980;* associated with CTCL *JAAD 32:124–125, 1995; Int J Derm 29:519–520, 1990;* ichthyosis, ichthyosiform erythroderma, acanthosis nigricans, Darier's disease

Lichen sclerosus et atrophicus – personal observation

Lichen simplex chronicus

Mamillary fistula

Mammary duct ectasia – bloody nipple discharge of infancy with hemorrhagic nodule *Ped Derm 34:361–362, 2017; AD 145:1068–1069, 2009*

    Differential diagnosis includes:
        Cystic mastitis
        Epithelial hyperplasia
        Intraductal carcinoma
        Intraductal papilloma
        Hemangioma

Acute mastitis – personal observation

Melanosis of nipple and areola *JAMA Derm 149:357–362, 2013*

Morphea

Nevus anelasticus *J Cut Pathol 41:519–523, 2014*

Nipple hyperpigmentation
    Addison's disease
    Androgen excess
    Curcumin supplements
    Hormone replacement therapy
    Melanosis of nipple and areola *Int J Derm, 2015; JAMADerm 149:357–363, 2013*
    Nevoid hyperkeratosis

Pigmented epidermotropic breast metastases

Pigmented Paget's disease

Pregnancy

Seborrheic keratosis

Nipple retraction (inverted nipple) – normal *JAAD 80:1467–1481, 2019; Ann Plast Surg 25:457–460, 1990*

Nevoid hyperkeratosis of the nipple *Ped Derm 36:247–248, 2019; JAAD 46:414–418, 2002*

Papillary adenomatosis – personal observation

Periareolar perforating pseudoxanthoma elasticum *An Bras Dermatol 85:705–707, 2010*

Phylloid hypermelanosis – cicatricial alopecia, onychodystrophy, deafness, malformed ear, mental retardation, umbilicated nipples *JAAD 19:1037–1044, 1988; Rev Neurol (Paris)95:48–54, 1956*

Pseudo-acanthosis nigricans – personal observation

Psoriasis

Sebaceous glands – ectopic sebaceous glands (Fordyce spots) – areola of nipple *J Dermatol 21:524–526, 1994*

Vitiligo *JAAD 38:647–666, 1998*

PSYCHOCUTANEOUS DISORDERS

Factitial dermatitis

SYNDROMES

Ablepharon macrostomia syndrome – absent eyelids, ectropion, abnormal ears, hypertelorism, aplasia or rudimentary nipples, dry, lax, redundant skin, macrostomia, ambiguous genitalia *Hum Genet 97:532–536, 1996; Am J Med Genet 31:299–304, 1988*

ACC with nipple and breast hypoplasia, nail dysplasia, delayed dentition *Am J Med Genet 14:381–384, 1983*

Accessory nipples associated with the following syndromes and abnormalities *Cutis 87:300–304, 2011:*

Arthrogryposis multiplex – articular rigidity with absent or incomplete muscles

Simpson-Golabi- Behmel syndrome – X-linked recessive; prenatal or post-natal overgrowth, facial dysmorphism, polythelia, heart malformations, cleft palate, post-axial polydactyly

Pallister-Killian mosaic syndrome – tetrasomy 12p; severe neonatal hypotonia, decreased bitemporal hair growth, prominent forehead, coarse face, pigmentary anomalies, mental retardation, seizures, diaphragmatic defects, supernumerary nipples

Acrofacial dysostosis – oligodactyly, accessory nipples

Adams-Oliver syndrome – autosomal dominant; terminal transverse limb anomalies, aplasia cutis congenita, cutis marmorata telangiectatica congenita, severe growth retardation, aplasia cutis congenita of knee, short palpebral fissures, dilated scalp veins, simple pinnae, skin tags on toes, hemangioma, undescended testes, supernumerary nipples, hypoplastic optic nerve, congenital heart defects *Ped Derm 24:651–653, 2007*

Acro-dermato-ungual-lacrimal-tooth syndrome (ADULT syndrome) – ectrodactyly or syndactyly, freckling and dry skin, dysplastic nails, superficial blisters and desquamation of hands and feet; lacrimal duct atresia, primary hypodontia, conical teeth, and early loss of permanent teeth; small ears hooked nose, sparse thin blond hair, frontal alopecia, hypohidrosis, lacrimal duct atresia, hypoplastic breasts and nipples, urinary tract anomalies; mutation in *TP63* gene (encodes transcription factor p63); p63 mutations also responsible for EEC, AEC, limb mammary, and Rapp-Hodgkin syndromes *BJD 172:276–278, 2015; Ped Derm 27:643–645, 2010; Hum Mol Genet 11:799–804, 2002; Am J Med Genet 45:642–648, 1993*

AEC syndrome (Hay-Wells syndrome) – ankyloblepharon, ectodermal dysplasia, cleft lip/palate syndrome – blepharitis, eyelid papillomas, periorbital wrinkling; microcephaly, widespread congenital scalp erosions; alopecic ulcerated plaques of scalp, trunk, groin; alopecia of scalp and eyebrows; congenital erythroderma; depigmented patches; syndactyly; bony abnormalities; widely spaced nipples; TP63 mutation *Ped Derm 26:617–618, 2009; AD 141:1591–1594, 2005; AD 141:1567–1573, 2005; AD 134:1121–1124, 1998; Ped Derm 14:149–150, 1997;* generalized fissured erosions of trunk *BJD 149:395–399, 2003;* TP63 mutations seen in AEC syndrome, EEC syndrome, Rapp-Hodgkin syndrome, limb-mammary syndrome, split-hand split-foot malformation type 4, acro-dermato-ungual-lacrimal-tooth syndrome *AD 141:1567–1573, 2005*

Aghei-Dasthgeib syndrome – generalized hypertrichosis, bilateral nipple retraction, unilateral left-sided accessory nipple *BJD 174:741–752, 2016; Dermatol Online J 12: 19, 2006*

Anhidrotic ectodermal dysplasia with amastia and palmoplantar keratoderma – *EDAR* mutation *BJD 168:1353–1355, 2013*

Bannayan-Riley-Ruvalcaba-Zonana syndrome (PTEN phosphatase and tensin homolog hamartoma) – accessory nipple, dolichocephaly, frontal bossing, macrocephaly, ocular hypertelorism, long philtrum, thin upper lip, broad mouth, relative micrognathia, lipomas, penile or vulvar lentigines, facial verruca-like or acanthosis nigricans-like papules, multiple acrochordons, angiokeratomas, transverse palmar crease, syndactyly, brachydactyly, vascular malformations, arteriovenous malformations, lymphangiokeratoma, goiter, hamartomatous intestinal polyposis *JAAD 53:639–643, 2005*

Barber-Say syndrome – generalized hypertrichosis, dysmorphic facies (bilateral ectropion, hypertelorism, macrostomia, abnormal ears, bulbous nose, sparse eyebrows and eyelashes), hypoplasia of nipples with absence of mammary glands, transposition of scrotum, club feet, short neck, lax skin, premature aged appearance, cleft palate, conductive hearing loss *Ped Derm 23:183–184, 2006; Am J Med Genet 86:54–56, 1999; Syndrome Ident 8:6–9, 1982*

Becker's nevus syndrome – breast hypoplasia *Am J Med Genet 68:357–361, 1997;* supernumerary nipples *BJD 136:471–472, 1997; Clin Exp Dermatol 22:240–241, 1997;* hypoplastic nipples *Am J Med Genet 77:76–77, 1998*

CANDLE syndrome (chronic atypical neutrophilic dermatosis with lipodystrophy and elevated temperature) – annular erythematous edematous plaques of face and trunk which become purpuric and result in residual annular hyperpigmentation; limitation of range of motion with plaques over interphalangeal joints; periorbital edema with violaceous swollen eyelids, edema of lips (thick lips), lipoatrophy of cheeks, nose, and arms, chondritis with progressive ear and saddle nose deformities, hypertrichosis of lateral forehead, gynecomastia, wide spaced nipples, nodular episcleritis and conjunctivitis, epididymitis, myositis, aseptic meningitis; short stature, anemia, abnormal liver functions, splenomegaly, protuberant abdomen *Ped Derm 28:538–541, 2011; JAAD 62:487–495, 2010*

Cardiofaciocutaneous syndrome – hyperplastic nipples; low set ears with linear earlobe creases; brittle, dark, sparse curly hair; increased numbers of melanocytic nevi; characteristic facies with thick facial appearance, broad nose, frontal bossing, ulerythema ophryogenes, sparse eyebrows; 1–2 café au lait macules; palmoplantar keratoderma; pulmonic stenosis, hypertrophic cardiomyopathy, congenital heart defects, psychomotor delay, failure to thrive; *RASopathy (BRAF, MAP2K1, MAP2K2, KRAS* mutations) *BJD 164:521–529, 2011*

CEDNIK syndrome (cerebral dysgenesis-neuropathy-ichthyosis-keratoderma) – microcephaly; dysmorphic face with small anterior fontanelles; pointed prominent nasal tip, small chin, inverted nipples and long toes, high palate, thick gingivae, cradle cap, sparse brittle coarse hair, scarring alopecia, fixed flexion posture; decreased SNAP 29 protein; mutation in SNARE proteins mediating vesicle trafficking; mutation in ABCA12 gene *BJD 164:610–616, 2011; AD 144:334–340, 2008*

Cornelia de Lange (Brachmann-de Lange) syndrome – hypoplastic nipples and umbilicus, generalized hypertrichosis, confluent eyebrows, low hairline, hairy forehead and ears, hair whorls of trunk, single palmar crease, cutis marmorata, psychomotor and growth retardation with short stature, specific facies, hypertrichosis of forehead, face, back, shoulders, and extremities, bushy arched eyebrows with synophrys; long delicate eyelashes, skin around eyes and nose with bluish tinge, small nose with depressed root, prominent philtrum, thin upper lip with crescent shaped mouth, widely spaced, sparse teeth, hypertrichosis of forehead, posterior neck, and arms, low set ears, arched palate, antimongoloid palpebrae; congenital eyelashes; xerosis, especially over hands and feet, nevi, facial cyanosis, lymphedema *Ped Derm 24:421–423, 2007; JAAD 56:541–564, 2007; JAAD 48:161–179, 2003; JAAD 37:295–297, 1997; Am J Med Genet 47:959–964, 1993*

Ectrodactyly-ectodermal dysplasia-clefting syndrome – alopecia of scalp, eyebrows, and eyelashes, xerosis, atopic dermatitis, nail dystrophy, hypodontia with peg shaped teeth, reduced sweat glands and salivary glands, syndactyly, mammary gland and nipple hypoplasia, conductive or sensorineural hearing loss, urogenital anomalies, lacrimal duct abnormalities; *TP63* mutations *BJD 162:201–207, 2010; Ped Derm 20:113–118, 2003; BJD 146:216–220, 2002; Dermatologica 169:80–85, 1984*

Hereditary acrolabial telangiectasia – blue lips, blue nails, blue nipples, telangiectasia of the chest, elbows, knees, dorsa of hands, varicosities of the legs, migraine headaches *AD 115:474–478, 1979*

Birt-Hogg-Dube – trichodiscomas *JAAD 16:452–457, 1987*

Carney complex – cutaneous myxomas of the nipples (papules) *JAAD 43:377–379, 2000; Cutis 62:275–280, 1998*

Gardner's syndrome – epidermoid cysts

Finlay-Marks syndrome (scalp-ear-nipple syndrome) – nipple or breast hypoplasia or aplasia, aplasia cutis congenita of scalp, cleft lip/palate, cardiac malformations, polydactyly, narrow convex nails

Hutchinson-Gilford syndrome (progeria) – hypoplastic nipples *Am J Med Genet 82:242–248, 1999; J Pediatr 80:697–724, 1972*

Incontinentia pigmenti – inverted nipples *JAAD 64:508–515, 2011;* hyperpigmented nipples; supernumerary nipples; nipple hypoplasia *AD 139:1163–1170, 2003; JAAD 47:169–187, 2002;* incontinentia pigmenti in boys with supernumerary nipple *Ped Derm 23:523–527, 2006*

Johanson-Blizzard syndrome – autosomal recessive; growth retardation, microcephaly, ACC of scalp, sparse hair, hypoplastic ala nasi, CALMs, hypoplastic nipples and areolae, hypothyroidism, sensorineural deafness *Clin Genet 14:247–250, 1978*

Keratitis-ichthyosis-deafness (KID) syndrome – acanthosis nigricans-like change of the nipple *AD 123:777–782, 1987;* hypoplasia of nipples *Ped Derm 19:513–516, 2002*

Limb mammary syndrome – ectrodactyly, mammary gland/nipple hypoplasia, cleft palate *Am J Hum Genet 64:481–492, 2001*

Lumpy scalp, odd ears, and rudimentary nipples *BJD 99:423–430, 1978*

Neurofibromatosis – personal observation

NAME/LAMB syndrome *AD 122:790–798, 1986*

Oculo-osteocutaneous syndrome – sparse, fair hair, limb and digit abnormalities, hypoplastic nipples, abnormal genitalia *Ped Derm 19:226, 2002*

Pallister-Killian syndrome – supernumerary nipples, mental retardation, coarse facies with hypertelorism and prominent forehead, sparse temporal hair and high frontal hairline, hypo- and hyperpigmentation, Blaschko linear hypopigmented bands of face and shoulder; i(12p) (tetrasomy 12p); tissue mosaicism; pigmentary mosaicism and localized alopecia *Ped Derm 23:382–385, 2006; Ped Derm 22:270–275, 2005*

Rapp-Hodgkin hypohidrotic ectodermal dysplasia – autosomal dominant; alopecia of wide area of scalp in frontal to crown area, short eyebrows and eyelashes, coarse wiry sparse hypopigmented scalp hair, sparse body hair, scalp dermatitis, ankyloblepharon, syndactyly, nipple anomalies, cleft lip and/or palate; nails narrow and dystrophic, small stature, hypospadias, conical teeth and anodontia or hypodontia; distinctive facies, *JAAD 53:729–735, 2005; Ped Derm 7:126–131, 1990; J Med Genet 15:269–272, 1968*

Rubinstein-Taybi syndrome – supernumerary nipples *JAAD 46:159, 2002*

Scalp-ear-nipple syndrome – autosomal dominant; aplasia cutis congenita of the scalp, irregularly shaped pinna, hypoplastic nipple, widely spaced teeth, partial syndactyly *Am J Med Genet 50:247–250, 1994*

Simpson-Golabi-Behmel syndrome – X-linked; increased growth, accessory nipples, coarse facies, polydactyly, midline defects, mental retardation *Am J Med Genet 46:606–607, 1993*

Trichorhinophalangeal syndrome type I – autosomal dominant; receding frontotemporal hairline with high bossed forehead; facial pallor, pear-shaped nose, long philtrum, thin upper lip, receding chin, tubercle of normal skin below the lower lip, distension and deviation with fusiform swelling of the PIP joints; hip malformation, brachydactyly, prognathism, fine brittle slow growing sparse hair, eyebrows sparse laterally, dense medially, short stature; dental malocclusion mutation in zinc finger nuclear transcription factor *BJD 157:1021–1024, 2007; AD 137:1429–1434, 2001; Am J Hum Genet 68:81–91, 2001; Dermatology 193:349–352, 1996;JAAD 31:331–336, 1994; Ped Derm 10:385–387, 1993; Hum Genet 74:188–189, 1986*

Trichorhinophalangeal syndrome type III – like type I (alopecia) (receding frontotemporal hairline), facial dysmorphism, high bossed forehead, bone deformities, brachydactyly, facial pallor, protruding low set ears, bulbous distal nose, elongated philtrum, thin upper lip, prognathism, micrognathia, dental malocclusion, high arched palate, supernumerary teeth, koilonychias, leukonychia, flat feet) with severe growth retardation; shortening of all phalanges *BJD 157:1021–1024, 2007*

Turner's syndrome – shield chest with widely spaced nipples *JAAD 50:767–776, 2004*

Ulnar-mammary syndrome – autosomal dominant; ulnar defects, nipple or apocrine gland hypoplasia; wide face, nasal base and tip, protruding chin; cardiac abnormalities *TXB3* mutation *Eplasty 27:14:ic35, e collection 2014, 2014 September*

TRAUMA

Guitar nipple – cystic swelling at base of nipple *Br Med J 2:226, 1974*

VASCULAR DISEASES

Acrocyanosis – blue nipples *JAAD S207–208, 2001*

Lymphangioma circumscriptum (microcystic lymphatic malformation) – supernumerary nipple-like lesion *Case Rep Dermatol Med Feb 11, 2018*

Peripheral symmetric gangrene

Raynaud's phenomenon *Br Med J 314:644–645, 1997;* Raynaud's phenomenon in breast feeding – white blanching of nipple *JAMADerm 149:300–306, 2013*

Thrombosed angioma

NO FINGERPRINT SYNDROMES (ADERMATOGLYPHIA, ABSENT DERMATOGLYPHICS)

Ped Derm 29:527–529, 2012; JAAD 64:974–980, 2011; JAAD 64:801–808, 2011; JAAD 50:782, 2004; Am J Med Genet 16:81–88, 1983; J Pediatr 64:621–631, 1964

Absent dermatoglyphics – autosomal dominant *JAAD 65:974–980, 2011*

Absent dermatoglyphics and transient facial milia *JAAD 32:315–318, 1995*; digital flexion contractures, webbed toes, palmoplantar hypohidrosis, painful fissured calluses, acral blistering, simian crease *JAAD 59:1050–1063, 2008*

Acro-dermato-ungual-lacrimal-tooth syndrome (ADULT syndrome)

Adermatoglyphia – hypohidrosis, skin blistering, congenital milia *J Pediatr 64:621–631, 1964*

AEC syndrome (ankyloblepharon-ectodermal dysplasia-clefting syndrome)

Baird syndrome – absence of dermatoglyphics; familial skin fragility, heterozygous deletion involving *SMARCD1 J Ped 194:248–252, 2018*

Basan syndrome (ectodermal dysplasia) – congenital facial milia, nail dystrophy, progressive palmoplantar callosities, absent dermatoglyphics; transient neonatal acral bullae *Ped Derm 29:684–685, 2012; Ped Derm 29:527–529, 2012; JAAD 59:1050–1063, 2008; JAAD 32:315–318, 1995; J Pediatr 64:621–631, 1964*

CEDNIK syndrome – autosomal recessive; cerebral dysgenesis, neuropathy, ichthyosis, keratoderma, microcephaly, facial dysmorphism, absent dermatoglyphics, deafness *Ped Derm 36:372–376, 2019*

Dermatopathia pigmentosa reticularis – autosomal dominant; reticulate pigmentation of trunk, neck, and proximal extremities, alopecia, nail changes (mild onychodystrophy), palmoplantar hyperkeratosis, loss of dermatoglyphics, hyperpigmented tongue, hypo- or hyperhidrosis, non-scarring blisters of dorsal hands and feet, dark areolae, thin eyebrows; keratin 14 mutation *Ped Derm 24:566–570, 2007; J Dermatol 24:266–269, 1997; Semin Cut Med Surg 16:72–80, 1997; JAAD 26:298–301, 1992; AD 126:935–939, 1990; Hautarzt 6:262, 1960; Dermatol Wochenschr 138:1337, 1958*

Dyskeratosis congenita – absent dermatoglyphics *JAAD 77:1194–1196, 2017*

Ectodermal dysplasia, absent dermatoglyphics, nail changes, simian crease, milia *Ped Derm 25:474–476, 2008*

Epidermolysis bullosa simplex with cardiomyopathy – loss of dermatoglyphics, hypohidrosis; mutation in KLHL24 *BJD 179:1181–1183, 2018*

Epidermolysis bullosa progressiva (Ogna Gedde-Dahl) – autosomal recessive; delayed onset; bullae with surrounding atrophic (cigarette paper) wrinkled skin, absent nail plates, palmoplantar keratoderma, absent dermal finger ridges, tooth and enamel defects *JAAD 16:195–200, 1987*

Hidrotic ectodermal dysplasia – pachydermic dermatoglyphics *Am J Med Genet 38:552–556, 1991*

Hypohidrotic ectodermal dysplasia – X-linked recessive; ridge flattening

Jorgenson-Lenz syndrome

Junctional epidermolysis bullosa of late onset (skin fragility in childhood) – speckled hyperpigmentation of elbows; hemorrhagic

bullae, teeth and nail abnormalities, oral blisters, disappearance of dermatoglyphics, palmoplantar keratoderma, small vesicles, atrophy of skin of hands *BJD 169:714–716, 2013*

Ichthyosis en confetti (congenital reticulated ichthyosiform erythroderma) – reticulated erythroderma with guttate hypopigmentation, palmoplantar keratoderma; loss of dermatoglyphics; temporary hypertrichosis of normal skin *BJD 166:434–439, 2012; JAAD 63:607–641, 2010*

Junctional epidermolysis bullosa of late onset (formerly junctional epidermolysis bullosa progressive) (skin fragility in childhood) – loss of dermatoglyphics, waxy hyperkeratosis of dorsal hand, atrophic skin of lower leg, transverse ridging and enamel pits of teeth, nail atrophy, amelogenesis imperfect, hyperhidrosis, blisters on elbows, knees, and oral cavity *BJD 169:714–716, 2013; BJD 164:1280–1284, 2011*

Keratosis-ichthyosis-deafness (KID) syndrome – pachydermic dermatoglyphics

Kindler's syndrome – absent dermatoglyphics *An Bras Dermatol 90:592–593, 2015*

Naegeli-Franceschetti-Jadassohn syndrome – autosomal dominant; absent dermatoglyphics; reticulated hyperpigmentation, palmoplantar keratoderma, dental abnormalities, abnormal sweating SASH1 related lentigines, hyper- and hypopigmentation, alopecia, nail dystrophy, palmoplantar keratoderma, skin cancer;

keratin 14 mutation *BJD 177:945–959, 2017*

Rapp-Hodgkin syndrome – hypoplastic dermatoglyphics *Clin Dysmorphol 8:101–110, 1999*

Schopf-Schulz-Passarge syndrome (congenital ectodermal dysplasia) – acral papules of syringocystadenoma papilliferum and syringofibroadenoma; reticulated palmoplantar keratoderma, hypodontia, hypotrichosis, nail dystrophy, multiple eyelid apocrine hidrocystomas, no dermatoglyphics of fingertips; mutation in WNT10A *JAAD 65:1066–169, 2011*

NODULES, CONGENITAL

Ped Derm 9:301, 1991

Adipose plantar nodules *BJD 142:1262–1264, 2000*

Arteriovenous malformation *JAAD 46:934–941, 2002*

Benign and/or disseminated neonatal hemangiomatosis *JAAD 24:816–818, 1991; Ped Derm 8:140–146, 1991*

Blueberry muffin lesions of congenital infections or ABO/Rh incompatibility *Ann DV 125:199–201, 1998*; hemophagocytic lymphohistiocytosis *Ped Derm 34:e150–151, 2017*; Langerhans cell histiocytosis *Ann DV 141:130–133, 2014*

Branchial sinus and/or cyst

Cartilaginous rest of the neck – nodule over medial clavicle *Cutis 58:293–294, 1996; AD 127:1309–1310, 1991*

Cephalocele – includes encephalocele, meningocele (rudimentary meningocele), meningoencephalocele, meningomyelocele; blue nodule with overlying hypertrichosis *JAAD 46:934–941, 2002; AD 137:45–50, 2001*

Cephalohematoma (cephalohematoma deformans) – blood between outer table of skull and periosteum; fixed *Ped Clin North Amer 6:1151–1160, 1993*

Cervical thyroid

Congenital complex corneal choristoma – associated with bilateral subcutaneous vascular nodules *JAAPOS 19:185–188, 2015*

Congenital self-healing Langerhans cell histiocytosis (Hashimoto-Pritzker disease) – multiple congenital red-brown nodules *Ped Derm*

23:273–275, 2006; JAAD 48:S75–77, 2003; Ped Derm 17:322–324, 2000

Dacryocystocele – congenital blue/red firm nodule of medial canthus or medial lower eyelid due to congenital obstruction of nasolacrimal duct *Ped Derm 34:209–211, 2017; Ped Derm 28:70–72, 2011; JAAD 61:1088–1090, 2009*

   vs. Encephalocele
      Nasal glioma
      Infantile hemangioma
      Congenital hemangioma
      Dermoid cyst

Dermatofibrosarcoma protuberans – oval pink nodule *JAAD 61:1014–1023, 2009;* deep red plaque *Cutis 90:285–288, 2012; Ped Derm 25:317–325, 2008*

Dermoid cyst *AD 135:463–468, 1999*

Desmoplastic trichoepithelioma – firm skin colored scalp nodule *Ped Derm 34:189–190, 2017*

Eccrine angiomatous hamartoma *Ped Derm 36:909–912, 2019; JAAD 47:429–435, 2002; Ped Derm 14:401–402, 1997; Ped Derm 13:139–142, 1996;* skin-colored nodule with blue papules *JAAD 41:109–111, 1999*

Embryonal rhabdomyosarcoma – orbit, nasopharynx, nose

Encephalocele

Epithelioid blue nevi- multiple congenital blue-gray nodules *J Cut Pathol 46:954–959, 2019*

Ewing's sarcoma

Fibroblastic connective tissue nevus *Ped Derm 3:644–650, 2018*

Fibrodysplasia ossificans progressiva – multiple neonatal scalp nodules associated with malformation of the great toes (hallux valgus) *JAAD 64:97–101, 2011*

Fibromatosis – congenital generalized fibromatosis *Ped Derm 8:306–309, 1991; AD 122:89–94, 1986; JAAD 10:365–371, 1984*

Fibrosarcoma, neonatal *Ped Derm 23:330–334, 2006; JAAD 50:S23–25, 2004; Ped Derm 14:241–243, 1997*

Fibrous hamartoma of infancy – benign, single, soft to firm ill-defined subcutaneous mass present at birth or before 2 years of age; more common in boys, freely movable, most commonly located on the shoulder, arm or axillary region *JAAD 54:800–803, 2006; JAAD 41:857–859, 1999; Ped Derm 13:171–172, 1996; AD 125:88, 1989; J Pathol Bacteriol 72:149–154, 1956*

Glomangioma *Ped Derm 12:242–244, 1995*

Glomangiomyoma – congenital multiple plaque-like glomangio-myoma *Am J Dermatopathol 21:454–457, 1999*

Gonorrhea – newborn with gonococcal scalp abscess *South Med J 73:396–397, 1980; Am J Obstet Gynecol 127:437–438, 1977*

Non-neural congenital granular cell tumor – soft tumors of the forearm *Ann Dermatol 29:776–778, 2017*

Hamartoma with ectopic meningothelial elements – simulates angiosarcoma *Am J Surg Pathol 14:1–11, 1990*

Hemangiomas *JAAD 46:934–941, 2002*

Hemangiopericytoma – violaceous nodule *Ped Derm 23:335–337, 2006; J Bone Joint Surg Br 83:269–272, 2001*

Heterotopic brain tissue (heterotopic meningeal nodules) – blue-red cystic mass with overlying alopecia *JAAD 46:934–941, 2002;* bald cyst of scalp with surrounding hypertrichosis

AD 131:731, 1995; JAAD 28:1015, 1993; BJD 129:183–185, 1993; AD 125:1253–1256, 1989; cyst with collar of hair (heterotopic meningeal nodules) *JAAD 28:1015–1017, 1993; AD 123:1253–1256, 1989*

Langerhans cell histiocytosis *J Dermatol 46:812–815, 2019*

Congenital immune deficiencies with cutaneous granulomas *Ann DV 122:501–506, 1995*

Infantile myofibromatosis – painless nodules, solitary or multicentric *JAAD 7:264–270, 2014; Pediatrics 104:113–115, 1999;* solitary nodule *S Afr Med J 64:590–591, 1983*

Juvenile xanthogranuloma – giant congenital form *J Cut Med Surg 22:488–494, 2018; Ann DV 122:678–681, 1995*

Kaposiform hemangioendothelioma *Am J Surg Pathol 17:321–328, 1993*

Leiomyoma *Ped Derm 3:158–160, 1986*

Leukemia – congenital leukemia (AML) (purpuric papules or nodules in the neonate) *Ped Derm 25:34–37, 2008; JAAD 54:S22–27, 2006;* neonatal monoblastic leukemia *Ped Derm 27:651–652, 2010; Ann DV 126:157–159, 1999;* lymphoblastic leukemia *JAAD 34:375–378, 1996; AD 129:1301–1306, 1993;* neonatal myelomono-cytic leukemia

Lipoblastomatosis – congenital lipoblastomatosis *Ped Derm 15:210–213, 1998*

Lipoma – deep forehead lipoma *Ped Derm 37:520–523, 2020;* vulvar *AD 118:447, 1982*

Lymphatic malformation *Ped Derm 23:330–334, 2006*

Lymphoma

Malignant fibrous histiocytoma *Ped Derm 23:330–334, 2006*

Malignant hemangiopericytoma *West Afr J Med 19:317–318, 2000*

Malignant peripheral nerve sheath tumor *Ped Derm 23:330–334, 2006*

Malignant rhabdoid tumor *Arch Pathol Lab Med 122:1099–1102, 1998*

Mastocytosis

Melanocytic nevi with nodules *J Dermatol 23:828–831, 1996;* giant congenital melanocytic nevus with proliferative nodules *Ann Dermatol 26:554–556, 2014*

Melanoma – with congenital melanocytic nevus syndrome *Ped Derm 35:e281–285, 2018*

Meningioma – scalp nodule *Eur J Pediatr Surg 10:387–389, 2000*

Meningocele

Midline raphe cyst of the scrotum

Nasal glioma – red or bluish nodules; resemble hemangiomas, nasal encephalocele, meningoencephalocele, extracranial menin-gioma, dermoid cyst, lacrimal duct cyst, neuroblastoma, rhabdo-myosarcoma *Ear Nose Throat J 80:410–411, 2001; Arch Otolaryngol 107:550–554, 1981*

Nerve sheath myxoma (neurothekeoma) of the tongue *Oral Surg Oral Med Oral Pathol Oral Radiol Endod 90:74–77, 2000*

Neuroblastoma, metastatic *Ped Derm 37:565–567, 2020; Neonatal Netw 38:341–347, 2019; J Formos Med Assoc 90:422–425, 1991*

Neurocristic cutaneous hamartoma *Mod Pathol 11:573–578, 1998;* malignant melanotic neurocristic tumors arising in neurocristic hamartomas *Am J Surg Pathol 20:665–677, 1996*

Neurofibroma

Peripheral primitive neuroectodermal tumor *Med Pediatr Onco30:357–363, 1998*

Precalcaneal congenital fibrolipomatous hamartoma – skin colored nodule of medial foot *J Cut Pathol 46:277–279, 2019; Ped Derm 24:74–75, 2007*

Pyogenic granuloma – presenting as congenital epulis *Arch Pediatr Adolesc Med 154:603–605, 2000*

Pyramidal lobe of thyroid gland

Rapidly involuting congenital hemangioma (RICH) – violaceous large mass with central telangiectasia *JAAD 50:875–882, 2004*

Rhabdomyosarcoma – embryonal rhabdomyosarcoma *Ped Derm 23:330–334, 2006*

Sinus pericranii – alopecic red nodule of scalp *JAAD 46:934–941, 2002*

Subcutaneous fat necrosis, congenital *Glob Pediatr Health Oct 1, 2018*

Subepicranial hygromas *JAAD 46:934–941, 2002*

Tufted angioma *Ped Derm 23:330–334, 2006*

Venous cavernoma (venous malformation) *JAAD 46:934–941, 2002; Zentralbl Neurochir 59:274–277, 1998*

Wattle; cutaneous cervical tag *AD 121:22–23, 1985*

Wilms' tumor

NODULES, FOOT

AUTOIMMUNE DISEASES AND DISEASES OF IMMUNE DYSFUNCTION

Behcet's disease *J Rheumatol 25:2469–2472, 1998*

Chronic granulomatous disease – chilblains *JAAD 36:899–907, 1997;* X-linked chronic granulomatous disease – photosensitivity, chilblain lupus of fingertips and toes *Ped Derm 3:376–379, 1986*

Common variable immunodeficiency (Gottron-like papules) – granulomas presenting as acral red papules and plaques with central scaling, scarring, atrophy, ulceration *Cutis 52:221–222, 1993*

Gain of function mutation of NLRC4 (inflammasome) – fever, periodic urticarial rash, conjunctivitis, arthralgias, painful red nodules of foot or leg, enterocolitis, splenomegaly, macrophage activation syndrome; increased IL-18 *BJD 176:244–248, 2017; Nat Genet 46:1135–1139, 2014; Nat Genet 46:1140–1146, 2014; J Exp Med 211:2385–2396, 2014*

Rheumatoid nodule – painful plantar nodule *J Gen Int Med 32:955–956, 2017; J Dermatol 24:798, 1997;* plantar nodule *JAAD 53:191–209, 2005;* rheumatoid nodulosis *Foot (Edinb)24:37–41, 2014*

Lupus erythematosus, systemic – digital vasculitis; painful nodule *Rev Bras Rheumatol Engl Ed 57:583–589, 2017*

CONGENITAL ANOMALIES

Congenital infantile digital fibromatosis *Ped Derm 19:370–371, 2002*

Congenital pedal papules

Infantile plantar nodules – personal observation

Precalcaneal congenital fibrolipomatous hamartoma – skin colored nodule of medial foot *J Cut Pathol 46:277–279, 2019; Ped Derm 24:74–75, 2007*

DEGENERATIVE DISEASES

Dupuytren's contracture – in children *Br J Plast Surg 41:313–315, 1988*

DRUG REACTIONS

Hydantoin – thickening of the heel pad due to long term hydantoin therapy *Am J Roentgenol Radium Ther Nucl Med 124:52–56, 1975*

Neutrophilic eccrine hidradenitis, chemotherapy-induced

EXOGENOUS AGENTS

Foreign body granuloma

Sea urchin spine – plantar nodule

INFECTIONS AND INFESTATIONS

Alternariosis – red nodule of foot *Clin Inf Dis 30:13,174–175, 2000*

Anthrax

Arthropod bites

Bacillary angiomatosis

Brucellosis

Cat scratch fever

Chromomycosis *JAAD 32:390–392, 1995*

Coccidioidomycosis – granuloma of foot

Cryptococcosis – cryptococcal panniculitis *Cutis 85:303–306, 2010*

Diphtheria

Ecthyma

Endocarditis – Osler's nodes *Am J Cardiol 118:1094, 2016*

Filariasis (*Dirofilaria immitis*) – blue papule; zoonotic deep cutaneous filariasis *Ped Derm 25:230–232, 2008*

Herpes simplex, chronic

Herpes zoster, chronic

Insect bites – plantar nodule *Ped Derm 15:97–102, 1998*

Leishmaniasis – post kala-azar dermal leishmaniasis *Clin Med (Lond)15:304–306, 2015*

Leprosy *Int J Lepr Other Mycobact Dis 68:272–276, 2001*

Mycetoma *J Orthp Case Rep 7:12–15, 2017; JAAD 53:931–951, 2005; JAAD 32:311–315, 1995; Cutis 49:107–110, 1992; Australas J Dermatol 31:33–36, 1990; JAAD 6:107–111, 1982; Sabouraudia 18:91–95, 1980; AD 99:215–225, 1969*

Mycobacterium abscessus – hand, foot disease in children *Ped Derm 31:292–297, 2014*

Mycobacterium avium-intracellulare AD 124:1545–1549, 1988

Mycobacterium chelonei JAAD 28:809–810, 812–813, 1993

Mycobacterium haemophilum JAAD 59:139–142, 2008

Mycobacterium kansasii JAAD 24:208–215, 1991

Mycobacterium marinum – nodule or papule of hands, elbows, knees becomes crusted ulcer or abscess; or verrucous papule; sporotrichoid; rarely widespread lesions *Br Med J 300:1069–1070, 1990; AD 122:698–703, 1986; J Hyg 94:135–149, 1985*

Mycobacterium tuberculosis – lupus vulgaris *Int J Derm 40:336–339, 2001;* tuberculous abscess *Am J Case Rep 20:503–507, 2019*

Nocardiosis – *N. otitidiscaviarum* actinomycetoma; red nodules of the foot with sinus tracts *AD 142:101–106, 2006*

North American blastomycosis – verrucous nodules of toes *AD 143:653–658, 2007*

Paecilomyces variotii Transpl Infec Dis 20:e12871, 2018

Phaeohyphomycosis (*Exophiala*) – nodules of finger and multiple subcutaneous nodules of the foot *JAAD 61:977–985, 2009*

Pseudomonas hot tub folliculitis – palmoplantar red nodules; *pseudomonas* hot-foot syndrome – 1–2 cm plantar nodules; spontaneous resolution in 14 days *NEJM 345:335–338, 2001*

Rocky Mountain spotted fever – palmoplantar red nodules

Scabies, nodular *J Cutan Pathol 19:124–127, 1992;*

crusted (Norwegian) scabies presenting with hyperkeratotic nodules of the soles *AD 134:1019–1024, 1998*

Scedosporium apiospermum – sporotrichoid nodules of foot and leg *Australas J Dermatol 56:e39–42, 2015*

Schizophyllum commune BMC Infec Dis 18:286, 2018

Septic emboli

Trichophyton rubrum – invasive in immunocompromised host *JAAD 39:379–380, 1998;* mimicking Kaposi's sarcoma *Int J Dermatol 18:751–752, 1979*

Tungiasis (*Tunga penetrans*) (toe-tip or subungual nodule) – crusted or ulcerated *Acta Dermatovenerol (Stockh)76:495, 1996; JAAD 20:941–944, 1989; AD 124:429–434, 1988*

Warts, including human papillomavirus type 60-associated plantar wart; myrmecia (deep periungual or plantar warts) *BMJ 1:912–915, 1951*

INFILTRATIVE DISEASES

Amyloidosis *Cutis 59:142, 1997;* nodular amyloidosis of the toe *AD 139:1157–1159, 2003;* bilateral foot nodules *Cutis 93:89–94, 2014*

Juvenile xanthogranuloma of sole – brown nodule with rim of hyperkeratosis *Ped Derm 17:460–462, 2000; Ped Derm 15:203–206, 1998*

INFLAMMATORY DISEASES

Erythema multiforme – plantar nodules *Ped Derm 15:97–102, 1998*

Erythema nodosum – plantar nodules *Dermatology 199:190, 1999; JAAD 40:654–655, 1994*

Neutrophilic eccrine hidradenitis of the palms and soles – idiopathic in children *JAAD 79:987–1006, 2018; Eur J Pediatr 160:189–191, 2001; AD 134:76–79, 1998; J Cutan Pathol 21:289–296, 1994;*idiopathic recurrent palmoplantar eccrine hidradenitis – often post-traumatic *Ped Derm 21:466–468, 2004; BJD 142:1048–1050, 2000*

Panniculitis – due to blind loop syndrome *JAAD 37:824–827, 1997;* plantar nodule *Ped Derm 15:97–102, 1998*

Relapsing eosinophilic perimyositis – fever, fatigue, and episodic muscle swelling; erythema over swollen muscles *BJD 133:109–114, 1995*

Sarcoid – plantar nodules *JAAD 54:360–361, 2006;* painful palmoplantar nodules *Med Cutan Ibero Lat Am 15:384–386, 1987*

METABOLIC DISEASES

Calcinosis cutis – tumoral calcinosis; calcified cutaneous nodules – heels of children due to heel sticks as a neonate *J Foot Ankle Surg Nov 12, 2019; Ped Derm 18:138–140, 2001*

Gout *Dermatol J Online Jan 15, 2015; Cutis 48:445–451, 1991; Ann Rheum Dis 29:461–468, 1970*

Pancreatic panniculitis – red nodules of ankle and dorsolateral foot *JAMA 311:615–616, 2014*

Thyroid acropachy

Xanthomas – tendinous, tuberous xanthomas – personal observation

NEOPLASTIC DISORDERS

Acquired fibrokeratoma *Dermatol Online J Sept 15, 2017*

Acral calcified vascular leiomyoma – swollen fingertip; plantar or heel nodule *JAAD 59:1000–1004, 2008*

Adipose plantar nodules (congenital) *BJD 142:1262–1264, 2000*

Aggressive digital papillary adenocarcinoma *Am J Dermatopathol 38:910–914, 2010*

Angioleiomyoma - pink nodule of heel *Cutis 81:123,140–141, 2008; J Foot Surg 31:372–377, 1992*

Angiolipoma *J Foot Surg 31:17–24, 1992*

Atypical fibroxanthoma

Childhood fibrous hamartoma – plantar nodule *Ped Derm 17:429–431, 2000*

Chondroid syringoma *J Am Podiatr Med Assoc 79:563–565, 1989;* malignant chondroid syringoma of the foot *An Bras Dermatol 88:997–999, 2013; Am J Clin Oncol 23:227–232, 2000*

Clear cell hidradenoma (nodular hidradenoma, eccrine sweat gland adenoma of the clear cell type, solid cystic hidradenoma, eccrine acrospiroma) *Dermatol Surg 26:685–686, 2000*

Combined type blue nevus *Ped Derm 14:358–360, 1994*

Connective tissue nevus, including eruptive collagenoma – personal observation

Dermatofibroma – dorsum of foot; plantar nodule *Ped Derm 21:506–507, 2004*

Dermatofibrosarcoma protuberans *J Cutan Pathol 44:794–797, 2017*

Digital fibrous tumor of childhood – toe nodule *AD 131:1195–1198, 1995*

Eccrine acrospiroma

Eccrine angiomatous hamartoma – toes, fingers, palms and soles- skin-colored to blue *Cutis 71:449–455, 2003; JAAD 47:429–435, 2002; Ped Derm 13:139–142, 1996; JAAD 37:523–549, 1997; Ped Derm 14:401–402, 1997; Ped Derm 18:117–119, 2001; Ped Derm 14:401–402, 1997;* skin-colored nodule with blue papules *JAAD 41:109–111, 1999; AD 74:511–521, 1956*

Eccrine syringofibroadenoma (acrosyringeal hamartoma) *JAAD 41:650–651, 1999*

Elastoma – isolated, Buschke-Ollendorf

Embryonal rhabdomyosarcoma – plantar nodule *Ped Derm 21:506–507, 2004*

Enchondromas

Epidermoid cysts, plantar – HPV-60-related *BJD 152:961–967, 2005*

Fibrosarcoma, congenital – plantar nodule *Ped Derm 21:506–507, 2004*

Fibrous hamartoma of infancy – congenital plantar nodule *Ped Derm 21:506–507, 2004*

Fibrous histiocytoma, benign *Cutis 46:223–226, 1990*

Ganglion cyst

Giant cell tumor of the tendon sheath *J Bone Joint Surg Am 66:76–94, 1984*

Glomus tumor, extradigital *Mol Clin Oncol 2:237–239, 2014*

Granular cell tumor – plantar skin colored nodule *Ped Derm 28:473–474, 2011*

Infantile histiocytic nodules *J R Soc Med 77 Suppl:19–21, 1984*

Kaposi's sarcoma – classic *JAAD 38:143–175, 1998; Int J Dermatol 36:735–740, 1997; Dermatology 190:324–326, 1995;* anaplastic Kaposi's sarcoma – yellow hyperkeratotic plantar nodules *BJD 164:209–211, 2011*

Keloids

Leiomyoma, vascular *J Clin Diagn Res 7:571–572, 2013*

Lipoma – plantar nodule *Ped Derm 21:506–507, 2004*

Lymphocytoma cutis

Lymphoma, including cutaneous T-cell lymphoma; diffuse large B-cell lymphoma, leg type *Clin Nuc Med 41:65–68, 2016*

Lymphomatoid papulosis – personal observation

Malignant fibrous histiocytoma, myxoid variant – papule or nodule of ankle *JAAD 48:S39–40, 2003; JAAD 43:892, 2000;*

Malignant giant cell tumor of soft parts *Am J Dermatopathol 11:197–201, 1989*

Malignant melanoma of the soft parts (clear-cell sarcoma) – nodule of tendons of foot *Cancer 65:367–374, 1990*

Melanoma *Derm Surg 27:591–593, 2001*

Mesenchymal hamartoma *J Dermatol 25:406–408, 1998*

Myeloid sarcoma *Transpl Proc 47:2227–2232, 2015*

Myofibroma – plantar nodule *Ped Derm 21:506–507, 2004*

Myopericytoma *Am J Surg Pathol 4:1034–1044, 2017*

Myxoid cyst *G Ital DV 153:847–854, 2018*

Neurofibroma *Cleve Clin J Med 83:414–416, 2016*

Nevus lipomatosis

Neurilemmoma (schwannoma) – pink or vascular nodule of the foot *Cutis 67:127–129, 2001*

Neuromas *Am J Podiatr Med Assoc 90:252–255, 2000*

Nodular fasciitis *Ped Derm 21:506–507, 2004*

Plantar aponeurotic fibroma *Ped Derm 17:429–431, 2000;* anteromedial plantar fibromatosis of childhood *Ped Derm 17:472–474, 2000*

Plantar fibromatosis (Ledderhose's disease) – red plantar nodule; painful; may ulcerate *Cutis 68:219–222, 2001; Curr Prob in Derm 8:137–188, 1996*

Plexiform schwannoma of the foot *BMC Musculoskel Disord 15:342, 2014; Eur Radiol 9:1653–1655, 1999*

Precalcaneal congenital fibrolipomatous hamartoma – benign anteromedial plantar nodule of childhood- a distinct form of plantar fibromatosis *Ped Derm 17:429–431, 2000*

Reticulohistiocytoma *An Bras Dermatol 93:595–597, 2018*

Schwannoma (neurilemmoma) – vascular nodule of the foot *Cutis 67:127–129, 2001*

Spindle cell hemangioendothelioma -hyperkeratotic nodules of soles *BJD 142:1238–1239, 2000; J Dermatol 18:104–111, 1991*

Squamous cell carcinoma

Superficial acral fibromyxoma – fingers, toes, palms and soles *Am J Dermatopathol 39:14–22, 2017; BJD 159:1315–1321, 2008*

Verrucous carcinoma (epithelioma cuniculatum)

Waldenstrom's macroglobulinemia – cutaneous macroglobulinosis – painful plantar nodules *JAAD 71;e251–252, 2014*

PRIMARY CUTANEOUS DISEASES

Granuloma annulare – deep granuloma annulare *Arch Pediatr 2:858–860, 1995(Fr);* perforating granuloma annulare – palmoplantar red nodule *JAAD 32:126–127, 1995;* congenital granuloma annulare *Ped Derm 22:234–236, 2005*

Lichen sclerosus et atrophicus – ankle nodule *JAAD 31:817–818, 1994*

Macrodactyly, primary – giant nodule of plantar surface

Migratory angioedema – plantar nodule *Ped Derm 15:97–102, 1998*

Piezogenic nodules

Primary macrodactyly

Prurigo nodularis

SYNDROMES

Blue rubber bleb nevus syndrome – plantar blue nodules

Ehlers-Danlos syndrome

Familial cutaneous collagenoma

Fibroblastic rheumatism *J Rheumatol 25:2261–2266, 1998*

Focal dermal hypoplasia

Hemihyperplasia-Multiple Lipomatosis syndrome – extensive congenital vascular stain, compressible blue nodule, multiple subcutaneous nodules, hemihypertrophy, syndactyly, thickened but not cerebriform soles, dermatomyofibroma *Soc Ped Derm Annual Meeting, July 2005; Am J Med Genet 130A–111–122, 2004; Am J Med Genet 79:311–318, 1998*

IgG4 disease (retractile mesenteritis) – fasciitis and panniculitis – personal observation

Infantile digital fibromatosis *J Dermatol 25:523–526, 1998*

Multicentric reticulohistiocytosis *Am J Roentgenol Radium Ther Nucl Med 124:610–624, 1975*

Multiple exostoses syndrome *JAAD 25:333–335, 1991*

Multiple symmetric lipomatosis of the soles *JAAD 26:860–862, 1992*

Neurofibromatosis *Ped Derm 21:506–507, 2004*

Ollier syndrome – multiple enchondromas

Olmsted syndrome – plantar squamous cell carcinoma *BJD 145:685–686, 2001*

Reactive arthritis – keratoderma blenorrhagicum *Semin Arthritis Rheum 3:253–286, 1974*

Sweet's syndrome – plantar red nodules *AD 134:76–79, 1998*

Tuberous sclerosis – shagreen patch

TRAUMA

Athlete's nodules – sports-related collagenomas *AD 143:417–422, 2007; Cutis 50:131–135, 1992; JAAD 24:317–318, 1991*

Bunion

Chilblains – plantar or dorsal red papules or nodules *AD 134:76–79, 1998*

Delayed pressure urticaria – nodules of soles *JAAD 29:954–958, 1993*

Hypertrophic scar – plantar giant nodule *BJD 145:1005–1007, 2001*

Piezogenic nodules or papules – plantar *Ped Derm 17:429–431, 2000; Hautarzt 24:114–118, 1973*

Prayer nodules *Clin Exp Dermatol 9:97–98, 1984*

Surfer's nodules of anterior tibial prominence, dorsum of feet, knuckles *Radiol Case Rep 11:201–206, 2016; Cutis 50:131–135, 1992*

Traumatic plantar urticaria – red nodules *JAAD 18:144–146, 1988*

Vibratory angioedema – palmoplantar red nodules

VASCULAR DISORDERS

Angiosarcoma – in chronic lymphedema *BJD 138:692–694, 1998*

Emboli – plantar nodule *Ped Derm 15:97–102, 1998;* atrial myxoma – acral papule; painful pink or purpuric papules as a manifestation of Carney complex *JAAD 55:551–553, 2006; BJD 147:379–382, 2002*

Epithelioid hemangioma – plantar nodule *JAAD 49:113–116, 2003*

Erythema elevatum diutinum *Am J Dermatopathol 40:442–444, 2018*

Glomus tumor *Foot Ankle Int 18:672–674, 1997*

Lymphostasis verrucosa cutis

Plantar thrombotic nodules of diabetes *J Dermatol 24:405–409, 1997*

Polyarteritis nodosa – palmar and plantar nodules *AD 130:884–889, 1994; Ped Derm 15:103–107, 1998;* nodules along the course of superficial arteries around knee, anterior lower leg and dorsum of foot *Ann Int Med 89:666–676, 1978;* cutaneous infarcts presenting as tender nodules

Pseudo-Kaposi's sarcoma

Pseudomyogenic hemangioendothelioma (cutaneous epithelioid sarcoma-like) *Dermatol Ther 31:e12715, 2018; JAMADerm 149:459–465, 2013*

Pyogenic granuloma

Spindle cell hemangioma -multilobulated violaceous nodule *AD 142:641–646, 2006*

Thrombosis of deep plantar vein – plantar nodule *Ped Derm 15:97–102, 1998; Clin Podiatr Med Surg 13:85–89, 1996*

Vascular hamartomas

Vasculitis – plantar nodule JAAD 47:S263–265, 2002;

Ped Derm 15:97–102, 1998

Venous malformation

NODULES, JUXTA-ARTICULAR

AUTOIMMUNE DISEASES AND DISEASES OF IMMUNE DYSFUNCTION

Common variable immunodeficiency *J Drugs Dermatol 5:370–372, 2006*

Dermatomyositis – Gottron's papules *Curr Opin Rheum 11:475–482, 1999;* calcinosis cutis – nodules of elbows and forearms *JAMA 305:183–190, 2011*

Epidermolysis bullosa acquisita

Graft vs host disease *J Immunol 134:1475–1482, 1985*

Jaccoud's arthritis – non-erosive arthritis following repeated bouts of rheumatic fever or systemic lupus erythematosus

Lupus erythematosus – systemic lupus – mimic rheumatoid nodules *AD 72:49–58, 1970;* rheumatoid nodules

Rheumatoid arthritis – rheumatoid nodules *Eur J Radiol 27 Suppl 1:S18–24, 1998; J Rheumatol 6:286–292, 1979;* palisaded neutrophilic granulomatous dermatitis of rheumatoid arthritis (rheumatoid neutrophilic dermatosis) – nodules over joints *Cutis 78:133–136, 2006; JAAD 47:251–257, 2002; AD 133:757–760, 1997; AD 125:1105–1108, 1989;* bursal cyst with cholesterol crystals of left elbow *NEJM 369:1945, 2013;* rheumatoid nodulosis – personal observation

Sclerederma – soft cystic nodules (focal mucinosis) over interphalangeal joints *BJD 136:598–600, 1997;* nodules of necrotic fibrinous material *BJD 101:93–96, 1979;* CREST syndrome; rheumatoid nodules

Sclerodermatomyositis – Gottron's papules, periorbital erythema, Raynaud's phenomenon, acrosteolysis, dysphagia, digital ulcers; high risk of interstitial lung disease *Arthr Research Therapy 16:R111, 2014; AD 144:1351–1359, 2008; Arthr Rheum 50:565–569, 2004; J Clin Immunol 4:40–44, 1984*

DEGENERATIVE DISEASES

Bouchard's nodes – osteoarthritis; proximal interphalangeal joints *Ann Rheum Dis 48:523–527, 1953*

Heberden's nodes – distal interphalangeal joints *Br Med J i:181–187, 1952*

DRUG REACTIONS

Acral dysesthesia syndrome

Bleomycin-induced dermatomyositis-like rash *JAAD 48:439–441, 2003*

Hydroxyurea – dermatomyositis-like eruption – personal observation

Tegafur – knuckle pad-like keratoderma *Int J Dermatol 37:315–317, 1998*

Voriconazole-induced fluoride excess; periostitis with swollen joints of hands *Clin Inf Dis 57:562–563,616–617, 2013*

EXOGENOUS AGENTS

Foreign body granuloma

Plant thorns – common blackthorn; persistent nodules of wrists and fingers *Lancet i:309–310, 1960*

INFECTIONS AND INFESTATIONS

Bejel

Cryptococcosis – cryptococcal panniculitis

Dracunculosis (*Dracunculus medinensis*) *(Guinea worm)* – subcutaneous nodule of ankle *JAAD 54:154, 2006*

Gianotti-Crosti syndrome – personal observation

Gonococcemia – periarticular lesions appear in crops with red macules, papules, vesicles with red halo, pustules, bullae becoming hemorrhagic and necrotic; suppurative arthritis and tenosynovitis *Ann Int Med 102:229–243, 1985*

Leishmaniasis – AIDS-related visceral leishmaniasis *BJD 143:1316–1318, 2000*

Leprosy – digital papule *JAAD 11:713–723, 1984*

Lyme borreliosis – juxta-articular fibroid nodules *Hautarzt 51:345–348, 2000; AD 131:1341–1342, 1995; Clin Exp Dermatol 19:394–398, 1994; BJD 128:674–678, 1993*

Meningococcemia – chronic *Rev Inf Dis 8:1–11, 1986*

Molluscum contagiosum

Mycetoma *JAAD 32:311–315, 1995; Cutis 49:107–110, 1992; Australas J Dermatol 31:33–36, 1990; JAAD 6:107–111, 1982; Sabouraudia 18:91–95, 1980; AD 99:215–225, 1969*

Mycobacterium avium complex – wrist nodule *Clin Exp Dermatol 23:214–221, 1998*

Mycobacterium haemophilum Ped Derm 23:481–483, 2006; BJD 149:200–202, 2003

Mycobacterium marinum – nodule or papule of hands, elbows, knees becomes crusted ulcer or abscess; or verrucous papule; sporotrichoid; rarely widespread lesions *Br Med J 300:1069–1070, 1990; AD 122:698–703, 1986; J Hyg 94:135–149, 1985*

Mycobacterium tuberculosis – scrofuloderma – infected lymph node, bone, joint, lacrimal gland with overlying red-blue nodule which breaks down, ulcerates, forms fistulae, scarring with adherent fibrous masses which may be fluctuant and draining *BJD 134:350–352, 1996*

Nocardia – red nodule overlying wrist in patient with chronic granulomatous disease *Clin Inf Dis 33:235–239, 2001*

Parvovirus B19 – dermatomyositis-like Gottron's papules *Hum Pathol 31:488–497, 2000*

Pinta – Lutz-Jeanselme disease *Gaz Med Port 6:109–112, 1953*

Rheumatic fever – papules on extensor extremities near joints subcutaneous nodules around elbows or knees *Rheumatol Rehab 21:195–200, 1982*

Sporotrichosis – personal observation

Syphilis – juxta-articular nodes *Gaz Med Port 6:109–112, 1953*

Verruca vulgaris – knuckle papules *Derm Surg 27:591–593, 2001;* myrmecia – personal observation

Yaws – tertiary – juxta-articular nodes *JAAD 54:559–578, 2006; Ann Trop Med Parasitol 55:309–313, 1961*

INFILTRATIVE DISEASES

Acral persistent papular mucinosis – mimicking knuckle pads *AD 140:121–126, 2004; JAAD 27:1026–1029, 1992*

Amyloidosis

Juxta-articular myxoma – rare variant in vicinity of large joints *Eur Radiol 20:764–768, 2010; Skeletal Radiology 24:389–391, 1995*

Lichen myxedematosus – resembling acral persistent papular mucinosis *BJD 144:594–596, 2001; Dermatology 185:81, 1992*

Mastocytoma knuckle pads

Self-healing (papular) juvenile cutaneous mucinosis – juxta-articular painless nodules; also nodules of face, neck, scalp, abdomen, and thighs; arthralgias; white papules of head, neck, trunk, periarticular; deeper nodules of face and periarticular areas; periorbital edema *Ped Derm 31:515–516, 2014; Ped Derm 26:91–92, 2009; JAAD 55:1036–1043, 2006; JAAD 50:S97–100, 2004; Ped Derm 20:35–39, 2003; JAAD 44:273–281, 2001; Ped Derm 14:460–462, 1997; AD 131:459–461, 1995; JAAD 11:327–332, 1984; Ann DV 107:51–57, 1980;* of adult *JAAD 50:121–123, 2004, BJD 143:650–651, 2000; Dermatology 192:268–270, 1996; Lyon Med 230:474–475, 1973*

INFLAMMATORY DISEASES

Bunion

Extravascular necrotizing palisaded granulomas – found in systemic lupus erythematosus, Churg-Strauss disease, Wegener's granulomatosis, lymphoproliferative disease, hepatitis, inflammatory bowel disease, Takayasu's arteritis *BJD 147:371–374, 2002*

Interstitial granulomatous dermatitis – personal observation

Sarcoidosis (Darier-Roussy sarcoid) *JAAD 44:725–743, 2001; AD 133:882–888, 1997; Am J Med 85:731–736, 1988;* nodules of DIP joints *BJD 142:1052–1053, 2000*

Seronegative ankylosing spondylitis – rheumatoid nodules

METABOLIC DISEASES

Calcinosis cutis – metastatic or dystrophic calcinosis *Cutis 63:149–153, 1999; JAAD 39:527–544, 1998;* tumoral calcinosis – around hip, elbow, ankle, and scapula *Seminars in Dermatol 3:53–61, 1984;* in ESRD *JAAD 40:975–986, 2000*

Calciphylaxis (vascular calcification cutaneous necrosis syndrome) – papules or nodules around large joints or flexures *J Dermatol 28:27–31, 2001; Br J Plast Surg 53:253–255, 2000; JAAD 40:979–987, 1999; J Cutan Med Surg 2:245–248, 1998; JAAD 33:53–58,* *1995; JAAD 33:954–962, 1995; JAAD 33:954–962, 1995; AD 127:225–230, 1991;* tumoral calcinosis – progressively growing lobulated masses

Diabetic finger pebbling (Huntley's papules) *Cutis 69:298–300, 2002*

Erythropoietic protoporphyria

Gout *J Cut Aesthet Surg 10:223–225, 2017; Cutis 48:445–451, 1991; Ann Rheum Dis 29:461–468, 1970*

Pancreatic panniculitis – periarticular subcutaneous nodules; *JAAD 34:362–364, 1996; Arthritis Rheum 22:547–553, 1979*

Pseudogout – pseudotophi

Sitosterolemia – tuberous and tendon xanthomas *Ped Derm 17:447–449, 2000*

Xanthomas, especially tendinous and tuberous xanthomas – cerebrotendinous xanthomatosis – mutation in sterol 27-hydroxylase; increased serum cholestanol and urinary bile alcohols; normal serum cholesterol; familial hypercholesterolemia – increased cholesterol and LDL *Ped Derm 24:230–234, 2007;* tendon xanthomas also seen in heterozygous familial hypercholesterolemia, familial defective lipoprotein B100, familial dysbetalipoproteinemia, beta sitosterolemia *JAAD 45:292–295, 2001;* phytosterolemia – excessive absorption of plant sterols – normal LDL *Clin Biochem Rev 25:49–68, 2004;* tuberous xanthomas

NEOPLASTIC DISEASES

Dupuytren's contracture – personal observation

Eccrine angiomatous hamartoma *Ped Derm 18:117–119, 2001; Ped Derm 13:139–142, 1996; Ped Derm 14:401–402, 1997;* skin-colored nodule with blue papules *JAAD 41:109–111, 1999*

Eccrine poroma and eccrine porocarcinoma – red nodule of ankle *BJD 150:1232–1233, 2004*

Fibromas

Giant cell tumor of the tendon sheath – single or multiple *JAAD 43:892, 2000;* nodules of the fingers *J Dermatol 23:290–292, 1996; J Bone Joint Surg Am 66:76–94, 1984*

Keloids

Lymphoma – cutaneous T-cell lymphoma; primary cutaneous marginal zone lymphoma *J Cut Pathol 40:477–484, 2013*

Malignant melanoma of the soft parts (clear-cell sarcoma) – nodule of tendons of foot or knee *Cancer 65:367–374, 1990*

Myxoid cyst

Neurofibroma

Osteochondromatosis of the ankle *J Foot Surg 29:330–333, 1990*

Osteoma cutis

Synovial cyst or ganglion

PARANEOPLASTIC DISEASES

Necrobiotic xanthogranuloma with paraproteinemia *AD 133:97–102, 1997;* nodules of knees *JAAD 52:729–731, 2005*

Paraneoplastic pemphigus – periarticular plaques *Ped Derm 29:656–657, 2012*

Paraneoplastic sclerederma

PRIMARY CUTANEOUS DISEASES

Acanthosis nigricans

Acrodermatitis chronica atrophicans – juxta-articular fibroid nodule *AD 131:1341–1342, 1995*

Acrokeratoelastoidosis of Costa – knuckle pads *Ped Derm 19:320–322, 2002; JAAD 22:468–476, 1990; Acta DV 60:149–153, 1980; Dermatologica 107:164–168, 1953*

Acrokeratosis verruciformis of Hopf

Cutis laxa, acquired – fibrotic nodules over bony prominences

Dercum's disease (adiposis dolorosa) – painful peri-articular lipomas and ecchymoses; lipomas feel like "bag of worms" *JAAD 44:132–136, 2001*

Epidermolysis bullosa

Epidermolytic hyperkeratosis

Erythema elevatum diutinum – violaceous knuckle pads (juxta-articular nodules) *Cutis 101:462–465, 2018; JAAD 49:764–767, 2003; JAAD 28:394–398, 1994; AD 129:1043–1044, 1046–1047, 1993;* ankles, knees *JAMADerm 153:315–316, 2017; Cutis 78:129–132, 2006; AD 129:1043–1044, 1046–1047, 1993;* HIV – *JAAD 28:919–922, 1993*

Granuloma annulare – subcutaneous granuloma annulare mimicking knuckle pads *Acta DV Croat 25:292–294, 2017; JAAD 3:217–230, 1980;* in adults *Am J Dermatopathol 27:1–5, 2005*

Hidrotic ectodermal dysplasia

Id reactions

Juvenile fibromatosis

Knuckle pads – idiopathic (fibromatosis), keratotic knuckle pads unassociated with palmoplantar keratoderma *AJDC 140:915–917, 1986;* trauma-induced, associated with Dupuytren's contracture, Ledderhose's disease, Peyronie's disease, Bart-Pumphrey syndrome – sensorineural deafness, leukonychia, and knuckle pads; autosomal dominant *Ped Derm 17:450–452, 2000; NEJM 276:202–207, 1967*

Lichen nitidus – knuckle pads *AD 134:1302–1303, 1998*

Lichen simplex chronicus

Pachydermodactyly – digital fibromatosis; bilateral asymptomatic swelling of soft tissues lateral aspects of the PIP joints of second and fourth fingers; benign fibromatosis of fingers of young men; thought to be trauma-related (poultry processing workers); large knuckles *AD 148:925–928, 2012; AD 144:1651–1656, 2008; Clin Rheumatol 26:962–964, 2007; Clin Exp Dermatol 28:674–675,2003; Ann DV 125:247–250, 1998; BJD 133:433–437, 1995; AD 111:524, 1975; Bull Soc Fr Dermatol Syphiligr 80:455–458, 1973;*

Papular urticaria – personal observation

Prurigo nodularis

Psoriasis

PSYCHOCUTANEOUS DISEASES

Bulimia nervosa – Russell's sign (crusted knuckle nodules) *Clin Orthop 343:107–109, 1997; JAAD 12:725–726, 1985;* perniosis *Clin Sci 61:559–567, 1981;* pseudo knuckle pads (calluses on second fifth MCP joints) *Psychol Med 9;429–48, 1979*

SYNDROMES

Albright's hereditary osteodystrophy – ectopic bone formation

Bart-Pumphrey syndrome – knuckle pads, leukonychia, sensorineural deafness, and diffuse palmoplantar hyperkeratosis; autosomal dominant *JAAD 51:292, 2004; Curr Prob Derm 14:71–116, 2002; NEJM 276:202–207, 1967*

Cerebrotendinous xanthomatosis – autosomal recessive; tendon (Achilles tendon) and tuberous xanthomas *Ped Derm 17:447–449, 2000*

Distal pachydermodactyly (acquired digital fibrosis) – skin colored nodule of the elbow *JAAD 38:359–362, 1998*

Ehlers-Danlos syndrome (molluscum pseudotumor) – knuckle pads; personal observation

Familial histiocytic dermatoarthritis – knuckle pads

Familial Mediterranean fever

Farber's disease (disseminated lipogranulomatosis) – autosomal recessive; lysosomal acid ceramidase deficiency (*N*-acylsphingosine amidohydrolase) (chromosome 8p22–21.2); red papules and nodules of joints and tendons of hands and feet; deforming arthritis; papules, plaques, and nodules of ears, back of scalp and trunk (proximal and distal interphalangeal joints, wrist, elbow, knees, ankles, metatarsals); progressive hoarseness; rarely nodules seen in conjunctivae, nostrils, ears, mouth; heart, liver, spleen, lung; progressive psychomotor retardation *Ped Derm 26:44–46, 2009; Ped Derm 21:154–159, 2004; Eur J Ped 157:515–516, 1998; AD 130:1350–1354, 1994; Am J Dis Child 84:449–500, 1952*

Fibroblastic rheumatism – symmetrical polyarthritis, nodules over joints and on palms, elbows, knees, ears, neck, Raynaud's phenomenon, sclerodactyly; joint contractures, thick palmar fascia; scalp nodules, red tender swelling of toe tips, periarticular nodule; skin lesions resolve spontaneously *JAAD 66:959–965, 2012; Ped Derm 19:532–535, 2002; AD 139:657–662, 2003; AD 131:710–712, 1995; Clin Exp Dermatol 19:268–270, 1994; Rev Rheum Ed Fr 47:345–351, 1980*

Francois syndrome (dermochondrocorneal dystrophy) – knuckle pads; nodules on hands, nose, and ears *Ann DV 104:475–478, 1977; AD 124:424–428, 1988*

Hunter syndrome – MPS II *Ped Derm 12:370–372, 1995*

Infantile digital fibromatosis

Juvenile hyaline fibromatosis (infantile systemic hyalinosis) (Murray-Puretic-Drescher syndrome) – autosomal recessive; gingival fibromatosis with hypertrophy, focal skin nodularity with multiple subcutaneous tumors (nodular perianal lesions, facial red or pearly papules (paranasal, periauricular), dusky red plaques of buttocks, ears, lips), synophrys, thickened skin with sclerodermiform atrophy, osteolytic (osteoporotic) skeletal lesions, stiff muscles with massive stiffness, flexural joint contractures, hyperpigmentation, flexion contractures of joints, juxta-articular nodules (knuckle pads), nodules of ears, diarrhea, recurrent suppurative infections failure to thrive with stunted growth (growth failure) and death in infancy; CMG2 (capillary morphogenesis protein 2) (transmembrane protein); deposition of collagen type VI (bound to laminin and collagen 4) mutation (chromosome 4q21) *Ped Derm 25:557–558, 2008; JAAD 58:303–307, 2008; Ped Derm 21:154–159, 2004; JAAD 50:S61–64, 2004; Ped Derm 18:534–536, 2001; Ped Derm 18:400–402, 2001; Dermatology 198:18–25, 1999; Int J Paediatr Dent 6:39–43, 1996; J Periodontol 67:451–453, 1996; Dermatology 190:148–151, 1995; Ped Derm 11:52–60, 1994; Ped Derm 6:68–75, 1989; Oral Surg 63:71–77, 1987; Arch Fr Pediatr 35:1063–1074, 1978*

Knuckle pads, leukonychia, and deafness syndrome

Knuckle pads with palmoplantar keratoderma and acrokeratoelastoidosis

Ledderhose's nodules (plantar fibromatosis) *JAAD 41:106–108, 1999;* Dupuytren's contracture (palmar fibromatosis) and/or Peyronie's disease – knuckle pads

Lipoid proteinosis – xanthoma-like nodules of elbows; nodules of finger joints, knees *BJD 151:413–423, 2004; JID 120:345–350, 2003; BJD 148:180–182, 2003; Hum Molec Genet 11:833–840, 2002; Acta Paediatr 85:1003–1005, 1996; JAAD 27:293–297, 1992*

Mal de Meleda (recessive transgressive palmoplantar keratoderma) – knuckle pads *Curr Prob Derm 14:71–116, 2002; Ped Derm 14:186–191, 1997*

Multicentric reticulohistiocytosis – elbow nodules *BJD 161:470–472, 2009; JAAD 58:541–543, 2008; AD 140:919–921, 2004; BJD 133:71–76, 1995; AD 126:251–252, 1990; Clin Exp Dermatol 15:1–6, 1990; Oral Surg Oral Med Oral Pathol 65:721–725, 1988; Pathology 17:601–608, 1985; JAAD 11:713–723, 1984; AD 97:543–547, 1968; Proc R. Soc Med 30:522–526, 1937;* mimicking dermatomyositis *JAAD 48:S11–14, 2003*

Neurofibromatosis

Pachydermoperiostosis – knuckle pads *J Dermatol 27:106–109, 2000*

Palmoplantar keratoderma, Vorner – knuckle pads; papules on knuckles *BJD 125:496, 1991*Penttinen syndrome – progeroid disorder with overgrowth; resembles mandibuloacral dysplasia (which has micrognathia); hypertelorism, malar hypoplasia, prognathia, narrow nose; open font, shallow orbits, lipoatrophy with thin translucent skin; scars overlying joints; acroosteolysis *Am J Med Genet A 161A:1786–1791, 2013; Am J Med Genet 69:182–187, 1997*

Polyfibromatosis syndrome – Dupuytren's contracture, knuckle pads, Peyronie's disease, keloids, or plantar fibromatosis; stimulation by phenytoin *BJD 100:335–341, 1979*

Pseudohypoparathyroidism – periarticular calcified nodules *JAAD 15:353–356, 1986*

Reflex sympathetic dystrophy with chilblain-like lesions – digital papule

Rowell's syndrome – lupus erythematosus and erythema multiforme-like syndrome – perniotic lesions *JAAD 21:374–377, 1989*

Stiff skin syndrome – knuckle pads *Ped Derm 3:48–53, 1985*

Vohwinkel's syndrome – knuckle papules, palmoplantar keratoderma, ichthyosis, pseudoainhum *JAAD 44:376–378, 2001*

TRAUMA

Callosities, occupational (carpenters, live chicken hangers *Contact Derm 17:13–16, 1987*), frictional, bulimic; tight shoes *Dermatol Clin 33:207–241, 2015*

Chilblains – tender, pruritic red or purple digital papules *JAAD 45:924–929, 2001*

Garrod's pads – violinist's knuckles (second and third knuckles) – thickened skin over the interphalangeal joints from intense flexion of tendons of fingers *Cutis 62:261–262, 1998*

Piezogenic wrist papules

Scars – mimic knuckle pads

Skier's thumb *Acta Orthop Belg 65:440–446, 1999*

Surfer's nodules of anterior tibial prominence, dorsum of feet, knuckles *Cutis 50:131–135, 1992*

VASCULAR DISEASES

Eosinophilic granulomatosis with polyangiitis – elbow papules and nodules *JAAD 37:199–203, 1997;* umbilicated nodules of elbows *BJD 150:598–600, 2004*

Vasculitis

Granulomatosis with polyangiitis – herpetiform necrotic purpuric papules over joints (ankles, elbows) *AD 148:849–854, 2012*

NODULES, KNEE

AUTOIMMUNE DISEASES AND DISORDERS OF IMMUNE DYSREGULATION

Dermatomyositis – calcinosis cutis *Ann Dermatol 28:375–380, 2016*

Epidermolysis bullosa acquisita

Rheumatoid nodule

DRUG REACTIONS

Acral dysesthesia syndrome

EXOGENOUS AGENTS

Foreign body granuloma

INFECTIONS AND INFESTATIONS

Coccidioidomycosis – interstitial granulomatous dermatitis *JAAD 55:929–942, 2006*

Exophiala spinifera Med Mycol 50:207–213, 2012

Fusarium Dermatol Online J 18:6 April 15, 2012

Leishmaniasis – diffuse cutaneous leishmaniasis – multiple red verrucous nodules of knees; multilobulated skin colored nodules of ears *BJD 156:1328–1335, 2007*

Leprosy

Lobomycosis

Mycobacterium chelonae JAAD 43:333–336, 2000

Mycobacterium marinum – nodule or papule of hands, elbows, knees becomes crusted ulcer or abscess; or verrucous papule; sporotrichoid; rarely widespread lesions *Br Med J 300:1069–1070, 1990; AD 122:698–703, 1986; J Hyg 94:135–149, 1985*

North American blastomycosis – *Blastomyces dermatitidis* Am J Trop Med Hyg 27:1203–1205, 1978

Paecilomyces lilacinus Transpl Infec Dis 10:117–122, 2008

Pine moth caterpillar disease – skin nodules and arthritis *Skeletal Radiol 15:422–427, 1986*

Scedosporium apiospermum Transpl Proc 39:2033–2035, 2007

Staphylococcus aureus – abscess *Ann DV 144:275–278, 2017*

INFILTRATIVE DISORDERS

Amyloidosis *Dermatol Online J 19:20711, Dec 16, 2013*

Intralymphatic histiocytosis *BJD 158:402–404, 2008*

INFLAMMATORY DISORDERS

Bursitis

Fibroblastic rheumatism – papulonodules on elbows and knees

Panniculitis, pancreatic *Ann Dermatol 23:225–228, 2011;*

Int J Dermatol 35:39–41, 1996

Sarcoid – scar sarcoid; subcutaneous nodules (Darier-Roussy sarcoid) *Exp Ther Med 13:1535–1537, 2017*

METABOLIC DISORDERS

Calcinosis cutis *J Orthop Case Rep 6:78–79, 2016;* subepidermal calcified nodule *J Dermatol 39:965–966, 2012; West Indian Med J 52:255–256, 2003;*

Gout *Cutis 48:445–451, 1991; Ann Rheum Dis 29:461–468, 1970*

Xanthomas – tuberous xanthomas

NEOPLASTIC DISORDERS

Connective tissue nevi

Giant dermatofibroma *JAAD 30:714–718, 1994*

Elastoma

Enchondromas

Epithelioid hemangioendothelioma *Am J Dermatopathol 20:541–546, 1998*

Ganglion cyst

Kaposi's sarcoma – purple nodule

Keloids

Keratoacanthoma *Australas J Dermatol 50:194–197, 2009*

Lymphoma – primary cutaneous B-cell lymphoma *Int J Clin Exp Pathol 15:1193–1199, 2014*

Malignant melanoma of the soft parts (clear-cell sarcoma) – nodule of knee *J Clin Oncol 36:1649–1653, 2018; Cancer 65:367–374, 1990*

Merkel cell carcinoma – violaceous nodule of knee *AD 145:715–720, 2009*

Metastasis – osteogenic sarcoma *JAAD 49:757–760, 2003*

Nevus lipomatosis superficialis

Nodular macroglobulinosis – violaceous nodule of knee *JAAD 77:1145–1158, 2017*

Pleomorphic angioleiomyoma *Am J Dermatopathol 22:268–271, 2000*

Primary cutaneous cribriform carcinoma – rare apocrine tumor *J Cutan Pathol 32:577–580, 2005*

Sclerosing perineurioma *Am J Dermatopathol 41:436–437, 2019*

PRIMARY CUTANEOUS DISORDERS

Acrodermatitis chronica atrophicans *Ned Tikdschr Geneeskd 201:154.A2012.PMID 20699042*

Elastosis perforans serpiginosa

Epidermolysis bullosa dystrophica

Erythema elevatum diutinum *Ann DV 135:575–579, 2008; Cutis 78:129–132, 2006; AD 129:1043–1044, 1046–1047, 1993*

Granuloma annulare

IgM storage papule – pink or skin colored

Papular urticaria

Prurigo nodularis

SYNDROMES

Ehlers-Danlos syndrome (molluscoid tumors)

Juvenile hyaline fibromatosis *J Pediatr Orthop B7:235–238, 1998; AD 112:86–88, 1976*

Multicentric reticulohistiocytosis *BJD 133:71–76, 1995; AD 126:251–252, 1990; Clin Exp Dermatol 15:1–6, 1990; Oral Surg Oral Med Oral Pathol 65:721–725, 1988; Pathology 17:601–608, 1985; JAAD 11:713–723, 1984;; JAAD 11:713–723, 1984; AD 97:543–547, 1968;* with recurrent breast cancer *JAAD 39:864–866, 1988*

TRAUMA

Callosities

Islamic prayer nodules – on knees and ankles of Shi'ite Muslims *Cutis 38:281–286, 1986*

Hypertrophic scar

Surfer's nodules *JAMA 201:134–136, 1967*

VASCULAR LESIONS

Leukocytoclastic vasculitis with antiphospholipid antibody syndrome *J Dermatol 32:1032–1037, 2005*

Pyogenic granuloma *Am J Dermatopathol 8:379–385, 1986*

Vascular hamartomas

NODULES, MULTILOBULATED

AUTOIMMUNE DISEASES AND DISEASES OF IMMUNE DYSFUNCTION

Adenosine deaminase deficiency (SCID) – dermatofibrosarcoma protuberans *BJD 178:335–349, 2018*

CREST syndrome – calcinosis cutis – personal observation

Dermatomyositis with cutaneous mucinosis *AD 126:1639–1644, 1990;* calcinosis cutis – multilobulated subcutaneous nodules *JAMADerm 150:724–729, 2014; AD 148:455–462, 2012*

Lupus erythematosus – nodular episcleritis

Morphea – keloidal (Addisonian keloid) *Ped Derm 29:111–112, 2012; Int J Dermatol 31:422–423, 1992; Med Chir Trans 37:27–47, 1854;* generalized morphea – keloidal nodules

Rheumatoid arthritis – rheumatoid nodules *J Rheumatol 6:286–292, 1979; Eur J Radiol 27 Suppl 1:S18–24, 1998*

CONGENITAL

Accessory tragus

Congenital circumferential skin folds – mountain range appearance; dysmorphic features, ear abnormalities, prominent philtrum with central ridge *Ped Derm 29:89–95, 2012*

Congenital fibroblastic connective tissue nevi – multilobulated keloid-like plaque of chest *Ped Derm 35:644–650, 2018*

Congenital cutaneous plate-like osteoma cutis – mountain range-like topography *Ped Derm 10:371–376, 1993*

Congenital lipoblastomatosis *Ped Derm 15:210–213, 1998*

Congenital papillated apocrine cystadenoma *JAAD 11:374–376, 1984*

Dermoid cyst – lobulated scalp nodule *Ped Derm 30:706–711, 2013*

Torus mandibularis *Cutis 71:363–364, 2003*

Torus palatinus *NEJM 368:1434, 2013*

DRUG-INDUCED LESIONS

Iododerma *JAAD 36:1014–1016, 1997*

EXOGENOUS AGENTS

Cutaneous geode – nodular crateriform scar *JAAD 14:1085–1086, 1986*

Podoconiosis – multilobulated hyperkeratotic nodules of feet; cobblestoned; bare feet exposed to red clay from alkaline volcanic rock *BJD 168:550–554, 2013; JAAD 65:214–215, 2011*

Foreign body granuloma – intralymphatic histiocytosis due to molybdenum – red multilobulated nodule *BJD 158:402–404, 2008*

Organochlorine exposure (agent orange) – chloracne with comedones, gray dyschromia, hypertrichosis, folliculitis, porphyria cutanea tarda, melanoma and non-melanoma skin cancer, non-Hodgkin's lymphoma, dermatofibrosarcoma protuberans *JAAD 74:143–170, 2016*

Tattoo – granulomatous reaction *Dermatol Clin 33:509–630, 2015*

INFECTIONS AND INFESTATIONS

Actinomycetoma *NEJM 372:264, 2015*

Actinomycetoma – due to *Nocardia brasiliensis;* pustules, scarring, sinus tracts, multilobulated nodules, grains *JAAD 62:239–246, 2010*

Adiaspiromycosis – cutaneous adiaspiromycosis (*Chrysosporium species*) – hyperpigmented plaque with white-yellow papules, ulcerated nodules, hyperkeratotic nodules, crusted nodules, multilobulated nodules *JAAD S113–117, 2004*

African histoplasmosis (*Histoplasma capsulatum var duboisii*) *J Mycol Med 26:265–270, 2016*

Alternariosis *Dermatol Online Dec 15, 2019; Transplant Inf Dis 12:242–250, 2010*

Aspergillosis – primary cutaneous aspergillosis; cauliflower-like lesion *Am J Dermatopathol 23:224–226, 2001*

Bacillary angiomatosis *SKINmed 4:215, 2005*

Botryomycosis – *Staphylococcus aureus*; cutaneous granular bacteriosis *Ped Derm 33:253–263, 2016; Clin Exp Dermatol 34:887–889, 2009*

Burkholderia fungorum (actinomycetoma) – fungating multinodular tumid mass *BJD 171:1261–1263, 2014*

Candida albicans – in immunosuppressed host *Intern Med 53:1385–1390, 2014; JAAD 28(pt2)315–317, 1993*

Carbuncle

Chromomycosis – mountain range appearance *Cutis 101:442,447–448, 2018; BJD 146:704, 2002; AD 133:1027–1032, 1997; BJD 96:454–458, 1977; AD 104:476–485, 1971;* multinodular annular brown plaque of thigh; *Fonsacaea pedrosoi JAAD 63:1083–1087, 2010*

Coccidioidomycosis *Cutis 85:25–27, 2010; AD 144:933–938, 2008; An Circulo Med Argent 15:585–597, 1892*

Dermatophyte infection – deep dermatophytosis in inherited autosomal recessive CARD9 deficiency; vegetative plaques, verrucous plaques and nodules; perianal vegetative plaques *NEJM 1704–1714, 2013*

Furuncle

Giant condyloma of Buschke and Lowenstein – cerebriform, multilobulated giant tumor; HPV6 with huge grape-like nodule composed of multiple small nodules *BJD 166:247–251, 2012; J Dermatol 20:773–778, 1993*

Herpes simplex, hypertrophic – personal observation

Keloidal blastomycosis (lobomycosis) – *Lacazia (Loboa) loboi;* Amazon rain forest of South America; legs, arms, face *Cutis 83:67–68, 2009; BJD 159:234–236, 2008; JAAD 53:931–951, 2006; JAAD 29:134–136, 139–140, 1993; Cutis 46:227–234, 1990; Int J Dermatol 27:481–484, 1988*

Leishmaniasis – diffuse cutaneous leishmaniasis – multilobulated skin colored nodules of ears *BJD 156:1328–1335, 2007;* leishmaniasis recidivans (lupoid leishmaniasis) – brown-red or brown-yellow papules close to scar of previously healed lesion; resemble lupus vulgaris; may ulcerate or form concentric rings; keloidal form, verrucous form of legs, extensive psoriasiform dermatitis; diffuse cutaneous (*L. aethiopica, L. mexicana*) *Int J Dermatol 49:295–297, 2010; Int J Dermatol 46:711–714, 2007JAAD 23:368–371, 1990*

Lagochilascariasis – rare nematode; tropical and subtropical zones; affecting rural inhabitants; Mexico to Argentina; wild felines are natural reservoir (jaguar)

Emerging Inf Dis 25:2331–2332, 2019

Leprosy – *AD 148:1096–1097, 2012;* Wirchowian leprosy *Annual Meeting AAD 2000;* type 1 leprosy reactions – edema of hands, feet, face; mountain range-like swelling of prior lesions *BJD 167:29035, 2012*

Lyme disease – lymphocytoma cutis, *Borrelia*-associated *JAAD 23:401–410, 1990*

Milker's nodule

Molluscum contagiosum, giant *AD 147:652–654, 2011; Clin Inf Dis 52:1029–1030,1077–1078, 2011 Cutis 60:29–34, 1997*

Mucormycosis – personal observation

Mucor irregularis – multilobulated red nodule covering orbital skin *BJD 180:213–214, 2019*

Mycetoma, *Acremonium* – personal observation

Mycobacterium tuberculosis – multilobulated tumor of the earlobe *BJD 150:370–371, 2004;* Pott's disease – giant subcutaneous multilobulated mass of lower back *Cutis 85:85–89, 2010*

Paracoccidioidomycosis – verrucous multinodular plaque of nose *Clin Dermatol 38:152–159, 2020*

Phaeohyphomycotic cyst – *Exophiala dermatitidis* – multilobulated red nodules of elbow *JAMADerm 152:567–568, 2016*

Rhinosporidiosis – vascular nodules; *Arch Otolaryngol 102:308–312, 1976*

Schistosoma mansoni – anal fissure with multilobulated giant anal polyp *AD 144:950–952, 2008*

Syphilis – granulomatous, tertiary *AD 125:551–556, 1989*

Tinea capitis – presenting as acne keloidalis *JAAD 56:699–701, 2007*

Warts – condylomata acuminate – personal observation

Yaws *Int J Derm 21:220–3, 1982*

INFILTRATIVE DISEASES

Amyloidosis – nodular (tumefactive) amyloidosis; of great toe *JAAD 49:307–310, 2003;* nodular primary localized cutaneous amyloidosis *JAAD 71:1035–1037, 2014; Cutis 91:271,283–284, 2014; JAAD 57:S26–29, 2007*

Langerhans cell histiocytosis

Lymphocytoma cutis – personal observation

Mastocytosis *Diagnostic Challenges Vol V25–27, 1994; AD 127:405–410, 1991*

Pretibial mucinosis – multilobulated plaques of legs *Cutis 88:300–302, 2012; AD 129:1152–1156, 1993*

Pretibial myxedema *BJD 166:457–459, 2012*

Rosai-Dorfman disease (sinus histiocytosis with massive lymphadenopathy)– multinodular tumor with cobblestoning *AD 142:428–430, 2006; AD 114:191–197, 1978;* multilobular facial red nodules with yellow centers *AD 144:120–121, 2008;* keloidal nodule *JAAD 68:346–348, 2013;* red plaque with multinodular areas *JAAD 65:890–892, 2011;* multilobulated nodules of ear *JAMADerm 150:81–82, 2014*

Scleromyxedema – mountain range lesions of post-auricular crease *JAAD 69:66–72, 2013*

Verruciform xanthoma of toes in patient with Milroy's disease due to persistent leg edema *Ped Derm 20:44–47, 2003; JAAD 20:313–317, 1989*

Xanthoma disseminatum – mountain range-like topography *AD 121:1313–1317, 1985*

INFLAMMATORY DISEASES

Crohn's disease, metastatic *Ped Derm 13:25–28, 1996*

Dissecting cellulitis of the scalp

Hidradenitis suppurativa

Lipomembranous fat necrosis in mixed connective tissue disease – subcutaneous multinodular plaques *JAAD 64:1010–1011, 2011*

Malacoplakia *JAAD 23:947–948, 1990*

Sarcoid – keloid-like lesions; subcutaneous nodules *Clin Nuc Med 36:584–586, 2011; Clin Rheumatol 30:1123–1128, 2011; Am J Med 85:731–736, 1988*

METABOLIC DISEASES

Calcinosis cutis, dystrophic *Cutis 60:259–262, 1997;* calcinosis universalis in dermatomyositis *NEJM 349:1246, 2003;* idiopathic calcinosis of the scrotum *NEJM 369:965, 2013;* tumoral calcinosis – progressively growing red-yellow lobulated masses *Ped Derm 27:299–300, 2010*

Cushing's syndrome – buffalo hump

Endometriosis – cutaneous deciduosis *JAAD 43:102–107, 2000*

Goiter

Gout *Cutis 48:445–451, 1991; Ann Rheum Dis 29:461–468, 1970*

Osteoma cutis – platelet osteoma cutis presenting as cutis verticis gyrata *JAAD 64:613–615, 2011*

Xanthomas – tuberous xanthomas *JAAD 19:95–111, 1988; Cutis 59:315–317, 1997*

NEOPLASTIC DISEASES

Acrochordon, giant

Aggressive digital papillary adenocarcinoma – exophytic friable multilobulated tumor *JAAD 60:331–339, 2009*

Angiomyofibroblastoma of vulva *Ginecol Obstet Mex 81:345–348, 2013*

Angiomyxomas *AD 144:1217–1222, 2008*

Apocrine cystadenoma – congenital papillated apocrine cystadenoma *JAAD 11:374–376, 1984*

Apocrine gland carcinoma – axillary mass *Am J Med 115:677–679, 2003*

Atypical fibroxanthoma *AD 135:1113–1118, 1999; JAAD 35:262–264, 1996;* multilobulated, ulcerated, scalp nodule *JAAD 67:1091–1092, 2012*

Basal cell carcinoma *JAAD 54:S50–52, 2006; JAAD 52:149–151, 2005; Cutis 58:289–292, 1996; Neuroradiology 38:575–577, 1996; BJD 127:164–167, 1992; J Derm Surg Oncol 12:459–464, 1986*

Buschke-Lowenstein tumor – giant, multilobulated, disfiguring, exophytic cauliflower-like tumor *JAAD 66:867–880, 2012*

Cervical cysts – branchial cleft anomalies, dermoid cyst, median ectopic thyroid, cervical teratomas, midline cervical clefts *Surg Clin NA 92:583–597, 2012*

Chordoma *AD 133:179–1584, 1997*

Clear cell acanthoma *JAAD 44:314–316, 2001*

Clear cell eccrine porocarcinoma *BJD 149:1059–1063, 2003*

Clear cell hidradenoma (eccrine acrospiroma) – head, neck, upper extremities *Ped Derm 18:356–358, 2001;* giant eccrine acrospiroma *JAAD 23:663–668, 1990*

Clear cell hidradenocarcinoma *JAAD 12:15–20, 1985*

Connective tissue nevus – mountain range-like plaque *JAAD 67:233–239, 2012*

Cylindrocarcinoma *BJD 145:653–656, 2001*

Cylindroma *JAAD 33:199–206, 1995; BJD 145:653–656, 2001; JAAD 19:397–400, 1988;* Blaschko distribution *BJD 166:1376–1378, 2012*

Dermatofibroma – multinodular hemosiderotic dermatofibroma *Dermatologica 181:320–323, 1990*

Dermatofibrosarcoma protuberans *JAAD 65:564–575, 2011; JAAD 64:212–214, 2011; Dermatol Ther 21:428–432, 2008; Cutis 82:325, 343–344, 2008; JAAD 57:548–550, 2007; Sem Cut Med Surg 21:159–165, 2002; JAAD 35:355–374, 1996; Dermatol Z 43:1–28, 1925; Ann Dermatol Syphiligr 5:545–562, 1924;* perianal DFSP *Cutis 87:85–88, 2011;* multilobulated scalp nodule *JAAD 67:861–866, 2012;* subcutaneous DFSP *JAAD 77:503–511, 2017*

Eccrine gland carcinoma *JAAD 20:693–696, 1989*

Eccrine porocarcinoma – multilobulated or cauliflower-like nodule *BJD 152:1051–1055, 2005; JAAD 49:S252–254, 2003; J Derm Surg 25:733–735, 1999; JAAD 35:860–864, 1996*

Eccrine poroma *JAAD 53:539–541, 2005;* giant eccrine poroma *Cutis 88:227–229, 2011; AMA Arch Derm 74:511–521, 1956*

Epidermal nevus – personal observation

Epidermoid cyst – ruptured with scarring; multiloculated epidermoid cyst *BJD 151:943–945, 2004;* proliferating *AD 144:547–552, 2008; Cutan Pathol 22:394–406, 1995*

Exophytic Schneiderian papilloma – frond-like mass within nostril; gray, pink, tan, exophytic, polypoid, verrucous *JAMADerm 153:709–710, 2017*

Fibrous hamartoma of infancy – occurs within first year of life (23% congenital); male:female ratio of 2.4:1; painless shoulder girdle or neck; solitary with rapid growth; 3–5 cm *JAAD 64:579–586, 2011*
Differentiate from:
   Infantile myofibromatosis – 50% congenital; occur within first 2 years of life; male>female; neck>extremities>viscera; solitary; affects skin, bone, soft tissues; generalized myofibromatosis with visceral involvement
   Infantile fibrosarcoma – in first year of life; male>female; deep tissues of extremities; large solitary red painless dome shaped 10–15 cm tumor; vascular and ulcerated appearance; metastases uncommon

Folliculosebaceous cystic hamartoma – multilobulated lesion of nose *The Dermatologist April 2018:47–50*

Ganglion cyst overlying acromioclavicular joint – verrucous multilobulated tumor *JAAD 64:1206–1208, 2011; AJR Roentgenol 178:1445–1449, 2002*

Giant cell fibroblastoma *JAMADerm 150:323–324, 2014*

Giant cell tumor of soft tissue *Cutis 93:278, 286–288, 2014*

Giant cell tumor of the tendon sheath – multilobulated single or multiple *JAAD 43:892, 2000;* nodules of the fingers *J Dermatol 23:290–292, 1996; J Bone Joint Surg Am 66:76–94, 1984*

Giant folliculosebaceous cystic hamartoma – multinodular plaque of scalp *AD 141:1035–1040, 2005*

Hibernoma – giant multilobulated tumor of neck *NEJM 367:1636, 2012*

Infantile digital fibromatosis – pink multilobulated nodule of toe *Ped Dem 26:347–348, 2009*

Intradermal nevus, lobulated *JAAD 24:74–77, 1991*

Kaposi's sarcoma – keloidal Kaposi's sarcoma *JAAD 59:179–206, 2008; AD 141:1311–1316, 2005; BJD 145:847–849, 2001; JAAD 38:143–175, 1998; Dermatology 190:324–326, 1995;* keloidal Kaposi's sarcoma *Dermatology (Basel) 189:271–274, 1994;* lymphangioma-like variant of KS *AD 139:381–386, 2003*

Keloids *J Drugs Dermatol 10:468–480, 2011; Ped Derm 24:280–284, 2007;;* keloids in Ehlers-Danlos syndrome, progeria, Rubinstein-Taybi syndrome *Ped Derm 12:387–389, 1995;* plantar keloid *JAAD 48:131–134, 2003*

Keratoacanthoma *JAAD 19:826–830, 1988;* keratoacanthoma centrifugum marginatum *BJD 163:633–637, 2010*

Leiomyosarcoma *Ped Derm 26:477–479, 2009; J D Surg Oncol 9:283–287, 1983*

Leukemia cutis, including congenital leukemia cutis *JAAD 34:375–378, 1996;* chronic lymphocytic leukemia – multilobulated helices *AD 147:1443–1448, 2011;* acute myelogenous leukemia – mountain range lesions with leonine facies *Cutis 102:266,271–272, 2018*

Lipoblastomatosis *Ped Derm 23:152–156, 2006*

Lipomas, multiple

Lymphocytoma cutis

Lymphoma – cutaneous T-cell lymphoma *JAAD 70:205–220, 2014;; JAAD 25:345–349, 1991;* HTLV-1 (keloid-like) *JAAD 34:69–76, 1996;* cutaneous type adult T-cell leukemia/lymphoma – multilobulated giant purple tumor *JAAD 57:S115–117, 2007;* pilotropic (follicular) CTCL *AD 138:191–198, 2002;* gamma/delta T cell lymphoma *AD 136:1024–1032, 2000;* CD30+ lymphoma of AIDS; primary cutaneous follicle center lymphoma *JAAD 69:343–354, 2013; JAAD 64:135–143, 2011; AD 143:1520–1526, 2007; BJD 157:1205–1211, 2007;* cutaneous B-cell lymphoma – multilobulated red nodules *BJD 177:287–289, 2017; Cutis 94:3217,249–251, 2014;* B-cell lymphoma *JAAD 29:359–362, 1993; JAAD 16:518–526, 1987;* large B-cell lymphoma *BJD 149:542–553, 2003;* primary cutaneous large B-cell lymphoma of the legs *BJD 159:145–151, 2008; AD 132:1304–1308, 1996;* primary cutaneous marginal zone B-cell lymphoma *AD 145:1183–1188, 2009;* reticulohistiocytoma of the dorsum (B-cell lymphoma) *JAAD 18:259–272, 1988;* primary cutaneous epidermotropic CD8+ T-cell lymphoma – mixture of patches, plaques, papulonodules with central ulceration, necrosis, and hemorrhage *JAAD 62:300–307, 2010;* primary cutaneous follicle center lymphoma with diffuse CD 30 expression – papules, plaques, nodules, multilobulated scalp tumor *JAAD 71:548–554, 2014;* Burkitt's lymphoma – multiple subcutaneous mountain range nodules *JAAD 64:1196–1197, 2011;;* primary cutaneous follicle center cell lymphoma – multilobulated nodules, red plaques of scalp, nodules of head and neck,

papules of head and neck *JAAD 70:1010–1020, 2014;* extranodal NK/T-cell lymphoma, nasal type – multilobulated giant tumor of leg *JAMADerm 150:1109–1110, 2014;* Epstein-Barr virus associated plasmablastic lymphoma (HIV-defining lesion) – ulcerated fungating giant perianal tumor *Cutis 103:328,333–334, 2019; BJD 174:398–401, 2016*

Malignant blue nevus; *JAAD 19:712–722, 1988*

Malignant fibrous histiocytoma

Malignant histiocytosis X *Cancer 54:347–352, 1984*

Malignant proliferating trichilemmal tumor *BJD 150:156–157, 2004;* of scalp *Indian J Surg 78:493–495, 2016*

Melanocytic nevus – giant congenital melanocytic nevi with benign proliferative nodules *BJD 176:1131–1143, 2017; AD 140:83–88, 2004;* atypical proliferative nodules in congenital melanocytic nevi of scalp *BJD 165:1138–1142, 2011*

Melanoma *Curr Prob Derm 14:41–70, 2002; Cutis 69:353–356, 2002; Semin Oncol 2:5–118, 1975;* polypoid melanoma *JAAD 23:880–884, 1990;* animal type melanoma *AD 145:55–62, 2009;* amelanotic melanoma arising in large congenital melanocytic nevus – multilobulated vascular nodule *JAAD 68:913–925, 2013;* anal mucosal melanoma – perianal multilobulated skin colored nodule *Cutis 89:112, 116, 2012;* amelanotic melanoma – multilobulated red nodules of lower lip *Cutis 92:250–252, 2013*

Melanoma of the soft parts (clear cell sarcoma) *JAAD 38:815–819, 1998*

Merkel cell carcinoma – multilobulated red nodules of scalp *AD 145:494–495, 2009;* of nose *AD 149:501–502, 2013*

Metastases – carcinoma telangiectoides; lung cancer with emboli in pulmonary venous circulation; nodules of scalp resembling cylindromas; *Cancer 19:162–168, 1966;* cutaneous metastases (adenocarcinoma) – lymphangioma-like lesions *JAAD 30:1031–1032, 1994;* metastatic prostate carcinoma mimicking cylindromas *JAAD 33:161–182, 1995;* rhinophyma-like metastatic carcinoma *Cutis 57:33–36, 1996;* breast carcinoma; Sister Mary Joseph nodule – multilobulated nodule of umbilicus; metastatic gastric adenocarcinoma *Cutis 85:90–92, 2010*

Mucinous carcinoma of skin *JAAD 49:941–943, 2003; JAAD 36:323–326, 1997*

Mucinous nevus (connective tissue hamartoma) *AD 141:897–902, 2005*

Multiple myeloma – multinodular violaceous fungating tumor *JAAD 74:878–884, 2016*

Myofibroma – personal observation

Myxoid dermatofibrosarcoma protuberans – multilobulated or sessile nodule *AD 147:857–862, 2011*

Nerve sheath myxoma *AD 145:195–200, 2009* Neural fibrolipoma *AD 135:707–712, 1999*

Neuroectodermal tumors – multiple primitive neuroectodermal tumors *JAAD 31:356–361, 1994*

Neurofibroma – diffuse neurofibroma *JAAD 48:938–940, 2003;* plexiform neurofibroma

Neurogenic sarcoma

Nevus lipomatosis superficialis – mountain range-like lesions *Ped Derm 37:352–354, 2020; BJD 156:380–381, 2007; Cutis 72:237–238, 2003; AD 128:1395–1400, 1992*

Nevus sebaceous – personal observation

Nevus sebaceous with tubular apocrine adenoma and syringocystadenoma papilliferum – velvety, grouped nodules of breast *BJD 156:1397–1399, 2007;* trichoblastoma, basal cell carcinoma, eccrine poroma, sebaceous carcinoma, leiomyosarcoma, syringocystadenoma papilliferum

Pilomatrixoma

Plaque-like myofibroblastic tumor of infancy – multinodular red-brown plaque *Ped Derm 34:176–179, 2017*

Plasmacytoma – trauma-induced secondary cutaneous plasmacytoma *AD 146:1301–1306, 2010*

Pleomorphic fibrohistiocytoma – personal observation

Plexiform schwannoma of the foot *Eur Radiol 9:1653–1655, 1999*

Polymorphous sweat gland carcinoma *JAAD 46:914–916, 2002*

Primary cutaneous alveolar rhabdomyosarcoma – annular multinodular mass of chest *Ped Derm 37:184–186, 2020*

Primitive myxoid mesenchymal tumor of infancy – multilobulated plaque/tumor *Ped Derm 27:635–637, 2010*; differential diagnosis includes rhabdomyosarcoma, infantile desmoids fibromatosis, fibromyxoid sarcoma, low grade myofibrosarcoma, congenital infantile fibrosarcoma

Proliferative fasciitis *SKINmed 12:111–112, 2014*

Proliferating pilar cyst *JAAD 69:849–850, 2013; Cutis 48:49–52, 1991*

Regressing atypical histiocytosis *AD 126:1609–1616, 1990*

Rhabdomyomatous mesenchymal hamartoma – papillomatous lesion *Ped Derm 32:256–262, 2015*

Alveolar rhabdomyosarcoma, metastatic red multinodular ulcerated plaque *Ped Derm 33:225–226, 2016*

Congenital rhabdomyosarcoma – multilobulated cobblestoned nodule of bridge of nose *Ped Derm 36:747–749, 2019*

Salivary pleomorphic adenoma *Cutis 63:167–168, 1999*

Malignant schwannoma – personal observation

Sclerotic fibroma – personal observation

Sebaceous carcinoma *Cutis 91:169,175–176, 2013; JAAD 47:950–953, 2002;* cystic sebaceous carcinoma *J Drugs Dermatol 6:540–543, 2007*

Sebaceoma – multilobulated facial nodule *AD 145:1325–1330, 2009*
Seborrheic keratosis

Spindle cell tumor

Squamous cell carcinoma – multiloculated milia *Cutis 89:45–47, 2012;* squamous cell carcinoma associated with lichen planus – multilobulated, ulcerated, red nodule and plaque *JAAD 71:698–707, 2014;* genital squamous cell carcinoma – cerebriform (mulberry-like); multilobulated nodules *BJD 171:779–785, 2014;* cauliflower-like tumor; complicating venous stasis ulcers *South Med J 58:779–781, 1965*

Stewart-Treves angiosarcoma – reddish-blue macules and/or nodules which become polypoid; pachydermatous changes, blue nodules, telangiectasias, palpable subcutaneous mass, ulcer; red-brown or ecchymotic patch, nodules, plaques in lymphedematous limb *Cancer 1:64–81, 1948; JAAD 77:1009–1020, 2017; JAAD 67:1342–1348, 2012*

Syringocystadenoma papilliferum – cerebriform multilobulated pink nodules of legs *AD 148:1411–1416, 2012;* giant multilobulated linear tumor *Ped Derm 26:758–759, 2009;* linear multilobulated verrucous plaque *Ped Derm 28:61–62, 2011*

Syringomatous carcinoma – multilobulated digital nodule *BJD 144:438–439, 2001*

Torus palatinus

Tumoral melanosis – multilobulated nodule as marker of regressed melanoma *BJD 175:391–393, 2016*

PARANEOPLASTIC DISORDERS

Necrobiotic xanthogranuloma with paraproteinemia *JAAD 52:729–731, 2005*

PRIMARY CUTANEOUS DISEASES

Acne conglobata *JAAD 62:861–863, 2010*

Acne keloidalis *JAAD 56:699–701, 2007*

Acne rosacea – rhinophyma *NEJM 367:1838, 2012*

Cutis verticis gyrata – acromegaly, Apert syndrome, amyloidosis, leukemia, myxedema, syphilis, pachydermoperiostosis, tuberous sclerosis

Cystic acne – exophytic abscesses of chin in follicular occlusion triad *JAAD 48:S47–50, 2003*

Endometriosis (villar nodule) – umbilical multilobulated red nodule *AD 148:1331–1332, 2012*

Erythema elevatum diutinum *JAMADerm 153:315–316, 2017; BJD 143:415–420, 2000;* keloid-like lesions of erythema elevatum diutinum in AIDS *AD 144:933–938, 2008; JAAD 28:919–922, 1993*

Follicular mucinosis *JAAD 20:441–446, 1989*

Granuloma annulare, including subcutaneous granuloma annulare

Hailey-Hailey disease – vegetative multilobulated malodorous friable plaques of cheek *JAAD 65:223–224, 2011*

Lichen simplex chronicus – personal observation

Myospherulosis (subcutaneous spherulocystic disease) – multilobulated abdominal nodule *AD 138:1309–1314, 2002*

Periumbilical pseudoxanthoma elasticum *JAAD 39:338–344, 1998*

Pseudofolliculitis barbae with keloids

SYNDROMES

Benign symmetrical lipomatosis *AD 126:235–240, 1990; JAAD 18:359–362, 1988*

Birt-Hogg-Dube syndrome – trichoblastoma; multilobulated scalp nodule *BJD 160:1350–1353, 2009*

Blue rubber bleb nevus syndrome – personal observation

Buschke-Ollendorff syndrome – connective tissue nevi and osteopoikilosis; single or multiple yellow, white, or skin colored papules, nodules, plaques of extremities; mountain range skin colored nodules; *LEMD3* mutation *BJD 166:900–903, 2012; Ped Derm 28:447–450, 2011; JAAD 48:600–601, 2003; Derm Wochenschr 86:257–262, 1928*

Carney complex – cutaneous myxoma *AD 141:916–918, 2005*

Delleman-Oorthuys syndrome *Clin Genet 25:470–472, 1984*

Dercum's disease (adiposis dolorosa) – painful peri-articular lipomas and ecchymoses; lipomas feel like "bag of worms" *JAAD 44:132–136, 2001*

Encephalocranial lipomatosis (nevus psiloliparus) – hairless with abundant fatty tissue *JAAD 63:1–22, 2010*

Familial multiple lipomatosis *JAAD 15:275–279, 1986*

Goeminne syndrome – X-linked; torticollis, keloids, cryptorchidism, renal dysplasia *AD 137:1429–1434, 2001; Acta Genet Med (Roma) 17:439–467, 1968*

Goltz's syndrome – raspberry-like papillomas of lips, perineum, ears, fingers, toes, buccal mucosa, and esophagus

Hennekam syndrome – autosomal recessive; intestinal lymphangiectasia, lymphedema of legs and genitalia, gigantic scrotum and penis, multilobulated lymphatic ectasias, small mouth, narrow palate, gingival hypertrophy, tooth anomalies, thick lips, agenesis of ear, pre-auricular pits, wide flat nasal bridge, frontal upsweep, platybasia, hypertelorism, pterygium colli, hirsutism, bilateral single palmar crease, mild mental retardation, facial anomalies, growth retardation, pulmonary, cardiac, hypogammaglobulinemia *Ped Derm 23:239–242, 2006*

Infantile myofibromatosis *Ped Derm 27:29–33, 2010*

Juvenile hyaline fibromatosis – infiltration and multinodularity of nose; mutation of capillary morphogenesis protein 2 gene *BJD 157:1037–1039, 2007*

Multiple lipomas due to intracranial lesions (Frohlich syndrome)

Lipomas, multiple Lipomatosis of Touraine and Renault

Maffucci's syndrome– multilobulated blue lesion; deformed hands; post-zygotic somatic mutations in isocitrate dehydrogenase (*IDH1*); enchondromas and spindle cell hemangioendotheliomas; cancers associated in Maffucci's syndrome include lymphangiosarcoma, fibrosarcoma, angiosarcoma, osteosarcoma, mesenchymal ovarian tumors, gliomas, breast cancer, pancreatic cancer, and liver adenocarcinoma *Ped Derm 36:947–948, 2019*

Michelin tire baby syndrome – smooth muscle hamartomas *JAAD 28:364–370, 1993;* nevus lipomatosis superficialis *AD 115:978–979, 1979; AD 100:320–323, 1969*

Muir-Torre syndrome – personal observation

Multicentric reticulohistiocytosis – digital papule; knuckle pads; yellow papules and plaques *JAAD 44:373–375, 2001;*

AD 126:251–252, 1990; Oral Surg Oral Med Oral Pathol 65:721–725, 1988; Pathology 17:601–608, 1985; JAAD 11:713–723, 1984; AD 97:543–547, 1968

Muscular dystrophy – pseudo-athletic appearance

Neurofibromatosis type I – plexiform neurofibromas ("bag of worms") *JAAD 61:1–14, 2009*

Neurolipomatosis Alsberg

Nodular lipomatosis of Krabbe and Bartels

Noonan's syndrome – webbed neck, short stature, malformed ears, nevi, keloids, transient lymphedema, ulerythema ophryogenes, keratosis follicularis spinulosa decalvans *JAAD 46:161–183, 2002; J Med Genet 24:9–13, 1987*

Phakomatosis pigmentokeratotica – multilobulated pink nodules representing connective tissue nevus *Ped Derm 25:76–80, 2008*

Proteus syndrome – multiple lipomas, connective tissue nevi of palms and soles; somatic mosaic mutation of *AKT1 NEJM 365:611–619, 2011;Ped Derm 11:222–226, 1994;* multilobulated cerebriform scalp nodule (connective tissue nevus) *JAAD 67:890–897, 2012*

Pseudolipomatosis of Verneuil and Patain

Rubinstein-Taybi syndrome – keloids; CREB-binding protein (transcriptional coactivator) *AD 137:1429–1434, 2001*

SOLAMEN syndrome (segmental overgrowth, lipomatosis, arteriovenous malformation, and epidermal nevus) *Eur J Hum Genet 15:767–773, 2007*

Steatocystoma multiplex

Tuberous sclerosis – fibrous cephalic plaque of scalp – multipapillated firm plaque *JAMADerm 155:1071–1072, 2019;* giant angiofibromas *JAAD 67:1319–1326, 2012;* adenoma sebaceum *JAAD 20:918–920, 1989;* non-symmetrical subcutaneous lipomatosis; Koenen's tumors; folliculocystic and collagen hamartoma – comedo-like openings, multilobulated cysts, scalp cysts and nodules *JAAD 66:617–621, 2012*

Turner's syndrome – keloids *JAAD 74:231–244, 2016; JAAD 46:161–183, 2002; West J Med 137:32–44, 1982;* multiple piloma-

trixomas; facial papules; may be multilobulated *JAMA Derm 149:559–564, 2013*

TRAUMA

Verrucous hyperplasia of the stump

Verruciform xanthoma – red-orange plaque; multilobulated, vegetative, cobblestoned; perigenital; seen in KID, CHILD, syndromes and recessive dystrophic epidermolysis bullosa; usually at site of friction or frequent trauma *Ped Derm 37:176–179, 2020*

VASCULAR

Agminated eruptive pyogenic granuloma-like lesions over congenital vascular stains (capillary malformations) *Ped Derm 29:186–190, 2012*

Angiokeratoma *AD 143:318–325, 2007*

Angiosarcoma *Cutis 83:91–94, 2009;* violaceous multilobulated tumor *JAAD 65:448–449, 2011*

Angiolymphoid hyperplasia with eosinophilia *AD 136:837–839, 2000; JAAD 37:887–920, 1997; Cutis 60:281–282, 1997*

Blue rubber bleb nevus syndrome – perianal vascular lesions *Ped Derm 16:222–227, 1999;* adult onset *SKINMed 13:406–409, 2015; Case Rep Surg 2014; 683684*

Elephantiasis nostras of penis *AD 137:1095–1100, 2001*

Glomus tumors – multiple or plaque type; hemi-facial *JAAD 45:239–245, 2001; Ped Derm 18:223–226, 2001; AD 127:1717–1722, 1991*

Granulomatosis with polyangiitis *Dermatol Clin 33:509–630, 2015*

Hemangioma

Hemolymphangioma

Klippel-Trenaunay-Weber syndrome – aneurysmal venous dilatation *JAAD 18:1169–1172, 1988*

Lipomyxangioma

Lymphangiectasia (acquired lymphangioma) – due to scarring processes such as recurrent infections, radiotherapy, scrofuloderma, sclerederma, keloids, tumors, tuberculosis, repeated trauma *BJD 132:1014–1016, 1996*

Lymphangioma circumscriptum – frog spawn-like appearance *BJD 83:519–527, 1970*

Lymphatic malformation – multilobulated nodule with edematous vulva *Cutis 93:297–300, 2014;* superficial microcystic lymphatic malformation – pigmented, multinodular sessile tumor of leg *Ped Derm 32:867–868, 2015*

Lymphedema of vulva – chronic infection, recurrent streptococcal cellulitis *Genital Skin Disorders, Fischer and Margesson, CV Mosby, 1998, p. 222–223*

Lymphostasis verrucosa cutis

PHACES syndrome – giant multilobulated hemangioma with hemihypertrophy of face

Port wine stain with epithelial and mesenchymal hamartomas *JAAD 50:608–612, 2004*

Pyogenic granuloma

Spindle cell hemangioma – multilobulated violeaceous nodule *AD 142:641–646, 2006*

Tufted angioma *Advances in Dermatol 24:105–124, 2008*

Venous malformations *BJD 162:350–356, 2010; AD 139:1409–1416, 2003*

NODULES, MULTIPLE, SUBCUTANEOUS

AUTOIMMUNE DISEASES AND DISEASES OF IMMUNE DYSFUNCTION

Dermatomyositis – calcinosis cutis *AD 140:365–366, 2004;* juvenile dermatomyositis with calcinosis cutis *BJD 144:894–897, 2001;* panniculitis *Pan Afr Med J 33:149, 2016*

Lupus erythematosus – nodular mucinosis of SLE *Cutis 72:366–371, 2003; BJD 137:450–453, 1997; J Rheumatol 21:940–941, 1994; JAAD 27:312–315, 1992; Int J Derm 31:649–652, 1992;* panniculitis *Cureus 12:e6790, 2020*

Morphea profunda *J Dermatol 46:354–357, 2019*

Rheumatoid arthritis – rheumatoid nodules *JAAD 46:161–183, 2002;* rheumatoid nodulosis *Arthritis Rheum 29:1278–1283, 1986; J Rheumatol 6:286–292, 1979;* rheumatoid vasculitis *BJD 147:905–913, 2002*

Still's disease (juvenile rheumatoid nodule) *Ann Rheum Dis 17:278–283, 1958*

CONGENITAL LESIONS

Congenital cartilaginous rests of the neck *Cutis 58:293–294, 1996*

Fibrous hamartoma of infancy – multiple subcutaneous nodules *AD 144:547–552, 2008*

DRUG-INDUCED

DRESS – lymphadenopathy *Cutis 89:180–182, 2012*

Exenatide *AACE Clin Case Rep 5:e197–200, 2019*

HAART – induction of multiple lipomas *AD 143:1596–1597, 2007*

Imatinib-induced Epstein-Barr virus and B-cell lymphoproliferative disease *AD 143:1222–1223, 2007*

Indinavir – multiple angiolipomas due to protease inhibitors *JAAD 42:129–131, 2000; BJD 143:1113–1114, 2000*

L-asparaginase – acute pancreatitis *Ped Derm 26:47–49, 2009*

Methotrexate-induced accelerated rheumatoid nodulosis *Medicine 80:271–278, 2001; J Dermatol 26:46–464, 1999; JAAD 39:359–362, 1998*

Minocycline-induced p-ANCA+ cutaneous polyarteritis nodosa – multiple subcutaneous nodules of the legs *Eur J Dermatol 13:366–368, 2003; JAAD 44:198–206, 2001*

Zidovudine – multiple subcutaneous nodules due to insect bites *JAAD 46:284–293, 2002*

EXOGENOUS AGENTS

Aluminum-containing allergen extracts *Eur J Dermatol 11:138–140, 2001*

Facial lipogranulomas – self-injection of Vitamin A oil – facial nodules *Int J Womens Dermatol 5:126–128, 2018*

Iatrogenic calcium deposits – calcium infusion for tetany *Arch Pediatr 53:215–223, 1936;* pitressin tannate *Br J Radiol 57:921–922, 1984*

Iodide mumps – iodine contrast agent; giant acute inflammatory swelling of submandibular, sublingual, or parotid glands *Ann Int Med 145:155–156, 2006; Circulation 104:2384, 2001; Acta Radiol 36:82–84, 1995; Am J Roentgenol 159:1099–1100, 1992; JAMA 213:2271–2272, 1970; NEJM 255:433–434, 1956*

Oleomas – multiple subcutaneous oleomas due to injection with sesame seed oil *BJD 149:1289–1290, 2003; JAAD 42:292–294, 2000*

Polyvinyl pyrrolidone injections

Siliconomas – distant migration following breast implant rupture *Plast Reconstr Surg Glob Open 4:e1011, 2016*

INFECTIONS

Acanthamoeba J Clin Inf Dis 20:1207–1216, 1995

Actinomycetoma (actinomycosis) (*A. israelii*) – primary cutaneous – subcutaneous nodules with draining sinuses *NEJM 372:264, 2015; Hum Pathol 4:319–330, 1973*

African histoplasmosis

Alveolar echinococcosis *JAAD 34:873–877, 1996*

Bacillary angiomatosis *BJD 126:535–541, 1992*

Botryomycosis *Indian Dermatol Online J 10:311–315, 2019*

Candida sepsis *JAAD 80:869–880, 2019*

Cat scratch disease *AIDS 3:751–753, 1989*

Chagas' disease – painful subcutaneous nodules *Transplant Proc 37:2793–2798, 2005*

Chromomycosis *Mycoses 31:343–352, 1988*

Cryptococcosis – renal transplant recipient

Cysticercosis *Indian Dermatol Online J 10:574–576, 2019; JAAD 50:S14–17, 2004; Int J Dermatol 34:574–579, 1995*

Fusarium solani, disseminated *JAAD 47:659–666, 2002; J Med Vet Mycol 24:105–111, 1986*

Leishmania JAAD 36:847–849, 1997; Int J Dermatol 26:300–304, 1987; diffuse cutaneous leishmaniasis; *L. martiniquensis* – multiple subcutaneous fibrotic *BJD 173:663–670, 2015*

Leprosy – reactional state in tuberculoid leprosy *JAMADerm 153:313–314, 2017; Indian J Lepr 65:239–242, 1993*

Loiasis *Clin Infect Dis 29:680–682, 1999*

Lymphogranuloma venereum – sign of the groove

Mucormycosis *J Cut Pathol 41:483–486, 2014*

Mycetoma

Mycobacterium abscesses J Cut Med Surg 5:28–32, 2001

Mycobacterium avium complex – subcutaneous nodules *Rev Inf Dis 11:625–628, 1989*

Mycobacterium avium-intracellulare BJD 142:789–793, 2000; J Dermatol 25:384–390, 1998; BJD 130:785–790, 1994

Mycobacterium chelonae AD 123:1603–1604, 1987; kansasii, haemophilum BJD 131:379, 1994; scrofulaceum, marinum, fortuitum, abscessus, avium-intracellulare Clin Inf Dis 19:263–273, 1994

Mycobacterium tuberculosis – tuberculous cervical adenitis *Ped Derm 37:29–39, 2020;* renal transplant recipient *Transplant Proc 51:1618–1520, 2019;* nodular tuberculid *Ann Dermatol 29:95–99, 2017*

Nocardia – abscesses *J Dermatol 26:829–833, 1999;* lymphocutaneous nocardiosis *Acta DV 74:447–448, 1994;* actinomycetomas – multiple subcutaneous nodules; *N. brasiliensis; Actinomadura madurae BJD 158:698–674, 2008*

Onchocerciasis – onchocercomas *AD 140:1161–1166, 2004; BJD 121:187–198, 1989*

Paragonimiasis westermani – subcutaneous migratory masses *AXXCBFZZZ 31:200–203, 2019*

Phaeohyphomycosis (*Exophiala*) – nodules of finger and multiple subcutaneous nodules of the foot *JAAD 61:977–985, 2009*

Pseudomonas aeruginosa Cutis 63:161–163, 1999

Rheumatic fever *JAAD 8:724–728, 1983*

Rhinosporidiosis *Indian Heart J 45:463–467, 1993; Indian J Pathol Microbiol 40:95–98, 1997*

Sporotrichosis – multiple disseminated subcutaneous nodules *Rev Soc Bras Med Trop 50:871–873, 2017*

Streptocerciasis – *Mansonella streptocerca* – similar rash to onchocerciasis; acute or lichenified papules with widespread lichenification and hypopigmented macules

Syphilis – subcutaneous secondary syphilis *J Dermatol 44:1401–1403, 2017*; scalp nodules *Int J Dermatol 58:e203–204, 2019; Clin Dermatol 23:555–564, 2005*

Toxocariasis – (*T. canis, T. cati, T. leonensis*) visceral larva migrans – migrating panniculitis *JAAD 59:1031–1042, 2008; Dermatologica 144:129–143, 1972*

Trichophyton rubrum – numerous lower extremity subcutaneous nodules *BMC Inf Dis 19:271, 2019*

Yaws – tertiary – gumma; multiple subcutaneous nodules; overlying skin ulcerates with purulent discharge; atrophic pigmented scars

· Zygomycosis – subcutaneous zygomycosis *JAAD 30:904–908, 1994*

INFILTRATIVE LESIONS

Amyloidosis – subcutaneous nodular amyloidosis *Hum Pathol 32:346–348, 2001;* beta-2 microglobulin amyloidosis – shoulder pain, carpal tunnel syndrome, flexor tendon deposits of hands, lichenoid papules, hyperpigmentation, subcutaneous nodules (amyloidomas) *Int J Exp Clin Inves 4:187–211, 1997; South Med J 88:876–878, 1995; Arch Pathol Lab Med 118:651–653, 1994; J Clin Pathol 46:771–772, 1993; Nephron 55:312–315, 1990; Nephron 53:73–75, 1989;* dialysis-related beta-2 microglobulin amyloidosis of buttocks *BJD 149:400–404, 2003;* bilateral popliteal tumors *Am J Kidney dis 12:323–325, 1988;* multiple primary cutaneous nodular amyloidosis *Dermatol Online J May 15, 2017*

Atypical cutaneous mucinosis *SKINMed 16:428–431, 2018*

Cutaneous mucinosis of infancy – skin colored rubbery nodules *Ped Derm 27:299–300, 2010; AD 116:198–200, 1980*

Hereditary progressive mucinous histiocytosis – infantile dermal nodules of scalp, trunk, and extremities *Dermatology 36:958–960, 1997*

Juvenile hyaline fibromatosis (infantile systemic hyalinosis) *Ped Derm 23:458–464, 2006*

Langerhans cell histiocytosis *Int Med Case Rep J 11:65–68, 2018; Clin Exp Dermatol 27:135–137, 2002*

Mastocytosis – vulvar nodules *J Ped Adolesc Gyn 31:156–157, 2018*

Self-healing juvenile cutaneous mucinosis – red nodules of face, scalp, hand; macrodactyly (enlarged thumbs); periarticular papules and nodules, painful polyarthritis; linear ivory white papules, multiple subcutaneous nodules, indurated edema of periorbital and zygomatic areas *JAAD 55:1036–1043, 2006; JAAD 44:273–281, 2001; AD 131:459–461, 1995; Ann DV 107:51–57, 1980; Lyon Med 230:470–474, 1973;* in adulthood *Am J Dermatopathol 41:60–64, 2019*

Juvenile xanthogranuloma, micronodular *AD 148:531–536, 2012*

INFLAMMATORY DISEASES

Fat necrosis – nodular cystic fat necrosis *JAAD 21:493–498, 1989;* membranous fat necrosis *AD 129:1331, 1334, 1993*

Hidradenitis suppurativa *Derm Surg 26:638–643, 2000; BJD 141:231–239, 1999*

IgG4 disease *J Dermatol 44:288–296, 2017; JAAD 75:197–202, 2016*

Lymphadenopathy, reactive

Proliferative fasciitis – multiple rapidly growing painful subcutaneous nodules in children following trauma; spontaneous resolution *AD 144:255–260, 2008; JAAD 55:1036–1043, 2006;*

Cancer 36:1450–1458, 1975

Proliferative myositis *Clin Exp Dermatol 22:101–103, 1997*

Relapsing polychondritis – nodules of limbs *Medicine 80:173–179, 2000*

Rosai-Dorfman disease (sinus histiocytosis with massive lymphadenopathy) *Int J Derm 37:271–274, 1998*

Sarcoidosis (Darier-Roussy sarcoid) *JAAD 72:924–926, 2015; JAAD 54:55–60, 2006; Clin Exp Dermatol 19:356–358, 1994; Ann Dermatol Syphil 5:144–149, 1904*Subcutaneous fat necrosis of the newborn – red to bluish-red firm nodules and/or plaques; buttocks, thighs, shoulders, back, cheeks, and arms *Clin Pediatr 20:748–750, 1981*

Whipple's disease – multiple subcutaneous nodules mimicking rheumatoid nodules; macular and reticulated erythema; Addisonian hyperpigmentation; *Tropheryma whipplei JAAD 60:277–288, 2009*

METABOLIC DISEASES

Albright's osteodystrophy – with osteoma cutis; painful subcutaneous nodules and shortened digits *Ped Derm 36: 944–945, 2019*

Calciphylaxis *Case Rep Nephrol Dial 9:119–125, 2019*

Cerebrotendinous xanthomatosis – mutation of sterol 27-hydroxylas (mitochondrial enzyme); increased cholestanol *BJD 142:378–380, 2000*

Dermal hematopoiesis, neonatal *Ped Derm 14:383–386, 1997;* extramedullary hematopoiesis *JAAD 58:703–706, 2008*

Gout *AD 134:499–504, 1998; Arthritis Care Res 9:74–77, 1996*

Nephrogenic fibrosing dermopathy (nephrogenic systemic fibrosis) *BJD 158:607–610, 2008; JAAD 48:42–47, 2003*

Oxalate granulomas *BJD 128:690–692, 1993*

Pancreatic fat necrosis *Am J Med Sci 319:68–72, 2000*

Pretibial myxedema

Primary osteoma cutis – generalized osteomas; unilateral anodontia, hemihypertrophy, linear basal cell nevus

Pseudohypothyroidism type 1A – osteoma cutis *World J Clin Cases 8:589–593, 2020*

Tendinous xanthomas/tuberous xanthomas

Cerebrotendinous xanthomatosis – periarticular tendon xanthomas; mutation in sterol 27-hydroxylase; increased serum cholestanol and urinary bile alcohols; normal serum cholesterol *JAAD 45:292–295, 2001*

   Phytosterolemia (beta sitosterolemia)
   Familial hypercholesterolemia
   Familial combined hyperlipidemia
   Familial type III hyperlipoproteinemia

Weber-Christian disease or recurrent nodular panniculitis *Rev Clin Esp 196:405–406, 410, 1996(Sp)*

NEOPLASTIC DISEASES

Angiolipoma – arms, legs, abdomen *AD 126:666–667, 669, 1990; AD 82:924–931, 1960*

Carcinoid tumors *Tumori 76:44–47, 1990*

Cylindromas *AD 145:1277–1284, 2009*

Dermatofibroma – metastasizing cellular dermatofibroma *Am J Surg Pathol 20:1361–1367, 1996*

Dermatofibrosarcoma protuberans *J Pak Med Assoc 69:113–115, 2019*

Elastofibromas *JAAD 50:126–129, 2004*

Folliculosebaceous cystic hamartomas *AD 139:803–808, 2003*

Granular cell tumors *AD 140:353–358, 2004; AD 140:353–358, 2004; JAAD 47:S180–182, 2002; BJD 143:906–907, 2000; JAAD 36:327–330, 1997; AD 126:1051–1056, 1990*

Infantile myofibromatosis – single or multiple (hundreds); head, neck, trunk *Ped Derm 18:305–307, 2001; JAAD 41:508, 1999; AD 134:625–630, 1998; Cancer 48:1807–1818, 1981*

Kaposi's sarcoma – African endemic lymphadenopathic KS *AD 144:1217–1222, 2008*

Keratoacanthomas of Ferguson-Smith

Leiomyomas

Leiomyosarcomas *J Exp Clin Cancer Res 17:405–407, 1998; Am J Pediatr Hematol Oncol 14:265–268, 1992*

Leukemia – leukemia cutis (AML, AMML) *AD 134:1477–1482, 1998;* chronic lymphocytic leukemia – multiple lymph nodes; chronic myelogenous leukemia – neutrophilic panniculitis *BMJ Case Rep Oct 8, 2019*

Lipoblastomas, including congenital lipoblastomatosis *BJD 143:694, 2000; Ped Derm 15:210–213, 1998*

Familial lipomatosis *Acta Chir Belg 110:98–100, 2010; JAAD 15:275–279, 1986; Acta DV 60:509–513, 1980; Br J Clin Pract 28:101–102, 1974;* of shoulder girdle *Ann Int Med 117:749–752, 1992;* spindle cell lipomas *JAAD 48:82–85, 2003;* familial multiple lipomatosis *Cutis 79:227–232, 2007*

Lymphoma – Sezary syndrome – lymphadenopathy *NEJM 369:559–569, 2013;* intravascular B-cell lymphoma mimicking erythema nodosum *J Cutan Pathol 27:413–418, 2000;* subcutaneous panniculitis-like T-cell lymphoma *JAAD 50:465–459, 2004;* cytophagic histiocytic panniculitis and subcutaneous panniculitis-like T-cell lymphoma *JAAD 50:S18–22, 2004; AD 136:889–896, 2000;* gamma/delta T-cell lymphoma *AD 136:1024–1032, 2000;* CD8+ T-cell lymphoma *JAAD 53:1093–1095, 2005;* lymphadenopathy; primary cutaneous natural killer/T-cell nasal type *BJD 160:205–207, 2009;* intravascular B-cell lymphoma – red patch overlying multiple subcutaneous nodules *JAAD 61:885–888, 2009;;* Burkitt's lymphoma – multiple subcutaneous mountain range nodules *JAAD 64:1196–1197, 2011;* cutaneous extranodal natural killer T-cell lymphoma – multiple violaceous or red nodules of extremities, subcutaneous nodules, cellulitis, abscess-like lesions *JAAD 70:1002–1009, 2014;* diffuse large cell B-cell lymphoma – multiple red subcutaneous nodules of neck *BJD 173:134–145, 2015*

Melanoma, metastatic *SKINmed 10:373–383, 2012*

Metastases – multiple primary sites; squamous cell carcinoma of the cervix *Int J Gynecol Cancer 11:78–80, 2001;* metastatic carcinoid *AD 141:93–98, 2005;* prostate *AD 143:937–942, 2007; Dermatology Online J 11:24, 2005;* lymphadenopathy; lung cancer *Proc (Baylor Univ Med Ctr)33:67–68, 2019*

Multiple calcifying aponeurotic fibroma *Ter Arkh 90:91–95, 2018*

Multiple myeloma *Clin Nuc Med 44:746–747, 2019*

Neurilemmomatosis *BJD 125:466–468, 1991*

Neuromas – multiple palisaded encapsulated neuromas *JAAD 62:358–359, 2010*

Pilomatrixomas – multiple pilomatrixomas associated with myotonic dystrophy (Curschmann-Batten-Steinert disease) *Ped Derm 28:74–76, 2011;* Gardner's syndrome *Ped Derm 12:331–335, 1995;* Turner's syndrome; Trisomy 9; Rubenstein-Taybi syndrome *Ped Derm 11:21–25, 1994;* Sotos syndrome, Kabuki syndrome

Plantar fibromatosis *Cutis 68:219–222, 2001*

Post-transplantation lymphoproliferative disorder *AD 140:1140–1164, 2004*

Progressive nodular fibrosis of the skin *Ann DV 104:141–146, 1977*

Pseudo-cutaneous T-cell lymphoma in HIV disease – deep nodules *AD 131:1281–1288, 1995*

Schwannomatosis *BJD 148:804–809, 2003*

Spindle cell hemangioendothelioma – multiple subcutaneous nodules; palmar giant cobblestoning; hypertrophy of hand *Cutis 79:125–128, 2007*

Squamous cell carcinoma/keratoacanthoma – recurrent on legs of elderly women

Stewart-Treves tumor (angiosarcoma post-lymphedema) *Int J Clin Exp Pathol 12:680–688, 2019*

Trichilemmal cyst nevus – multiple subcutaneous nodules with cystic lesions with and without comedones in Blaschko distribution, filiform hyperkeratoses *JAAD 57:S72–77, 2007*

Undifferentiated pleomorphic sarcoma *J Cutan Pathol 44:477–479, 2017*

PRIMARY CUTANEOUS DISEASES

Adiposis dolorosa (Dercum's disease) *JAAD 56:901–916, 2007*

Granuloma annulare, subcutaneous ("pseudorheumatoid nodule") *Acta DV Croat 25:292–294, 2017; Pediatr 100:965–967, 1997;* of forehead *Ped Derm 5:407–408, 2008*

Kimura's disease – multiple large subcutaneous or salivary gland masses; young Asian men *JAAD 43:905–907, 2000; J Rheumatol 22:774–776, 1995*

Multiple symmetric lipomatosis (benign symmetric lipomatosis) (Launois-Bensaude syndrome) *Int J Obesity 26:253–261, 2002; Int J Dermatol 44:236–237, 2005; Medicine 63:56, 1984*

Painful piezogenic pedal papules *JAAD 36:780–781, 1997*

SYNDROMES

Adiposis dolorosa (Dercum's disease) – multiple painful periarticular lipomas *JAAD 56:901–916, 2007; JAAD 44:132–136, 2001*

Autoimmune lymphoproliferative syndrome *NEJM 351:1409–1418, 2004*

Bannayan-Riley-Ruvalcaba-Zonana syndrome (PTEN phosphatase and tensin homolog hamartoma) (PTEN hamartoma-tumor syndrome) – lipomas and vascular malformations, macrosomia at birth, hypotonia, lipoid storage myopathy, dolichocephaly, frontal bossing, megalencephaly (macrocephaly), subcutaneous and visceral lipomas, ocular hypertelorism, long philtrum, thin upper lip, broad mouth, relative micrognathia, lipomas, penile or vulvar lentigines, facial verruca-like or acanthosis nigricans-like papules, multiple acrochordons, angiokeratomas, transverse palmar crease, accessory nipple, syndactyly, brachydactyly, capillary (vascular) café au lait macules, malformations, arteriovenous malformations, lymphangiokeratoma, goiter, hamartomatous intestinal polyposis *JAAD 56:541–564, 2007; AD 142:625–632, 2006; JAAD 53:639–643, 2005*

Benign symmetrical lipomatosis (horse-collar neck) (Madelung's deformity) (multiple symmetric lipomatosis) – autosomal dominant; male alcoholics; lipomas of head, neck, shoulder girdle, proximal extremities; neuropathy *BJD 143:684–686, 2000; Skeletel Radiol 24:72–73, 1995;* of the lower abdomen, thighs *Int J Dermatol 32:594–597, 1993;* of the soles *JAAD 26:860–862, 1992*

Birt-Hogg-Dube syndrome – giant disfiguring lipomas *JAAD 50:810–812, 2004*

Buschke-Ollendorff syndrome *JAMADerm 152:844–845, 2016*

CLOVES syndrome – truncal lipomas, vascular malformations, and acral musculoskeletal anomalies (scoliosis, spinal high flow lesions, neural tube defects, tethered cord, spasticity), bony overgrowth and deformity, macrodactyly *Ped Derm 28:215–216, 2011*

Congenital generalized myofibromatosis – autosomal recessive or dominant *Ped Derm 21:154–159, 2004; Pediatr Pathol Lab Med 15:571–587, 1995*

Congenital self-healing reticulohistiocytosis (Hashimoto-Pritzker disease) – multiple congenital purple nodules

Cowden's syndrome (PTEN hamartoma-tumor syndrome) – sclerotic fibromas; megalencephaly (macrocephaly), dysplastic ganglioyctoma of the cerebellum (Lhermitte-Duclos disease), hamartomatous intestinal polyposis *AD 142:625–632, 2006; J Cut Pathol 19:346–351, 1992;* type 2 segmental Cowden's disease – keratinocytic soft, thick papillomatous nevus, connective tissue nevi, vascular nevi (including cutis marmorata), angiomas, varicosities, lymphatic hamartomas, lipomas, lipoblastomatosis, hydrocephalus, seizures, hemihypertrophy of limbs, ballooning of toes, bowel polyps, glomerulosclerosis, macrocephaly *BJD 156:1089–1090, 2007; Eur J Dermatol 17:133–136, 2007*

Diffuse infiltrative lymphocytosis syndrome (DILS) – autoimmune syndrome with oligoclonal expansion of CD8+ T lymphocytes in response to HIV antigens; lymphocytic infiltration of salivary glands (parotid glands) and viscera *Clin Lab Haem 27:278–282, 2005*

Ekbom's syndrome (myoclonic epilepsy and ragged muscle fibers) (mitochondrial syndrome) – cervical lipomas *JAAD 39:819–823, 1998*

Encephalocraniocutaneous lipomatosis – unilateral or bilateral skin-colored or yellow domed papules or nodules of scalp (hairless plaque), head, and neck; ipsilateral cranial and facial asymmetry, cranial and ocular abnormalities, spasticity, mental retardation *Ped Derm 10:164–168, 1993; Arch Neurol 22:144–155, 1970*

Familial histiocytic dermatoarthritis syndrome – uveitis, destructive arthritis; papulonodular eruption *Am J Med 54:793–800, 1973*

Familial multiple lipomatosis *NEJM 371:1237, 2014;* familial angiolipomatosis *Arch Pathol Lab Med 123:946–948, 1999*

Farber's disease (lipogranulomatosis) – lysosomal acid ceramidase deficiency (*N*-acylsphingosine amidohydrolase) (chromosome 8p22–21.2); deformed or stiff joints with painful limb contractures and red periarticular subcutaneous nodules(proximal and distal interphalangeal joints, wrist, elbow, knees, ankles, metatarsals), and progressive hoarseness; rarely nodules seen in conjunctivae, nostrils, ears, mouth; heart, liver, spleen, lung; progressive psychomotor retardation *Ped Derm 26:44–46, 2009; Eur J Ped 157:515–516, 1998; AD 130:1350–1354, 1994*

Fibrodysplasia ossificans progressiva – heterotopic bone formation within soft tissues; multiple neonatal scalp nodules associated with malformation of the great toes (hallux valgus); hypoplastic great toes; development of tumors is cranial to caudal, dorsal to ventral and proximal to distal; ossification after infections or trauma; scalp nodules large, firm, and immobile; mutation in *ACVR1* gene *JAAD 64:97–101, 2011*

Hypereosinophilic syndrome *Case Rep Med Nov 18, 2019*

Gardner's syndrome – multiple epidermoid cysts, osteomas (especially of facial bones), lipomas, fibromas *Am J Surg 143:405–408, 1982; Clin Exp Dermatol 1:75–82, 1976;* nuchal fibroma – multiple lesions associated with Gardner's syndrome *JAAD 66:959–965, 2012*

Goltz's syndrome (focal dermal hypoplasia) – giant fat herniations *Ped Derm 22:420–423, 2005*

Hemihyperplasia-Multiple Lipomatosis syndrome – hemihyperplasia at birth, moderate overgrowth, extensive congenital vascular stain (superficial capillary malformation), compressible blue nodule, multiple subcutaneous nodules, hemihypertrophy, syndactyly, thickened but not cerebriform soles, dermatomyofibroma *JAAD 56:541–564, 2007; Soc Ped Derm Annual Meeting, July 2005; Am J Med Genet 130A–111–122, 2004; Am J Med Genet 79:311–318, 1998*

Infantile myofibromatosis (multicentric infantile myofibromatosis) – gingival and joints are spared compared with Winchester syndrome and juvenile hyaline fibromatosis and infantile systemic hyalinosis *J Dermatol 28:379–382, 2001; AD 136:597–600, 2000; JAAD 41:508, 1999*

Infantile systemic hyalinosis – large subcutaneous nodules *AD 144:1351–1359, 2008*

Juvenile hyaline fibromatosis – large subcutaneous nodules of scalp, trunk, and extremities *Hum Mut 39:1752–1763, 2018; AD 144:1351–1359, 2008; Ped Derm 18:400–402, 2001; Pathol Int 48:230–236, 1998*

Leri-Weill dyschondrosteosis – mesomelic short stature syndrome with Madelung's deformity; SHOX haploinsufficiency like Turner's syndrome *JAAD 50:767–776, 2004*

Maffucci's syndrome (enchondromatosis) – enchondromas and multiple venous malformations; spindle cell hemangioendothelioma; oral and intra-abdominal venous and lymphatic anomalies; short stature, shortened long bones with pathologic fractures; enchondromas undergo sarcomatous change in 30–40%; breast, ovarian, pancreatic, parathyroid, pituitary tumors *JAAD 56:541–564, 2007; Cutis 69:21–22, 2002; Ped Derm 17:270–276, 2000; Ped Derm 12:55–58, 1995; Dermatologic Clinics 13:73–78, 1995; JAAD 29:894–899, 1993*

Multiple endocrine neoplasia syndrome (MEN I) – lipomas *JAAD 56:877–880, 2007; AD 133:853–857, 1997;* collagenomas *JAAD 42:939–969, 2000*

Mandibuloacral dysplasia – autosomal recessive; progeroid facies; facial asymmetry, micrognathia, small nose, prominent eyes, large open fontanelles; congenital brown pigmentation of ankles progresses to mottled pigmentation; hypoplastic clavicles; contractures of lower extremities; failure to thrive; progressive glomerulopathy; subcutaneous calcified nodules; mutation in *ZMPSTE24* (lamin) *JAMADerm 151:561–562, 2015*

Mucopolysaccharidosis type IX – autosomal recessive; hyaluronidase 1 deficiency; soft tissue masses, short stature, coarse facies, hypertrichosis, synophrys; accumulation of hyaluronic acid *Ped Derm 33:594–601, 2016*

Neurofibromatosis type I *NEJM 365:2020, 2011; Dermatol Clinics 13:105–111, 1995; Curr Prob Cancer 7:1–34, 1982; NEJM 305:1617–1627, 1981*

Nevoid basal cell carcinoma syndrome – multiple epidermal inclusions cysts

Pachyonychia congenita – multiple epidermoid cysts of volar upper extremities; keratin 17 mutation *BJD 159:730–732, 2008*

Penchaszadeh syndrome (nasopalpebral lipoma-coloboma syndrome) – eyelid lipoma *Am J Med Genet 11:397–410, 1982*

Polyneuropathy with nerve angiomatosis and multiple soft tissue tumors *Am J Surg Pathol 19:1325–1332, 1995*

Proteus syndrome – soft tissue and bony hypertrophy of hands and feet, hemihypertrophy, exostosis, cranial hyperostosis, visceral hamartomas, lipomas, vascular malformations, linear epidermal nevi, connective tissue nevus, gigantism, mosaic distribution of lesions; cerebriform thickening of palms and soles, capillary, venous, lymphatic and combined slow-flow malformations (like Klippel-Trenaunay syndrome); mosaic distribution, progressive course, sporadic occurrence; bilateral ovarian cystadenomas, parotid monomorphic adenoma, lipomas, lung cysts, facial phenotype *JAAD 56:541–564, 2007; Eur J Pediatr 140:5–12, 1983;*

multiple lipomas *JAAD 52:834–838, 2005; BJD 151:953–960, 2004; AD 140:947–953, 2004; JAMA 285:2240–2243, 2001;* lipomatosis with hemihypertrophy

Pseudohypoparathyroidism – dry, scaly, hyperkeratotic puffy skin; multiple subcutaneous osteomas, collagenoma *BJD 143:1122–1124, 2000*

Pseudoxanthoma elasticum – multiple calcified cutaneous nodules *Am J Med 31:488–489, 1961*

SOLAMEN syndrome (segmental overgrowth, lipomatosis, arteriovenous malformation, and epidermal nevus) *Eur J Hum Genet 15:767–773, 2007*

Steatocystoma multiplex *SKINmed 12:267–269, 2014; JAAD 43:396–399, 2000; AD Syphilol 36:31–36, 1937*

Sweet's syndrome – secondary to melioidosis *BMC Dermatol 19:16, 2019*

Wells' syndrome – eosinophilic panniculitis *Eur J Dermatol 28:700–701, 2018*

Winchester syndrome (hereditary contractures with sclerodermoid changes of skin) – scleredema-like skin changes, widespread nodules, joint contractures, gingival hyperplasia, hypertrichosis, dwarfism, arthritis of small joints (RA-like), osteolysis, corneal opacities *JAAD 55:1036–143, 2006; JAAD 50:S53–56, 2004; Am J Med Genet 26:123–131, 1987; J Pediatr 84:701–709, 1974; Pediatrics 47:360–369, 1971*

TRAUMA

Intravenous drug abuse – foreign body granulomas or nonspecific nongranulomatous inflammation; panniculitis *BJD 150:1–10, 2004*

VASCULAR DISEASES

Angiolymphoid hyperplasia with eosinophilia *J Clin Diagn Res 11:2D21–2D23, 2017*

Arteriovenous malformation – mountain range appearance *AD 143:1043–1045, 2007*

Eosinophilic granulomatosis with polyangiitis *JAAD 47:209–216, 2002; Mayo Clinic Proc 52:477–484, 1977*

Congenital fibromuscular dysplasia – aneurysm in skin *BJD 163:1362–1364, 2010; JAAD 27:883–885, 1992*

Diffuse neonatal hemangiomatosis *Ped Derm 14:383–386, 1997*

Generalized lymphangiomatosis *Ped Derm 15:296–298, 1998*

Glomus tumors – multiple or plaque type; hemi-facial *Cutis 83:24–27, 2009; JAAD 45:239–245, 2001; Ped Derm 18:223–226, 2001; AD 127:1717–1722, 1991*

Henoch-Schonlein purpura *Leung, Robson, 2000*

Kaposiform hemangioendothelioma *JAAD 38:799–802, 1998*

Klippel-Trenaunay-Weber syndrome

Polyarteritis nodosa, systemic; cutaneous (livedo with nodules) – painful or asymptomatic red or skin colored multiple nodules with livedo reticularis of feet, legs, forearms face, scalp, shoulders, trunk *Ped Derm 15:103–107, 1998; AD 130:884–889, 1994; JAAD 31:561–566, 1994; JAAD 31:493–495, 1994*

Takayasu's arteritis *NEJM 349:160–169, 2003*

Giant varicosities, cirrhosis – personal observation

NODULES, RED, EXTREMITIES

AUTOIMMUNE DISEASES AND DISEASES OF IMMUNE DYSFUNCTION

Deficiency of adenosine deaminase – ADA 1 – autosomal recessive; severe combined immunodeficiency; ADA 2 – loss of function mutation in cat eye syndrome chromosome candidate 1 gene (*CECR1*); painless leg nodules with intermittent livedo reticularis, Raynaud's phenomenon, cutaneous ulcers, morbilliform rashes, Raynaud's phenomenon, digital gangrene, oral aphthae; vasculitis of small and medium arteries with necrosis, fever, early recurrent ischemic and hemorrhagic strokes, peripheral and cranial neuropathy, and gastrointestinal involvement (diarrhea); hepatosplenomegaly, systemic vasculopathy, stenosis of abdominal arteries *Ped Derm 37:199–201, 2020;*

NEJM 380:1582–1584, 2019; Ped Derm 33:602–614, 2016; NEJM 370:911–920, 2014; NEJM 370:921–931, 2014

Bowel arthritis dermatitis syndrome – erythema nodosum-like lesions *Ped Derm 25:509–519, 2008; AD 135:1409–1414, 1999; Cutis 63:17–20, 1999; JAAD 14:792–796, 1986; Mayo Clin Proc 59:43–46, 1984; AD 115:837–839, 1979*

Bullous pemphigoid without blisters – pemphigoid nodularis *JAAD 81:355:363, 2019; JAMA Derm 149:950–953, 2013*

Chronic granulomatous disease *JAAD 36:899–907, 1997;* suppurative cutaneous granulomas in chronic granulomatous disease (Microascus cinereus) *Clin Inf Dis 20:110–114, 1995;* also *Aspergillus, Candida, Paecilomyces, Exophiala dermatitidis, Acremonium strictum, Sarcinosporon inkin*

Complement deficiency – low serum complement with SLE-like illness *Clin Res 22:416(Abstract), 1974*

Dermatitis herpetiformis – prurigo nodularis-like lesions *J Eur Acad Dermatol Venereol 16:88–89, 2002*

Dermatomyositis – calcinosis of elbows and forearms *JAMA 305:183–190, 2011;* panniculitis which may ulcerate and form sinuses *Ped Derm 16:270–272, 1999; BJD 128:451–453, 1993; AD 119:336–344, 1983;* nodular panniculitis *AD 148:740–744, 2012;* nodules and plaques on arms, thighs, buttocks, abdomen with lipoatrophy *AD 127:1846–1847, 1991; JAAD 23:127–128, 1990;* erythema nodosum

Fogo selvagem (endemic pemphigus) – prurigo nodularis-like lesions *JID 107:68–75, 1996; JAAD 32:949–956, 1995*

Gain of function mutation of NLRC4 (inflammasome) – fever, periodic urticarial rash, conjunctivitis, arthralgias, painful red nodules of foot or leg, enterocolitis, splenomegaly, macrophage activation syndrome; increased IL-18 *BJD 176:244–248, 2017; Nat*

Genet 46:1135–1139, 2014; Nat Genet 46:1140–1146, 2014; J Exp Med 211:2385–2396, 2014

GATA2 deficiency (includes MONOMAC syndrome, DCML, Emberger syndrome) (lymphedema and myelodysplasia) (familial acute leukemia and myelodysplasia) – monocytopenia, B-cell and natural killer cell lymphopenia, myeloid leukemias, disseminated mycobacterial infection, human papilloma virus infection, fungal infection; GATA2-transcription factor in early hematopoietic differentiation and lymphatic and vascular development; primary alveolar proteinosis; panniculitis; erythema nodosum-like lesions; primary lymphedema; skin tumors, Sweet's syndrome with myelodysplastic syndrome *BJD 178:593–594, 2018; JAAD 73:367–381, 2015; JAAD 71:577–580, 2014; BJD 170:1182–1186, 2014*

Hyper-IgD syndrome – recurrent transient and fixed pink plaques and nodules of face and extremities; cephalic pustulosis; mevalonate kinase deficiency *Ped Derm 35:482–485, 2018*

Lupus erythematosus – lupus panniculitis (lupus profundus) – thighs, buttocks, arms, breasts, face *AD 122:576, 1986; AD 103:231–242, 1971;* LE hypertrophicus et profundus – mimicking thrombophlebitis *J Rheumatol 16:1400, 1989;* chilblain lupus – chilblain-like lesions of legs

Pemphigoid nodularis *JAAD 53:S101–104, 2005; JAAD 29:293–299, 1993; JAAD 21:1099–1104, 1989*

Rheumatoid arthritis – neutrophilic lobular panniculitis *JAAD 45:325–361, 2001; J R Soc Med 84:307–308, 1991;* palisaded neutrophilic granulomatous dermatitis of rheumatoid arthritis (rheumatoid neutrophilic dermatosis) *Cutis 78:133–136, 2006; JAAD 47:251–257, 2002; JAAD 45:596–600, 2001; AD 133:757–760, 1997; AD 125:1105–1108, 1989*

Sjogren's syndrome – plasma cell panniculitis *J Cutan Pathol 23:170–174, 1996;* red nodules of legs *JAAD 48:311–340, 2003*

CONGENITAL LESIONS

Dermoid cyst – red cystic nodule of back *Ped Derm 30:706–711, 2013*

Leukemia cutis *Dermatol Therapy 18:104–116, 2005;* red-violaceous nodule; neonatal B-cell leukemia *Ped Derm 36:988–989, 2019*

Sacrococcygeal teratoma – masquerading as infantile hemangioma; red vascular plaque; red subcutaneous nodule of medial buttock *Ped Derm 30:112–116, 2013*

Subcutaneous fat necrosis of newborn *AD 146:882–885, 2010; Ped Derm 27:317–318, 2010*
  Neonatal subcutaneous nodules
    Infection
    Congenital leukemia
    Dermoid cysts
    Hemangiomas
    Infantile myofibromatosis
    Rhabdomyosarcoma
    Infantile fibrosarcoma
    Neuroblastoma
    Sclerema neonatorum

DRUG-INDUCED

All-trans-retinoic acid – Sweet's syndrome-like neutrophilic panniculitis; solitary red nodule *JAAD 56:690—693, 2007;* All-retinoic acid syndrome; fever, respiratory distress, weight gain, leg edema, pleural effusions, renal failure, pericardial effusions, hypotension, vasculitis, hypercalcemia, bone marrow necrosis and

fibrosis, thromboembolic events, erythema nodosum *Leuk Lymphoma 44:547–548, 2003*

Azathioprine – erythema nodosum-like nodules of legs in patients with inflammatory bowel disease *AD 143:744–748, 2007;* azathioprine hypersensitivity reaction – occurs within first four weeks of treatment; fever, malaise, arthralgias, myalgias, nausea, vomiting, diarrhea; morbilliform eruption, leukocytoclastic vasculitis, acute generalized exanthematous pustulosis, erythema nodosum, Sweet's syndrome; red papulonodules with pustules *JAAD 65:184–191, 2011*

Bortezomib (proteasome inhibitor for treatment of myeloma) – red nodules of trunk, face, neck, and extremities *JAAD 71:217–227, 2014; JAAD 55:897–900, 2006*

Calcium gluconate – calcinosis cutis; red nodules along veins *Ped Derm 34:356–358, 2017*

Corticosteroids – post-steroid panniculitis *Ped Derm 5:92–93, 1988; AD 90:387–391, 1964;* topical corticosteroid-induced infantile gluteal granuloma *Clin Exp Dermatol 6:23–29, 1981*

Enfuvirtide – injection site reaction *JAAD 49:826–831, 2003*

Erythema nodosum – drug-induced erythema nodosum – sulfonamides, other antibiotics, analgesics, antipyretics, birth control pill, granulocyte colony-stimulating factor, all-trans retinoic acid *Rook p. 3393, 1998, Sixth Edition*

5-fluorouracil, capecitabine, tegafur – granulomatous septal panniculitis *JAAD 71:203–214, 2014*

FLT3 inhibitor in acute myelogenous leukemia – neutrophilic dermatosis *JAMADerm 152:480–482, 2016*

Furosemide – Sweet's like *JAAD 21:339–343, 1989*

G-CSF – Sweet's syndrome, pyoderma gangrenosum *Ped Derm 17:205–207, 2000;* neutrophilic dermatosis of legs and buttocks *Ped Derm 18:417–421, 2001*

Glatiramer acetate – injected for multiple sclerosis; panniculitis *JAAD 55:968–974, 2006*

Imatinib (Gleevec) *BJD 149:678–678, 2003;* imatinib-associated Sweet's syndrome *AD 141:368–370, 2005*

Immunization granuloma

Influenza vaccine – hypersensitivity to influenza vaccine in Epstein-Barr virus-associated T-lymphoproliferative disorder *BJD 172:1686–1688, 2015*

Interleukin 2 injections – lobular panniculitis *Br J Cancer 66:698–699, 1992*

Iododerma – scaly red papules and nodules; secondary to amiodarone *JAMADerm 151:891–892, 2015; Australas J Dermatol 28:119–122, 1987*

Kit and BCR-ABL inhibitors – imatinib, nilotinib, dasatinib – facial edema morbilliform eruptions, pigmentary changes, lichenoid reactions, psoriasis, pityriasis rosea, pustular eruptions, DRESS, Stevens-Johnson syndrome, urticarial, neutrophilic dermatoses, photosensitivity, pseudolymphoma, porphyria cutanea tarda, small vessel vasculitis, panniculitis, perforating folliculitis, erythroderma *JAAD 72:203–218, 2015*

Leukocyte colony stimulating factors *AD 130:77–81, 1994*

Meperidine *AD 110:747–750, 1974*

Methotrexate-related lymphoproliferative disorder – linear perilymphatic nodules of leg; linear bands; ulcerated and non-ulcerated red nodules *JAMADerm 154:490–492, 2018; JAAD 61:126–129, 2009*

Pembrolizumab – granulomatous panniculitis *JAMADerm 153:721–722, 2017*

Pentazocine *AD 110:747–750, 1974*

Sorafenib – erythema nodosum *JAMADerm 154:369–370, 2018*

Sulindac-induced pancreatitis *JAAD 45:325–361, 2001*

Vasculitis secondary to various drugs; propylthiouracil nodular vasculitis *Cutis 49:253–255, 1992*

Vemurafenib – panniculitis (erythema nodosum-like; violaceous leg nodules) with arthralgias *Ped Derm 34:337–341, 2017; Ped Derm 32:153–154, 2015; BJD 167:987–994, 2012; AD 148:363–366, 2012*

EXOGENOUS AGENTS

Aluminum hypersensitivity – vaccination sites

Aspartame (Nutra-Sweet) – lobular panniculitis *JAAD 24:298–300, 1991*

BCG granulomas *AD 142:249–250, 2006*

BRAF inhibitors (vemurafenib or dabrafenib) – panniculitis and arthralgia *AD 148:357–361, 2012*

Bromoderma – multiple red nodules of forehead, upper back, arms, and legs *BJD 158:427–429, 2008*

Contact dermatitis, irritant

Mercury ingestion *JAAD 37:131–133, 1997;* mercury granulomas due to injections – violaceous nodules and plaques *Cutis 88:189–193, 2011*

Paraffinoma *Plast Reconstr Surg 65:517–524, 1980*

Povidone panniculitis *AD 116:704–706, 1980*

RAF inhibitors (MAPK pathway) – vemurafenib and dabrafenib – exanthema warts and other hyperkeratotic lesions, keratoacanthomas, squamous cell carcinoma, melanocytic nevi, keratosis pilaris, seborrheic dermatitis, hyperkeratotic hand-foot reactions, photosensitivity, panniculitis with arthralgias, alopecia *JAAD 72:221–236, 2015*

Sea urchin spine *Cutis 98:303–305, 2016*

Silicone granuloma *AD 117:366–367, 1981*

Zyderm test site

INFECTIONS AND INFESTATIONS

Abscess

Acanthamebiasis – in AIDS *JAAD 42:351–354, 2000; Arch Int Med 157:569–572, 1997; AD 131:1291–1296, 1995; Cutis 56:285–287, 1995; NEJM 331:85–87, 1994; Ped Inf Dis 11:404–407, 1992;* tender red nodules of trunk and extremities with necrosis and eschars *AD 147:857–862, 2011;* associated with CPAP machine *BJD 174: 625–628, 2016*

Actinomycetoma – *Nocardiopsis dassonvillei AD 121:1332–1334, 1985*

Actinomycosis – panniculitis *J Cutan Pathol 16:183–193, 1989*

African histoplasmosis (*Histoplasma capsulatum* var. *duboisii*) -exclusively in Central and West Africa and Madagascar *Clin Inf Dis 48:441, 493–494, 2009*

AIDS – neutrophilic eccrine hidradenitis in HIV infection *J Dermatol 25:199–200, 1998; Int J Dermatol 35:651–652, 1996*

Alternariosis – *Alternaria chartarum BJD 142:1261–1262, 2000; A. alternate* – pink crusted nodule of leg *AD 143:1583–1588, 2007; A. tenuissima AD 143:1583–1588, 2007*

Amebiasis – red nodules of extremities *JAAD 147:735–740, 2011*

Aspergillosis – primary cutaneous aspergillosis *JAAD 38:797–798, 1998; A. fumigatus* – red nodules of legs *AD 143:535–540, 2007*

Bacterial sepsis

Bartonellosis – verruga peruana; bacillary angiomatosis

Bacille-Calmette-Guerin (BCG) infection, disseminated – nodules of scalp, back, and legs *Ped Derm 36:672–676, 2019*

Bacillus species in subacute combined immunodeficiency *JAAD 39:285–287, 1998*

Bartonella bacilliformis – Oroya fever with verruga peruana – red papules in crops become nodular, hemangiomatous or pedunculated; face, neck, extremities, mucosal lesions *Ann Rev Microbiol 35:325–338, 1981*

Bed bug bites (*Cimex lectularius*) *NEJM 359:1047, 2008*

Borrelia burgdorferi – nodular panniculitis *J Infect Dis 160:596–597, 1992;* Lyme borreliosis – acrodermatitis chronica atrophicans – red to blue nodules or plaques; tissue-paper-like wrinkling; pigmented; poikilodermatous; hands, feet, elbows, knees *BJD 121:263–269, 1989: Int J Derm 18:595–601, 1979*

Brucellosis – red papulonodules of legs (erythema nodosum-like lesions) *JAAD 48:474–476, 2003; Cutis 63:25–27, 1999; AD 117:40–42, 1981*

Botryomycosis – prurigo nodularis-like lesions; *Staphylococcus aureus Cutis 80:45–47, 2007*

Buruli ulcer (*Mycobacteria ulcerans subspecies shinshuense*) – ulcerated red nodule of arm *JAMA Derm 150:64–67, 2014*

Campylobacter jejuni – in HIV disease *Rev Med Interne 18:257–258, 1998*

Candida sepsis – papules and nodules with pale centers *Am J Dermatopathol 8:501–504, 1986; JAMA 229:1466–1468, 1974;* septic panniculitis in infancy *Textbook of Neonatal Dermatology, p.425, 2001; Candida kefyr* – unilateral red nodules of leg, bullae, pustules; arterial thrombus of left iliac artery *Cutis 91:137–140, 2013*

Cat scratch disease – erythema nodosum *Pediatrics 81:559–561, 1988*

Chagas' disease (American trypanosomiasis; *T. cruzi*) – reactivation chagoma *Dermatol Clinics 29:53–62, 2011; AD 139:104–105, 2003;* acute infection (chagoma) *Dermatol Therapy 17:513–516, 2004*

Chromomycosis *JAAD 8:1–16, 1983*

Coccidioidomycosis – red nodule of arm *JAAD 49:944–949, 2003;* of legs *AD 143:548–549, 2007*

Corynebacterium jeikeium

Cryptococcosis – cryptococcal panniculitis *J Drugs Dermatol 14:519–522, 2015;* indurated edematous nodules *Cutis 84:93–96, 2009; AD 144:1651–1656, 2008;* erythema nodosum-like (cryptococcal panniculitis) *Cutis 85:303–306, 2010; AD 112:1734–1740, 1976; Arch Int Med 136:670–677, 1976; BJD 74:43–49, 1962*

Cysticercosis

Dematiaceous fungal infections in organ transplant recipients – all lesions on extremities
Alternaria
Bipolaris hawaiiensis
Exophiala jeanselmei, E. spinifera, E. pesciphera, E. castellani
Exserohilum rostratum
Fonsacaea pedrosoi
Phialophora parasitica

Deep dermatophytosis – dermal and subcutaneous tissue invasion; *CARD9* mutation *NEJM 369:1704–1714, 2013*

Dirofilaria tenuis (raccoon heartworm) – red nodule of leg *JAAD 73:929–944, 2015; Cutis 80:125–128, 2007*

Fascioliasis – *Fasciola hepatica* (fluke parasite) – eosinophilic panniculitis *JAAD 42:900–902, 2000*

Fusarium – red nodule with central pallor *Sabouradis 17:219–223, 1979;* dusky nodules with central necrosis *AD 146:1037–1042, 2010;* dark nodules of leg *Clin Inf Dis 32:1237–1240, 2001; F.*

falciforme – starts as red nodule with or without central necrosis *BJD 157:407–409, 2007*

Fusobacterium – septic panniculitis in infancy

Glanders – nodules with lymphangitis *JAAD 54:559–578, 2006*

Gnathostomiasis – red migratory swellings *JAAD 68:301–305, 2013; BJD 145:487–489, 2001; JAAD 33:825–8, 1995;* eosinophilic migratory panniculitis (larva migrans profundus – *Gnathostoma doloresi* or *G. spinigerum*) *JAAD 11:738–740, 1984*

Gonococcemia *Am J Med Sci 260:150–159, 1970*

Helicobacter cinaedi – erythema nodosum-like eruption *Ann Intern Med 121:90–93, 1994*

Hepatitis B – erythema nodosum *JAAD 9:602–603, 1983;* hepatitis A – nodular panniculitis *Cutis 32:543–547, 1983;* polyarteritis nodosa

Herpes simplex – chronic HSV infection in AIDS – red nodule resembling basal cell carcinoma *JAAD 36:831–833, 1997*

Histoplasmosis – personal observation; *Diagnostic Challenges V 77–79, 1994; AD 121:914–916, 1985*

Insect bite reactions – personal observation

Klebsiella species – septic panniculitis in infancy

Leishmaniasis – papulotuberous lesions *JAAD 60:897–925, 2009; Clinics in Dermatology 14:425–431, 1996;* post-kala azar dermal leishmaniasis

Leprosy – lepromatous leprosy including erythema nodosum leprosum (vasculitis) *AD 138:1607–1612, 2002; AD 111:1575–1580, 1975;* subcutaneous lepromas erythema nodosum leprosum – new painful dermal or subcutaneous nodules with fever, anorexia, malaise, arthralgias and myalgias, epididymitis, orchitis, periostitis, dactylitis, lymphadenitis, hepatosplenomegaly, glomerulonephritis, iridocyclitis, panniculitis, edema of dermis *JAAD 71:795–803, 2014; AD 111:1575–1580, 1975;* targetoid red nodules with central necrosis *AD 144:821–822, 2008*

Lobomycosis – *Lacazio(Loboa)loboi* – legs, arms, face *JAAD 53:931–951, 2005; Mycoses 55:298–309, 2012*

Loiasis

Meningococcemia, chronic *BJD 153:669–671, 2005; Rev Infect Dis 8:1–11, 1986;* acute *Am J Med Sci 260:150–159, 1970*

Microascus cinereus in chronic granulomatous disease *J Clin Inf Dis 20:110–114, 1995*

Milker's nodules

Mucormycosis – *Mucor racemosus;* mimicking panniculitis *JAAD 66:975–984, 2012*

Mycetoma *JAAD 53:931–951, 2005; JAAD 49:S170–173, 2003; JAAD 32:311–315, 1995; Cutis 49:107–110, 1992; Australas J Dermatol 31:33–36, 1990; JAAD 6:107–111, 1982; Sabouraudia 18:91–95, 1980; AD 99:215–225, 1969*

   Eumycetoma
      Pseudallescheria boydii
      Madurella mycetomatis
      Madurella grisea
      Exophiala jeanselmei
      Pyrenochaeta romeroi
      Leptosphaeria senegalensis
      Curvularia lunata
      Neotestudina rosatii
      Aspergillus nidulans
      Aspergillus flavus
      Fusarium spp
      Cylindrocarpon spp
   Bacterial mycetoma – aerobic actinomycetes
      Actinomadura madurae

Actinomadura pelletieri
Streptomyces somaliensis
Nocardia brasiliensis
Nocardia caviae
Nocardia asteroides
Nocardia otitidiscaviarum

Mycobacterium abscessus – personal observation

Mycobacterium avium complex – panniculitis *Cutis 89:175–179, 2012*

Mycobacterium chelonae JAAD 60:177–179, 2009; JAAD 36:495–496, 1997; Ped Derm 14:370, 1994; panniculitis *AD 126:1064–1067, 1990;* from pedicure whirlpool footbath *AD 139:629–634, 2003*

Mycobacterium fortuitum Dermatol Clin 33:509–630, 2015; AD 139:629–634, 2003; following pedicures *JAAD 54:520–524, 2006;* draining cystic nodule of leg *J Drugs in Dermatol 10:914–916, 2011*

Mycobacterium gordonae

Mycobacterium haemophilum AD 138:229–230, 2002; Clin Inf Dis 33–330–337, 2001

Mycobacterium interjectum – leg nodules *BJD 159:1382–1384, 2008*

Mycobacterium kansasii Cutis 67:241–242, 2001; JAAD 36:497–499, 1997

Mycobacterium malmoense

Mycobacterium marinum – nodule or papule of hands, elbows, knees becomes crusted ulcer or abscess; or verrucous papule; sporotrichoid; rarely widespread lesions *Clin Inf Dis 31:439–443, 2000; Br Med J 300:1069–1070, 1990; AD 122:698–703, 1986; J Hyg 94:135–149, 1985*

Mycobacterium massiliense – red brown nodules of posterior calves mimicking erythema induratum *BJD 173:235–238, 2015*

Mycobacterium scrofulaceum Clin Inf Dis 20:549–556, 1995

Mycobacterium tuberculosis – erythema induratum of Bazin (nodular vasculitis) – tuberculid; nodules on backs of erythrocyanotic lower legs; ulcerate *Clin Inf Dis 70:1254–1257, 2020; AD 147:949–952, 2011; BJD 157:1293–1294, 2007; JAAD 45:325–361, 2001; AD 133:457–462, 1997; JAAD 14:738–342, 1986;* panniculitis *J Cutan Pathol 20:177–179, 1993; Ped Derm 13:386–388, 1996;* miliary TB; nodular tuberculid – red to blue-red nodules *JAAD 53:S154–156, 2005; Ped Derm 17:183–188, 2000; Mycobacterium tuberculosis –*
nodular granulomatous phlebitis (phlebitic tuberculid) – nonulcerative subcutaneous nodules along anterior and medial leg veins *Am J Clin Dermatol 3:319–328, 2002; Histopathology 30:129–134, 1997*

Mycobacterium vaccae J Clin Inf Dis 23:173–175, 1996

Myiasis – furuncular myiasis; true flies, 2-winged flies, botflies (*Dermatobia hominis* (human botfly) (*Cuterebra polita, C. latifrons*) (rodent or rabbit botfly)), warble flies (*Hypoderma bovis, H. lineatum*), flesh flies (*Wohlfahrtia vigil, W. opaca*), tumbu fly (*Cordylobia anthropophaga, C. rodhaini*) *Cutis 94:281–284, 2014; JAAD 58:907–926, 2008; JAAD 50:S26–30, 2004;* carbuncular plaque – *Cordylobia JAAD 58:907–926, 2008;* migratory myiasis – *Gasterophilus intestinalis, Hypoderma spp. JAAD 58:907–926, 2008*

Nocardia – sporotrichoid painful nodules of extremities *Cutis 89:75–77, 2012; J Cutan Pathol 16:183–193, 1989;* wrist nodule in chronic granulomatous disease *Clin Inf Dis 33:235–239, 2001; Nocardia* eccrine hidradenitis *JAAD 50:315–318, 2004;* septic panniculitis in infancy; *Nocardia beijingensis* – ulcerated nodules of legs *BJD 166:216–218, 2012*

North American blastomycosis – disseminated *NEJM 356:1456–1462, 2007*

Onchocerciasis – red nodules of legs *JAAD 73:929–944, 2015*

Osteomyelitis – palpable painful mass of thigh

Paecilomyces lilacinus – nodules on legs *Clin Inf Dis 34:1415–1417, 2002; JAAD 39:401–409, 1998; JAAD 37:270–271, 1997;* red nodules with necrotic centers *Ann Int Med 125:799–806, 1996*

Panniculitis – infectious; *Streptococcus pyogenes, Staphylococcus aureus, Pseudomonas spp., Klebsiella spp., Nocardia,* atypical mycobacteria, tuberculosis, *Candida, Fusarium, Histoplasma capsulatum, Cryptococcus neoformans, Actinomycosis, Sporothrix schenckii, Aspergillus fumigatus,* chromoblastomycosis *JAAD 45:325–361, 2001*

Pediculosis – body lice; generalized prurigo nodularis *JAAD 82:551–569, 2020*

Penicillium marneffei

Phaeohyphomycosis – *Exophiala J Clin Inf Dis 19:339–341, 1994*

Phlegmon – personal observation

Pythium insidiosum (pythiosis) (alga) (aquatic oocyte) – necrotizing hemorrhagic plaque; ascending gangrene of legs; Thailand; painful subcutaneous nodules, eyelid swelling and periorbital cellulitis, facial swelling, ulcer of arm or leg, pustules evolving into ulcers *BJD 175:394–397, 2016; J Infect Dis 159:274–280, 1989*

Post-streptococcal suppurative panniculitis

Prototecosis *BJD 146:688–693, 2002; JAAD 32:758–764, 1995; AD 125:1249–1252, 1989; Am J Clin Pathol 61:10–19, 1974*

Pseudomonas aeruginosa – nodular ecthyma gangrenosum; in HIV *JAAD 32:279–80, 1995;* nodular panniculitis *JAMADerm 1 50:628–632, 2014; J Eur Acad Dermatol Venereol 4:166–169, 1995;* septic panniculitis in infancy; *Pseudomonas* sepsis – red nodules with bullae atop several *Ped Derm 28:204–205, 2011; Ped Derm 23:243–246, 2006; Clin Inf Dis 26:188–189, 1998; AD 116:446–447, 1980*

Psittacosis – erythema nodosum *J Hyg 92:9–19, 1984*

Pyomyositis – palpable painful mass of thigh

Salmonella enteritis – erythema nodosum – <u>personal observation</u>

Scabies – in babies – red nodules of trunk and extremities *JAMA 321:604–605, 2019; Ped Derm 4:690–694, 2017;* pseudo-CTCL *BJD 124:277–278, 1991*

Serratia marcescens – sepsis *JAAD 58:S55–56, 2008;* neutrophilic eccrine hidradenitis *BJD 142:784–788, 2000; AD 121:1106–1107, 1985*

Sparganosis – application sparganosis; painful red nodules

Sporotrichosis *Cutis 54:279–286, 1994; Dermatologica 172:203–213, 1986;* fixed cutaneous

Staphylococcal aureus – abscess, sepsis *Hautarzt 16:453–455, 1965;* panniculitis *J Cutan Pathol 16:183–193, 1989;* septic panniculitis in infancy; nodular lymphangitis *Ped Derm 34:103–104, 2017*

Staphylococcus epidermidis – septic panniculitis in infancy

Streptococcal species – septic panniculitis in infancy Group A streptococcal panniculitis – multiple red nodules of extremities *Ped Derm 31:256–258, 2014*

Syphilis – nodular syphilis; deep red oval nodules *JAAD 82:1–14, 2020; JAMADerm 152:83–84, 2016; JAAD 57:S57–58, 2007; Sex Transm Dis 14:52–53, 1987;* Jarisch-Herxheimer reaction; syphilis in AIDS *Clin Inf Dis 23:462–467, 1996;* syphilitic panniculitis – purple subcutaneous nodules of lower legs *AD 148:269–270, 2012;* tertiary – nodular (tubercular) form – firm, coppery, red nodules; often on arms; may be cyanotic on legs; late congenital syphilis – nodular syphilids, gummata

Tinea corporis – *Trichophyton rubrum* – Majocchi's granuloma (nodular folliculitis) invasive *JAAD 21:167–179, 1989; AD 81:779–785, 1960; AD 64:258–277, 1954;* invasive tinea corporis (*T.*

violaceum) *BJD 101:177–183, 1979; T. rubrum* – violaceous nodules of thighs and lower legs – personal observation; *T. mentagrophytes* – violaceous nodules (pseudomycetoma) *BJD 155:628–629, 2006*

Toxocariasis *JAAD 33:8 JAAD 75:19–30, 2016; 25–828, 1995*

Toxoplasma gondii *AD 136:791–796, 2000*

Trypanosomiasis – African trypanosomiasis *AD 13:1178–1182, 1995;* trypanosomal chancre – red tender 2–5 cm nodule with blister on surface of forearm or leg

Trichophyton rubrum –Majocchi's granuloma (nodular folliculitis); invasive *Trichophyton rubrum* – hemorrhagic purpuric leg nodules in transplant patient *AD 149:475–480, 2013*

Trypanosoma brucei rhodesiense (African trypanosomiasis) – ulcerated nodule of leg; transmitted by tsetse fly in Tanzania, Malawi, Zambia, Zimbabwe; causes sleeping sickness; 2–5 cm trypanosomal chancre at site of bite with regional lymphadenopathy; chancres rare in Gambian sleeping sickness *NEJM 369:763, 2013*

Tularemia – *Francisella tularensis*; skin, eye, respiratory, gastrointestinal portals of entry; ulceroglandular, oculoglandular, glandular types; toxemic stage heralds generalized morbilliform eruption, erythema multiforme-like rash, crops of red nodules on extremities *Cutis 54:279–286, 1994; Medicine 54:252–269, 1985*

Tunga penetrans

Yaws – secondary *JAAD 54:559–578, 2006;* tertiary – nodules, tuberous lesions

Zygomycosis – violaceous necrotic and crusted nodules; *Rhizopus spp. AD 143:417–422, 2007*

INFILTRATIVE DISEASES

Amyloidosis – red translucent nodules of legs *JAAD 71:1035–1037, 2014*

Angioplasmocellular hyperplasia – red nodule with red rim, ulcerated nodule, vascular nodule of face, scalp, neck, trunk, and leg *JAAD 64:542–547, 2011*

Cutaneous lymphoid hyperplasia *JAAD 65:112–124, 2011*

Generalized eruptive histiocytoma

Erdheim-Chester disease (non-Langerhans cell histiocytosis) – multiple pink exophytic nodules – skin, pulmonary, vocal cord; bone, retro-orbital tissues, central nervous system, pituitary gland, large vessels, kidneys, retroperitoneum, heart; CD68+, CD1a *BJD 173:540–543, 2015; Virchows Arch Pathol Anat 173:561–602, 1930*

Histiocytosis

Indeterminate cell histiocytosis – red nodule; multiple red papulonodules *JAAD 57:1031–1045, 2007*

Intralymphatic histiocytosis – red patch overlying swollen knee; livedo reticularis, papules, nodules, urticaria, unilateral eyelid edema *AD 146:1037–1042, 2010*

Jessner's lymphocytic infiltrate

Langerhans cell histiocytosis – Hashimoto-Pritzker disease; congenital single yellow-red nodule with central ulceration *Ped Derm 26:121–126, 2009*

Progressive mucinous histiocytosis *BJD 142:133–137, 2000*

Progressive nodular histiocytomas – dermal dendrocytes; red nodules of face, trunk, and extremities *BJD 143:628–631, 2000; JAAD 29:278–280, 1993; AD 114:1505–1508, 1978*

Self-healing juvenile cutaneous mucinosis – red nodules of face, scalp, hand; macrodactyly (enlarged thumbs); periarticular papules and nodules, painful polyarthritis; linear ivory white papules, multiple subcutaneous nodules, indurated edema of periorbital and zygomatic areas *JAAD 55:1036–1043, 2006; AD 131:459–461, 1995; Ann DV 107:51–57, 1980; Lyon Med 230:470–474, 1973*

Xanthoma disseminatum – red nodules in flexures *NEJM 338:1138–1143, 1998*

INFLAMMATORY DISEASES

Atypical lymphocytic lobular panniculitis (T cell dyscrasia) – spontaneously resolves; red plaques and nodules of arms and legs with associated edema; identical presentation as subcutaneous panniculitis-like T-cell lymphoma with hemophagocytosis *JAAD 61:875–881, 2009; J Cutan Pathol 31:300–306, 2004*

Cytophagic histiocytic panniculitis (nodule) *AD 121:910–913, 1985*

Eosinophilic fasciitis

Eosinophilic panniculitis *Ped Derm 12:35–38, 1995; J Dermatol 20:185–187, 1993*

Equestrian cold panniculitis

Erythema induratum (Whitfield) – nodules with edematous ankles

Erythema nodosum *JAMA 316:91–92, 2016; On Cutaneous Diseases. London:Johnson 1798*

ERYTHEMA NODOSUM-ASSOCIATED CAUSES

Semin Cutan Med Surg 26:114–125, 2007; Sem Arth Rheum 4:1, 1974

Acne fulminans *Clin Exp Dermatol 2:351–354, 1977*

Acupuncture therapy

Adenocarcinoma of the colon, stomach

African trypanosomiasis

Amebiasis

Ankylosing spondylitis

Antiphospholipid antibody syndrome

Ascariasis

Aspergillosis

Atypical mycobacterial infections

Azathioprine *JAMA 316:91–92, 2016*

Behcet's syndrome

Borrelia burgdorferi infections

Boutonneuse fever

Breast abscesses

Brucellosis

Campylobacter Q J Med 28:109–124, 1959; asymptomatic *campylobacter coli* infection *JAAD 24:285, 1991*

Carcinoid – primary cutaneous carcinoid *Histopathology 36:566–567, 2000*

Carcinoma of the uterine cervix

Cat scratch disease *AD 100:148–154, 1969*

Celiac disease

Chancroid

Chlamydia psittaci Proc R Soc Med 75:262–267, 1982

Chronic active hepatitis

Crohn's disease

Coccidioidomycosis *JAAD 55:929, 942, 2006*

Corynebacterium diphtheriae infections

Cytomegalovirus infections

Dermatophyte infections

Diverticulosis (itis) of the colon

Drugs
  Acetaminophen
  Actinomycin D
  All-trans retinoic acid
  Aminopyrine
  Amiodarone
  Ampicillin
  Antimony
  Arsphenamine
  Azathioprine
  Bromides
  Busulfan
  Carbamazepine
  Carbenicillin
  Carbimazole
  Cefdinir
  Chlordiazepoxide
  Chlorotrianisene
  Chlorpropamide
  Ciprofloxacin
  Clomiphene
  Codeine
  Cotrimoxazole
  D-penicillamine
  Dapsone
  Diclofenac
  Dicloxacillin
  Diethylstilbestrol
  Disopyramide
  Echinacea herbal therapy
  Enoxacin
  Erythromycin
  Estrogens
  Fluoxetine
  Furosemide
  Glucagon
  Gold salts *AD 107:602–604, 1973*
  Granulocyte colony-stimulating factor
  Hepatitis B vaccine
  Hydralazine
  Ibuprofen
  Indomethacin
  Interleukin-2
  Iodides
  Isotretinoin
  Leukotriene modifying agents (zileuton and zafirlukast)
  Levofloxacin
  Meclofenamate
  Medroxyprogesterone
  Meprobamate
  Mesalamine
  Methicillin
  Methimazole
  Methyldopa
  Mezlocillin
  Minocycline
  Naproxen
  Nifedipine
  Nitrofurantoin
  Ofloxacin
  Omeprazole
  Oral contraceptives *AD 98:634–635, 1968*

Oxacillin
Paroxetine
Penicillin
Phenylbutazone
Phenytoin
Piperacillin
Progestins
Propylthiouracil
Pyritinol
Sorafenib *JAMADerm 154:369–370, 2018*
Sparfloxacin
Streptomycin
Sulfamethoxazole
Sulfisoxazole
Sulfonamides
Sulfones
Sulfonylureas
Sulfasalazine
Thalidomide
Ticarcillin
Trimethoprim
Typhoid vaccination
Vaccines
Verapamil

Escherichia coli

Factitial dermatitis

Giardiasis

Gonococcal disease

Granulomatous mastitis

Hepatitis B *JAAD 9:602, 1983*

Hepatitis C *AD 131:1185–1193, 1995*

Hepatocellular carcinoma

Herpes simplex

Hidradenitis suppurativa – personal observation

Histoplasmosis *Am Rev Resp Dis 117:929–956, 1978*

HIV infection

Hookworm infestation

Hyalohyphomycosis – *Paecilomyces lilacinus BJD 143:873–875, 2000*

Hydatidosis

Idiopathic

Idiopathic granulomatous mastitis *Ann DV 146:571, 2019;* with erythema nodosum *J Eur Acad DV 31:e391–393, 2017;* arthritis *Rheumatol Int 31:1093–1095, 2011*

IgA nephropathy

Infectious mononucleosis *Br Med J ii:1263, 1979*

Intestinal bypass for obesity

Intestinal parasitosis

Jellyfish sting

Kerion *Ped Derm 29:479–482, 2012*

Klebsiella pneumoniae infections

Leishmaniasis

Leprosy

Leptospirosis *Br Med J 285:937–940, 1982*

Leukemia *AD 110:415–418, 1974*

Lupus erythematosus, including C4 deficiency SLE

Lymphogranuloma venereum *Acta DV (Stockh) 60:319–322, 1980*

Lymphoma – Hodgkin's disease *BJD 106:593–595, 1982;* non-Hodgkin's lymphoma

Measles

Meningococcal disease

Milkers' nodules *Acta DV (Stockh) 56:69–72, 1976*

Moraxella catarrhalis

Mycobacterium szulgai in MonoMAC syndrome *Clin Inf Dis 57:6978–699, 2013*

Mycoplasma pneumoniae infections

Myiasis, furuncular *Med Cutan Ibero Lat Am 13:411–418, 1985*

North American blastomycosis *Am J Med 27:750–766, 1959*

Pancreatic carcinoma

Parvovirus B19

Pasteurella pseudotuberculosis infections

Pertussis

Post-radiation therapy for pelvic carcinoma

Pregnancy

Propionibacterium acnes

Pseudomonas aeruginosa sepsis *Am J Med 80:528–529, 1986*

Psittacosis (Bateman's syndrome) *Br Med J ii:1469–1470, 1965*

Q fever

Radiation *BJD 142:188, 2000; BJD 140:372–373, 1999*

Relapsing polychondritis

Reiter's syndrome

Renal carcinoma

Rheumatoid arthritis

Salmonella Br Med J 102:339–340, 1980

Sarcoidosis – Lofgren's syndrome – erythema nodosum with sarcoidosis and arthralgias *Ped Derm 22:366–368, 2005*

Schistosomiasis

Sarcoma

Shigella infections

Sjogren's syndrome

Smoke inhalation

South American blastomycosis

Sparganum larva

Staphylococcus aureus – abscess (furuncle)

Still's disease, adult

Streptococcal infection – pharyngitis and tonsillitis, erysipelas, rheumatic fever

Sweet's syndrome

Syphilis

Takayasu's arteritis

Thromboangiitis obliterans (Buerger's disease) *Am J Med Sci 136:567–580, 1908*

Toxoplasmosis

Trichomoniasis

Trichophyton infections *Pediatrics 59:912–915, 1977*

Tropical eosinophilia

Tuberculosis

Tularemia *JAAD 49:363–392, 2003*

Ulcerative colitis *Gut 5:1–22, 1964*

Varicella

Vogt-Koyanagi disease

Wegener's granulomatosis

Yersinia enterocolitica BJD 93:719–720, 1975; asymptomatic dog vector

Erythema nodosum in children
Streptococcal infections most common cause

Erythema nodosum in adults
Infections, drugs, sarcoidosis, autoimmune disorders, inflammatory bowel disease most common

Febrile idiopathic lobar panniculitis of childhood – abdominal pain, arthralgia, fever, red nodules of face, legs, trunk, lipoatrophy *Ped Derm 31:652, 2014*

Granulomatous nodules – after mastectomy for breast carcinoma *BJD 146:891–894, 2002*

Histiocytic phagocytic panniculitis – red nodules of the forearms *JAAD 44:120–123, 2001*

Interstitial granulomatous dermatitis – personal observation

IgG4 disease – multisystem inflammatory disease with papules, plaques, and nodules; parotitis with parotid gland swelling, lacrimal gland swelling, dacryoadenitis, sialadenitis, proptosis; idiopathic pancreatitis, retroperitoneal fibrosis, aortitis; Mikuliczs syndrome, angiolymphadenopathy with eosinophilia, Riedel's thyroiditis, biliary tract disease, renal disease, meningeal disease, pituitary gland; Kuttner tumor, Rosai-Dorfman disease; elevated IgG4 with plasma cell dyscrasia, diffuse or localized swelling or masses; lymphocytic and plasma cell infiltrates with storiform fibrosis *JAAD 75:177–185, 2016*

Intralymphatic histiocytosis – red nodules associated with livedo reticularis *J Drugs in Dermatol 10:1208–1209, 2011; Am J Dermatopathol 31:140–151, 2009; Am J Dermatopathol 29:165–168, 2007*

Kaposi's sarcoma – HIV

Lipoatrophic panniculitis

Lipophagic panniculitis of childhood

Malacoplakia *JAAD 34:325–332, 1996*

Membranous fat necrosis *AD 129:1331, 1334, 1993*

Membranous lipodystrophy

Myositis – systemic or focal myositis – palpable painful mass of thigh

Neutrophilic eccrine hidradenitis *Ped Derm 6:33–38, 1989; AD 118:263–266, 1982*

Neutrophilic panniculitis – not a diagnosis but a histologic pattern
Alpha-1 anti-trypsin deficiency
Familial Mediterranean fever
Infectious panniculitis
Pancreatic panniculitis
Panniculitic bacterid
Subcutaneous Sweet's syndrome
Ulcerative colitis

Palmoplantar hidradenitis in children *AD 131:817–820, 1995*

Panniculitis
1) Enzyme panniculitis
Alpha-1 antitrypsin deficiency *JAAD 18:684–692, 1988*
Pancreatic panniculitis – acute alcoholic pancreatitis *NEJM 368:465, 2013*
2) Immunologic panniculitis
Complement deficiency
Cytophagic histiocytic panniculitis
Erythema nodosum, including familial erythema nodosum *Arthr Rheum 34:1177–1179, 1991*
Lipoatrophic panniculitis

Lipophagic panniculitis of childhood *JAAD 21:971–978, 1989*
Lupus panniculitis
3) Neoplastic
Lymphoma, leukemia
Histiocytosis
4) Cold panniculitis, including cold panniculitis of neonate – red nodules of cheeks; equestrian cold panniculitis
5) Factitial panniculitis
6) Post-steroid panniculitis
7) Crystal panniculitis
8) Eosinophilic panniculitis
9) Idiopathic nodular panniculitis (Weber-Christian disease) *Medicine 64:181–191, 1985;* relapsing idiopathic nodular panniculitis *BJD 152:582–583, 2005*
10) Associations with Sweet's syndrome, sarcoid, Behcet's disease, familial Mediterranean fever, Whipple's disease, relapsing polychondritis
11) Lipomembranous panniculitis with nodular fat necrosis
12) Subcutaneous fat necrosis after hypothermic cardiac surgery *JAAD 15:331–336, 1986*
13) Subcutaneous fat necrosis of newborn
14) Sweet's syndrome panniculitis *JAAD 56:S61–62, 2007; Am J Dermatopathol 11:99–111, 1989*
15) Neutrophilic panniculitis of infancy *JAAD 57:S65–68, 2007*
15a) Neutrophilic panniculitis – associated with:
Familial Mediterranean fever
Infections – *Staphylococcus, Streptococcus, Klebsiella, Nocardia, Candida, Fusarium, Histoplasmosis, Cryptococcus, Actinomyces*
Panniculitic bacterid – associated with intranasal aspergilloma, streptococcal tonsillitis, viral pharyngitis, dental abscess, impetiginized dermatitis, breast abscess, staphylococcal cellulitis
Pseudomonas pneumonia
Ulcerative colitis
16) Granulomatous panniculitis in Sjogren's syndrome – red nodules and plaques *AD 144:815–816, 2008*
17) Lipoatrophic panniculitis (lipophagic panniculitis of childhood; annular atrophy of the ankles, annular atrophic panniculitis of the ankles) – red nodules and red plaques of extremities; annular atrophy of ankle and/or dorsal foot *Ped Derm 28:146–148, 2011; AD 146:877–881, 2010*
18) Annular atrophic connective tissue panniculitis – erythematous nodules and plaques of ankles followed by circumferential band of atrophy *Ped Derm 28:146–148, 2011; Ped Derm 28:142–145, 2011; J Cut Pathol 38:270–274, 2011; AD 146:877–881, 2010*

Lymphocytoma cutis (pseudolymphoma) *JAAD 38:877–905, 1998; Acta DV 62:119–124, 1982*
Allergen injections
Carbamazepine
Cowpox vaccination
Gold hypersensitivity
Idiopathic
Insect bites
Lyme borreliosis
Phenytoin
Tattoos
Trauma

Pyoderma gangrenosum *Br J Plast Surg 53:441–443, 2000; JAAD 18:559–568, 1988*

Relapsing polychondritis – erythema nodosum-like lesions; superficial thrombophlebitis *Medicine 80:173–179, 2000*

Rosai-Dorfman disease (sinus histiocytosis with massive lymphadenopathy) – xanthoma-like lesions with grouped yellow-red papules and nodules of head, neck, ears, trunk, arms and legs; cervical lymphadenopathy; also axillary, inguinal, and mediastinal adenopathy; hypergammaglobulinemia; emperipolesis (histiocytes with intracellular inflammatory cells and debris) *JAAD 65:1069–1071, 2011; Int J Derm 37:271–174, 1998; Am J Dermatopathol 17:384–388, 1995; Semin Diagn Pathol 7:19–73, 1990; Cancer 30:1174–1188, 1972;* red nodules *JAMADerm 150:177–181, 2014;* disseminated red papules and nodules of extremities *JAMA 310:199–200, 2013*

Sarcoid (Darier-Roussy sarcoid) *JAAD 72:924–926, 2015; JAAD 54:55–60, 2006; Ann Dermatol Syphil 5:144–149, 1904;* syringotropic sarcoid – localized hypohidrosis *JAAD 68:1016–1021, 2013*

Subacute nodular migratory panniculitis of Villanova and Pinol-Aguade (erythema nodosum migrans) *Acta DV (Stockh) 53:313–317, 1973; AD 89:170–179, 1964*

Subcutaneous fat necrosis of the newborn *J Cutan Pathol 5:193–199, 1978; AD 134:425–426, 1998*

Sweet's syndrome – edematous red nodules, hemorrhagic bullae, subcutaneous red nodule *JAAD 79:987–1006, 2018*

Ulcerative colitis with nodular panniculitis *J Gastroenterol 29:84–87, 1994*

Whipple's disease – red nodules indicating immune reconstitution; macular and reticulated erythema; Addisonian hyperpigmentation; *Tropheryma whipplei JAAD 60:277–288, 2009*

METABOLIC DISEASES

Acquired depletion of C1-esterase inhibitor – lobular panniculitis *Am J Med 8:959–962, 1987*

Alpha-1 antitrypsin deficiency-associated panniculitis – red nodules of legs *NEJM 382:1443–1455, 2020; JAAD 65:227–229, 2011; JAAD 51:645–655, 2004; Cutis 71:205–209, 2003; AD 123:1655–1661, 1987*

Blueberry muffin baby in hereditary spherocytosis – red nodules, generalized *Cutis 101:111–114, 2018*

Calcinosis cutis (dystrophic calcification) *Cutis 60:259–262, 1997*

Calciphylaxis *Cutis 51:245–247, 1993; JAAD 22:743–747, 1990*

Crohn's disease – metastatic Crohn's disease – red nodules of lower legs *JAAD 10:33–38, 1984;* granulomatous ulcer *JAAD 41:476–479, 1999*

Crystal panniculitis

Cystic fibrosis-associated episodic arthritis – pink macules, urticarial papules, arthritis, purpura of legs, erythema nodosum, cutaneous vasculitis *JAMADerm 155:375–376, 2019; Respir Med 88:567–570, 1994; Am J Dis Child 143:1030–1032, 1989; Ann Rheum Dis 47:218–223, 1988; Arch Dis Child 59:377–379, 1984*

Diabetic muscle infarction – palpable painful mass of thigh *Am J Med 101:245–250, 1996*

Gout – gouty panniculitis with urate crystal deposition *Cutis 76:54–56, 2005; Am J Dermatopathol 9:334–338, 1987; AD 113:655–656, 1977*

Intrahepatic cholestasis of pregnancy – prurigo nodularis-like lesions *AD 143:757–762, 2007*

Nodular obesity-associated lymphedematous mucinosis – red nodules of legs *JAMA Derm 149:867–868, 2013*

Pancreatic panniculitis – periarticular subcutaneous nodules of lower legs; post-traumatic pancreatitis, acute and chronic pancreatitis, pancreatic carcinoma, pancreatic pseudocyst, anatomical ductal anomaly of pancreas, pancreas divisum, vasculopancreatic fistulae *JAMADerm 154:471–472, 2018; NEJM*

375:1972–1981, 2016; JAMADerm 151:95–96, 2015; NEJM 368:465, 2013; JAAD 45:325–361, 2001; JAAD 34:362–364, 1996; Arthritis Rheum 22:547–553, 1979; Am J Med 58:417–423, 1975; HIV infection and hemophagocytic syndrome *BJD 134:804–807, 1996*

Pretibial myxedema – personal observation

Vascular calcification – cutaneous necrosis syndrome *JAAD 33:53–8, 1995*

Whipple's disease – subcutaneous Whipple's disease; leg nodules or erythema nodosum

Xanthoma

NEOPLASTIC DISEASES

Acrospiroma *Cutis 58:349–351, 1996*

Aneurysmal fibrous histiocytoma – red nodule of wrist *Ped Derm 23:591–592, 2006; Cancer 47:2053–2061, 1981*

Angioimmunoblastic T-cell lymphoma

Angiosarcoma – Stewart-Treves tumor; hemorrhagic ulcerated plaque and nodule in chronic lymphedema *JAAD 77:995–1006, 2017; AD 146:337–342, 2010*

Atypical Spitzoid melanocytic tumors – bright pink nodule *JAAD 64:919–935, 2011*

Basal cell carcinoma – metastatic *JAAD 59:S1–3, 2008*

Blastic plasmacytoid dendritic cell neoplasm – violaceous nodule *Ped Derm 30:142, 144, 2013;* violaceous nodule with golden contusiform rim *JAMA Derm 150:73–76, 2014*

Cartilaginous matrix-producing apocrine carcinoma – pink papulonodule *BJD 163:215–218, 2010*

CD 30+ lymphoproliferative disorders – red tumors, red plaques with or without necrosis, giant tumor *JAAD 72:508–515, 2015*

Cellular dermatofibroma – purple nodule of arm *Ped Derm 35:403–405, 2018*

Chondroid syringoma

Clear cell acanthoma – personal observation

Clear cell hidradenoma – brown-red nodule *JAAD 54:S248–249, 2006; Ped Derm 22:450–452, 2005*

Combined squamous cell carcinoma and Merkel cell carcinoma – crusted papule, red facial nodule, red papule, red nodule of wrist *JAAD 73:968–975, 2015*

Crystal-storing histiocytosis associated with lymphoplasmacytic lymphoma – panniculitis *Hum Pathol 27:84–87, 1996*

Cytophagic histiocytic panniculitis – manifestation of hemophagocytic syndrome; red tender nodules; T-cell lymphoma, B-cell lymphoma, histiocytic lymphoma, sinus histiocytosis with massive lymphadenopathy (Rosai-Dorfman disease) *JAAD 4:181–194, 1981; Arch Int Med 140:1460–1463, 1980*

Dermal duct tumor – red nodule of head, neck, arms, legs, or back *AD 140:609–614, 2004*

Dermatofibrosarcoma protuberans – early, red papule/nodule *Ped Derm 36:400–401, 2019; JAAD 57:548–550, 2007; JAAD 35:355–374, 1996;* nodules of leg *Ped Derm 31:676–682, 2014*

Dermatomyofibroma – red nodule or plaque *Ped Derm 16:154–156, 1999;* pink nodule of shoulder *AD 148:113–118, 2012*

Eccrine angiomatous hamartoma *Ped Derm 14:401–402, 1997*

Eccrine porocarcinoma *JAAD 49:S252–254, 2003*

Eccrine poroma and eccrine porocarcinoma – red nodule of ankle *BJD 150:1232–1233, 2004*

Eccrine spiradenocarcinoma – red nodule of arm; tender, solitary subcutaneous nodule *Cutis 92:285–287, 2013; Pol Med J 11:388–396, 1972*

Eccrine syringofibroadenoma *BJD 142:1050–1051, 2000*

Epithelioid sarcoma – personal observation

Eruptive infundibulomas *Ann DV 114:551–6, 1987*

Extramedullary hematopoiesis in chronic idiopathic myelofibrosis with myelodysplasia *JAAD 55:S28–31, 2006*

Fibrosarcoma/spindle cell sarcoma – red or violaceous nodule

Fibrous tumors of infants
  Calcifying aponeurotic fibroma
  Digital fibromatosis
  Fibromatosis colli
  Fibrous hamartoma of infancy
  Hyaline fibromatosis
  Infantile myofibromatosis *AD 134:625–630, 1998*
  Intravascular fasciitis

Fibrous histiocytoma

Granular cell schwannoma – including prurigo nodularis-like lesions *Int J Derm 20:126–129, 1981*

Granulocytic sarcoma – violaceous nodule with green halo *Cutis 94:65, 81–82, 2014*

Hidradenocarcinoma, metastatic *AD 142:1366–1367, 2006*

Histiocytic lymphoma (true histiocytic lymphoma) *JAAD 50:S9–10, 2004*

Infantile myofibromatosis – purple nodules of legs *Ped Derm 19:520–522, 2002; Curr Prob Derm 14:41–70, 2002*

Kaposi's sarcoma *Dermatol Clin 24:509–520, 2006; AD 141:1311–1316, 2005*

Keratoacanthoma

Leiomyoma – pink, red, dusky brown papules or nodules *Cancer 54:126–130, 1984*

Leiomyosarcoma *JAAD 48:S51–53, 2003; JAAD 38:137–142, 1998; J Exp Clin Cancer Res 17:405–407, 1998; JAAD 21:1156–1160, 1989*

Leukemia – acute lymphoblastic – purple nodules *JAAD 38:620–621, 1998;* leukemia cutis – AML violaceous nodules *Ped Derm 36:658–663, 2019; AD 110:415–418, 1974;* monocytic leukemia – red, brown, violaceous nodule *Cutis 85:31–36, 2010; AD 123:225–231, 1971;* eosinophilic leukemia *AD 140:584–588, 2004;* congenital leukemia cutis (AML) *Ped Derm 25:34–37, 2008;* natural killer cell CD 56- large granular lymphocytic leukemia – panniculitis *JAAD 62:496–501, 2010;* aleukemic leukemic cutis – purple nodule of thigh *JAAD 63:539–541, 2010*

Lipoblastoma

Lymphadenoma, cutaneous – pink nodule of face or leg *AD 144:255–260, 2008; J EurAcad Dermatol Venereol 15:481–483, 2001; Am J Dermatopathol 18:186–191, 1996; Am J Surg Pathol 15:101–110, 1991*

Lymphangiosarcoma (Stewart-Treves tumor) – red-brown or ecchymotic patch, nodules, plaques in lymphedematous limb *Arch Surg 94:223–230, 1967; Cancer 1:64–81, 1948*

Lymphoma/leukemia – subcutaneous panniculitic T-cell lymphoma; *JAAD 79:892–898, 2018; The Dermatologist, October 2014, pp.42–44; JAAD 50:S18–22, 2004; BJD 148:516–525, 2003; AD 138:740–742, 2002; JAAD 36:285–289, 1997; AD 132:1345–1350, 1996; AD 129:1171–1176, 1993;* subcutaneous panniculitis-like T-cell lymphoma alpha/beta *Ped Derm 32:526–532, 2015; BJD 163:1136–1138, 2010;* subcutaneous panniculitis-like T-cell lymphoma (with hemophagocytic syndrome) – blue-red nodules of

extremities and face with edema of legs *JAAD 61:875–881, 2009; Ped Derm 23:537–540, 2006; Am J Surg Pathol 15:17–27, 1991;;* EBV-associated natural killer/T-cell lymphoproliferative disorder – painful red subcutaneous nodules of legs *AD 147:216–220, 2011;* primary cutaneous follicle center lymphoma with diffuse CD 30 expression – papules, plaques, nodules, multilobulated scalp tumor *JAAD 71:548–554, 2014;* folliculocentric cutaneous T-cell lymphoma – prurigo lesions *JAAD 70:205–220, 2014;* gamma/delta T-cell lymphoma *JAAD 56:643–647, 2007; JAAD 34:904–910, 1996;* lymphomatoid granulomatosis – angiocentric T-cell lymphoma *AD 127:1693–1698, 1991; AD 132:1464–1470, 1996;* CD30- CTCL *AD 1331:1009–1015, 1995;* primary cutaneous anaplastic large cell lymphoma CD 30+ –– red nodule of the arm *JAAD 70:374–376, 2014; AD 145:1399–1404, 2009; AD 145:667–674, 2009; BJD 157:1060–1061, 2007;* post-transplant lymphoma *JAAD 81:600–602, 2019;* B cell lymphoma overlying acrodermatitis chronica atrophicans associated with Borrelia burgdorferi infection *JAAD 24:584–590, 1991;* nasal NK/T-cell lymphoma *JAAD 46:451–456, 2002;* NK/T-cell lymphoma – ulcerated red nodule of leg *BJD 173:134–145, 2015;* CD 30+ CTCL (Ki+anaplastic large cell lymphoma) – isolated red nodule *Ann Oncol 5(Suppl.1)25–30, 1994;* primary B-cell lymphoma *AD 130: 1551–1556, 1994;* primary cutaneous diffuse large B-cell lymphoma, leg type; Bcl-2 expression – red to bluish nodules of one or both legs and ankles *JAAD 69:329–340, 2013; JAAD 66:650–654, 2012; BJD 160:713–716, 2009; AD 143:1520–1526, 2007; AD 143:1144–1150, 2007;* and primary cutaneous large B-cell lymphoma of the legs *AD 132:1304–1308, 1996;* large cell B-cell lymphoma of the leg *JAAD 49:223–228, 2003;* primary cutaneous marginal zone B-cell lymphoma – red nodules with surrounding erythema or pink papules or nodules *BJD 176:1010–1020, 2017; JAMADerm 150:412–418, 2014; JAAD 59:179–1206, 2008; AD 141:1139–1145, 2005; BJD 147:1147–1158, 2002;* intravascular B-cell (malignant angioendotheliomatosis) lymphoma mimicking erythema nodosum *J Cutan Pathol 27:413–418, 2000; JAAD 39:318–321, 1998; Cancer 3:1738–1745, 1994;* intravascular lymphoma – painful gray-brown, red, blue-livid patches, plaques, nodules, with telangiectasia and underlying induration; 40% of patients with intravascular lymphoma present with cutaneous lesions *BJD 157:16–25, 2007;* angiotropic B-cell lymphoma (malignant angioendotheliomatosis); lymphoplasmacytic lymphoma *JAAD 38:820–824, 1998;* plasmablastic lymphoma (HIV- and EBV-associated) – skin-colored-pink, purple nodules of legs *JAAD 58:676–678, 2008;* follicular-center B-cell lymphoma – nodules of face, scalp, trunk, extremities *AD 132:1376–1377, 1996;* immunocytoma (low grade B- cell lymphoma) – reddish-brown papules, red nodules, plaques and/or tumors on the extremities *JAAD 44:324–329, 2001;* CD56+ lymphoma *AD 140:427–436, 2004;* HTLV-1 lymphoma *BJD 128:483–492, 1993; Am J Med 84:919–928, 1988;* plasmacytoid dendritic cell neoplasm (lymphoblastoid natural killer-cell lymphoma) – purple nodule of leg; nodule of face or scalp *BJD 162:74–79, 2010; BJD 146:148–153, 2002;* histiocytic lymphoma (reticulum cell sarcoma) – blue-red nodules *Am J Dermatopathol 14:511–517, 1992; Cancer 62:1970–1980, 1988;* Epstein-Barr virus and natural killer T-cell lymphoma *JAAD 59:157–161, 2008;* cutaneous Richter syndrome (CLL rapidly developing into large cell lymphoma) *BJD 140:708–714, 1999; Clin Exp Dermatol 18:263–267, 1993; Am J Med 68:539–548, 1980;* primary cutaneous marginal zone B-cell lymphoma *JAAD 69:329–340, 2013;* on back *BJD 157:591–595, 2007;* in children *BJD 161:140–147, 2009;* plasmablastic post-transplant lymphoproliferative disorder *Ped Derm 26:713–716, 2009;* anetodermic primary cutaneous B-cell lymphoma – associated with anti-phospholipid antibodies *AD 146:175–182, 2010; Arthritis Rheum 36:133–134, 2010; Clin Exp Dermatol 31:130–131, 2006; Actas Dermosifiligr 94:243–246, 2003; Am J Dermatopathol 23:124–132, 2001; BJD 143:165–170, 2000;* angioimmunoblastic T-cell lymphoma (angioimmunoblastic lymphadenopathy with dysproteinemia) – morbilliform eruption; arthralgias, purpura, petechiae, urticaria, nodules *JAAD 65:855–862, 2011; NEJM 361:900–911, 2009; BJD 144:878–884, 2001; JAAD 36:290–295, 1997; JAAD 1:227–32, 1979;* metastatic testicular lymphoma *JAAD 66:650–654, 2012;* primary cutaneous diffuse large cell B-cell lymphoma, leg type – red-violaceous sporotrichoid nodules of leg *AD 148:1199–1204, 2012;* primary cutaneous follicular center B-cell lymphoma *JAAD 69:343–354, 2013;* cutaneous extranodal natural killer T-cell lymphoma – multiple violaceous or red nodules of extremities, subcutaneous nodules, cellulitis, abscess-like lesions *JAAD 70:1002–1009, 2014;* HTLV-1 leukemia/lymphoma – nodulotumoral lesions, nodules, ulcerated nodules, multipapular lesions, red plaques, red patches, erythroderma *JAAD 72:293–301, 2015;* Richter transformation – transformation of chronic lymphocytic leukemia to high grade lymphoma – red nodules and plaques of arm with generalized lymphadenopathy *BJD 172:513–521, 2015;* primary cutaneous aggressive cytotoxic epidermotropic CD8+ T-cell lymphoma – necrotic nodules *BJD 173:869–871, 2015;* cutaneous peripheral T-cell lymphoma *JAAD 75:992–999, 2016;* multifocal primary cutaneous anaplastic large cell lymphoma *BJD 179:724–731, 2018*

Lymphomatoid granulomatosis (angiocentric lymphoma) – violaceous nodules *Ped Derm 17:369–372, 2000*

Lymphomatoid papulosis *JAAD 49:1049–1058, 2003;* red nodule with scale *AD 147:943–947, 2011*

Malignant fibrous histiocytoma *Cutis 69:211–214, 2002*

Malignant histiocytosis – single red or violaceous nodules or diffuse papulonodular eruption of legs and/or buttocks *JAAD 56:302–316, 2007; Hum Pathol 15:368–377, 1984*

Malignant nodular hidradenoma (aka clear cell eccrine carcinoma, clear cell hidradenocarcinoma, malignant acrospiroma, malignant clear cell acrospiroma, malignant clear cell hidradenoma, malignant clear cell myoepithelioma, solid cystic hidradenocarcinoma) – nodule of head, trunk, distal extremities *Cutis 68:273–278, 2001;* deep red nodule of leg *Cutis 88:173–174, 2011*

Malignant schwannoma

Melanocytic nevus – congenital nevus presenting as proliferative red nodule without underlying pigmentation *BJD 176:1131–1143, 2017; Society Pediatric Dermatology Annual Meeting, July, 2015*

Melanoma, including amelanotic melanoma *NEJM 368:1536, 2013; AD 144:560–561, 2008; Semin Oncol 2:5–118, 1975;* metastatic uveal melanoma *BJD 169:160–161, 2013;* spitzoid melanoma – purple nodule of leg *Cutis 90:180,187–188, 2012*

Merkel cell carcinoma – red nodule of arm *Cutis 87:81–84, 2011;* red nodules of legs *JAAD 81:1–21, 2019; J Drugs in Dermatol 9:779–784, 2010; Cutis 90: 183–185, 2012; Dermatol Ther 21:447–451, 2008; JAAD 58:375–381, 2008;* violaceous nodule of knee *AD 145:715–720, 2009*

Metaplastic synovial cysts – red nodules of buttocks *JAAD 41:330–332, 1999*

Metastases – testicular carcinoma *JAAD 65:455–456, 2011*

Multiple myeloma *JAAD 76:S71–72, 2017; AD 139:475–486, 2003*

Muscle tumors – primary or metastatic tumors of muscle; palpable painful mass of thigh

Myelodysplastic syndromes – prurigo nodularis-like lesions *JAAD 33:187–191, 1995;* neutrophilic panniculitis *BJD 136:142–144, 1997*

Myeloid sarcoma, de novo – diffuse red-brown nodules *Ped Derm 36:509–510, 2019*

Myoepithelioma, cutaneous *AD 147:499–504, 2011*

Myofibromatosis

Nerve sheath myxoma *AD 145:195–200, 2009*

Neurofibroma

Neurothekeoma *Ped Derm 37:187–189, 2020; AD 139:531–536, 2003*

Nevus comedonicus, inflammatory *JAAD 38:834–836, 1998*

Nodular hidradenoma (clear cell hidradenoma, eccrine acrospiroma, clear cell myoepithelioma) *AD 136:1409–1414, 2000; JAAD 42:693–695, 2000*

Nodular subepidermal fibroma *Cutis 69:173–174, 2002*

Peripheral neuroepithelioma *Curr Prob Derm 14:41–70, 2002*

Pilar cyst

Pilomatrixoma *Cutis 69:173–174, 2002*

Plasmacytoma – extramedullary plasmacytoma – violaceous brown nodule *JAAD 49:S255–258, 2003;* primary plasmacytoma *JAAD 38:820–834, 1998;* trauma-induced secondary cutaneous plasmacytoma *AD 146:1301–1306, 2010*

Plasmacytosis, systemic *JAAD 38:629–631, 1998*

Porocarcinoma *AD 136:1409–1414, 2000*

Poroid hidradenoma – painful deep red, blue, brown or violaceous nodule of arm, scalp, face, or trunk *Ped Derm 28:60–61, 2011; AD 146:557–562, 2010*

Post-transplantation lymphoproliferative disorder – annular violaceous nodules *JAMADerm 155:619–620, 2019; JAAD 72: 1016–1020, 2015; JAAD 54:657–663, 2006; JAAD 52:S123–124, 2005; AD 140:1140–1164, 2004; JAAD 51:778–780, 2004*

Primary cutaneous perivascular epithelioid cell tumor – red nodule of legs and abdomen *JAAD 71:1127–1136, 2014*

Progressive eruptive histiocytomas (brown) *JAAD 35:323–325, 1996*

Rhabdomyosarcoma

Soft tissue sarcoma

Solitary fibrous tumor – purple nodule of thigh, scalp or face *AD 142:921–926, 2006*

Spitz nevus – *BAP-1* loss in epithelioid Spitz nevus

Squamous cell carcinoma – complicating venous stasis ulcers *South Med J 58:779–781, 1965;* complicating non-Herlitz junctional epidermolysis bullosa – beefy red nodules *JAAD 65:780–789, 2011*

Stewart-Treves lymphosarcoma – personal observation

Subcutaneous myeloid sarcoma *AD 141:104–106, 2005* Transplant-associated hematolymphoid neoplasm – p16 hypermethylation and Epstein-Barr virus infection; skin colored nodules; red nodules of legs *JAAD 55:794–798, 2006*

Syringofibroadenoma – multiple erythematous nodules of legs; associated with chronic skin ulcers, burn scars, venous stasis, elephantiasis, lepromatous neuropathy *Skin and Allergy News, Sep 2014; pp.35*

PARANEOPLASTIC DISEASES

Eosinophilic dermatosis of myeloproliferative disease – face, scalp; scaly red nodules; trunk – red nodules; extremities – red nodules and hemorrhagic papules *AD 137:1378–1380, 2001*

Erythema nodosum associated with acute myelogenous leukemia, chronic myelogenous leukemia, chronic myelomonocytic leukemia

Exaggerated arthropod bite reactions – chronic lymphocytic leukemia

Necrobiotic xanthogranuloma with paraproteinemia *Medicine (Baltimore) 65:376–388, 1986*

Neutrophilic panniculitis of myelodysplasia – red nodules of legs and soles; *MYSM1* deficiency; short stature *Ped Derm 36:258–259, 2019; JAAD 50:280–285, 2004*

Pancreatic panniculitis – pancreatic carcinoma *Cutis 80:289–294, 2007;* acinar cell carcinoma – fever and arthritis *Cutis 91:186–190, 2013*

Paraneoplastic septal panniculitis associated with acute myelog-enous leukemia *BJD 144:905–906, 2001*

Paraneoplastic vasculitis – nodules, panniculitis *J Rheumatol 18:721–727, 1991*

Polyarteritis nodosa – associated with hairy cell leukemia, and chronic myelomonocytic leukemia

Thrombophlebitis migrans (Trousseau's sign) – association with internal malignancy *Circulation 22:780, 1960*

Thrombosed veins at IV sites with squamous cell carcinoma of the kidney – personal observation

PRIMARY CUTANEOUS DISEASE

Anetoderma of Jadassohn *AD 102:697–698, 1970*

Epidermolysis bullosa pruriginosa – dominant dystrophic or recessive dystrophic; mild acral blistering at birth or early childhood; violaceous papular and nodular lesions in linear array on shins, forearms, trunk; lichenified hypertrophic and verrucous plaques in adults, reticulate scarring, dermatitis with lichenified plaques, violaceous linear scars, albopapuloid lesions of the trunk, prurigo nodularis-like lesions, milia *Ped Derm 26:115–117, 2009; BJD 152:1332–1334, 2005; BJD 146:267–274, 2002; BJD 130:617–625, 1994*

Epidermolysis bullosa – junctional epidermolysis bullosa – abnor-mal teeth with papular prurigo-like lesions *BJD 169:195–198, 2013*

Erythema elevatum diutinum *Cutis 68:41–42, 55, 2001; Cutis 34:41–43, 1984*

Granuloma annulare

Keratosis lichenoides chronica – extremities and buttocks *JAAD 38:306–309, 1998; JAAD 37:263–264, 1997; AD 131:609–614, 1995; AD 105:739–743, 1972*

Nodular erythrocyanosis – calves, knees, thighs, buttocks of women with paralysis

Prurigo nodularis – idiopathic or associated with lymphoma, peripheral T-cell lymphoma (Lennert's lymphoma) *Cutis 51:355–358, 1993;* Hodgkin's disease *Dermatologica 182:243–246, 1991; Ped Derm 7:136–139, 1990;* gluten sensitive enteropathy *BJD 95:89–92, 1976;* AIDS *JAAD 33:837–838, 1995;* uremia *South Med J 68:138–141, 1975;* depression, liver disease, alpha-1 antitrypsin deficiency *Australas J Dermatol 32:151–157, 1991;* malabsorption *Dermatologica 169:211–214, 1984*

PSYCHOCUTANEOUS DISEASES

Factitial panniculitis – lipomembranous traumatic panniculitis with overlying hypertrichosis *SKINmed 12:127–130, 2014*

SYNDROMES

Behcet's disease – erythema nodosum-like lesions (superficial vein thrombophlebitis extending to subcutaneous fat) *AD 145:171–175, 2009; BJD 159:555–560, 2008; BJD 147:331–336, 2002; JAAD 40:1–18, 1999; JAAD 36:689–696, 1997; Ped Derm 11:95–101, 1995;* subcutaneous red nodules (vasculitis) *JAAD 31:493–495,* *1994;* Behcet's disease *JAAD 41:540–545, 1999; NEJM 341:1284–1290, 1999;* neutrophilic eccrine hidradenitis *Cutis 68:107–111, 2001*

CANDLE syndrome (chronic atypical neutrophilic dermatosis with lipodystrophy and elevated temperature) – fever, recurrent annular violaceous plaques and nodules, violaceous eyelid edema, low weight and height, lipodystrophy, hepatosplenomegaly, and inflammation *Ped Derm 26:654, 2009*

Congenital self-healing reticulohistiocytosis – Hashimoto-Pritzker type *AD 134:625–630, 1998*

DADA2 (deficiency of adenosine deaminase 2) – autosomal recessive; recurrent fevers, early onset stroke, livedo racemosa, polyarteritis nodosa, hepatosplenomegaly; mutation in *CECR1 JAAD 75:449–453, 2016*

Disseminated lipogranulomatosis (Farber's disease)

Familial Mediterranean fever – panniculitis *AD 134:929–931, 1998;* erythema nodosum-like lesions *AD 112:364–366, 1976;* neutrophilic lobular panniculitis – subcutaneous red nodules of extremities with contusiform changes *JAMADerm 150:213–214, 2014*

Farber's disease (lipogranulomatosis) – deformed or stiff joints with painful limb contractures and red periarticular subcutaneous nodules *Ped Derm 26:44–46, 2009; Eur J Ped 157:515–516, 1998; AD 130:1350–1354, 1994*

Fibrodysplasia ossificans progressiva

Hemophagocytic lymphohistiocytosis syndrome *AD 128:193–200, 1992*

Histiophagocytic syndrome – panniculitis *Ryumachi 41:31–36, 2001; Ann DV 128:1339–1342, 2001; J Rheumatol 26:927–930, 1999*

Hypereosinophilic syndrome – red macules, red papules, plaques, and nodules, urticaria, angioedema *Allergy 59:673–689, 2004; Am J Hematol 80:148–157, 2005; AD 132:535–541, 1996; Medicine 54:1–27, 1975*

Hyper IgD syndrome – red macules or papules, urticaria, red nodules, combinations of fever, arthritis, and rash, annular ery-thema, and pustules – autosomal recessive; mevalonate kinase deficiency *AD 136:1487–1494, 2000; AD 130:59–65, 1994*

Hyper IgM syndrome – X-linked; sarcoid-like granulomas; multiple papulonodules of face, buttocks, arms *Ped Derm 21:39–43, 2004*

IgG4 disease – papules, plaques, nodules, parotid gland swelling (parotitis), lacrimal gland swelling, dacryoadenitis, sialadenitis, proptosis, idiopathic pancreatitis, retroperitoneal fibrosis, aortitis *JAAD 75:197–202, 2016*

IPEX syndrome – X-linked; immune dysregulation, polyendocrinop-athy (diabetes mellitus, thyroiditis), autoimmune enteropathy; mutation of FOXP3 gene encodes DNA-binding protein that suppresses transcription of multiple genes involved in cytokine production and T cell proliferation; atopic-like or nummular dermati-tis, urticaria, scaly psoriasiform plaques of trunk and extremities, penile rash, alopecia universalis, trachyonychia, bullae; pemphigoid nodularis (bullae and prurigo nodularis) *JAAD 55:143–148, 2006; AD 140:466–472, 2004; J Pediatr 100:731–737, 1982*

Nakajo syndrome – nodular erythema with digital changes

Neurofibromatosis type 1

Noonan's syndrome – multiple granular cell tumors (pink nodules) *Ped Derm 27:209–211, 2010*

Relapsing polychondritis – panniculitis *Dermatology 193:266–268, 1996*

Rosai-Dorfman disease (sinus histiocytosis with massive lymphade-nopathy *JAAD 56:302–316, 2007; Arch Pathol 87:63–70, 1969*

Sweet's syndrome *JAAD 31:535–536, 1994;* septal erythema nodosum-like panniculitis *AD 121:785–788, 1985;* subcutaneous

Sweet's syndrome *AD 138:1551–1554, 2002; Ann DV 128:641–643, 2001; BJD 136:142–144, 1997; JAAD 23:247–249, 1990;* subcutaneous Sweet's syndrome associated with myeloid disorders *JAAD 68:1006–1015, 2013*

TRAUMA

Athletes' nodules – pink-red nodules (collagenomas) above ankles *AD 143:417–422, 2007*

Carpenter's calluses – personal observation

Cold panniculitis – in two month old – red nodules of back and legs *Ped Derm 34:614–615, 2017;* including equestrian cold panniculitis in women *AD 116:1025–1027, 1980;* cold panniculitis from ice packs *Cutis 95:21–24, 2015*

Hematoma – palpable painful mass of thigh

Intravenous drug abuse (IVDA) – tracks

Islamic prayer nodules of knees – personal observation

Lymphoid hyperplasia secondary to cat scratches – red subcutaneous nodules *Ped Derm 27:294–297, 2010*

VASCULAR DISEASES

Angiokeratoma circumscriptum

Angiosarcoma – purple nodules *BJD 138:692–694, 1998; AD 124:263–264, 266–267, 1988*

Arteriovenous fistulae – congenital or acquired; red pulsating nodules with overlying telangiectasia – extremities, head, neck, trunk

Benign (reactive) angioendotheliomatosis – red-brown or violaceous nodules on arms or legs *JAAD 38:143–175, 1998*

Cholesterol emboli *JAAD 55:786–793, 2006; BJD 146:511–517, 2002; Medicine 74:350–358, 1995; Angiology 38:769–784, 1987; AD 122:1194–1198, 1986*

Eosinophilic granulomatosis with polyangiitis – elbow nodules *JAAD 37:199–203, 1997;* subcutaneous red nodules (vasculitis) *JAAD 31:493–495, 1994*

Cutaneous polyarteritis nodosa – atrophie blanche lesions, acrocyanosis, Raynaud's phenomenon, peripheral gangrene, red plaques and peripheral nodules, myalgias; macular lymphocytic arteritis – red or hyperpigmented reticulated patches of legs *JAAD 73:1013–1020, 2015*

Deep vein thrombophlebitis – personal observation

Degos' disease – red papules with yellow centers *JAAD 38:852–856, 1998; Ann DV 79:410–417, 1954*

Epithelioid angiosarcoma – red nodule of leg *JAAD 38:143–175, 1998*

Epithelioid hemangioendothelioma – purple subcutaneous nodule of forearm *JAAD 58:519–521, 2008*

Erythema induratum of Whitfield (nodular vasculitis) – nodules with edematous ankles

Erythrocyanosis – may have ulceration, erythema, keratosis pilaris, desquamation, nodular lesions, edema, and fibrosis

Fat emboli

Glomus tumor, solitary – painful pink, purple nodule *Ann Plast Surg 43:436–438, 1999*

Granulomatosis with polyangiitis – subcutaneous red nodules *JAAD 31:493–495, 1994*

Infantile hemangioma with minimal or arrested growth *Ped Derm 36:125–131, 2019*

Intravascular microemboli from polymer coats of intravascular device – hemorrhagic panniculitis presenting as ecchymosis; nodules of buttocks, arms, and trunk *JAMADerm 151:204–207, 2015*

Intravascular papillary endothelial hyperplasia – pseudo-Kaposi's sarcoma – red or purple papules and nodules of the legs *JAAD 10:110–113, 1984*

Lipodermatosclerosis, acute *JAAD 35:566–568, 1996*

Leukocytoclastic vasculitis – subcutaneous red nodules *JAAD 31:493–495, 1994*

Lymphocytic thrombophilic arteritis – painless non-ulcerating livedo reticularis, reticulated hyperpigmentation, red nodules *AD 144:1175–1182, 2008*

Lymphostasis verrucosa cutis – personal observation

Malignant angioendotheliomatosis (intravascular lymphomatosis) – red to purple nodules and plaques on trunk and extremities with prominent telangiectasias over lesions *JAAD 38:143–175, 1998*

Multifocal lymphangioendotheliomatosis with thrombocytopenia – red-brown plaques, nodules, and tumors *JAAD 67:898–903, 2012*

Necrotizing vasculitis

Nodular vasculitis (leukocytoclastic vasculitis) *JAAD 45:163–183, 2001*

Non-involuting capillary hemangioma (NICH) – red patch; blue patch; red nodules *JAAD 70:899–903, 2014;* large purple tumor *Ped Derm 29:182–185, 2012*

Papillary intralymphatic angioendothelioma/retiform hemangioendothelioma spectrum – subcutaneous purple nodules or deep red plaques *BJD 171:474–484, 2014; Cancer 24:503–510, 1969*

Perniosis – due to cold therapy system; red nodules of legs *AD 148:1101–1102, 2012*

Polyarteritis nodosa, systemic *BJD 159:615–620, 2008;*

Ann Int Med 89:66–676, 1978; cutaneous infarcts presenting as tender nodules; cutaneous (microscopic polyangiitis) (livedo with nodules) – painful or asymptomatic red or skin colored multiple nodules with livedo reticularis of feet, legs, forearms face, scalp, shoulders, trunk *BJD 159:615–620, 2008; JAAD 53:724–728, 2005; BJD 146:694–699, 2002; Ped Derm 15:103–107, 1998; Ann Rheum Dis 54:134–136, 1995; AD 130:884–889, 1994; JAAD 31:561–566, 1994; JAAD 31:493–495, 1994; Acta Med Scand 76:183–225, 1931;* cutaneous associated with Crohn's disease *Dis Colon Rectum 23:258–262, 1980;* familial polyarteritis nodosa of Georgian Jewish, German, and Turkish ancestry – oral aphthae, livedo reticularis, leg ulcers, Raynaud's phenomenon, digital necrosis, nodules, purpura, erythema nodosum; systemic manifestations include fever, myalgias, arthralgias, gastrointestinal symptoms, renal disease, central and peripheral neurologic manifestations; mutation in adenosine deaminase 2 (*CECR1*) *NEJM 370:921–931, 2014*

Post-thrombotic periphlebitis

Pustular vasculitis of hands *JAAD 32:192–198, 1995; JAAD 31:493–495, 1994*

Pyogenic granuloma

Retiform hemangioendothelioma – exophytic masses of arms or legs *JAAD 38:143–175, 1998*

Spindle cell hemangioendothelioma – purple nodule *Cutis 53:134–136, 1994*

Superficial migratory thrombophlebitis – oval tender red nodules of the legs, abdomen, arms *JAAD 45:163–183, 2001; JAAD 23:975–985, 1990;* associated with acute pancreatitis – personal observation; reticulated hyperpigmented patches with red subcutaneous nodules *Cutis 101:322,325–326, 2018*

Superficial thrombophlebitis

Takayasu's arteritis – subcutaneous red nodules *JAAD 31:493–495, 1994*

Temporal arteritis – granulomatous lipophagic panniculitis *Ann Rheum Dis 51:812–814, 1992*

Thromboangiitis obliterans (Buerger's disease) – palpable painful mass of thigh; superficial thrombophlebitis (leg nodule); acute thrombophlebitis; red nodules of sides of feet and lateral legs; associated with peripheral arterial disease *Am J Med Sci 136:567–580, 1908*

Thrombophlebitis, idiopathic – livid painful nodules *NEJM 344:1222–1231, 2001*

Tufted angioma – red nodule *Ped Derm 35:808–816, 2018; AD 142:745–751, 2006; Ped Derm 19:394–401, 2002; JAAD 20:214–225, 1989*

Vasculitis – large and/or small vessel – leukocytoclastic vasculitis; urticarial vasculitis *AD 134:231–236, 1998*

Venous thrombosis – swelling and pain of calf *NEJM 344:1222–1231, 2001; BMJ 320:1453–1456, 2000*

NODULES, RED, FACE

AUTOIMMUNE DISEASES AND DISEASES OF IMMUNE DYSFUNCTION

Chronic granulomatous disease – granulomas, furuncles, suppurative nodules *NEJM 317:687–694, 1987*

Hyper IgD syndrome – recurrent transient and fixed pink plaques and nodules of face and extremities; cephalic pustulosis; mevalonate kinase deficiency *Ped Derm 35:482–485, 2018*

Lupus erythematosus – discoid lupus erythematosus; lupus profundus (lupus panniculitis) *AD 122:576, 1986; AD 103:231–242, 1971*

CONGENITAL LESIONS

Microcystic adnexal carcinoma *Ped Derm 28:35–38, 2011*

Nasal glioma – midline nasal nodule *Dermatol Therapy 18:104–116, 2005*

Neuroglial heterotopia (encephaloceles that lost intracranial connection) – red nodule of nasal root; skin colored nodule; red blue firm non-compressible nodule (nasal glioma); intranasal polypoid masses; and rudimentary or atretic encephaloceles *Ped Derm 32:161–170, 2015*

DRUG-INDUCED

Anti-PD-1 therapy – lichen planus follicularis tumidus *JAMADerm 155:1197–1198, 2019*

Bortezomib (proteasome inhibitor for treatment of myeloma) – red nodules of trunk, face, neck, and extremities *JAAD 55:897–900, 2006*

Drug-induced pseudolymphoma syndrome *JAAD 38:877–905, 1998*

Ipilimumab – reactivation of dermal filler foreign body reaction after treatment with ipilimumab *BJD 175:1351–1353, 2016*

Voriconazole-induced squamous cell carcinomas *Clin Inf Dis 58:839,901–902, 2014*

EXOGENOUS AGENTS

BCG granuloma

Bromoderma – multiple red nodules of forehead, upper back, arms, and legs *BJD 158:427–429, 2008*

Foreign body granuloma *AD 139:17–20, 2003*

Halogenoderma

Hyaluronic acid plus dextranomer microparticles (Matridex), injectable *JAAD 64:1–34, 2011*

Paraffinoma – facial nodules and eyelid edema *JAAD 56:S127–128, 2007;* nodule of glabella with recurrent facial edema; hepatosplenomegaly, pulmonary fibrosis *AD 148:385–390, 2012*

Self-injection with dermal fillers *BJD 172:782–783, 2015*

Silica granulomas from mine explosion – red nodules of face, neck, chest *JAMADerm 154:953–954, 2018*

Silicone gel, injectable – red nodule of chin *JAAD 64:1–34, 2011*

INFECTIONS

Abscess, carbuncle, furuncle

Actinomycosis, cervicofacial – nodule of cheek or submaxillary area; board-like induration; multiple sinuses with puckered scarring; sulfur granules discharged *Arch Int Med 135:1562–1568, 1975*

African blastomycosis

Anthrax

Bacillary angiomatosis

Bejel

Botryomycosis

Candida sepsis – papules and nodules with pale centers *Am J Dermatopathol 8:501–504, 1986; JAMA 229:1466–1468, 1974*

Chromomycosis – *Aureobasidium pullulans AD 133:663–664, 1997*

Coccidioidomycosis *AD 144:933–938, 2008; JAAD 46:743–747, 2002; An Circulo Med Argent 15:585–597, 1892;* crateriform nasal nodule *AD 146:789–794, 2010*

Cryptococcosis – umbilicated nodule *NEJM 370:1741, 2014; Clin Inf Dis 33:700–705, 2001*

Demodicidosis – nodulocystic lesions of face *BJD 170:1219–1225, 2014*

Dental sinus – ulcerated nodule of lower cheek *Ped Derm 27:410–411, 2010*

Dracunculosis

Ecthyma

Emmonsia pasteuriana – dimorphic fungus; disseminated infection in South Africa; lichenoid diffuse papulosquamous eruption; crusted verrucous facial nodules and plaques *NEJM 369:1416–1424, 2013*

Epstein-Barr virus (HHV4) – primary cutaneous Epstein-Barr virus-related lymphoproliferative disorders; violaceous nodule *JAAD 58:74–80, 2008*

Erysipelas

Fusarium – sepsis; red nodule with central pallor *Rhinology 34(4):237–241, 1996*

Gnathostomiasis – migratory tender red nodules *JAAD 68:301–305, 2013*

Herpes simplex – pseudolymphoma appearance – violaceous nodule *Am J Dermatopathol 13:234–240, 1991*

Insect bite

Kerion

Lacrimal gland abscess – adjacent to medial canthus

Leishmaniasis – acute cutaneous leishmaniasis *JAMADerm 150:201–202, 2014; Clin Inf Dis 33:815,897–898, 2001; J Clin Inf Dis 22:1–13, 1996; AD 128:83–87, 1992; L. tropica* – ulcerated nodule of face *JAAD 71:271–277, 2014; JAAD 53:810–815, 2005;* post-kala-azar dermal leishmaniasis *BJD 165:411–414, 2011; BJD 163:870–874, 2010;* ulcerated facial nodules *JAAD 73:897–908, 2015*

Leprosy – lepromatous leprosy; Souza Campos nodule of leprosy *JAAD 54:559–578, 2006;* subcutaneous lepromas *Rook p.1224–1227, 1998, Sixth Edition;* erythema nodosum leprosum (vasculitis) – painful facial nodules with fever, arthralgias, dactylitis, iritis, uveitis, orchitis, adenitis, glomerulonephritis, tibial periostitis; ulcerated nodules *JAAD 83:17–30, 2020; JAAD 51:416–426, 2004; AD 138:1607–1612, 2002;* histoid leprosy – centrofacial distribution *BJD 160:305–310, 2009*

Milker's nodule

Molluscum contagiosum, giant

Mycobacterium abscessus – facial nodules after soft tissue augmentation *Dermatol Surg 29:97–973, 2003*

Mycobacterium avium-intracellulare – cervicofacial lymphadenitis in children *Ped Derm 21:24–29, 2004*

Mycobacterium chelonae – facial lesions; red papules and nodules *BJD 170:471–473, 2014*

Mycobacterium malmoense – cervicofacial lymphadenitis in children *Ped Derm 21:24–29, 2004*

Mycobacterium marinum

Mycobacterium mucogenicum – following cosmetic use of poly-L-lactic acid *SKINmed 12:353–357, 2013;* red nodule of medial canthus following dacryocystorhinostomy and Cranford tube replacement *JAMADerm 150:981–983, 2014*

Mycobacterium scrofulaceum – ulcerated nodule of cheek *Ped Derm 22:476–479, 2005*

Mycobacterium tuberculosis – scrofuloderma – infected lymph node, bone, joint, lacrimal gland with overlying red-blue nodule which breaks down, ulcerates, forms fistulae, scarring with adherent fibrous masses which may be fluctuant and draining *BJD 134:350–352, 1996;* BCG granuloma; lupus vulgaris

Myiasis – cuterebrid myiasis *Ped Derm 21:515–516, 2004; Hypoderma tarandi;* bumblebee-like fly of subarctic regions; eggs deposited on reindeer (caribou); larvae penetrate skin, hatch, and result in migratory swellings; ophthalmomyiasis may result in blindness *NEJM 367:2456–2457, 2012*

Nocardiosis, primary cutaneous *AD 146:81–86, 2010*

North American blastomycosis – pustulonodular infiltration of nose *JAMA 312:2564–2565, 2014;* disseminated – red facial scaly nodule *Ped Derm 35:673–675, 2018; NEJM 356:1456–1462, 2007*

Onchocerciasis (*Onchocerca volvulus*) – facial nodules *JAAD 73:929–944, 2015*

Orf *Clin Dermatol 32:715–733, 2014; JAAD 40:815–817, 1999*

Paecilomyces lilacinus – red nodules with necrotic centers *Ann Int Med 125:799–806, 1996*

Papular urticaria

Paracoccidioidomycosis *JAAD 53:931–951, 2005*

Preauricular cyst *Curr Prob in Dermatol 13:249–300, 2002*

Pseudomonas sepsis *JAAD 32:279–280, 1995; Am J Med 80:528–529, 1986*

Rhinoscleroma (*Klebsiella pneumonia subspecies rhinoscleromatis*) – facial perioral nodule *JAAD 69:1066–1067, 2013*

Scabies – in elderly and infants *JAAD 82:533–548, 2020*

Sporotrichosis, fixed cutaneous *Cutis 54:279–286, 1994; Dermatologica 172:203–213, 1986; Sporothrix schenckii var brasiliensis* – red nodule of cheek with conjunctivitis *BJD 172:1116–1119, 2015*

Staphylococcus aureus – abscess (furuncle) *Rook p.1119, Sixth Edition*

Syphilis – nodular secondary *JAAD 82:1–14, 2020; AD 133:1027–1032, 1997;* in AIDS *Clin Dermatol 38:152–159, 2020; J Clin Inf Dis 23:462–467, 1996;* tertiary (gumma); ulcerated nodules of face – malignant secondary syphilis *JAMADerm 152:829–830, 2016; AD 99:70–73, 1969; BJD 9:11–26, 1897*

Tropical ulcer

Tularemia

Warts

Yaws

INFILTRATIVE DISORDERS

Amyloidosis – nodular primary localized cutaneous amyloidosis *JAAD 57:S26–29, 2007*

Cutaneous lymphoid hyperplasia *JAAD 65:112–124, 2011*

Hashimoto-Pritzker disease (congenital self-healing reticulohistiocytosis) – red facial nodule *JAAD 53:838–844, 2005*

IgG4-related skin disease – plasma cells and fibrosis; FoxP3+ cells *JAMA Derm 149:742747, 2013*

Jessner's lymphocytic infiltrate

Juvenile xanthogranuloma – personal observation

Lymphocytoma cutis – personal observation

Progressive nodular histiocytosis – dermal dendrocytes; red nodules of face, trunk, and extremities *BJD 143:628–631, 2000*

Rosai-Dorfman disease (sinus histiocytosis with massive lymphadenopathy) – multiple multilobular red nodules with yellow centers *JAMA Derm 149:992–994, 2013; BJD 164:213–215, 2011; AD 144:120–121, 2008*

Sea blue histiocytosis – facial macular brown hyperpigmentation; nodules of face, trunk, hands, and feet; eyelid infiltration; puffy face; leonine facies *JAAD 57:1031–1045, 2007*

Self-healing juvenile cutaneous mucinosis – red nodules of face, scalp, hand; macrodactyly (enlarged thumbs); periarticular papules and nodules, painful polyarthritis; linear ivory white papules, multiple subcutaneous nodules, indurated edema of periorbital and zygomatic areas *JAAD 55:1036–1043, 2006; AD 131:459–461, 1995; Ann DV 107:51–57, 1980; Lyon Med 230:470–474, 1973*

INFLAMMATORY DISORDERS

Erythema nodosum in children *Ped Derm 13:447–450, 1996*

Febrile idiopathic lobar panniculitis of childhood – abdominal pain, arthralgia, fever, red nodules of face, legs, trunk, lipoatrophy *Ped Derm 31:652, 2014*

Idiopathic aseptic facial granuloma – purple facial nodules in infants and toddlers *Ped Derm 35:397–400, 2018; Ped Derm 35:490–493, 2018*

Hidradenitis suppurativa – personal observation

Idiopathic facial granuloma of children – red or violaceous nodule of cheek *Ped Derm 31:729–730, 2014; Ped Derm 30:394–395, 2013*

Lymphocytoma cutis (cutaneous lymphoid hyperplasia) *AD 142:1561–1566, 2006; Cancer 69:717–724, 1992; Acta DV (Stockh)62:119–124, 1982;* eyebrow nodule *Ped Derm 30:628–629, 2013*

Nodular fasciitis *AD 137:719–721, 2001*

Panniculitis – personal observation

Pseudolymphomatous folliculitis – solitary red dome shaped or flat elevated nodule of cheek, nose, eyelid, forehead *Am J Surg Pathol 23:1313–1319, 1999; Am J Pathol 24:367–387, 1948;* differential diagnosis includes T cell-rich B-cell lymphoma, primary cutaneous follicular center lymphoma, folliculotropic CTCL, cutaneous B-cell lymphoid hyperplasia, cutaneous T-cell pseudolymphoma, granulomatous rosacea

Cutaneous Rosai-Dorfman disease – facial nodules *JAMADerm 150:787–788, 2014*

Sarcoid – lupus pernio *JAAD 48:290–293, 2003; JAAD 16:534–540, 1987; BJD 112:315–322, 1985; Clin Exp Dermatol 9:614–617, 1984*

Sinus histiocytosis with massive lymphadenopathy (Rosai-Dorfman disease) – violaceous, red papules and nodules; cervical lymphadenopathy; also axillary, inguinal, and mediastinal adenopathy *JAAD 41:335–337, 1999; Int J Derm 37:271–274, 1998;*

Am J Dermatopathol 17:384–388, 1995; Cancer 30:1174–1188, 1972

Subcutaneous fat necrosis of the newborn *AD 134:425–426, 1998*

METABOLIC DISEASES

Blueberry muffin baby in hereditary spherocytosis – red nodules, generalized *Cutis 101:111–114, 2018*

Verrucous xanthoma – nodule of nose *J Laryngol Otol 113:79–81, 1999; Am J Dermatopathol 8:237–240, 1986*

NEOPLASTIC DISEASES

Adenoid cystic carcinoma

Angiolipoma

Apocrine hidrocystoma *AD 137:657–662, 2001*

Atypical fibroxanthoma *AD 137:719–721, 2001; Cutis 51:47–48, 1993; BJD 97:167, 1977; Cancer 31:1541–1552, 1973; Tex St J Med 59:664–667, 1963*

Basal cell carcinoma *Acta Pathol Microbiol Scand 88A:5–9, 1980;* basal cell carcinomas in nevoid basal cell carcinoma syndrome *JAAD 55:S86–89, 2006*

Benign nodular hidradenoma *AD 140:609–614, 2004*

Blastic plasmacytoid dendritic cell neoplasm – "purple plum" nodule of face *BJD 169:579–586, 2013*

Carcinosarcoma (basal cell carcinoma with sarcomatous component) *JAAD 59:627–632, 2008*

CD4 + CD56+ hematodermic neoplasm – vascular nodule of forehead; red plaques of face; tumor of plasmacytoid dendritic cells *Cutis 89:278–283, 2012*

Chondroid syringoma *AD 84:835–847, 1961;* purple nodule *AD 140:751–756, 2004*

Clear cell hidradenoma (eccrine acrospiroma)

Combined squamous cell carcinoma and Merkel cell carcinoma – crusted papule, red facial nodule, red papule, red nodule of wrist *JAAD 73:968–975, 2015*

Congenital self-healing reticulohistiocytosis (Hashimoto-Pritzker disease) *Int J Dermatol 38:693–696, 1999*

Cylindroma *Am J Dermatopathol 17:260–265, 1995*

Dermal duct tumor – red nodule of head, neck, arms, legs, or back *AD 140:609–614, 2004*

Dermatofibrosarcoma protuberans *Dermatol Ther 21:428–432, 2008*

Eccrine porocarcinoma *Dermatol Ther 21:433–438, 2008*

Eccrine poroma

Eccrine sweat gland carcinoma – face, scalp, palm *J Cutan Pathol 14:65–86, 1987*

Embryonal rhabdomyosarcoma *Ped Derm 15:403–405, 1998*

Epidermoid cyst, ruptured or infected – personal observation

Epithelioid fibrohistiocytoma – red nodule of nose *Ped Derm 35:678–680, 2018*

Hidradenocarcinoma, metastases – red nodules of face and scalp *AD 147:998–999, 2011*

Hidrocystoma

Infantile myofibromatosis *AD 134:625–630, 1998*

Kaposi's sarcoma

Keloids

Keratoacanthoma – giant keratoacanthoma in xeroderma pigmentosum – personal observation

Leiomyoma (pilar), congenital *JAAD 59:S102–104, 2008*

Leukemia, including congenital monocytic leukemia; monocytic leukemia – red, brown, violaceous nodule *AD 123:225–231, 1971*

Lipoma, including subgaleal lipoma – personal observation

Lymphadenoma – preauricular red nodule *AD 141:633–638, 2005*

Lymphoepithelioma-like carcinoma of the skin *AD 134:1627–1632, 1998;* associated with Epstein-Barr virus infection – ulcerated red nodule of lateral cheek *JAAD 62:681–684, 2010*

Lymphoma – cutaneous T-cell lymphoma – ulcerated nodule *JAAD 82:634–641, 2020;* multiple facial nodules *AD 145:92–94, 2009;* CTCL – ulcerated nodule of temple *BJD 156:1379–1381, 2007;* primary cutaneous CD4+ small-sized pleomorphic T-cell lymphoma *JAMA Derm 149:956–959, 2013;* B-cell, T-cell, angiotropic B-cell lymphoma (malignant angioendotheliomatosis), Hodgkin's disease, immunocytoma (low grade B-cell lymphoma) – reddish-brown papules *AD 145:92–94, 2009; JAAD 44:324–329, 2001;* primary cutaneous marginal zone B-cell lymphoma (immunocytoma) (MALT) *Ped Derm 37:228–229, 2020; JAAD 58:S62–63, 2008; AD 141:1139–1145, 2005;* primary cutaneous follicle center B-cell lymphoma *JAAD 69:343–354, 2013;* plasmacytoid dendritic cell neoplasm (lymphoblastoid natural killer-cell lymphoma) – purple nodule of leg; nodule of face or scalp *BJD 162:74–79, 2010;* HTLV-1 lymphoma *BJD 128:483–492, 1993; Am J Med 84:919–928, 1988;* post-transplant lymphoma *JAAD 81:600–602, 2019;* red-orange papulonodules – HTLV-1 granulomatous T cell lymphoma *JAAD 44:525–529, 2001;* Hodgkin's disease *AD 116:1038–1040, 1980;* follicular CTCL *JAAD 48:448–452, 2003;* primary cutaneous anaplastic large cell lymphoma *BJD 150:1202–1207, 2004;* subcutaneous panniculitis-like T-cell lymphoma (with hemophagocytic syndrome) – blue-red nodules of extremities and face; nodules of head and neck, legs, trunk, cheeks, lips *Ped Derm 32:526–532, 2015; Ped Derm 23:537–540, 2006; Am J Surg Pathol 15:17–27, 1991;* cutaneous Richter syndrome (CLL rapidly developing into large cell lymphoma) *Ann DV 122:530–533, 1995;* primary cutaneous anaplastic large cell lymphoma – ulcerated purpuric nodule of nasal tip *Ped Derm 28:570–575, 2011;* anaplastic large cell lymphoma – umbilicated nodule of cheek *Cutis 98:253–256, 2016;* cutaneous B-cell lymphoblastic lymphoma *JAAD 66:51–57, 2012;* primary cutaneous anaplastic large cell lymphoma *J Drugs Dermatol 18:460–462, 2019*

Lymphomatoid papulosis *JAAD 33:741–748, 1995*

Malignant cylindrocarcinoma *BJD 145:653–656, 2001*

Melanocytic nevus

Melanoma, including amelanotic melanoma *AD 149:413–421, 2013; Semin Oncol 2:5–118, 1975*

Merkel cell carcinoma – red or purple nodule *SKINmed 12:120–121, 2014;* red-pink vascular nodule of face *JAAD 65:983–990, 2011; JAAD 49:832–841, 2003; JAAD 43:755–767, 2000; JAAD 36:727–732, 1997; J Maxillofac Surg 13:39–43, 1985;* red nodule of chin *Sem Cut Med Surg 30:48–56, 2011;* multiple nodules *BJD 146:895–898, 2002;* verrucous nodule of cheek *Cutis 97:290–295, 2016*

Metastases – prostate carcinoma – vascular nodule *AD 146:206–208, 2010*

Mixed tumor (chondroid syringoma) *AD 125:1127, 1989*

Mucinous carcinoma – multilobulated facial tumor *AD 144:1383–1388, 2008*

Multiple myeloma *AD 139:475–486, 2003*

Neurilemmoma (schwannoma) – pink-gray or yellowish nodules of head and neck

Neuroectodermal tumors – congenital primitive neuroectodermal tumors

Neurothekeoma – red nodule of face, nose *AD 139:531–536, 2003*

Osteoma – personal observation

Pilomatrixoma *Ped Derm 26:195–196, 2009*

Porocarcinoma *AD 136:1409–1414, 2000*

Poroid hidradenoma – painful deep red nodule of arm, scalp, face, or trunk *AD 146:557–562, 2010*

Post-transplant lymphoproliferative disorder – violaceous macules, facial nodules *Ped Derm 36:681–685, 2019*

Primary cutaneous adenoid cystic carcinoma – violaceous nodules of face and neck *JAAD 58:636–641, 2008*

Progressive nodular histiocytosis – red-brown facial nodules *JAMA Derm 149:1229–1230, 2013*

Rhabdomyomatous mesenchymal hamartoma *Am J Dermatopathol 11:58–63, 1989*

Rhabdomyosarcoma *AD 124:1687, 1988*

Undifferentiated pleomorphic sarcoma – skin colored nodule *JAAD 79:853—859, 2018*

Sebaceous gland carcinoma – ulcerated brown nodule of lateral eyebrow *Ped Derm 24:501–504, 2007;* cystic sebaceous carcinoma - multilobulated nodule of nose *J Drugs Dermatol 6:540–543, 2007*

Spindle cell liposarcoma *BJD 163:638–640, 2010*

Spitz nevus – ulcerated nodule of face *Ped Derm 32:148–150, 2015*

Squamous cell carcinoma – squamous cell carcinoma, metastatic, of face due to long-term voriconazole therapy – multiple facial ulcerated nodules *Clin Inf Dis 58:839, 901–902, 2014*

Trichoepithelioma

Verrucous carcinoma – hyperkeratotic nodule of cheek *BJD 165:694–696, 2011*

Warty dyskeratoma – face, neck, scalp, axillae

PARANEOPLASTIC DISORDERS

Necrobiotic xanthogranuloma with paraproteinemia *J Cutan Pathol 27:374–378, 2000; Medicine (Baltimore) 65:376–388, 1986*

Neutrophilic panniculitis associated with myelodysplastic syndrome *JAAD 50:280–285, 2004*

PRIMARY CUTANEOUS DISEASES

Acne rosacea – pediatric granulomatous rosacea *Ped Derm 30:109–111, 2013*

Acne vulgaris – inflammatory nodulocystic lesion

Alopecia mucinosa – personal observation

Darier's disease – comedonal Darier's disease; nodules, cysts, ice pick scars *BJD 162:687–689, 2010*

Erythema elevatum diutinum – violaceous nodules of face *JAMADerm 152:331–332, 2016*

Granuloma faciale *Int J Dermatol 36:548–551, 1997; AD 129:634–635, 637, 1993*

Infantile acne *Ped Derm 30:513–518, 2013;* cyst *Ped Derm 22:166–169, 2005*

Lichen planus follicularis tumidus – due to anti-PD-1 therapy *JAMADerm 155:1197–1198, 2019*

Malakoplakia *Ped Derm 29:541–543, 2012*

Pyoderma faciale (form of acne rosacea) – sudden onset of nodules, abscesses, sinuses *AD 128:1611–1617, 1992*

SYNDROMES

Activated STING in Vascular and Pulmonary syndrome – autoinflammatory disease; butterfly telangiectatic facies; acral violaceous psoriasiform, papulosquamous and atrophic plaques of vasculitis of hands; nodules of face, nose, and ears; fingertip ulcers with necrosis; nail dystrophy; nasal septal perforation; interstitial lung disease with fibrosis; polyarthritis; myositis *NEJM 371:507–518, 2014*

Familial histiocytic dermatoarthritis *Am J Med 54:793–800, 1973*

Hereditary progressive mucinous histiocytosis

Hyper IgM syndrome – X-linked; sarcoid-like granulomas; multiple papulonodules of face, buttocks, arms *Ped Derm 21:39–43, 2004*

Muir-Torre syndrome

Neurofibromatosis types I and II – plexiform Schwannoma *Ped Derm 29:536–538, 2012*

Rosai-Dorfman disease (sinus histiocytosis with massive lymphadenopathy *JAAD 56:302–316, 2007; Arch Pathol 87:63–70, 1969*

Sea-blue histiocyte syndrome – nodular facial lesions; brown hyperpigmentation of face *JAAD 56:302–316, 2007*

Xeroderma pigmentosum – multiple cancers *JAAD 75:855–870, 2016*

TRAUMA

Cold panniculitis (Haxthausen's disease) *Burns Incl Therm Inj 14:51–52, 1988; AD 94:720–721, 1966; BJD 53:83–89, 1941;* popsicle panniculitis *Ped Derm 25:502–503, 2008; Pediatr Emerg Care 8:91–93, 1992*

Hematoma – personal observation

Islamic prayer nodule – personal observation

VASCULAR DISORDERS

Arteriovenous malformation – <u>personal observation</u>

Angiofibroma

Benign (reactive) angioendotheliomatosis – red-brown to violaceous nodules or plaques *JAAD 38:143–175, 1998*

Blue rubber bleb nevus syndrome – personal observation

Diffuse neonatal hemangiomatosis – personal observation

Facial hemangioma – ulcerated nodule *JAAD 64:827–832, 2011; JAAD 64:833–838, 2011*

Granulomatosis with polyangiitis

Juvenile temporal arteritis – forehead nodule *JAAD 62:308–314, 2010*

Kimura's disease – periauricular red nodule *JAAD 38:143–175, 1998*

Lymphatic malformation – giant tumor of cheek *JAAD 70:1050–1057, 2014*

Phakomatosis pigmentokeratotica – multilobulated pink nodules representing connective tissue nevus *Ped Derm 25:76–80, 2008*

Polyarteritis nodosa – in children; fever, peripheral gangrene, black necrosis, livedo reticularis, ulcers, nodules, vesiculobullous lesions, arthralgia, nodules of face and extremities, conjunctivitis *JAAD 53:724–728, 2005; Ann Rheum Dis 54:134–136, 1995*

Pyogenic granuloma

Tufted angioma

NODULES, RED, HAND

AUTOIMMUNE DISEASES AND DISEASES OF IMMUNE DYSFUNCTION

IgG-4 related skin disease *BJD 171:959–967, 2014*

Pemphigoid nodularis *BJD 142:143–147, 2000*

Rheumatoid arthritis – neutrophilic dermatosis *J Dermatol 27:782–787, 2000;* rheumatoid nodules *Clin Dermatol 38:3041–3048, 2019*

Systemic lupus erythematosus – vasculitis *Rev Bras Rheumatol Engl Ed 57:583–589, 2017*

DRUG-INDUCED

Imatinib-associated Sweet's syndrome *AD 141:368–370, 2005*

Lenalidomide-associated Sweet's syndrome *AD 142:1070–1071, 2006*

Neutrophilic eccrine hidradenitis – chemotherapy-induced *JAAD 40:367–398, 1999*

Sorafenib – interstitial granulomatous dermatitis; red papules, nodules, and plaques of palms *AD 147:1118–1119, 2011*

EXOGENOUS AGENTS

Barber's sinus *J Hand Surg AM 15:652–655, 1991*

Calcium hydroxyapatite *Aesthet Surg 38:S24–28, 2018*

Foreign body granuloma

Halogenoderma

Mercury granuloma *JAAD 43:81–90, 2000*

Milker's sinus – tender nodules with discharging sinuses

Paraffinoma – grease gun injury; nodule, plaque, sinus of hand *BJD 115:379–381, 1986*

Silicone granulomas of face and hands – personal observation

INFECTIONS AND INFESTATIONS

Abscesses

Anthrax

Bacillary angiomatosis *Acta DV Croat 22:294–297, 2014; Ann Plast Surg 70:652–653,; J Hand Surg AM 21:307–308, 1996*

Bacterial sepsis – septic emboli – palmoplantar red nodule

Chancriform pyoderma

Chromomycosis – red papules on dorsum of hand (*Chaetomium funicola*) *Mycopathologica 180:123–129, 2015; BJD 157:1025–1029, 2007*

Cryptococcosis *Infection 42:771–774, 2014*

Dirofilaria – hand nodule *Cutis 72:269–272, 2003*

Fusarium – red nodule with central pallor

Gram negative sepsis – personal observation

Insect bite

Leishmaniasis – chancre (ulcerated nodule) *JAAD 60:897–925, 2009;* necrotic red nodule of dorsum of hand *BJD 160:311–318, 2009*

Leprosy – lepromatous leprosy including erythema nodosum leprosum (vasculitis), subcutaneous lepromas *JAMADerm 153:313–314, 2017; J Eur Acad DV 20:344–345, 2006;* histoid leprosy *Biomedica 35:165–170, 2015*

Lyme borreliosis (*Borrelia burgdorferi*) – acrodermatitis chronica atrophicans – red to blue nodules or plaques; tissue-paper-like wrinkling; pigmented; poikilodermatous; hands, feet, elbows, knees *BJD 121:263–269, 1989: Int J Derm 18:595–601, 1979*

Milker's nodule – parapoxvirus species endemic to cattle; starts as flat red papule on fingers or face, progresses to red-blue tender nodule, which crusts; zone of erythema; may resemble pyogenic granulomas *JAAD 49:910–911, 2003; AD 111:1307–1311, 1975*

Mycetoma *JAAD 53:931–951, 2005*

Mycobacterium chelonae J Clin Inf Dis 23:1189–1191, 1996

Mycobacterium gordonae Int J Dermatol 26:181–184, 1987

Mycobacterium haemophilum JAAD 59:139–142, 2008

*Mycobacterium marinum Dermatol Online J Feb 15, 2019, march 15, 2019; Microbiol Spectr April 5, 2017 doi:*https://doi.org/10.1128/microbiolspec.TNM17-0038-2016*; Clin Inf Dis 31:439–443, 2000*

Mycobacterium tuberculosis Int J Mycobacteriol 8:205–207, 2019

Nocardia asteroides – after a cat scratch *BJD 145:684–685, 2001; N. yamanashiensis Tumor 99:e156–158, 2013*

Orf – parapoxvirus endemic to sheep and goats *Acta DV Croat 27:280–281, 2019; Am Fam Physician 86:77–78, 2012; Transpl Infect 23:e62–64, 2010; JAAD 1172–1174, 1984*

Osteomyelitis

Phaeohyphomycotic cyst (*Exophiala jeanselmei*) *JAAD 12:207–212, 1985; Phialophora, Cladosporium, and Alternaria JAAD 8:1–16, 1983; E. oligosperma Med Mycol 54:297–301, 2013; Alternaria rosae Transpl Infect Dis June 2017 19(3):doi:*https://doi.org/10.1111/tid.12698

Prototothecosis – sporangia with cartwheel-like appearance *JAAD Case Rep 5:846–848, 2019*

Pseudomonas hot tub folliculitis – palmoplantar red nodules

Rocky Mountain spotted fever – palmoplantar red nodules

Sealpox (parapoxvirus) – gray concentric nodule with superimposed bulla on dorsum of hand *BJD 152:791–793, 2005*

Sporotrichosis – primary chancre *Cutis 54:279–286, 1994; Dermatologica 172:203–213, 1986*

Staphylococcus aureus – abscess (furuncle)

Streptococcal suppurative panniculitis – personal observation

Subacute bacterial endocarditis – Janeway lesion *Med News 75:257–262, 1899;* Osler's node *Korean J Intern Med 33:1034–1035, 2018*

Syphilis – primary (chancre), nodular secondary *JAAD 82:1–14, 2020; Dermatologica Sinica 36:36–41, 2018; BMJ Case Rep 2013:bcr2013009130.doi:*https://doi.org/10.1136/bcr-2013-009130*; BJD 115:495–496, 1986,* tertiary (gumma) – palmoplantar red nodules

Trichophyton rubrum – invasive tinea corporis – personal observation; Majocchi's granuloma

Tanapox – red nodule with headache and backache *Bull WHO 63:1027–1035, 1985*

INFILTRATIVE DISEASES

Acral histiocytic nodules *Clin Exp Dermatol 37:245–248, 2012*

Langerhans cell histiocytosis resembling cherry angiomas *Ped Derm 3:304–310, 1986*

Mastocytoma – palmar nodule *Ped Derm 15:386–387, 1998*

Myxoid cyst *G Ital DV 153:847–854, 2018*

Self-healing juvenile cutaneous mucinosis – red nodules of face, scalp, hand; macrodactyly (enlarged thumbs); periarticular papules and nodules, painful polyarthritis; linear ivory white papules, multiple subcutaneous nodules, indurated edema of periorbital and zygomatic areas *JAAD 55:1036–1043, 2006; AD 131:459–461, 1995; Ann DV 107:51–57, 1980; Lyon Med 230:470–474, 1973*

INFLAMMATORY DISEASES

Erythema elevatum diutinum *J Hand Surg Am 44:522ei-522e5, 2019; Cutis 34:41–43, 1984;* palmoplantar nodules *BJD 142:116–119, 2000*

Erythema multiforme – palmoplantar red nodules

Erythema nodosum – palmoplantar red nodules *J Dermatol 27:420–421, 2000*

Fibroblastic rheumatism *JAAD 66:959–965, 2012*

Idiopathic palmoplantar hidradenitis of children *AD 131:817–820, 1995; J Cut Path 21:289–296, 1994;* palmar eccrine hidradenitis *Ped Derm 34:e283–285, 2017*

Panniculitis – palmoplantar red nodule

Pseudosarcomatous nodular fasciitis

Pyoderma gangrenosum *Arch Bone Jt Surg 4:83–86, 2016*

Relapsing eosinophilic perimyositis – fever, fatigue, and episodic muscle swelling; erythema over swollen muscles *BJD 133:109–114, 1995*

Sarcoid

METABOLIC DISEASES

Calcinosis cutis – tumoral calcinosis

Cryoproteinemia – reactive angiomatosis with cryoproteinemia *JAAD 27:969–973, 1992*

Gout – tophi *Indian J Med Res 149:682–683, 2019; BMJ Case Rep Oct 28, 2018*

Low IL-2 level *JAAD 29:473–477, 1993*

NEOPLASTIC DISORDERS

Acquired digital fibrokeratoma *Int J Dermatol 58:151–158, 2019*

Aggressive digital papillary adenocarcinoma – exophytic friable multilobulated tumor arising from sweat glands *Dermatol Online J April 15, 2018; JAAD 60:331–339, 2009*

Angioleiomyoma *Cureus 12:e7530, 2020*

Angiomatoid malignant fibrous histiocytoma *AD 121:275–276, 1985*

Angiosarcoma

Apocrine nevus

Juvenile aponeurotic palmoplantar fibroma

Basal cell carcinoma

Bony exostosis *Dermatol Online J 10:15 July 15, 2004*

Chloroma

Chondroid syringoma *Pathol Res Pract 198:755–764, 2002*

Chondroma – solitary chondroma of skin *Dermatol Online J 19:18176 may 15, 2013*

Clear cell acanthoma *JAAD 14:918–927, 1986*

Dermatofibrosarcoma protuberans

Eccrine porocarcinoma *JAAD 35:860–864, 1996*

Eccrine poroma *AD 74:511–512, 1956*

Eccrine spiradenoma

Eccrine syringofibroadenoma

Epithelioid sarcoma *Hautarzt 63:278–282, 2012*

Fibrosarcoma

Fibrous hamartoma of infancy – nodules of hands and feet *J Hand Surg 22A:740–742, 1997*

Giant cell tumor of the tendon sheath *Case Rep Orthop 2016:1834740:doi.https://doi.org/10.1155/2016/1834940; J Clin Diagn Res 8:170–171, 2014*

Granular cell tumor *Indian Dermatol Online J 4:33–36, 2013*

Kaposi's sarcoma – classic type *JAAD 38:143–175, 1998; Int J Dermatol 36:735–740, 1997; Dermatology 190:324–326, 1995*

Keratoacanthoma

Leiomyosarcoma

Lymphoma – B-cell, T-cell, angiotropic B cell lymphoma (malignant angioendotheliomatosis), Hodgkin's disease, immunocytoma (low grade B cell lymphoma) – reddish-brown papules *JAAD 44:324–329, 2001;* HTLV-1 lymphoma *BJD 128:483–492, 1993; Am J Med 84:919–928, 1988;* red-orange papulonodules – HTLV-1 granulomatous T cell lymphoma *JAAD 44:525–529, 2001;* pityriasis lichenoides-like CTCL *BJD 142:347–352, 2000*

Lymphomatoid papulosis

Malignant eccrine poroma

Malignant fibrous histiocytoma

Melanoma, including amelanotic melanoma *Semin Oncol 2:5–118, 1975;* acral lentiginous melanoma *Clin Exp Dermatol 36:174–177, 2011*

Merkel cell tumor *JAAD Case Rep 4:507–508, 2018; Hand (NY)11:Np24–29, 2016; JAAD 58:375–381, 2008; AD 123:1368–1370, 1987*

Metaplastic synovial cyst *Iran Red Crescent Med J 17:e22467. doi:https://doi.org/10.5812/ircmj.22467*

Metastatic carcinoma – thyroid, renal cell or GI tract, prostate *AD 128:1533–1538, 1992;* breast *Indian J DV Lerol 77:695–698, 2011;* hepatocellular carcinoma *Hand Surg 17:131–134, 2012*

Myelofibrosis – extramedullary hematopoiesis in myelofibrosis *AD 112:1302–1303, 1976*

Myxoid neurothekeoma *Niger J Surg 19:32–34, 2013*

Nodular hidradenoma *Cutis 95:E1–3, 2015*

Ossifying plexiform tumor *J Cutan Pathol 42:61–65, 2015*

Osteochondroma

Plantar and palmar fibromatosis *J Dtsch Dermatol Ges 17:393–397, 2019*

Sarcomatoid carcinoma *Clin Exp Dermatol 37:505–508, 2012*

Schwannomas *Medicine (Balt)98:e14605, 2019*

Sebaceous adenoma in AIDS *AD 124:489–490, 1988*

Spitz nevi mimicking pyogenic granulomas in black children *JAAD 23:842–845, 1990*

Squamous cell carcinoma

Superficial acral fibromyxoma *Int J Dermatol 54:499–508, 2015*

Sweat gland tumor

Verrucous carcinoma

PRIMARY CUTANEOUS DISEASES

Angiolymphoid hyperplasia with eosinophilia *J Med Case Rep 13:87, March 27, 2019; Int J Surg Case Rep 39:84–87, 2017*

Granuloma annulare – perforating granuloma annulare – palmoplantar red nodule *JAAD 32:126–127, 1995;* subcutaneous granuloma annulare *Acta DV Croat 25:292–294, 2017; Seminar Cut Med Surg 26:96–99, 2007;* "pseudorheumatoid nodules" *Am J Dermatopathol 27:1–5, 2005*

Granuloma faciale – extrafacial granuloma faciale

SYNDROMES

Acral dysesthesia syndrome

Behcet's syndrome *J Rheumatol 25:2469–2472, 1998*

Bowel bypass syndrome

Blue rubber bleb nevus syndrome – phlebectasias *Ped Derm 3:75–78, 1985*

Fibroblastic rheumatism *J Dermatol 45:e1142–1143, 2018*

Maffucci's syndrome *Actas Dermsifiliogr 108:861–862, 2017*

Multicentric reticulohistiocytosis *J Hand Surg Am 45:457.e1–457. e5, 2020; Rheumatol (Oxford) Nov 19, 2019*

POEMS syndrome (glomeruloid hemangioma) *JAAD 21:1061–1068, 1989; JAAD 12:961–964, 1985*

Pseudo-Kaposi's sarcoma in reflex sympathetic dystrophy *JAAD 22:513–520, 1990*

Relapsing eosinophilic perimyositis – fever, fatigue, and episodic muscle swelling; erythema over swollen muscles *BJD 133:109–114, 1995*

RS3PE – remitting seronegative synovitis with pitting edema *BMJ Case Rep April 22, 2020*

Sweet's syndrome *JAAD 31:535–536, 1994* including drug-induced Sweet's syndrome – all-trans retinoic acid, furosemide *JAAD 21:339–343, 1989;* G-CSF, GM-CSF, hydralazine, minocycline, trimethoprim-sulfamethoxazole, triphasil

TRAUMA

Delayed pressure urticaria – palmoplantar red nodules

Perniosis (chilblains)

Vibratory angioedema – palmoplantar red nodules

VASCULAR DISORDERS

Acral pseudolymphomatous angiokeratoma of children (APACHE) *BJD 124:387–388, 1991; AD 126:1524–1525, 1990*

Acroangiodermatitis (pseudo-Kaposi's sarcoma) after A-V shunt *JAAD 21:499–505, 1989; Arch Derm Res 281:35- 39, 1989*

Angiokeratoma

Cholesterol emboli – palmoplantar red nodules

Disseminated neonatal hemangiomatosis *JAAD 24:816–818, 1991; Ped Derm 8:140–146, 1991*

Eruptive pseudoangiomatosis *JAAD 29:857–859, 1993*

Glomus tumor *J med Case Rep 12:302, Oct 18, 2018; Mol Clin Oncol 2:237–239, 2014; Ann Plast Surg 43:436–438, 1999*

Granulomatosis with polyangiitis *Immun Infekt 18:89–90, 1990*

Hemangioma *Skeletal Radiol 39:1097–1102, 2010*

Hemangiopericytoma

Intravascular papillary endothelial hyperplasia *Skeletal Radiol 45:235–242, 2016; Cutis 59:148, 1997; JAAD 10:110–113, 1984;* vascular nodule of palmar third finger *BJD 166:1147–1149, 2012*

Kaposi's sarcoma including Kaposi's sarcoma in Castleman's disease *JAAD 26:105–109, 1992*

Polyarteritis nodosa

Pustular vasculitis of the hands (neutrophilic dermatosis of the dorsal hands *AD 138:361–365, 2002; JAAD 32:192–198, 1995*

Pyogenic granuloma *JAAPA 31:27–29, 2018; J Eur Acad DV 31:e512–513m 2017*

Self-healing pseudoangiosarcoma *AD 124:695–698, 1988*

Targetoid hemosiderotic hemangioma *JAAD 19:550–558, 1988*

Tufted angioma, acquired *Int J Dermatol 57:e54–55, 2018*

Vasculitis

NODULES, RED OR VIOLACEOUS, VASCULAR APPEARANCE

AUTOIMMUNE DISEASES AND DISEASES OF IMMUNE DYSFUNCTION

Dermatomyositis – presenting as panniculitis *JAAD 23:127–128, 1990*

Graft vs. host disease, chronic – chronic sclerotic graft vs. host disease-associated angiomatosis (eruptive violaceous vascular nodules) *BJD 174:782–784, 2016; JAAD 71:745–753, 2014; BJD 149:667–668, 2003; JAAD 10:918–921, 1984*
  Differential diagnosis:
  Reactive angioendotheliomatosis – brown to violaceous ulcerated patches and plaques
  Diffuse dermal angiomatosis – brown to violaceous ulcerated patches and plaques over legs, pannus, or breast associated with obesity
  Acroangiomatosis
  Atypical vascular lesions following breast radiation
  Pyogenic granuloma
  Cavernous hemangioma
  Tufted angioma – deep red to violaceous plaque or nodule

Low interleukin 2 level – vascular nodules and plaques *JAAD 29:473–477, 1993*

Lupus erythematosus – lupus profundus *JAAD 14:910–914, 1986*

Pemphigoid nodularis (purple) *AD 126:1522–1523, 1990; JAAD 21:1099–1104, 1989;* nonbullous pemphigoid *JAAD 29:293, 1993*

Pemphigus vulgaris *JAAD 23:522–523, 1990*

Rheumatoid nodule

CONGENITAL LESIONS

Benign and/or disseminated (diffuse) neonatal hemangiomatosis – diffuse (visceral involvement) or benign (only cutaneous involvement) *Ped Derm 21:469–472, 2004; JAAD 37:887–920, 1997; JAAD 24:816–818, 1991; Ped Derm 8:140–146, 1991*

Congenital infantile fibrosarcoma – ulcerated vascular nodule *Cutis 89:61–64, 2012*

Encephalocele *Soc Ped Derm Annual Meeting, 2005*

Epulis 10850508

Hamartoma with ectopic meningothelial elements – simulates angiosarcoma *Am J Surg Pathol 14:1–11, 1990*

Hemangiomatous branchial clefts, lip pseudoclefts, unusual facies – hemangiomatous branchial clefts in retroauricular areas extending down along the sternocleidomastoid muscle *Am J Med Genet 14:135–138, 1983*

Meningocele – sequestrated meningocele *Ped Derm 14:315–318, 1994*

Nasal glioma

Neonatal purple tumors or plaques – RICH, fibrosarcoma, malignant hemangiopericytoma, dermatofibrosarcoma protuberans *Ped Derm 19:5–11, 2002*

Omphalomesenteric duct remnants (vitelline duct remnant) – completely patent, peripheral portion – cherry red nodule; combined omphalomesenteric and urachal remnants differential diagnosis includes pyogenic granuloma (umbilical granuloma), sarcomas, congenital hemangiomas, patent urachus (passage of urine through umbilicus), ligated umbilical hernia *Ped Derm 24:65–68, 2007; Cutis 76:224, 233–235, 2005*

Patent vitello-intestinal duct (persistent urachal fistula) – vascular nodule of umbilicus of infancy *AD 145:1447–1452, 2009*

Pyogenic granulomas, congenital disseminated *Ped Derm 26:323–327, 2009*

Sacrococcygeal teratoma – masquerading as infantile hemangioma; red vascular plaque; red subcutaneous nodule of medial buttock *Ped Derm 30:112–116, 2013*

Spinal dysraphism with overlying protrusion, dimple, sinus, lipoma, faun tail nevus, dermoid cyst, hemangioma, port wine stain *AD 114:573–577, 1978; AD 112:1724–1728, 1976*

Thyroglossal duct cyst

Umbilical granuloma – vascular nodule *Ped Derm 36:393–394, 2019;* congenital *Ped Derm 28:404–407, 2011*

Urachus – complete or partial patency of urachus

DRUG-INDUCED

Capecitabine – pyogenic granuloma-like paronychial lesions *BJD 147:1270–1272, 2002*

Cyclosporine-induced T cell infiltrates

5-fluorouracil, capecitabine, tegafur – pyogenic granulomas *JAAD 71:203–214, 2014*

Furosemide-induced Sweet's eruption *JAAD 21:339–343, 1989*

Gefitinib (epidermal growth factor receptor inhibitor) – pyogenic granulomas of proximal nail folds *AD 142:939, 2006*

Indinavir (protease inhibitor)-induced paronychial pyogenic granuloma *JAAD 46:284–293, 2002; BJD 140:1165–1168, 1999; NEJM 338:1776–1777, 1998*

Lisinopril – associated with development of Kaposi's sarcoma *BJD 147:1042–1044, 2002*

Neuroleptics – pseudolymphoma *AD 128:121–123, 1992*

Retinoids, systemic – pyogenic granulomas

Sulindac – pancreatitis and subcutaneous fat necrosis *JAAD 13:366–369, 1985*

Vemurafenib – pyogenic granuloma *NEJM 371:1265–1267, 2014*

EXOGENOUS AGENTS

Aspartame-induced lobular panniculitis *JAAD 24:298–300, 1991*

Duoderm-induced exuberant granulation tissue

Foreign body granuloma – silk or polymer sutures, talc, starch, oily material, silicone, hair, silica, tattoo, zirconium, beryllium, wood splinter

Mercury granuloma *JAAD 12:296–303, 1985*

Silicone granuloma *AD 130:787–792, 1994*

INFECTIONS AND INFESTATIONS

Alternariosis

Amebiasis, including Acanthamoeba in AIDS *JAAD 26:352–355, 1992*

Aspergillosis, primary cutaneous – purple or brown *AD 129:1189–1194, 1993; AD 124:121–126, 1988*

Bacillary angiomatosis (*Bartonella henselae*) *Clin Inf Dis 33:772–779, 2001; BJD 136:60–65, 1997; J Hand Surg (Am) 21:307–308, 1996; JAMA 269:770–775, 1993; Hautarzt 44:361–364, 1993; JAAD 24:802–803, 807–808, 1991; JAAD 22:501–512, 1990;* vascular papules or nodules on gingival, palate or floor of mouth *J Oral Pathol 22:235–239, 1993*

Bartonellosis – *Bartonella bacilliformis;* bacillary angiomatosis; Andes mountains, Peru, Colombia, Ecuador; Oroya fever with verruga peruana; sandflies and fleas as vectors; red papules in crops become nodular, hemangiomatous or pedunculated; face, neck, extremities, mucosal lesions; 1–4 mm pruritic red papules; massive hemolytic anemia, high fever, muscle pain, delirium, coma *JAAD 59:179–1206, 2008; JAAD 54:559–578, 2006; Clin Inf Dis 33:772–779, 2001; Ann Rev Microbiol 35:325–338, 1981; 22:501–512, 1990*

Bipolaris spicifera (dematiaceous fungus)

Botryomycosis *JAAD 21:1312–1314, 1989;* intraoral botryomycosis 10530188

Brucellosis – erythema nodosum-like *AD 125:380–383, 1989*

Candida – sepsis, chronic mucocutaneous candidiasis

Cat scratch disease *JAAD 31:535–536, 1994*

Cave tick (*Ornithodoros tholozani*) bite *JAAD 27:1025–1026, 1992*

Chancriform pyoderma

Chromomycosis *AD 123:519–524, 1987*

Co-existent infections of Kaposi's sarcoma in HIV disease – cytomegalovirus, molluscum contagiosum, *Candida albicans, Cryptococcus neoformans, Histoplasma capsulatum, Mycobacterium avium-intracellulare, Mycobacterium tuberculosis Clin Inf Dis 58:540,596–597, 2014; Pathol Res Int 2011:398546; Am J Dermatopathol 34:e7–9, 2012; JAAD 62:676–680, 2010*

Cryptococcosis *JAAD 26:122–124, 1992;* cryptococcosis and Kaposi's sarcoma, coexistent – giant purple tumor of lower face in HIV disease; satellite papules *Clin Inf Dis 58:540,596–597, 2014*

Cytomegalovirus *JAAD 18:1333–1338, 1988*

Dental sinus

Dirofilariasis

Echovirus infection – eruptive pseudoangiomatosis *JAAD 29:857–859, 1993;* vascular papules or nodules; Echovirus 25, 32; Coxsackie B virus *Ped Derm 19:76–77, 2002*

Furunculosis – *Staphylococcus aureus*

Fusarium

Glanders

Gnathostomiasis *JAAD 13:835–836, 1985*

Histoplasmosis *JAAD 29:311–313, 1993, JAAD 23:422–428, 1990;* histoplasma panniculitis *AD 121:914–916, 1985*

Insect bites, including exaggerated insect bite reaction in AIDS *JAAD 29:269–272, 1993*

Leishmaniasis – AIDS-related visceral leishmaniasis *BJD 143:1316–1318, 2000;* diffuse cutaneous leishmaniasis; mucocutaneous leishmaniasis *J Emerg Med 20:353–356, 2001; AD 134:193–198, 1998; J Clin Inf Dis 22:1–13, 1996*

Leprosy, including erythema nodosum leprosum *JAAD 14:59–69, 1986*

Lyme disease *AD 120:1520–1521, 1984*

Lymphogranuloma venereum

Malacoplakia due to *Escherichia coli*

Meningococcus

Milker's nodule – starts as flat red papule on fingers or face, progresses to red-blue tender nodule, which crusts; zone of erythema; may resemble pyogenic granulomas *AD 111:1307–1311, 1975*

Mucormycosis

Mycetoma

Mycobacterium avium-intracellulare

Mycobacterium chelonae JAAD 28:352–355, 1993

Mycobacterium fortuitum

Mycobacterium haemophilum

Mycobacterium intracellulare (erythema nodosum-like nodule) *JAAD 27:1019–1021, 1992*

Mycobacterium kansasii

Mycobacterium malmoense

Mycobacterium marinum

Mycobacterium tuberculosis – acute miliary, erythema induratum, lupus vulgaris

Mycobacterium ulcerans

Myiasis, cuterebrid myiasis *JAAD 763–772, 1989*

Nocardiosis *AD 130:243–248, 1994; JAAD 26:1132–133, 1992; N. brasiliensis Ped Derm 2:49–51, 1985*

North American blastomycosis

Onchocercoma

Orf – vascular nodule of fingertip with or without ulceration *JAMADerm 151:1032–1033, 2015;JAAD 29:256–257, 1993; AD 126:356–358, 1990; JAAD 11:72–74, 1984*

Osteomyelitis

Papular urticaria

Phaeohyphomycosis *AD 123:1346–1350, 1987;* phaeohyphomycotic cyst (Exophiala jeanselmei) *JAAD 12:207–212, 1985*

Phialophora repens

Phlegmon (*Serratia*)

Pneumocystis carinii

Porto-caval shunt, infected

Protothecosis – keratoacanthoma-like *AD 121:1066–1069, 1985;* purple subcutaneous nodules *Cutis 63:185–188, 1999*

Pseudomonas sepsis *Ped Derm 4:18–20, 1987*

Rhinosporidiosis – vascular nodules of nose, extending to pharynx or lips *NEJM 380:1359, 2019; Mycopathologica 73:79–82, 1981; Arch Otolaryngol 102:308–312, 1976*

Scabies – apple jelly *JAAD 32:758–764, 1995*

Scolecobasidium constrictum (dematiaceous fungus)

Sparganosis

Sporotrichosis – primary chancre

Syphilis – primary (chancre), extragenital chancre, nodular and nodulo-ulcerative secondary *AD 113:1027–1032, 1997;* tertiary (gumma)

Tick bite granuloma

Toxoplasmosis *JAAD 14:600–605, 1986*

Trichophyton rubrum, invasive *JAAD 51:s101–104, 2004; Cutis 67:457–462, 2001;* Majocchi's granuloma

Trichosporon beigelii

Trypanosomiasis – primary lesion

Tularemia

Tungiasis

Typhoid fever

Verruca vulgaris

Xanthomonas maltophilia

Yaws – "crab yaws" – raspberry like; primary red papule, ulcerates, crusted; satellite papules; become round ulcers, papillomatous or vegetative friable nodules which bleed easily (framboesia)

Zygomycosis

INFILTRATIVE DISEASES

Primary amyloidosis – in Campbell de Morgan spots; targetoid lesions of amyloid in pre-existent capillary hemangioma *BJD 112:209–211, 1985;* tumefactive amyloid *Cutis 46:255–259, 1990;* nodular primary cutaneous amyloidosis *JAAD 14:1058–1062, 1986*

Angioplasmocellular hyperplasia – red nodule with red rim, ulcerated nodule, vascular nodule of face, scalp, neck, trunk, and leg *JAAD 64:542–547, 2011*

Jessner's lymphocytic infiltrate

Langerhans cell histiocytosis *Ped Derm 26:751–753, 2009; Australas J Dermatol 50:77–97, 2009; Ped Derm 3:75–8, 1985;* resembling cherry angiomas *Ped Derm 3:75–78, 1985;* eosinophilic granuloma; self-healing Langerhans cell histiocytosis *Cutis 102:309,316,321, 2018*

Xanthoma disseminatum *AD 127:1717–1722, 1991; AD 86:582–589, 1962*

INFLAMMATORY DISEASES

Adiposis dolorosa

Crohn's disease, metastatic (with or without ulceration) *AD 126:645–648, 1990; JAAD 19:421–425, 1988*

Endometriosis – (32% of all umbilical tumors, most common); cutaneous endometrioma – blue-red nodule *AD 147:1317–1322, 2011; AD 112:1435–1436, 1976; JAMA 191:167, 1965; duVivier p.686, 2003; AD 135:1113–1118, 1999*

Hidradenitis suppurativa

Membranous fat necrosis *AD 129:1331–1336, 1993*

Neutrophilic eccrine hidradenitis *JAAD 28:775–776, 1993; JAAD 26:793–794, 797, 1992; JAAD 11:584–590, 1984*

Pilonidal cyst and sinus

Pseudolymphomatous folliculitis

Pseudosarcomatous nodular fasciitis *Cancer 49:1668–1678, 1982*

Pyoderma gangrenosum

Rosai-Dorfman disease (sinus histiocytosis with massive lymphadenopathy; histiocytic lymphophagocytic panniculitis *AD*

124:1246–1249, 1988, JAAD 18:1322–1332, 1988; Ped Derm 4:247–253, 1987; mimicking pyogenic granuloma *Semin Diagn Pathol 7:19–73, 1990*

Sarcoid *AD 120:1239–1240, 1984*

METABOLIC

Angiokeratoma corporis diffusum
  Adult type neuraminidase deficiency
  Fabry's disease
  Fucosidosis type II
  Sialidosis type II
  Late infantile galactosialidosis
  Aspartyl glycosaminuria
  Adult onset GM1 gangliosidosis
  alpha N-acetyl galactosaminidase deficiency
  beta mannosidase deficiency
  normal variant

Blueberry muffin baby – widespread blue, purple, or red macules papules or nodules of trunk, head, and neck; may develop petechiae on surface
  Dermal erythropoiesis
    Congenital infections
      Rubella
      Cytomegalovirus
      Coxsackie B2
      Syphilis
      Toxoplasmosis
      Hereditary spherocytosis
    Rh incompatibility
      ABO blood-group incompatibility
      Twin-twin transfusion syndrome
    Neoplastic infiltrates
      Congenital leukemia
      Neuroblastoma
      Congenital rhabdomyosarcoma
    Other disorders
      Neonatal lupus erythematosus

Calcinosis cutis – tumoral calcinosis

Congenital disorders of glycosylation (CDG-Ie) – eyelid telangiectasia, hemangiomas, inverted nipples, microcephaly; dolichol-phosphate-mannose synthase *Ped Derm 22:457–460, 2005*

Primary umbilical endometriosis – solitary vascular appearing umbilical nodule *JAMADerm 156:339–340, 2020*
  Differential diagnosis includes:
    Keloid
    Urachal duct cyst
    Omphalomesenteric duct remnant
    Metastatic adenocarcinoma
    Abdominal hernia
    Nodular melanoma

Gamma heavy chain disease *JAAD 23:988–991, 1990*

Gout – tophi

Primary hyperoxalosis

IgA benign monoclonal gammopathy – violaceous nodules *JAAD 21:1303–1304, 1989*

Nodular pretibial myxedema *AD 129:365–370, 1993*

Pregnancy – pyogenic granulomas; small hemangiomas *Cutis 13:82–86, 1974*

Reactive angiomatosis with cryoproteinemia *JAAD 27:969–973, 1992*

NEOPLASTIC DISEASES

Acrospiroma (clear cell, nodular, or solid-cystic hidradenoma) *JAAD 21:271–277, 1989*

Adenosquamous carcinoma *Cutis 94:231–233, 2014*

Aggressive digital papillary adenocarcinoma – exophytic friable tumor *JAAD 60:331–339, 2009*

Alveolar rhabdomyosarcoma *Ped Derm 5:254–256, 1988;* neonatal tongue lesion with massive macroglossia *Soc Ped Derm Annual Meeting, July 2005*

Aneurysmal benign fibrous histiocytoma *Histopathology 26:323–331, 1995*

Angiokeratoma – personal observation

Angiolipoleiomyoma, periungual *JAAD 23:1093–1098, 1990;*

Angioleiomyoma – digital *JAAD 29:1043–1044, 1993*

Angiomatous nevus; angiomatous nevus following radiation

Angiomatoid malignant fibrous histiocytoma *AD 121:275–276, 1985*

Angiomyxoma *JAAD 33:352–355, 1995*

Angiosarcoma including Stewart-Treves tumor *Cancer 77:2400–2406, 1996; AD 124:263–268, 1988;* angiosarcoma of the face and scalp (Wilson-Jones angiosarcoma) *BJD 172:1156–1158, 2015; JAAD 38:143–175, 1998;* red-black breast nodules following breast irradiation for breast cancer *JAAD 54:499–504, 2006;* angiosarcoma in clotted A-V shunt *JAAD 65:882–883, 2011*

Apocrine adenoma

Apocrine nevus *JAAD 18:579–581, 1988*

Juvenile aponeurotic palmoplantar fibroma

Atrial myxoma *BJD 115:239–242, 1986*

Atypical fibroxanthoma *AD 135:1113–1118, 1999;* pyogenic granuloma-like lesion *AD 146:1399–1404, 2010; AD 112:1155–1157, 1976; Cancer 31:1541–1542, 1973*

Basal cell carcinoma *Acta Pathol Microbiol Scand 88A:5–9, 1980*

Blastic plasmacytoid dendritic cell neoplasm – purple nodules of back, vascular nodule of trunk; "purple plum" nodule of face *JAMADerm 154:492–494, 2018; BJD 169:579–586, 2013*

Bony exostosis

Carcinoid, primary cutaneous *JAAD 22:366–370, 1990*

Caruncle – vascular papillary growth of urinary meatus *JAAD 57:371–392, 2007*

Castleman's disease (giant lymph node hyperplasia) *JAAD 29:778–780, 1993*

CD4 + CD56+ hematodermic neoplasm – vascular nodule of forehead; red plaques of face; tumor of plasmacytoid dendritic cells *Cutis 89:278–283, 2012*

Chondroblastoma, subungual – toe tip *Ped Derm 21:452–453, 2004*

Chondroma, solitary

Chondroid syringoma *AD 84:835–847, 1961*

Clear cell acanthoma *JAAD 16:1075–1078, 1987*

Clear cell variant of mucoepidermoid carcinoma *JAAD 29:642–644, 1993*

Cylindroma *Cutis 56:239–240, 1995*

Dermal dendrocytoma (keratotic) *AD 126:689–690, 1990*

Dermatofibroma – dermatofibroma with spreading satellitosis *JAAD 27:1017–1019, 1992*

Dermatofibrosarcoma protuberans – congenital *AD 139:207–211, 2003; Pre-AAD Pediatric Derm Meeting, March 2000*

Eccrine acrospiroma – purple nodule *Cutis 49:49–50, 1992; Ped Derm 6:53–54, 1989*

Eccrine angiomatous hamartoma – vascular nodule; macule, red plaque, acral nodule of infants or neonates; painful, red, purple, blue, yellow, brown, skin-colored *JAAD 47:429–435, 2002; JAAD 37:523–549, 1997; Ped Derm 13:139–142, 1996*

Eccrine poroma *Cutis 54:183–184, 1994*

Eccrine spiradenoma *Int J Dermatol 37:221–223, 1998; J Cut Pathol 10:312–320, 1983*

Eccrine sweat gland carcinoma *AD 122:585–590, 1986;* metastatic eccrine gland carcinoma

Eccrine syringofibroadenoma *AD 126:945–949, 1990*

Embryonal rhabdomyosarcoma *Ped Derm 22:218–221, 2005*

Endometriosis – brown *JAAD 21:155, 1989*

Epidermoid inclusion cyst – ruptured or with hemorrhage

Epithelioid cell histiocytoma *BJD 120:185–195, 1989*

Epithelioid sarcoma *JAAD 26:302–305, 1992*

Erythema nodosum with B cell lymphoma infiltrate *JAAD 32:361–363, 1995*

Extramedullary hematopoiesis in chronic idiopathic myelofibrosis with myelodysplasia *JAAD 55:S28–31, 2006*

Fibroma

Fibrosarcoma/spindle cell sarcoma – red or violaceous nodule; fibrosarcoma, neonatal – ulcerated vascular nodule *Ped Derm 25:141–143, 2008; Ped Derm 23:330–334, 2006; Soc Ped Derm Annual Meeting, July 2005; JAAD 50:S23–25, 2004*

Giant cell tumor of the tendon sheath (finger nodules) *Cancer 57:875–884, 1986*

Glomangiosarcoma 18521375

Glomus tumor – single or multiple; malignant glomus tumor *Derm Surg 27:837–840, 2001*

Granular cell myoblastoma – benign or malignant *AD 126:1051–1056, 1990; AD 130:913–918, 1994*

Hemophagocytic syndrome – purple nodule *JAAD 25:919–924, 1991; AD 128:193–200, 1992*

Hibernoma – neck, axilla, central back; vascular dilatation overlying lesion *AD 73:149–157, 1956*

Indeterminate cell tumor *JAAD 15:591–597, 1986*

Infantile choriocarcinoma *JAAD 14:918–927, 1986*

Infantile myofibromatosis – resembling hemangioma *JAAD 71:264–270, 2014; Ped Derm 27:29–33, 2010; JAAD 41:508, 1999;* red nodule *Curr Prob Derm 14:41–70, 2002; Ped Derm 18:305–307, 2001; Ped Derm 8:306–309, 1991*

Inverted follicular keratosis 11411260

Juvenile xanthogranuloma *JAAD 29:868–870, 1993*

Kaposi's sarcoma *Dermatol Clin 24:509–520, 2006; Cutis 54:275–260, 1994;* of the nasal mucosa *J Laryngol Otol 112:280–282, 1998;* in Castleman's disease *JAAD 26:105–109, 1992;* violaceous eyelid papules and pulmonary infiltrates in HIV disease with immune reconstitution syndrome *NEJM 369;1152–1161, 2013;*

Keratoacanthoma

Leiomyomas

Leiomyosarcoma *Ped Derm 14:281–283, 1997*

Leukemia cutis *JAAD 11:121–128, 1984;* granulocytic sarcoma *AD 120:1341–1343, 1984;* congenital leukemia cutis *AD 129:1301–1306, 1993*

Lipoblastoma – mimicking hemangioma *Pediatrics 105:123–128, 2000; Ped Derm 16:77–83, 1999;* ulcerated vascular nodule *Ped Derm 34:180–186, 2017*

Lymphocytoma cutis

Lymphoma – cutaneous T-cell lymphoma, immunoblastoma, lymphoplasmacytic lymphoma *JAAD 16:1106–110,1987;* HTLV-1 lymphoma, Ki-1+, CD 8+ lymphoepithelioid lymphoma *JAAD 29:871–875, 1993;* cytophagic panniculitis (B-cell lymphoma) *JAAD 13:882–885, 1985;* primary cutaneous anaplastic large cell lymphoma – vascular nodules or plaques *JAAD 70:724–735, 2014; BJD 150:1202–1207, 2004;* large cell lymphoma resembling sarcoid *JAAD 28:327–330, 1993;* CD 30+ anaplastic large cell lymphoma *Ped Derm 21:525–533, 2004; AD 139:1075–1080, 2003;* primary cutaneous CD30+ lymphoproliferative disorder (CD8+/CD4+) *JAAD 51:304–308, 2004;* primary cutaneous anaplastic large cell lymphoma *JAAD 74:1135–1143, 2016;* plasmablastic lymphoma after transplant *BJD 149:889–890, 2003;* primary cutaneous follicle center B-cell lymphoma *BJD 157:1205–1211, 2007*

Lymphomatoid granulomatosis (angiocentric lymphoma) *AD 127:1693–1698, 1991*

Lymphomatoid papulosis

Malignant eccrine poroma

Malignant fibrous histiocytoma resembling mycetoma – vascular nodule of leg *Sem Cut Med Surg 21:159–165, 2002;* purple *JAAD 29:318–321, 1993*

Malignant histiocytosis

Malignant rhabdoid tumor *Ped Derm 13:468–471, 1997*

Malignant synovioma

Mammary duct ectasia – bloody nipple discharge of infancy with hemorrhagic nodule *Ped Derm 34:361–362, 2017; AD 145:1068–1069, 2009*

Differential diagnosis includes:
  Cystic mastitis
  Epithelial hyperplasia
  Intraductal carcinoma
  Intraductal papilloma
  Hemangioma

Melanocytic nevi – giant congenital melanocytic nevi with proliferative nodules *AD 140:83–88, 2004;* irritated nevus

Melanoma – primary cutaneous *BJD 172:662–668, 2015; NEJM 368:1536, 2013; Ped Derm 27:201–203, 2010;* giant vascular tumor *JAMADerm 150:574–575, 2014;* bright red vascular nodule of helix *JAMADerm 151:105–106, 2015;* primary dermal melanoma *JAAD 75:1263–1265, 2016;* melanotic melanoma *Semin Oncol 2:5–118, 1975;* amelanotic subungual melanoma mimicking pyogenic granuloma *J R Coll surg Edinb 47:638–640, 2002;* amelanotic acral lentiginous melanoma *BJD 155:561–569, 2006;* metastatic melanoma *Cutis 69:353–356, 2002;* amelanotic acral melanoma – red plaque of toe tip *JAAD 69:700–707, 2013;* spindle cell amelanotic melanoma *BJD 155:81–88, 2006;* amelanotic melanoma arising in large congenital melanocytic nevus – multilobulated vascular nodule *JAAD 68:913–925, 2013*

Merkel cell tumor *BJD 174:158–164, 2016; AD 140:609–614, 2004; JAAD 31:271–272, 1994; AD 127:571–576, 1991; AD 123:1368–1370, 1987;* cherry red nodules with shiny surface *J Drugs in Dermatol 9:779–784, 2010; BJD 169:294–297, 2013;* red-pink vascular nodule of face *JAAD 65:983–990, 2011;* mimicking angiosarcoma; eyelid papule *Eyelid and Conjunctival Tumors, Shields JA and Shields CL, Lippincott Williams and Wilkins, 1999, p.101;* purple plum

Metastases – renal cell (purple) (red vascular) *Cutis 101:78, 117–118, 2018; Cutis 98:376,383–384, 2016; Derm Surg 27:192–194, 2001;* vascular red papule of nipple (renal cell carcinoma) *Cutis 90:196–199, 2012; Cutis 86:69, 73–74, 2010;* oat cell carcinoma, anaplastic carcinoma, carcinoid, GI tract, retinoblastoma, Ewing's sarcoma, neuroblastoma, and leukemia cutis, thyroid, bronchogenic carcinoma *AD 126:665–670, 1990*; others *AD 127:571, 1991*; prostate *AD 146:206–208, 2010; AD 128:1533–1538, 1992; J Urol 113:734–735, 1975*; testicular choriocarcinoma *Cutis 67:117–120, 2001;* Sister Mary Joseph nodule (umbilical metastatic carcinoma) *JAAD 10:610–615, 1984;* colon *Cutis 80:469–472, 2007;* bladder carcinoma *AD 145:213–215, 2009;* endometrial carcinoma; metastatic serous adenocarcinoma of the ovary – peristomal red nodule *JAMA 319:1158–1159, 2018;* serous papillary carcinoma *JAMADerm 155:956, 2019;* metastatic endometrial carcinoma *Cutis 103:217–218, 2019*

Multinucleate cell angiohistiocytoma *Cutis 59:190–192, 1997*

Multiple neurilemmomatosis *JAAD 10:744–754, 1984*

Myelodysplastic syndrome – subcutaneous eosinophilic necrosis with myelodysplastic syndrome *JAAD 20:320–323, 1989*

Myelofibrosis – extramedullary hematopoiesis *JAAD 32:805, 1995; JAAD 22:334–337, 1990; AD 112:1302–1303, 1976*

Myeloma *Ann DV 128:753–755, 2001;* extramedullary plasmacytoma in myeloma *AD 127:69–74, 1991*

Myofibroma

Myopericytoma

Myxoid cyst

Nasal polyp 98306

Neural hamartoma

Neurilemmoma (Schwannoma) – pink or vascular nodule of the foot *Cutis 67:127–129, 2001*

Neuroblastoma, metastatic *Dermatol Therapy 18:104–116, 2005; JAAD 24:1025–1027, 1991*

Neurothekeoma *JAAD 25:80–88, 1991; AD 129:1505–1510, 1993, Ped Derm 9:272–274, 1992*

Neurovascular hamartoma – marker for renal tumors

Nodular hidradenoma (clear cell hidradenoma, eccrine acrospiroma, clear cell myoepithelioma) – ulcerated vascular appearing nodule *JAAD 76:S46–48, 2017; AD 136:1409–1414, 2000*

Non-X histiocytosis *AD 124:1254–1257, 1988*

Osteosarcoma – primary cutaneous osteosarcoma *JAAD 51:S94–96, 2004*

Pilomatrixoma – papule of face *Ped Derm 26:195–196, 2009; Eyelid and Conjunctival Tumors, Shields JA and Shields CL, Lippincott Williams and Wilkins, 1999, p.71;*

Cutis 50:290–292, 1995; Prog Med 8:826, 1880; including perforating pilomatrixoma (draining nodule) *Cutis 44:130–132, 1989; JAAD 35:116–118, 1996;* proliferating trichilemmal tumor

Plasmacytoma – simulates hemangioma *Arch Pathol Lab Med 124:628–631, 2000;* eyelid papule *Eyelid and Conjunctival Tumors, Shields JA and Shields CL, Lippincott Williams and Wilkins, 1999, p.133; JAAD 19:879–890, 1988*

Plexiform fibrohistiocytic tumor *AD 131:211–216, 1995*

Plexiform neurofibroma

Plexiform schwannoma – mimics giant hemangioma *BJD 157:838–839, 2007*

Porocarcinoma *AD 136:1409–1414, 2000*

Progressive nodular histiocytosis *Ped Derm 10:64–68, 1993*

Proliferating trichilemmal cyst *Cancer 48:1207–1214, 1981*

Reticulohistiocytoma, solitary *AD 126:665–670, 1990*

Reticulohistiocytoma of the dorsum (Crosti's syndrome) – red nodule; low grade B-cell lymphoma

Rhabdoid tumor – ulcerated vascular nodule *Ped Derm 28:295–298, 2011; J Cutan Pathol 26:509–515, 1999; Ped Derm 13:468, 1996*

Rhabdomyomatous mesenchymal hamartoma – red vascular polypoid mass of labia majora *Ped Derm 26:753–755, 2009;*

Rhabdomyosarcoma *Curr Prob Derm 14:41–70, 2002;* congenital *Ped Derm 20:335–338, 2003;* vascular plaque of vulva *Ped Derm 34:352–355, 2017*

Sclerosing sweat duct carcinoma *The Dermatologist November 2013,pp. 47–49*

Sebaceous adenoma in AIDS *AD 124:489–490, 1988;* pedunculated vascular nodule of dorsal penis *JAAD 57:S42–43, 2007*

Sebaceous epithelioma

Sebaceous gland carcinoma – ulcerated violaceous nodule *BJD 166:222–224, 2012; JAAD 61:549–560, 2009; Dermatol Ther 21:459–466, 2008; AD 137:1367–1372, 2001; Nippon Ganka Gakkai Zasshi 104:740–745, 2000*

Seborrheic keratosis, irritated

Self-healing reticulohistiocytosis *JAAD 48:S75–77, 2003; JAAD 13:383–404, 1985*

Skin tag, irritated – personal observation

Spitz nevi, including Spitz nevi mimicking pyogenic granulomas in black children *JAAD 23:842–845, 1990;* multiple epithelioid Spitz nevi with loss of *BAP1* expression – red vascular papules *JAMA Derm 149:333–339, 2013*

Squamous cell carcinoma – complicating non-Herlitz junctional epidermolysis bullosa – beefy red nodules *JAAD 65:780–789, 2011;* beefy red nodule of groin – HPV-16+ *BJD 170:753–754, 2014;* vascular papule of proximal nailfold *JAAD 69:253–261, 2013*

Stewart-Treves angiosarcoma – personal observation

Subungual myxoid pleomorphic fibroma 9790115

Sweat gland adenocarcinoma – beefy red nodule *BJD 161:694–696, 2009* Syringocystadenoma papilliferum – pre-auricular vascular nodule; linear vascular appearing nodules of neck *Ped Derm 35:511–512,2018; AD 144:1509–1514, 2008*

Trichoblastic carcinoma – giant red beefy tumor *BJD 173:1059–1062, 2015*

Umbilical mucosal polyp – vascular umbilical polyp *JAMADerm 153:597–598, 2017*

Verrucous acanthoma – personal observation

Verrucous carcinoma *JAAD 32:1–21, 1995*

Xanthogranuloma – vascular nodule of sole *AD 135:707–712, 1999*

PARANEOPLASTIC

Cytophagic histiocytic panniculitis – associated with malignant histiocytic syndromes *AD 121:910–913, 1985*

Eruptive hemangiomatosis – associated with multi-centric Castleman's disease *JAMA Derm 149:204–208, 2013*

Granulomatous vasculitis with lymphocytic lymphoma *JAAD 14:492–501, 1986*

Neutrophilic dermatosis in chronic myelogenous leukemia *JAAD 29:290–292, 1993*

PRIMARY CUTANEOUS DISEASES

Acne conglobata

Acne fulminans

Acne keloidalis

Acne rosacea

Acne vulgaris

Angiolymphoid hyperplasia with eosinophilia – ear lesions *AD 143:841–844, 2007; Cutis 44:147–150, 1989; JAAD 12:781–796, 1985; BJD 81:1–14, 1969*

Endometriosis (villar nodule) – umbilical multilobulated red nodule *AD 148:1331–1332, 2012*

Endosalpingosis – ectopic fallopian tube epithelium; umbilical nodule *BJD 151:924–925, 2004*

Epidermolysis bullosa – excess granulation tissue; junctional EB, Herlitz type, laryngo-onycho-cutaneous syndrome *JAAD 58:931–950, 2008;* autosomal dominant epidermolysis bullosa – excess granulation tissue of external auditory canals; mutation in *ITGB4 JAMADerm 152:558–562, 2016*

Erythema elevatum diutinum *JAAD 49:764–767, 2003; AD 129:1043–148, 1993*

Granuloma faciale

Granuloma gluteale infantum *Ped Derm 7:196–198, 1990*

Lichen planus

Lichen sclerosus et atrophicus – angiokeratoma-like lesions (red-violaceous papules) *AD 145:1458–1460, 2009*

Membranous lipodystrophy *JAAD 24:844–847, 1991*

MOTT *JAAD 24:208–215, 1991*

Progressive nodular fibrosis of the skin *JID 87:210–216, 1986*

Prurigo nodularis

Urethral prolapse – polypoid, edematous, vascular-appearing, violaceous mass at urethral opening *JAAD 57:371–392, 2007*

SYNDROMES

Antiphospholipid antibody syndrome *AD 128:847–852, 1992*

Bannayan-Riley-Ruvalcaba-Zonana syndrome – hemangiomas, vascular malformations, lipomas, genital hyperpigmentation, supernumerary nipples *JAAD 68:189–209, 2013; AD 142:625–632, 2006; AD 132:1214–1218, 1996; Am J Med Genet 44:307–314, 1992*

Beckwith-Wiedemann syndrome – hemangiomas; diagonal linear grooves of the ear lobes, preauricular tags or pits, nevus flammeus of central forehead and upper eyelids, macroglossia, macrosomia, omphalocele or other umbilical anomalies *Syndromes of the Head and Neck 1990:323–328*

Behcet's syndrome – erythema nodosum-like lesions

Blue rubber bleb nevus syndrome – vascular malformation *AD 116:924–929, 1996;* with phlebectasias *Ped Derm 3:304–310, 1986*

C syndrome – hemangiomas *Birth Defects 5:161–166, 1969*

Cardiofaciocutaneous syndrome (Noonan-like short stature syndrome) (NS) – xerosis/ichthyosis, eczematous dermatitis, growth failure, hyperkeratotic papules, ulerythema ophryogenes, seborrheic dermatitis, CALMs, nevi, keratosis pilaris, autosomal dominant, patchy or widespread ichthyosiform eruption, sparse curly short scalp hair and eyebrows and lashes, hemangiomas, acanthosis nigricans, congenital lymphedema of the hands, redundant skin of the hands, short stature, abnormal facies, cardiac defects; gain of function sporadic missense mutations in *BRAF, KRAS, MEK1,* or *MEK2 BJD 164:521–529, 2011; Ped Derm 27:274–278, 2010; JAAD 46:161–183, 2002; Ped Derm 17:231–234, 2000; JAAD 22:920–922, 1990; JAAD 28:815–819, 1993; AD 129:46–47, 1993;* port wine stain *Clin Genet 42:206–209, 1992*

CHILD syndrome – X-linked dominant; strawberry-like papillomatous lesions of toes; linear hyperkeratosis with brownish scaling of fingers and toes *AD 142:348–351, 2006;* linear hyperkeratotic plaques of feet (unilateral inflammatory ichthyosiform nevus)with spontaneous involution; macrodactyly; ptychotropism, shortening and absence of limbs, short stature; ipsilateral involvement of bones, lung, kidney, heart, brain; epiphyseal stippling (chondrodysplasia punctata); short stature, scoliosis, clefting of hand or foot, hexadactyly; lateralization and mutations in *NSDHL* gene which encodes 3-beta hydroxysteroid dehydrogenase *JAAD 63:1–22, 2010; BJD 161:714–715, 2009*

Classic arthrogryposis:amyoplasia – extensive proliferative hemangioma of the face

Congenital generalized fibromatosis *JAAD 10:365–371, 1984*

Cowden's syndrome (multiple hamartoma syndrome) – angiomas *JAAD 17:342–346, 1987;* type 2 segmental Cowden's disease – keratinocytic soft, thick papillomatous nevus, connective tissue nevi, vascular nevi (including cutis marmorata), angiomas, varicosities, lymphatic hamartomas, lipomas, lipoblastomatosis, hydrocephalus, seizures, hemihypertrophy of limbs, ballooning of toes, bowel polyps, glomerulosclerosis, macrocephaly *BJD 156:1089–1090, 2007; Eur J Dermatol 17:133–136, 2007*

Cutaneous cavernous malformations with cutaneous angiokeratomas and hemangiomas – mutation in *KRIT1 (CCMI) Cutis 96:329–332, 2015*

Edward's syndrome (Trisomy 18) – capillary hemangiomas *J Med Genet 15:48–60, 1978*

Epidermal nevus syndrome – hemangiomas *Ped Derm 6:316–320, 1989*

Fetal alcohol syndrome – short stature, angiomas, hypertrichosis *JAAD 46:161–183, 2002; Ped Derm 11:178–180, 1994*

Goltz's syndrome (focal dermal hypoplasia) – painful exophytic granulation tissue *BJD 160:1103–1109, 2009;* asymmetric linear and reticulated streaks of atrophy and telangiectasia; yellow-red nodules; raspberry-like papillomas of lips, perineum, acrally, at perineum, buccal mucosa; xerosis; scalp and pubic hair sparse and brittle; short stature; asymmetric face; syndactyly, polydactyly; ocular, dental, and skeletal abnormalities with osteopathia striata of long bones *JAAD 25:879–881, 1991;* raspberry-like papillomas; mutation in PORCN gene (encodes transmembrane endoplasmic reticulum proteins that target WNT signaling proteins

Gorham's syndrome (hemangiomas with osteolysis) (disappearing bone disease) – violaceous vascular plaque with overlying telangiectasias of back, neck, and chest; cutaneous vascular lesions with replacement of bone by venous malformations *JAAD 56:S21–25, 2007; JAMA 252:1449–1451, 1984; Am J Dis Child 132:715–716, 1978; AD 92:501–508, 1965;* with Kasabach-Merritt syndrome *JAAD 29:117–119, 1993*

Hemangiomas of the face and anterior trunk associated with sternal clefting, median abdominal raphe (sternal malformation vascular dysplasia syndrome) *Ped Derm 10:71–76, 1993; Am J Med Genet 21:177–186, 1985*

Hereditary hemorrhagic telangiectasia (Osler-Weber-Rendu syndrome) *Am J Med 82:989–997, 1987; NEJM 257:105–109, 1957*

Hereditary neurocutaneous angioma (vascular malformations) – hemangiomas, macular vascular anomalies; intracranial arteriovenous malformations *Clin Genet 33:44–48, 1988*

Hereditary phlebectasia of the lips

Hypomelia, hypotrichosis, facial hemangioma syndrome (pseudothalidomide syndrome) – sparse silvery blond hair *Am J Dis Child 123:602–606, 1972*

IgG4-related disease – cutaneous plasmacytosis (papulonodules); pseudolymphoma; angiolymphoid hyperplasia with eosinophilia; Mikulicz's disease; psoriasiform dermatitis; morbilliform eruption; hypergammaglobulinemic purpura; urticarial vasculitis; ischemic digits; Raynaud's disease and digital gangrene *BJD 171:929,959–967, 2014*

Infantile hemangiomatosis

Kasabach-Merritt syndrome – associated with Kaposiform hemangioendothelioma or tufted angioma; enlargement, tenderness, induration, and ecchymosis occur within the vascular lesion; consumptive coagulopathy with hemorrhage *Ped Derm 11:79–81, 1994*

Klippel-Trenaunay-Weber syndrome *Clin Exp Derm 12:12–17, 1987*

Laryngo-onycho-cutaneous syndrome – autosomal recessive type of junctional epidermolysis bullosa; skin ulceration with prominent granulation tissue, early hoarseness and laryngeal stenosis; scarred nares; chronic erosion of corners of mouth (giant perleche); paronychia with periungual inflammation and erosions; onycholysis with subungual granulation tissue and loss of nails with granulation tissue of nail bed, conjunctival inflammation with polypoid granulation tissue, and dental enamel hypoplasia and hypodontia; only in Punjabi families; mutation in laminin alpha-3 (*LAMA3A*) *BJD 169:1353–1356, 2013; Ped Derm 23:75–77, 2006; Biomedica 2:15–25, 1986; Ped Derm 24:306–308, 2007; Ped Derm 23:75–77, 2006; Cornea 20:753–756, 2001; Arch Dis Child 70:319–326, 1994; JAAD 29:906–909, 1993; Clin Dysmorphol 1:3–14, 1992; Eye 5:717–722, 1991;*

Lipoid proteinosis

Lumbosacral hemangiomas, tethered cord, and multiple congenital anomalies (occult spinal dysraphism) *Pediatrics 83:977–980, 1989; AD 122:684–687, 1986;* sacral hemangiomas, imperforate anus, genitourinary developmental defects *AD 122:684–687, 1986*

Macrocephaly with cutis marmorata, hemangioma, and syndactyly syndrome – macrocephaly, hypotonia, hemihypertrophy, hemangioma, cutis marmorata telangiectatica congenita, internal arteriovenous malformations, syndactyly, joint laxity, hyperelastic skin, thickened subcutaneous tissue, developmental delay, short stature, hydrocephalus *Ped Derm 16:235–237, 1999; Clin Dysmorphol 6:291–302, 1997*

Maffucci's syndrome – enchondromas and hemangiomas *Ped Derm 12:55–58, 1995; BJD 96:317–322, 1977*

Melorheostosis – cutaneous lesions resemble linear morphea overlying bony lesions (endosteal bony densities resembling candle wax) with angiomas and arteriovenous abnormalities *J Bone and Joint Surg 61:415–418, 1979; BJD 86:297–301, 1972*

Muir-Torre syndrome

Multiple cutaneous hemangiomas, right aortic arch, and coarctation of the aorta

Neurofibromatosis *Neurofibromatosis 1:137–145, 1988*

Ollier's syndrome – enchondromas only *J Neurol 235:376–378, 1988*

Pallister-Hall syndrome – hemangiomas *Am J Med Genet 7:75–83, 1980*

Patau syndrome (Trisomy 13) – hemangiomas of forehead; localized scalp defects *G Ital DV 121:25–28, 1986; J Genet Hum 23:83–109, 1975*

PHACES syndrome – posterior fossa malformation (Dandy-Walker malformation), large facial hemangiomas, arterial anomalies, coarctation of the aorta and other cardiac defects (atrial septal defect), eye abnormalities, sternal clefting or supraumbilical raphe *J Pediatr 139:117–123, 2001; AD 132:307–311, 1996; J Pediatr 122:379–384, 1993; Ped Derm 5:263–265, 1988;* temporal vascular papules *BJD 155:192–194, 2006*

Phakomatosis pigmentovascularis type IV A *AD 121:651–5, 1985*

POEMS syndrome (Crow-Fukase syndrome, Takatsuki syndrome) (PEP syndrome – plasma cell dyscrasia, endocrinopathy,

polyneuropathy) – plethora, angiomas (cherry, globular, glomeruloid) presenting as red nodules of face, trunk, and extremities, diffuse hyperpigmentation, hypertrichosis, sclerederma-like changes, either generalized or localized (legs), hyperhidrosis, clubbing, leukonychia, papilledema, pleural effusion, peripheral edema, ascites, pulmonary hypertension, weight loss, fatigue, diarrhea, thrombocytosis, polycythemia, fever, renal disease, arthralgias; osteosclerotic myeloma (IgG or IgA lambda) bone lesions, progressive symmetric sensorimotor peripheral polyneuropathy, hypothyroidism, and hypogonadism; peripheral edema, thrombocytosis, cutaneous angiomas, blue dermal papules associated with Castleman's disease (benign reactive angioendotheliomatosis), maculopapular brown-violaceous lesions, purple nodules; papilledema *JAAD 58:671–675, 2008; JAAD 55:149–152, 2006; JAAD 44:324–329, 2001, JAAD 40:808–812, 1999; AD 124:695–698, 1988, Cutis 61:329–334, 1998; JAAD 21:1061–1068, 1989; JAAD 12:961–964, 1985; Nippon Shinson 26:2444–2456, 1968; JAAD 55:149–152,2006; JAAD 44:324–329, 2001; JAAD 21:1061–1068, 1989; JAAD 12:961–964, 1985, AD 124:695–698, 1988, Cutis 61:329–334, 1998; JAAD 40:808–812, 1999;* glomeruloid hemangioma – lesion of multicentric Castleman's disease associated with POEMS syndrome; intralesional protein deposits *BJD 148:1276–1278, 2003; Am J Surg Pathol 14:1036–1046, 1990*

Proteus syndrome – port wine stains, subcutaneous hemangiomas and lymphangiomas, lymphangioma circumscriptum, hemihypertrophy of the face, limbs, trunk; macrodactyly, cerebriform hypertrophy of palmar and/or plantar surfaces, macrocephaly; verrucous epidermal nevi, sebaceous nevi with hyper- or hypopigmentation *AD 140:947–953, 2004; Am J Med Genet 27:99–117, 1987;* vascular nevi, soft subcutaneous masses; lipodystrophy, café au lait macules, linear and whorled macular pigmentation *JAAD 25:377–383, 1991; Pediatrics 76:984–989, 1985; Am J Med Genet 27:87–97, 1987; Eur J Pediatr 140:5–12, 1983*

Reflex sympathetic dystrophy – pseudo-Kaposi's sarcoma *Cutis 68:179–182, 2001*

Roberts pseudothalidomide syndrome – superficial capillary hemangiomas of the midface, forehead, ears *Prog Clin Biol Res 104:351–356, 1982*

Rubinstein-Taybi syndrome – multiple hemangiomas; hypogonadotropic hypogonadism; autosomal dominant; mutations or deletions of chromosome 16p13.3; human cAMP response element binding protein *Ped Derm 21:44–47, 2004; JAAD 46:161–183, 2002; JAAD 46:159, 2002*

Sweet's syndrome; with septal granulomatous or neutrophilic lobular panniculitis *AD 121:785–788, 1985*

Thrombocytopenia-absent radius syndrome (TAR syndrome) – extensive proliferative hemangioma of the face

Trichothiodystrophy syndromes – BIDS, IBIDS, PIBIDS – hemangiomas, sparse or absent eyelashes and eyebrows, brittle hair, premature aging, sexual immaturity, ichthyosis, dysmyelination, bird-like facies, dental caries; trichothiodystrophy with ichthyosis, urologic malformations, hypercalciuria and mental and physical retardation *JAAD 44:891–920, 2001; Ped Derm 14:441–445, 1997*

Partial trisomy 2P – hemangiomas

Tuberous sclerosis – angiofibromas *Syndromes of the Head and Neck, p. 410–415, 1990*

Von Hippel-Lindau syndrome – hemangiomas

X-linked hyper IgM syndrome treated with G-CSF – disseminated pyogenic granulomas *JAAD 49:105–108, 2003*

XXYY syndrome – features of Klinefelter's; sparse body hair; also multiple angiomas, acrocyanosis, and premature peripheral vascular disease *AD 94:695–698, 1966*

Xeroderma pigmentosum – short stature, conjunctivitis, photophobia, pyogenic granulomas in toddlers *BJD 168:1109–1113, 2013*

TRAUMA

Chondrodermatitis nodularis chronica helicis

Fiddler's neck *JAAD 22:657–663, 1990*

Nose piercing with pyogenic granuloma

Perniosis

Picker's papule

Post-radiation vascular proliferations of breast (atypical vascular lesions of the breast) – erythema; erythema with underlying induration or ulceration, telangiectasias, papules, plaques, nodules, *JAAD 57:126–133, 2007*

Pseudoaneurysm of face and forehead – pulsatile subcutaneous mass; hematoma with sinus tract communicating with lumen; following Mohs' surgery *JAMADerm 150:546–549, 2014*

Pseudo-Kaposi's sarcoma in reflex sympathetic dystrophy *JAAD 22:513–520, 1990*

VASCULAR

Acquired digital arteriovenous malformation – periungual vascular papule *JAAD 56:S122–124, 2007*

Acral pseudolymphomatous angiokeratoma of children (APACHE) – unilateral multiple persistent vascular papules on hands and feet; may have keratotic surface or collar *JAAD 38:143–175, 1998; BJD 124:387–388, 1991; AD 126:1524–1525, 1990; BJD 119(Suppl):135, 1988*

Acroangiodermatitis of Mali – violaceous papules, nodules, and plaques *Cutis 86:239–240, 2010; JAAD 37:887–920, 1997; Int J Dermatol 33:179–183, 1994;* due to A-V shunts *JAAD 21:499–505, 1989; Arch Derm Res 281:35–39, 1989; AD 110:907, 1974; AD 111:1656, 1975; AD 100:297, 1969;* associated with chronic venous insufficiency *Eur J Vasc Endovasc Surg 24:558–560, 2002; AD 96:176, 1967; AD 92:515–518, 1965*

Agminated eruptive pyogenic granuloma-like lesions over congenital vascular stains (capillary malformations) or hemangioma *JAMADerm 150:781–783, 2014; Ped Derm 29:186–190, 2012*

Angiokeratoma – solitary *AD 143:318–325, 2007;* acral angiokeratomas of Mibelli in Turner's syndrome – blue-black keratotic vascular papules *Ped Derm 27:662–664, 2010;*

circumscriptum; angiokeratoma of Fordyce; Mibelli – acral vascular papules *JAAD 45:764–766, 2001;* solitary papular, of scrotum or vulva; angiokeratoma corporis diffusum (Fabry's disease (alpha galactosidase A) *NEJM 276:1163–1167, 1967;* fucosidosis (alpha-I-fucosidase) – autosomal recessive *Rook p. 2639, 1998, Sixth Edition; AD 107:754–757, 1973;* Kanzaki's disease (alpha-N-acetylgalactosidase) – lesions on face and extremities *AD 129:460–465, 1993;* beta-mannosidase deficiency; neuraminidase deficiency (sialidosis); aspartylglycosaminuria (aspartylglycosaminidase) *Paediatr Acta 36:179–189, 1991;* adult-onset GM1 gangliosidosis (beta galactosidase) *Clin Genet 17:21–26, 1980;* galactosialidosis (combined beta-galactosidase and sialidase) *AD 120:1344–1346, 1984;* no enzyme deficiency *AD 123:1125–1127, 1987; JAAD 12:885–886, 1985;* – telangiectasias or small angiokeratomas; and arteriovenous fistulae without metabolic disorders – papules *AD 131:57–62, 1995;* eruptive unilateral angiokeratomas *AD 144:1663–1664, 2008*

Angiolymphoid hyperplasia with eosinophilia (Kimura's disease) – papules and/or nodules along hairline *AD 136:837–839, 2000;*

JAAD 38: 143–175, 1998; JAAD 12:781–796, 1985; following earlobe piercing *Ped Derm 31:738–741, 2014*

Arteriovenous aneurysms

Arteriovenous fistula with venous hypertension and pseudo-Kaposi's sarcoma *Clin Exp Dermatol 14:289–290, 1989*

Arteriovenous hemangioma (cirsoid aneurysm or acral arteriovenous tumor) – associated with chronic liver disease *BJD 144:604–609, 2001*

Arteriovenous malformation – vascular nodule with congenital swelling of toe *Ped Derm 31:103–104, 2014*

Atypical vascular lesion (lymphatic type) – vascular papule of breast *JAMA Derm 149:1341–1342, 2013; Am J Clin Pathol 102:757–763, 1994*

Benign (reactive) angioendotheliomatosis (benign lymphangioendothelioma, acquired progressive lymphangioma, multifocal lymphangioendotheliomatosis) – present at birth; red brown or violaceous nodules or plaques on face, arms, legs with petechiae, ecchymoses, and small areas of necrosis *AD 140:599–606, 2004; JAAD 38:143–175, 1998; AD 114:1512, 1978*

Bossed hemangioma with telangiectasia and peripheral pallor *AD 134:1145–1150, 1998*

Cherry angiomas (Campbell de Morgan spots)

Eosinophilic granulomatosis with polyangiitis

Combined Kaposiform hemangioendothelioma and combined capillary-venous-lymphatic malformation *Ped Derm 28:439–443, 2011*

Composite hemangioendothelioma – purple nodule *BJD 171:474–484, 2014*

Congenital hemangioma – GNA11 mutation *JAMADerm 152:1015–1020, 2016*

Congenital infiltrating giant cell angioblastoma *JAAD 37:887–920, 1997*

Congenital nonprogressive hemangiomas – blue nodules *AD 137:1607–1620, 2001*

Congenital plaque type glomuvenous malformations – glomulin gene on 1p21; loss of function mutation; atrophic at birth; livedoid plaques, blue plaques, vascular nodules, red patches, cerebriform, targetoid *AD 142:892–896, 2006*

Deep vein thrombosis

Diffuse neonatal hemangiomatosis (multifocal infantile hemangiomas) *JAAD 67:898–903, 2012*

Endovascular papillary angioendothelioma (Dabska's tumor) – vascular nodule *JAAD 38:143–175, 1998*

Epithelioid angiosarcoma – legs – resembles angiosarcoma *JAAD 38:143–175, 1998*

Epithelioid hemangioendothelioma *JAAD 20:362–366, 1989*

Epithelioma hemangioma – entrance of external auditory canal *NEJM 373:2070–2077, 2015*

Eruptive pseudoangiomatosis – red papules *Ped Derm 19:243–245, 2002; BJD 143:435–438, 2000; JAAD 29:857–859, 1993*

Erythema induratum

Extravascular papillary angioendothelioma *Ped Derm 4:332–335, 1987*

Exuberant granulation tissue

Familial cutaneo-cerebral capillary malformations – hyperkeratotic cutaneous vascular malformations *Hum Molec Genet 9:1351–1355, 2000; Ann Neurol 45:250–254, 1999*

Familial multiple mucocutaneous venous malformations *Human Molec Genet 8:1279–1289, 199; Cell 87:1181–1190, 1996*

5q14.3 microdeletions – capillary malformations, arteriovenous malformations, neurologic findings *Ped Derm 34:156–159, 2017*

Glomangiomyoma – congenital multiple plaque-like glomangio-myoma *Am J Dermatopathol 21:454–457, 1999*

Glomangiopericytoma

Glomus tumor, solitary (glomangioma) – painful pink, purple nodule; multiple or plaque type; hemi-facial *JAAD 45:239–245, 2001; Ped Derm 18:223–226, 2001; AD 127:1717–1722, 1991*

Granulation tissue

Hemangioendothelioma

Infantile hemangioma, proliferative (thrombosed); hemangioma of lower lateral cheek associated with airway obstruction; large facial hemangiomas of PHACES syndrome; sacral hemangiomas associated with spinal dysraphism; benign neonatal hemangiomato-sis, disseminated neonatal hemangiomatosis *Ped Derm 29:64–67, 2012; BJD 169:20–30, 2013; Ped Derm 28:502–506, 2011; Ped Derm 28:267–275, 2011; JAAD 48:477–493, 2003;* infantile hemangiomas with unusually prolonged growth phase *AD 144:1632–1637, 2008;* hemangioma and nevus – personal observation

Differential diagnosis of hemangioma of infancy *Ped Derm 34:331–336, 2017; JAAD 48:477–493, 2003*
    Arteriovenous malformation
    Capillary malformation
    Dermatofibrosarcoma protuberans
    Encephalocele
    Fibrosarcoma
    Giant cell fibroblastoma
    Kaposiform hemangioendothelioma
    Lipoblastoma
    Lymphatic malformation
    Myofibromatosis
    Nasal glioma
    Neurofibroma
    Non-involuting congenital hemangioma
    Pyogenic granuloma
    Rapidly-involuting congenital hemangioma
    Rhabdomyosarcoma
    Spindle cell hemangioendothelioma
    Tufted angioma
    Venous malformation

Hemangiopericytoma – violaceous nodule *Ped Derm 23:335–337, 2006; J Bone Joint Surg Br 83:269–272, 2001; AD 116:806, 1980;* familial *Cancer 61:841–844, 1988*

Hemolymphangioma

Histiocytoid hemangioma *Dermatology 189:87–89, 1994*

Hobnail hemangioma – vascular papules of the nose *BJD 146:162–164, 2002*

Intravascular papular endothelial hyperplasia (Masson's intravascu-lar papillary endothelial hyperplasia (pseudoangiosarcoma)) – red or purple papules and nodules of the legs *Cutis 59:148–150, 1997; JAAD 10:110–113, 1984;* vascular nodule of palmar third finger *BJD 166:1147–1149, 2012*

Kaposiform hemangioendothelioma of infancy – red-blue tumid swelling; red plaque or nodule with ecchymotic or purpuric border *Ped Derm 19:388–393, 2002; JAAD 38:799–802, 1998; AD 133:1573–1578, 1997; Am J Surg Pathol 17:321–328, 1993*

Klippel-Trenaunay syndrome – microcystic lymphatic malformation *JAMADerm 152:1058–1059, 2016*

Lichen aureus

LUMBAR syndrome (PELVIS syndrome) – cutaneous infantile hemangiomas of lower body; myelopathy, cutaneous defects, urogenital abnormalities, bony deformities, anorectal abnormalities, arterial anomalies, renal anomalies *JAAD 68:885–896, 2013; Ped*

Derm 27:588, 2010; J Pediatr 157:795–801, 2010; AD 42:884–888, 2006; Dermatology 214:40–45, 2007

Lymphangioendothelioma (red macules and plaques) *J Cut Pathol 19:502–505, 1992*

Lymphangioma circumscriptum

Lymphangiosarcoma

Lymphangiosarcoma of Stewart-Treves

Lymphostasis verrucosa cutis – Milroy's, etc.

Malignant angioendotheliomatosis (intravascular malignant lymphoma) (Dabska-type hemangioendothelioma) – red to purple nodules and plaques on trunk and extremities with prominent telangiectasias overlying the lesion *JAAD 18:407, 1988; JAAD 38:143–175, 1998; AD 104:320, 1971; AD 84:22, 1961*

Microvenular hemangioma *AD 131:483–488, 1995*

Multifocal infantile hemangiomas *Ped Derm 33:621–626, 2016*

Multifocal lymphangioendotheliomatosis – congenital appearance of hundreds of flat vascular papules and plaques associated with gastrointestinal bleeding, thrombocytopenia with bone and joint involvement; spontaneous resolution *J Pediatr Orthop 24:87–91, 2004*

Multiple vascular malformations

Glomuvenous malformations

Blue rubber bleb nevus syndrome

Capillary malformation-arteriovenous malformation syndrome

Multinucleate cell angiohistiocytoma – red to purple dome shaped 2–15 mm vascular papules, grouped on hands, wrists, and thighs; mimics Kaposi's sarcoma *AD 139:933–938, 2003; JAAD 38:143–175, 1998*

Multiple vascular lesions *BJD 171:466–473, 2014*
    Eruptive pseudoangiomatosis – small red papules following viral infection (Echovirus, cytomegalovirus, Epstein-Barr virus)
    Neonatal hemangiomatosis
    Blue rubber bleb nevus
    Glomuvenous malformations
    Maffucci's syndrome
    Hereditary hemorrhagic telangiectasia
    Familial mucocutaneous venous malformations
    Multifocal lymphangioendotheliomatosis with thrombocytopenia

Non-involuting congenital hemangioma (NICH) – warm high-flow lesion with coarse telangiectasias over surface; less commonly ulcerated *Plast Reconstr Surg 107:1647–1654, 2001;* multiple vascular papules *Ped Derm 36:720–722, 2019*

Papular angioplasia *AD 79:17–31, 1959*

Partially involuting congenital hemangioma *JAAD 70:75–79, 2014*

PELVIS syndrome (may be part of urorectal septum malformation sequence) – macular telangiectatic patch; larger perineal hemangio-mas, external genitalia malformations, lipomyelomeningocele, vesicorenal abnormalities, imperforate anus, and skin tags *AD 142:884–888, 2006*

Progressive lymphangioma

Polyarteritis nodosa, including cutaneous PAN *AD 130:884–889, 1994*

Port wine stain – may be associated with underlying vascular malformation; or have pyogenic granuloma, angiokeratoma, arteriovenous malformation, or angiosarcoma develop within it *BJD 144:644–645, 2001; AD 120:1453–1455, 1984*

Progressive multiple angioma *Acta DV 31:304–307, 1951*

Pseudo-Kaposi's sarcoma – Bluefarb-Stewart syndrome *JAAD 37:887–920, 1997;* after A-V shunt *JAAD 21:499–505, 1989; Arch Dermatol Res 281:35–39, 1989;* pseudo-Kaposi's sarcoma – due to acquired arteriovenous fistula *J Dermatol 24:28–33, 1997*

Pseudoangiosarcoma

Pyogenic granuloma *BJD 171:466–473, 2014;* pedunculated nodule of scalp *Ped Derm 26:615–616, 2009;* disseminated pyogenic granulomas after exfoliative erythroderma *JAAD 32:280–282, 1995;* eruptive pyogenic granulomas *JAAD 21:391–394, 1989; Acta DV 50:134–136, 1970; BJD 80:218–227, 1968;* due to trauma, retinoids *J Dermatol Treat 1:151–154, 1990;* after burn and hypogammaglobulinemia *BJD 98:461–465, 1978;* cyclosporine *BJD 132:829–830, 1995;* alcoholic cirrhosis *Am J Dermatopathol 8:379–385, 1986;* of nail bed *BJD 163:941–953, 2010;* of gingiva *JAAD 81:43–56, 2019*

Rapidly involuting congenital hemangioma (RICH) – palpable tumor with pale rim, coarse overlying telangiectasia with central depression or ulcer *BJD 158:1363–1370, 2008; Ped Dev Pathol 6:495–510, 2003; Ped Derm 19:5–11, 2002*

Reactive diffuse dermal angioendotheliomatosis *JAAD 45:601–605, 2001*

Recurrent lobular capillary hemangioma with satellitosis (metastatic pyogenic granulomas) (Warner and Wilson-Jones syndrome) – large central vascular papule surrounded by multiple small vascular papules *Cutis 93:125,132, 2014*

Retiform hemangioendothelioma – *JAAD 42:290–292, 2000;* red plaque of scalp, arms, legs, and penis *JAAD 38:143–175, 1998*

Self-healing pseudoangiosarcoma *AD 124:695–698, 1988*

Sinusoidal hemangioma

Spindle cell hemangioendotheliomas (hemangioma) – multilobulated violaceous nodule *AD 142:641–646, 2006; Cutis 62:23–26, 1998*

Subungual vascular nodules
  Glomus tumor
  Pyogenic granuloma
  Angiomatous nevus

Superficial spreading capillary hemangioma

Symplastic hemangioma – vascular nodule growing atop an infantile hemangioma *Ped Derm 36:961–962, 2019*

Takayasu's arteritis – erythema nodosum or pyoderma gangrenosum *AD 123:796–800, 1987;* Churg-Strauss granuloma in Takayasu's arteritis *JAAD 17:998–1005, 1987*

Targetoid hemosiderotic hemangioma – brown to violaceous nodule with ecchymotic halo *AD 138:117–122, 2002; AD 136:1571–1572, 2000; J Cutan Pathol 26:279–286, 1999; JAAD 32:282–284, 1995; JAAD 41:215–224, 1999*

Thrombosed capillary aneurysm – personal observation

Tufted angioma – nodularity *AD 142:745–751, 2006;* of neck *Ped Derm 29:778, 2012*

Superficial migratory thrombophlebitis

Thrombosed capillary aneurysm

Tufted angioma *AD 145:847–848, 2009; Ped Derm 19:388–393, 2002; JAAD 20:214–225, 1989; Am J Dermatopathol 9:299–300, 1987*

Varicocele

Vasculitis – small, medium or large vessel vasculitis

Vascular malformation

Venous lake

Verrucous hemangioma *Ped Derm 17:213–217, 2000; AD 132:703–708, 1996; Int J Surg Pathol 2:171–176, 1995; J Derm Surg Oncol 13:1089–1092, 1987; Ped Derm 2:191–193, 1985; AD 96:247–253, 1967;* linear *JAAD 42:516–518, 2000*

NODULES, SKIN COLORED

AUTOIMMUNE DISEASES AND DISEASES OF IMMUNE DYSFUNCTION

Chronic granulomatous disease (at immunization site)

Connective tissue panniculitis – nodules, atrophic linear plaques of face, upper trunk, or extremities *AD 116:291–294, 1980*

CREST – plate-like calcinosis cutis – personal observation

Dermatitis herpetiformis *Clin Exp Dermatol 24:283–285, 1999*

Dermatomyositis – plate-like calcinosis cutis; calcinosis cutis *AD 148:455–462, 2012;*

panniculitis *JAAD 46:S148–150, 2002;* nodular cystic fat necrosis *Ped Derm 31:588–590, 2014*

Lupus erythematosus – papulonodular mucinosis – hypopigmented or skin colored papules and nodules *Ped Derm 24:585–586, 2007; AD 140:121–126, 2004; Int J Derm 35:72–73, 1996; JAAD 32:199–205, 1995; AD 114:432–435, 1978;* lymphadenopathy

Morphea – nodular, keloidal (Addisonian keloid) *Int J Dermatol 31:422–423, 1992;* generalized morphea – keloidal nodules

Rheumatoid arthritis – rheumatoid nodules *Eur J Radiol 27 Suppl 1:S18–24, 1998; J Rheumatol 6:286–292, 1979;* mucinous nodules *J Dermatol 26:229–235, 1999;* pustular panniculitis *J R Soc Med 84:307–308, 1991;* rheumatoid vasculitis *JAAD 48:311–340, 2003*

Sclerederma – nodular sclerederma *JAAD 32:343–345, 1995;* sclerederma with subcutaneous nodules *BJD 101:93–96, 1979;* with osteoma cutis

Serum sickness – lymphadenopathy

Sjogren's syndrome- parotid swelling

Still's disease (juvenile rheumatoid nodule) *Ann Rheum Dis 17:278–283, 1958*

CONGENITAL LESIONS

Branchial cleft sinus and/or cyst

Bronchogenic cyst (overlying the suprasternal notch or manubrium sterni, scapular) – may drain mucoid fluid; may be either sinus tract or subcutaneous nodule *AD 142:1221–1226, 2006; JAAD 46:S16–18, 2002; AD 136:925–930, 2000; Ped Derm 16:285–287, 1999; Ped Derm 12:304–306, 1995; Am J Dermatopathol 13:509–517, 1991; Ann DV 115:855–858, 1988; J Cutan Pathol 12:404–409, 1985; Am J Roentgenol Radium Ther Nucl Med 70:771–785, 1953; J Thoracic Cardiovasc Surg 14:217–220, 1945;* skin-colored nodule of chin *BJD 143:1353–1355, 2000;* papilloma *JAAD 11:367–371, 1984*

Cervical thyroid (ectopic thyroid gland) *NEJM 363:1351, 2010*

Chordoma – arise from notochord; skin of perineum, sacrum, buttocks; single or multiple nodules; resemble sacral cysts *JAAD 29:63–66, 1993*

Congenital cartilaginous rest of the neck – nodule over medial clavicle *AD 127:1309–1310, 1991*

Congenital cranial fasciitis – giant skin colored nodule *Ped Derm 24:263–266, 2007*

Congenital fibromatosis of the palm

Congenital generalized fibromatosis *JAAD 10:365–371, 1984*

Congenital lipomatosis – adipose tissue malformation *Skeletal Radiol 9:248–254, 1983; J Pediatr Surg 6:742–744, 1971*

Congenital neurilemmomatosis *JAAD 26:786–787, 1992*

Cutaneous ciliated cyst – on legs of women *AD 136:925–930, 2000*

Darwinian tubercle

Dermoid cyst – nodule above medial eyebrow *Ped Derm 37:40–51, 2020*

Ectopic or christomatous salivary gland (heterotopic salivary gland tissue) – skin colored nodule along lower surface of the sternocleidomastoid muscle *JAAD 58:251–256, 2008*

Fibrosarcoma – congenital subcutaneous nodule *Ped Derm 27:525–526, 2010*

Fibrous hamartoma of infancy – skin colored plaque with hypertrichosis and hyperhidrosis *Ped Derm 32:533–535, 2015;* congenital subcutaneous nodule *Ped Derm 27:525–526, 2010;* solitary nodule on shoulder, arm, axilla *JAAD 54:800–803, 2006; JAAD 41:857–859, 1999; Ped Derm 13:171–172, 1996; AD 125:88, 1989; J Pathol Bacteriol 72:149–154, 1956*

   Differential diagnosis includes: *Ped Derm 32:533–535, 2015*
   Infantile fibromatosis
   Fibrolipoma
   Calcifying aponeurotic fibroma
   Myofibroma
   Rhabdomyosarcoma
   Infantile fibrosarcoma
   Inclusion body fibromatosis
   Juvenile hyaline fibromatosis
   Histiocytoma
   Dermatofibrosarcoma protuberans
   Gardner syndrome-associated fibroma
   Dermatomyofibroma
   Fibroblastic connective tissue nevus

Foregut cystic developmental malformation of scapula – soft skin colored nodule of scapula *Ped Derm 29:363–364, 2012*

Hemangioma – congenital subcutaneous nodule *Ped Derm 27:525–526, 2010*

Heterotopic brain tissue – skin colored scalp nodule *Dermatol Therapy 18:104–116, 2005*

Congenital xanthogranulomas *Ped Derm 35:582–587, 2018*
   Yellow scalp nodule
   Ulcerated pink nodule
   Subcutaneous nodule with pink papules
   Brown-gray patch with pink yellow papules
   Atrophic patch with yellow macules and papules

Juvenile xanthogranuloma – congenital plaque *Ped Derm 29:217–218, 2012*

Leiomyoma – congenital subcutaneous nodule *Ped Derm 27:525–526, 2010*

Leiomyosarcoma – congenital subcutaneous nodule *Ped Derm 27:525–526, 2010*

Lipoma – deep forehead lipoma *Ped Derm 37:520–523, 2020;* congenital vulvar lipoma with accessory labioscrotal fold – labial enlargement with subcutaneous nodule *Ped Derm 28:424–428, 2011*

Lipomyelomeningocele (lower back) *Ped Derm 26:688–695, 2009*
   vs. Angiomatous nevi
      True tail in newborn *Ped Derm 12:263–266, 1995*
      Perirectal inflammatory lesions
      Giant cell tumors of the sacrum

Meningocele

Myelomeningocele *Ped Derm 26:688–695, 2009*

Myofibroma – congenital subcutaneous nodule *Ped Derm 27:525–526, 2010*

Myopericytoma – congenital subcutaneous nodule *Ped Derm 27:525–526, 2010*

Myxoid neurothekeoma – skin colored scalp nodules *Ped Derm 28:333–334, 2011*

Neuroblastoma – congenital subcutaneous nodule *Ped Derm 27:525–526, 2010*

Neurofibroma – congenital subcutaneous nodule *Ped Derm 27:525–526, 2010*

Neuroglial heterotopia (encephaloceles that lost intracranial connection) – red nodule of nasal root; skin colored nodule; red blue firm non-compressible nodule (nasal glioma); intranasal polypoid masses; and rudimentary or atretic encephaloceles *Ped Derm 32:161–170, 2015*

Nevus lipomatosus superficialis – congenital exophytic nodule *Ped Derm 34:367–368, 2017; Arch Dermatol Syphil 130:327–333, 1921*

Nodular macroglobulinosis *JAAD 77:1145–1158, 2017*

Palisaded encapsulated neuroma – skin colored papule of face *Cutis 92:167, 177–178, 2013*

Pyramidal lobe of thyroid gland

Rhabdomyosarcoma – congenital subcutaneous nodule *Ped Derm 27:525–526, 2010*

Solitary congenital calcified nodule of ear

Spinal dysraphism, occult – with overlying connective tissue nevus (skin colored plaque), protrusion, dimple, sinus, lipoma, faun tail nevus, dermoid cyst, hemangioma, port wine stain *BJD 156:1065–1066, 2007; AD 114:573–577, 1978; AD 112:1724–1728, 1976*

Striated muscle hamartoma (rhabdomyomatous mesenchymal hamartoma) – skin colored papule of upper chest; may be single or multiple, dome-shaped, pedunculated or filiform *Ped Derm 16:65–67, 1999*

Subcutaneous fat necrosis – subcutaneous tumid mass *Ped Derm 30:120–123, 2013*

Supernumerary breast – accessory supernumerary axillary breast and nipple with breast carcinoma *Cutis 87:300–304, 2011*

Vestigial tail *Arch J Dis Child 104:72–73, 1962*

Wattle (cutaneous cervical tag) *AD 121:22–23, 1985*

DEGENERATIVE DISORDERS

Baker's cyst

Frontal mucocele – skin colored nodule of forehead *JAAD 51:1030–1031, 2004*

Groin hernia
   Direct (acquired) hernia
   Femoral hernia
   Indirect (congenital)hernia
   Obturator hernia
   Perineal hernia

Linea alba (epigastric)hernia

Muscle herniation – anterior tibialis muscle herniation – pretibial skin colored compressible nodule *Ped Derm 36:664–667, 741–742, 2019*

Spigelian (linea semilunaris) hernia

Transsternal gastric hernia *NEJM 370:1440, 2014*

Umbilical hernia (abdominal hernia)

DRUG-INDUCED

Anti-HIV drugs, including nucleoside reverse transcriptase inhibitors, protease inhibitors, and non-nucleoside reverse transcriptase inhibitors – lipoatrophy, lipohypertrophy, gynecomastia; with metabolic syndrome *JAAD 63:549–561, 2010*

Anti-retroviral agents – scalp nodules *NEJM 352:63, 2005*

BCG – disseminated BCG infection *AD 143:1323–1328, 2007*

Corticosteroid – corticosteroid granuloma, resembling rheumatoid nodule *Am J Dermatopathol 4:199–203, 1982;* steroid atrophy

Drug reaction with eosinophilia and systemic symptoms (DRESS) – lymphadenopathy, morbilliform eruption, cheilitis (crusted hemorrhagic lips), diffuse desquamation, areolar erosion, periorbital dermatitis, vesicles, bullae, targetoid plaques, purpura, pustules, exfoliative erythroderma, facial edema *JAAD 68:693–705, 2013;*

Efavirenz – HIV and HAART; bullfrog neck (HIV lipodystrophy) *AD 146:1279–1282, 2010*

Insulin – insulin granuloma, zinc-induced *Clin Exp Dermatol 14:227–229, 1989;* lipohypertrophic insulin lipodystrophy *JAAD 19:570, 1988*

Interferon beta 1a – calcified subcutaneous nodules *BJD 157:624–625, 2007*

Iodide mumps – giant acute inflammatory swelling of submandibular, sublingual, or parotid glands *Ann Int Med 145:155–156, 2006; Circulation 104:2384, 2001; Acta Radiol 36:82–84, 1995; Am J Roentgenol 159:1099–1100, 1992; JAMA 213:2271–2272, 1970; NEJM 255:433–434, 1956*

Leuprorelin acetate granulomas *BJD 152:1045–1047, 2005*

Methotrexate nodulosis *J Dermatol 26:46–464, 1999; JAAD 39:359–362, 1998*

Minocycline-induced p-ANCA+ cutaneous polyarteritis nodosa (vasculitis) – subcutaneous nodules of extremities *JAAD 48:311–340, 2003; JAAD 44:198–206, 2001*

Protease inhibitor (saquinavir, nelfinavir, indinavir) – buffalo hump, supraclavicular fat pads, angiolipomas *JAAD 46:284–293, 2002*

EXOGENOUS AGENTS

Aluminum – persistent subcutaneous nodules at the injection site (hypersensitivity to vaccine aluminum adjuvant) *Ped Derm 35:234–236, 2018;* immunization site granuloma – due to aluminum hydroxide *JAAD 52:623–629, 2005; AD 131:1421–1424, 1995; AD 120:1318–1322, 1984*

Bovine collagen implant *J Derm Surg Oncol 9:377–380, 1983*

Bullet foreign body reaction – personal observation

Foreign body granuloma from IVDA *JAAD 13:869–872, 1985*

Hair granuloma

Hyaluronic acid (Captique) – hypersensitivity reaction to non-animal stabilized hyaluronic acid; facial nodules *JAAD 55:128–131, 2006*

Implanted stones, glass beads of penis *JAAD 20:852, 1989*

Oleomas – multiple subcutaneous oleomas due to injection with sesame seed oil *JAAD 42:292–294, 2000*

Paraffinoma (sclerosing lipogranuloma) – face, breast, thighs, buttocks *Acta Chir Plast 33:163–165, 1991; Plast Reconstr Surg 65:517–524, 1980*

Plant thorns – common blackthorn; persistent nodules of wrists and fingers *Lancet i:309–310, 1960*

Poly L-lactic microspheres (New-Fill), injectable – skin-colored nodules of cheek *JAAD 64:1–34, 2011*

Povidone panniculitis (polyvinyl pyrrolidone) *AD 116:704–706, 1980*

Silica granuloma *AD 127:692–694, 1991*

Silicone – silicone granulomas with facial nodules at crow's feet *BJD 152:1064–1065, 2005; Derm Surg 29:429–432, 2003;* skin colored nodules of lower legs – liquid silicone migration from augmentation to buttocks *JAAD 64:1–34, 2011;* firm skin colored papules of dorsum of hand after rupture of breast implants *AD 147:1215–1220, 2011*

INFECTIONS AND INFESTATIONS

Acanthamoeba – subcutaneous nodule *J Clin Inf Dis 20:1207–1216, 1995*

Actinomycosis, disseminated *Arch Int Med 134:688–693, 1974;* primary cutaneous – subcutaneous nodules with draining sinuses *Hum Pathol 4:319–330, 1973*

African trypanosomiasis – enlargement of posterior cervical lymph nodes (Winterbottom's sign)

AIDS – diffuse infiltrative lymphocytosis syndrome (DILS) – personal observation

Alternaria alternata JAAD 52:653–659, 2005; BJD 143:910–912, 2000

Amebiasis

Aspergillosis – primary cutaneous aspergillosis *JAAD 31:344–347, 1994;* subcutaneous granuloma *BJD 85(suppl 17):95–97, 1971*

Bacillary angiomatosis (*Bartonella henselae*) *Hautarzt 44:361–364, 1993; JAAD 22:501–512, 1990*

Bartonellosis (*Bartonella bacilliformis*) *Clin Inf Dis 33:772–779, 2001*

BCG – disseminated BCG in X-linked severe combined immunodeficiency *Ped Derm 23:560–563, 2006*

Botryomycosis *Cutis 80:45–47, 2007*

Brodie abscess of tibia – *Aggregatibacter aphrophilus* (facultative gram-negative bacillus anaerobe of oral cavity) *Clin Inf Dis 63:1360,1388–1389, 2016*

Calymmatobacterium granulomatis (Donovanosis) *J Clin Inf Dis 25:24–32, 1997*

Candida – deep subcutaneous nodules *JAAD 80:869–880, 2019; Clin Exp Dermatol 34:106–110, 2009;* chronic mucocutaneous candidiasis *Ann Rev Med 32:491–497, 1981*

Cat scratch disease – lymphadenopathy

Cestodes (tapeworms) (*Echinococcus* and cysticercosis) – slow growing solitary subcutaneous nodule of anterior abdominal wall *JAAD 73:929–944, 2015*

Chagas' disease (*Trypanosoma cruzi*) – chagoma *NEJM 373:456–466, 2016*

Chromobacterium violaceum – subcutaneous nodules *JAAD 54:S224–228, 2006*

Coccidioidomycosis – primary inoculation *Am Rev Resp Dis 117:559–585; 727–771, 1978*

Coenurosis – metacestode larval stage (coenurus) of tapeworms *Taenia multiceps, Taenia serialis, Taenia brauni Clin Inf Dis 56:1293,1347–1348, 2013*

Corynebacterium jeikeium – ulcers, subcutaneous nodules *Scand J Infect Dis 27:581–584, 1995; JAAD 16:444–447, 1987*

Cryptococcosis *JAAD 37:116–117, 1997*

Cysticercosis (*Taenia solium*) (*Cysticercus cellulosae*) – undercooked pork; multiple asymptomatic subcutaneous nodules; multiple red painless nodules of legs; abdominal pain, muscle edema and pain; diarrhea; neurocysticercosis *JAAD 73:929–944, 2015; JAAD 43:538–540, 2000; JAAD 25:409–414, 1991; NEJM 330:1887, 1994; JAAD 12:304–307, 1985*

Dermatophilus congolensis – contact with infected animals *BJD 145:170–171, 2001*

Dipetalonemiasis

Dirofilariasis, subcutaneous (migratory nodules) – eyelid, scrotum, breast, arm, leg, conjunctiva *JAAD 73:929–944, 2015; Cutis 72:269–272, 2003; JAAD 35:260–262, 1996*

Echinococcosis – dog tapeworm; hydatid cyst; urticaria, subcutaneous nodules *JAAD 73:929–944, 2015; BJD 147:807, 2002;* giant intraperitoneal cyst

Fascioliasis – *(Fasciola hepatica, F. gigantica)* – liver fluke; urticarial, jaundice, diarrhea, serpiginous tracts, subcutaneous nodules *JAAD 73:929–944, 2015*

Filariasis – *Wuchereria bancrofti, Brugia malayi, Brugia timori;* mosquito vector – first sign is edema, pain, and erythema with swellings of arms, legs, or scrotum *Dermatol Clin 7:313–321, 1989*

Gnathostomiasis – including urticarial migratory lesions; intermittent migratory swellings and nodules; subcutaneous hemorrhages along tracks of migration; abdominal pain, nausea and vomiting, diarrhea; South East Asia *JAAD 73:929–944, 2015; JAAD 73:929–944, 2015; JAAD 11:738–740, 1984; AD 120:508–510, 1984*

Granuloma inguinale (donovanosis) ("serpiginous ulcer") – *Calymmatobacterium granulomatis* – starts as skin colored subcutaneous nodule which breaks down into vulvar ulcer, vegetative perianal plaques with fistula formation, mutilation, and elephantine changes *JAAD 54:559–578, 2006*

Histoplasmosis – breast mass *NEJM 375:1172–1180, 2016*

HIV/AIDS – parotid lymphoepithelial cysts

Infectious mononucleosis – cervical lymphadenopathy

Leishmaniasis – disseminated cutaneous leishmaniasis – multilobulated skin colored nodules of ears *BJD 156:1328–1335, 2007; JAAD 34:257–272, 1996;* AIDS-related visceral leishmaniasis *BJD 143:1316–1318, 2000*

Leprosy – lepromatous leprosy

primary neuritic leprosy with nerve abscesses *AD 130:243–248, 1994;* erythema nodosum leprosum; Lucio's phenomenon – firm subcutaneous nodules *AD 114:1023–1028, 1978;* histoid lesions of relapse of lepromatous leprosy *Int J Lepr 31:129–142, 1963*

Loiasis – Calabar swellings; temporary of arm and hand, and elsewhere; angioedema

Lobomycosis (*Lacazia loboi*)

Lyme borreliosis – juxta-articular fibroid nodule in acrodermatitis chronica atrophicans *AD 131:1341–1342, 1995*

Mansonella perstans – pericardial inflammation, subcutaneous nodules, peritoneal or pleural cavity involvement, angioedema, pruritus, fever, headaches, arthralgias, neurologic symptoms *JAAD 75:19–30, 2016*

Molluscum contagiosum, giant

Mumps – presternal swelling *Cutis 39:139–140, 1987;* parotid swelling

Mycetoma

Mycobacterium avium complex – traumatic inoculation panniculitis; disseminated infection in AIDS – nodules, panniculitis *BJD 130:785–790, 1994;* subcutaneous nodule *J Dermatol 25:384–390, 1998*

Mycobacterium chelonae-fortuitum – disseminated nodules *AD 123:1603–1604, 1987;* single nodule following navel piercing *Ped Derm 25:219–222, 2008*

Mycobacterium szulgai – diffuse cellulitis, nodules, and sinuses *Am Rev Respir Dis 115:695–698, 1977;* subcutaneous nodule *BJD 142:838–840, 2000*

Mycobacterium tuberculosis – tuberculous gumma (metastatic tuberculous ulcer) – firm subcutaneous nodule or fluctuant swelling breaks down to form undermined ulcer; bluish surrounding skin bound to the inflammatory mass; sporotrichoid lesions along draining lymphatics; extremities more than trunk *Scand J Infect Dis 32:37–40, 2000; JAAD 6:101–106, 1982; Semin Hosp Paris 43:868–888, 1967;* parasternal pulsatile nodule *J Clin Inf Dis 22:871–872, 1996;* parotid swelling; miliary tuberculosis *JAAD 33:433–440, 1995*

Mycobacterium ulcerans (Buruli ulcer) – subcutaneous nodule of legs *JAAD 54:559–578, 2006; Aust J Dermatol 26:67–73, 1985*

Myiasis, furuncular – house fly *BJD 76:218–222, 1964;* New World screw worm (*Cochliomyia*), Old World screw worm (*Chrysomya*), Tumbu fly (*Cordylobia*) *BJD 85:226–231, 1971;* black blowflies (*Phormia*) *J Med Entomol 23:578–579, 1986;* green bottle (*Lucilia*), bluebottle (*Calliphora*), flesh flies (*Sarcophaga, Wohlfahrtia*) *Neurosurgery 18:361–362, 1986;* rodent botflies (*Cuterebra*) *JAAD 21:763–772, 1989;* human botflies (*Dermatobia hominis*) *Clin Inf Dis 37:542, 591–592, 2003; AD 126:199–202, 1990; AD 121:1195–1196, 1985; Hypoderma tarandi;* bumblebee-like fly of subarctic regions; eggs deposited on reindeer (caribou); larvae penetrate skin, hatch, and result in migratory swellings; ophthalmomyiasis may result in blindness *NEJM 367:2456–2457, 2012*

North American blastomycosis – subcutaneous nodule *AD 143:1323–1328, 2007*

Onchocerciasis – onchocercomas *AD 140:1161–1166, 2004; Cutis 72:297–302, 2003; JAAD 45:435–437, 2001; Cutis 65:293–297, 2000*

Paragonimiasis (*Paragonimus westermani, P. szechuanensis, P. bueitunensis*) – lung fluke; undercooked crustaceans; painless migratory subcutaneous nodules of abdominal wall, inguinal area, proximal legs; eosinophilic meningitis and encephalitis *JAAD 73:929–944, 2015*

   Migratory subcutaneous nodules *JAAD 73:929–944, 2015*
     Paragonimiasis
     Sparganosis
     Onchocerciasis

Phaeohyphomycosis, subcutaneous *JAAD 36:863–866, 1997; J Clin Inf Dis 25:1195, 1997*

Plague (*Yersinia pestis*) – bubonic plague (subcutaneous nodule) *JAAD 54:559–578, 2006*

Pneumocystis carinii (jirovecii) – classified as fungus (not protozoan); red or skin-colored papules or nodules *JAAD 60:897–925, 2009*

Polyacrylamide hydrogel fillers in cosmetic surgery – biofilms of *Staphylococcus epidermidis and Propionibacterium acnes;* nodules and granulomas at sites of injections of fillers *Clin Inf Dis 56:1438–1444, 2013*

Protothecosis *JAAD 55:S122–123, 2006; AD 142:921–926, 2006; Am J Clin Pathol 77:485–488, 1982; Am J Clin Pathol 61:10–19, 1974*

Pseudomonas aeruginosa Cutis 63:161–163, 1999

Rheumatic fever – nodules of occiput, wrist, backs of forearms *Indian Heart J 45:463–467, 1993; JAAD 8:724–728, 1983; Arch Pathol 30:70–89, 1940*

Rubella – cervical lymphadenopathy

Scarlet fever – cervical lymphadenopathy

Sparganosis (larvae of tapeworm) – ingestion sparganosis – edematous painful nodules *JAMADerm 152:831–832, 2016; Adv Parasitol 72:351–408, 2010; JAAD 15:1145–1148, 1986; S. proliferum* – subcutaneous nodules and pruritic papules *JAAD 73:929–944, 2015; Am J Trop Med Hyg 30:625–637, 1981;* spirometra – muscle, skin, orbits, and brain *JAAD 73:929–944, 2015*

Sternoclavicular joint septic arthritis *J Clin Inf Dis 19:964–966, 1994*

Streptocerciasis – *Mansonella streptocerca* – similar rash to onchocerciasis; acute or lichenified papules with widespread lichenification and hypopigmented macules

Subcutaneous phaeohyphomycosis – *Exophiala jeanselmei;* nodule of leg *BJD 150:597–598, 2004*

Subperiosteal abscess – skin colored nodule overlying tibia *JAMADerm 150:663–664, 2014*

Syphilis – secondary – facial nodule *J Clin Inf Dis 23:462–467, 1996;* osteitis of the skull *JAAD 40:793–794, 1994;* tertiary *Cutis 59:135–137, 1997;* lymphadenopathy; parotid swelling

Toxoplasmosis – lymphadenopathy

Trichophyton rubrum, invasive – subcutaneous nodule *Cutis 67:457–462, 2001*

Tropical pyomyositis – *Staphylococcus aureus JAAD 54:559–578, 2006*

Tularemia – bubo; lymphadenopathy

Tungiasis – *Tunga penetrans JAAD 20:941–944, 1989*

Visceral larva migrans – *Toxocara canis*

Warts

Whipple's disease – subcutaneous Whipple's disease *JAAD 16:188–190, 1987*

Yaws – tertiary – gumma; subcutaneous nodule; overlying skin ulcerates with purulent discharge; atrophic pigmented scars

Zygomycosis – subcutaneous zygomycosis (Basidiobolus ranarum) – subcutaneous nodule with edema *Derm Clinics 17:151–185, 1999; JAAD 30:904–908, 1994*

INFILTRATIVE DISEASES

Amyloidosis – nodular tumefactive amyloid; articular amyloid (amyloid arthropathy) – shoulder pad sign *NEJM 351:e23, 2004; Scand J Immunol 54:4048, 2001; NEJM 288:354–355, 1973*

Cutaneous focal mucinosis (superficial angiomyxoma) – face, trunk, or extremities *Am J Surg Pathol 12:519–530, 1988; AD 93:13–20, 1966*

Cutaneous mucinosis of infancy – skin-colored rubbery nodules *Ped Derm 27:299–300, 2010; AD 116:198–200, 1980*

Generalized eruptive histiocytosis

Indeterminate cell histiocytosis *BJD 153:206–207, 2005*

Juvenile xanthogranuloma – subcutaneous nodule of heel *Am J Surg Pathol 15:150–159, 1991*

Langerhans cell histiocytosis – eosinophilic granuloma

Lichen myxedematosus *JAAD 33:37–43, 1995*

Papular mucinosis – personal observation

Reticulohistiocytoma cutis – solitary reticulohistiocytoma *Hifuka Gakkai Zasshi 101, 735–742, 1991;* destructive arthritis with rheumatoid-like nodules *Clin Exp Dermatol 15:1–6, 1990*

Self-healing juvenile cutaneous mucinosis – skin-colored papules and nodules of face and acral areas, arthralgias; periarticular papules *Ped Derm 31:515–516, 2014; AD 148:755–760, 2012;*

periorbital edema *AD 148:755–760, 2012;* myalgias, swelling of joints with refusal to walk; erythema and edema of upper and lower eyelids, violaceous periarticular nodules, skin colored nodules of neck and abdomen *Am J Dermatopathol 34:699–705, 2012; AD 145:211–212, 2009; JAAD 55:1036–1043, 2006; JAAD 50:S97–100, 2004; AD 131:459–461, 1995*

Subcutaneous xanthogranulomatosis *JAAD 21:924–929, 1989*

INFLAMMATORY DISORDERS

Acne keloidalis nuchae *Dermatol Clin 6:387–395, 1988;*

Dissecting cellulitis of the scalp

Fibroblastic rheumatism *JAAD 66:959–965, 2012*

IgG4 disease – multisystem inflammatory disease with papules, plaques, and nodules; parotitis with parotid gland swelling, lacrimal gland swelling, dacryoadenitis, sialadenitis, proptosis; idiopathic pancreatitis, retroperitoneal fibrosis, aortitis; Mikuliczs syndrome, angiolymphadenopathy with eosinophilia, Riedel's thyroiditis, biliary tract disease, renal disease, meningeal disease, pituitary gland; Kuttner tumor, Rosai-Dorfman disease; elevated IgG4 with plasma cell dyscrasia, diffuse or localized swelling or masses; sclerosing mesenteritis; lymphocytic and plasma cell infiltrates with storiform fibrosis *JAAD 75:177–185, 2016*

Interstitial granulomatous dermatitis – multiple skin colored papules *JAAD 51:S105–107, 2004*

Kimura's disease (angiolymphoid hyperplasia with eosinophilia) – large subcutaneous swellings of face, neck, extremities *Cutis 70:57–61, 2002;* large subcutaneous nodule *AD 136:837–839, 2000; JAAD 27:954–958, 1992; JAAD 38:143–175, 1998; JAAD 16:143–145, 1987; JAAD 12:781–796, 1985*

Lymph node – lymphadenitis; lymphadenopathy

Lymphocytoma cutis – skin colored to plum-red dermal or subcutaneous nodules; idiopathic or due to insect bites, *Borrelia burgdorferi,* trauma, vaccinations, injected drugs or antigens for hyposensitization, injection of arthropod venom, acupuncture, gold pierced earrings, tattoos, post-zoster scars *JAAD 38:877–905, 1998*

Malacoplakia

Masseter spasm due to hypersensitive mastication muscle syndrome

Myositis, focal – painful nodule *Cutis 54:189–190, 1994*

Myospherulosis *JAAD 38:274–275, 1998; AD 127:88–90, 1991; JAAD 21:400–403, 1989*

Nodular cystic fat necrosis *JAAD 21:493–498, 1989*

Nodular fasciitis – of popliteal fossa *Cutis 102:26, 31–32, 2018;* painful subcutaneous nodule *Cutis 92:199–202, 2013; JAAD 40:490–492, 1999;* on the head and neck, extremities, or trunk *AD 137:719–721, 2001*

Nodular pseudosarcomatous fasciitis *AD 124:1559–1564, 1988; Arch Pathol Lab Med 73:437–444, 1962*

Proliferative fasciitis – multiple rapidly growing painful subcutaneous nodules in children following trauma; spontaneous resolution *AD 144:255–260, 2008; JAAD 55:1036–1043, 2006; Cancer 36:1450–1458, 1975*

Cutaneous sinus histiocytosis with lymphadenopathy (Rosai-Dorfman disease) *AD 133:231–236, 1977*

Sarcoid – panniculitis *JAAD 45:325–361, 2001;* subcutaneous (Darier-Roussy) sarcoid *Practical Dermatol March 2019:67–70; JAAD 66:699–716, 2012; JAAD 54:55–60, 2006;*

BJD 153:790–794, 2005; JAAD 44:725–743, 2001; AD 133:882–888, 1997; Am J Med 85:731–736, 1988; AD 120:1028–1031,

1984; Ann Dermatol Syphil 5:144–149, 1904; pretibial subcutaneous nodule *JAMADerm 150:663–664, 2014;* subcutaneous sarcoid mimicking breast cancer *BJD 146:924, 2002;* lymphadenopathy; uveoparotid fever (Heerfordt's syndrome) – parotid swelling

Sclerosing mesenteritis (retractile mesenteritis) – sclerodermoid changes with subcutaneous nodules; now renamed IgG4 disease *AD 146:1009–1013, 2010*

Sialadenosis – swelling of parotid gland

Subcutaneous fat necrosis of the newborn *AD 117:36–37, 1981*

Tietze's disease

METABOLIC DISORDERS

Abetalipoproteinemia

Adiposis dolorosa (Dercum's disease) – obesity; multiple painful subcutaneous lipomas, acral edema, telangiectasias *JAAD 81:1037–1057, 2019*

Albright's hereditary osteodystrophy

Alcoholism – parotid enlargement

Benign symmetrical lipomatosis

Calcinosis cutis – idiopathic; papular or nodular calcinosis cutis secondary to heel sticks *Ped Derm 18:138–140, 2001;* cutaneous calculus *BJD 75:1–11, 1963;* extravasation of calcium carbonate solution; metastatic calcification *JAAD 33:693–706, 1995; Cutis 32:463–465, 1983;* tumoral calcinosis

Calciphylaxis (vascular calcification cutaneous necrosis syndrome) – papules or nodules around large joints or flexures *JAAD 40:979–987, 1999; JAAD 33:53–58, 1995; JAAD 33:954–962, 1995;J Dermatol 28:27–31, 2001; Br J Plast Surg 53:253–255, 2000; J Cutan Med Surg 2:245–248, 1998; JAAD 33:954–962, 1995; AD 127:225–230, 1991*

Cerebrotendinous xanthomatosis (cholestanosis)

Chronic renal failure – benign nodular calcification of chronic renal failure *JAAD 33:693–706, 1995*

Cryoglobulinemia – dermal nodules *JAAD 48:311–340, 2003*

Cushing's disease – buffalo hump, supraclavicular fat pads – personal observation

Cystinosis – subcutaneous plaque; skin atrophy and telangiectasia mimicking premature aging; normal skin *JAAD 62:AB26, 2010*

Diabetic lipohypertrophy – giant skin colored tumid mass *BJD 171:1402–1406, 2014*

Diabetes mellitus – parotid gland enlargement – personal observation

Endometriosis, primary cutaneous *AD 145:605–606, 2009; Cutis 81:124–126, 2008*

Extramedullary hematopoiesis *JAAD 58:703–706, 2008*

Gout- tophi *Semin Arthritis Rheum 29:56–63, 1999; AD 113:655–656, 1977*

Hyperoxalosis, primary *JAAD 46:S16–18, 2002; AD 131:821–823, 1995; AD 125:380–383, 1989;* secondary hyperoxalosis – calcified nodules or miliary papules *JAAD 49:725–728, 2003*

IgM storage papule – knee, elbow *AD 128:377–380, 1992; BJD 106:217–222, 1982*

Miliaria profunda – skin-colored papules

Osteoma cutis – primary miliary osteoma cutis *Ped Derm 29:483–484, 2012; JAAD 24:878–881, 1991;* congenital plate-like osteoma cutis; primary multiple miliary osteomas *AD 134:641–643, 1998;* differential diagnosis of primary osteoma

Albright's hereditary osteodystrophy
Fibrodysplasia ossificans progressiva
Congenital plate-like osteomatosis
Progressive osseous dysplasia

Oxalate granulomas *BJD 128:690–692, 1993*

Pretibial myxedema *Cutis 58:211–214, 1996*

Progressive osseous heteroplasia *Ped Derm 16:74–75, 1999; AD 132:787–791, 1996; J Bone Joint Surg Am 76:425–436, 1994*

Sickle cell anemia – parotid swelling

Sitosterolemia – subcutaneous tuberous and tendon xanthomas *Ped Derm 17:447–449, 2000*

Verrucous xanthoma – skin colored verrucous papule of earlobe *Cutis 91:198–202, 2013*

Xanthomas with or without fibrosis

NEOPLASTIC DISORDERS

Acrochordon, giant

Acrospiroma *Cutis 58:349–351, 1996*

Adenoid cystic carcinoma – scalp papules or nodules *Cutis 77:157–160, 2006; JAAD 40:640–642, 1999;* giant tumor *Cutis 87:237–239, 2011*

Adenolipoma *JAAD 29:82, 1993*

Aggressive angiomyxoma – greater than 5 cm subcutaneous nodule *Am J Surg Pathol 7:463–475, 1983*

Alveolar soft part sarcoma – tumor of muscle or fascial planes *Clin Exp Dermatol 10:523–539, 1985*

Angiokeratoma – personal observation

Angioleiomyoma *JAAD 46:477–490, 2002;* subcutaneous nodule of leg, face, trunk, or oral cavity *JAAD 38:143–175, 1998* Epstein-Barr virus positive angioleiomyomas in AIDS *BJD 147:563–567, 2002*

Angiolipoleiomyoma *JAAD 54:167–171, 2006*

Angiomatoid fibrous histiocytoma *Ped Derm 26:636–638, 2009; BJD 142:537–539, 2000*

Angiomyolipoma (angiolipoleiomyoma) (face, ear, elbow, toe) *AD 139:381–386, 2003; JAAD 29:115–116, 1993; JAAD 23:1093–1098, 1990*

Angiolipoma – arms, legs, abdomen *JAAD 38:143–175, 1998; AD 126:666–667, 669, 1990; AD 82:924–931, 1960*

Angiosarcoma *AD 133:1303–1308, 1997*

Apocrine hamartoma *Ped Derm 24:346–347, 2007*

Apocrine hidrocystomas, congenital – axillary papules in infancy *Ped Derm 30:491–492, 2013*

Apocrine nevus *Ped Derm 12:248–251, 1995*

Atypical fibroxanthoma *Cancer 55:172–180, 1985*

Baker's cyst

Basal cell carcinoma, including multiple hereditary infundibulocystic basal cell carcinomas *AD 135:1227–1235, 1999*

Blastic plasmacytoid dendritic cell neoplasm (blastic natural killer cell lymphoma) – skin colored nodule of scalp *JAMA Derm 149:971–972, 2013*

Carcinoid tumors *Tumori 76:44–47, 1990;* primary cutaneous carcinoid *JAAD 51:S74–76, 2004*

Castleman's syndrome

Chondroid syringoma *AD 140:751–756, 2004; Cutis 71:49–55, 2003*

Chondromyxoid fibroma – skin colored nodule overlying tibia *JAMADerm 150:663–664, 2014*

Chordoma, metastatic *AD 133:1579–1584, 1997*

Clear cell hidradenoma *Ped Derm 22:450–452, 2005*

Clear cell sarcoma (malignant melanoma of soft parts) – deep subcutaneous nodule *BJD 169:1346–1352, 2013*

Collagenous fibroma (desmoplastic fibroblastoma) *JAAD 41:292–294, 1999*

Connective tissue nevus (collagenoma) *JAAD 67:890–897, 2012; JAAD 3:441–446, 1980;* familial collagenoma *BJD 101:185–195, 1979; Cutis 10:283–288, 1972; AD 98:23–27, 1968*
   Birt-Hogg-Dube syndrome
   Buschke-Ollendorff syndrome
   Cowden's syndrome
   Familial cutaneous collagenomas
   Down's syndrome
   Tuberous sclerosis

Cribriform apocrine carcinoma – skin colored nodule of extremities *JAAD 61:644–651, 2009*

Cutaneous ciliated cyst *JAAD 56:159–160, 2008; AD 49:70–73, 1978*

Cylindromas – scalp, face, nose, around ears and neck *BJD 155:182–186, 2006*

Dendritic fibromyxolipoma – skin colored pedunculated giant tumor *AD 144:795–800, 2008*

Dermatofibroma – deep fibrous histiocytoma *Cutis 65:243–245, 2000*

Dermatofibrosarcoma protuberans *Ped Derm 29:707–713, 2012; Ped Derm 25:317–325, 2008; Sem Cut Med Surg 21:159–165, 2002; JAAD 35:355–374, 1996;* subcutaneous DFSP *JAAD 77:503–511, 2017*

Dermatomyofibroma – oval nodule or firm skin colored plaque of shoulders, axillae, upper arms, neck, or abdomen *Ped Derm 31:249–250, 2014; Clin Exp Dermatol 21:307–309, 1996*

Dermoid cyst – presternal subcutaneous nodule *Ped Derm 30:128–130, 2013;* dermoid cyst in adult – skin colored nodule of nose *JAMA Derm 149:609–614, 2013*

Desmoid tumor – subcutaneous mass in subumbilical paramedian region

Digital mucous cyst

Dupuytren's contractures – palmar, plantar

Eccrine angiomatous hamartoma – acral skin colored nodule *Ped Derm 27:93–94, 2010; Ped Derm 23:365–368, 2006; Ped Derm 23:516–517, 2006; Ped Derm 18:117–119, 2001; Ped Derm 14:401–402, 1997; Ped Derm 13:139–142, 1996;* skin-colored nodule with blue papules *JAAD 41:109–111, 1999*

Eccrine nevi *JAAD 51:301–304, 2004*

Eccrine poroma – personal observation

Eccrine porocarcinoma *JAAD 35:860–864, 1996*

Eccrine spiradenoma

Eccrine syringofibroadenoma – skin colored nodule of distal extremity *BJD 143:591–594, 2000*

Elastofibroma dorsi – back, over deltoid muscle, ischial tuberosity, greater trochanter, olecranon, stomach, cornea, foot *JAAD 51:1–21, 2004; JAAD 21:1142–1144, 1989*

Elastoma

Embryonal rhabdomyosarcoma *AD 138:689–694, 2002; Ped Derm 15:403–405, 1998*

Ependymoma – lumbosacral nodule *Pathology 12:237–243, 1980*

Epidermoid cyst

Epithelioid cell sarcoma – skin colored nodule of hands or digits *JAAD 38:815–819, 1998; AD 121:394–395, 1985; Cancer 26:1029–1041, 1970;* proximal type epithelioid sarcoma *Ped Derm 21:117–120, 2004*

Ewing's sarcoma – primary cutaneous Ewing's sarcoma; subcutaneous nodule *BJD 171:660–662, 2014*

Subcutaneous fibrohistiocytic tumors
   Angiomatoid malignant fibrous histiocytoma
   Cutaneous solitary fibrous tumor with myxoid stroma *BJD 147:1267–1269, 2002*
   Neural hamartoma
   Plexiform fibrohistiocytic tumor
   Recurrent adult myofibromatosis
   Soft tissue sarcomas

Fibroepithelioma of Pinkus – skin colored plaque; pedunculated, polypoid; gray-brown papule or plaque; pink papule *AD 142:1318–1322, 2006;* abdomen or groin *AD 126:953–958, 1990; AD 67:598, 1953*

Fibrolipoma

Fibrolipomatous hamartomas – subcutaneous of heels and hypothenar eminence of hand *Ped Derm 36:728–729, 2019*

Fibroma

Fibromatosis *Cutis 65:243–245, 2000*

Fibromatosis colli

Fibrosarcoma *JAAD 38:815–819, 1998;* congenital fibrosarcoma *AD 134:625–630, 1998*

Fibrous hamartoma of infancy *Ped Derm 17:429–431, 2000; AD 125:88–91, 1989*

Solitary fibrous tumors of soft tissue *Am J Surg Pathol 19:1257–1266, 1995*

Folliculosebaceous cystic hamartoma – skin colored papule or nodule of central face or scalp; pedunculated or dome-shaped and umbilicated *BJD 157:833–835, 2007; Clin Exp Dermatol 31:68–79, 2006; AD 139:803–808, 2003; JAAD 34:77–81, 1996; Am J Dermatopathol 13:213–220, 1991; J Cutan Pathol 7:394–403, 1980*

Frontalis-associated sarcoma – forehead nodule *JAAD 31:1048–1049, 1994*

Ganglion cyst of the ankle *JAAD 13:873–877, 1985;* of the knee

Ganglioneuroma *JAAD 35:353–354, 1996*

Giant cell fibroblastoma of soft tissue – neck and trunk *Ped Derm 19:28–32, 2002; Ped Derm 18:255–257, 2001*

Giant cell tumors of the sacrum – lumbosacral nodule

Giant cell tumor of skin or soft tissue *AD 147:359–361, 2011*

Giant cell tumor of the tendon sheath – single or multiple *JAAD 43:892, 2000;* nodules of the fingers *J Dermatol 23:290–292, 1996; J Bone Joint Surg Am 66:76–94, 1984*

Giant folliculosebaceous cystic hamartoma – skin colored exophytic papules *AD 141:1035–1040, 2005; Am J Dermatopathol 13:213–220, 1991*

Glandular congenital lymphadenoma (benign lymphoepithelial tumor of the skin) *Ped Derm 24:547–550, 2007*

Granular cell tumor (nodule) (Abrikossoff tumor) *JAAD 47:S180–182, 2002; Cutis 69:343–346, 2002; Cutis 62:147–148, 1998; Cutis 43:548–550, 1989;* multiple granular cell tumors *JAAD 24:359–363, 1991;* plantar skin colored nodule *Ped Derm 28:473–474, 2011*

Hair follicle hamartoma

Hibernoma – neck, axilla, central back, scapular region; vascular dilatation overlying lesion *AD 73:149–157, 1956*

Hidradenoma papilliferum; nodular hidradenoma *JAAD 48:S20–21, 2003; JAAD 12:15–20, 1985*; poroid hidradenoma *Cutis 50:43–46, 1992;* scalp *JAAD 19:133–135, 1988;* eyelid *AD 117:55–56, 1981;* nipple *Hautarzt 19:101–109, 1968;* external auditory canal *J Laryngol Otol 95:843–848, 1981*

Hidrocystoma

Intramuscular hydatid cyst – giant skin colored subcutaneous tumor (25x15cm) *Clin Inf Dis 61:1707, 1759–1760, 2015*

Infantile desmoid type fibromatosis – deep nodule *Skeletal Radiol 23(5):380–384, 1994*

Infantile digital fibromatosis *Ped Derm 8:137–139, 1991; J Cut Pathol 5:339–346, 1978*

Infantile systemic fibromatosis *Textbook of Neonatal Dermatology, p.395, 2001*

Infantile myofibromatosis – single or multiple; head, neck, trunk *Ped Derm 22:281–282, 2005; JAAD 41:508, 1999; AD 134:625–630, 1998* vs. soft tissue sarcomas
 Hemangioendotheliomas
 Fibrosarcomas
 Lipomas
 Fibrous histiocytomas
 Lipoblastomas
 metastatic neuroblastoma
 neurofibromas
 rhabdomyosarcomas

Juvenile xanthogranuloma *JAAD 36:355–367, 1997*

Kaposi's sarcoma – skin colored nodule of penis *BJD 142:153–156, 2000*

Keloid

Leiomyoma – angiomyoma; leg, trunk, face

Leiomyosarcoma *JAAD 71:919–925, 2014; JAAD 21:1156–1160, 1989; JAAD 38:137–142, 1998; J Exp Clin Cancer Res 17:405–407, 1998*

Leukemia – parotid swelling

Leukemia/lymphoma – adult T-cell leukemia/lymphoma (HTLV-1 leukemia/lymphoma) *JAAD 65:432–434, 2011*

Lipoblastoma – subcutaneous mass *Ped Derm 34:180–186, 2017;* lipoblastoma of infancy – rapidly growing tumor of cheek mimicking malignancy *Ped Derm 23:514–515, 2006; Cutis 65:243–245, 2000;* lipoblastomatosis *Ped Derm 12:82, 1995*

Lipofibromatosis (non-desmoid infantile fibromatosis) – subcutaneous nodule with bands of arms; mass of distal extremities *Ped Derm 31:298–304, 2014*
 Differential diagnosis:
 Lipoblastoma
 Calcifying aponeurotic fibroma
 Myofibromas (purple)
 Fibrous hamartoma of infancy) (hypertrichosis, axillae, proximal extremities, groin)
 Lipofibromatous hamartoma (intra-neural tumor) (macrodactyly) (third decade)
 Diffuse lipofibromatosis
 Venolymphatic malformations

Lipoma – lipoma of forehead; frontalis-associated lipoma *JAAD 20:462–468, 1989;* subgaleal lipoma of forehead *AD 125:384–385, 1989;* mobile encapsulated lipomas *Cutis 49:63–64, 1992;* congenital infiltrating lipoma *BJD 143:180–182, 2000;* multiple palmar lipomas *BJD 159:757–758, 2008*

Lipomatous variant of eccrine angiomatous hamartoma

Liposarcoma – diffuse nodular infiltration of leg or buttock *JAMA 321:1718–1719, 2019; JAAD 38:815–819, 1998;* giant subcutaneous nodule *JAAD 64:1202–1203, 2011*

Lymphoepithelioma *JAAD 22:691–693, 1990*

Lymphoepithelioma-like carcinoma of the skin *AD 134:1627–1632, 1998;* subcutaneous skin colored nodule of face *Cutis 101:170, 183–184, 2018*

Lymphoepithelioid cysts of the parotid gland

Lymphoma – Burkitt's lymphoma; cutaneous T-cell lymphoma *Rook p.2376–2378, 1998, Sixth Edition;* adult T-cell lymphoma/leukemia (HTLV-1) *JAAD 46:S137–141, 2002;*

AD 134:439–444, 1998; JAAD 34:69–76, 1996; BJD 128:483–492, 1993; Am J Med 84:919–928, 1988; angiocentric T-cell lymphoma *AD 132:1105–1110, 1996;* Hodgkin's disease – parotid swelling; non-B-cell large cell lymphoma of AIDS; painful skin colored nodules – granulomatous cutaneous T-cell lymphoma *BJD 163:1129–1132, 2010;* subcutaneous nodule – primary cutaneous diffuse large B-cell lymphoma, leg type; Bcl-2 expression *AD 143:1144–1150, 2007;* primary cutaneous marginal zone B-cell lymphoma *BJD 157:1205–1211, 2007;* lymphadenopathy; hemato-dermic/plasmacytoid dendritic cell CD4+ CD56+ lymphoma – subcutaneous nodule *JAAD 58:480–484, 2008; Blood 99:1556–1563, 2002;* Epstein-Barr virus-associated hydroa vacciniforme-like cutaneous lymphoma; variant of extranodal NK/T cell lymphoma, nasal type/-CD8+ cytotoxic T cells – recurrent papulovesicles, necrosis, ulceration, facial edema, atrophic scars, lip ulcers, edema of hands, subcutaneous nodules; systemic manifestations; occurs on both sun-exposed and non-sun-exposed skin *Ped Derm 27:463–469, 2010; AD 142:587–595, 2006; BJD 151:372–380, 2004; JAAD 38:574–579, 1998;* CD4+ small/medium pleomorphic T-cell lymphoma – skin colored nodule of face, red nodule of scalp, red plaque of neck *JAAD 65:739–748, 2011;* cutaneous B-cell lymphoblastic lymphoma *JAAD 66:51–57, 2012*

Lymphomatoid granulomatosis – Epstein-Barr-related T-cell rich B-cell lymphoproliferative disorder; papules and dermal nodules with or without ulceration, folliculitis-like lesions, maculopapules, indurated plaques, ulcers *BJD 157:426–429, 2007; JAAD 54:657–663, 2006*

Malignant fibrous histiocytoma *JAAD 67:1335–1341, 2012; Sem Cut Med Surg 21:159–165, 2002; JAAD 42:371–373, 2000; AD 135:1113–1118, 1999; JAAD 38:815–819, 1998*

Malignant giant cell tumor of soft parts *Am J Dermatopathol 11:197–201, 1989*

Malignant histiocytosis – skin colored nodule(s) *JAAD 56:302–316, 2007; BJD 113:355–361, 1985; Hum Pathol 15:368–377, 1984*

Malignant schwannoma (neurofibrosarcoma) – nodule which enlarges and becomes painful *JAAD 38:815–819, 1998; Am J Dermatopathol 11:213–221, 1989*

Melanocytic nevi; intradermal nevus

Melanoma – amelanotic melanoma; anal mucosal melanoma – skin colored multilobulated perianal nodule *Cutis 89:112,116,140, 2012;* desmoplastic melanoma *JAAD 26:704–709, 1992;* metastatic melanoma; melanoma of the soft parts (clear cell sarcoma) – nodule of the foot, ankle, knee, hand, wrist *JAAD 38:815–819, 1998*

Meningioma – intracranial malignant meningioma *JAAD 34:306–3077, 1996;* primary cutaneous meningioma – scalp or paraspinal region of children and teenagers *Cancer 34:728–744, 1974*

Merkel cell tumor *JAAD 29:143, 1993*

Mesenchymal tumor – subcutaneous hyperpigmented nodule; phosphaturic mesenchymal tumor, mixed connective tissue type; tumor induced osteomalacia (TIO) (low serum phosphate, increased urinary phosphate excretion, low 1,25 dihydroxy vitamin D levels, and elevated serum FGF-23); observe acquired renal phosphate wasting (hypophosphatemia); prominent bony osteoid formation and unmineralized bone; progressive weakness and bone pain *JAAD 57:509–512, 2007*

Metastases *JAAD 31:319–321, 1994;* including scalp nodules due to metastases – lung and kidney in men; breast in women; also ovaries, uterus, gallbladder, prostate, testis, gastrointestinal, melanoma, leukemia, lymphoma, thyroid; subungual nodule – metastatic renal cell carcinoma *JAAD 36:531–537, 1997; AD 130:913–918, 1994;* lymphadenopathy

Microcystic adnexal carcinoma *Derm Surg 27:979–984, 2001; JAAD 45:283–285, 2001; JAAD 41:225–231, 1999*

Mixed tumor

Monophasic synovial sarcoma *Cutis 93:13–16, 2014*

Mucinous carcinoma *AD 103:68–78, 1971*

Mucinous nevus (localized or familial) – skin colored papules or plaque *JAAD 67:890–897, 2012; Ped Derm 25:288–289, 2008; AD 132:1522–1523, 1996; JAAD 28:797–798, 1993*

Mucoepidermoid carcinoma – skin colored nodule of scalp *Ped Derm 24:452–453, 2007*

Multiple myeloma – personal observation

Musculoaponeurotic fibromatosis (extraabdominal desmoid) *Ped Derm 10:49–53, 1993*

Myofibroma – skin-colored to hyperpigmented nodules of hand, mouth, genitals, shoulders *JAAD 46:477–490, 2002; J Cutan Pathol 23:445–457, 1996; Histopathol 22:335–341, 1993*

Myxoid liposarcoma *Ped Derm 17:129–132, 2000*

Myxoinflammatory fibroblastic sarcoma – painful subcutaneous nodule *JAAD 62:711–712, 2010*

Myxoma (intramuscular) *JAAD 34:928–930, 1996*

Nerve sheath myxoma

Neurilemmomas (Schwannomas) *JAAD 38:106–108, 1998*

Neuroblastoma, metastatic *AD 134:625–630, 1998*

Neurofibroma

Neurolipomatosis (fibrolipomatous hamartoma of nerve) *Am J Surg Pathol 9:7–14, 1985*

Neuroma – traumatic neuroma; interdigital neuroma *JAAD 38:815–819, 1998;* multiple palisaded encapsulated neuromas *JAAD 62:358–359, 2010*

Neurothekeoma – skin-colored scalp nodule *BJD 144:1273–1274, 2001;* head and neck *JAAD 50:129–134, 2004*

Neuromuscular hamartoma (triton tumor) *Cancer 55:43–54, 1985*

Nevus lipomatosis superficialis *AD 120:376–379, 1984*

Nevus lipomatosis superficialis – skin colored grouped papulonodules *Ped Derm 28:189–190, 2011*

Ossifying fibromyxoid tumor of the skin *JAAD 52:644–647, 2005*

Osteochondroma – personal observation

Osteoma cutis

Osteosarcoma of mandible

Palisaded encapsulated neuroma

Palmar fibromatosis

Papillary eccrine adenoma (arm or leg) *JAAD 19:1111–1114, 1988*

Parotid tumors

PEComas – perivascular epithelioid cell neoplasm – *TFE3* mutation *BJD 17 4:617–620, 2016*

Periosteal aneurysmal bone cyst – pretibial skin colored nodule *JAMADerm 150:663–664, 2014*

Periosteal chondroma – skin colored nodule overlying tibia *JAMADerm 150:663–664, 2014*

Periosteal ganglia – skin colored nodule overlying tibia *JAMADerm 150:663–664, 2014*
    Differential diagnosis:

Erythema nodosum
Nodular pretibial myxedema
Subcutaneous sarcoidosis
Periosteal chondroma
Periosteal lipoma
Subperiosteal hematoma
Subperiosteal abscess
Periosteal aneurysmal bone cyst
Chondromyxoid fibroma
Periosteal osteosarcoma

Subperiosteal hematoma – skin colored nodule overlying tibia *JAMADerm 150:663–664, 2014*

Periosteal lipoma – skin colored nodule overlying tibia *JAMADerm 150:663–664, 2014*

Periosteal osteosarcoma – pretibial skin colored nodule *JAMADerm 150:663–664, 2014*

Pheochromocytoma, metastatic *JAAD 55:341–344, 2006*

Phosphaturic mesenchymal tumor, mixed connective tissue variant; tumor secretes fibroblast growth factor 23 (FGF23) resulting in renal phosphate wasting and low vitamin 1, 25 dihydroxy vitamin D3 and subsequent osteomalacia *BJD 157:198–200, 2007*

Pilar cyst

Pilomatrixoma – multiple pilomatrixomas associated with myotonic dystrophy and familial gastrointestinal polyps *Ped Derm 32:97–101, 2015; AD 106:41–44, 1972;* with Gardner's syndrome *Ped Derm 12:331–335, 1995;* with Sotos syndrome *Ped Derm 25:122–125, 1995;* with trisomy 9 *Ped Derm 26:482–484, 2009*

Plantar aponeurotic fibroma *Ped Derm 17:429–431, 2000*

Plasmacytoma – extramedullary plasmacytoma *AD 129:1331–1336, 1993; AD 127:69–74, 1991; JAAD 19:879–890, 1988*

Pleomorphic adenoma of parotid gland

Plexiform fibrohistiocytic tumor *Ped Derm 28:26–29, 2011; Ped Derm 23:71–12, 2006; Derm Surg 27:768–771, 2001*

Polyfibromatosis syndrome – Dupuytren's contracture (palmar fibromatosis), Peyronie's disease (penile fibromatosis), Ledderhose's nodules (plantar fibromatosis), knuckle pads, keloids *JAAD 41:106–108, 1999;* stimulation by phenytoin *BJD 100:335–341, 1979*

Polymorphous sweat gland carcinoma *JAAD 46:914–916, 2002*

Polypoid eccrine nevus – coccygeal papule overlying a depression *BJD 157:614–615, 2007*

Porocarcinoma *BJD 152:1051–1055, 2005*

Post-transplantation lymphoproliferative disorder – lymphadenopathy of head and neck *JAAD 54:657–663, 2006*

Precalcaneal congenital fibrolipomatous hamartoma – benign anteromedial plantar nodule of childhood – a distinct form of plantar fibromatosis *Ped Derm 21:655–656, 2004; Ped Derm 17:429–431, 2000; Med Cut Ibero Lat Am 18:9–12, 1990*

Pretibial bursal cyst – personal observation

Progressive nodular fibrosis

Progressive nodular histiocytosis *JAAD 29:278–280, 1993*

Pseudolipoma – inflammation of subcutaneous fat with encapsulation *Medical Ultrasonography 14:2012*

Rhabdomyomatous mesenchymal hamartoma (striated muscle hamartoma) (congenital) – associated with Dellemann's syndrome – multiple skin tag-like lesions (pedunculated and snake-like) of infancy *Ped Derm 15:274–276, 1998; Ped Derm 14:370, 1994;* skin colored nodule *Ped Derm 32:256–262, 2015;* skin colored plaque of upper chest *Ped Derm 37:64–68, 2020*

Rhabdomyosarcoma *Cutis 73:39–43, 2004; JAAD 38:815–819, 1998;* large solitary tumor of the head and neck; differential diagnosis includes infantile hemangioma, lymphatic malformation, myofibroma, lipoblastoma, teratoma, fibrosarcoma *Acta Oncol 35:494–495, 1996; Hautkr 53:887–892, 1978;* congenital – giant skin colored tumor *Ped Derm 28:299–301, 2011; Ped Derm 20:335–338, 2003*

Malignant schwannoma

Undifferentiated pleomorphic sarcoma – skin colored nodule *JAAD 79:853—859, 2018*

Schwannoma – lateral neck nodule *Ped Derm 353–354, 2016*

Sebaceous carcinoma *JAAD 61:549–560, 2009; Dermatol Ther 21:459–466, 2008*

Smooth muscle hamartoma

Solitary fibrous tumor of the skin – facial, scalp, posterior neck nodule *JAAD 46:S37–40, 2002*

Spindle cell hemangioendothelioma *JAAD 18:393–395, 1988*

Spindle cell lipoma – subcutaneous nodule of posterior neck *AD 142:921–926, 2006*

Squamous cell carcinoma

Steatocystomas (steatocystoma multiplex)

Stewart-Treves angiosarcoma – reddish-blue macules and/or nodules which become polypoid; pachydermatous changes, blue nodules, telangiectasias, palpable subcutaneous mass, ulcer *JAAD 67:1342–1348, 2012*

Storiform collagenoma (sclerotic fibroma) *Cutis 64:203–204, 1999*

Striated muscle hamartoma (like a soft fibroma) *AD 136:1263–1268, 2000; Ped Derm 3:153–157, 1986*

Subdermal fibrous hamartoma *Cutis 65:243–245, 2000*

Synovial sarcoma *JAAD 51:1–21, 2004*

Syringocystadenoma papilliferum *AD 71:361–372, 1955*

Syringoma *JAAD 10:291–292, 1984*

Syringomatous carcinoma – skin-colored nodule of face *Cutis 77:19–24, 2006*

Teratoma *Cutis 65:243–245, 2000*

Transplant-associated hematolymphoid neoplasm – p16 hypermethylation and Epstein-Barr virus infection; skin-colored nodules; red nodules of legs *JAAD 55:794–798, 2006*

Trichoblastoma *J Cutan Pathol 26:490–496, 1999*

Trichoepithelioma

Trichofolliculoma

Waldenstrom's IgM storage papules

Warthin's tumor, extraparotid – skin-colored neck nodule *JAAD 40:468–470, 1999*

Virchow's node (Troisier's node) – left supraclavicular adenopathy associated with gastrointestinal and pelvic malignancies; abdominal and pelvic tumors uniformly metastasized to left supraclavicular lymph node; malignancies of the head and neck, thorax, breast, skin, and lymphoma show no significant difference in laterality

PARANEOPLASTIC DISORDERS

Crystal-storing histiocytosis (composed of monoclonal immunoglobulins) – multiple subcutaneous nodules *AD 130:484–488, 1994*

Eruptive segmental neurofibromas – esophageal, lung, colon, gastric cancer *JAAD 60:880–881, 2009; Clin Exp Dermatol 32:43–44, 2007; Dermatology 209:342, 2004; J Dermatol 29:350–353, 2002*

Necrobiotic xanthogranuloma with paraproteinemia *JAAD 52:729–731, 2005*

Neurofibromatosis, juvenile xanthogranulomas, and juvenile myelomonocytic leukemia *Ped Derm 36:114–118, 2017*

PRIMARY CUTANEOUS DISEASES

Axillary accessory breast tissue *JAAD 49:1154–1156, 2003; AD 137:1367–1372, 2001*

Acne necrotica varioliformis (KA-like) *JAAD 16:1007–1014, 1987*

Acne vulgaris – multiple miliary osteoma cutis *AD 110:113–114, 1974;* acne cyst with osteoma cutis

Adiposis dolorosa (Dercum's disease) *JAAD 56:901–916, 2007*

Anetoderma, neurofibroma-like appearance (outpouching) *Cutis 81:501–506, 2008; AD 120:1032–1039, 1984*

Angiolymphoid hyperplasia with eosinophilia

Benign rheumatoid nodules – healthy children; pretibial areas, feet, scalp *Aust NZ J Med 9:697–701, 1979*

Cutis anserina (goosebumps)

Dupuytren's contracture

Epidermolysis bullosa – dominant dystrophic epidermolysis bullosa, albopapuloidea (Pasini) – pretibial nodules and plaques *BJD 146:267–274, 2002*

Fascial hernias of the legs *JAMA 145:548–549, 1951*

Granuloma annulare – including subcutaneous granuloma annulare (head, hands, buttock, shins) (pseudorheumatoid nodule) *JAAD 75:457–465, 2016; Curr Prob Derm 14:41–70, 2002; JAAD 45:163–183, 2001; JAAD 3:217–230, 1980;* of forehead *Ped Derm 5:407–408, 2008*

Granuloma faciale, extrafacial – skin-colored papule of earlobe *JAMADerm 156:94–95, 2020*

Infantile perianal pyramidal protrusion *AD 132:1481–1484, 1996*

Kimura's disease (eosinophilic pustular folliculitis) – subcutaneous nodule *BJD 157:420–421, 2007; Hautarzt 27:309–317, 1976*

Knuckle pads *AD 129:1043–1048, 1993*

Lipofascial hernia in natal or perianal region – mimics lipoma

Malakoplakia – perianal nodules, vulvar nodules, skin colored nodules, ulcerations, abscesses, red papules, masses *Arch Pathol Lab Med 132:113–117, 2008*

Lumbar hernia – personal observation

Muscle herniation – nodules of legs *Ped Derm 36:741–742, 2019*

Pachydermodactyly, distal *JAAD 38:359–362, 1998*

Painful piezogenic leg nodules – personal observation

Temporalis muscle hypertrophy – personal observation

Umbilical hernia – personal observation

PSYCHOCUTANEOUS DISORDERS

Factitial dermatitis – dermal nodules *JAAD 1:391–407, 1979*

SYNDROMES

Adenosine deaminase type 2 deficiency (DADA2) – painless nodules with intermittent livedo reticularis *Ped Derm 37:199–201, 2020*

Adiposis dolorosa – multiple painful lipomas *JAAD 56:901–916, 2007*

Aesop syndrome – extensive red violaceous skin patch or plaque of chest overlying a solitary bone plasmacytoma with regional adenopathy; dermal mucin and vascular hyperplasia (mucinous angiomatosis) *JAAD 55:909–910, 2006; Medicine 82:51–59, 2003; JAAD 40:808–812, 1999; JAAD 21:1061–1068, 1989; J Neurol Neurosurgery Psychiatry 41:177–184, 1978; Br J Dis Chest 68:65–70, 1974;* due to malignant blue cell tumor *AD 148:1431–1437, 2012*

Albright's hereditary osteodystrophy (pseudohypoparathyroidism) – osteoma cutis – periarticular calcified or ossified nodules (ectopic ossification); short stocky build; round face; low flat nasal bridge; short neck, brachymetaphalangism and brachydactyly; developmental delay, cataracts, hearing loss, seizures, poor dentition, basal ganglia calcification, osteomalacia, rickets, osteoporosis *JAMA Derm 149:975–976, 2013; JAAD 15:353–356, 1986; AD 104:636–642, 1971; Medicine 37:317–352, 1958*

Atrichia with papular lesions – autosomal recessive; follicular cysts *AD 139:1591–1596, 2003; JAAD 47:519–523, 2002*

Autoimmune lymphoproliferative syndrome *NEJM 351:1409–1418, 2004*

Bannayan-Riley-Ruvalcaba syndrome (macrocephaly and subcutaneous hamartomas) (lipomas and hemangiomas) – autosomal dominant *JAAD 68:189–209, 2013; AD 132:1214–1218, 1996; Eur J Ped 148:122–125, 1988;* lipoangiomas (perigenital pigmented macules, macrocephaly) *AD 128:1378–1386, 1992;* lipomas in Ruvalcaba-Myhre-Smith syndrome *Ped Derm 5:28–32, 1988*

Beckwith-Wiedemann syndrome (Exomphalos-Macroglossia-Gigantism) (EMG) syndrome – autosomal dominant; umbilical hernia, zosteriform rash at birth, exomphalos, macrosomia, macroglossia, visceromegaly, facial salmon patch of forehead, upper eyelids, nose, and upper lip and gigantism; linear earlobe grooves, circular depressions of helices; increased risk of Wilms' tumor, adrenal carcinoma, hepatoblastoma, and rhabdomyosarcoma; neonatal hypoglycemia *Am J Med Genet 79:268–273, 1998; JAAD 37:523–549, 1997; Am J Dis Child 122:515–519, 1971*

Benign symmetric lipomatosis (Launois-Bensaude) (Madelung disease) *JAAD 17:663–674, 1987*

vs. Familial multiple lipomatosis *JAAD 15:275–279, 1986*
    Lipomatosis (adiposis) dolorosa (Dercum's disease)
    Michelin tire baby syndrome – folded skin with lipomatous nevus
    Multiple angiolipomas
        Neurolipomatosis
        Multiple lipomas due to intracranial lesions (Froehlich syndrome)
        Hereditary lipomas
        NF-1
        Buffalo neck (Cushing)
        Muscular dystrophy with pseudoathletic appearance
        Lymphoma
        Cervical cysts

Blue rubber bleb nevus syndrome (Bean syndrome) – large subcutaneous venous malformations; blue lesions of skin and mucous membranes *JAAD 50:S101–106, 2004*

Buschke-Ollendorff syndrome – connective tissue nevi and osteopoikilosis; single or multiple yellow, white, or skin-colored papules, nodules, plaques of extremities; mountain range skin-colored nodules; *LEMD3* mutation *BJD 166:900–903, 2012; Ped Derm 28:447–450, 2011; JAAD 48:600–601, 2003; Derm Wochenschr 86:257–262, 1928*

Carbohydrate-deficient glycoprotein syndrome – emaciated appearance; lipoatrophy over buttocks; lipoatrophic streaks extend down legs; high nasal bridge, prominent jaw, large ears, inverted nipples, fat over suprapubic area and labia majora, fat pads over buttocks; hypotonia

Carney complex – subcutaneous myxomas *JAAD 46:161–183, 2002;* acromegaly, facial lentigines, cutaneous myxoma, blue nevus of

vulva; gain of function mutation of *PRKACB* (catalytic subunit alpha of cAMP-dependent protein kinase) *NEJM 370:1065–1067, 2014*

Cleft lip-palate, sensorineural hearing loss, sacral lipomas, aberrant fingerlike appendages *Syndromes of the Head and Neck, p. 773, 1990*

CLOVE syndrome – congenital lipomatous overgrowth; capillary, venous, and mixed vascular malformations, epidermal nevi; hemihypertrophy (milder than that of Proteus syndrome) *Ped Derm 27:311–312, 2010; Am J Med Genet 143A:2944–2958, 2007*

COPS syndrome – poikiloderma, calcinosis cutis, osteoma cutis, skeletal abnormalities

Cowden's syndrome – sclerotic fibroma of skin *JAAD 24:508–509, 1991;* ganglioneuromas, lipomas, angiolipomas, epidermoid cysts

Cutaneous nodules with urinary tract abnormalities *Cancer 26:1256–1260, 1970*

Dermo-chondro-corneal dystrophy

Diffuse cutaneous reticulohistiocytosis *JAAD 25:948–951, 1991*

Down's syndrome – generalized connective tissue nevus *AD 115:623–624, 1979*

Ehlers-Danlos syndrome – cutaneous calcification; painful piezogenic pedal papules; molluscoid pseudotumors *JAAD 17:205–209, 1987;* firm cyst-like nodules (spheroids) of shins and forearms *JAAD 46:161–183, 2002*

Ekbom's syndrome (myoclonic epilepsy and ragged muscle fibers) (mitochondrial syndrome) – cervical lipomas *JAAD 39:819–823, 1998*

Encephalocraniocutaneous lipomatosis (Haberland syndrome) – red soft plaque of bulbar conjunctiva (limbal dermoids) (pterygium like lesion)lipomatous hamartomas of scalp and eyelids; linear yellow papules of forehead extending to eyelids; alopecia and ocular christomas; scalp nodules, skin colored nodules, facial and eyelid papules, lipomas, and fibrolipomas; subcutaneous fatty masses of frontotemporal or zygomatic region; nodular tags from outer canthus to tragus; nevus psiloliparus – well-demarcated, smooth alopecic plaque of scalp; mesodermal nevus with paucity of hair and excess fat tissue; appears in encephalocranial lipomatosis *Ped Derm 22:206–209, 2005;* ophthalmologic manifestations; seizures, mental retardation; mandibular or maxillary ossifying fibromas and odontomas; cranial asymmetry; developmental delay, mental retardation, seizures, spasms of contralateral limbs; unilateral porocephalic cysts with cortical atrophy *Ped Derm 30:491–492, 2013; Ped Derm 23:27–30, 2006; Ped Derm 22:206–209, 2005; JAAD 47:S196–200, 2002; Am J Med Genet 191:261–266, 2000; JAAD 37:102–104, 1998; BJD 104:89–96, 1981; Arch Neurol 22:144–155, 1970; AD 144:266–268, 2008; Ped Derm 23:27–30, 2006; JAAD 37:102–104, 1998; JAAD 32:387–389, 1995; Ped Derm 10:164–168, 1993; Arch Neurol 22:144–155, 1970*

Familial histiocytic dermatoarthritis

Farber's disease (lipogranulomatosis)

Fibroblastic rheumatism – symmetrical polyarthritis, nodules over joints and on palms, elbows, knees, ears, neck, Raynaud's phenomenon, sclerodactyly; skin lesions resolve spontaneously *AD 131:710–712, 1995*

Fibrodysplasia ossificans progressiva – heterotopic bone formation within soft tissues; multiple neonatal scalp nodules associated with malformation of the great toes (hallux valgus); hypoplastic great toes; development of tumors is cranial to caudal, dorsal to ventral and proximal to distal; ossification after infections or trauma; scalp nodules large, firm, and immobile; mutation in *ACVR1* gene *JAAD 64:97–101, 2011*

Gardner's syndrome – epidermoid cysts, osteomas, desmoid tumors – arise in incisional scars of abdomen; supernumerary or unerupted teeth *JAAD 68:189–209, 2013; Curr Prob Derm 14:41–70, 2002; Cancer 36:2327–2333, 1975; AD 90:20–30, 1964;* multiple pilomatrixomas *Ped Derm 12:112–115, 1995*

Goeminne syndrome – multiple spontaneous keloids

Goltz's syndrome (focal dermal hypoplasia) – giant fat herniations *Ped Derm 22:420–423, 2005;* giant cell tumor of bone (large subcutaneous nodule) *BJD 160:1103–1109, 2009*

Hereditary progressive mucinous histiocytosis – autosomal dominant; skin-colored or red-brown papules; nose, hands, forearms, thighs *JAAD 35:298–303, 1996; AD 130:1300–1304, 1994*

Hunter's syndrome (mucopolysaccharidosis IIb) – X-linked recessive; MPS type II; iduronate-2 sulfatase deficiency; lysosomal accumulation of heparin sulfate and dermatan sulfate; linear and reticulated 2–10 mm skin colored papules over and between scapulae, chest, neck, arms; also posterior axillary lines, upper arms, forearms, chest, outer thighs; rough thickened skin, coarse scalp hair, and hirsutism; short stature, full lips, coarse facies with frontal bossing, hypertelorism, and thick tongue (macroglossia); dysostosis multiplex; hunched shoulders and characteristic posturing; widely spaced teeth, dolichocephaly, deafness, retinal degeneration, inguinal and umbilical hernias hepatosplenomegaly; upper and lower respiratory infections due to laryngeal or tracheal stenosis; mental retardation; deafness; retinal degeneration and corneal clouding; umbilical and inguinal hernias; valvular and ischemic heart disease with thickened heart valves lead to congestive heart failure; clear corneas (unlike Hurler's syndrome), progressive neurodegeneration, communicating hydrocephalus; adenotonsillar hypertrophy, otitis media, obstructive sleep apnea, diarrhea *Ped Derm 21:679–681, 2004; Clin Exp Dermatol 24:179–182, 1999; Ped Derm 7:150–152, 1990*

Hunter syndrome – skin colored papules *Ped Derm 29:369–370, 2012*

Hurler's syndrome – scapular papules; also posterior axillary lines, upper arms, forearms, chest, outer thighs *Acta Paediatr 41:161–167, 1952;* hernias; disorder of glycosaminoglycans accumulation; autosomal recessive; coarse facies, macroglossia, short stature, macrocephaly, hepatosplenomegaly, hernias, corneal clouding, vision and hearing loss; cardiac anomalies; respiratory infections; alpha-l-iduronate deficiency *Ped Derm 33:594–601, 2016*

Infantile myofibromatosis *Ped Derm 27:29–33, 2010*

Juvenile hyaline fibromatosis (systemic hyalinosis) – translucent papules or nodules of scalp, face, neck, trunk, gingival hypertrophy, flexion contractures of large and small joints

JAAD 16:881–883, 1987

Kawasaki's syndrome – cervical lymphadenopathy

Keratosis-ichthyosis-deafness syndrome (KID syndrome) – autosomal dominant; congenital generalized erythema; hyperkeratotic papules with follicular spiny projections, verrucous plaques of forehead, cheeks, perioral region, elbows, knees, and scalp; scarring alopecia of scalp and eyebrows; red-orange reticulated plaques, scalp cysts, follicular occlusion triad, paronychia with chronic mucocutaneous candidiasis, nodules (trichilemmal tumors, squamous cell carcinomas), progressive corneal scarring with blindness; bilateral deafness; mutation in *GJB2* (connexin 26) *JAAD 69:127–134, 2013; Ped Derm 27:651–652, 2010; Ped Derm 26:427–431, 2009; Ped Derm 23:81–83, 2006; Ped Derm 15:219–221, 1998; AD 117:285–289, 1981; J Cutan Dis 33:255–260, 1915*

    Disorders with mutations in *GJB2* (connexin 26) *JID 127:2713–2725, 2007*

        Bart-Pumphrey syndrome
        Deafness with Clouston-type phenotype
        Hystrix-like ichthyosis-deafness syndrome
        Non-syndromic deafness

        Sensorineural hearing loss with keratoderma
        Vohwinkel's syndrome

Leri-Weill dyschondrosteosis – mesomelic short stature syndrome with Madelung's deformity; SHOX haploinsufficiency like Turner's syndrome *JAAD 50:767–776, 2004*

MEN I – skin colored plaque; connective tissue nevus *JAAD 67:890–897, 2012*

Mikulicz's syndrome – swelling of major salivary glands

Mitochondrial DNA syndrome – lipomas *JAAD 39:819–823, 1998*

Mucolipidosis (pseudo-Hurler polydystrophy) – connective tissue nevus *BJD 130:528–533, 1994*

Multicentric reticulohistiocytosis *Cutis 85:153–155, 2010; BJD 161:470–472, 2009; AD 144:1383–1388, 2008; AD 144:1360–1366, 2008; AD 144:105–110, 2008; JAAD 58:541–543, 2008; JAAD 56:302–316, 2007; JAAD 53:1075–1079, 2005; AD 140:919–921, 2004; JAAD 49:1125–1127, 2003; JAAD 25:948–951, 1991; AD 126:251–252, 1990; Oral Surg Oral Med Oral Pathol 65:721–725, 1988; Pathology 17:601–608, 1985; JAAD 11:713–723, 1984; Clin Exp Dermatol 5:267–279, 1980; AD 97:543–547, 1968*

Multiple endocrine neoplasia syndrome (MEN I) (Wermer's syndrome) – autosomal dominant; lipomas *AD 148:1317–1322, 2012; JAAD 56:877–880, 2007; J Clin Endocrinol Metab 89:5328–5336, 2004; AD 133:853–857, 1997;* collagenomas *JAAD 42:939–969, 2000;* angiofibromas of vermilion border; facial angiofibromas, lipomas, abdominal collagenomas, cutis verticis gyrata, pedunculated skin tags, acanthosis nigricans, red gingival papules, confetti-like hypopigmented macules; café au lait macules; primary hyperparathyroidism with hypercalcemia, kidney stones, prolactinoma, gastrinoma, bilateral adrenal hyperplasia *JAAD 61:319–324, 2009; J Clin Endocrinol Metab 89:5328–5336, 2004; AD 133:853–857, 1997*

Multiple mucosal neuroma syndrome (MEN IIB) – skin-colored neuromas of oral mucosa, tongue, eyelids, conjunctivae, perioral or periocular lentigines, freckles, or hyperpigmentation; multiple sclerotic fibromas – elongated papules of trunk, heel nodules *JAMADerm 153:1298–1301, 2017*

Neurofibromatosis type 1 – neurofibromas; patients with whole gene deletion have more neurofibromas, severe cognitive impairment, large hands, dysmorphic facies, higher risk o malignant peripheral nerve sheath tumors *JAAD 61:1–14, 2009; Lancet Neurol 6:340–351, 2006; Ann Int Med 144:842–849, 2006; Lancet 361:1552–1554, 2003*

Nodular fibromatosis

Novel fibrosing disorder – subcutaneous fibrotic nodules, progressive distal joint contractures, marfanoid stature, forehead nodules, skin tightening (sclerodermoid changes), palmoplantar nodules, nodules of elbows and knees, linear arrays of nodules later in course; differentiate from Marfan's syndrome, congenital contractural arachnodactyly, Winchester syndrome, multicentric osteolysis nodulosis and arthropathy (MONA) syndrome *BJD 163:1102–1115, 2010*

Penchaszadeh syndrome (nasopalpebral lipoma-coloboma syndrome) – eyelid lipoma *Am J Med Genet 11:397–410, 1982*

Polyneuropathy with nerve angiomatosis and multiple soft tissue tumors *Am J Surg Pathol 19:1325–1332, 1995*

Proteus syndrome – lipomas, connective tissue nevi, lymphatic malformations *AD 140:947–953, 2004; AD 125:1109–1114, 1989*

Pseudoxanthoma elasticum – multiple calcified cutaneous nodules *Am J Med 31:488–489, 1961*

Pseudohypoparathyroidism type IA (Albright's hereditary osteodystrophy) – subcutaneous nodule (osteoma cutis); short stature, round face, obesity, subcutaneous ossifications, bilateral brachydactyly, mental retardation, hypothyroidism, saddle nose deformity *Ped Derm 33:675–676, 2016*

PTEN syndromes – sclerotic fibromas; Cowden's syndrome, Bannayan-Ruvalcaba syndrome, Lhermitte-Duclos syndrome, autism spectrum with macrocephaly *JAMADerm 153:1298–1301, 2017*

Reed syndrome (cutaneous leiomyomatosis) *Cutis 87:65, 76–77, 2011*

Rubinstein-Taybi syndrome – keloids, hypertrichosis, long eye-lashes, thick eyebrows, keratosis pilaris or ulerythema ophryogenes, low set ears, very short stature, broad terminal phalanges of thumbs and great toes, hemangiomas, nevus flammeus, café au lait macules, pilomatrixomas, cardiac anomalies, mental retardation *Ped Derm 19:177–179, 2002; Ped Derm 11:21–25, 1994; Am J Dis Child 105:588–608, 1963*

Schnitzler's syndrome – lymphadenopathy *JAAD 68:834–853, 2013*

Steatocystoma multiplex

Self-healing infantile familial cutaneous mucinosis *Ped Derm 14:460–462, 1997*; self-healing juvenile cutaneous mucinosis – papules, plaques, and nodules of head and trunk *JAAD 31:815–816, 1994*

Multiple trichoepitheliomas

Tuberous sclerosis – shagreen patch – <u>personal observation</u>

Turner's syndrome – macrocystic lymphatic malformation *JAAD 74:231–244, 2016*

Wells' syndrome *Ped Derm 14:312–315, 1997*

Williams' syndrome with granular cell tumors

Winchester syndrome – dwarfism, osteolysis, corneal opacities, rheumatoid-like joint destruction, hypertrichosis, thickening of skin, widespread nodular lesions *JAAD 50:S53–56, 2004*

Wiskott-Aldrich syndrome – parotid gland enlargement

TOXINS

Iodine poisoning – parotid swelling

Lead poisoning – parotid swelling

Mercury – oral *JAAD 39:131–133, 1997;* intravenous – surreptitious injection of liquid mercury; subcutaneous nodules along veins; embolic to lungs with numerous diffuse high density opacities *NEJM 369:2031, 2013*

TRAUMA

Athletes' nodules – foot/knee/knuckle (collagenomas); skin-colored nodules of ankle and dorsal foot *AD 145:1325–1330, 2009*

Cutis 50:131–135, 1992

Dermabrasion with osteoma cutis

Fascial hernias of the legs *JAMA 145:548–549, 1951*

Fat necrosis following cardiac surgery – personal observation

Hematoma with osteoma cutis

Incisional hernia

Lipomas – following soft tissue trauma *BJD 157:92–99, 2007*

Lipomembranous panniculitis after air bag deployment *AD 140:231–236, 2004*

Paradoxical adipose hyperplasia after cryolipolysis *JAMADerm150:317–319, 2014*

Piezogenic papules or leg nodules; piezogenic wrist papules

Pseudocyst of the auricle

Puncture sites with osteoma cutis

Surfer's nodules of anterior tibial prominence, dorsum of feet, knuckles *Cutis 50:131–135, 1992*

Weightlifters nodule – subcutaneous nodules of upper back *SkinMed 13:246–249, 2015*

VASCULAR DISORDERS

Aneurysm of the superficial temporal artery

Angiomyxoma *JAAD 38:143–175, 1998*

Arterial fibromuscular dysplasia; cutaneous aneurysm; pulsatile subcutaneous nodule *JAAD 27:883–885, 1992*

Benign lymphangiomatous papules of the skin – skin-colored papules *JAAD 52:912–913, 2005*

Cerebral cavernous malformation (familial cerebral cavernomas) – venous malformation *BJD 157:210–212, 2007;* red hyperkeratotic plaques; cutaneous venous malformations *Lancet 352:1892–1897, 1998*

Eosinophilic granulomatosis with polyangiitis – "Churg-Strauss granuloma" *Autoimmunol Rev 14:341–348, 2015; JAAD 48:311–340, 2003; JAAD 37:199–203, 1997; JAAD 27:821–824, 1992; JID 17:349–359, 1951; Am J Pathol 25:817, 1949*

Cystic hygroma (lymphatic malformation) *NEJM 309:822–825, 1983;* lymphatic malformation

Dabska's tumor (papillary intralymphatic angioendothelioma) *Bolognia, p.1828, 2003*

Endoleak – complication pf endovascular aneurysm repair with persistent blood flow within aneurysm sac; nontender skin colored subcutaneous mass of right midsternum *Cutis 96:97–99, 2015*

Epithelioid hemangioendothelioma *JAAD 38:143–175, 1998*

Fibrofatty residua following involution of infantile hemangioma *JAMADerm 154:735–737, 2018*

Gorham syndrome *Ped Derm 30:391–394, 2013*

Hemangioma, including sinusoidal hemangioma; fibrous remnant of resolved proliferating hemangioma; deep infantile hemangioma – skin colored nodule with red dots *Ped Derm 31:286–291, 2014*

Hemangiopericytoma *JAAD 37:887–920, 1997; AD 134:625–630, 1998*

Hunter syndrome (mucopolysaccharidosis type II) – accumulation of glycosaminoglycans; X-linked recessive; iduronate 2-sulfatase deficiency; recurrent otitis media, respiratory infections, hepato-splenomegaly, hernias, cardiomyopathy *Ped Derm 33:594–601, 2016*

Intravascular papillary endothelial hyperplasia *AD 124:263–268, 1988*

Lipodermatosclerosis – chronic venous insufficiency with hyperpig-mentation, induration, inflammation *Lancet ii:243–245, 1982*

Lymphangiectasia (acquired lymphangioma) – due to scarring processes such as recurrent infections, radiotherapy, scrofulo-derma, sclerederma, keloids, tumors, tuberculosis, repeated trauma *BJD 132:1014–1016, 1996*

Lymphangioma circumscriptum with underlying lymphatic malforma-tion *BJD 83:519–527, 1970;* acquired lymphangioma (lymphangiec-tasia) – due to scarring processes such as recurrent infections, radiotherapy, scrofuloderma, sclerederma, keloids, tumors, tuberculosis, repeated trauma *BJD 132:1014–1016, 1996*

Lymphatic malformation *JAAD 56:353–370, 2007*

Lymphostasis

Malignant glomus tumors *JAAD 38:143–165, 1998*

Massive localized lymphedema in the morbidly obese – giant pendulous masses of the medial thighs *Lymphology 39:181–184, 2006; Obes Surg 16:1126–1130, 2006; Obes Surg 16:88–93, 2006; Plast Surg Reconstr Surg 106:1663–1664, 2000; Human Pathol 31:1162–1168, 2000; Am J Surg Pathol 22:1277–1283, 1998*

Methylenetetrahydrofolate reductase (MTHFR) polymorphisms – thrombophilia and vasculopathy; leg nodules and leg ulcers; treated with folic acid, vitamins B6 and B12 *AD 147:450–453, 2011; Int J Dermatol 46:431–434, 2007; AD 142:75–78, 2006; J Endocrinol Metab 91:2021–2026, 2006;* livedo vasculopathy and MTHFR polymorphisms *BJD 155:850–852, 2006*

Neuroma of the supraorbital nerve – subcutaneous nodule of the forehead *JAAD 49:S286–288, 2003*

Polyangiitis with granulomatosis *JAAD 48:311–340, 2003; AD 130:861–867, 1994*

Polyarteritis nodosa, systemic; cutaneous (livedo with nodules) – painful or asymptomatic red or skin-colored multiple nodules along arteries with livedo reticularis of feet, legs, forearms face, scalp, shoulders, trunk; nodules of cutaneous PAN around malleoli *JAAD 48:311–340, 2003; Ped Derm 15:103–107, 1998; AD 130:884–889, 1994; JAAD 31:561–566, 1994; JAAD 31:493–495, 1994*

Pseudoaneurysm of the superficial temporal artery – subcutaneous nodule of the forehead *JAAD 49:S286–288, 2003*

Retiform hemangioendothelioma *JAAD 38:143–175, 1998*

Seroma (lymphocele)

Spindle cell hemangioendotheliomas *Cutis 62:23–26, 1998*

Spontaneous superficial venous aneurysm – soft, compressible, non-pulsatile mobile subcutaneous nodule *The Dermatologist April 2020, pp 48–50*

Takayasu's arteritis *Clin Exp Rheumatol 12:381–388, 1994*

Traumatic aneurysm

Vascular malformation

Venous malformation *Ped Derm 37:40–1, 2020*

NODULES, ULCERATED

AUTOIMMUNE DISEASES AND DISEASES OF IMMUNE DYSFUNCTION

Chronic granulomatous disease *AD 130:105–110, 1994;* of scalp *AD 103:351–357, 1971*

Common variable immunodeficiency – ulcerated papulonodular lesions of legs *BJD 147:364–367, 2002; Dermatology 198:156–158, 1999*

Dermatitis herpetiformis – prurigo nodularis-like lesions *J Eur Acad Dermatol Venereol 16:88–89, 2002*

Graft vs. host disease

Leukocyte adhesion deficiency (beta-2 integrin deficiency) – (congenital deficiency of leucocyte-adherence glycoproteins (CD11a (LFA-1), CD11b, CD11c, CD18)) – pyoderma gangrenosum-like lesions; necrotic cutaneous abscesses, psoriasiform dermatitis, gingivitis, periodontitis, septicemia, ulcerative stomatitis, pharyngitis, otitis, pneumonia, peritonitis *BJD 139:1064–1067, 1998; BJD 123:395–401, 1990*

Lupus erythematosus – discoid LE, tumid LE – personal observation

Pemphigoid nodularis *JAAD 27:863–867, 1992*

Rheumatoid arthritis – superficial ulcerating necrobiosis *AD 118:255–259, 1982;* ulcerated rheumatoid nodule; ulcerated

rheumatoid nodule of the vulva *J Clin Pathol 49:85–87, 1996;* ulcerated rheumatoid nodule of sacrum *Br Med J iv:92–93, 1975;* pyoderma gangrenosum *AD 111:1020–1023, 1975;* rheumatoid neutrophilic dermatosis; neutrophilic lobular panniculitis *JAAD 45:325–361, 2001; J R Soc Med 84:307–308, 1991*

CONGENITAL LESIONS

Congenital infantile fibrosarcoma – ulcerated vascular nodule *Cutis 89:61–64, 2012*

Langerhans cell histiocytosis – eroded red papule in newborn *Ped Derm 34:363–364, 2017*

Congenital xanthogranulomas *Ped Derm 35:582–587, 2018*
  Yellow scalp nodule
  Ulcerated pink nodule
  Subcutaneous nodule with pink papules
  Brown-gray patch with pink yellow papules
  Atrophic patch with yellow macules and papules

DRUG-INDUCED

G-CSF – pyoderma gangrenosum *Ped Derm 17:205–207, 2000*

Interferon alpha – pyoderma gangrenosum at injection site *JAAD 46:611–616, 2002*

Lenalidomide – neutrophilic dermatosis; crusted hemorrhagic ulcerated nodules *JAAD 61:709–710, 2009*

Methotrexate-related lymphoproliferative disorder – linear perilymphatic nodules of leg; linear bands; ulcerated and non-ulcerated red nodules *JAAD 61:126–129, 2009*

Non-selective antiangiogenic multikinase inhibitors – sorafenib, sunitinib, pazopanib – hyperkeratotic hand foot skin reactions with knuckle papules, inflammatory reactions, alopecia, kinking of hair, depigmentation of hair; chloracne-like eruptions, erythema multiforme, toxic epidermal necrolysis, drug hypersensitivity, red scrotum with erosions, yellow skin, eruptive nevi, pyoderma gangrenosum-like lesions *JAAD 72:203–218, 2015*

Trastuzumab (Herceptin) – necrotizing c-ANCA+ panniculitis *JAAD 54:S249–251, 2006*

Voriconazole-induced squamous cell carcinomas of temples *Clin Inf Dis 58:839,901–902, 2014*

EXOGENOUS AGENTS

Benzocaine – erosive papulonodular vulvar dermatitis *JAAD 55:S74–80, 2006*

Drug abuse *NEJM 277:473–475, 1967*

Bromoderma – ingestion of soft drink (Ruby Red Squirt) *NEJM 348:1932–1934, 2003*

Foreign body granuloma

Irritant contact dermatitis – urostomy *JAAD 19:623–628, 1988; Scand J Urol Nephrol 13:201–204, 1979*

Paraffinoma (sclerosing lipogranuloma) *Acta Chir Plast 33:163–165, 1991; Plast Reconstr Surg 65:517–524, 1980*

INFECTIONS AND INFESTATIONS

Actinomycosis

Adiaspiromycosis (*Chrysosporium* species) – hyperpigmented plaque with white-yellow papules, ulcerated nodules, hyperkeratotic nodules, crusted nodules, multilobulated nodules *JAAD S113–117, 2004*

African histoplasmosis (*Histoplasma capsulatum* var. *duboisii*) – ulceropolypoid lesions; exclusively in Central and West Africa and Madagascar *Clin Inf Dis 48:441, 493–494, 2009*

African trypanosomiasis *AD 131:1178–1182, 1995*

AIDS – cutaneous CD8+ T cell infiltrates in advanced HIV disease *JAAD 41:722–727, 1999*

Allescheria boydii – personal observation

Alternariosis *BJD 143:910–912, 2000; A. tenuissima* – ulcerated verrucous nodule *BJD 142:840–841, 2000; A. tenuissima* – ulcerated nodule of foot *Cutis 93:237–240, 2014; Alternaria alternata* – ulcerated plaque *JAAD 75:19–30, 2016*

Alveolar echinococcosis *JAAD 34:873–877, 1996*

Amebiasis, including *Acanthamoeba* in AIDS *Cutis 73:241–248, 2004; Clin Inf Dis 20:1207–1216, 1995*

Anthrax – *Bacillus anthracis*; malignant pustule; face, neck, hands, arms; starts as papule then evolves into bulla on red base; then hemorrhagic crust with edema and erythema with small vesicles; edema of surrounding skin *Am J Dermatopathol 19:79–82, 1997; J Clin Inf Dis 19:1009–1014, 1994; Br J Opthalmol 76:753–754, 1992; J Trop Med Hyg 89:43–45, 1986; Bol Med Hosp Infant Mex 38:355–361, 1981*

Aspergillosis, primary cutaneous *Dermatol Ther 18:44–57, 2005*

Bacillary angiomatosis *JAAD 35:285–287, 1996; Am J Clin Pathol 80:714–718, 1983;* giant tumor with ulceration in HIV disease *JAMADerm 150:1015–1016, 2014*

Bejel

Bipolaris spicifera AD 125:1383–1386, 1989

Buruli ulcer (*Mycobacterium ulcerans subspecies shinshuense*) – ulcerated red nodule of arm and hand *JAMA Derm 150:64–67, 2014*

Candidal sepsis – ecthyma gangrenosum-like lesion

Cat scratch disease *AD 135:983–988, 1999*

Chancriform pyoderma

Chancroid

Chromomycosis – feet, legs, arms, face, and neck *AD 133:1027–1032, 1997; BJD 96:454–458, 1977; AD 104:476–485, 1971*

Coccidioidomycosis *AD 129:1589–1593, 1993;* primary inoculation coccidioidomycosis *Int J Derm 33:720–722, 1994*

Cowpox

Cryptococcosis *Cutis 78:53–56, 2006; JAAD 32:844–850, 1995*

Cytomegalovirus infection – perinatal CMV *JAAD 54:536–539, 2006;* ulcerated red papules in immunocompetent adult *AD 145:1030–1036, 2009*

Dental sinus – ulcerated nodule of lower cheek *Ped Derm 27:410–411, 2010*

Diphtheria – ulcerated nodules of the feet *JAMADerm 151:1247–1248, 2015*

Ecthyma

Ecthyma gangrenosum *JAAD 11:781–787, 1984*

Epstein-Barr virus (HHV4) – primary cutaneous Epstein-Barr virus-related lymphoproliferative disorders *JAAD 58:74–80, 2008*

Erythema induratum *Clin Inf Dis 70:1254–1257, 2020; AD 133:457–462, 1997; JAAD 738–742, 1986*

Fire coral granulomas

Fusarium – ecthyma gangrenosum-like lesions *Ped Derm 13:118–121, 1996;* violaceous nodules with central necrosis *Clin Inf Dis 32:1237–1240, 2001*

Gonorrhea – chancre as primary lesion on thighs of women *Bull Soc Fr Dermatol Syphilol 81:159–160, 1974*

Granuloma inguinale *JAAD 32:153–154, 1995*

Herpes simplex virus – hypertrophic HSV *AD 146:124–126, 2010*

Histoplasmosis *BJD 133:472–474, 1995; AD 114:1197–1198, 1978;* mimicking pyoderma gangrenosum *Int J Dermatol 40:518–521, 2001*

Insect bites

Klebsiella sepsis

Kerion

Leishmaniasis – Old World leishmaniasis – ulcerated red plaque *Ped Derm 35:384–387, 2018; JAAD 73:897–908, 2015; J Drugs in Dermatol 12:476–478, 2013; JAAD 60:897–925, 2009; AD 142:1368–1369, 2006; JAAD 46:803, 2002;* KA-like lesions *Clin Inf Dis 22:1–13, 1996; JAAD 16:1183–1189, 1987; L. tropica* – ulcerated nodule of face *JAAD 71:271–277, 2014; JAAD 53:810–815, 2005;* Old World leishmaniasis *Cutis 93:67,69–70, 2014; L. brasiliensis BJD 153:203–205, 2005; J Clin Inf Dis 22:1–13, 1996;* multiple ulcerated plaques – New World leishmaniasis *Ped Derm 24:657–658, 2007;* ulcerated nodule of buttock; *L. Mexicana, L. venezuelensis; L. amazonensis, L. braziliensis. L. peruviana, L. guyanensis, L. panamensis;* lip ulcers, crusted ulcer of face; ulcers of nasal septum, palate, lips, pharynx, larynx can develop months to years after initial infection; *L infantum, L. mexicana (Lutzomyia)* – ulcerated papule *JAAD 58:650–652, 2008;* leishmaniasis recidivans (lupoid leishmaniasis) – brown-red or brown-yellow papules close to scar of previously healed lesion; resemble lupus vulgaris; may ulcerate or form concentric rings; keloidal form, verrucous form of legs, extensive psoriasiform dermatitis *Cutis 77:25–28, 2006*

Leprosy – lepromatous leprosy of legs; ulcerative erythema nodosum leprosum *BJD 144:175–181, 2001; AD 128:1643–1648, 1992;* Lucio's phenomenon; type 1 reaction in borderline leprosy; histoid leprosy *BJD 160:305–310, 2009*

Lobomycosis

Mucormycosis – pyoderma gangrenosum-like lesion; *Mucor, Rhizopus oryzae, Rhizomucor, Lichtheimia, Saksenaea, Cunninghamella, Apophysomyces JAAD 80:869–880, 2019*

Mycetoma *JAAD 53:931–951, 2005; JAAD 32:311–315, 1995; Cutis 49:107–110, 1992; Australas J Dermatol 31:33–36, 1990; JAAD 6:107–111, 1982; AD 99:215–225, 1969*

Mycobacterium abscessus – ulcerated nodules of lower legs *JAAD 57:413–420, 2007*

Mycobacterium avium complex – traumatic inoculation *BJD 130:785–790, 1994;* multiple subcutaneous nodules which ulcerate *Dermatol Therapy 17:491–498, 2004*

Mycobacterium bovis – chancre *JAAD 43:535–537, 2000*

Mycobacterium chelonae Dermatol Clin 33:563–577, 2015; AD 139:629–634, 2003; BJD 147:781–784, 2002; Clin Inf Dis 33:1433–1434, 2001

Mycobacterium fortuitum AD 139:629–634, 2003; BJD 147:781–784, 2002; draining cystic nodule of leg *J Drugs in Dermatol 10:914–916, 2011*

Mycobacterium gordonae – crusted nodule; prurigo nodularis-like *J Clin Inf Dis 25:1490–1491, 1997*

Mycobacterium haemophilum Ped Derm 23:481–483, 2006; Clin Inf Dis 14:1195–1200, 1992

Mycobacterium kansasii BJD 152:727–734, 2005; JAAD 40:359–363, 1999

Mycobacterium marinum – ulcerated nodule of distal arm *Cutis 100:331–336, 2017;* ulcerated digital papule or nodule *Clin Inf Dis 31:439–443, 2000*

Mycobacterium scrofulaceum – ulcerated nodule of cheek *Ped Derm 22:476–479, 2005*

Mycobacterium tuberculosis – primary (chancre) – begins as red-brown papulonodular lesion with well demarcated ulcer with red, blue, or undermined borders *Am J Clin Dermatol 3:319–328, 2002;*, tuberculous gumma *Clin Dermatol 38:152–159, 2020; BJD 144:601–603, 2001;* multilocular inoculation tuberculosis *BJD 143:226–228, 2000;* erythema induratum of Bazin (nodular vasculitis) – tuberculid; nodules on backs of erythrocyanotic lower legs; ulcerate *Clin Inf Dis 70:1254–1257, 2020; JAAD 45:325–361, 2001; JAAD 14:738–342, 1986;* scrofuloderma – infected lymph node, bone, joint, lacrimal gland with overlying red-blue nodule which breaks down, ulcerates, forms fistulae, scarring with adherent fibrous masses which may be fluctuant and draining *BJD 134:350–352, 1996;* noduloulcerative tuberculid *BJD 141:554–557, 1999*

Mycobacterium ulcerans

Myiasis *JAAD 28:254–256, 1993*

Nocardiosis – chancriform syndrome with sporotrichoid lymphangitic spread *J Inf Dis 134:286–289, 1976;* disseminated nocardiosis or nocardial mycetoma *JAAD 13:125–133, 1985; Nocardia beijingensis* – ulcerated nodules of legs *BJD 166:216–218, 2012*

North American blastomycosis – inoculation chancre *Cutis 19:334–335, 1977;* disseminated blastomycosis *NEJM 356:1456–1462, 2007; Clin Infect Dis 33:1706, 1770–1771, 2001; Am Rev Resp Dis 120:911–938, 1979; Medicine 47:169–200, 1968;* ulcerated verrucous plaque *Ped Derm 30:23–28, 2013*

Orf *BJD 178:547–550, 2018; AD 145:607–608, 2009; AD 126:356–358, 1990;* of scalp *AD 145:1053–1058, 2009*

Paracoccidioidomycosis, disseminated (*Paracoccidioides brasiliensis*) – disseminated purpuric ulcerated nodules in HIV disease; ulcerated nodule of dorsal hand *Clin Inf Dis 58:1431–1432,2014*

Phaeohyphomycosis (*Phoma species*) *JAAD 34:679–680, 1996;* subcutaneous phaeohyphomycosis – *Exophiala jeanselmii Cutis 72:132–134, 2003; Exserohilum JAMADerm 152:85–86, 2016*

Phaeohyphomycosis – *Alternaria > Exophiala > Exserohilum*

Prototechosis *AD 130:243–248, 1994; AD 125:1249–1252, 1989*

Pseudomonas mesophilica AD 128:273–274, 1992

Rat bite fever (*Spirillum minor*)

Rhodococcus species *JAAD 24:328–332, 1991*

Scopulariopsis – *S. brevicaulis* – vegetative ulcerative nodule of forearm *Clin Inf Dis 30:820–823, 2000; S. brumptii* – ulcerating granulomas of perineum, inguinal area, and buttock *Clin Inf Dis 19:198–200, 1994*

Schistosomiasis – ectopic cutaneous granuloma – skin colored papule, 2–-3 mm; group to form mamillated plaques; nodules develop with overlying dark pigmentation, scale, and ulceration *Dermatol Clin 7:291–300, 1989; BJD 114:597–602, 1986*

Screwworm infection (*Chrysomya bezziana* (Old World screwworm); *Cochliomyia hominivorax* (New World screwworm) – draining nodules *Annual Meeting AAD 2000*

Sporotrichosis – fixed cutaneous sporotrichosis *JAAD 53:931–951, 2005;* disseminated *JAAD 27:463–464, 1992;* pyoderma gangrenosum-like; solitary lesion *Cutis 33:549–551, 1984;* multiple ulcerated nodules in AIDS *JAAD 40:350–355, 1999*

Staphylococcal botryomycosis with hyper-IgE syndrome *JAAD 28:109–111, 1993*

Syphilis – primary chancre of genitalia, arm, neck, nipple, lips; secondary (noduloulcerative) (lues maligna) in AIDS – necrotic papules and nodules *JAAD 82:1–145, 2020; JAMADerm 152:829–830, 2016; JAMA Derm 149:1429–1430, 2013; Int J STDs and AIDS 23:599, 2012; Sex Trans Dis 36:512–514, 2009; AD 141:1311–1316,* *2005; AIDS Patient Care STDs 12:921–925, 1998; Clin Inf Dis 25:1343, 1447, 1997; Clin Inf Dis 20:387–390, 1995; JAAD 22:1061–1067, 1990;* tertiary (gumma) *AD 134:365–370, 1998; AD 99:70–73, 1969; BJD 9:11–26, 1897;* tertiary serpiginous noduloulcerative lesions (gummas) *Dermatol Clin 24:497–507, 2006;* endemic (Bejel); condyloma lata – personal observation; syphilitic gumma – ulcerated plaque of forehead and scalp

Tanapox virus – few pruritic papules undergoing central necrosis, then evolving into ulcerated nodules, healing with scarring *AD 140:656, 2004*

Trichophyton rubrum – invasive; in AIDS *JAAD 34:1090–1091, 1996*

Trichosporon beigelii

Trypanosoma brucei rhodesiense (African trypanosomiasis) – transmitted by tsetse fly in Tanzania, Malawi, Zambia, Zimbabwe; causes sleeping sickness; 2–5 cm trypanosomal chancre at site of bite with regional lymphadenopathy; chancres rare in Gambian sleeping sickness *NEJM 369:763, 2013; JAAD 60:897–925, 2009; J Clin Inf Dis 23:847–848, 1996*

Tularemia – *Francisella tularensis*; skin, eye, respiratory, gastrointestinal portals of entry; ulceroglandular, oculoglandular, glandular types; toxemic stage heralds generalized morbilliform eruption, erythema multiforme-like rash, crops of red nodules on extremities *Medicine 54:252–269, 1985*

Yaws – ulcerated primary stage (mother yaw) – ulcerated nodule of glans;

secondary; tertiary – ulcerated nodules, tuberous lesions gumma; multiple subcutaneous nodules; overlying skin ulcerates with purulent discharge; atrophic pigmented scars

INFILTRATIVE

Angioplasmocellular hyperplasia – red nodule with red rim, ulcerated nodule, vascular nodule of face, scalp, neck, trunk, and leg *JAAD 64:542–547, 2011*

Juvenile xanthogranuloma *Acta DV 82:210–211, 2002; JAAD 36:355–367, 1997; JAAD 24:1005–1009, 1991*

Langerhans cell histiocytosis – ulcerated nodule of groin *Curr Prob Derm 14:41–70, 2002;* solitary Langerhans cell histiocytoma *AD 122:1033–1037, 1986;* vulvar *JAAD 13:383–404, 1985;* granulomatous ulcerative nodules *JAAD 13:481–496, 1985;* Hashimoto-Pritzker disease; congenital single yellow-red nodule with central ulceration *Ped Derm 26:121–126, 2009*

INFLAMMATORY DISEASES

Crohn's disease – metastatic Crohn's *AD 132:928–932, 1996;* pyoderma gangrenosum

Cytophagic histiocytic panniculitis – personal observation

Dissecting cellulitis of the scalp

Erythema of Jacquet – eroded violaceous nodules of vulva and pubic area *AD 149:475–480, 2013*

Gout – personal observation

Idiopathic granulomatous mastitis – red ulcerated nodules of breast *Cutis 103:38–42, 2019*

Malacoplakia *JAAD 34:325–332, 1996*

Pancreatic panniculitis *JAAD 34:362–364, 1996; Arthritis Rheum 22:547–553, 1979*

Pyoderma gangrenosum *AD 22:655–680, 1930;* in infancy *Ped Derm 26:65–69, 2009; Ann Dermatol Syphil (Paris) 6:1–39, 1916*
    Associations in childhood include:
        Asymmetric seronegative arthritis *AD 120:757–761, 1984*

Behcet's disease *Int J Derm 44:257–258, 2005*

Chronic granulomatous disease with hyper IgE syndrome *Am J Med 73:63–70, 1982*

Crohn's disease *Ped Derm 23:43–48, 2006; AD 120:757–761, 1984*

Hypogammaglobulinemia *Ann DV 106:695–696, 1979*

Leukemia *AD 120:757–761, 1984*

Leukocyte adhesion deficiency *BJD 139:1064–1067, 1998;bjd 123:395–401, 1990*

PAPA (pyogenic arthritis, pyoderma gangrenosum, acne vulgaris) syndrome; autosomal dominant; mutation in proline serine threonine phosphatase-interacting protein 1 (PSTPIP1) *BJD 161:1199–1201, 2009; Mayo Clin Proc 72:611–615, 1997*

Peristomal pyoderma gangrenosum *BJD 1206–1207, 2009*

Sterile multifocal osteomyelitis *Turk J Pediatr 48:159–161, 2006*

Takayasu's arteritis *JAAD 25:109–110, 1991*

Ulcerative colitis *AD 120:757–761, 1984*

Relapsing idiopathic nodular panniculitis *BJD 152:582–583, 2005*

Rosai-Dorfman disease (sinus histiocytosis with massive lymphadenopathy) *JAAD 51:931–939, 2004*

Sarcoid *Cutis 100:312–316, 2017; AD 142:17–19, 2006; AD 133:215–219, 1997; BJD 67:255–260, 1955*

Subcutaneous fat necrosis of the newborn *Dermatology 197:261–263, 1998*

Weber-Christian disease

METABOLIC DISORDERS

Alpha-1 antitrypsin deficiency panniculitis – red plaque, ulcerated nodule; trunk and proximal extremities *BJD 174:753–762, 2016; Cutis 93:303–306, 2014; JAAD 51:645–655, 2004; Cutis 71:205–209, 2003; JAAD 18:684–692, 1988; AD 123:1655–1661, 1987;* anasarca, generalized edema, pulmonary embolus, and hypogammaglobulinemia; violaceous nodule with yellow pseudovesicles and telangiectasias; ulcerated red nodules *BJD 173:289–291, 2015*

Calcinosis cutis – idiopathic; papular or nodular calcinosis cutis secondary to heel sticks *Ped Derm 18:138–140, 2001;* cutaneous calculus *BJD 75:1–11, 1963;* extravasation of calcium carbonate solution; metastatic calcification *JAAD 33:693–706, 1995; Cutis 32:463–465, 1983*

Cryoglobulinemia

Gout- tophaceous gout *AD 134:499–504, 1998; Cutis 48:445–451, 1991; Am J Pathol 32:871–895, 1956;* ulcerative fungating mass *Arthr Rheum 35:1399–1340, 1992;* gouty panniculitis with urate crystal deposition; ulcerated hyperpigmented nodules of legs *JAAD 57:S52–54, 2007; Cutis 76:54–56, 2005*

Hyperoxalosis, primary *JAAD 46:S16–18, 2002; AD 131:821–823, 1995; AD 125:380–383, 1989*

Necrobiosis lipoidica diabeticorum – yellow ulcerated plaques *JAAD 69:783–791, 2013*

Porphyria cutanea tarda with calcinosis

Thrombocythemia – livedo reticularis, acrocyanosis, erythromelalgia, gangrene, pyoderma gangrenosum *Leuk Lymphoma 22 Suppl 1:47–56, 1996; Br J Haematol 36:553–564, 1977; AD 87:302–305, 1963*

Tuberous xanthomas – personal observation

NEOPLASTIC DISORDERS

Adenocarcinoma with fistula

Angiosarcoma *AD 142:1059–1064, 2006*

Adenoma of the anogenital mammary-like glands – pedunculated; lobulated, tan-brown or gray-pink or white papules or nodules of vulva or perianal area; may ulcerate *JAAD 57:896–898, 2007; Breast J 9:113–116, 2003; J Reprod Med 47:949–951, 2002; Eur J Gynaecol Oncol 23:21–24, 2002; Gynecol Oncol 73:155–159, 1999*

Atypical fibroxanthoma *AD 143:653–658, 2007; Sem Cut Med Surg 21:159–165, 2002; Cutis 51:47–48, 1993; Cancer 31:1541–1552, 1973;* multilobulated, ulcerated, scalp nodule *JAAD 67:1091–1092, 2012*

Atypical granular cell schwannoma – oval red ulcerated plaque *Ped Derm 31:729–731, 2014*

Atypical piloleiomyoma *Cutis 57:168–170, 1996*

Basal cell carcinoma *Cutis 103:288–289, 2019; Cutis 92:247–249, 2013; Acta Pathol Microbiol Scand 88A:5–9, 1980*

Basaloid squamous cell carcinoma of the skin – ulcerated plaque of inguinal crease; necrotic linear ulcer of inguinal crease *JAAD 64:144–151, 2011*

Carcinosarcoma – ulcerated nodule or red plaque of scalp *Cutis 92:247–249, 2013*

CD 30+ lymphoproliferative disorders – red tumors, red plaques with or without necrosis, giant tumor *JAAD 72:508–515, 2015*

Clear cell hidradenoma *Ped Derm 17:235–237, 2000; JAAD 12:15–20, 1985; Cancer 23:641–657, 1969*

Cutaneous lymphoproliferative disease associated with Epstein-Barr virus *JAAD 57:S69–71, 2007;* cutaneous lymphoproliferative disorder associated with infectious mononucleosis – ulcerated eyelid nodule *Ped Derm 28:149–155, 2011*

Cylindroma *NEJM 351:2530, 2004*

Cytophagic histiocytic panniculitis – manifestation of hemophagocytic syndrome; red tender nodules; T-cell lymphoma, B-cell lymphoma, histiocytic lymphoma, sinus histiocytosis with massive lymphadenopathy (Rosai-Dorfman disease) *JAAD 4:181–194, 1981; Arch Int Med 140:1460–1463, 1980*

Dermatofibrosarcoma protuberans *JAAD 35:355–374, 1996*

Eccrine epithelioma *JAAD 6:514–518, 1982*

Eccrine hidradenoma – dermal nodule with or without ulceration; face, scalp, anterior trunk *AD 97:651–661, 1968*

Eccrine porocarcinoma *JAAD 49:S252–254, 2003*

Eccrine poroma – blue-black pedunculated tumor of chin *BJD 152:1070–1072, 2005*

Eccrine sweat gland carcinoma *AD 122:585–590, 1986*

Embryonal rhabdomyosarcoma *Ped Derm 15:403–405, 1998*

Epidermoid cyst, ruptured

Epithelioid hemangioendothelioma *JAAD 26:352–355, 1992*

Epithelioid cell sarcoma *JAAD 38:815–819, 1998; AD 121:394–395, 1985*

Exostosis, subungual *JAAD 45:S200–201, 2001*

Fibrosarcoma/spindle cell sarcoma – ulcerated red or violaceous nodule; congenital *Ped Derm 25:141–143, 2008; Ped Derm 23:330–334, 2006; JAAD 50:S23–25, 2004; Ped Derm 14:241–243, 1997*

Granular cell myoblastoma *JAAD 61:916–917, 2009*

Granular cell schwannoma – personal observation

Hidradenocarcinoma *JAAD 52:101–108, 2005*

Hidradenoma papilliferum – vulvar or perianal nodule *AD 83:965–967, 1961*

Hidroacanthoma simplex

Histiocytic lymphoma (true histiocytic lymphoma) *JAAD 50:S9–10, 2004*

Histiocytoma – congenital solitary histiocytoma (monolesional variant of congenital self-healing Langerhans cell histiocytosis) *Ped Derm 26:473–474, 2009*

Kaposi's sarcoma *JAAD 59:179–206, 2008; JAAD 38:143–175, 1998; Dermatology 190:324–326, 1995*

Keloids – suppurative necrosis

Keratoacanthomas – multiple self-healing keratoacanthomas of Ferguson-Smith – cluster around ears, nose, scalp; red nodule becomes ulcerated, resolve with crenellated scar; develop singly or in crops *Cancer 5:539–550, 1952;* one reported unilateral case *AD 97:615–623, 1968*

Leiomyosarcoma *Sem Cut Med Surg 21:159–165, 2002; JAAD 38:137–142, 1998; Ped Derm 14:281–283, 1997*

Leukemia – large granular lymphocytic leukemia *JAAD 31:251–255, 1994;* monocytic leukemia – ulcerated violaceous papules and nodules *Cutis 85:31–36, 2010;* aleukemic leukemia cutis with T-cell acute lymphoblastic leukemia *Ped Derm 28:535–537, 2011;* chronic lymphocytic leukemia – leukemia cutis of lower legs

Lipoblastoma – ulcerated vascular nodule *Ped Derm 34:180–186, 2017*

Lymphangiosarcoma (Stewart-Treves tumor) – ulcerated nodules in lymphedematous extremity *Arch Surg 94:223–230, 1967; Cancer 1:64–81, 1948*

Lymphoma – cutaneous T- and B-cell lymphomas *JAAD 70:205–220, 2014; JAAD 60:359–375, 2009; Curr Prob Dermatol 19:203–220, 1990, JAAD 29:549–554, 1993;* CTCL *AD 145:677–682, 2009;* CTCL – ulcerated nodule of temple *BJD 156:1379–1381, 2007;* CD8+ cytotoxic cutaneous T-cell lymphoma *NEJM 357:2496–2505, 2007;* CTCL – ulcerated tumor of forearm *JAAD 66:661–663, 2012;* CTCL of T–/null cells – erythroderma and ulcerated nodules *BJD 172:1637–1641, 2015;* cytophagic histiocytic panniculitis and subcutaneous panniculitis-like T cell lymphoma *JAAD 50:465–459, 2004; AD 136:889–896, 2000; JAAD 34:904–910, 1996;* gamma/delta T-cell lymphoma *JAAD 56:643–647, 2007;* primary cutaneous epidermotropic CD8+ T-cell lymphoma – mixture of patches, plaques, papulonodules with central ulceration, necrosis, and hemorrhage *JAAD 62:300–307, 2010;* angioimmunoblastic lymphadenopathy with dysproteinemia (angioimmunoblastic T-cell lymphoma) *JAAD 36:290–295, 1997;* lymphomatoid granulomatosis (angiocentric lymphoma) *JAAD 17:621–631, 1987; Hum Pathol 3:457–458, 1972;* CTCL with malignancy of FOXP3 regulatory cells – erosive and ulcerative hemorrhagic pyoderma gangrenosum-like lesions; ulcerated papulonodular lesions *JAAD 61:348–355, 2009;* extranodal nasal and nasal type natural killer T-cell lymphoma (angiocentric lymphoma) – ulcerated hyperpigmented plaque *JAAD 72:21–34, 2015; BJD 160:333–337, 2009; JAAD 54:S192–197, 2006; JAAD 40:268–272, 1999;* NK/T-cell lymphoma *BJD 173:134–145, 2015;* Ki-1+ anaplastic large cell lymphoma *JAAD 29:696–700, 1993; JAAD 26:813–817, 1992;* CD 30+ lymphoma *JAAD 44:239–247, 2001;* regressing CTCL or CD30+ anaplastic large-cell lymphoma (regressing atypical histiocytosis) – thighs and buttocks *Cancer 70:476–483, 1992;* Ki-1 (CD30+) positive anaplastic large cell lymphoma *JAAD 74:1135–1143, 2016; JAAD 57:S92–96, 2007; JAAD 51:103–110, 2004; JAAD 49:1049–1058, 2003; JAAD 47:S201–204, 2002;* CD30+ Ki-1+ anaplastic large cell lymphoma (associated with hepatitis C cryoglobulinemias) *BJD 151:941–943, 2004;* cutaneous anaplastic large cell lymphoma – facial ulcerated nodules *JAAD 145:1399–1404, 2009;* primary cutaneous CD30+ lymphoproliferative disorder (CD8+/CD4+) *JAAD 51:304–308, 2004;* gamma/delta T-cell lymphoma *AD 136:1024–1032, 2000;* Hodgkin's disease – ulcerated papules, plaques, and nodules of the scalp and face *AD 127:405–408, 1991;* ulcerated chest nodule *JAAD 58:295–298, 2008; AD 133:1454–1458, 1997;* lymphoblastoid natural killer-cell lymphoma *BJD 146:148–153, 2002;* large cell

B-cell lymphoma of the leg *JAAD 49:223–228, 2003;* peripheral T-cell lymphoma of breast *Ped Derm 23:193–195, 2006;* plasmablastic lymphoma (HIV and EBV-associated) *BJD 149:889–891, 2003;* cutaneous Richter syndrome (CLL rapidly developing into large cell lymphoma) *Ann DV 122:530–533, 1995; BJD 140:708–714, 1999;* primary cutaneous anaplastic large cell lymphoma – ulcerated purpuric nodule of nasal tip *Ped Derm 28:570–575, 2011;* primary cutaneous epidermotropic aggressive CD8+ T-cell lymphoma – red plaques with central necrosis (targetoid); ulcerated nodule *JAAD 67:748–759, 2012;* CD8+ transformation of cutaneous T-cell lymphoma *BJD 175:830–833, 2016;* HTLV-1 leukemia/lymphoma – nodulotumoral lesions, nodules, ulcerated nodules, multipapular lesions, red plaques, red patches, erythroderma *JAAD 81:23–41, 2019; JAAD 72:293–301, 2015;* Epstein-Barr virus associated plasmablastic lymphoma (HIV-defining lesion) – ulcerated fungating giant perianal tumor *BJD 174:398–401, 2016*

Lymphomatoid granulomatosis – Epstein-Barr-related angiocentric T-cell rich B-cell lymphoproliferative disorder; presents as urticarial dermatitis; papules and dermal nodules with or without ulceration, folliculitis-like lesions, maculopapules, indurated plaques, ulcers *BJD 157:426–429, 2007; JAAD 54:657–663, 2006*

Lymphomatoid papulosis *JAAD 55:903–906, 2006; JAAD 33:741–748, 1995*

Macroglobulinosis – Waldenstrom's macroglobulinemia; ulcerated nodules and plaques with central necrosis; skin colored papules of dorsal hands with central crusts; peripheral neuropathy *AD 146:165–169, 2010*

Malignant eccrine spiradenoma *AD 121:1445–1448, 1985*

Malignant fibrous histiocytoma *JAAD 52:101–108, 2005*

Malignant histiocytosis – ulcerated skin colored to violaceous nodules *Hum Pathol 15:368–377, 1984*

Malignant proliferating trichilemmal cyst *JAAD 32:870–873, 1995*

Melanocytic nevi – giant congenital melanocytic nevi with proliferative nodules *AD 140:83–88, 2004; Ped Derm 17:299–301, 2000*

Melanoma – primary nodular melanoma; amelanotic melanoma *AD 138:1246–1251, 2002; Semin Oncol 2:5–118, 1975;* acral lentiginous melanoma; primary scrotal melanoma *AD 145:1071–1072, 2009;* congenital pigment synthesizing melanoma of the scalp (animal type melanoma); black, pedunculated, ulcerated scalp nodule *JAAD 62:324–329, 2010;* subungual amelanotic melanoma – ulcerated nodule of nail bed *JAMA 319:713–714, 2018*

Meningioma – primary cutaneous meningioma – scalp or paraspinal region of children and teenagers *Cancer 34:728–744, 1974*

Metastases – tumid ulceration; metastatic mucoepidermoid carcinoma *JAAD 37:340–342, 1997;* Sister Mary Joseph nodule; stomach *AD 111:1478–1479, 1975;* renal cell carcinoma *AD 140:1393–1398, 2004; J Comput Assist Tomogr 22:756–757, 1998;* ovarian *JAAD 10:610–615, 1984;* pancreas *Cutis 31:555–558, 1983;* uterus *Br J Clin Pract 46:69–70, 1992;* leiomyosarcoma *AD 120:402–403, 1984;* peritoneal mesothelioma *Am J Dermatopathol 13:300–303, 1991;* cervical carcinoma *JAAD 45:133–135, 2001;* prostate *AD 143:937–942, 2007*

Mucinous carcinoma of skin *JAAD 49:941–943, 2003; JAAD 36:323–326, 1997*

Metastases – ulcerated pigmented nodules secondary to metastatic breast cancer *JAAD 64:994–996, 2011*

Multiple myeloma *Int J Derm 29:562–566, 1990*

Myelodysplastic syndromes *JAAD 33:187–191, 1995;* neutrophilic dermatosis with myelodysplastic syndrome *JAAD 23:247–249, 1990*

Myofibromatosis – solitary or multiple *Ped Derm 20:345–349, 2003;* solitary congenital infantile myofibroma/myopericytoma – most common juvenile fibrous tumor *AD 144:405–410, 2008;* recurrent infantile myofibromatosis *SkinMed 11:371–373, 2013*

Nevus lipomatosis superficialis *Int J Dermatol 14:273–276, 1975*

Nodular hidradenoma – ulcerated vascular appearing nodule *JAAD 76:S46–48, 2017; AD 136:1409–1414, 2000; JAAD 42:693–695, 2000*

Pilar cyst, ruptured

Piloleiomyoma *Cutis 57:168–170, 1996*

Pilomatrixoma, perforating *JAAD S146–147, 2003; JAAD 18:754–755, 1988;* pilomatrix carcinoma (trichilemmal carcinoma) *Dermatol Surg 28:284–286, 2002; BJD 143:646–647, 2000; JAAD 36:107–109, 1997; JAAD 17:264–270, 1987*

Plantar fibromatosis (Ledderhose's disease) – red plantar nodule; painful; may ulcerate *Curr Prob in Derm 8:137–188, 1996*

Plasmacytoma – extramedullary plasmacytoma *JAAD 49:S255–258, 2003; Am J Clin Oncol 20:467–470, 1997; Clin Exp Dermatol 21:367–369, 1996; AD 127:69–74, 1991; JAAD 19:879–890, 1988*

Plexiform fibrohistiocytic tumor *Ann Plast Surg 38:-307–306, 1997*

Primary trichilemmal tumor of the scalp – ulcerated nodule *BJD 159:483–485, 2008*

Progressive nodular histiocytoma *AD 114:1505–1508, 1978*

Proliferating trichilemmal cyst *Cancer 48:1207–1214, 1981*

Rhabdoid tumor – ulcerated vascular nodule *Ped Derm 28:295–298, 2011; J Cutan Pathol 26:509–515, 1999; Ped Derm 13:468, 1996*

Rhabdomyosarcoma – ulcerated perianal nodule *Ped Derm 30:97–99, 2013;* alveolar rhabdomyosarcoma, metastatic – red multinodular ulcerated plaque *Ped Derm 33:225–226, 2016*

Sebaceoma (sebaceous epithelioma) – yellow ulcerated papules *J Cut Pathol 11:396–414, 1984*

Sebaceous adenoma *Cancer 33:82–102, 1974*

Sebaceous gland carcinoma – ulcerated violaceous nodule *AD 137:1367–1372, 2001; Nippon Ganka Gakkai Zasshi 104:740–745, 2000;* ulcerated brown nodule of lateral eyebrow *Ped Derm 24:501–504, 2007*

Seborrheic keratosis – personal observation

Skin tag

Solitary congenital indeterminate cell histiocytoma *AD 129:81–85, 1993*

Spiradenoma, malignant *JAAD 44:395–398, 2001*

Spitz nevus – ulcerated nodule of face *Ped Derm 32:148–150, 2015;*

Great Cases from the South, AAD Meeting; March 2000

Squamous cell carcinoma *AD 143:889–892, 2007;* squamous cell carcinoma associated with lichen planus – multilobulated, ulcerated, red nodule and plaque *JAAD 71:698–707, 2014;*

perianal squamous cell carcinoma *J Clin Inf Dis 21:603–607, 1995;* squamous cell carcinoma of inguinal crease – HPV-16+ *BJD 170:753–754, 2014;* squamous cell carcinoma of the external auditory canal – ulcerated nodule with extensive destruction and purulent discharge *Cancer 59:156–160, 1987;* squamous cell carcinoma, metastatic, of face due to long-term voriconazole therapy – multiple facial ulcerated nodules *Clin Inf Dis 58:839, 901–902, 2014*

Suppurative keloidosis *JAAD 15:1090–1092, 1986*

Syringocystadenoma papilliferum – post-auricular eroded red papule in Goltz's syndrome *AD 145:218–219, 2009;* eyelid *Eyelid and Conjunctival Tumors, Shields JA and Shields CL, Lippincott Williams and Wilkins, 1999, p.5*Woringer-Kolopp disease (pagetoid reticulosis) *JAAD 59:706–712, 2008; Ann Dermatol Syph 10:945–958, 1939*

PARANEOPLASTIC DISEASES

Carcinoid syndrome – pyoderma gangrenosum *Cutis 18:791–794, 1976*

Insect bite-like reactions associated with hematologic malignancies *AD 135:1503–1507, 1999*

Necrobiotic xanthogranuloma with paraproteinemia *AD 133:97–102, 1997; Medicine (Baltimore) 65:376–388, 1986; BJD 113:339–343, 1985; JAAD 3:257–270, 1980*

Neutrophilic dermatosis with myelodysplastic syndrome *JAAD 23:247–249, 1990*

PRIMARY CUTANEOUS DISEASE

Alopecia mucinosa (follicular mucinosis) *Dermatology 197:178–180, 1998; AD 125:287–292, 1989; JAAD 10:760–768, 1984; AD 76:419–426, 1957*

Erythema elevatum diutinum *AD 129:1043–1044;1046–1048, 1993, JAAD 28:846–849, 1993*

Febrile ulceronecrotic Mucha-Habermann disease – crusted ulcerated red plaques; diarrhea, pulmonary involvement, abdominal pain, CNS symptoms, arthritis *Ped Derm 29:53–58, 2012*

Knuckle pad – personal observation

Lichen sclerosus et atrophicus

Neurotic excoriations *Cutis 85:149–152, 2010*

Painful piezogenic pedal papule *JAAD 36:780–781, 1997*

Prurigo nodularis

Reactive perforating collagenosis and other perforating disorders

PSYCHOCUTANEOUS DISORDERS

Factitial dermatitis (Munchhausen syndrome) – ulcerated nodules; necrosis of legs; injection of paint thinner *JAAD 71:376–381, 2014; Lancet 1:339–341, 1951*

SYNDROMES

Alport's syndrome – tophi

Antiphospholipid antibody syndrome – pyoderma gangrenosum-like lesions *BJD 120:419–429, 1989*

Ataxia telangiectasia – granulomas *Ped Derm 31:703–707, 2014*

Behcet's disease – pyoderma gangrenosum-like lesions *JAAD 41:540–545, 1999; JAAD 40:1–18, 1999; NEJM 341:1284–1290, 1999; JAAD 36:689–696, 1997*

Congenital self-healing reticulohistiocytosis (Hashimoto-Pritzker disease) *Curr Prob Dermatol 14:41–70, 2002; AD 134:625–630, 1998; Ped Derm 3:230–236, 1986*

Familial chilblain lupus – paronychia, acral erythema, acral papules, necrotic ulcers, facial ulcers, mutilation of fingers, ear lesions; mutation of exonuclease III domain of 3' repair exonuclease 1 (*TREX1*) *JAMADerm 151:426–431, 2015*

Hemophagocytic syndrome *AD 128:193–200, 1992*

Infantile myofibromatosis – solitary or multicentric *Curr Prob Derm 14:41–70, 2002; Ped Derm 8:306–309, 1991; Cancer 48:1807–1818, 1981;* giant necrotic pedunculated nodule *Ped Derm 27:29–33, 2010*

vs. Calcifying aponeurotic fibroma
    Digital fibromatosis
    Fibrous hamartoma of infancy
    Fibromatosis colli

Hyaline fibromatosis

Intravascular fasciitis

Juvenile hyaline fibromatosis

Muir-Torre syndrome – *JAAD 74:558–566, 2016;* personal observation

Neurofibromatosis – ulcerated neurofibromas, neurofibrosarcomas *Ann DV 114:807–811, 1987*

Noonan's syndrome – keloids

PAPA (pyogenic arthritis, pyoderma gangrenosum, acne vulgaris) syndrome – autosomal dominant; mutation in proline serine threonine phosphatase-interacting protein 1 (*PSTPIP1*) (*CD2BP1*) *JAAD 68:834–853, 2013; BJD 161:1199–1201, 2009; Mayo Clin Proc 72:611–615, 1997*

PAPASH syndrome – pyogenic arthritis, pyoderma gangrenosum, acne, hidradenitis suppurativa; autoinflammatory syndrome; mutation in *PSTPIP1* gene *JAMA Derm 149:762–764, 2013*

Regressing atypical histiocytosis *AD 123:1183–1187, 1987; Dermatologica 174:253–7, 1987*

SAPHO syndrome – palmoplantar pustulosis with sternoclavicular hyperostosis; non-palmoplantar pustulosis, acne fulminans, acne conglobata, hidradenitis suppurativa, psoriasis, multifocal osteitis *Cutis 71:63–67, 2003; Cutis 62:75–76, 1998; Rev Rheum Mol Osteoarthritic 54:187–196, 1987; Ann Rev Rheum Dis 40:547–553, 1981;* with neutrophilic dermatosis (ulceronecrotic bullous Sweet's syndrome) *AD 143:275–276, 2007*

Sweet's syndrome

Turner's syndrome – keloids

TRAUMA

Chondrodermatitis nodularis chronica helicis

Equestrian cold panniculitis – personal observation

Granuloma fissuratum

Post-operative pressure and cold panniculitis – personal observation

VASCULAR

Angiosarcoma *BJD 162:697–699, 2010; JAAD 49:530–531, 2003; JAAD 40:872–876, 1999;* including angiosarcoma of Stewart-Treves *AD 146:337–342, 2010;* radiation-induced angiosarcoma – ulcerated nodules and plaques *JAAD 38:143–175, 1998; JAAD 38:837–840, 1998*

Cholesterol emboli – ulcerated plaques of buttocks with livedo reticularis *JAMADerm 150:903–905, 2014*

Endovascular papillary angioendothelioma (Dabska's tumor) *JAAD 38:143–175, 1998*

Epithelioid hemangioendothelioma *JAAD 49:113–116, 2003; Eur J Dermatol 9:487–490, 1999*

Granulomatosis with polyangiitis – ulcerated plaque of forehead *Ped Derm 33:551–552, 2016*

Infantile hemangioma *BJD 169:20–30, 2013;* segmental hemangiomas of the head and neck, lip, and perineum *BJD 156:1050–1052, 2007;* facial hemangioma *JAAD 64:827–832, 2011; JAAD 64:833–838, 2011*

Hemangiopericytoma *Ped Derm 23:335–337, 2006*

Lymphangiosarcoma

Polyangiitis with granulomatosis – pyoderma gangrenosum-like lesions *JAAD 31:605–612, 1994*

Polyarteritis nodosa, systemic or cutaneous *JAAD 48:311–340, 2003; Ped Derm 15:103–107, 1998*

Pustular vasculitis of hands (Sweet's-like) *JAAD 32:192–198, 1995*

Pyogenic granuloma

Rapidly involuting congenital hemangioma (RICH) – palpable tumor with pale rim, coarse overlying telangiectasia with central depression or ulcer *JAMADerm 151:422–425, 2015; BJD 158:1363–1370, 2008; Ped Dev Pathol 6:495–510, 2003; Ped Derm 19:5–11, 2002*

NODULES, UNSPECIFIED LOCATION

AUTOIMMUNE DISEASES AND DISEASES OF IMMUNE DYSFUNCTION

Bowel-associated dermatitis-arthritis syndrome – red nodules *AD 135:1409–1414, 1999*

Chronic granulomatous disease – granulomas, furuncles, suppurative nodules *NEJM 317:687–694, 1987*

Graft vs. host disease – chronic; hyperpigmented nodules which soften and atrophy

Morphea *Dermatology 218:63–66, 2009; AD 122:76–79, 1986*

Nodular sclerederma *Australas J Dermatol 61:e269–273, 2020; Case Rep Dermatol 8:303–310, 2018; JAAD 32:343–5, 1995; JAAD 11:1111–1114, 1984*

CONGENITAL ANOMALIES

Congenital self-healing Langerhans cell histiocytosis – multiple congenital red-brown nodules *Ped Derm 17:322–324, 2000*

Congenital leukemia – generalized neonatal purple nodules *Ped Derm 26:139–142, 2009*

Dermatofibrosarcoma protuberans – oval pink nodule *JAAD 61:1014–1023, 2009*

DRUGS

Calcium gluconate – soft tissue calcification

Corticosteroids – peristomal granulomas due to fluorinated corticosteroids *J Cutan Pathol 8:361–364, 1981*

Drug-induced panniculitis *G Ital DV 149:263–270, 2014*

Drug-induced pseudolymphoma – red nodules *AD 132:1315–1321, 1996*

Glatiramer – for multiple sclerosis *J Cutan Pathol 35:407–410, 2008; JAAD 55:968–974, 2006*

Vemurafenib – neutrophilic panniculitis *Dermatol Online J 19:16, 2013*

EXOGENOUS AGENTS

Aluminum hypersensitivity – vaccination sites

Foreign body granuloma, including cutaneous reaction to broken thermometer *JAAD 25:915–919, 1991*

Metal sutures – red nodule

INFECTIONS AND INFESTATIONS

AIDS – cutaneous CD8+ T cell infiltrates in advanced HIV disease – red nodules *JAAD 41:722–727, 1999*

Aspergillosis *AD 129:1189–1194, 1993*

Bacillary angiomatosis *An Bras Dermatol 94:594–602, 2019; Transpl Infect Dis 14:403–409, 2012*

Botryomycosis *ID Cases Jan 30, 2020; Dermatopathol (Basel))1:81–85, 2014*

Candida – candidal granuloma; disseminated candidiasis in immunosuppressed host – red nodule

Cat scratch disease

Chancroid – inguinal buboe, purulent *Clin Inf Dis 22:233–239, 1996*

Chromomycosis – red nodule *Mycopathologia 181:379–385, 2016*

Coccidioidal granuloma – red nodule

Covid-19 – eosinophilic panniculitis *Actas Dermsifiliogr 2020 May, 22:S0001–7310(20)30163–0.doi:*https://doi.org/10.1016/jaa 2020.05.003

Cryptococcosis *Mycopathologia 180:219–225, 2015; Actas Dermosifiliogr 102:221–223, 2011*

Cutaneous larva migrans – red nodules of buttocks *BJD 145:434–437, 2001*

Cysticercosis – *Taenia solium NEJM 330:1887, 1994*

Fusarium solani sepsis – red nodule *Semin Resp Crit Care Med 36:706–714, 2015; Dermatol Online J 18:6, 2012*

Gnathostomiasis – nodular migratory eosinophilic panniculitis *JAAD 13:835–836, 1985*

Herpes simplex *Am J Dermatopathol 35:371–376, 2013*

Histoplasmosis *AD 132:341–346, 1996*

Insect bite granuloma

Leeches – hyperpigmented papules and nodules due to application of *Hirudo medicinalis* (leeches) *JAAD 43:867–869, 2000*

Leishmaniasis, acute or chronic, disseminated cutaneous leishmaniasis (diffuse nodules) *Ped Derm 13:455–463, 1996*

Leprosy – sporotrichoid nerve abscesses *Indian J Lepr 86:103–113, 2014*

Lobomycosis (keloidal blastomycosis) *Med Sante Trop 29:377–380, 2019; An Bras Dermatol 93:279–281, 2018; Ther Adv Infect Dis 2:91–96, 2014*

Lymphogranuloma venereum – inguinal buboes *Clin Inf Dis 22:233–239, 1996*

Malacoplakia – violaceous nodules *AD 134:244–245, 1998; Am J Dermatopathol 20:185–188, 1998; JAAD 34:325–332, 1996; JAAD 30:834–836, 1994;* perianal red nodule *AD 143:1441–1446, 2007*

Mucormycosis *Mycopatholgia 184:677–682, 2019; Rhizopus Med Mycol 60:17–21, 2019; Saksenaea vasiformis Mycopatholgia 185:577–581, 2020*

Mycetoma

Myiasis (*Dermatobia hominis*) – red nodule of back *Cutis 84:81–83, 2009;* painful red nodule – tumbu fly (*Cordylobia anthropophaga*) *JAMADerm 150:791–792, 2014;* New World screwworm *Trans R Soc Trop Med Hyg 84:747–748, 1990Mycobacterium kansasii JAAD 16:1122–1128, 1987*

Mycobacterium (TB, non-tuberculous) (*scrofulaceum, chelonei, marinum, ulcerans*) *Derm Clinics 17:151–185, 1999*); tuberculous chancre – brown papule or nodule, ragged undermined ulcer with granular hemorrhagic base; face; paronychia; surrounded by lupoid nodules; occurs after circumcision *Semin Hosp Paris 43:868–888, 1967;* traumatic wounds, surgical wounds *Rev Bras Oftel 23:183–192, 1964;* tattoos *AD 121:648–650, 1985;* massive tuberculous lymphadenopathy (red nodule) of lower neck in paradoxical response to anti-tuberculous therapy associated with infliximab treatment *Clin Inf Dis 40:756–759, 2005*

North American blastomycosis *Respiration 96:283–301, 2018; Curr Infect Dis Rep 15:440–449, 2013*

Onchocercoma

Octopus bite *J Cutan Pathol 35:1066–1072, 2008*

Paecilomyces lilacinus – violaceous nodules *JAAD 39:401–409, 1998*

Papular urticaria – red-brown nodules *Ped Derm 19:409–411, 2002*

Paracoccidioidomycosis

*Talaromyces (*formerly *Penicillium) marneffei* – nodules *Lancet 344:110–113, 1994; Mycoses 34:245–249, 1991*

Phaeohyphomycosis *JAAD 40:364–366, 1999; Derm Clinics 17:151–185, 1999*

Protothecosis *JAAD Case Rep 5:846–848, 2019; Mycopathologia 183:821–828, 2018*

Pseudomonas sepsis – red nodule *Clin Infect Dis 26:188–189, 1998; Am J Med 80:528–529, 1986*

Q fever – red nodule of buttock with granulomatous panniculitis *BJD 151:685–687, 2004*

Salmonella abscess *Ostomy Wound Manage 62:46–49, 2016; BMJ Case Rep July 13, 2012*

Sparganosis – *Spirometra mansonoides* – subcutaneous nodule *Derm Clinics 17:151–185, 1999* Sporotrichosis – fixed nodular type

Staphylococcal abscess

Strongyloides stercoralis – prurigo nodularis *Cutis 71:22–24, 2003*

Syphilis – secondary *Sex Trans Infec 94:192–193, 2018; BMJ Case Rep May 8, 2013;* lues maligna *BMJ Case Rep July 7, 2011;* tertiary *AD 134:365–370, 1998*

Trichophyton rubrum, invasive – red nodule *JAAD 33:315–318, 1995*

Yaws *Stat Pearls Nov 16, 2019*

INFILTRATIVE

Amyloidosis, primary systemic *JAAD 24:139, 1991*

Colloid milium, nodular *Cutis 10:355–358, 1985*

Eosinophilic granuloma

Jessner's lymphocytic infiltrate – red nodule

Juvenile xanthogranuloma – red nodule *Rev Pocul Pediatr 37:257–260, 2019*

Langerhans cell histiocytosis *JAAD 13:481–496, 1985*

Rosai-Dorfman disease *BJD 154:277–286, 2006*

Xanthoma disseminatum – brown nodule *J Postgrad Med 60:69–71, 2014*

INFLAMMATORY DISEASES

Crohn's disease – metastatic Crohn's disease – red papules and plaques with overlying scale/crust; red scaly plaque with shallow ulcer; red plaques and nodules; abscess-like lesions *JAAD 71:804–813, 2014; J Eur Acad Dermatol Venereol 15:343–345, 2001; JAAD 36:986–988, 1996*

Kikuchi's disease (histiocytic necrotizing lymphadenitis) (subacute necrotizing lymphadenitis) – morbilliform eruption, urticarial, and rubella-like exanthems; red papules of face, back, arms; red plaques; erythema and acneiform lesions of face; exanthem overlying involved lymph nodes; red or ulcerated pharynx; cervical adenopathy; associations with SLE, lymphoma, tuberculous adenitis, viral lymphadenitis, infectious mononucleosis, and drug eruptions *AD 142:641–646, 2006; Ped Derm 18:403–405, 2001; JAAD 22:909–912, 1990; Am J Surg Pathol 14:872–876, 1990;*

rubella-like eruption, generalized erythema and papules *BJD 146:167–168, 2002*

Lymphocytoma cutis – skin colored to plum-red dermal or subcutaneous nodules; idiopathic or due to insect bites, Borrelia burgdorferi, trauma, vaccinations, injected drugs or antigens for hyposensitization, injection of arthropod venom, acupuncture, gold pierced earrings, tattoos, post-zoster scars *JAAD 38:877–905, 1998*

Panniculitis
1) Enzyme panniculitis
   Pancreatic panniculitis *G Ital DV 148:419–425, 2013*
   Alpha-1 antitrypsin deficiency *Int J Dermatol 57:952–958, 2018; BJD 174:753–762, 2016; JAAD 18:684–692, 1988*
2) Immunologic panniculitis
   Erythema nodosum, including familial erythema nodosum *Dermatol Online J 20:22376, 2014; Arthr Rheum 34:1177–1179, 1991*
   Lupus panniculitis *Adv Rheumatol 59:3, 2019; Medicine (Balt)95:e3429, 2016*
   Complement deficiency *AD 122:576–582, 1986*
   Lipoatrophic panniculitis *Ann DV 138:681–685, 2011*
   Lipophagic panniculitis of childhood *JAAD 21:971–978, 1989*
   Rheumatoid arthritis *Clin Exp Rheumatol 34:126–128, 2016; Am J Dermatopathol 21:247–25, 1999*
   Cytophagic histiocytic panniculitis
3) Neoplastic
   Lymphoma, leukemia – subcutaneous panniculitis-like T-cell lymphoma *Diagn Pathol 14:80, 2019; J Cutan Pathol 46:44–51, 2019; Ped Derm 32:526–532, 2015;* gamma-delta T-cell lymphoma *J Cutan Pathol 40:896–892, 2013*
   Histiocytosis, including cytophagic histiocytic panniculitis
4) Cold panniculitis, including cold panniculitis of neonate – red nodules of cheeks *Am J Dermatopathol 40:291–294, 2018;* equestrian cold panniculitis *J Cutan Pathol 40:485–490, 2013*
5) Factitial panniculitis *Dermatol Online J May 15, 2019; Clin Exp Dermatol 34:e170–173, 2009*
6) Post-steroid panniculitis *Indian Dermatol Online J 4:318–320, 2013; Acta DV Alp Pannonica Adriat 21:77–78, 2012*
7) Crystal panniculitis – crystal storing histiocytosis, gouty panniculitis, subcutaneous fat necrosis of the newborn, post-steroid panniculitis; etanercept injection *J Cutan Pathol 42:413–415, 2015*
8) Eosinophilic panniculitis *JAAD 34:229–234, 1996; Ped Derm 12:35–38, 1995; JAAD 12:161–164, 1985*
9) Idiopathic nodular panniculitis
10) Associations with Sweet's syndrome – histiocytoid Sweet's syndrome *Case Rep Dermatol May, 2014.954254doi.101155/2014/954254;,* sarcoid, Behcet's disease *Front Pediatr 6:377, 2018; Rheumatol Int 30:1657–1659, 2010;,* familial Mediterranean fever, Whipple's disease *Am J Dermatopathol 36:344–346, 2014;,* relapsing polychondritis
11) Lipomembranous panniculitis with nodular fat necrosis – systemic sclerederma *J Cut Pathol 37:1170–1173, 2010;* dermatomyositis, morphea, lupus profundus, peripheral vascular disease *Ann Diagn Pathol 11:282–284, 2007*
12) Subcutaneous fat necrosis after hypothermic cardiac surgery *JAAD 15:331–336, 1986*
13) Subcutaneous fat necrosis of newborn *J Cut Med Surg 22:223–225, 2018*

Proliferative fasciitis – hyperpigmented and red nodules of abdomen *SKINmed 12:111–112, 2014*

Rosai-Dorfman disease (sinus histiocytosis with massive lymphadenopathy) – cutaneous nodules *Ped Derm 17:377–380, 2000*

Sarcoidosis – Darier-Roussy sarcoid *Am J Med 85:731–736, 1988*

METABOLIC

Calcinosis cutis – tumoral calcinosis

Gout (tophus) – foot nodule *Cutis 62:239–241, 1998;* panniculitis *J Cut Aesthetic Surg 10:223–225, 2017; Case Rep Rheumatol 2014.320940 doi:https://doi.org/10.1155/2014/320940; Rheumatol Int 31:831–835, 2011*

Primary hyperoxalosis *AD 131:821–823, 1995*

Pretibial myxedema *Dermatopathol (Basel)3:61–67, 2016*

Xanthomas (tuberous)

NEOPLASTIC DISEASES

Adenoid cystic carcinoma

Anal carcinoma – perianal nodule *BJD 1621269–1277, 2010*

Atypical fibroxanthoma

Atypical histiocytoma – red nodule

Basal cell carcinoma

Carcinoid – metastatic cutaneous carcinoid *JAAD 13:363–366, 1985*

Chondroid syringoma

Chordoma, metastatic – red nodules *JAAD 55:S6–10, 2006; Derm Surg 26:259–262, 2000*

Cutaneous blastic plasmacytoid dendritic cell neoplasm – ulceronecrotic lesions of scalp; red nodules of back *BJD 172:298–300, 2015*

Dermal duct tumor – red nodule of back *AD 140:609–614, 2004*

Dermatofibroma – brown-yellow papules, nodules

Dermatofibrosarcoma protuberans – violaceous nodule of back *Ped Derm 36:163–165, 2019*

Desmoid tumor *JAAD 34:352–356, 1996*

Eccrine angiomatous nevus – brown to yellow nodule

Eccrine poroma

Eccrine spiradenoma

Elastofibroma dorsi – red nodule of the back *AD 135:341346, 1999*

Fibroepithelioma of Pinkus

Fibroma

Fibrosarcoma

Fibrous hamartoma of infancy – hypertrichotic pink nodule of back *BJD 156:1052–1055, 2007*

Folliculosebaceous cystic hamartoma *JAAD 34:77–81, 1996*

Glomus tumor

Granular cell myoblastoma – red, hyperpigmented *Ped Derm 14:489–490, 1997*

Hidradenoma papilliferum

Hidrocystoma

Kaposi's sarcoma

Keratoacanthoma

Leiomyoma – multiple pink nodules *JAAD 62:904–906, 2010*

Leiomyosarcoma – brown nodule *AD 135:341–346, 1999*

Leukemia cutis (chloroma) – large truncal nodules *BJD 143:773–779, 2000*

Lipoma

Liposarcoma

Lymphoepithelioma-like carcinoma of the skin – red nodule of trunk, face, or scalp *AD 134:1627–1632, 1998*

Lymphoma – including angioimmunoblastic lymphadenopathy with dysproteinemia (angioimmunoblastic T-cell lymphoma) *JAAD 36:290–295, 1997;* Lennert's lymphoma *Am J Dermatopathol 11:549–554, 1989;* T-zone lymphoma – subcutaneous nodules of lower abdomen and groin *BJD 146:1096–1100, 2002;* primary cutaneous B-cell lymphoma *AD 143:1520–1526, 2007;* folliculotropic cutaneous T-cell lymphoma *AD 144:738–746, 2008;* large cell transformation of cutaneous T-cell lymphoma – nodule within CTCL *JAAD 67:665–672, 2012;* primary large cell anaplastic lymphoma – purple nodules *JAMADerm 151:1030–1031, 2015;* cutaneous T-cell lymphoma of face *JAAD 82:634–641, 2020*

Malignant fibrous histiocytoma

Melanoma, including metastatic melanoma; red perianal nodule *JAAD 71:366–375, 2014*

Merkel cell tumor

Metastatic carcinoma – red truncal nodules – endometrial carcinoma *Cutis 84:33–38, 2009*

Mucoepidermoid carcinoma

Multiple myeloma *JAAD 78:471–478, 2018; SkinMed 15:153–155, 2017; Am J Dermatopathol 35:377–380, 2016; Blood 117:2088, 2011*

Myxoma

Neurilemmoma

Neurofibroma

Neuroma

Nevus, melanocytic

Plexiform fibrohistiocytic tumor – tender red nodule of chest *Ped Derm 36:490–496, 2019*

Rhabdoid tumor

Rhabdomyosarcoma

Spitz nevus

Squamous cell carcinoma

Sweat gland adenoma

Synovial sarcoma – skin colored subcutaneous nodule on one leg in woman with congenital lymphedema of both legs – personal observation

Syringocystadenoma papilliferum – pink, brown linear plaques or nodules *AD 71:361–372, 1955*

Waldenstrom's macroglobulinemia *AD 134:1127–1131, 1998*

PHOTOSENSITIVITY DISORDERS

Actinic reticuloid – red nodules *JAAD 38:877–905, 1998*

PRIMARY CUTANEOUS DISEASES

Acne vulgaris – keloidal scarring

Pilonidal fistula – red nodule above gluteal crease *JAAD 62:247–256, 2010*

SYNDROMES

Antiphospholipid antibody syndrome *JAAD 36:149–168, 1997; JAAD 36:970–982, 1997*

Blue rubber bleb nevus syndrome

Familial Mediterranean fever *J Dermatol 41:827–820, 2014*

Hypereosinophilic syndrome *AD 132:535–541, 1996*

Hyper IgD syndrome – periodic fever, red macules, urticaria, annular erythema, nodules, arthralgias, abdominal pain, lymphadenopathy *AD 130:59–65, 1994*

Infantile systemic hyalinosis – autosomal recessive; synophrys, thickened skin, perianal nodules, dusky red plaques of buttocks, gingival hypertrophy, joint contractures, juxta-articular nodules (knuckle pads), osteopenia, growth failure, diarrhea, frequent infections, facial red papules *JAAD 50:S61–64, 2004*

Maffucci's syndrome

Muir-Torre syndrome – red subcutaneous nodule of shoulder *JAAD 73:889–891, 2015*

Multicentric reticulohistiocytosis *BMC Res Notes 11:647, 2018*

Myofibromatosis – red nodules

POEMS syndrome – cutaneous angiomas, blue dermal papules associated with Castleman's disease (benign reactive angioendotheliomatosis), diffuse hyperpigmentation, morphea-like changes, maculopapular brown-violaceous lesions, purple nodules *JAAD 44:324–329, 2001, JAAD 21:1061–1068, 1989; JAAD 12:961–964, 1985, AD 124:695–698, 1988, Cutis 61:329–334, 1998; JAAD 40:808–812, 1999*

Proteus syndrome

Pseudoxanthoma elasticum – chronic granulomatous nodules in skin lesions *AD 96:528–531, 1967*

Relapsing polychondritis *Clin Exp Rheumatol 20:89–91, 2002*

Rosai-Dorfman disease (sinus histiocytosis with massive lymphadenopathy – red papules and/or nodules on any cutaneous surface *JAAD 56:302–316, 2007; Arch Pathol 87:63–70, 1969*

Rubinstein-Taybi syndrome – keloids

Turner's syndrome – keloids *JAAD 36:1002–1004, 1996*

Xanthogranuloma

TRAUMA

Bicycle rider's nodule (athlete's nodule) – red nodule over sacrococcygeal area *BJD 143:1124–1126, 2000*

Contusion

Hypertrophic scar

Keloid

Traumatic panniculitis *Dermatol Clin 26:481–483, 2008*

VASCULAR

Angiokeratoma

Angiosarcoma

Cutaneous polyarteritis nodosa *Int J Dermatol 49:750–756, 2010*

Degos' disease (malignant atrophic papulosis) – gumma-like nodules

Granulomatosis with polyangiitis *Adv Exp Mol Biol 2013:755:307–310 doi.https://doi.org/10.1007/978-94-007-4546-9_39; AD 130:861–867, 1994*

Hemangioma

Intravascular microemboli from polymer coats of intravascular device – hemorrhagic panniculitis presenting as ecchymosis; nodules of buttocks, arms, and trunk *JAMADerm 151:204–207, 2015*

Leukocytoclastic vasculitis *AD 134:309–315, 1998*

Lipodermatosclerosis *JAAD 62:1005–1012, 2010*

Lymphangioma

Polyarteritis nodosa *Stat Pearls Jan 31, 2019*

Portocaval shunt, infected – red nodule *Am J Gastroenterol 84:1335–1336, 1989*

Pyogenic granuloma

Stewart-Treves syndrome – red nodules

NORMAL SKIN (BARELY PERCEPTIBLE PLAQUE)

AUTOIMMUNE DISEASES

Morphea

CONGENITAL LESIONS

Meningeal heterotopia (ectopic rests of meningeal tissue that have lost central nervous system connection) and rudimentary or atretic meningoceles – exophytic nodular or cystic mass of occipital or parietal scalp – normal skin; glistening or bullous appearance, alopecia, hair collar *Ped Derm 32:161–170, 2015*

INFECTIONS AND INFESTATIONS

Dental sinus, quiescent

Leprosy bonita *JAAD 42:324–328, 2000*

Lichen scrofulosorum

Syphilid – macular syphilid in dark-skinned persons

Tinea incognito – personal observation

Verruca plana

INFILTRATIVE DISEASES

Amyloidosis

Amyloid elastosis *JAAD 42:324–328, 2000*

Papular mucinosis

Pretibial myxedema

Solitary mucinosis

INFLAMMATORY DISEASES

Sarcoid *JAAD 42:324–328, 2000*

METABOLIC DISORDERS

Cystinosis – normal skin; subcutaneous plaques; skin atrophy and telangiectasia mimicking premature aging *JAAD 62:AB26, 2010; JAAD 68:e111–116, 2013*

Erythropoietic protoporphyria

Myxedema

Nephrogenic fibrosing dermopathy *BJD 152:531–536, 2005*

Pretibial myxedema *JAAD 42:324–328, 2000*

Xanthomas – plane xanthomas

NEOPLASTIC DISEASES

Acne-free nevus – region of normal skin in patient with severe acne *BJD 96:287–290, 1977*

Connective tissue nevus

Eruptive vellus hair cysts

Hamartoma moniliformis

Lymphoma – cutaneous T-cell lymphoma – normal skin with pruritus *JAAD 47:S168–171, 2002; JAAD 42:324–328, 2000; JAAD 16:61–74, 1987;* intravascular B-cell lymphoma *JAAD 59:148–151, 2008*

Syringomas

Trichodiscoma

NORMAL VARIANTS

Juxtaclavicular beaded lines

PRIMARY CUTANEOUS DISEASES

Aquadynia – pain on exposure to water *Ped Derm 27:646–649, 2010; Ann DV 130:195–198, 2003; JAAD 38:357–358, 1998; BJD 136:980–981, 1997*

Atopic dermatitis

Frontal fibrosing alopecia – facial follicular papules *AD 147:1424–1427, 2011*

Futcher's lines – pigmentary line of demarcation

Ichthyosis en confetti (congenital reticulated ichthyosiform erythroderma) – reticulated erythroderma with guttate hypopigmentation, palmoplantar keratoderma; loss of dermatoglyphics; temporary hypertrichosis of normal skin *BJD 166:434–439, 2012; JAAD 63:607–641, 2010*

Idiopathic unilateral circumscribed hyperhidrosis *AD 137:1241–1246, 2001; Ped Derm 17:25–28, 2000*

Lichen nitidus

Lichen planus *JAAD 42:324–328, 2000;* Graham-Little syndrome (lichen planopilaris) – personal observation

Linea alba

Linea nigra

Perifollicular elastolysis

Pseudoxanthoma elasticum-like papillary dermal elastolysis *AD 136:791–796, 2000; JAAD 26:648–650, 1992*

Scleredema adultorum – personal observation

Vulvodynia (vulvar vestibulitis) *Dermatologic Clin 10:435–444, 1992*

White fibrous papulosis of the neck *JAAD 20:1073–1077,1989*

SYNDROMES

Buschke-Ollendorff syndrome – personal observation

Ehlers-Danlos syndrome – personal observation

Hunter syndrome – personal observation

Proctalgia fugax (chronic idiopathic anal pain, coccygodynia) *J R Soc Med 75:96–101, 1982*

Pseudoxanthoma elasticum *JAAD 42:324–328, 2000; Dermatology 199:3–7, 1999*

Red scrotum syndrome *BJD 104:611–619, 1981*

Tuberous sclerosis – hypopigmentation

Williams' syndrome – skin with soft texture, abnormal smoothness, easy mobility from underlying subcutaneous tissue, growth retardation, elfin-like facies, mental retardation, hoarse voice, supravalvular aortic stenosis; deletion of elastin gene *BJD 156:1052–1055, 2007*

TOXINS

Eosinophilia myalgia syndrome

VASCULAR

Angiokeratoma

Glomus tumor

OBESITY SYNDROMES/PROTUBERANT ABDOMEN

Abdominal hernia

Achondrogenesis type 1B *Gene Reviews Nov 14, 2013*

Ascites

Atelosteogenesis type 2 *Gene Reviews Jan 23, 2014*

Bardet-Biedl syndrome *Atlas of Clinical Syndromes: A Visual Aid to Diagnosis, 1992, pp. 288–289*

Beckwith-Wiedemann syndrome (exomphalos-macroglossia-gigantism syndrome) *Atlas of Clinical Syndromes: A Visual Aid to Diagnosis, 1992, pp. 136–137*

CANDLE syndrome *Best Practice and Res Clin Rheum 31:441–459, 2017*

Canities – obesity related to canities *JAAD 72:321–327, 2015*

Celiac disease – in children with persistent diarrhea, failure to thrive *J Coll Physicians Surg Pak 17:554–557, 2007*; "pseudoascites" *Am J Gastroenterol 78:730–731, 1983*

Childhood acquired lipodystrophy *JAAD 55:947–950, 2006*

Cirrhosis, hepatic

Cohen syndrome *Atlas of Clinical Syndromes: A Visual Aid to Diagnosis, 1992, pp. 290–291*

Coffin-Siris syndrome – mutation in *ARID1B*; extreme obesity, macrocephaly, hepatomegaly, hyperinsulinemia, polycystic ovarian syndrome, hypertrichosis, hypoplastic or absent fifth distal phalanx or nail *Eur J Hum Genet 22:1327–1329, 2014*

Cranioectodermal dysplasia 1

Crix belly

Fanconi-Bickel syndrome *Indian J Ped 81:1237–1239, 2014*

Fibrosarcoma *J Coll Physicians Surg Pak 15:728–770, 2005*

Gaucher's disease types I and II *Atlas of Clinical Syndromes: A Visual Aid to Diagnosis, 1992, pp. 114–115*

Glycogen storage disease type I *Atlas of Clinical Syndromes: A Visual Aid to Diagnosis, 1992, pp. 110–111; Eur J Obstet Gynecol Reprod Bio 66: 69–70, 1990*; type 1A (von Gierke's disease) *Cureus 9:e1548, 2017*

Jarcho-Levin syndrome – with splenic herniation *Am J Case Rep 17:745–748, 2016*

Klinefelter's syndrome *Atlas of Clinical Syndromes: A Visual Aid to Diagnosis, 1992, pp. 544–545*

Mannosidosis *Atlas of Clinical Syndromes: A Visual Aid to Diagnosis, 1992, pp. 130–131*

Mauriac's syndrome *Ital J Ped Jan 7, 2019*

Mucopolysaccharidosis (MPS) type VI; Maroteaux-Lamy *Mol Syndromol 10:275, 2020*

Niemann-Pick disease *Atlas of Clinical Syndromes: A Visual Aid to Diagnosis, 1992, pp. 112–113*

Ovarian tumor

Polycystic kidney disease *Atlas of Clinical Syndromes: A Visual Aid to Diagnosis, 1992, p. 302*

Polycystic ovarian disease – obesity in children *Ped Derm 32:579–592, 2015*

Prader-Willi syndrome *Atlas of Clinical Syndromes: A Visual Aid to Diagnosis, 1992, pp. 286–287*

Pregnancy

Proteus syndrome *Atlas of Clinical Syndromes: A Visual Aid to Diagnosis, 1992, pp. 352–355*

Prune belly syndrome *Atlas of Clinical Syndromes: A Visual Aid to Diagnosis, 1992, pp. 300–301*

Pseudoascites – recent food binging *WMJ 99:32–34, 2000*

Pseudohypoparathyroidism type Ia (Albright's hereditary osteodystrophy) – subcutaneous nodule (osteoma cutis); short stature, round face, obesity, subcutaneous ossifications, bilateral brachydactyly, mental retardation, hypothyroidism, saddle nose deformity *Ped Derm 33:675–676, 2016; Atlas of Clinical Syndromes: A Visual Aid to Diagnosis, 1992, pp. 188–189*

Rectus muscle diastasis *Plast Reconstr Surg 101:1685–1689, 1998*

Sanfilippo syndrome type A *J Inherit Metab Dis 37:431–437, 2014*

Short rib polydactyly syndrome *Arch Gynecol Obstet 272:173–175, 2005*

Sialuria

Thanatophoric dysplasia *J Clin Diagn Res 9:QD1–3, 2015*

Uterine leiomyomata

Vitamin D-dependent rickets types 1 and 2

ONYCHOLYSIS

AUTOIMMUNE DISEASES AND DISEASES OF IMMUNE DYSFUNCTION

Allergic contact dermatitis – nail polish, acrylic cements *Clin Exp Dermatol 44:599–605, 2019; Eur J Dermatol 10:223–225, 2000; Int J Dermatol 37:31–36, 1998*; hydroxylamine in color developer *Contact Derm 24:158, 1991*; formaldehyde nail hardeners; tulips *Cutis 71:347–348, 2003*

Alopecia areata *Int J Dermatol 57:776–783, 2018*

Lupus erythematosus, systemic *Ann DV 147:18–28, 2020*

Pemphigus vulgaris *Rev Hosp Clin Fac Sao Paolo 57:229–234, 2002; BJD 146:836–839, 2002*

Scleroderma – rarely onycholysis *JAAD 76:1115–1123, 2017*

Vitiligo *An Bras Dermatol 91:442–445, 2016*

CONGENITAL LESIONS

Congenital malalignment of the great toenails – personal observation

DRUG-INDUCED

Acridine

Adriamycin

Bleomycin

Captopril *Ann Int Med 105:305–306, 1986*

Capecitabine *Cutis 72:234–236, 2003; BJD 145:521–522, 2001*

Cephaloridine

Cetuximab (epidermal growth factor receptor inhibitor) *BJD 161:515–521, 2009*

Chloramphenicol

Chlorazepate dipotassium

Cloxacillin

Cyclophosphamide *Cutis 71:229–232, 2003*

Demethylchlortetracycline

Docetaxel *Cutis 71:229–232, 2003*

Dovitinib (selective pan-FGF-R inhibitor) – oncholysis, trichomegaly, straightening of the scalp hair, hyperkeratosis of heels, xerostomia *JAMADerm 153:723–725, 2017*

Doxorubicin *AD 126:1244, 1990*

Doxycycline – photo-onycholysis *Therapie Jan 13, 2020*

Epidermal growth factor receptor inhibitors – cetuximab and panitumumab; erlotinib and gefitinib; lapatinib; canertinib; vandetanib *JAAD 72:203–218, 2015*

Erlotinib (epidermal growth factor receptor inhibitor) *BJD 161:515–521, 2009*

Etoposide *JAAD 40:367–398, 1999; Gynecol Oncol 57:436, 1995*

5-Fluorouracil, topical *Acta DV 52:320–322, 1972*

Fluoroquinolones

Gefitinib (epidermal growth factor receptor inhibitor) *JAAD 55:657–670, 2006; J Clin Oncol 21:1980–1987, 2003*

Griseofulvin – photo-onycholysis *Presse Med 41(pt 1)879–881, 2012*

Hydroxyurea *Cutis 71:229–232, 2003*

Indomethacin *Textbook of Neonatal Dermatology, p. 512, 2001*

Isotretinoin *J Dermatol Treat 12:115–116, 2001*

Lucitanib (selective pan-FGF-R inhibitor) – oncholysis, trichomegaly, straightening of the scalp hair, hyperkeratosis of heels, xerostomia *JAMADerm 153:723–725, 2017*

Mercaptopurine

Methotrexate *AD 123:990–992, 1987*

Minocycline

Mitoxantrone *Clin Exp Dermatol 20:459–461, 1995*

Mycophenolate *Ann Int Med 133:921–922, 2000*

Oral contraceptives (norethindrone and mestranol)

Paclitaxel *Cutis 71:229–232, 2003; Cancer 88:2367–2371, 2000*

Phenothiazines

Photo-onycholysis – psoralens, demethylchlortetracyline, doxycycline *JAAD 33:551–73, 1995*; including benoxaprofen, chlorpromazine, chloramphenicol, cephaloridine, clorazepate dipotassium *JAAD 21:1304–1305, 1989*; cloxacillin, fluoroquinolones, PUVA *Photodermatol 1:202–203, 1984*; quinine *Clin Exp Dermatol 14:335, 1989*; tetracycline *Cutis 23:657–658, 1979*; thiazide diuretics, trypaflavine

Practolol

Psoralens

Quinine *Clin Exp Dermatol 14:335, 1989*

Retinoids

Sodium valproate *Eur Neurol 42:64–65, 1999*

Sulfonamides

Taxol and other taxanes *JAAD 71:787–794, 2014*

Tetracycline – photo-onycholysis *Clin Exp Dermatol 39:746–747, 2014*

Thiazides

Vincristine *Cutis 71:229–232, 2003*

EXOGENOUS AGENTS

Irritant contact dermatitis

Hair cosmetics

Nail cosmetics – nail hardener *Contact Derm 57:280–281, 2007*; acrylates *J Eur Acad DV 21:169–174, 2007; Dermatol Clin 24:233–239, 2006*

Subungual trichogranuloma

Water exposure (soap and water)

Weed killers

INFECTIONS AND INFESTATIONS

Acremonium species – distal and lateral onychomycosis *JAAD 66:494–502, 2012*; hand, foot, and mouth disease – onycholysis with splinter hemorrhages *BJD 170:748–749, 2014*

Beta papillomavirus – toenail *Am J Dermatopathol 37: 329–333, 2015*

Candida *Indian J Med Microbiol 22:258–259, 2004; BJD 118:47–58, 1988*

Coxsackie virus – hand, foot, and mouth disease *Int J Dermatol 56:e61–62, 2017*

Dermatophyte infection – *Trichophyton rubrum, T. mentagrophytes; T. violaceum BJD 144:212–213, 2001*

Herpes zoster

Leprosy *Int J Leprol Other Mycobact Dis 71:320–327, 2003; AD 88:117–185, 1963*

Onychomycosis

Paronychia *BJD 118:47–58, 1988*

Poliomyelitis

Pseudomonas Derm Ther 15:99–106, 2002

Syphilis – secondary, tertiary *AD 88:117–185, 1963*

Trichosporon inkin Skin Appendage Disorders 1:144–146, 2016

Verrucae vulgaris

INFILTRATIVE DISORDERS

Amyloidosis *Rev Med Interne 36:356–358, 2015*

Langerhans cell histiocytosis – onycholysis, subungual hyperkeratosis, and hemorrhage *Ped Derm 25:247–251, 2008; Ped Hematol Oncol 24:45–51, 2007; BJD 130:523–527, 1994; AD 120:1052–1056, 1984*

INFLAMMATORY DISEASES

Neuritis

Sarcoidosis *J Clin Diagn Res 11:WD01–03, 2017; BJD 135:340, 1996*; linear striations, thinning, and onycholysis *JAAD 60:1050–1052, 2009*

METABOLIC DISORDERS

Chronic renal failure in hemodialysis *ISRN Dermatol 2012;679619*

Congenital erythropoietic porphyria – onycholysis, milia of the nose, facial hypertrichosis, bullae of the hand, hyper- and hypopigmentation with scarring *BJD 171:422–423, 2014*

Erythropoietic protoporphyria photo-onycholysis *Proc R Soc Med 70:572–574, 1977*

Acquired hypoparathyroidism *Indian J Endocrinol Metab 16:819–820, 2012*

Iron deficiency anemia

Pellagra

Porphyria cutanea tarda – induced by birth control pills *Postgrad Med J 52:535–538, 1976*

Pregnancy

Scurvy

Thyroid disease – hyper- or hypothyroidism; Plummer's nails *Intern Med 57:3055–3056, 2018; Pan Afr Med J 32:31, 2019; Thyroid 11:707, 2001*

NEOPLASTIC DISORDERS

Bowen's disease *AD 130:204–209, 1994*

Leiomyoma, subungual *J Cut Pathol 43:379–382, 2016*

Lung cancer *JAMA 238:1246–1247, 1977*

Lymphoma – cutaneous T-cell lymphoma with complete onycholysis, trachyonychia, and subungual hyperkeratosis *AD 142:1071–1073, 2006; Sezary syndrome J Cut Med Surg 23:380–387, 2019*

Melanoma – amelanotic subungual melanoma *AD 148:947–952, 2012*

Metastases – distal phalangeal metastases of chondrosarcoma *Clin Exp Dermatol 17:463–465, 1992*

Myeloma

Onycholemmal carcinoma – paronychia, crusted ulcer of the nail fold, onycholysis *JAAD 68:290–295, 2013; J Cut Pathol 33:577–580, 2006*

Onychomatrixoma – onycholysis with linear yellow band *JAAD 70:395–397, 2014*

Onychopapilloma – V-shaped distal split of the nail, longitudinal erythronychia, longitudinal leukonychia, onycholysis, longitudinal melanonychia, splinter hemorrhages, distal subungual hyperkeratotic mass *JAAD 74:521–526, 2016*

Squamous cell carcinoma *Dermatol Pract Concept 31:238–244, 2018; J Derm Surg Oncol 8:853–855, 1982*

Subungual exostosis – hyperkeratotic subungual papule of the fingertip *Cutis 98:128–129, 2016*

Subungual onycholemmal cyst – pressure-induced onycholysis overlying blue discoloration *Cutis 98:107–110, 2016*

PARANEOPLASTIC DISORDERS

Bazex syndrome *Case Rep Dermatol Med 2016;7137691; AD 113:1613, 1977*

Carcinoma of the lung *Clin Exp Dermatol 21:244, 1996; JAMA 238:1246–1247, 1977*

Glucagonoma syndrome – onycholysis; periorbital and perioral erythema; alpha cell tumor in the tail of the pancreas; 50% of cases have metastasized by the time of diagnosis; skin rash, angular stomatitis, cheilosis, beefy red glossitis, blepharitis, conjunctivitis, alopecia, crumbling nails; rarely, associated with MEN I or IIA syndromes *BJD 174:1092–1095, 2016; JAMADerm 345–347, 2016; JAAD 54:745–762, 2006; JAAD 12:1032–1039, 1985; Int J Derm 43:12–18, 2004; AD 133:909, 912, 1997; JAAD 12:1032–1039, 1985; Ann Int Med 91:213–215, 1979; AD 45:1069–1080, 1942*

PHOTODERMATOSES

Chronic actinic dermatitis (actinic reticuloid)

Drug-induced photodermatoses

PUVA *Clin Case Rep 22:267–268, 2017*

PRIMARY CUTANEOUS DISEASES

Acrodermatitis continua of Hallopeau *Clin Exp Dermatol 32:619–620, 2007*

Acropustulosis repens *Int J Dermatol 45:389–393, 2006*

Atopic dermatitis *Int J Dermatol Dec 3, 2019*

Epidermolysis bullosa

Epidermolysis bullosa, autosomal recessive – blisters and erosions, mild skin fragility, fatal interstitial lung disease, nephrotic syndrome, sparse fine hair, large dystrophic toenails with distal onycholysis; integrin alpha6-beta4 integrin mutation *NEJM 366:1508–1514, 2012*

Hand dermatitis

Hereditary distal onycholysis *Clin Exp Dermatol 15:146–148, 1990*

Hyperhidrosis

Kawasaki's disease *J Clin Rheumatol Feb 19, 2019*

Lichen planus

Lichen striatus *Ann DV 106:885–891, 1979*

Palmoplantar pustulosis *BJD 134:1079–1080, 1996*

Primary onycholysis (idiopathic or simple) *JAAD 70:793–794, 2014*

Pseudoporphyria – hemodialysis-related *Ann DV 117:723–725, 1990*

Psoriasis, including pustular psoriasis *Acta DV 80:209, 2000; psoriatic arthritis J Rheumatol 39:1441–1444, 2012*

PSYCHOCUTANEOUS DISEASES

Factitial

SYNDROMES

Amelo-onychohypohidrotic dysplasia (amelogenesis imperfecta and terminal onycholysis) *Oral Surg 39:71086, 1975*

CHILD syndrome – onychodystrophy *AD 142:348–351, 2006*

Cronkhite-Canada syndrome *Turk J Gastroenterol 24:277–285, 2013*

Hereditary onychodysplasia of the fifth toenails

Hereditary partial onycholysis associated with hard nails *Dermatol Wochenschr 152:766–768, 1966*

Hidrotic ectodermal dysplasia (Clouston syndrome)

J Dermatol March 27, 2020

Hypoplastic enamel-onycholysis-hypohidrosis (Witkop-Brearley-Gentry syndrome) – marked facial hypohidrosis, dry skin with keratosis pilaris, scaling and crusting of the scalp, onycholysis and subungual hyperkeratosis, hypoplastic enamel of teeth *Oral Surg 39:71–86, 1975*

Laryngo-onycho-cutaneous syndrome – autosomal recessive type of junctional epidermolysis bullosa; skin ulceration with prominent granulation tissue, early hoarseness and laryngeal stenosis; scarred nares; chronic erosion of corners of the mouth (giant perleche); paronychia with periungual inflammation and erosions; onycholysis with subungual granulation tissue and loss of nails with granulation tissue of the nail bed, conjunctival inflammation with polypoid granulation tissue, and dental enamel hypoplasia and hypodontia; only in Punjabi families; mutation in laminin alpha-3 (*LAMA3A*) *BJD 169:1353–1356, 2013; Ped Derm 23:75–77, 2006; Biomedica 2:15–25, 1986*

Leuko-onycholysis paradentotica (Schuppli syndrome)

Leprechaunism

Multicentric reticulohistiocytosis

Naegeli-Franceschetti-Jadassohn syndrome

Pachyonychia congenita

Partial hereditary onycholysis with scleronychia

PATEO syndrome *Acta Oncol 57:991–992, 2018*

Periodic shedding of the nails

Pseudoglucagonoma syndrome – periorificial erythema, crusted migratory plaques, hair loss, brittle nails, diarrhea, poor weight gain, onycholysis; associated with cirrhosis, celiac disease, inflammatory bowel disease, small cell lung cancers *Am J Med 126:387–389, 2013*

Reactive arthritis

Shell nail syndrome – clubbing with atrophy of underlying bone and nail bed *AD 96:694–695, 1967*

Yellow nail syndrome – bronchiectasis *Curr Opin Pulm Med 15:371–375, 2009; JAAD 22:605–611, 1990*

TRAUMA

Barber's hair sinus *Int J Dermatol 46:suppl 3:48–49, 2007*

French manicure – not onycholysis *Dermatol Online J Sept 16, 2014*

Infantile finger sucking *J Hand Surg Am 30:620–622, 2005*

Microwaves

Nail treatments

Physical trauma – overzealous manicure, water, occupational, leisure activities; housewife's onycholysis *Saudi Med J 26:1439–1441, 2005*

Playstation thumb *AD 142:1664–1665, 2006*

Pressure onycholysis – slaughterhouse workers *Acta DV Suppl 120:88–89, 1985*

Skier's toe *BMJ Case Rep 2009*

Thermal injury

VASCULAR DISEASES

Peripheral vascular disease with ischemia *Cutis 87:287–288, 2011; BJD 74:165–173, 1962*

Raynaud's disease

ORAL MUCOSAL HYPERPIGMENTATION

JAAD 16:431–434, 1987; Br Dent J 158:9–12, 1985

AUTOIMMUNE DISEASES AND DISEASES OF IMMUNE DYSFUNCTION

Graft vs. host disease *J Periodontol 74:552–556, 2003*

Lupus erythematosus – discoid lupus erythematosus; subacute cutaneous LE (SCLE) *Lupus 24:111–112, 2015*

CONGENITAL LESIONS

Congenital melanotic macules of the tongue *Ped Derm 32:109–112, 2015*

DRUGS

ACTH – soft palate, buccal mucosa, at sites of trauma *Br J Dent 158:297–305, 1985*

Amiodarone

Amlodipine *Saudi Med J 25:103–105, 2004*

Antimalarials *Oral Surg Oral Med Oral Pathol Oral Radiol Endod 90:189–194, 2000*; amodiaquine – blue-black; hydroxychloroquine *OSOMOPOR 124:e54–66, 2018*

Arsenic

Azathioprine *JAAD 56:828–834, 2007*

AZT (azidothymidine) *Am J Med 86:469–470, 1989*

Bismuth

Busulfan – brown hyperpigmentation

Capecitabine *Cureus March 30, 2018*

Chloroquine *JAAD 56:828–834, 2007*

Chlorpromazine – blue-black oral pigmentation *Clin in Derm 37:468–486, 2019*

Clofazimine – brown hyperpigmentation *JAAD 56:828–834, 2007*; blue-black oral pigmentation *Clin in Derm 37:468–486, 2019*

Cyclophosphamide *JAAD 56:828–834, 2007*

Doxorubicin *JAAD 56:828–834, 2007*

Estrogen – gingival hyperpigmentation *JAAD 56:828–834, 2007; J Am Dent Assoc 100:713–714, 1980*

5-Fluorouracil – mucosal hyperpigmentation *JAAD 71:203–214, 2014; JAAD 56:828–834, 2007*

Fixed drug eruption *Ped Derm 12:51–52, 1995; JAAD 17:399–402, 1987*

Gold – purplish-red hyperpigmentation

Hydroxyurea *Dermatol Online J Oct 15, 2019*

Imatinib – hard palate hyperpigmentation *JAAD 77:902–910, 2017*

Interferon alpha – treatment for chronic hepatitis C; melanonychia, facial hyperpigmentation, hyperpigmentation of the tongue and buccal mucosa *JAMADerm 149:675–677, 2013*

Ketoconazole *JAAD 56:828–834, 2007*

Mephenytoin

Minocycline – blue-gray staining of the gingiva *JAAD 56:828–834, 2007*; lip lentigines *JAAD 30:802–803, 1994*; gray pigmentation of teeth

Oral contraceptives *Cutis 48:61–64, 1991*

Oxabolone *Acta DV 75:158:1995*

Palifermin *Acta Hematol 124:185–187, 2010*

Premarin *Cutis 48:61–64, 1991*

Phenothiazines

Phenolphthalein

Plaquenil *JAAD 56:828–834, 2007*

Quinacrine *JAAD 56:828–834, 2007*

Quinidine – blue-black oral pigmentation *Clin in Derm 37:468–486, 2019*

Tetracycline teeth *Int J Dermatol 43:709–715, 2004*

Zidovudine – blue-black oral pigmentation *Clin in Derm 37:468–486, 2019*

EXOGENOUS AGENTS

Amalgam tattoos – silver, tin, mercury, copper, and zinc *JAAD 81:43–56, 2019; JAAD 56:828–834, 2007; AD 110:727–728, 1974*; gingival and tongue hyperpigmentation from silver amalgams *Quintessence Int 26:553–557, 1995*

Betel nut – chewing betel nut – gingival, oral mucosal, and dental hyperpigmentation – red to black *JAAD 37:81–88, 1998*

Bismuth salicylate – pseudo-black hairy tongue *Cutis 105:288, 293, 2020*

Blackberries

Blue grapes

Brass

Cadmium

Carbon tattoo

Chloracne – halogenated aromatic hydrocarbons – chloronaphthalenes, chlorobiphenyls, chlorobiphenyl oxides used as dielectrics in conductors and insulators, chlorophenols in insecticides, fungicides, herbicides, and wood preservatives *Am J Ind Med 5:119–125, 1989*

Chrome

Copper

Coloring agents

Contact mucositis

Dyes

Eritrean soot tattooing *AD 124:1018–1019, 1988*

Heavy metals – blue-black oral pigmentation *Clin in Derm 37:468–486, 2019*

Ink

Juglans regia – chewing bark of plant *Juglans regia*

Lead *JAAD 81:43–56, 2019; Oral Surg 52:143–149, 1981*

Manganese

Mercury *JAAD 43(pt 1)81–90, 2000; JAAD 5:1–18, 1981*

Phenolphthalein

Silver – gingival hyperpigmentation *JAAD 30:350–354, 1994*

Smoking (smoker's melanosis) *JAAD 81:43–56, 2019; J Natl Med Assoc 83:434–438, 1991; J Oral Pathol Med 20:8–12, 1991; AD 113:1533–1538, 1977*

Tattoos – intentional gingival tattoo *J Oral Med 41:130–133, 1986*; graphite tattoo *Oral Surg 62:73–76, 1986*

Tin

Tobacco chewing *Am J Med Sci 326:179–182, 2003*

INFECTIONS

Golden tongue syndrome – *Ramichloridium schulzeri*

HIV infection – *Ann DV 124:460–462, 1997; Oral Surg Oral Med Oral Pathol 70:748–755, 1990*

INFILTRATIVE LESIONS

Erdheim-Chester disease (non-Langerhans cell histiocytosis) – CD68+ and factor XIIIa+; negative for CD1a and S100; xanthoma and xanthelasma-like lesions (red-brown-yellow papules and plaques); flat wart-like papules of the face; lesions occur in folds; skin becomes slack with atrophy of folds and face; also lesions of eyelids, axillae, groin, neck; pretibial dermopathy, pigmented lesions of the lips and buccal mucosa; long bone sclerosis; diabetes insipidus, painless exophthalmos, retroperitoneal fibrosis, renal (hairy kidneys), cerebellar syndrome, and pulmonary histiocytic infiltration; differential diagnosis includes Graves' disease, Hashimoto's thyroiditis, sarcoid *J Cutan Pathol 38:280–285, 2011; Int J Urol 15:455–456, 2008; Austral J Dermatol 44:194–198, 2003; JAAD 57:1031–1045, 2007; AD 143:952–953, 2007; Hautarzt 52:510–517, 2001; Medicine (Baltimore) 75:157–169, 1996; Virchow Arch Pathol Anat 279:541–542, 1930*

INFLAMMATORY DISORDERS

Periodontitis – melanotic blue macules with periodontitis

Post-inflammatory hyperpigmentation *JAAD 81:43–56, 2019*

Sarcoid

METABOLIC DISEASES

Acromegaly

Addison's disease – spots or patches *JAAD 81:43–56, 2019; JAAD 56:828–834, 2007; Cutis 76:97–99, 2005; Cutis 66:72–74, 2000*; hyperpigmentation of the vermilion border of the lips, tongue, gingiva *Ped Derm 25:215–218, 2008*; gingival hyperpigmentation

Congenital erythropoietic porphyria – erythrodontia *Ped Derm 30:484–489, 2013*

Cushing's syndrome

Graves' disease – Addisonian hyperpigmentation; gingiva, buccal mucosa *JAAD 48:641–659, 2003*

Hemochromatosis – Addisonian hyperpigmentation of the oral mucosa *Clin Dermatol 23:457–464, 2005; AD 113:161–165, 1977*

Nelson's syndrome *J Oral Med 1:13–17, 1982*

Niemann-Pick disease – black macules

Ochronosis – hyperpigmentation of the buccal mucosa, nails

Porphyria

Thalassemia beta

Vitamin B12 deficiency *Clin Exp Dermatol 40:626–628, 2015; J Dermatol 28:54–57, 2001*

NEOPLASTIC DISORDERS

Blue nevus *Oral Surg Oral Med Oral Pathol 49:55–62, 1980*

Ephelis *JAAD 81:43–56, 2019*

Granular cell tumor *JAAD 56:828–834, 2007*

Kaposi's sarcoma – gingival hyperpigmentation

Labial melanotic macule *JAAD 81:43–56, 2019*

Lentigo maligna – hyperpigmented lips and oral mucosa *AD 138:1216–1220, 2002*

Melanoacanthoma in blacks – buccal mucosa *JAAD 81:43–56, 2019; JAAD 56:828–834, 2007; Oral Surg Oral Med Oral Pathol Oral Radiol Endod 84:492–494, 1997*; multiple pigmented macules of the gingiva *JAMADerm 153:1045–1046, 2017*; pigmented papule on maxillary labial gingival surfaces *Ped Derm 27:384–387, 2010*

Melanocytic nevus *JAAD 81:43–56, 2019; Cutis 86:89–93, 2010; JAAD 56:828–834, 2007; Oral Surg Oral Med Oral Pathol 49:55–62, 1980; Cancer 25:812–823, 1970*

Melanoma – black-brown to red-purple *JAAD 81:59–71, 2019; NEJM 372:1944, 2015; JAAD 71:366–375, 2014*; gingival *NEJM 369:1452, 2013; AD 144:558–560, 2008; JAAD 56:828–834, 2007; Oral Oncol 36:152–169, 2000; J Oral Maxillofac Surg 48:732–734,*

1990; Am J Surg 148:362–366, 1984; Oral Surg Oral Med Oral Pathol 36:701–706, 1973; Cancer 25:812–823, 1970; misdiagnosed as racial pigmentation Dermatopathol (Basel) 26:1–7, 2016

Melanotic macule (ephelis, lentigo) – vermilion of the lips, gingiva, buccal mucosa, palate Oral Surg Oral Med Oral Pathol 48:244–249, 1979; congenital melanocytic macule of the tongue Ped Derm 32:536–538, 2015

Melanotic neuroectodermal tumor of infancy (pigmented neuroectodermal tumor of infancy) blue-black oral pigmentation Clin in Derm 37:468–486, 2019

Nevus of Ota (nevus fuscoceruleus ophthalmomaxillaris) J Med Case Reports 13:174, 2019; BJD 67:317–319, 1955

Pigmented mucoepithelioid carcinoma Int J Surg Pathol 13:295–297, 2005

PARANEOPLASTIC DISEASES

Acanthosis nigricans, malignant JAAD 42:357–362, 2000

Ectopic ACTH (bronchogenic carcinoma) – soft palate hyperpigmentation Oral Surg 41:726–733, 1976

Peutz-Jeghers-like mucocutaneous pigmentation – associated with breast and gynecologic carcinomas in women Medicine (Baltimore) 79:293–298, 2000

PHOTOSENSITIVITY DISORDERS

Melasma

PRIMARY CUTANEOUS DISEASES

Acanthosis nigricans World J Surg Oncol 15:208, 2017

Ashy dermatosis (erythema dyschromicum perstans) An Bras Dermatol 92(suppl 1)17–20, 2017

Becker's nevi, segmental Ped Derm 29:670–671, 2012

Benign melanotic macules JAAD 56:828–834, 2007

Black hairy tongue

Epidermal choristoma (hamartoma of the epidermis of the tongue) – hyperpigmented macule of the tongue; mimics congenital melanocytic macule of the tongue Ped Derm 32:536–538, 2015

Focal melanosis JAAD 56:828–834, 2007

Idiopathic lenticular mucocutaneous pigmentation AD 132:844–845, 1996

Lentiginosis in blacks

Generalized lentiginosis

Lentigo

Lichen planus Int J Derm 32:76, 1993; lichen planus pigmentosus Dermatologica 162:61–3, 1982; J Pharm Bioallied Sci 7(suppl 2) S495–498, 2015

Oral melanotic macules – 1 cm or less; young white women; lip, hard palate, tongue, buccal mucosa (mucosal melanotic macule) OSOMOPOR Endod 112:e21–25, 2011

Physiologic pigmentation – benign racial pigmentation JAAD 81:43–56, 2019; OSOMOPOR Endod 105:606–616, 2008; Clin Dermatol 18: 579–587, 2000

Pigmented fungiform papillae of the tongue AD 140:1275–1280, 2004; JAMA 45:588–594, 1905

Racial oral pigmentation – gingiva, hard palate, buccal mucosa, tongue JAAD 71:1030–1033, 2014; J Prosthet Dent 4:392–396, 1980

SYNDROMES

Albright's syndrome JAMADerm 15):760–763; J Med Genetics 48:458–461, 2011

Bandler syndrome – autosomal dominant; perioral, oral hyperpigmented macules; pigmentation of the hands and nails; associated with intestinal vascular malformations JAAD 62:171–173, 2010

Carney complex (LAMB, NAME syndrome) – oral lentigines common NEJM 370:2229–2236, 2014; JAAD 56:828–834, 2007; JAAD 46:161–183, 2002; Oral Surg 63:175–183, 1987

Centrofacial lentiginosis BJD 94:39–43, 1976

Dyskeratosis congenita

Fanconi's anemia – autosomal recessive; endocrine abnormalities with hypothyroidism, decreased growth hormone, diabetes mellitus, café au lait macules, diffuse hyperpigmented macules, guttate hypopigmented macules, intertriginous hyperpigmentation, skeletal anomalies (thumb hypoplasia, absent thumbs, radii, carpal bones), oral/genital erythroplasia with development of squamous cell carcinoma, hepatic tumors, microphthalmia, ectopic or horseshoe kidney, broad nose, epicanthal folds, micrognathia, bone marrow failure, acute myelogenous leukemia, solid organ malignancies (brain tumors, Wilms' tumor) BJD 164:245–256, 2011; JAAD 54:1056–1059, 2006; black hyperpigmentation of the buccal mucosa, tongue, and palate SADJ 63:O28–31, 2008

Incontinentia pigmenti

Laugier-Hunziker syndrome AD 143:631–633, 2007; J Dermatol 28:54–57, 2001; Cutis 42:325–326, 1988

LEOPARD syndrome – oral hyperpigmentation is unusual JAAD 56:828–834, 2007; Clin Dysmorphol 16:277–278, 2007; Ped Derm 21:139–145, 2004

Nelson's syndrome

Neurofibromatosis

Peutz-Jeghers syndrome JAAD 81:43–56, 2019; NEJM 370:2229–2236, 2014; JAAD 56:828–834, 2007; JAAD 53:660–662, 2005

Pseudoxanthoma elasticum

Wilson's disease – most common of the inner lower lip; yellow white streaks OSOMOPOR 121:E6–9, 2016; Case Rep Dermatol 2013:490785 Ann DV 135:183–186, 2008

Xeroderma pigmentosum JAAD 75:855–870, 2016

X-linked adrenoleukodystrophy – mutations in ABCD1; generalized hyperpigmentation with accentuation of elbows, knees, and gingivae and palate; accumulation of long-chain fatty acids; adrenal insufficiency, myelopathy, cerebral demyelinization BJD 182:239–240, 2020

TOXINS

Arsenic Dermatol Clinics 29:45–51, 2011

TRAUMA

Leukokeratosis/leukedema

Mechanical trauma

Radiation therapy *Oral Surg Oral Med Oral Pathol 77:431–434, 1994*

Tobacco smoking – irritation; smoker's palate, smoker's melanosis *Am J Med 326:179–182, 2003; J Oral Pathol Med 22:228–230, 1993*

VASCULAR DISORDERS

Bleeding diathesis

Blue rubber bleb nevus

Facial port-wine stain – red-stained gums *JAAD 67:687–693, 2012*

Thrombosed varix

ORAL MUCOSA, BLUE PIGMENTATION

AUTOIMMUNE DISEASES AND DISEASES OF IMMUNE DYSFUNCTION

Systemic lupus erythematosus

DRUG-INDUCED

Amiodarone *Circulation 113:d63, 2006*

Antimalarials *Oral Surg Oral Med Oral Pathol Oral Radiol Endod 90:189–194, 2000*; amodiaquine – blue-black

Argyria *Cutis 89:221–224, 2012; Med Clin (Barc) 73:386–388, 1979*

Arsenic

Bismuth *AD 129:474–476, 1993*

Chlorpromazine *Clin in Derm 37:468–486, 2019*

Clofazimine *JAAD 17:867–871, 1987*

Doxorubicin

Estrogen *Cutis 48:61–64, 1991*

Gold (chrysiasis) *BJD 133:671–678, 1995*

Haloperidol *Clin in Derm 37:468–486, 2019*

Hydroxychloroquine *OSOMOPORE 90:189–194, 2000*

Imatinib *Int J Dermatol 57:784–790, 2019*

Ketoconazole *Clin in Derm 37:468–486, 2019*

Metoclopramide *Clin in Derm 37:468–486, 2019*

Minocycline – blue-gray staining of the gingiva *Br Dent J 215:71–73, 2013; J Clin Periodontol 32:119–122, 2005*

Mitoxantrone *Clin in Derm 37:468–486, 2019*

Oral contraceptives *Clin in Derm 37:468–486, 2019*

Quinidine *AD 122:1062–1064, 1986*

Risperidone

Retigabine (ezogabine) *BMC Oral Health 15:122, 2015*

Steroid atrophy

Tetracycline *Clin in Derm 37:468–486, 2019*

Zidovudine

EXOGENOUS AGENTS

Amalgam tattoo *Quintessence Int 23:805–810, 1992; J Am Dent Assoc 110:52–54, 1985; Oral Surg 49:139–147, 1980*

Arsenic *Clin Dermatol 37:468–486, 2019*

Bismuth *Clin Dermatol 37:468–486, 2019*

Black and blue dye *Clin in Derm 37:468–486, 2019*

Ethnobotanical *Clin in Derm 37:468–486, 2019*

Graphite tattoo *Oral Surg 62:73–76, 1986*

India ink *Clin in Derm 37:468–486, 2019*

Lead intoxication (Burtonian line) – blue-black line along the gingival margin *J Pharm Bioallied Sci 7(suppl2)S403–408, 2015; AD 129:474–476, 1993*

Mercury intoxication *AD 122:1062–1064, 1986*

Tattoo – metal tattoo from dental instruments

METABOLIC

Addison's disease *Ped Derm 9:123–125, 1992*

Hemochromatosis *OSOMOP 33:186–190, 1972*

Methemoglobinemia *BMJ Case Rep 2012: Am J Med Sci 353:603–604, 2017*

Ochronosis *J Cut Med Surg 16:357–360, 2012*

NEOPLASTIC

Angioleiomyoma *Gen Dent 52:53–54, 2004*

Blue nevus *Oral Surg Oral Med Oral Pathol 49:55–62, 1980*; cellular blue nevus *Cutis 80:189–192, 2007*

Diffuse melanosis cutis *JAAD 68:482–488, 2013*

Kaposi's sarcoma *J Nat Sci Biol Med 6:459–461, 2015; JAAD 38:143–175, 1998; Dermatology 190:324–326, 1995*

Lentigo maligna

Leukemia – chloroma *AD 123:251–256, 1987*

Lymphoma

Melanocytic neuroectodermal tumor of infancy *Clin in Derm 37:468–486, 2019*

Melanocytic nevi *J Oral Pathol Med 19:197–201, 1990*

Melanotic macule *JAAD 44:1048–1049, 2001*

Melanoma *J Assoc Physicians India 60:50–53, 2012; Oral Oncol 36:152–169, 2000; Oral Surg Oral Med Oral Pathol 36:701–706, 1973*; diffuse melanosis of metastatic melanoma

Melanotic neuroectodermal tumor of infancy (odontoameloblastoma) – pigmented oral mass of early infancy – blue or black *Braz Dent J 29:400–404, 2018; Acta Pathol Jpn 39:465–468, 1989; Cancer 22:151–161, 1968*

Mucocele *J Oral Maxillofac Surg 69:1086–1093, 2011*

Mucocele of the sublingual gland (ranula) *J Oral Maxillofac Path 18(suppl1):S72–77, 2014*

Mucoepidermoid carcinoma – blue-red nodule *JAAD 81:59–71, 2019*

Nevus of Ota (nevus fuscoceruleus ophthalmomaxillaris) *J Med Case Rep 13:174, 2019; BJD 67:317–319, 1955*

Oral cyst

PRIMARY CUTANEOUS DISEASES

Lichen sclerosus et atrophicus – bluish-white plaques of the mouth

SYNDROMES

Albright's syndrome

Blue rubber bleb nevus syndrome *Arch Neurol 38:784–785, 1981*

Hemoglobin M disease *Bull Yamaguchi Med Sch 14:141, 1967*

Hereditary acrolabial telangiectasias *AD 115:474–478, 1979*

Maffucci's syndrome (enchondromatosis) – enchondromas and multiple venous malformations; spindle cell hemangioendothelioma; oral and intra-abdominal venous and lymphatic anomalies; short stature, shortened long bones with pathologic fractures; enchondromas undergo sarcomatous change in 30–40%; breast, ovarian, pancreatic, parathyroid, pituitary tumors *JAAD 56:541–564, 2007; Ped Derm 17:270–276, 2000; Ped Derm 12:55–58, 1995*

Neurofibromatosis

Niemann-Pick disease – Mongolian spots of the skin and oral mucosa

Peutz-Jeghers syndrome *Romanian J Morph Embryol 49:241–245, 2008*

Pseudoxanthoma elasticum

TRAUMA

Hematoma *Clin in Derm 37:468–486, 2019*

VASCULAR DISEASES

Cyanosis *Isr Med Assoc J 3:286–287, 2001*

Hemangioma *Pediatr Dent 35:E75–78, 2013*

Hemangiosarcoma

Intravascular papillary endothelial hyperplasia *Oral Dis 5:175–178, 1999*

Lymphangioma

Malignant angioendotheliomatosis *JAAD 18:407–412, 1988*

Sublingual varices

Varicosity *Clin in Derm 37:468–486, 2019*

Vascular malformation *JAAD 81:43–56, 2019*

ORAL MUCOSA, CYSTS

Ped Derm 1:301–306, 1984

CONGENITAL ANOMALIES

Alimentary duplication cyst of the floor of the mouth *Z Kinderchir 41:45–48, 1986*

Bohn's nodules – yellowish-white keratinous cysts of the alveolar ridge

Branchial cyst

Branchiogenic cyst, pseudocyst

Dermoid cyst of the floor of the mouth *Ped Derm 25:308–311, 2008*

Epstein's pearls (palatal cysts) – yellowish-white keratinous cysts in midline of junction of the hard and soft palate *Stat Pearls Aug 17, 2019; JAAD 23:77–81, 1990*

Eruption cyst, congenital – fluctuant swelling; blue-red to black translucent, elevated compressible over alveolar ridge; overlie teeth about to erupt; epithelial cyst of the oral mucosa on the gingival margin *Ped Derm 27:671–672, 2010; Braz Dent J 21:259–262, 2010*

Gingival cyst of the newborn *J UOEHS:163–168, 1983; Am J Dis Child 116:44–48, 1968*

Ranula – mucocele of the anterior floor of the mouth *J Clin Pediatr Dent 34:263–266, 2010*

EXOGENOUS AGENTS

Dermal filler injection *Br Dent J 227:281–284, 2019*

INFECTIONS AND INFESTATIONS

Cysticercosis *Oral Surg Oral Med Oral Pathol Oral Radiol Endod 79:572–577, 1995*

INFILTRATIVE LESIONS

Oral focal mucinosis *Int J Oral Maxillofac Surg 19:337–340, 1990*

INFLAMMATORY DISEASES

Sarcoid

NEOPLASTIC DISEASES

Cystic choristomas (teratoid cyst) *J Oral Maxillofac Surg 71:1706–1711, 2013; Pediatr Pathol 12:835–838, 1992*

Dental lamina cyst – on crest of the alveolar ridge

Dentigerous cyst

Dermoid cyst of the floor of the mouth (sublingual) *Med J Armed Forces India 71(supp2)S389–394, 2015*

Epidermoid cyst *Med Oral Pathol Oral Cir Bucal l19:e308–312, 2014; Oral Surg Oral Med Oral Pathol 67:181–184, 1989*

Gingival cyst of adult *Gen Dent 65:42–44, 2017*

Heterotopic intestinal cyst – most lined with gastric mucosa and involve the tongue *Korean J Pathol 47:279–283, 2013*

Hydatid cyst (*Echinococcus* tapeworm) *Indian J Dent 6:157–160, 2015*

Kaposi's sarcoma

Lipoma of the floor of the mouth

Lymphoepithelial cysts of the floor of the mouth (sublingual) *Indian J Pathol Microbiol 6:473–474, 2013*

Lymphoma, MALT type *J Pediatr Surg 46:2414–2416, 2011*

Mucocele of the lip, tongue – on labial mucosa, ventral surface of the tip of the tongue, buccal mucosa, floor of the mouth *Ped Derm 32:647–650, 2015; Ped Derm 25:308–311, 2008; Oral Surg Oral Med Oral Pathol Oral Radiol Endod 88:469–472, 1999*; congenital oral mucous extravasation cysts *Pediatr Dent 21:285–288, 1999*

Nasolabial cyst in buccal mucosa *Indian J Dent Res 30:957–959, 2019*

Neurilemmoma of the tongue

Odontogenic keratocyst of the buccal mucosa *SAGE Open Med Case Rep May 19, 2019*

Palatine papilla cyst

Salivary duct cyst *J Oral Maxillofac Pathol 23:429–431, 2019; Head Neck Pathol 11:469–476, 2017*

Salivary gland cyst *Compendium 12:150, 152, 154–156, 1991*

Salivary gland tumor

Sialolithiasis

Sublingual gland cysts

Thyroglossal duct cyst of the dorsum of the tongue

VASCULAR LESIONS

Cystic hygroma of the floor of the mouth *Ped Derm 25:308–311, 2008*

Hemangioma of the floor of the mouth *Ped Derm 25:308–311, 2008*

ORAL MUCOSA, NODULES

AUTOIMMUNE DISEASES AND DISEASES OF IMMUNE DYSFUNCTION

Angioedema

Rheumatoid nodule *J Oral Maxillofac Surg 72:1532, 2014; J Oral Pathol 16:403–405, 1987*

CONGENITAL LESIONS

Bohn's nodules – buccal and lingual sides of alveolar ridges

Dermoid cyst *Case Rep Pathol 2014;389752; Plast Reconstr Surg 11:1560–1565, 2003*

Developmental cysts

Epstein's pearls

Epulis (congenital epulis) – soft nodule of the gingival margin of the maxillary ridge; tumor of granular cells; 10 female:1 male; differential diagnosis includes infantile hemangioma, lymphatic malformation, fibroma, rhabdomyoma, heterotopic gastrointestinal cysts *Ped Derm 28:577–578, 2011; J Oral Surg 30: 30–35, 1972*

Fibrous developmental malformation of maxillary tuberosities

Lingual thyroid *NEJM 358:1712, 2008; Dermatol Clin 21:157–170, 2003; Br J Oral Surg 24:58–62, 1986*

Lingual tonsil – on posterior third of the tongue *Dermatol Clin 21:157–170, 2003; J Laryngol Otol 103:922–925, 1989*

Odontomas *Case Rep Dent 2015:835171*

DRUGS

Gingival hyperplasia secondary to phenytoin, cyclosporine, nifedipine

Oral contraceptive – pill gingivitis

Hypertrophy of fungiform papillae of the tongue – after transplant *Ped Derm 8:194–198, 1991*

EXOGENOUS AGENTS

Denture-induced granuloma (epulis fissuratum) – buccal or labial vestibule *J Oral Pathol 10:65–80, 1981*

Filler cosmetic injections – granulomatous foreign body reaction with intraoral migration *J Am Geriatr Soc 62:587–588, 2014; OSOMOPOR 117:105–110, 2014*

Foreign body, including body piercing (sarcoid-like) *Oral Surg Oral Med Oral Pathol Oral Radiol Endod 84:28–31, 1997*; tongue nodule *AD 142:385–390, 2006*

Pulse granuloma – embedded vegetables *Br J Oral Surg 23:346–350, 1985*

INFECTIONS

Abscess of the buccal mucosa

Actinomycosis; abscess *Br J Oral Surg 27:249–253, 1989*

Aspergillosis – aspergilloma

Bacillary angiomatosis – vascular papules or nodules on the gingiva, palate, or floor of the mouth *J Oral Pathol 22:235–239, 1993*

Bartonella henselae-related pseudoangiomatous papillomatosis of the tongue accompanying graft vs. host disease; yellow-pink pseudomembranous pedunculated vegetations of the tongue *BJD 157:174–178, 2007*

Cysticercosis (*C. cellulosae*) (larval form of *Toxocara solium*) – papulonodules, subcutaneous cysts, cysts in skeletal muscles, mucous membranes, seizures (neurocysticercosis) *JAAD 75:19–30, 2016*; intraoral solitary nodule *Natl J Maxillofac Surg 7:209–212, 2016*

Epstein-Barr virus infection – mucocutaneous lymphocytic infiltration *Dermatologica 183:139–142, 1991*

Filariasis *Contemp Clin Dent 4:254–257, 2013*

Gongylonema pulchrum – parasite of pigs, bears, hedgehogs, monkeys – migratory nodules of the pharynx

Herpes zoster – tongue nodule

Histoplasmosis – oral mucosal nodules; tongue nodule *Cutis 55:104–106, 1995*

Human papillomavirus – buccal filiform white papules *JAMADerm 151:1359–1363, 2015*

Infectious mononucleosis (Epstein-Barr virus) – pedunculated papule of the tongue (lymphoid hyperplasia) *JAAD 67:e113–114, 2012*

Leishmaniasis – post-kala-azar dermal leishmaniasis – papules of the cheeks, chin, ears, extensor forearms, buttocks, lower legs; in India, hypopigmented macules; nodules develop after years; tongue, palate, genitalia *E Afr Med J 63:365–371, 1986*; New World leishmaniasis – gingival yellow papules *Ped Derm 24:657–658, 2007*; ulcerated oral nodules *Gerodontology 29:e1168–1171, 2012*

Leprosy – lepromatous leprosy – palate, uvula, tongue, gingivae; histoid nodules of the lip *Int J Lepr Other Mycobact Dis 65:374–375, 1997*

Molluscum contagiosum *OSOMOPOR 114:E57–60, 2012; OSOMOP 72:334–336, 1991*

Mycobacterium tuberculosis – lupus vulgaris; starts as red-brown plaque, vegetative and ulcerative lesions of the buccal mucosa, palate, gingiva, oropharynx *Int J Dermatol 26:578–581, 1987; Acta Tuberc Scand 39(Suppl 49):1–137, 1960*

Nocardiosis – abscess

North American blastomycosis *Gen Dent 50:561–564, 2002; OSOMOP 47:157–160, 1979*

Onchocerciasis *Oral Surg Oral Med Oral Pathol 62:560–563, 1986*

Oroya fever with verruga peruana – *Bartonella bacilliformis*; red papules in crops become nodular, hemangiomatous, or pedunculated; face, neck, extremities, mucosal lesions *Ann Rev Microbiol 35:325–338, 1981*

Paracoccidioidomycosis (South American blastomycosis) (*Paracoccidioides brasiliensis*) – oral and perioral lesions; mulberry-like ulcerated swellings *JAAD 53:931–951, 2005; Oral Surg 75:461–465, 1993; Oral Surg 72:430–435, 1991*

Talaromyces (Penicillium) marneffei – pharyngeal papules *JAAD 49:344–346, 2003*; umbilicated papules *Curr Opin Infec Dis 13:129–134, 2000*

Rhinoscleroma – *Klebsiella rhinoscleromatis* (Frisch bacillus) exudative stage with rhinorrhea; then proliferative stage with exuberant friable granulation tissue of the nose, pharynx, larynx; progresses to nodules; then fibrotic stage *Acta Otolaryngol 105:494–499, 1988; Cutis 40:101–103, 1987*

Rhinosporidium seeberi

Syphilis – secondary syphilis with tongue nodules *NEJM 368:561, 2013; JAAD 54:S59–60, 2006*; mucosal-colored papules of the anterior tongue *Oral Surg Oral Med Oral Pathol 45:540–542, 1978*; red plaque of the hard palate *AD 147:869–870, 2011*; granulomatous secondary syphilis – personal observation; tertiary – gumma – white nodule of the hard palate

Wart (papilloma) *Oral Surg 65:526–532, 1988*

INFILTRATIVE DISORDERS

Amyloidosis; solitary intraoral amyloid *Ann Otol Rhinol Laryngol 101:794–796, 1992*; red nodule of the tongue in primary systemic amyloidosis *AD 126:235–240, 1990*; multiple nodules of the buccal mucosa *Contemp Clin Dent 6(suppl 1:)S282–284, 2015*

Juvenile colloid milium – eyelids, nose, gingiva, conjunctiva *Clin Exp Dermatol 25:138–140, 2000*

Juvenile xanthogranuloma *BJD 144:909–911, 2001; AD 135:707–712, 1999*; tongue nodule *Am J Otolaryngol 20:241–244, 1999; JAAD 36:355–367, 1997*

Langerhans cell histiocytosis *Curr Prob Dermatol 14:41–70, 2002*

Lichen myxedematosus – oral papules

Progressive nodular histiocytosis *JAAD 57:1031–1045, 2007; BJD 143:628–631, 2000*

Verruciform xanthoma of the tongue or gingiva – pale, red, or keratotic surface *Oral Surg 51:619–625, 1981; Oral Surg 49:429–434, 1980*

Xanthoma disseminatum *NEJM 338:1138–1143, 1998*; disseminated verruciform xanthoma *BJD 151:717–719, 2004; Oral Surg Oral Med Oral Pathol 31:784–789, 1971*; tongue papules *Ped Derm 22:550–553, 2005*

INFLAMMATORY DISORDERS

Acute gingivitis – oral papular eruption *AD 120:1451–1455, 1984*

Acute lymphonodular pharyngitis

Crohn's disease – gingival nodules *JAAD 36:697–704, 1997; Oral Surg 49:131–138, 1980*; pseudopolyps of the buccal mucosa (mucosal tags) *AD 135:439–442, 1999*

Fistula granuloma – at opening of the duct of the dental fistula

Necrotizing sialometaplasia *AD 122:208–210, 1986*

Nodular fasciitis *Br J Oral Surg 27:147–151, 1989*

Orofacial granulomatosis – facial edema with swelling of the lips, cheeks, eyelids, forehead, mucosal tags, mucosal cobbling, gingivitis, oral aphthae *BJD 143:1119–1121, 2000*

Parotitis – acute suppurative parotitis *Arch Otolaryngol Head Neck Surg 118:469–471, 1992*

Peripheral giant cell granuloma *Contemp Clin Dent 2:41–44, 2011*

Pseudolymphoma – palatal nodule *Oral Surg 55:162–168, 1983*

Sarcoid – nodules, ulcers, mostly solitary *BMJ Case Rep Dec 1, 2019; JAAD 77:809–830, 2017; QJM 105:755–767, 2012; J Oral Surg 34:237–244, 1976*; tongue papules *JAAD 66:699–716, 2012*

METABOLIC DISEASES

Calcinosis – gingival calcified nodule *OSOMOP 73:472–475, 1992*; calcified nodule of the buccal mucosa *B-ENT 7:215–218, 2011*

Gout – tophus *Am J Pathol 32:871–895, 1956; AD 134:499–504, 1998*

Hyperparathyroidism, primary – brown giant cell tumor of the palate

Osteitis fibrosa (renal osteodystrophy) – nodule of the hard palate *NEJM 359:74, 2008*

Tangier disease – yellow-orange tonsils and adenoids *Pediatr Int 56:777–779, 2014*

Verrucous xanthoma *Oral Oncol 37:326–331, 2001; AD 117:563–565, 1981*

Xanthomas – eruptive xanthomas

NEOPLASTIC DISORDERS

Acanthoma, pale (clear) cell of the palate *Head Neck Pathol June 22, 2019*

Acinar cell carcinoma, buccal mucosa *Gen Dent 56:e43–45, 2008; Quintessence Int 38:289–294, 2007*

Adenocarcinoma of the minor salivary gland

Adenocarcinoma of the palate

Adenoid cystic carcinoma – palatal nodule *JAAD 81:59–71, 2019*

Adenoid squamous cell carcinoma

Angiofibroma *J Cut Aesthet Surg 74:227–228, 2014; Med Oral Path Oral Cir Bucal 13:e540–543, 2008*

Angiomyoma – bluish-purple color *Int J Health Sci (Qassim)13:47–49, 2019*

Basal cell carcinoma

Benign fibrous histiocytoma *JAAD 41:860–862, 1999*; of the tongue

Benign lymphoepithelial tumor *Int J Oral Maxillofac Surg 45:1626–1629, 2016*

Blastic plasmacytoid dendritic cell neoplasm – vascular plaque under the tongue; violaceous plaque of the posterior pharynx *BJD 169:579–586, 2013*

Canalicular adenomas *Oral Surg Oral Med Oral Pathol Oral Radiol Endod 87:346–350, 1999*

Carcinoma of the parotid gland duct

Cartilaginous choristoma – tongue nodule *AD 143:653–658, 2007*; buccal mucosa *Br J Plast Surg 36:395–397, 1983*; soft palate *Oral Surg Oral Med Oral Pathol 26:601–604, 1968*; gingival *Ann Dent 53:19–27, 1994*

Chloroma (granulocytic sarcoma) – swollen maxilla *Br J Oral Surg 26:124–128, 1988*

Chondrosarcoma *Anticancer Res 32:3345–3350, 2012*

Clear cell adenocarcinoma *Med Mol Morphol 50:117–121, 2017; J Laryngol Otol 116:851–853, 2002*

Cutaneous epithelioid sarcoma-like hemangioendothelioma – gingival papule *AD 149:459–465, 2013*

Cysts, developmental

Dental lamina cyst – on crest of the alveolar ridge

Dermatofibrosarcoma protuberans *JAAD 41:860–862, 1999*

Epidermal nevus (verrucous nevus) – red papules of the uvula, soft palate, and gingiva *AD 141:515–520, 2005*

Epidermoid cyst *J Maxillofac Oral Surg 12:90–93, 2013*

Epithelioid sarcoma of the tongue *J Clin Pathol 50:869–870, 1997;* of the gingiva *OSOMOPOR Endod 111:e25–28, 2011*

Fibroepithelial hyperplasia *Oral Surg Oral Med Oral Pathol 46:34–39, 1978*; multifocal *Int J Appl Basic Med Res 9:253–255, 2019*

Fibroepithelial polyp *Periodontics 6:277–299, 1986*

Fibrofolliculomas, Birt-Hogg-Dube syndrome

Solitary fibrous tumor of the oral cavity (fibroma) *J Oral Pathol Med 49:14–20, 2020*

Fibrosarcoma *JAAD 41:860–862, 1999*; of the tongue

Fibromatosis of the tongue – aggressive tumor of musculoaponeurotic tissue *Oral Surg Oral Med Oral Pathol Oral Radiol Endod 100:e31—34, 2005*

Fibrous hyperplasia of the tongue *AD 142:385–390, 2006*

Giant cell epulis *J Oral Surg 27:787–791, 1969*

Giant cell fibroma – mucosal-colored papule; of the tongue *AD 143:1583–1588, 2007; Oral Surg Oral Med Oral Pathol 37:374–384, 1974*; on the mandibular gingiva or buccal mucosa *AD 143:1583–1588, 2007*

Gingival fibromatosis

Granular cell tumor of the gingiva (congenital epulis) *Ped Derm 18:234–237, 2001; Ped Derm 15:318–320, 1998*; of the tongue (Abrikossoff tumor) *JAAD 60:537–538, 2009; AD 142:385–390, 2006*

Inclusion cysts in newborn, dental lamina cysts *J Med Case Rep Sept 21, 2014*

Kaposi's sarcoma – usually on the palate *JAMA 313:514–515, 2015; JAAD 59:179–206, 2008*; red, purple, brown, or bluish nodule *NEJM 346:1207–1210, 2002; JAAD 41:860–862, 1999; JAAD 38:143–175, 1998; Dermatology 190:324–326, 1995; Oral Surg 71:38–41, 1991*

Keratin-filled pseudocysts of sebaceous gland ducts of the vermilion border *J Oral Pathol 3:279–283, 1974*

Keratoacanthoma; *AD 120:736–740, 1984*; tongue papules – eruptive KAs *JAAD 29:299–304, 1993*

Leiomyoma – tongue or palate; pedunculated congenital leiomyoma of the tongue *Int J Pediatr Otorhinolaryngol 29:139–145, 1994*

Leiomyosarcoma *JAAD 41:860–862, 1999*

Leukemia – violaceous plaque of the oral mucosa *Cutis 104:326–330, 2019*; macrocheilia *Cutis 64:46–48, 1999*; gingival enlargement *K Oral Maxillofacial Pathol 22(suppl 1)S77–81, 2018*

Lipoma *Head Neck Surg 3:145–168, 1980*

Lymphoepithelial carcinoma *Head Neck Pathol 5:327–334, 2011*

Lymphoepithelial cysts of the oral mucosa *Oral Surg Oral Med Oral Pathol 35:77–84, 1973*

Lymphoma – nodules (occasionally ulcerated) – pharynx, palate, tongue, gingiva, lips; cutaneous T-cell lymphoma *Oral Surg 75:700–705, 1993*; non-Hodgkin's lymphoma in AIDS *NEJM 311:565–570, 1984*; Epstein-Barr virus-associated lymphoma *Tyring, p. 155, 2002*; primary cutaneous CD30+ lymphoproliferative disorder (CD8+/CD4+) – tongue nodule *AD 142:385–390, 2006; JAAD 51:304–308, 2004*; Epstein-Barr virus-associated plasmablastic lymphoma (HIV-defining lesion) *Oral Oncol 38:96–102, 2013*

Lymphomatoid papulosis – tongue nodule *Am J Dermatopathol 20:522–526, 1998*; ulcerated nodules *Acta DV 93:250–251, 2013*

Malignant fibrous histiocytoma *JAAD 41:860–862, 1999*

Carcinoma ex-pleomorphic adenoma *Rare Tumors 8:6138, 2016; Ann Diagn Pathol 19:164–168, 2015*

Mandibular tori – personal observation

Maxillary antral carcinoma

Melanoma *JAMADerm 151:797–798, 2015*; desmoplastic melanoma *JAAD 41:860–862, 1999*; amelanotic melanoma *AD 138:1607–1612, 2002*

Melanotic neuroectodermal tumor of infancy (odontoameloblastoma) – pigmented oral mass of early infancy *Can J Plast Surg 16:41–44, 2008; J Oral Maxillogac Surg 65:1595–1599, 2007; Acta Pathol Jpn 39:465–468, 1989; Cancer 22:151–161, 1968; Beitr Pathol Anat 82:165–169, 1918*; gingival and maxillary mass in 7-month-old *AD 146:337–342, 2010*; gingival nodule *Ped Derm 29:633–636, 2012*

Differential diagnosis of rapidly growing mass of the anterior maxilla in an infant: *AD 146:337–342, 2010*

Congenital epulis
Ewing sarcoma
Lymphoma
Melanoma
Melanotic neuroectodermal tumor
Metastatic retinoblastoma
Neuroblastoma
Rhabdomyosarcoma
Teratoma

Metastatic carcinoma – breast, lung, kidney, stomach, liver *J Maxillofac Surg 10:253–258, 1982*; metastatic chondrosarcoma *J Periodontol 62:223–226, 1991*; metastatic hepatocellular carcinoma – vascular nodule mimicking pyogenic granuloma *JAAD 49:342–343, 2003*

Mucocele

Mucoepidermoid carcinoma *OSOMOPOR 121:576–582, 2016*

Mucosal horn of the tongue

Multiple idiopathic mucocutaneous neuromas *BJD 145:826–829, 2001*

Myeloma *Oral Surg 57:267–271, 1984*

Myofibroma – skin-colored to hyperpigmented nodules of the hand, mouth, genitals, shoulders *JAAD 46:477–490, 2002*

Myxoma *J Clin Diagn Res 8:KD 01–02, 2014*

Nerve sheath tumors (oral neural tumors) *J Clin Exp Dent 11:e721—731, 2019; JAAD 41:860–862, 1999*

Neurofibroma of the tongue *AD 142:385–390, 2006*

Neuroma (mucosal neuroma) – palisaded encapsulated neuroma *AD 140:1003–1008, 2004*; solitary, circumscribed *J Dent (Shiraz)18:314–317, 2017*

Neurothekeoma *Case Reports Otolaryngol 2016:4709753; JAAD 50:129–134, 2004*

Nevus sebaceus with intraoral fibroepitheliomatous nodules *Oral Surg 34:774–780, 1972*

Odontogenic cysts

Odontogenic tumors (odontomas)

Osteoma mucosae (osseous choristoma) *J Med Case Rep March 17, 2016; OSOMOP 72:337–339, 1991*

Osteosarcoma *Quintessence 44:783–791, 2013*; sclerosing epithelioid fibrosarcoma *Head Neck Pathol 1:13–20, 2007*

Papillary cystadenoma lymphomatosum – of the salivary gland, lip, buccal mucosa, and palate *Oral Maxillofac Surg 17:161–164, 2013*

Papilloma

Peripheral ossifying fibroma *AD 143:1583–1588, 2007*

Plasmacytoma *Cancer 43:2340–2343, 1979*

Pleomorphic adenoma of the minor salivary gland of the hard palate *AD 144:1077–1078, 2008*

Pterygoid hamulus – a hook-shaped bony process on each medial pterygoid plate of the sphenoid bone, rare intraoral pain syndrome (bursitis) *J Craniofac Surg 30:e643–645, 2019*

Reactive fibrous papule of the oral mucosa (giant-cell fibroma) – fingers and palms *Oral Surg Med Pathol 37:374–384, 1974*; giant cell fibroma of the tongue

Recurrent infantile digital fibromatosis – tongue papule *Am J Surg Pathol 8:787–790, 1984*

Reticulohistiocytoma *BJD 62:351–355, 1984*

Rhabdomyoma *Br J Oral Surg 23:284–291, 1985; Oral Surg 48:525–531, 1979*

Rhabdomyosarcoma *Med Oral Patol Oral Cir Bucal 11:e136–140, 2006; Oral Surg 64:585–596, 1987*

Salivary gland tumors

Sarcoma

Schwannoma – of the tongue; gingival nodule *AD 144:689–690, 2008*; palatal nodule *Gen Dent 65:58–61, 2017*

Sialolithiasis *J Clin Diagn Res 10:ZD06–07, 2016*

Spindle cell carcinoma

Squamous cell carcinoma *J Oral Maxillofac Surg 53:144–147, 1995; Oral Oncol 31B:16–26, 1995; Crit Rev Oncol Hematol 21:63–75, 1995*; tongue nodule *NEJM 369:2437, 2013*; squamous cell carcinoma in oral lichen planus *BJD 169:106–114, 2013*; verrucous carcinoma in oral lichen planus *Indian J Dent Res 29:525–528, 2018*

Submucosal nodular chondrometaplasia *J Prosth Dent 54:237–240, 1985*

Verrucous carcinoma – oral florid papillomatosis *Int J Derm 18:608–622, 1979; JAAD 14:947–950, 1986; JAAD 32:1–21, 1995*

Warty dyskeratoma – papule or nodule of the gingiva, palate, alveolar ridge *Int J Dermatol 23:123–130, 1984; AD 116:929–931, 1980*

PARANEOPLASTIC DISEASES

Necrobiotic xanthogranuloma with IgA paraproteinemia – painful oral nodules and hoarseness *Am J Dermatopathol 12:579–584, 1990*

PRIMARY CUTANEOUS DISEASES

Acanthosis nigricans – papillomatosis *Am J Dermatopathol 10:68–73, 1988*

Angiolymphoid hyperplasia with eosinophilia (epithelioid hemangioma) – oral nodule *JAAD 74:506–512, 2016*; of the tongue *JAAD 11:333–339, 1984*; multiple red nodules *Slep Arth Celok Lek 144:535–540, 2016*

Epidermolysis bullosa *Oral Surg Oral Med Oral Pathol 40:385–390, 1975*

Epulis fissuratum *Dermatol Online J Aug 15, 2010*; osteoma of the maxilla presenting as epulis fissuratum *J Dent Res Dent Clinic Dent Prospects 7:177–181, 2013*

Foliate lingual papilla

Heck's disease – lip and tongue papules; HPV-13 or HPV-32 *Ped Derm 33:91–92, 2016*

Kimura's disease (angiolymphoid hyperplasia with eosinophilia) – papules and/or nodules *BJD 145:365, 2001; JAAD 43:905–907, 2000; BJD 134:744–748, 1996*; epithelioid hemangioma (angiolymphoid hyperplasia with eosinophilia) *Oral Oncol 35:435–438, 1999; BJD 134:744–748, 1996*

Lingual thyroid *NEJM 358:1712, 2008*

Median rhomboid glossitis *AD 135:593–598, 1999*

Occluded sublingual duct – personal observation

Parotid papillae

Polyp of the lingual frenulum – personal observation

Sialolith *OSOMOPOR Endod 100:345–348, 2005*; hard nodule lower lip *NTS Dent J 75:40–42, 2019*

Torus mandibularis; maxillaris *Cutis 71:350, 363, 2003; Scand J Dent Res 94:233–240, 1986*

Torus palatinus *Compend Contin Educ Dent 6:149–152, 1985*

Unerupted teeth

SYNDROMES

Birt-Hogg-Dube syndrome – oral fibromas of the lips, gingiva, tongue, buccal mucosa *JAAD 74:231–244, 2016; JAAD 50:810–812, 2004*

Blue rubber bleb nevus syndrome *Case Rep Dermatol 7:194–198, 2015; Br J Oral Surg 26:160–164, 1988*

Byars-Jurkiewicz syndrome – gingival fibromatosis, hypertrichosis, fibroadenomas of the breast

Carney complex (NAME/LAMB) – oral myxomas of the palate or tongue *Oral Surg 63:175–183, 1987; JAAD 10:72–82, 1984*

Cowden's disease – lipomas, angiolipomas, tongue papillomas *JAAD 11:1127–1141, 1984; AD 106:682–690, 1972*; lip and gingival papillomas *BJD 160:1116–1118, 2009*

Cross syndrome – gingival fibromatosis with hypopigmentation, seizures, and mental retardation *Clin Genet 51:118–121, 1997*

Farber's disease (lipogranulomatosis) – lysosomal acid ceramidase deficiency (*N*-acylsphingosine amidohydrolase) (chromosome 8p22-21.2); deformed or stiff joints with painful limb contractures and red periarticular subcutaneous nodules (proximal and distal interphalangeal joints, wrist, elbow, knees, ankles, metatarsals), and progressive hoarseness; rarely nodules seen in conjunctivae, nostrils, ears, mouth; heart, liver, spleen, lung; progressive psychomotor retardation *Ped Derm 26:44–46, 2009; Eur J Ped 157:515–516, 1998; AD 130:1350–1354, 1994*

Focal epithelial hyperplasia (Heck's disease) – multiple pink lip, gingival, hard palate, and buccal mucosal papules; tongue papule; cobblestoned appearance; common in native Americans and Eskimo populations; HPV-13 or HPV-32; *Ped Derm 26:465–468, 2009; Ped Derm 26:87–89, 2009; Oral Surg Oral Med Oral Pathol 20:201–212, 1965*

Gardner's syndrome – osteoma of the mandible *Int J Med Sci 9:137–41, 2012; Pathol Int 5f4:523–526, 2004*

Hereditary gingival fibromatosis; with ear, nose, bone, nail defects, and hepatosplenomegaly; with progressive deafness; with hypertrichosis *Orphanet J Rare Dis Jan 17, 2016*

Goltz's syndrome (focal dermal hypoplasia) – asymmetric linear and reticulated streaks of atrophy and telangiectasia; yellow-red nodules; raspberry-like papillomas of the lips, perineum, acrally, buccal mucosa; xerosis; scalp and pubic hair sparse and brittle; short stature; asymmetric face; syndactyly, polydactyly; ocular, dental, and skeletal abnormalities with osteopathia striata of long bones *JAAD 25:879–881, 1991*

Hereditary gingival fibromatosis – autosomal dominant *Oral Surg 78:452–454, 1994*

Hereditary hemorrhagic telangiectasia (Osler-Weber-Rendu syndrome) – red vascular papules of the tongue *JAMA 312:741–742, 2014*

Hereditary mucoepithelial dysplasia – papules of the palate or gingiva *JAAD 21:351–357, 1989*

Hereditary progressive mucinous histiocytosis – yellow dome-shaped papules of the face, gingiva, hard palate *BJD 141:1101–1105, 1999*

Juvenile hyaline fibromatosis – gingival enlargement *Oral Surg 63:71–77, 1987*

Klippel-Trenaunay-Weber syndrome – hemangiomas of the buccal mucosa and tongue *Oral Surg 63:208–215, 1987*

Laband syndrome – gingival fibromatosis, aplasia or dysplasia of fingernails, hypertrophy of the nasal tip and ears, hypermobility

Laryngo-onycho-cutaneous syndrome (Shabbir syndrome) – autosomal recessive; symblepharon, crusted erosions of elbows, anonychia with granulation tissue of the nail bed, mucosal nodule of the hard palate; hoarse cry and laryngeal stenosis, chronic granulation tissue, conjunctival inflammation with polypoid granulation tissue, tooth enamel hypoplasia; laminin alpha 3A mutation (*LAMA 3A*) with N-terminal deletion of LAMA 3A *Ped Derm 24:306–308, 2007; Ped Derm 23:75–77, 2006; Cornea 20:753–756, 2001; Arch Dis Child 70:319–326, 1994; JAAD 29:906–909, 1993; Clin Dysmorphol 1:3–14, 1992; Eye 5:717–722, 1991; Biomedica 2:15–25, 1986*

Lipoid proteinosis – sublingual papules *AD 144:1383–1388, 2008;* oral mucosa nodules *J Clin Ped Dent 33:171–174, 2008*

Maffucci's syndrome – intraoral hemangioma *Oral Surg 57:263–266, 1984*

Multicentric reticulohistiocytosis *Clin Rheumatol 15:62–66, 1996*

Multiple endocrine neoplasia syndrome (MEN I) – gingival papules *JAAD 42:939–969, 2000*

Multiple endocrine neoplasia type 2B syndrome – autosomal dominant; papules of eyelids, lips, and tongue; medullary carcinoma of the thyroid, mucosal neuromas, intestinal ganglioneuromas, marfanoid body habitus; RET proto-oncogene *NEJM 364, 870, 2011*

Multiple mucosal neuroma syndrome (MEN IIB) (Gorlin's syndrome) (Wagenmann-Froboese syndrome) – skin-colored papules of the cheeks and nodules of the lips, tongue, oral mucosa (buccal mucosa, gingiva, palate, pharynx); medullary carcinoma of the thyroid; adrenal medulla pheochromocytoma; eversion of the lips and eyelids, widened nasal base; marfanoid features; RET proto-oncogene *JAMADerm 152:939–940, 2016; NEJM 373:756, 2015; NEJM 364:870, 2011; Ped Derm 25:477–478, 2008; JAAD 55:341–344, 2006; Curr Prob Derm 14:41–70, 2002; Am J Med 31:163–166, 1961*

Neurofibromatosis – papillomatous tumors of the palate, buccal mucosa, tongue, and lips *J Dent Child 47:255–260, 1980*

Nevoid basal cell carcinoma syndrome – intraoral malignancies – fibrosarcoma, ameloblastoma, squamous cell carcinoma *Br J Oral Surg 25:280–284, 1987*

Olmsted syndrome – white papules of the tongue *Ped Derm 10:376–381, 1993;* rare genodermatosis; leukokeratosis of the oral mucosa; rare periodontal disease *Odontology 103:241–245, 2015*

Oral-facial-digital syndrome type 1 (Papillon-Leage-Psaume syndrome) – X-linked dominant; congenital facial milia which resolve with pitted scars; milia of the face, scalp, pinnae, and dorsal hands; short stature, hypotrichosis with dry and brittle hair, short upper lip, hypoplastic ala nasi and lower jaw, pseudoclefting of the upper lip, hooked pug nose, hypertrophied labial frenulae, bifid or multilobed tongue with small white tumors within clefts, ankyloglossia, multiple soft hamartomas of the oral cavity, clefting of the hard and soft palate, teeth widely spaced with dental caries, trident hand or brachydactyly, syndactyly, clinodactyly, ulnar deviation of the index finger, or polydactyly; hair dry and brittle, alopecic, numerous milia of the face, ears, backs of the hands, mental retardation with multiple central nervous system abnormalities, frontal bossing, hypertelorism, telecanthus, broad depressed nasal bridge; polycystic renal disease; combination of polycystic renal disease, milia, and hypotrichosis is highly suggestive of OFD1 *Ped Derm 27:669–670, 2010; JAAD 59:1050–1063, 2008; Ped Derm 25:474–476, 2008; Ped Derm 9:52–56, 1992; Am J Med Genet 86:269–273, 1999; JAAD 31:157–190, 1994; Ped Derm 9:52–56, 1992; Pediatrics 29:985–995, 1962; Rev Stomatol 55:209–227, 1954*

PTEN-hamartoma-tumor syndrome – mucocutaneous neuromas *AD 142:625–632, 2006*

Ramon syndrome – cherubism, gingival fibromatosis, epilepsy, mental deficiency, hypertrichosis, and stunted growth

Rutherford syndrome (congenital hypertrophy of the gingiva (fibromatosis), altered eruption of teeth, and corneal dystrophy)

Tuberous sclerosis – fibromatous nodules (oral fibromas) of gums and palate *Ped Derm 32:563–570, 2015; JAAD 56:786–790, 2007; Oral Med Oral Surg Oral Pathol 39:578–582, 1975*

Xeroderma pigmentosum – squamous cell carcinoma of the tongue *JAAD 12:515–521, 1985*

TRAUMA

Acanthoma fissuratum secondary to dentures

Herniation of the buccal fat pad *Int J Ped Otolaryngol 38:175–179, 1996; J Oral Surg 24:265–268, 1986*

Irritation hyperplasia – mucosal-colored papule of the buccal mucosa in elderly *AD 143:1583–1588, 2007;* denture-induced granuloma

Papillary hyperplasia of the palate *Br Dent J 118:77–80, 1965*

Post-extraction granuloma *J Indian Soc Periodontol 23:580–583, 2019*

Post-traumatic spindle cell nodule *Oral Oncol 36:121–124, 2000*

VASCULAR DISORDERS

Angiokeratoma circumscriptum – tongue lesions *Ped Derm 20:180–182, 2003*

Angioleiomyoma *JAAD 38:143–175, 1998*

Glomus tumors *J Dermatol 27:211–213, 2000*

Granulomatosis with polyangiitis *OSOMOPOR Endod 85:153–157, 1998;* and strawberry gingivae and palatal perforation

Hematoma *OSOMOPOR 121:576–582, 2016*

Infantile hemangioma *Otolaryngol Clin North Am 19:769–796, 1986;* of the tongue *AD 142:385–390, 2006*

Hemangiopericytoma *JAAD 41:860–862, 1999*

Hemolymphangioma – red papules of the tongue *JAAD 52:1088–1090, 2005*

Hereditary hemorrhagic telangiectasia – red papules of the tongue in patients with hemiparesis due to brain abscess *JAMA 312:741–742, 2014*

Lymphangioma (cystic hygroma) *Head Neck Pathol Dec 10, 2019*

Phlebolith

Polyarteritis nodosa – submucosal oral nodules along the path of vessels *Oral Surg 56:597–601, 1983*

Pyogenic granuloma, including pregnancy tumor *Br J Oral Surg 24:376–382, 1986*; tongue nodule *JAAD 58:S52–53, 2008*

Spindle cell hemangioendotheliomas *Cutis 62:23–26, 1998*; epithelioid hemangioendothelioma – painless solitary mass *Oral Dis 13:244–250, 2007*

Tufted angioma – red or blue papule of the labial mucosa *BJD 142:794–799, 2000*; blue papule of the floor of the mouth

Vascular malformation *OSOMOPOR 121:578–582, 2016*

ORAL MUCOSA, ULCERATION

AUTOIMMUNE DISEASES AND DISEASES OF IMMUNE DYSFUNCTION

Allergic contact stomatitis to propolis *AD 134:511–513, 1998*; allergic contact stomatitis to dental materials (mercuric chloride, copper sulfate) *Contact Dermatitis 27:157–160, 1992*

Antiepidermal growth factor receptor antibody C225 – aphthae *BJD 144:1169–1176, 2001*

Antineutrophil cytoplasmic antibody syndrome – purpuric vasculitis, orogenital ulceration, fingertip necrosis, pyoderma gangrenosum-like ulcers *BJD 134:924–928, 1996*

Aphthous stomatitis – minor, major, herpetiform

Brunsting-Perry cicatricial pemphigoid – scalp erosions, bullae, oral bullae and ulcers, scarring alopecia *BJD 170:743–745, 2014*

Bullous disease with IgA vs. collagen VII and IgG vs. laminin 332 – urticarial plaques and bullae and oral erosions *BJD 167:938–941, 2012*

Bullous pemphigoid; anti-p200 and anti-alpha3 chain of laminin 5 – lip ulcers *JAAD 52:S90–92, 2005*; anti-p200 bullous pemphigoid – oral ulcers *JAMADerm 152:897–904, 2016*; *BJD 160:462–464, 2009*; bullous pemphigoid associated with renal allograft rejection *JAAD 65:217–219, 2011*

C4 deficiency and intraoral herpes simplex virus type 1 *Clin Inf Dis 33:1604–1607, 2001*

Chediak-Higashi syndrome – oral ulcers, gingivitis *BJD 178:335–349, 2018*

Chronic granulomatous disease – perioral and/or intraoral ulcers *JAAD 36:899–907, 1997*; *AD 130:105–110, 1994*; DLE-like lesions and stomatitis in female carriers *BJD 104:495–505, 1981*; *Oral Surg Oral Med Oral Pathol 46:815–819, 1978*

Chronic ulcerative stomatitis with stratified epithelium-specific ANA *JAAD 22:215–220, 1990*

Cicatricial pemphigoid (mucous membrane pemphigoid) – desquamative gingivitis, oral ulcers *Ped Derm 36:953–954, 2019*; *JAAD 77:795–806, 2017*; *BJD 174:436–438, 2016*; *JAAD 64:1199–1200, 2011*; *Acta DV 89:101–102, 2009*; *AD 138:370–379, 2002*; *JAAD 43:571–591, 2000*; *J Periodontol 71:1620–1629, 2000*; *BJD 118:209–217, 1988*; *Oral Surg 54:656–662, 1982*; anti-laminin 332 mucous membrane pemphigoid – lip ulcers *BJD 165:815–822, 2011*; palatal ulcers *Clin Dermatol 32:817–826, 2014*; anti-laminin gamma 1 and anti-laminin 332 mucous membrane pemphigoid – lip erosions, nasal erosions, conjunctival erosions, scrotal ulcers *BJD 171:1257–1259, 2014*; gingival erosions – antibodies to alpha6-beta4 integrin *BJD 171:1555–1556, 2014*

Common variable immunodeficiency *J Oral Pathol Med 22:157–158*

Deficiency of interleukin-1 receptor antagonist (DIRA) (IL-1 receptor deficiency) – loss-of-function mutation of *IL1RN*; neutrophilic pustular dermatosis with confluent pustules and lakes of pus; infantile pustulosis and exfoliative erythroderma; oral ulcers, joint swelling; periostitis, aseptic multifocal osteomyelitis; increased acute

phase reactants *Ped Derm 30:758–760, 2013*; *AD 148:747–752, 2012*; *NEJM 360:2426–2437, 2009*

Dermatitis herpetiformis *AD 134:736–738, 1998*; *Oral Surg 62:77–80, 1986*

Dermatomyositis*; Update 33:94–96, 1986*; oral ulcers; tender hyperkeratotic palmar papules in palmar creases of fingers with central white coloration; dermatomyositis with MDA-5 (CADM-40) (melanoma differentiation-associated gene 5) MDA 5 – RNA-specific helicase; all with interstitial lung disease; ulcers of nail folds, Gottron's papules, and elbows; these patients demonstrate hair loss, hand edema, arthritis/arthralgia, diffuse hair loss, punched-out ulcers of the shoulder or metacarpophalangeal joints, digital necrosis, erythema of elbows and knees (Gottron's sign), and tender gingiva *JAAD 78:776–785, 2018*; *JAAD 65:25–34, 2011*

Epidermolysis bullosa acquisita *BJD 157:417–419, 2007*; *AD 135:954–959, 1999*; *Ped Derm 12:16–20, 1995*; *AD 123:772–776, 1987*

Food sensitivities

Good syndrome – adult acquired primary immunodeficiency in context of past or current thymoma; sinopulmonary infections; lichen planus, oral lichen planus of the tongue, gingivitis, oral erosions *BJD 172:774–777, 2015*; *Am J Med Genet 66:378–398, 1996*

Graft vs. host reaction – acute graft vs. host reaction *Biol Blood Marrow Transplant 20:1717–1721, 2014*; *AD 120:1461–1465, 1984*; chronic *JAAD 38:369–392, 1998*; *AD 134:602–612, 1998*

Herpes gestationes – IgA herpes gestationes *JAAD 47:780–784, 2002*

Hyper-IgD syndrome – combination of periodic fever, arthritis, and rash; annular erythema and pustules; oral aphthae (ulcers); morbilliform eruption, urticaria red macules or papules, red nodules, urticaria myositis, myalgias; urticarial plaques; lymphadenopathy; abdominal pain, vomiting, diarrhea; arthralgias; recurrent transient and fixed pink plaques and nodules of the face and extremities; cephalic pustulosis; mevalonate kinase deficiency *Ped Derm 35:482–485, 2018*; *AD 136:1487–1494, 2000*; *Ann DV 123:314–321, 1996*; *AD 130:59–65, 1994*

IgA pemphigus – oral and perianal ulcers *Cutis 80:218–220, 2007*; *JAAD 20:89–97, 1989*

IgG4-related disease *J Clin Pathol 68:802–807, 2015*

Immunoglobulin deficiency with hyper-IgM and neutropenia (hyper-IgM immunodeficiency syndromes, hypogammaglobulinemia with hyper-IgM – ulcers of the palate, tongue, buccal mucosa, and lips; *JAAD 38:191–196, 1998*

Leukocyte adhesion deficiency (beta 2 integrin deficiency) (congenital deficiency of leukocyte-adherence glycoproteins (CD11a (LFA-1), CD11b, CD11c, CD18)) – necrotic cutaneous abscesses, cellulitis, skin ulcerations (pyoderma gangrenosum-like ulcer), gingivitis, periodontitis, septicemia, ulcerative stomatitis, pharyngitis, otitis, pneumonia, peritonitis; delayed separation of umbilical stump and omphalitis *JAAD 72:1066–1073, 2015*; *JAAD 31:316–319, 1994*; *BJD 139:1064–1067, 1998*; *J Pediatr 119:343–354, 1991*; *BJD 123:395–401, 1990*; *Ann Rev Med 38: 175–194, 1987*; *J Infect Dis 152:668–689, 1985*

Lichenoid reactions with antibodies to desmoplakins I and II – ulcers of the hard palate and tongue *JAAD 48:433–438, 2003*

Linear IgA disease – desquamative gingivitis *JAAD 77:795–806, 2017*; *J Periodontol 74:879–882, 2003*; lip erosions, oropharyngeal ulcers *Ped Derm 26:28–33, 2009*; *Oral Surg Oral Med Oral Pathol Oral Radiol Endo 88:196–201, 1999*; *JAAD 22:362–465, 1990*; mimicking Stevens-Johnson syndrome *BJD 178:786–789, 2018*

Linear IgA/IgG bullous dermatosis – dyshidrosiform bullae of the palms, herpetiform bullae, cutaneous erosions, tongue erosions *JAMADerm 149:1308–1313, 2013*

Lupus erythematosus – systemic lupus erythematosus – lesions of the palate, buccal mucosa, gums; red or purpuric areas with red halos break down to form shallow ulcers *BJD 135:355–362, 1996; BJD 121:727–741, 1989*; bullous dermatosis of SLE (annular bullae) – face, neck, upper trunk, oral bullae *JAAD 77:795–806, 2017; JAAD 27:389–394, 1992; Ann Int Med 97:165–170, 1982; Arthritis Rheum 21:58–61, 1978*; discoid lupus erythematosus *BJD 121:727–741, 1989*; subacute cutaneous lupus erythematosus – palatal ulcers *Med Clin North Am 73:1073–1090, 1989; JAAD 19:1957–1062, 1988*; drug-induced lupus with C1q deficiency *BJD 142:521–524, 2000*; aphthous ulcers *JAAD 57:S38–41, 2007*

Mixed connective tissue disease – orogenital ulcers *Am J Med 52:148–159, 1972*

Mucous membrane pemphigoid *Sem Cut Med Surg 34:171–177, 2015; NEJM 369:265–274, 2013*

Neutropenia – cyclic, chronic benign or idiopathic neutropenia *J Pediatr 129:551–558, 1996*; autoimmune cyclic neutropenia *AD 132:1399–1400, 1996*; congenital neutropenia *BJD 178:335–349, 2018*; cyclic neutropenia – oral aphthae, gingivitis, weakness, fever, sepsis, diarrhea, gangrenous enterocolitis *Ped Derm 20:519–523, 2003; Ped Derm 18:426–432, 2001; Am J Med 61:849–861, 1976; JAAD 57:538–541, 2007*; chronic benign neutropenia interdental ulcers in leukopenic patients

Pemphigus foliaceus (anti-Dsg 1 positive, anti-Dsg 3 negative) – oral ulcers *BJD 166:976–980, 2012*

Pemphigus vegetans, Neumann type – giant cobblestoning with vegetative intertriginous plaques and blisters; oral bullae *JAMA 314:2296–2297, 2015; AD 145:715–720, 2009*

Pemphigus vulgaris *Sem Cut Med Surg 34:171–177, 2015; JAMADerm 151:878–882, 2015; Clin Dermatol 31:374–381, 2013; JID 132:776–784, 2012; BJD 166:154–160, 2012; BJD 161:313–319, 2009; BJD 156:352–356, 2007; Acta Odontol Scand 40:403–414, 1982; AD 110:862–865, 1974*; palatal ulcers *Clin Dermatol 32:817–826, 2014*; gingival ulcers *JAAD 77:795–806, 2017*

Periodic fever, immunodeficiency, and thrombocytopenia – severe oral ulcers leading to scarring and microstomy; fever, poor growth, infections, thrombocytopenia *Ped Derm 33:602–614, 2016*

Rheumatoid arthritis with Felty's syndrome

Selective IgA deficiency

Severe combined immunodeficiency *J Clin Immunol 11:369–377, 1991*; severe combined immunodeficiency in Athabascan American-Indian children; deep punched-out oral ulcers of the neonate *AD 135:927–931, 1999*

Sjögren's syndrome *Postepy Dermatol Alergol 33:23–27, 2016*

X-linked agammaglobulinemia – oral ulcers, oral leukokeratosis *BJD 178:335–349, 2018*

CONGENITAL LESIONS

Congenital palatal ulcers associated with cleft lip and palate *Cleft Palate Craniofac J 33:262–263, 1996*

Noma neonatorum – deep ulcers with bone loss, mutilation of the nose, lips, intraorally, anus, genitalia; *Pseudomonas*, malnutrition, immunodeficiency

DEGENERATIVE DISEASES

Neurotrophic ulcer; palatal ulcer *Proc Finn Dent Soc 72:23–26, 1976*; trigeminal neurotrophic ulcer *Arch Stomatol (Napoli) 30:1197–1208, 1989*

DRUG-INDUCED

Alendronate – osteonecrosis of the mandible; halitosis, hypesthesia of the lower lip, submental sinus; necrosis of the mandible underlying gingiva *NEJM 367:551, 2012; J Oral Pathol Med 29:514–518, 2000*

Amitriptyline

Aspirin burn

Beta-blockers – aphthous ulcers *BJD 143:1261–1265, 2000*

Bisphosphonate-related osteonecrosis of the jaw – gingival ulceration *AD 146:1301–1306, 2010*; palatal ulcer *Clin Dermatol 32:817–826, 2014*; stomatitis *NEJM 25:355, 2006*; oral ulcer *Dermatology 232:117–121, 2016*; alendronate oral ulcers *J Oral Maxillofac Surg 70:830–836, 2012*

Bleomycin *JAAD 40:367–398, 1999*

Calcium channel blockers *J Am Dent Assoc 130:1611–1618, 1999*

Captopril *Ann Int Med 94:659, 1981*

Cefaclor

Cancer chemotherapeutic agents – stomatitis with ulceration; actinomycin D, Adriamycin, amsacrine, bleomycin, busulfan, chlorambucil, cyclophosphamide, dactinomycin, daunorubicin, doxorubicin, fluorouracil, IL-2, mercaptopurine, methotrexate, mithramycin, mitomycin, nitrosoureas, procarbazine, vincristine *JAAD 40:367–398, 1999; NCI Monogr (9):61–71, 1990; Semin Dermatol 8:173–181, 1989; Oral Surg Oral Med Oral Pathol 63:424–428, 1987*; chemotherapy-induced neutropenia *Int J Paed Dentistry 2:73–79, 1992*

Cetuximab (epidermal growth factor receptor inhibitor) *BJD 161:515–521, 2009*

Chlorpromazine

Corticosteroids – inhaled *Respir Med 88:159–160, 1994*

ddC in AIDS *JAAD 21:1213–1217, 1989*

Doxepin

Doxorubicin *Dermatol Clin 21:1–15, 2003*

DRESS (drug reaction with eosinophilia and systemic symptoms) syndrome – cheilitis, facial edema, exanthem, erythroderma, oral erosions *BJD 169:1071–1080, 2013*

Drug reactions

Emepromium bromide *Lancet 30:1442, 1972*

Epidermal growth factor inhibitors – oral aphthae; stomatitis *JAAD 72:203–218, 2015; JAAD 55:657–670, 2006*

Ergotamine tartrate in temporal arteritis – tongue ulcer *AD 130:261–262, 1994*

Erlotinib (epidermal growth factor receptor inhibitor) *BJD 161:515–521, 2009*

Estrogen

5-BUDR *JAAD 21:1235–1240, 1989*

5-Fluorouracil, capecitabine, tegafur – stomatitis *JAAD 71:203–214, 2014*

Fixed drug eruption *Ped Derm 36:531–532, 2019*

Foscarnet *JAAD 27:124–126, 1992*

Gold *JAAD 16:845–854, 1987; Quintessence Int 18:703–706, 1987; Oral Surg 58:52–56, 1984*

Hepatitis B vaccine *Ann Derm Vener 123:657–659, 1996*

Hydralazine

Hydroxyurea *JAAD 36:178–182, 1997*; oral erythema *AD 135:818–820, 1999*

Idelalisib *Int J Dermatol 56:e180–181, 2017*

IL-2 – aphthous ulcers *JAMA 258:1624–1629, 1987*

Imipramine

Imiquimod – intraoral aphthous ulcers when imiquimod applied to lip *JAAD S35–37, 2005*

Indomethacin *J Am Dent Assoc 90:632–634, 1975*

Interferon alpha *M I Med 158:126–127, 1993*

Lithium

Losartan *Clin Nephrol 50:197, 1998*

6-Mercaptopurine (6-MP)

Methotrexate – oral ulcers *JAAD 77:247–255, 2017; Cancer Chemother Pharmacol 2:225–226, 1979*; methotrexate lip necrosis *JAAD 77:247–255, 2017; Cutis 92:121–124, 2013*; palatal ulcer *Clin Dermatol 32:817–826, 2014*

Methyldopa

mTOR inhibitors – rapamycin, everolimus, temsirolimus – stomatitis, rash *JAAD 72:221–236, 2015*

Mycophenolate mofetil *JAAD Case Reports 1:261–263, 2015; Transpl Proc 39:612–614, 2007; Transplantation 77:1911–1912, 2004*

Naproxen

Narcotics – palatal ulcers *Clin Dermatol 32:817–826, 2014*

Nicorandil *JAAD 56:S116–117, 2007; BJD 138:712–713, 1998; Eur J Dermatol 7:132–133, 1997*

Nivolumab (PD-1 inhibitor) *JAMADerm 153:235–237, 2017*

Nonsteroidal anti-inflammatory drugs – erosive lichenoid eruptions *Oral Surg Oral Med Oral Pathol 64:541–543, 1987*

Nortriptyline *Mental Health Clinic 8:309–312, 2018*

Pralatrexate mucositis – personal observation

Pellagrous dermatitis – carbamazepine, phenobarbital, hydantoins, INH, 6-mercaptopurine, azathioprine, 5-fluorouracil, chloramphenicol, ethionamide, protionamide; aphthous ulcers and fissured cheilitis *JAAD 67:1113–1127, 2012; JAAD 46:597–599, 2002*

Pembrolizumab-induced mucous membrane pemphigoid – tongue ulcers, oral ulcers *BJD 179:993–994, 2018*

Penicillamine *JAAD 8:548, 1983; Oral Surg 45:385–395, 1978*

Potassium – slow-release tablets *Br Med J Oct 19;4(5937):164–165, 1974*

Prochlorperazine – lip ulceration

Sorafenib – severe mucositis *BJD 161:1045–1051, 2009*

Sunitinib – multikinase inhibitor; bullous palmoplantar erythrodysesthesia, periungual erythema, perianal erythema, severe mucositis *AD 144:123–124, 2008*

Tacrolimus

Tetracycline *Ann Pharmacother 30:547–548, 1996*

Valproic acid

Vancomycin – linear IgA disease *JAAD 48:S56–57, 2003*; oral bullae *Cutis 73:65–67, 2004*

Zalcitabine *JAAD 46:284–293, 2002*

Zomepirac

EXOGENOUS AGENTS

Acrylic resin burn

Amalgam *Br J Dent 160:434–437, 1986*; lichenoid amalgam reaction *Ped Derm 26:458–464, 2009*

Antiseptics

Betel chewing *Cutis 71:307–311, 2003; J Oral Pathol Med 27:239–242, 1998*

Bone marrow transplantation *Bone Marrow Transplant 4:89–95, 1989*

Cementation of adhesive bridges – sublingual ulceration *Dent Update 23:389–390, 1996*

Cinnamon dermatitis *Ped Derm 26:458–464, 2009*

Cocaine abuse – palatal perforation *JAAD 59:483–487, 2008; Otolaryngol Head Neck Surg 116:565–566, 1997*

Cyanamide *JAAD 23:1168–1169, 1990*

Denture cleanser tablets – mucosal injury *Oral Surg Oral Med Oral Pathol Oral Radiol Endod 80:756–758, 1995*

Ecstasy *J Craniofac Surg 30:e189–191, 2019*

Foreign bodies

Gluten-sensitive recurrent oral ulceration without gastrointestinal abnormalities *J Oral Pathol Med 20:476–478, 1991*

Hydrogen peroxide *J Periodontol 57:689–692, 1986*

Irritant contact stomatitis

Marijuana vaping *Ped Derm 37:347–349, 2020*

Oral hygiene products *NEJM 347:429–436, 2002*

Orthodontic

Phenol

Silver nitrate

Smokeless tobacco

Smoking cessation *Press Med 25:2043, 1996*

Stem cell transplantation *J Clin Oncol 19:2201–2205, 2001*

INFECTIONS AND INFESTATIONS

Abscess – palatal necrosis – personal observation

Acanthamebiasis in AIDS *AD 131:1291–1296, 1995*

Actinomycosis – ulcerated plaque of the palate and gingiva *JAAD 65:1135–1136, 2011*; necrotic oral plaques *Ped Derm 29:519–520, 2012*

AIDS – HIV infection; acute retroviral syndrome – oral erythema with palatal and buccal erosions *Sem Cut Med Surg 34:171–177, 2015; AD 138:117–122, 2002; AD 134:1279–1284, 1998*

Aphthae of AIDS – major aphthae *BJD 142:171–176, 2000*; HIV gingivitis/periodontitis *Oral Dis 3Suppl 1:S141–148, 1997*; linear gingival erythema of HIV; necrotizing stomatitis

Anthrax – ingestion of contaminated meat *Clin Inf Dis 19:1009–1014, 1994*

Aspergillosis – invasive aspergillus stomatitis in acute leukemia (*Aspergillus flavus*); gingival ulcer with or without necrosis of the alveolar bone *Clin Inf Dis 33:1975–1980, 2001*; rhinocerebral aspergillus with palatal necrosis *Clin Dermatol 32:817–826, 2014; Periodontol 49:39–59, 2009*

Bejel – primary chancre *J Oral Maxillofac Surg 49:532–534, 1991*

Calymmatobacterium granulomatis (donovanosis) *J Clin Inf Dis 25:24–32, 1997*

Cancrum oris (noma) – *Fusobacterium necrophorum, Prevotella intermedia Am J Trop Med Hyg 60:150–156, 1999; Br J Plast Surg 45:193–198, 1992; Cutis 39:501–502, 1987; S Afr Med J 46:392–394, 1972*

Candidiasis *Mycoses 53:168–172, 2010*

Capnocytophaga canimorsus

Cat scratch disease

Chancroid

Chikungunya fever – oral aphthae *Ped Derm 35:408–409, 2018; JAAD 75:1–16, 2016*

Coccidioidomycosis – palatal ulcers; intraoral ulcers *JAAD 77:197–218, 2017; Clin Dermatol 32:817–826, 2014*; tongue ulcer *Arch Pathol Lab Med 129:4–6, 2005*

Cowpox – tongue ulcer, targetoid and umbilicated indurated papules, vesicles, pustules with central necrosis; exposure to pet rat *Clin Inf Dis 68:1063–1064, 2019*

Coxsackie B5

Cryptococcosis *Oral Surg Oral Med Oral Pathol 64:449–453,454–459, 1987*; stellate ulcerated plaque of the hard palate *AD 144:1651–1656, 2008; Periodontol 49:39–59, 2000*

Cytomegalovirus *Dermatology 200:189–195, 2000; J Oral Pathol Med 24:14–17, 1995; Oral Surg Oral Med Oral Pathol 77:248–253, 1994; JAAD 18:1333–1338, 1988; Oral Surg 64:183–189, 1987*; lip ulcer *J Transpl Sci 1:26–28, 2015; Infection 42:235, 2014*; tongue ulcer *NEJM 383:67, 2020; Bone Marrow Transplant 14:99–104, 1994*

Dental sinus

Diphtheria – palatal ulcers *Clin Dermatol 32:817–826, 2014*

Ebola virus hemorrhagic fever (filovirus) – dark red discoloration of the soft palate, pharyngitis, oral ulcers, glossitis, gingivitis; morbilliform exanthem which becomes purpuric with desquamation of the palms and soles; high fever, body aches, myalgia, arthralgias, prostration, abdominal pain, watery diarrhea; disseminated intravascular coagulation *Int J Dermatol 51:1037–1043, 2012; JAMA 287:2391–2002; Int J Dermatol 51:1037–1043, 2012; JAAD 65:1213–1218, 2011; MMWR 44, No. 19, 382, 1995*

Echovirus (Boston exanthem)

Enterobacter cloacae Cutis 59:281–283, 1997

Epstein-Barr virus (infectious mononucleosis) – aphthosis *Am J Surg Pathol 34:405–417, 2010; Am J Surg Pathol 43:201–219, 2019*; Epstein-Barr virus-positive mucocutaneous ulcers as pseudomalignancies *J Clin Exp Hematol 59:64–71, 2019*; EBV and self-remitting CD30+ lymphoproliferative disorder *Ann Diagn Pathol 37:57–61, 2018*

Escherichia coli

Exanthem subitum – human herpesvirus 6 – uvulo-palatoglossal junctional ulcers *Sem Cut Med Surg 34:171–177, 2015; J Clin Virol 17:83–90, 2000; Med J Malaysia 54:32–36, 1999*

Fusarium – necrotic ulceration of the gingiva to bone in acute myelogenous leukemia *J Oral Pathol Med 24:237–240, 1995*

Generalized juvenile periodontitis

Giardia lamblia infection – aphthous ulcer *B J Dent 166:457, 1989*

Glanders (*Burkholderia mallei*) – palatal ulcers *Clin Dermatol 32:817–826, 2014*

Gonococcal stomatitis *Pediatrics 84:623–625, 1989*

Granuloma inguinale – palatal ulcers *Clin Dermatol 32:817–826, 2014*

Hand, foot, and mouth disease (*Coxsackie A5, A10, A16; Coxsackie A6*) – vesicular *NEJM 369:265–274, 2013*; Coxsackie A16, *JAAD 75:1–16, 2016; BJD 79:309–317, 1967*; Enterovirus 71 *Clin Inf Dis 32:236–242, 2001*; Enterovirus 71 – myocarditis, encephalitis, aseptic meningitis, pulmonary edema *BJD 160:890–892, 2009; NEJM 341:929–935, 1999*

Herpangina – soft palatal ulcers *Oral Medicine/Oral Pathology Forum; AAD Annual Meeting, Feb 2002*; Coxsackie A1, A6, A10, A22, B1-5, Echovirus types 9, 11, 17 *J Infect Dis 15:191, 1987; Prog Med Virol 24:114–157, 1978*

Herpes simplex virus infection – primary herpetic gingivostomatitis *Sem Cut Med Surg 34:171–177, 2015; JAAD 57:737–763, 2007; Infection 25:310–312, 1997*; recurrent herpes simplex *JAMA 311:1152–1153, 2014; JAAD 18:169–172, 1988; NEJM 314:686–691, 1986; NEJM 314:749–757, 1986*; palatal ulcer *Clin Dermatol 32:817–826, 2014*

Herpes zoster – palatal ulcer *Clin Dermatol 32:817–826, 2014*

Histoplasmosis *Periodontol 49:39–59, 2009; JAAD 56:871–873, 2007; OSOMOP 47:157–160, 2002; AD 132:341–346, 1996; Int J Dermatol 30:614–622, 1991; JAAD 22:1088–1090, 1990*; in AIDS *JAAD 23:422–428, 1990*; palatal ulcer *Clin Dermatol 32:817–826, 2014*; tongue ulcer *JAMADerm 151:333–334, 2015*

Infectious mononucleosis – palatal ulcers *Clin Dermatol 32:817–826, 2014*

Klebsiella pneumoniae Cutis 59:281–283, 1997; lip ulcer *Braz Dent J 11:161–165, 2000*

Kyasanur Forest disease (*Flavivirus*) – hemorrhagic exanthem, papulovesicular palatine lesions

Lassa fever – capillary leak syndrome with severe swelling of the head and neck, oral ulcers, tonsillar patches *JAAD 65:1213–1218, 2011*

Leishmaniasis – espundia (mucocutaneous leishmaniasis) – ulcers of the mouth and lips *Oral Surg 73:583–584, 1992; Int J Derm 21:291–303, 1982*; ulcer of the hard palate in AIDS *BJD 160:311–318, 2009*; multiple ulcerated plaques – New World leishmaniasis *Ped Derm 24:657–658, 2007*; ulcerated nodule of the buttock; *L. mexicana, L. venezuelensis; L. amazonensis, L. braziliensis, L. peruviana, L. guyanensis, L. panamensis*; lip ulcers, crusted ulcer of the face; ulcers of the nasal septum, palate, lips, pharynx, larynx can develop months to years after initial infection

Leprosy – palatal ulcer *Clin Dermatol 32:817–826, 2014*

Lymphogranuloma venereum – tongue ulcer in men having sex with men *Sex Transm Infect 95:169–170, 2019*

Measles *J Clin Periodontol 30:665–668, 2003*

Meleney's ulcer – palatal ulcer *Clin Dermatol 32:817–826, 2014*

Monkeypox – exanthem indistinguishable from smallpox (papulovesiculopustular) (vesicles, umbilicated pustules, crusts) but is centrifugal; fever, chills, headache, back pain, sore throat, myalgias, diaphoresis, cough, nausea, vomiting, nasal congestion, blepharitis, oral ulcers, centrifugally clustered umbilicated papules and pustules, lymphadenopathy; heal with varioliform scarring *JAAD 55:478–481, 2006; JAAD 55:478–481, 2006; NEJM 355:962–963, 2006; CDC Health Advisory, June 7,2003; JAAD 44:1–14, 2001; J Infect Dis 156:293–298, 1987; Bull World Health Organ 46:593–597, 1972*

Mucormycosis – palatal ulcer *Clin Dermatol 32:827–838, 2014; Contemp Clin Dent 2:119–123, 2011; Oral Surg 68:624–627, 1989*; fatal palatal ulcer in diabetic ketoacidosis *OSOMOP 68:32–36, 1969*

Mumps

Mycobacterium avium complex (MAC) JAAD 37:450–472, 1997

Mycobacterium chelonae Br J Oral Surg 13:278–281, 1976

Mycobacterium kansasii Ped Derm 18:131–134, 2001

Mycobacterium tuberculosis – tuberculosis cutis orificialis (acute tuberculous ulcer) – oral ulcers; lip ulcers, floor of the mouth, soft palate, anterior tonsillar pillar, and uvula; *Clin Inf Dis 19:200–202,*

1994; J Oral Surg 36:387–389, 1978; tongue ulcer *Cutis 60:201–202, 1997*; lupus vulgaris; palatal ulcer *Clin Dermatol 32:817–826, 2014*

Mycoplasma pneumoniae-induced rash (*Mycoplasma*-induced rash and mucositis (MIRM)) – oral ulcers, lip ulcers, penile ulcers *JAMA 322, 2019*; sparse oval papules and mucositis *JAAD 72:239–245, 2015*

Myospherulosis *Int J Oral Maxillofacial Surg 22:234–235, 1993*

North American blastomycosis – palatal ulcers *Clin Dermatol 32:817–826, 2014; Oral Surg Oral Med Oral Pathol 47:157–160, 1979*; ulceration of the lip *OSOMOP 47:157–160, 1979; OSOMOP 28:914–923, 1969*

Omsk hemorrhagic fever – papulovesicular eruption of the soft palate

Orf – oral bullae and erosions as part of generalized severe blistering eruptions *JAAD 58:49–55, 2008*

Paecilomyces sinusitis – eroded hard palate *Clin Inf Dis 23:391–393, 1996*

Paracoccidioidomycosis (South American blastomycosis) (*Paracoccidioides brasiliensis*) – oral and perioral lesions; mulberry-like ulcerated swellings – painful ulcerative stomatitis with punctuate vascular pattern over a granulomatous base (Aguiar-Pupo stomatitis) *JAAD 53:931–951, 2005; Cutis 40:214–216, 1987*; ulceration of the lip, palatal ulcers *Clin Dermatol 32:817–826, 2014*

Parvovirus B19, including papular-purpuric "gloves and socks" syndrome – oral erosions *JAAD 41:793–796, 1999; AD 120:891–896, 1984*; bullous papular-purpuric gloves and socks syndrome with oral aphthae of the tongue *JAAD 60:691–695, 2009*

Periapical abscess – palatal ulcer *Clin Dermatol 32:817–826, 2014*

Periodontitis

Proteus infections

Pseudomonas
　　Oral ulcers with severe cutaneous infection with *Pseudomonas* in primary immunodeficiency syndromes *BJD 178:335–349, 2018*
　　　　CD40 ligand (CD154) deficiency (hyper-IgM syndrome)
　　　　CD40 deficiency (HIGM3)

Relapsing fever

Rhinoscleroma – palatal ulcer *Clin Dermatol 32:817–826, 2014*

Rhinosporidiosis – palatal ulcer *Clin Dermatol 32:817–826, 2014*

Rickettsialpox *AD 139:1545–1552, 2003*

Rubella

Salmonella colitis *Am J Roent 158:918, 1992*

Schizophyllum – palatal ulcer *Sabouraudia 11:201–204, 1973*

Serratia

Smallpox

Sporotrichosis – palatal ulcers *Clin Dermatol 32:817–826, 2014*

Stenotrophomonas maltophilia – lip edema with ulcers *AD 149:495–497, 2013*; acute necrotizing ulcerative gingivitis (ANUG) *Ped Inf Dis J 24:181–183, 2008*

Streptococcal gingivostomatitis

Syphilis, primary – chancre inside lower lip *NEJM 374:372, 2016; Sem Cut Med Surg 34:171–177, 2015; Rev Stomatol Chir Maxillofac 85:391–398, 1984*; ulcerated tonsil *Rook p. 1244, 1998, Sixth Edition*; secondary – painful shallow ulcers; may be

serpiginous or snail track ulcers *NEJM 380:1062–1071, 2019; NEJM 362:740–748, 2010; Clinics (Sao Paulo) 61:161–166, 2006; AD 131:833, 1995; J Clin Inf Dis 21:1361–1371, 1995; Br J Dent 160:237–238, 1986*; gingival erosion *AD 147:869–870, 2011*; tertiary – gumma – ulcers of the palate with palatal perforation; endemic (Bejel); congenital

Toxic shock syndrome

Trichosporon beigelii – palatal ulcer *Clin Dermatol 32:817–826, 2014*

Tularemia – palatal ulcers *Clin Dermatol 32:817–826, 2014*

Vaccinia *Arch Otorhinolaryngol 213:333–362, 1976 (German)*

Varicella

Vesicular stomatitis virus – vesicles of fingers, gums, buccal, and pharyngeal mucosa *NEJM 277:989–994, 1967*

Vincent's disease – acute necrotizing ulcerative gingivitis (ANUG)

Stenotrophomonas maltophilia

Yaws – palatal ulcers *Clin Dermatol 32:817–826, 2014*

Yersinia

Zygomycosis, mucormycosis

INFILTRATIVE DISEASES

Langerhans cell histiocytosis including Hand-Schuller-Christian disease; eosinophilic granuloma *JAAD 78:1035–1044, 2018; AD 121:770–774, 1985*; oral and palatal ulcerations *Clin Dermatol 38:223–234, 2020; JAAD 60:289–298, 2009; J Clin Periodontol 25:340–342, 1998; J Periodontol 60:57–66, 1989*

INFLAMMATORY DISEASES

Acute gingivitis *AD 120:1461–1465, 1984*

Acute necrotizing ulcerative gingivitis (ANUG) – rapid onset of painful friable gingivae, punched-out ulcers of interdental papillae, and marginal gingiva *BMJ Case Rep 12:e22983, 2019; Ann Periodontol 4:65–73, 1999; J Periodont 66:990–998, 1995*

Chronic marginal gingivitis *Eur J Oral Sci 105:562–570, 1997*

Circumorificial plasmacytosis *J Dermatol 46:48–51, 2019*

Crohn's disease – linear ulcers of sulci, aphthae-like ulcers, angular cheilitis and ulceration *JAAD 57:S38–41, 2007; AD 135:439–442, 1999; JAAD 36:697–704, 1997*; buccal space abscesses *Oral Surg Oral Med Oral Pathol Oral Radiol Endod 88:33–36, 1999*; palatal ulcers *Clin Dermatol 32:817–826, 2014;*

Cyclic neutropenia, congenital *BJD 178:335–349, 2018; JAAD 57:S38–41, 2007*

Cytophagic histiocytic panniculitis *Ped Derm 21:246–249, 2004*

Desquamative gingivitis *JAAD 78:839–848, 2018*

Eosinophilic ulcer of the lip, tongue, or buccal mucosa *AD 137:815–820, 2001; Cutis 57:349–351, 1996; JAAD 33:734–740, 1995*

Erythema multiforme *Sem Cut Med Surg 34:171–177, 2015; NEJM 369:265–274, 2013; NEJM 362:740–748, 2010; Medicine 68:133–140, 1989; JAAD 8:763–765, 1983*; Stevens-Johnson syndrome *BJD 174:1194–1227, 2016; Ped Derm 23:546–555, 2006; Am J Dis Child 24:526–533, 1922*

Gingivitis secondary to mouth breathing *Compendium 8:20–22, 1987*

Idiopathic midline destructive disease – palatal necrosis and ulceration *Am J Clin Pathol 77:162–167, 1982*

Impacted tooth – palatal ulcer *Clin Dermatol 32:817–826, 2014*

Inflammatory bowel disease – deep granulomatous ulcers of the buccal mucosa, lips, palate, gingiva *NEJM 362:740–748, 2010*

Kikuchi's disease (histiocytic necrotizing lymphadenitis) – red papules of the face, back, arms; red plaques; erythema and acneiform lesions of the face; morbilliform, urticarial, and rubella-like exanthems; red or ulcerated pharynx; cervical adenopathy; associations with SLE, lymphoma, tuberculous adenitis, viral lymphadenitis, infectious mononucleosis, and drug eruptions *JAAD 36:342–346, 1997; Am J Surg Pathol 14:872–876, 1990*; gingival ulcers *BJD 144:885–889, 2001*

Necrotizing sialometaplasia – palatal ulcer *Histopathol 40:200, 2002; JADA 127:1087–1092, 1996; Oral Surg Oral Med Oral Pathol 72:3170325, 1991; Cutis 41:97, 1988; AD 122:208–10, 1986; Plast Reconstr Surg 41:325–328, 1983; Ann Otol Rhinol Laryngol 87:409–411, 1978; Cancer 32:130, 1973*; ulcer of the posterior hard palate *JAAD 77:809–830,2017; Cutis 41:97, 1988; AD 122:208–210, 1986*

Necrotizing stomatitis – palatal ulcers *Clin Dermatol 32:817–826, 2014*

Orofacial granulomatosis – facial edema with swelling of the lips, cheeks, eyelids, forehead, mucosal tags, mucosal cobblestoning, gingivitis, oral aphthae *JAAD 62:611–620, 2010; BJD 143:1119–1121, 2000*

Periadenitis mucosa necrotica recurrens (Sutton's disease) *AD 133:1161–1166, 1997*

Plasma cell mucositis *Clin Exp Dermatol 41:951–952, 2016*

Pyoderma gangrenosum – oral ulcers *Head Neck Pathol 11:427–441, 2017; BJD 144:393–396, 2001*; orogenital ulcers *AD 94:732–738, 1966*; lip ulcer *Ped Derm 30:497–499, 2013*

Pyostomatitis vegetans – deep fissures, pustules, papillary projections *JAAD 50:785–788, 2004; Oral Surg Oral Med Oral Pathol 75:220–224, 1993; J Oral Pathol Med 21:128–133, 1992; Gastroenterology 103:668–674, 1992; JAAD 21:381–387, 1989; AD 121:94–98, 1985*; lip ulcers; lip swelling with cobblestoning, micropustules *NEJM 368:1918, 2013*

Relapsing polychondritis – aphthosis *Medicine 80:173–179, 2000*; MAGIC syndrome *J Clin Rheumatol 13:221–223, 2007*

Sarcoid – deep granulomatous ulcers on the gingiva and palate *JAAD 77:809–830, 2017; NEJM 362:740–748, 2010*; ulcers of the buccal mucosa, palate, larynx, tongue *Clin Dermatol 32:817–826, 2014*; aphthae *J Indian Soc Periodontol 20:627–629, 2016*

Toxic epidermal necrolysis *Oral Maxillofac Surg 40:59–61, 1982*

Ulcerative colitis *Clin Gastroenterol 9:307, 1980; Gut 5:1, 1964*

METABOLIC DISEASES

Acrodermatitis enteropathica – stomatitis *Ped Derm 19:426–431, 2002*; acquired zinc deficiency stomatitis *JAAD 69:616–624, 2013*

Acatalasia (acatalasemia) – Takahara's disease; ulceration, gangrene, and necrosis of soft tissues of the mouth and nose *Lancet 2:1101–1104, 1952*

Agranulocytosis (neutropenic ulcers) – interdental ulcers *AD 132:1399–1400, 1996*

Anemia

Cryoglobulinemia *JAAD 25:21–27, 1991*

Erythropoietic porphyria *BJD 167:901–913, 2012*

Folate deficiency – aphthosis *Med Clin (Barc) 109:85–87, 1997*

Gluten-sensitive enteropathy – celiac disease *Oral Medicine/Oral Pathology Forum; AAD Annual Meeting, Feb 2002*

Heavy chain disease (Franklin's disease) *AD 124:1538–1540, 1988*

Hypoplasminogenemia – autosomal recessive; red eyes, oral ulcers, gingival edema; ligneous conjunctivitis with red eyes, ligneous periodontitis, blindness, tooth loss; decreased wound healing *JAMADerm 150:1227–12228, 2014*

Hypothyroidism *Oral Surg Oral Med Oral Pathol 46:216–219, 1978*

Iron deficiency – aphthosis *Med Clin (Barc) 109:85–87, 1997*

Kwashiorkor *Cutis 67:321–327, 2001*

Kynureninase deficiency (xanthurenic aciduria)

Malabsorption

Menses – cyclic aphthosis; PFAPA *J Ped Adolesc Gyn March 26, 2020*

Neutropenia *J Periodontol 58:51–55, 1987*

Nutritional disorders

Pernicious anemia (B12 deficiency) – aphthosis *SMJ 83:475–477, 1990*; severe stomatitis with recurrent ulcers

Pregnancy

Scurvy *Aust Dent J 47:82, 2002*

Ulcerative colitis – aphthous ulcers *JAAD 57:S38–41, 2007*

Uremic stomatitis – friable gingivae, ulcerative stomatitis, uremic glossitis, xerostomia *OSOMOPOR Endod 101:608–613, 2006*

Vitamin B1 deficiency (thiamine) – beriberi; edema, burning red tongue, vesicles of the oral mucosa *Oral Surg Oral Pathol Oral Med Oral Radiol Endod 82:634–636, 1996*

Vitamin B12 deficiency – linear erosions of lateral or dorsal tongue; linear erosions of the hard and soft palate *JAAD 60:498–500, 2009*

Type 1B glycogen storage disease *Oral Surg Oral Med Oral Pathol 69:174–176, 1990*

NEOPLASTIC DISEASES

Adenocarcinoma – palatal ulcers *Clin Dermatol 32:817–826, 2014*

Anaplastic carcinoma – palatal ulcers *Clin Dermatol 32:817–826, 2014*

Angiofibroma – ulcerated hard palatal mass *OSOMOPOR Endod 94:228–238, 2002*

Basal cell carcinoma of the lip – personal observation

Benign accessory salivary gland neoplasm – palatal ulcer *Clin Dermatol 32:817–826, 2014*

Benign lymphoid hyperplasia – palatal ulcers *Clin Dermatol 32:817–826, 2014*

Canalicular adenomas *J Oral Pathol Med 27:388–394, 1998*

Carcinoma of the parotid gland duct

Chondrosarcoma *BMJ Case Rep Dec 22, 2017*

Erythroplasia (erythroplakia) *Oral Oncol 41:551–561, 2005*

Invasive canal cyst (nasopalatine duct cyst) – palatal ulcer *Clin Dermatol 32:817–826, 2014*

Kaposi's sarcoma – palatal ulcers *Clin Dermatol 32:817–826, 2014*

Keratoacanthoma – oral ulcer with rolled margin on the gingiva *Br J Oral Surg 24:438–441, 1986*; of the lip

Leukemia – acute lymphocytic leukemia; acute myelomonocytic leukemia; chronic myelogenous leukemia *Oral Oncol 30B:346–350, 1994*; acute lymphoblastic leukemia with eosinophilia *Ped Derm 20:502–505, 2003*; T-cell large granular lymphocytic leukemia – complex aphthosis *JAAD 57:S60–61, 2007*; HTLV-1 leukemia/

lymphoma – ulcers of the lips, hard palate, tongue *AD 146:804–805, 2010*

Lymphoma – AIDS-associated *Cutis 59:281–283, 1997; NEJM 311:565–570, 1984*; Hodgkin's/non-Hodgkin's lymphoma *NEJM 362:740–748, 2010; J Oral Med 29:45–48, 1974*; lymphomatoid granulomatosis – palatal ulcer *Arch Otolaryngol 107:141–146, 1981*; nasal and nasal-type natural killer/T-cell lymphoma (angiocentric lymphoma) – necrotic ulcer of the gingiva and hard palate *NEJM 371:1629, 2014; JAAD 40:268–272, 1999*; lethal midline granuloma; extranodal natural killer cell/T-cell lymphoma, nasal type – ulcers of the hard palate and gingiva *NEJM 371:1629, 2014*; lethal midline granuloma (NK/T-cell lymphoma) *Indian J Otolaryngol Head Neck Surg 71(suppl 3)2140–2142, 2019*

Lymphomatoid papulosis *Ann Diagn Pathol 31:50–55, 2017*

Melanoma – neurotropic desmoplastic melanoma; lip ulcers *JAAD 53:S120–122, 2005*; palatal ulcer *Clin Dermatol 32:817–826, 2014*

Metastatic carcinoma – gastric cancer *BMC Cancer 5:117, 2005*; colon adenocarcinoma *Case Rep Dent 2011;357518*

Mucoceles, superficial *Oral Surg 66:318–322, 1988*

Mucoepidermoid carcinoma – palatal ulcer *Clin Dermatol 32:817–826, 2014*

Multiple myeloma – bullous lichenoid lesions *Oral Surg Oral Med Oral Pathol 70:587–589, 1990*; plasmacytic ulcerative stomatitis (myeloma) – bulla *Oral Surg 75:483–487, 1993; Oral Surg 70:587–589, 1990*

Myelodysplastic syndrome *Eur J Cancer B Oral Oncol 30B:346–350, 1994; Oral Surg Oral Med Oral Pathol 70:579–583, 1990; Oral Surg 61:466–470, 1986*; trisomy 8-positive myelodysplastic syndrome – aphthous ulcers *JAAD 57:S38–41, 2007*

Odontogenic and salivary gland tumors

Palatal pleomorphic adenoma palate *J Craniofac Surg 30:e50–582, 2019*

Plasmacytoma, extramedullary *OSOMOP 75:483–487, 1983; J Mass Dent Soc 57:53–58, 2008*

Polycythemia vera *Blood 90:3370–3377, 1997*

Sarcomas – palatal ulcers *Clin Dermatol 32:817–826, 2014*

Sebaceous carcinoma – ulcerated buccal mucosa *J Laryngol Otol 110:500–502, 1996*

Sickle cell anemia

Squamous cell carcinoma *Sem Cut Med Surg 34:171–177, 2015; NEJM 362:740–748, 2010; J Oral Maxillofac Surg 53:144–147, 1995; Oral Oncol 31B:16–26, 1995; Crit Rev Oncol Hematol 21:63–75, 1995*; lip ulcer *JAAD 59:175–177, 2008*

Waldenström's macroglobulinemia

PARANEOPLASTIC DISEASES

Paraneoplastic pemphigus – extensive erosions and ulcers of the lips, intraoral surfaces; acral bullae; associated with non-Hodgkin's B-cell lymphoma, chronic lymphocytic leukemia, Waldenström's macroglobulinemia, Hodgkin's disease, T-cell lymphoma, Castleman's disease, thymoma, poorly differentiated sarcoma, round-cell liposarcoma, inflammatory fibrosarcoma, uterine adenosarcoma *JAAD 77:795–806, 2017; BJD 176:1406–1408, 2017; BJD 176:824–826, 2017; BJD 174:930–932, 2016; JAMADerm 151:439–440, 2015; NEJM 369:265–274, 2013; AD 141:1285–1293, 2005; BJD 149:1143–1151, 2003; JAAD 48:S69–72, 2003; JAAD 40:649–671, 1999; JAAD 39:867–871, 1998; AD 129:866–869, 1993; NEJM 323:1729–1735, 1990*

PHOTODERMATOSES

Hydroa vacciniforme *Cutis 88:245–253, 2011*; cheilitis with ulcers of the lip *Ped Derm 21:555–557, 2004*; oral mucosal ulcers *Acta DV 90:498–501, 2010*

PRIMARY CUTANEOUS DISEASES

Acute parapsoriasis (pityriasis lichenoides et varioliformis acuta) (Mucha-Habermann disease) – red and necrotic lesions *AD 123:1335–1339, 1987; AD 118:478, 1982; Oral Surg 53:596–601, 1982*

Angina bullosa hemorrhagica (blood blisters) *Br Dent J 180:24–25, 1996; JAAD 31:316–319, 1994*

Aphthous stomatitis – major (Sutton's ulcer), minor (Mikulicz ulcers), herpetiform *Sem Cut Med Surg 34:171–177, 2015; NEJM 362:740–748, 2010; AD 139:1259–1262, 2003; Oral Surg Oral Med Oral Pathol Oral Radiol Endod 81:141–147, 1996*; palatal ulcers *Clin Dermatol 32:817–826, 2014*; recurrent aphthous stomatitis *Ped Derm 32:476–480, 2015*

   AIDS
   Behcet's syndrome *JAAD 79:987–1006, 2018; BJD 159:555–560, 2008*
   Crohn's disease *JAAD 57:538–571, 2007*
   Celiac disease *BJD 103:111, 1980; BMJ 1:11–13, 1976*
   Cyclic neutropenia *Sem Cut Med Surg 34:171–177, 2015*
   FAPA syndrome
   Folate deficiency *Med Clin (Barc)109:85–87, 1997*
   Foreign bodies at distant locations
     IUD
     Contact lenses *Lancet 1:857, 1974*
   Herpes simplex
   Idiopathic
   IgA deficiency *Sem Cut Med Surg 34:171–177, 2015*
   Iron deficiency
   Luteal phase of menstrual cycle
   MAGIC syndrome *Sem Cut Med Surg 34:171–177, 2015*
   Neutropenia
     Cyclic
     Chemotherapy-induced
   Reactive arthritis
   Sweet's syndrome *Dermatologica 169:102–103, 1984*
   Toothpaste – sodium lauryl sulfate
   Trauma
   Ulcerative colitis
   Vitamin B1, B2, B6, B12 deficiency
   Zinc deficiency

Bullous dermolysis of the newborn (form of autosomal dominant epidermolysis bullosa or recessive dystrophic epidermolysis bullosa) – hypopigmented patches; giant bullae of the hand and foot; erosions, tongue erosions, milia *Ped Derm 30:736–740, 2013*

Chronic ulcerative stomatitis – resembles ulcerative lichen planus *JAAD 22:215–220, 1990; JAAD 38:1005–1006, 1998*

Congenital insensitivity to pain – ulcers of fingers, lips, tongue, excoriations of the face *BJD 179:1135–1140,2018*

Epidermolysis bullosa simplex *Epidermolysis Bullosa: Basic and Clinical Aspects. New York: Springer, 1992: 89–117*; oral bullae with epidermolysis bullosa; simplex – generalized, herpetiform (Dowling-Meara) *Cutis 70:19–21, 2002*; superficialis *AD 125:633–638, 1989*; junctional – Herlitz, generalized mild, localized, inverse, progressive; dominant dystrophic – hyperplastic, albopapuloid, and polydysplastic dystrophic type; junctional, non-Herlitz type;

COL17A1 mutations (GABEB); enamel hypoplasia *JAAD 77:809–830, 2017; BJD 156:861–870, 2007*; recessive dystrophic – localized, generalized, mutilating, inverse; *Oral Surg 43:859–872, 1977*; variants *Oral Surg Oral Med Oral Pathol 71:440–446, 1991; Oral Surg 67:555–563, 1989*; dystrophic epidermolysis bullosa inversa – flexural bullae, oral ulcers, dental caries, milia *Ped Derm 20:243–248, 2003*; junctional epidermolysis bullosa of late onset (formerly junctional epidermolysis bullosa progressiva) – loss of dermatoglyphs, waxy hyperkeratosis of the dorsal hand, atrophic skin of the lower leg, transverse ridging and enamel pits of teeth, nail atrophy, amelogenesis imperfecta, hyperhidrosis, blisters on elbows, knees, and oral cavity *BJD 164:1280–1284, 2011*

Erythema elevatum diutinum – *BJD 166:222–224, 2012*

Hailey-Hailey disease *BJD Nov 19, 2019*

Junctional epidermolysis bullosa of late onset (skin fragility in childhood) – speckled hyperpigmentation of elbows; hemorrhagic bullae, teeth and nail abnormalities, oral blisters, disappearance of dermatoglyphs, palmoplantar keratoderma, small vesicles, atrophy of the skin of the hands *BJD 169:714–716, 2013*

Keratosis lichenoides chronica (Nekam's disease) – reticulated flat-topped keratotic papules, linear arrays, atrophy, comedo-like lesions, prominent telangiectasia; conjunctival injection, seborrheic dermatitis-like eruption; acral dermatitis over toes; punctate keratotic papules of palmar creases; scaly red papules of the face; seborrheic dermatitis-like rash of the face; nail dystrophy; oral and genital erosions, conjunctivitis *AD 147:1317–1322, 2011; Cutis 86:245–248, 2010; Ped Derm 26:615–616, 2009; AD 145:867–69, 2009; AD 144:405–410, 2008; JAAD 56:S1–5, 2007; Am J Dermatopathol 28:260–275, 2006; JAAD 49:511–513, 2003; Dermatology 201:261–264, 2000; JAAD 38:306–309, 1998; JAAD 37:263–264, 1997; Dermatopathol Pract Concept 3:310–312, 1997; AD 131:609–614, 1995; Dermatology 191:188–192, 1995; AD 105:739–743, 1972; Presse Med 51:1000–1003, 1938; Arch Dermatol Syph (Berlin) 31:1–32, 1895*; in children *JAAD 56:S1–5, 2007*

Kikuchi's disease – red macules, malar erythema, oral ulcers, photosensitivity, conjunctival injection, lymphadenopathy, fever, arthralgia *JAAD 59:130–136, 2008*; morbilliform eruption *Ped Derm 24:459–460, 2007*

Kimura's disease (angiolymphoid hyperplasia with eosinophilia) *BJD 145:365, 2001; JAAD 43:905–907, 2000*

Kindler's syndrome – autosomal recessive; photosensitivity, cigarette paper atrophy, atrophied gingiva, poikiloderma, mucosal fragility, gingivitis, periodontitis; fermitin family homolog 1 mutation *JAAD 67:113–1127, 2012; BJD 160:233–242, 2009; Ped Derm 23:586–588, 2006; AD 142:1619–1624, 2006; AD 142:620–624, 2006; AD 140:939–944, 2004; BJD 144:1284–1286, 2001; AD 132:1487–1490, 1996; Ped Derm 13:397–402, 1996; Ped Derm 6:91–101, 1989; Ped Derm 6:82–90, 1989; BJD 66:104–111, 1954*; oral bullae, lip ulcer *BJD 157:1281–1284, 2007*

Lethal acantholytic epidermolysis bullosa – autosomal recessive, universal alopecia, cutaneous and mucosal shedding, skin fragility, erythroderma, blistering, anonychia, malformed ears, cardiomyopathy; mutation in desmoplakin (*DSP*) *BJD 162:1388–1394, 2010; JID 130:2680–2683, 2010; BJD 162:1388–1394, 2010; Dermatol Clin 28:131–135, 2010*; mutation in *JUP* gene *Hum Med Genet 20:1811–1819, 2011*

Lichen planus *Sem Cut Med Surg 34:171–177, 2015; NEJM 369:265–274, 2013; JAAD 66:761–766, 2012; Ped Derm 26:458–464, 2009; JAAD 46:207–214, 2002; J Oral Maxillofac Surg 50:116–118, 1992; J Oral Pathol 14:431–458, 1985*; isolated lip erosions *Cutis 71–210–212, 2003*; palatal ulcers *Clin Dermatol 32:817–826, 2014*; vulvo-vaginal-gingival syndrome *Dermatol Clin 21:91–98, 2003*

Lichen planus pemphigoides – oral bullae and erosions, flat-topped papules, cutaneous bullae *BJD 171:1230–1235, 2014*

Lichen sclerosus et atrophicus – bluish-white plaques of the mouth; *BJD 131:118–123, 1994; Br J Oral Maxillofac Surg 89:64–65, 1991*

Orofacial granulomatosis *Indian Dermatol Online J 81:32–34, 2017*

Pityriasis rosea – oral erythematomacular, papular, erythematovesicular, petechial lesions *JAAD 77:833–837, 2017; AD 121:1449–1451, 1985; JAMA 205:597, 1968; Cutis 50:276, 1992*; vesicular pityriasis rosea; oral hemorrhage, erosions or ulcers, red macules and plaques *JAAD 61:303–318, 2009*

Toxic epidermal necrolysis, idiopathic *Ped Derm 36:550–551, 2019*

Transient acantholytic dermatosis (Grover's disease) *JAAD 35:653–666, 1996*

Reactive perforating collagenosis *JAAD 25:1079–1081, 1991*

PSYCHOCUTANEOUS DISEASES

Fabricated or induced (Munchausen by proxy) *Central Eur J Immunol 40:109–114, 2015*

Factitial *J Periodontol 66:241–245, 1995; Oral Surg Oral Med Oral Pathol 65:685–688, 1988*; gingival ulcers *J Periodont 65:442–447, 1994*; palatal ulcers *Clin Dermatol 32:817–826, 2014*

Self-mutilation *J Periodontol 66:241–245, 1995*; in Lesch-Nyhan syndrome *Oral Maxillofac Surg 23:37–38, 1994*

SYNDROMES

Ataxia telangiectasia *OSOMOP 75:791–797, 1993*

Behcet's disease *Ped Derm 25:509–519, 2008; BJD 157:901–906, 2007; JAAD 41:540–545, 1999; JAAD 40:1–18, 1999; NEJM 341:1284–1290, 1999; JAAD 36:689–696, 1997*; palatal ulcers *Clin Dermatol 32:817–826, 2014*; in children *Ped Derm 32:714–717, 2015*

CANDLE syndrome (chronic atypical neutrophilic dermatosis with lipodystrophy and elevated temperature) – annular erythematous edematous plaques of the face (periorbital erythema) and trunk which become purpuric and result in residual annular hyperpigmentation; urticarial papules; limitation of range of motion with plaques over interphalangeal joints; periorbital edema with violaceous swollen eyelids, edema of the lips (thick lips), lipoatrophy of the cheeks, nose, and arms, chondritis with progressive ear and saddle nose deformities, hypertrichosis of lateral forehead, gynecomastia, wide-spaced nipples, nodular episcleritis and conjunctivitis, epididymitis, myositis, aseptic meningitis; short stature, anemia, abnormal liver functions, splenomegaly, protuberant abdomen; pleuritic chest pain; lymphadenopathy; arthralgia/oral ulcers *BJD 170:215–217, 2014; JAAD 68:834–853, 2013; Ped Derm 28:538–541, 2011; JAAD 62:487–495, 2010*

Chediak-Higashi syndrome

Dyskeratosis congenita (Zinsser-Engman-Cole syndrome) – Xq28; oral bullae and erosions, oral leukokeratosis *BJD 178:335–349, 2018; J Med Genet 33:993–995, 1996; Dermatol Clin 13:33–39, 1995; BJD 105:321–325, 1981*

Ehlers-Danlos syndrome *Int Med 35:200–202, 1996*

FAPA syndrome (fever, aphthosis, pharyngitis, and adenitis) *JAAD 57:S38–41, 2007*

Fuchs syndrome – Stevens-Johnson syndrome without skin lesions *Ped Derm 28:474–476, 2011; Klin Monatsbl Augenheilkd 14:333–351, 1876*

Glucagonoma syndrome *South Med J 75:222–224, 1982*

Hereditary sensory and autonomic neuropathy *Istanb Univ Fac Dent 50:49–53, 2016*

Hypereosinophilic syndrome – erosions of the buccal, gingival, or labial mucosa *Lancet 359:1577–1578, 2002; AD 132:535–541, 1996; Semin Dermatol 14:122–128, 1995; Blood 83:2759–2779, 1994; JAMA 247:1018–1020, 1982*

Hyper-IgM syndrome (hypogammaglobulinemia with hyper-IgM) – X-linked with mutation in CD40 ligand gene; low IgA and IgG; sarcoid-like granulomas; multiple papulonodules of the face, buttocks, arms *Ped Derm 21:39–43, 2004; Ped Derm 18:48–50, 2001*

Kawasaki's disease *Oral Surg 67:569–572, 1989*

Keratosis-ichthyosis-deafness (KID) syndrome *AD 113:1701–1704, 1977*

KID syndrome with fissured lips – paronychial pustules, blepharitis without keratitis, perineal psoriasiform plaques, tongue erosions, honeycomb palmoplantar keratoderma; red gingivae; mutation in connexin 26(N14K)*GJB2*

Lesch-Nyhan syndrome, self-mutilation *Neurology 65:E25, 2005; J Oral Pathol Med 34:573–575, 2005*

Lipoid proteinosis – oral erosions *BJD 151:413–423, 2004; JID 120:345–350, 2003; Hum Molec Genet 11:833–840, 2002*

MAGIC syndrome (relapsing polychondritis + Behcet's) *Am J Med 79:665, 1985; J Rheum 4:559, 1984*

Muckle-Wells syndrome *Am J Med Genet 53:72–74, 1994; AD 126:940–944, 1990*

Periodic fever, aphthous stomatitis, pharyngitis, and cervical adenopathy syndrome (PFAPA) *Ped Derm 28:290–294, 2011; J Pediatr 135:98–101, 1999; J Ped Hem Onc 25:212–218, 1996; Ped Inf Dis J 8:186–187, 1989; J Pediatr 110:43–46, 1987*

Reactive arthritis syndrome – erosions with marginal erythema; circinate erosions *JAAD 59:113–121, 2008; NEJM 309:1606–1615, 1983; Semin Arthritis Rheum 3:253–286, 1974; Dtsch Med Wochenschr 42:1535–1536, 1916*

Riley-Day syndrome (familial dysautonomia) – dental and soft tissue self-mutilation *Harefuah 155:490–494, 2016(Hebrew)*

Rowell's syndrome – lupus erythematosus and erythema multiforme-like syndrome – papules, annular targetoid lesions, vesicles, bullae, necrosis, ulceration, oral ulcers; perniotic lesions *JAAD 21:374–377, 1989*

Shedding oral mucosa syndrome *Cutis 54:323–326, 1996; peeling Brit Dent J 214:374, 2013*

Sweet's syndrome *JAAD 31:535–556, 1994; JAAD 23:503–507, 1990; palatal ulcer Clin Dermatol 32:817–826, 2014*

TOXINS

Arsenic poisoning – acute; stomatitis *BJD 149:757–762, 2003*

Mercury poisoning (acrodynia) – oral, perioral ulceration *AD 124:107–109, 1988*

Thallium – anagen effluvium *JAAD 50:258–261, 2004; nausea, vomiting, stomatitis, painful glossitis, diarrhea; severe dysesthesias and paresthesias in distal extremities, facial rashes* of the cheeks and perioral region, acneiform eruptions of the face, hyperkeratosis of the palms and soles, hair loss, Mees' lines *AD 143:93–98, 2007*

TRAUMA

Angina bullosa hemorrhagica *J Pak Med Assoc 68:1527–1530, 2018*

Bednar's aphthae – repetitive trauma in infant, pacifier, narrow nipple holes requiring vigorous sucking *Ped Derm 37:213–214, 2020*

Thermal burns – pizza burn of the tongue or palate; microwaved food *Burns 25:465–466, 1999*

Chemical burn *Br Dent J 208:297–300, 2010*

Cheek biting *J Prosthet Dent 67:581–582, 1992*

Child abuse and neglect – ulcer of the upper labial frenulum *Oral Implantol (Rome)8:68–73, 2016*

Dental materials – restorative materials, sodium hypochlorite, formocresol, topical aspirin

Dentures *J Oral Pathol 10:65–80, 1981; denture cleaners*

Electrical burn *Burns 44:1065–1076, 2018; Int J Ped Otorhinolaryngol 77:1325–1328, 2013; Chest 174:317–318, 1978*

Endotracheal tube insertion – lip ulcer, oral ulcer *Chest 74:317–318, 1978; lip ulcer*

Exploding electronic cigarettes *J Am Dent Assoc 147:891–896, 2016*

Facial trauma

Injection

Lye

Maxillectomy, septoplasty, intubation, tooth extraction, radiation therapy – palatal ulcers *Clin Dermatol 32:817–826, 2014*

Neurolytic mandibular nerve block *Reg Anesth Pain Med 24:188–189, 1999*

Oral sex *Am J Forensic Med Pathol 2:217–219, 1981*

Orthodontic treatment – traumatic ulcers *Community Dent Oral Epidemiol 17:154–157, 1989*

Overuse of mouthwash *Cutis 64:131–134, 1999*

Radiation stomatitis *Clin Oncol 8:15–24, 1996; J Oral Pathol Med 18:167–171, 1989*

Radiation recall stomatitis

Radiation, ionizing *Mutat Res 77:(pt B)292–298, 2016*

Riga-Fede disease (traumatic oral granuloma) – oral ulcer of the labial mucosa; affects teething infants aged less than 2 years and is always associated with local trauma (teeth); clinically and histopathologically resembles traumatic eosinophilic ulcer of the oral mucosa *Ped Derm 24:663–664, 2007; JAAD 47:445–447, 2002; J Ped 116:1742–1743, 1990*

Seizure

Smoking – palatal erosions

Trauma *Sem Cut Med Surg 34:171–177, 2015*

Traumatic eosinophilic ulcer of the oral mucosa (traumatic ulcerative granuloma with stromal eosinophilia (TUGSE)) – rarely recognized in clinical practice, it presents as a painless ulcer or indurated lesion on the tongue or buccal mucosa which heals spontaneously within 1 month; easily confused with squamous cell carcinoma; cause is unknown, but it is often associated with local trauma; mixed cell inflammatory infiltrate, mainly eosinophils beneath the ulcerated surface *World J Surg Oncol 17:184, 2019; Oral Oncol 33:375–379, 1997; Cutis 57:349–351, 1996*

VASCULAR DISEASES

Caliber-persistent artery of the lip – persistent ulcer of the lip *JAAD 46:256–259, 2002; BJD 113:757–760, 1985; J Oral Pathol 9:137–144, 1980*

Allergic granulomatous vasculitis with eosinophilia – palatal ulcers, refractory oral ulcers *J Dermatol 46:e377–378, 2019; Clin Dermatol 32:817–826, 2014*

Giant cell arteritis – ulcer of the lip *J Oral Maxillofac Surg 51:581–583, 1993*

Granulomatosis with polyangiitis (formerly Wegener's granulomatosis) – oral erosions, large and necrotic oral ulcers, perforation of the nasal septum, ulcers or perforation of the hard palate *Sem Cut Med Surg 34:171–177, 2015; NEJM 369:265–274, 2013; NEJM 362:740–748, 2010; JAAD 48:311–340, 2003; JAAD 49:335–337, 2003; Ann Otol Rhinol Laryngol 107:439–445, 1998; AD 130:861–867, 1994; Oral Surg Oral Med Oral Pathol 46:53–63, 1978*; palatal ulcers and unilateral eyelid edema *Caspian J Intern Med 10:343–346, 2019*

Lymphatic malformations – palatal ulcers *Clin Dermatol 32:817–826, 2014*

Necrotizing vasculitis with HIV disease *J Oral Maxillofac Surg 50:1000–1003, 1992*

Polyarteritis nodosa *Oral Surg 56:597–601, 1983*; familial polyarteritis nodosa of Georgian Jewish, German, and Turkish ancestry – oral aphthae, livedo reticularis, leg ulcers, Raynaud's phenomenon, digital necrosis, nodules, purpura, erythema nodosum; systemic manifestations include fever, myalgias, arthralgias, gastrointestinal symptoms, renal disease, central and peripheral neurologic manifestations; mutation in adenosine deaminase 2 (*CECR1*) *NEJM 370:921–931, 2014;* palatal ulcers *Clin Dermatol 32:817–826, 2014*

Takayasu's arteritis – recurrent oral ulcers *Clin Exp Rheum Jan 14, 2020*

ORAL MUCOSA, VERRUCOUS AND VEGETATING LESIONS

AUTOIMMUNE DISEASES AND DISEASES OF IMMUNE DYSFUNCTION

Lupus erythematosus – discoid lupus erythematosus *BJD 121:727–741, 1989*; pseudolymphomatous tumid lupus *Am J Dermatopathol 32:704–707, 2010*

Mucous membrane pemphigoid *Int Wound J 15:903–913, 2018*

Pemphigus vegetans *Stat Pearls Dec 8, 2019; Case Rep Dermatol 27:145–150, 2017; Ann Dermatol 23(suppl3)S310–313, 2011; Int J Dermatol 45:425–428, 2006*

DRUGS

Black hairy tongue

BRAF inhibitors – oral hyperkeratotic lesions *BJD 172:1680–1682, 2015*

Bromides

Iodides

INFECTIONS

Bacillary angiomatosis *Rev Int Med Trop Sao Paolo Aug 24, 2017; Acta DV Croat 22:294–297, 2014*

Bartonella *BJD 157:174–178, 2007*

Bejel

Candida – chronic hyperplastic candidiasis *Oral Surg Oral Med Oral Pathol 56:388–395, 1983*; chronic mucocutaneous candidiasis *Ann Rev Med 32:491–497, 1981*; verrucous Candida *J Cutan Pathol 44:815–818, 2017*

Coccidioidomycosis *Acta DV suppl(Stockh)121:57–72, 1986*

Histoplasmosis *BJD 133:472–474, 1995*

Human papillomavirus (HPV) *Head Neck Pathol 13:80–90, 2019*; verruca vulgaris *J Cancer Res Ther 14:454–456, 2018*

Leishmaniasis *Oral Dis 8:59–61, 2002*

Leprosy *Egyptian J DV 35:37–44, 2015; Indian J DV Leprol 69:381–385, 2003*

Mucormycosis *Acta Stomatol Croat 53:274–277, 2019; Med Mycol 49:400–405, 2011*

Mycobacterium tuberculosis – tuberculosis verrucosa *Postepy Dermatol Alergol 32:302–306, 2015*

Oral hairy leukoplakia *Oral Dis 22:suppl 1:120–127, 2016; OSOMOPOR 119:326–332, 2015*; no immunosuppression *J Can Dent Assoc 84:4 May 2018*

Paracoccidioidomycosis – granulomatous friable lesions (blackberry stomatitis) *Oral Dis 24:1492–1502, 2018; Mycoses 56:189–199, 2013; Oral Dis 7:56–60, 2001*

Pinta

Rhinoscleroma – *Klebsiella rhinoscleromatous* (Frisch bacillus) exudative stage with rhinorrhea; then proliferative stage with exuberant friable granulation tissue of the nose, pharynx, larynx; progresses to nodules; then fibrotic stage *Acta Otolaryngol 105:494–499, 1988; Cutis 40:101–103, 1987*

Sporotrichosis *Case Rep Dermatol 24:231–237, 2018; Med Mycol 50:170–178, 2012; Acta Cytol 54:648–650, 2007*

Syphilis
  Chancre
  Secondary lesions – warty mucosal lesions, oral condylomata lata *Indian J DV Leprol 83:277, 2017*
  Interstitial glossitis

Verrucae *J Cancer Res Ther 14:454–456, 2018*

Yaws

INFILTRATIVE DISEASES

Verruciform xanthoma (disseminated verruciform xanthoma) – alveolar ridge, palate, floor of the mouth *BJD 151:717–719, 2004; Oral Oncol 37:326–331, 2001; Int J Oral Maxillofac Surg 8:62–66, 1999; Oral Surg Oral Med Oral Pathol 31:784–789, 1971*

INFLAMMATORY DISEASES

Crohn's disease *Oral Surg Oral Med Oral Pathol 75:220–224, 1993*

Median rhomboid glossitis

Pyostomatitis vegetans – marker of inflammatory bowel disease *JAMADerm 156:335, 2020; J Cut Med Surg 20:163–165, 2016; Acta DV 81:134–136, 2001; JAAD 31:336–341, 1994*

Sarcoidosis *BMJ Case Reports Dec 1, 2019*

Plasma cell mucositis *Clin Exp Dermatol 41:951–952, 2016*

METABOLIC DISEASES

Tyrosinemia type II (Richner-Hanhart syndrome) – hyperkeratosis of the tongue *Ann DV 106:53–62, 1979*

NEOPLASTIC DISEASES

Bowen's disease *OSOMOPOR Endod 90:466–473, 2000*

Epithelioma *Oral Surg Oral Med Oral Pathol Oral Radiol Endod 87:197–208, 1999*

Kaposi's sarcoma *J Periodontol 77:523–533, 2006*

Linear verrucous epidermal nevus *Head Neck Pathol 4:139–143, 2010; Dermatol Online J Jan 15, 2020*

Lymphoma – cutaneous T-cell lymphoma

Plasmoacanthoma *An Bras Dermatol 91:128–130, 2016*

Proliferative verrucous leukoplakia *J Calif Dent Assoc 27:300–305, 308–309, 1999; Oral Surg Oral Med Oral Pathol Oral Radiol Endod 83:471–477, 1997*

Squamous cell carcinoma

Verrucous carcinoma (oral florid papillomatosis) *JAAD 81:59–71, 2019; NEJM 372:2049, 2015; Cancer 89:2597–2606, 2000; Dermatology 192:217–221, 1996; J Craniomaxillofac Surg 17:309–314, 1989; Surg 23:670–678, 1948;* of the lip *BJD 157:813–815, 2007*

Verrucous hyperplasia *J Oral Pathol Med 49:404–408, 2020; J Invest Clin Dent 7:417–423, 2016; J Oral Biol Craniofac Res 2:163–169, 2012; J Maxillofac Surg 11:13–19, 1983; Cancer 46:1855–1862, 1980*

Warty dyskeratoma *J Oral Pathol Med 41:261–267, 2012; Br J Oral Maxillofac Surg 23:371–375, 1985*

PARANEOPLASTIC DISORDERS

Acanthosis nigricans, malignant *World J Surg Oncol 15:208, 2017; BJD 176:e99, 2017; Am J Dermatopathol 10:68–73, 1988;* florid papillary oral lesions *OSOMOPORE 81:445–449, 1996*

PRIMARY CUTANEOUS DISEASES

Acanthosis nigricans *Acta DV Croat 16:91–95, 2008; Int J Dermatol 43:530–532, 2004; JAAD 31:1–19, 1994*

Acquired epidermodysplasia verruciformis – personal observation

Darier's disease *JAAD 77:809–830, 2017; Indian J Dent Research 22:843–846, 2011; OSOMOPORE 102:e29–33, 2006; Int J Dermatol 43:835–839, 2004*

Keratosis lichenoides chronica *Dermatology 191:188–192, 1995; AD 131:609–614, 1995*

Lichen planus

SYNDROMES

Cowden's syndrome – oral papillomatous fibromatosis *Quintessence Int 48:413–418, 2017; Case Reps in Dentistry Sept 16, 2013 Article 10315109; OSOMOP 59:264–268, 1985;* oral cobblestoning *An Bras Dermatol 88(suppl 1):52–55, 2013*

Focal epithelial hyperplasia (Heck's disease) *SKINMed 14:395–397, 2016; J Oral Pathol Med 18:419–421, 1989*

Hereditary mucoepithelial dysplasia

Riga-Fede disease – white oral verrucous plaque of the mucosal surface of the lip, tongue, frenulum due to trauma; sign of infantile or natal teeth or sensory neuropathies *JAAD 47:445–447, 2002*

TRAUMA

Dentures

VASCULAR DISEASES

Lymphangioma circumscriptum

Pyogenic granuloma *Braz J Otorhinolaryngol 85:399–407, 2019; pregnancy Clin Dermatol 34:353–358, 2015;* upper lip *J Taibab Univ Med Sch Sc 14:95–98, 2018*

OSTEOMA CUTIS

Cureus 10:e3170, 2018; BJD 146:1075–1080, 2002; Arch Pathol 76:44–54, 1963

Primary osteoma cutis
   Albright's hereditary osteodystrophy
   Fibrodysplasia ossificans progressiva
   Myositis ossificans progressiva
   Plate-like osteoma cutis (congenital or acquired)
   Progressive osseous heteroplasia
   Pseudohypoparathyroidism
   Pseudo-pseudohypoparathyroidism

Secondary osteoma cutis
   Acne vulgaris
   Actinic keratosis
   Atypical fibroxanthoma
   Basal cell carcinoma *Cureus 2018 Aug:10(8):;e3170*
   Bronchogenic carcinoma, metastatic
   Chondroid syringoma
   Chondroma
   Dermatofibroma
   Dermatomyositis
   Desmoid tumor
   Epidermal nevi
   Folliculitis
   Gardner's syndrome
   Hemangioma
   Infantile fibromatosis
   Infundibular cyst
   Lipoma
   Lupus erythematosus
   Melanocytic nevus
   Melanoma
   Mixed tumor of the skin
   Morphea profunda
   Myositis ossificans
   Neurilemmoma
   Pilar cyst
   Pilomatrixoma
   Pseudoxanthoma elasticum
   Pyogenic granuloma
   Scar
   Scleroderma
   Syphilis
   Trauma

Trichoepithelioma
Trichofolliculoma
Venous insufficiency, chronic

OVERGROWTH SYNDROMES

Bannayan-Riley-Ruvalcaba syndrome – macrocephaly, café au lait macules, pigmented macules of the penis, lipomas, vascular malformations, hamartomatous polyps of the distal ileum, colon; PTEN hamartoma syndrome

Beckwith-Wiedemann syndrome (hemihypertrophy-lipomatosis syndrome) – congenital overgrowth syndrome; abdominal wall defects, macroglossia, gigantism, glabellar nevus simplex, exomphalos, macroglossia, hypoglycemia, pre- and postnatal overgrowth, limb hemihypertrophy, embryonal cancers *JAAD 69:589–594, 2013; Cutis 80: 297–302, 2007; Am J Med Genet 79:274–278, 1998; Clin Genet 46:168–174, 1994*

MCAP – megalencephaly and capillary malformation – *PIK3CA* mutation *Ped Derm 35:681–682, 2018*

CLAPO syndrome – capillary malformation of the lower lip; lymphatic malformation of the face and neck; swollen lip, prominent veins of the neck, jaw, and scalp, asymmetry of the face and limbs, partial or generalized overgrowth reticulate erythema of the neck; PIK3CA mutation *Ped Derm 35:681–682, 2018*

CLOVES syndrome (congenital lipomatous overgrowth with vascular, epidermal, and spinal and skeletal abnormalities); lipoatrophy – somatic activating mutation in *PIK3CA Ped Derm 35:681–682, 2018; Ped Derm 34:735–736, 2017; Clin Genet 91:14–21, 2017; JAAD 68:885–896, 2013; Am J Hum Genet 90:1108–1115, 2012*

Cowden's syndrome

Diffuse capillary malformation with overgrowth – reticulated red patch with hemihypertrophy (nonprogressive proportionate overgrowth) *JAAD 69:589–594, 2013*

Encephalocraniocutaneous lipomatosis syndrome – cranial asymmetry; lipomas, connective tissue nevi *Cutis 80: 297–302, 2007*

Hemihyperplasia multiple lipomatosis syndrome (familial lipomatosis/hemihyperplasia syndrome) – hemihyperplasia at birth, moderate overgrowth with subcutaneous lipomas, superficial capillary malformations *JAAD 56:541–564, 2007; Cutis 80: 297–302, 2007; Overgrowth Syndromes. New York. Oxford Univ. Press, 2002, pp. 5–110; Am J Med Genet 79:311–318, 1998*

High flow vascular lesions – warmth, multifocal, soft tissue fullness or overgrowth, peripheral pallor *Ped Derm 35:723–724, 2018*

Klippel-Trenaunay syndrome (capillary-lymphatic-venous malformation) – varicose veins with or without venous malformations; port-wine stain; hemihypertrophy (limb hypertrophy) (bony or soft tissue hyperplasia); may involve spleen, liver, bladder, colon *JAAD 66:71–77, 2012; AD 146:1347–1352, 2010; JAAD 61:621–628, 2009; JAAD 56:541–564, 2007; JAAD 56:242–249, 2007; Arch Gen Med (Paris) 3:641–672, 1900*

Kosaki overgrowth syndrome *Am J Med Genet A173:2422–2427, 2017*

Luscan-Lumish syndrome *J Autism Dev Disorders 45:3764–3770, 2015; J Med Genet 51:512—517, 2014*

Macrocephaly-CMTC (cutis marmorata telangiectatica congenita syndrome) – renamed "macrocephaly-capillary malformation syndrome" – macrocephalic neonatal hypotonia and developmental delay; frontal bossing, segmental overgrowth, syndactyly,

asymmetry, distended linear and serpiginous abdominal wall veins, patchy reticulated vascular stain without atrophy; telangiectasias of the face and ears; midline reticulated facial nevus flammeus (capillary malformation) (vascular stains), hydrocephalus, skin and joint hypermobility, hyperelastic skin, thickened subcutaneous tissue, polydactyly, 2–3 toe syndactyly, postaxial polydactyly, hydrocephalus, frontal bossing, hemihypertrophy with segmental overgrowth; neonatal hypotonia, developmental delay; *PIK5CA* mutation *JAAD 63:805–814, 2010; Ped Derm 26:342–346, 2009; AD 145:287–293, 2009; JAAD 58:697–702, 2008; Ped Derm 24:555–556, 2007; JAAD 56:541–564, 2007; Ped Derm 16:235–237, 1999; Genet Couns 9:245–253, 1998; Am J Med Genet 70:67–73, 1997; Clin Dysmorphol 6:291–302, 1997* (Note: Beckwith-Wiedemann syndrome demonstrates dysmorphic ears, macroglossia, body asymmetry, midfacial vascular stains, visceromegaly with omphalocele, neonatal hypoglycemia, *but no macrocephaly*)

Maffucci's syndrome *Br J Radiol 89(1067)20160521.Nov 2016*

Malan syndrome *J Ped Genet 4:136–143, 2015*

Marshall-Smith syndrome

McCune-Albright syndrome (polyostotic fibrous dysplasia)

Neurofibromatosis

Nevus sebaceus syndrome – facial hemihypertrophy; hemimegalencephaly; neuronal and glial proliferation leading to enlargement of the cerebral hemisphere *Ped Derm 24:428–429, 2007*

Parkes-Weber syndrome – arteriovenous malformation with multiple arteriovenous fistulae along the extremity with limb (usually leg) overgrowth; arteriovenous shunting; cutaneous red stain; lymphedema; high-output congestive heart failure, hypertrophied digits with severe deformity; red foot *JAAD 56:541–564, 2007*

Perlman syndrome – characteristic facial dysmorphology; micropenis; nephroblastoma, renal hamartoma, facial dysmorphism, fetal gigantism *Am J Med Genet C Semin Med Genet 163C:106–113, 2013*

PHACES syndrome – multilobulated giant hemangioma with hemihypertrophy of the face

Primrose syndrome – calcified ears *Mol Syndromol 9:70–82, 2018*

Proteus syndrome – soft tissue and bony hypertrophy of the hands and feet, hemihypertrophy, exostosis, cranial hyperostosis, visceral hamartomas, lipomas, vascular anomalies, port-wine stains, linear epidermal nevi, connective tissue nevus, gigantism, mosaic distribution of lesions; cerebriform thickening of the palms and soles, capillary, venous, lymphatic, and combined slow-flow malformations (like Klippel-Trenaunay syndrome); lipohypoplasia; mosaic distribution, progressive course, sporadic occurrence; bilateral ovarian cystadenomas, parotid monomorphic adenoma, lipomas, vascular malformations, lung cysts, facial phenotype; somatic mosaic mutation of *AKT1 NEJM 365:611–619, 2011; Cutis 83:255–261, 2009; JAAD 56:541–564, 2007; Cutis 80: 297–302, 2007; Eur J Pediatr 140:5–12, 1983; Birth Defects 15:291–296, 1979*

PTEN-hamartoma-tumor syndrome – grossly enlarged head; recurrent arteriovenous malformations of the hand and forearm; macrocephaly, frontal bossing, café au lait macules, congenital nevi, low-set ears, downward slanting eyebrows and palpebral fissures *Ped Derm 28:466–467, 2011*

Simpson-Golabi-Behmel syndrome – generalized somatic overgrowth; coarse facial features, hypertelorism, downslanting palpebral fissures, epicanthal folds, short nose with broad nasal bridge, macrostomia, macroglossia, central groove of the lower lip and/or tongue; short broad hands, fingernail hypoplasia of the index finger, supernumerary nipples *Cutis 83:255–261, 2009*

SOLAMEN syndrome (segmental overgrowth, lipomatosis, arteriovenous malformation, and epidermal nevus) – segmental overgrowth, lipomatosis, arteriovenous malformation, epidermal nevus; loss of wild-type *PTEN* allele in Cowden families; phenotype mimics Proteus patients *Eur J Hum Genet 15:767–773, 2007*

Sotos syndrome – generalized somatic overgrowth; prominent forehead, downslanting palpebral fissures, malar flushing *J Pediatr Genet 4:136–143, 2015 Cutis 83:255–261, 2009*

Sturge-Weber syndrome

Tatton-Brown syndrome – tall stature, macrocephaly, characteristic facies – round face, heavy horizontal eyebrows, narrow, small or downslanting palpebral fissures, marked philtrum, triangular interpillar space, low tone joint hypermobility

Thaurin-Robinet-Faivre syndrome *Clin Genet 2016:89:e1–4*

Weaver syndrome – generalized somatic overgrowth; macrocephaly, broad forehead, flattened occiput, large low-set ears, hypertelorism; soft loose skin, redundant nuchal skin folds; umbilical hernia; thin deep set nails *J Ped Genet 4:136–143, 2015; Cutis 83:255–261, 2009*

P63-ASSOCIATED DISORDERS

Ped Derm 28:15–19, 2011

Acro-dermato-ungual-lacrimal-tooth syndrome (ADULT syndrome) – excessive freckling in sun-exposed areas; decreased sweating; hypoplastic, dysplastic, absent or ridged nails; fine hair, dry skin; lacrimal punctae absent in many; breast and/or nipple hypoplasia

Ankyloblepharon ectodermal dysplasia clefting syndrome (AEC) – rare autosomal dominant; congenital erythroderma, skin fragility, atrophy, palmoplantar hyperkeratosis, extensive/long lasting erosions, eyelid fusion, lacrimal duct obstruction *Hum Mol Genet 22:531–543, 2013*

Ectrodactyly ectodermal dysplasia clefting syndrome (EEC) – triad of lacrimal tract anomalies, urogenital anomalies, conductive hearing loss; thin, dry skin; sparse silvery blond hair *Cell Mol Life Sci 75:1179–1190, 2018*

Isolated orofacial clefting (isolated cleft lip, NSCL)

Limb mammary syndrome (LMS) – nail and lacrimal duct defects; hypohidrosis, breast and nipple hypoplasia, orofacial clefting *Gene Reviews Dec 5, 2019 PMID 20556892*

Split hand-foot malformation (SHFM4) – split hand/foot with or without syndactyly; aplasia or hypoplasia of phalanges and metacarpals; ectodermal abnormalities with cleft lip/palate rare *Gene Reviews Dec 5, 2019 PMID 20556892; Cell Cycle 6:161–168, 2007*

Rapp-Hodgkin syndrome (Hay-Wells syndrome part of spectrum of AEC) – severe skin erosions, teeth and hair defects and/or alopecia, lacrimal duct obstruction, orofacial clefting, anhidrotic ectodermal dysplasia

PAINFUL TUMORS

EXOGENOUS AGENTS

Iododerma *Australas J Dermatol 29:179–180, 1988*

INFLAMMATORY DISEASES

Myositis – focal myositis presenting as painful nodules *Cutis 54:189–190, 1994*

Nodular fasciitis – skin-colored nodules (tender or painful) on the head and neck, extremities, or trunk *Cutis 92:199–202, 2013; AD 137:719–721, 2001*

Palmoplantar eccrine hidradenitis *Ped Derm 18 (Suppl):60, 2001*

METABOLIC DISORDERS

Albright's osteodystrophy – with osteoma cutis; painful subcutaneous nodules and shortened digits *Ped Derm 36: 944–945, 2019*

Calcinosis cutis *Actas Dermosifilogr 106:785–794, 2015*

Osteoma cutis *Actas Dermosifilogr 92: (suppl 1)113–114, 2017*

Perineural xanthoma in diabetes mellitus – tender red nodule of back *Cutis 92:299–302, 2013*

NEOPLASTIC DISEASES

Actinic keratosis

Adenoid cystic carcinoma – head and neck *JAAD 17:113–118, 1987*

Aggressive digital papillary adenocarcinoma *AD 146:191–196, 2010*

Angioleiomyomas *J Hand Surg (Br) 20:479–483, 1995; AD 79:32–41, 1959;* pink nodule of heel *Cutis 81:123,140–141, 2008*

Angiolipoma *Am J Surg Pathol 14:75–81, 1990;* cellular angiolipoma *Clin Exp Dermatol 42:104–105, 2017*

Angiomyofibroblastoma – painful red nodule of vulva *Ped Derm 29:217–218, 2012; BJD 157:189–191, 2007; Histopathology 40:505–509, 2002*

"Blend an egg" or "Calm hog fled pen and gets back" *Indian J DV Leprol 85:231–234, 2020; Clin Cosmetic Inv Derm 12:123–132, 2019; JAAD 28:298–300, 1993*

Carcinoid, metastatic

Clear cell hidradenoma *Ped Derm 17:235–237, 2000; Cancer 23:641–657, 1969*

Dermatofibroma *AD 142:1351–1356, 2006*

Eccrine angiomatous hamartoma *Ped Derm 26:316–319, 2009; AD 142:1351–1356, 2006; Ped Derm 23:365–368, 2006; Ped Derm 22:175–176, 2005; Cutis 71:449–455, 2003; JAAD 47:429–435, 2002; Ped Derm 18:117–119, 2001; JAAD 41:109–111, 1999; JAAD 37:523–549, 1997; Ped Derm 14:401–402, 1997; Ped Derm 13:139–142, 1996; AD 129:105–110, 1993; Virchow Arch Pathol Anat 16:160, 1859;* skin-colored nodule with blue papules

Eccrine epithelioma *JAAD 6:514–518, 1982*

Eccrine hidrocystoma

Eccrine porocarcinoma – painful violaceous papule of temple *Cutis 92:67–70, 2013*

Eccrine poroma *AD 128:1530, 1533, 1992*

Eccrine spiradenocarcinoma – tender, solitary, subcutaneous nodule *Cutis 92:285–287, 2013*

Eccrine spiradenoma *AD 138:973–978, 2002; J Eur Acad DV 15:163–166, 2000; BJD 140:154–157, 1999*

Eccrine sweat gland carcinoma *J Cutan Pathol 14:65–86, 1987*

Enchondroma, subungual *Derm Surg 27:591–593, 2001*

Endometrioma *AD 142:1351–1356, 2006*

Epithelioma cuniculatum *AD 128:106–107, 109–110, 1992*

Fibromyxoma *Am J Surg Pathol 36:789–798, 2012*

Fibrous histiocytoma – aneurysmal variant; dark brown-black tender nodular mass of thigh *Ped Derm 35:836–838, 2018*

Granular cell tumor *AD 142:1351–1356, 2006*

Hidradenoma *Dermatol Online J 22 (9)13–30, 2016*

Keloid

Keratoacanthomas *Int J Dermatol 35:648–650, 1996*

Leiomyomas *AD 144:1217–1222, 2008; JAAD 38:272–273, 1998; Dermatology 191:295–298, 1995;* cold-induced pain *BJD 118:255–260, 1988;* multiple pink painful nodules associated with renal cell carcinoma; fumarate hydratase deficiency *JAAD 55:683–686, 2006; Am J Hum Genet 10:48–52, 1958;* Reed syndrome – cutaneous and uterine leiomyomas; fumarate hydratase deficiency *Acta DV 53:409–416, 1973;* unilateral red painful papules *JAMA Derm 149:865–866, 2013*

Leiomyosarcoma *Acta DV 95:633–634, 2015*

Lymphoma – immunocytoma (low grade B-cell lymphoma) – blue or reddish-brown papules *JAAD 44:324–329, 2001;* marginal zone B-cell lymphoma of MALT type *JAAD S86–88, 2003;* intravascular lymphoma – painful nodules and plaques *Cutis 82:267–272, 2008;* painful skin colored nodules – granulomatous cutaneous T-cell lymphoma *BJD 163:1129–1132, 2010;* EBV-associated natural killer/T-cell lymphoproliferative disorder – painful red subcutaneous nodules of legs *AD 147:216–220, 2011*

Malignant schwannoma (neurofibrosarcoma) – nodule which enlarges and becomes painful *JAAD 38:815–819, 1998; Am J Dermatopathol 11:213–221, 1989*

Metastases – esophageal carcinoma (scalp nodule) *Cutis 70:230–232, 2002;* transitional cell carcinoma of renal pelvis *JAAD 42:867868, 2000;* colon cancer *Cutis 60:297–298, 1997;* carcinoid *JAAD 36:997–998, 1996;* gastric carcinoid *Am J Dermatopathol 14:263–269, 1992;* chondrosarcoma (scapula) *AD 114:584–586, 1978;* breast cancer – painful erythematous nodules of palms *Indian J DV Leprol 77:695–698, 2011*

Morton's neuroma – damage to plantar digital nerve with fibrosis; pain between third and fourth metatarsals

Myxoinflammatory fibroblastic sarcoma – painful subcutaneous nodule *JAAD 62:711–712, 2010*

Neurilemmoma (schwannoma) – pink- gray or yellowish nodules of head and neck *AD 142:1351–1356, 2006*

Neuroma *J Bone Joint Surg Br 76:474–476, 1994*

Neuromatous hyperplasia

Neurothekeoma (nerve sheath myxoma) *J Korean Med Sci 7:85–89, 1992*

Osteoid osteomas – nocturnal pain *Derm Surg 27:591–593, 2001*

Paraganglioma, metastatic *JAAD 44:321–323, 2001*

Plexiform fibrohistiocytic tumor – tender red nodule of chest *Ped Derm 36:490–496, 2019*

Plexiform Schwannomas – painful plantar nodules *BMC Musculoskelet Disord Oct 11, 2014*

Poroid hidradenoma – painful deep red nodule of arm, scalp, face, or trunk *AD 146:557–562, 2010*

Proliferating trichilemmal tumor *AD 124:936, 938–939, 1988*

Congenital smooth muscle hamartoma – painful 5 cm hyperpigmented plaque of posterior thigh *Clin Exp Dermatol 45:490–492, 2020*

Spiradenoma *JAAD 2:59–62, 1980*

Squamous cell carcinoma of the scalp *JAAPA 13:125–126, 2000;* painful scar *Br J Plast Surg 41:197–199, 1988*

PRIMARY CUTANEOUS DISEASES

Dercum's disease (adiposis dolorosa) – painful peri-articular lipomas *JAAD 44:132–136, 2001*

Pacinian corpuscle hyperplasia with foreign body giant cell reaction – painful blue macule on palmar thumb *JAMA Derm 149:97–102, 2013*

Piezogenic pedal papule

Scar

SYNDROMES

Blue rubber bleb nevus syndrome – vascular malformation *AD 116:924–929, 1996*

Incontinentia pigmenti – painful subungual dyskeratotic tumors *Ann Dermatol Syphiligr (Paris) 100:159–168, 1973*

TRAUMA

Chondrodermatitis nodularis helicis chronicus *Cureus 10:e2367, 2018*

VASCULAR TUMORS

Angioendotheliomatosis *Clin Exp Dermatol 32:45–47, 2007*

Angioma *Int J Dermatol 44:1045–1047, 2005*

Epithelioid hemangioendothelioma – painful brown-pink nodule *AD 143:937–942, 2007*

Glomuvenous malformation (plaque-type glomus tumor) – blue macules, papules, plaques; may be hyperkeratotic; mutation in glomulin gene (*GLMN*) *Ped Derm 26:70–74, 2009; Ped Derm 25:381–382, 2008; JAAD 58:S92–93, 2008; BJD 154:450–452, 2006; Ped Derm 18:223–226, 2001; AD 132:704–705, 707–708, 1996; Lyon Chir 21:257–280, 1924;* blue-purple nodules with pebbly surface *JAAD 56:353–370, 2007;* congenital plaque type glomuvenous malformation – may resemble capillary malformation (red patch), venous malformation, or blue nevus *JAAD 56:353–370, 2007;* familial GVM *Bull Soc Fr Dermatol Syphiligr 43:736–740, 1936*

Intravascular papillary endothelial hyperplasia

Thrombosed vein – plantar *Clin Podiatr Med Surg 13:85–89, 1996*

Thrombosis of palmar digital vein – painful firm blue nodule *Ann Dermatol 24:351–354, 2012*

Thrombus *AD 104:427–430, 1971; AD 93:670–673, 1966*

Tufted angioma *Ped Derm 19:388–393, 2002; JAAD 31:307–311, 1994; Int J Dermatol 33:675–676, 1994; Clin Exp Dermatol 17:344–345, 1992*

Venous aneurysm – painful blue nodule of hand *AD 140:1393–1398, 2004*

Venous malformation – discrete mass with soft tissue swelling; may be blue or with skin discoloration *Ped Derm 30:534–540, 2013; JAAD 56:353–370, 2007*

PALATAL NECROSIS (NECROTIC ULCERS OF THE PALATE)

DRUG REACTIONS

Intranasal abuse of acetaminophen *Ear Nose Throat J 94:E40–42, 2015*

Rituximab *Mult Scler Relat Disord 37:101429, 2020*

EXOGENOUS AGENTS

Cocaine – nasal cocaine abuse; cocaine-induced midline destructive lesions (CIMDL) *Dermatol Online J Sept 15, 2016;* levamisole-tainted cocaine *Ann Oto Rhino Laryngol 124:30–34, 2015; Eur Arch Otorhinolaryngol 255:446–447, 1998*

Heroin snorting *Subst Abuse 34:409–414, 2013*

INFECTIONS AND INFESTATIONS

Actinomycosis *J Craniofac Surg 30:e645–646, 2019*

Aspergillosis *Cutis 66:15–18, 2000;* rhinocerebral aspergillosis with palatal necrosis

Glanders – *Burkholderia mallei* – cellulitis which ulcerates with purulent foul-smelling discharge, regional lymphatics become abscesses; nasal and palatal necrosis and destruction; metastatic papules, pustules, bullae over joints and face, then ulcerate; deep abscesses with sinus tracts occur; polyarthritis, meningitis, pneumonia

Herpes zoster *Cutis 66:15–18, 2000*

Leprosy *Med Oral Patol Oral Cir Bucal 11:E474–479, 2006*

Mucormycosis *J Gen Intern Med 33:1815, 2018; J Craniofac Surg 28:e4–5, 2017; Indian J Dermatol 59:423, 2014; Cut Infec Dis Rep 14:423–434, 2012; J Coll Physicians Surg Pak 15:182–183, 2005; Cutis 66:15–18, 2000*

Mycobacteria, atypical Cutis 66:15–18, 2000

Mycobacterium tuberculosis Emedicine, March 28, 2002

Noma (cancrum oris) – non-hemolytic streptococci, Staphylococcus aureus, Bacteroides saccharolyticus, *Fusobacterium necrophorum, Prevotella intermedia Cutis 66:15–18, 2000*

Paecilomyces sinusitis – eroded hard palate *Clin Inf Dis 23:391–393, 1996*

Paracoccidioidomycosis – palatal perforation *JAAD 53:931–951, 2005*

Talaromyces marneffei Oral Dis 5:286–293, 1999

Pseudomonas – suppurative medial otitis, palatal necrosis *Cir Pediatr 19L115–116, 2006*

Syphilis *Emedicine, March 28, 2002*

INFLAMMATORY DISORDERS

Necrotizing sialometaplasia – reactive condition of minor or occasionally major salivary glands; probably due to ischemia or vasculitis *Spec Care Dentist 30:160–162, 2010; Med Oral 9:304–308, 2004; J Am Dent Assoc 101:823–824, 1980*

Necrotizing stomatitis *Cutis 66:15–18, 2000*

Sarcoid

NEOPLASTIC DISORDERS

Kaposi's sarcoma *Cutis 66:15–18, 2000*

Lymphoma – HIV-associated *Cutis 66:15–18, 2000;* midline malignant B-cell lymphoma *Cancer 70:2958–2962, 1992;* extranodal NK-T-cell lymphoma *Head Neck Pathol 13:624–634, 2019;* post-transplant lymphoproliferative disorder *J Ped Hematol Oncol 39:e97–99, 2017*

Mucoepidermoid carcinoma

Pleomorphic adenoma of palate – with extensive necrosis *Oral Dis 10:54–59, 2004*

Squamous cell carcinoma *Emedicine 39:e97–99, 2017; Emedicine, March 28, 2002*

PRIMARY CUTANEOUS DISEASES

Aphthous stomatitis *Emedicine, March 28, 2002*

Idiopathic midline destructive disease *Am J Clin Pathol 77:162–167, 1982*

SYNDROMES

Behcet's disease *Emedicine, September 24, 2004*

TRAUMA

Radiation therapy

Trauma – bottle feeding in a child *Int J Paediatr Dent 5:109–111, 1995*

VASCULAR LESIONS

Granulomatosis with polyangiitis – perforation of palate *J Clin Rheumatol 26:e54, 2020; Oral Disease 6:259–261, 2000; Emedicine, March 28, 2002*

Palantine artery embolization for epistaxis *J Craniofac Surg 29:e437–438, 2018*

Polyarteritis nodosa *J Med Case Rep March 18, 2013*

Post-anesthesia necrosis – dentistry *Contemp Clin Dent 8:501–505, 2017*

PALMAR AND/OR PLANTAR ERYTHEMA

AUTOIMMUNE DISEASES AND DISEASES OF IMMUNE DYSFUNCTION

Allergic contact dermatitis – SLIME *Ped Derm 36:139–141, 2019*

Angioedema

Atopic dermatitis *Allergy 61:1392–1396, 2006*

Dermatitis herpetiformis – red palmoplantar plaques *Cutis 37:184–187, 1986*

Dermatomyositis *Cutis 89:84–88, 2012; Dermatol Online J 15:2, 2009;* anti-synthetase syndrome *QJM 111:329–330, 2018*

Graft vs. host disease – red palms and soles; TEN-like erosions, flat-topped papules *Ped Derm 30:335–341, 2013 An Bras Dermatol 80:69–80, 2005; JAAD 38:369–392, 1998; AD 134:602–612, 1998; Int J Derm 20:249, 1981; Cutis 46:397–404, 1990;* chronic GVHD – erythema and fissuring of palms *JAAD 66:515–532, 2012*

Linear IgA disease – annular psoriasiform, serpiginous red plaques of palms *JAAD 51:S112–117, 2004*

Lupus erythematosus – systemic – reticulated telangiectatic erythema of thenar and hypothenar eminences, finger pulps, toes, lateral feet, and heels; bluish red with small white scars *Cutis 89:84–88, 2012; Br J Derm 135:355–362, 1996;* discoid lupus erythematosus *NEJM 269:1155–1161, 1963;* systemic lupus erythematosus with anti-phospholipid antibodies – erythema of thenar and hypothenar eminences and fingertips *BJD 168:213–215, 2013*

Mixed connective tissue disease

Rheumatoid arthritis (Dawson's palms) *JAAD 53:191–209, 2005; Clin Rheumatol 4:449–451, 1985;* rheumatoid neutrophilic dermatitis

Scleroderma *Cutis 89:84–88, 2012*

Serum sickness – personal observation

Sjogren's syndrome *Br J Rheumatol 33:745–748, 1994*

Urticaria

CONGENITAL LESIONS

Syringomyelia

DEGENERATIVE

Neurotrophic erythema – neuropathy-associated acral paresthesia and vasodilatation

DRUGS

Allopurinol hypersensitivity syndrome

Bromocriptine ingestion – mimics erythromelalgia *Neurology 31:1368–1370, 1981*

Chemotherapy-induced acral dysesthesia syndrome (palmoplantar erythrodysesthesia syndrome) *JAAD 24:457–461, 1991; Cutis 46:397–404, 1990; AD 122:1023–1027, 1986; Ann Int Med 101:12, 1984*
  Capecitabine (Xeloda)
  Cytosine arabinoside
Docetaxel
  Doxorubicin
  Fluorouracil
  Vinblastine

Chemotherapy-induced Raynaud's phenomenon

Chemotherapy-induced eccrine squamous syringometaplasia – cytarabine, mitoxantrone, fluorouracil, cisplatin, doxorubicin, cyclophosphamide, etoposide, methotrexate, busulfan, melphalan, carmustine, thiotepa *AD 133:873–878, 1997;* acral edematous erythema of palm – docetaxel *BJD 146:524–525, 2002*

Corticosteroids – systemic or topical – personal observation

Cytosine arabinoside *AD 121:1240–1241, 1985; AD 121:102–104, 1985*

Dilantin hypersensitivity

Docetaxel *Am J Clin Oncol 25:599–602, 2002*

Doxorubicin *AD 121:102–104, 1985; Ann Int Med 101:798–799, 1984*

Drug eruption, morbilliform – many agents

Etoposide *Cancer 71:3153–3155, 1993*

Fluorouracil *Ann Int Med 101:798–799, 1984*

Hydroxyurea – dermatomyositis-like lesions *JAAD 21:797–799, 1989;* lichenoid eruption *JAAD 36:178–182, 1997*

Mercaptopurine *AD 122:1413–1414, 1986*

Methotrexate *Ann Int Med 98:611–612, 1983*

Nifedipine – mimics erythromelalgia *Neurology 31:1368–1370, 1981*

Oral contraceptives (estrogens)

Roquinimex (cytokine inducer) *AD 133:873–878, 1997*

Salbutamol *Ann DV 119:293–294, 1992*

Sorafenib – personal observation

Sympathomimetics in pregnancy *BJD 124:210, 1991*

Thalidomide *JAAD 35:976, 1996*

Topiramate *J Drugs Dermatol 3:321–322, 2004*

Vandetanib – erythema of palms and soles *AD 148:1418–1420, 2012*

Vemurafenib – cystic lesions of face, keratosis pilaris-like eruptions, hyperkeratotic plantar papules, squamous cell carcinoma; multiple nodules of cheeks; follicular plugging; exuberant seborrheic dermatitis-like hyperkeratosis of face; hand and foot reaction; diffuse spiny follicular hyperkeratosis; cobblestoning of forehead *JAAD 67:1375–1379, 2012;*

AD 148:357–361, 2012

EXOGENOUS AGENTS

Irritant contact dermatitis *Am J Ind Med 8:265–271, 1985*

INFECTIONS

Brucellosis *Int J Dermatol 40:434–438, 2001*

Cellulitis

Clostridial sepsis

Coxsackie virus A6 (atypical hand, foot, and mouth disease) – red papulovesicles of fingers, palmar erythema, red papules of ears, red papules of antecubital fossa, perioral papulovesicles, vesicles of posterior pharynx *JAAD 69:736–741, 2013*

Dengue fever *Indian J Crit Care Med 19:661–664, 2015*

Endocarditis, including acute and subacute bacterial endocarditis *JAMA 119:1417–1418, 1942*

Erysipelas

Erysipeloid

Hepatitis C virus *CMAJ 174:1450, 2006*

HIV – acute HIV infection – acral erythema *Cutis 40:171–175, 1987*

Human Parechovirus 3 (HPeV-3) – sepsis-like illness *Korean J Ped 59:308–311, 2016; Ped Infect Dis J 32:233–236, 2013*

Human T-lymphotrophic virus 1-associated myelopathy *Am J Clin Dermatol 8:347–356, 2007*

Leprosy

Measles – atypical measles

Meningococcemia

Mycobacterium tuberculosis – pulmonary tuberculosis

Parvovirus B19 (erythema infectiosum) *Hum Pathol 31:488–497, 2000;* including papular pruritic petechial glove and sock syndrome *Cutis 54:335–340, 1994*

Rat bite fever

Rocky Mountain spotted fever

Scabies

Scarlet fever and scarlatiniform

Septic emboli

Syphilis – secondary

Tinea manuum – steroid treated; 2 foot 1 hand syndrome – personal observation

Toxic shock syndrome, either staphylococcal or streptococcal – erythema and edema of the palms and soles *JAAD 39:383–398, 1998; JAAD 8:343–347, 1983;* association with tampon use (Rely tampons) and *Staphylococcus aureus NEJM 303:1436, 1442, 198*

Trichinellosis *Parasite 13:65–70, 2006*

Viral exanthem

INFILTRATIVE DISORDERS

Mastocytosis

INFLAMMATORY DISEASES

Crohn's disease *JAAD 36:697–704, 1997*

Erythema multiforme

Erythema nodosum – palmar *JAAD 29:284, 1993; AD 129:1064–1065, 1993*

Recurrent palmoplantar hidradenitis in children (neutrophilic eccrine hidradenitis) *AD 131:817–20, 1995*

Sarcoid *J Med Aust 178:75–76, 2003; Clin Exp Dermatol 23:123–124, 1998; AD 133:882–888, 1997*

Toxic epidermal necrolysis

METABOLIC DISEASES

Acrodermatitis enteropathica *Cutis 81:314, 324–326, 2008*

Chronic febrile disease

Cold agglutinins

Cryofibrinogenemia

Cryoglobulinemia

Diabetes mellitus *Cutis 89:84–88, 2012; Cutis 89:84–88, 2012*

Hemochromatosis *AD 113:161–165, 1977; Medicine 34:381–430, 1955*

Hyperthyroidism (Graves' disease) *Cutis 89:84–88, 2012;JAAD 26:885–902, 1992*

Liver disease, chronic – hyperestrogenic state *Cutis 89:84–88, 2012; Am J Clin Dermatol 8:347–356, 2007* cirrhosis, Wilson's disease, hemochromatosis, hepatitis B, C infection, portal hypertension

Lung disease, chronic – obstructive pulmonary disease

Polycythemia vera

Pregnancy – hyperestrogenic state *Cutis 89:84–88, 2012; Am J Clin Dermatol 7:65–69, 2006; Ann DV 121:227–231, 1994; Cutis 3:120–125, 1967*

Pseudoglucagonoma syndrome due to malnutrition *AD 141:914–916, 2005*

Thrombocythemia – livedo reticularis, acrocyanosis, erythromelalgia, gangrene, pyoderma gangrenosum *Leuk Lymphoma 22 Suppl 1:47–56, 1996; Br J Haematol 36:553–564, 1977; AD 87:302–305, 1963*

Puberty *Cutis 89:84–88, 2012; Am J Clin Dermatol 8:347–356, 2007*

Steatohepatitis *Transl Gastroenterol Hepatol Sept, 2019*

Thyrotoxicosis *J Pak Assoc Derm 13:17–20, 2003*

Tyrosinemia type II – hepatic failure – personal observation

Zinc deficiency, chronic alcoholism – personal observation

NEOPLASTIC DISEASES

Angioimmunoblastic B- or T-cell lymphoma

Atrial myxoma *Br Heart J 36:839–840, 1974*

Basal cell carcinoma *Cutis 89:84–88, 2012*

Eccrine angiomatous hamartoma – painful erythema *AD 125:1489–1490, 1989*

Kaposi's sarcoma *BJD 148:1061–1063, 2003;* plantar erythema

Leukemia – hyperleukocytosis – acral lividosis; chronic myelogenous leukemia with leukostasis – livedo *AD 123:921–924, 1987*

Lung cancer *Cutis 89:84–88, 2012*

Lymphoma – Woringer-Kolopp disease *AD 131:325–329, 1995;* Hodgkin's disease *Ann DV 105:349, 1978*

Metastatic cancer

Multinucleate cell angiohistiocytoma – personal observation

Plantar fibromatosis *JAAD 12:212–214, 1985*

Waldenstrom's macroglobulinemia

PARANEOPLASTIC DISEASES

Bazex syndrome *Hautarzt 66:342–344, 2015*

Lymphoma – red papules and plaques on palmar aspects of fingers *JAAD 51:600–605, 2004*

Palmar fasciitis and polyarthritis syndrome – pancreatic cancer *J Clin Rheumatol 19:203–205, 2013;* metastatic ovarian carcinoma *Gulf J Oncol 12:59–61, 2012;* indurated reticulate palmar erythema *Australas J Dermatol 50:198–201, 2009*

Paraneoplastic autoimmune multiorgan syndrome (paraneoplastic pemphigus) – arciform and polycyclic lesions *AD 137:193–206, 2001*

Paraneoplastic palmar erythema – metastatic and primary brain tumors; gastric adenocarcinoma *Dermatology 204:209–213, 2002; Med Cutan Ibero Lat Am 13:487–490, 1985;* Hodgkin's disease *Ann DV 105:349, 1978;* myeloproliferative disease *AD 121:1240, 1985*

PRIMARY CUTANEOUS DISEASES

Acral localized acquired cutis laxa *JAAD 21:33–40, 1989*

Atopic hand and/or foot dermatitis

Circumscribed palmar or plantar hypokeratosis – red atrophic patch *JAAD 51:319–321, 2004; JAAD 49:1197–1198, 2003; JAAD 47:21–27, 2002*

Ectodermal dysplasia

Epidermolytic hyperkeratosis

Erythema elevatum diutinum *Presse Med 41:1041–1042, 2012*

Erythema palmare hereditarium – Lane disease *Ped Derm 34:590–594, 2017; Hautarzt 51:264–265, 2000; Arch Dermatol Syphilol 20:445–448, 1929*

Erythroderma, multiple causes

Erythrokeratoderma variabilis

Erythrokeratolysis hiemalis (Oudtshoorn disease) (keratolytic winter erythema) – palmoplantar erythema, cyclical and centrifugal peeling of affected sites, targetoid lesions of the hands and feet – seen in South African whites; precipitated by cold weather or fever *BJD 98:491–495, 1978*

Follicular mucinosis, erythrodermic

Granuloma annulare, generalized *JAAD 20:39–47, 1989*

Greither's palmoplantar keratoderma (transgrediens et progrediens palmoplantar keratoderma) – red hands and feet; hyperkeratoses extending over Achilles tendon, backs of hands, elbows, knees; livid erythema at margins *Ped Derm 20:272–275, 2003; Cutis 65:141–145, 2000*

Hand dermatitis, including hand dermatitis treated with topical steroids

Healthy female

Idiopathic

Juvenile plantar dermatosis

Kawasaki's disease *Ped Rheumatol Online J July 3, 2018;* in adult *Medicine 89:149–158, 2010*

Keratolysis exfoliativa – personal observation

Lamellar ichthyosis

Lichen planus – personal observation

Mal de Meleda – autosomal dominant, autosomal recessive transgrediens with acral erythema in glove-like distribution *Dermatology 203:7–13, 2001; AD 136:1247–1252, 2000; J Dermatol 27:664–668, 2000; Dermatologica 171:30–37, 1985*

Mal de Meleda – in infancy *AD 136:1247–1252, 2000*

Necrolytic acral erythema – acral velvety hyperpigmented and hyperkeratotic plaques of distal dorsal feet; red palms with desquamation, erythroderma with flaccid bullae, edema and desquamation of face, onychodystrophy and onycho madesis; hepatitis C *Cutis 84:301–304, 2009*

Pityriasis rubra pilaris

Progressive symmetric erythrokeratoderma

Psoriasis *JAAD 65:137–174, 2011*

Recurrent non-toxic erythema – personal observation

Stasis dermatitis with id reaction

SYNDROMES

Anti-phospholipid antibody syndrome

Familial cerebral malformation *Cutis 89:84–88, 2012*

Familial erythromelalgia *AD 118:953, 1982*

Familial Mediterranean fever – erysipelas-like lesions *Arch Ped 20:382–385, 2013; QJM 75:607–616, 1990*

Goodpasture's syndrome – annular erythematous macule *AD 121:1442–1444, 1985*

Goltz's syndrome *Cutis 89:84–88, 2012*

Hypereosinophilic syndrome – palmoplantar erythema *JAAD 46:s133–136, 2002*

Ichthyosis follicularis with atrichia and photophobia (IFAP) – palmoplantar erythema; collodion membrane and erythema at birth; ichthyosis, spiny (keratotic) follicular papules (generalized follicular keratoses), non-scarring alopecia, keratotic papules of elbows, knees, fingers, extensor surfaces, xerosis; punctate keratitis, photophobia; nail dystrophy, psychomotor delay, short stature; enamel dysplasia, beefy red tongue and gingiva, angular stomatitis, atopy, lamellar scales, psoriasiform plaques *Curr Prob Derm 14:71–116, 2002; JAAD 46:S156–158, 2002; BJD 142:157–162, 2000; AD 125:103–106, 1989; Ped Derm 12:195, 1995; Dermatologica 177:341–347, 1988; Am J Med Genet 85:365–368, 1999*

Keratolytic erythema – rare; autosomal dominant; recurrent episodes of palmoplantar erythema and keratolytic peeling *Am J Hum Genet 100:737–750, 2017*

Netherton's syndrome

Olmsted syndrome– palmoplantar keratoderma with erythromelalgia; mutation in *TRFV3 JAMA Derm 150:303–306, 2014*

Papillon-Lefevre syndrome – palmar erythema precedes development of palmoplantar keratoderma *JAAD 49:S240–243, 2003*

Peeling skin syndrome type B – *BJD 169:1322–1325, 2013*

Reflex sympathetic dystrophy (causalgia) (complex regional pain syndrome) *JAAD 22:513–520, 1990*

Schopf-Schulz-Passarge syndrome (hypotrichosis, palmoplantar hyperkeratosis, apocrine hidrocystomas of eyelid margins, nail dystrophy) – oligodontia; red palms and soles with focal dryness; maceration with hyperhidrosis; finger and toenail dystrophy; mutation in *WNT10A BJD 171:1211–1214, 2014; Ped Derm 30:491–492, 2013; JAAD 65:1066–1069, 2011; AD 140:231–236, 2004; Acta DV 88:607–612, 2008; JAAD 10:922–925, 1984*

TOXINS

Acrodynia, infantile (pink disease) – mercury poisoning; erythema with or without exfoliation *Ped Derm 21:254–259, 2004; JAAD*

46:1109–1111, 2003; Arch Dis Child 86:453, 2002 Ann DV 121:309–314, 1994; AD 124:107–109, 1988

Alcoholic liver disease

Chronic radiation dermatitis

Eosinophilia myalgia syndrome *JAAD 23:1063–1069, 1990*

Thallium intoxication *J Rheumatol 16:171–174, 1989*

TRAUMA

Chilblains *JAAD 23:257–262, 1990*

Chronic radiation dermatitis – personal observation

Cold erythema *JAMA 180:639–42, 1962*

Computer palms *JAAD 42:1073–1075, 2000*

Delayed pressure urticaria

Erythema ab igne *Am J Clin Dermatol 8:347–356, 2007*

Frostbite – recovery phase *JAAD 23:166, 1990*

Heat exposure

Pool palms and soles *Ped Derm 24:95, 2007*

Urticaria – traumatic plantar urticaria *JAAD 18:144–146, 1988*

Vibratory urticaria *Am J Ind Med 8:266–271, 1985*

VASCULAR DISORDERS

Acrocyanosis

Acrocyanosis with atrophy *AD 124:263–268, 1988*

Arteriosclerotic peripheral vascular disease *JAAD 50:456–460, 2004*

Arteriovenous fistula *Clin Nephrol 36:158, 1991*

Cholesterol emboli

Cutis marmorata telangiectatica congenita (plantar erythema)

Erythrocyanosis

Erythromelalgia – associations include essential thrombocythemia, polycythemia vera, diabetes mellitus, peripheral neuropathy, systemic lupus erythematosus, rheumatoid arthritis, hypertension, frostbite, colon cancer, gout, calcium channel blockers, bromocriptine *BJD 153:174–177, 2005; JAAD 50:456–460, 2004;* all types exacerbated by warmth; may affect one finger or toe; ischemic necrosis *JAAD 22:107–111, 1990;* primary (idiopathic) – lower legs, no ischemia *JAAD 21:1128–1130, 1989;* secondary to peripheral vascular disease *JAAD 43:841–847, 2000; AD 136:330–336, 2000;* following influenza vaccine *Clin Exp Rheumatol 15:111–113, 1997;* erythromelalgia with thrombocythemia *JAAD 24:59–63, 1991*

Fat emboli

Hemangioma

Henoch-Schonlein purpura

Klippel-Trenaunay-Weber syndrome

Livedo reticularis *Am J Clin Dermatol 8:347–356, 2007; JAAD 20:453–457, 1989*

Pigmented purpuric eruption

Polyarteritis

Port wine stain

Raynaud's disease – hyperperfusion phase

Recurrent cutaneous eosinophilic vasculitis *BJD 149:901–902, 2003*

Thoracic outlet syndrome – unilateral palmar erythema *Ann Indian Acad Neuro 15:323–325, 2012*

Thromboangiitis obliterans

Urticarial vasculitis

Vascular malformation

Vasculitis – leukocytoclastic, other

Venous gangrene – plantar erythema *AD 123:933–936, 1987*

Venous stasis

PALMAR AND/OR PLANTAR NODULES

AUTOIMMUNE DISEASES AND DISORDERS OF IMMUNE DYSREGULATION

Rheumatoid arthritis – rheumatoid nodule (digital papule) *Clin Rheumatol 14:592–593, 1995; Ann Rheum Dis 51:1005–116, 1992; JAAD 11:713–723, 1984;* rheumatoid papules (rheumatoid neutrophilic dermatitis) *JAAD 20:348–352, 1988;* rheumatoid neutrophilic dermatitis – nodules over joints *AD 133:757–760, 1997; AD 125:1105–1108, 1989;* plantar nodules *J Gen Intern Med 32:955–956, 2017*

EXOGENOUS AGENTS

Foreign body granuloma – digital papule; cactus spine (Opuntia cactus) granulomas *Cutis 65:290–292, 2000;*

Sea urchin spine (granuloma) – plantar nodule

INFECTIONS AND INFESTATIONS

Cellulitis – plantar nodule *Ped Derm 15:97–102, 1998*

Dirofilariasis *Chir Main 30:66–68, 2011*

HPV type 60 infection *AD 130:1418–1420, 1994*

Mycobacterium scrofulaceum – palmar nodule *AD 138:689–694, 2002*

Phaeohyphomycotic cyst *J Clin Microbiol 25:605–608, 1987*

Pseudomonas – hot foot syndrome – painful plantar erythematous nodules *Klin Pediatr 224–225, 2012; NEJM 345:1643–1644, 2001*

Scabies ; crusted (Norwegian) scabies presenting with hyperkeratotic nodules of the soles *AD 134:1019–1024, 1998*

INFILTRATIVE DISORDERS

Nodular amyloid, plantar *JAAD 49:307–310, 2003*

INFLAMMATORY DISORDERS

Erythema multiforme *Medicine 68:133–140, 1989; JAAD 8:763–765, 1983;* plantar nodules *Ped Derm 15:97–102, 1998*

Erythema nodosum *JAAD 26:259–260, 1992; JAAD 20:701–702, 1989*

Palmoplantar eccrine neutrophilic hidradenitis (idiopathic recurrent palmoplantar hidradenitis) (idiopathic plantar hidradenitis) *Ped Derm 21:30–32, 2004; JAAD 47:S263–265, 2002; J Pediatr 160:189–191, 2001; J Pediatr 160:189–191, 2001; AD 134:76–79, 1998; Ped Derm 15:97–102, 1998; J Eur Acad Dermatovenereol 10:257–261, 1998; AD 131:817–820, 1995*

Panniculitis – plantar nodule *Ped Derm 15:97–102, 1998*

METABOLIC DISORDERS

Dystrophic calcification – plantar, posterior heel stick *Australas J Dermatol 51:206–207, 2010; Clin Exp Dermatol 28:502–503, 2003*

NEOPLASTIC DISORDERS

Acquired fibrokeratoma – multiple plantar nodules *Dermatol Online J 16:5, 2010*

Aggressive digital papillary adenocarcinoma – asymptomatic dome shaped skin colored nodule *J Dermatol 35:468–470, 2008*

Atypical palmar fibromatosis – with giant fibrous nodule *J Hand Surg Am 29:159, 2004; J Hand Surg Am 28:525–527, 2003*

Basal cell carcinoma – palmar papule in nevoid basal cell carcinoma syndrome *AD 143:813–814, 2007*

Chondroid syringoma *Pathol Res Pract 198755–764, 2002*

Cutaneous fibroma

Dermatofibroma *SKINMed 7:41–43, 2008*

Dupuytren's contracture (palmar fibromatosis) – starts as palmar nodule *J Hand Surg Am March 14, 2020; Am J Surg Pathol 1:255–270, 1977*

Eccrine angiomatous hamartoma – toes, fingers, palms and soles-skin-colored to blue *Cutis 71:449–455, 2003; JAAD 47:429–435, 2002; Ped Derm 13:139–142, 1996; JAAD 37:523–549, 1997; Ped Derm 14:401–402, 1997; Ped Derm 18:117–119, 2001; Ped Derm 14:401–402, 1997;* skin-colored nodule with blue papules *JAAD 41:109–111, 1999*

Eccrine poroma – plantar red nodule; *AD 74:511–521, 1956;* digital papule *AD 74:511–512, 1956*

Epithelioid neurofibroma

Epithelioid sarcoma – nodule of flexor finger or palm *JAAD 14:893–898, 1986; AD 121:389–393, 1985;* of sole

Fibroma of tendon sheath

Fibrous hamartoma of infancy – congenital plantar nodule *Ped Derm 21:506–507, 2004;* palmar cutaneous hamartoma *Am J Dermatopathol 20:65–68, 1998*

Giant cell tumor of tendon sheath – one of the most common neoplasmas of hand; solitary, painless *Chir Main 26:165–169, 2007*

Late fibrosing stage of tenosynovial giant cell tumor

Granular cell tumor – red nodule of palm *Ped Derm 27:656–657, 2010*

Hypertrophic scar – plantar giant nodule *BJD 145:1005–1007, 2001*

Ledderhose's nodules (plantar fibromatosis) *Indian Dermatol Online J 6:422–424, 2015; JAAD 41:106–108, 1999*

Lipofibromatosis – rare benign tumor of childhood *Ann DV 138:391–394, 2011*

Lipoma – adipose plantar nodules (congenital) *BJD 142:1262–1264, 2000;* palmar subcutaneous lipoma *Cutis 40:29–32, 1987*

Metastasis – breast cancer – painful erythematous nodules *Indian J DV Leprol 77:695–698, 2011;* squamous cell lung cancer *AD 126:665–666, 1990*

Nerve sheath myxoma – painless, firm slow growing nodule of the palm *Oman Med J 27:e305, 2012*

Painful piezogenic pedal papules or nodules *Dermatol Monatsschr 161:43–45, 1975*

Plantar fibromatosis or palmar fibromatosis *Clin Podiatr Med Surg 22:11–18, 2005; Am J Surg Pathol 29:1095–1105, 2005*

Plexiform Schwannomas – painful plantar nodules *BMC Musculoskelet Disord Oct 11, 2014*

Precalcaneal congenital fibrolipomatous hamartoma (pedal papules of the newborn) – plantar nodule over medial plantar heel *J Cut Pathol 46:277–279, 2019; Ped Derm 24:74–75, 2007; Ped Derm 21:655–656, 2004; Med Cut Ibero Lat Am 18:9–12, 1990*

Sclerosing perineuroma – palmar nodule, digital nodule *Int J Surg Pathol 26:195–197, 2018; Ped Derm 21:606–607, 2004; BJD 146:129–133, 2002*

Sclerotic adnexal tumor

Traumatic neuroma

Waldenstrom's macroglobulinemia – cutaneous macroglobulinosis *JAAD 71:e251–252, 2014*

PRIMARY CUTANEOUS DISEASES

Delayed pressure urticaria – nodules of soles *JAAD 29:954–958, 1993*

Granuloma annulare – red palmar papule or nodule *AD 142:49–54, 2006; JAAD 3:217–230, 1980*

Migratory angioedema – plantar nodule *Ped Derm 15:97–102, 1998*

SYNDROMES

Blue rubber bleb nevus syndrome – plantar blue nodules

Maffucci's syndrome – enchondromas, angiomas, cartilaginous nodules *Dermatologic Clinics 13:73–78, 1995; JAAD 29:894–899, 1993*

Neurofibromatosis – linear, segmental; multiple soft nodules of plantar surface *J Cut Med Surg 16:436–437, 2012*

Reactive arthritis – keratoderma blenorrhagicum *Semin Arthritis Rheum 3:253–286, 1974*

Scleroatrophic syndrome of Huriez – palmar nodule, scleroatrophy of the hands *BJD 137:114–118, 1997*

TRAUMA

Callosities – occupational (carpenters, live chicken hangers, frictional) *Contact Derm 17:13–16, 1987*

VASCULAR LESIONS

Epithelioid hemangioendothelioma

Glomus tumor – painful on the plantar arch *Foot Ankle Int 18:672–674, 1999*

Plantar thrombotic nodules *J Dermatol 24:405–409, 1997*

Spindle cell hemangioendothelioma – hyperkeratotic nodules of soles *BJD 142:1238–1239, 2000*

Thrombosis of palmar digital vein – painful firm blue nodule *Ann Dermatol 24:351–354, 2012*

Vasculitis – plantar nodule *JAAD 47:S263–265, 2002; Ped Derm 15:97–102, 1998*

Venous aneurysm – painful blue nodule of hand *AD 140:1393–1398, 2004*

PALMAR PITS AND PUNCTATE KERATOSES/DYSHIDROSIS-LIKE LESIONS

AUTOIMMUNE DISEASES AND DISEASES OF IMMUNE DYSFUNCTION

Discoid lupus erythematosus

Mixed connective tissue disease

Scleroderma – acrokeratoelastoidosis-like lesions *JAAD 46:767–770, 2002;* CREST syndrome – acral pits

DRUG-INDUCED

PUVA – punctate keratoses *JAAD 42:476–479, 2000*

INFECTIONS

Epidermodysplasia verruciformis *Indian J DV Leprol 78:501–503, 2012; Cutis 5253–55, 1993;* acquired epidermodysplasia verruciformis *JAAD 60:315–320, 2009*

Mycobacterium tuberculosis – miliary tuberculosis in AIDS *JAAD 23:381–385, 1990;* punctate palmoplantar keratoses acuminata (papulonecrotic tuberculid) *J Cut Med Surg 12:198–202, 2008; Int J Derm 8:470–471, 1982*

Paracoccidioidomycosis – punctate palmoplantar keratoderma *J Clin Inf Dis 23:1026–1032, 1996*

Pitted keratolysis – *Corynebacterium* species (now *Kytococcus sedentarius) Case Reports Dermatol 2:146–148, 2010; Cutis 79:371–377, 2007;* white hyperkeratosis with circular erosions in malodorous feet *JAAD 7:787–791, 1982; Dermatophilus congolensis* – due to contact with infected animals *BJD 145:170–171, 2001; BJD 137:282, 1997; JAAD 7:752–757, 1982; SkinMed 11:201–203, 2013; Dermatologia CMQ 10:90–92, 2012;* original description by Castellani in 1910 – "keratome plantare sulcatum" *Med Cut Ibero Lat Am 15:151–160, 10987*

Scabies

Syphilis – secondary; minute craters surrounded by hyperkeratotic papules; syphilitic clavi *JAAD 70:E131–132, 2014; Sex Transm Infec 85:484, 2009; AD Syphilology 25:3–34, 1893*

Warts *Cutis 74:173–179, 2004*

Yaws – minute craters surrounded by hyperkeratotic papules (hormoguillo); *JAAD 29:519–535, 1993;* palmoplantar keratoderma; primary mother yaw; papule enlarging with satellite nodules, ulcerates to form crusted lesion; secondary yaws has disseminated lesions (daughter yaws) which expand, ulcerate and weep; healing in circinate and annular patterns; painful osteoperiostitis and polydactylitis; all lesions non-scarring; tertiary yaws – destructive hyperkeratotic, nodular, plaque-like, and ulcerated lesions with deforming bone and joint lesions with prominent palmoplantar keratoderma

INFILTRATIVE DISEASES

Nodular amyloid

INFLAMMATORY DISEASE

Eosinophilic pustular folliculitis

Prurigo nodularis – increased numbers of calcitonin gene-related peptide and substance P-containing nerve fibers.

Sarcoid – erythroderma with keratotic spines and palmar pits *BJD 95:93–97, 1976*

METABOLIC

Calcified milia – in patient with milia-like syringomas *Ped Derm 27:370–372, 2010*

Cystic fibrosis – transient papulotranslucent acrokeratoderma *Australas J Dermatol 41:172–174, 2000*

Gouty tophi *Challenges in Derm 13:6–7, 1988*

Tyrosinemia type II (Richner-Hanhart syndrome) *Arch Int Med 145:1697–1700, 1985*

Xanthoma – punctate xanthoma *JAAD 22:468–476, 1990; Cutis 43:169–171, 1988*

NEOPLASTIC DISEASES

Bowen's disease

Eccrine poromas *JAAD 3:43–49, 1980; AD 101:606, 1970*

Eccrine syringofibroadenomatosis – dyshidrosiform lesions *AD 130:933–934, 1994*

Epidermal nevus, linear

Lymphoma, including cutaneous T-cell lymphoma *JAAD 7:792–796, 1982*

Lymphomatoid papulosis *JAAD 27:627–628, 1992*

Nevus comedonicus *BJD 145:682–684, 2001; JAAD 12:185–188, 1985*

Porokeratosis of Mantoux – crateriform lesions of palms

Porokeratosis of Mibelli

Porokeratosis palmaris et plantaris et disseminata (punctate porokeratosis) *Indian Dermatol Online J 7:290–292, 2016; JAAD 21:415–418, 1989; JAAD 11:454–460, 1984*

Porokeratosis punctata plantaris or palmaris – music box spicules *AD 125:1715, 1989; AD 120:263–264, 1984; J Cutan Pathol 4:338–341, 1977*

Porokeratotic eccrine ostial and dermal duct nevus – linear punctate pits of sole mofrten filled with comedo-like plugs, or palmoplantar papules; mutation in connexin 26 (GJB2) *Ped Derm 37:373–374, 2020; AD 138:1309–1314, 2002; Ped Derm 15:140–142, 1998; JAAD 20:924–927, 1989; BJD 101:717–722, 1979*

Porokeratotic hamartoma (porokeratotic adnexal ostial nevus, variant of porokeratotic eccrine hamartoma) *Indian J DV Leprol 85:546–548, 2019;* personal observation

Proliferating trichilemmal cysts and cicatricial alopecia *AD 107:435–8, 1973*

Squamous cell carcinoma with arsenical keratoses *Dermatol Online J Dec 15, 2016; Dermatol Online J 14:24, 2008*

Trichoepitheliomas – multiple trichoepitheliomas *JAAD 22:1109–1110, 1990*

PARANEOPLASTIC DISEASES

Hereditary punctate keratoderma and internal malignancy (punctate keratoses of the palms and soles) – associated with lung and bladder carcinomas *JAAD 22:468–476, 1990;* colon cancer *JAAD 10:587–591, 1984*

Punctate palmoplantar keratoderma *BJD 134:720–726, 1996*

Punctate porokeratotic keratoderma *Clin Exp Dermatol 19:139–141, 1994*

PHOTODERMATOSES

Degenerative collagenous plaques of the hands (keratoelastoidosis marginalis of the hands) – hyperkeratotic plaques/papules of hands in elderly; chronic sun damage, trauma, heavy physical work *Hautarzt 69 (suppl 1)37–38, 2018; Indian Dermatol Online J 7:195–197, 2016; AD 82:362–366, 1960; Dermatologica 131:169–175, 1954*

PRIMARY CUTANEOUS DISEASES

Acrokeratoelastoidosis of Costa *Cutis 74:173–179, 2004;*

Ped Derm 19:320–322, 2002; JAAD 22:468–476, 1990; Acta DV 60:149–153, 1980; Dermatologica 107:164–168, 1953

Acrokeratoelastoidosis and knuckle pads *Cutis 102:344–346, 2018*

Acrokeratoelastoidosis lichenoides *JAAD 58:344–348, 2008*

Acrokeratosis verruciformis of Hopf – associated with Darier's disease and Cowden's syndrome *Clin Exp Dermatol 31:558–563, 2006*

Benign familial pemphigus (Hailey-Hailey disease) – autosomal dominant; photo- and/or heat exacerbated; erosive intertriginous dermatitis; may have oral, esophageal or vaginal erosions *AD 96:254–258, 1967; BJD 81:77, 1969*

Buschke-Fischer-Brauer keratoderma (punctate palmoplantar keratoderma) (keratodermia palmo-plantaris papulosa) (keratodermia palmoplantare papuloverrucoides progressiva) (keratoma dissipatum hereditarium palmare et plantare (Brauer)) – autosomal dominant; clinical subtypes include pinhead papules, spiky filiform lesions, dense round 1–2 mm papules, clavus-like lesions, hard warty masses, cupuliform lesions, and focal translucent lesions; mutation in *AAGAB Case Rep Dermatol 11:292–296, 2019; BJD 171:433–436, 2014; BJD 152:874–878, 2005; JAAD 49:1166–1169, 2003; Curr Prob Derm 14:71–116, 2002; BJD 128:104–105, 1993; JAAD 8:700–702, 1983; Hum Genet 60:14–19, 1982; JAAD 3:43–49, 1980* with ainhum *Actas Dermosifiliogr 73:105–110, 1982*

Collie-Davies PPK (punctate palmoplantar keratoderma) (palmoplantar papular keratoderma of Davies-Colley) – keratosis palmoplantaris maculosa seu papulosa *Cutis 78:42–46, 2006; Hautarzt 48:577–580, 1997; Trans Pathol Soc Lond 30:451, 1879*

Darier's disease (keratosis follicularis) – punctate or filiform palmar keratoses or pits *J Ayub Med Coll Abbottabad 22:230–233, 2010; Clin Dermatol 19:193–205, 1994; JAAD 27:40–50, 1992*

Delayed onset palmoplantar keratoderma – personal observation

Dowling-Degos disease, generalized *JAAD 57:327334, 2007*

Dupuytren's contracture – presenting as palmar pits *J Cut Med Surg 12:198–202, 2008; J Med 9:347–350, 1978*

Dyshidrosis

Epidermolysis bullosa, autosomal recessive – diffuse palmoplantar keratoderma with pitting, pitted palmar keratoderma, dystrophic toenails, blistering, generalized reticulated hyperpigmentation; dental caries with squamous cell carcinoma of tongue; keratin 14 mutation; must be differentiated from EBS with mottled pigmentation (keratin 5 mutation), Kindler's syndrome, Naegeli syndrome – inflammatory blisters and hypohidrosis (keratin 14 mutation), and dyskeratosis congenita (telomerase mutation) *BJD 162:880–882, 2010*

Epidermolysis bullosa simplex with mottled pigmentation of neck, upper trunk, arms and leg with or without keratoderma (punctate palmoplantar keratoses); cutaneous atrophy, nail dystrophy; wart-like hyperkeratotic papules of axillae, wrists, dorsae of hands, palms and soles; P25L mutation of keratin 5 *JAAD 52:172–173, 2005; BJD 150:609–611, 2004; Clin Genet 15:228–238, 1979*

Epidermolysis bullosa simplex with mottled pigmentation with keratoderma (Dowling-Meara type) – focal punctate palmoplantar keratoderma; acral blistering, hemorrhagic bullae, dystrophic thick nails *BJD 144:40–45, 2001; JID 111:893–895, 1998; Ped Derm 13:306–309, 1996;* punctate keratoderma *AD 122:900–908, 1986*

Erythrokeratoderma variabilis

Familial dyskeratotic comedones *JAAD 17:808–814, 1987*

Focal acral hyperkeratosis (acrokeratoelastoidosis without elastorrhexis) – autosomal dominant; crateriform papules of the sides of the hands and feet *JAAD 47:448–451, 2002; AD 120:263–264, 1984; BJD 109:97–103, 1983*

Hereditary painful calluses *AD 114:591–592, 1978*

Hyperkeratosis lenticularis perstans (Flegel's disease) – smaller lesions than Kyrle's disease *Actas Dermosifiliogr 100:157–159, 2009;* punctate pits *Med Trop (mars)62:85–88, 2002*

Hyperkeratotic dermatitis of the palms *BJD 107:195–202, 1982*

Guttate hypopigmentation with punctate palmoplantar keratoderma *AD 145495–497, 2009; Ped Derm 19:302–306, 2002*

Keratosis lichenoides chronica – punctate keratotic papules of palmar creases *AD 105:739–743, 1972;* keratotic linear and reticulated plaques of flexures *Arch Dermatol Syphil 31:1–29, 1895;* seborrheic dermatitis-like eruption face *Ped Derm 26:615–616, 2009; JAAD 38:306–309, 1998;* acral dermatitis of toes *Ped Derm 26:615–616, 2009*

Keratosis palmoplantaris papulosa seu maculosa (punctate keratoderma)

Keratosis papulosa *JAAD 58:344–348, 2008*

Keratosis punctata et plantaris *Acta DV 56:105–110, 1976*

Kyrle's disease – atypical in palmoplantar areas *Z Hautkr 64:286–291, 1989*

Lichen nitidus – palmar hyperkeratosis *Clin Exp Dermatol 18:381–383, 1993;* minute papules *AD 104:538–540, 1971*

Lichen planus *AD 140:1275–1280, 2004; Int J Dermatol 25:592–593, 1986*

Mal de Meleda – pits within PPK *Cutis 56:235–238, 1995*

Marginal papular keratodermas *Ped Derm 19:320–322, 2002*
  Acrokeratoelastoidosis of Costa *Ped Derm 19:320–322, 2002; JAAD 22:468–476, 1990; Acta DV 60:149–153, 1980; Dermatologica 107:164–168, 1953*
  Focal acral hyperkeratosis
  Keratoelastoidosis marginalis of the hands
  Palmar xanthomas
  Flat warts
  Porokeratosis
  Mosaic acral keratosis

Palmoplantar keratoderma – circumscriptum

Palmoplantar keratoderma of the punctate type (keratosis palmoplantaris varians et punctata) (familial punctate keratoderma) *BJD 145:682–684, 2001; Hautarzt 47:858–859, 1996; JAAD 18:75–86, 1988*

Pitted palmoplantar keratoderma in palmar creases (keratosis punctata of palmar creases of black patients) (keratotic pits of palmar creases) – racial variant *Cutis 74:173–179, 2004; JAAD 22:468–70, 1990; Cutis 33:394–396, 1984*

Prurigo nodularis

Psoriasis

Punctate porokeratotic keratoderma (punctate porokeratosis of the palms and soles) – punctate pits and keratotic papules scattered diffusely on palms and occasionally the soles *JAAD 22:468–476, 1990; Acta DV 70:478–482, 1990; AD 125:816–819, 1989; AD 124:1678–1682, 1988; JAAD 13:908–912, 1985; AD 120:263–264, 1984; AD 104:682–683, 1971*

Reticulate acropigmentation of Kitamura (milia-like keratotic papules) – palmar pits *AD 139:657–662, 2003; JAAD 37:884–886, 1997; J Dermatol 27:745–747, 2000; JAAD 40:462–467, 1999; BJD 109:105–110, 1983; BJD 95:437–443, 1976;* pigmented palmar pits *Indian Dermatol Online J 11:108–110, 2020*

Spiny-filiform hyperkeratosis of palms and soles *JAAD 58:344–348, 2008;* classification of filiform hyperkeratosis (spiny keratoderma)
  Palmoplantar porokeratotic filiform hyperkeratosis
  Palmoplantar parakeratotic spiny keratosis
  Disseminated porokeratotic filiform hyperkeratosis
  Disseminated parakeratotic spiny keratosis
  Palmoplantar orthokeratotic filiform hyperkeratosis
  Palmoplantar orthokeratotic spiny keratosis
  Disseminated orthokeratotic filiform hyperkeratosis
  Disseminated orthokeratotic spiny keratosis
  Filiform hyperkeratosis in eccrine hamartoma – aka porokeratotic eccrine ostial and dermal duct nevus
  Spiny keratosis in eccrine hamartoma – aka porokeratotic eccrine ostial and dermal duct nevus

Spiny keratoderma (multiple minute palmar-plantar digitate hyperkeratoses) (music box keratoderma) (punctuate/spiny keratoderma) – spiny, filiform, spiked, minute aggregate; palmar pits and digitate hyperkeratosis to the palms and soles *JAAD 58:344–348, 2008; Cutis 54:389–394, 1994; BJD 121:239–242, 1989; JAAD 18:431–436, 1988; BJD 95:93–97, 1976; AD 104:682–683, 1971;* autosomal dominant; may remit with topical 5-fluorouracil; may be associated with autosomal dominant polycystic kidney disease *JAAD 34:935–936, 1996; JAAD 26:879–881, 1992;* acquired form with questionable paraneoplastic associations *Dermatology 201:379–380, 2000;* digestive adenocarcinoma *Ann DV 124:707–709, 1997;* breast cancer *Ann DV 117:834–836, 1990*

SYNDROMES

Alagille syndrome *Ped Derm 31:599–602, 2014*

Alopecia-onychodysplasia-hypohidrosis-deafness syndrome (ectodermal dysplasia)

Basaloid follicular hamartoma syndrome – autosomal dominant; milia, comedone-like lesions, dermatosis papulosa nigra, skin tag-like lesions, hypotrichosis, multiple skin-colored, red, and hyperpigmented papules of the face in periorificial distribution, neck chest, back, proximal extremities, and eyelids; syndrome includes milia-like cysts, comedones, sparse scalp hair, palmar pits, and parallel bands of papules of the neck (zebra stripes); hypohidrosis *Dermatopathol 2014, Apr 2; AD 144:933–938, 2008; Cutis 78:42–*

46, 2006; JAAD 49:698–705, 2003; BJD 146:1068–1070, 2002; JAAD 45:644–645, 2001; BJD 143:1103–1105, 2000; JAAD 43:189–206, 2000; JAAD 27:237–240, 1992; AD 107:435–438, 1973

Brooke-Spiegler syndrome *Clin Exp Dermatol 28:539–541, 2003*

Cole's disease – generalized hypopigmented macules with punctate keratoses of the palms and soles; mutation in *ENPP1* encoding endonucleotide pyrophosphatase/phosphodiesterase *BJD 174:1152–1156, 2016; Ped Derm 19:302–306, 2002; JID 67:72–89, 1976*

Congenital poikiloderma with traumatic bullae, anhidrosis, and pitted PPK

Conradi-Hunermann syndrome – X-linked dominant chondrodysplasia punctata

Curry-Jones syndrome – linear hypo- or hyperpigmented lesions, palmoplantar pitting, atrophoderma, hypertrichosis, trichoblastomas and nevus sebaceous, polydactyly of syndactyly, dysmorphic facies, macrocephaly, microcephaly, dental anomalies, craniosynostosis, anal stenosis, myofibromas and smooth muscle hamartomas, medulloblastomas, cerebral malformations, developmental delay, cataracts, microphthalmia, coloboma, glaucoma, cryptorchidism; mutation in SMOc.1234C>T *BJD 182:212–217, 2020*

Cowden's syndrome – punctate translucent keratoses *AD 146:337–342, 2010; Cutis 74:173–179, 2004; Nat Genet 13:114–116, 1996; J Med Genet 32:117–119, 1995; Dermatol Clin 13:27–31, 1995; AD 122:821, 824–825, 1986; Ann Intern Med 58:136–142, 1963*

Dermatopathia pigmentosa retularis – autosomal dominant, reticulate hyperpigmentation of trunk, onychodystrophy, alopecia, oral hyperpigmentation, punctate hyperkeratosis of palms and soles, hypohidrosis; atrophic macules over joints with hypertrophic scarring *Semin Cut Med Surg 16:72–80, 1997; AD 126:935–939, 1990; Hautarzt 6:262, 1960*

Focal dermal hypoplasia, morning glory anomaly, and polymicrogyria – swirling pattern of hypopigmentation, papular hypopigmented and herniated skin lesions of face, head, hands, and feet, basaloid follicular hamartomas, mild mental retardation, macrocephaly, microphthalmia, unilateral morning glory optic disc anomaly, palmar and lip pits, and polysyndactyly *Am J Med Genet 124A:202–208, 2004*

Greither's ectodermal dysplasia

Happle-Tinschert syndrome – basaloid follicular hamartomas, basal cell carcinomas, linear hypo- or hyperpigmented lesions, palmoplantar pitting, atrophoderma, hypertrichosis, hypotrichosis; polydactyly, syndactyly, rudimentary ribs, limb length disparities, dysmorphic facies, macrocephaly, jaw ameloblastomas, dental anomalies, imperforate anus, colon adenocarcinoma; medulloblastoma cerebral manifestation, developmental delay, optic glioma or meningioma, cataracts, microphthalmia , coloboma; mutation in *SMOc.1234C>T BJD 182:212–217, 2020*

Hereditary acral keratotic poikiloderma of Weary *Ped Derm 13:427–429, 1996*

Hereditary papulotranslucent acrokeratoderma (punctate keratoderma) *JAMA Derm 150:1001–1002, 2014; Cutis 61:29–30, 1998; AD 34:686–688, 1996*

Hidrotic ectodermal dysplasia

HOPP syndrome – hypotrichosis, striate, reticulated pitted palmoplantar keratoderma, acro-osteolysis, psoriasiform plaques, lingua plicata, onychogryphosis, ventricular arrhythmias, periodontitis *BJD 150:1032–1033, 2004; BJD 147:575–581, 2002*

Keratoderma with mental retardation and spastic paraplegia

Lipoid proteinosis – punctate keratoderma of palms and soles *Indian J DV Leprol 55:200–201, 1989*

Naegeli- Franceschetti-Jadassohn syndrome – autosomal dominant, reticulate gray to brown pigmentation of neck, upper trunk and flexures, punctate or diffuse palmoplantar keratoderma, onycholysis, subungual hyperkeratosis, yellow tooth enamel *JAAD 28:942–950, 1993*

Nevoid basal cell carcinoma syndrome (Gorlin's syndrome) – autosomal dominant; basal cell carcinomas, basaloid follicular hamartomas, linear hypo- or hyperpigmented lesions; macrocephaly, frontal bossing, hypertelorism, cleft lip or palate, papules of the face, neck, and trunk, facial milia, lamellar calcification of the falx cerebri and tentorium cerebelli, cerebral cysts, calcifications of the brain, palmoplantar pits, mandibular keratocysts, skeletal anomalies, including enlarged mandibular coronoid, bifid ribs, kyphosis, spina bifida, polydactyly of the hands or feet, syndactyly; basal cell carcinomas; multiple eye anomalies – congenital cataract, microphthalmia, coloboma of the iris, choroid, and optic nerve; strabismus, nystagmus, keratin-filled cysts of the palpebral conjunctivae; also medulloblastomas, ovarian tumors (fibromas), mesenteric cysts, cardiac fibromas, fetal rhabdomyomas, astrocytomas, meningiomas, craniopharyngiomas, fibrosarcomas, ameloblastomas; renal anomalies; hypogonadotropic hypogonadism, *BJD 182:212–217, 2020; BJD 165:30–34, 2011; JAAD 39:853–857, 1998; Dermatol Clin 13:113–125, 1995; JAAD 11:98–104, 1984; NEJM 262:908–912, 1960;* linear unilateral nevoid basal cell nevus syndrome *JAAD 50:489–494, 2004; BJD 174:68–76, 2016; Pediatr Int 56:667–674, 2014; Summer Meeting, American Academy of Dermatology, July 31, 2004; Int J Oral Maxillofac Surg 33:117–124, 2004; Clin Genet 55:34–40, 1999; Am J Med Genet 69:299–308, 1997; Am J Med Genet 69:299–308, 1997; Dermatol Clin 13:113–125, 1995; Medicine 66:98–113, 1987;* with type 2 mosaicism; linear palmar pits *BJD 169:1342–1345, 2013*

Pachyonychia congenita *Cutis 78:42–46, 2006*

Palmoplantar keratoderma with leukoplakia – focal palmoplantar keratoderma and leukokeratosis anogenitalis *J Eur Acad DV 29:612–613, 2015*

Palmoplantar keratoderma with scleroatrophy of the extremities (Huriez syndrome)

Papillon-Lefevre syndrome – punctate hyperkeratosis of palms and soles (pitted on heels and forefoot) *Ped Derm 30:749–750, 2013; JAAD 48:345–351, 2003*

Punctate acrokeratoderma with pigmentary disorder *BJD 128:693–695, 1993*

Reactive arthritis

Reticulate acropigmentation of Kitamura – reticulate pigmentation of dorsal hands and feet with palmoplantar pits; differs from acropigmentation symmetrica of Dohi by the absence of hypopigmented macules *BJD 144:162–168, 2001; Semin Cut Med Surg 16:72–80, 1997; AD 115:760, 1979; BJD 95:437–443, 1976; Rinsho No Hifu Hitsunyo 1943:201;* pigmented palmar pits *Indian Dermatol Online J 11:108–110, 2020*

Schopf-Schulze-Passarge syndrome – hidrocystomas, hyperkeratoses of palms and soles, hypoplastic teeth, hypotrichosis

Soto's syndrome *Am J Med Genet C Semin Med Genet 181:502–508, 2019*

Speckled hyperpigmentation palmoplantar punctate keratoses, childhood blistering *BJD 105:579–585, 1981*

TOXIC AGENTS

Arsenical keratoses – punctate palmar keratoses with hyperkeratosis of the soles *Dermatol Clinics 29:45–51, 2011; BJD 159:169–174, 2008; Cutis 80:305–308, 2007; Postgrad Med J 79:391–396, 2003; Int J Derm 36:241–250, 1997; Dermatol Surg 22:301–304, 1996; JID 4:365–383, 1941*

Chloracne due to dioxin – punctate keratoderma-like lesions on the palms and soles *BJD 143:1067–1071, 2000*

TRAUMA

Calluses

Clavi, clavus, corn *Stat Pearls Sept 13, 2019*

Mechanical

PALMOPLANTAR KERATODERMAS

Clin in Dermatol 23:15–22, 2005; Int J Derm 32:493–498, 1993

AUTOIMMUNE DISEASES AND DISEASES OF IMMUNE DYSFUNCTION

Allergic contact dermatitis

Bullous pemphigoid – transient palmoplantar keratoderma *JAMA Derm 155:216–220, 2019*

Dermatitis herpetiformis – acquired palmoplantar keratoderma *BJD 149:1300–1302, 2003*

Dermatomyositis – presenting as a pityriasis pilaris-like eruption *Ped Derm 24:151–154, 2007; BJD 136:768–771, 1997;* juvenile dermatomyositis *BJD 36:917–919, 1997;* mechanic's hands *Ann Int Med 91:577–578, 1979*

Graft vs. host disease *Ped Derm 12:311–313, 1995;* exfoliative erythroderma with palmoplantar keratoderma *AD 143:1157–1162, 2007*

Lupus erythematosus – discoid lupus erythematosus *NEJM 269:1155–1161, 1963*

Pemphigus – striate palmoplantar keratoderma of endemic pemphigus of El Bagre region of Colombia *JAAD 49:599–608, 2003*

Pemphigus- and pemphigoid-like lesions with acquired palmoplantar keratoderma with tripe pattern – antibodies to desmocollin 3 *BJD 157:168–173, 2007*

CONGENITAL LESIONS

Ichthyosis prematurity syndrome – autosomal recessive; premature birth, ichthyosis, scaly erythroderma, neonatal asphyxia; hyperkeratotic thick caseous lesions of hands, feet, and scalp; eosinophilia; Norway and Sweden; mutation in fatty acid transport protein 4 (*FATP4*) *Ped Derm 31:517–518, 2014; AD 147:750–752, 2011*

DEGENERATIVE DISEASES

Disuse hyperkeratosis

Keratoderma climactericum of Haxthausen *Can Fam Physician 42:629, 631, 1996; Dermatologica 172:258–262, 1986; J Am Podiatry Assoc 68:595–597, 1978; BJD 46:161–167, 1934*

DRUG-INDUCED

Acral dysesthesia syndrome – capecitabine; hyperpigmentation and hyperkeratosis of the dorsal and palmar surfaces of the hands and feet of black patients *Cutis 73:101–106, 2004*

Alpha methyldopa *Semin Derm 14:152–161, 1995*

Aspirin – aquagenic palmoplantar keratoderma (aquagenic palmar hyperwrinkling) (acquired aquagenic keratoderma) (aquagenic syringeal acrokeratoderma) *AD 142:1661–1662, 2006*

Bleomycin

Celecoxib – aquagenic palmoplantar keratoderma (aquagenic palmar hyperwrinkling) (acquired aquagenic keratoderma) (aquagenic syringeal acrokeratoderma) *Acta Dermosifiliogr 96:537–539, 2005*

5-fluorouracil

Glucan-induced keratoderma *AD 123:751–756,1987*

Gold salts *Semin Derm 14:152–161, 1995*

Hydroxyurea – long-term therapy *JAAD 49:339–341, 2003; Rook p. 3481, 1998, Sixth Edition; Semin Derm 14:152–161, 1995*

Lithium *J Clin Psychopharmacol 11:149–150, 1991*

Mepacrine *Semin Derm 14:152–161, 1995*

Mexiletine *Semin Derm 14:152–161, 1995*

Practolol *Semin Derm 14:152–161, 1995*

Proguanil *Semin Derm 14:152–161, 1995*

Quinacrine

Rofecoxib – aquagenic palmoplantar keratoderma (aquagenic palmar hyperwrinkling) (acquired aquagenic keratoderma) (aquagenic syringeal acrokeratoderma) *Ped Derm 19:353–355, 2002*

Retinoids *Semin Derm 14:152–161, 1995*

Sorafenib – hand-foot syndrome; hyperkeratotic with or without livedoid erythema *AD 144:886–892, 2008*

Tegafur – chronic acral erythema leading to palmoplantar keratoderma *AD 131:364–365, 1995*

Tumor necrosis factor alpha antagonists – lichen planus-like palmar hyperkeratotic dermatitis *JAAD 61:104–111, 2009;* palmoplantar keratoderma *BJD 161:1081–1088, 2009*

Vemurafenib – palmoplantar hyperkeratosis *JAAD 67:1265–1272, 2012*

EXOGENOUS AGENTS

Aquagenic palmoplantar keratoderma (aquagenic palmar hyperwrinkling) (acquired aquagenic keratoderma) (aquagenic syringeal acrokeratoderma) *The Dermatologist January, 2015, pp. 47–49, 2015; BJD 167:575–582, 2012; JAAD 59:S112–113, 2008; Ped Derm 24:197–198, 2007; Ped Derm 23:39–42, 2006; Cutis 78:317–318, 2006; Dermatology 204:8, 2002; JAAD 45:124–126, 2001; JAAD 44:696–699, 2001;* in cystic fibrosis *BJD 163:162–166, 2010; AD 145:1296–1299, 2009; Ped Derm 26:660–661, 2009; Australas J Dermatol 49:19–20, 2008; Dermatology 216:222–226, 2008; AD 141:621–624, 2005; Lancet ii:108:1974*

Chloracne with punctate keratoderma *BJD 143:1067–1071, 2000*

Crack cocaine smoking – hyperkeratotic palms *Cutis 50:193–194, 1992*

Pesticides – weed sprayer with sclerodactyly of fingers and toes with hyperkeratosis of palms and chloracne *Clin Exp Dermatol 19:264–267, 1994*

INFECTIONS AND/OR INFESTATIONS

AIDS – may be with or without associated pustules; seen with T cell count under 100 cells/mm3; may have concomitant Trichophyton rubrum infection or may be seen with AIDS-associated Reiter's syndrome *JAAD 22:1270–1277, 1990*

Chronic mucocutaneous candidiasis – sporadic, autosomal dominant, or autosomal recessive; associated with other immunodeficiencies, endocrinopathies, abnormalities of iron metabolism; keratotic candidal granulomas with skin and scalp involvement, paronychia, mucous membrane involvement; may be seen with multiple carboxylase deficiencies or ectodermal dysplasia *Ann Rev Med 32:491, 1981*

Cutaneous larva migrans, generalized – personal observation

Leprosy – symmetric palmoplantar keratoderma *Hansenol Int 10:32–37, 1985 (Italian)*

Mycobacterium tuberculosis – papulonecrotic tuberculid – punctate palmoplantar lesions *Int J Derm 21:470–471, 1982*

Paracoccidioidomycosis – punctate palmoplantar keratoderma *J Clin Inf Dis 23:1026–1032, 1996*

Pinta – tertiary (late phase) – hyperkeratoses of palms and soles

Pitted keratolysis *AD 117:609, 1981*

Scabies, crusted *Can Fam Physician 45:1455, 1462, 1999*

Syphilis, secondary – syphilitic keratoderma resembles reactive arthritis, psoriasis, lichen planus, Bazex, Unna-Thost and Howell-Evans syndromes *AD 144:255–260, 2008*

Tinea manuum *Acta DV (Stockh) 36:272–278, 1956*

Tinea pedis (*Trichophyton rubrum*)

Tungiasis – focal plantar keratoderma *BJD 144:118–124, 2001*

Verrucae in AIDS; papilloma virus-infected cells may have small eosinophilic granules and dense clumps of basophilic keratohyalin granules composed of E4 (E1-4) protein, a viral protein which collapses the cytoplasmic keratin filament network enabling release of other virions *JAAD 19:401–405, 1988*

Yaws – secondary – hyperkeratotic plantar lesions fissure and can cause crablike gait, hence "crab yaws" *Clin Dermatol 18:687–700, 2000; JAAD 29:519–535, 1993*; tertiary – keratoderma of palms and soles *Ped Derm 27:364–367, 2010*

METABOLIC

Hypothyroidism – keratoderma of myxedema *Aust Fam Physician 28:1217–1222, 1999; BJD 139:741–742, 1998; Clin Exp Derm 13:339–41, 1988; Acta DV 66:354–357, 1986*

Malnutrition

Menopause

Mitochondrial respiratory chain disorders

Necrolytic acral erythema – cutaneous marker for hepatitis C infection; psoriasiform hyperpigmented, hyperkeratotic plaques of acral palmar, plantar, dorsal surfaces of hands and feet; darker, more velvety and verrucous than psoriasis *JAAD 53:247–251, 2005; AD 141:85–87, 2005; Int J Derm 44:916–921, 2005; JAAD 50:s121–124, 2004, Int J Derm 35:252–256, 1996*

Obesity – thick palms and soles *JAAD 81:1037–1057, 2019*

Pheochromocytoma

Porphyria – erythropoietic protoporphyria with homozygous mutation of ferrochelatase gene *BJD 160:1330–1334, 2009; JID 129:599–605, 2009;* seasonal palmar keratoderma; autosomal recessive EPP; decreased risk of liver disease; neurologic symp-toms; relatively low protoporphyrin level *BJD 161:966–967, 2009; JID 129:599, 2009; BJD 155:574–581, 2006*

Tyrosinemia type II (Richner-Hanhart syndrome) – autosomal recessive; painful focal palmoplantar keratoderma, photophobia, dendritic (herpetiform) corneal erosions, mental retardation; severe nail dystrophy due to onychophagia, diagnosis by tandem mass spectrometry; increased serum and urine tyrosine and no succinyl-acetone in urine (only seen in type I tyrosinemia) *BJD 160:704–706, 2009; Ped Derm 25:378–380, 2008; Curr Prob Derm 14:71–116, 2002; Ped Derm 14:110–112, 1997; JAAD 35:857–859, 1996*

Zinc deficiency

NEOPLASTIC

Eccrine syringofibroadenomatosis (psoriasiform keratoderma) – papules, plaques, or palmoplantar keratoderma, red papules and nodules, solitary vegetating nodule, pyogenic granuloma-like papule, crusted papules, flat red lesions, opalescent papules and plaques, keratotic papules, tapioca pudding pattern on palms and soles *JAAD 26:805–813, 1992;* diffuse unilateral plantar hyperkeratosis *BJD 149:885–886, 2003*

Epidermal nevus – systematized, linear (ichthyosis hystrix) – may also be acquired

Epithelioma cuniculatum (verrucous carcinoma) – slowly enlarging cauliflower-like mass; distinctive foul smell

Kaposi's sarcoma – hyperkeratosis of palms and soles (palmoplantar keratoderma-like) *JAAD 59:179–206, 2008*

Leukemia cutis – macules, papules, plaques, chloroma, nodules, ecchymoses, palpable purpura, ulcers, erythroderma, bullae, gingival hyperplasia (AML or AMML); associated with a grave prognosis *JAAD 11:121–128, 1984*

Lymphoma – cutaneous T-cell lymphoma; *JAAD 70:205–220, 2014; BJD 161:826–830, 2009; AD 143:109–114, 2007; AD 134:1019–1024, 1998; AD 136:971, 1996; AD 131:1052–1056, 1995; JAAD 13:897–899, 1985; JAAD 7:792–796, 1982; Ann Int Med 83:534–552, 1975;* fissured palmoplantar keratoderma *BJD 161:1420–1422, 2009;* non-cutaneous T-cell lymphoma *Int J Dermatol 30:871–872, 1991;* syringotropic CTCL – palmoplantar hyperkeratosis *JAAD 71:926–934, 2014; JAAD 61:133–138, 2009;* Sezary syndrome; CTCL with focal palmoplantar keratoderma

Punctate palmoplantar porokeratosis

Porokeratosis of Mantoux – crateriform lesions of palms

Porokeratosis plantaris, palmaris, et disseminata – autosomal dominant; painful papules on soles, porokeratosis lesions on both sun and non-sun exposed skin *Curr Prob Derm 14:71–116, 2002; JAAD 13:598–603, 1985;* may be circumscribed PPK

Porokeratotic eccrine ostial and dermal duct nevus – linear or band-like plantar or palmar area with multiple punctate pits and comedo-like plugs; almost always present at birth *AD 127:1219–1224, 1991; JAAD 20:924–927, 1989*

PARANEOPLASTIC

Acanthosis nigricans

Acquired diffuse palmoplantar keratoderma with bronchial carcinoma *AD 124:497–498, 1988; Acta DV 62:313–316, 1982;* gastric adenocarcinoma *Dermatologica 165:660–663, 1982*

Acquired palmoplantar keratoderma with diffuse plane xanthomatosis associated with myeloma *BJD 132:286–289, 1995*

Bazex syndrome (acrokeratosis paraneoplastica) – violaceous keratoderma; scaling of fingertips, nailfolds, nose, ears; psoriasiform; upper aerodigestive malignancies *JAAD 54:745–762, 2006; AD 141: 389–394, 2005; Cutis 49:265–268, 1992; AD 119:820–826, 1983; BJD 102:301–306, 1980*

Epidermolytic palmoplantar keratoderma – breast and ovarian carcinoma *BJD 117:363–370, 1987*

Florid cutaneous papillomatosis

Howell-Evans syndrome (tylosis (smooth pattern)) – autosomal dominant; focal PPK; oral leukokeratosis, carcinoma of the esophagus; esophageal strictures, oral leukoplakia, squamous cell carcinoma of the tylotic skin, carcinoma of larynx and stomach *Curr Prob Derm 14:71–116, 2002; Dis Esophagus 12:173–176, 1999; Eur J Cancer B Oral Oncol 30B:102–112, 1994; JAAD 28:295–297, 1993; Q J Med 155:317–333, 1970; QJMed 27:413–429, 1958; QJ Med 27:415–429, 1950;* envoplakin on TOCG (tylosis oesophageal gene) chromosome 17q25 *Genomics 37:381–385, 1996*

Non-familial PPK (cobblestone pattern) – carcinoma of esophagus and bronchus *JAAD 28:295–297, 1993;* breast, urinary bladder, stomach

Palmoplantar keratoderma and malignancy (palmoplantar ectodermal dysplasia type III) – 17q24 *AD 132:640–651, 1996*

Porokeratosis plantaris

Punctate keratoderma – carcinoma of breast, uterus, lung, bladder, colon *BJD 134:720–726, 1996; J Clin Oncol 7:669–678, 1989; JAAD 10:587–591, 1984; AD 92:553–556, 1965*

Punctate porokeratotic keratoderma *Clin Exp Dermatol 19:139–141, 1994*

Tripe palms – tripe is the rugose surface of bovine foregut; gastric, pulmonary, bladder, breast, cervix, ovary, kidney, colon, gallbladder, sarcoma, tongue, uterus, brain, melanoma, lymphoma, pancreas, prostate; occurs alone in 25% or with acanthosis nigricans in 75 *BJD 138:698–703, 1998; J Dermatol 22:492–495, 1995; Clin Dermatol 11:165–173, 1993; JAAD 27:271–272, 1992; Dermatology 185:151–153, 1992; J Clin Oncol 7:669–678, 1989; Clin Exp Dermatol 5:181–189, 1980*

PRIMARY CUTANEOUS DISEASE

Absorption reaction – personal observation

Acanthosis nigricans – hereditary benign *Int J Dermatol 35:126–127, 1996;* benign *Am J Public Health 84:1839–1842, 1994;* pseudo-acanthosis nigricans *Am J Med 87:269–272, 1989;* drug-induced (nicotinic acid *Dermatology 189:203–206, 1994;* fusidic acid *JAAD 28:501–502, 1993;* stilbestrol *AD 109:545–546, 1974;* triazinate *AD 121:232–236, 1985);* malignant acanthosis nigricans; nevoid acanthosis nigricans – unilateral and localized *Int J Dermatol 30:452–453, 1991*

Adolescent onset ichthyosiform erythroderma *BJD 144:1063–1066, 2001*

Atopic dermatitis

Atypical epidermolytic hyperkeratosis with palmoplantar keratoderma with keratin 1 mutation – palmoplantar keratoderma with psoriasiform plaques of elbows and antecubital fossae *BJD 150:1129–1135, 2004*

Darier's disease (keratosis follicularis) – autosomal dominant with variable penetrance; skin colored to yellow brown papules in seborrheic distribution; associated with acrokeratosis verruciformis of Hopf; palmar punctate keratoses and/or pits; hemorrhagic macules on hands and feet; cobblestoning of mucous membranes;

nail changes of red and white longitudinal bands with distal V-shaped nicks; photosensitive; characteristic odor

Epidermodysplasia verruciformis – severe palmoplantar keratoderma *AD 146:667–672, 2010; Arch Dermatol Syph 141:193–203, 1922*

Epidermolysis bullosa *JAAD 58:931–950, 2008*; EBS, plakophilin deficiency; focal keratoderma with fissuring; EBS, localized – focal keratoderma in adulthood; EBS, Dowling-Meara – diffuse palmoplantar keratoderma; EBS other generalized – focal keratoderma; EBS, autosomal recessive – focal keratoderma; EBS with mottled pigmentation – focal; junctional EB, non-Herlitz type, generalized – focal

Epidermolysis bullosa, autosomal recessive – diffuse palmoplantar keratoderma with pitting, pitted palmar keratoderma, dystrophic toenails, blistering, generalized reticulated hyperpigmentation; dental caries with squamous cell carcinoma of tongue; keratin 14 mutation; must be differentiated from EBS with mottled pigmentation (keratin 5 mutation), Kindler's syndrome, Naegeli syndrome – inflammatory blisters and hypohidrosis (keratin 14 mutation), and dyskeratosis congenita (telomerase mutation) *BJD 162:880–882, 2010*

Epidermolysis bullosa simplex with punctate keratoderma *JAAD 15:1040–1044, 1985; Derm Clinics 11:549–563, 1993*

    EBS – clumped tonofilaments and basal layer blisters. Keratin 5 or 14, chromosome 12q or 17q

    EB junctional – hemidesmosomal proteins

    EB dystrophic – scarce or absent anchoring fibrils. Collagen type VII A abnormal; chromosome 3p21.1

    Epidermolytic hyperkeratosis – clumping of tonofilaments. Keratin 1 or 10; chromosome 12q or 17q

    Epidermolytic epidermolysis bullosa- Kobliner, Weber-Cockayne, Ogna Gedde-Dahl, Fischer and Gedde-Dahl (with mottled pigmentation), herpetiformis with mottled pigmentation, and herpetiformis *JAAD 42:1051–1066, 2000*

    Dominant dystrophic epidermolysis bullosa with punctate keratoderma *JAAD 15:1289–1291, 1986*

    Epidermolysis bullosa, mottled pigmentation, and punctate keratoses *BJD 105:579–585, 1981*

    Epidermolysis bullosa simplex with muscular dystrophy – plectin mutation (premature termination codon) *JAAD 41:950–956, 1999*

Epidermolysis bullosa, dominant dystrophic hyperplastique – Cockayne-Touraine

Epidermolysis bullosa, progressive junctional type – autosomal recessive; palmoplantar hyperkeratosis (non-lethal localized junctional EB) – legs and feet only; hyperkeratosis with erosions of soles *J R Soc Med 78 (Suppl 11); 32–33, 1985;* Ogna Gedde-Dahl – delayed onset; bullae with surrounding atrophic (cigarette paper) wrinkled skin, absent nail plates, palmoplantar keratoderma, absent dermal finger ridges, tooth and enamel defects *JAAD 16:195–200, 1987*

Epidermolysis bullosa; non-Herlitz junctional epidermolysis bullosa with collagen XVII mutation – palmoplantar callosities *JAAD 52:371–373, 2005; AD 122:704–710, 1986; Dermatologica 152:72–86, 1976*

Epidermolysis bullosa simplex – palmoplantar callosities *JAAD 42:1051–1066, 2000*

Epidermolysis bullosa simplex herpetiformis with mottled pigmentation with keratoderma (Dowling-Meara type) – autosomal dominant; focal punctate palmoplantar keratoderma; acral blistering, hemorrhagic bullae, dystrophic thick nails;

BJD 144:40–45, 2001; JID 111:893–895, 1998; Ped Derm 13:306–309, 1996; punctate keratoderma *AD 122:900–908, 1986; Bull Soc Fr Dermatol Syph 45:26–29, 1938*

Erythema elevatum diutinum – hyperkeratotic palmar papules

Erythema gyratum repens with ichthyosis and palmoplantar hyperkeratosis *Clin Exp Dermatol 14:223–226, 1989*

Erythrokeratoderma variabilis – psoriasiform plaques, urticarial plaques and palmoplantar keratoderma *BJD 173:309–311, 2015; BJD 157:410–411, 2007; BJD 152:1143–1148, 2005; Ped Derm 19:285–292, 2002; AD 122:441–445, 1986; AD 101:68–73, 1970*

Focal acral hyperkeratosis – yellow papules on lateral aspect of palms *AD 132:1365, 1368, 1996*

Hand or foot dermatitis, chronic

Hyperkeratotic dermatosis of the palms *BJD 107:195–201, 1982*

Hypomelanosis of Ito – autosomal dominant; Blaschko-esque depigmentation; unilateral or bilateral; no prior inflammatory stages; 75% present at birth; CNS, musculoskeletal, ophthalmologic abnormalities, diffuse alopecia, nail and dental anomalies; decrease in pigmented melanosomes *JAAD 19:217–255, 1988*

Hypotrichosis, striate, reticulated pitted palmoplantar keratoderma, acro-osteolysis, psoriasiform plaques, periodontitis, lingua plicata, ventricular arrhythmias *BJD 147:575–581, 2002*

Ichthyosis cerebriformis – keratotic plugs, depressions, thick skin, palmoplantar keratoderma *JAAD 58:505–507, 2008*

Ichthyosis en confetti (congenital reticulated ichthyosiform erythroderma) – reticulated erythroderma with guttate hypopigmentation, palmoplantar kertoderma; loss of dermatoglyphics; temporary hypertrichosis of normal skin *JAMA Derm 151:64–69, 2015; BJD 166:434–439, 2012; JAAD 63:607–641, 2010*

Ichthyosis hystrix – epidermolytic hyperkeratosis with diffuse or striate PPK

Ichthyosis hystrix, Curth-Macklin type – hyperkeratotic lesions of elbows, knees in parallel grooves (zebra stripe pattern); palmoplantar keratoderma; spiky hyperkeratosis; *KRT1* mutation *BJD 175:1372–1375, 2016; AD 147:999–1001, 2011; AD 141:779–784, 2005; Am J Hum Genet 6:371–382, 1954*

Ichthyosis vulgaris palmaris et plantaris dominans – form of ichthyosis vulgaris *Dermatologica 165:627–635, 1982*

Junctional epidermolysis bullosa of late onset (skin fragility in childhood) – speckled hyperpigmentation of elbows; hemorrhagic bullae, teeth and nail abnormalities, oral blisters, disappearance of dermatoglyphics, palmoplantar keratoderma, small vesicles, atrophy of skin of hands *BJD 169:714–716, 2013*

Juvenile plantar dermatosis

Keratosis follicularis spinulosa decalvans – X-linked dominant, X-linked recessive or autosomal dominant; one of spectrum of keratosis pilaris atrophicans (others are KP atrophicans facei, atrophoderma vermiculatum); diffuse KP and scarring alopecia of scalp; atopy, palmoplantar keratoderma, photophobia, corneal abnormalities *JAAD 47:S275–278, 2002; AD 128:397–402, 1992; Dermatol Monatsschr 174:736–740, 1988; AD 119:22–26, 1983; Acta DV 51:146,1971; AD 114:761,1978*

Nekam's disease (keratosis lichenoides chronica) – isolated palmoplantar hyperkeratosis; violaceous papular and nodular lesions in linear and reticular arrays, especially on hands and feet with seborrheic dermatitis-like rash on face *JAAD 56:S1–5, 2007; JAAD 49:511–513, 2003; AD 131:609–614, 1995; AD 105:739–743, 1972; JAAD 37:263–264, 1997; JAAD 38:306–309, 1998*

Eur J Dermatol 9:497–499, 1999; AD 105:739–743, 1972; Presse Med 46:1000, 1938

Keratosis plantaris discreta

Lamellar ichthyosis – autosomal dominant, autosomal recessive

Lichen nitidus – palmoplantar hyperkeratosis and nail dystrophy *Clin Exp Dermatol 18:381–383, 1993*

Lichen planus *AD 140:1275–1280, 2004; BJD 142:310–314, 2000;* may be yellowish papules or plaques; may mimic tylosis

Lichen simplex chronicus – personal observation

Neutral lipid storage disease (Dorfman-Chanarin syndrome) – autosomal recessive; at birth collodion baby or ichthyosiform erythroderma; thereafter pattern resembles non-bullous ichthyosiform erythroderma; hypohidrosis; ectropion; palmoplantar hyperkeratosis, WBC vacuoles, myopathy, fatty liver, CNS disease, deafness *JAAD 17:801–808, 1987; AD 121:1000–1008, 1985*

Non-bullous CIE (congenital ichthyosiform erythroderma) (erythrodermic lamellar ichthyosis) – autosomal recessive; hyperkeratosis of palms and soles *AD 121:477–488, 1985*

Non-striate palmoplantar keratoderma – autosomal dominant; mutation in desmoglein-1 *BJD 166:36–45, 2012*

Pachydermoperiostosis (Touraine-Solente-Gole syndrome) – primary pachydermoperiostosis; autosomal dominant; skin of face, forehead, scalp folded and thickened; weary expression; cutis verticis gyrata of scalp; skin of hands and feet thickened; hyperhidrosis; spade-like hands; clubbing, mental retardation common *NEJM 272:923–931, 1956*

Peeling skin syndrome *JAAD 31:291–292, 1994*

Pityriasis rubra pilaris *J Dermatol 27:174–177, 2000; JAAD 31:997–999, 1994;* juvenile PRP *JAAD 59:943–948, 2008*

Porokeratotic palmoplantar keratoderma discreta *Clin Exp Dermatol 21:451–453, 1996*

Progressive symmetric keratoderma – personal observation

Psoriasis

Punctate keratoses of the palms and soles – 1–3 mm round to oval yellow to flesh colored papules scattered on palms and soles *JAAD 22:468–476, 1990*

HEREDITARY KERATODERMAS

HEREDITARY DIFFUSE PALMOPLANTAR KERATODERMAS

Unna Thost (Vorner) – autosomal dominant palmoplantar keratoderma; *KRT1, KRT9* mutations; begins in infancy as patchy hyperkeratosis and is well developed by 3–4 years of age as thick diffuse, yellowish hyperkeratosis with sharply demarcated erythematous lateral margin (non-transgradiens); no nail changes, hyperhidrosis; secondary dermatophyte infection and pitted keratolysis with pruritus and malodor; epidermolytic (Vorner) and non-epidermolytic (Unna-Thost) hyperkeratosis; acral blistering in infancy rare *Ped Derm 20:195–198, 2003; Arch Dermatol Res 294:268–272, 2002; BJD 140:486–490, 1999; JID 103:764–769, 1994; JID 103:474, 1994; Acta DV 72:120–122, 1992;* familial association with internal malignancies (breast, ovary) *BJD 117:363–370, 1987;* with pseudoainhum *AD 145:609–610, 2009;* epidermolytic PPK, knuckle pads, digital mutilation; *KRT9* mutation *BJD 165:199–201, 2011*

Vorner-like PPK – tonotubular keratin clumps; mutation in 1B domain of keratin 1 *BJD 160:446–449, 2009; JID 126:607–613, 2006; JAAD 24:638–642, 1991*

Diffuse PPK with DSG-1 mutation – autosomal dominant; thick hyperkeratosis (no transgradiens); mild onycholysis with yellow discoloration, no hyperhidrosis, enlarged intercellular spaces and partial keratinocyte separation

Nagashima PPK – autosomal recessive; Japan and China; non-epidermolytic PPK similar to mal de Meleda but milder phenotype; *SERPINB7* mutation; mild diffuse hyperkeratosis with erythema and transgradiens, hyperhidrosis; no nail changes; lesions over knees, elbows, Achilles tendon, and ears; maceration, foul odor, white spongy changes of water-soaked skin is diagnostic clue; no mutilation; constricting bands, spontaneous amputations and contractures *BJD 173:1288–1290, 2015; BJD 171:847–853, 2014; Am J Hum Gene 93:945–956, 2013; AD 144:375–379, 2008*

Bothnian PPK – autosomal dominant; *AQP5* mutation; mild to thick diffuse hyperkeratosis, transgradiens, hyperhidrosis, curved nails, ragged cuticles, nonprogressive; white spongy changes of water-soaked skin; diffuse non-epidermolytic PPK, pitted keratolysis, malodor *BMC Dermtol 16:7, 2016; BJD 174:430–432, 2016*

Greither's PPK – autosomal dominant; *KRT1* mutation; thick diffuse hyperkeratosis, partial transgradiens, hyperhidrosis, no nail changes, lesions over flexures, elbows, knees, Achilles tendon area; onset in infancy, develops fully in childhood; transient blistering in infancy; progressive; may regress in 4th or 5th decade; spontaneous amputations; orthohyperkeratosis, acanthosis, with prominent irregular keratohyalin granules *JAAD 53:S225–230, 2005; Ped Derm 20:272–275, 2003; Cutis 65:141–145, 2000*

Sybert syndrome – autosomal dominant; unknown mutation; thick hyperkeratotic; transgradiens, no nail changes nor hyperhidrosis; resembles Greither's PPK but more severe and widespread hyperkeratosis; lesions over elbows, knees, natal cleft, and groin; periorbital and perioral erythema; progressive; spontaneous amputations *Indian J Dermatol 55:297–299, 2010; Dermatol Online J 9:30, 2003; Prob Derm 14:71–116, 2002; JAAD 18:75–86, 1988*

Gamborg-Nielsen PPK – autosomal recessive; *SLURP1* mutation; thick hyperkeratosis, transgradiens; no hyperhidrosis or nail changes; knuckle pads over dorsal hands *Arch Dermatol Res 282:363–370, 1990; Clin Genet 28:361–366, 1985*

Acral keratoderma – autosomal recessive; unknown mutation; thick diffuse and striate hyperkeratosis, transgradiens, no nail changes nor hyperhidrosis; linear hyperkeratotic lesions over knees, elbows, ankles, Achilles tendon area *BJD 163:711–718, 2010; AD 111:763–768, 1975*

Huriez syndrome – autosomal dominant; unknown mutation; triad of diffuse PPK, nail dystrophy/hypoplasia with onset in infancy, and congenital scleroatrophy of extremities; pseudosclerodermatous hands; PPK is mild an diffuse with involvement of palms > soles; parchment-like dry hyperkeratotic skin over dorsal feet, hands, delayed growth affecting hands; atrophic plaques with increased risk of developing squamous cell carcinoma (15% cases by third or fourth decade with early metastases); poikilodermatous nose *AD 146:1419–1424, 2010; BJD 143:1091–1096, 2000; BJD 137:114–118, 1997; BJD 134:512–516, 1996; Ped Derm 15:207–209, 1998; JAAD 26:855–857, 1992; Dem Hop Paris 44:481–488, 1968*

Keratosis-ichthyosis-deafness (KID) syndrome – autosomal dominant; *GJB2 (GJB6), Cx26 (Cx30);* diffuse PPK dotted waxy, fine granular stippled or reticulated surface pattern of PPK of palms and soles; no transgradiens, no hyperhidrosis, or nail dystrophies; ichthyosiform erythroderma in infancy; hypotrichosis of scalp, eyebrows and eyelashes; acrofacial verruciform hyperkeratosis, perioral furrows, leukoplakia, sensorineural deafness, photophobia with vascularizing keratitis, blindness; increase risk of bacterial infections and squamous cell carcinoma *Ped Derm 29:349–357, 2012; Ped Derm 27:651–652, 2010; JAAD 69:127–134, 2013; Ped Derm 23:81–83, 2006; JAAD 51:377–382, 2004; BJD 148:649–653, 2003*

Bart-Pumphrey syndrome – autosomal dominant; *GJB2 (Cx26);* diffuse focal or punctate keratosis, no transgradiens, no hyperhidrosis; leukonychia, sensorineural hearing loss, knuckle pads, breast and axillary cysts *Clin Dermatol 23:23–32, 2005; Curr Prob Derm 14:71–116, 2002; NEJM 276:202–207, 1967;* mutation in *GJD6* encoding connexin 30 *BJD 161:452–455, 2009*

Howell-Evans syndrome – autosomal dominant; focal PPK; *RHBDF2* mutation; diffuse yellow callosities, no transgradiens, no nail changes; hyperhidrosis, keratosis pilaris, fissuring and infections; chronic rhinitis, maxillary decalcification, alveolysis and tooth loss; oral leukoplakia; esophageal carcinoma in mid- or late life; esophageal strictures *JAAD 52:403–409; 2005; Dis Esophagus 12:173–176, 1999; Genomics 37:381–385, 1996; JAAD 28:295–297, 1993; Q J Med 155:317–333, 1970*

SAM syndrome – severe dermatitis, allergies, metabolic wasting, palmoplantar keratoderma *Ped Derm 37:576–578, 2020; BJD 172:257–261, 2015*

DIFFUSE MUTILATING PALMOPLANTAR KERATODERMAS

Mal de Meleda (Gamborg-Nielsen/Norrbotten) PPK – autosomal recessive; *SLURP* (Ly6/Upar family); severe diffuse mutilating thick yellow-brown hyperkeratosis with prominent erythematous border, massive transgradiens and progradiens in a glove/stocking pattern; nail dystrophy; hyperhidrosis, nonepidermolytic hyperkeratosis, prominent stratum lucidum, perivascular inflammatory infiltrate, lesions over flexures, elbows, knee, Achilles tendon area; digital tapering, joint stiffness/contractures; psoriasiform lesions of elbows, knees, with severe mutilation, contractures, constricting bands around digits; pseudoainhum and digital amputation are features of progressive disease; fissuring, maceration, foul odor, and infections; high arched palate, perioral erythema, angular cheilitis *Am J Clin Dermatol 17:63–70, 2016; BJD 168:1372–1374, 2013; AD 147:748–750, 2011; BJD 160:878–880, 2009; AD 144:375–379, 2008; Hum Mol Genet 10:875–880, 2001; AD 136:1247–1252, 2000; BJD 128:207–212, 1993*

Vohwinkel syndrome (keratoderma hereditaria mutilans) – autosomal dominant; *GJB2 (Cx26)* mutation; diffuse yellowish severe mutilating PPK presents at birth and more evident in adulthood; honeycomb appearance of PPK with fine discernible superficial pattern replacing normal dermatoglyphics; transgradiens, nail dystrophy, hyperhidrosis; starfish keratotic plaques of knuckles, wrists, elbows, and knees; over time affect children develop constricting fibrosing bands, pseudoainhum and autoamputation of fingers and toes, particularly 5th digit; sensorineural deafness, alopecia, myopathy (spastic paraplegia possible), mental retardation, acanthosis nigricans, ichthyosiform dermatitis, focal epilepsy *BJD 164:197–199, 2011; Clin Dermatol 23:23–32, 2005; Curr Prob Dermatol 14:71–116, JAAD 44:376–378, 2001; BJD 145:657–660, 2001*

Loricrin keratoderma – ichthyosiform variant of Vohwinkel syndrome (Camisa disease) (congenital ichthyosiform erythroderma with collodion baby) – autosomal dominant; loricrin mutation, diffuse yellow, severe mutilating honeycomb PPK, nail dystrophies; no sensorineural deafness (no gap junction protein mutation), nor star shaped keratoses; mild ichthyosis, pseudoainhum *BJD 172:1158–1162, Ped Derm 19:285–292, 2002; BJD 145:657–660, 2001*

Olmsted syndrome – most cases sporadic; autosomal dominant; *TRPV3* mutation; X-linked recessive with *MBTPS2* mutation and autosomal recessive; diffuse yellow-brown, mutilating PPK, fissures, transgradiens, contractures, constrictions, pseudoainhum and autoamputation of digits over time; severe pruritus; nail dystrophies, hyperhidrosis or anhidrosis; hyperkeratotic plaques periorally, around nostrils, ears, anogenital region, neck, upper thorax abdomen, inguinal folds, thighs, elbows, knees; histological inflammatory infiltrate with mast cells; alopecia universalis, infections oral leukokeratosis, chronic blepharitis, corneal dystrophies, delayed growth, hi tone hearing loss, abnormal dentition, bone deformities, hyper IgE, eosinophilia (rare), foul odor, and recurrent infections *Orphanet J Rare Dis 10:33, 2015; ;BJD 167:440–442, 2012; Ped Derm 25:223–229, 2008; JAAD 53:S266–272, 2005; Ped Derm 21:603–605, 2004; Ped Derm 20:323–326, 2003; BJD 136:935–938, 1997; AD 132:797–800, 1996; AD 131;738–739, 1995; JAAD 31:508–510, 1994; Ped Derm 10:376–381, 1993; BJD 122:245–252, 1990; JAAD 10:600–610, 1984;* follicular hyperkeratosis of buttocks and knees *BJD 136:935–938, 1997;* with erythromelalgia; mutation in *TRFV3 Ped Derm 36:942–943, 2019;* as *JAMA Derm 150:303–306, 2014;* associated hypotrichosis

KLICK syndrome (keratosis linearis with ichthyosis and sclerosing keratoderma) – autosomal recessive; *POMP* mutation; diffuse mutilating PPK, no transgradiens, no hyperhidrosis, nor nail changes; hyperkeratotic plaque, ichthyosis and papules in linear patterns over arm flexors and wrists; linear keratosis of skin folds; erythroderma; red elbows and knees *JAAD 67:1362–1374, 2012; JAAD 63:607–641, 2010; BJD 153:461, 2005; Acta DV 77:225–227, 1997; Am J Hum Genet 1:581–589, 1997*

FOCAL PALMOPLANTAR KERATODERMAS

PPK nummularis – autosomal dominant; *KRT16, KRT6c, DSG1, TRPV3* mutations; circumscribed painful callosities, no transgradiens, no hyperhidrosis, no or minimal nail changes (5th toenail hypertrophy with splinter hemorrhages); childhood onset, appears when infant starts to walk; may be induced by mechanical stress, pressure and becomes painful; follicular hyperkeratosis; plantar blistering; no spontaneous amputation; minimal oral or anogenital leukokeratosis *JID 130:425–429, 2010; AD 142:1074–1076, 2006; Dermatology 193:47–49, 1996; Acta DV 75:405–406, 1995; JAAD 25:113–114, 1991; JAAD 9:204–209, 1983; AD 114:591–592, 1978*

Focal palmoplantar keratoderma and gingival hyperkeratosis – autosomal dominant; painful hyperkeratosis over weight-bearing plantar skin since infancy; leukokeratosis attached gingiva; leukokeratosis of glans penis; no nail changes, epidermolytic hyperkeratosis on biopsy *JAAD (pt 1)52:403–409, 2005; Am J Med Genet 104:339–341, 2001; Arch Int Med 113:866–871, 1974*

STRIATE PALMOPLANTAR KERATODERMA

Striate PPK I, II, III (Brunauer-Fohs-Siemens syndrome Wachter-type focal nonepidermolytic palmoplantar keratoderma) – autosomal dominant; striate PPK I – *DSG1* (desmoglein 1), striate PPK II – *DSP (*desmoplakin), and striate PPK III *KET 1 (*keratin 1); linear skin thickening over flexor aspects of digits and pressure points of soles (diffuse on soles in striate PPK III), no transgradiens, no nail changes; hyperhidrosis in type I, classification of type I-III base on responsible gene mutation; knee, elbow hyperkeratosis is rare, foul odor, plantar pain in type I improves with age *BJD 176:1345–1350, 2017;* striate PPK mutation desmoplakin II *BJD 166-36–45, 2-012;* PPK I mutation *DSG1 JAAD 62:107–113, 2010; BJD 150:878–891, 2004; Int J Dermatol 40:644–645, 2004*

HOPP syndrome – hypotrichosis, acro-osteolysis, striate palmoplantar keratoderma; periodontitis, psoriasis-like skin lesions *BJD 147:575–581, 2002;* resembles Papillon-Lefevre and Haim Munk

PPK varians type (Wachter's type) – autosomal dominant; striate palmoplantar keratoderma (linear hyperkeratosis of fingers and focal islands or plaques of hyperkeratosis of feet with sparing of central sole *J Eur Acad DV 12:33–37, 1999;* regression of symptoms *Dermatology 186:245–247, 1993; Med Cutan Ibero Lat Am 16:66–69, 1988*

PPK with cutaneous horns *Int J Dermatol 31:369–370, 1992;* combination of striate and diffuse

PPK and Charcot-Marie-Tooth disease – autosomal dominant *AD 116:789–790, 1980*

PPK with clinodactyly – autosomal dominant *Birth Defects Orig Art Ser 18 (3B):207–210, 1982; Dermatologica 162:300–303, 1981*

SAM syndrome – severe dermatitis, allergies, and metabolic wasting *Ped Derm 37:576–578, 2020;* mutation in *DSG1 BJD 179:755–757, 2018*

PUNCTATE PALMOPLANTAR KERATODERMA

Type-1A (Buschke-Fischer-Brauer syndrome) – autosomal dominant; *AAGAB* mutation *Clin Exp Dermatol 42:316–319, 2017;* presents between ages 12 and 30; multiple asymptomatic palmoplantar punctate keratoses; no transgradiens, no hyperhidrosis; clinical subtypes include pinhead sized papules, spiky filiform lesions, dense 1-2 mm papules, callus-like lesions, hard warty mass, cupuliform lesions, and focal translucent lesions; no or rare nail changes, onset late childhood or adolescence; increase in number and size with age; worsen with soaking in water; ankylosing spondylitis, spastic paralysis, sebaceous hyperplasia, and association with gastrointestinal and pulmonary malignancy *BJD 171:433–436, 2014; BJD 152:874–878, 2005; JID 122:1121–1125, 2004; JAAD 49:1166–1169, 2003; J Med Genet 40:872–878, 2003; BJD 134:720–726, 1996; BJD 128:104–105, 1993; JAAD 8:700–702, 1983;* with ainhum *JAAD 3:43–49, 1980;* possible link with cancer in 18 Canadian families *Cut Med Surg 24:28–32, 2020; Case Rep Dermatol 11:292–296, 2019*

Type 1B – *COL14A1* – classification of type 1A and 1B is base on responsible gene mutation *J Med Genet 49:563–568, 2012*

Type 2 (porokeratotic type or spiny keratoderma) – autosomal dominant; unknown mutation; early onset of tiny punctate spiny palmoplantar keratoses; late onset pits with keratotic plugs, no transgradiens, no hyperhidrosis, no nail changes; columnar parakeratosis overlying reduced or absent granular layer; onset early 20s; sebaceous hyperplasia in men

Type 3 (acrokeratoelastoidosis of Costa) – autosomal dominant; unknown mutation; keratotic papules along margins of hands and feet; small round or oval smooth shiny or umbilicated papules of dorsal hands, knuckles in first interdigital space and along lateral margins of hands and wrists; transgradiens rare; rare nail dystrophy, no hyperhidrosis; hyperkeratosis, hypergranulosis, elastorrhexis; onset in adolescence or adult life *JAAD 27:881–882, 1997; Semin Derm 14:152–161, 1995; JAAD 22:468–476, 1990; BJD 106:337–344, 1982*

Focal acral hyperkeratosis (acrokeratoelastoidosis without elastorrhexia) – autosomal dominant; crateriform papules of sides of hands and feet *JAAD 47:448–451, 2002: AD 120:63–264, 1984; BJD 109:97–103, 1983*

Acrokeratoelastoidosis and knuckle pads *Cutis 102:344–346, 2018*

Degenerative collagenous plaques of hands (keratoelastoidosis marginalis)- linear bands around thumb and index fingers *AD 93:202–203, 1966*

Cole disease – autosomal dominant; punctate keratoses of palms and sole; guttate hypopigmentation *J Eur Acad DV 29:2492–2493, 2015; Acta DV 91:737–738, 2011; AD 145:495–497, 2009; Ped Derm 19:302–306, 2002*

Collie-Davies (punctate keratoderma palmoplantaris maculosa seu papulose) *Hautarzt 48:577–580, 1997*

Keratosis punctata of palmar creases – autosomal dominant; African Americans *JAAD 13:381–382, 1995; Cutis 33:394–396, 1984; Cutis 32:75–76, 1983; AD 116:669–671, 1980;* in Caucasians *Dermatology 188:200–202, 1994*

Punctate acrokeratoderma – autosomal dominant; keratotic papules of hands and feet; pronounced hyperkeratosis of palms and soles; freckle-like pigmentation of dorsal hands and feet *BJD 128:693–695, 1993*

PALMOPLANTAR KERATODERMA WITH SYNDROMES OF ECTODERMAL DYSPLASIA

Pachyonychia congenita – autosomal dominant; mutation in one of four keratin genes – *KRT6A/KRT6B/KRT16/KRT17;* diffuse plantar keratoderma, fissures, blisters, ulcerations; thickened toenails in 90% before age 5; hyperhidrosis; oral leukokeratosis present at birth in 54% and by one year of age in 73%; steatocystomas *JAAD 67:680–686, 2012; JAAD 52:403–409, 2005; JID Symp Proc 10:3–17, 2005*

Type 1 – Jadassohn-Lewandowsky syndrome – keratin 16 mutation

Type 2 – Jackson-Lawler syndrome – type 1 plus bullae of palms and soles; hyperhidrosis, natal or neonatal teeth and steatocystomas or epidermoid cysts; keratin 17 mutation *BJD 159:730–732, 2008*

Type 3 – types 1 and 2 plus angular cheilitis, corneal dyskeratosis, and cataracts

Type 4 – types 1,2, and 3 plus laryngeal lesions, hoarseness, mental retardation; hair anomalies and alopecia *BJD 152:800–802, 2005; Clin Exp Dermatol 28:434–436, 2003; JID 117:1391–1396, 2001; JAAD 19:705–711, 1988*

Clouston syndrome (hidrotic ectodermal dysplasia) – autosomal dominant; *GJB6* gene encoding Cx30; progressive diffuse palmoplantar keratoderma with transgradiens with punctiform accentuation; pebbled appearance on dorsum; hypotrichosis with sparse, brittle hair, alopecia, nail dystrophy; milky white in infancy and gradually thicken with short easily shed nail plates; periungual swelling, oral leukoplakia; potophobia, cataracts, strabismus, tufted terminal phalanges, normal teeth, normal sweating *JAMA Derm 149:1350–1351, 2013; BJD 142:24252, 2000; Nature Genet 26:142–144, 2000; Can Med J 21:18–31, 1929;* associated eccrine syringofibroadenoma *Ann Bras Dermatol 89:504–506, 2014; AD 125:1715, 1989;* sweat glands, sebaceous glands, and teeth are normal distinguishing this syndrome from hypophidrotic ectodermal dysplasia

Papillon-Lefevre syndrome – autosomal recessive; *CTSC* (cathepsin C) gene mutation; diffuse palmoplantar keratoderma with painful callosities, trangradiens characteristic; early onset sever periodontitis of primary and permanent dentition (edentulous by age 14–15); radiologically see loss or resorption of both maxillary and mandibular alveolar ridges; susceptibility to cutaneous and systemic infections (liver) mostly *Staphylococcus aureus;* manifests at birth or early infancy with appearance of palmoplantar keratoderma which may be preceded by erythema; soles more severely affected than palms and malodorous hyperhidrosis common; scaly psoriasiform plaques over interphalangeal joints, elbows, knees, Achilles tendon area and lateral malleoli; hypotrichosis, nail fragility; ectopic calcification of falx cerebri and choroid plexus *Int J Dermatol 55:898–902, 2016; Ped Derm 30:749–750, 2013; Eur J Ped 170:689–691, 2011; BMC Med Genet 4:5, 2003*

Haim-Munk syndrome – autosomal recessive; *CTSC* (cathepsin C) gene mutation; resembles Papillon-Lefevre syndrome (variants of the same disease) with acro-osteolysis, arachnodactyly, and pes planus; congenital diffuse palmoplantar kertoderma, periodontitis, severe alveolar bone destruction and tooth loss, deformities of digits with claw-like deformity of terminal phalanges and atrophic nail changes *JAAD 66:339–341, 2012; BJD 152:353–356, 2005; J Med Genet 37:88–94, 2003; BJD 147:575–581, 2002; Eur J Hum Genet 5:156–160, 1997; BJD 115:243–248, 1986*

Striate palmoplantar keratoderma, periodontitis, acro-osteolysis, psoriasis-like skin lesions resembling Papillon-Lefevre syndrome and Haim-Munk syndrome but no cathepsin C gene mutation; hypotrichosis, ventricular arrhythmias *BJD 147:575–581, 2002*

Oculo-dento-digital dysplasia syndrome (ODD) – autosomal dominant; *GJA1* mutation encoding Cx43; diffuse palmoplantar keratoderma, typical facies, narrow pinched nose with hypoplastic alae nasi, hyper/hypotelorism; microphthalmia, microcornea, glaucoma; complete syndactyly of 4th and 5th fingers; brittle nails; hypotrichosis, dental abnormalities, neurologic defects, lymphedema *Clin Genet 84:378–381, 2013; JAAD 57:732–733, 2007*

Odonto-onycho-dermal dysplasia – autosomal recessive; *WNT-10A* gene mutation; diffuse palmoplantar keratoderma with hyperhidrosis; oligodontia with widely spaced peg-shaped teeth; absence of secondary teeth; onychodysplasia; hair may be sparse; facial lesions atrophic, erythematous, telangiectatic, reticulated with atrophic malar and ala nasal patches with vermiculate scarring; benign adnexal tumors (eccrine poroma, apocrine hidrocystoma, syringofibroadenoma) *JAAD 57:332–333, 2007; Am J Med Genet 14:335–346, 1983*

Schopf-Schulz-Passarge syndrome – autosomal recessive; *WNT10A* gene mutation; diffuse palmoplantar keratoderma with hyperhidrosis; features of odonto-onycho-dermal dysplasia and eyelid margin hidrocystomas; increased risk of squamous cell carcinoma; hypodontia with conical teeth, thin scalp hair, hypoplastic eyelids, facial telangiectasias, brittle and furrowed nails *BJD 171:1211–1214, 2014; Ped Derm 30:491–492, 2013; JAAD 65:1066–1069, 2011; JAAD 36:569–576, 1997; BJD 120:131–132, 1989; Birth Defects 12:219–221, 1971;* eccrine syringofibroadenoma of palms and soles *BJD 143:591–594, 2000*

Naegali-Franceschetti syndrome (dermatopathia pigmentosa reticularis syndrome – diffuse and punctate keratoderma; autosomal dominant; *K14* (non-helical E!/V1 domain); diffuse palmoplantar keratoderma, other patterns are localized – punctate keratoses of palmar creases, linear; adermatoglyphia, reticulate pigmentary abnormality which fades after puberty; hypohidrosis, hyperpyrexia; early loss of teeth, dental enamel defects; hair abnormalities *BJD 177:945–959, 2017; Am J Hum Genet 79:724–830, 2006; Curr Prob Derm 14:71–116, 2002; JAAD 28:942–950, 1993*

Ectodermal dysplasia with skin fragility (McGrath syndrome) – autosomal recessive; *PKP1* mutation (plakophilin-1); severe disabling focal palmoplantar keratoderma; generalized superficial erosions; perioral and tongue fissures; abnormal nails, hypotrichosis, esophageal strictures, constipation, sparse eyelashes, blepharitis *Dermatol Clin 28:125–129, 2010;* cardiac function normal *J Med Genet 53:289–295, 2016*

Christ-Siemens-Touraine syndrome (anhidrotic ectodermal dysplasia) – X-linked recessive (female carriers); ectodysplasia A; mild diffuse palmoplantar keratoderma; anhidrosis with hyperpyrexia, conical, pointed spaced teeth; dystrophic nails in 50%; madarosis, alopecia, abnormal facies with saddle nose, prominent frontal ridge and chin, sunken eyes, large lips

SYNDROMES AND DERMATOSES WITH DIFFUSE OR PUNCTATE PALMOPLANTAR KERATODERMA

Erythrokeratoderma variabilis – first described by Mendes de Costa in 1925; relatively fixed patches of hyperkeratosis with erythematous areas "characterized by capriciously formed outlines, like the boundary lines of seacoasts on maps"; autosomal dominant; erythematous areas move from hour to hour; usually evident at birth or within first year of life; face, buttocks and extremities; palmoplantar keratoderma

Progressive symmetric erythrokeratoderma – autosomal dominant in 50%; other case sporadic or autosomal recessive *Am J Hum Genet 100:978–984, 2017;* mutation in *KDSR* in ceramide synthesis pathway; sharply marginated non-migratory symmetrical keratotic or psoriasiform plaques shortly after birth of dorsal hands, elbows, feet, buttocks, sometimes face; typically spares the trunk; with palmoplantar keratoderma *BJD 173:309–311, 2015; BJD 157:410–415, 2005; Ped Derm 19:285–292, 2002; AD 12:434–440,441–445, 1986*

Pityriasis rubra pilaris – sharply demarcated reddish-orange diffuse thick palmoplantar keratoderma with fissuring (PRP sandal); juvenile PRP with circumscribed, psoriasiform dermatitis of knees and ankles with palmoplantar keratoderma *Ped Derm 31:138–145, 2014; JAAD 59:943–948, 2008; JAAD 31:997–999, 1994*

SAM syndrome – severe dermatitis, allergies and metabolic wasting; focal or diffuse palmoplantar keratoderma, rarely striate pattern; mutation in *DSB1* gene *Ped Derm 37:576–578, 2020; Nat Genet 45:1244–1248, 2013*

CONGENITAL ICHTHYOSIS

Ichthyosis vulgaris – rough palms and soles, hyperlinearity, mosaic scaling shins, keratosis pilaris, atopy

Ichthyosis palmaris et plantaris – yellow brown hyperkeratosis, ill-defined border, no erythematous or pigmented halo; absence of eccrine sweat glands *Dermatologica 165:627–635, 1982*

Autosomal recessive congenital ichthyosis (ARCI) *Hum Mutat 39:1305–1313, 2018*

ABCA 12

ALOX12B, ALOXE3 – severe diffuse palmoplantar keratoderma *J Med Genet 44:615–620, 2007; Hum Mol Genet 13:2473–2482, 2004*

NIPAL4, *ICHTHYIN* mutation – diffuse yellow palmoplantar keratoderma

CERS3 mutation – mild palmoplantar keratoderma with hyperlinearity

TGNI, CYP4F22, PNPLA1, SDR9C7, SULT2B1

Epidermolytic hyperkeratosis (epidermolytic ichthyosis) (bullous congenital ichthyosiform erythroderma) – palmoplantar keratoderma and mild fine slae in body folds; mutation in L12 domain of keratin 1 *BJD 162:875–879, 2010*

Ichthyosis en confetti (congenital reticular ichthyosiform erythroderma) (ichthyosis variegate) – autosomal dominant; reticulated erythroderma with guttate hypopigmentation; palmoplantar keratoderma, orange red; loss of dermatoglyphics; mutation in keratin 10 *BJD 166:434–439, 2012; JAAD 63:607–641, 2010;* PPK *JAMA Derm 151:64–69, 2015*

Lamellar ichthyosis – *TGM1* mutation; palmoplantar keratoderma *J Dermatol 45:1463–1467, 2018;* ectropion, hair loss, hypohidrosis, constriction of fingers; bathing suit distribution unique to Africans *Dermatol Clin 12:787–796, 1994*

EPIDERMOLYSIS BULLOSA

Kindler syndrome (bullous acrokeratotic poikiloderma of Kindler and Weary) – autosomal recessive; acral bullae in infancy; progressive poikiloderma with photosensitivity; nail dystrophy; webbing of digits; esophageal and urethral stenosis; ectropion; poor dentition, gingival fragility; aged hands with fine wrinkling and scarring; palmoplantar hyperkeratosis; mutation in *FERMT1* (formerly *KIND1*) gene *Ped Derm 37:337–341, 2020; BJD 157:1252–1256, 2007; AD 142:620–624, 2006; Ped Derm 23:586–588, 2006; AD 140:939–944, 2004; AD 132:1487–1490, 1996*

Dowling-Meara type (generalized severe form) (epidermolysis bullosa herpetiformis) – autosomal dominant; diffuse palmoplantar keratoderma with mottled pigmentation; acral blistering, hemorrhagic bullae; dystrophic thick nails *BJD 144:40–45, 2001; Ped Derm 13:306–309, 1996; AD 122:900–908, 1986*

K5, 14 gene; *KRT5* mutation; punctate palmoplantar keratoderma, mottled pigmentation of limbs, localized skin blistering and fragility mostly during childhood (EBS) *Eur J Dermatol 20:698–700, 2010; Proc Natl Acad Sci USA 93:9079–9084, 1996*

Lethal acantholytic epidermolysis bullosa – palmoplantar keratoderma, cardiomyopathy, mutation in desmoplakin *J Cosme Dermatol 18:371–376, 2019;* autosomal recessive alopecia *BJD 166;36–45, 2012; Am J Hum Genet 77:653–660, 2005*

Epidermolysis bullosa simplex – keratin 5 or 14 mutations; *KRT5* – severe blistering in childhood with improvement over time and to palmoplantar keratoderma and nail dysplasia *Ped Derm 36:1007–1009, 2019; Acta DV 97:1114–1119, 2017; KRT5P. E477K* mutation-associate keratoconus

Darier's disease – autosomal dominant with variable penetrance; punctate keratoses or tiny pits present over palms and soles; associated with acrokeratosis verruciformis of Hopf; cobblestoning of mucous membranes; nail changes of red, white, blue longitudinal bands with distal V-shaped nicks; characteristic odor; skin colored to yellow-brown crusted papules in seborrheic distribution *JAAD 27:40–50, 1982*

Acrokeratosis of Hopf – diffuse thickening, small keratoses; palmar papules with central depressions and punctiform breaks in dermatoglyphic; skin colored warty, keratotic papules over dorsal hands and feet *Clin Exp Dermatol 31:558–563, 2006*

Cowden's disease – (multiple hamartoma syndrome) – translucent punctate keratoses and acrokeratosis verruciformis-like lesions over dorsal hands and feet; facial trichilemmomas; multiple angiomas and lipomas; café au lait macules; fibrocystic breast disease with breast cancer; goiter, thyroid cancer *JAAD 68:189–209, 2013; Int J Clin Pract 61:645–652, 2007; JAAD 17:343–346, 1987; JAAD 11:1127–1141, 1984*

Nevoid basal cell carcinoma syndrome (Gorlin's syndrome) – autosomal dominant; punctate hyperkeratosis or characteristic pits *Dermmatol Surg 39:1557–1572, 2013;* odontogenic keratocysts, defective dentition, bifid ribs, kyphoscoliosis, broad nasal root, hypertelorism, frontal bossing, calcification

of falx cerebri, epidermoid cysts and milia *Am J Med Genet 50:282–290, 1994; Medicine 66:98–113, 1987*

Spiny keratoderma (multiple minute palmoplantar digitate hyperkeratosis) (music box spicules, music box keratoderma, palmar filiform hyperkeratosis) (porokeratosis palmaris et plantaris, punctate porokeratotic keratoderma, punctate keratoderma) – discrete keratotic plugs arising from palms, soles or both; spiny filiform spiked minute aggregates *Int J Dermatol 56:915–919, 2017; JAAD 58:344–348, 2008; JAAD 26 (pt 2)879–881, 1992; JAAD 18:431–436, 1988; AD 104:682–683, 1971;* associated with autosomal dominant polystic kidney disease *JAAD 34:935–936, 1986;* questionable paraneoplastic associations in non-familial spiny keratoderma *Dermatology 201:379–380, 2000;* gastrointestinal adenocarcinoma *Ann DV 124:707–709, 1997;* breast cancer *Ann DV 117:834–836, 1990;* familial *Dermatol Online J 18:8, 2012*

SASH1 variants – autosomal dominant palmoplantar keratoderma, alopecia, nail dystrophy, recurrent squamous cell carcinomas, acrofacial hyper- and hypopigmentation *BJD 177:945–959, 2017; Eur J Hum Genet 23:957–962, 2015*

Palmoplantar keratoderma and woolly hair; KANK2 (KN motif and ankyrin repeat domain) gene mutation; autosomal recessive, striate keratoderma, woolly hair, leukonychia, pseudoainhum, follicular papules over extensors, cheeks; sparse scalp and body/eye hairs; nephrotic syndrome *J Med Genet 51:338–394, 2014*

Oudtshoorn disease (keratolytic winter erythema; erythrokeratolysis hiemalis) – autosomal dominant; diffuse palmoplantar keratoderma; thickening preceded by erythema, dry blister and centrifugal peeling of palms and soles with recurrences in winter *J Eur Acad DV 32:704–719, 2018; AD 142:1073–1074, 2006; Curr Prob Dermatol 14:71–116, 2002*

Tyrosinemia type II (keratosis palmoplantaris with corneal dystrophy, Richner-Hanhart syndrome) – autosomal recessive; yellowish-white, hyperkeratotic papules and plaques; painful, friction-related; no transgradiens; bullae may occur; developmental/growth delay; onset at early infancy or adolescence; hyperhidrosis, photophobia, tearing, redness and pain progressing to dendritic herpetiform corneal erosions, ulcers, dystrophy, opacities, and scarring; severe nail dystrophy due to onychophagia; elevated serum and urine tyrosine levels *J Eur Acad DV 32:899–925, 2018; Ped Derm 25:378–380, 2008; Ped Derm 23:259–261, 2006; JAAD 35:857–859, 1996; Pediatr 126:266–269, 1995; AD 130:507–511, 1994; Ann DV 120:139–142, 1993; Dermatol 182:168–171, 1991; AD 126:1342–1346, 1990*

Cystic fibrosis – *CFTR* gene mutation; autosomal recessive; aquagenic palmoplantar keratoderma in 40–84% of cases; transient palmoplantar whitish papules after water immersion *Acta DV 96:848–849, 2016;* transient reactive papulotranslucent acrokeratoderma *Ped Derm 24:564–566, 2007; Australas J Dermatol 41:172–174, 2000; JAAD 34:686–687, 1996; AD 108:108–110, 1993;* aquagenic acrosyringeal keratoderma *JAMA Derm 150:1001–1002, 2014; JAAD 45:124–126, 2001;* aquagenic wrinkling of palms *BJD 163:162–166, 2010; AD 145:1296–1299, 2009; Ped Derm 26:660–661, 2009*

Palmoplantar keratoderma with anogenital leukokeratosis – diffuse palmoplantar keratoderma with slowly progressive anogenital leukokeratosis; nails normal, no ectodermal dysplasia or signs of pachyonychia congenita *Dermatology 197:300–302, 1998*

Palmoplantar keratoderma with ankylosing spondylitis – ankylosing vertebral hyperostosis with tylosis *Acta DV (Stockh)68;346–350, 1988*

Palmoplantar keratoderma with acrocyanosis and livedo reticularis *Acta DV 75:331, 1995; Acta DV 69:156–161, 1981*

CONGENITAL DIFFUSE PALMOPLANTAR KERATODERMA ASSOCIATED WITH SYSTEMIC ABNORMALITIES

Indian Dermatol Online J 10:365–379, 2019

CARDIAC DISEASE

Naxos disease (plakoglobin) – autosomal recessive; focal palmoplantar keratoderma, arrhythmogenic right ventricular dysplasia;

cardiomegaly and ventricular tachycardia due to focal myocarditis or cardiomyopathy; woolly hair *Ped Derm 34:724–725, 2017; JAAD 44:309–322, 2011; JAAD 34:1021, 2001; AD 136:1247–1252, 2000;* recessive mutation in desmoplakin *BJD 166:36–45, 2012; BJD 165:917–921, 2011; Hum Mol Genet 9:2761–2766, 2000;* desmocollin 2 mutation, woolly hair nevus, mild palmoplantar keratoderma, arrhythmogenic right ventricular cardiomyopathy *BJD 166:36–45, 2012;* non-fragile skin

Carvajal-Huerta syndrome (desmoplakin) – autosomal recessive; striate palmoplantar keratoderma with woolly hair and sparse hair and arrhythmogenic left ventricular dilated cardiomyopathy *BJD 166:36–45, 2012;* nail dystrophy, follicular hyperkeratosis with hyperpigmented plaques of elbows *Ped Derm 32:282–288, 2015;* non-fragile skin; autosomal recessive; focal striate palmoplantar keratoderma, woolly hair, dilated cardiomyopathy *Curr Prob Dermatol 14:71–116, 2002;* epidermolytic palmoplantar keratoderma, woolly hair, dilated cardiomyopathy *Orphanet J Rare Dis 13:74, May 2018; JAAD 39:418–421, 1998*

CAPK syndrome – cardiomyopathy, alopecia, and palmoplantar keratoderma *J Med Genet 53:289–295, 2016;* autosomal recessive arrhythmogenic right ventricular cardiomyopathy, alopecia and palmoplantar keratoderma *BJD 165:917–921, 2011*

Desmocollin 2 mutations (*DSC2*) – autosomal recessive; mild palmoplantar keratoderma, arrhythmogenic left cardiomyopathy, woolly hair

Desmoplakin mutation, congenital alopecia, with persistent hypotrichosis of scalp, sparse eyebrows, eyelashes; striate palmoplantar keratoderma, cardiomyopathy requiring orhtotopic heart transplant *Ped Derm 36:1010–1011, 2019*

HEARING DEFECTS

Vohwinkel syndrome – autosomal dominant; *GJB2, Cx 26*

Bart-Pumphrey syndrome – autosomal dominant; *GJB2, Cx 26*

KID syndrome – autosomal dominant; *GJB2>GJB6, Cx 26*

Ichthyosis hystrix (Curth-Macklin) – hyperkeratotic lesions of elbows, knees in parallel grooves (zebra stripe pattern); palmoplantar keratoderma and spiky hyperkeratosis; *KRT1* mutation *BJD 175:1372–1375, 2016; AD 147:999–1001, 2011; AD 141:779–784, 2005; Am J Hum Genet 6:371–382, 1954; GJB2, Cx 26 –* sensorineural hearing loss

Palmoplantar keratoderma, short stature, facial dysmorphism, hypodontia, deafness, epilepsy *Ped Dent 11:145–150, 1989*

Palmoplantar keratoderma with deafness – *GJB2, Cx 26;* autosomal dominant; sensorineural deafness *Semin Cell Dev Biol 50:4–12, 2016*

Oculo-dental-digital dysplasia syndrome – autosomal dominant; *GJA1, Cx 43;* conductive hearing loss

Palmoplantar keratoderma, papulopustular acne, sensorineural hearing loss with age – periorificial erythematous patches, angular cheilitis, psoriasiform plaques; *GJB2* mutation *Acta DV 99:1192–1194, 2019*

Focal palmoplantar keratoderma with sensorineural deafness *BJD 143:8760883, 2000*

NEUROPATHY

CEDNIK (cerebral dysgenesis, neuropathy, ichthyosis, keratoderma) – decreased SNAP29 protein; mutation in *ABCA12* gene; microcephaly, dysmorphic face with small anterior fontanelles; pointed prominent nasal tip, small chin, inverted nipples, and long toes; high palate, thick gingivae, cradle cap, sparse, brittle coarse hair, scarring alopecia; fixed flexion posture *BJD 164:610–616, 2011; JAAD 63L607–641, 2010; AD 144:334–340, 2008; Am J Hum Genet 77:242–251, 2005*

MEDNIK (mental retardation, enteropathy, deafness, neuropathy, ichthyosis, keratoderma) – *AP1S1*

Oculo-dental-digital dysplasia

OPHTHALMIC DEFECTS

Tyrosinemia type II (Richner-Hanhart syndrome0

Olmsted syndrome

Schopf-Schulz-Passarge syndrome

KID syndrome

Oculo-dental-digital dysplasia

MALIGNANCY

Howell-Evans syndrome

Huriez syndrome

Hereditary punctate keratoderma and internal malignancy *JAAD 10:587–591, 1984;* hereditary epidermolytic palmoplantar keratoderma – breast and ovarian cancer *BJD 117; 363–370, 1987;* breast, uterus, lung, bladder, colon *BJD 134:720–726, 1996;* palmoplantar keratoderma – esophageal cancer *Turkey BMC Cancer July 28, 2005;* spiny keratoderma of palms and soles, acquired *Hautarzt 63:923–926, 2012*

Oral florid papillomatosis, leukoplakia of esophagus, palmoplantar keratoderma, and transepidermal elimination *J Dermatol 21:974–978, 1994*

PALMOPLANTAR KERATODERMAS WITH SYSTEMIC MANIFESTATIONS OR ASSOCIATED FEATURES

Acro-osteolysis with keratoderma (Bureau-Barriere syndrome) – diffuse palmoplantar keratoderma *Hautarzt 44:5–13, 1993; Acta DV (Stockh)52:278–280, 1972*

Cantu's syndrome – autosomal dominant; hyperpigmented macules of face, forearms, feet; hyperkeratotic palms and soles *Clin Genet 14:165–168, 1978*

Congenital atrichia, palmoplantar keratoderma (Bazex-like), mental retardation, early loss of teeth *JAAD 30:893–898, 1994*

Hereditary palmoplantar keratoderma, type papulose – in Croatia; rare autosomal dominant; Slovenia; no malignancies *Acta DV alp Pannonica Adriat 18: 114–116, 2009; JAAD 29:435–437, 1993*

Hereditary palmoplantar keratoderma, nail dystrophy, motor and sensory neuropathy; autosomal dominant *J Med Genet 25:765–757, 1988*

Hyperkeratosis-hyperpigmentation syndrome – autosomal dominant; mild palmoplantar keratoderma; hyperpigmented spots *TIG 13:229, 1997; Clin Genet 43:73–75, 1993; Rev Neurol (Paris)144:421–424, 1988; Clin Genet 23:329–335, 1983; Clin Genet 14:165–168, 1978*

Palmoplantar keratoderma, mental retardation, spastic paraplegia *Am J Med Genet A 161A:1390–1393, 2013; Clin Genet 23:329–335, 1983;* striate keratoderma of palms; X-linked *Clin Genet 23:329–335, 1983; BJD 109:589–596, 1983*

Palmoplantar keratoderma, clubbing, skeletal deformity of terminal phalanges *Acta DV 52:278–280, 1972*

Palmoplantar keratoderma, large ears, sparse hypopigmented hair, frontal bossing *Ped Derm 19:224–228, 2002*

Sjogren-Larsson syndrome – autosomal recessive; congenital ichthyosis, mental retardation, spastic diplegia, diffuse palmoplantar keratoderma; deficiency of fatty aldehyde dehydrogenase *Ped Derm 22:569–571, 2005; Ped Derm 8:217–220, 1991*

Symmetrical interdigital keratoderma of the hands *Clin Exp Dermatol 93:193–198, 2014; Dermatol Online J 11:26, 2005; Clin Exp Dermatol 20:240–241, 1995; Acta DV 73:459–460, 1993*

Diffuse progressive palmoplantar keratoderma – transgradiens, hypotrichosis, trichorrhexis nodosa, keratosis pilaris, leukonychia totalis; hyperkeratotic lesions of knees, elbows, and perianal region *BJD 133:633–638, 1995*

TRANSGRADIENS PALMOPLANTAR KERATODERMAS

AD 147:748–750, 2011; Cutis 93:193–198, 2014

Acral keratoderma *BJD 171:847–853, 2014*

Bothnian

Clouston syndrome

Gamborg-Nielsen keratoderma

Greither's palmoplantar keratoderma

Haim-Munk syndrome

Loricrin keratoderma *BJD 172:262–264, 2015*

Mal de Meleda

Nagashima type palmoplantar keratoderma *BJD 171:847–853, 2014*

Olmsted syndrome

Papillon-Lefevre syndrome

Sybert's palmoplantar keratoderma

Vohwinkel syndrome

MUTILATING PALMOPLANTAR KERATODERMAS

Stat Pearls Feb 5, 2020

Olmsted syndrome

Papillon-Lefevre syndrome

Loricrin keratoderma

Mal de Meleda

SYNDROMES

Acantholytic ectodermal dysplasia (similar to McGrath syndrome) – curly hair, palmoplantar keratoderma, skin fragility, hyperkeratotic fissured plaques with perioral involvement, red fissured lips, nail dystrophy *BJD 160:868–874, 2009*

Alagille's syndrome (arteriohepatic dysplasia) with keratoderma *J R Soc Med 82:297–298, 1989*

Albers-Schonberg – PPK with cirrhosis

Anhidrotic ectodermal dysplasia – alopecia or sparse hair, tooth abnormalities, periorbital wrinkling and/or hyperpigmentation, facial sebaceous hyperplasias *New England Dermatological Society Conference, Sept 15, 2007*

Alopecia-onychodysplasia-hypohidrosis-deafness syndrome – small teeth, thick dystrophic toenails, hypohidrosis, hyperkeratosis of palms and soles, elbows and knees, sensorineural deafness *Human Hered 27:127–337, 1977*

Anhidrotic ectodermal dysplasia with amastia and palmoplantar keratoderma – *EDAR* mutation *BJD 168:1353–1355, 2013*

Ankyloblepharon-ectrodactyly-cleft lip/palate (AEC) syndrome – palmar hyperkeratosis with erosions *AD 141:1591–1594, 2005*

Apert's syndrome – plantar hyperkeratoses *Cutis 52:205–208, 1993*

Autosomal recessive epidermolytic palmoplantar keratoderma *J Med Genet 27:519–522, 1990*

Cardio-facio-cutaneous syndrome – abnormal hair, sparse eyebrows and lashes, ichthyosiform hyperkeratosis, widespread keratosis pilaris-like papules, seborrheic dermatitis, hemangiomas, nail dystrophy, bromhidrosis, lymphedema; characteristic facies with large head, high forehead, bitemporal constriction, antimongoloid slant of palpebral fissures, depressed nasal bridge, low set ears with thick helices psychomotor and growth retardation; pulmonic stenosis and atrial septal defects *JAAD 28:815–819, 1993*

Carvajal syndrome (ectodermal dysplasia/skin fragility syndrome) – autosomal recessive (Carvajal-Huerta syndrome); skin peeling; generalized erythema and peeling at birth; very short stature, superficial skin fragility with crusts of face, knees, alopecia of scalp and eyebrows, perioral hyperkeratosis with fissuring and cheilitis, thick dystrophic cracking finger- and toenail dystrophy, keratotic plaques on limbs, diffuse or focal striate palmoplantar keratoderma with painful fissuring; mutation in *PKP1* gene (encoding plakophilin 1) or *DSP* (encoding desmoplakin); follicular hyperkeratosis of knees; woolly hair; perianal erythema and erosions; cardiomyopathy associated with mutation in desmoplakin not with plakophilin *Ped Derm 32:641–646, 2015; BJD 166:36–45, 2012; Derm Clin 28:125–129, 2010; BJD 160: 692–697, 2009; JAAD 55:157–161, 2006; Acta DV 85:394–399, 2005; JID 122:1321–1324, 2004; Curr Prob Derm 14:71–116, 2002; Hum Molec Genet 9:2761–2766, 2000; Hum Molec Genet 8:143–148, 1999*

Charcot-Marie-Tooth disease *TIG 13:229, 1997*

Carvajal-like syndrome – autosomal recessive; blisters, woolly hair, palmoplantar kertoderma, cardiac abnormalities (left ventricular abnormalities); hypodontia, oligodontia, leukonychia (autosomal dominant); follicular keratotic papules, clubbing, blisters, psoriasiform plaques, unilateral deafness, pharyngitis; heterozygotes of *DSP* (desmoplakin) *Ped Derm 34:724–725, 2017; Int J Trihology 8:53–55, 2016; BJD 166:894–896, 2012; Clin Genet 80:50–58, 2011; J Cutan Pathol 36:553–559, 2009*

CEDNIK syndrome (cerebral dysgenesis-neuropathy-ichthyosis-keratoderma) – microcephaly; dysmorphic face with small anterior fontanelles; pointed prominent nasal tip, small chin, inverted nipples and long toes, high palate, thick gingivae, cradle cap, sparse brittle coarse hair, scarring alopecia, fixed flexion posture; decreased SNAP 29 protein; mutation in SNARE proteins mediating vesicle trafficking; mutation in ABCA12 gene *BJD 164:610–616, 2011; JAAD 63:607–641, 2010; AD 144:334–340, 2008; Am J Hum Genet 77:242–251, 2005*

Cole's disease – guttate hypopigmentation and punctate palmoplantar keratoderma *AD 145:495–497, 2009; Ped Derm 19:302–306, 2002; AD 112:998–1000, 1976*

Collodion baby with palmoplantar keratoderma *J Med Assoc Thai 76:17–22, 1993*

Congenital ichthyosiform dermatosis with linear flexural papules and sclerosing PPK *AD 125:103–106, 1989*

Congenital insensitivity to pain – autosomal recessive; anhidrosis with palmoplantar keratoderma; unilateral plantar ulcer; mutation in *NTRK1 Ped Derm 30:754–756, 2013*

Conradi-Hunermann syndrome – X-linked dominant chondrodysplasia punctata; cataracts, whorled ichthyosiform eruption, palmoplantar keratoderma, Blaschko-distributed pigmentation; follicular

atrophoderma and patchy cicatricial alopecia *AD 121:1064–1065, 1985*

Corneodermatoosseous syndrome – autosomal dominant; diffuse PPK; photophobia, corneal dystrophy, distal onycholysis, brachydactyly, short stature, medullary narrowing of digits, dental decay *Curr Prob Derm 14:71–116, 2002; Am J Hum Genet 18:67–77, 1984*

Costello syndrome – palmar hyperkeratosis *Ped Derm 34:160–162, 2017; JAAD 32:904–907, 1995;* palmoplantar keratoderma, hyperpigmentation, warty papules around nose and mouth, legs, perianal skin; loose skin of neck, hands, and feet, thick, redundant palmoplantar surfaces, hypoplastic nails, short stature, craniofacial abnormalities *Ped Derm 30:665–673, 2013; BJD 168:903–904, 2013; Am J Med Genet 117:42–48, 2003;Eur J Dermatol 11:453–457, 2001; Am J Med Genet 82:187–193, 1999; Clin Genet 50:244–257, 1996; JAAD 32:904–907, 1995; Am J Med Genet 47:176–183, 1993; Aust Paediat J 13:114–118, 1977;* linear papillomatous papules of upper lip *Eur J Dermatol 11:453–457, 2001*

Cutis laxa (dermatochalasis connata) – autosomal dominant; mild disease of late onset *Ped Derm 21:167–170, 2004;* bloodhound appearance of premature aging *Ped Derm 19:412–414, 2002; JAAD 29:846–848, 1993; Clin Genet 39:321–329, 1991; Ped Derm 2:282–288, 1985*

Cowden's syndrome (multiple hamartoma syndrome) – punctate palmar papules with central depressions; autosomal dominant with variable penetrance; facial trichilemmomas with cobblestone appearance around eyes and mouth; acrokeratosis verruciformis; punctate palmoplantar keratoderma; multiple angiomas and lipomas; café au lait macules; mucous membrane papillomas; craniomegaly; fibrocystic breast disease with associated breast cancer; goiter with thyroid carcinoma; other adenocarcinomas and melanoma *JAAD 68:189–209, 2013; JAAD 17:342–346, 1987; JAAD 11:1127–1141, 1984*

Dermatopathia pigmentosa reticularis – autosomal dominant; reticulate pigmentation, alopecia, nail changes, palmoplantar punctate hyperkeratosis, loss of dermatoglyphics *Int J Dermatol 34:645–646, 1995; JAAD 26:298–301, 1992; AD 126:935–939, 1990*

Chanarin-Dorfman syndrome (neutral lipid storage disease) – nonbullous congenital ichthyosiform erythroderma, hyperkeratosis of the palms and soles, ichthyosiform eruption, lipid vacuoles within neutrophils, liver, muscle, and CNS involvement *Ped Derm 26:40–43, 2009; BJD 144:430–432, 2001*

Desmoplakin mutations – syndrome of dilated cardiomyopathy with severe left ventricular dysfunction, congenital alopecia, striate palmoplantar keratoderma, nail dystrophy, follicular hyperkeratosis with hyperpigmented plaques of elbows *Ped Derm 32:102–108, 2015*

Diffuse palmoplantar keratoderma with recurrent nonsense mutation of *DSG1 AD 141:625–628, 2005*

Down's syndrome – keratosis palmaris et plantaris *Ped Derm 24:317–320, 2007*

Dyskeratosis benigna intraepithelialis mucosae et cutis hereditaria – conjunctivitis, umbilicated keratotic nodules of scrotum, buttocks, trunk; palmoplantar verruca-like lesions, leukoplakia of buccal mucosa, hypertrophic gingivitis, tooth loss *J Cutan Pathol 5:105–115, 1978*

Dyskeratosis congenita – X-linked recessive or autosomal dominant; reticulate gray-brown pigmentation, poikilodermatous appearance; leukoplakia, periodontal disease and premature caries; canities and cicatricial alopecia; nail dystrophy; associated malignancies include lymphomas and adenocarcinomas; Fanconi's anemia *JAAD 77:1194–1196, 2017; J Med Genet 12:339–354, 1975*

Ectodermal dysplasia – autosomal recessive ectodermal dysplasia with corkscrew hairs *JAAD 27:917–921, 1992*

Ectodermal dysplasia/skin fragility syndrome – autosomal recessive (Carvajal-Huerta syndrome); skin peeling; generalized erythema and peeling at birth; very short stature, superficial skin fragility with crusts of face, knees, alopecia of scalp and eyebrows, perioral papules with hyperkeratosis with fissuring and cheilitis, thick dystrophic cracking finger- and toenail dystrophy, keratotic plaques on limbs, diffuse or focal striate palmoplantar keratoderma with painful fissuring; loss of function of *PKP1* gene (encoding plakophilin 1) or *DSP* (encoding desmoplakin); follicular hyperkeratosis of knees; woolly hair; perianal erythema and erosions; cardiomyopathy associated with mutation in desmoplakin not with plakophilin *Ped Derm 36:255–257, 2019; BJD 166:36–45, 2012; Derm Clin 28:125–129, 2010; BJD 160: 692–697, 2009; JAAD 55:157–161, 2006; Acta DV 85:394–399, 2005; JID 122:1321–1324, 2004; Curr Prob Derm 14:71–116, 2002; Hum Molec Genet 9:2761–2766, 2000; Hum Molec Genet 8:143–148, 1999*

Ellis-van Creveld syndrome (chondroplastic dwarf with defective teeth and nails, and polydactyly) – autosomal recessive; chondrodysplasia, polydactyly, peg-shaped teeth or hypodontia, short upper lip bound down by multiple frenulae; nail dystrophy, hair may be normal or sparse and brittle; cardiac defects; ichthyosis, palmoplantar keratoderma *Ped Derm 18:485–489, 2001; J Med Genet 17:349–356, 1980; Arch Dis Child 15:65–84, 1940*

Epidermolytic palmoplantar keratoderma – palmoplantar keratoderma and knuckle pads; *KRT9* gene mutation *Ped Derm 30:354–358, 2013*

Familial dyskeratotic comedones *JAAD 17:808–814, 1987*

Fitzsimmons syndrome *Clin Genet 23:329–335, 1983*

Fibroblastic rheumatism – palmar thickening *Cutis 100:354, 356–357, 2017*

Focal palmoplantar and oral mucosa (gingival) hyperkeratosis syndrome (MIM:148730) (hereditary painful callosities) – palmoplantar keratoderma, leukoplakia (gingival keratosis), and cutaneous horn of the lips *JAAD 52:403–409, 2005; BJD 146:680–683, 2002; Oral Surg 50:250, 1980; Birth Defects 12:239–242, 1976; Arch Int Med 113:866–871, 1964*

Haber's syndrome – rosacea-like acneiform eruption, verrucous papules (seborrheic keratosis-like) of flexures, palmoplantar keratoderma, perioral pitted scars *BJD 160:215–217, 2009*Hereditary acrokeratotic poikiloderma *AD 114:1207–1210, 1978; AD 103:409–422, 1971*

Hidrotic ectodermal dysplasia with diffuse eccrine syringofibroadenomatosis *AD 125:1715, 1989*

Hereditary focal transgressive palmoplantar keratoderma – autosomal recessive; hyperkeratotic lichenoid papules of elbows and knees, psoriasiform lesions of scalp and groin, spotty and reticulate hyperpigmentation of face, trunk, and extremities, alopecia of eyebrows and eyelashes *BJD 146:490–494, 2002*

Hyperkeratosis-hyperpigmentation syndrome *Clin Genet 43:73–75, 1993*

Hypereosinophilic syndrome, idiopathic; red macules, red papules, plaques, and nodules, urticaria, angioedema *AD 142:1215–1218, 2006; Am J Hematol 80:148–157, 2005; AD 132:535–541, 1996; AD 114:531–535, 1978; Medicine 54:1–27, 1975; BJD 143:641–644, 2000; BJD 144:639, 2001; AD 132:583–585, 1996; Blood 83:2759–2779, 1994; AD 114:531–535, 1978;* urticaria and/or angioedema *Med Clin (Barc)106:304–306, 1996; AD 132:535–541, 1996; Sem Derm 14:122–128, 1995; Blood 83:2759–2779, 1994;* palmoplantar keratoderma with exfoliative erythroderma *Allergy 59:673–689, 2004*

Incontinentia pigmenti – plantar hyperkeratosis *JAAD 47:169–187, 2002*

Jakac-Wolf syndrome – palmoplantar keratoderma with squamous cell carcinoma, gingival dental anomalies, hyperhidrosis *JAAD 53:S234–239, 2005*

Keratolytic winter keratoderma (Oudtshoorn syndrome) – autosomal dominant; diffuse PPK, may be hyperkeratotic with seasonal centrifugal desquamation of the palms and soles *AD 142:1073–1074, 2006; Curr Prob Derm 14:71–116, 2002*

Keratoma dissipatum hereditarium palmare et plantare (Brauer) (punctate keratoderma)

Keratosis follicularis spinulosa decalvans – X-linked dominant and autosomal dominant; alopecia, xerosis, thickened nails, photophobia, spiny follicular papules (keratosis pilaris), scalp pustules, palmoplantar keratoderma *Ped Derm 22:170–174, 2005; JAAD 47:S275–278, 2002*

Keratosis-ichthyosis-deafness (KID) syndrome – autosomal recessive; dotted waxy, fine granular, stippled, or reticulated surface pattern of severe diffuse hyperkeratosis of palms and soles (palmoplantar keratoderma), ichthyosis with well marginated, serpiginous erythematous verrucous plaques, hyperkeratotic elbows and knees, perioral furrows, leukoplakia, follicular occlusion triad, scalp cysts, nodules (trichilemmal tumors, squamous cell carcinoma), bilateral sensorineural deafness, photophobia with vascularizing keratitis, blindness, hypotrichosis of scalp, eyebrows, and eyelashes, dystrophic nails, chronic mucocutaneous candidiasis, otitis externa, abscesses, blepharitis; connexin 26 mutation *JAAD 69:127–134, 2013; Ped Derm 27:651–652, 2010; Ped Derm 23:81–83, 2006; JAAD 51:377–382, 2004; BJD 148:649–653, 2003; Cutis 72:229–230, 2003; Ped Derm 19:285–292, 2002; Ped Derm 15:219–221, 1998; Ped Derm 13:105–113, 1996; JAAD 19:1124–1126, 1988; AD 123:777–782, 1987; AD 117:285–289, 1981; J Cutaneous Dis 33:255–260, 1915;* red gingivae; mutation in connexin 26 (N14K) GJB2

Kindler's syndrome – acral bullae in infancy; progressive poikiloderma with photosensitivity; nail dystrophy, webbing of digits, esophageal and urethral stenosis, ectropion, poor dentition, gingival fragility, aged hands with fine wrinkling and scarring, hyperkeratosis of hands and palms and soles, dyspigmentation, diffuse telangiectasias; short arm chromosome 20; Kind 1; actin cytoskeleton-extracellular matrix interactions (membrane associated structural and signaling protein) *BJD 157:1252–1256, 2007; Ped Derm 23:586–588, 2006; AD 142:620–624, 2006; AD 140:939–944, 2004; AD 132:1487–1490, 1996*

Lelis syndrome – acanthosis nigricans with hypohidrosis, hypotrichosis, hypodontia, furrowed tongue, nail dystrophy, palmoplantar keratoderma *Genetic Skin Disorders, Second Edition, 2010, pp.94–97*

Lipoid proteinosis

Loricrin keratoderma – honeycomb or non-honeycomb palmoplantar keratoderma, ichthyosis, hyperkeratosis of the dorsal hands *BJD 159:714–719, 2008*

Mental retardation-enteropathy-deafness-neuropathy-ichthyosis-keratodermia syndrome *JAAD 63:607–641, 2010; Proc Natl Acad Sci USA 4:1–9, 2009*

Naegeli-Franceschetti-Jadassohn syndrome (diffuse and punctate PPK) – autosomal dominant; subtype of ectodermal dysplasia; reticulate pigmentation which fades after puberty, bullae of hands and feet, palmoplantar keratoderma, hypohidrosis, nail dystrophy, dental enamel defects, hypoplasia or aplasia of dermatoglyphics, malaligned great toe nails, blistering in first week of life; differential diagnosis includes dermatopathia pigmentosa reticularis, hereditary bullous acrokeratotic poikiloderma (Weary-Kindler), and pachyonychia congenita *BJD 177:945–959, 2017; Curr Prob Derm*

14:71–116, 2002; JAAD 28:942–950, 1994; JAAD 28:942–950, 1993

Naxos disease (mal de Naxos) – autosomal recessive – focal palmoplantar keratoderma, arrhythmogenic right ventricular dysplasia; cardiomegaly and ventricular tachycardia due to focal myocarditis or cardiomyopathy, woolly hair *Ped Derm 34:724–725, 2017; Curr Prob Derm 14:71–116, 2002; BJD 147:575–581, 2002; JAAD 44:309–311, 2001; AD 136:1247–1252, 2000; Br Heart J 56:321–326, 1986; JAAD 134:1021, 1024, 1998;* recessive mutation in desmoplakin *Hum Molec Genet 9:2761–2766, 2000*

Nevoid basal cell carcinoma syndrome (Gorlin's syndrome) – autosomal dominant; smooth surfaced rounded papules 1–15 mm; epidermoid cysts and milia; diffuse palmoplantar hyperkeratosis; palmoplantar punctate hyperkeratosis with pits; odontogenic keratocysts; bifid ribs; spina bifida occulta, kyphoscoliosis; broad nasal root, hypertelorism, frontal bossing, syndactyly, calcification of falx cerebri, defective dentition, neurologic and eye abnormalities; abnormal renal resorption of phosphate *Am J Med Genet 50:282–290, 1994; Medicine 66:98–113, 1987*

Noonan's syndrome – short stature, webbed neck, hypertelorism, blepharoptosis, epicanthal folds, small chin; skeletal defects, pulmonary stenosis; lymphedema of legs and feet; undescended testes; coarse hair with low posterior hairline; ulerythema oophyrogenes is a cutaneous marker *Am J Med Genet 21:493–506, 1985*

Odonto-onycho-dermal dyplasia – oligodontia with small widely spaced conical peg-shaped teeth, hypodontia, absence of secondary teeth; palmoplantar keratoderma, hyperhidrosis, dystrophic nails, erythematous telangiectatic, reticulated atrophic malar and ala nasal patches with vermiculate scarring *JAAD 57:732–733, 2007; Am J Med Genet 14:335–346, 1983*

Olmsted syndrome – autosomal dominant; mutilating palmoplantar focal or diffuse palmoplantar keratoderma, hypotrichosis, perioral periorificial, nasal, and anal keratotic papules and plaques; abnormal connexin 26; follicular hyperkeratosis of buttocks and knees; follicular papules; intertrigo (keratotic lesions of flexures), linear streaky hyperkeratosis, leukokeratosis of the tongue, sparse hair anteriorly or diffusely, onychodystrophy; mutation in *TRPV-3* (transient receptor potential vanilloid-3 gene) *JAMA Derm 156:191–195, 2020; Ped Derm 36:942–943, 2019; BJD 174:209–211, 2016; Ped Derm 25:223–229, 2008; JAAD 53:S266–272, 2005; Ped Derm 21:603–605, 2004; Ped Derm 20:323–326, 2003; Eur J Derm 13:524–528, 2003; J Dermatol 27: 557–568, 2000; BJD 136:935–938, 1997; AD 132:797–800, 1996; AD 131:738–739, 1995; Semin Derm 14:145–151, 1995; JAAD 31:508–510, 1994; Ped Derm 10:376–381, 1993; BJD 122:245–252, 1990;JAAD 10:600–610, 1984; Am J Dis Child 33:757–764, 1927;* follicular hyperkeratosis of buttocks and knees *BJD 136:935–938, 1997;* Olmsted syndrome with erythromelalgia – palmoplantar keratoderma with erythromelalgia; mutation in *TRFV3 JAMA Derm 150:303–306, 2014*Pachydermoperiostosis – personal observation

Pachyonychia congenita – autosomal dominant. Type 1 (Jadassohn-Lewandosky syndrome) (56%)- autosomal dominant; thick hyperkeratoses of pressure areas of soles (focal palmoplantar keratoderma), thickened finger and toenails, keratosis pilaris, follicular keratoses of elbows and knees, oral leukokeratosis, symmetric subungual hyperkeratosis; occasional hyperhidrosis; mutation in keratin 6A (*KRT6A*) *Ped Derm 33:337–342, 2016; JAAD 72:879–889, 2015; BJD 171:343–355, 2014; JAMA Derm 150:146–153, 2014; BJD 169:1357–1360, 2013; BJD 166:875–878, 2012; JAAD 67:680–686, 2012; BJD 161:139–145, 2009; BJD 160:1327–1329, 2009; Cutis 84:269–271, 2009; Clin in Dermatol 23:6–14, 2005; J Dermatol 26:677–681, 1999; Ped Derm 14:491–493, 1997; Semin Dermatol 14:129–134, 1995; Ped Derm 7:33–38, 1990;* type 1 – keratin 16 mutations *Exp Dermatol 9:170–177, 2000; Prenat*

Diagn 19:941–946, 1999; mutation in keratin 6a *Nat Genet 10:363–365, 1995;* with steatocystoma multiplex *J Dermatol 25:479–491, 1998;* facial steatocystoma multiplex and palmoplantar keratoderma; mutation in keratin 17 *BJD 171:1565–1567, 2014;* pachyonychia congenita tarda *Clin Exp Dermatol 20:226–229, 1995; AD 127:701–703, 1991;* Type 2 (Jackson-Lawlor syndrome) (24%)- Type 1 plus bullae of palms and soles, palmoplantar hyperhidrosis, natal or neonatal teeth and steatocystoma multiplex or epidermoid cysts; keratin 17 mutation *BJD 159:730–732, 2008;* Type 3 (11%)-Types 1 and 2 plus angular cheilosis, corneal dyskeratosis (leukokeratosis), and cataracts. Type 4 (7%)-Types 1, 2, and 3 plus laryngeal lesions, hoarseness, mental retardation, hair anomalies, and alopecia *BJD 152:800–802, 2005; Clin Exp Dermatol 28:434–436, 2003; JID 117:1391–1396, 2001; JAAD 19:705–711, 1988;* with focal palmoplantar keratoderma *BJD 165:1145–1147, 2011*

Reactive arthritis – keratoderma blenorrhagicum *Semin Arthritis Rheum 3:253–286, 1974*

Palmoplantar and perioroficial keratoderma with corneal epithelial dysplasia *BJD 125:186–188, 1991*

Poikiloderma with neutropenia – autosomal recessive; Navajo Indians; erythematous rash of limbs, trunk, and face beginning in infancy; evolves into poikiloderma; recurrent infections; palmoplantar keratoderma; pachyonychia of great toenails, photosensitivity; growth retardation; dental caries; atrophic scars; mutation in *C16orf57 BJD 163:866–869, 2010; Am J Med Genet A 146A:2762–2769, 2008; Am J Hum Genet 86:72–76, 1991*

Progressive symmetric erythrokeratoderma – autosomal dominant with variable penetrance; erythematokeratotic plaques on extremities, medial buttocks, sparing chest and abdomen; palmoplantar keratoderma *Dermatologica 1982; AD 122:434–440, 1986*

Rapp-Hodgkin ectodermal dysplasia – autosomal dominant; palmoplantar keratoderma; ectodermal dysplasia, cleft lip/palate and distinct facies (mild frontal prominence, midfacial hypoplasia, small mouth), glossy tongue, congenital absence of lingual frenum and of sublingual caruncles; scalp ulcers, scalp dermatitis, hair abnormalities *Am J Med Genet 79:343–346, 1998*

Ectodermal dysplasias in association with cleft lip and/or palate include: (1) Rapp-Hodgkin syndrome (2) EEC syndrome (ectodermal dysplasia, ectrodactyly, cleft lip/palate) (3) Hay-Wells (AEC) syndrome (ankyloblepharon, ectodermal defects, cleft lip and palate, with extensive scalp dermatitis) *JAAD 27:249–256, 1992*

Refsum's disease – heredopathia atactica polyneuritiformis

Rothmund-Thomson syndrome (poikiloderma congenitale) – autosomal recessive; poikiloderma of face and extremities, alopecia, dystrophic teeth and nails, juvenile cataracts, retarded physical development, hypogonadism, bony malformations, cutaneous and non-cutaneous malignancies; erythematous patches and plaques with or without blistering on cheeks, forehead, ears and neck, extensor extremities, buttocks; flexural sparing; these progress to photodistributed poikiloderma; hyperkeratotic lesions and calcinosis may occur *JAAD 75:855–870, 2016*

SAM syndrome (severe dermatitis, multiple allergies, metabolic wasting) – biallelic loss of function mutations in desmoglein1 (Dsg1); palmoplantar keratoderma, psoriasiform plaques, multiple allergies; autosomal recessive *BJD 444–448, 2016; BJD 172:257–261, 2015*

SASH1 related lentigines, hyper- and hypopigmentation, alopecia, nail dystrophy, palmoplantar keratoderma, skin cancer *BJD 177:945–959, 2017*

Schopf-Schulz-Passarge syndrome – autosomal recessive; hidrocystomas of eyelid margins, hypoplastic eyelids, facial telangiectasia, hypodontia with conical teeth, alopecia (thin scalp hair), diffuse fissured palmoplantar keratoderma, brittle and furrowed nails, multiple squamous cell carcinomas; mutation in *WNT10A BJD 171:1211–1214, 2014; Ped Derm 30:491–492, 2013; JAAD 65:1066–1069, 2011; Acta DV 88:607–612, 2008; AD 140:231–236, 2004; Dermatology 196:463–466, 1998; JAAD 36:569–576, 1997; BJD 127:33–35, 1992; BJD 120:131–132, 1989; Birth Defects XII:219–221, 1971;* eccrine syringofibroadenoma of palms and soles – rough palms and soles *BJD 143:591–594, 2000*

Schwachman syndrome – autosomal recessive; malabsorption, failure to thrive, neutropenia; dry face with perioral dermatitis, palmoplantar hyperkeratosis; generalized xerosis, follicular hyperkeratosis, widespread dermatitis *Ped Derm 9:57–61, 1992; Arch Dis Child 55:531–547, 1980; J Pediatr 65:645–663, 1964*

Sclerodactyly, non-epidermolytic palmoplantar keratoderma, multiple cutaneous squamous cell carcinomas, periodontal disease with loss of teeth, hypogenitalism with hypospadias, altered sex hormone levels, hypertriglyceridemia, 46XX *JAAD 53:S234–239, 2005*

Sjogren-Larsson syndrome – autosomal recessive; ichthyosis at birth; hyperkeratotic scale, thickened red skin with accentuated flexural skin markings, palmoplantar keratoderma; spastic diplegia, tetraplegia, mental retardation; fatty aldehyde dehydrogenase *Cutis 100:452–455, 2017; Ped Derm 22:569–571, 2005; Dermatology 193:77–82, 1996; Semin Dermatol 12:210–218, 1993*

Skin fragility-ectodermal dysplasia syndrome – autosomal recessive; mutation in plakophilin 1 (*PKP1*); widespread superficial scale crust, erosions, painful thickening and fissuring of palms and soles, anomalies of hair and nails *BJD 154:546–550, 2006*

Tay's syndrome – IBIDS

Transgradiens pachyonychia congenital – palmoplantar keratoderma with psoriasiform plaques *BJD 166:124–128, 2012*

Tricho-oculo-dermo-vertebral syndrome (Alves syndrome) – plantar keratoderma *Am J Med Genet 46:313–315, 1993*

Tricho-oculo-dermo-vertebral syndrome (Alves syndrome) – dry, sparse, brittle hair, dystrophic nails, plantar keratoderma, short stature, cataracts *Am J Med Genet 46:313–315, 1993*

Tricho-odonto-onychodysplasia syndrome – autosomal recessive; alopecia of vertex; hair dry, brittle, and sparse, enamel hypoplasia of teeth, nail dystrophy, supernumerary nipples, palmoplantar hyperkeratosis, melanocytic nevi *Am J Med Genet 15:67–70, 1983*

Trichothiodystrophy – PIBIDS *Ped Derm 32:865–866, 2015*

Woolly hair and skin fragility syndrome – blistering of heels and lower legs, focal and diffuse palmoplantar keratoderma; mutation in desmoplakin *JAAD 59:1–22, 2008*

Woolly hair and striate palmoplantar keratoderma – mutation in *KANK2;* leukonychia, pseudoainhum of 5th toe; no cardiac abnormalities *Ped Derm 34:724–725, 2017*

Woolly hair, mild palmoplantar keratoderma, and arrhythmogenic right ventricular cardiomyopathy – *DSC2* (desmocollin 2) mutation *BJD 166:36–45, 2012*

TOXINS

Arsenic – diffuse palmoplantar keratoderma; arsenic toxicity due to contaminated ground water consumption; especially in Bangladesh and West Bengal, India; also in India, Argentina, China, Chile, Thailand, and Mexico *SkinMed 11:211–216, 2013; Dermatol Clinics 29:45–51, 2011; Cutis 80:305–308, 2007; J Envir Sci Health Part A Tox Hazard Subst Environ Eng 38:141:163, 2003*

papular punctate palmoplantar hyperkeratosis *Cutis 80:305–308, 2007; Acta DV 80:292–293, 2000; J Am Podiatry Assoc 66:91–94, 1976;* multiple palmoplantar keratoses *Hautarzt 46:198–201, 1995*

TRAUMATIC

Callosities – occupational, recreational – weight lifter's calluses, surfer's nodules *Cutis 50:131–135, 1992; JAAD 24pt 1 317–318, 1991; JID 85:394–397, 1985*

Hyperkeratosis of the heel secondary to a foreign body *AD 74:469–470, 1956;* shoes *Semin Dermatol 10:112–114, 1991*

Pool palms *JAAD 27:111, 1992*

VASCULAR DISEASES

Lymphedema and keratoderma *Hautarzt 42:518–522, 1991*

Polyarteritis nodosa *Rev Clin Esp 149:379–381, 1978*

Stasis dermatitis with id reaction – personal observation

PALMOPLANTAR KERATODERMA WITH ATRICHIA OR HYPOTRICHOSIS

1. Atrichia, PPK (Bazex-like), mental retardation, and early loss of teeth *Ped Derm 19:226, 2002; JAAD 30:89–898, 1994*
2. Alopecia congenita with keratosis palmoplantaris *Act Genet Statis Med 9:127–132, 1959*
3. Clouston syndrome *Can Med Assoc J 40:1–7, 1939*
4. Fitzsimmons syndrome *Clin Genet 23:329–335, 1983*
5. Schopf syndrome *Birth Defects 7:219–221 1971*
6. Richner Hanhart syndrome
7. Olmsted syndrome
8. Alopecia, onychodysplasia, hypohidrosis, deafness *Hum Hered 27:127–133, 1977*
9. Hereditary PPK, congenital alopecia, onychodystrophy, enamel dysplasia *Hautarzt 25:8–16, 1970*
10. Hereditary focal transgressive palmoplantar keratoderma – autosomal recessive; hyperkeratotic lichenoid papules of elbows and knees, psoriasiform lesions of scalp and groin, spotty and reticulate hyperpigmentation of face, trunk, and extremities, alopecia of eyebrows and eyelashes *BJD 146:490–494, 2002*
11. PPK, hypotrichosis, leukonychia totalis *BJD 133:636–638, 1995*
12. Punctate palmoplantar keratoderma – fine scalp hair *Ped Derm 19:226, 2002*
13. Keratoderma, hypotrichosis, and leukonychia totalis – dry, brittle, sparse hair *Ped Derm 19:226, 2002*

PAPULES, CRUSTED

AUTOIMMUNE DISEASES AND DISEASES OF IMMUNE DYSFUNCTION

Bowel-associated dermatosis-arthritis syndrome *JAAD 14:792–796, 1986*

Bullous pemphigoid – crusts *JAAD 81:355:363, 2019*

Dermatitis herpetiformis – elbows, knees, buttocks, face *Ped Derm 31:511–514, 2014; JAAD 64:1017–1024, 2011*

Dermatomyositis – amyopathic necrotizing dermatomyositis; crusted Gottron's papules *Cutis 82:407–413, 2008;* vesiculobullous *SKINMed11:185–187, 2013*

IgA pemphigus foliaceus *JAAD 20:89–97, 1989*

IL-1 receptor-associated kinase 4 gene (IRAK-4) mutations – cellulitis, abscesses, impetigo *JAAD 54:951–983, 2006; Science 299:2076–2079, 2003*

Job's syndrome (hyper IgE syndrome) – autosomal dominant or sporadic; atrophoderma vermiculatum; coarse facial features with broad nose, rough thickened skin with prominent follicular ostia; papular and papulopustular folliculitis-like eruptions; oral candidiasis; chronic paronychia; cold abscesses of neck and trunk; otitis media common; mutation in *STAT3* (transcription 3 gene activator and signal transducer *JAAD 65:1167–1172, 2011*

Lupus erythematosus – systemic lupus erythematosus – crusted facial papules *Ped Derm 35:808–816, 2018;* non-bullous histiocytoid neutrophilic dermatosis; crusted red plaques *AD 144:1495–1498, 2008;* papules of the elbows *Lupus 21:84–88, 2012;* leukocytoclastic vasculitis and palisaded neutrophilic granulomatous dermatitis *Dermatol Online J 9 (4)1 Oct, 2013*

Pemphigoid (herpes) gestationis

Pemphigoid nodularis – crusted papules and nodules *BJD 147:343–349, 2002*

Pemphigus erythematosus *JAAD 10:215–222, 1984*

Pemphigus foliaceus – starts in seborrheic distribution (scalp, face, chest, upper back)

Perforating neutrophilic and granulomatous dermatitis of the newborn – cutaneous eruption of immunodeficiency; papules, plaques, vesicles, crusts, ulcers; prominent involvement of palms and soles; sparing of trunk *Ped Derm 24:211–215, 2007*

Rheumatoid arthritis – vasculitis – papulonecrotic lesions *JAAD 48:311–340, 2003;* rheumatoid neutrophilic dermatitis *JAAD 45:596–600, 2001; Cutis 60:203–205, 1997*

Adult onset Still's disease *JAAD 52:1003–1008, 2005*

Systemic lupus erythematosus

CONGENITAL LESIONS

Hair collar sign – with protruding scalp mass – aplasia cutis with sinus pericranii; irregular plaque of aplasia with yellow crusts and prominent blood vessels *Ped Derm 37:40–51, 2020*

DRUG ERUPTION

Checkpoint inhibitors – Grover's disease *JAAD 80:990–997, 2019*

DRESS *J Drugs Dermatol 18:207–209, 2019*

Ipilimumab – transient acantholytic dermatosis *BJD 171:1236–1237, 2014*

Lenalidomide – neutrophilic dermatosis; crusted hemorrhagic ulcerated nodules *JAAD 61:709–710, 2009*

Lichenoid drug eruption

Drug-induced subacute cutaneous lupus erythematosus - crusted and necrotic annular and polycyclic lesions

Syringosquamous metaplasia – red, blanching, crusted papules; due to cancer chemotherapy *AD 126:73–77, 1990; Am J Dermatopathol 12:1–6, 1990*

Targeted anti-cancer therapies – pruritus and excoriations *JAAD 69:708–720, 2013*

EXOGENOUS AGENTS

Bindii (Jo-Jo) dermatitis *JAAD 10:768–773, 1984*

Blasting cap explosion

Cocaine abuse – excoriated papules ("coke bugs") *JAAD 59:483–487, 2008*

Fiberglass dermatitis

Weed wacker purpura – personal observation

INFECTIONS AND INFESTATIONS

Acanthamoeba *Transpl Infec Dis April 19, 2017; Am J Clin Pathol 145:266–270, 2016; Transpl Infect Dis 12:529–537, 2010; Clin Infect Dis 35:e43–49, 2002; JAAD 42 (pt2)351–354, 2000;* crusted nodules in HIV disease *AD 139:1647–1652, 2003*

Adiaspiromycosis (*Chrysosporium species*) – hyperpigmented plaque with white-yellow papules, ulcerated nodules, hyperkeratotic nodules, crusted nodules, multilobulated nodules *JAAD S113–117, 2004*

African histoplasmosis

AIDS – papular dermatitis of AIDS *Int J Dermatol 57:746–751, 2014; Dermatol Clinics 32:211–225, 2014; JAAD 24 (pt1)231–235, 1991*

Alternariosis *J Formos Med Assoc 91:462–466, 1992; AD 124:1421–1426, 1988*

Anthrax – *Bacillus anthracis*; malignant pustule; face, neck, hands, arms; starts as papule then evolves into bulla on red base; then hemorrhagic crust with edema and erythema with small vesicles; edema of surrounding skin *Am J Dermatopathol 19:79–82, 1997; J Clin Inf Dis 19:1009–1014, 1994; Br J Opthalmol 76:753–754, 1992; J Trop Med Hyg 89:43–45, 1986; Bol Med Hosp Infant Mex 38:355–361, 1981*

Aspergillosis, primary cutaneous *JAMA Pediatr 169:1173–1174, 2015*

Beetle dermatitis *Indian J DV Leprol 73:333–335, 2007*

Botryomycosis – *Staphylococcus aureus Cutis 80:45–47, 2007*

Brucellosis *NEJM 380;275–283, 2019*

Campylobacter jejuni – in X-linked agammaglobulinemia *J Clin Inf Dis 23:526–531, 1996*

Candidal sepsis; *Candida parapsilosis* – personal observation

Cat scratch disease *Cutis 49:318–320, 1992*

Cheyletiella mites ("walking dandruff") – cats

Chromomycosis – earliest lesion is ulcerated papule *JAAD 53:931–951, 2005*

Coccidioidomycosis *JAAD 26:79–85, 1992*

Cowpox – generalized cowpox in Darier's disease – crusted papules, pustules, and vesicles; cobblestoned appearance; with massive periorbital edema *BJD 164:1116–1118, 2011; Clin Exp Dermatol 12:286–287, 1987*

Coxsackie virus A6 (atypical hand, foot, and mouth disease) – red papulovesicles of fingers, palmar erythema, red papules of ears, red papules of antecubital fossa, perioral papulovesicles, vesicles of posterior pharynx; crusted papules of scalp, ears, and face; purpuric targetoid painful vesicular lesions of hands and feet, arthritis, fissured scrotum *MMWR 65:678–680, 2016; JAMA Derm 149:1419–1421, 2013; JAAD 69:736–741, 2013*

Coxsackie virus A9, B13 – purpuric exanthem

Cryptococcosis *Med Mycol 57:E5–9, 2016; Int J Dermatol 41:773–774, 2002*

Curvularia spp. – crusted nodule of arm *BJD 158:1374–1375, 2008*

Cutaneous larva migrans *J Clin Diagn Res 7:2313, 2013; Int J Dermatol 52:327–330, 2013*

Cytomegalovirus infection *Dermatology 200:189–195, 2000*

Demodex folliculorum – papulonodular demodicidosis in AIDS *Clin Pediatr 58:478–481, 2019; JAAD 20:197–201, 1989;* pustular rosacea in immunocompromised patient *Case Rep Dermatol Med 2014:458046*

Dental sinus *Am Fam Physician 40:113–116, 1989; Cutis 43:22–24, 1989*

Dirofilaria – crusted papule of forehead *Trop Doct 35:181–182, 2005*

Echo *virus 4, 9, 11*

Ecthyma *Medicine (Balt)96:e6244, 2017*

Eczema herpeticum – atopic dermatitis, Hailey-Hailey disease, congenital ichthyosiform erythroderma, Darier's disease, CTCL, pemphigus foliaceus, burn, Wiskott-Aldrich syndrome

Epidemic typhus *Infect Dis Clin NA 8:689–712, 1994; JAAD 2:359–373, 1980*

Fire ant bites *J Cutan Pathol 44:1012–1017, 2017*

Fusarium sepsis Ped Derm 9:255–258, 1992; Fusarium solani JAAD 32:346–351, 1995

Gianotti-Crosti syndrome

Gonococcemia

Herpes simplex – herpetic folliculitis *ID Cases 19:e00663 Nov 6, 2019; BJD 142:555–559, 2000;* Kaposi's varicelliform eruption in Darier's disease *JAMA Derm 153:317–318, 2017*

Herpes zoster – V1 herpes zoster – confluent hypertrophic crusting of scalp, forehead, and eyelids *NEJM 362:1128, 2010*

Histoplasmosis, disseminated – crusted papulonodules *Clin Dermatol 30:592–598, 2012; Ped Derm 27:549–551, 2010; AD 145:1447–1452, 2009;* facial papules, crusted papules, muscle weakness, pulmonary infiltrates; morbilliform rash with scale *BJD 173:797–800, 2015*

Hot tub folliculitis – personal observation

Insect bite reactions *The Clinical Management of Itching; Parthenon Publishing, 2000; p. xiii*

Kerion – crusted nodules and abscess of scalp *Ped Derm 28:655–657, 2011*

Kytococcus schroeteri sepsis – crusted papules and distinctive histologic plump tetrads *AD 147:1119–1121, 2011*

Leishmaniasis – impetigo- and ecthyma-like lesions of legs (Bauru ulcers) *JAAD 60:897–925, 2009;* hands, face, neck, arms *JAAD 51:S125–128, 2004; Clin Inf Dis 33:815,897–898, 2001; AD 125:1540–1542, 1989; JAAD 12:985–992, 1985;* chronic lupoid leishmaniasis *AD 132:198–202, 1996; Leishmania panamensis* – crusted eroded plaque *JAAD 73:897–908, 2015; Leishmania braziliensis* – crusted plaques and papules of nose and neck *JAMA 312:1250–1251, 2014*

Leprosy – tuberculoid leprosy

Majocchi's granuloma – crusted papules and pustules of leg *JAMA Derm 153:205–206, 2017*

Meningococcemia *J Clin Inf Dis 21:1023–1025, 1995*

Milker's nodule (paravaccinia virus (parapoxvirus) – erythema multiforme, erythema nodosum, Gianotti-Crosti syndrome *Cutis 74:316–318, 2004*

Mite bites- Grocer's itch, coolie itch, copra mite, wheat-pollard mite, baker's itch, dried fruit itch, Cheyletiella; *Dermanyssus gallinae* infestation *AD 147:1458–1459, 2011*

Molluscum contagiosum

Mycobacterium haemophilum – crusted nodule *BJD 168:446–447, 2013*

Mycobacterium immunogenum Dermatol Online J 23 (10):13030/ qt92g5r07t Oct 15, 2017

Mycobacteria kansasii Ped Derm 18:131–134, 2001; papulonecrotic tuberculid *JAAD 36:497–499, 1997*

Mycobacterium marinum – crusted papules of dorsal foot *NEJM 373:1761, 2015*

Mycobacterium mucogenicum – crusted papules *Dermatol Online J 14:5, 2008*

Mycobacterium tuberculosis – miliary tuberculosis; large crops of blue papules, crusted papules, vesicles, pustules, hemorrhagic papules; red nodules; vesicles become necrotic to form ulcers *Practitioner 222:390–393, 1979; Am J Med 56:459–505; AD 99:64–69, 1969;* congenital tuberculosis – red papule with central necrosis *AD 117:460–464, 1981;* papulonecrotic tuberculid – dusky red crusted or ulcerated papules occur in crops on elbows, hands, feet, knees, legs; also ears, face, buttock, and penis; may evolve into pustules *NEJM 380:275–283, 2019; Dermatol Clin 33:541–562, 2015; Dermatol Therapy 21:154–161, 2008; Am J Clin Dermatol 3:319–328, 2002; Int J Dermatol 30:487–490, 1991; JAAD 14:815–826, 1986;* lupus vulgaris; lichen scrofulosorum *Ped Derm 17:373–376, 2000; AD 124:1421–1426, 1988; Clin Exp Dermatol 1:391–394, 1976*

Myiasis – tumbu fly myiasis *AD 131:951–956, 1995*

Nocardia *BMC Clin Pathol Oct 1, 2018*

North American blastomycosis – disseminated blastomycosis *Am Rev Resp Dis 120:911–938, 1979; Medicine 47:169–200, 1968*

Onchocerciasis (*Onchecerca volvulus*)- transmitted by Simuliidae (humpbacked black fly) localized acute dermatitis or chronic generalized dermatitis; papules, crusted papules, lichenified plaques; often with hyperpigmented nodules *JAAD 45:435–437, 2001; Cutis 65:293–297, 2000; BJD 121:187–198, 1989*

Ornithodoriasis – tick bites

Orf *Acta DV Croat 27:280–281, 2019*

Paecilomyces lilacinus JAAD 37:270–271, 1997

Paracoccidioides brasiliensis – umbilicated crusted papules of face *Clin in Dermatol 38:52–62, 2020*

Papular urticaria *Cutis 68:89–91, 2001: Semin Dermatol 12:53–56, 1993*

Paracoccidioidomycosis – near mouth, anus, or genitalia *JAAD 53:931–951, 2005; J Clin Inf Dis 23:1026–1032, 1996*

Pediculosis – crusts behind ears *JAAD 25 (pt 1)248–251, 1991*

Portuguese man o' war sting *Cutis 80:186–188, 2007*

Protothecosis – pyoderma-like lesions *BJD 146:688–693, 2002*

Rat bite fever (*Streptobacillus moniliformis* (pleomorphic facultative anaerobic bacillus) or *Spirillum minor* (Sodoku) – macular, petechial, or morbilliform widespread exanthem; palmoplantar rash; arthralgia and chronic arthritis; Haverhill fever (raw milk) – papules, crusted papules, vesicles, pustules; chronic abscesses *Cleveland Clin Q 52 (2):203–205, 1985; Pediatr Clin N Am 26:377–411, 1979*

Rhinosporidiosis – hemorrhagic crusted papule of shoulders *SKINMed 16:63–65, 2018*

Rickettsia africae Infect Dis Clin NA 33:213–229, 2019

Rickettsia slovaca (Hungary) – *Dermacentor marginatus* or *D. reticulatus* tick bite; erythema marginatum-like lesions; scalp papules, crusted scalp papules and subsequent alopecia; tick-borne lymphadenopathy *Clin Inf Dis 34:1331–1336, 2002*

Rickettsialpox (*Rickettsia akari*) (house mouse mite bite) – generalized papules, vesicles, papulovesicles, crusts *NEJM 331:1612–1617, 1994; Clin Inf Dis 18:624–626, 1994*

Rocky Mountain spotted fever

Sandfly bites

Scabies crusted *Case Rep Pediatr 2019:9542857 Oct 20, 2019; S Med J 87:352–356, 1994; Semin Dermatol 12:15–21, 1993;* canine scabies (sarcoptic mange) *Dermatology 223:104–106, 2011*

Schistosomiasis – ectopic cutaneous schistosomiasis *An Bras Dermatol 91:109–110, 2016; An Bras Dermatol 89:646–648, 2014; An Bras Dermatol 88:820–821, 2013 AD 115:869–870, 1979*

Septic emboli

Sporotrichosis *Dermatol Online J 38:760–761, 2016*

Staphylococcal sepsis

Syphilis, palisading granuloma *JAAD 12:957–60, 1985*; nodular syphilis *AD 126:1666–9, 1989;* lues maligna – necrotic papules and nodules *JAMA Derm 149:1429–1430, 2013; JAAD 22:1061–1067, 1990;* malignant lues *World J Clin Cases 7:2406–2412, 2019;* congenital syphilis *J Cut Med Surg 22:97–99, 2018*

Talaromyces marneffei – necrotic papules *JAAD 37:450–472, 1997*

Tinea capitis – favus; yellowish cup-shaped crusts (scutula) *Dermatologica 125:369–381, 1962* Tinea corporis, invasive – disseminated *Trichophyton rubrum* – purple papules with central black hemorrhagic crusting *JAMA Derm 152:941–942, 2016*

Toxoplasmosis, congenital – necrotic papules *JAAD 60:897–925, 2009*

Trench fever – *Bartonella Quintana An Bras Dermatol 94:594–602, 2019; Lancet Infect Dis 16:e164–172, 2016*

Tungiasis (*Tunga penetrans*) – hemorrhagic crusted umbilicated papule of heel *JAMA Derm 149:1235–1236, 2013*

Tularemia – necrotic papule *Cutis 54:276–286, 1994*

Varicella

Viral exanthem

Yaws – primary (mother yaw) – crusted papule; secondary (daughter yaws, pianomas, framboesiomas) – small papules which ulcerate, become crusted; resemble raspberries; periorificial (around mouth, nose, penis, anus, vulva); extend peripherally (circinate yaws); hyperkeratotic plantar plaques (crab yaws); periungual

Zygomycosis *JAAD 23:346–351, 1995*

INFILTRATIVE

Eosinophilic histiocytosis *JAAD 13:952–958, 1985*

Primary and secondary intralymphatic histiocytosis – excoriated papules *Am J Dermatopathol 31:140–151, 2009;* red patch of back; livedo reticularis *JAAD 70:927–933, 2014*

Indeterminate cell histiocytosis *Am J Dermatopathol 39:542–544, 2017*

Juvenile xanthogranuloma, congenital *Ped Derm 13:65–68, 1996*

Langerhans cell histiocytosis – in adults or children *JAAD 13:383–404, 1985;* congenital self-healing reticulohistiocytosis (Hashimoto-Pritzker disease) – hypopigmented macules of trunk, solitary papules with necrosis, erosive and ulcerated papules, keratotic plantar papules *Child World J Ped 15:536–545, 2019; JAAD 78:1035–1044, 2018; Int J Dermtol 56:1182–1185, 2017; AD 146:149–156, 2010; Ped Derm 23:273–275, 2006; JAAD 48:S75–77, 2003;* self-healing Langerhans cell histiocytosis *Cutis 102:309,316,321, 2018*

INFLAMMATORY

Erythema multiforme with epidermal necrosis

Chondrodermatitis nodularis chronicus helicis *Ped Derm 24:337–339, 2007; AD 68:241–255, 1953*

Eosinophilic pustular folliculitis – 2–3 months following stem-cell transplantation *Ped Derm 34:326–330, 2017*

Kikuchi's histiocytic necrotizing lymphadenitis *JAAD 36:342–346, 1997*

Perforating folliculitis *Ann DV 117:515–520, 1990; Am J Dermatopathol 4:101–108, 1982*

Pyoderma gangrenosum – mimicking transient acantholytic dermatosis *Acta DV (Stockh) 61:77–79, 1981*

Sarcoid – resembling papulonecrotic tuberculid *Arch Dermatol Syphilol 13:675–676, 1926*

METABOLIC

Congenital erythropoietic porphyria – sclerodactyly with crusted papules on dorsal hands; atrophic scars, erythrodontia *BJD 166:697–699, 2012*

Miliarial gout *QJM 109:811–812, 2016*

Hepatoerythropoietic porphyria *Ped Derm 4:229–233, 1987*

Prurigo of pregnancy (Besnier's prurigo) – multiple excoriated papules of abdomena and extensor extremities *Australas J Dermatol 9:258–267, 1968*

Xanthomas, eruptive *Medicine (Bat)95:e4866, 2016*

NEOPLASTIC

Adult T-cell leukemia/lymphoma *Indian J Dermatol 57:219–221, 2012*

Angioimmunoblastic T-cell lymphoma *Clin Case Rep 3:483–488, 2015; Am J Dermatopathol 37:274–283, 2015; J Clin Oncol 31:240–246, 2013; J Drugs Dermatol 9:851–855, 2010*

Angiosarcoma – black crusted nodules and plaques *Dermatol Online J 25:13030, Dec 15, 2019*

Aneurysmal fibrous histiocytomas (variant of dermatofibroma) *BJD 153:664–665, 2005*

Atypical fibroxanthoma – crusted pink papule of neck *Ped Derm 24:450–452, 2007*

Basal cell carcinoma – crusted papule of vulva *Dermatol Surg 23:207–209, 1997*

Bowen's disease *Indian J DV Leprol 79:227–230, 2013*

Combined squamous cell carcinoma and Merkel cell carcinoma – crusted papule, red facial nodule, red papule, red nodule of wrist *JAAD 73:968–975, 2015*

Eruptive keratoacanthomas of Grzybowski *Int J Dermatol 53:131–136, 2014*

Infantile choriocarcinoma *JAAD 14:918–927, 1986*

Leukemia

Lymphoma – cutaneous T-cell lymphoma; pityriasis lichenoides chronica-like lesions in CTCL *BJD 142:347–352, 2000;* CD8+ CTCL *AD 126:801–804, 1990;* lymphomatoid granulomatosis *AD 127:1693–98, 1991; AD 126:801–804, 1990;* pemphigus foliaceus-like disorder in chronic T-cell leukemia *JAAD 18:1197–1202, 1988;* Epstein-Barr virus-associated T-cell lymphoma – necrotic, crusted papules; eyelid edema and intramuscular infiltration mimicking dermatomyositis *BJD 147:1244–1248, 2002;* hydroa vacciniforme-like cutaneous T-cell lymphoma, Epstein-Barr virus-related – edema, blisters, vesicles, ulcers, scarring, facial scars, swollen nose, lips, and periorbital edema, crusts with central hemorrhagic necrosis, facial dermatitis, photodermatitis, facial edema, facial papules and plaques, crusting of ears, fever *JAAD 81:23–41, 2019; JAAD 69:112–119, 2013; Ped Derm 96–100, 2012; BJD 151:372–380, 2004*

Lymphomatoid granulomatosis – Epstein-Barr-related angiocentric T-cell rich B-cell lymphoproliferative disorder; presents as urticarial dermatitis; papules and dermal nodules with or without ulceration, folliculitis-like lesions, maculopapules, indurated plaques, ulcers *NEJM 372:650–659, 2015; BJD 157:426–429, 2007; JAAD 54:657–663, 2006;* in children *BJD 171:138–146, 2014*

Lymphomatoid papulosis – papules or nodules with central crust and/or necrosis *BJD 169:1157–1159, 2013; AD 147:1340–1342, 2011; Am J Dermatopathol 18:221–235, 1996; JAAD 17:632–636, 1987; JAAD 13:736–743, 1985*

Melanocytic nevi – inflammatory nevi evolving into halo nevi in children *BJD 152:357–360, 2005*

Melanoma, verrucous – crusted pigmented papule *AD 124:1534–1538, 1988*

Metastatic breast cancer

Piloleiomyoma – crusted *Indian J Dermatol 54:75–76, 2009*

Poroma *JAAD 44:48–52, 2001*

Spitz nevus *JAAD 27:901–913, 1992*

Squamous cell carcinoma

Transient myeloproliferative disorder associated with mosaicism for trisomy 21 – vesiculopustular rash *Ped Derm 36:702–706, 2019; NEJM 348:2557–2566, 2003;* in trisomy 21 or normal patients; periorbital vesiculopustules, red papules, crusted papules, and ulcers; with periorbital edema *Ped Derm 21:551–554, 2004*

Waldenstrom's IgM storage papules – skin-colored translucent papules on extensor extremities, buttocks, trunk; may be hemorrhagic, crusted, or umbilicated *JAAD 45:S202–206, 2001;* macroglobulinosis – Waldenstrom's macroglobulinemia; ulcerated nodules and plaques with central necrosis; skin colored papules of dorsal hands with central crusts *AD 146:165–169, 2010; AD 128:372–376, 1992*

Warty dyskeratoma *Cutis 29:79–81, 1982*

PARANEOPLASTIC DISORDERS

Cutaneous granulomas in myelodysplasia with acute myelogenous leukemia – personal observation

Necrolytic migratory erythema (glucagonoma syndrome) *JAMA Derm 155:1180, 2019; Int J Dermatol 57:642–645, 2018; Int J Dermatol 49:24–29, 2010; J Eur Acad Dermatol 18:591–595, 2004;* crusted plaques of lower legs *Cutis 87:78–80, 2011*

Reactive perforating collagenosis *BJD 142:190–191, 2000*

Paraneoplastic leukocytoclastic vasculitis in chronic lymphocytic leukemia *J Cancer Res Ther 2:206–208, 2006*

Paraneoplastic pemphigus *Am J Med 99:207–216, 1995*

Solid pseudopapillary tumor of pancreas – produced GCSF; pustules of legs, palms and soles; evolve into crusted plaques *BJD 177:1122–1126, 2017*

Sterile suppurative folliculitis associated with acute myelogenous leukemia *BJD 146:904–907, 2002*

PHOTODERMATOSES

Actinic prurigo *JAAD 44:952–956, 2001; Australas J Dermatol 42:192–195, 2001; Photodermatol Photoimmunol Photomed 15:183–187, 1999; Int J Dermatol 34:380–384, 1995; JAAD 26:683–692, 1992; JAAD 5:183–190, 1981; Clin Exp Dermatol 2:365–372, 1977;* familial, in North American Indians *Int J Dermatol 10:107–114, 1971;* in Caucasians *BJD 144:194–196, 2001;* occurrence in non-Indians *JAAD 34:612–617, 1996;* Southeast Asian *Photodermatol Photoimmunol Photomed 9:225–228, 1992*

Disseminated superficial actinic porokeratosis *JAAD 40:479–480, 1999; Int J Derm 38:204–206, 1999*

Hydroa aestivale

Hydroa vacciniforme (Epstein-Barr virus-related) – red macules progress to tender papules or vesiculopapules, hemorrhagic vesicles or bullae, umbilication and crusting; pock-like scars; edema of cheeks, eyelids, ears, and lips *AD 142:587–595, 2006;* crusted papules, facial necrosis, ulcers *BJD 173:801–805, 2015*

PRIMARY CUTANEOUS DISEASE

Acne excoriee

Acne keloidalis *JAAD 53:1–37, 2005*

Acne necrotica miliaris

Acne necrotica varioliformis – necrotizing lymphocytic folliculitis *Australas J Dermatol 59:e53–58, 2018; AD 132:1367, 1370, 1996*

Acrodermatitis continua – crusted plaques *JAMA Derm 154:1346, 2018*

Acute parapsoriasis (pityriasis lichenoides et varioliformis acuta) (Mucha-Habermann disease) *Ped Derm 32:579–592, 2015; Int J Dermatol 49:257–261, 2010; BJD 157:941–945, 2007; Am J Clin Dermatol 8:29–36, 2007; JAAD 55:557–572, 2006; AD 123:1335–1339, 1987; AD 118:478, 1982; Dermtol Z 45:42–48, 1925; Arch Dermatol Syph (Wien) 123:586–592, 1916; Verh Dtsch Dermatol Ges 4:495–499, 1894*

Atopic dermatitis *Allergy Asthma Proc 40:433–436, 2019*

Darier's disease *Clin Inf Dis 32:1643–1647, 2001;* linear *JAAD Case Rep 6:441–443, 2020*

Degos's disease – personal observation

Dermatofibrosis lenticularis disseminata – Buschke-Ollendorff syndrome

Dowling-Degos disease – autosomal dominant; reticulated hyperpigmented scaly plaques, red-brown macules, crusted papules, perioral pitted scars, comedones; mutation in *KRT5* and *POFUT-1* (protein O-fucotransferase 1) and *POGLUT-1* (protein o-glucosyltransferase-1) *BJD 176:270–274, 2017; JAMA Derm 152:461–462, 2016*

Elastosis perforans serpiginosa *Ann Dermatol 26:103–106, 2014*

Epidermolysis bullosa – dystrophic epidermolysis bullosa pruriginosa (epidermolysis bullosa pruriginosa) – red, crusted, and lichenified papules *Ped Derm 29:725–731, 2012; BJD 159:464–469, 2008; BJD 130:617–625, 1994*

Erythema elevatum diutinum – red nodules, crusted papules *Cutis 68:41–42,55, 2001*

Estrogen auto dermatitis *Australas J Dermatol 40:96–98, 1999*

Fabry's disease *Ped Derm 22:334–337, 2005*

Febrile ulceronecrotic pityriasis lichenoides et varioliformis acuta *Ped Derm 31:525–527, 2014; JAAD 29:903–906, 1993; J Rheumatol 16:387–389, 1989*

Folliculitis decalvans

Galli-Galli disease – autosomal dominant; reticulated hyperpigmented scaly plaques, red-brown macules, crusted papules, perioral pitted scars, comedones; mutation in *KRT5* and *POFUT-1* (protein O-fucotransferase 1) and *POGLUT-1* (protein o-glucosyltransferase-1) *BJD 176:270–274, 2017; JAMA Derm 152:461–462, 2016*

Granuloma annulare, perforating *Int J Derm 36:340–348, 1997;* generalized perforating granuloma annulare *JAAD 27:319–322, 1992*

Grover's disease (transient or persistent acantholytic dermatosis) *JAAD 77:952–957, 2017; Am J Dermatopathol 33:e41–43, 2011; JAAD 55:263–268, 2006; JAAD 35:653–666, 1996; AD 101:426–434, 1970;* folliculitis *JAAD 11:253–256, 1984;* precipitating factors include ribavirin, irritation, occlusion, sunlight, heat and sweating, xerosis, malignancy, pregnancy, ionizing radiation, interleukin-4, membranous glomerulonephritis *BJD 142:1257–1258, 2000;* pseudoherpetic *Am J Dermatopathol 40:445–448, 2018*

Guttate parapsoriasis

Hailey-Hailey disease *JAMA Derm 150:97–99, 2014; BJD 126:275–282, 1992; Arch Dermatol Syphilol 39:679–685, 1939*

Hyperkeratosis lenticularis perstans (Flegel's disease) *JAAD 27:812–816, 1992*

Keratosis lichenoides chronica *BJD 144:422–424, 2001*

Kyrle's disease *J Fam Med Prim Care 4:284–286, 2015*

Lichen planus

Pityriasis lichenoides chronica

Pityriasis rosea

Pityriasis rubra pilaris

Prurigo nodularis

Prurigo pigmentosa – red papules with vesiculation and crusting arranged in reticulated pattern or reticulate plaques; heals with reticulated hyperpigmentation; urticarial red pruritic papules, papulovesicles, vesicles, crusted papules, and plaques with reticulated hyperpigmentation *Ped Derm 35:239–241, 2018; Ped Derm 24:277–279, 2007; JAAD 55:131–136, 2006; Cutis 63:99–102, 1999; JAAD 34:509–11, 1996; AD 130:507–12, 1994; BJD 120:705–708, 1989; AD 125:1551–1554, 1989; JAAD 12:165–169, 1985; J Dermatol 5:61–67, 1978; Jpn J Dermatol 81:78–91, 1971;* zosteriform reticulated crusted papules *Ped Derm 31:523–525, 2014*

Psoriasis

Reactive perforating collagenosis and other perforating disorders *Dermatologica 171:255–258, 1985;* acquired perforating dermatosis *BJD 135:671–677, 1996; BJD 129:211, 1993;* perforating folliculitis

Relapsing linear acantholytic dermatosis *JAAD 33:920–922, 1995; BJD 112:349–355, 1985*

Trichodysplasia spinulosa – follicular crusted papules with keratotic spines; lesions of face, neck with eyebrow alopecia; trichodysplasia spinulosa-associated polyoma virus *Ped Transpl 23:e13394, 2019; BJD 180:1302–1311, 2019; Ped Derm 36:723–724, 2019; AD 147:1215–1220, 2011*

PSYCHOCUTANEOUS

Factitial dermatitis

Neurotic excoriations

SYNDROMES

Behcet's disease *SKINMed 15:97–104, 2017; Clin Exp Rheumatol 33 (suppl 94) S101–106, 2015; Dermatol Online J 10:14 Nov 30, 2004*

Congenital self-healing histiocytosis (Hashimoto-Pritzker disease) – congenital crusted red or blue nodules *Skin and Allergy News, Feb 2001, p.31*

Degos' disease – flat, white papules with erythematous telangiectatic halos *NEJM 370:2327–2337, 2014; J Dermatol 31:666–670, 2004*

Down's syndrome (trisomy 21) – clue to transient myeloproliferative disorder (leukemoid reactions) – neonatal pustules, vesicles, papulovesicles, vesicopustules; crusted papules *Ped Derm 36:702–706, 2019; Cutis 85:286–288, 2010; Ped Derm 20:232–237, 2003; AD 137:760–763, 2001*

Hypereosinophilic syndrome – excoriated red papules *JAAD 56:S68–72, 2007*

Kawasaki's disease – erythema, crusting, or necrosis of BCG inoculation sites *JAAD 69:501–510, 2013*

Lipoid proteinosis – crusted red papules of face heal with scarring *Ped Derm 22:266–267, 2005; BJD 151:413–423, 2004; JID*

120:345–350, 2003; Hum Molec Genet 11:833–840, 2002; JAAD 39:149–171, 1998; Arch Pathol Anat 273:286–319, 1929

Prader-Willi syndrome – picker's papules *AD 128:1623–1625, 1992*

Reflex sympathetic dystrophy – ulcerating papules *Cutis 68:179–182, 2001*

TOXIC

Dioxin exposure – late manifestation *JAAD 19:812–819, 1988*

Potato poisoning – rash of lower abdomen and medial thighs consisting of red papules which progress to pustules and crusted lesions; facial and abdominal edema; headache, vomiting, diarrhea *J R Coll Physicians Edinb 36:336–339, 2007*

TRAUMA

Chondrodermatitis nodularis chronicus helicis – papule of helix or antihelix *JAAD 2:148–154, 1980*

Walkman dermatosis – crusted papules on arm and trunk *AD 123:1225–1226, 1228–1229, 1987*

VASCULAR

Eosinophilic granulomatosis with polyangiitis – papulonecrotic lesions *Autoimmun Rev 14:341–348, 2015; Clin Exp Nephrol 17:603–606, 2013; JAAD 48:311–340, 2003*

Granulomatosis with polyangiitis – acneiform facial and truncal lesions with crusted necrotic papules, ulcers; palpable purpura *JAAD 72:859–867, 2015;* papulonecrotic lesions *JAAD 48:311–340, 2003; JAAD 28:710–718, 1993*

Leukocytoclastic vasculitis

Lymphangiectasia *SAGE Open Med Case Rep Oct 9, 2018:6:2050313X18802137*

Polyarteritis nodosa

Pyogenic granuloma

Takayasu's arteritis – papulonecrotic tuberculid-like lesions *AD 123:796–800, 1987*

PAPULES, DIGITAL

AUTOIMMUNE DISEASES AND DISEASES OF IMMUNE DYSFUNCTION

Anti-phospholipid antibody syndrome *BJD 140:725–729, 1999*

Chronic granulomatous disease – chilblains *JAAD 36:899–907, 1997;* X-linked chronic granulomatous disease – photosensitivity, chilblain lupus of fingertips and toes *Ped Derm 3:376–379, 1986;* finger papules of DLE in carriers *J Invest Allergol Clin Immunol 7:57–61, 1997*

Dermatomyositis – Gottron's papules; inverse Gottron's papules in MDA-5 dermatomyositis *J Clin Rheumatol 22:274–275, 2016;* mechanic's hands, anti-synthetase syndrome *Ann DV 146:19–25, 2019*

Lupus erythematosus – acral papulonodular dermal mucinosis *JAAD 27:312–315, 1992;* chilblain lupus – fingers, toes, elbows, knees, calves, knuckles, nose, ears *BJD 143:1050–1054, 2000; BJD 98:497–506, 1978;* systemic lupus – recurrent Osler's nodes *Angiology 20:33–37, 1969*

Rheumatoid arthritis – rheumatoid nodules *JAAD 11:713–723, 1984;* rheumatoid vasculitis- Bywater's lesions; purpuric papules *Cutis 71:462, 464, 2003; BJD 77:207–210, 1965;* rheumatoid neutrophilic dermatitis *JAAD 22 (pt2)922–925, 1990*

Scleroderma – CREST syndrome with calcinosis cutis – digital papule

CONGENITAL ANOMALY

Congenital infantile digital fibromatosis *Ped Derm 19:370–371, 2002*

Supernumerary digit – digital papule *Ped Derm 20:108–112, 2003*

22q11.2 deletion syndrome – DiGeorge syndrome (conotruncal cardiac defects, hypoparathyroidism and thymic aplasia) or velocardiofacial syndrome (pharyngeal defects, dysmorphic facies, learning disabilities and cardiac anomalies) and juvenile dermato-myositis *JAAD 69:326–328, 2013*

DEGENERATIVE

Carpal tunnel syndrome – chilblain-like lesions with necrosis

Heberden's nodes of knuckles – degenerative joint disease *JAAD 43:892, 2000*

DRUG

Acral dysesthesia syndrome

EXOGENOUS AGENTS

Cactus spine granuloma – pink palmar distal digital papules *Cutis 79:208–210, 2007; J Dermatol 20:424–427, 1993*

Fiberglass dermatitis *Int J Dermatol 58:1107–1111, 2019; J Formos Med Assoc 92:755–758, 1993*

Foreign body granulomas, including cactus spine (Opuntia cactus) granulomas *Cutis 65:290–292, 2000;* sea urchin granulomas

Phenytoin reaction – keratotic finger papules *Cutis 61:101–102, 1998*

INFECTIONS

AIDS – erythema elevatum diutinum in AIDS *JAAD 28:919–922, 1993, JAAD 26:38–44, 1992*

Anthrax – slaughtering dead bullock *West Bengal J Assoc Physicians India 60:86–93, 2012*

Bacillary angiomatosis *Indian J Dermatol 60:523, 2015*

Camelpox infection *Vet Microbiol 152:29–38, 2011*

Cat scratch disease, inoculation papule *Ped Derm 5:1–9, 1988*

Covid-19 infection – painful acral red-purple papules *J Dermatol Sci April 29, 2020;* covid toes – chilblain-like – personal observation

Coxsackie virus A6 (atypical hand, foot, and mouth disease) – red papulovesicles of fingers, palmar erythema, red papules of ears, red papules of antecubital fossa, perioral papulovesicles, vesicles of posterior pharynx *JAAD 69:736–741, 2013*

Gianotti-Crosti syndrome – acral papules *Pediatr Am 36:800–804, 2007*

Gonococcemia *Dermatol Online J Jan 15, 2017*

Histoplasmosis *JAAD 43:1155–1160, 2016*

HTLV-1 associated adult T-cell leukemia/lymphoma *J Cutan Pathol 45:171–175, 2018*

Leishmaniasis – post kala-azar dermal leishmaniasis

Leprosy, lepromatous *JAAD 11:713–723, 1984*

Milker's nodules *JAAD 49:910–911, 2003;* digital papule

Mycobacterium marinum Clin Inf Dis 31:439–443, 2000

Orf – Parapoxvirus (genus); Family Poxviridae *Cutis 71:288–290, 2003; AD 126:235–240, 1990*

Osler's node (subacute bacterial endocarditis) – small, red papules on distal finger and toe pads *Acta DV Croat 27:280–281, 2019; Clin Inf Dis 32:63,149, 2001; NEJM 295:1500–1505, 1976*

Parvovirus B19 – dermatomyositis-like Gottron's papules *Hum Pathol 31:488–497, 2000*

Puss caterpillar *Cutis 60:125–126, 1997*

Rat bite fever – *Streptobacillus moniliformis; Clin Inf Dis 43:1585–1586, 2006*

Scabies *Am J Clin Dermatol 3:9–18, 2002*

Scedosporium apiospermum – red nodules of dorsal hand and fingers *Clin Inf Dis 51:255–257, 2010*

Septic emboli JAAD 47:S263–265, 2002

Sporotrichosis *Intern Emerg Med 11:481–482, 2016*

Staphylococcal sepsis *JAAD 47:S263–265, 2002*

Syphilis – primary chancre; secondary; condyloma lata of toe webs *Cutis 57:38–40, 1996*

Talaromyces marneffei – brown papules of fingers *JAAD 49:344–346, 2003*

Trichophyton rubrum – invasive *T. rubrum* in immunosuppressed patients

Tularemia

Tungiasis (Tunga penetrans) (toe-tip or subungual nodule) – crusted or ulcerated *JAAD 82:551–569, 2020; Acta Dermatovenerol (Stockh)76:495, 1996; JAAD 20:941–944, 1989; AD 124:429–434, 1988*

Verruca vulgaris – digital papule, knuckle pads *Derm Surg 27:591–593, 2001;* flat warts

INFILTRATIVE DISEASES

Acral persistent papular mucinosis *Clin Case Rep 8:344–346, 2020; Cutis 87:143–145, 2011; JAAD 51:982–988, 2004; AD 122:1237–1239, 1986;* mimicking knuckle pads *AD 140:121–126, 2004; JAAD 27:1026–1029, 1992*

Amyloidosis – nodular amyloidosis of the toe *AD 139:1157–1159, 2003*

Juvenile xanthogranuloma *Actas Dermosifiliogr 110:855–856, 2019; Ann Dermatol 20:200–203, 2008*

Lichen myxedematosus (scleromyxedema) – resembling acral persistent papular mucinosis *BJD 144:594–596, 2001; Dermatology 185:81, 1992;* mimicking knuckle pads

Recurrent self-healing cutaneous mucinosis – red papules of palms and fingertips with pustules and vesicles *BJD 143:650–652, 2000*

Self-healing juvenile cutaneous mucinosis – knuckle nodules *JAAD 11:327–332, 1984; JAAD 31:815–816, 1994; Dermatology 189:93–94, 1994*

INFLAMMATORY DISEASES

Erythema multiforme *Medicine 68:133–140, 1989; JAAD 8:763–765, 1983;* plantar nodules *Ped Derm 15:97–102, 1998*

Interstitial granulomatous dermatitis *J Dermatol 38:382–385, 2011*

Palmoplantar eccrine neutrophilic hidradenitis *Ped Derm 15:97–102, 1998; AD 131:817–820, 1995*

Sarcoid – fingertip nodules *Indian J DV Leprol 76:448, 2010; JAAD 44:725–743, 2001; JAAD 11:713–723, 1984*

Verruciform xanthoma of toes in patient with Milroy's disease due to persistent leg edema *Ped Derm 20:44–47, 2003; JAAD 20:313–317, 1989*

METABOLIC DISEASES

Alkaptonuria – hyperchromic papules *An Bras Dermatol 89:799–801, 2014*

Calcinosis cutis – digital papules *Cutis 66:465–467, 2000;* plate-like calcinosis cutis; digital papular calcific elastosis *J Cutan Pathol 17:358–370, 1990*

Diabetes mellitus – Huntley's papules *Int J Dermatol 44:755–756, 2005*

Erythropoietic protoporphyria – lichenoid papules in sun exposed areas *JAMA Derm 152:937–938, 2016; Hautarzt 67:479–482, 2016*

Gout – tophus – digital papule(s) *Cutis 64:233–236, 1999; AD 134:499–504, 1998*

Oxalosis – calcium oxalate *Am J Dermatopathol 40:e78–79, 2018; Am J Kid Dis 25:492–497, 1995;* secondary oxalosis – papules on palmar skin of fingers *JAAD 31:368–372, 1994*

Xanthomas – type II hypercholesterolemia

NEOPLASTIC DISEASES

Acquired digital fibrokeratoma – digital papule *Cutis 79:129–132, 2007; AD 124:1559–1564, 1988; JAAD 12:816–821, 1985*

Acquired reactive digital fibroma – subungual tumor with enlarged paronychium and macrodactyly *JAAD 69:603–608, 2013*
   Differential diagnosis
      Fibro-osseous pseudotumor of the digits; myofibroblastic proliferation in females; affects flexor digits and palms *Chir Main 28:107–112, 2009; Cancer 58:2103–2109, 1986*
      Superficial acral fibromyxoma (cellular digital fibroma)– slow growing, painful solitary subungual tumor *Clin Dermatol 35:85–98, 2017; JAAD 69:603–608, 2013; Am J Surg Pathol 36:789–798, 2012*

Acquired subungual exostoses *JAAD 26:295–298, 1992*

Acral pseudolymphomatous angiokeratoma of children (APACHE) *Dermatol Online J July 15, 2015; JAAD 45:S209–211, 2001*

Actinic keratoses; in transplant patients *JAAD 47:1–17, 2002*

Aggressive digital papillary adenocarcinoma – occur on fingers and toes *Cutis 72:145–147, 2003; Dermatol Surg 26:580–583, 2000; JAAD 23:331–334, 1990;*

Aggressive digital papillary adenoma *Cutis 69:179–182, 2002; AD 120:1612, 1984*

Aggressive infantile fibromatosis *AD 107:574–579, 1973*

Angiokeratoma of Mibelli – autosomal dominant; associated with chilblains; on dorsum of fingers, toes, hands, feet *AD 106:726–728, 1972*

Atrial myxoma – tender red fingertip papule *JAAD 21:1080–1084, 1989;* violaceous papules *Eur J Dermatol 91650–1, 1999; BJD 147:379–382, 2002*

Basal cell carcinoma – periungual – basal cell carcinoma of toenail unit *JAAD 48:277–278, 2003;* Gorlin's syndrome *BJD 171:1227–1229, 2014*

Blue nevus – of nail fold

Bowen's disease, pigmented *An Bras Dermatol 92:686–688, 2017; J Fam Pract 98:149–151, 2009*

Chondroblastoma, subungual – toe tip *Ped Derm 21:452–453, 2004*

Clear cell syringofibroadenoma of Mascaro – subungual papule *BJD 144:625–627, 2001*

Dermatofibroma – digital papule; papule of foot fibrous dermatofibroma – periungual fibroma

Digital fibrous tumor of childhood – toe nodule *AD 131:1195, 1198, 1995*

Digital myxoid cyst *J Cutan Pathol 42:974–977, 2015; Derm Surg 27:591–593, 2001;* herpetiform appearance *Ann Dermatol 22:194–195, 2010*

Eccrine angiomatous hamartoma – toes, fingers, palms and soles-skin-colored to blue *JAAD 47:429–435, 2002; Ped Derm 13:139–142, 1996; JAAD 37:523–549, 1997; Ped Derm 14:401–402, 1997; Ped Derm 18:117–119, 2001; Ped Derm 14:401–402, 1997;* skin-colored nodule with blue papules *JAAD 41:109–111, 1999*

Eccrine poroma – digital papule *AD 74:511–512, 1956*

Eccrine spiradenoma – papule of proximal nail fold *AD 140:1003–1008, 2004*

Enchondroma *Derm Surg 27:591–593, 2001;* may be subungual

Epidermal nevus – digital papule

Epidermoid cyst – digital papule *JAAD 43:892, 2000*

Epidermolytic acanthoma – on fingers mimicking flat warts *Case Rep Dermatol 14:98–101, 2017*

Epithelioid sarcoma – nodule of flexor finger or palm *AD 121:389–393, 1985; JAAD 14:893–898, 1986*

Exostosis, subungual (bony exostosis) (variant of osteochondroma) *JAAD 45:S200–201, 2001; Derm Surg 27:591–593, 2001;* subungual exostosis *Cutis 68:57–58, 2001; AD 128:847–852, 1992;* differentiate from carcinoma of the nailbed, Koenen's tumor, pyogenic granuloma, verruca, glomus tumor, melanoma

Fibroma – digital papule or subungual fibroma *Derm Surg 27:591–593, 2001*

Fibroma of the tendon sheath *JAAD 11:625–628, 1984*

Garlic clove tumor (fibroma) (acquired periungual fibrokeratoma); *AD 97:120–129, 1968*

Giant cell tumor of the tendon sheath – single or multiple *BJD 147:403–405, 2002; JAAD 43:892, 2000;* nodules of the fingers *J Dermatol 23:290–292, 1996;* overlying dorsal digital interphalangeal crease *J Hand Surg 5:39–50, 1980;* subungual giant cell tumor of the tendon sheath *Cutis 58:273–275, 1996 (*nail dystrophy and swelling)

Granular cell tumor – digital papule, paronychial nodule *Cutis 62:147–148, 1998; Cutis 35:355–356, 1985*

Infantile digital fibromatosis – multiple soft fibromas on dorsal digits *JAAD 49:974–975, 2003; AD 138:1245–1251, 2002; BJD 143:1107–1108, 2000; Ped Derm 8:137–139, 1991; J Cut Pathol 5:339–346, 1978;* on lateral fifth finger *AD 141:549–550, 2005*

Infantile myofibromatosis – skin colored to purple-red multiple nodules or papules *Cutis 73:229–231, 2004; Cancer 7:953–978, 1954*

Infundibular follicular cyst

Intraosseous epidermoid cysts *JAAD 27:454–455, 1992*

Kaposi's sarcoma *Int J Health Sci (Qassim)2:153–156, 2008*

Keratoacanthoma – digital papule *AD 120:736–740, 1984*

Leukemia cutis – digital papule; preleukemic state of monocytosis and neutropenia – perniotic lesions *BJD 81:327–332, 1969;* chronic myelomonocytic leukemia – chilblain-like lesions *BJD 115:607–609, 1986; AD 121:1048–1052, 1985;* chronic myelomonocytic leukemia – chilblain-like lesions *JAAD 50:S42–44, 2004*

Lipoma – periungual lipoma *JAAD 51:S91–93, 2004;* subungual lipoma *BJD 149:418, 2003*

Malignant proliferating onycholemmal cyst *J Cut Pathol 21:183, 1994*

Melanocytic nevus

Melanoma – acral lentiginous *Surg Pathol Clin 2:535–541, 2009*

Metastatic tumors – plantar nodule of toe; pancreatic carcinoma *AD 139:1497–1502, 2003;* bronchogenic carcinoma – subungual papule *Cutis 35:121–124, 1985;* squamous cell carcinoma – palmar nodule; papules of fingers/toes – hepatocellular carcinoma *Ahonghua Yi Zue Zhi (Taipei) 64:253–257, 2001*

Multinucleate giant cell angiohistiocytoma – multiple grouped asymptomatic; middle aged and elderly women *Clin Exp Dermatol 35:e203–204, 2010*

Nerve sheath myxoma – most common on hands, fingers, knees *AD 145:195–200, 2009*

Neurofibroma *AD 124:1185–1186, 1988;* myxoid neurofibroma, periungual *Cutis 69:54–56, 2002*

Neurofibrosarcoma *J Pediatr 51:566–70, 1957*

Neurothekeoma, subungual *JAAD 52:159–162, 2005*

Osteochondroma, subungual *Derm Surg 27:591–593, 2001*

Osteoma cutis *JAAD 39:527–544, 1998; JAAD 20:973–978, 1989*

Panfollicular nevus *J Cutan Pathol 34:Suppl 1 14–17, 2007*

Porokeratotic eccrine ostial and dermal duct nevus *Dermatol Online J Sept 16, 2014*

Progressive nodular fibrosis of the skin – nodules on fingers *JID 87:210–216, 1986*

Reactive fibrous papule of the fingers (giant-cell fibroma) – fingers and palms *Dermatologica 143:368–375, 1971*

Sclerosing perineuroma – painless skin colored papule *An Bras Dermatol 84:643–649, 2009; Am J Surg Pathol 21:1433–1442, 1997*

Squamous cell carcinoma *Derm Surg 27:591–593, 2001*

Syringomas *Case Rep Dermatol Med Jan 11, 2020; J Cut Med Surg 13:169–171, 2009*

Syringomatous carcinoma – multilobulated digital nodule *BJD 144:438–439, 2001*

Unilateral punctate porokeratosis *An Bras Dermatol 88:441–443, 2013*

Vascular and myxoid fibromas of the fingers – multiple warty lesions of palms and fingers *JAAD 2:425–431, 1980*

Verrucous acanthoma

PHOTODERMATOSES

Degenerative collagenous plaques of the hands – digital papular calcific elastosis *J Cutan Pathol 17:358–370, 1990;* keratoelastoidosis marginalis *Hautarzt 69 (suppl 1) 37–38, 2016*

PRIMARY CUTANEOUS DISEASES

Accessory digit

Acrodermatitis continua of Hallopeau *J Dermatol Treat 18:315–318, 2007*

Acrokeratoelastoidosis *Int J Dermatol 44:406–407, 2005; Dermatology 188:28–31, 1994*

Acrokeratosis verruciformis of Hopf *J Drugs Dermatol 3:687–688, 2004*

Anetoderma *BMC Dermatol Aug 19, 2004*

Congenital hypertrophy of the lateral nail folds of the hallux *Ped Derm 5:243–245, 1989*

Erythema elevatum diutinum – knuckle pads (juxta-articular nodules), papules *JAAD 49:764–767, 2003; Cutis 67:381–384, 2001; Ped Derm 15:411–412, 1998;* including EED associated with HIV disease – digital papule; of feet *Caputo, 2000, p.29;* papules of proximal nail fold

Focal acral hyperkeratosis *Dermatology 188:28–31, 1994*

Granuloma annulare *J Hand Surg Am 36::1039–1041, 2011; JAAD 3:217–230, 1980;* mimicking dorsal knuckle pads; acute onset, painful *AD 142:49–54, 2006*

Greither's palmoplantar keratoderma (transgradiens et progradiens palmoplantar keratoderma) *Cutis 65:141–145, 2000*

Idiopathic non-familial acro-osteolysis – yellow digital papules *Indian J Dermatol 57:486–488, 2012*

Knuckle pads (heloderma); *AD 129:1043–1048, 1993;* sports-related *Int J Dermatol 41:291–293, 2002*

Lichen nitidus – digital papule, knuckle pads *Cutis 103:E3–5, 2019; AD 134:1302–1303, 1998*

Lichen sclerosus et atrophicus – ivory white papules *Ann DV 135:201–204, 2008*

Lichen simplex chronicus – knuckle pads

Lichen striatus *Ann DV 136:883–886, 2009*

Palisaded neutrophilic and granulomatous dermatitis *Am J Dermatopathol 35:847–850, 2013*

Palmoplantar keratoderma, epidermolytic – papules on knuckles *BJD 125:496, 1991*

Pityriasis lichenoides et varioliformis acuta *Dermatol Pract Concept 31:27–34, 2017*

Psoriasis

Punctate porokeratotic keratoderma – keratotic papules of fingers and toes *Dermatol Online J Jan 15, 2010*

Reactive perforating collagenosis *SKINMed 16:390–396, 2018*

PSYCHOCUTANEOUS DISEASES

Bulimia nervosa – Russell's sign (crusted knuckle nodules) *Clin Orthop 343:107–109, 1997; JAAD 12:725–726, 1985;*

perniosis *Clin Sci 61:559–567, 1981;* pseudo knuckle pads (calluses on 2nd 5th MCP joints) *Psychol Med 9;429–48, 1979*

SYNDROMES

Alport's syndrome – gouty tophi, nephritis, deafness

Bart-Pumphrey syndrome – knuckle pads, leukonychia, deafness, and palmoplantar hyperkeratosis; connexin mutation *Int J Dermatol 52:192–205, 2014*

Blue rubber bleb nevus syndrome – nail fold lesions

Ehlers-Danlos syndrome (molluscum pseudotumor) – knuckle pads, chilblains, acrocyanosis, elastosis perforans serpiginosa, piezogenic papules, scars, fragile skin

Ellis van Creveld syndrome – polydactyly *JAAD 46:161–183, 2002; Ped Derm 18:68–70, 2001*

Familial multiple acral mucinous fibrokeratomas – verrucous papules of the fingers *JAAD 38:999–1001, 1998*

Familial histiocytic dermatoarthritis – knuckle pads *Am J Dermatopathol 9:491–496, 1987*

Farber's disease (disseminated lipogranulomatosis) – red papules and nodules of joints and tendons of hands and feet; deforming arthritis; papules, plaques, and nodules of ears, back of scalp and trunk; *Am J Dis Child 84:449–500, 1952;* acid ceramide deficiency; *ASAH1* mutation *Orphanet J Rare Dis 183:121, July, 2018*

Fibroblastic rheumatism – symmetrical polyarthritis, nodules over joints and on palms, elbows, knees, ears, neck, Raynaud's phenomenon, sclerodactyly; skin lesions resolve spontaneously *AD 139:657–662, 2003; Ped Derm 19:532–535, 2002; AD 131:710–712, 1995; Clin Exp Dermatol 19:268–270, 1994; JAAD 14:1086–1088, 1986; Rev Rheum Ed Fr 47:345–351, 1980;* periungual papules *Ped Derm 19:532–535, 2002*

Francois syndrome (dermochondrocorneal dystrophy) – knuckle pads; nodules on hands, nose, and ears *Ann DV 104:475–478, 1977; AD 124:424–428, 1988*

Goltz's syndrome – papillomas of toes and lips *AD 145:218–219, 2009*

Hereditary progressive mucinous histiocytosis *Acta DV 90:65–67, 2010; BJD 141:1101–1105, 1999*

Hunter's syndrome – MPS II – knuckle pads *Ped Derm 12:370–372, 1995*

Incontinentia pigmenti – painful subungual keratotic tumor of IP *JAAD 50:S45–52, 2004; JAAD 47:169–187, 2002; J Hand Surg 18B:667–669, 1993; AD 124:29–30, 1988*

Infantile systemic hyalinosis – knuckle pads *Ped Derm 11:52–60, 1994*

Juvenile hyaline fibromatosis – pearly white papules of face and neck; larger papules and nodules around nose, behind ears, on fingertips, knuckle pads; multiple subcutaneous nodules of scalp, trunk, and extremities, papillomatous perianal papules; joint contractures, skeletal lesions, gingival hyperplasia, stunted growth *AD 121:1062–1063, 1985; AD 107:574–579, 1973*

Knuckle pads with marginal palmoplantar papular keratoderma and acrokeratoelastoidosis *Cutis 102:344–346, 2018*

Ledderhose's nodules (plantar fibromatosis) *JAAD 41:106–108, 1999;* Dupuytren's contracture (palmar fibromatosis) and/or Peyronie's disease – knuckle pads

Lipoid proteinosis – acral papules *BJD 151:413–423, 2004; JID 120:345–350, 2003; BJD 148:180–182, 2003; Hum Molec Genet 11:833–840, 2002;* digital papule *AD 132:1239–1244, 1996*

Maffucci's syndrome – enchondromas, angiomas, cartilaginous nodules; *Dermatologic Clinics 13:73–78, 1995; JAAD 29:894–899, 1993*

Mal de Meleda – knuckle pads *Ped Derm 14:186–191, 1997*

Mucocutaneous neuromas, PTEN hamartoma-tumor syndrome *AD 142:625–632, 2006*

Multicentric reticulohistiocytosis – digital papule; knuckle pads; yellow papules and plaques *AD 140:919–921, 2004; JAAD 49:1125–1127, 2003; AD 126:251–252, 1990; Oral Surg Oral Med Oral Pathol 65:721–725, 1988; Pathology 17:601–608, 1985; JAAD 11:713–723, 1984; AD 97:543–547, 1968*

Multiple exostoses syndrome *JAAD 25:333–335, 1991*

Neurofibromatosis – digital papule, knuckle pads

Ollier syndrome – multiple enchondromas

Pachydermodactyly – benign fibromatosis of fingers of young men *AD 129:247–248, 1993; JAAD 27:303–305, 1992; AD 111:524, 1975*

Pachyonychia congenita – papules on the fingers

Palmoplantar keratoderma, Vorner – knuckle pads

Proteus syndrome *Ped Derm 5:14–21, 1988*

Reflex sympathetic dystrophy with chilblain-like lesions

Rowell's syndrome – lupus erythematosus and erythema multiforme-like syndrome – papules, annular targetoid lesions, vesicles, bullae, necrosis, ulceration, oral ulcers; perniotic lesions *JAAD 21:374–377, 1989*

Stiff skin syndrome – knuckle pads *Ped Derm 3:48–53, 1985*

Sweet's syndrome – neutrophilic dermatosis of the hands *J Hand Surg Am 43:e1–185, 2018; Clin Dermatol 35:81–84, 2017*

Trichorhinophalangeal dysplasia syndrome (Laugier-Gideon syndrome) *Ped Derm 13:212–218, 1996*

Tuberous sclerosis – periungual angiofibromas (Koenen's tumors) *JAAD 18:369–372, 1988;* digital papules *J Clin Neurol 7:221–224, 1992*

TOXINS

Arsenical keratoses – palms and soles; resemble corns; fingers, backs of hands; *JID 4:365–383, 1941*

TRAUMA

Chilblains (perniosis) – tender, pruritic red or purple digital papules *Dermatol Online J Dec 15, 2016; JAAD 47:S263–265, 2002; JAAD 45:924–929, 2001 AD 117:26–28, 1981*

Dermatophagia ("wolf-biter") *Cutis 59:19–20, 1997*

Garrod's pads (knuckle pad syndrome) – violinist's knuckles – thickened skin over the interphalangeal joints from intense flexion of the tendons of the fingers *JAAD 22:657–663, 1990; Annals Rheum Dis 46:169–170, 1987*

Neuroma, traumatic – digital papule; palisaded encapsulated neuroma *AD 140:1003–1008, 2004;* interdigital neuroma *JAAD 38:815–819, 1998;* traumatic neuroma due to treatment of supernumerary digit *Ped Derm 20:108–112, 2003*

Writer's callus

VASCULAR DISEASES

Acral hemosiderotic lymphatic malformation *J Cutan Pathol 40:657–660, 2013*

Acroangiodermatitis of Mali – pseudo-Kaposi's sarcoma; chronic venous insufficiency, arteriovenous malformations, paralysis – tops of first and second toes *Acta DV (Stockh) 75:475–478, 1995; Int J Dermatol 33:179–183, 1994;*

Angiofibroma, acral – acquired digital fibrokeratoma, garlic clove fibroma; tuberous sclerosis *Clin Dermatol 35:85–98, 2017*

Angiokeratoma – of nail fold

Angiolipoleiomyoma – ears, fingers, toes *JAAD 38:143–175, 1998*

Cholesterol emboli *AD 122:1194–1198, 1986*

Chylous lymphedema – xanthomas of toes and feet *BJD 146:134–137, 2002*

Digital verrucous fibroangioma *Acta DV 72:303–304, 1992*

Glomus tumors – digital papule, subungual *J Eur Acad DV 25:1392–1397, 2011; Derm Surg 27:591–593, 2001*

Hemangioma – of foot or toes

Neonatal hemangiomatosis

Polyangiitis with granulomatosis *AD 130:861–867, 1994*

Pyogenic granuloma – digital papule *Derm Surg 27:591–593, 2001;*

PAPULES, DIRTY BROWN

AUTOIMMUNE DISEASES AND DISEASES OF IMMUNE DYSFUNCTION

Adult onset Still's disease – dirty brown exanthema *JAAD 73:294–303, 2015*

Lupus erythematosus – discoid lupus erythematosus *NEJM 269:1155–1161, 1963*

Pemphigus foliaceus *J Drugs Dermatol 1:333–334, 2002*

Rheumatoid neutrophilic dermatitis *JAAD 45:596–600, 2001*

INFECTIONS AND INFESTATIONS

Epidermodysplasia verruciformis *BJD 121:463–469, 1989; Arch Dermatol Res 278:153–160, 1985*

Gianotti-Crosti syndrome *Asia Pac Allergy 2:223–226, 2012*

Scabies, Norwegian (crusted)

Syphilis, secondary *Oxf Med Case Reports Feb 1, 2018*

Tinea versicolor

Tinea nigra

Tuberculosis – lupus vulgaris *Int J Dermatol 40:336–339, 2001;* lichen scrofulosorum *Indian Dermatol Online J 3:190–192, 2012;* papulonecrotic tuberculid *Clin Exp Dermatol 45:238–240, 2020*

Verrucae planae

INFILTRATIVE DISEASES

Amyloidosis – lichen amyloidosis

Benign cephalic histiocytosis *JAAD 47:908–913, 2002*

Generalized eruptive histiocytosis *Australas J Dermatol 60:e314–316, 2019*

Langerhans cell histiocytosis *World J Pediatr 15:536–545, 2019*

Urticaria pigmentosa *Pen Child Health 22:33–34, 2017*

INFLAMMATORY DISEASES

Rosai-Dorfman disease *BJD 134:749–753, 1996*

METABOLIC DISEASES

Diabetes mellitus – diabetic pretibial pigmented patches

Necrolytic acral erythema *Clin Cosmet Invest Dermatol 1:275–281, 2020*

NEOPLASTIC DISEASES

Actinic keratosis

Becker's nevus, follicular – a new clinical variant *Indian J Dermatol 65:130–132, 2020*

Bowen's disease, pigmented *Dermatologica 157:229–237, 1978*

Bowenoid papulosis *Cutis 102:151–154, 2018; Dis Colon Rectum 30:62–64, 1987*

Clear cell acanthoma – pigmented keratotic papule *Am J Dermatopathol 16:134–139, 1994*

Dermatosis papulosa nigra *J Cosmet Dermatol Jan 28, 2020*

Eccrine porocarcinoma, dark brown *AD 131:211–216, 1995*

Eruptive keratoacanthomas *Int J Dermatol 53:131–136, 2014*

Leukemia cutis , therapy related *JAMA 314:2182–2183, 2015*

Lymphomatoid papulosis *Acta DV Croat 27:202–204, 2019*

Piloleiomyoma *An Bras Dermatol 90:178–180, 2015*

Plasmacytosis, cutaneous and systemic *Oncol Lett 11:1923–2925, 2016*

Syringomas *Ann DV 143:521–528, 2016; Cutis 66:259–262, 2000; AD 126:954–955, 957–958, 1990*

Warty dyskeratoma

PHOTODERMATOSES

Disseminated superficial actinic porokeratosis

PRIMARY CUTANEOUS DISEASES

Acrokeratosis verruciformis of Hopf *Am J Dermatopathol 39:370–373, 2017*

Confluent and reticulated papillomatosis *Actas Dermosifiliogr 109:e7–11, 2018; BJD 154:287–293, 2006*

Darier's disease *SKINmed 13:313–315, 2015; Ann Dermatol 10:597, 1889; J Cutan Genitourin Dis 7:201, 1889;* linear Darier's disease *Cutis 86:224,237–238, 2010*

Dowling-Degos disease *Int J Dermatol 30:39–42, 1991*

Erythema elevatum diutinum *Stat Pearls Dec 20, 2019 PMID:28846276; JAAD 26:38–44, 1992*

Flegel's disease (hyperkeratosis lenticularis perstans) – autosomal dominant *JAAD 73:346–348, 2015; An Bras Dermatol 86:576–577, 2011; Int J Dermatol 47:38–41, 2008; JAAD 16:190–195, 1987; BJD 116:681–691, 1987; Hautarzt 9:363–364, 1958*

Fox-Fordyce disease *Hautarzt 69:373–375, 2018; Dermatol Online J 18:28, 2012*

Galli-Galli disease *Acta DV Croat 25:300–302, 2017*

Granular parakeratosis *JAAD 52:863–867, 2005*

Grover's disease – personal observation

Hailey-Hailey disease *Dermatol Ther 32:e12945, 2019*

Ichthyosis or ichthyosiform eruption, including X-linked ichthyosis

Ig G4-related disease *Mod Rheumatol 23:986–993, 2013*

Keratosis lichenoides chronica *SKINMed 15:211–213, 2017*

Lichen amyloidosis – familial and non-familial

Lichen planus and lichen planus pigmentosus *J Dermatol 24:193–197, 1997*

Lupus miliaris disseminate faciei *Dermatol Ther April 3, 2020; BMJ Case Rep July 14, 2017; bcr 2017221118; SKINMed 4:234–238, 2005*

Pityriasis rubra pilaris

Reactive perforating collagenosis *SKINMed 16:390–396, 2018*

PSYCHOCUTANEOUS DISEASES

Cutaneous dirt-adherent disease (severe terra firme) – brown plaques of face *AD 145:1070–1071, 2009;* terra firme *Case Rep Dermatol 11:108–112, 2019; Dermatol Pract Concepts 31:29–33, 2015*

SYNDROMES

Bazex syndrome – dirty brown papules of back *JAMA Derm 150:1368–1370, 2014*

Congenital self-healing histiocytosis – with hemosiderin deposits *Ann DV 128:238–240, 2001*

Generalized basaloid follicular hamartoma syndrome – autosomal dominant; milia, comedone-like lesions, dermatosis papulosa nigra, skin tag-like lesions, hypotrichosis, palmar pits *J Clin Aesthet Dermatol 11:39–41, 2018; JAAD 45:644–645, 2001*

Phakomatosis pigmentokeratotica *Dermatology 197:377–380, 1998*

VASCULAR DISEASES

Granulomatous pigmented purpuric eruption *J Dermatol 23:551–555, 1996*

PAPULES, DISTAL DIGITAL, WHITE

Calcium oxalate

Calcium phosphate

Calcium pyrophosphate

Dystrophic calcification

Iatrogenic calcification

Idiopathic calcification

Metastatic calcification – deposition of calcium in the media of blood vessels of the kidneys, myocardium, stomach, lungs, and skin

Monosodium urate

Pustules

PAPULES, SOLITARY FACIAL

CONGENITAL LESIONS

Accessory tragus – facial, glabellar papule – isolated, Treacher Collins syndrome (mandibulofacial dysostosis; autosomal dominant), Goldenhar syndrome (oculo-auriculo-vertebral syndrome) – macroglossia, preauricular tags, abnormal pinnae, facial asymmetry, macrostomia, epibulbar dermoids, facial weakness, central nervous system, renal, and skeletal anomalies, Nagers syndrome, Wolf-Hirschhorn syndrome (chromosome 4 deletion syndrome), oculocerebrocutaneous syndrome *Ped Derm 17:391–394, 2000;* Townes-Brocks syndrome *Am J Med Genet 18:147–152, 1984;* VACTERL syndrome *J Pediatr 93:270–273, 1978;* Hurson syndrome
Differential diagnosis of accessory tragus includes:
Acrochordon
Adnexal tumor
Auricular fistula
Branchial cleft cyst and/or fistula
Cartilaginous remnants
Congenital midline hamartoma
Epidermoid cyst
Hair follicle nevus
Lipoma
Skin tags
Thyroglossal duct cyst
Wattle

Bronchogenic cyst – skin-colored nodule of chin *BJD 143:1353–1355, 2000*

Congenital midline hamartoma – polypoid nodule of chin *Ped Derm 7:199–201, 1990*

Congenital vellus hamartoma (hair follicle nevus) – skin colored papule of face *Int J Dermatol 31:578–581, 1992*

Dermoid cyst (midline) *Pediatr Rev 11 (9):262–267, 1990*

Lacrimal duct cyst

Meningocele

Nasal glioma – blue or red nodule *J Neurosurg 64:516–519. 1986; Pediatr Rev 11 (9):262–267, 1990;* papule of nose *AD 137:1095–1100, 2001*

Neuroblastoma

Rhabdomyosarcoma

EXOGENOUS AGENTS

Poly-L-lactic acid injection *Ann Plast Surg 4:435–441, 2010*

Silicone – metastatic silicone granuloma *AD 138:537–538, 2002*

INFECTIONS AND INFESTATIONS

Abscess

Acremonium sepsis JAAD 37:1006–1008, 1997

Actinomycosis, cervicofacial *Laryngoscope 94:1198–1217, 1984*

Anthrax – *Bacillus anthracis;* malignant pustule; face, neck, hands, arms; starts as papule then evolves into bulla on red base; then hemorrhagic crust with edema and erythema with small vesicles; edema of surrounding skin *Br J Opthalmol 76:753–754, 1992; J Trop Med Hyg 89:43–45, 1986; Bol Med Hosp Infant Mex 38:355–361, 1981*

Bacillary angiomatosis – *Bartonella henselae AD 131:933–936, 1995*

Botryomycosis

Candidal sepsis

Chromomycosis – *Aureobasidium pullulans AD 133:663–664, 1997*

Dental sinus *Am Fam Physician 40:113–116, 1989*

Fusarium sepsis JAAD 37:1006–1008, 1997

Herpes simplex – pseudolymphoma appearance – violaceous nodule *Am J Dermatopathol 13:234–240, 1991*

Insect bite

Kerion

Leishmaniasis *Iran J Parasitol 12:544–553, 2017*

Leprosy *J Cut Med Surg 12:139–141, 2008*

Milker's nodule

Molluscum contagiosum *BJD 115:131–138, 1987*

Mycobacterium tuberculosis – scrofuloderma – infected lymph node, bone, joint, lacrimal gland with overlying red-blue nodule which breaks down, ulcerates, forms fistulae, scarring with adherent fibrous masses which may be fluctuant and draining *BJD 134:350–352, 1996;* BCG granuloma; lupus vulgaris

Myiasis – cuterebrid myiasis *Ped Derm 21:515–516, 2004*

North American blastomycosis

Pseudomonas sepsis JAAD 32:279–280, 1995; Am J Med 80:528–529, 1986

Rhinosporidiosis – nasal polyp

Rickettsial pox

Syphilis

Wart

INFILTRATIVE DISORDERS

Amyloidosis – nodular tumefactive amyloid

Cutaneous focal mucinosis (superficial angiomyxoma) – face, trunk, or extremities *Am J Surg Pathol 12:519–530, 1988; AD 93:13–20, 1966*

Jessner's lymphocytic *AD 124:1091–1093, 1988*

Papular xanthoma *JAAD 22:1052–1056, 1990; Ped Derm 15:65–67, 1998*

Urticaria pigmentosa – solitary mastocytoma *Acta Clin Croat 48:59–64, 2009*

Xanthogranuloma *AD 112:43–44, 1976*

INFLAMMATORY DISEASES

Erythema nodosum

Foreign body granuloma – reaction to ruptured hair follicle

Idiopathic facial aseptic granuloma – facial papulonodule *AD 137:1253–1255, 2001*

Lymphocytoma cutis; *Cancer 69:717–724, 1992; Acta DV (Stockh)62:119–124, 1982; Cancer 24:487–502, 1969*

Nodular fasciitis – subcutaneous facial nodule *AD 137:719–721, 2001*

Sarcoid; *AD 133:882–888, 1997; NEJM 336:1224–1234, 1997; Clinics in Chest Medicine 18:663–679, 1997*

Subcutaneous fat necrosis of the newborn – facial nodule *AD 134:425–426, 1998*

METABOLIC DISEASES

Cutaneous calculus *BJD 75:1–11, 1963*

Ossifying fasciitis – red nodule of the nose *JAAD 37:357–361, 1997*

Osteoma cutis

NEOPLASTIC DISORDERS

Acrochordon

Actinic keratosis

Adenoid cystic carcinoma

Angiolipoma

Apocrine carcinoma *Cancer 71:375–381, 1993*

Apocrine hidrocystoma *AD 137:657–662, 2001*

Atypical fibroxanthoma *Cutis 51:47–48, 1993; Cancer 31:1541–1552, 1973; subcutaneous facial nodule AD 137:719–721, 2001*

Basal cell carcinoma – single or multiple *Acta Pathol Mibrobiol Scand 88A:5–9, 1980*

Basaloid follicular hamartoma *JAAD 27:237–240, 1992*

Blue nevus

CD 34+ fibrous papule of the nose *JAAD 35:342–345, 1996*

Chondroid syringoma – solitary papule *AD 125:1127–1132, 1989*

Clear cell acanthoma – pink papule *Stat Pearls July 13, 2020; Ann Dermatol Syphilol 89:361–371, 1962*

Clear cell hidradenoma (eccrine acrospiroma)

Cylindroma – red nodule *AD 129:495–500, 1993;* plum colored *AD 129:499–500, 1993*

Dermal dendrocytoma *AD 126:689–690, 1990*

Desmoplastic trichoepithelioma *J Cutan Pathol 17:45–52, 1990*

Eccrine hidroadenoma – dermal nodule with or without ulceration; face, scalp, anterior trunk *AD 97:651–661, 1968*

Eccrine poroma

Eccrine sweat gland carcinoma – face, scalp, palm *J Cutan Pathol 14:65–86, 1987*

Embryonal rhabdomyosarcoma *Ped Derm 15:403–405, 1998*

Epidermoid cyst

Epidermolytic acanthoma, solitary – keratotic papule *AD 101:220–223, 1970*

Epithelioid sarcoma – nose *J Cutan Pathol 27:186–190, 2000*

Facial neuroma

Fibrofolliculoma *JAAD 11:361–363, 1984; JAAD 17:493–496, 1987*

Fibrous papule of the face (nose) (angiofibroma) *JAAD 10:670–671, 1984*

Folliculosebaceous cystic hamartoma *JAAD 34:77–81, 1996; JAAD 32:814–816, 1995*

Hidradenoma, benign nodular *AD 140:609–614, 2004*

Hidradenoma papilliferum *JAAD 41:115–118, 1999*

Pigmented hidrocystoma of nasal epithelium (PHONE) *Dermatol Online J May 15, 2016*

Inverted follicular keratosis *J Clin Pathol 28:465–471, 1975*

Juvenile xanthogranuloma *Pediatr Ann 43:e22–24, 2014*

Kaposi's sarcoma *JAAD 41:860–862, 1999; JAAD 40:312–314, 1999; JAAD 38:143–175, 1998; Dermatology 190:324–326, 1995*

Keloid

Keratoacanthoma

Large cell acanthoma *Ann DV 143:118–123, 2016*

Leiomyoma – angiomyoma

Leukemia cutis *BJD 143:773–779, 2000*

Lichen planus-like keratosis

Lymphoepithelioma-like carcinoma (flesh-colored or red purple)

Lymphoma

Melanocytic nevus

Melanoma, including metastatic melanoma

Merkel cell carcinoma

Metastases

Microcystic adnexal carcinoma *Am J Dermatopathol 19:358–362, 1997*

Milia, including multiple eruptive milia – face, earlobe; *JAAD 37:353–356, 1997; Cutis 60:183–184, 1997; Clin Exp Dermatol 21:58–60, 1996*

Mixed tumor of the face *J Dermatol 23:369–371, 1996*

Multinucleate cell angiohistiocytoma *BJD 133:308–310, 1995*

Multiple myeloma *AD 139:475–486, 2003*

Neurofibroma

Neurothekeoma – red nodule of face, nose *J Drugs Dermatol 11:252–255, 2012; AD 139:531–536, 2003*

Osteonevus of Wanta *J Craniofac Surg 27:e543–544, 2016*

Palisaded encapsulated neuroma (solitary circumscribed) *Int J Surg Pathol 27:506–515, 2019; AD 125:386–389, 1989*

Perifollicular fibroma *Ann Dermatol 23:236–238, 2011; AD 100:66–69, 1969*

Pilar sheath acanthoma – umbilicated skin colored papule with central keratinous plug of moustache area *AD 114:1495–1497, 1978*

Pilar tumor of nose *Cutis 36:251–252, 1985*

Pilomatrixoma *Curr Prob Derm 14:41–70, 2002; Pediatr Rev 11 (9):262–267, 1990; Cancer 45:2368–2373, 1980*

Porocarcinoma *AD 136:1409–1414, 2000*

Rhabdomyomatous mesenchymal hamartoma *Am J Dermatopathol 11:58–63, 1989*

Rhabdomyosarcoma *Curr Prob Derm 14:41–70, 2002; JAAD 30:243–249, 1994; AD 124:1687, 1988*

Schwannoma, superficial malignant *J Laryngol Otol 103:316–318, 1989*

Sebaceous carcinoma *Br J Ophthalmol 82:1049–1055, 1998; Br J Plast Surg 48:93–96, 1995; JAAD 25:685–690, 1991; J Derm Surg Oncol 11:260–264, 1985;* papule *Eyelid and Conjunctival Tumors, Shields JA and Shields CL, Lippincott Williams and Wilkins, 1999, p.40–41;* morpheic plaque, blepharitis *JAAD 14:668–673, 1986*

Sebaceous hyperplasia

Seborrheic keratosis

Solitary fibrous tumor of the skin – facial nodule *JAAD 46:S37–40, 2002*

Spitz nevus – *Pediatr Rev 11 (9):262–267, 1990*

Squamous cell carcinoma

Striated muscle hamartoma *AD 136:1263–1268, 2000; Ped Derm 16:65–67, 1999; Ped Derm 3:153–157, 1986*

Superficial epithelioma with sebaceous differentiation *Acta DV Alp Pannonica Adriat 26:63–66, 2017*

Syringocystadenoma papilliferum – solitary papule

Syringoma *Am J Dermatopathol 17:465–470, 1995*

Trichilemmal carcinoma *JAAD 36:1021–1023, 1997*

Trichilemmoma

Trichoblastic fibroma *AD 131:198–201, 1995*

Trichodiscoma *J Cut Pathol 31:398–400, 2004*

Trichoepithelioma

Trichofolliculoma

Tumor of follicular infundibulum *JAAD 33:979–984, 1995*

Verrucous acanthoma

Warty dyskeratoma *Iran J Public Health 43:1145–1147, 2014*

PRIMARY CUTANEOUS DISEASES

Acne rosacea *AD 134:679–683, 1998*

Acne vulgaris

Granuloma faciale *Stat Pearls Jan 20, 2020*

SYNDROMES

Behcet's syndrome – erythema nodosum; nodule *AD 138:467–471, 2002*

Carney complex – myxoma

Cri du chat syndrome (chromosome 5, short arm deletion syndrome) – premature greying of the hair, pre-auricular skin tag with low-set malformed ears *J Pediatr 102:528–533, 1983*

Muir-Torre syndrome – sebaceous adenomas, sebaceous carcinomas, keratoacanthomas *Curr Prob Derm 14:41–70, 2002; BJD 136:913–917, 1997; JAAD 33:90–104, 1995; JAAD 10:803, 1984*

Proteus syndrome – facial nodule

Sakati syndrome – patchy alopecia with atrophic skin above ears, submental linear scars, acrocephalopolysyndactyly, short limbs, congenital heart disease, abnormally shaped low-set ears, ear tag, short neck with low hairline *J Pediatr 79:104–109, 1971*

Wolf-Hirschhorn syndrome – del (4p) syndrome – preauricular tag or dimple, craniofacial asymmetry, mental and growth retardation, eye lesions, cleft lip and palate, cardiac defects *Eur J Hum Genet 8:519–526, 2000*

TRAUMA

Cold panniculitis (Haxthausen's disease) *Burns Incl Therm Inj 14:51–52, 1988; AD 94:720–721, 1966; BJD 53:83–89, 1941;* popsicle panniculitis *Pediatr Emerg Care 8:91–93, 1992*

Extruding tooth – white papule *Cutis 54:253–254, 1994*

Granuloma fissuratum of the nose *AD 97:34–37, 1968*

VASCULAR DISORDERS

Angiofibroma *JAAD 38:143–175, 1998*

Angioleiomyoma *JAAD 38:143–175, 1998*

Angiolymphoid hyperplasia with eosinophilia – papules and/or nodules along hairline *AD 136:837–839, 2000;* angiofibroma like lesions *JAAD 12:781–796, 1985*

Angiomatous nevus

Hemangioma

Hemangiopericytoma

Hobnail hemangioma – vascular papules of the nose *BJD 146:162–164, 2002*

Kimura's disease – periauricular or submandibular subcutaneous nodule *JAAD 38:143–175, 1998*

Microvenular hemangioma *Dermatol Pract Concept 31:7–11, 2018*

Polyangiitis with granulomatosis

Pyogenic granuloma

Spindle cell hemangioendothelioma – pink papule of nose *AD 138:259–264, 2002*

Tufted angioma

PAPULES, FLAT-TOPPED

AUTOIMMUNE DISEASES AND DISEASES OF IMMUNE DYSFUNCTION

Allergic contact dermatitis – lichenoid eruptions due to p-phenylene-diamine in color developers *Contact Dermatitis 10:280–285, 1984;* nickel allergic contact dermatitis in children with lichenoid id eruption *Ped Derm 19:106–109, 2002*

Chronic graft vs host disease – lichen planus-like eruption *Ped Derm 35:343–353, 2018*

Dermatomyositis – Gottron's papules and papules over joints *Dermatol Online J Dec 30, 2005*

Good syndrome – adult acquired primary immunodeficiency in context of past or current thymoma; sinopulmonary infections; lichen planus, oral lichen planus of tongue, gingivitis, oral erosions *BJD 172:774–777, 2015; Am J Med Genet 66:378–398, 1996*

Graft vs. host disease, acute of adult – macular erythema starts on face, neck and shoulders, becomes generalized; may become lichenoid or bullous *Rook p. 2756, 1998, Sixth Edition*; chronic – lichen planus-like eruptions; lichen sclerosus-like eruptions; plantar erythema, TEN-like erosions, flat-topped papules *Ped Derm 30:335–341, 2013; JAAD 66:515–532, 2012; AD 126:1324–1329, 1990; AD 132:1161–1163, 1996; JAAD 38:369–392, 1998; AD 134:602– 612, 1998*

Influenza vaccine – widespread lichenoid eruption *J Drugs Dermatol 13:873–875, 2014*

Lichen planus pemphigoides – bullae and flat topped papules *Cutis 100:415–418, 2017; BJD 171:1230–1235, 2014; Ped Derm 26:569–574, 2009*

Pemphigus foliaceus presenting as multiple seborrheic keratoses *JAAD 11:299–300, 1984*

Rheumatoid arthritis – velvet hands; papules *J Dermatol 22:324–329, 1995*

Severe combined immunodeficiency syndrome – desquamative erythematous, morbilliform or vesiculopapular eruption of newborn (3 weeks); erythroderma, seborrheic dermatitis-like eruption; morbilliform eruptions, lichen planus-like eruptions, dermatitis; mutations in cytokine common gamma chain, JAK3, RAG1 or RAG2, IL-7Rgamma, adenosine deaminase *JAAD 66:292–311, 2012; Ped Derm 26:213–214, 2009; AD 144:342–346, 2008; Dermatol Therapy 18:176–183, 2005; Ped Derm 17:91–96, 2000; AD 136:875–880, 2000; J Pediatr 123:564–572, 1993; Ped Derm 8:314–321, 1991*

Still's disease in the adult – brown coalescent scaly papules; persistent psoriasiform papular lesions *JAAD 52:1003–1008, 2005*; persistent pruritic flat-topped papules *Aem Arthr Rheum 42:317–326, 2012*

DRUG-INDUCED

Anti-PD-1 therapy (nivolumab/pembrolizumab – lichenoid eruptions, vitiligo, dermatitis, red papules with scale, red papules and nodules, inflammation surrounding seborrheic keratosis, dyshidrosiform palmar lesions, penile erosions *JAMA Derm 152:1128–1136, 2016; JAAD 74:455–461, 2016*

BCG vaccination – lichenoid and red papules and papulopustules *Ped Derm 13:451–454, 1996*; lichenoid eruption after BCG vaccine (lichen scrofulosorum-like) *JAAD 21:1119–1122, 1989*

Captopril lichen planus – personal observation

Checkpoint inhibitors – lichenoid eruptions *JAAD 80:990–997, 2019*

Crizotinib-induced lichenoid eruption *Cutis 102:403–406, 2018*

Influenza vaccine – widespread lichenoid eruption *J Drugs Dermatol 13:873–875, 2014; Dermatology 221:296–299, 2010; J Drugs Dermatol 29:1067–1069, 2011*

Kit and BCR-ABL inhibitors – imatinib, nilotinib, dasatinib – facial edema morbilliform eruptions, pigmentary changes, lichenoid reactions, psoriasis, pityriasis rosea, pustular eruptions, DRESS, Stevens-Johnson syndrome, urticarial, neutrophilic dermatoses, photosensitivity, pseudolymphoma, porphyria cutanea tarda, small vessel vasculitis, panniculitis, perforating folliculitis, erythroderma *JAAD 72:203–218, 2015*

Lichenoid drug eruption *SKINmed 10:373–383, 2012*; amiphenazole, captopril, gold *AD 109:372–376, 1974*; isoniazid, levamisole *J R Soc Med 73:208–211, 1980*; levopromazine, methyldopa, metropromazine, propranolol, exprenolol, labetalol

(beta-blockers), chlorpropamide, enalapril, pyrimethamine *Clin Exp Dermatol 5:253–256, 1980*; antimalarials, quinidine, penicillamine, thiazide diuretics, streptomycin, hydroxyurea, tiopronin, naproxen, carbamazepine, ethambutol, simvastatin, PAS, pravastatin *JAAD 29:249–255, 1993; Cutis 61:98–100, 1998*; glyburide *Cutis 76:41–45, 2005*; photo-induced lichen planus (demeclocycline *AD 109:97–98, 1974*) oral LP, and contact LP; quinacrine – lichenoid dermatitis *JAAD 4:239–248, 1981*; quinine – lichenoid photodermatitis *Clin Exp Dermatol 19:246–248, 1994*; hepatitis B vaccine *JAAD 45:61–615, 2001*; indomethacin, naproxen, fenclofenac, diflunisal, flurbiprofen, ibuprofen, benoxaprofen, aspirin, salsalate *JAAD 45:616–619, 2001*; amlodipine *BJD 144:920–921, 2001*; hydroxyurea *JAAD 36:178–182, 1997*; arsenicals, dapsone, furosemide, methyldopa, penicillamine, phenytoin, streptomycin, sulfonylurea, thiazides; amlodipine *BJD 144:920–921, 2001*; p-aminosalicylic acid, griseofulvin, ketoconazole, tetracyclines, trovofloxacin, labetalol, doxazosin, prazosin, chloroquine, hydroxychloroquine, quinidine, amitriptyline, chlorpromazine, imipramine, laevonepromazine, lorazepam, clonazepam, diazepam, temazepam, methopromazine, phenytoin, furosemide, spironolactone, tolazamide, tolbutamide, gold salts, arsenic, bismuth, mercury, palladium, sulindac, allopurinol, amiphenazole, cinnarizine, cyanamide, dapsone, gemfibrozil, hydroxyurea, interferon-alpha, iodides, lithium, mercaptopropionylglycine, mesalamine, methyracan, nifedipine, omeprazole, penicillamine, procainamide, pyrimethamine, pyrithioxin, simvastatin, quinine, sulfasalazine, trihexyphenidyl; dactinomycin *Ped Derm 23:503–506, 2006*; infliximab *AD 138:1258–1259, 2002*; terazosin – photolichenoid dermatitis *BJD 158:426–427, 2008*; tumor necrosis factor alpha antagonists – lichen planus-like eruptions *JAAD 61:104–111, 2009*; tricyclic antidepressants, HIV medications, carbamazepine, oxcarbazepine, phenytoin, valproate sodium, insulin, aspirin, fenclofenac, ibuprofen, rofecoxib, lithium, dactinomycin, thyroxine, rifampin, cimetidine, ranitidine, omeprazole *Ped Derm 26:458–464, 2009*; guanfacine *Ped Derm 31:614–615, 2014*; imatinib mesylate – hyperpigmented flat-topped papules of trunk and lips *Cutis 99:189–192, 2017*

EXOGENOUS AGENTS

Fire corals – urticarial lesions followed by vesiculobullous rash, chronic granulomatous and lichenoid lesions *Contact Dermatitis 29:285–286, 1993; Int J Dermatol 30:271–273, 1991*

Hydrocarbon (tar) keratosis – flat-topped papules of face and hands; keratoacanthoma-like lesions on scrotum *JAAD 35:223–242, 1996*

Jellyfish, coral, and sea urchin spines – pruritic lichenoid papules and plaques; linear flagellate patterns *Am Fam Physician 40:97–106, 1989*

Sweet vermouth – oral lichenoid eruption *Dermatitis 29:89–91, 2018*

INFECTIONS AND INFESTATIONS

AIDS – pruritic papular eruption of AIDS; firm discrete red, hyperpigmented urticarial papules *JAMA 292:2614–2621, 2004*; mucinosis of HIV disease *Clin Exp Dermatol 35:801–802, 2010; BJD 1077–1080, 1998*

Coxsackie A16 – Gianotti-Crosti-like rash *JAAD 6:862–866, 1982*

Dengue fever – hyperpigmentation of nose (chik sign); transient flushing, purpuric lesions, scleral injection, morbilliform exanthem with circular islands of sparing, aphthous ulcers, lichenoid papules, flagellated pigmentation, urticarial lesions, erythema multiforme-like *Ped Derm 36:737–739, 2019; Indian Dermatol Online J 8:336–342, 2017; Indian J DV Leprol 76:671–676, 2010*

Dermatophytid *Pediatr 128:e453–457, 2011*

Emmonsia pasteuriana – dimorphic fungus; disseminated infection in South Africa; lichenoid diffuse papulosquamous eruption; crusted verrucous facial nodules and plaques *NEJM 369:1416–1424, 2013*

Epidermodysplasia verruciformis *JAAD 76:1161–1175, 2017; BJD 175:803–806, 2016; JAAD 74:437–451, 2016; Cutis 96:114–118, 2015; Ped Derm 20:176–178, 2003; AD 131:1312–1318, 1995; BJD 121:463–469, 1989; Arch Dermatol Res 278:153–160, 1985; Arch Dermatol Syphilol 141:193–203, 1922;* acquired epidermodysplasia verruciformis of HIV – flat topped papules of hand, forehead, scalp *JAMA Derm 150:327–328, 2014; AD 146:903–905, 2010;* lichen planus-like appearance *Summer AAD Meeting, New York, New York;* acquired epidermodysplasia verruciformis in HIV disease – lichenoid hyperpigmented, pink flat warts, tinea versicolor-like *Dermatol Surg 39:974–980, 2013; Clin Inf Dis 54:e119–123, 2012; AD 148:128–130, 2012; AD 147:590–596, 2011; JAAD 60:315–320, 2009;* hypopigmented guttate macules in immunocompromised patients *JAAD 76:1161–1175, 2017; JAAD 74:437–451, 2016;* flat topped red papules of face *J Drugs Dermatol 15:350–352, 2016;* epidermodysplasia verruciformis with squamous cell carcinoma; *TMC6, TMC8, RHOH, CORO1A, IL-7, MST-1 JAAD 56:882–886, 2007;* flat-topped red papules of face *J Drugs Dermatol 15:350–352, 2016*

Gianotti-Crosti syndrome (papular acrodermatitis of childhood) *Ped Derm 28:733–734, 2011; JAAD 65:876–877, 2011; JAAD 51:606–624, 2004; Cutis 67:291–294, 2001; Am J Dermatopathol 22:162–165, 2000; JAAD 18:239–259, 1988*

HIV-1 dermatitis – lichenoid photodermatitis *JAAD 28:167–173, 1993*

Leprosy *Indian J DV Leprol 84:703–705, 2018*

Milker's nodule – starts as flat red papule on fingers or face, progresses to red-blue tender nodule, which crusts; zone of erythema; may resemble pyogenic granulomas *AD 111:1307–1311, 1975*

Mycobacteria chelonae – flat-topped papules *JAAD 62:501–506, 2010*

Mycobacterium tuberculosis – lichen scrofulosorum – yellow to red-brown flat-topped papules, slightly scaly, surmounted with minute pustule; trunk *Dermatol Clin 33:541–562, 2015; AD 142:385–390, 2006; Ped Derm 19:122–126, 2002; Am J Clin Dermatol 3:319–328, 2002; Ped Derm 17:373–376, 2000; AD 124:1421–1426, 1988; Clin Exp Dermatol 1:391–394, 1976;* lichen scrofulosorum – red, lichenoid, firm follicular and parafollicular papules; resemble keratosis pilaris, lichen nitidus, lichen spinulosus, or pityriasis rubra pilaris *BJD 136:483–489, 1997;* miliary tuberculosis *JAAD 50:S110–113, 2004*

Onchocerciasis (*Onchocerca volvulus*) – chronic dermatitis with flat-topped papules *JAAD 73:929–944, 2015*

Phaeohyphomycosis – seborrheic keratosis-like lesion *AD 123:1597–1598, 1987*

Syphilis – secondary; lichenoid papules *JAAD 82:1–14, 2020; NEJM 374:372, 2016*

Warts, flat *Dermatol Onlin J 25 (3)13030/qt19g49405 March 15, 2019*

INFILTRATIVE DISEASES

Acral papular mucinosis *JAAD 51:982–988, 2004*

Amyloidosis – hemodialysis-induced cutaneous amyloid – lichenoid papules *BJD 128:686–689, 1993;* lichen amyloid *BJD 161:1217–1224, 2009;* beta-2 microglobulin amyloidosis – shoulder pain, carpal tunnel syndrome, flexor tendon deposits of hands, lichenoid papules, hyperpigmentation, subcutaneous nodules (amyloidomas) *Int J Exp Clin Invest 4:187–211, 1997*

Benign cephalic histiocytosis – red-brown papules of cheeks, forehead, earlobes, neck *Ped Derm 36:411–413, 2019; Ped Derm 11:265–267, 1994; Ped Derm 6:198–201, 1989; AD 122:1038–43, 1986; JAAD 13:383–404, 1985;* flat topped papules of face *Int J Dermatol 57:529–530, 2018*

Erdheim-Chester disease (non-Langerhans cell histiocytosis) – CD68+ and factor XIIIa+; negative for CD1a and S100; flat wart-like papules of face *AD 143:952–953, 2007*

Focal mucinosis – solitary asymptomatic skin colored to white papule, nodule or plaque anywhere on body or oral mucosa *An Bras Dermatol 94:334–336, 2019*

Juvenile xanthogranuloma (generalized lichenoid juvenile xanthogranuloma) – face, neck, scalp, upper trunk *BJD 126:66–70, 1992*

Langerhans cell histiocytosis – Letterer-Siwe disease *Curr Prob Derm 14:41–70, 2002; JAAD 13:481–496, 1985; Acta DV 61:447–451, 1981*

Papular xanthoma – disseminated primary papular xanthoma *AD 143:667–669, 2007*

Scleromyxedema (papular mucinosis, lichen myxedematosis) *Case Rep Dermatol 11:64–70, 2019; Int J Dermatol 53:971–974, 2014; JAAD 33:37–43, 1995*

Self-healing reticulohistiocytosis – hypopigmented flat topped papules *J Med Assoc Thai 97:993–997, 2014*

Verruciform xanthoma of scrotum – red or yellow flat-topped papules *J Dermatol 16:397–401, 1989*

INFLAMMATORY DISEASES

Chronic erythema multiforme – personal observation

Sarcoidosis *JAAD 66:699–716, 2012; JAAD 51:606–624, 2004; Ped Derm 20:416–418, 2003; Ped Derm 18:384–387, 2001; AD 133:882–888, 1997; Cutis 20:651–658, 1977;* pigmented purpuric dermatosis-like *J Dermatol 42:629–631, 2015*

METABOLIC DISORDERS

Zinc deficiency in HIV disease – personal observation

NEOPLASTIC DISEASES

Atrial myxoma *J Dermatol 22:600–605, 1995*

Basal cell carcinoma – single or multiple *Stat Pearls Dec 16, 2019 PMID 29494046; Acta Pathol Mibrobiol Scand 88A:5–9, 1980*

Bowen's disease, including pigmented Bowen's disease *JAAD 23:440–444, 1990;* vulvar *Ann DV 109:811–812, 1982; Cancer 14:318–329, 1961*

Bowenoid papulosis (penile intraepithelial neoplasia) – hyperpigmented flat topped papules of penis *Cutis 102:151–152,4, 2018; AD 147:1001–1002, 2011; Cancer 57:823–836, 1986;* vulvar verrucous, lichenoid, dry, brown, whitish papules or plaques *Cancer 57:823–836, 1986*

Epidermal nevus, including divided epidermal nevi *JAAD 29:281–282, 1993*

Epidermolytic acanthoma *Case Rep Dermatol 9:98–101, 2017*

Fibroepithelioma of Pinkus – flat-topped, gray-brown or hypopigmented papule *JAAD 52:168–169, 2005*

Giant lymph node hyperplasia – Castleman's disease

Intraepidermal epithelioma of Borst-Jadassohn *AD 131:1329–1334, 1995*

Juvenile xanthogranulomas – lichenoid JXGs *Ped Derm 26:238–240, 2009*

Large cell acanthomas – white to red flat-topped papules *JAAD 53:335–337, 2005; JAAD 8:840–845, 1983*

Lichen planus-like keratosis *AD 116:780–782, 1980; Dermatologica 132:386–392, 1966*

Leukemia – HTLV-1 lymphoma/leukemia *J Cutan Pathol 45:171–175, 2018; J Dermatol 42:967–974, 2015; Int J Dermatol 47:359–362, 2008;* T-cell prolymphocytic leukemia *J Dermatol 46:65–69, 2019*

Lymphoma – cutaneous T-cell lymphoma – lichenoid papules *JAAD 23:653–662, 1990;* CTCL resembling keratosis lichenoides chronica *JAAD 47:914–918, 2002; BJD 138:1067–1069, 1998;* HTLV-1 leukemia/lymphoma – multiple papules, cobblestoned skin *JAMA Derm 151:443–444, 2015*

Multinucleated atypia of the vulva – white flat-topped papules *Cutis 75:118–120, 2005*

Multinucleate cell angiohistiocytoma *Clin Exp Dermatol 35:e203–204, 2010; Cutis 59:190–192, 1997*

Nevus anelasticus *JAAD 51:165–185, 2004*

Papular epidermal nevus with skyline basal cell layer (PENS) – flat topped hyperkeratotic papules, some annular *Ped Derm 33:296–300, 2016; JAAD 64:888–892, 2011*

Seborrheic keratoses, including stucco keratoses; familial hypochromatic seborrheic keratoses *SKINMed 15:77–78, 2017*

Syringomas, including eruptive syringomas *Iran J Public Health 48:1161–1164, 2019;* vulvar – lichenoid papules *JAAD 48:735–739, 2003*

Trichodiscomas – flat-topped papules of central face *JAAD 15:603–607, 1986*

Verrucous acanthomas

Vulvar intraepithelial neoplasia

PARANEOPLASTIC DISORDERS

Diffuse plane xanthomatosis – flat yellow plaques of eyelids, neck, trunk, buttocks, flexures *AD 93:639–646, 1966*

Lichenoid vasculitis associated with myeloproliferative disorders *BJD 145:359–360, 2001*

Paraneoplastic pemphigus – lichenoid lesions of non-mucosal surfaces *AD 141:1285–1293, 2005; BJD 150:1018–1024, 2004; BJD 149:1143–1151, 2003;* in children *BJD 147:725–732, 2002*

PHOTODERMATOSES

Actinic prurigo *Dermatol Clin 32:335–344, 2014*

Actinic reticuloid *Semin Diagn Pathol 8:109–116, 1991*

Disseminated superficial actinic porokeratosis *Stat Pearls Nov 13, 2019 PMID 29083728*

Juvenile spring eruption – pruritic papules on red ears *BJD 168:1066–172, 2013*

Lichen planus actinicus – personal observation

Polymorphous light eruption *JAAD 3:329–343, 1980*

PRIMARY CUTANEOUS DISEASES

Acanthosis nigricans

Acrokeratoelastoidosis of Costa *JAAD 12:832–836, 1985*

Acrokeratosis verruciformis of Hopf *Ped Derm 27:93–94, 2010; AD 141:515–520, 2005; AD 130:508–509, 511–512, 1994; Ann DV 115:1229–1232, 1988; Dermatol Zeitschr 60:227–250, 1931*

Aquagenic syringeal acrokeratoderma *JAAD 45:124–126, 2001*

Asteatotic dermatitis

Atopic dermatitis

Blaschkitis *J Cutan Pathol 41:950–954, 2014; An Bras Dermatol 86:142–143, 2011*

Clear cell papulosis – hypopigmented macules and slightly elevated 1–10 mm papules along milk line on lower abdomen and pubic area of young children *Dermatol Online J 24 (1) pii 13030 Jan 15, 2018; JAAD 63:266–273, 2010; AD 145:1066–1068, 2009;AD 143:358–360, 2007: Ped Derm 22:268–269, 2005; Ped Derm 14:380–382, 1997; Am J Surg Path 11:827–834, 1987*

Darier's disease *Int J Dermatol 40:278–280, 2001*

Epidermolysis bullosa – albopapuloid epidermolysis bullosa (Pasini variant) *JAAD 29:785–786, 1993;* simplex, Dowling-Meara; pretibial epidermolysis bullosa – lichenoid papules *JID 104:803–805, 1995;* dominant dystrophic epidermolysis bullosa; dystrophic epidermolysis bullosa pruriginosa – red, crusted, and lichenified papules *BJD 159:464–469, 2008*

Epidermolysis bullosa pruriginosa – flat topped papules, crusted papules, linear violaceous scars *SKINmed 11:308–309, 2013; Ped Derm 29:725–731, 2012; Indian J Dermatol Venereol Leprol 71:109–111, 2005; Indian J Dermatol Venereol Leprol 66:249–250, 2000*

Flegel's disease (hyperkeratosis lenticularis perstans) – 3 mm flat-topped hyperkeratotic generalized papules; hyperkeratotic pointy spicules of legs (chronic keratotic papules of extremities) *AD 144:1509–1514, 2008; Int J Dermatol 47 Suppl 1:38–41, 2008; AD 133:909–914, 1997; Acta DV 68:341–345, 1988; JAAD 16:190–195, 1987; Hautarzt 9:363–364, 1958*

Granuloma annulare, including generalized granuloma annulare

Hailey-Hailey disease – lichenoid papules of thighs *SKINMed 15:387–388, 2017*

Keratosis lichenoides chronica (Nekam's disease) – reticulated flat-topped keratotic papules, linear arrays, atrophy, comedo-like lesions, prominent telangiectasia; conjunctival injection, seborrheic dermatitis-like eruption; acral dermatitis over toes; punctate keratotic papules of palmar creases *Cutis 86:245–248, 2010; Ped Derm 26:615–616, 2009; AD 145:867–69, 2009; AD 144:405–410, 2008;JAAD 49:511–513, 2003; BJD 144:422–424, 2001; Dermatology 201:261–264, 2000; JAAD 38:306–309, 1998; JAAD 37:263–264, 1997; AD 131:609–614, 1995; AD 105:739–743, 1972; Presse Med 51:1000–1003, 1938; Arch Dermatol Syph (Berlin) 31:1–32, 1895;* in children *JAAD 56:S1–5, 2007*

Lichen nitidus *Stat Pearls Dec 3, 2019*

Lichen planus *Ped Derm 27:34–38, 2010;* lichen planus precipitated by radiation therapy *JAAD 46:604–605, 2002;* lichen planus actinicus – violaceous plaques of dorsal hands *JAMA Derm 151:1121–1122, 2015*

Lichen ruber moniliformis *AD 34:830–849, 1936*

Lichen sclerosus et atrophicus – extragenital simulating lichen planus *Indian J Dermatol 60:105, 2015*

Lichen simplex chronicus

Lichen spinulosis *JAAD 22 (pt 1)261–264, 1990*

Lichen striatus *Pediatr Child Health 23:260–261, 2018*

Mal de Meleda – autosomal dominant, autosomal recessive; lichenoid plaques; diffuse PPK; transgrediens with acral erythema in glove-like distribution; perioral erythema and hyperkeratosis;

hyperhidrosis; knuckle pads; pseudo-ainhum with amputation; lingua plicata, brachydactyly, syndactyly, hairy palms and soles, nail anomalies, high arched palate, lefthandedness; mutations in SLURP1 *Dermatology 203:7–13, 2001; AD 136:1247–1252, 2000; J Dermatol 27:664–668, 2000; Dermatologica 171:30–37, 1985*

Papular acantholytic dyskeratosis of the vulva *AD 148:755–760, 2012; Ped Derm 22:237–239, 2005; Am J Dermatopathol 6:557–560, 1984;* papular acantholytic dyskeratosis of the penis *J Dermatol 36:427–429, 2009; Am J Dermatopathol 8:365–366, 1986*

Papuloerythroderma of Ofuji *Stat Pearls Nov 15, 2019–2020; AD 127:96–98, 1991*

Perianal pseudoverrucous papules and nodules *Ped Derm 34:e3434, 2017; Indian J Sex Trans Dis AIDS 34:44–46, 2013*

Pigmented purpuric eruption – personal observation

Pityriasis lichenoides chronica (chronic guttate parapsoriasis) *Am J Clin Dermatol 8:29–36, 2007*

Pityriasis rosea – lichenoid papules at the edges of the lesions *S Afr Med J 30:210–218, 1956*

Pityriasis rubra pilaris – follicular or flat topped *Am J Clin Dermatol 19:377–379, 2018*

Progressive symmetric erythrokeratoderma – personal observation

Psoriasis – lichenoid variant of flexures *Br Med J ii:823–828, 1954;* keratoses in psoriatics on therapy *JAAD 23:52–55, 1990;* multiple benign eruptive keratoses in psoriatic treated with cyclosporine *JAAD 26:128–129, 1992*

Unilateral laterothoracic exanthem of childhood *AD 138:1371–1376, 2002*

SYNDROMES

Blau or Jabs syndrome (familial juvenile systemic granulomatosis) – autosomal dominant; onset under 4 years of age; generalized papular rash of infancy; translucent skin-colored papules (noncaseating granulomas) of trunk and extremities or dense lichenoid yellow to red-brown papules with grainy surface with anterior or panuveitis, synovitis, symmetric polyarthritis; polyarteritis, multiple synovial cysts; red papular rash in early childhood; exanthema resolves with pitted scars; camptodactyly (flexion contractures of PIP joints); no involvement of lung or hilar nodes; activating mutations in NOD2 (nucleotide-binding oligomerization domain 2) (caspase recruitment domain family, member 15; CARD 15) *Clin Exp Dermatol 44:811–813, 2019; Ped Rheumatol Online J Aug 6, 2014; Ped Derm 27:69–73, 2010; AD 143:386–391, 2007; Clin Exp Dermatol 21:445–448, 1996; J Pediatr 107:689–693, 1985*

Buschke-Ollendorff syndrome (dermatofibrosis lenticularis disseminata) – uniform, small lichenoid papules resembling pseudoxanthoma elasticum *AD 100:465–470, 1969*

Clouston's syndrome (hidrotic ectodermal dysplasia) – syringofibroadenomas – flat-topped coalescing papules (acral)

JAAD 40:259–262, 1999

Cowden's syndrome (multiple hamartoma syndrome) – trichilemmomas *Case Rep Dent 2013:315109; JAAD 11:1127–1141, 1984; AD 114:743–746, 1978*

Hereditary focal transgressive palmoplantar keratoderma – autosomal recessive; hyperkeratotic lichenoid papules of elbows and knees, psoriasiform lesions of scalp and groin, spotty and reticulate hyperpigmentation of face, trunk, and extremities, alopecia of eyebrows and eyelashes *BJD 146:490–494, 2002*

Multicentric reticulohistiocytosis – mimicking dermatomyositis *JAAD 48:S11–14, 2003*

POEMS syndrome – eruptive seborrheic keratoses *JAAD 19:979–982, 1988;* glomeruloid hemangiomas with Castleman's disease *Pathol Int 58:390–395, 2008; Indian J DV Leprol 74:364–366, 2008*

Trichoepitheliomas – solitary non-familial or multiple familial form *Acta DV Croat 26:162–165, 2018*

Van den Bosch syndrome – acrokeratosis verruciformis with anhidrosis, skeletal deformities, mental deficiency and choroideremia – X-linked recessive

Vohwinkel's syndrome – verruciform hyperkeratotic papules on dorsum of hand *Clin Dermatol 23:23–32, 2005*

Wiskott-Aldrich syndrome – flat warts

TOXINS

Arsenical keratoses *Cancer 21:312–339, 1968;* Bowen's disease, single or multiple lesions; arsenic toxicity due to contaminated ground water consumption; especially in Bangladesh and West Bengal, India; also in India, Argentina, China, Chile, Thailand, and Mexico *SkinMed 11:211–216, 2013*

TRAUMA

Frictional lichenoid dermatitis (Sutton's summer prurigo) *JAAD 51:606–624, 2004; Ped Derm 7:111–115, 1990; AD 94:592–593, 1966*

VASCULAR LESIONS

Lymphangioma circumscriptum *Iran J Public Health 48:1161–1164, 2019*

Pigmented purpuric eruption – lichenoid of Gougerot-Blum *AD 144:405–410, 2008*

Multifocal lymphangioendotheliomatosis – congenital appearance of hundreds of flat vascular papules and plaques associated with gastrointestinal bleeding, thrombocytopenia with bone and joint involvement; spontaneous resolution *J Pediatr Orthop 24:87–91, 2004*

Takayasu's arteritis – lichenoid chest papules *AD 123:796–800, 1987*

PAPULES, FOLLICULAR (FOLLICULOCENTRIC, INCLUDING FOLLICULITIS)

AUTOIMMUNE DISEASES AND DISEASES OF IMMUNE DYSFUNCTION

Allergic contact dermatitis to nickel with id reaction – follicular facial dermatitis *Ped Derm 28:276–280, 2011;* follicular contact dermatitis

Chronic granulomatous disease – scalp folliculitis *Dermatol Therapy 18:176–183, 2005; AD 130:105–110, 1994*

Contact dermatitis to nickel, polyoxyethylene lauryl-ether, formaldehyde, chrome, copper, fluoride, homomenthylsalicylate, methyl glucose sesquistearate *JAAD 42:879–880, 2000;* folliculitis *Contact Derm 32:309–310, 1995;* to tocopheryl linoleate *Dermatology 189:225–233, 1994;* to sodium fusidate *Contact Derm 23:186–187, 1990*

Cyclic neutropenia – folliculitis *Ped Derm 18:426–432, 2001; Am J Med 61:849–861, 1976*

Dermatomyositis – presenting as a pityriasis rubra pilaris- like eruption (type Wong dermatomyositis) – follicular hyperkeratotic papules of face, back of neck, trunk, linear lesions of backs of hands and feet, palms, soles in Chinese patients *Clin Dermatol 32:839–872, 2014; JAAD 43:908–912, 2000; BJD 136:768–771, 1997; BJD 81:544–547, 1969;* follicular hyperkeratosis *BJD 81:544, 1969;* juvenile dermatomyositis *Ped Derm 17:37–40, 2000;* follicular papules – phrynoderma and perforating folliculitis in dermatomyositis *JAMA Derm 150:891–892, 2014*

Graft vs. host disease, acute – red macules or folliculocentric papules of face, ears, palms and soles, periungual areas, upper back and neck *AD 143:67–71, 2007;* follicular papules *JAAD 38:369–392, 1998; AD 134:602–612, 1998; AD 124:688–691, 1442, 1988;* red plaque with follicular papules *AD 142:1237–1238, 2006;* chronic with follicular involvement *J Derm 20:242–246, 1993;* chronic – follicular keratosis and plugs *JAAD 72:690–695, 2015; AD 138:924–934, 2002;* keratosis pilaris-like GVHD *Biol Blood Marrow Transplant 12:1101–1113, 2006;* follicular GVHD *Indian J Dermatol 64:324–327, 2019*

IL-10 defects – folliculitis *BJD 178:335–349, 2018*

IL-17 deficiency – folliculitis *BJD 178:335–349, 2018;*

Job's syndrome (hyper IgE syndrome) – autosomal dominant or sporadic; atrophoderma vermiculatum; coarse facial features with broad nose, rough thickened skin with prominent follicular ostia; papular and papulopustular folliculitis-like eruptions; oral candidiasis; chronic paronychia; cold abscesses of neck and trunk; otitis media common; mutation in *STAT3* (transcription 3 gene activator and signal transducer *JAAD 65:1167–1172, 2011*

Linear IgM dermatosis of pregnancy *JAAD 18:412–415, 1988*

Lupus erythematosus – systemic lupus – hyperkeratotic follicular papules of trunk and extremities in Chinese; discoid lupus erythematosus – umbilicated papular eruption of the back with acneiform hypertrophic follicular scars *BJD 87:642–649, 1972;* subacute lupus erythematosus *JAAD 35:147–169, 1996;* follicular erythema and petechiae in SLE *BJD 147:157–158, 2002;* papular mucinosis of SLE – perifollicular skin colored to red papules *AD 146:789–794, 2010; JAAD 27:312–315, 1992; BJD 66:429–433, 1954;* atypical acneiform and comedonal plaque *Lupus 27:853–857, 2018*

NLRP 1-associated autoinflammatory arthritis and dyskeratosis – phrynoderma; increased caspase 1 function; increased IL-18 *Ped Derm 33:602–614, 2016*

Rheumatoid vasculitis – folliculitis *JAAD 53:191–209, 2005*

DRUG-INDUCED

Allopurinol and timedium-induced eosinophilic pustular folliculitis *JAAD 54:729–730, 2006*

Antiepidermal growth factor receptor antibody C225 *BJD 144:1169–1176, 2001;* other antiepidermal growth factor receptor antibody *J Clin Oncol 20:2240–2250, 2002*

Anti-epileptic drugs – acne keloidalis-like lesions *Int J Derm 29:559–560, 1990*

Carbamazepine – eosinophilic pustular folliculitis *JAAD 38:641–643, 1998*

CD 30+ lymphomatoid drug reaction *Am J Dermatopathol 39:e62–65, 2019*

Certolizumab – folliculitis-like, lichenoid sarcoid *Case Rep Dermatol 11:158–163, 2017*

Cetuximab (epidermal growth factor receptor inhibitor) – follicular papules and pustules *BJD 161:515–521, 2009; JAAD 58:545–570, 2008; JAAD 55:429–437, 2006; AD 138:129–131, 2002*

Chemotherapy-induced eosinophilic pustular folliculitis *JAAD 54:729–730, 2006*

Corticosteroid folliculitis *Int J Derm 37:772–777, 1998*

Cyclophosphamide – folliculitis of face and chest *JAAD 65:657–659, 2011*

Cyclosporine –hyperplastic pseudofolliculitis barbae *BJD 136:132–133, 1997; Dermatologica 172:24–30, 1986;* folliculitis *Hautarzt 44:521–523, 1993;* tufted folliculitis *AD 142:251–252, 2006;* keratosis pilaris *Dermatologica 172:24–31, 1986*

Dabrafenib – folliculitis *JAMA Derm 151:1103–1109, 2015*

Doxorubicin – polyethylene glycol-coated liposomal doxorubicin; scaly erythema with follicular accentuation *AD 136:1475–1480, 2000;* doxorubicin/daunorubicin – follicular rash *JAAD 71:203–214, 2014*

DRESS syndrome (drug reaction with eosinophilia and systemic symptoms) – facial edema, exfoliative dermatitis, follicular eruptions; association with HHV-6; lymphadenopathy, circulating atypical lymphocytes, abnormal liver function tests *AD 137:301–304, 2001*

Drug eruption, multiple agents

Epidermal growth factor receptor inhibitors – follicular papules, pustules, acneiform eruption *JAAD 56:460–465, 2007*

Erlotinib (epidermal growth factor receptor inhibitor) – papules and pustules *J Drugs in Dermatol 13:1410–1411, 2014; BJD 161:515–521, 2009; JAAD 58:545–570, 2008; JAAD 55:429–437, 2006;* after discontinuation of erlotinib *J Drugs Dermatol 13:1410–1411, 2014*

Etanercept – perforating folliculitis *BJD 156:368–371, 2007*

5-fluorouracil – forehead folliculitis *JAAD 25:905–908, 1991*

Gefitinib – follicular papulopustular eruptions *JAAD 58:545–570, 2008*

Human granulocyte colony stimulating factor – folliculitis *AD 134:111–112, 1998; BJD 127:193–194, 1992*

Infliximab – perforating folliculitis *BJD 156:368–371, 2007*

Isotretinoin – pseudofolliculitis – personal observation

Lithium – follicular hyperkeratosis *Clin Exp Derm 21:296–298, 1996*

Minocycline-induced eosinophilic pustular folliculitis *JAAD 54:729–730, 2006*

Nivolumab – lichen nitidus-like eruption *JAMA Derm 154:367–369, 2018*

Phenytoin hypersensitivity – follicular accentuation *AD 114:1350–1353, 1978*

Ponitinib – pityriasis rubra pilaris-like changes, eyebrow thinning, ichthyosiform changes *BJD 173:574–577, 2015*

RAF inhibitors (MAPK pathway) – vemurafenib and dabrafenib – exanthema warts and other hyperkeratotic lesions, keratoacanthomas, squamous cell carcinoma, melanocytic nevi, keratosis pilaris, seborrheic dermatitis, hyperkeratotic hand-foot reactions, photosensitivity, panniculitis with arthralgias, alopecia *JAAD 72:221–236, 2015*

Smallpox vaccination – focal and generalized folliculitis *JAMA 289:3290–3294, 2003*

Sorafenib – keratosis pilaris lesions *JAAD 71:217–227, 2014; JAAD 61:360–361, 2009;* red scaly plaque with follicular papules (pityriasis rubra pilaris-like) *JAAD 65:452–453, 2011*

Trametinib – folliculitis *Ped Derm 34:90–94, 2017; JAMA Derm 151:1103–1109, 2015*

Vemurafenib (BRAF inhibitor) – erythematous eruption with spiny keratosis pilaris *BJD 169:934–938, 2013;* cystic lesions of face, hidradenitis suppurativa, keratosis pilaris-like eruptions, eruptive melanocytic nevi; hyperkeratotic plantar papules, squamous cell carcinoma; multiple nodules of cheeks; follicular plugging; exuberant seborrheic dermatitis-like hyperkeratosis of face; hand and foot reaction; diffuse spiny follicular hyperkeratosis; cobblestoning of forehead *BJD 173:1024–1031, 2015; BJD 167:987–994, 2012; AD 148:1428–1429, 2012; JAAD 67:1375–1379, 2012; AD 148:357–361, 2012*

EXOGENOUS AGENTS

Antimony melting workers – folliculitis *J Occup Med 35:39–44, 1993*

Automotive oil folliculitis – personal observation

Bone marrow autograft – eosinophilic folliculitis *Cancer 73:2512–2514, 1994*

Chloracne – folliculitis of thighs and forearms *Clin Exp Derm 18:523–525, 1993*

Coal tar products – pitch, asphalt, creosote – diffuse melanosis of exposed skin; evolves to atrophy, telangiectasia, lichenoid papules, follicular keratosis; tar keratoses *Clin Dermatol 32:839–872, 2014*

Contact epilating folliculitis *Cutis 54:12–13, 1994*

Exogenous ochronosis (follicular accentuation) *JAAD 19:942–946, 1988; JAAD 10:1072–1073, 1984; BJD 93:613–622m 1975*

Fiberglass dermatitis *Kao Hsiung I Hsueh 12:491–494, 1996*

Irritant folliculitis

Localized perifollicular cold urticaria *JAAD 26:306–308, 1992*

Mineral oils – folliculitis

Mudi-chood – due to oils applied to hair; papulosquamous eruption of nape of neck and upper back; begin as follicular pustules then brown-black papules with keratinous rim *Int J Dermatol 31:396–397, 1992*

Oil field mud – calcinosis cutis from percutaneous penetration of oil field drilling mud *JAAD 12:172–175, 1985*

Synthetic opioid MT-45 – painful intertrigo, folliculitis, dry eyes, hair depigmentation, hair loss, Mees' lines, abnormal liver function tests *BJD 176:1021–1027, 2017*

Organochlorine exposure (agent orange) – chloracne with comedones, gray dyschromia, hypertrichosis, folliculitis, porphyria cutanea tarda, melanoma and non-melanoma skin cancer, non-Hodgkin's lymphoma, dermatofibrosarcoma protuberans *JAAD 74:143–170, 2016*

Polycyclic hydrocarbons – folliculitis *G Ital Med Lav Ergon 19:152–163, 1997*

Sock – hemorrhagic folliculitis – personal observation

Sugar cane worker folliculitis *Cutis 54:12–13, 1994*

Synthetic sport shorts folliculitis *Arch Ped Adolesc Med 148:1230–1231, 1994*

Tar keratosis *Clin Dermatol 32:839–872, 2014*

INFECTIONS AND INFESTATIONS

Aeromonas hydrophila folliculitis – mimicking hot tub folliculitis *Ped Derm 26:601–603, 2009;* due to inflatable swimming pool *Australas J Dermatol 49:39–41, 2008*

AIDS – pruritic follicular papular eruption of HIV disease *Int J Derm 32:784–789, 1993;* AIDS-associated eosinophilic pustular folliculitis *NEJM 318:1183–1186, 1988; Sex Transm Infec 4 (3):229–230, 1987;* necrotizing folliculitis in AIDS *BJD 116:581–584, 1987;* HIV-associated follicular syndrome – acne, pityriasis rubra pilaris-like lesions and follicular spicules *BJD 179;774–775, 2018Ancylostoma caninum* larvae folliculitis *AD 127:247–250, 1991*

Bacterial folliculitis, usually Staphylococcal *J Dermatol25:563–568, 1998*

Brucellosis – contact brucellosis

Candidiasis, disseminated – nodular folliculitis; Candida folliculitis mimicking tinea barbae *Int J Derm 36:295–297, 1997; Candida krusei* in acute myelogenous leukemia – fever, neutropenia, disseminated folliculocentric eruption *Dermatol Online J Nov 18, 2015*

Citrobacter freundii – folliculitis, cellulitis, ecthyma, ulcers, red plaque with central ulceration and caseation *AD 143:124–125, 2007*

Cheyletiella dermatitis *AD 116:435–437, 1980*

Clostridium perfringens – facial folliculitis *Clin Inf Dis 26:501–502, 1998*

Coccidioidomycosis *Clin Exp Dermatol 43:336–338, 2018*

Cryptococcosis *Clin Dermatol 32:839–872, 2014*

Cutaneous larva migrans – folliculitis *BJD 146:314–316, 2002;* folliculotropic papules *Int J Dermatol 52:327–330, 2013*

Demodex folliculitis *Am J Dermatopathol 20:536–537, 1998; J Med Assoc Thai 74:116–119, 1991; JAAD 21:81–84, 1989;* of scalp *Cutis 76:321–324, 2005;* papulo-pustular rosacea and demodicidosis *Acta DV 99:47–52, 2019*

Dermatophytids – associated with kerion; widespread eruption follicular papules sometimes with keratotic spines *J Dermatol 21:31–34, 1994*

Ebola hemorrhagic fever – perifollicular papules *JAAD 75:1–16, 2016*

Epidermodysplasia verruciformis – brown follicular papules in GVHD *JAAD 37:578–580, 2007*

Erysipelothrix rhusiopathiae – rare systemic form with perifollicular papules

Gram negative folliculitis complicating acne therapy *Fortschr Med 115:42–44, 1997*

Herpes simplex infection – sycosis, folliculitis *AD 113:983–986, 1997*

Herpes zoster – red plaque with follicular prominence *AD 113:983–986, 1997;* verrucous follicular papules of face in patient with B-cell lymphoma *AD 148:405, 2012*

Histoplasmosis *AD 132:341–346, 1996*

Hot tub folliculitis – personal observation

Leishmaniasis – post kala-azar leishmaniasis – nodular *J Cutan Pathol 25:95–99, 1998*

Leprosy, histoid *Int J Dermatol 59:365–368, 2020*

Lupoid sycosis *BJD 138:199–200, 1998*

Measles *Clin Dermatol 32:839–872, 2014*

Merkel cell polyoma virus – widespread follicular papules; alopecia *BJD 175:1410, 2016*

Molluscum contagiosum *JAAD 51:478–479, 2004; AD 113:983–986, 1997; BJD 113:493–495, 1985*

Mycobacterium avium complex – traumatic inoculation folliculitis, *BJD 130:785–790, 1994*

Mycobacterium chelonae – folliculitis *Rev Clin Esp 196:606–609, 1996*

Mycobacterium fortuitum – folliculitis *An Bras Dermtol 88:102–104, 2013*

Mycobacterial infection, rapid growers (*M.fortuitum, M. chelonae, M. abscessus*) – folliculitis and/or furunculosis *BJD 152:727–734, 2005*

Mycobacterium tuberculosis – lichen scrofulosorum – red, lichenoid, firm follicular and parafollicular papules; resemble keratosis pilaris, lichen nitidus, lichen spinulosus, or pityriasis rubra pilaris *Clin Exp Dermatol 42:369–372, 2017; SKINmed 10:28–33, 2012; Ped Derm 30:7–16, 2013; Am J Clin Dermatol 3:319–328, 2002; BJD 136:483–489, 1997;* acne scrofulosorum – follicular papules heal with scarring; domed papulopustular follicular lesions *Clin Exp*

Dermatol 6:339–344, 1981; BJD 7:341–351, 1895; lupus vulgaris presenting as granulomatous folliculitis *Int J Derm 28:388–392, 1989;* acute miliary, in AIDS *Eur J Clin Micro Infect Dis 14:911–914, 1995; JAAD 26:356–359, 1992;* lichen scrofulosorum *BJD 94:319–325, 1976; AD 124:1421–1426, 1988;* papulonecrotic tuberculid – folliculitis *Amer J Derm 16:474–485, 1994*

Peloderma strongyloides (nematode larvae) *JAAD 51:S181–184, 2004; JAAD 51:S109–112, 2004; JAAD 51:S109–112, 2004; Cutis 48:123–126, 1991; Ped Derm 2:33–37, 1984; BJD 98:107–112, 1978*

Talaromyces (Penicillium) marneffei – folliculitis *BMC Infec Dis 19:707, 2019; Lancet 344:110–113, 1994; Mycoses 34:245–249, 1991*

Pinworm infestation (*Enterobius vermicularis*) – folliculitis of buttocks *Sex Transm Dis 13:45–46, 1986*

Pityrosporum folliculitis – upper trunk and upper arms *Int J Derm 38:453–456, 1999; Int J Derm 37:772–777, 1998; JAAD 12:56–61, 1985; AD 107:388–391, 1973;* Splendore-Hoeppli phenomenon in pityrosporum folliculitis *J Cutan Pathol 18:293–297, 1991*

Pseudomonas – *Pseudomonas* diving suit folliculitis *Cutis 59:245–246, 1997; JAAD 31:1055–1056, 1994; Pseudomonas* hot tub folliculitis *Cutis 45:97–98, 1990; AD 120:1304–1307, 1984; Pseudomonas* folliculitis in HIV *JAAD 32:279–280, 1995;* Pseudomonas folliculitis with non-0:11 serogroups *J Clin Inf Dis 21:437–439, 1995;* pseudomonas folliculitis after depilation *Ann Derm Venereol 123:268–270, 1996*

Rhodotorula mucilaginosa folliculitis *BJD 164:1120–1122, 2011*

Scabies – diffuse papular folliculitis

Schistosoma haematobium folliculitis *Amer J Derm 16:442–446, 1994*

Staphylococcus aureus – folliculitis chronic folliculitis of the legs of Indian males *Indian J DV 39:35–39, 1973;* folliculitis in AIDS *JAAD 21:1024–1026, 1989*

Syphilis – secondary *JAAD 82:1–14, 2020; Cutis 35:259–261, 1985;* syphilitic folliculitis *Med Clin North Amer 82:1081–1104, 1998;* alopecia of secondary syphilis *Am J Dermatopathol 17 (2):158–162, 1995*

Tinea capitis, corporis, barbae *Indian J Dermatol 64:266–271, 2019; Int J Derm 33:255–257, 1994*

Tinea versicolor *Cureus 12:e6531, 2020*

Trichodysplasia spinulosa (trichodysplasia of immunosuppression, viral-associated trichodysplasia spinulosa, pilomatrix dysplasia, cyclosporine-induced folliculodystrophy) – DNA polyoma virus in renal transplant patient; alopecia, particulate matter, keratosis pilaris like appearance (follicular papules), thickened skin, eyebrow alopecia, leonine facies *BJD 174:629–632, 2016; Ped Derm 32: 545–546, 2015; Australasian J Dermatol 55:e33–e36, 2014; AD 148:726–733, 2012; AD 146:871–874, 2010; JAAD 60:169–172, 2009; J Cutan Pathol 34:721–725, 2007; AD 142:1643–1648, 2006; JAAD 52:540–541, 2005; Am J Surg Pathol 29:241–246, 2005; JAAD 52:540, 2005; JAAD 50:318–322, 2004; JAAD 50:310–315, 2004; JAAD 43:118–122, 2000; J Invest Dermatol Symp Proc 4:268–271, 1999; Hautarzt 46:871–874, 1995*

Trichophytid, lichenoid

Trichosporon beigelii folliculitis *Derm Clinics 14:57–67, 1996*

Tufted folliculitis of the scalp – *Staphylococcus aureus BJD 138:799–805, 1998; JAAD 38:857–859, 1998*

Tumbu fly myiasis – folliculitis *AD 13:951, 1995*

Vaccinia – sycosis vaccinatum – folliculocentric pustules of bearded region *JAMA Derm 151:799–800, 2015*

Warts – filiform verrucae, flat warts *Clin Dermatol 32:839–872, 2014*

West Nile virus – scattered red papules resembling folliculitis *JAAD 51:820–823, 2004*

Yaws – follicular pustules

INFILTRATIVE DISEASES

Benign cephalic histiocytosis *JAAD 12:328–331, 1985*

Follicular mucinosis of childhood – red facial plaques, hypopigmented facial plaques, follicular papules; alopecic scaly plaque of face (follicular mucinosis in childhood) *Ped Derm 30:192–198, 2013;* hypopigmented follicular papules *JAAD 67:1174–1181, 2012*

Langerhans cell histiocytosis in adults – in scalp and groin – follicular pustules *JAAD 28:166–170, 1993;* presenting as scalp folliculitis *AD 13:719–720, 1995*

Papular mucinosis – localized papular mucinosis associated with IgA nephropathy; cobblestoned shiny grouped follicular papules of the neck *AD 147:599–602, 2011*

INFLAMMATORY

Dermatophytid reaction *Clin Dermatol 32:839–872, 2014*

Eosinophilic pustular folliculitis *Clin Dermatol 32:839–872, 2014*

Hidradenitis suppurativa *AD 133:967–970, 1997*

Inflammatory bowel disease – folliculitis *BJD 178:335–349, 2018*

Necrotizing infundibular crystalline folliculitis – follicular papules with waxy keratotic plugs *BJD 145:165–168, 2001*

Perforating folliculitis – keratotic papules *JAAD 63:179–182, 2010; Am J Dermatopathol 20:147–154, 1998; AD 97:394–399, 1968*

Perifolliculitis capitis abscedens et suffodiens (dissecting cellulitis of the scalp) *Ann DV 121:328–330, 1994*

Pseudofolliculitis barbae *Clin Dermatol 32:839–872, 2014*

Sarcoid *Eur J Dermatol 10:303–305, 2000;* folliculitis-like lichenoid sarcoid *Case Rep Dermatol 9:158–163, 2017*

Sterile neutrophilic folliculitis with perifollicular vasculopathy *J Cutan Pathol 25:215–221, 1998*

METABOLIC DISEASES

Biotin deficiency

Cholinergic/adrenergic urticaria

Essential fatty acid deficiency

Hereditary LDH M-subunit deficiency *AD 122:1420–1424, 1986*

Hypothyroidism *Ped Derm 22:447–449, 2005*

Kwashiorkor

Liver disease – vesiculopustular eruption of hepatobiliary disease *Int J Derm 36:837–844, 1997*

Miliaria *Acta DV 77:1–3, 1997;* miliaria profunda

Nutritional follicular keratoses *Clin Dermatol 32:839–872, 2014*

Ochronosis – follicular accentuation *Clin Dermatol 32:839–872, 2014*

Papular dermatitis of pregnancy – folliculitis *Semin Derm 8:23–25, 1989*

Pellagra *Clin Dermatol 32:839–872, 2014*

Phrynoderma – Vitamin A deficiency; – hyperkeratotic follicular papules (umbilicated) of elbows, knees, neck, posterior axillary folds, xerosis, patchy hyperpigmentation *AD 144:1509–1514, 2008; Ped Derm 28:346–349, 2006; JAAD 41:322–324, 1999; AD*

120:919–921, 1984; Indian Med Gazette 68:681–687, 1933; folliculitis JAAD 29:447–461, 1993; phrynoderma as sign of general malnutrition not specific for Vitamins A, B, E or essential fatty acid deficiency Ped Derm 22:60–63, 2005; in Crohn's disease – hyperkeratotic follicular papules Ped Derm 32:234–236, 2015

Pretibial myxedema

Pruritic folliculitis of pregnancy – limbs and abdomen An Bras Dermatol 91 (Suppl 1)66–68, 2016; JAAD 43:132–134, 2000; Semin Derm 8:23–25, 1989; AD 117:20–22, 1981

Riboflavin deficiency (Vitamin B2 deficiency) – "dyssebacea" Clin Dermatol 32:839–872, 2014

Scurvy – follicular hyperkeratosis or perifollicular hemorrhagic keratotic papules AD 142:658, 2006; JAAD 41:895–906, 1999; JAAD 29:447–461, 1993; NEJM 314:892–902, 1986; follicular red papules Ped Derm 28:444–446, 2011

Uremic follicular hyperkeratosis JAAD 26:782–783, 1992; Vitamin A intoxication – follicular keratoses NEJM 315:1250–1254, 1986

Vitamin B12-induced folliculitis DICP 23:1033–1034, 1989

NEOPLASTIC DISEASES

Basaloid follicular hamartoma Indian J Dermatol 65:130–132, 2020; JAAD 43:189–206, 2000; Ped Derm 16:281–284, 1999; AD 131:454–458, 1995; JAAD 27:237–240, 1992

Becker's nevus

Congenital smooth muscle hamartoma with follicular accentuation J Pediatr 110:742–724, 1987; JAAD 13:837–838, 1985

Epidermal nevus

Epidermoid cysts, follicular – following isotretinoin therapy for acne BJD 144:919, 2001; BJD 143:228–229, 2000

Eruptive infundibulomas JAAD 21:361–366, 1989

Florid cutaneous papillomatosis Clin Dermatol 32:839–872, 2014

Follicular hamartoma – personal observation

Folliculosebaceous cystic hamartoma JAAD 34:77–81, 1996

Generalized follicular harmatoma (S) AD 131:454–8, 1995; AD 107:435–440, 1973; AD 99:478–493, 1969

Hamartoma moniliformis Clin Exp Derm 13:34–35, 1988

Inverted follicular keratosis

Keratoacanthomas – multiple keratoacanthomas JAAD 23:862–866, 1990; generalized eruptive keratoacanthoma of Grzybowski – skin-colored to red, dome-shape follicular papules of face (confluent), trunk, proximal extremities; ectropion, narrowing of mouth with keratosis of face; oral involvement BJD 142:800–803, 2000; JAAD 37:786–787, 1997; BJD 91:461–463, 1974; AD 97:615–623, 1968

Lymphoma – follicular (pilotropic) cutaneous T-cell lymphoma BJD 152:193–194, 2005; JAAD 48:448–452, 2003; JAAD 48:238–243, 2003; AD 138:191–198, 2002; AD 137:657–662, 2001; BJD 141:315–322, 1999; Ann DV 126:243–246, 1999; JAAD 36:563–568, 1997; AD 132:683–687, 1996; JAAD 29:330–334, 1993; Am J Dermatopathol 16:52–55, 1994; JAAD 31:819–822, 1994; umbilicated follicular papules AD 146:607–613, 2010; keratosis pilaris-like AD 132:683–687, 1996; CTCL with alopecia mucinosa; Sezary syndrome – follicular hyperkeratosis (spinulosis) BJD 162:695–696, 2010; lymphomatoid granulomatosis – folliculitis-like eruptions AD 127:1693–1698, 1991; HTLV-1 JAAD 34:69–76, 1996; syringotropic CTCL – hypopigmented alopecic plaque with follicular papules JAAD 60:152–154, 2009; primary cutaneous follicle center lymphoma with follicular mucinosis – skin colored follicular papules JAMA Derm 150:906–907, 2014; B-cell lymphoma – facial papules J Dtsch Dermatol Ges 16:1493–1495, 2018

Lymphomatoid granulomatosis – Epstein-Barr-related T-cell rich B-cell lymphoproliferative disorder; papules and dermal nodules with or without ulceration, folliculitis-like lesions, maculopapules, indurated plaques, ulcers BJD 157:426–429, 2007; JAAD 54:657–663, 2006

Lymphomatoid papulosis Am J Dermatopathol 19:189–196, 1997

Medallion-like dendritic hamartoma – personal observation

Melanocytic nevi, follicular Clin Exp Dermatol 37:871–873, 2012

Melanoma – follicular melanoma Clin Dermatol 32:839–872, 2014

metastatic melanoma; mimicking folliculitis Z Hautkr 60:1682, 1685–1689, 1985

Metastases, folliculotropic Acta DV Croat 24:154–157, 2016

Milia Clin Dermatol 32:839–872, 2014

Myeloma with cryoglobulinemia – follicular spicules JAAD 32:834–839, 1995; myeloma – hyperkeratotic papules with filiform follicular spicules JAMA Derm 151:82–84, 2015; JAAD 49:736–740, 2003; JAAD 36:476–477, 1997

Nevoid follicular epidermolytic hyperkeratosis AD 111:221–222, 1975

Nevus anelasticus JAAD 51:165–185, 2004

Nevus comedonicus Clin Dermatol 32:839–872, 2014

Nevus sebaceus

Multiple miliary osteomas Clin Dermatol 32:839–872, 2014

Pigmented follicular cysts BJD 134:758–762, 1996

Porokeratosis, follicular Am J Dermatopathol 37:e134–136, 2015; Clin Dermatol 32:839–872, 2014; J Cutan Pathol 36:1195–1199, 2009

Porokeratotic eccrine ostial dermal duct nevus Clin Dermatol 32:839–872, 2014

Sebaceous casts – nasolabial follicular sebaceous casts; filiform projections BJD 143:228–229, 2000

Sebaceous gland hyperplasia Am J Dermatopathol 18:296–301, 1996

Smooth muscle hamartoma – transient piloerection; linear, follicular spotted appearance Ped Derm 24:628–631, 2007; JAAD 46:477–490, 2002; BJD 142:138–142, 2000; JAAD 13:837–838, 1985; J Dermatol Surg Oncol 11:714–717, 1985; J Cutan Pathol 9:33–42, 1982; AD 114:104–106, 1978

Steatocystoma multiplex

Trichilemmal cyst – folliculitis J Cutan Pathol 17:185–188, 1990

Trichodiscomas Acta DV 68:163–165, 1988

Vellus hair cysts – eruptive Eur J Dermatol 10:487–489, 2000; familial eruptive vellus hair cysts (keratosis pilaris-like) Ped Derm 5:94–96, 1988; on extremities Indian Online J 4:2213–215, 2013

Warty dyskeratoma Clin Dermatol 32:839–872, 2014; Am J Dermatopathol 34:674–675, 2012; JAAD 47:423–428, 2002

PARANEOPLASTIC DISORDERS

Glucagonoma Indian J DV Leprol Aug 1, 2019; Int J Dermatol 57:642–645, 2018

Palmoplantar keratoderma and malignancy AD 132:640–645, 1996

Paraneoplastic pityriasis rubra pilaris – isolated cases of metastatic adenocarcinoma, hepatocellular carcinoma, and leukemia

Sterile suppurative folliculitis associated with acute myelogenous leukemia BJD 146:904–907, 2002

PHOTODERMATITIS

Actinic superficial folliculitis *BJD 139:359–360, 1998; BJD 138:1070–1074, 1998; Clin Exp Dermatol 14:69–71, 1989; BJD 113:630–631, 1985*

Polymorphic light eruption, follicular *Clin Dermatol 32:839–872, 2014*

PRIMARY CUTANEOUS DISEASES

Acne keloidalis nuchae *JAAD 53:1–37, 2005; JAAD 39:661, 1998; Dermatol Clin 6:387–395, 1988*

Acne necrotica miliaris

Acne necrotica varioliformis (necrotizing lymphocytic folliculitis) *AD 132:1367, 1370, 1996; JAAD 16:1007–1014, 1987*

Acne rosacea; *AD 134:679–683, 1998;* acne agminata (granulomatous rosacea) – monomorphic brown papules of chin, cheeks, eyelids *BJD 134:1098–1100, 1996*

Acne vulgaris *Curr Probl Derm 8:237–268, 1996;* follicular white papular scarring of the back *AD 126:797–800, 1990*

Alopecia and follicular papules *Int J Derm 38 (Suppl 1):31, 1999*
   Alopecia, keratosis pilaris, cataracts and psoriasis
   Alopecia mucinosa (follicular mucinosis) *Dermatology 197:178–180, 1998; AD 125:287–292, 1989; JAAD 10:760–768, 1984; AD 76:419–426, 1957;* with hematologic malignancies *JAAD 80:1704–1711, 2019*
   Atrichia with papular lesions *JAAD 47:519–523, 2002; AD 121:1167–1174, 1985*
   Down's syndrome
   Hayden's disease
   Ichthyosis follicularis with atrichia and photophobia (IFAP) – collodion membrane and erythema at birth; generalized follicular keratoses, non-scarring alopecia, keratotic papules of elbows, knees, fingers, extensor surfaces, xerosis; punctate keratitis *JAAD 46:S156–158, 2002; Am J Med Genet 85:365–368, 1999; AD 125:103–106, 1989; Dermatologica 177:341–347, 1988*
   Monilethrix
   Noonan's syndrome
   Pachyonychia congenita
   Resistant Vitamin D dependent rickets type II – autosomal recessive, partial or total alopecia, follicular papules of face, scalp, extremities, short stature *Acta Dermosifilogr 108:859–860, 2017*
   Schopf-Schulz-Passarge syndrome
Alopecia, keratosis pilaris, cataracts and psoriasis

Alopecia mucinosa (follicular mucinosis) *Dermatology 197:178–180, 1998; AD 125:287–292, 1989; JAAD 10:760–768, 1984; AD 76:419–426, 1957*

Acquired perforating dermatosis – folliculitis *J Derm 20:329–340, 1993*

Atopic dermatitis, follicular *Clin Dermatol 32:839–872, 2014; Acta DV Suppl 171:1–37, 1992;* "follicular eczema"

Atrophoderma vermiculatum – autosomal recessive *Ped Derm 26:427–431, 2009; Ped Derm 15:285–286, 1998*

Axillary granular parakeratosis – folliculitis *JAAD 37:789–790, 1997*

Blaschkitis – personal observation

Cutis anserina (gooseflesh)

Darier's disease (keratosis follicularis) – dirty yellow brown papules; autosomal dominant; mutations in ATP2A2 *Curr Prob Derm 14:71–116, 2002;* linear Darier's disease *J Derm 25:469–475, 1998*

Dermatitis palaestrae limosae *JAMA 269:502–504, 1993*

Dermographism, follicular *Cutis 32:244–245, 254, 260, 1983*

Dilated pore of Winer

Dissecting folliculitis of the scalp *J Derm Surg Oncol 18:877–880, 1992*

Disseminated and recurrent infundibulofolliculitis – neck, trunk, extremities; resembles follicular atopic dermatitis in darkly pigmented skin *J Derm 25:51–53, 1998; Dermatol Clin 6:353–362, 1988; AD 105:580–583, 1972*

Dowling-Degos disease *JAAD 24:888–892, 1991*

Elastosis perforans serpiginosa – folliculitis *Clin Dermatol 32:839–872, 2014; J Derm 20:329–340, 1993*
   Reactive – Down's syndrome, Ehlers-Danlos syndrome, osteogenesis imperfect, scleroderma, acrogeria, pseudoxanthoma elasticum
   Drug-induced – penicillamine
   Idiopathic

Eosinophilic pustular folliculitis (Ofuji's disease) *Eur J Dermatol 12:600–602, 2002; Clin Exp Dermatol 26:179–181, 2001;* HIV-associated *J Dermatol 25:178–184, 1998; J Derm 25:742–746, 1998; AD 127:206–209, 1991;* Ofuji's disease – follicular plugs *Ann DV 124:540–543, 1997; JAAD 29:259–260, 1993; JAAD 12:268–273, 1985; AD 121:921–923, 1985*

Eosinophilic pustular folliculitis of infancy/childhood *Am J Dis Child 147:197–200, 1993*

Erosive pustular dermatitis of the scalp – folliculitis-like *Hautarzt 43:576–579, 1992*

Erythema toxicum neonatorum

Erythromelanosis follicularis faciei et colli (keratosis rubra pilaris faciei atrophicans) – facial erythema, keratosis pilaris, follicular atrophy, hyperpigmentation , – follicular plugging of cheeks, arms, and pre-auricular area *Ped Derm 35:e70–71, 2018; Clin Dermatol 32:839–872, 2014; AD 147:235–240, 2011; Ped Derm 23:31–34, 2006; JAAD 34:714, 1996; JAAD 32:863–866, 1995; JAAD 25:430–432, 1991; Cutis 34:163–170, 1984; JAAD 5:533–534, 1981; BJD 102:323–325, 1980; Dermatologica 132:269–287, 1966; Hautarzt 9:391–393, 1960*

Erythrose peribuccale pigmentale of Brocq

Facial Afro-Caribbean childhood eruption – folliculitis *Clin Exp Derm 15:163–166, 1990*

Familial dyskeratotic comedones

Flegel's disease (hyperkeratosis lenticularis perstans) – keratinous papules of calves *BJD 116:681–691, 1987*

Folliculitis decalvans – follicular plugging of scalp, inflammation, and pustules; scarring *Cutis 98:175–178, 2016; Ped Derm 26:427–431, 2009; J Dermatol 28:329–331, 2001;*

Follicular ichthyosis – X-linked; triad of follicular ichthyosis, atrichia of scalp and photophobia *Clin Dermatol 32:839–872, 2014; BJD 111:101–109,1984*

Fox-Fordyce disease *Dermatol Ther 33:e13223, 2020; An Bras Dermatol 93:562–565, 2018; AD 147:573–576, 2011*

Frontal fibrosing alopecia – facial follicular papules *AD 147:1424–1427, 2011;* miniscule red dots of glabella *BJD 170:745–746, 2014;* facial lesions – skin colored facial papules, follicular red dots, perifollicular and diffuse erythema with reticulated pattern, pigmented macules *JAAD 73:987–990, 2015*

Granuloma annulare – follicular, pustular granuloma annulare *Dermatol Online J Dec 16, 2015; BJD 138:1075–1078, 1998*

Granuloma faciale – follicular prominence *Int J Dermatol 36:548–551, 1997; AD 129:634–635, 637, 1993*

Granulosis rubral nasi *Clin Dermatol 32:839–872, 2014*

Ichthyosis congenita type IV – erythrodermic infant with follicular hyperkeratosis *BJD 136:377–379, 1997*

Juxtaclavicular beaded lines *Dermatol Online J 15:14, 2009; Dermatology 197:94–95, 1998*

Keratosis circumscripta – age 3–5; plaques of follicular keratoses of elbows, knees, hips, posterior axillary folds, and sacrum with palmoplantar thickening (possible childhood PRP) *Int J Dermatol 50:1259–1261, 2011; Cutis 79:363–366, 2007; Dermatologica 159:182–183, 1980; Dermatologica 156:342–350, 1978; AD 93:408–410, 1966*

Keratosis follicularis contagiosa (Brooks' syndrome) – personal observation

Keratosis follicularis spinulosa decalvans – personal observation

Keratosis follicularis squamosa – follicular hyperkeratotic papule; annular with scale; "lotus leaves on water" *J Dermatol Sci 60:193–196, 2010; BJD 144:1070–1072, 2001*

Keratosis pilaris *JAAD 72:890–900, 2015; JAAD 39:891–893, 1998*; papular profuse and precocious keratosis pilaris *Ped Derm 29:285–288, 2012*

Keratosis pilaris atrophicans *AD 130:469–475, 1994*; ulerythema ophryogenes *Ped Derm 11:172–175, 1994*; keratosis pilaris decalvans non-atrophicans *Clin Exp Dermatol 18:45–46, 1993*; keratosis follicularis spinulosa decalvans *AD Syphilol 151:384–387, 1926*; folliculitis decalvans *Acta DV (Stockh) 43:14–24, 1963*; atrophoderma vermiculatum – cheeks and pre-auricular regions *JAAD 18:538–542, 1988; J Cutan Dis 36:339–352, 1918*

keratosis pilaris atrophicans facei *JAAD 39:891–893, 1998*;

associated with Noonan's syndrome *BJD 100:409–416, 1979*;

associated with Woolly hair *BJD 110:357–362, 1984*; rubra faciei

Keratosis pilaris, ulerythema ophryogenes, koilonychia, and monilethrix *JAAD 45:627–629, 2001; Ped Derm 16:297–300, 1999*

Keratosis pilaris rubra (keratosis rubra pilaris) *J Cutan Pathol 45:958–961, 2018; Clin Dermatol 32:839–872, 2014; AD 142:1611–1616, 2006; Ped Derm 23:31–34, 2006; BJD 147:822–824, 2002*

Kyrle's disease (hyperkeratosis follicularis et parafollicularis in cutem penetrans); *J Derm 20:329–340, 1993; JAAD 16:117–123, 1987*

Lichen myxedematosus *J Eur Acad DV 31:45–52, 2017*

Lichen nitidus *J Cutan Pathol Apr 14, 2020; Cutis 62:247–248, 1998; JAAD 12:597–624, 1985*

Lichen planopilaris (Graham-Little syndrome) (follicular lichen planus); *Dermatol Clin 14:773–782, 1996; JAAD 27:935–942, 1992; JAAD 22:594–598, 1990; AD Syphilol 5:102–113, 1922*; lichen planus faceie of Brocq

Lichen planus follicularis tumidus – plaques with follicular papules of retroauricular area *Clin Dermatol 32:839–872, 2014*

Lichen sclerosus et atrophicus

Lichen simplex chronicus

Lichen spinulosus *AD 136:1165–1170, 2000; JAAD 22:261–264, 1990; Int J Derm 34:670–671, 1985*; generalized lichen spinulosus *Ped Derm 27:299–300, 2010*

Lupus miliaris disseminata faciei *Clin Exp Dermatol 39:500–502, 2014*

Mid-dermal elastolysis (perifollicular atrophy) (finely wrinkled skin) – well-circumscribed patches of fine wrinkling of trunk and proximal extremities of young women; perifollicular papular protrusions; persistent reticular erythema and fine wrinkling *AD 146:1167–1172, 2010; Arch Dermatol Res 302:85–93, 2010; BJD 161:203–205, 2009; J Dtsch Dermatol Ges 7:68–69, 2009; JAAD 51:165–185, 2004; JAAD 48:846–851, 2003; JAAD 48:846–851, 2003; Cutis 71:312–314, 2003; J Cut Med Surg 4:40–44, 2000; BJD 132:487, 1995; JAAD 26:490–492, 1992; JAAD 26:169–173, 1992; AD 125:950–951, 1989; BJD 97:441–445, 1977*; perifollicular protrusions

Monilethrix – horny follicular papules *AD 132:577–582, 1996*; alopecia, keratosis pilaris, xerosis; autosomal recessive – *Dsg4* mutation; autosomal dominant *KRT81,KRT83, KRT86 BJD 165:425–431, 2011*

Multiple minute digitate keratoses – follicular keratoses *JAAD 31:802–803, 1994*

Necrotizing infundibular crystalline folliculitis – calcium palmitate *Am J Dermatopathol 40:e9–11, 2018; JAAD 66:823–826, 2012*

Neurofollicular hamartoma *Clin Dermatol 32:839–872, 2014*

Nevus anelasticus – pink-red perifollicular papules *Ped Derm 22:153–157, 2005* Palmoplantar keratoderma – epidermolytic palmoplantar keratoderma, woolly hair, and dilated cardiomyopathy – striated palmoplantar keratoderma, follicular keratosis, clubbing, vesicles and bullae on trunk, psoriasiform keratoses on knees, legs, and feet *JAAD 39:418–421, 1998*

Perforating folliculitis

Perifollicular elastolysis – gray or white follicular papules of neck, earlobes *JAAD 51:165–185, 2004*

Perioral dermatitis *Derm 195:235–238, 1997*

Pityriasis alba *Int J Derm 32:870–873, 1993*; follicular *Clin Dermatol 32:839–872, 2014*

Pityriasis rosea

Pityriasis rubra pilaris – erythematous perifollicular papules; grouped; scaly scalp; orange palmoplantar keratoderma; islands of sparing; resembles seborrheic dermatitis *Clin Dermatol 37:657–662, 2019; BJD 133:990–993, 1995; Eur J Dermatol 4:593–597, 1994; JAAD 20:801–807, 1989*

Prurigo nodularis *J Cutan Pathol 15:208–211, 1988*

Pseudofolliculitis barbae *Clin Cosmet Investig Dermatol April 16, 2019;12:241–247; Derm Surg 26:737–742, 2000; Cutis 61:351–356, 1998; J Emerg Med 4:283–286, 1986; Dermatol Clin 6:387–395, 1988*; pubis; of scalp *AD 113:328–329, 1977*; of nasal hairs *AD 117:368–369, 1981*

Psoriasis, follicular *Ped Derm 34:e65–68, 2017; BJD 137:988–991, 1997*; herpetiform follicular papules *JAMA Derm 152:1043–1044, 2016*

Pustular eruption of striae – folliculitis-like *Cutis 50:225–228, 1992*

Pyoderma vegetans – folliculitis *J Derm 19:61–63, 1992*

Reactive perforating collagenosis – folliculitis-like lesions *J Derm 20:329–340, 1993; AD 96:277–282, 1967*

Rhinophyma *Clin Exp Dermatol 15:282–284, 1990*

Seborrheic dermatitis – perifollicular *Clin Dermatol 32:839–872, 2014*

Syringolymphoid hyperplasia *JAAD 49:1177–1180, 2003*

Syringoma *Clin Dermatol 32:839–872, 2014*

Transient or persistent acantholytic dermatosis (Grover's disease) *JAAD 35:653–666, 1996*; folliculitis *JAAD 11:253–256, 1984*

Trichoepithelioma *Clin Dermatol 32:839–872, 2014*

Trichostasis spinulosa *Clin Dermatol 32:839–872, 2014*

Woolly hair hypotrichosis – keratosis pilaris; mutations in *LPAR6 (PZRY5)* or *LIPH* genes *BJD 165:425–431, 2011*

White fibrous papulosis of the neck *Clin Exp Derm 16:224–225, 1991*

PSYCHOCUTANEOUS DISORDERS

Trichotillomania – follicular hyperkeratosis *BJD 145:1034–1035, 2001*

SYNDROMES

Alagille syndrome (arteriohepatic dysplasia) – follicular hyperkeratosis *BJD 138:150–154, 1998*

Behcet's disease – folliculitis *Cutis 60:159–161, 1997; Ann Hematol 74:45–48, 1997;* pseudofolliculitis *BJD 159:555–560, 2008*

Birt-Hogg-Dube syndrome *Dermatol Sci 89:177–184, 2018*

Blau or Jabs syndrome (familial juvenile systemic granulomatosis) – autosomal dominant; translucent skin-colored papules (non-caseating granulomas) of trunk and extremities; may resolve with pitted scars with follicular atrophoderma; with uveitis, synovitis, arthritis; polyarteritis, multiple synovial cysts; red papular rash in early childhood; camptodactyly (flexion contractures of PIP joints) mutations in NOD2 (nucleotide-binding oligomerization domain 2) (caspase recruitment domain family, member 15; *CARD* 15) *AD 143:386–391, 2007; Clin Exp Dermatol 21:445–448, 1996*

Brook's syndrome (keratosis follicularis contagiosa)

Buschke-Ollendorf syndrome – keratosis pilaris lesions; osteopoikilosis, connective tissue nevus; elastomas, dermatofibrosis lenticularis; *LEMD3* gene *Case Rep Dermatol Med 2016:2483041*

Cardio-facio-cutaneous syndrome – autosomal dominant, xerosis/ichthyosis, eczematous dermatitis, alopecia, growth failure, hyperkeratotic papules, ulerythema ophyrogenes (decreased or absent eyebrows), seborrheic dermatitis, CALMs, nevi, hemangiomas, follicular hyperkeratosis of arms, legs, face; keratosis pilaris, patchy or widespread ichthyosiform eruption, sparse curly scalp hair and sparse eyebrows and lashes, congenital lymphedema of the hands, redundant skin of the hands, short stature, abnormal facies with macrocephaly, broad forehead, bitemporal narrowing, hypoplasia of supraorbital ridges, short nose with depressed nasal bridge, high arched palate, low set posteriorly rotated ears with prominent helices, cardiac defects; gain of function sporadic missense mutations in *BRAF, KRAS, MEK1,* or *MEK2, MAP2K1/MAP2K2 BJD 180:172–180, 2019; Ped Derm 30:665–673, 2013; BJD 164:521–529, 2011; BJD 163:881–884, 2010; Ped Derm 27:274–278, 2010; Ped Derm 17:231–234, 2000; JAAD 28:815–819, 1993; AD 129:46–47, 1993; JAAD 22:920–922, 1990;* port wine stain *Clin Genet 42:206–209, 1992*

Conradi-Hunermann syndrome (chondrodysplasia punctata – X-linked dominant) – linear and whorled hyperkeratosis, keratotic follicular plugs with calcification, follicular atrophoderma of forearms in Blaschko distribution; linear atrophic lesions with follicular plugging of scalp; cicatricial alopecia of scalp; patchy patterned alopecia, generalized xerosis; cataracts, chondrodysplasia punctata; asymmetric shortening of long bones epiphyseal stippling, short stature, short limbs, kyphoscoliosis, craniofacial abnormalities); short arms and legs; cataracts; X-linked; mutation in emopamil binding protein (EBP) *BJD 173:1316–1318, 2015; Ped Derm 31:493–496, 2014; BJD 160:1335–1337, 2009; Curr Prob in Derm VII:143–198, 1995; AD 121:1064–1065, 1985;* ichthyotic and psoriasiform lesions (Blaschko hyperkeratotic scaling), nail defects, cicatricial alopecia, follicular pitted scars, skeletal anomalies *JAAD 33:356–360, 1995; Hum Genet 53:65–73, 1979;* neonatal transient scaly plaques of limbs, trunk, and scalp; scaly rash disappears in months leaving hypo- or hyperpigmented streaks with follicular atrophoderma and patchy scarring alopecia; *CDPX2* – X-linked lethal in males; X-linked dominant (mosaic for emopamil-binding protein); X-linked recessive – male EBP disorder with neurologic defects *BJD 166:1309–1313, 2012*

Cornelia de Lange syndrome – with ulerythema ophyrogenes; specific facies, hypertrichosis of forehead, face, back, shoulders, and extremities, synophrys; long delicate eyelashes, cutis marmorata, skin around eyes and nose with bluish tinge, red nose *Ped Derm 19:42–45, 2002; JAAD 37:295–297, 1997*

Deletion short arm chromosome 18 (18p-) – ulerythema ophyrogenes *Ped Derm 11:172–175, 1994*

Desmoplakin mutations – syndrome of dilated cardiomyopathy with severe left ventricular dysfunction, congenital alopecia, striate palmoplantar keratoderma, nail dystrophy, follicular hyperkeratosis with hyperpigmented plaques of elbows *Ped Derm 32:102–108, 2015*

Down's syndrome – presternal and interscapular follicular papules; keratosis pilaris; pityrosporum folliculitis *BJD 129:696–699, 1993;* deep folliculitis of posterior neck; folliculitis *Ped Derm 37:219–221, 2020;* acquired reactive perforating collagenosis *Ped Derm 28:53–54, 2011*

Ectodermal dysplasia/skin fragility syndrome – autosomal recessive (Carvajal-Huerta syndrome); skin peeling; generalized erythema and peeling at birth; very short stature, superficial skin fragility with crusts of face, knees, alopecia of scalp and eyebrows, perioral hyperkeratosis with fissuring and cheilitis, thick dystrophic cracking finger- and toenail dystrophy, keratotic plaques on limbs, diffuse or focal striate palmoplantar keratoderma with painful fissuring; *PKP1* gene (encoding plakophilin 1) or *DSP* (encoding desmoplakin); follicular hyperkeratosis of knees; woolly hair; perianal erythema and erosions; cardiomyopathy associated with mutation in desmoplakin not with plakophilin *BJD 160: 692–697, 2009; JAAD 55:157–161, 2006; Acta DV 85:394–399, 2005; JID 122:1321–1324, 2004; Curr Prob Derm 14:71–116, 2002; Hum Molec Genet 9:2761–2766, 2000; Hum Molec Genet 8:143–148, 1999*

Epidermodysplasia verruciformis – brown perifollicular papules in the setting of graft vs. host disease *JAAD 57:S78–80, 2007; BJD 149:627–633, 2003*

Focal palmoplantar and oral mucosa (gingival) hyperkeratosis syndrome (MIM:148730) (hereditary painful callosities) – palmoplantar keratoderma, follicular hyperkeratosis, leukoplakia (gingival keratosis), and cutaneous horn of the lips *JAAD 52:403–409, 2005; BJD 146:680–683, 2002; Oral Surg 50:250, 1980; Birth Defects 12:239–242, 1976; Arch Int Med 113:866–871, 1964*

Follicular keratotic papules with distal limb polyneuropathy *Am J Dermatopathol 39:e83–84, 2017; Am J Dermatopathol 39:549–550, 2017*

Gall-Galli syndrome – Dowling-Degos disease with acantholysis – hyperkeratotic follicular papules *JAAD 45:760–763, 2001*

Haber's syndrome – early onset rosacea-like erythema, multiple truncal keratotic lesions *Australas 38:82–84, 1997*

Hereditary mucoepithelial dystrophy (dysplasia) (dyskeratosis) (Gap junction disease, Witkop disease) – autosomal dominant; red eyes (childhood keratitis and cataracts), photophobia with infantile nystagmus, non-scarring alopecia, keratosis pilaris, chronic red macules (erythema) of oral (hard palate, gingival, tongue) and nasal mucous membranes, cervix, vagina, and urethra; perineal and perigenital psoriasiform dermatitis; increased risk of infections, fibrocystic lung disease *Ped Derm 26:427–431, 2009; BJD 153:310–318, 2005; Ped Derm 11:133–138, 1994; Am J Med Genet 39:338–341, 1991; JAAD 21:351–357, 1989; Am J Hum Genet 31:414–427, 1979; Oral Surg Oral Med Oral Pathol 46:645–657, 1978*

Hidrotic ectodermal dysplasia

Hypereosinophilic syndrome *Dermatology 227:67–71, 2013; Curr Allergy Asthma Rep 12:85–98, 2012*

Hyper IgE syndrome – autosomal dominant; *STAT3* mutation; *Staphylococcus aureus* folliculitis *Allergol 61:191–196, 2012; JAAD 65:1167–1172, 2011; JAAD 54:855–865, 2006*

Hypohidrotic ectodermal dysplasia (Christ-Siemens-Touraine), syndrome 10A, 10B – smooth dry skin, periorbital pigmentation, hypotrichosis, hypohidrosis, hypodontia, craniofacial dysmorphology *Am J Med Genet A 179:442–447, 2019*

Hypoplastic enamel-onycholysis-hypohidrosis (Witkop-Brearley-Gentry syndrome) – marked facial hypohidrosis, dry skin with keratosis pilaris, scaling and crusting of the scalp, onycholysis and subungual hyperkeratosis, hypoplastic enamel of teeth *Oral Surg 39:71–86, 1975*

Ichthyosis follicularis with atrichia and photophobia (IFAP) – X-linked recessive; hyperkeratotic plaques overlying Achilles tendons; atopic dermatitis; collodion membrane and erythema at birth; ichthyosis, spiny (keratotic) follicular papules (generalized follicular keratoses), non-scarring alopecia totalis, keratotic papules of elbows, knees, fingers, extensor surfaces, xerosis; punctate keratitis, photophobia with progressive corneal scarring; nail dystrophy, paronychia, psychomotor delay, short stature; enamel dysplasia, beefy red tongue and gingiva, angular stomatitis (angular cheilitis), lamellar scales, psoriasiform plaques, palmoplantar erythema; mutation of *MBTPS2* (intramembrane zinc metalloproteinase needed for cholesterol homeostasis and endoplasmic reticulum stress response) *Ped Derm 30:e263–264, 2013; JAAD 64:716–722,2011; BJD 163:886–889, 2010; Ped Derm 26:427–431, 2009; Curr Prob Derm 14:71–116, 2002; JAAD 46:S156–158, 2002; BJD 142:157–162, 2000; Am J Med Genet 85:365–368, 1999; Ped Derm 12:195, 1995; AD 125:103–106, 1989; Dermatologica 177:341–347, 1988; BJD 21:165–189, 1909*

Ichthyosis prematurity syndrome ("self-healing congenital verruciform hyperkeratosis") – autosomal recessive; erythrodermic infant with caseous vernix-like desquamation; evolves into generalized xerosis and mild flexural hyperkeratosis and of lower back; cutaneous cobblestoning; keratosis pilaris-like changes; fine desquamation of ankles; focal erythema, diffuse alopecia, fine scaling of scalp, red and white dermatographism; in utero polyhydramnios with premature birth, thick caseous desquamating skin (thick vernix caseosa-like covering) (hyperkeratotic scalp) neonatal asphyxia; later in childhood, dry skin with follicular keratosis; mutation in fatty acid transporter protein 4 (FATP4) *JAAD 66:606–616, 2012; JAAD 63:607–641, 2010; JAAD 59:S71–74, 2008*

Jung syndrome – pyoderma, folliculitis, atopic dermatitis, response to histamine-1 antagonist, blepharitis *Am J Med Genet 66:378–398, 1996; Lancet ii:185–187, 1983*

Kartagener's syndrome – autosomal recessive; folliculitis; primary ciliary dyskinesia, triad of chronic sinusitis, bronchiectasis, and situs inversus *Dermatology 186:269–271, 1993; Dermatologica 183:251–254, 1991*

Keratoderma, woolly hair, follicular keratoses, blistering *Retinoids Today Tomorrow 37:15–19, 1994;* keratosis pilaris atrophicans follicularis and woolly hair *Ped Derm 7:202–204, 1990*

Keratosis-ichthyosis-deafness syndrome (KID syndrome) – autosomal dominant; congenital generalized erythema; hyperkeratotic papules with follicular spiny projections, verrucous plaques of forehead, cheeks, perioral region, elbows, knees, and scalp; scarring alopecia of scalp and eyebrows; progressive corneal scarring; bilateral deafness; most mutations connexin 26 *Ped Derm 29:349–357, 2012; Ped Derm 27:653, 2010; Ped Derm 26:427–431, 2009; Ped Derm 23:81–83, 2006; Ped Derm 15:219–221, 1998*

Keratosis follicularis spinulosa decalvans (Siemens syndrome) – autosomal recessive; X-linked dominant; X-linked recessive; and autosomal dominant; alopecia with keratotic follicular papules of scalp, eyebrows; punctate keratitis, photophobia which remits at puberty; xerosis, thickened nails, spiny follicular papules (keratosis pilaris); scalp pustules, variable palmoplantar keratoderma; unlike IFAP alopecia is progressive and not congenital; no involvement of eyebrows or lashes; *MBTPS2* mutation *Clin Exp Dermatol 37:631–*

634, 2012; JAAD 58:499–502, 2008; Ped Derm 22:170–174, 2005; JAAD 47:S275–278, 2002; JAAD 39:891–893, 1998; BJD 134:138–142, 1996; AD 128:397–402, 1992; Dermatol Monatsschr 174:736–740, 1988; Arch Dermatol Syphilol 151:384–387, 1926

Keratosis-ichthyosis-deafness (KID) syndrome – follicular hyperkeratoses; reticulated severe diffuse hyperkeratosis of palms and soles, well marginated, serpiginous erythematous verrucous plaques, perioral furrows, leukoplakia, sensory deafness, photophobia with vascularizing keratitis, blindness *JAAD 39:891–893, 1998; Ped Derm 13:105–113, 1996; BJD 122:689–697, 1990; JAAD 23:385–388, 1990; AD 123:777–782, 1987; AD 117:285–289, 1981*

Keratosis spinulosa decalvans (KFSD variant) – follicular inflammation at puberty with scarring *Ped Derm 26:427–431, 2009*

Loeys-Dietz syndrome – dysmorphic facies; atrophoderma vermiculatum, milia; wide aortic root and pulmonary artery; patent ductus arteriosus, sagittal craniosynostosis, thoracic scoliosis, lordosis, pectus excavatum, long extremities, vertical talus, varus deformity, hyperlaxity, amelogenesis imperfect, high arched palate, lobulated uvula; mutation in *TGFBR2 JAMA Derm 151:675–676, 2015*

Myhre syndrome – autosomal dominant; low birth weight, short stature, muscular build, limited joint mobility, cardiac defects, pericarditis, laryngotracheal stenosis, deafness, skeletal abnormalities, facial dysmorphism, thick skin, keratosis pilaris, coarse facies; mutation in *SMAD4 Eur J Pediatr 175:1307–1315, 2016*

Neurofibromatosis type 1 – congenital reddish neurofibromatosis dermal hypoplasia with follicular papules *Cutis 68:253–256, 2001*

Noonan's syndrome – malformed ears, nevi, keloids, transient lymphedema, ulerythema ophyrogenes, keratosis follicularis spinulosa decalvans, joint hyperextensibility, hypertelorism, webbed neck, down slanting of palpebral fissures, keratosis pilaris atrophicans, short stature, chest deformity (pectus carinatum and pectus excavatum), cubitus valgus, radioulnar synostosis, clinobrachydactyly, congenital heart disease; PTPN 11 gene on chromosome 12; gain of function of non-receptor protein tyrosine phosphate SHP-2 or KRAS gene *Ped Derm 24:417–418, 2007; JAAD 46:161–183, 2002; Ped Derm 15:18–22, 1998; Ann DV 115:303–310, 1988; J Med Genet 24:9–13, 1987; J Pediatr 63:468–470, 1963;* ulerythema ophyrogenes *Ped Derm 7:77–78, 1990; BJD 100:409–416, 1979;* extremities *Cutis 46:242–246, 1990*

Olmsted syndrome – follicular hyperkeratosis of buttocks and knees; follicular papules; intertrigo, mutilating palmoplantar keratoderma, linear streaky hyperkeratosis, leukokeratosis of the tongue, sparse hair anteriorly *JAAD 53:S266–272, 2005; Ped Derm 21:603–605, 2004; Ped Derm 20:323–326, 2003; Eur J Derm 13:524–528, 2003; BJD 136:935–938, 1997; AD 132:797–800, 1996; AD 131:738–739, 1995; Semin Derm 14:145–151, 1995; JAAD 10:600–610, 1984; Am J Dis Child 33:757–764, 1927*

Pachyonychia congenita type I – follicular hyperkeratotic papules of elbows and knees *JAMA Derm 150:146–153, 2014; AD 147:1077–1080, 2011; Cutis 72:143–144, 2003; Ped Derm 14:491–493, 1997; JAAD 19:705–711, 1988, AD 122:919–923, 1986;* generalized follicular hyperkeratotic papules – mutation of *KRT 6A Ped Derm 33:337–342, 2016*

Pachyonychia congenita type II – natal teeth, bushy eyebrows, follicular keratoses, angular cheilitis, unruly hair *BJD 159:500–501, 2008;* follicular hyperkeratosis of lower back and buttocks; mutation in keratin 6A (*KRT6A*) *BJD 171:343–355, 2014; BJD 160:1327–1329, 2009*

Pili torti, enamel hypoplasia syndrome – keratosis pilaris, dry fair hair, enamel hypoplasia, widely spaced abnormal teeth *BJD 145:157–161, 2001*

Reflex sympathetic dystrophy – folliculitis *JAAD 35:843–845, 1996*

Reticular erythematous mucinosis (REM) syndrome *Int J Dermatol 51:903–909, 2012; Photodermatol Photoimmunol Photomed 20:235–238, 2004*

Rubinstein-Taybi syndrome – ulerythema ophyrogenes *Ped Derm 16:134–136, 1999*

Sabinas syndrome – trichothiodystrophy with folliculitis *Clin Exp Dermatol 34:e94–98, 2009; Am J Med Genet 33:957–967, 1981*

Schwachman's syndrome – neutropenia, malabsorption, failure to thrive; generalized xerosis, follicular hyperkeratosis, widespread dermatitis, palmoplantar hyperkeratosis *Ped Derm 9:57–61, 1992; Arch Dis Child 55:531–547, 1980; J Pediatr 65:645–663, 1964*

Trichothiodystrophy syndromes – BIDS, IBIDS, PIBIDS – follicular keratotic papules, sparse or absent eyelashes and eyebrows, brittle hair, premature aging, sexual immaturity, ichthyosis, dysmyelination, bird-like facies, dental caries; trichothiodystrophy with ichthyosis, urologic malformations, hypercalciuria and mental and physical retardation *Ped Derm 32:865–866, 2015; Ped Derm 14:441–445, 1997; JAAD 44:891–920, 2001*

Tuberous sclerosis – adenoma sebaceum *Clin Dermatol 32:839–872, 2014*

TRAUMA

Amputation stump frictional follicular hyperkeratosis *Clin Exp Dermatol 31:600–601, 2006; BJD 130:770–772, 1994*

Follicular keratosis of the chin – frictional dermatitis; yellow-white to skin colored papules *Clin Dermatol 32:839–872, 2014; Ped Derm 24:412–414, 2007; JAAD 26:134–135, 1992; Int J Dermatol 24:320–321, 1985; J Cutan Pathol 10:376, 1983; J Dermatol 6:365–369, 1979*

Frictional follicular dermatitis – personal observation

Loofah sponge folliculitis *J Clin Microbiol 31:480–483, 1993*

Occlusion folliculitis – beneath adhesive dressings or plasters *JAMA Derm 150:329–330, 2014*

Perniosis

Physical or chemical trauma – folliculitis

Radiation dermatitis, chronic – peau d'orange appearance *JAAD 54:28–46, 2006*

Traction folliculitis – papules and pustules *Cutis 79:26–26–30, 2007*

Traumatic folliculitis due to home epilating device *JAAD 27:771–772, 1992*

Wax epilation – severe folliculitis with keloidal scarring *Cutis 59:41–42, 1997*

VASCULAR

Leukocytoclastic vasculitis with follicular accentuation *JAAD 24:898–902, 1991*

PAPULES, HYPERKERATOTIC

AUTOIMMUNE DISEASES AND DISEASES OF IMMUNE DYSFUNCTION

CD 40L deficiency – X-linked hyper IgM syndrome

Dermatomyositis – follicular hyperkeratosis *BJD 81:544–547, 1969;* juvenile dermatomyositis *Ped Derm 17:37–40, 2000;* Wong's dermatomyositis; holster sign; TIF-18 *JAAD 72:449–455, 2015*

Dermatophytids – associated with kerion; widespread eruption of follicular papules sometimes with keratotic spines *J Dermatol 21:31–34, 1994*

Epidermodysplasia verruciformis-like lesions in common variable immunodeficiency *Clin Inf Dis 51:195–196, 248–249, 2010*

Graft vs. host disease – annular scaly papules of epithelioid granulomas *J Cutan Pathol 43:236 244, 2016; BJD 149:898–899, 2003*

HUMAN PAPILLOMA VIRUS-ASSOCIATED IMMUNODEFICIENCY SYNDROMES

JAAD 73:367–381, 2015

Combined variable immunodeficiency

DOCK8 deficiency – autosomal recessive hyper IgE syndrome

Idiopathic CD4 lymphocytopenia *JAAD 76:1161–1175, 2017*

Gain of function of *STAT1* mutation

    Decreased Th17 cells with increased response to type 1 interferons

GATA2 deficiency – autosomal dominant; human papilloma virus, herpes simplex, varicella-zoster, non-tuberculous mycobacterial, *Clostridium dificile* infections, myeloid dysplasia, acute myelogenous leukemia; panniculitis, congenital lymphedema, clubbing, embolic stroke, bony infarcts, deep venous thrombosis; melanoma and non-melanoma skin cancers; sensorineural deafness, thyroid disease; normal immunoglobulins *Curr Opinion Allergy Clin Immunol 15:104–109, 2015*

    GATA2 cytopenias

        Monocyte

        B cell

        NK cell

        CD4+

        Neutropenia

HIV disease *JAAD 76:1161–1175, 2017*

MST 1 deficiency

    Neutropenia

    B and T cell lymphopenia

WHIM syndrome – warts, hypogammaglobulinemia, infections, and myelokathesis; CXCR deficiency *JAAD 76:1161–1175, 2017*

    Cytopenias

        Neutropenia

        B and T cell lymphopenia

    Decreased IgG and IgA

    Normal IgM

Immunosuppression – multiple verrucous acanthomas

Interleukin-7 (IL-7) deficiency, inherited – CD4 lymphopenia with generalized warts (HPV-3) *JAAD 72:1082–1084, 2015*

Leukocyte adhesion deficiency (LAD-1) – DD18 deficiency

Lupus erythematosus – systemic lupus – hyperkeratotic follicular papules of trunk and extremities in Chinese hypertrophic DLE *JAAD 19:961–965, 1988;* discoid lupus erythematosus – warty papules, resemble prurigo nodularis *NEJM 269:1155–1161, 1963*

MST1 (MST or STK4 deficiency)

NEMO

NLRP 1-associated autoinflammatory arthritis and dyskeratosis – phyrynoderma; increased caspase 1 function; increased IL-18 *Ped Derm 33:602–614, 2016*

Pemphigoid nodularis *JAAD 27:863–867, 1992; AD 118:937–939, 1982*

Pemphigus erythematosus *JAAD 10:215–222, 1984*

Pemphigus foliaceus resembling seborrheic keratoses *AD 126:543–544, 1990*

Rheumatoid nodules – perforating variant

Severe combined immunodeficiency – multiple warts of hands *JAAD 76:1161–1175, 2017; AD 148:659–660, 2012*

WHIM syndrome – warts, hypoglobulinemia, infections, myelokathexis; mutation in *CXCR4 AD 146:931–932, 2010*

WILD syndrome – warts, immunodeficiency, lymphedema and anogenital dysplasia *JAAD 76:1161–1175, 2017*

CONGENITAL LESIONS

Bronchogenic cyst – keratotic papule *Ped Derm 15:277–281, 1998*

Ectopic nail *JAAD 35:484–485, 1996*

Supernumerary digit *Ped Derm 11:181–182, 1994*

DRUG-INDUCED

Capecitabine activation of actinic keratosis – personal observation

Captopril – lichen planus – personal observation

Drug eruption, including lichenoid drug eruption

Etanercept – perforating folliculitis *BJD 156:368–371, 2007*

Etretinate – digitate keratoses induced in treatment of disseminated superficial actinic porokeratosis *Clin Exp Dermatol 15:370–371, 1990*

Infliximab – perforating folliculitis *BJD 156:368–371, 2007*

Iododerma *J Drugs Dermatol 12:574–576, 2013*

Lithium *J Clin Psychopharmacol 11:149–150, 1991*

Phenytoin reaction – keratotic finger papules *Cutis 61:101–102, 1998*

RAF inhibitors (MAPK pathway) – vemurafenib and dabrafenib – exanthema warts and other hyperkeratotic lesions, keratoacanthomas, squamous cell carcinoma, melanocytic nevi, keratosis pilaris, seborrheic dermatitis, hyperkeratotic hand-foot reactions, photosensitivity, panniculitis with arthralgias, alopecia *JAAD 72:221–236, 2015*

Ruxolitinib (Janus kinase inhibitor) – eruptive keratoacanthomas *BJD 173:1098–1099, 2015*

Sorafenib – keratosis pilaris lesions; inflamed seborrheic keratoses *JAAD 61:360–361, 2009*

Tegafur *AD 131:364–365, 1995*

Tofacitinib – multiple warts *JAMA Derm 155:629–631, 2019*

Vemurafenib – warty dyskeratomas, Grover's disease *JAAD 67:1265–1272, 2012;* cystic lesions of face, keratosis pilaris-like eruptions, seborrheic dermatitis rashes, painful hyperkeratosis of soles, squamous cell carcinoma, morbilliform eruptions *BJD 173:1024–1031, 2015; JAMA Derm 151:1103–1109, 2015; AD 148:357–361, 2012;* palmoplantar hyperkeratosis *JAAD 67:1265–1272, 2012*

EXOGENOUS

Arsenical keratosis *J Cut Med Surg 20:67–71, 2016; Dermatology 186:303–305, 1993*

Calcium-containing EEG paste – papules with central umbilication due to perforation of calcium *Neurology 15:477–480, 1965*

Caustic drilling fluid in petrochemical industry – papules with central umbilication due to perforation of calcium *JAAD 14:605–611, 1986*

Foreign body granulomas from lava lamp – umbilicated keratotic papules *Ped Derm 31:623–624, 2014*

Halogenated aromatic weedkiller *Clin Exp Dermatol 19:264–267, 1994*

Hydrocarbon (tar) keratosis – flat-topped papules of face and hands; keratoacanthoma-like lesions on scrotum *JAAD 35:223–242, 1996;* pitch, asphalt, creosote – diffuse melanosis of exposed skin; evolves to atrophy, telangiectasia, lichenoid papules, follicular keratosis

Injected steroid or foreign material

Scar keratosis

INFECTIONS AND INFESTATIONS

Adiaspiromycosis – cutaneous adiaspiromycosis (*Chrysosporium species*) – hyperpigmented plaque with white-yellow papules, ulcerated nodules, hyperkeratotic nodules, crusted nodules, multilobulated nodules *JAAD S113–117, 2004*

Amoebiasis (*Entamoeba histolytica*) – verrucous papules *Int J Dermatol 41:676–680, 2002*

Bacillary angiomatosis *BJD 126:535–541, 1992*

Coccidioidomycosis *AD 140:609–614, 2004; JAAD 46:743–747, 2002; AD 134:365–370, 1998*

Condyloma acuminatum *JAAD 66:867–880, 2012*

Cryptococcosis *JAAD 44:391–394, 2001*

Cytomegalovirus *JAAD 44:391–394, 2001*

Demodex folliculitis – hyperkeratotic papules of face *Ped Derm 33:671–672, 2016*

Erythrasma, petalloid

Herpes simplex, chronic

Herpes zoster, chronic *JAAD 44:391–394, 2001; JAAD 28:306–308, 1993;* verrucous follicular papules of face in patient with B-cell lymphoma *AD 148:405, 2012*

Histoplasmosis in AIDS *JAAD 44:391–394, 2001; Int J Dermatol 30:614–622, 1991;* transepidermal elimination *Cutis 47:397–400, 1991*

HIV-associated follicular syndrome – disseminated follicular spicules *BJD 179;774–775, 2018*

Leishmaniasis – personal observation

Leprosy *Indian J Leprosy 64:183–187, 1992*

Molluscum contagiosum *JAAD 44:391–394, 2001*

Mycobacterium kansasii JAAD 41:854–856, 1999

Mycobacterium tuberculosis – tuberculosis verrucosa cutis, lichen scrofulosorum *Clin Exp Dermatol 42:369–373, 2017;* papular tuberculid *Acta DV 99:123–124, 2019;* tuberculosis cutis miliaris disseminate – personal observation

Paracoccidioidomycosis – near mouth, anus, or genitalia *Clin Inf Dis 23:1026–1032, 1996*

Phaeohyphomycosis, by inoculation – seborrheic keratosis-like lesion *AD 123:1597–1598, 1987*

Pinta

Pneumocystis pneumoniae JAAD 44:391–394, 2001

Rhinosporidiosis

Scabies, crusted (Norwegian) *Case Rep Ped Oct 20, 2019; AD 124:121–126, 1988;* hyperkeratotic nodule of the soles *AD 134:1019–1024, 1998;* scabies-associated acquired perforating dermatosis *JAAD 51:665–667, 2004*

Schistosomiasis – ectopic cutaneous granuloma – skin colored papule, 2–3 mm; group to form mamillated plaques; nodules develop with overlying dark pigmentation, scale, and ulceration *Dermatol Clin 7:291–300, 1989; BJD 114:597–602, 1986*

Strongyloides stercoralis – hyperkeratotic papules (prurigo nodularis-like) *JAAD 41:357–361, 1999*

Syphilis – secondary *Presse Med 19:369–371, 1990;* malignant lues

Tinea versicolor

Trichodysplasia of immunosuppression (trichodysplasia spinulosa, viral-associated trichodysplasia spinulosa, pilomatrix dysplasia, cyclosporine-induced folliculodystrophy); filiform, folliculocentric spiny papules; polyoma virus *Ped Derm 32:545–546, 2015; JAAD 60:169–171, 2009; AD 142:1643–1648, 2006; JAAD 52:540–541, 2005; Am J Surg Pathol 29:241–246, 2005; JAAD 52:540, 2005; JAAD 50:318–322, 2004; JAAD 50:310–315, 2004; JAAD 43:118–122, 2000; J Invest Dermatol Symp Proc 4:268–271, 1999; Hautarzt 46:841–846, 1995;* eyebrow alopecia *Transplantation 101:e314, 2017; Ped Derm 32:e296–297, 2015; AD 147:1215–1220, 2011*

Trichophytosis

Varicella-zoster virus, chronic – in AIDS *JAAD 20:637–642, 1989*

Verruca vulgaris; associated with immune disorders – Wiskott Aldrich syndrome, isolated primary IgM deficiency, X-linked immunodeficiency with hyper-IgM, Hodgkin's disease, lymphoma, chronic lymphocytic leukemia; flat wart *Indian Ped 53:757, 2016*

Verruga peruana

Yaws, including clavus of yaws on the soles

INFILTRATIVE LESIONS

Amyloidosis – lichen amyloidosis *Dermatol Online J March 7, 2018; BJD 177:e143–144, 2017*

Colloid milium, papuloverrucous variant *BJD 143:884–887, 2000*

Langerhans cell histiocytosis *Pediatr Ann 43:e9–12, 2014*

Lichen myxedematosis – lichenoid waxy papules *Int J Dermatol 53:971–974, 2014; Case Rep Dermatol 5:168–175, 2013*

INFLAMMATORY

Chondrodermatitis nodularis chronicus helicis

Crohn's disease

Cryoglobulinemia – follicular spinulosus (hyperkeratotic follicular papules) *JAAD 32:834–839, 1995*

Folliculitis spinulosa decalvans – pustules, keratotic papules of scalp, scarring alopecia *Ped Derm 23:255–258, 2006*

Perforating folliculitis – keratotic papules *JAAD 63:179–182, 2010; Am J Dermatopathol 20:147–154, 1998; AD 97:394–399, 1968*

Rosai-Dorfman disease, cutaneous (sinus histiocytosis with massive lymphadenopathy) – multiple hyperkeratotic papulonodules *JAAD 65:890–892, 2011*

Sarcoid – keratotic lesions of palms resembling psoriasis or syphilis *J Dermatol 45:246–247, 2018*

METABOLIC DISEASES

Calcinosis cutis, including cutaneous calculus

Fabry's disease – angiokeratomas; alpha galactosidase A deficiency *AD 140:1440–1446, 2004; Ped Derm 19:85–87, 2002*

Gout – tophi; ear *Nose Throat J 96:52–55, 2017; Dermatol Online J Oct 15, 2016; Indian J DV Leprol 76:393–396, 2010*

Monoclonal gammopathy – papules, follicular spicules *J Eur Acad DV 31:45–52, 2017*

Necrobiosis lipoidica diabeticorum – perforating variant

Osteoma cutis *Eur J Dermatol 28:434–439, 2018*

Phrynoderma – Vitamin A deficiency; follicular hyperkeratotic papules, xerosis, patchy hyperpigmentation *Ped Derm 28:346–349, 2006;* elbows, knees, neck, posterior axillary folds *AD 144:1509–1514, 2008; JAAD 41:322–324, 1999; AD 120:919–921, 1984; Indian Med Gazette 68:681–687, 1933;* phrynoderma as sign of general malnutrition not specific for Vitamins A, B, E or essential fatty acid deficiency *Ped Derm 22:60–63, 2005;* in Crohn's disease; hyperkeratotic follicular papules *Ped Derm 32:234–236, 2015*

Pretibial myxedema – thyroid acropathy

Renal disease – chronic renal failure – acquired perforating disease of chronic renal failure *Int J Derm 32:874–876, 1993; Int J Dermatol 31:117–118, 1992; AD 125:1074–1078, 1989*

Scurvy – follicular hyperkeratosis or perifollicular hemorrhagic keratotic papules *JAAD 41:895–906, 1999; JAAD 29:447–461, 1993; NEJM 314:892–902, 1986*

Tyrosinemia type II – elbows and knees

Uremic follicular hyperkeratosis *JAAD 26:782–783, 1992*

Vitamin A intoxication – follicular keratoses *NEJM 315:1250–1254, 1986*

Zinc deficiency *J Podiatr 163:1222, 2013*

NEOPLASTIC DISEASES

Acantholytic acanthoma *AD 131:211–216, 1995*

Acquired digital fibrokeratoma – digital papule *Cutis 79:129–132, 2007; AD 124:1559–1564, 1988; JAAD 12:816–821, 1985;* of the nail bed *Dermatology 190:169–171, 1995*

Acquired fibrokeratoma of the heel *AD 121:386–388, 1985*

Acquired periungual fibrokeratoma *AD 97:120–129, 1968*

Actinic keratosis *Stat Pearls April 22, 2020*

Adenosquamous carcinoma of the skin – red keratotic papule or plaque of head, neck or shoulder; extensive local invasion *AD 145:1152–1158, 2009*

Basal cell carcinoma – single or multiple *Acta Pathol Mibrobiol Scand 88A:5–9, 1980;* basal cell carcinoma of the palm

Bowen's disease pigmented *Dermatologica 157:229–237, 1978*

Bowenoid papulosis *Curr Urol Rep 18:62, 2017*

Clear cell acanthoma *Am J Dermatopathol 16:134–139, 1994; BJD 83:248–254, 1970*

Cutaneous horn

Dermal dendrocytoma – keratotic papules *AD 126:689–690, 1990*

Dermatofibroma

Dermatosis papulosa nigra *Cutis 32:385–392, 1983; AD 89:655–658, 1964*

Digital myxoid cyst

Disseminated superficial actinic porokeratosis *JAAD 11:724–730, 1984*

Eccrine angiokeratomatous hamartoma – red-violaceous keratotic nodule of lateral malleolus *JAAD 55:S104–106, 2006*

Eccrine dermal duct tumor – dermal nodule with overlying verrucous changes *AD 94:50–55, 1966*

Eccrine poroma

Epidermal nevus – papular with skyline basal cell layer (PENS) *Case Rep Dermatol 10:1–5, 2017; JAAD 64:888–892, 2011*

Epidermolytic acanthoma *J Eur Acad DV 25:175–180, 2011; BJD 141:728–730, 1999*

Exostosis, subungual *JAAD 45:S200–201, 2001*

Familial dyskeratotic comedones – discreet black papules with firm central keratotic plugs *SkinMed 16:273–274, 2018; Indian Dermatol Online J 7:46–48, 2016*

Intra-epidermal carcinoma of the eyelid margin *BJD 93:239–252, 1975*

Inverted follicular keratosis *J Clin Pathol 28:465–471, 1975*

Isolated epidermolytic acanthoma *AD 101:220–223, 1970*

Eruptive vellus hair cysts *AD 131:341–346, 1995*

Fibrokeratoma

Garlic clove tumor (fibroma) (acquired periungual fibrokeratoma); *AD 97:120–129, 1968*

Generalized eruptive histiocytoma – brown scaly papules *AD 139:933–938, 2003; AD 88:586–593, 1963*

Glomus tumor – hyperkeratotic papule of palm *JAAD Case Rep 18:38–40, 2017*

Granular cell tumor *Cutis 62:147–148, 1998;* prurigo nodularis-like lesions *Int J Derm 20:126–129, 1981*

Intraepidermal epithelioma of Jadassohn *Cutis 37:339–341, 1986*

Juvenile xanthogranuloma *Dis Chest 50:325–329, 1966*

Keratoacanthoma – single or multiple *AD 120:736–740, 1984*

Kaposi's sarcoma *JAAD 38:143–175, 1998*

Large cell acanthoma *J Cutan Pathol 17:182–184, 1990*

Lichen planus-like keratosis *Am J Surg Pathol 17:259–263, 1993*

Lymphoma – cutaneous T cell lymphoma – pityriasis lichenoides-like *BJD 142:347–352, 2000; JAAD 31:819–822, 1994;* Woringer-Kolopp disease *AD 120:1045–1051, 1984; ;* syringotropic cutaneous T-cell lymphoma – punctate red papules; hyperkeratotic follicular papules, punctate red papules; anhidrosis; palmoplantar keratoderma; poikiloderma vasculare atrophicans *JAAD 71:926–934, 2014; Am J Surg Pathol 35:100–109, 2011; Eur J Dermatol 15:262–264, 2005;* HTLV-1 granulomatous T cell lymphoma – hyperkeratotic and/or umbilicated red-orange papulonodules *JAAD 44:525–529, 2001;* Sezary syndrome – follicular hyperkeratosis (spinulosis) *BJD 162:695–696, 2010;*

Lymphomatoid keratosis *AD 143:53–59, 2007*

Lymphomatoid papulosis *Am J Clin Dermatol 17:319–317, 2016*

Melanoacanthoma

Melanocytic nevus – keratotic melanocytic nevus *J Cutan Pathol 27:344–350, 2000*

Melanoma – verrucous and keratotic melanoma *Histopathology 23:453–458, 1993;* amelanotic melanoma *AD 144:416–417, 2008*

Metastasis – renal cell carcinoma – keratotic papule of the eyelid *and Conjunctival Tumors, Shields JA and Shields CL, Lippincott Williams and Wilkins, 1999, p.135;* breast cancer *Am J Dermatopathol 38:302–304, 2016*

Mucinous nevus *AD 132:1522–1523, 1996*

Nevoid follicular epidermolytic hyperkeratosis *AD 111:221–222, 1975*

Nevus corniculatus *BJD 122:107–112, 1990*

Nevus sebaceus

Papular CD8+ lymphoproliferative disorder – acral sites in renal transplant patient *Clin Exp Dermatol 42:902–905, 2017*

Papular epidermal nevus with skyline basal cell layer (PENS) – 1–7 mm polygonal keratotic papules present at birth *Ped Derm 33:296–300, 2016; JAAD 64:888–892, 2011*

Pilar sheath acanthoma *AD 114:1495–1496, 1978*

Pilomatrixoma – keratoacanthoma-like *JAAD 39:191–195, 1998*

Plasma-acanthoma of the lip *An Bras Dermatol 91:suppl 1:128–130, 2016*

Porokeratosis – of Mibelli *AD 122:586–587, 1986;* giant porokeratosis *Hautarzt 41:633–635, 1990;* hyperkeratotic porokeratosis *Int J Dermatol 32:902–903, 1993;* linear porokeratosis *Ped Derm 21:682–683, 2004; AD 135:1544–1555,1547–1548, 1999; Cutis 44:216–219, 1989; Int J Dermatol 27:589–590, 1988; Ped Derm 4:209, 1987; AD 109:526–528, 1974;* palmoplantar porokeratosis *JAAD 21:415–418, 1989;* palmaris et plantaris et disseminata; disseminated superficial actinic porokeratosis – multiple 3–4 mm keratotic papules *JAAD 11:724–730, 1984*

Punctate porokeratosis *AD 120:263–264, 1984*

Porokeratotic eccrine ostial and dermal duct nevus – mutation in GJB2 *JAMA Derm 151:638–641, 2015; Ped Derm 24:162–167, 2007; Ped Derm 23:465–466, 2006; J Cutan Pathol 15:393–395, 1988; BJD 101:717–722, 1979;* seen in KID syndrome *Ped Derm 27:514–517, 2010*

Seboacanthoma – verrucous sessile papules *AD 84:642–644, 1961*

Seborrheic keratosis; eruptive seborrheic keratoses associated with erythroderma (psoriasis, pityriasis rubra pilaris, allergic contact dermatitis, drug eruption) *JAAD 45:S212–214, 2001*

Squamous cell carcinoma

Stucco keratosis *AD 105:859–861, 1972*

Syringoacanthoma – seborrheic keratosis-like *AD 120:751–756, 1984*

Syringocystadenoma papilliferum – verrucous papules of upper lip *Sultan Qaboos Univ Med J 14:e575–577, 2014*

Trichilemmal carcinoma *Dermatol Surg 28:284–286, 2002;* with cutaneous horn *JAAD 36:107–109, 1997*

Trichilemmal cyst with horn

Trichilemmal horn *JAAD 39:368–371, 1998*

Trichilemmoma – eyelash margin – PTEN hamartoma syndrome (Cowden's syndrome)

Vascular and myxoid fibromas of the fingers – multiple warty lesions of palms and fingers *JAAD 2:425–431, 1980*

Verrucous acanthoma *Eur J Dermatol 21:436–438, 2011*

Verrucous carcinoma (epithelioma cuniculatum) *Histopathology 5:425–436, 1986*

Verrucous perforating collagenoma *Dermatologica 152:65–66, 1976*

Warty dyskeratoma *Plast Reconstr Surg 111:1562–1563, 2003*

PARANEOPLASTIC DISEASES

Eosinophilic dermatosis of myeloproliferative disease – face, scalp; scaly red nodules; trunk – red nodules; extremities – red nodules and hemorrhagic papules *AD 137:1378–1380, 2001*

Florid cutaneous papillomatosis – multiple acuminate keratotic papules; commonly associated gastric adenocarcinoma *Indian J DV 71:195–196, 2005; Int J Dermatol 32:56–58, 1993; AD 114:1803–1806, 1978; Dermatol Online J Aug 15, 2018*

Sign of Leser-Trelat *Cutis 89:33–35, 2012*

PHOTODERMATITIS

Disseminated superficial actinic porokeratosis *Int J Derm 38:204–206, 1999; Int J Dermatol 34:71–72, 1998; BJD 123:249–254, 1996; Cutis 42:345–348, 1988;*

PRIMARY CUTANEOUS DISEASES

Acanthosis nigricans – hereditary benign *Int J Dermatol 35:126–127, 1996*; benign *Am J Public Health 84:1839–1842, 1994*; pseudo-acanthosis nigricans *Am J Med 87:269–272, 1989*; drug-induced (nicotinic acid *Dermatology 189:203–206, 1994*; fusidic acid *JAAD 28:501–502, 1993*; stilbestrol *AD 109:545–546, 1974*; triazinate *AD 121:232–236, 1985*); malignant acanthosis nigricans – bladder *Int J Dermatol 33:433–435, 1994*; kidney *Int J Dermatol 32:893–894, 1993*; bile-duct *Acta DV (Stockh) 32:893–894, 1993*; thyroid, esophagus, bronchus, rectum

Acquired perforating dermatosis – hyperpigmented hyperkeratotic papule *AD 148:160–162, 2012*

Acrokeratoelastoidosis of Costa – crateriform hyperkeratotic papules of the lateral palms and soles *Cutis 99:E7–8, 2017; AD 140:479–484, 2004*; of legs *Clin Exp Derm 26:263–265, 2001*

Acrokeratosis verruciformis of Hopf *AD 130:508–509, 511–512, 1994; Ann DV 115:1229–1232, 1988; Dermatol Zeitschr 60:227–250, 1931*; along Blaschko's lines *Indian J Dermatol 58:406, 2013*

Acrosyringeal epidermolytic papulosis neviformis *Dermatologica 171:122–125, 1985*

Acquired ichthyosis

Acquired perforating collagenosis – hyperpigmented hyperkeratotic nodules; linear, targetoid *AD 143:1201–1206, 2007*

Alopecia mucinosa – scaly red papules *AD 138:244–246, 2002*

Angiolymphoid hyperplasia with eosinophilia – prurigo nodularis-like lesions *J Dermatol 20:660–661, 1993*

Atopic dermatitis – legs, periumbilical region *Ped Derm 16:436–438 1999*

Confluent and reticulated papillomatosis of Gougerot and Carteaud *Pan Afr Med J 26:207, 2017; AD 148:505–508, 2012; Int J Derm 31:480–483, 1992*

Darier's disease (keratosis follicularis) – follicular skin-colored, brown papule *Dermatol Online J Dec 15, 2016; JID 134:1961–1970, 2014; JCI 115:2656–2664, 2005; Am J Clin Dermatol 4:97–105, 2003; Clin Dermatol 19:193–205, 1994; JAAD 27:40–50, 1992*; zosteriform Darier's disease *Mt Sinai J Med 68:339–341, 2001*

Disseminated and recurrent infundibulofolliculitis *Indian Dermatol Online J 8:39–41, 2017; Ped Derm 32:e5–7, 2015*

Ectopic plantar nail *BJD 149:1071–1074, 2003*

Elastosis perforans serpiginosa *JAAD 51:1–21, 2004; Hautarzt 43:640–644, 1992; AD 97:381–393, 1968*; in Ehlers-Danlos syndrome *Dermatol Online J March 15, 2019*; osteogenesis imperfect, Down's syndrome *Clin Exp Dermatol 26:521–524, 2001*; penicillamine

Epidermolysis bullosa with mottled pigmentation – wart-like hyperkeratotic papules of axillae, wrists, dorsae of hands, palms and soles; P25L mutation of keratin 5 *JAAD 52:172–173, 2005*

Epidermolysis bullosa pruriginosa – dominant dystrophic or recessive dystrophic; mild acral blistering at birth or early childhood; violaceous papular and nodular lesions in linear array on shins, forearms, trunk; red, crusted, and lichenified papules; lichenified hypertrophic and verrucous plaques in adults *BJD 159:464–469, 2008; BJD 146:267–274, 2002; BJD 130:617–625, 1994*

Epidermolytic acanthoma *BJD 141:728–730, 1999*

Erythema elevatum diutinum – personal observation

Flegel's disease (hyperkeratosis lenticularis perstans) – 3 mm flat-topped hyperkeratotic generalized papules; hyperkeratotic pointy spicules of legs (chronic keratotic papules of extremities); spiky papules of dorsal feet *Cutis 105:123–125, 2020; JAMA Derm*

155:739–740, 2019; AD 144:1509–1514, 2008; Int J Dermatol 47 Suppl 1:38–41, 2008; AD 133:909–914, 1997; Acta DV 68:341–345, 1988; JAAD 16:190–195, 1987; Hautarzt 9:363–364, 1958

Focal acral hyperkeratosis *Ped Derm 21:128–130, 2004; BJD 142:340–342, 2000; Hautarzt 50:586–589, 1999; AD 132:1365–1370, 1996; Dermatology 188:28–31, 1994; AD 123:1225, 1228, 1987; BJD 109:97–103, 1983; Hautarzt 9:362–364, 1958*

Fox-Fordyce disease *Dermatol Online J 18:28, 2012*

Granular parakeratosis (axillary granular parakeratosis) – brownish red keratotic papules *Am J Clin Dermatol 16:495–500, 2015AD 140:1161–1166, 2004*; submammary granular parakeratosis *JAAD 40:813–814, 1999*; hyperkeratotic papules and plaques in the intertriginous areas *Ped Derm 19:146–147, 2002*

Granuloma annulare, perforating – personal observation

Grover's disease (transient acantholytic dermatosis)
   Drug-induced by IL-4 infusion *JAAD 29:206–209, 1993*

Hailey-Hailey disease – genital papules *JAAD 26:951–955, 1992*; lichenoid papules of thigh *SkinMed 15:387–388, 2017*

Hereditary callosities

Hereditary papulotranslucent acrokeratoderma *Z Hautkr 60:211–214, 1985*

Hyperkeratosis of the nipple and areola *JAAD 32:124–125, 1995; AD 113:1691–1692, 1977*

Ichthyosis congenita type IV – erythrodermic infant with follicular hyperkeratosis *BJD 136:377–379, 1997*

Idiopathic disseminated comedones *Ped Derm 23:163–166, 2006*

Interstitial granulomatous dermatitis – skin colored papules *J Biol Regul Homeost Agents 30:49–52, 2016*

Keratosis circumscripta – age 3–5; plaques of follicular keratoses of elbows, knees, hips, posterior axillary folds, and sacrum with palmoplantar thickening (possible childhood PRP) *Cutis 79:363–366, 2007; Dermatologica 159:182–183, 1980; AD 93:408–410, 1966*

Keratosis follicularis spinulosa decalvans – X-linked dominant; follicular hyperkeratosis, corneal degeneration, alopecia, alopecia of eyebrows *Clin Exp Dermatol 37:631–634, 2012; Curr Prob Derm 14:71–116, 2002*

Keratosis follicularis squamosa – follicular hyperkeratotic papule; annular with scale *BJD 144:1070–1072, 2001*

Keratosis lichenoides chronica (Nekam's disease) – reticulated keratotic papules, linear arrays, atrophy, comedo-like lesions, prominent telangiectasia *AD 144:405–410, 2008; JAD 56:51–55, 2007; Dermatology 201:261–264, 2000; Dermatology 191:264–267, 1995; AD 131:609–614, 1995; AD 105:739–743, 1972; JAAD 37:263–264, 1997; JAAD 38:306–309, 1998*

Keratosis palmoplantaris papulosa *Hautarzt 63:368–369, 2012*

Keratosis pilaris – autosomal dominant *JAAD 72:890–900, 2015; Curr Prob Derm 14:71–116, 2002; JAAD 39:891–893, 1998*

Keratosis pilaris atrophicans *AD 130:469–475, 1994*; ulerythema ophryogenes *Ped Derm 11:172–175, 1994*; keratosis pilaris decalvans non-atrophicans *Clin Exp Dermatol 18:45–46, 1993*; keratosis follicularis spinulosa decalvans *AD Syphilol 151:384–387, 1926*; folliculitis decalvans *Acta DV (Stockh) 43:14–24, 1963*; atrophoderma vermiculatum – cheeks and pre-auricular regions *JAAD 18:538–542, 1988; J Cutan Dis 36:339–352, 1918*

Keratosis pilaris rubra (keratosis rubra pilaris) *AD 142:1611–1616, 2006; BJD 147:822–824, 2002*

Knuckle pads (heloderma) *AD 129:1043–1048, 1993*; keratotic knuckle pads unassociated with palmoplantar keratoderma

Kyrle's disease (hyperkeratosis follicularis et parafollicularis in cutem penetrans) *Stat Pearls Nov 14, 2019; J Derm 20:329–340, 1993; JAAD 16:117–123, 1987*

Lenticular acral keratosis in washerwomen *Int J Derm 37:532–537, 1998*

Lichen nitidus *Dermatol Online J Oct 15, 2017; Clin Exp Dermatol 18:381–383, 1993*

Lichen planus/lichen planopilaris (Graham-Little syndrome) *Stat Pearls Dec 20, 2019;* with keratosis pilaris *BJD 27:183–190, 1915;* hypertrophic lichen planus *Ned Tijdschr Geneeskd 159:A7868, 2015*

Lichen spinulosus *JAAD 22:261–264, 1990; Cutis 43:557–560, 1989*

Lichen striatus *Clin Dermatol 33:631–643, 2015*

Minute aggregate keratoses *Clin Exp Dermatol 10:566–571, 1985*

Multiple minute digitate hyperkeratosis – disseminated spiked hyperkeratosis – after X-ray therapy *Clin Exp Dermatol 20:425–427, 1995;* sporadic *AD 111:1176–1177, 1975;* familial (autosomal dominant) *JAAD 18:431–436, 1988;* associated with laryngeal carcinoma *Med Cutan Ibero Lat Am 6:279–283, 1978;* filiform keratoses (spiked, filiform, or hairy keratoses) – sporadic *Int J Dermatol 32:446–447, 1993;* familial *AD 117:412–414, 1981;* cyclosporine-induced *Hautarzt 46:841–846, 1995;* myeloma-associated *JAAD 33:346–351, 1995*

Pachydermatous eosinophilic dermatitis *Arch DV Croat 19:31–35, 2011; BJD 134:469–474, 1996*

Papular acantholytic dyskeratosis of the vulva *Ped Derm 22:237–239, 2005*

Parapsoriasis – acute (PLEVA), pityriasis lichenoides chronica (guttate parapsoriasis) *JAAD 56:205–210, 2007*

Perforating folliculitis – in cystic fibrosis; scaly papules of legs *Ped Derm 27:660–661, 2010*

Periumbilical pseudoxanthoma elasticum (acquired perforating pseudoxanthoma elasticum) – flat, well-demarcated, hyperpigmented, reticulated, atrophic central plaque with raised scaly border *An Bras Dermatol 85:705–707, 2010; JAAD 51:1–21, 2004; JAAD 39:338–344, 1998*

Persistent acantholytic dermatosis *Ann Acad Med Singapore 29:770–772, 2000*

Pityriasis rosea

Pityriasis rubra pilaris – erythematous perifollicular papules; grouped; scaly scalp; orange palmoplantar keratoderma; islands of sparing; resembles seborrheic dermatitis *Am J Clin Dermatol 19:377–390, 2018; BJD 133:990–993, 1995; Eur J Dermatol 4:593–597, 1994; JAAD 20:801–807, 1989*

Poikiloderma vasculare atrophicans *Ann Dermatol 23:548–552, 2011*

Postpemphigus acanthomata *Int J Derm 36:194–196, 1997*

Progressive symmetric erythrokeratoderma – elbows, knees, hands, and feet – personal observation

Prurigo nodularis – idiopathic *AD 148:794–796, 2012;* or associated with lymphoma, peripheral T-cell lymphoma (Lennert's lymphoma) *Cutis 51:355–358, 1993;* Hodgkin's disease *Dermatologica 182:243–246, 1991; Ped Derm 7:136–139, 1990;* gluten sensitive enteropathy *BJD 95:89–92, 1976;* AIDS *JAAD 33:837–838, 1995;* uremia *South Med J 68:138–141, 1975;* depression, liver disease, alpha-1 antitrypsin deficiency *Australas J Dermatol 32:151–157, 1991;* malabsorption

Dermatologica 169:211–214, 1984

Psoriasis – guttate, small plaques; rupioid, elephantine, ostraceous (oyster-like)

Punctate porokeratotic keratoderma *Dermatol Online J 16:9, 2010*

Reactive perforating collagenosis – early childhood, precipitated by trauma; skin colored umbilicated papules; heal with hypopigmentation or scar *Stat Pearls Jan 24, 2020; AD 121:1554–1555, 1557–1558, 1985*

Spiny keratoderma (palmoplantar parakeratotic spiny keratoderma, disseminated parakeratotic spiny keratoderma, palmoplantar orthokeratotic spiny keratoderma, Disseminated orthokeratotic spiny keratoderma, spiny keratoderma in eccrine hamartoma) *Cureus 11:e5609 Sept 9, 2019; Cutis 54:389–394, 1996*

Terra firme

Transient reactive papulotranslucent acrokeratoderma *Australas J Dermatol 41:172–174, 2000*

Trichostasis spinulosa *AD 133:1579,1582, 1997*

Urostomy site – pseudoverrucous peristomal lesions – warty papules at mucocutaneous junction *JAAD 19:623–632, 1988*

Waxy keratoses of childhood (disseminated hypopigmented keratoses) – generalized dome-shaped yellow or skin-colored keratotic papules *Ped Derm 18:415–416, 2001; Clin Exp Dermatol 19:173–176, 1994*

Warty dyskeratoma *JAAD 75:e97–98, 2016*

X-linked ichthyosis *Cutis 102:402,414–415, 2018*

PSYCHOCUTANEOUS DISORDERS

"Neglected nipples" – acanthosis nigricans like papules; avoidance of cleansing *Dermatol Pract Concept 4:81–84, 2014*

Trichotillomania – follicular hyperkeratosis *BJD 145:1034–1035, 2001*

SYNDROMES

Alagille syndrome (arteriohepatic dysplasia) – follicular hyperkeratosis *BJD 138:150–154, 1998*

Ataxia telangiectasia – ATM deficiency

Atrichia with keratin cysts – horny papules of face, neck, scalp; then trunk and extremities *Ann DV 121:802–804, 1994*

Cardio-facio-cutaneous syndrome – xerosis/ichthyosis, eczematous dermatitis, alopecia, growth failure, hyperkeratotic papules, ulerythema ophryogenes, seborrheic dermatitis, CALMs, nevi, keratosis pilaris *Ped Derm 17:231–234, 2000;* KRAS and BRAF mutations *Nat Genet 38:294–296, 2006*

CHILD syndrome

Costello syndrome – verrucous papillomas of nose and arms; growth and mental retardation, sociable, depressed nasal bridge, low set ears with thick earlobes, short neck, limited joint mobility, cardiac abnormalities, malignancies (rhabdomyosarcoma, ganglioneuroblastoma, neuroblastoma, bladder carcinoma), loose redundant skin of neck, hands and feet with deep creases of palms and soles, acanthosis nigricans, pigmented acral nevi, vascular birthmarks, hyperkeratosis, hyperpigmentation of skin, thin nails, thick eyebrows, sparse curly scalp hair; mutation in HRAS gene *Am J Med Genet 117:42–48, 2003*

Cowden's syndrome

Desmoplakin mutations – syndrome of dilated cardiomyopathy with severe left ventricular dysfunction, congenital alopecia, striate palmoplantar keratoderma, nail dystrophy, follicular hyperkeratosis with hyperpigmented plaques of elbows *Ped Derm 32:102–108, 2015*

Down's syndrome – keratosis pilaris; elastosis perforans serpiginosa *Clin Exp Dermatol 31:623–629, 2006; J Cut Med Surg 5:289–293, 2001*

Dyskeratosis benigna intraepithelialis mucosae et cutis hereditaria – conjunctivitis, umbilicated keratotic nodules of scrotum, buttocks, trunk; palmoplantar verruca-like lesions, leukoplakia of buccal mucosa, hypertrophic gingivitis, tooth loss *J Cutan Pathol 5:105–115, 1978*

Ectodermal dysplasia–skin fragility syndrome – autosomal recessive; plakophilin gene mutation (PKP1) – follicular hyperkeratosis; widespread skin fragility, alopecia of scalp and eyebrows, focal palmoplantar keratoderma with painful fissures, hypohidrosis; skin peeling; generalized erythema and peeling at birth; perioral fissuring and cheilitis; perianal erythema and erosions *JAAD 55:157–161, 2006; Acta DV 85:394–399, 2005; JID 122:1321–1324, 2004*

Epidermodysplasia verruciformis – seborrheic keratosis-like lesions; EVER 1 and EVER 2 deficiency *TMC6, TMC8, RHOH, CORO1A, IL-7, MST-1 JAAD 76:1161–1175, 2017; J Cutan Pathol 20:237–241, 1993*

Gall-Galli syndrome – Dowling-Degos disease with acantholysis – hyperkeratotic follicular papules *JAAD 45:760–763, 2001*

Greither's syndrome – warty keratoses of hands and feet with poikiloderma

Haber's syndrome – keratotic axillary papules *JAAD 40:462–467, 1999;* rosacea-like acneiform eruption, verrucous papules (seborrheic keratosis-like) of flexures, palmoplantar keratoderma, perioral pitted scars *BJD 160:215–217, 2009*

Hereditary acrokeratotic poikiloderma – vesicopustules of hands and feet at 1–3 months of age; widespread dermatitis; keratotic papules of hands, feet, elbows, and knees *AD 103:409–422, 1971*

Hereditary focal transgressive palmoplantar keratoderma – autosomal recessive; hyperkeratotic lichenoid papules of elbows and knees, psoriasiform lesions of scalp and groin, spotty and reticulate hyperpigmentation of face, trunk, and extremities, alopecia of eyebrows and eyelashes *BJD 146:490–494, 2002*

Ichthyosis follicularis with atrichia and photophobia (IFAP) – X-linked recessive; hyperkeratotic plaques overlying Achilles tendons; atopic dermatitis; collodion membrane and erythema at birth; ichthyosis, spiny (keratotic) follicular papules (generalized follicular keratoses), non-scarring alopecia totalis, keratotic papules of elbows, knees, fingers, extensor surfaces, xerosis; punctate keratitis, photophobia with progressive corneal scarring; nail dystrophy, paronychia, psychomotor delay, short stature; enamel dysplasia, beefy red tongue and gingiva, angular stomatitis (angular cheilitis), lamellar scales, psoriasiform plaques, palmoplantar erythema; mutation of *MBTPS2* (intramembrane zinc metalloproteinase needed for cholesterol homeostasis and endoplasmic reticulum stress response) *BJD 163:886–889, 2010; Ped Derm 26:427–431, 2009; Curr Prob Derm 14:71–116, 2002; JAAD 46:S156–158, 2002; BJD 142:157–162, 2000; Ped Derm 12:195, 1995; AD 125:103–106, 1989; Dermatologica 177:341–347, 1988; Am J Med Genet 85:365–368, 1999; BJD 21:165–189, 1909*

Incontinentia pigmenti – solitary keratotic papule on finger *Ped Derm 13:47–50, 1996*

Keratosis-ichthyosis-deafness (KID) syndrome – red scaly papules of palms and soles at birth *Ped Derm 23:81–83, 2006*

Kindler's syndrome – acral keratoses

Klippel-Trenaunay-Weber syndrome – angiokeratomous nodules; venous malformation, arteriovenous fistula, or mixed venous lymphatic malformation *Cutis 83:255–261, 2009; Br J Surg 72:232–236, 1985; Archives Generales de Medecine 3:641–672, 1900*

Lipoid proteinosis *Int J Dermatol 39:203–204, 2000; JAAD 39:149–171, 1998*

Maffucci's syndrome

Mal de Meleda – hyperkeratotic plaques

Netherton's syndrome – SPINK 5 deficiency

Noonan's syndrome – webbed neck, short stature, malformed ears, nevi, keloids, transient lymphedema, ulerythema ophyrogenes, keratosis follicularis spinulosa decalvans *JAAD 46:161–183, 2002; Ped Derm 15:18–22, 1998; J Med Genet 24:9–13, 1987;* extremities *Cutis 46:242–246, 1990*

Olmsted syndrome – periorificial keratotic papules and plaques; follicular hyperkeratosis of buttocks and knees; intertrigo, mutilating palmoplantar keratoderma, linear streaky hyperkeratosis, leukokeratosis of the tongue, sparse hair anteriorly *JAAD 53:S266–272, 2005; Eur J Derm 13:524–528, 2003; Ped Derm 20:323–326, 2003; BJD 136:935–938, 1997; Semin Derm 14:145–151, 1995; Am J Dis Child 33:757–764, 1927*

Pachyonychia congenita – keratotic papules on dorsa of fingers, elbows, and knees *BJD 171:343–355, 2014; Ped Derm 14:491–493, 1997;* follicular hyperkeratosis of lower back and buttocks; mutation in keratin 6A (*KRT6A*) *BJD 160:1327–1329, 2009*

Papillon-Lefevre syndrome – keratotic papules over knuckles (metacarpophalangeal and proximal interphalangeal joints); palmoplantar keratoderma, pitted on heels and forefoot; cathepsin C mutation *Ped Derm 30:749–750, 2013*

Phakomatosis pigmentokeratotica *Dermatology 197:377–380, 1998*

Pili torti, enamel hypoplasia syndrome – keratosis pilaris, dry fair hair, enamel hypoplasia, widely spaced abnormal teeth *BJD 145:157–161, 2001*

POEMS syndrome – multiple seborrheic keratoses

Proteus syndrome – epidermal nevus, eruptive seborrheic keratoses, depigmented nevi; (Takatsuki syndrome, Crowe-Fukase syndrome) – osteosclerotic bone lesions, peripheral polyneuropathy, hypothyroidism, and hypogonadism *JAAD 25:377–383, 1991; JAAD 21:1061–1068, 1989, Cutis 61:329–334, 1998*

Reactive arthritis syndrome – keratotic papules of palms and soles *J Family Med Prim Care 8:1250–1252, 2019*

Rothmund-Thomson syndrome – warty keratoses of hands, wrists, feet, and ankles

Tuberous sclerosis

Wiskott-aldrich syndrome – WASP deficiency

TRAUMA

Callosities from clothing and appliances

Chondrodermatitis nodularis chronicus helicis

Clavus

Carpenter's calluses

Ectopic nail – post-traumatic *JAAD 50:323–324, 2004*

Habit tics – callosities

Plantar calluses

Prayer nodules – forehead, knees, and ankles

Radiation – post irradiation keratoses post-irradiation digitate keratosis; keratotic miliaria secondary to radiotherapy *AD 124:855–856, 1988*

Thermal keratoses and squamous cell carcinoma in situ with erythema ab igne *AD 115:1226–1228, 1979*

VASCULAR

APACHE (acral pseudolymphomatous angiokeratoma of children) – linear scaly red papules of hand *BJD 145:512–514, 2001; BJD 124:387–388, 1991*

Angiokeratoma circumscriptum *AD 117:138–139, 1981*

Angiokeratoma corporis diffusum without metabolic abnormalities *AD 142:615–618, 2006*

Angiokeratoma of Fordyce – scrotal angiokeratomas

Angiokeratoma of Mibelli – autosomal dominant; associated with chilblains; on dorsum of fingers, toes, hands, feet *AD 106:726–728, 1972*

Angiokeratoma, solitary papular – occur after trauma in adult life – red to blue-black; may rapidly enlarge or bleed and simulate melanoma *AD 117:138–139, 1981; AD 95:166–175, 1967*

Angiokeratoma corporis diffusum (Fabry's disease (alpha galactosidase A) – X-linked recessive *NEJM 276:1163–1167, 1967;* fucosidosis (alpha-l-fucosidase) *AD 107:754–757, 1973;* Kanzaki's disease (alpha-N-acetylgalactosidase) *AD 129:460–465, 1993;* aspartylglycosaminuria (aspartylglycosaminidase) *Paediatr Acta 36:179–189, 1991;* adult-onset GM1 gangliosidosis (beta galactosidase) *Clin Genet 17:21–26, 1980;* galactosialidosis (combined beta–galactosidase and sialidase)*; AD 120:1344–1346, 1984;* no enzyme deficiency *AD 123:1125–1127, 1987; JAAD 12:885–886, 1985*) – telangiectasias or small angiokeratomas; acid sphingomyelinase deficiency *Ped Derm 36:906–908, 2019;* angiokeratomas corporis diffusum without enzyme deficiency *AD 142:615–618, 2006*

Cobb syndrome – angiokeratoma circumscriptum; nevus flammeus, angioma in spinal cord *Indian Dermatol Online J 11:212–219, 2020*

Degos' disease

Digital verrucous fibroangioma *Acta DV 72:303–304, 1992*

Hemangioma, including cutaneous keratotic hemangioma *AD 132:703–708, 1996*

Lymphangioma circumscriptum *BJD 83:519–527, 1970;* acquired vulvar lymphangioma mimicking genital warts *J Cutan Pathol 26:150–154, 1999*

Lymphangiectasia (acquired lymphangioma) – due to scarring processes such as recurrent infections, radiotherapy, scrofuloderma, scleroderma, keloids, tumors, tuberculosis, repeated trauma *BJD 132:1014–1016, 1996;* acquired lymphangiectasis S/P mastectomy *Cutis 58:276–278, 1996*

Lymphostasis verrucosa cutis (lymphedematous keratoderma) *BJD 127:411–416, 1992; Int J Dermatol 20:177–187, 1981*

Pyogenic granuloma

Verrucous hemangiomas, including eruptive verrucous hemangiomas *Ped Derm 2:191–193, 1985; Dermatologica 171:106–111, 1985*

PAPULES, HYPERPIGMENTED WITH HYPERTRICHOSIS (HYPERPIGMENTED HAIRY PAPULES)

CONGENITAL LESIONS

Congenital hypertrophy with hypertrichosis

Congenital smooth muscle hamartoma *Ped Derm 25:236–239, 2008; JAAD 48:161–179, 2003; JAAD 46:477–490, 2002; Curr Prob Derm 14:41–70, 2002; Ped Derm 13:431–433, 1996; AD 125:820–822, 1989; AD 121:1200–1201, 1985; AD 114:104–106, 1978*

Supernumerary nipples (accessory nipple or nipple nevus) *Cutis 62:235–237, 1998*

Transient thickening of the skin with hypertrichosis

DRUG ERUPTIONS

Vaccines – DPT or BCG immunizations

INFILTRATIVE DISEASES

Lichen amyloidosis

Pretibial myxedema *JAAD 46:723–726, 2002; AD 122:85–88, 1986*

Xanthoma disseminatum – mimicking melanocytic nevi *AD 128:1207–1212, 1992*

INFLAMMATORY DISEASES

Casting

Local inflammation – friction, gonococcal arthritis,

recurrent thrombophlebitis, melorheostatic scleroderma, chewing, burn, bug bites

NEOPLASTIC

Becker's nevi

Eccrine angiomatous hamartoma – vascular nodule; macule, red plaque, acral nodule of infants or neonates; painful, red, purple, blue, yellow, brown, skin-colored *JAAD 47:429–435, 2002; JAAD 37:523–549, 1997; Ped Derm 13:139–142, 1996*

Granular cell tumor *Cutis 69:343–346, 2002*

Hairy Pacinian neurofibroma (nerve sheath myxoma*) JAAD 18:416–419, 1988*

Melanocytic nevi – intradermal nevi; congenital melanocytic nevi *JAAD 48:161–179, 2003 JAAD 36:409–416, 1997;* eruptive atypical nevi in AIDS *AD 125:397–401, 1989*

Neurofibroma resembling congenital melanocytic nevus *JAAD 201358–362, 1989*

Nevus spilus *Ped Derm 30:100–104, 2013*

Spitz nevi – eruptive Spitz nevi *JAAD 15:1155–1159, 1986;* pigmented spindle cell nevus (Spitz nevus) *JAAD 28:565–571, 1993*

PRIMARY CUTANEOUS DISEASES

Epidermolysis bullosa, dystrophic types *Ann Ital Dermatol 10:195–196, 1995*

Lichen simplex chronicus *JAAD 48:161–179, 2003;*

SYNDROMES

Neurofibromatosis type I – schwannomas

Neurofibromatosis type II – schwannomas *J Med Genet 37:897–904, 2000*

Syndromes associated with nevi *JAAD 29:374–388, 1993*

PAPULES AND NODULES, HYPERPIGMENTED (WITH OR WITHOUT HYPERKERATOSIS)

AUTOIMMUNE DISEASES AND DISEASES OF IMMUNE DYSFUNCTION

Allergic contact dermatitis – pigmented poison ivy allergic contact dermatitis

Graft vs. host disease – chronic; hyperpigmented nodules which soften and atrophy

Morphea *AD 122:76–79, 1986;* pansclerotic morphea – hyperpigmented sclerodermoid plaques *JAMA Derm 155:388–389, 2019*

Pemphigus foliaceus resembling seborrheic keratoses *AD 126: 543–544, 1990*

Scleroderma, nodular *JAAD 32:343–5, 1995*

Sjogren's syndrome – annular urticarial-like erythema, localized cutaneous nodular amyloidosis (brown nodule), leukocytoclastic vasculitis, photosensitivity *JAAD 79:736–745, 2018*

Still's disease in the adult – brown coalescent scaly papules *JAAD 52:1003–1008, 2005*

CONGENITAL

Accessory tragi

Congenital hypertrichotic melanoneurocytoma – congenital hypertrichotic hyperpigmented plaque *JAAD 67:799–801, 2012*

Congenital pigmented nevus with cartilaginous differentiation – congenital pigmented nevus with giant pedunculated pink tumor *Ped Derm 30:501–502, 2013*

Congenital self-healing Langerhans cell histiocytosis – multiple congenital red-brown nodules *JAAD 56:290–294, 2007; Ped Derm 17:322–324, 2000*

Myelomeningocele *Ped Derm 26:688–695, 2009*

Supernumerary nipple *Cutis 71:344–346, 2003*

Transient neonatal pustular melanosis – brown papules of scrotum *Ped Derm 35:845–846, 2018*

DRUG-INDUCED

Chemotherapy – epidermal dysmaturation; brown papules *JAAD 43:358–360, 2000*

Imatinib mesylate – hyperpigmented lichenoid flat-topped papules of trunk and lips *Cutis 99:189–192, 2017*

Lichenoid drug eruption

Minocycline pigmentation of scar *Cutis 74:293–298, 2004*

Nadroparin-calcium injections – calcifying panniculitis *BJD 153:657–660, 2005*

Voriconazole – melanoma *AD 146:300–304, 2010*

EXOGENOUS

Foreign body granuloma

Mudi-chood – due to oils applied to hair; papulosquamous eruption of nape of neck and upper back; begin as follicular pustules then brown-black papules with keratinous rim *Int J Dermatol 31:396–397, 1992*

Stockings mimicking nevi

INFECTIONS AND INFESTATIONS

AIDS – photo-induced lichen planus or lichenoid eruption; pruritic papular eruption with HIV in Uganda *JAMA 292:2614–2621, 2004; JAAD 24 (pt 1)231–235, 1991*

Alternariosis, cutaneous – hyperkeratotic hyperpigmented plaque of leg ulcer; following laceration *Ped Derm 27:99–101, 2010*

Aspergillosis – primary cutaneous – purple or brown papulonodules *AD 129:1189–1194, 1993; AD 124:121–126, 1988; BJD 85 (suppl 17)95–97, 1971*

Botryomycosis in AIDS *JAAD 16:238–242, 1987*

Cat scratch fever

Condyloma acuminatum *JAAD 66:867–880, 2012*

Cunninghamella bertholletiae – mucormycosis *Clin Inf Dis 66:154–157, 2017*

Cytomegalovirus infection – hyperpigmented nodules of plaques *JAAD 7:545–548, 1982*

Dermatophyte infection, invasive *Clin Exp Dermatol 57:1344–1350, 2018*

Epidermodysplasia verruciformis *Int J Dermatol 57:1344–1350, 2018; ; Dermatol Online J 15:1, 2009;* brown follicular papules in GVHD *JAAD 37:578–580, 2007*

Hepatitis C infection – necrolytic acral erythema; red to hyperpigmented psoriasiform plaques with variable scale or erosions *JAAD 53:247–251, 2005; Int J Derm 35:252–256, 1996*

Herpes zoster, chronic in AIDS *AD 126:1048–1050, 1990; JAAD 20:637–642, 1989*

Histoplasmosis, disseminated in AIDS – brown papule *AD 132:341–346, 1996; AD 125:689–694, 1989*

Lobomycosis) – *Lacazia (Loboa) loboi* (keloidal blastomycosis); Amazon rain forest of South America; legs, arms, face *JAAD 53:931–951, 2006; JAAD 29:134–136, 139–140, 1993; Cutis 46:227–234, 1990; Int J Dermatol 27:481–484, 1988*

Leeches – hyperpigmented papules and nodules due to application of *Hirudo medicinalis* (leeches) *JAAD 43:867–869, 2000*

Leishmaniasis – Old World leishmaniasis – brown plaque of scalp with alopecia *AD 147:1097–1102, 2011;* disseminated leishmaniasis with dermatofibroma-like lesions *BJD 148:185–187, 2003;* hyperpigmented scar *Arch Dermatol Res 256:127–136, 1976*

Leprosy – lepromatous leprosy *JAAD 60:181–182, 2009;* borderline leprosy – coppery-brown plaque *JAAD 54:559–578, 2006;* targetoid red–brown plaques *Cutis 92:187–189, 2013*

Malacoplakia – violaceous nodules *AD 134:244–245, 1998; Am J Dermatopathol 20:185–188, 1998; JAAD 34:325–332, 1996; JAAD 30:834–836, 1994*

Mycobacterium massiliensis – red brown nodules of posterior calves mimicking erythema induratum *BJD 173:235–238, 2015*

Mycobacterium tuberculosis – miliary *JAAD 23:381–385, 1990;* lichen scrofulosorum; lupus vulgaris; nodular tuberculid *JAAD 53:S154–156, 2005;* erythema induratum of Bazin – brown nodules with ulceration and scarring *Clin Inf Dis 70:1254–1257, 2020*

Onchocerciasis (*Onchecerca volvulus*)- transmitted by Simuliidae (humpbacked black fly) localized acute dermatitis or chronic generalized dermatitis; papules, crusted papules, lichenified plaques; often with hyperpigmented nodules *JAAD 45:435–437, 2001; Cutis 65:293–297, 2000; BJD 121:187–198, 1989*

Papular urticaria – red-brown nodules *Ped Derm 19:409–411, 2002*

Paragonimiasis – pulmonary nodule and brown chest nodule *Clin Inf Dis 60:1532,1582–1583, 2015*

Talaromyces (Penicillium) marneffei – brown papules and nodules *JAAD 49:344–346, 2003*

Phaeohyphomycosis – diffuse infiltrated pigmented plaques; subcutaneous cysts, abscesses, ulcerated plaques, hemorrhagic pustules, necrotic papulonodules, cellulitis *JAAD 75:19–30, 2016*

Syphilis, secondary; nodular

Scabies – red-brown nodules *Ped Derm 19:409–411, 2002;* Norwegian scabies *AD 124:121–126, 1988*

Varicella – hyperpigmented scar *Ped Derm 18:378–380, 2001*

Verrucae – pigmented wart – HPV 4,60,65 *BJD 148:187–188, 2003;* verruca vulgaris; flat warts

Yaws

INFILTRATIVE

Amyloidosis – amyloid elastosis *AD 121:498–502, 1985;* lichen amyloidosis; nodular localized primary cutaneous amyloid – brown facial plaque *BJD 158:860–862, 2008; Cutis 82:55–59, 2008;* brown plantar nodule *AD 146:557–562, 2010;* brown papules of conchal bowl *JAAD 62:1078–1079, 2010*

Benign cephalic histiocytosis – red–brown nodules *Ped Derm 19:409–411, 2002*

Congenital self-healing histiocytosis – red–brown nodules *Ped Derm 19:409–411, 2002*

Eosinophilic granuloma – brown papule of pre-tragus *Ped Derm 36:251–252, 2019*

Erdheim-Chester disease (multisystem non-Langerhans cell histiocytosis) – CD68+ and factor XIIIa+; negative for CD1a and S100; xanthoma and xanthelasma-like lesions (red–brown–yellow papules and plaques) (resemble xanthoma disseminatum); flat wart-like papules of face; lesions occur in folds; skin becomes slack with atrophy of folds and face; also lesions of eyelids, axillae, groin, neck; bony lesions; involvement of heart (congestive heart failure), lungs (pulmonary fibrosis), central nervous system, gastrointestinal tract, endocrine; death; diabetes insipidus and exophthalmos *JAAD 57:1031–1045, 2007; AD 143:952–953, 2007; Hautarzt 52:510–517, 2001; Medicine (Baltimore) 75:157–169, 1996; Virchow Arch Pathol Anat 279:541–542, 1930;* infiltration of vulva and clitoris *Cut Opin Rheumatol 24:53–59, 2012*

Hereditary progressive mucinous histiocytosis – red–brown or skin colored papules *JAAD 57:1031–1045, 2007*

Langerhans cell histiocytosis – red–brown nodules *Ped Derm 19:409–411, 2002;* red–brown papules of scalp *AD 143:1067–1072, 2007*

Urticaria pigmentosa (mastocytosis) – red–brown nodules *Curr Ped Rev 15:42–46, 2019; Am J Hematol 88:612–624, 2013; Am J Clin Dermatol 12:259–270, 2011; Ped Derm 19:409–411, 2002;* diffuse cutaneous mastocytosis *J Investig Dermatol Symp Proc 6:143–147, 2001; BJD 144:682–695, 2001;* familial mastocytosis – R634Wc-kit mutation *Ped Derm 32:267–270, 2015*

Xanthogranuloma – red–brown nodules *Ped Derm 19:409–411, 2002;* micronodular juvenile xanthogranuloma *AD 148:531–536, 2012*

Xanthoma disseminatum – nevi-like red–brownish–yellow papulo-nodules *JAAD 56:302–316, 2007; AD 128:1207–1212, 1992*

INFLAMMATORY DISEASES

Kikuchi's disease (histiocytic necrotizing lymphadenitis) – multiple red to red–brown papules of face, scalp, chest, back, arms; red

plaques; erythema and acneiform lesions of face; morbilliform, urticarial, and rubella-like exanthems; red or ulcerated pharynx; cervical adenopathy; associations with SLE, lymphoma, tuberculous adenitis, viral lymphadenitis, infectious mononucleosis, and drug eruptions *AD 142:641–646, 2006; BJD 144:885–889, 2001; JAAD 36:342–346, 1997; Am J Surg Pathol 14:872–876, 1990*

Neutrophilic eccrine hidradenitis – hyperpigmented plaques *Cancer 62:2532–2536, 1988*

Proliferative fasciitis – hyperpigmented and red nodules of abdomen *SKINmed 12:111–112, 2014*

Pseudolymphoma – red–brown nodules *Ped Derm 19:409–411, 2002*

Rosai-Dorfman disease (sinus histiocytosis with massive lymphadenopathy) – keloidal nodule *JAAD 68:346–348, 2013*

Ped Derm 17:377–380, 2000

Sarcoidosis (Darier-Roussy sarcoid) *JAAD 54:55–60, 2006; Ann Dermatol Syphil 5:144–149, 1904*

METABOLIC

Addison's disease – scarring *Cutis 66:72–74, 2000*

Calcinosis cutis – personal observation

Endometriosis – in caesarian section scar *Z Hautkr 61:940–942, 1986;* brown nodule *JAAD 21:155, 1989*

Gouty panniculitis – ulcerated hyperpigmented nodules of legs *JAAD 57:S52–54, 2007;* miliary gout – brown plaques and milky white fluid *JAMA Derm 150:569–570, 2014*

Osteoclastic activity due to tertiary hyperparathyroidism – brown tumor of fingertip *Annual Meeting AAD 2000*

NEOPLASTIC

Acantholytic acanthoma *JAAD 19:783–786, 1988*

Acquired digital fibrokeratoma – hyperpigmented nodule of palm *Ped Derm 29:111–112, 2012*

Acrochordon (skin tag)

Actinic keratosis

Aneurysmal fibrous histiocytomas (variant of dermatofibroma) *BJD 153:664–665, 2005*

Angioleiomyoma, congenital – gray and pink nodule with depression *Ped Derm 28:460–462, 2011*

Angiosarcoma

Agminated fibroblastic connective tissue nevus – brown herpetiform nodules *Ped Derm 36:997–998, 2019*

Apocrine hidrocystoma *AD 127:571–576, 1991*

Apocrine nevus *JAAD 18:579–581, 1988*

BAP-1 inactivated melanocytic tumors – pink-brown symmetric macules and papules with peripheral nodule *JAAD 89:1585–1583, 2019; BJD 179:973–975, 2018*

Basal cell carcinoma

Blastic plasmacytoid dendritic cell neoplasm – purple brown nodules of face, scalp, and legs; confluent brown-red plaques of trunk *Arch Pathol Lab Med 138:564, 2014; Haematologica 92:2, 2013; BJD 169:579–586, 2013*

Blue nevus – cellular blue nevus – light brown papule

Bowen's disease, pigmented *BJD 138:515–518, 1998; AD 129:1043–1048, 1993; J Derm Surg Oncol 14:765–769, 1988;* HPV type 56-associated Bowen's disease – longitudinal melanonychia;

pigmented hyperkeratotic plaque *BJD 167:1161–1164, 2012;* mimicking malignant melanoma *Derm Surg 27:673–674, 2001;* of scrotum *J Derm Surg Oncol 12:1114–1115, 1986*

Bowenoid papulosis – hyperpigmented flat-topped papules of penis *JAAD 81:1–21, 2019; Cutis 102; 151–152,4, 2018; Cutis 86:278,295–296, 2010*

Multicentric Castleman's disease – hyperpigmented plaques of back *The Dermatologist March 2015, pp39–41*

Chordoma, metastatic *J Eur Acad DV 11:85–86, 1998*

Clear cell acanthoma (Degos' acanthoma) – brown shiny papule of lower leg *AD 143:255–260, 2007*

Clear cell eccrine porocarcinoma *BJD 149:1059–1063, 2003*

Clear cell hidradenoma – brown–red nodule *JAAD 54:S248–249, 2006*

Clear cell sarcoma (clear cell sarcoma of tendons and aponeuroses) (malignant melanoma of soft parts) – tan pink–brown papule of thigh *AD 147:609–614, 2011;* brown indurated tumor of thigh *BJD 169:1346–1352, 2013*

Connective tissue nevus

Dermal dendrocyte hamartoma (dermal dendrocytoma) – medallion-like; annular brown or red congenital lesion of central chest with slightly atrophic wrinkled surface *JAAD 51:359–363, 2004; AD 126:689–690, 1990*

Dermatofibroma – brown–yellow papules, nodules *SKINmed 13:308–309, 2015; Rook p. 2350, 1998, Sixth Edition;* multiple eruptive dermatofibromas associated with systemic lupus erythematosus, dermatomyositis, HIV disease, hematologic malignancy, pregnancy *JAAD 57:S81–84, 2007*

Dermatofibrosarcoma protuberans – in adenosine deaminase deficiency; mimicking dermal dendritic hamartoma; 3–6 mm atrophic hyperpigmented papules *Ped Derm 33:359–360, 2016*

Congenital multiple clustered dermatofibroma – hyperpigmented patch with papules and some depressed areas *Ped Derm 31:105–106, 2014; J Cutan Pathol 37:e42–45, 2010; BJD 142:1040–1043, 2000*

Deep penetrating nevus – black or darkly pigmented nevus of head, neck, and scalp *JAAD 71:1234–1240, 2014*

Dermatofibrosarcoma protuberans, pigmented (Bednar's tumor) – blue–brown nodule of dorsal foot *Ped Derm 28:583–585, 2011; JAAD 57:548–550, 2007; Am J Surg Pathol 9:630–639, 1985*

Dermatomyofibroma – red neck plaque, hyperpigmented papule *Ped Derm 34:347–351, 2017*

Dermatosis papulosa nigra *Cutis 32:385–392, 1983; AD 89:655–658, 1964*

Desmoid fibromatosis

Eccrine angiomatous hamartoma – congenital red–brown papules and plaques *Ped Derm36:909–912, 2019;* brown and pink plaque of superior gluteal crease *AD 145:241–243, 2009;* hyperpigmented plaque and violaceous patches *Ped Derm 26:662–663, 2009;* vascular nodule; macule, red plaque, acral nodule of infants or neonates; painful, red, purple, blue, yellow, brown, skin-colored *Ped Derm 22:175–176, 2005; JAAD 47:429–435, 2002; JAAD 37:523–549, 1997; Ped Derm 13:139–142, 1996*

Eccrine nevus – brown papule *JAAD 51:301–304, 2004*

Eccrine poroma – mimicking melanoma *Cutis 59:43–46, 1997*

Eccrine porocarcinoma *AD 131:211–216, 1995*

Eccrine sweat gland carcinoma

Eccrine syringofibroadenoma *JAAD 13:433–436, 1985*

Epidermal nevus

Eruptive vellus hair cysts *Ped Derm 5:94–96, 1988; BJD 116:465–466, 1987;* dark brown papules *Ped Derm 31:515–516, 2014*

Extramammary Paget's disease – red brown plaque of lower back *Cutis 101:422–424, 2018*

Fibroepithelioma of Pinkus (variant of basal cell carcinoma) *BJD 150:1208–1209, 2004;* gray–brown papule or plaque; skin colored plaque; pedunculated, polypoid; pink papule *AD 142:1318–1322, 2006; JAAD 52:168–169, 2005*

Fibrokeratoma

Fibro-osseous pseudotumor of the digit – hyperkeratotic brown papule of the toe tip *AD 147:975–980, 2011; Cancer 58:2103–2109, 1986*

Fibrous hamartoma of infancy – hyperpigmented hypertrichotic hyperhidrotic plaque *JAAD 64:579–586, 2011; J Pediatr Surg 46:753–755, 2011; J Cutan Pathol 34:39–43, 2007; Ped Pathol 14:39–52, 1994*

Generalized eruptive histiocytoma (progressive eruptive histiocytomas) – hundreds of skin-colored, brown, blue–red papules; resolve with macular pigmentation; face, trunk, proximal extremities; brown scaly papules *AD 139:933–938, 2003; JAAD 35:323–325, 1996; JAAD 31:322–326, 1994; JAAD 20:958–964, 1989; JAAD 17:499–454, 1987; AD 117:216–221, 1981; AD 116:565–567, 1980; AD 96:11–17, 1967; AD 88:586–593, 1963;* progressive nodular histiocytoma – red–brown nodules *Ped Derm 19:409–411, 2002*

Granular cell myoblastoma – red, hyperpigmented *Cutis 75:21,23–24, 2005; Ped Derm 14:489–490, 1997; AD 126:1051–1056, 1990*

Multiple granular cell tumors – personal observation

Hair follicle hamartoma – hyperpigmented plaque – personal observation

Infantile myofibromatosis – brown plaque with central necrosis *JAAD 71:264–270, 2014*

Kaposi's sarcoma – personal observation

Keloid *JAAD 46:S63, 2002; Dermatol Surg 25:631–638, 1999*

Leiomyomas – red–brown *AD 88:510–520, 1963*

Leiomyosarcoma – brown nodule *AD 135:341–346, 1999*

Leukemia – acute myelogenous leukemia – red–brown papules and plaques *JAMA3142182–2183, 2015;* granulocytic sarcoma (chloroma) – personal observation

Lipoblastomas – multiple subcutaneous nodules with overlying hyperpigmentation and hypertrichosis *BJD 143:694, 2000*

Lymphoma – ichthyosiform cutaneous T-cell lymphoma with brown papulonodules *JAMA Derm 155:1195–1197, 2019;* red–brown nodules *Ped Derm 19:409–411, 2002;* cutaneous T-cell lymphoma *Ped Derm 21:558–560, 2004;* cutaneous T-cell lymphoma mimicking lipodermatosclerosis *JAMA Derm 152:487–488, 2016;* granulomatous cutaneous T-cell lymphoma *AD 144:1609–1617, 2008;* immunocytoma (low grade B-cell lymphoma) – blue or reddish-brown papules *JAAD 44:324–329, 2001;* extranodal nasal type natural killer T-cell lymphoma – ulcerated hyperpigmented plaque of arm *JAAD 72:21–34, 2015; JAAD 54:S192–197, 2006;* intravascular lymphoma – painful gray–brown, red, blue–livid patches, plaques, nodules, with telangiectasia and underlying duration; 40% of patients with intravascular lymphoma present with cutaneous lesions *BJD 157:16–25, 2007*

Melanoacanthoma – pink and hyperpigmented nodule *JAMA Derm 151:1129–1130, 2015*

Melanocytic nevus, including congenital melanocytic nevus *Cutis 83:69–72, 2009;* giant congenital melanocytic nevi with benign proliferative nodules – hyperpigmented plaques and nodules *BJD*

176:1131–1143, 2017; giant congenital melanocytic nevus sparing nipple *Ped Derm 32:514–517, 2015;* congenital dermal melanocytic nevus – widespread hyperpigmented nodules *JAAD 49:732–735, 2003;* congenital melanocytic nevus – hyperpigmented plaque *BJD 167:1085–1091, 2012;* atypical nevi; eruptive atypical nevi in AIDS *AD 125:397–401, 1989;* eruptive nevi associated with chronic myelogenous leukemia *JAAD 35:326–329, 1996;* eruptive nevi associated with immunosuppression *JAAD 54:338–340, 2006; BJD 154:880–886, 2006; Melanoma Res 15:223–224, 2005; JAAD 49:1020–1022, 2003;* eruptive melanocytic nevi following Stevens-Johnson syndrome *AD 143:1555–1557, 2007*

Melanoma – primary; pigmented papules and nodules *AD 147:549–555, 2011; JAMA 292:2771–2776, 2004; Semin Oncol 2:5–118, 1975;* thin nodular *AD 146:311–318, 2010;* metastatic melanoma – 2 mm brown papules of face and neck *Ped Derm 27:201–203, 2010;* hyperpigmented plaque *JAAD 73:645–654, 2015;* primary dermal melanoma – pedunculated pink papule, dark macule, blue pigmented nevus, dome-shaped hemorrhagic papule, changing pigmented nevus *JAAD 71:1083–1091, 2014*

Melanotrichoblastoma – pedunculated pigmented papule *Cutis 100:243–246, 2017*

Mesenchymal tumor – subcutaneous hyperpigmented nodule; phosphaturic mesenchymal tumor, mixed connective tissue type; tumor induced osteomalacia (TIO) (low serum phosphate, increased urinary phosphate excretion, low 1,25 dihydroxy vitamin D levels, and elevated serum FGF-23); observe acquired renal phosphate wasting (hypophosphatemia); prominent bony osteoid formation and unmineralized bone; progressive weakness and bone pain *JAAD 57:509–512, 2007*

Metastases – metastatic breast carcinoma as pigmented papule *JAAD 31:1058–1060, 1994; AD 125:536–539, 1989*

Mucinous nevus *BJD 148:1064–1066, 2003;* congenital mucinous nevus – brown-skin colored plaques *Ped Derm 20:229–231, 2003*

Mucinous eccrine nevus *Ped Derm 20:137–139, 2003*

Multinucleate cell angiohistiocytoma – multiple dark brown papules and nodules of extremities *JAAD 35:320–322, 1996; AD 132:703–708, 1996; JAAD 30:417–422, 1994*

Myeloid sarcoma – diffuse red brown nodules *Ped Derm 36:509–510, 2019*

Neurilemmomatosis *JAAD 10:344–354, 1984*

Neurocutaneous melanosis *BJD 157:397–398, 2007; JAAD 24:747–755, 1991*

Neurofibroma resembling congenital melanocytic nevus *JAAD 20:358–362, 1989*

Neurothekeoma

Nevus – giant bathing trunk nevus; brown plaque *BJD 157:99–601, 2007*

Nevus spilus

Olfactory neuroblastoma, pigmented – pigmented polypoid lesion of nasal cavity; confused with mucosal melanoma *AD 144:270–272, 2008*

Ossifying fibromyxoid tumor of the skin – tan-brown, dark brown nodule *JAAD 52:644–647, 2005*

Paget's disease in male – hyperpigmented plaque *AD 144:1660–1662, 2008*

Pigmented hamartomatous lesions including acanthosis nigricans, epidermal nevus, melanoacanthoma, nevus verrucosus, nevus sebaceus *JAAD 10:1–16, 1984*

Pigmented spindle cell nevus *Clin Derm 37:447–467, 2019*

Pinkus tumor – flesh, pink, or brown; sessile or pedunculated *Cutis 54:85–92, 1994*

Plasmacytosis – brown papule or plaque; extracellular crystal deposition in cutaneous plasmacytosis *JAMA Derm 156:217–218, 2020*

Plexiform schwannoma – hyperpigmented annular plaque in neurofibromatosis type II *JAMA Derm 154:341–346, 2018*

Poikiloderma vasculare atrophicans with CTCL

Poroid hidradenoma – painful deep red, blue, brown or violaceous nodule of arm, scalp, face, or trunk *Ped Derm 28:60–61, 2011; AD 146:557–562, 2010*

Porokeratosis – disseminated superficial actinic porokeratosis *JAAD 58:657–660, 2008;* porokeratosis ptychotropica – hyperpigmented verrucous plaques of intertriginous areas *JAMA Derm 149:1099–1100, 2013*

Progressive nodular histiocytosis – red–brown nodules, including facial nodules *JAMA Derm 149:1229–1230, 2013*

Reed nevus (pigmented spindle cell nevus) – brown–black papule or nodule *JAAD 71:1234–1240, 2014*

Scars, pigmented
    Spontaneously regressing melanoma *Pathology 7:91–99, 1975*
    Hemorrhage within scar *Cutis 74:293–298, 2004*

Seborrheic keratoses

Seborrheic keratosis with trichilemmomas masquerading as melanoma *Cutis 54:351–353, 1994*

Self-healing reticulohistiocytosis *JAAD 13:383–404, 1985*

Spitz nevi *JAAD 65:1073–1074, 2011; JAAD 27:901–913, 1992;* agminated Spitz nevi *Ped Derm 22:546–549, 2005; BJD 117:511–512, 1987;* eruptive Spitz nevi *BJD 164:873–877, 2011; JAAD 15:1155–1159, 1986;* congenital Spitz nevus mimicking melanoma *JAAD 47:441–444, 2002;* combined Spitz nevus – pink, red, tan, or dark brown *AD 125:1703–1708, 1989; AD 82:325–335, 1960;* multiple Pagetoid Spitz nevi *AD 148:37—374, 2012*

Smooth muscle hamartoma – patchy hyperpigmented plaque *AD 147:1234–1235, 2011*

Pigmented spindle cell nevus; pigmented Spitz and Reed nevus *AD 143:549–550, 2007*

Spitz nevus – pink–brown papule or nodule *JAAD 71:1241–1249, 2014;* eruptive disseminated Spitz nevi *JAAD 57:519–523, 2007;* agminated Spitz nevi on a nevus spilus, induced by chemotherapy *Ped Derm 27:411–413, 2010;* desmoplastic Spitz nevus *Ped Derm 32:727–728, 2015*

Squamous cell carcinoma *BJD 149:1292–1308, 2003; J Cutan Pathol 27:381–386, 2000;* hyperpigmented plaque of proximal nail fold *BJD 161:1262–1269, 2009*

Syringoacanthoma – seborrheic keratosis-like *AD 120:751–756, 1984*

Syringomas, including eruptive syringomas *Cutis 76:267; – 269, 2005; AD 140:1161–1166, 2004; J Eur Acad Dermatol Venereol 15:242–246, 2001; AD 125:1119–1120, 1989;* generalized eruptive clear cell syringomas – brown *AD 125:1716–1717, 1989*

Trichoblastoma – arising in a nevus sebaceus *BJD 149:1067–1070, 2003*

Vellus hair cysts, eruptive

Waldenstrom's macroglobulinemia – neoplastic B-cell infiltrates; red–brown or violaceous papulonodules *Ann DV 129:53–55, 2002; JAAD 45:S202–206, 2001; Ann DV 112:509–516, 1985*

PARANEOPLASTIC DISORDERS

Necrolytic acral erythema – hyperpigmented hyperkeratotic plaques of feet and shins *JAAD 67:962–968, 2012*

Necrobiotic xanthogranuloma with paraproteinemia

Reed syndrome (hereditary leimyomatosis and renal cell cancer) *Fam Cancer 13:637–644, 2014; Cutis 81:41–48, 2008*

Sign of Leser-Trelat

PHOTODERMATITIS

Colloid milium – orange brown translucent facial papules *AD 142:784–785, 2006*

PRIMARY CUTANEOUS DISEASES

Acanthosis nigricans, including generalized acanthosis nigricans

Acquired perforating collagenosis – hyperpigmented hyperkeratotic nodules *AD 143:1201–1206, 2007*

Acquired perforating dermatosis – hyperpigmented hyperkeratotic papule *AD 148:160–162, 2012*

Axillary granular parakeratosis – brownish red keratotic papules *AD 140:1161–1166, 2004*

Blaschkitis – acquired self-healing Blaschko dermatitis; personal observation

Confluent and reticulated papillomatosis

Darier's disease

Distal subungual corn – tender acral pigmented keratotic subungual papule *BJD 171:69–72, 2014*

Dowling-Degos disease (reticulated pigmented anomaly of the flexures)

Endosalpingosis – ectopic fallopian tube epithelium; umbilical nodule *BJD 151:924–925, 2004*

Erythema elevatum diutinum – red–brown patches of extremities in HIV disease *Acta Rheumatol Port 42:324–328, 2017; Clin in Dermatol 37:679–683, 2019;* red–brown plaques of fingers and knees *JAAD 65:469–471, 2011; JAAD 49:764–767, 2003*

Flegel's disease (hyperkeratosis lenticularis) *JAAD 16:190–195, 1987; Cutis 48:201–204, 1991*

Galli–Galli disease – lentigines and papules *AD 148:641–646, 2012;* reticulate, hyper- and hypopigmented macules and papules; intertrigo; mutation in keratin 5 *BJD 170:1362–1365, 2014*

Disseminated granuloma annulare – personal observation

Granuloma faciale – red, brown, violaceous, yellowish *JAMA Derm 154:1312–1315, 2018; JAAD 53:1002–1009, 2005*

Kyrle's disease

Lichen aureus – red–brown papules *AD 144:1169–1173, 2008*

Lichen nitidus

Lichen planus – hyperpigmented plaque – personal observation; lichen planus pigmentosus *JAAD 21:815, 1989; Dermatologica 149:43–50, 1974*

Lichen planus tropicus

Lichen sclerosus et atrophicus – personal observation

Lichen simplex chronicus – in blacks

Lupus miliaris disseminata faciei

Necrolytic acral erythema – acral hyperkeratotic hyperpigmented plaques with red to violaceous centers *JAAD 81:23–41, 2019; Cutis 98: 16,19–20, 2016; Int J Derm 35:252–256, 2016; Ped Derm 28:701–706, 2011*

Periumbilical perforating pseudoxanthoma elasticum *JAAD 39:338–344, 1998; JAAD 26:642–644, 1992; AD 115:300–303, 1979*

Pityriasis rubra pilaris

Pseudoacanthosis nigricans

Reactive perforating collagenosis *Rev Med Chil 138:1281–1284, 2010*

Symmetrical acrokeratoderma (?acanthosis nigricans) – hyperpigmented hyperkeratotic flexural regions and dorsal hands; wrists, knees, ankles *BJD 170:948–951, 2014; JAAD 70:533–538, 2014*

Terra firme *Case Rep Dermatol 11:108–112, 2019; Ped Derm 28:79–81, 2011*

SYNDROMES

Albright's hereditary osteodystrophy – pseudohypoparathyroidism, round face, short neck, osteomas of skin with overlying hyperpigmentation, short stature, hypogonadism, macrocephaly, psychomotor retardation, endocrinologic abnormalities; mutation in *GNAS1 Ped Derm 28:135–137, 2011; Endocrinology 30:922–932, 1942*

Bannayan-Riley-Ruvalcaba- Zonana syndrome – supernumerary nipples, hemangiomas, genital hyperpigmentation *AD 132:1214–1218, 1996; Am J Med Genet 44:307–314, 1992*

Basaloid follicular hamartoma syndrome – autosomal dominant; milia, comedone-like lesions, dermatosis papulosa nigra, skin tag-like lesions, hypotrichosis, multiple skin-colored, red, and hyperpigmented papules of the face in periorificial distribution, neck chest, back, proximal extremities, and eyelids; syndrome includes milia-like cysts, comedones, sparse scalp hair, palmar pits, and parallel bands of papules of the neck (zebra stripes); hypohidrosis *Cutis 78:42–46, 2006; JAAD 49:698–705, 2003; BJD 146:1068–1070, 2002; JAAD 45:644–645, 2001; JAAD 43:189–206, 2000; JAAD 27:237–240, 1992;* segmental *Int J Derm 17:745–749, 1978*

Blue rubber bleb nevus syndrome

Desmoplakin mutations – syndrome of dilated cardiomyopathy with severe left ventricular dysfunction, congenital alopecia, striate palmoplantar keratoderma, nail dystrophy, follicular hyperkeratosis with hyperpigmented plaques of elbows *Ped Derm 32:102–108, 2015*

Dyskeratosis congenita

Ehlers-Danlos syndrome, type IV – keloids *JAAD 56:53–54, 2007*

Epidermodysplasia verruciformis – flat-topped facial and hyperpigmented papules *BJD 175:803–806, 2016; AD 131:1312–1318, 1995;* atypical EDV with *LCK* mutation *BJD 175:1204–1209, 2017*

Greither's syndrome – warty keratoses on the hands and feet with poikiloderma

H syndrome – autosomal recessive; hyperpigmented indurated plaques of legs with hypertrichosis, periorbital hyperpigmentation, diabetes mellitus, proptosis, sensorineural hearing loss, hemorrhage, hypogonadotropic hypogonadism, hallux valgus, flexion contractures; loss of function mutation of *SLC29A3* (same mutation as in cutaneous Rosai-Dorfman syndrome); gene encodes human equilibrative nuclear transporter3 (hENT3) protein which transports hydrophilic nucleoside, nucleobases, and nucleoside analog drugs across cell membranes and interacts with insulin signaling pathway *Ped Derm 32:731–732, 2015*

Hypereosinophilic syndrome – personal observation

Infantile myofibromatosis – brown nodule *Ped Derm 27:29–33, 2010*

Infantile systemic hyalinosis – hyperpigmented papules and plaques overlying joints; mimics atopic dermatitis; joint contractures, short stature, thickened skin and hyperpigmentation, pearly papules of face, perianal nodules, gingival hyperplasia, increased susceptibility to infection, osteopenia, protein losing enteropathy (diarrhea); death by age 2; mutation in CMG2 (capillary morphogenesis protein 2)

JAAD 61:629–638, 2009; JAAD 58:303–307, 2008; Pediatr Pathol 6:55–79, 1986

LEOPARD (Moynahan's) syndrome – CALMs, granular cell myoblastomas, steatocystoma multiplex, small penis, hyperelastic skin, low set ears, short webbed neck, short stature, syndactyly *JAAD 46:161–183, 2002; Am J Med 60:447–456, 1976; JAAD 40:877–890, 1999; J Dermatol 25:341–343, 1998; Am J Med 60:447–456, 1976; AD 107:259–261, 1973; Proc R Soc Med 55:959–960, 1962*

Li-Fraumeni syndrome – multiple melanomas *AD 147:248–250, 2011*

Multicentric reticulohistiocytosis *AD 140:919–921, 2004*

Neurofibromatosis – type I – plexiform neurofibromas *JAAD 61:1–14, 2009;* type II, or segmental; schwannoma – personal observation

Neurofibromatosis type II – plexiform schwannoma – hyperpigmented annular plaque in neurofibromatosis type II *JAMA Derm 154:341–346, 2018*

Nevoid basal cell carcinoma syndrome – personal observation

Phakomatosis pigmentokeratotica – 3 mm pigmented papules of neck (melanocytic nevi); Blaschko epidermal nevus; *HRAS* mosaic mutation; tendency for squamous cell carcinoma *NEJM 381:1458, 2019*

Phacomatosis pigmentovascularis – nevus spilus in phacomatosis pigmentovascularis Type IIIb *AD 125:1284–1285, 1989;* segmental neurofibromatosis *NEJM 372:963, 2015*

POEMS syndrome – cutaneous angiomas, blue dermal papules associated with Castleman's disease (benign reactive angioendotheliomatosis), diffuse hyperpigmentation, morphea-like changes, maculopapular brown-violaceous lesions, purple nodules *JAAD 44:324–329, 2001; JAAD 40:808–812, 1999; Cutis 61:329–334, 1998; JAAD 21:1061–1068, 1989; AD 124:695–698, 1988; JAAD 12:961–964, 1985*

SCALP syndrome – sebaceous nevus syndrome, central nervous system malformations, aplasia cutis congenital, limbal dermoid, pigmented nevus (giant congenital melanocytic nevus) with neurocutaneous melanosis *JAAD 58:884–888, 2008*

Steatocystoma multiplex

Tuberous sclerosis – pigmented papules and nodules; fibrous cephalic plaques in tuberous sclerosis *JAAD 78:717–724 , 2018*

TOXINS

Arsenic *JGH Open 4:259–300, 2019*

TRAUMA

Burn scar *Surgery 121:654–661, 1997*

Scar

VASCULAR DISEASES

Acquired progressive lymphangioma *AD 131:341–346, 1995*

Acroangiodermatitis – personal observation

Angiolymphoid hyperplasia with eosinophilia and follicular mucinosis *Indian J Dermatol 58:159, 2013*

Benign (reactive) angioendotheliomatosis (benign lymphangioendothelioma, acquired progressive lymphangioma, multifocal lymphangioendotheliomatosis) – present at birth; red brown or violaceous nodules or plaques on face, arms, legs with petechiae, ecchymoses,

and small areas of necrosis *AD 140:599–606, 2004; JAAD 38:143–175, 1998; AD 114:1512, 1978*

Epithelioid hemangioendothelioma – painful brown–pink nodule *AD 143:937–942, 2007*

Glomus tumors – plaque type glomus tumors

Lymphatic malformation, superficial microcystic – pigmented, multinodular sessile tumor of leg *Ped Derm 32:867–868, 2015*

Lymphedema with solid papules – personal observation

Multifocal lymphangioendotheliomatosis with thrombocytopenia – flat or indurated red–brown or burgundy papules, plaques, nodules, and tumors; involvement of gastrointestinal tract, lungs, brain, spleen, synovium, muscle *BJD 171:474–484, 2014; JAAD 67:898–903, 2012*

Pigmented purpuric eruption overlying arteriovenous malformation – personal observation

Superficial hemosiderotic lymphovascular malformation (hobnail hemangioma) (targetoid hemosiderotic hemangioma) – red–brown papule; blue–purple papule; yellow/green blue/papule *Ped Derm 31:281–285, 2014*

Targetoid hemosiderotic hemangioma – brown to violaceous nodule with ecchymotic halo *AD 138:117–122, 2002; AD 136:1571–1572, 2000; JAAD 41:215–224, 1999; J Cutan Pathol 26:279–286, 1999; JAAD 32:282–284, 1995*

Tufted angioma – brown nodule *Ped Derm 35:808–816, 2018*

PAPULES, PERIORBITAL

AUTOIMMUNE DISEASES AND DISEASES OF IMMUNE DYSFUNCTION

Allergic contact dermatitis

Graft vs. host reaction *JAAD 26:49–55, 1992*

Lupus erythematosus – discoid lupus *J Dermatol 38:486–488, 2011*

CONGENITAL LESIONS

Blueberry muffin baby

DRUG–INDUCED

Corticosteroid-induced periorbital dermatitis – personal observation

Drug eruption

EXOGENOUS AGENTS

Irritant contact dermatitis

INFECTIONS AND INFESTATIONS

Anthrax *BMC Res Notes 6:313, 2013*

Cat scratch disease

Coccidioides imitis Ann Ophthalmol 20:391–393, 1988

Gianotti-Crosti syndrome

Insect bite

Leishmaniasis

Lepidopterism

Leprosy

Measles

Molluscum contagiosum *J Ped Ophthalmol Strabismus 30:58–59, 1993; Ann Ophthalmol 20:391–393, 1988*

North American blastomycosis

Papular urticaria

Roseola infantum

Scabies, nodular

Sporotrichosis

Stye

Syphilis – primary, secondary

Tinea faciei *Ann Ophthalmol 20:391–393, 1988; AD 114:250–252, 1978*

Verrucae

Viral exanthem

INFILTRATIVE DISORDERS

Amyloidosis, primary systemic *NEJM 349:583–596, 2003;* AL amyloid papules presenting sign of multiple myeloma *BMJ Case Rep Feb 20, 2017*

Benign cephalic histiocytosis

Colloid milium

Erdheim-Chester disease (non Langerhans cell histiocytosis) – xanthelasma-like periorbital yellow papules and plaques; CD68+, CD163+, CD1a-, Langerin (CD207)-; BRAF mutations *BJD 178:261–264, 2018; JAAD 74:513–520, 2016*

Langerhans cell histiocytosis

Mucinosis *Clin Dermatol 29:151–156, 2011*

Rosai-Dorfman disease *Am J Dermatopathol 36:357–363, 2014*

Xanthogranulomas, including juvenile xanthogranuloma *Clin Exp Derm 18:462–463, 1993*

Xanthoma disseminatum *JAAD 15:433–436, 1991*

INFLAMMATORY DISEASES

Blepharitis granulomatosa *AD 120:1141, 1984*

Erythema multiforme

Neutrophilic eccrine hidradenitis *JAAD 28:775, 1993; AD 131:1141–1145, 1995*

Sarcoid

METABOLIC DISEASES

Calcinosis cutis – dystrophic calcification due to intralesional corticosteroids for infantile periocular hemangiomas *Ped Derm 15:23–26, 1998*

Xanthelasma *JAAD 77:728–734, 2017*

NEOPLASTIC DISORDERS

Actinic keratosis

Apocrine hidrocystomas *Cutis 105:169, 172–173, 2020; AD 134:1627–1632, 1998*

Basal cell carcinoma

Bowen's disease

Dermoid cyst

Dermatosis papulosa nigra

Eccrine hidrocystomas *J Dermatol 23:652–654, 1996*

Embryonal rhabdomyosarcoma

Epidermal inclusion cyst

Eruptive hidradenoma *Cutis 46:69–72, 1990*

Eruptive vellus hair cysts – skin colored, red, white, blue, yellow *Ped Derm 19:26–27, 2002*

Hidrocystomas *Dermatol Online J May 15, 2016*

Kaposi's sarcoma *JAAD 40:312–314, 1999*

Leiomyoma

Leukemia

Lymphoma – cutaneous T-cell lymphoma; HTLV-1

Melanocytic nevus, including divided nevus

Melanoma

Merkel cell tumor

Metastatic breast cancer

Microcystic adnexal carcinoma – periorbital papule or nodule *Derm Surg 27:979–984, 2001*

Milium

Milia en plaque *Dermatol Surg 28:291–295, 2002*

Mucinous eccrine carcinoma (mucinous carcinoma of skin) *AD 136:1409–1414, 2000; Dermatol Surg 25:566–568, 1999; JAAD 36:323–326, 1997; AD 133:1161–1166, 1997*

Myeloma – cutaneous crystalline deposits *AD 130:484–488, 1994*

Myxomas *JAAD 34:928–930, 1995*

Nevus, melanocytic

Nevus sebaceous – papule *Eyelid and Conjunctival Tumors, Shields JA and Shields CL, Lippincott Williams and Wilkins, 1999, p.21*

Oncocytoma – bright red or yellow papule of eyelid *Arch Ophthalmol 102:263–265, 1984*

Orbital tumors (ethmoid sinus carcinoma)

Preauricular cyst, inflamed

Sebaceous carcinoma

Seborrheic keratosis – papule

Sweat gland carcinoma

Syringomas – papule *Dermatol Surg 43:381–388, 2017*

Trichoepitheliomas

PARANEOPLASTIC DISEASES

Lichen myxedematosus *Indian Dermatol Online J 8:198–200, 2017*

Necrobiotic xanthogranuloma with paraproteinemia *JAMA Derm 156:270–279, 2020; Hautarzt 61:902–906, 2016; AD 133:99, 102, 1997*

Normolipemic plane xanthomas

PHOTODERMATOSES

Chronic actinic dermatitis

Favre-Racouchot *An Bras Dermatol 90:185–187, 2015*

Photo-induced drug eruption

Polymorphic light eruption

PRIMARY CUTANEOUS DISEASES

Acne vulgaris

Alopecia mucinosa

Atopic dermatitis

Colloid milium

Granuloma annulare – periorbital *AD 118:190–191, 1982;* of the eyelid *Ped Derm 16:373–376, 1999*

Lichen planus

Lichen sclerosus et atrophicus

Lichen striatus

Periorbital "perioral" dermatitis *Semin Cutan Med Surg 18:206–209, 1999;* granulomatous periorificial dermatitis of childhood *Indian J DV Leprol 77:703–706, 2011*

Psoriasis

Rosacea, including granulomatous rosacea

Seborrheic dermatitis

SYNDROMES

Ankyloblepharon-ectrodactyly-cleft lip, palate syndrome (AEC syndrome) – eyelid papillomas

Atrichia with papular lesions – autosomal recessive; follicular cysts *AD 139:1591–1596, 2003; JAAD 47:519–523, 2002*

Carney complex – cutaneous myxomas of the *eyelids Cutis 62:275–280, 1998*

Down's syndrome – syringomas

Fabry's disease

Familial sea blue histiocytosis

Kawasaki's disease

Lipoid proteinosis *Orbit 30:242–244, 2011*

Multicentric reticulohistiocytosis

Sly syndrome

Sweet's syndrome

TRAUMA

Granuloma fissuratum

VASCULAR DISORDERS

Angiolymphoid hyperplasia with eosinophilia *Ann Allergy 69:101–105, 1992*

Angiosarcoma *JAAD 34:308–310, 1996*

Disseminated neonatal hemangiomatosis

Granulomatosis with polyangiitis

Hemangiomas

Pyogenic granuloma

Vasculitis

PAPULES, RED

AUTOIMMUNE DISEASES AND DISEASES OF IMMUNE DYSFUNCTION

Adrenergic urticaria *JAAD 70:763–766, 2014*

Allergic contact dermatitis – spandex waistband – personal observation

Atopic dermatitis – red papules of chest, antecubital fossa *BJD 162:472–477, 2010;* elbow papules *Ped Derm 29:395–402, 2012*

Autoeczematization reaction

Bowel arthritis dermatitis syndrome – papular and pustular vasculitis, erythema nodosum-like lesions; tenosynovitis, non-destructive polyarthritis *Ped Derm 25:509–519, 2008; AD 138:973–978, 2002; BJD 142:373–374, 2000; AD 135:1409–1414, 1999; Cutis 63:17–20, 1999; JAAD 14:792–796, 1986; Mayo Clin Proc 59:43–46, 1984; AD 115:837–839, 1979*

Bullous pemphigoid without blisters – pemphigoid nodularis *JAMA Derm 149:950–953, 2013*

Chronic granulomatous disease – suppurative granuloma – *Microascus cinereus Clin Inf Dis 20:110–114, 1995*

Common variable immune deficiency – granulomas *JAAD 37:499–500, 1997*

Congenital combined immunodeficiency – cutaneous granulomas of elbows and hands *Mt Sinai J Med 68:326–330, 2001*

Dermatitis herpetiformis – elbows, knees, buttocks, face *JAAD 64:1017–1024, 2011*

Dermatomyositis – Gottron's papules

DOCK8 deficiency syndrome (dedicator of cytokinesis 8 gene) (aka autosomal recessive hyper-IgE syndrome) DOCK8 – involved in T cell polarization and activation; atypical guanine exchange factor; interacts with Rho GTPases (CDC42 and RAC) which mediate actin cytoskeletal reorganization; hematologic stem cell homing and mobilization – immunodeficiency; resembles Job's syndrome; decrease T and B cells; increased IgE, decreased IgM, increased eosinophilia; recurrent sinopulmonary infections, severe cutaneous viral infections and lymphopenia; red papules of neck – molluscum contagiosum; warts, widespread dermatitis (atopic dermatitis-like (24% at birth; Job's 81% dermatitis at birth), asthma, cutaneous staphylococcal abscesses; malignancies – aggressive T-cell lymphoma vulvar squamous cell carcinoma, diffuse large B-cell lymphoma; Job's syndrome may be differentiated by presence of pneumatoceles and bronchiectasis, rash at birth, osteoporosis, scoliosis, craniosynostosis, minimal trauma fractures, joint hyperex-tensibility; dominant negative STAT3 mutation *AD 148:79–84, 2012*

Estrogen dermatitis *J Dermatol 30:719–722, 2003*

Graft vs host disease *J Dermatol 20:242–246, 1993*

Hyper IgD syndrome – autosomal recessive; red macules or papules, urticaria, red nodules, combinations of fever, arthritis, and rash, annular erythema, and pustules; mevalonate kinase deficiency *Ped Derm 22:138–141, 2005; AD 136:1487–1494, 2000; AD 130:59–65, 1994; Ann DV 123:314–321, 1996; Medicine 73:133–144, 1994; Lancet 1:1084–1090, 1984;*

abdominal pain with vomiting and diarrhea, lymphadenopathy; elevated IgD and IgA

Interstitial granulomatous dermatitis with arthritis *JAAD 34:957–961, 1996; Dermatopathol Prac Concept 1:3–6, 1995*

Juvenile rheumatoid arthritis – Still's disease; evanescent rash; persistent pruritic papules and plaques; urticarial and urticarial-like rash, vesiculopustular eruptions, edema of the eyelids, widespread non-pruritic persistent erythema *Medicine 96:e6318, 2017*

Linear IgA disease, adulthood *Cutis 81:336–338, 2008*

Lupus erythematosus – chilblain lupus – fingers, toes, elbows, knees, calves, knuckles, nose, ears *Cutis 69:183–184, 190, 2002; BJD 98:497–506, 1978;* papulonodular dermal mucinosis of SLE – perifollicular skin colored to red papules *AD 146:789–794, 2010; AD 140:121–126, 2004; Int J Derm 35:72–73, 1996; JAAD 32:199–205, 1995; JAAD 27:312–315, 1992; AD 114:432–435,*

1978; BJD 66:429–433, 1954; discoid lupus erythematosus *Clin Case Rep 8:155–158, 2019*

Pemphigoid gestationis *JAAD 40:847–849, 1999*

Perforating neutrophilic and granulomatous dermatitis of the newborn – cutaneous eruption of immunodeficiency; papules, plaques, vesicles, crusts, ulcers; boggy pustular masses; purpuric lesions; prominent involvement of palms and soles; sparing of trunk *Ped Derm 24:211–215, 2007*

Rheumatoid arthritis – palisaded neutrophilic granulomatous dermatitis of rheumatoid arthritis (rheumatoid neutrophilic dermatosis) *JAAD 47:251–257, 2002; JAAD 45:596–600, 2001; JAAD 22:922–925, 1990; AD 133:757–760, 1997*

Still's disease – adult onset; persistent plaques and linear pigmentation; flagellate erythema *JAMA Derm 149:1425–1426, 2013; J Eur Acad Dermatol Venereol 19:360–363, 2005; Dermatology 188:241–242, 1994*

Urticaria

X-linked agammaglobulinemia – caseating granulomas *JAAD 24:629–633, 1991*

CONGENITAL LESIONS

Congenital candidiasis – neonatal papules and vesicles; pneumonia *Cutis 93:229–232, 2014*

Congenital neurovascular hamartoma – papillomatous red–brown lesion

Meningocele

Perineal pyramidal protrusion

Neutrophil rich subcutaneous fat necrosis of the newborn – red papules and plaques *JAAD 75:177–185, 2016*

Umbilical granuloma *J Pediatr Child Health 55:857–859, 2019*

Umbilical polyp – failure of regression of omphalomesenteric duct at peripheral cutaneous pole *Clin Exp Dermatol 4:367–369, 2020*

DRUG-INDUCED

Anti-PD-1 therapy (nivolumab/pembrolizumab – lichenoid eruptions, vitiligo, dermatitis, red papules with scale, red papules and nodules, inflammation surrounding seborrheic keratosis, dyshidrosiform palmar lesions, penile erosions *JAMA Derm 152:1128–1136, 2016; JAAD 74:455–461, 2016*

Arsenic trioxide – treatment for promyelocytic leukemia; flexural red papules *JAMA Derm 155:389–390, 2019*

Azathioprine – neutrophilic dermatosis (azathioprine hypersensitivity syndrome) – palpebral conjunctival erythema, pink macules, pink or red plaques *JAMA Derm 149:592–597, 2013*

BCG – disseminated BCG infection *AD 143:1323–1328, 2007*

BRAF inhibitors – granulomas *JAMA Derm 150:307–311, 2014*

Carboplatin and docetaxel – inflammation of actinic keratosis *Cases Journal 9:6946–6948, 2009*

Corticosteroids – peristomal granulomas due to fluorinated corticosteroids *J Cutan Pathol 8:361–364, 1981*

Cytarabine – intertriginous eruption begins as erythematous papules *JAAD 73:821–828, 2015*

Drug-induced pseudolymphoma syndrome *JAAD 38:877–905, 1998*

Drug rash, morbilliform

G-CSF – neutrophilic dermatosis *Ped Derm 18:417–421, 2001*

Gemcitabine – red papules in groin; pseudolymphoma *BJD 145:650–652, 2001*

Imatinib – eccrine squamous syringometaplasia; red facial and eyelid papules *JAAD 55:S58–59, 2006*

Interferon alpha – sarcoidal papules *BJD 146:320–324, 2002*

Interferon alpha (pegylated) and ribavirin as treatment for hepatitis C infection – sarcoidosis *AD 141:865–868, 2005*

Methotrexate-induced rheumatoid papules – red papules on arms and buttocks *JAAD 40:702–707, 1999;* methotrexate-associated lymphoproliferative disorder – red papules and plaques of nose, cheeks, eyelids *JAAD 56:686–690, 2007*

Sirolimus – drug-induced vasculitis *Transplantation 74:739–743, 2002*

Subacute cutaneous lupus erythematosus – drug-induced including hydrochlorothiazide, ACE inhibitors, calcium channel blockers *Ann Int Med 103:49–51, 1985*

Telaprevir *Dermatol Online J Jan 15, 2015*

Ustekinumab – lymphomatoid drug reaction; pink papules and nodules of trunk *AD 147:992–993, 2011*

Vemurafenib – multiple eruptive keratoacanthomas *AD 148:363–366, 2012*

Vincristine/vinblastine/vinorelbine – erythema multiforme-like lesions *JAAD 71:203–214, 2014*

Zoledronic acid (bisphosphonate) – pseudolymphoma *JAAD 65:1138–1140, 2011*

EXOGENOUS AGENTS

Acrylic or nylon fibers form dust or carpet *BJD 96:673–677, 1977*

BCG vaccine – granulomas *JAAD 21:1119–1122, 1989*

Bromoderma *Int J Dermatol 42:370–371, 2003*

Coral contact dermatitis *Int J Derm 30:271–273, 1991*

Fiberglass dermatitis

Foreign body granuloma – talc, kaolin, quartz in slate, brick, gravel, coal; silica; beryllium – sarcoidal granulomas

Iododerma – scaly red papules and nodules; secondary to amiodarone *JAMA Derm 151:891–892, 2015; Australas J Dermatol 28:119–122, 1987*

Irritant contact dermatitis – from squirrel monkey – personal observation

Pyrethroid insecticides *Br J Ind Med 45:548–551, 1988*

Red tattoos *Dermatology 233:100–109, 2017*

Sea urchin spine – sarcoidal granuloma *BJD 77:335–343, 1965*

Surgical staples – hypertrophic scars; multiple red papules *JAAD 62:157–158, 2010*

Zirconium – axillary sarcoidal granuloma from deodorants *J Dermatol 38:223–232, 1962; BJD 70:75–101, 1958*

INFECTIONS AND INFESTATIONS

African histoplasmosis (*Histoplasma capsulatum* var. *duboisii*) -exclusively in Central and West Africa and Madagascar *Clin Inf Dis 48:441, 493–494, 2009*

African tick-bite fever – *Rickettsia africae Clin Inf Dis 39:700–701, 741–742, 2004*

Alternariosis *JAAD 52:653–659, 2005; BJD 143:910–912, 2000; AD 94:201–207, 1976*

Amebiasis – *Acanthamoeba Ped Inf Dis J 22:197–199, 2003; JAAD 42:351–354, 2000; Clin Inf Dis 25:267–272, 1997;* red nodules and crusted nodules in HIV disease *AD 139:1647–1652, 2003*

Ancylostomiasis – papular or papulovesicular rash; feet; generalized urticaria; late changes resemble kwashiorkor *Dermatol Clin 7:275–290, 1989*

Anthrax – papule develops central vesicle with surrounding brawny edema becomes hemorrhagic, necrotic with satellite vesicles; black eschar, painless ulcer *JAAD 65; 1213–1218, 2011; JAMA 260:616, 1987; J Clin Inf Dis 19:1009–1014, 1994*

Ants – bullet ant (*Tocandira*); *Paraponers spp.; Pseudomyrmex ants* – painful stings *JAAD 67:331–344, 2012*

Aquarium dermatitis – cercarial dermatitis *Dermatology 197:84–86, 1998*

Arthropod bites – persistent nodular arthropod reactions on elbows, abdomen, genitalia, and axillae (pseudolymphoma syndrome) *JAAD 38:877–905, 1998;* avian mites from pet gerbils – itchy red bumps *AD 137:167, 2001*

Aspergillosis *BJD 85 (suppl 17):95–97, 1971;* primary cutaneous aspergillosis *JAAD 31:344–347, 1994;* disseminated (red) *JAAD 20:989–1003, 1989; Aspergillus fumigatus* – painful, purpuric necrotic papules and pustules in tattoo *BJD 170:1373–1375, 2014; J Ped Surg 22:504–505, 1987*

Bacillary angiomatosis (*Bartonella henselae*) – starts as pinpoint erythematous papule *BJD 143:609–611, 2000; Bol Assoc Med PR 88:46–51, 1996; Hautarzt 44:361–364, 1993; JAAD 22:501–512, 1990*

Bartonellosis – *Bartonella bacilliformis;* bacillary angiomatosis; Andes mountains, Peru, Colombia, Ecuador; Oroya fever with verruga peruana sandflies and fleas as vectors; red papules in crops become nodular, hemangiomatous or pedunculated; face, neck, extremities, mucosal lesions; 1–4 mm pruritic red papules; massive hemolytic anemia, high fever, muscle pain, delirium, coma *JAAD 54:559–578, 2006; Clin Inf Dis 33:772–779, 2001; Ann Rev Microbiol 35:325–338, 1981*

Bed bugs (*Cimex lectularis*) *JAAD 67:331–344, 2012*

Bird mites *Commun Dis Intell Q Rep 27:259–261, 2003*

Botryomycosis – granulomatous reaction to bacteria with granule formation; single or multiple abscesses of skin and subcutaneous tissue break down to yield multiple sinus tracts; small papule; extremities, perianal sinus tracts, face; papule at base of great toe; *Staphylococcus aureus JAMA Derm 153:321–322, 2017;*

Cutis 80:45–47, 2007; Int J Dermatol 22:455–459, 1983; AD 115:609–610, 1979

Brown recluse spider bite *JAAD 55:888–890, 2006*

Brucellosis *JAAD 48:474–476, 2003*

Cactus spines *J Med Case Rep 4:152 May 25, 2010*

Calymmatobacterium granulomatis (Donovanosis) – papules of upper arms and chest *J Clin Inf Dis 25:24–32, 1997*

Candida sepsis – papules and nodules with pale centers *Am J Dermatopathol 8:501–504, 1986; JAMA 229:1466–1468, 1974; Candida tropicalis Cutis 71:466–468, 2003;* targetoid lesions with central necrosis *J Hosp Infect 50:316–319, 2002; Mycoses 40:17–20, 1997; AD 115:234–235, 1979; C. krusei AD 143:1583–1588, 2007;* congenital cutaneous candidiasis *AJDC 135:273–275, 1981; Candida albicans, Candida parapsilosis* – personal observation

Cat scratch disease – *Bartonella henselae;* red papule, becomes vesicle, crusts, ulcerates, heals with scar *Am J Dis Child 139:1124–1133, 1985; JAMA 154:1247–1251, 1954*

Caterpillars – puss caterpillar (larval stage of flannel moth, Megalopyge opercularis) *Cutis 71:445–448, 2003;* airborne disease due to oak processionary caterpillar *Ped Derm 23:64–66, 2006;* gypsy moth caterpillar (*Lymantra dispar*) dermatitis – severe itch with red papules *Cutis 80:110–112, 2007;* poison ivy-like dermatitis – hickory tussock moth, hickory tiger moth (*Lophocampa caryae*)

Cutis 80:110–112, 2007; caripito itch – setae of *Hylesia* moths *JAAD 62:1–10, 2010*

Cercarial dermatitis – schistosomes; pruritic red papules; fresh water avian cercarial dermatitis (swimmer's itch) *Cutis 19:461–467, 1977;* papules of forehead, cheeks, shoulders, upper extremities *JAAD 60:174–176, 2009;* sea water avian cercarial dermatitis *Bull Marine Sci Gulf Coast 2:346–348, 1952;* fresh water mammalian cercarial dermatitis *Trans R Soc Trop Med Hyg 66:21–24, 1972;* cercarial dermatitis from snail (Lymnaea stagnalis) in aquarium tank *BJD 145:638–640, 2001*

Cheyletiella mites – dogs, cats, rabbits; papules, papulovesicles, pustules, necrosis *JAAD 50:819–842, 2004; AD 116:435–437, 1980*

Chigger bites *Cutis 99:386–388, 2017; Cutis 77:350–352, 2006*

Chromomycosis – red papules on dorsum of hand (*Chaetomium funicola*) *BJD 157:1025–1029, 2007*

Coccidioidomycosis *Cutis 70:70–72, 2002;* acute pulmonary coccidioidomycosis with interstitial granulomatous dermatitis *JAAD 45:840–845, 2001*

Coral dermatitis *Int J Dermatol 30:271–273, 1991*

Corythuca ciliate (lace bug) – lace bug infestation *JAMA Derm 151:909–910, 2015*

Covid-19 coronavirus infection *J Dermatol Sci 98:75–81, 2020; Clin Exp Dermatol May 9, 2020*

Cowpox – papule progresses to vesicle to hemorrhagic vesicle to umbilicated pustule, then eschar with ulcer *JAAD 49:513–518, 2003; JAAD 44:1–14, 2001; BJD 1331:598–607, 1994*

Coxsackie virus A6 (atypical hand, foot, and mouth disease) – red papulovesicles of fingers, palmar erythema, red papules of ears, red papules of antecubital fossa, perioral papulovesicles, vesicles of posterior pharynx *JAAD 69:736–741, 2013*

Cryptococcosis *Hautarzt 61:980–984, 2010; Clin Inf Dis 33:700–705, 2001; JAAD 32:844–850, 1995*

Cutaneous larva migrans – urticarial papules *AD 146:557–562, 2010*

Cysticercosis (*C. cellulosae*) (larval form of *Toxocara solium*) – papulonodules, subcutaneous cysts, cysts in skeletal muscles, mucous membranes, seizures (neurocysticercosis) *JAAD 75:19–30, 2016*

Cytomegalovirus *JAAD 38:349–351, 1998;* pruritic papules *JAAD 11:743–747, 1984;* ulcerated red papules *AD 145:1030–1036, 2009*

Dematiaceous fungal infections in organ transplant recipients – all lesions on extremities
  Alternaria
  Bipolaris hawaiiensis
  Exophiala jeanselmei, E. spinifera, E. pisciphera, E. castellani
  Exserohilum rostratum
  Fonsacaea pedrosoi
  Phialophora parasitica

Dental sinus *Am Fam Physician 40:113–116, 1989*

Dermatophytosis – invasive dermatophyte; Majocchi's granuloma *Med Mycol 47:312–316, 2009;* disseminated dermatophyte infection; *J Clin Microbiol 34:460–462, 1996; Mycopathologica 82:77–82, 1983; Trichophyton rubrum,* invasive *Cutis 67:457–462, 2001;* disseminated *Trichophyton rubrum* – purple papules with central black hemorrhagic crusting *JAMA Derm 152:941–942, 2016*

Dracunculosis – small papule or vesicle which ruptures *Dermatol Clinic 7:323–330, 1989; Dracuncula medinensis* (Guinea worm) – stagnant water with copepods; painful papular lesions, nausea and vomiting, fever, syncope, urticarial, red papulonodular lesions which become vesiculobullous, cellulitis lesions *JAAD 73:929–944, 2015*

Ebola virus hemorrhagic fever – non-specific macules and papules *JAAD 75:1–16, 2016*

Epidermodysplasia verruciformis, acquired, in HIV disease – lichenoid hyperpigmented, pink flat warts, tinea versicolor-like *AD 147:590–596, 2011*

Eruptive pseudoangiomatosis – vascular papules or nodules; *Echovirus 25, 32; Coxsackie B virus Ped Derm 19:76–77, 2002*

Fire ant stings *Cutis 83:17–20, 2009*

Fire corals – urticarial lesions followed by vesiculobullous rash, chronic granulomatous and lichenoid lesions *Contact Dermatitis 29:285–286, 1993; Int J Dermatol 30:271–273, 1991*

Folliculitis – various organisms

Fusarium – sepsis with red/gray papules *JAAD 47:659–666, 2002*

Gianotti-Crosti syndrome – red papules on elbows *AD 148:1257–1264, 2012; Ped Derm 21:542–547, 2004;* pink papules coalescing into plaques *Ped Derm 30:137–138, 2013;* in adult *Cutis 89:169–172, 2012*

Glanders (farcy) – *Burkholderia (Pseudomonas) mallei* – cellulitis which ulcerates with purulent foul-smelling discharge, regional lymphatics become abscesses; nasal and palatal necrosis and destruction; metastatic papules, pustules, bullae over joints and face, then ulcerate; deep abscesses with sinus tracts occur; polyarthritis, meningitis, pneumonia *JAAD 54:559–578, 2006;*

Gnathostomiasis

Gonococcemia – periarticular lesions appear in crops with red macules, papules, vesicles with red halo, pustules, bullae becoming hemorrhagic and necrotic; suppurative arthritis and tenosynovitis *Ann Int Med 102:229–243, 1985*

Gypsy moth caterpillar dermatitis *JAAD 24:979–981, 1991; NEJM 306:1301–1302, 1982*

Hand, foot, and mouth disease – personal observation

Helminth infection – *Enterobius vermicularis Clin Colon Rectal Surg 32:364–371, 2019*

Herpes simplex – disseminated red papules and pustules *BJD 172:278–280, 2015*

Herpes zoster – disseminated zoster, hyponatremia, severe abdominal pain, and leukemia relapse *BJD 149:862–865, 2003;* granulomas at site of herpes zoster *BJD 156:1369–1371, 2007*

Histoplasmosis – disseminated histoplasmosis *AD 143:255–260, 2007; BJD 144:205–207, 2001; J Eur Acad Dermatol Venereol 10:182–185, 1998; Int J Dermatol 36:599–603, 1997; Diagnostic Challenges Vol V:77–79, 1994; JAAD 29:311–313, 1993; JAAD 23:422–428, 1990; BJD 113:345–348, 1985*

Hot tub folliculitis *Ann DV 144:290–294, 2017; JAAD 57:596–600, 2007; JAAD 8:153–156, 1983*

Insect bites – bed bug bites *JAMA 301:1358–1366, 2009;* mites including avian mite bites (*Dermanyssus gallinae*) (gamasoidosis, acariasis); other bird mites (*Ornithonyssus sylviarum* and *O. bursa*); tropical rat mite dermatitis *AD 146:1419–1424, 2010;* baker's itch (*Acarus siro*); grocer's itch (*Glycophagus domesticus*); coolie itch (onions, plant bulbs, tea) (*Rhizoglyphus parasiticus*); dried fruit itch (dried fruit, feathers, skin) (*Carpoglyphus lactis*); from pet gerbils *AD 137:167–170, 2001;* mites – barley itch, grain-shoveller's itch, grain itch (*Pyemotes tritici*), straw itch, cotton seed dermatitis *Rook p.1468, 1998, Sixth Edition;* chiggers *Cutis 77:353–357, 2006;* ;trombiculid mites (*Eutromicula*) (chiggers (*E.alfreddugusi*)); *Pyemotes ventricosus* (wood mite) *The Clinical Management of Itching; Parthenon; p. 61, 2000;* tropical rat mite (*O. baconi*) *Cutis 42:414–416, 1988;* cheese mite (*Glyciphagus*) bites – papulovesicles and pustules *Dermatol Clin 8:265–275, 1990;* fleas – human flea (*Pulex irritans*); cat flea (*Ctenocephalides felis*) *Cutis 85:10–11, 2010;* dog flea (*C. canis*); bird flea (*Ceratophyllus gallinae*); beetles (*Paederus fuscipes*) – blisters, papules *Eur J Ped 152:6–8, 1993;* carpet beetle (*Anthrenus verbasci*) *JAAD 5:428–432, 1981;*

bedbugs (*Cimex lectularis, C. hemipterus*); mosquitoes *The Clinical Management of Itching; Parthenon; p. 63, 2000;* sandflies (*Phlebotomus, Lutzomyia*) – harara, urticaria multiformis endemica in Middle East *The Clinical Management of Itching; Parthenon; p. 64, 2000; Amblyomma americanum (lone star tick) larvae bites AD 142:491–494, 2006;* oak leaf itch mite (*Pyomotes herfsi*) *Cutis 88:114–116, 2011*

Janeway lesion *Stat Pearls May 31, 2020; Clin Dermatol 29:S11–22, 2011; Med News 75:257–262, 1899*

Jellyfish stings

Leishmaniasis *BJD 160:311–318, 2009; Clin Inf Dis 33:815,897–898, 2001; AD 134:193–198, 1998; J Clin Inf Dis 22:1–13, 1996;* plaque containing multiple agminated red papules *NEJM 371:1736, 2014;* post-kala azar dermal leishmaniasis – papules of cheeks, chin, ears, extensor forearms, buttocks, lower legs; in India, hypopigmented macules; nodules develop after years; tongue, palate, genitalia *E Afr Med J 63:365–371, 1986; L. mexicana (Lutzomyia) JAAD 58:650–652, 2008*

Lepidopterism – butterflies and moths

Leprosy – lepromatous leprosy; erythema nodosum leprosum in histoid leprosy – numerous papulonodules of trunk *BJD 160:305–310, 2009;* histoid leprosy – multiple dusky red nodules *AD 148:947–952, 2012; AD 140:751–756, 2004;* pink papules with surrounding hyperpigmentation – de novo histoid leprosy *Ped Derm 31:387–388, 2014*

Listeriosis

Lobomycosis (*Lacazio loboi*) – papules *Mycoses 55:298–309, 2012*

Lyme disease – papular variant *JAAD 49:363–392, 2003*

Malacoplakia *AD 134:244–245, 1998*

Mansonelliasis (filariasis) (*M. ozzardi*) – biting midges or black flies; angioedema, chronic pruritus with hyperpigmentation, papular eruption *JAAD 75:19–30, 2016*

Meningococcemia – acute or chronic *BJD 153:669–671, 2005; Rev Infect Dis 8:1–11, 1986;* chronic – necrotic papule *AD 144:770–773, 2008;* chronic – red papules *JAMA Derm 150:752–755, 2014*

Mites and ticks – erythema, edema, papules *JAAD 67:347–354, 2012*

Molluscum contagiosum, including giant molluscum contagiosum; inflammatory reaction surrounding molluscum contagiosum lesions due to immune reconstitution inflammatory syndrome (IRIS) *Ped Derm 27:631–634, 2010*

Moths – *Hylesia* moths – contact with bristles results in erythematous papules, conjunctivitis, iritis, and keratitis *JAAD 67:331–344, 2012*

Mucormycosis – *Mucor, Rhizopus oryzi, Rhizomucor, Lichtheimia, Saksenaea, Cunninhghamella, Apophysomyces* pink papules *JAAD 80:869–880, 2019*

Murine typhus *Clin Inf Dis 21:859, 1995*

Mycobacterium avium complex – traumatic inoculation papules *BJD 130:785–790, 1994*

Mycobacterium chelonae BJD 171:79–89, 2014; in tattoos *JAAD 62:501–506, 2010*

Mycobacterium haemophilum Clin Inf Dis 33-330–337, 2001

Mycobacteria kansasii Ped Derm 18:131–134, 2001

Mycobacterium tuberculosis – tuberculosis cutis orificialis (acute tuberculous ulcer) – red edematous papules break down to form shallow ulcers of mouth, tongue, dental sockets, genitalia, perianal region; miliary *J Clin Inf Dis 23:706–710, 1996;* lupus vulgaris; papulonecrotic tuberculid *Ped Derm 7:191–195, 1990; Ped Derm 15:450–455, 1998;* lichen scrofulosorum – red, lichenoid, firm follicular and parafollicular papules; resemble keratosis pilaris, lichen nitidus, lichen spinulosus, or pityriasis rubra pilaris *BJD 136:483–489, 1997;* papulonecrotic tuberculid *Arthr Rheum 41:1884–1888, 1998*

*Mycoplasma pneumonia-*induced rash – sparse oval papules and mucositis *JAAD 72:239–245, 2015*

Myiasis – starts as a red papule *J Travel Med 10:293–295, 2003; Cutis 55:47–48, 1995*

Neutrophilic eccrine hidradenitis – infectious etiology – *Serratia, Enterobacter cloacae, Staphylococcus aureus JAAD 38:1–17, 1998*

Nocardia *BMC Clin Pathol Oct 1, 2018; J Coll Physicians Surg Pak 24:Suppl 3:S176–177, 2014*

North American blastomycosis – disseminated blastomycosis *Clin Infect Dis 33:1706, 1770–1771, 2001; Am Rev Resp Dis 120:911–938, 1979; Medicine 47:169–200, 1968*

Onchocerciasis (*Onchocerca volvulus*) – presents with blotchy erythema and urticarial papules *BJD 121:187–198, 1989;* acute papular onchodermatitis – papules, vesicles, pustules *JAAD 73:929–944, 2015*

Orf – reddish-blue papule becomes hemorrhagic umbilicated pustule or bulla surrounded by gray-white or violaceous rim which is surrounded by a rim of erythema *Acta DV Croat 27:280–281, 2019; AD 126:356–358, 1990;* large lesions may resemble pyogenic granulomas or lymphoma; rarely widespread papulovesicular or bullous lesions occur *Int J Dermatol 19:340–341, 1980*

Osler's node (subacute bacterial endocarditis) – small, red papules on distal finger and toe pads *NEJM 295:1500–1505, 1976*

Paecilomyces lalacinus (cutaneous hyalohyphomycosis) *JAAD 35:779–781, 1996; JAAD 39:401–409, 1998*

Paederus beetle dermatitis – linear papular, vesicular, and pustular dermatitis *JAAD 57:297–300, 2007; Cutis 69:277–279, 2002*

Papular urticaria *Semin Dermatol 12:53–56, 1993*

Paragonimus

Pediculosis – head lice – pruritic papules of nape of neck; generalized pruritic eruption *NEJM 234:665–666, 1946;* body lice *Cutis 105:118–120, 2020*

Peloderma strongyloides (nematode larvae) – exanthem of papules and pustules *JAAD 51:S181–184, 2004; JAAD 51:S109–112, 2004; JAAD 51:S109–112, 2004; Cutis 48:123–126, 1991; Ped Derm 2:33–37, 1984; BJD 98:107–112, 1978*

Phaeohyphomycotic cyst – fluctuant papules *JAAD 28:34–44, 1993*

Pinta – primary *AD 135:685–688, 1999*

Pityrosporum folliculitis *J Dermatol 27:49–51, 2000; Int J Dermatol 38:453–456, 1999; JAAD 234:693–696, 1991; Ann Int Med 108:560–563, 1988; JAAD 12:56–61, 1985*

Plague (*Yersinia pestis*) *JAAD 2011:65 (6)1213.e15.doi:10.1016/jaad.2010.08.040*

Portuguese man-of-war stings *J Emerg Med 10:71–77, 1992*

Prototothecosis – pink or red papules *Dermatol Online J 17:2, Sept 15, 2011; AD 142:921–926, 2006; AD 125:1249–1252, 1999; Cutis 63:185–188, 1999; JAAD 32:758–764, 1995*

Pseudomonas – swimming pool or hot tub folliculitis; macules, papules, pustules, urticarial lesions *JAMA 239:2362–2364, 1978; JAMA 235:2205–2206, 1976; Pseudomonas* wet suit dermatitis – pustules and papules *Ped Derm 458–459, 2003*

Rat bite fever (*Streptobacillus moniliformis* (pleomorphic facultative anaerobic bacillus) or *Spirillum minor* (Sudoku)) – macular, petechial, or morbilliform widespread exanthem; palmoplantar rash; arthralgia and chronic arthritis; Haverhill fever (raw milk) – papules, crusted papules, vesicles, pustules; chronic abscesses *Clin Inf Dis*

43:1585–1586;1616–1617, 2006; JAAD 38:330–332, 1998; Cleveland Clin Q 52 (2):203–205, 1985; Pediatr Clin N Am 26:377–411, 1979

Rheumatic fever – papules on extensor extremities near joints *AD 89:334–338, 1964*

Rhinosporidiosis (*Rhinosporidium seeberi*) – intranasal and conjunctival red polypoid lesions *JAAD 53:931–951, 2005;* strawberry shaped papule of forehead *SkinMed 16:63–65, 2018*

Rickettsia slovaca (Hungary) – *Dermacentor marginatus or D. reticulatus* tick bite; erythema marginatum-like lesions; scalp papules, crusted scalp papules and subsequent alopecia; tick-borne lymphadenopathy *Clin Inf Dis 34:1331–1336, 2002*

Rickettsial pox – personal observation

Salmonella typhimurium – rose spots on abdomen, chest, and back seen in typhoid fever *NEJM 340:869–876, 1999; Lancet 1:1211–1213, 1975; AD 105:252–253, 1972*

Scabies – persistent nodular arthropod reactions on elbows, abdomen, genitalia, and axillae (pseudolymphoma syndrome) *J Eur Acad DV 31:1248–1253, 2017; JAAD 38:877–905, 1998; Int J Dermatol 30:703–706, 1991*

Schistosomal dermatitis – popular pruritic eruption identical to swimmer's itch *JAAD 73:929–944, 2015; Dermatol Clin 7:291–300, 1989; Schistosoma hematobium* – groin and back *JAAD 42:678–680, 2000; Am J Dermatopath 16:434–438, 1994*

Seabather's eruption – *Linuche planulae JAAD 44:624–628, 2001; Linuche* unguiculata (larvae of Cnidaria thimble jellyfish); *Edwardsia lineate* (larvae of sea anemone) *Cutis 77:151–152, 2006; AD 60:227–237, 1949*

Sea urchin sting – red rash on knees and ankles *Dermatologica 180:99–101, 1990;* sea urchin granuloma *Int J Derm 25:649–650, 1986; Hautarzt 31:159–160, 1980*

Serratia marcescens – papular eruption with pustules *AIDS 10:1179–1180, 1996*

Silkmoth stings (*Saturniidae*) (*Hemileuca*) – urticarial papules *JAAD 62:1–10, 2010*

Sporotrichosis, disseminated *Indian Dermatol Online J 10:303–306, 2019; Dermatol Online J Nov 15, 2018*

Staphylococcal sepsis

Straw mite itch (*Pyemotes ventricosus*) *JAMA Derm 153:686–688, 2017*

Swimmer's itch – cercaria of *Trichobiharzia ocellata, T. szidati, Diplostomum spathaceum, Schistosoma spindale Folia Parasitologica 39:399–400, 1992; Cutis 23:212–216, 1979;* Hawaiian swimmer's itch (stinging seaweed dermatitis) – olive-green or black algae (*Microcolus lyngbyaceus*) *Hawaii Med J 52:274–275, 1993*

Sycosis

Syphilis – secondary *Cutis 93:277, 301–302, 2014;* malignant lues *Rev Inst Med Trop Sao Paolo 62:e21, 2020; JAAD 22:1061–1067, 1990*

Talaromyces (Penicillium) marneffei Clin Inf Dis 18:246–247, 1994

Tanapox – pruritic papule, initially *SkinMed 1:156–157, 2002*

Tick, engorged – personal observation

Tick bites – bites of larvae of *Haemaphysalis longicornis AD 147:1333–1334, 2011*

Toxocariasis – (*Toxocara canis, T. cati, T. leonensis*) visceral larva migrans – papular rash of trunk and legs *Dermatologica 144:129–143, 1972*

Toxoplasmosis – papular dermatitis *JAMA 116:807–814, 1941;* purple papules *JAAD 59:781–784, 2008*

Trichodysplasia spinulosa – papovaviral infection of immunocomprised host; progressive alopecia of eyebrows initially, then scalp and body hair and red follicular papules of nose, ears, forehead; leonine facies *JID Symposium Proceedings 4:268–271, 1999*

Trichosporon beigelii sepsis *AD 129:1020–1023, 1993*

Trichosporon louberi – red papulue of palm; fever, leukopenia *AD 147:975–980, 2011*

Tropical rat bite dermatitis (*Ornithonyssus bacoti*) *Dermatology 215:66–81, 2007*

Trypanosomiasis

Tsukamurella paurometabolum J Clin Inf Dis 23:839–840, 1996

Tularemia – vesiculopapular lesions of trunk and extremities *Cutis 54:279–286, 1994; Photodermatology 2:122–123, 1985;*

Yaws – primary red papule (mother yaw), ulcerates, crusted; satellite papules; become round ulcers, papillomatous or vegetative friable nodules which bleed easily (raspberry-like) (framboesia); heals with large atrophic scar with white center with dark halo; secondary (daughter yaws, pianomas, framboesiomas) – small papules which ulcerate, become crusted; resemble raspberries; periorificial (around mouth, nose, penis, anus, vulva); extend peripherally (circinate yaws); hyperkeratotic plantar plaques (crab yaws); periungual *Rook p.1268–1271, 1998, Sixth Edition; JAAD 29:519–535, 1993*

Varicella – post-varicella granulomatous dermatitis *Cutis 93:50–54, 2014; J Dtsch Dermatol Ges 2:770–772, 2004; Hautarzt 52:1111–1114, 2001; BJD 138:161–168, 1998; Am J Dermatopathol 16:588–592, 1994; J Cutan Pathol 19:557, 1992; Int J Dermatol 29:652–654, 1990*

Viral exanthem

Water bugs (*Belostomidae*) – painful bites *JAAD 67:331–344, 2012*

West Nile virus – scattered red papules resembling folliculitis *JAAD 51:820–823, 2004*

Yaws *JAAD 54:559–578, 2006*

Zika virus – fever, pinpoint red papules coalescing into morbilliform (macular and papular exanthem) eruption, arthralgia, conjunctivitis, myalgia, headache, retro-orbital pain, edema; palatal petechiae; Africa, Asia, Yap Island, Micronesia; mosquito vector (*Aedes hensilli*) *JAMA Derm 152:691–693, 2016; Clin Inf Dis 61:1445,1485–1486, 2015; NEJM 360:2536–2543, 2009*

INFILTRATIVE DISORDERS

Amyloidosis – primary systemic amyloid; lichen amyloid; presents as papular pruritis *Dermatology 194:62–64, 1997*

Benign cephalic histiocytosis – red-brown papules of cheeks, forehead, earlobes, neck *Ped Derm 11:265–267, 1994; Ped Derm 6:198–201, 1989; AD 122:1038–43, 1986; JAAD 13:383–404, 1985*

Congenital self-healing histiocytosis (Hashimoto-Pritzker disease) – red or blue nodular lesions in generalized distribution including palms and soles in neonatal period; self-limited over a few weeks *Ped Derm 18:41–44, 2001; AD 134:625–630, 1998*

Erdheim-Chester disease (non-Langerhans cell histiocytosis) – CD68+ and factor XIIIa+; negative for CD1a and S100; xanthoma and xanthelasma-like lesions (red-brown-yellow papules and plaques); widespread red papules; flat wart-like papules of face; lesions occur in folds; skin becomes slack with atrophy of folds and face; also lesions of eyelids, axillae, groin, neck; bony lesions *JAAD 74:513–520, 2016; Orphanet J Rare Dis 8:137, 2013; J Cut Pathol 38:280–285, 2011; Nat Clin Pract Rheumatol 4:50–55, 2008; JAAD 57:1031–1045, 2007; AD 143:952–953, 2007; Australas J Dermatol 44:194–198, 2003; Hautarzt 52:510–517, 2001; Medicine (Baltimore) 75:157–169, 1996; Virchow Arch Pathol Anat 279:541–542, 1930*

Generalized eruptive histiocytosis *Am J Dermatopathol March, 2015; An Bras Dermatol 88:105–108, 2013; JAAD 50:116–120, 2004; Am J Dermatopathol 18:490–504, 1996; AD 88:586–596, 1963*

Hemophagocytic lymphohistiocytosis *JAMA Derm 152:950–952, 2016*

Hereditary progressive mucinous histiocytosis – red-brown or skin colored papules *JAAD 57:1031–1045, 2007*

Histiocytosis, cutaneous – papulonodular variant *BJD 133:444–448, 1995; ;* non-Langerhans cell histiocytosis – generalized eruptive – exanthem with recurrent crops of red-brown papules, including the face *Acta DV 87:533–536, 2007; JAAD 50:116–120, 2004; Am J Dermatopathol 18:490–504, 1996;* associated with acute myelogenous leukemia *JAAD 50:116–120, 2004;* indeterminate cell histiocytosis – firm red, yellow, brown papules; more on trunk than head and neck; S-100, CD1a, HAM 56, CD 68, MAC 387, lysozyme, alpha-1 anti-trypsin, HLA-DR, CD 11c, CD 14b, factor XIIIa positive; reported with acute myelogenous leukemia and low grade lymphoproliferative disorders *JAAD 50:116–120, 2004;* S100-CD1a+ histiocytosis; indeterminate and dermal dendritic cells; exanthem with multiple papules *AD 147:995–997, 2011;*

indeterminate cell histiocytosis – widespread erythematous papulonodular eruption *BJD 158:838–840, 2008;* facial pink papules *BJD 156:1357–1361, 2007*

Intralymphatic histiocytosis – red patch overlying swollen knee; livedo reticularis, papules, nodules, urticaria, unilateral eyelid edema *AD 146:1037–1042, 2010*

Jessner's lymphocytic infiltrate *Dermatology 213:15–22, 2006; Dermatology 207:276–284, 2003; Indian J Lepr 57:804–806, 1985*

Focal mucinosis

Langerhans cell histiocytosis *JAAD 13:481–496, 1985;* in adulthood – disseminated papular eruption *AD 145:949–950, 2009; BJD 157:1277–1279, 2007;* self-healing Langerhans cell histiocytosis – red papule on arm of infant *Cutis 102:309, 316– 317, 2018;* vulvar red papules *Eur J Gyn Onc 30:691–694, 2009*

Langerhans cell histiocytosis in the adult – scrotal ulcer; solitary pink papule; red papules of trunk; ulceronecrotic plaque of scalp; perianal plaque; perianal dermatitis *BJD 167:1287–1294, 2012*

Mastocytosis – urticaria pigmentosa; solitary mastocytoma *NEJM 373:163–172, 2015; Acta DV (Stockh) 42:433–439, 1962*

Non-Langerhans cell histiocytosis *Am J Dermatopathol 18:490–504, 1996*

Plasmacytosis – benign primary cutaneous plasmacytosis *AD 145:299–302, 2009*

Pretibial myxedema – translucent red papules *JAAD 48:641–659, 2003; Medicine 73:1–7, 1994*

Progressive mucinous histiocytosis *BJD 142:133–137, 2000*

Verruciform xanthoma – red or yellow cauliflower-like appearance *J Dermatol 16:397–401, 1989;* disseminated verruciform xanthoma – hyperkeratotic yellow plaques; subungual pink papules *Cutis 93:307–310, 2014*

Xanthogranulomas, including juvenile xanthogranuloma; spindle cell xanthogranuloma – dark red dome-shaped papule *Cureus 10:e2595, May 8, 2018;* eruptive juvenile xanthogranulomas *J Cut Pathol 35:50–54, 2008;* most JXGs are yellow-red

Xanthoma disseminatum *Iran J Otorhinolaryngol 29:365–368, 2017*

INFLAMMATORY DISORDERS

Crohn's disease – metastatic lesions – red papules and plaques with overlying scale/crust; red scaly plaque with shallow ulcer; red plaques and nodules; abscess-like lesions *JAAD 71:804–813, 2014; J Eur Acad Dermatol Venereol 15:343–345, 2001*

Diffuse cutaneous pseudolymphoma due to medicinal leeches (*Hirudo medicinalis*) *JAMA Derm 150:783–784, 2014*

Endometriosis *JAAD 41:327–329, 1999*

Eosinophilic pustular folliculitis of AIDS

Erythema multiforme *Medicine 68:133–140, 1989; JAAD 8:763–765, 1983*

Granuloma gluteale infantum *JAAD 85:439–440, 2019*

Hidradenitis suppurativa – papules, nodules, abscesses, sinus tracts *BJD 165:415–418, 2011*

IgG4 disease – multisystem inflammatory disease with papules, plaques, and nodules; parotitis with parotid gland swelling, lacrimal gland swelling, dacryoadenitis, sialadenitis, proptosis; idiopathic pancreatitis, retroperitoneal fibrosis, aortitis; Mikuliczs syndrome, angio lymphadenopathy with eosinophilia, Riedel's thyroiditis, biliary tract disease, renal disease, meningeal disease, pituitary gland; Kuttner tumor, Rosai-Dorfman disease; elevated IgG4 with plasma cell dyscrasia, diffuse or localized swelling or masses; lymphocytic and plasma cell infiltrates with storiform fibrosis *JAAD 75:177–185, 2016*

Interstitial granulomatous dermatitis with plaques (aka linear rheumatoid nodule, railway track dermatitis, linear granuloma annulare, palisaded neutrophilic granulomatous dermatitis) *JAAD 47:319–320, 2002*

Kikuchi's disease (histiocytic necrotizing lymphadenitis) – multiple red to red-brown papules of face, scalp, chest, back, arms; red plaques; erythema and acneform lesions of face; morbilliform, urticarial, and rubella-like exanthems; red or ulcerated pharynx; cervical adenopathy; associations with SLE, lymphoma, tuberculous adenitis, viral lymphadenitis, infectious mononucleosis, and drug eruptions *AD 142:641–646, 2006; BJD 144:885–889, 2001; JAAD 36:342–346, 1997; Am J Surg Pathol 14:872–876, 1990*

Lymphocytoma cutis (pseudolymphoma) *Acta DV 62:119–124, 1982;* CD30+ T-cell rich pseudolymphoma – induced by gold acupuncture *BJD 146:882–884, 2002*

Necrotizing infundibular crystalline folliculitis – red umbilicated follicular papules with waxy keratotic plugs of face, neck, and back *JAMA Derm 149:1233–1234, 2013; BJD 145:165–168, 2001; BJD 143:310–314, 1999*

Neutrophilic eccrine hidradenitis *BJD 142:784–788, 2000; JAAD 40:367–398, 1999; JAAD 38:1–17, 1998; JAAD 35:819–822, 1996; AD 118:263–266, 1982*

Pyoderma gangrenosum

Rosai-Dorfman disease (sinus histiocytosis with massive lymphadenopathy) – disseminated red papules and nodules of extremities *Cutis 103:171–173, 2019; JAMA 310:199–200, 2013; J Clin Aesthet Dermatol 3:34–36, 2010; JAAD 56:302–316, 2007; BJD 148:1060–1061, 2003;* clustered erythematous papules of thigh; associated with uveitis *Practical Dermatol August 2014, pp.56,60;–* violaceous, red papules and nodules; cervical lymphadenopathy; also axillary, inguinal, and mediastinal adenopathy *JAAD 41:335–337, 1999; Int J Derm 37:271–274, 1998; BJD 134:749–753, 1996; Am J Dermatopathol 17:384–388, 1995; AD 114:191–197, 1978; Cancer 30:1174–1188, 1972; Arch Pathol 87:63–70, 1969*

Sarcoid – erythrodermic sarcoid with multiple red papules *JAMA Derm 153:335–336, 2017AD 133:882–888, 1997; NEJM 336:1224–1234, 1997; Clinics in Chest Medicine 18:663–679, 1997*

Subacute necrotizing lymphadenitis *JAAD 22:909–912, 1990*

METABOLIC DISEASES

Angiokeratoma corporis diffusum *BJD 166:712–720, 2012; JAAD 57:407–412, 2007; AD 142:615–618, 2006; BJD 144:363–368, 2001; AD 132:1219, 1222, 1996; AD 129:460–465, 1993;* acid sphingomyelinase deficiency – red vascular papules *Ped Derm 36:906–908, 2019*

    All disorders below are autosomal recessive except for Fabry's disease with characteristic facies, central nervous system dysfunction, mental retardation, and organomegaly

    Acid sphingomyelinase deficiency – massive hepatosplenomegaly, pulmonary infiltrates and skeletal abnormalities *Ped Derm 36:906–908, 2019*

    Adult onset GM–1, gangliosidosis (beta D–galactosidase deficiency) *AD 142:615–618, 2006; Clin Genet 17:323–334, 1980*

    Alpha-N acetylgalactosaminidase deficiency (Kanzaki's disease) (Kanzaki-Schindler disease) (alpha-N-acetylgalactosaminidase) *AD 142:615–618, 2006; AD 129:460–465, 1993*

    Aspartylglucosaminuria (aspartylglycosaminidase deficiency) *BJD 147:760–764, 2002; J Med Genet 36:398–404, 1999; Paediatr Acta 36:179–189, 1991; Helv Paediatr Acta 36:179–189, 1981*

    Beta-galactosidase deficiency (GM-1 gangliosidosis)

    Beta-mannosidosis (beta mannosidase deficiency) – mental retardation, deafness, speech impairment, susceptibility to infections, hypotonia, epilepsy, peripheral neuropathy, facial dysmorphism, skeletal abnormalities *JAAD 57:407–412, 2007; BJD 152:177–178, 2005; J Dermatol 31:931–935, 2004; AD 132:1219–1222, 1996; J Inherit Metab Dis 11:17–29, 1988; NEJM 315:1231, 1986;* alpha and beta D-mannosidase = alpha and beta mannosidosis *AD 142:615–618, 2006*

    Fabry's disease (Anderson-Fabry disease) – alpha galactosidase A deficiency – X-linked accumulation of globotriaosylceramide *BJD 166:712–720, 2012; Ped Derm 28:727–728, 2011; Clin Exp Dermatol 36:506–508, 2011; BJD 157:331–337, 2007;NEJM 276:1163–1167, 1967; Arch Dermatol Syphil 43:187, 1898;* red papules of face and lips *BJD 166:712–720, 2012*

    Fucosidosis type II (alpha-L-fucosidase) – red papules, purpura, short stature *Ped Derm 24:442–443, 2007;*

AD 107:754–757, 1973; Science 176:420–427, 1972

Galactosialidosis (combined beta-galactosidase and sialidase deficiencies) *AD 120:1344–1346, 1984*
    Normal
    Idiopathic angiokeratoma corporis diffusum without metabolic abnormalities; – telangiectasias or small angiokeratomas

AD 123:1125–1127, 1987; JAAD 12:885–886, 1985; telangiectasias or small angiokeratomas; and arteriovenous fistulae without metabolic disorders – papules *AD 131:57–62, 1995; BJD 166:712–720, 2012; AD 142:615–618, 2006; Hautarzt 46:785–788, 1995*
    Schindler disease type II (Kanzaki disease)
    Sialidosis type II (sialidase) *AD 142:615–618, 2006; BJD 152:177–178, 2005; Ann Neurol 6:232–244, 1978*
    Solitary and localized angiokeratoma

Cryoglobulinemia *JAAD 48:311–340, 2003*

Cystic fibrosis – red papules of antecubital fossa; granulomatous dermatitis with PXE-like changes *AD 145:1292–1295, 2009*

Endometriosis *Acta Ob Gyn Scand 71:337–342, 1992*

Hepatocutaneous syndrome – in chronic active hepatitis; firm red papules leaving atrophic scars *Br Med J i:817, 1977*

Necrobiosis lipoidica diabeticorum – starts as red papule *Int J Derm 33:605–617, 1994; JAAD 18:530–537, 1988*

Nephrogenic systemic fibrosis *J Am Coll Radiol 5:40–44, 2008*

Osteoma cutis – congenital osteoma cutis *AD 133:775–780, 1997;*

progressive osseous heteroplasia – pink papules *AD 132:787–791, 1996*

Perineural xanthoma in diabetes mellitus – tender red nodule of back *Cutis 92:299–302, 2013*

Pregnancy – prurigo of pregnancy *Semin Derm 8:23–25, 1989;* pruritic urticarial papules and plaques of pregnancy *JAAD 10:473–480, 1984; Clin Exp Dermatol 7:65–73, 1982; JAMA 241:1696–1699, 1979*

Scurvy – follicular red papules *Ped Derm 28:444–446, 2011*

Whipple's disease – sarcoid-like granulomas *Ann DV 105:235–238, 1978*

Xanthomas – eruptive xanthomas *Cutis 89:141–144, 2012*

NEOPLASTIC LESIONS

Acquired digital fibrokeratoma *Cutis 79:129–132, 2007*

Acrochordon, irritated

Acrospiroma *Cutis 58:349–351, 1996*

Actinic keratosis; actinic keratoses inflamed by chemotherapy (capecitabine) *JAAD 55:S119–120, 2006;* 5-fluorouracil *BJD 74:229–236, 1962;* doxorubicin, dactinomycin-dacarbazine-vincristine sulfate, 2-deoxycoformycin, fludarabine, and cisplatin *AD 139:77–81, 2003;* actinic keratosis *Stat Pearls April 22, 2020*

Multinucleate cell angiohistiocytoma – red to red-brown papule *J Cutan Pathol 46:59–61, 2019; Cutis 63:145–148, 1999; Cutis 59:190–192, 1997; JAAD 30:417–422, 1994; BJD 113 (suppl 129):15, 1985;* generalized multinucleate cell angiohistiocytoma *JAAD 320–322, 1996*

Angioleiomyoma – pink nodule of heel *Cutis 81:123,140–141, 2008*

Angiosarcoma – lymphedematous leg *BJD 138:692–694, 1998;* radiation-induced – papulonodules *JAAD 38:143–175, 1998*

Aortic angiosarcoma with cutaneous metastases *JAAD 43:930–933, 2000*

Cutaneous radiation-associated angiosarcoma of the breast – livedoid violaceous plaques with nodules of the breast *JAMA Derm 149:973–974, 2013*

Atrial myxoma – red macules and papules *Cutis 62:275–280, 1998; JAAD 32:881–883, 1995; JAAD 21:1080–1084, 1989*

Atypical fibroxanthoma *Semin Cut Med Surg 38:E65–66, 2019' Dermatol Surg 37:146–157, 2011*

BAP-1 inactivated melanocytic tumors – pink dome-shaped papules *JAAD 89:1585–1586, 2019*

Basal cell carcinoma – superficial basal cell carcinomas in radiation port *AD 136:1007–1011, 2000; J Natl Cancer Inst 88:1848–1853, 1996; AD 131:484–488, 1995;* red dot basal cell carcinoma *J Clin Aesthet Dermtol 10:56–58, 2017; J Drugs Dermatol 15:645=647, 2016*

Basal cell nevus, linear unilateral *Cutis 78:122–124, 2006; Arch Dermatol Syphilol 65:471–476, 1952*

Basaloid follicular hamartoma – pink papule *AD 133:381–386, 1997*

Blue nevus – hypopigmented blue nevus of dorsum of foot; pink papule *AD 138:1091–1096, 2002; J Cutan Pathol 24:494–498, 1997*

Bowenoid papulosis *Actas Dermosifilogr 72:545–550, 1981*

Burkitt's lymphoma, disseminated – red macules and papules *BJD 174:184–186, 2016*

Cartilaginous matrix-producing apocrine carcinoma – pink papulonodule *BJD 163:215–218, 2010*

Chalazion – yellow, skin colored or red papule or nodule *Eyelid and Conjunctival Tumors, Shields JA and Shields CL, Lippincott Williams and Wilkins, 1999, p.165; Ophthalmology 87:218–221, 1980*

Cellular neurothekeoma *Ped Derm 37:320–325, 2020*

Chondroid syringoma

Clear cell acanthoma (Degos' acanthoma) (pale cell acanthoma) *The Dermatologist October 2016, pp47–49; Am J Dermatopathol 16:134–139, 1994; BJD 83:248–254, 1970; Ann Dermatol Syphilol 89:361–371, 1962;* multiple *J Dermatol Case Rep 4:25–27, 2010; AD 116:433–434, 1980*

Clear cell hidradenoma *The Dermatologist October 2016, pp47–49*

Dermal duct tumor *AD 114:1659–1664, 1978*

Dermatofibroma

Dermatofibrosarcoma protuberans – early, red papule/nodule *JAAD 35:355–374, 1996;* pediatric *J Surg Res 170:69–72, 2011*

Desmoplastic nevus *Histopathology 20:207–211, 1992*

Desmoplastic Spitz nevus – smudgy purple papule *Cutis 89:22, 2012*

Digital mucous cyst

Eccrine angiomatous hamartoma – congenital red-brown papules and plaques *Ped Derm 36:909–912, 2019*

Primary eccrine porocarcinoma – acral red papules *BJD 169:1059–1061, 2013*

Eccrine poroma – plantar red papule *BJD 145:830–833, 2001; JAAD 44:48–52, 2001; AD 74:511–521, 1956;* digital papule *AD 74:511–512, 1956;* eruptive eccrine poromas, 1–4 mm *Cutis 89:81–83, 2012*

Eccrine spiradenoma *J Dermatol 31:564–568, 2004; Hautarzt 41:692–695, 1990*

Eccrine syringofibroadenoma *BJD 143:591–594, 2000*

Epithelioid sarcoma – red papule in nasal septum of a child *J Cutan Pathol 27:186–190, 2000*

Eruptive vellus hair cysts *JAAD 3:425–429, 1980*

Erythroplasia of Queyrat

Exostosis, subungual *Derm Surg 27:591–593, 2001*

Extramammary Paget's disease – red papule of penile shaft *AD 142:515–520, 2006;* perigenital red nodules of scrotum and pubic region *Cutis 94:276–278, 2014*

Extramedullary hematopoiesis in chronic idiopathic myelofibrosis with myelodysplasia *JAAD 55:S28–31, 2006*

Facial apocrine fibroadenoma *Am J Dermatopathol 29:274–278, 2007*

Fibroepithelioma of Pinkus – skin-colored or red pedunculated nodule of trunk, groin, or thigh *BJD 150:1208–1209, 2004;* gray-brown papule or plaque; skin colored plaque; pedunculated, polypoid; pink papule *AD 142:1318–1322, 2006; JAAD 52:168–169, 2005*

Fibrofolliculomas

Fibrous papule of the face (nose) (angiofibroma) *JAAD 10:670–671, 1984*

Generalized eruptive histiocytoma – hundreds of skin-colored, brown, blue-red papules; resolve with macular pigmentation; face, trunk, proximal extremities *JAAD 31:322–326, 1994; JAAD 20:958–964, 1989; JAAD 17:499–454, 1987; AD 117:216–221, 1981; AD 116:565–567, 1980; AD 96:11–17, 1967*

Glomus tumor *Ann Plast Surg 43:436–438, 1999; Acta DV 66:161–164, 1986*

Granular cell tumor *Ped Derm 14:489–490, 1997*

Hidradenoma papilliferum *JAAD 41:115–118, 1999*

Histiocytoma – acquired mucosal indeterminate cell histiocytoma – red papule of glans penis *Ped Derm 24:253–256, 2007*

Kaposi's sarcoma – in pityriasis rosea-like distribution; in HIV disease with immune reconstitution syndrome *NEJM 369:1152–1161, 2013;* micronodular Kaposi's sarcoma *Dermatology 208:255–258, 2004*

Keloids

Keratoacanthoma – solitary; Grzybowski *AD 120:736–740, 1984*

Leiomyoma *AD 141:199–206, 2005;* multiple pink nodules *JAAD 62:904–906, 2010;* multiple pink painful nodules associated with renal cell carcinoma (Reed syndrome); fumarate hydratase deficiency *The Dermatologist, July 2016, pp.47–49; NEJM 369:1344–1355, 2013; JAMA Derm 149:22–228, 2013; JAAD 55:683–686, 2006; Am J Hum Genet 10:48–52, 1958;* Reed syndrome – cutaneous and uterine leiomyomas; type II papillary renal cell carcinoma of collecting duct carcinoma *JAAD 66:337–339, 2012; Acta DV 53:409–416, 1973;* oval pink papules in pityriasis rosea distribution *JAAD 62:168–170, 2010; AD 120:1618–1620, 1984;* agminated pink papules of buttock *JAAD 66:337–339, 2012;* unilateral red painful papules *JAMA Derm 149:865–866, 2013*

Leiomyosarcoma – blue-black; also red, brown, yellow or hypopigmented *JAAD 46:477–490, 2002*

Leukemic infiltrates, including AMML, ALL, CLL – red papules and violaceous plaque of skin and oral mucosa *Cutis 104:326–330, 2019; JAAD 35:849–850, 1996;* monocytic leukemia – red, brown, violaceous patch or nodule *AD 123:225–231, 1971;* preleukemic state of monocytosis and neutropenia – perniotic lesions *BJD 81:327–332, 1969;* congenital monocytic leukemia *Ped Derm 6:306–311, 1989;* adult T-cell leukemia/lymphoma *BJD 152:76–81, 2005;* aleukemic leukemia cutis *J Eur Acad DV 20:453–456, 2006*

Leukemid – personal observation

Lichen planus-like keratosis *AD 116:780–782, 1980*

Lymphangiosarcoma (Stewart-Treves tumor) – red papules in lymphedematous extremity *Arch Surg 94:223–230, 1967; Cancer 1:64–81, 1948*

Lymphoma – B-cell, primary cutaneous *Ped Derm 26:34–39, 2009;* cutaneous T-cell lymphoma *JAAD 52:694–698, 2005;* primary cutaneous marginal zone B-cell lymphoma – red or violaceous papules of back *JAAD 69:329–340, 2013; JAAD 64:135–143, 2011;* angiotropic B-cell lymphoma (malignant angioendotheliomatosis) – cherry angioma-like lesions *BJD 143:162–164, 2000;* Hodgkin's disease, immunocytoma (low grade B cell lymphoma) – reddish-brown papules *JAAD 44:324–329, 2001;* adult T-cell lymphoma/leukemia (HTLV-1) *JAAD 46:S137–141, 2002; AD 134:439–444, 1998; JAAD 34:69–76, 1996; BJD 128:483–492, 1993; Am J Med 84:919–928, 1988;* HTLV-1 leukemia/lymphoma (ATLL) – red brown annular patches, red papules and nodules *BJD 152:76–81, 2005;* red-orange papulonodules – HTLV-1 granulomatous T cell lymphoma *JAAD 44:525–529, 2001;* pityriasis lichenoides-like CTCL *BJD 142:347–352, 2000;* nasal NK/T-cell lymphoma *JAAD 46:451–456, 2002;* angioimmunoblastic lymphadenopathy (T-cell lymphoma) *BJD 144:878–884, 2001;* primary cutaneous follicle center lymphoma *JAAD 69:343–354, 2013;* primary cutaneous follicular helper T-cell lymphoma – red papules, red plaques, scalp nodule, facial plaques *AD 148:832–839, 2012;* primary cutaneous follicle center lymphoma with diffuse CD 30 expression – papules, plaques, nodules, multilobulated scalp tumor *JAAD 71:548–554, 2014;* primary cutaneous EBV diffuse large B-cell lymphoma *Cutis 102:421–424, 2018*

Lymphomatoid granulomatosis – pink papules *NEJM 372:650–659, 2015; JAAD 54:657–663, 2006; AD 139:803–808, 2003*

Lymphomatoid papulosis *Dermatol Online J May 15, 2018; J Cutan Pathol 34:584–587, 2007*

Mantleomas – multiple red papules *BJD 171:417–418, 2014; Hautarzt 52:43–46, 2001; Am J Dermatopathol 15:306–310, 1993*

Melanocytic nevus, including atypical nevus *JAAD 14:1044–1052, 1986*

Melanoma – primary, metastatic; thin nodular *AD 146:311–318, 2010;* amelanotic melanoma *JAAD 54:341–344, 2006;* amelanotic melanoma – red papule of penile shaft *AD 142:515–520, 2006*

Merkel cell carcinoma – red papule of eyelid mimicking chalazion *Am J Ophthalmol 121:331–332, 1996; Aust N Z J Ophthlmol 24:377–380, 1996; J R Coll Surg Edin 36:129–130, 1991;* red papules of leg *J Drugs in Dermatol 9:779–784, 2010;* epidermotropic Merkel cell carcinoma – red eyelid papules; papules of leg, neck, or hand *JAAD 62:463–468, 2010;* red papules *Cutis 100:103–104, 124, 2017; Indian J Dermatol 58:243, 2013;*

Metastases – induration, ulcer, or painless nodule *Arch Opthalmol 92:276–286, 1974;* breast cancer *Cutis 31:411–415, 1983;* testicular choriocarcinoma *Cutis 67:117–120, 2001;* lung *Eu J Derm 8:573–574, 1998;* carcinoma telangiectatica; renal cell carcinoma; osteosarcoma *JAAD 49:757–760, 2003;* well differentiated fetal adenocarcinoma – purple nodule *BJD 150:778–780, 2004;* carcinoma telangiectoides; melanoma with lymphangiectatic metastases *Cutis 84:151–158, 2009;* red nodule of chest – metastatic gastric carcinoma *JAMA 308:812812, 2012*

Mucinous nevus (connective tissue nevus of the proteoglycan type) – linear pink papules of chest *JAMA Derm 150:1018–1019, 2014; BJD 148:1064–1066, 2003; JAAD 37:312–313, 1997; AD 132:1522–1523, 1996; BJD 1331:368–370, 1994*

Mucoepidermoid carcinoma – red papule of scalp *Derm Surg 27:1046–1048, 2001*

Multinucleate cell angiohistiocytoma – women over 50 years old; thighs, knees, dorsal hands and fingers – grouped violaceous macules or soft red-purple papules *Cutis 100:429–431, 2017; JAMA Derm 149:357–362, 2013; J Cut Med Surg 14:178–180, 2010; New England Dermatological Society Conference, Sept 15, 2007; Cutis 63:145–148, 1999; JAAD 38:143–175, 1998; AD 132:703–708, 1996; JAAD 30:417–422, 1994; BJD 121:113–121, 1989; BJD 113:15, 1985*

Multiple mucocutaneous neuromas (palisaded encapsulated and non-encapsulated neuromas) – lip, palmar, dorsal hand red papules *AD 149:498–500, 2013*

Multiple myeloma, metastases *JAAD 74:878–884, 2016; J Drugs Dermatol 14:1485–1486, 2015*

Myelodysplastic syndrome – disseminated cutaneous granulomatous eruptions *Clin Exp Dermatol 18:559–563, 1993*

Myxoid cutaneous pleomorphic fibroma *AD 146:1037–1042, 2010*

Neurofibroma

Neuroma, including solitary encapsulated neuroma *BJD 142:1061–1062, 2000*

Neurothekeomas – pink papules on a background of a café au lait macule *Ped Derm 28:77–79, 2011*

Nevus comedonicus, inflammatory *JAAD 38:834–836, 1998*

Nevus elasticus *Int J Dermatol 25:171–173m 1986*

Nevus, melanocytic, hemorrhagic

Nevus sebaceus

Oncocytoma – bright red or yellow papule of eyelid *Arch Ophthalmol 102:263–265, 1984*

Pilomatrixoma – papule *Eyelid and Conjunctival Tumors, Shields JA and Shields CL, Lippincott Williams and Wilkins, 1999, p.71*

Pinkus tumors (fibroepithelioma of Pinkus) – variant of basal cell carcinoma *J Clin Aesthet Dermatol 1:42–44, 2008;* red papule of foot *Am Fam Physician 77:1449–1450*

Plasmacytoid dendritic cell neoplasm – purple macules, violaceous papules, nodules, tumefactions; highly pigmented dark red, purpuric, necrotic lesions of face, neck *JAAD 66:278–291, 2012; Turk J Hematol 28:312–316, 2011*

Plasmacytoma – extramedullary plasmacytoma *JAAD 19:879–890, 1988; AD 127:69–74, 1991;* systemic plasmacytosis *JAAD 38:629–631, 1998;* primary cutaneous plasmacytomas *J Dermtol 38:364–367, 2011; AD 145:299–302, 2009; Dermatology 189:251–255, 1994;* of penis *JAMA Derm 155:247–248, 2019;* red facial papule *J Dtsch Dermatol Ges 11:1161–1167, 2013*

Porocarcinoma *BJD 152:1051–1055, 2005*

Porokeratosis, disseminated superficial actinic *AD 99:408–412, 1969;* linear porokeratosis *AD 135:1544–1555,1547–1548, 1999; Ped Derm 4:209, 1987; AD 109:526–528, 1974;* porokeratosis palmaris et plantaris et disseminata

Post-transplant Epstein-Barr virus-associated lymphoproliferative disorder *JAAD 51:778–780, 2004;* red papules *JAAD 54:657–663, 2006*

Pseudo-cutaneous T-cell lymphoma in HIV disease *Int J Derm 38:111–118, 1999*

Pseudolymphoma *Arch Dermatol Res 279:552–554, 1987*

Reticulohistiocytoma – personal observation

Sebaceous carcinoma – red papule (mimics chalazion); late ulceration *Br J Ophthalmol 82:1049–1055, 1998; Br J Plast Surg 48:93–96, 1995; JAAD 25:685–690, 1991; J Derm Surg Oncol 11:260–264, 1985;* papule *Eyelid and Conjunctival Tumors, Shields JA and Shields CL, Lippincott Williams and Wilkins, 1999, p.40–41*

Rhabdomyosarcoma *AD 124:1687–1690, 1988*

Spitz nevus *JAAD 27:901–913, 1992;* eruptive disseminated Spitz nevi *JAAD 57:519–523, 2007;* multiple epithelioid Spitz nevi with loss of *BAP1* expression – red vascular papules *JAMA Derm 149:333–339, 2013;* agminated *Am J Dermatopathol 40:686–689, 2018*

Squamous cell carcinoma

Sweat gland adenoma – personal observation

Syringosquamous metaplasia *JAAD 38:1–17, 1998; AD 123:1202–1204, 1987*

Syringocystadenoma papilliferum – linear red papules *JAAD 45:139–141, 2001; AD 121:1197–1202, 1985*

Transient myeloproliferative disorder associated with mosaicism for trisomy 21 – vesiculopustular rash *NEJM 348:2557–2566, 2003;* in trisomy 21 or normal patients; periorbital vesiculopustules, red papules, crusted papules, and ulcers; with periorbital edema *Ped Derm 21:551–554, 2004*

Tumor of follicular infundibulum – single or multiple – associated with Cowden's, nevus sebaceus *JAAD 33:979–84, 1995*

Waldenstrom's IgM storage papules – skin-colored translucent papules on extensor extremities, buttocks, trunk; may be hemorrhagic, crusted, or umbilicated pruritic papules, vesicles, bullae, urticaria *JAAD 45:S202–206, 2001; BJD 106:217–222m 1982;* red papules of lower legs *AD 145:77–82, 2009*

Waldenstrom's macroglobulinemia with lymphoplasmacytoid B cells – chest, earlobes, facial papules *JAAD 45:S202–206, 2001;* red papule *AD 134:1127–1131, 1998; AD 128:372–376, 1992; AD 124:1851–1856, 1988; Acta Medica Scand 209:129–131, 1981;* Waldenstrom's macroglobulinemia with granulomatous dermatitis – personal observation

PHOTOSENSITIVITY DISORDERS

Actinic reticuloid (pseudolymphoma syndrome) *JAAD 38:877–905, 1998*

HIV photosensitivity

Papular elastolytic giant cell granuloma *J Eur Acad DV 18:365–368, 2004; Eur J Dermatol 9:647–649, 1999*

Polymorphic light eruption *Photodermatol Photoimmunol Photomed 18:303–306, 2002*

PARANEOPLASTIC DISEASES

Eosinophilic dermatosis of myeloproliferative disease – red papulonodules, red plaques *JAAD 81:246–249, 2019; AD 137:1378–1380, 2001*

Eruptive cherry angiomas *Clin Exp Dermatol 3:147–155, 1978*

Generalized eruptive histiocytosis associated with acute myelogenous leukemia *JAAD 49:S233–236, 2003*

Insect bite-like reactions associated with hematologic malignancies *AD 135:1503–1507, 1999*

Melanocytic BAP1-mutated atypical intradermal tumors (MBAIT) – pink-skin colored papules; sign of renal cell carcinoma and melanoma *JAMA Derm 153:999–1000, 2017*

Necrobiotic xanthogranuloma with paraproteinemia

Sign of Leser-Trelat – inflammatory seborrheic keratoses

PRIMARY CUTANEOUS DISEASES

Acne rosacea, including lupus miliaris disseminata faciei *Dermatol Online J Dec 16, 2015; Clin Exp Dermatol 39:500–502, 2014;* rosacea fulminans (pyoderma faciale) *An Bras Dermatol 91:S151–153, 2016*

Acne vulgaris

Acute parapsoriasis (pityriasis lichenoides et varioliformis acuta) (Mucha-Habermann disease) *JAAD 55:557–572, 2006; AD 123:1335–1339, 1987; AD 118:478, 1982; Dermtol Z 45:42–48, 1925; Arch Dermatol Syph (Wien) 123:586–592, 1916; Veth Dtsch Dermatol Ges 4:495–499, 1894*

Alopecia mucinosa (follicular mucinosis) *JAAD 38:803–805, 1998*

Angiolymphoid hyperplasia with eosinophilia – along scalp line *Clin Inf Dis 62:1419–1421, 2016;* disseminated papules over face, trunk and extremities *Cutis 72:323–326, 2003*

Axillary acne agminata – axillary red papules (form of granulomatous rosacea) *JAMA Derm 151:893–894, 2015*

Cholinergic urticarial – personal observation

Darier's disease – linear pink papules *AD 143:535–540, 2007*

Elastosis perforans serpiginosa – red papules in circinate pattern *Dermatol Online J March 15, 2019*

Eosinophilic pustular folliculitis of childhood *AD 133:775–780, 1997*

Epidermolysis bullosa – dystrophic epidermolysis bullosa pruriginosa – red, crusted, and lichenified papules *BJD 159:464–469, 2008*

Eruptive pseudoangiomatosis – bright red pinpoint lesions *JAAD 52:174–175, 2005; AD 140:757, 2004*

Erythema elevatum diutinum *Stat Pearls Dec 20, 2019; J Dtsch Dermatol Ges 6:303–305, 2008; Cutis 68:41–42, 55, 2001; Medicine (Baltimore) 56:443–455, 1977*

Erythema of Jacquet

Granular parakeratosis – scaly red papules *JAAD 52:863–867, 2005*

Granuloma annulare – of dorsal fingers and palms *AD 142:49–54, 2006; JAAD 3:217–230, 1980;* generalized granuloma annulare *JAAD 75:457–465, 2016;* perforating granuloma annulare *Ped Derm 20:131–133, 2003*

Granuloma faciale *Dermatol Online J Oct 9, 2003; Int J Dermatol 36:548–551, 1997; AD 129:634–635, 637, 1993;* extrafacial granuloma faciale *AD 79:42–52, 1959*

Granulomatous periorificial dermatitis – extrafacial and generalized periorificial dermatitis *AD 138:1354–1358, 2002*

Granulosis rubra nasi

Grover's disease (transient acantholytic dermatosis) *AD 101:426–434, 1970*

Keratosis pilaris

Keratosis pilaris rubra (keratosis rubra pilaris) *AD 142:1611–1616, 2006; Ped Derm 23:31–34, 2006; BJD 147:822–824, 2002*

Lichen nitidus

Lichen planus

Lichen planus pemphigoides *BJD 142:509–512, 2000*

Malakoplakia – perianal nodules, vulvar nodules, skin colored nodules, ulcerations, abscesses, red papules, masses *Arch Pathol Lab Med 132:113–117, 2008*

Miliaria rubra *BJD 99:117–137, 1978*

Papular elastorrhexis *Clin Cosmet Invertis Dermtol 26:541–544, 2018; JAAD 19:409–414, 1988*

Papular prurigo *J Dermatol 28:75–80, 2001; JAAD 24:697–702, 1991*

Perforating folliculitis

Perioral dermatitis including facial Afro-Caribbean childhood eruption (FACE) *BJD 91:435–438, 1976*

Pityriasis lichenoides chronica *JAAD 56:205–210, 2007; JAAD 55:557–572, 2006; BJD 129:353–354, 1993; AD 119:378–380, 1983; Ann Dermatol Syphiligr (Paris) 3433–468, 1902; AD Syphilol 50:359–374, 1899*

Pityriasis lichenoides et varioliformis acuta *Dermatol Pract Concepts 31:27–34, 2017; Am J Clin Dermatol 8:29–36, 2007*

Pityriasis rosea

Pityriasis rubra pilaris

Psoriasis

Prurigo pigmentosa – urticarial red pruritic papules, papulovesicles, vesicles, and plaques with reticulated hyperpigmentation *JAAD 55:131–136, 2006; Cutis 63:99–102, 1999; BJD 120:705–708, 1989; AD 125:1551–1554, 1989; JAAD 12:165–169, 1985*

Pseudoxanthoma elasticum

Reactive perforating collagenosis

Subacute prurigo (itchy red bump disease) *JAAD 24:697–702, 1991; JAAD 4:723–729, 1981*

SYNDROMES

Acral angiokeratoma-like pseudolymphoma (APACHE syndrome) – red papules *JAAD S209–211, 2001; BJD 124:387–388, 1991*

Ataxia-telangiectasia – granuloma *Clin Exp Dermatol 18:458–461, 1993*

Basaloid follicular hamartoma syndrome – multiple skin-colored, red, and hyperpigmented papules of the face, neck chest, back, proximal extremities, and eyelids; syndrome includes milia-like cysts, comedones, sparse scalp hair, palmar pits, and parallel bands of papules of the neck (zebra stripes) *JAAD 43:189–206, 2000*

Behcet's disease *JAAD 41:540–545, 1999; JAAD 40:1–18, 1999; NEJM 341:1284–1290, 1999; JAAD 36:689–696, 1997*

Blau or Jabs syndrome (familial juvenile systemic granulomatosis) – translucent skin-colored papules of trunk and extremities with uveitis, synovitis, arthritis; polyarteritis, multiple synovial cysts; red papular rash in early childhood; autosomal dominant; resembles childhood sarcoid – red papules; chromosome 16p12–q21 *JAAD 49:299–302, 2003; Am J Hum Genet 76:217–221, 1998; Am J Hum Genet 59:1097–1107, 1996; Clin Exp Dermatol 21:445–448, 1996*

Cardiofaciocutaneous syndrome – congenital heart defects, sparse and woolly hair , hyperkeratotic skin lesions (keratosis pilaris), generalized ichthyosis-like; KRAS and BRAF mutations *Nat Genet 38:294–296, 2006; Am J Med Genet 25:413–427, 1986*

Congenital self-healing reticulohistiocytosis *AD 134:625–630, 1998*

Cowden's syndrome – tumor of follicular infundibulum – single or multiple – associated with Cowden's – nevus sebaceus *JAAD 33:979–84, 1995;* angiomas

Eruptive familial lingual papillitis *Ped Derm 14:13–16, 1997*

Farber's disease (disseminated lipogranulomatosis) – red papules and nodules of joints and tendons of hands and feet; deforming arthritis; papules, plaques, and nodules of ears, back of scalp and trunk *Am J Dis Child 84:449–500, 1952*

Goltz's syndrome – raspberry papillomas *J Med Genet 27:180–187, 1990*

Hepatocutaneous syndrome

Hereditary progressive mucinous histiocytosis *JAAD 35:298–303, 1996; AD 124:1225–1229, 1988*

Hereditary hemorrhagic telangiectasia (Osler-Weber-Rendu disease)

Hereditary LDH M-subunit deficiency – annular red rash in summer, resolves in autumn; muscular symptoms; small papules and annular red centrifugal spread *AD 122:1420–1424, 1986*

Hereditary progressive mucinous histiocytosis – autosomal dominant; skin-colored or red-brown papules; nose, hands, forearms, thighs *JAAD 35:298–303, 1996; AD 130:1300–1304, 1994*

Hypereosinophilic syndrome – red papulonodules *Am J Hematol 80:148–157, 2005; BJD 144:639, 2001; AD 132:583–585, 1996; Med Clin (Barc)106:304–306, 1996; Blood 83:2759–2779, 1994; AD 114:531–535, 1978; Medicine 54:1–27, 1975*

Infantile systemic hyalinosis *Am J Med Genet 100:122–129, 2001*

Multicentric reticulohistiocytosis – generalized ruby red papules and hepatocellular carcinoma *Case Rep Dermatol 4:163–169m 2012*

Multiple endocrine neoplasia syndrome type 1 (MEN1) – red angiofibromas of face *Hered Cancer Clin Pract 15:10 July 21, 2017*

POEMS syndrome (Crowe-Fukase syndrome, Takatsuki syndrome) – plethora, angiomas (cherry, globular, glomeruloid) presenting as rd nodules of face, trunk, and extremities, diffuse hyperpigmentation, hypertrichosis, scleroderma-like changes, hyperhidrosis, clubbing, leukonychia, papilledema, sclerotic bone lesions, pleural effusion, peripheral edema, ascites, pulmonary hypertension, weight loss, fatigue, diarrhea, thrombocytosis, polycythemia, fever, renal disease, arthralgias *JAAD 55:149–152, 2006; JAAD 37:887–920, 1997*

Reactive arthritis

REM (reticular erythematous mucinosis) syndrome *JAAD 27:825–828, 1992; Ped Derm 7:1–10, 1990; Z Hautkr 63:986–998, 1988*

(German); JAAD 19:859–868, 1988; AD 115:1340–1342, 1979; BJD 91:191–199, 1974; Z Hautkr 49:235–238, 1974

Rowell's syndrome – lupus erythematosus and erythema multiforme-like syndrome – papules, annular targetoid lesions, vesicles, bullae, necrosis, ulceration, oral ulcers; perniotic lesions *JAAD 21:374–377, 1989*

Self-healing infantile familial cutaneous mucinosis *Ped Derm 14:460–462, 1997*

Sweet's syndrome – red papules of knees associated with human granulocytic anaplasmosis *AD 141:887–889, 2005;* red papules and plaques of neck *JAAD 69:557–564, 2013;* photodistributed red papules *Indian J Dermatol 59:186–189, 2014*

Torre's syndrome

Tuberous sclerosis – adenoma sebaceum *Plast Reconstr Surg 70:91–93, 1982*

Wells' syndrome – papulonodular variant *AD 142:1157–1161, 2006*

TOXINS

Eosinophilia myalgia syndrome (l-tryptophan related) – morphea, urticaria, papular lesions; arthralgia *BJD 127:138–146, 1992; Int J Dermatol 31:223–228, 1992; Mayo Clin Proc 66:457–463, 1991; Ann Int Med 112:758–762, 1990*

Potato poisoning – rash of lower abdomen and medial thighs consisting of red papules which progress to pustules and crusted lesions; facial and abdominal edema; headache, vomiting, diarrhea *J R Coll Physicians Edinb 36:336–339, 2007*

TRAUMA

Chilblains (perniosis) *AD 117:26–28, 1981*

Chondrodermatitis nodularis chronicus helicis

Cold panniculitis

Granuloma fissuratum

Mastectomy – granulomatous nodules after mastectomy for breast carcinoma *BJD 146:891–894, 2002*

Radiation therapy – eosinophilic polymorphic and pruritic eruption associated with radiotherapy (EPPER) – bullae, red papules, pruritic *JAAD 56:S60–61, 2007; JAAD 54:728–729, 2006; AD 137:821–822, 2001;* violaceous or red papules – post-radiation angiosarcoma

Scar

VASCULAR LESIONS

Acral angiokeratoma-like pseudolymphoma *J Cutan Pathol 44:878–881, 2017*

Acral arteriovenous hemangioma *Dermatologica 113:129–141, 1956*

Acroangiodermatitis *Indian J Dermatol 60:268–271, 2015*

Angiofibroma

Angiokeratoma
1. Circumscriptum – usually present at birth; may be part of Klippel-Trenaunay-Weber syndrome, mixed vascular malformations, or Cobb's syndrome *AD 117:138–139, 1981*
2. Mibelli – autosomal dominant; autosomal dominant; associated with acrocyanosis and chilblains; develop at age 10–15 on dorsum of fingers, toes, hands, feet *AD 106:726–728, 1972*
3. Acquired – solitary papule; occur after trauma in adult life – red to blue–black; may rapidly enlarge or bleed and simulate melanoma

AD 117:138–139, 1981; AD 95:166–175, 1967; strawberry glans penis due to multiple angiokeratomas *BJD 142:1256–1257, 2000*
4. Angiokeratoma of scrotum (Fordyce) – scrotal bleeding *Emerg Med J 23:e57, 2006*
5. Angiokeratoma corporis diffusum (Fabry's disease) *Dermatol Online J 11:8 Dec 30, 2005AD Syphilol 64:301–308, 1951*

Angiolymphoid hyperplasia with eosinophilia *The Dermatologist, June 2018, pp44–46*

Angioma – proliferating hemangioma, cherry angioma (Campbell de Morgan spots)

Angiomas, eruptive – treatment with cyclosporine in a patient with psoriasis *AD 134:1487–1488, 1998*

Angioma serpiginosum

Angiopericytomatosis (angiomatosis with cryoproteins) – painful red papules and ulcerated plaques acrally; necrotic plaques *JAAD 49:887–896, 2003*

Arteriovenous hemangioma (cirsoid aneurysm or acral arteriovenous tumor) – associated with chronic liver disease *BJD 144:604–609, 2001*

Benign (reactive) angioendotheliomatosis (benign lymphangioendothelioma, acquired progressive lymphangioma, multifocal lymphangioendotheliomatosis) – present at birth; red brown or violaceous nodules or plaques on face, arms, legs with petechiae, ecchymoses, and small areas of necrosis *AD 140:599–606, 2004; JAAD 38:143–175, 1998; AD 114:1512, 1978*

Benign lymphangiomatous papules of the skin *JAAD 52:912–913, 2005*

Cirsoid aneurysm *Indian J Dermatol 60:423, 2015*

Degos' disease (malignant atrophic papulosis) – generalized red papules *Clin Exp Dermatol 32:483–487, 2007; BJD 100:21–36, 1979; Ann DV 79:410–417, 1954*

Diffuse dermal angiomatosis of the breast *Dermatol Online J May 15, 2018*

Disseminated (diffuse) benign neonatal hemangiomatosis *J Ped Child Health 51:646,648, 2015; Ped Derm 21:469–472, 2004; Ped Derm 14:383–386, 1997*

Eosinophilic granulomatosis with polyangiitis – erythema multiforme-like exanthems *Autoimmun Rev 14:341–348, 2015; Dermatopathol 37:214–221, 2015; JAAD 37:199–203, 1997; JAAD 47:209–216, 2002; JID 17:349–359, 1951; Am J Pathol 25:817, 1949*

Eosinophilic vasculitis *AD 130:1159–1166, 1994;* in connective tissue diseases *JAAD 35:173–182, 1996;* cutaneous necrotizing eosinophilic vasculitis *AD 130:1159–66, 1994*

Epithelioid hemangioma *AD 137:365–370, 2001; JAAD 35:851–853, 1996*

Eruptive pseudoangiomatosis – 1.5 mm regular red vascular blanchable papules of face; probably a viral exanthema; sudden appearance of few to numerous bright red papules; transient dilatation of dermal capillaries; lasts 2–18 days in children, 1–3 months in adults *J Eur Acad Dermatol Venereol 18:387–389, 2004; Ped Derm 19:243–245, 2002; BJD 143:435–438, 2000; JAAD 29:857–859, 1993; Pediatr 44:498–502, 1969*

Glomeruloid hemangioma – vascular papule in POEMS syndrome *J Cutan Pathol 32:449–452, 2005; JAAD 49:887–896, 2003; Am J Med 97:543–553, 1994*

Granulomatosis with polyangiitis *NEJM 382:1750–1758, 2020*

Hemolymphangioma – red papules of tongue *JAAD 52:1088–1090, 2005*

Hobnail hemangioma *J Cutan Med Surg 21:164–166, 2017; J Nippon Med Sch 82:151–155, 2015*

Idiopathic systemic capillary leak syndrome – skin-colored or red papules of face, neck, abdomen, upper back, elbows, and hands; purpuric macules of lateral fingers, infiltrative edema of hands with sclerodermoid appearance, livedo reticularis of lower extremities; photodistributed eruption of face, neck, and arms *Dermatology 209:291–295, 2004*

Intravascular papillary endothelial hyperplasia – pseudo-Kaposi's sarcoma – red or purple papules and nodules of the legs *JAAD 10:110–113, 1984*

Kaposiform hemangioendothelioma *JAAD 38:799–802, 1998*

Lymphangiomas – benign lymphangiomatous papules (BLAP) often seen post radiation therapy or post-surgically *JAAD 52:912–913, 2005; Am J Surg Pathol 26:328–337, 2002; Histopathology 35:319–327, 1999; J Cutan Pathol 26:150–154, 1999*

Lymphohemangioma

Microvenular hemangioma *Dermatol Pract Concept 8:7–11, 2018; Am J Dermatopathol 32:837–840, 2010; AD 131:483–488, 1995*

Multifocal lymphangioendotheliomatosis – congenital appearance of hundreds of flat red–brown vascular papules and plaques associated with gastrointestinal bleeding, thrombocytopenia with bone and joint involvement; spontaneous resolution *JAAD 54:S214–217, 2006; J Pediatr Orthop 24:87–91, 2004*

Non-involuting congenital hemangioma – round to ovoid pink to purple papule or plaque with central or peripheral pallor, coarse telangiectasias *Ped Derm 36:466–470, 2019; JAAD 50: 875–882, 2004*

Polyarteritis nodosa, including cutaneous polyarteritis nodosa

Pyogenic granuloma *Stat Pearls April 12, 2020*

Spider telangiectasia

Targetoid hemosiderotic hemangioma – violaceous papule surrounded by pale brown halo *AD 136:1571–1572, 2000; J Cutan Pathol 26:279–286, 1999; JAAD 41:215–224, 1999; JAAD 32:282–284, 1995*

Tufted angioma – deep red papule, plaque, or nodule of back or neck *J Cutan Pathol 40:405–408, 2013; JAAD 52:616–622, 2005; Ped Derm 19:394–401, 2002; JAAD 20:214–225, 1989*

Vascular malformations

Vasculitis, including leukocytoclastic vasculitis, urticarial vasculitis

Verrucous hemangioma *Int J Dermatol 43:745–746, 2004*

Virus-associated hemosiderotic hemangioma

PAPULES, SKIN COLORED

AUTOIMMUNE DISEASES AND DISEASES OF IMMUNE DYSFUNCTION

Acantholytic acanthomas in immunosuppressed patients *JAAD 27:452–453, 1992*

Common variable immunodeficiency (Gottron-like papules) – granulomas presenting as acral skin colored papules *JAAD 73:350–352, 2015*

Bowel-associated dermatosis-arthritis syndrome *JAAD 14:792–796, 1986*

Lupus erythematosus – papulonodular dermal mucinosis of SLE – perifollicular skin colored to red papules *AD 146:789–794, 2010; AD 140:121–126, 2004; Int J Derm 35:72–73, 1996; JAAD 32:199–205, 1995; JAAD 27:312–315, 1992; AD 114:432–435, 1978; BJD 66:429–433, 1954*

Rheumatoid papules *JAAD 28:405–411 1993*

CONGENITAL LESIONS

Bronchogenic cyst with papilloma *JAAD 11:367–371, 1984*

Congenital rhabdomyomatous mesenchymal hamartoma

Wattle (cutaneous cervical tag) *AD 121:22–23, 1985*

DRUG-INDUCED

BCG vaccine – granulomas *JAAD 21:1119–1122, 1989*

EXOGENOUS AGENTS

Bovine collagen implant *J Derm Surg Oncol 9:377–380, 1983*

Foreign body granuloma

INFECTIONS AND INFESTATIONS

Brucellosis *AD 125:380–383, 1989*

Cat scratch disease, inoculation papule *Ped Derm 5:1–9, 1988; multiple leg papules Cutis 49:318–320, 1992*

Cheyletiella dermatitis *JAAD 15:1130–1133, 1986*

Coccidioidomycosis *JAAD 26:79–85, 1992*

Corynebacterium Group JK sepsis *JAAD 16:444–447, 1987*

Cowpox *JAAD 44:1–14, 2001*

Cytomegalovirus infection, generalized *JAAD 24:346–352,1991*

Demodex folliculorum – papulonodular demodicidosis in AIDS *JAAD 20:197–201, 1989*

Fusarium – papulovesicular *Ped Derm 962–965, 1992*

HIV exanthem *AD 125:629–632, 1989*

HTLV-1 *JAAD 24:633–637,1991*

Infectious eccrine hidradenitis *JAAD 22:1119–1120, 1990*

Insect bite granuloma

Leishmaniasis – localized cutaneous leishmaniasis *JAAD 34:257–272, 1996*

Lobomycosis (*Lacazia loboi*) – earliest lesion is a small pustule or papule *JAAD 53:931–951, 2006*

Meningococcemia *Ped Derm 3:414–416, 1986*

Milker's nodule – papilloma *JAAD 44:1–14, 2001*

Molluscum contagiosum

Monkeypox *JAAD 44:1–14, 2001*

Mycobacterium kansasii JAAD 40:359–363, 1999

Mycobacterium tuberculosis – miliary tuberculosis – papulovesicles *JAAD 23:1031–1035, 1990; papulonecrotic tuberculid JAAD 14:815–826, 1986*

Myiasis

Orf – papilloma *JAAD 44:1–14, 2001*

Pinta *AD 135:685–688, 1999*

Schistosomiasis – ectopic cutaneous granuloma – skin colored papule, 2–3 mm *Dermatol Clin 7:291–300, 1989; BJD 114:597–602, 1986*

Smallpox *JAAD 44:1–14, 2001*

Soil nematode, *Pelodera strongyloides Ped Derm 2:33–37, 1985*

Sparganosis – ingestion sparganosis; *Sparganum proliferum* – subcutaneous nodules and pruritic papules *Am J Trop Med Hyg 30:625–637, 1981*

Sporotrichosis, fixed cutaneous *JAAD 12:1007–1012, 1985*

Toxoplasmosis in AIDS *AD 124:1446–1447, 1988*

Verruca vulgaris

INFILTRATIVE DISEASES

Amyloidosis – primary cutaneous amyloidosis – lichenified dermatitis; dome-shaped skin colored 3–4 mm papules; autosomal dominant; mutation in oncostatin M receptor *BJD 161:944–947, 2009*

Benign cephalic histiocytosis

Cutaneous focal mucinosis *AD 93:13–20, 1966*

Cutaneous mucinosis of infancy – grouped skin-colored papules – resembles connective tissue nevus *BJD 144:590–593, 2001; Ped Derm 18:159–161, 2001; AD 116:198–200, 1980*

Disseminated xanthosiderohistiocytosis *JAAD 11:750–755, 1984*

Hereditary progressive mucinous histiocytosis *JAAD 57:1031–1045, 2007; AD 124:1225–1229, 1988*

Langerhans cell histiocytosis including Letterer-Siwe disease and xanthoma disseminatum *JAAD 25:433–436, 1991; JAAD 18:646–654, 1988*

Lichen myxedematosus *JAAD 14:878–888, 1986*

Non-X histiocytosis *JAAD 31:322–326, 1994*

Papular mucinosis *Cutis 55:174–176, 1995; AD 125:985–990, 1989*

Self healing juvenile cutaneous mucinosis

INFLAMMATORY DISEASES

Crohn's disease – anal skin tags, perianal ulcers, fissures, sinus tracts; rectal bleeding, perianal abscess, abdominal pain, perianal pustule, scrotal swelling and erythema, labial erythema and edema, perianal erythema, granulomatous cheilitis *Ped Derm 35:566–574, 2018*

Interstitial granulomatous dermatitis (palisaded neutrophilic granulomatous dermatitis) – annular plaques, skin colored papules, linear erythematous cords, urticarial lesions *JAAD 51:S105–107, 2004; JAAD 47:251–257, 2002*

Neutrophilic eccrine hidradenitis *J Dermatol 22:137–142, 1995; AD 126:527–532, 1990*

Sarcoid – lichen nitidus-like papules *AD 127:1049-1–54, 1991;* Darier-Roussy sarcoid

METABOLIC

Calcinosis cutis – idiopathic; papular or nodular calcinosis cutis secondary to heel sticks *Ped Derm 18:138–140, 2001;* cutaneous calculus *BJD 75:1–11, 1963;* extravasation of calcium carbonate solution; metastatic calcification *JAAD 33:693–706, 1995; Cutis 32:463–465, 1983*

Cutis anserina

Hunter syndrome – skin colored papules *Ped Derm 29:369–370, 2012*

Miliaria profunda – pale papules 1–3 mm *JAAD 35:854–856, 1996*

Papular dermatitis of pregnancy *JAAD 22:690–691, 1990*

Papular xanthoma *JAAD 22:1052–156,1990, AD 121:626–631, 1985*

X-linked infantile hypogammaglobulinemia (caseating granulomas) *JAAD 24:629–633, 1991*

NEOPLASTIC

Apocrine nevi – chest papules

Basal cell carcinoma – palmar *JAAD 33:823–824, 1995;* perianal *Clin Exp Dermatol 17:360–362, 1992*

Basaloid follicular hamartoma – solitary papule or generalized papules with alopecia and myasthenia gravis *BJD 146:1068–1070, 2002*

Clear cell acanthoma *AD 129:1505–1510, 1993*

Collagenoma (connective tissue nevus) – eruptive, familial cutaneous collagenomas *BJD 101:185–195, 1979*

Desmoplastic trichoepithelioma *AD 138:1091–1096, 2002; AD 132:1239–1240, 1996; Cancer 40:2979–2986, 1977*

Eccrine nevus – skin-colored perianal papule *AD 141:515–520, 2005*

Epidermal inclusion cyst

Eruptive hidradenoma *Cutis 46:69–72, 1990*

Eruptive infundibulomas – chest *JAAD 21:361–366, 1989*

Eruptive vellus hair cysts *AD 120:1191–1195, 1984*

Extramammary Paget's disease, perianal – resembles basal cell carcinoma *Clin Exp Dermatol 17:360–362, 1992*

Extramedullary hematopoiesis in acute myelofibrosis *AD 124:329–330, 1988*

Generalized eruptive histiocytoma – hundreds of skin-colored, brown, blue–red papules; resolve with macular pigmentation; face, trunk, proximal extremities *JAAD 31:322–326, 1994; JAAD 20:958–964, 1989; JAAD 17:499–454, 1987; AD 117:216–221, 1981; AD 116:565–567, 1980; AD 96:11–17, 1967*

Giant folliculosebaceous cystic hamartoma – skin colored exophytic papules *AD 141:1035–1040, 2005; Am J Dermatopathol 13:213–220, 1991*

Infantile choriocarcinoma *JAAD 14:918–927, 1986*

Juvenile xanthogranuloma *JAAD 14:405–411, 1986*

Kaposi's sarcoma in AIDS *JAAD 22:1237–1250, 1990*

Leukemia cutis – acute myelomonocytic leukemia *AD 126:653–656, 1990*

Lymphoma – generalized papular xanthomatosis in cutaneous T-cell lymphoma *JAAD 26:828–832, 1992;* HTLV-1 leukemia/lymphoma – multiple papules, cobblestoned skin *JAMA Derm 151:443–444, 2015*

Lymphomatoid granulomatosis *AD 127:1693–8, 1991*

Melanocytic nevus

Meningioma

Metastases – metastatic lung carcinoma – papule within a scar *JAAD 36:117–118, 1997*

Multiple cutaneous reticulohistiocytomas, including self-healing reticulohistiocytosis *JAAD 25:948–951, 1992*

Neurilemmomas

Neuroma, traumatic

Nevus elasticus

Osteoma cutis *JAAD 24:878–881, 1991*

Poroma – papilloma, especially of scalp *JAAD 44:48–52, 2001*

Progressive osseous heteroplasia – infants *JAAD 33:693–706, 1995*

Pilomatrixoma – multiple papules *Ped Derm 23:157–162, 2006*
    Multiple pilomatrixomas are seen in: *Ped Derm 37:9–17, 2020*
        Myotonic dystrophy

Familial adenomatous polyposis syndromes, including
Gardner's syndrome
Turner's syndrome
Rubinstein-Taybi syndrome

Pinkus tumor – skin colored, pink, or brown; sessile or pedunculated *Cutis 54:85–92, 1994*

Sclerotic fibromas *JAAD 20:266–271, 1989*

Sinus histiocytosis with massive lymphadenopathy *JAAD 13:383–404, 1985*

Skin tag lesions in epidermal nevi *JAAD 20:476–488, 1989*

Smooth muscle hamartoma – skin colored papules *Ped Derm 18:17–20, 2001*

Spitz nevus

Squamous cell carcinoma – vulvar squamous cell carcinoma – papular and polypoid lesions; verrucous white cobblestoned plaque *JAAD 66:867–880, 2012*

Steatocystoma multiplex

Superficial pigmented trichoblastoma arising in a nevus sebaceous *JAAD 42:263–268, 2000*

Syringomas, including eruptive syringoma *AD 125:1119–1120, 1989*

Syringocystadenoma papilliferum

Trichilemmal carcinoma *Dermatol Surg 28:284–286, 2002*

Trichoepithelioma, single or multiple

Urticaria pigmentosa

Waldenstrom's macroglobulinemia – skin colored translucent papule – IgM storage lesion *BJD 135:287–291, 1996*

PARANEOPLASTIC DISORDERS

Melanocytic BAP1-mutated atypical intradermal tumors (MBAIT) – pink-skin colored papules; sign of renal cell carcinoma and melanoma *JAMA Derm 153:999–1000, 2017*

PHOTODERMATOSES

Papular phytophotodermatitis – weed wacker dermatitis *AD 127:1419–1420, 1991*

PRIMARY CUTANEOUS DISEASES

Atrichia with papular lesions *AD 122:565–567, 1986*

Epidermolysis bullosa dystrophica et albopapuloidea (Pasini) *JAAD 16:891–893, 1987*

Fox-Fordyce disease

Frictional lichenoid dermatitis of childhood *AD 130:105–110, 1994*

Generalized perforating granuloma annulare *JAAD 27:319–322, 1992*

Hyperkeratosis lenticularis perstans (Flegel's disease) *JAAD 27:812–816, 1992*

Infantile perineal protrusion – differential diagnosis includes hemorrhoids, rectal prolapse, skin tags, sexual abuse, sentinel tag of anal fissure, inflammatory bowel disease, perineal midline malformation, hemangioma *JAAD 54:1046–1049, 2006*

Kikuchi's disease – histiocytic necrotizing lymphadenitis *JAAD 30:504–506, 1994*

Lichen nitidus – generalized lichen nitidus *AD 146:1419–1424, 2010; Ped Derm 26:109–111, 2009*

Papular elastorrhexis *Dermatology 205:198–200, 2002; Clin Exp Dermatol 27:454–457, 2002; JAAD 19:409–414, 1988; AD 123:433–434, 1987*

Perianal pyramidal protrusion – manifestation of lichen sclerosus et atrophicus *AD 134:1118–1120, 1998*

Pityriasis rosea, papular *Cutis 70:51–55, 2002*

Waxy keratoses of childhood (kerinokeratosis papulosa) – multiple shiny papules over entire skin surface *Ped Derm 18:415–416, 2001; JAAD 50:S84–85, 2004; Clin Exp Dermatol 19:173–176, 1994*

White fibrous papulosis of the neck *JAAD 20:1073–1077, 1989*

SYNDROMES

Atrichia congenita with papular lesions – autosomal recessive; infantile hair loss follicular papules; follicular cysts and milia-like lesions; no photophobia *Ped Derm 29:519–520, 2012; AD 139:1591–1596, 2003; JAAD 47:519–523, 2002; Ped Derm 19:155–158, 2002; Eur J Dermatol 11:375–377, 2001; Dermatology 185:284–288, 1992; Dermatologica 108:114–121, 1954;* atrichia with keratin cysts – face, neck, scalp then trunk and extremities *Ann DV 121:802–804, 1994*

Basaloid follicular hamartoma syndrome – multiple skin-colored, red, and hyperpigmented papules of the face, neck chest, back, proximal extremities, and eyelids; syndrome includes milia-like cysts, comedones, sparse scalp hair, palmar pits, and parallel bands of papules of the neck (zebra stripes) *JAAD 43:189–206, 2000*

Beare-Stevenson syndrome – skin tags, cutis gyrata (furrowed skin), corrugated forehead, acanthosis nigricans, macular hyperpigmentation of antecubital and popliteal fossae, hypertelorism, swollen lips, swollen fingers, prominent eyes, ear anomalies, and umbilical herniation *Ped Derm 20:358–360, 2003*

Birt-Hogg-Dube – collagenomas *JAAD 56:877–880, 2007; AD 135:1195–1202, 1999*

Blau syndrome (familial juvenile systemic granulomatosis) – translucent skin-colored papules of trunk and extremities with uveitis, synovitis, arthritis *Clin Exp Dermatol 21:445–448, 1996*

Brown-Crounse syndrome – 1–2 mm papules, plaques, and nodules, diffuse hypotrichosis resembling alopecia areata, basaloid follicular hamartomas, trichoepitheliomas, myasthenia gravis *AD 99:478–493, 1969*

Buschke-Ollendorf syndrome (dermatofibrosis lenticularis disseminata) – disseminated connective tissue nevi *Int J Dermatol 47:1159–1161, 2008; Eur J Dermtol 11:576–579, 2001*

Carney complex (NAME/LAMB) – myxomas

Cowden's syndrome – collagenomas (sclerotic fibromas) *JAAD 56:877–880, 2007; J Cutan Pathol 19:346–351, 1992*

Epidermodysplasia verruciformis – hypopigmented papules *Ped Derm 26:306–310, 2009*

Familial hemophagocytic lymphohistiocytosis – macules and papules with fever

Gardner's syndrome – multiple pilomatrixomas *Ped Derm 23:157–162, 2006; Ped Derm 12:331–335, 1995*

Giant lymph node hyperplasia (Castleman's syndrome) *JAAD 26:105–109, 1992*

Granulomatous synovitis, uveitis, and cranial neuropathies – JABS syndrome

Hereditary progressive mucinous histiocytosis *AD 124:1225–1229, 1988*

Hunter's syndrome (mucopolysaccharidosis IIb) – X-linked recessive; MPS type II; iduronate-2 sulfatase deficiency; lysosomal accumulation of heparin sulfate and dermatan sulfate; linear and reticulated 2–10 mm skin colored papules over and between scapulae, chest, neck, arms; also posterior axillary lines, upper arms, forearms, chest, outer thighs; rough thickened skin, coarse scalp hair, and hirsutism; short stature, full lips, coarse facies with frontal bossing, hypertelorism, and thick tongue (macroglossia); dysostosis multiplex; hunched shoulders and characteristic posturing; widely spaced teeth, dolichocephaly, deafness, retinal degeneration, inguinal and umbilical hernias hepatosplenomegaly; upper and lower respiratory infections due to laryngeal or tracheal stenosis; mental retardation; deafness; retinal degeneration and corneal clouding; umbilical and inguinal hernias; valvular and ischemic heart disease with thickened heart valves lead to congestive heart failure; clear corneas (unlike Hurler's syndrome), progressive neurodegeneration, communicating hydrocephalus; adenotonsillar hypertrophy, otitis media, obstructive sleep apnea, diarrhea *Ped Derm 21:679–681, 2004; Clin Exp Dermatol 24:179–182, 1999; Ped Derm 7:150–152, 1990*

Hurler-Scheie syndrome – deficient alpha-L-iduronidase *JAAD 35:868–870, 1996*

Infantile systemic hyalinosis – pearly papules *Ped Derm 11:52–60, 1994; Ped Derm 9:255–258, 1992*

Juvenile hyaline fibromatosis (systemic hyalinosis) – translucent papules or nodules of scalp, face, neck, trunk, gingival hypertrophy, flexion contractures of large and small joints; small papules of trunk, chin, ears, around nose *Ped Derm 18:400–402, 2001; JAAD 16:881–883, 1987*

MEN2A – multiple sclerotic fibromas presenting as elongated papules of trunk and heel nodules *JAMA Derm 153:1298–1301, 2017*

Mucolipidoses (pseudo-Hurler polydystrophy) – connective tissue nevus *BJD 130:528–533, 1994*

Multicentric reticulohistiocytosis

Multiple endocrine neoplasia syndrome (MEN I) – multiple dome shaped papules; collagenomas *JAAD 56:877–880, 2007; AD 133:853–857, 1997*

Multiple endocrine neoplasia syndrome (MEN II) – conjunctival papules *AD 139:1647–1652, 2003*

Myotonic dystrophy (Steinert) – multiple pilomatrixomas *Ped Derm 23:157–162, 2006; Ped Derm 12:331–335, 1995*

Niemann-Pick disease – autosomal recessive; sphingomyelinase deficiency; papular lesions *BJD 131:895–897, 1994*

Phakomatosis pigmentokeratotica – coexistence of an organoid nevus and a popular speckled lentiginous nevus *Skin and Allergy News, page 34, Sept 2000*

POEMS syndrome (Takatsuki syndrome, Crowe-Fukase syndrome) – generalized histiocytomas; osteosclerotic bone lesions, peripheral polyneuropathy, hypothyroidism, and hypogonadism *JAAD 21:1061–1068, 1989, Cutis 61:329–334, 1998*

Progressive nodular histiocytosis *AD 114:1505–1508, 1978*

Proteus syndrome – lipomas, connective tissue nevi, lymphatic malformations *AD 140:947–953, 2004; AD 125:1109–1114, 1989*

Raspberry-like papillomas on lips, perineum, fingers, toes, buccal mucosa and esophagus *Cutis 53:309–312, 1994*

Reflex sympathetic dystrophy *AD 127:1541–1544, 1991*

Rombo syndrome – papules and cysts of the face and trunk, basal cell carcinomas, vermiculate atrophoderma, milia, hypotrichosis, trichoepitheliomas, peripheral vasodilatation with cyanosis *JAAD 39:853–857, 1998; Acta DV 61:497–503, 1981*

Rubenstein-Taybi syndrome – multiple pilomatrixomas *Ped Derm 23:157–162, 2006*

Skull dysostosis – multiple pilomatrixomas *Ped Derm 23:157–162, 2006*

Tuberous sclerosis – collagenomas *JAAD 56:877–880, 2007; AD 135:1195–1202, 1999*

Turner's syndrome – multiple pilomatrixomas *Ped Derm 23:157–162, 2006*

TRAUMA

Dermabrasion with osteoma cutis

Radiation therapy – keratotic miliaria following radiotherapy *AD 124:855–856, 1988*

Scar

TOXINS

Acute dioxin exposure *JAAD 19:812–819, 1989*

Toxic oil syndrome – cutaneous mucinosis *JAAD 16:139–140, 1987*

VASCULAR

Polyangiitis with granulomatosis (necrotic or non-necrotic) *AD 130:861–867, 1994; JAAD 28:710–718, 1993*

Takayasu's arteritis – chest papules *AD 123:796–800, 1987*

Vascular malformation with underlying disappearing bone (Gorham-Stout disease) – skin colored papulovesicles along a vein of the thigh; dilated veins of foot *JAMA 289:1479–1480, 2003*

PAPULOSQUAMOUS ERUPTIONS

AUTOIMMUNE DISEASES AND DISEASES OF IMMUNE DYSFUNCTION

Allergic contact dermatitis

Amicrobial pustulosis associated with autoimmune disease treated with zinc *BJD 143:1306–1310, 2000*

Graft vs. host disease, chronic *Ped Derm 35:246–247, 2018; JAAD 66:515–532, 2012; JAAD 38:369–392, 1998;* annular scaly papules of epithelioid granulomas *BJD 149:898–899, 2003*

Lupus erythematosus – acute systemic *BJD 135:355–362, 1996;* annular, discoid, neonatal, psoriasiform; subacute cutaneous lupus erythematosus *AD 141:911–912, 2005; Med Clin North Am 73:1073–1090, 1989; JAAD 19:1957–1062, 1988*

DRUG-INDUCED DISEASES

Anti-seizure medications – cutaneous T cell lymphoma-like drug rash to phenytoin or carbamazepine *JAAD 24:216–220, 1991; AD 121:1181–1182, 1985*

Beta blocker-induced psoriasiform eruption *Int J Dermatol 27:619–627, 1988*

Drug eruptions

Infliximab – psoriasis *J Drugs Dermatol 12:939–943, 2013*

Lupus erythematosus – subacute cutaneous LE – annular scaly lesions in a photodistribution including the legs *AD 148:190–193, 2012;* – terbinafine, thiazides, piroxicam, D-penicillamine, sulfonylureas, procainamide, oxyprenolol, chrysotherapy, griseofulvin, naproxen, spironolactone, diltiazem, cinnarizine, captopril, cilazapril, verapamil, nifedipine, interferon beta, ranitidine *JAAD 44:925–931, 2001; Ann Int Med 103:49–51, 1985;* tiotropium bromide *AD 141:911–912, 2005*

Mogamulizumab granulomatous drug eruption – red macules and patches, scaly red plaques *JAMA Derm 155:968–971, 2019*

EXOGENOUS AGENTS

Mudi-chood – due to oils applied to hair; papulosquamous eruption of nape of neck and upper back; begin as follicular pustules then brown-black papules with keratinous rim *Int J Dermatol 31:396–397, 1992*

INFECTIONS AND INFESTATIONS

Bejel – secondary

Candidiasis

Covid-19 infection – digitate papulosquamous eruption *JAMA Derm 156:819–820, 2020*

Emmonsia pasteuriana – dimorphic fungus; disseminated infection in South Africa; lichenoid diffuse papulosquamous eruption; crusted verrucous facial nodules and plaques *NEJM 369:1416–1424, 2013*

Epidermodysplasia verruciformis

Erythrasma – red to brown irregularly shaped and sharply margin-ated scaly patches of groin, axillae, intergluteal, submammary flexures, toe webs *Rev Infect Dis 4:1220–1235, 1982*

Hepatitis C infection – necrolytic acral erythema; red to hyperpig-mented psoriasiform plaques with variable scale or erosions *JAAD 53:247–251, 2005; Int J Derm 35:252–256, 1996*

Histoplasmosis, disseminated

HIV-1 infection *JAAD 28:167–173, 1993*

Human polyoma virus 6 and 7 – pruritic and dyskeratotic dermato-ses – generalized hyperpigmented scaly dermatitis *JAAD 76:932–940, 2017*

Leishmaniasis – facial dermatitis resembling secondary syphilis *JAAD 60:897–925, 2009*

Lepromatous leprosy – brown hyperkeratotic plaques *AD 125:1569–1574, 1989;* pityriasis rosea-like *JAAD 15:204–208, 1986;* border-line tuberculoid leprosy

Mycoplasma avium complex – scaling papules *BJD 101:71074, 1979*

Mycobacteria chelonae – plaques with scale *JAAD 62:501–506, 2010*

Parvovirus B19 – subacute cutaneous lupus-like annular scaling erythematous rash *Hum Pathol 31:488–497, 2000*

Pinta – generalized cutaneous phase – erythematosquamous eruption; tertiary *Cutis 51:425–430, 1993*

Prototheca wickerhamii Am J Clin Path 77:485–493, 1982

Rubella congenital

Scabies – crusted – scaly abdomen and hand *Cutis 94:86–88,95, 2014*

Syphilis – congenital; secondary – morbilliform or papular (copper red) *JAAD 72:926–928, 2015; J Clin Inf Dis 21:1361–1371, 1995;* syphilis brephotrophica (non-sexually transmitted) *JAAD 38:638–639, 1998*

Tinea corporis – *Trichophyton rubrum, T. megninii, Epidermophyton floccosum;* Trichophyton verrucosum – extensive annular lesions of trunk and neck *AD 94:35–37, 1966*

Tinea versicolor *Semin Dermatol 4:173–184, 1985*

Toxoplasmosis – pityriasis lichenoides-like eruption *AD 100:196–199, 1969*

Viral exanthem

Yaws – secondary; superficial scaly patches *NEJM 372:693–695, 2015*

INFILTRATIVE DISEASES

Erdheim-Chester disease, pediatric – facial plaques, psoriasiform plaques, papulosquamous lesions, annular lesions, central atrophic scarring; osteolysis and osteosclerosis *BJD 178:261–264, 2018*

Langerhans cell histiocytosis

INFLAMMATORY DISEASES

Chronic erythema multiforme – personal observation

Sarcoidosis

METABOLIC DISEASES

Biotinidase deficiency

Hereditary LDH M-subunit deficiency *AD 122:1420–1424, 1986*

Kwashiorkor *AD 140:521–524, 2004*

Necrolytic acral erythema – cutaneous marker for hepatitis C infection; hyperkeratotic erythematous to violaceous scaly plaques; psoriasiform hyperpigmented, hyperkeratotic plaques of acral palmar, plantar, dorsal surfaces of hands and feet; darker, more velvety and verrucous than psoriasis *J Drugs in Dermatol 11:1370–1371, 2012; Int J Dermatol 49:24–29, 2010; ; JAAD 53:247–251, 2005; Int J Derm 44:916–921, 2005; JAAD 50:s121–124, 2004; AD 136:755–757, 2000; Int J Derm 35:252–256, 1996*

Necrolytic migratory erythema – recurrent seborrheic, serpiginous, annular papulosquamous eruptions; glucagonoma, chronic liver disease, inflammatory bowel disease, heroin abuse, pancreatitis, malabsorption syndromes

NEOPLASTIC DISEASES

Inflamed actinic keratoses due to systemic fluorouracil *AD 130:1193, 1994*

Kaposi's sarcoma *JAAD 28:371–395, 1993*

Lymphoma – HTLV-1 (adult T-cell lymphoma/leukemia) *JAAD 46:S137–141, 2002;* CTCL; pityriasis lichenoides chronica-like lesions in CTCL *BJD 142:347–352, 2000;* hypopigmented CTCL *Ped Derm 23:493–496, 2006*

Lymphomatoid papulosis – personal observation

PARANEOPLASTIC DISEASES

Bazex syndrome *JAAD 54:745–762, 2006; Cutis 49:265–268, 1992*

Necrolytic migratory erythema

Paraneoplastic pemphigus *JAAD 27:547–553, 1992;* lichenoid dermatitis *AD 136:652–656, 2000*

Thymoma-associated multiorgan autoimmunity GVH-like disease – generalized papulosquamous exanthem *JAAD 57:683–689, 2007; Eur J Gastroenterol 15:565–569, 2003; Clin Exp Dermatol 22:287–290, 1997*

PRIMARY CUTANEOUS DISEASES

Acanthosis nigricans *JAAD 21:461–469, 1989*

Acquired epidermodysplasia verruciformis – personal observation

Asteatotic dermatitis

Atopic dermatitis

Axillary granular parakeratosis *JAAD 24:541–544, 1991*

Blaschkitis – personal observation

CARD 14-associated papulosquamous eruption – features of psoriasis, pityriasis rubral pilaris, atopic dermatitis *JAAD 79:487–494, 2018*

Confluent and reticulated papillomatosis, including non-pigmenting variant *Ped Derm 23:497–499, 2006*

Digitate dermatosis

Erythema annulare centrifugum

Erythrokeratoderma variabilis *AD 101:68–73, 1970*

Ichthyosis

Keratosis follicularis squamosa of Dohi – scaly 3–10 mm patches symmetrical on trunk and thighs with central brown follicular plugs; margins slightly detached *BJD 150:603–605, 2004; Jpn J Dermatol 3:513–514, 1903;* associated with obesity *JAAD 81:1037–1057, 2019*

Keratosis lichenoides chronica – seborrheic dermatitis-like facial eruption *JAAD 49:511–513, 2003; JAAD 38:306–309, 1998; JAAD 28:870–873, 1993*

Lichen nitidus

Lichen planus – annular lichen planus *Cutis 100:199, 2017;*lichen planus pigmentosus – personal observation

Malignant disseminated porokeratosis *AD 123:1521–1526, 1987*

Necrolytic acral erythema – serpiginous, verrucous plaques of dorsal aspects of hands, legs; associated with hepatitis C infection *JAAD 50:S121–124, 2004; Int J Derm 35:252–256, 1996*

Papuloerythroderma of Ofuji

Parapsoriasis – digitate dermatosis, poikiloderma vasculare atrophicans; parapsoriasis en plaque; small plaque parapsoriasis *JAAD 59:474–482, 2008; Ann Dermatol Syphiligr (Paris)3:313–315, 1902*

Pityriasis lichenoides chronica *Ped Derm 32:579–592, 2015; The Dermatologist p.47–49, July, 2014; Dermatol Pract Concept 3:7–10, 2013; Am J Surg Pathol 36:1021–1029, 2012; JAAD 56:205–210, 2007; JAAD 55:557–572, 2006; BJD 129:353–354, 1993; AD 119:378–380, 1983; Ann Dermatol Syphiligr (Paris) 3433–468, 1902; AD Syphilol 50:359–374, 1899*

Pityriasis lichenoides et varioliformis acuta – personal observation; *The Clinical Management of Itching; Parthenon; p. 137, 2000*

Pityriasis rosea *JAAD 15:159–167, 1986*

Pityriasis rubra pilaris *JAAD 20:801–807, 1989*

Progressive symmetric erythrokeratoderma *Dermatologica 164:133–141, 1982*

Psoriasis – clearance of psoriasis after neurologic injury *BJD 172:988–993, 2015*

Seborrheic dermatitis, including AIDS-associated seborrheic dermatitis *BJD 111:603–607, 1984*

Vitiligo – serpiginous papulosquamous variant of inflammatory vitiligo *Dermatology 200:270–274, 2000*

SYNDROMES

Activated STING in Vascular and Pulmonary syndrome – autoinflammatory disease; butterfly telangiectatic facies; acral violaceous psoriasiform, papulosquamous and atrophic vasculitis of hands; nodules of face, nose, and ears; fingertip ulcers with necrosis; nail dystrophy; nasal septal perforation; interstitial lung disease with fibrosis; polyarthritis; myositis *NEJM 371:507–518, 2014*

Ataxia telangiectasia – autosomal recessive; telangiectasias of face, ocular telangiectasia, extensor surfaces of arms and bulbar conjunctiva; café au lait macules, hypopigmented macules, melanocytic nevi, facial papulosquamous rash, hypertrichosis, bird-like facies; immunodeficiency, increased risk of leukemia, lymphoma; cerebellar ataxia with eye movement signs, mental retardation, and other neurologic defects; cafe au lait macules *JAAD 68:932–936, 2013; Ann Int Med 99:367–379, 1983*

Congenital erosive and vesicular dermatosis – erosions at birth, blisters at birth, reticulated supple scarring, alopecia, hypohidrosis, anonychia, photosensitivity, cobblestoned scarring *AD 121:361–367, 1985*

Conradi-Hunermann-Happle syndrome – transient scaly plaques of limbs, trunk, and scalp; X-linked dominant (mosaic for emopamil-binding protein); X-linked recessive – male EBP disorder with neurologic defects *BJD 166:1309–1313, 2012*

Epidermodysplasia verruciformis – pityriasis rosea-like appearance *BJD 145:669–670, 2001;* multiple lichenoid papules *AD 138:649–654, 2002*

Glucagonoma syndrome

Netherton's syndrome – serpiginous papulosquamous ichthyosiform eruption *JAMA Derm 156:350–351, 2020; JAMA Derm 152:435–442, 2016*

Papillon-Lefevre syndrome – psoriasiform plaques of elbows *Ped Derm 6:222–225, 1989*

Reactive arthritis syndrome

VASCULAR DISORDERS

Granulomatosis with polyangiitis presenting as reactive arthritis – personal observation

PARANEOPLASTIC DERMATOSES

JAAD 54:745–762, 2006; Am J Med 99:662–671, 1995; JAAD 28:147–64, 1993

Acanthosis nigricans, malignant *Case Rep Dermatol 9:30–37, 2017; JAAD 25:361–365, 1991; Cancer 15:364–382, 1962* (Helen Ollendorff Curth);lips and/or palatal cobblestoning *AD 130:649–654, 1994*

Paraneoplastic acral vascular syndrome – acral cyanosis and gangrene *JAAD 70:393–395, 2014; JAAD 60:1–20, 2009; JAAD 47:47–52, 2002; AD 138:1296–1298, 2002; Br Med J iii:208–212, 1967;* Robboy's acral cyanosis – associated with gastric adenocarcinoma *Rev Esp Enferm Apar Dig 74:562–564, 1988;* myeloproliferative diseases – chronic myelogenous leukemia with leukostasis; *AD 123:921–924, 1987*

Acrochordons in Birt-Hogg-Dube syndrome *JAAD 49:698–705, 2003*

Adenosine deaminase severe combined immunodeficiency – increased risk of dermatofibrosarcoma protuberans *JAAD 74:437–451, 2016*

Alopecia – brain tumors of mid-brain and brainstem *Arch Dermatol Syphilol 176:196–199, 1937*

Amyloidosis, primary systemic

Angioedema – chronic lymphocytic leukemia; acute lymphoblastic leukemia with eosinophilia *Ped Derm 20:502–505, 2003;* myeloma, splenic marginal lymphoma *Am J Case Rep 20:1476–1481, 2019*

Angiomas, eruptive

Annular erythema, paraneoplastic – perigenital dermatitis

Anti-epiligrin cicatricial pemphigoid (anti-laminin 332) *Dermatol Pract Concept 9:119–125, 2019*

Anti-phospholipid antibody syndrome *Lupus 16:59–64, 2007; Semin Arthritis Rheum 35:322–332, 2006*

Arsenic – dyschromatosis with diffuse pigmentation, especially of trunk; with depigmentation yielding rain-drop appearance; lung, bladder cancer *Dermatol Clin 29:45–51, 2011*

Ataxia telangiectasia – pancreatic cancer *NEJM 371:1039–1049, 2014; J Ped Hemaol Oncol 40:483–486, 2018*

BAP1 tumor syndrome- melanoma, uveal melanoma, internal malignancy

Bazex syndrome (acrokeratosis paraneoplastica) – psoriasiform dermatitis of hands, feet, nose, ears *Ear Nose Throat J 96:413–414, 2017; JAAD 40:822–825, 1999; J Laryg Otol 110:899–900, 1996; Bull Soc Fr Dermatol Syphilol 72:182, 1965*

Beckwith-Wiedemann syndrome – pancreatoblastoma, adrenal cortical carcinoma, neuroblastoma, rhabdomyoblastoma, Wilms' tumor, hepatoblastoma *JAAD 74:231–244, 2016*

Birt-Hogg-Dube syndrome *Cancer Sci 111:15–22, 2020*

Bloom's syndrome – multiple internal malignancies *JAAD 75:855–870, 2016*

Bowens disease *Int J Dermatol 28:531–533, 1989*

Bullous pemphigoid

Bullous pyoderma gangrenosum *Leuk Lymphoma 47:147–150, 2008*

Breast cancer, increased risk *JAAD 80:1467–1481, 2019*
    Ataxia telangiectasia
    Cowden's syndrome
    Bloom's syndrome
    Down's syndrome
    Fanconi's anemia
    McCune-Albright syndrome
    Muir-Torre syndrome
    Nevoid basal cell carcinoma syndrome
    Peutz-Jegher's syndrome
    Poland syndrome
    Scalp-ear-nipple syndrome

Cachectic state associated with neoplasms

Carney complex – prolactinoma, thyroid neoplasms, Sertoli cell tumors, ovarian cysts and tumors *Ped Derm 36:160–162, 2019; NEJM 370:2229–2236, 2014*

Carcinoid syndrome – blue cyanotic nose and face *Gyn Oncol 61:259–265, 1996; Acta DV (Stockh) 41:264–276, 1961*; appendix, ileum, ovary, bronchus

Chediak-Higashi syndrome *Hematol Onc Stem Ther 9:71–75, 2016; Dermatol Clin 12:93–97, 1994*

CLOVES (congenital lipomatosis overgrowth, vascular malformations, epidermal nevi, skeletal anomalies – association with Wilms' tumor *JAAD 77:874–878, 2017*

Clubbing – non-small cell lung cancer *Postgrad Med 130:278–279, 2018; NEJM 375:1171, 2016*

CMMR-D syndrome – autosomal dominant; biallelic mutations in mismatch repair gene; café au lait macules and lentigines; early onset cancers; acute myelogenous leukemia, acute lymphoblastic leukemia, brain tumors, colorectal and endometrial cancer *NEJM 370:2229–2236, 2014*

Cowden's syndrome *Dermatol Online J Aug 15, 2017; J Natl Cancer Institute 105:1607–1616, 2013*

Cronkhite – Canada syndrome *World J Gastroenterol 20:7518–7522, 2014*

Cryoglubulinema

Cushing's syndrome – ectopic ACTH/carcinoid tumor/ovarian carcinoma *J Int Soc Gyn Endocrinol 30:192–196, 2014; Clin Endocrinol 45:775–778, 1996*

Cutis laxa – acquired cutis laxa *AD 147:323–328, 2011; JAAD 60:1052–1057, 2009; Cutis 69:114–118, 2002*

Cutis verticis gyrata *AD 125:434–435, 1989*

Cytophagic histiocytic panniculitis – associated with malignant histiocytic syndromes *AD 121:910–913, 1985*

Deep venous thrombosis *J Emerg Med 57:825–835, 2019*

Dermatitis – adult-onset recalcitrant eczema – marker of non-cutaneous lymphoma or leukemia *JAAD 43:207–210, 2000*

Dermatitis herpetiformis *Gastroenterol 123:1428–1435, 2002; Gut 38:528–530, 1996; BJD 133S:363–367, 1996; BMJ 308:13–15, 1994*

Dermatomyositis – erythroderma *JAAD 80:1364–1370, 2019; Clin Dermatol 36:450–458, 2018; CMAJ 190:E1453, 2018*

Digital ischemia *Br Med J iii:208–212, 1967*

Dyskeratosis congenita

Ectopic adrenocorticotropic hormone syndrome – adenocarcinoma of the lung *Arch Int Med 142:1387–1389, 1982;* soft palate hyperpigmentation *Oral Surg 41:726–733, 1976*

Eosinophilic dermatosis of myeloproliferative disease – face, scalp; scaly red nodules; trunk – red nodules; extremities – red nodules and hemorrhagic papules *JAAD 81:246–249, 2019; AD 137:1378–1380, 2001*

Epidermal nevus syndrome – ectodermal and mesodermal tumors

Epidermodysplasia verruciformis – *RHOH* deficient patients; bronchopulmonary disease and Burkitt's lymphoma *JAAD 76:1161–1175, 2017; CORO1A*-deficiency – molluscum contagiosum, bronchiectasis and lymphoma *JAAD 76:1161–1175, 2017*

Epidermolysis bullosa acquisita – with mantle cell lymphoma *Cutis 101:E13–15, 2018*

Erythema annulare centrifugum (PEACE) *Stat Pearls Jan 2020; 29486570*

Erythema elevatum diutinum – associated with hairy cell leukemia, chronic lymphocytic leukemia

Erythema gyratum repens – seen with malignancy, benign breast hypertrophy, CREST syndrome, ichthyosis, palmoplantar hyperkeratosis *JAMA Derm 156:912–2020; NEJM 380:e3, 2019; Int J Dermatol 58:408–415, 2019; JAAD 26:757–762, 1992; Am J Med Sci 2001;321 (5):302–305.doi.10.1097/00000441-200105000-00002; JAAD 26:757–762, 1992; J Eur Acad DV 28:112–115, 2012;* carcinoma of the breast *Arch Derm Syphilol 1952;66 (4);494–505. doi:10:1001/arch derm 1952.01530290070010*

Erythema multiforme

Erythema nodosum associated with acute myelogenous leukemia, chronic myelogenous leukemia, chronic myelomonocytic leukemia *Blood Reviews 31:370–388, 2017*

Erythrodermas – esophageal carcinoma *JAAD 13:311, 1985;* Fallopian tube carcinoma *Obstet Gynecol 71:1045–1047, 1988;* gastric carcinoma *Am J Gastroenterol 79:921–923, 1984;*

lymphoma – Hodgkin's disease *JAAD 49:772–773, 2003;*

others; lung cancer *An Bras Dermatol 95:67–70, 2020*

Erythromelalgia *Leuk Lymphoma 58:715–717, 2017; Arch Int Med 149:105–109, 1989*

Exaggerated arthropod reactions associated with chronic lymphocytic leukemia, diffuse large cell B-cell lymphoma *Am J Dermatopathol 41:303–308, 2019*

Extramammary Paget's disease *Dermatol Online J April 15, 2019*

Familial atypical multiple mole syndrome – melanoma; pancreatic cancer; mutation in *CDKN2A NEJM 371:1039–1049, 2014; Methods Mol Biol 1102:381–393, 2014; Genes Dev 28:1–7, 2014; Cancer J 18:485–491, 2012*

Familial melanoma

Fanconi's anemia *NEJM 370:2229–2236, 2014*

Florid cutaneous papillomatosis – related to acanthosis nigricans and sign of Leser-Trelat; sudden onset hyperkeratotic papules indistinguishable from viral warts; recurrent gastric adenocarcinoma *Dermatol Online J Aug 15, 2018*

Follicular mucinosis with hematologic malignancies *JAAD 80:1704–1711, 2019*

Folliculitis – sterile suppurative folliculitis associated with acute myelogenous leukemia *BJD 146:904–907, 2002*

Gardner's syndrome

GATA2 deficiency – autosomal dominant; human papilloma virus, herpes simplex, varicella-zoster, non-tuberculous mycobacterial, *Clostridium dificile* infections, myeloid dysplasia, acute myelogenous leukemia; panniculitis, congenital lymphedema, clubbing, embolic stroke, bony infarcts, deep venous thrombosis; melanoma and non-melanoma skin cancers; sensorineural deafness, thyroid disease; normal immunoglobulins with cytopenias of monocytes, B cells, BK cells, CD4+ cells, neutrophils *Blood 123:809–821, 2014*

Generalized eruptive histiocytosis associated with acute myelogenous leukemia *JAAD 49:S233–236, 2003*

Glucagonoma syndrome (necrolytic migratory erythema) *Am J Dermatopathol 41:e29–32, 2019; JAAD 24:473–477, 1991*

Granuloma annulare *JAAD 79:913–920, 2018; Clin Exp Dermatol 43:219–221, 2018*

Granulomas – annular scaly red and reticulated plaques due to cutaneous granulomas associated with systemic lymphoma *JAAD 51:600–605, 2004;* reactive granulomatous dermatitis with myelodysplastic syndrome *Blood Reviews 31:370–388, 2017*

Griscelli's syndrome

Hemochromatosis – hepatocellular carcinoma *JAMA 312:743–744, 2014*

Herpes zoster

Howel-Evans syndrome (tylosis) – esophageal cancer *Dermatol Online J June 15, 2018; Semin Oncol 43:341–346, 2016*

Hypercoagulable state

Hyperhidrosis, generalized

Hypertrichosis lanuginosa acquisita (malignant down) – in mild forms, confined to face – starts on nose and eyelids; lung, colon carcinomas most common; also breast, gall bladder, uterus, urinary bladder if accompanied by acanthosis nigricans, the malignancy is always an adenocarcinoma *BJD 157:1087–1092, 2007; Can Med Assoc 118:1090–1096, 1978*

Hypertrophic osteoarthropathy *Case Rep Med 2016:4259190; Best Pract Res Clin Rheumatol April 11, 2020; 101507*

Ichthyosis, acquired – multiple myeloma *AD Syphilol 72:506–522, 1955;* carcinoma of breast, lung, cervix *AD 111:1446–1447, 1975;* Kaposi's sarcoma *Dermatologica 147:348–351, 1973;* carcinoma of the breast, colon, lung, cervix, intestinal leiomyosarcoma *JAAD 40:862–865, 1999;* myeloma *JAAD 40:862–865, 1999;* leukemia *JAAD 40:862–865, 1999;* HTLV-1 (acute T-cell leukemia) (adult T-cell lymphoma/leukemia) *JAAD 49:979–1000, 2003; JAAD 46:S137–141, 2002;* lymphoma – Hodgkin's disease – ichthyosis vulgaris-like changes of legs or generalized (increased G-CSF levels) *JAAD 49:772–773, 2003; Br Med J*

1:763–764, 1955; non-Hodgkin's lymphoma, reticulolymphosarcoma, cutaneous T- cell lymphoma (CTCL) *JAAD 34:887–889, 1996;* B-cell lymphomas *JAAD 40:862–865, 1999;* CD 30+ cutaneous anaplastic large cell lymphoma *JAAD 42:914–920, 2000; Tumori 85:71–74, 1999;* metastatic male breast carcinoma – sclerodermoid ichthyosiform plaque of chest wall *AD 139:1497–1502, 2003;*

polycythemia rubra vera *JAAD 40:862–865, 1999;* rhabdomyosarcoma *JAAD 40:862–865, 1999;* spindle cell sarcoma *JAAD 40:862–865, 1999*

Keratoacanthoma visceral carcinoma syndrome – cancers of the genitourinary tract *AD 139:1363–1368, 2003; AD 120:123–124, 1984*

Leser-Trelat – eruptive inflammatory seborrheic keratoses *JAAD 35:88–95, 1996; JAAD 21:50–55, 1989*

Li-Fraumeni syndrome – pancreatic cancer *NEJM 371:1039–1049, 2014*

Linear IgA with Hodgkin's *JAAD 19:1122–4, 1988*

Lymphedema, unilateral

Maffucci's syndrome *J Neurosurg 131:1829–1834, 2018; Surg Pathol Clin 10:749–764, 2017; BMC Res Notes Feb 27, 2016*

Lynch syndrome (hereditary nonpolyposis colon cancer) – pancreatic cancer *NEJM 371:1039–1049, 2014*

Melanocytic BAP1-mutated atypical intradermal tumors (MBAIT) – pink-skin colored papules; sign of renal cell carcinoma and melanoma *JAMA Derm 153:999–1000, 2017*

Melanoma-astrocytoma syndrome

Merkel cell carcinoma *JAAD 75:541–547, 2016*
  Cerebellar degeneration with autonomic neuropathy
  Lambert-Eaton myasthenia syndrome
  Hyponatremia

Muir-Torre syndrome *JAAD 74:437–451, 2016*

Multiple endocrine neoplasia syndrome type 1

Multiple endocrine neoplasia syndrome type IIa

Multiple endocrine neoplasia syndrome type IIb/III

Multiple mucosal neuroma syndrome (MEN 2B) – enlarged lips, papules of tongue, Marfanoid habitus; medullary carcinoma of the thyroid; pheochromocytoma; missense gain of function mutation in RET proto-oncogene *JAMA Derm 152:939–940, 2016*

Multiple myeloma – follicular spicules *Dermatol Online J Oct 15, 2019*

Multicentric reticulohistiocytosis *Rheumatology (Oxford) Nov 19, 2019; Curr Rheum Rep 17:511, Jun 2015; Rheumatol Intl 31:1235–1238, 2011; JAAD 39 (pt2)864–866, 1998*

Necrobiotic xanthogranuloma with paraproteinemia – yellow eyelid papules *AD 145:279–284, 2009; Ann Hematol 86:303–306, 2007; Eyelid and Conjunctival Tumors, Shields JA and Shields CL, Lippincott Williams and Wilkins, 1999, p.143; Hautarzt 46:330–334, 1995; AD 128:94–100, 1992; JAAD 3:257–270, 1980;* extensive facial plaque *AD 146:957–960, 2010;* with giant cell myocardial disease *AD 133:97–102, 1997; Mayo Clin Proc 72:1028–1033, 1997; BJD 133:438–443, 1995*

Neuroendocrine syndromes

Neurofibromatosis

Neurofibromatosis, juvenile xanthogranulomas, and juvenile myelomonocytic leukemia *Ped Derm 34:114–118, 2017*

Neutrophilic dermatosis in chronic myelogenous leukemia *JAAD 29:290–292, 1993*

Neutrophilic eccrine hidradenitis – acute or chronic myelogenous leukemia *Blood Reviews 31:370–388, 2017*

Neutrophilic panniculitis of myelodysplasia – red nodules of legs and soles; *MYSM1* deficiency; short stature *Ped Derm 36:258–259, 2019*

Nevoid basal cell carcinoma syndrome

Neurofibromatosis type 1 *NEJM 370:2229–2236, 2014*

Noonan's syndrome – eightfold risk of acute myelogenous leukemia, acute lymphoblastic leukemia *NEJM 370:2229–2236, 2014*

Palmar fasciitis and polyarthritis syndrome *Clin Exp Dermatol 42:328–330, 2017; Semin Arth Rheumatol 14:105–111, 2014*

Palmar filiform hyperkeratosis *JAAD 33:337–340, 1995*

Palmoplantar keratoderma *Cutis 99:E32–35, 2017*

Panniculitis – paraneoplastic septal panniculitis associated with acute myelogenous leukemia *BJD 144:905–906, 2001;* neutrophilic panniculitis associated with myelodysplastic syndrome *JAAD 50:280–285, 2004;* pancreatic panniculitis *Australas J Dermatol 59:e269–276, 2018*

Papuloerythroderma of Ofuji – myelodysplastic syndrome *Australasian J Dermatol 59:e155–156, 2018*

Paraneoplastic autoimmune multiorgan syndrome (paraneoplastic pemphigus) – arciform and polycyclic lesions *Autoimmune Rev 17:1002–1010, 2018; JAAD 48:S69–72, 2003; AD 137:193–206, 2001*

Paraneoplastic hyperkeratosis *JAAD 31:157–190, 1994*

Porphyria cutanea tarda – hepatocellular carcinoma

Peutz-Jeghers syndrome *NEJM 370:2229–2236, 2014*

Peutz-Jeghers-like mucocutaneous pigmentation – associated with breast and gynecologic carcinomas in women *Medicine (Baltimore) 79:293–298, 2000;* pancreatic cancer *NEJM 371:1039–1049, 2014*

Phakomatosis pigmentokeratotica – 3 mm pigmented papules of neck (melanocytic nevi); Blaschko epidermal nevus; *HRAS* mosaic mutation; tendency for squamous cell carcinoma *NEJM 381:1458, 2019*

Pityriasis rotunda *Cutis 58:406–408, 1996; AD 119:607–6098, 1983*

Polyarteritis nodosa – associated with hairy cell leukemia, and chronic myelomonocytic leukemia *Blood Reviews 31:370–388, 2017*

Primary immune deficiency disorders

Pruritus, generalized *Acta DV 98:526–527, 2018; Curr Probl Dermatol 50:149–154, 2016*

Punctate keratoderma *Lancet i:530–533, 1984*

Pyoderma gangrenosum *Ann Hematol 98:2247–2248, 2019;* myelodysplastic syndrome *Dermatol Online J Jan 15, 2019;* bullous pyoderma gangrenosum – acute, chronic myelogenous leukemia, myelodysplastic syndrome, polycythemia vera, essential thrombocy-themia, myelofibrosis *Blood Reviews 31:370–388, 2017*

Raynaud's phenomenon

Reed syndrome – leiomyomatosis; renal cell carcinoma *JAAD 77:123–129, 2017; The Dermatologist July, 2016, pp47–49*

Rothmund-Thompson syndrome – osteosarcoma *JAAD 75:855–870, 2016*

Scleroderma, paraneoplastic *Acta Rheumatol Port 43:316–317, 2018; J Mal Vasc 41:365–370, 2016; NEJM 372:1056–167, 2015; Br J Rheumatol 28:65–69, 1989*

Scleromyxedema *Blood 135:1101–1110, 2020; Semin Oncol 43:395–400, 2016;* dermatoneuro syndrome *Clin Neuropathol 35:72–77, 2016; J Clin Oncol 30:e27–29, 2012*

Sjogren's syndrome – increased risk of lymphoma *A Clinician's Pearls and Myths in Rheumatology pp.107–130; ed John Stone; Springer 2009*

STAT1 gain-of-function mutation – chronic demodicidosis; recurrent staphylococcal infections of lungs and skin, mycobacterial infec-tions, cutaneous viral infections, invasive fungal infections; also cerebral aneurysms and cancers *J Clin Immunol 36:73–84, 2016; Ped Derm 37:153–155, 2020*

Sweet's syndrome – acute, chronic myelogenous leukemia, myelodysplastic syndrome, polycythemia vera, myelofibrosis *Blood Revies 31:37–388, 2017; Cancer 72:2723–2731, 1993; Clin Dermatol 11:149–157, 1993*

Tripe palms (acanthosis palmaris) *J Clin Oncol 7:669–678, 1989; JAAD 16:217–219, 1987*

Trousseau's sign (migratory thrombophlebitis) *J Women's Health 12:541–551, 2003; Circulation 22:780, 1960*

Tuberous sclerosis

Urticaria, chronic

Vasculitis – paraneoplastic vasculitis *J Rheumatol 18:721–727, 1991;* granulomatous vasculitis with lymphocytic lymphoma *JAAD 14:492–501, 1986;* large vessel vasculitis with myelodysplastic syndrome *Intern Med 57:2769–2771, 2018;* IgA vasculitis *Intern Med 57:1273–1276, 2018; Blood Reviews 31:370–388, 2017;* lung cancer and vasculitis *Lung Cancer 106:93–101, 2017*

Wells' syndrome – associated with lung cancer *BJD 145:678–679, 2001;* anal squamous cell carcinoma *Acta DV (Stockh)66:213–219, 1986;* nasopharyngeal carcinoma *Ann DV 111:777–778, 1984*

Werner's syndrome

Wiskott-Aldrich syndrome

Xanthomas, normolipemic – diffuse plane xanthomatosis – flat yellow plaques of eyelids, neck, trunk, buttocks, flexures *AD 93:639–646, 1966*

Xeroderma pigmentosum

Xerosis – generalized erythema craquele as a paraneoplastic phenomenon; lymphoma *BJD 97:323–326, 1977;* angioimmuno-blastic lymphadenopathy *AD 115:370, 1979;* gastric carcinoma *BJD 109:277–278, 1983;* breast cancer *BJD 110:246, 1984*

X-linked ichthyosis – testicular cancer

PARAPROTEINEMIAS, CUTANEOUS MANIFESTATIONS

JAAD 77:1145–1158, 2017; JAAD 20:206–11, 1989

Amyloidosis AL systemic

Angioedema (acquired inhibitor of complement deficiency)

Cryogobulinemia (purpura, cold urticaria, ulcers, Raynaud's phenomenon, livedo reticularis, cutaneous infarction, necrosis, hemorrhagic crusts) *Int J Dermatol 35:240–248, 1996; BJD 129:319–323, 1993; JAAD 25:21–27, 1991*

Cryokeratotic spicules of nose *JAMA Derm 151:457–458, 2015; Int J Dermatol 49:934–936, 2010; JAAD 49:736–740, 2003; JAAD 33:346–351, 1995; JAAD 32:834–839, 1995*

Crystal storing histiocytosis – facial swelling *Int J Surg Pathol 25:458–461, 2017; J Cutan Pathol 42:136–143, 2015; Head Neck Pathol 8:111–120, 2012; Int J Dermatol 45:1408–1411, 2006*

Crystalglobulinemia – purpura, necrotic ulcers, hemorrhagic blisters on distal extremities, painful papules, gangrenous ulcers) *Am J Kid Dis 67:787–791, 2016; Am J Dermatopathol 36:751–755, 2014*

Cutaneous AL amyloidoma – solitary waxy tan plaque or nodule with predilection for acral sites in absence of systemic AL amyloido-sis *Dermatol Online J 19:20711, 2013; AD 139:1157–1159, 2003*

Cutis laxa – heavy chain deposition disease *Case Rep Dermatol Med Feb 12, 2020; JAMA Derm 150:1192–1196, 2014; J Cut Med Surg 7:390–394, 2003*

Erythema elevatum diutinum *Int J Dermatol 58:408–415, 2019*

Hyperviscosity syndrome – ulcers *Eur J Intern Med 42:24–28, 2017*

Intravascular reactive glomeruloid angioendotheliomatosis *Clin Exp Dermatol 38:748–750, 2013; Dermatol Online J 19:20404, 2013; Am J Surg Pathol 26:685–697, 2002*

Light chain deposition disease

Necrobiotic xanthogranuloma with paraproteinemia *Eur J Dermatol 28:384–386, 2018*

Nodular macroglobulinosis (IgM storage papules) *JAAD 71:1145–1149, 2017; J Cut Pathol 40:440–444, 2013; JAAD 71:E251–252, 2017; AD 146:165–169, 2010; AD 114:280–281, 1978*

Papular mucinosis (scleromyxedema)

Plasmacytomas

POEMS syndrome (polyneuropathy, organomegaly, endocrinopathy, monoclonal gammopathy, skin changes) *AD 142:1501–1506, 2006; Clin Exp Dermatol 18:360–362, 1993*

Purpura (hyperviscosity, paraproteinemia, microangiopathy)

Pyoderma gangrenosum *Clin Exp Dermatol 44:e13–15, 2019; JAMA Derm 154:409–413, 2018; Clin Exp Dermatol 37:146–148, 2012; Ann Hematol 89:823–824, 2020*

Schnitzler's syndrome *JAAD Case Rep 5:312–316, 2019; BMJ Case Rep April 29, 2019; Rheumatology (Oxford)58 (suppl6) vi31–43, 2019*

Scleredema – secondary to paraproteinemia *JAMA Derm 150:788–789, 2014*

Sneddon-Wilkinson disease (subcorneal pustular dermatosis) *BJD 176:1341–1344, 2017; J Dtsch Dermatol Ges 7:893–896, 2009; Clin Exp Dermatol 33:229–233, 2008; Eur J Dermatol 16:687–690, 2006*

Sweet's syndrome

Systemic capillary leak syndrome

Urticaria-like neutrophilic dermatosis – with IgA gammopathy *BJD 170:1189–1191, 2014*

Vasculitis

Vasculitis without cryoglobulins *J Dermatol 45:1009–1012, 2018*

Waldenstrom's hyperglobulinemic purpura

Xanthomatosis – normolipemic plane xanthomas *Blood 118:3177–3184, 2011; JAAD 38:439–442, 1998; Am J Dermatopathol 15:572–575, 1993; BJD 101:711–716, 1979; AD 85:663–640, 1962*

PARATHYROID DISEASE, CUTANEOUS MANIFESTATIONS

CONGENITAL

Blueberry muffin baby – congenital transient neonatal hyperparathyroidism *Ped Derm 31:e91–93, 2014*

Calcinosis cutis of newborn – transient pseudohypoparathyroidism *Indian J Pediatr 78:1424–1426, 2011*

INFLAMMATORY LESIONS

Hypoparathyroidism (keratoconjunctivitis) – red eyes; paronychia, dry, rough, keratotic, and puffy skin; nails ridged, lusterless, and distally split *Clin Dermatol 24:281–286, 2006*

METABOLIC

Band keratopathy *Br J Ophthalmol 61:494–495, 1977*

Calcific uremic arteriolopathy *Saudi J Kidney Dis Transpl 27:1265–1269, 2016*

Calcinosis cutis *J Clin Rheumatol 20:330–331, 2014*

Calciphylaxis *NEJM 378:1704–1714, 2018*

Metastatic calcification *Clin Dermatol 24:281–288, 2006*

NEOPLASTIC DISORDERS

Hyperparathyroidism, primary – brown giant cell tumor of palate

Metastases – parathyroid carcinoma *Head Neck 38:E115–118, 2016*

Pseudohypoparathyroidism – dry, scaly, hyperkeratotic puffy skin; multiple subcutaneous osteomas, collagenoma *BJD 143:1122–1124, 2000*

PRIMARY CUTANEOUS DISEASES

Gingival hyperplasia – hyperparathyroidism

Leg ulcers – hyperparathyroidism *BJD 83:263–268, 1970*

Pruritus, generalized – hyperparathyroidism; hypoparathyroidism

Psoriasiform dermatitis – idiopathic hypoparathyroidism *Eur J Dermatol 9:574–576, 1999; Acta Med Scand (Suppl) 121:1–269, 1941*

Racket nails *Clin Exp Dermatol 9:267–269, 1984*

Urticaria – hyperparathyroidism *Lancet 1:1476, 1984*

Xerosis – hypoparathyroidism *JAAD 15:353–356, 1986*

SYNDROMES

Albright's hereditary osteodystrophy – pseudohypoparathyroidism, round face, short neck, osteomas of skin with overlying hyperpigmentation, short stature, hypogonadism, macrocephaly, psychomotor retardation, endocrinologic abnormalities; mutation in GNAS1 *Ped Derm 28:135–137, 2011; Endocrinology 30:922–932, 1942; plate-like osteoma cutis BMJ Case Rep May 5, 2014*

Autoimmune polyendocrinopathy-candidiasis-ectodermal dystrophy syndrome (APECED) – keratoconjunctivitis; enamel hypoplasia; sparse scalp, facial, and body hair, chronic mucocutaneous candidiasis, adrenal insufficiency, hypoparathyroidism, nail dystrophy, vitiligo; mutation in autoimmune regulator gene (AIRE) *Ped Derm 24:529–533, 2007*

DiGeorge's syndrome – pancreatic panniculitis; characteristic facial features *Dermatol Online J Nov 15, 2016; Ped Derm 33:e206–207, 2016*

IPEX syndrome – X-linked; immune dysregulation, polyendocrinopathy, enteropathy; mutation of FOXP3; nummular dermatitis, urticaria, scaly psoriasiform plaques of trunk and extremities, penile rash, alopecia universalis, bullae *AD 140:466–472, 2004*

Leukonychia, congenital hypoparathyroidism; hypoparathyroidism, onychorrhexis, and cataracts, LEOPARD syndrome *Int J Derm 29:535–541, 1990*

Maffucci's syndrome (enchondromatosis) – enchondromas and multiple venous malformations; spindle cell hemangioendothelioma; oral and intra-abdominal venous and lymphatic anomalies; short stature, shortened long bones with pathologic fractures; enchondromas undergo sarcomatous change in 30–40%; breast, ovarian, pancreatic, parathyroid, pituitary tumors *JAAD 56:541–564, 2007; Cutis 69:21–22, 2002; Ped Derm 17:270–276, 2000; Ped Derm*

12:55–58, 1995; Dermatologic Clinics 13:73–78, 1995; JAAD 29:894–899, 1993

Multiple endocrine neoplasia syndrome (MEN I) (Wermer's syndrome) – angiofibromas of face and nose JAAD 56:877–880, 2007; J Clin Endocrinol Metab 89:5328–5336, 2004; Endocr J 47:569–573, 2000; JAAD 42:939–969, 2000; JAAD 41:890–892, 1999; AD 133:853–857, 1997; angiofibromas of vermilion border; facial angiofibromas, lipomas, abdominal collagenomas, cutis verticis gyrate, pedunculated skin tags, acanthosis nigricans, red gingival papules, confetti-like hypopigmented macules; primary hyperparathyroidism with hypercalcemia, kidney stones, prolactinoma, gastrinoma, bilateral adrenal hyperplasia; mutation in menin, a nuclear protein involved in cell cycle regulation and proliferation JAAD 61:319–324, 2009; AD 133:853–857, 1997

VASCULAR LESIONS

Hyperparathyroidism – calcinosis cutis with venulitis

PARONYCHIA

AUTOIMMUNE DISEASES AND DISEASES OF IMMUNE DYSFUNCTION

Allergic contact dermatitis – latex Dermatol Clin 33:207–241, 2015; J Eur Acad DV 14:504–506, 2000; acrylic Contact Dermatitis 44:117–119, 2001; thymol Cutis 43:531–532, 1989; acrylic nails

Antiepidermal growth factor receptor antibody C225 – acute paronychia BJD 144:1169–1176, 2001

Bullous pemphigoid Dermatol Clin 33:207–241, 2015; JAAD 68:395–403, 2013; periungual blisters; anti-p200 and gamma2 subunit of laminin 5 BJD 158:1354–1357, 2008

Chronic granulomatous disease Ped Derm 21:646–651, 2004

Chronic granulomatous paronychia – pseudomegadactyly Dermatologica 169:86–87, 1984

Chronic mucocutaneous candidiasis Clin in Dermatol 23:68–77, 2005

Dermatomyositis – periungual erythema, telangiectasia, and ragged cuticles Dermatol Clin 33:207–241, 2015; anti-MDA 5 dermatomyositis – ulcers of nail folds JAAD 78:776–785, 2018

DiGeorge's syndrome

Graft vs. host disease – red macules or folliculocentric papules of face, ears, palms and soles, periungual areas, upper back and neck AD 143:67–71, 2007

Job's syndrome (hyper IgE syndrome) (Job's, Buckley's, Quie-Hill syndromes (allergic rhinitis)) – autosomal dominant or sporadic; atrophoderma vermiculatum; coarse facial features with broad nose, rough thickened skin with prominent follicular ostia; papular and papulopustular folliculitis-like eruptions; oral candidiasis; chronic paronychia; cold abscesses of neck and trunk; otitis media common; mutation in STAT3 (transcription 3 gene activator and signal transducer JAAD 65:1167–1172, 2011; Dermatol Therapy 18:176–183, 2005

Lupus erythematosus – systemic LE; discoid lupus erythematosus Clin Exp Dermatol 37:249–251, 2012; NEJM 269:1155–1161, 1963

Mucous membrane pemphigoid BMC Dermatol 19:3, 2019

Pemphigoid nodularis BJD 142:575–577, 2000

Pemphigus vegetans – verrucous paronychia Indian Dermatol Online J 11:87–89, 2019; Case Rep Med 11:5980937, 2018

Pemphigus vulgaris Skin Appendage Disord 5:362–365, 2019; Skin Appendage Disord 3:28–31, 2017; Dermatol Clin 33:207–241, 2015; Clin Exp Dermatol 21:315–317, 1996; JAAD 29:494–496, 1993; AD 126:1374–1375, 1990; hemorrhagic paronychia JAAD 43:529–535, 2000

Rheumatoid vasculitis – purpuric infarcts of paronychial areas (Bywater's lesions) BJD 77:207–210, 1965

Scleroderma J Rheumatol 19:1407–1414, 1992

STAT1 gain of function mutation – most common cause of chronic mucocutaneous candidiasis; demodicidosis with facial papulopustular eruptions, blepharitis, chalazion, dermatitis of the neck, nail dystrophy, congenital candidiasis Ped Derm 37:159–161, 2020

CONGENITAL DISORDERS

Congenital malalignment of the great toenails Ped Derm 33:e288–289, 2016

DRUGS

Acral dysesthesia syndrome Cutis 52:43–44, 1993

Acitretin Acta DV Alp Pannonica Adriat 20:217–218, 2011

Afatinib (epidermal growth factor receptor-tyrosine kinase inhibitors) – paronychia Onco Targets Ther 12:10897–10902, 2019; JAMA Derm 152:340–342, 2016

Capecitabine – pyogenic granuloma-like paronychial lesions BJD 147:1270–1272, 2002

Cetuximab (epidermal growth factor receptor antibody) – painful periungual granulation tissue BJD 161:515–521, 2009; JAAD 58:545–570, 2008; JAAD 56:317–326, 2007; JAAD 55:657–670, 2006; JAAD 55:429–437, 2006; JAAD 47:632–633, 2002

Cyclosporine BJD 132:829–830, 1995

Docetaxel – painful paronychia Cutis 71:229–232, 2003; Australas J Dermatol 42:293–296, 2002; Dermatology 198:288–290, 1999

Doxycycline – personal observation

Epidermal growth factor receptor inhibitors – cetuximab and panitumumab; erlotinib and gefitinib; lapatinib; canertinib; vandetanib Indian Dermatol Online J 9:293–298, 2018; JAAD 72:203–218, 2015

Erlotinib (epidermal growth factor receptor inhibitor) – painful periungual granulation tissue JAMA Derm 152:340–342, 2016; JAAD 69:463–472, 2013; BJD 161:515–521, 2009; JAAD 58:545–570, 2008; JAAD 56:317–326, 2007; JAAD 55:657–670, 2006; JAAD 55:429–437, 2006

Erythema multiforme SKINmed 11:265–268, 2013

Etanercept-induced dermatomyositis – paronychial erythema JAMA Derm 149:1204–1208, 2013

Etoposide/teniposide/amsacrine – paronychia JAAD 71:203–214, 2014

Fixed drug eruption – acute paronychia BJD 125:592–595, 1991; periungual and subungual erythema BJD 162:1397–1398, 2010

Gefitinib (epidermal growth factor receptor inhibitor) – pyogenic granulomas of proximal nail folds JAMA Derm 152:340–342, 2016; AD 148:1399–1402, 2012; JAAD 58:545–570, 2008; JAAD 56:317–326, 2007; AD 142:939, 2006

Gefitinib/erlotinib/cetuximab/panitumumab (epidermal growth factor receptor inhibitors) – paronychia JAAD 71:217–227, 2014;

Ibrutinib Skin Appendage Disord 6:32–36, 2020

Indinavir (protease inhibitors) – paronychia with or without pyogenic granulomas *JAAD 63:549–561, 2010; JAAD 46:284–293, 2002; Clin Inf Dis 32:140–143, 2001; BJD 142:1063–1064, 2000; NEJM 338:1776–1777, 1998*; indinavir/rotinavir combination *Ann Pharmacother 35:881–884, 2001*

Isotretinoin *An Bras Dermatol 91:223–225, 2016; Dermatol Clin 33:207–241, 2015*

Lamivudine *Lancet 351 (9111):1256, 1998*

Ledipasvir/sofosbuvir – for hepatitis C *J Clin Aesthet Dermatol 12:35–37, 2019*

Lenalidomide *J Dermatol 40:303–304, 2013*

MEK inhibitors – C1-1040, selumetinib, trametinib – morbilliform eruption, papulopustular eruptions, xerosis, paronychia *Indian Dermatol Online J 9:293–298, 2018; JAAD 72:221–236, 2015*

Methotrexate *AD 119:623–624, 1983*

Morbilliform drug eruption *SKINmed 11:265–268, 2013*

Neratinib *J Dermatol Treatment 30:487–488, 2019*

Retinoids, systemic – isotretinoin *JAAD 10:677–678, 1984; JAAD 9:708–713, 1983*; acitretin

Sunitinib – multikinase inhibitor; bullous palmoplantar erythrodyses-thesia, periungual erythema, perianal erythema, mucositis *AD 144:123–124, 2008*

Targeted therapy and immunotherapy *Am J Clin Dermatol 19 (suppl 1)31–39, 2018*

Taxane *Skin Appendage Disord 5:276–282, 2019*

Toxic epidermal necrolysis *SKINmed 11:265–268, 2013*

Trametinib (MAP kinase inhibitor) (MEK inhibitor) – angular cheilitis, xerosis, bacterial folliculitis, acneiform eruptions, paronychia, thinning hair *Dermatol Ther 30:e13164, 2020; Ped Derm 34:90–94, 2017*

Zidovudine *JAAD 46:284–293, 2002; JAAD 40:322–324, 1999*

EXOGENOUS AGENTS

Foods *JAAD 27:706–710, 1992*

Foreign body, hair – chronic paronychia *Int J Dermatol 14:661–663, 1975*

Levamisole-tainted cocaine – paronychial necrosis *BJD 140:948–951, 1999*

INFECTIONS AND INFESTATIONS

Abscess *Dermatol Clin 33:207–241, 2015*

Accidental inoculation – orf, leishmaniasis

Acute and chronic paronychia – *Staphylococcus aureus, Candida albicans, Pseudomonas aeruginosa, Serratia marcescens, Klebsiella pneumoniae*

Aspergillus *J Dermatol 45:1362–1366, 2018; Med Mycol J 57:e21–25, 2016*

Bacterial sepsis – hemorrhagic bullae of paronychial folds *Dermatol Clin 33:207–241, 2015*

Bartonella henselae *Lancet 350 (9084):1078, 1997*

Candida and/or *Pseudomonas* – chronic paronychia *Semin Dermatol 12:315–330, 1993*; acute paronychia *AD 129:786–787, 1993*; chronic mucocutaneous candidiasis *Clin Exp Dermatol 7:155–162, 1982*; congenital candidiasis *Textbook of Neonatal Dermatology, p.226, 2001; Candida albicans* acute paronychia *JAAD 70:120–126, 2014*

Citrobacter braaki Ann Dermatol 28:528–529, 2016

Cowpox

Curvularia lunata Mycopathologia 118:83–84, 1992

Dermatophyte infection – acute paronychia *JAAD 70:120–126, 2014*

Eikenella corrodens – chronic paronychia in children *Am J Surg 141:703–705, 1981*

Erysipeloid

Felon *Stat Pearls Nov 23, 2019*

Fusarium – red swollen toe with paronychia *J Dermatol 41:340–342, 2014; JAAD 65:235–237, 2011; JAAD 47:659–666, 2002*; purpuric paronychia *AD 147:1317–1322, 2011*

Herpes simplex – herpetic whitlow *JAAD 70:120–126, 2014; Eur J Rheumatol 46:46–47, 2014; Br Dent J 177:251–252, 1994; Am J Dis Child 137:861–863, 1983; Int J Dermatol 16:752–754, 1977; NEJM 283:804–805, 1970; AD 101:396–402, 1970*

Herpes zoster *Dermatol Clin 33:207–241, 2015*

Klebsiella pneumonia E FORT Open Rev 4:183–193, 2019

Leishmaniasis – ulcerated papular paronychia *An Bras Dermatol 92:268–269, 2017; Ped Derm 33:93–94, 2016; NEJM 371:1736, 2014*

Leprosy *Actas Dermosifiliogr 103:276–284, 2012*

Mixed infections *J Hand Surg (Am) 13:790, 1988*

Mycobacterium chelonae Acta Clin Belg 66:144–147, 2011

Mycobacterium marinum Dermatol Clin 33:509–630, 2015; Handchir Mikrochir Plast Chir 32:343–346, 2000

Mycobacterium tuberculosis – tuberculous chancre *AD 114:567–569, 1979*; primary inoculation *JAMA 245:1556–1557, 1981*; prosector's paronychia *AD 114:567–569, 1978; Arch Surg 103:757–758, 1971; Skin Appendage Disord 5:386–389, 2019; Ped Derm 30:e172–176, 2013*

Myrmecia (deep warts) – tender periungual nodules *AD 128:105–110, 1992*

Neisseria gonorrhea Stat Pearls Jan 7, 2020

North American blastomycosis *J Emerg Med 19:245–248, 2000*

Onychomycosis

Orf – acute paronychia *JAAD 70:120–126, 2014;*

Osteomyelitis of the fingertip; *Candida glabrata Case Rep Orthop 204:962575; Ned Tijdschr Geneeskd 154:A988, 2010*

Proteus vulgaris

Pseudomonas pyocyanea; Pseudomonas aeruginosa – proximal chronic non-tender paronychia *Clin Interv Aging 10:265–267, 2015*

Rat bite fever – personal observation

Scopulariopsis

Scytalidium dimidiatum – paronychia with onychomycosis *JAAD 65:1219–1227, 2011*

Staphylococcus aureus – acute paronychia *JAAD 70:120–126, 2014*; adults and children *Textbook of Neonatal Dermatology, p.183, 2001; Am J Dis Child 137:361–364, 1983*

Streptococcus, group A (GAS) *J Ped Infec Dis Soc Nov 29, 2019*

Syphilis, primary *Br J Vener Dis 59:167–171, 1983*; secondary – chronic paronychia *Khirurgiia (Mosk)12:93–94, 1975; AD 105:458, 1972*; congenital

Trichosporon beigelii Mykosen 28:601–606, 1985

Tularemia

Tungiasis (*Tunga penetrans, Tunga trimamillata*) *JAAD 82:551–559, 2020; SKINmed 13:264–266, 2015; JAAD 26:513–515, 519–520, 1992*

Varicella *Dermatol Clin 33:207–241, 2015*

Veillonella – anaerobic gram negative coccus; in neonates *Clin Pediatr 11:690–692, 1972*

Verruca vulgaris *Dermatol Clin 33:207–241, 2015*

Yaws – secondary (daughter yaws, pianomas, framboesiomas) – small papules which ulcerate, become crusted; resemble raspberries; periorificial (around mouth, nose, penis, anus, vulva); extend peripherally (circinate yaws); hyperkeratotic plantar plaques (crab yaws); periungual

INFILTRATIVE DISEASES

Amyloidosis, primary systemic *JAAD 42:339–342, 2000*

Langerhans cell histiocytosis *BJD 145:137–140, 2001; JAAD 13:522–524, 1985;* purpuric nail striae with paronychia *Ped Derm 37:18–183, 2020*

INFLAMMATORY DISEASES

Chronic recurrent multifocal osteomyelitis *JAAD 71:e218–219, 2014*

Erythema multiforme, Stevens-Johnson syndrome

METABOLIC DISEASES

Acrodermatitis enteropathica – pustulous paronychia *Acta DV 23:127–169, 1942;* periorificial dermatitis, generalized dermatitis, vesicular, bullous, pustular, desquamative dermatitis, psoriasiform dermatitis, alopecia, paronychia, perleche; solute carrier family 39 (zinc transporter) member 4 gene (*SLC39A4*) encodes histidine-rich protein Hzip4 *JAAD 56:116–124, 2008; Ped Derm 19:426–431, 2002; Ped Derm 19:426–431, 2002; Ped Derm 19:180–182, 2002; AD 116:562–564, 1980; Dermatologica 156:155–166, 1978; Lancet 1:676–677, 1973; Acta DV 17:513–546, 1936*

Celiac disease

Cryoglobulinemia with leukocytoclastic vasculitis – personal observation

Disseminated intravascular coagulations – personal observation

Hypoparathyroidism

Renal disease, chronic – hyperpigmentation of proximal nail folds *Dermatol Clin 33:207–241, 2015*

Zinc deficiency, acquired zinc deficiency – due to intestinal malabsorption; extensive burns, Crohn's disease, sickle cell anemia, sprue, systemic malignancies, pancreatic insufficiency, renal tubular dysfunction, drugs, defect of mammary zinc secretion, blind loop syndrome, diets high in phytates and calcium *JAAD 69:616–624, 2013;*

Am J Dis Child 135:968–969, 1981; total parenteral nutrition *Am J Clin Nutr 29:197–204, 1976;* prematurity *BJD 104:459–464, 1980;* alcoholism *Cutis 82:60–62, 2008*

NEOPLASTIC DISEASES

Acquired reactive digital fibroma – subungual tumor with enlarged paronychium and macrodactyly *JAAD 69:603–608, 2013*
   Differential diagnosis
      Fibro-osseous pseudotumor of the digits; myofibroblastic proliferation in females; affects flexor digits and palms *Chir Main 28:107–112, 2009; Cancer 58:2103–2109, 1986*
      Superficial acral fibromyxoma – subungual tumor *Am J Surg Pathol 36:789–798, 2012*

Cellular digital fibromas – resemble acquired digital fibrokeratoma and superficial acral fibromyxoma *JAAD 69:603–608, 2013*

Acral fibromyxoma – paronychial nodule *Int J Dermatol 54:499–508, 2015; JAAD 50:134–136, 2004*

Basal cell carcinoma of nail fold and nail unit – chronic paronychia *JAAD 56:811–814, 2007; Foot Ankle Int 22:675–678, 2001; Int J Derm 39:397–398, 2000; JAAD 37:791–793, 1997; AD 108:828, 1973*

Bowen's disease *JAAD 71:e65–67, 2014; AD 130:204–209, 1994;* pigmented paronychia *BJD 169:722–723, 2013*

Eccrine poroma *JAAD 54:733–734, 2006*

Eccrine spiradenoma – papule of proximal nail fold *AD 140:1003–1008, 2004*

Enchondroma

Intraosseous epidermal inclusion cyst *J Am Podiatr Med Assoc 100:133–137, 2010*

Kaposi's sarcoma *J Hand Surg (Am) 11:410–413, 1986*

Keratoacanthoma, subungual – chronic paronychia *Eur J Dermatol 29:246–247, 2019; Ann Plast Surg 34:84–87, 1995*

Leukemia – red swollen nail folds in chronic lymphocytic leukemia *Br J Haematol 112:1, 2001; Int J Dermatol 24:595–597, 1985*

Lymphoma – angioimmunoblastic T-cell lymphoma – personal observation; primary cutaneous CD8+ T-cell lymphoma *Am J Dermatopathol 40:e52–56, 2018;* Sezary syndrome *J Cutan Med Surg 23:380–387, 2019*

Melanoma – personal observation *Khirurgiia (Mosk) 9:150–151, 1990; Hand 9:49–51, 1977*

Metastatic squamous cell carcinoma *JAAD 31:259–263, 1994;* bronchogenic carcinoma *J Foot Ankle Surg 36:115–119, 1997;* small cell lung cancer; breast cancer mimicking acute paronychia *Am J Clin Oncol 16:86–91, 1993;* osteosarcoma *Int J Dermatol 56:104–105, 2017; BJD 171:663–665, 2014*

Myopericytoma, periungual *JAAD 54:1107–1108, 2006*

Onycholemmal carcinoma – paronychia, crusted ulcer of nailfold, onycholysis *JAAD 68:290–295, 2013*

Onychomatrixoma *Acta DV Croat 21:198–201, 2013*

Squamous cell carcinoma, subungual – chronic paronychia *World J Clin Cases 7:3590–3594, 2019; J Dermatol 46:e460–461, 2019; Dermatol Online J Nov 18, 2015; Eur J Dermatol 10:149–150, 2000; Cutis 36:189–191, 1985*

Subungual exostosis – periungual papules

PARANEOPLASTIC DISEASES

Bazex syndrome – periungual erythema *JAAD 55:1103–1105, 2006; JAMA 248:2882–2884, 1982; Bull Soc Fr Dermatol Syph 72:182–185, 1965*

Paraneoplastic pemphigus – erosive paronychia *BJD 147:725–732, 2002;* paronychial erythema *Ped Derm 29:656–657, 2012*

PRIMARY CUTANEOUS DISEASES

Acrodermatitis continua of Hallopeau – periungual acral erythema *J Dermatol Treat 25:489–494, 2014; Ped Derm 26:105–106, 2009; BJD 157:1073–1074, 2007; Clin Inf Dis 32:431,505, 2001; Dtsch Med Wochenschr 123:386–390, 1998*

Alopecia mucinosa *Clin Exp Dermatol 12:50–52, 1987*

Amicrobial pustulosis – exudative erythema, erosions, pustules, diffuse alopecia with dermatitis; associated with systemic autoimmune disorders; scalp, axillae, ears, thighs *BJD 154:568–569, 2006*

Atopic dermatitis *Dermatol Clin 33:207–241, 2015*

Chronic paronychia *BJD 160:858–860, 2009*

Dual toenails – chronic paronychia *J Derm Surg Oncol 12:1328–1329, 1986*

Dyshidrotic eczema – personal observation

Epidermolysis bullosa, junctional and dystrophic forms – paronychia at birth

Hand dermatitis *Dermatol Clin 33:207–241, 2015*

Granuloma annulare

Ingrown nails, including congenital ingrown nails *Clin Pediatr (Phila) 21:424–426, 1982; Clin Pediatr 18:247–248, 1979*

Keratoderma of Jadassohn and Lewandowski – congenital paronychia *Bull Soc Fr Dermatol Syphiligr 76:411–412, 1969*

Keratosis lichenoides chronica *AD 120:1471–1474, 1984*

Lichen planus *SKINMed 14:56–60, 2016; Int J Dermatol 52:684–687, 2013*

Lichen simplex chronicus *Dermatol Clin 33:207–241, 2015*

Parakeratosis pustulosa – psoriasiform dermatitis of children; paronychial skin with thickening of nail edges *BJD 79:527–532, 1967*

Psoriasis and pustular psoriasis – subacute and chronic paronychia *Dermatol Clin 33:207–241, 2015; J Hand Surg (Br) 11:265–268, 1986; BJD 92:685–688, 1975*

Racial hyperpigmentation of nail folds *Dermatol Clin 33:207–241, 2015*

Retronychia (embedding of proximal nail due to trauma) – swollen paronychial area *Ped Derm 35:e144–146, 2018, Dermatol Online J July 15, 2017; JAAD 70:388–390, 2014;* nail fold granulation tissue *JAAD 58:978–983, 2008*

PSYCHOCUTANEOUS DISEASES

Dermatophagia – body focused repetitive behavior disorder *JAAD 76:779–791, 2017*

Eating disorders *Clin Dermatol 31:80–85, 2013;* anorexia nervosa *Dermatoendocrinol 1:268–270, 2009*

Factitial paronychia *J R Coll Physicians Lond 17:199–205, 1983*

SYNDROMES

Anhidrotic ectodermal dysplasia (Clouston syndrome) *Cutis 71-224–225, 2003*

Apert's syndrome *Cutis 52:205–208, 1993*

Carpal tunnel syndrome *JAAD March 18, 2020*

CHILD syndrome – periungual hyperkeratosis *AD 142:348–351, 2006*

Familial chilblain lupus – paronychia, acral erythema, acral papules, necrotic ulcers, facial ulcers, mutilation of fingers, ear lesions; mutation of exonuclease III domain of 3' repair exonuclease 1 (*TREX1*) *JAMA Derm 151:426–431, 2015*

Fibroblastic rheumatism – periungual papules *Ped Derm 19:532–535, 2002;* symmetrical polyarthritis, nodules over joints and on palms, elbows, knees, ears, neck, Raynaud's phenomenon, sclerodactyly; joint contractures, thick palmar fascia; scalp nodules, red tender swelling of toe tips, periarticular nodule; skin lesions resolve spontaneously *JAAD 66:959–965, 2012; AD 139:657–662, 2003; Ped Derm 19:532–535, 2002; AD 139:657–662, 2003; AD 131:710–712, 1995; Clin Exp Dermatol 19:268–270, 1994; AD 131:710–712, 1995; Clin Exp Dermatol 19:268–270, 1994; JAAD 14:1086–1088, 1986; Rev Rheum Ed Fr 47:345–351, 1980*

Hereditary sensory and autonomic neuropathies – painless paronychia *JAAD 21:736–739, 1989*

Ichthyosis follicularis with atrichia and photophobia (IFAP) – X-linked recessive; atopic dermatitis; collodion membrane and erythema at birth; ichthyosis, spiny (keratotic) follicular papules (generalized follicular keratoses), non-scarring alopecia totalis, keratotic papules of elbows, knees, fingers, Achilles tendons; extensor surfaces, xerosis; punctate keratitis, photophobia with progressive corneal scarring; nail dystrophy, paronychia, psychomotor delay, short stature; enamel dysplasia, beefy red tongue and gingiva, angular stomatitis (angular cheilitis), lamellar scales, psoriasiform plaques, palmoplantar erythema; mutation of MBTPS2 (intramembrane zinc metalloproteinase needed for cholesterol homeostasis and endoplasmic reticulum stress response) *Ped Derm 26:427–431, 2009; Curr Prob Derm 14:71–116, 2002; JAAD 46:S156–158, 2002; BJD 142:157–162, 2000; AD 125:103–106, 1989; Ped Derm 12:195, 1995; Dermatologica 177:341–347, 1988; Am J Med Genet 85:365–368, 1999; BJD 21:165–189, 1909*

Incontinentia pigmenti – painful subungual tumors *J Hand Surg (Br) 18:667–669, 1993; JAAD 13:913–918, 1985*

Keratosis-ichthyosis-deafness (KID) syndrome – autosomal recessive; dotted waxy, fine granular, stippled, or reticulated surface pattern of severe diffuse hyperkeratosis of palms and soles (palmoplantar keratoderma), ichthyosis with well marginated, serpiginous erythematous verrucous plaques, hyperkeratotic elbows and knees, perioral furrows, leukoplakia, follicular occlusion triad, scalp cysts, nodules (trichilemmal tumors, squamous cell carcinoma), bilateral sensorineural deafness, photophobia with vascularizing keratitis, blindness, hypotrichosis of scalp, eyebrows, and eyelashes, dystrophic nails, chronic mucocutaneous candidiasis, otitis externa, abscesses, blepharitis; connexin 26 mutation *JAAD 69:127–134, 2013; Ped Derm 27:651–652, 2010; Ped Derm 23:81–83, 2006; JAAD 51:377–382, 2004; BJD 148:649–653, 2003; Cutis 72:229–230, 2003; Ped Derm 19:285–292, 2002; Ped Derm 15:219–221, 1998; Ped Derm 13:105–113, 1996; JAAD 19:1124–1126, 1988; AD 123:777–782, 1987; AD 117:285–289, 1981; J Cutaneous Dis 33:255–260, 1915*

KID syndrome with fissured lips – paronychial pustules, blepharitis without keratitis, perineal psoriasiform plaques, tongue erosions, honeycomb palmoplantar keratoderma; red gingivae; mutation in connexin 26 (*N14K*) *GJB2*

Laryngo-onycho-cutaneous syndrome – autosomal recessive type of junctional epidermolysis bullosa; skin ulceration with prominent granulation tissue, early hoarseness and laryngeal stenosis; scarred nares; chronic erosion of corners of mouth (giant perleche); paronychia with periungual inflammation and erosions; onycholysis with subungual granulation tissue and loss of nails with granulation tissue of nail bed, conjunctival inflammation with polypoid granulation tissue, and dental enamel hypoplasia and hypodontia; only in Punjabi families; mutation in laminin alpha-3 (*LAMA3A*) *BJD 169:1353–1356, 2013; Ped Derm 23:75–77, 2006; Biomedica 2:15–25, 1986*

Multicentric reticulohistiocytosis – coral beading around nail folds *AD 126:251–252, 1990; Oral Surg Oral Med Oral Pathol 65:721–725, 1988; Pathology 17:601–608, 1985; JAAD 11:713–723, 1984; AD 97:543–547, 1968*

Olmsted syndrome – leukokeratosis of oral mucosa, periorificial keratotic plaques; congenital diffuse sharply marginated transgradient keratoderma of palms and soles, onychodystrophy, constriction of digits (ainhum), diffuse alopecia, thin nails, chronic paronychia, linear keratotic streaks, follicular keratosis, anhidrosis, small stature; differential diagnostic considerations include Clouston hidrotic ectodermal dysplasia, pachyonychia congenita, acrodermatitis enteropathica, Vohwinkel's keratoderma, mal de Meleda, and other palmoplantar keratodermas *Ped Derm 20:323–326, 2003; AD 132:797–800, 1996; JAAD 10:600–610, 1984*

Pachyonychia congenita *JAAD 30:275–276, 1994*

Reflex sympathetic dystrophy *JAAD 29:865–868, 1993*

Reactive arthritis syndrome *BJD 102:480–482, 1980*

Tuberous sclerosis – periungual fibromas *Ped Derm 32:563–570, 2015*

Yellow nail syndrome *BJD 76:153–157, 1964*

TRAUMA

Accidental trauma

Artificial nails

Chilblains – personal observation

Fractures of the terminal phalanx *Arch Emerg Med 10:301–305, 1993*

Corrective casting *Foot Ankle Surg 22:229–232, 2016*

Harpists' fingers – paronychia with calluses of the sides and tips of fingers with onycholysis and subungual hemorrhage

Hematoma – from pulse oximetry

Manicures

Manipulating a hangnail (shred of eponychium) *Am Fam Physician 96:44–51, 2017*

Nailbiting (onychophagia) *Clin Pediatr (Phila) 29:690–692, 1990*

Occupational trauma – bartenders, housekeepers, dishwashers, laundry workers

Thumb sucking *Stat Pearls March 14, 2020;* finger sucking *Hand (NY)12:NP99–100, 2017*

VASCULAR DISEASES

Pyogenic granuloma *Dermatol Clin 33:207–241, 2015*

Raynaud's disease *Med Princ Pract 28:394–396, 2019*

Thromboangiitis obliterans (Buerger's disease) – necrosis around nails *Am J Med Sci 136:567–580, 1908;* chronic sterile paronychia *Australas J Dermatol 55:e9–11, 2014*

Vasculitis, drug-induced *Dermatol Clin 33:207–241, 2015*

PAROTID GLAND ENLARGEMENT

BILATERAL ENLARGEMENT (SIALOSIS)

AUTOIMMUNE DISEASES AND DISORDERS OF IMMUNE DYSREGULATION

Diffuse infiltrative lymphocytosis syndrome (DILS) – autoimmune syndrome with oligoclonal expansion of CD8+ T lymphocytes in response to HIV antigens; lymphocytic infiltration of salivary glands (parotid glands) and viscera *Clin Lab Haem 27:278–282, 2005; Ann Int Med 112:3–10, 1990*

IgG4-related disease – cutaneous plasmacytosis (papulonodules); pseudolymphoma; angiolymphoid hyperplasia with eosinophilia; Mikulicz's disease; psoriasiform dermatitis; morbilliform eruption; hypergammaglobulinemic purpura; urticarial vasculitis; ischemic digits; Raynaud's disease and digital gangrene *BJD 171:929, 959–967, 2014;* sclerosing mesenteritis – papules, plaques, nodules, parotid gland swelling (parotitis), lacrimal gland swelling, dacryoadenitis, sialadenitis, proptosis, idiopathic pancreatitis, sclerosing

mesenteritis (retroperitoneal fibrosis), aortitis *JAAD 75:197–202, 2016*

Lupus erythematosus – discoid LE; bilateral parotid gland enlargement

Selective IgA deficiency

Sjogren's syndrome – parotitis *Ped Dent 23:140–142, 2001; Eur J Pediatr 148:414–416, 1989; Radiology 169:749–751, 1988;* lymphoma *Arthritis Case Rep (Hoboken) April 5, 2020;* HIV Sjogren-like illness *Gesichtschir 1:82–85, 1997*

DRUG REACTIONS

Drugs
　Catecholamines
　Chlorhexidine
　Dextropropoxyphene
　High dose estrogen
　Iododerma –"iodine mumps" (iodide-associated sialadenitis); *Acad Radiol 27:428–435, 2020; NEJM 376:868, 2017; JAAD 36:1014–1016, 1997;* potassium iodide therapy *JAAD 53:931–951, 2005;*
　Methyldopa
　Nifedipine *Am J Cardiol 61:874, 1988*
　Nivolumab – sarcoid-like parotid enlargement, pulmonary granulomas *BJD 176:1060–1063, 2017*
　Phenothiazines
　Phenylbutazone
　Sulfonamides
　Thiouracil
　Thiourea diuretics

EXOGENOUS AGENTS

Alcohol abuse

Heavy metals

INFECTIONS AND INFESTATIONS

Abscesses, bilateral parotid *Dentomaxillofacial Radiology 40:403–414, 2011*

Ascariasis – parotid enlargement, forehead edema *Am J Clin Nutr 30:2117–2121, 1977*

Bungarus caeruleus bite (common krait bite) *Indian J Crit Care Med 22:809–810, 2018*

Cytomegalovirus sialadenitis *J Clin Inf Dis 22:1117–1118, 1996*

Foot and mouth disease

Malaria – nutritional consequence *Am J Clin Nutr 30:2117–2121, 1977*

Mumps *NEJM 371:2018–2027, 2014*

Mycobacterium tuberculosis

Parotitis – recurrent in adults; children *OSOMOPOR Endod 93:221–237, 2002*
　Actinomycosis *Br J Oral Maxillofac Surg 23:128–134, 1985*
　Acute bacterial suppurative parotitis
　Adenovirus parotitis in AIDS – unilateral or bilateral *Rev Soc Bras Med 29:503–506, 1996; Clin Inf Dis 19:1045–1048, 1994*
　Arachnia species
　Candida albicans Acta Otolaryngol 126:334–336, 2006
　Cat scratch disease *Turk Arch Otorhinolaryngol 58:48–51, 2020; Laryngorhinootologie 79:471–477, 2000*
　Chronic recurrent parotitis *J Comput Assist Tomogr 25:269–271, 2001*
　Coxsackie virus

Cytomegalovirus Clin Inf Dis 22:1117–1118, 1996; Arch Otolaryngol Head Neck Surg 120:414–416, 1994
Echo virus
Eikenella corrodens Arch Otolaryngol 109:772–773, 1983
Epstein-Barr virus – recurrent parotitis
Fungal parotitis
Hemophilus influenzae J Rheumatol 6:185–188, 1979
Human immunodeficiency virus
Human T-lymphotrophic virus-1
Influenza virus *J Infect Dis 152:853, 1985*
Leprosy
Lymphadenitis (HIV) *Laryngoscope 99 (6 Pt 1):590–595, 1989*
Measles *Mund Kiefer Gesichtchir 4:249–252, 2000*
Mumps *NEJM 371:2018–1027, 2014; Am J Dis Child 132:678–680, 1978*
Mycobacterium avium, and others *Am J Otolaryngol 16:428–432, 1995*
Mycobacterium tuberculosis Br J Oral Maxillofac Surg 39:320–323, 2001
Parainfluenza virus *South Med J 88:230–231, 1995*
Suppurative, preterminal bacterial (*Staphylococcus aureus*) *NEJM 345:662,*
Torulopsis glabrata J Clin Inf Dis 21:1342–1343, 1995
Treponema pallidum Br J Vener Dis 60:121–122, 1984
Tularemia
Viper snake bite *Asian Pac J Trop Biomed 3:154–155, 2013; J Assoc Physicians India 58:460, 2010*

INFILTRATIVE DISORDERS

Amyloidosis

Diffuse follicular lymphoid hyperplasia

Kimura's disease

Langerhans cell histiocytosis *SAGE Open Med Case Rep April 7, 2014; J Ped Hematol Oncol 26:276–278, 2004*

INFLAMMATORY DISORDERS

Kimura's disease *OSOMOPOR Endod 93:221–237, 2002*

Pancreatitis – acute *J Ped Surg 29:719–722, 1994;*

chronic pancreatitis *Gastroenterol 33:443–446, 1998; Australas Radiol 36:343–346, 1992*

Pneumoparotitis *J Laryngol Otol 106:178–179, 1992*

Recurrent parotitis of childhood

Sarcoid (Heerfordt's syndrome, bilateral parotomegaly, bilateral hilar adenopathy, uveitis) *JAAD 77:809–830, 2017; NEJM 369:458, 2013; Nuklearmedizin 34:47–49, 1995; Proc R Soc Med 68:651–652, 1975; Van Graefe's Arch Clin Exp Ophthalmol 70:254–265, 1909;* giant parotomegaly *Cutis 68:199–200, 2001*

METABOLIC DISORDERS

Acromegaly

Cirrhosis *Gastroenterology 96 (2 Pt 1):510–518, 1989*

Cystic fibrosis

Diabetes mellitus *Braz Dent J 6:131–136, 1995; Oral Surg Oral Med Oral Pathol 52:594–598, 1981; JAMA 232:20, 1975*

Gout *Arch Interam Rheumatol 8:272–278, 1965*

Hypothyroidism

Hyperlipidemia *JAMA 211:2016, 1970*

Pellagra

Starvation, anorexia, bulimia *Postgrad Med J 70:27–30, 1994*

NEOPLASTIC DISORDERS

Kaposi's sarcoma *J Otolaryngol 20:243–246, 1991*

Adnexotropic T-cell lymphoma *JAAD 38:493–497, 1998*

Lymphoepithelioid cysts (AIDS) *JAMA 278:166–167, 1997; Pathologica 82:287–295, 1990; Int J Radiat Oncol Biol Phys 23:1045–1050, 1992; Rheum Dis Clin North Am 17:99–115, 1991; Laryngoscope 98:772–775, 1988;* diffuse infiltrative lymphocytosis syndrome of HIV disease

Lymphoma – Hodgkin's disease *Lin Chung Es Bi Yan Hou Tou Jing Wai Ke Za Zhi 3:1852–1853, 2017;* MALT lymphoma – most frequently observed parotid lymphoma in Sjogren's syndrome and HIV disease *OSOMOPOR Endod 93:221–227, 2002Rev Stomatol Chir Maxillofac 82:7–10, 1981;* granulomatous slack skin *Int J Dermatol 39:374–376, 2000*

Leukemia – acute lymphoblastic leukemia *Natl J Maxillofac Surg 8:55–57, 2017;* chronic myelomonocytic leukemia *JAAD 35:804–807, 1996*

Metastases – gastric signet ring cell carcinoma *Tumor 104:NP10–13, 2018*

Papillary cystadenoma lymphomatosum (Warthin tumor)

Polycystic disease of the parotids *AJNR 16:1128–1131, 1995*

Salivary tumors – bilateral primary salivary tumor (5% of pleomorphic adenomata; papillary cystadenoma lymphomatosum *OSOMOPOR Endod 93:221–237, 2002*

Tumor infiltration (lung)

Waldenstrom's macroglobulinemia *Oral Surg Oral Med Oral Pathol 67:689–693, 1989*

PRIMARY CUTANEOUS DISEASES

Age-related asteatosis with pseudoparotomegaly

Masseter muscle hypertrophy (pseudoparotomegaly) *J Assoc Physicians India 68:83–84, 2020; Dentomaxillofac Radiol 28:52–54, 1999; Br J Oral Maxillofac Surg 37:405–408, 1999*

Scleredema of Buschke *Am J Med 9:707–713, 1950*

Sialectasis *Dentomaxillofac Radiol 22:159–160, 1993*

Sialolithiasis *Am J Dent 13:342–343, 2000*

Sialosis *J Cytol 34:51–52, 2017*

PSYCHOCUTANEOUS DISORDERS

Bulimia *J Drugs in Dermatol 8:577–579, 2009; Arch Otolaryngol Head Neck Surg 119:787–788, 1993;* anorexia nervosa *Clin Radiol 53:623, 1998; Oral Surg Oral Med Oral Pathol 53:567–573, 1982; Lancet 1 (7591):426, 1969*

SYNDROMES

H syndrome *Curr Res Transl Med 67:72–75, 2019*

Hemophagocytic syndrome – personal observation

Lipoid proteinosis – parotitis with parotid gland enlargement *Ped Derm 14:22–25, 1997; Acta DV (Stockh) 53 (Suppl.71):1–56, 1973*

Mikulicz's syndrome

Parana hard skin syndrome

TOXINS

Chronic alcoholism *Ariz Med 28:261–262, 1971*

Vinyl chloride disease *Br Med J 291:1094, 1985*

TRAUMA

Vomiting (Valsalva maneuver) *South Med J 74:251, 1981*

UNILATERAL ENLARGEMENT

AUTOIMMUNE DISORDERS

Sjogren's syndrome *NEJM 371:2018–2027, 2014*

DEGENERATIVE DISORDERS

Aplasia of parotid gland – compensatory hypertrophy due to aplasia of contralateral parotid gland *J Craniofac Surg 25:e265–267, 2014*

DRUG REACTIONS

Anesthesia mumps *Chang Gung Med J 30:453–457, 2007*

INFECTIONS

Actinomycosis

Adenovirus parotitis of AIDS *Clin Inf Dis 19:1045–1048, 1994*

Cryptococcus neoformans Diagn Cytopathol 33:36–38, 2005

Lymphoepithelioid cysts (HIV)

Bacterial sialadenitis

Leprosy

Melioidosis – *Burkholderia pseudomallei* – acute suppurative parotitis in children; pustules or subcutaneous abscesses *JAAD 75:1–16, 2016; JAAD 54:559–578, 2006*

Mumps *NEJM 371:2018–2027, 2014*

Staphylococcus aureus, including MRSA, abscess

Suppurative parotitis (abscess)
    Salmonella parotitis *J Clin Inf Dis 24:1009–1010, 1997*
    Staphylococcus aureus
    Streptococcus pneumonia Case Rep Med 2009:627170

Torulopsis glabrata *Clin Inf Dis 21:1342–1343, 1995*

Tuberculosis *Laryngol Otol 119:311–313, 2005*

Tularemia

INFLAMMATORY DISORDERS

Pneumoparotitis *Head Neck 35:E55–59, 2013*

Rosai-Dorfman disease *J Surg Case Rep June 1, 2012*

Sarcoidosis *Medicine 98:e18172, 2019*

METABOLIC DISORDERS

Acromegaly *J Oral Maxillofac Surg 78:564–567, 2020*

Calculus – with duct obstruction

Sialolithiasis *Spec Case Dentist March 11, 2020*

NEOPLASTIC DISORDERS

Cysts
  Adenolymphoma
  Branchial clefts #1, 2 *Arch Otolaryngol Head Neck Surg 124:291–295, 1998*
  Dermoid *Diagnostic Cytopathol 20:387–388, 1999*
  Hamartoma *Br J Radiol 55:182–188, 1982*
  Mucoepidermoid *Histopathol 33:379–386, 1998*
  Pleomorphic adenoma *J Otolaryngol 30:361–365, 2001*

Facial nerve neuroma

Kaposi's sarcoma – AIDS *Am Surg 64:259–260, 1998*

Lipomata *Dentomaxillofac Radiol 30:235–238, 2001*

Lymphoma *J Laryngol Otol 90:381–392, 1976*; mantle cell lymphoma *J Med Case Rep March 30, 3010*

Masseter hypertrophy *NY State Dent J 76:46–48, 2010*

Metastasis – renal cell carcinoma *Laryngoscope 120:Suppl 4:S128, 2010*

Primary tumor
  Benign (most to least frequent in parotid)
    Oxyphil adenoma *HNO 49:109–117, 2001*
    Pleomorphic adenoma *J Craniofac Surg 24:2197–2198, 2013; Acta Cytol 45:1008–1010, 2001*
    Warthin's tumor (adenolymphoma) *Eur Radiol 11:2472–2478, 2001; Ann Ital Chir 67:537–547, 1996*

Primary parotid tumor
  Malignant (most to least frequent in parotid)
    Acinic cell *HNO Oct 2001; p. 49*
    Adenocarcinoma *J Exp Clin Cancer Res 20:189–194, 2001*
    Adenoid cystic carcinoma *Hinyokika Kiyo 47:785–787, 2001*
    Kaposi's sarcoma

    Metastatic
    Mucoepidermoid carcinoma *Am J Surg Pathol 25:835–845, 2001*
    Oncocytoma *J Laryngol Otol 115:57–59, 2001*
    Primary lymphoma *Leuk Lymphoma 26:49–56, 1997*
    Squamous cell carcinoma *Aust NZ J Surg 71:345–348, 2001*

Rhabdomyosarcoma – parotid gland mass *Cancer 84:245–251, 1998*

TRAUMA

Acute masseteric band, obstructive parotitis *ORL J Otorhinolaryngol Relat Spec 74:12–15, 2012*

Orthodontic parotitis *J Orthod 39:314–316, 2012*

Pierced-ear lymphadenitis

Radiation sialadenitis

VASCULAR LESIONS

Angiolymphoid hyperplasia with eosinophilia *JAAD 74:506–512, 2016*

Infantile hemangiomas – intraparotid hemangiomas; unilateral or bilateral *Sem Cut Med Surg 35:108–116, 2016*

Lemierre's syndrome – swollen red eyelid; due to *Fusobacterium necrophorum;* cavernous sinus thrombophlebitis, carotid artery thromboarteritis, abscess of parotid gland and subperiosteal orbit *NEJM 371:2018–2027, 2014*

Granulomatosis with polyangiitis *J Oral Maxillofac Surg 78:564–567, 2020; Indian J Otolaryngol Head Neck Surg 71 (suppl 1)21–24, 2019; Singapore Med J 54:e196–198, 2013; Int J Oral Maxillofacial Surg 29:450–452, 2000; Am J Med 85 (5):741–742, 1988*

Temporal artery aneurysm

PARTICULATE MATTER/EXFOLIATION

AUTOIMMUNE DISORDERS AND DISEASES OF IMMUNE DYSFUNCTION

Allergic contact dermatitis

Systemic lupus erythematosus

DRUG-INDUCED

Cyclosporine-induced folliculodystrophy – small spicules of vellus hair emanating from follicular papules of face *JAAD 50:310–315, 2004*

Pustular drug eruption

EXOGENOUS AGENTS

Contact dermatitis – irritant

Airborne ragweed dermatitis

Fiberglass dermatitis *JAAD 80:e141–142, 2019; JAAD 80:e157, 2019; Int J Dermatol 40:258–261, 2001; J Formos Med Assoc 92:755–758, 1993*

Residual zinc oxide ointment

INFECTIONS AND INFESTATIONS

Actinomycosis (actinomycetoma) – yellow, white, or red granules *Cutis 60:191–193, 1997;* due to *Nocardia brasiliensis JAAD 62:239–246, 2010*

Black piedra (*Piedraia hortae*) *Clin Dermatol 28:140–145, 2010*

Demodectic frost – white frost of earlobe *JAMA Derm 153:356–357, 2017; Acta DV 84:407–408, 2004; BJD 138:901–903, 1998*

Dermatophytosis, generalized

Desquamation following viral exanthem, drug eruption, scarlet fever, Kawasaki's disease

Lagochilascariasis – contracted by eating undercooked or raw meat; Mexico to South America; worms issuing from the external auditory canal *Am J Trop Med Hyg pii:15–0792, 2016; Clin Inf Dis 63:iv, 2016*

Maggots – wound myiasis; *Cochliomyia hominivorax (*New World screwworm) (Central and South America), *Chrysomya bezziana* (Old World screwworm) (Africa, India, Southeast Asia), *Wohlfahrtia magnifica* (Wohlfart's wound myiasis fly) (Southeastern Europe, southern and Asiatic Russia, North Africa, Middle East), *Lucilia sericata, Phormia regina JAAD 58:907–926, 2008*

Mycetoma – *Pseudallescheria boydii, Acremonium falciforme, Acremonium kiliense, Acremonium recifei, Cylindrocarpon destructans, Fusarium moniliforme, Fusarium solani, Neotestudina rosati, Aspergillus nidulans, Aspergillus flavus, Polycytella hominis* – white and yellow grains; *Actinomadura madurae, Nocardia asteroides* – white grains; *Madurella mycetomatis Exophiala jeanselmei, Madurella grisea, Leptosphaeria tompkinsii, Leptosphaera senegalensis, Corynespora cassilicola, Pyrenochaeta mackinnonii, Pyronochaeta, romeroi, Plenodomus auramii, Curvularia spp,*

Phialophora verrucosa – brown or black grains; *Nocardia brasiliensis* – white or orange grains; *Nocardiopsis dassonvillei* – white or yellow; *Actinomadura pelletieri* – red grains; *Streptomyces somaliensis* – yellow grains *JAAD 53:931–951, 2005; Cutis 60:191–193, 1997;* eumycetoma – *Phaeoacremonium sphinctrophorum* – white grains *JAMA Derm 152: 1063–1065, 2016*

Pediculosis – pubic (nits (pubic hair, eyelashes)), head and body lice *JAMA Derm 155:1416 2019; Cutis 81:109–114, 2008;* body lice in seams of clothing *Cutis 80:397–398, 2007*

Scabies, crusted *AD 124:121–126, 1988*

Trichodysplasia spinulosa (trichodysplasia of immunosuppression) – DNA polyoma virus in renal transplant patient; alopecia, particulate matter, follicular papules, thickened skin, eyebrow alopecia, leonine facies; acneiform eruptions; inflammatory papules and pustules *Ped Derm 36:723–724, 2019; JAMA Derm 154:1342–1343, 2018; AD 148:726–733, 2012; AD 146:871–874, 2010; Ped Derm 27:509–513, 2010; JAAD 60:169–172, 2009; J Cutan Pathol 34:721–725, 2007; AD 142:1643–1648, 2006; JAAD 52:540–541, 2005; JAAD 50:310–315, 2004; J Invest Dermatol Symp Proc 4:268–271, 1999; Hautarzt 46:871–874, 1995*

Trichomycosis axillaris (*Corynebacterium tenuis*) (*C. propinquim*) – yellow concretions *JAMA Derm 151:1023–1024, 2015; NEJM 369:1735, 2013*

White piedra – *Trichosporon Clin Dermatol 28:140–145, 2010*

INFLAMMATORY DISORDERS

Erosive pustular dermatosis of the scalp – with urate-like crystals *Case Rep Dermatol Med 2017:1536434*

METABOLIC

Tumoral calcinosis – personal observation

Crohn's disease – with phrynoderma *Ped Derm 32:234–236, 2015*

Gouty tophi

Hypovitaminosis A (phrynoderma) *Ped Derm 22:60–63, 2005; AD 120:919–921, 1984*

Methylmalonic acidemia, cobalamin C type – desquamation *AD 133:1563–1566, 1997*

Miliaria crystallina

Monoclonal gammopathy – spicules *JAAD 33:346–351, 1995*

Porphyria cutanea tarda – calcinosis cutis of scalp – personal observation

Uremic frost *Kidney International 73:790, 2008*

Urostomy site – encrustations of crystals of phosphates and uric acid

NEOPLASTIC DISEASES

Acral angioosteoma cutis – tiny spicules of woven bone *Indian J DV Leprol 84:685–686, 2018; Am J Dermatopathol 32:477–478, 2010*

Lymphoma – cutaneous T-cell lymphoma, spiky follicular *Cut Pathol 42:164–172, 2015*

Multiple myeloma with cryoglobulinemia – follicular hyperkeratotic spicules (cyto-keratotic spicules of nose) *Dermatol Online J Oct 15, 2019; JAAD 77:1145–1158, 2017; JAAD 32:834–839, 1995; AD 126:509–513, 1990; AD 121:795–798, 1985;* monoclonal protein with yellowish-white hair casts of eyelashes and scalp hair and cutaneous spicules of nose *AD 142:1665–1666, 2006; JAAD*

49:736–740, 2003; follicular spicules associated with myeloma with monoclonal type 1 cryoglobulins *AD 145:479–484, 2009*

Nevus corniculatus *JAAD 31;157–190, 1994*

Perforating follicular hybrid cyst (pilomatrixoma and steatocystoma) of inner eyelid (tarsus) – chalky material *JAAD 48:S33–34, 2003*

PARANEOPLASTIC

Paraneoplastic hyperkeratosis *JAAD 31:157–190, 1994*

Skin spicules – paraneoplastic filiform seborrheic keratoses associated with marginal zone B-cell lymphoma *JAAD 60:852–855, 2009*

PHOTODERMATOSES

Photodermatitis of AIDS

PRIMARY CUTANEOUS DISEASES

Darier's disease

Epidermolysis bullosa superficialis resembling peeling skin syndrome *AD 125:633–638, 1989*

Hair casts (peripilar hair casts, pseudonits) *JAAD 75:e147–148, 2016; Cutis 60:251–252, 1997*

Ichthyosiform eruption

Idiopathic follicular hyperkeratotic spicules *Case Rep Dermatol 11:278–285, 2019*

Lichen nitidus, generalized

Lichen spinulosis in AIDS *JAAD 26:1013–1014, 1992*

Multiple milia

Multiple minute digitate hyperkeratosis *AD 144:1051–1056, 2008; BJD 142:1044–1046, 2000; JAAD 18:431–436, 1988;* status-post radiotherapy *Clin Exp Dermatol 11:646–649, 1986*

Pityriasis capitis (dandruff)

Pityriasis rubra pilaris with follicular spines *JAAD 23:526–527, 1990;* spiny hyperkeratoses

Psoriasis – personal observation

Pustular psoriasis

Seborrheic dermatitis

Spiny hyperkeratosis *JAAD 31:157–190, 1994*

Subcorneal pustular dermatosis

Tinea amientacea *Clin Exp Dermatol 2:137–144, 1977*

PSYCHOCUTANEOUS DISEASE

Delusions of parasitosis – "infesting organisms" brought to physician

Morgellon's disease – "protruding fibers or threads" *Clin Dermatol 36:714–718, 2018;* match box sign *Acta DV 90:517–519, 2010*

SYNDROMES

Kawasaki's disease

Keratosis-ichthyosis- deafness (KID) syndrome – spiny follicular plugs of nose

Continual skin peeling syndrome *AD 122:71–75, 1986; BJD 81:191–195, 1969; AD 121:545–546, 1985; Cutis 53:255–257, 1994*

TRAUMA

Radiation therapy – keratotic miliaria following radiotherapy *AD 124:855–856, 1988*

Traction alopecia – hair casts as a sign of traction alopecia *Ped Derm 30:614–615, 2013; BJD 163:1353–1355, 2010*

PEDUNCULATED (POLYPOID) LESIONS

JAAD 31:235–240, 1994

CONGENITAL LESIONS

Accessory scrotum with perineal lipoma *Ped Derm 29:521–524, 2012*

Accessory tragi – accessory tragus at nasal vestibule in nasal rim *Ped Derm 37:383–384, 2020*

Anterior cephalocele – intranasal polypoid lesion with broad nasal bridge *Ped Derm 32:161–170, 2015*

Bronchogenic cyst with papilloma *JAAD 11:367–371, 1984;* cutaneous bronchogenic cyst of abdominal wall *Pathol Int 51:970–973, 2001*

Congenital accessory skin appendage of the nasal columella *Surg Radiol Anat 40:923–926, 2018*

Congenital cartilaginous rests of the neck (wattles) *Dermatol Surg 31:1349–1350, 2005; Cutis 58:293–294, 1996*

Congenital pigmented nevus with cartilaginous differentiation – congenital pigmented nevus with giant pedunculated pink tumor *Ped Derm 30:501–502, 2013*

Ectopic immature renal tissue – pedunculated sacral mass in newborn *Ped Derm 36:542–543, 2019*

Epulis – soft nodule of gingival margin or alveolar mucosa *Pediodontics 6:277–299, 1986*

Human tail *Curr Prob in Dermatol 13:249–300, 2002;* vestigial tail *Arch J Dis Child 104:72–73, 1962*

Myxo-papillary ependymal rest – skin-colored pedunculated papule near gluteal cleft; heterotopic neuroglial tissue *JAAD 65:851–854, 2011*

Omphalomesenteric duct remnant – violaceous polypoid papule in umbilical depression *SKINMed 5:154–155, 2006*

Persistent vitelline duct and polyp – umbilical polyp *Dermatologica 150:111–115, 1975*

Rhabdomyomatous mesenchymal hamartoma (striated muscle hamartoma) (congenital) – associated with Dellemann's syndrome – multiple skin tag-like lesions of infancy *Ped Derm 37:64–68, 2020; Ped Derm 16:65–67, 1999; Ped Derm 15:274–276, 1998;* red vascular polypoid mass *Ped Derm 26:753–755, 2009;* differentiate from disorganization syndrome – filiform worm-like projections, syndactyly, popliteal pterygium, polydactyly, cleft lip/palate; ear abnormalities *Ped Derm 24:90–92, 2007; J Med Genet 26:417–420, 1989;* pedunculated papule associated with a midline cervical cleft *AD 141:1161–1166, 2005*

DRUGS

Dabrafenib (BRAF inhibitor) – acrochordons *JAMA Derm 150:575–576, 2014*

INFECTIONS

Bacillary angiomatosis (*Bartonella henselae*) *J Clin Inf Dis 21 (Suppl 1):S99–102, 1995*

Bartonella henselae-related pseudoangiomatous papillomatosis of the tongue accompanying graft vs. host disease; yellow-pink pseudomembranous pedunculated vegetations of the tongue *BJD 157:174–178, 2007*

Condyloma acuminate – personal observation

Molluscum contagiosum in a soft fibroma *Cutis 61:153–154, 1998*

Phaeohyphomycosis (*Veronaea botryose*) – multilobulated, pedunculated *Mycopathologica 175:497–503, 2013*

Pneumocystis, cutaneous *Ann Int Med 106:396–398, 1987;* polyps within external auditory canal *Am J Med 85:250–252, 1988*

Rhinosporidiosis (*Rhinosporidium seeberi*) – intranasal and conjunctival red polypoid lesions *Indian J Radiol Imaging 23:212–218, 2013; An Bras Dermatol 86:795–796, 2011; JAAD 53:931–951, 2005*

Schistosomiasis – perianal polyps; *Schistosoma mansoni* – anal fissure with multilobulated giant anal polyp *AD 144:950–952, 2008*

Syphilis – condyloma lata of buttock *JAMA Derm 335–336, 2015*

Verruga peruana (*Bartonella bacilliformis*) – Oroya fever; red papules in crops become nodular, hemangiomatous or pedunculated; face, neck, extremities, mucosal lesions *Ann Rev Microbiol 35:325–338, 1981*

Verrucae vulgaris

INFILTRATIVE DISORDERS

Cutaneous focal mucinosis *J Dermatol 44:335–338, 2017*

Juvenile xanthogranuloma *Dis Chest 50:325–329, 1966;* finger-like pedunculated papule *Ped Derm 24:576–577, 2007;* scalp *Am J Dermatopathol 39:773–775, 2017*

Langerhans cell histiocytosis – polypoid involvement of external auditory canal; *Curr Prob Derm VI Jan/Feb 1994; Clin Exp Derm 11:183–187, 1986; JAAD 13:481–496, 1985*

Verruciform xanthoma *AD 138:689–694, 2002;* verruciform xanthoma of scrotum – pedunculated red or yellow cauliflower-like appearance *BJD 150:161–163, 2004; J Dermatol 16:397–401, 1989*

Xanthoma disseminatum (Montgomery's syndrome) – red-yellow-brown skin tag-like papules of axilla *JAMA Derm 152:715–716, 2016*

INFLAMMATORY DISORDERS

Crohn's disease – perianal skin tags *Ped Derm 23:43–48, 2006*

Fibrous umbilical polyp – fasciitis-like proliferation; early childhood; male predominance *Am J Surg Pathol 25:1438–1442, 2001*

METABOLIC DISEASES

Calcinosis cutis – scrotal calcinosis, polypoid *South Med J 89:896–897, 1996;* subepidermal calcified nodule *Ped Derm 18:238–240, 2001*

Crohn's disease – perianal polypoid lesions (pseudo-acrochordons) *JAAD 68:189–209, 2013; Int J Dermatol 39:616–618, 2000; JAAD 36:697–704, 1997*

Endometriosis, umbilical – reddish-brown polypoid nodule within umbilicus *Gynecol Endocrinol 18:114–116, 2004*

NEOPLASTIC LESIONS

Acquired digital fibrokeratoma *Dermatol Online J 14:10, 2008; Cutis 79:129–132, 2007; AD 124:1559–1564, 1988; JAAD 12:816–821, 1985*

Acquired fibrokeratoma – pedunculated lesion of the foot *Dermatol Online J Sept 15, 2017*

Acrochordon (skin tag); normal finding *Dermatologica 174:180–183, 1987;* giant lumbar polypoid tumor with bullae *Acta DV Croat 27:127–128, 2019*

Associations with multiple acrochordons:
Acanthosis nigricans with insulin resistance *Indian J Dermatol 65:112–117, 2020*
Acromegaly *Clin Dermatol 24:256–259, 2006*
Aicardi-Gouteris syndrome – infantile spasms, agenesis of corpus callosum, chorioretinal lacunae; multiple nevi, skin tags, hemangiomas, angiosarcoma *Am J Med Genet A 138:254–258, 2005*
Bannayan-Riley-Ruvalcaba syndrome *JAAD 53:639–643, 2005*
Beare-Stevenson cutis gyrate syndrome – corrugated skin furrows, acanthosis nigricans, craniofacial anomalies, skin tags, prominent umbilical stump *Am J Med Genet 44:82–89, 1992*
Birt-Hogg-Dube syndrome *Am J Clin Dermatol 19:87–101, 2018*
Cowden's syndrome – personal observation
Crohn's disease – perianal skin tags *Br J Surg 91:801–814, 2004*
Duane anomaly, familial and urogenital abnormalities with bisatellited marker derived from chromosome 22 – Duane retraction syndrome – congenital cranial dysinnervation disorder with paradoxical lateral rectus muscle innervation of the affected eye by aons meant to innervate the ipsilateral medial rectus muscle (resultant varying degrees of cocontraction); sensorineural deafness and preauricular skin tags *Am J Med Genet 47:925–930, 1993*
Familial idiopathic fibroepithelial skin tags
Multiple basaloid follicular hamartoma syndrome – chondrosarcoma, acrochordons, and seborrheic keratosis *BJD 146:1068–1070, 2002*
Nevoid basal cell carcinoma syndrome *JAAD 44:789–794, 2001*
Obesity – metabolic syndrome *JAAD 81:1037–1057, 2019; JAAD 56:901–916, 2007*
Oculocerebrocutaneous syndrome – orbital cyst, cerebral malformations, skin tags, focal hypoplasia skin lesions *Am J Ophthalmol 99:142–148, 1985*
Sign of Leser-Trelat *NEJM 317:1582–1587, 1987*
Tuberous sclerosis – pancreatic islet-cell tumors and acrochordons; *TSC2* mutations *J Eur Acad DV 31:e507–508, 2017; Am J Med Genet A 140:1669–1672, 2006*

Adenoma of anogenital mammary-like glands – pedunculated; lobulated, tan-brown or gray-pink or white papules or nodules of vulva or perianal area; may ulcerate *JAAD 57:896–898, 2007; Breast J 9:113–116, 2003; J Reprod Med 47:949–951, 2002; Eur J Gynaecol Oncol 23:21–24, 2002; Gynecol Oncol 73:155–159, 1999*

Adnexal polyp, neonatal – firm, pink, polyp, 1 mm; near nipple; resolve in few days *BJD 92:659–662, 1975*

Aggressive angiomyxoma – vulvar, perineal, pelvic, scrotal polypoid masses *JAAD 58:S40–41, 2008; JAAD 38:143–175, 1998*

Angiomyofibroblastoma of vulva *BJD 157:189–191, 2007*

Angiomyxoma, superficial – exophytic nodule of scalp *JAMA Derm 149:751–756, 2013;* pink polypoid scrotal mass; may be associated with Carney complex *Ped Derm 28:200–201, 2011*

Apocrine acrosyringeal keratosis arising in syringocystadenoma papilliferum *BJD 142:543–547, 2000*

Apocrine gland carcinoma *Am J Med 115:677–679, 2003*

Atypical fibroxanthoma *AD 143:653–658, 2007*

Basal cell carcinomas – of buttock *J Derm Surg Oncol 11:115–117, 1985;* skin tag-like lesions in children with nevoid basal cell carcinoma syndrome *JAAD 47:792–794, 2002; JAAD 44:789–794, 2001;* perineal in adult with nevoid basal cell carcinoma syndrome *JAAD 57:S36–37, 2007;* giant polypoid basal cell carcinoma *Cutis 58:289–292, 1996;* polypoid perianal basal cell carcinoma *J Dermatol 31:51–55, 2004*

Basaloid tumors

Clear cell acanthoma *Am J Dermatopathol 12:393–395, 1990;* polypoid lesion of scalp *Cutis 67:149–151, 2001;* polypoid pigmented giant or cystic clear cell acanthoma *Dermatol Online J July 15, 2018*

Cutaneous hamartoma of adnexa and mesenchyma – skin tag-like papule *Ped Derm 16:65–67, 1999*

Cylindroma *Am J Dermatopathol 17:260–265, 1995;* dome shaped pedunculated cylindromas in Brooke-Spiegler syndrome *Indian J DV Leprol 74:632–634, 2008*

Dendritic fibromyxolipoma – skin colored pedunculated giant tumor; differential diagnosis includes solitary fibrous tumor, spindle cell lipoma, myxolipoma, myxoid liposarcoma *AD 144:795–800, 2008*

Dermal dendrocytic hamartoma – pedunculated red nodule with stubby hairs *JAAD 32:318–321, 1995*

Dermatofibroma *JAAD 30:714–718, 1994;* pseudosarcomatous dermatofibroma *AD 88:276–280, 1963;* atypical polypoid dermatofibroma *JAAD 24:561–565, 1991;* aneurysmal benign fibrous histiocytoma presenting as giant acrochordon *Indian Dermatol Online J 6:436–438, 2005*

Dermatofibrosarcoma protuberans *JAAD 49:1139–1141, 2003*

Eccrine nevus – perianal skin tag *AD 141:515–520, 2005; JAAD 51:301–304, 2004;* polypoid eccrine nevus – coccygeal papule overlying a depression *Arch Pathol Lab Med 143:890–892, 2019; BJD 157:614–615, 2007*

Eccrine porocarcinoma *JAAD 49:S252–254, 2003; JAAD 35:860–864, 1996; AD 131:211–216, 1995*

Eccrine poroma *AD 135:463–468, 1999;* blue-black pedunculated tumor of chin *BJD 152:1070–1072, 2005*

Eccrine syringofibroadenoma – reactive peristomal eccrine syringofibroadenoma – polypoid *Int J Surg Pathol 11:61–63, 2003*

Epidermal nevus

Epidermoid cyst

Epithelioid cell histiocytoma – pink polypoid leg nodule *BJD 172:1427–1429, 2015;* red pedunculated papule *AD 144:105–110, 2008*

Fibroepithelial polyp of gingiva (epulides) *Periodontics 6:277–299, 1986*

Fibroepithelioma of Pinkus – skin colored or red pedunculated nodule of trunk, groin, or thigh *BJD 150:1208–1209, 2004;* gray-brown papule or plaque; skin colored plaque; pedunculated, polypoid; pink papule *AD 142:1318–1322, 2006; JAAD 52:168–169, 2005*

Fibrolipoma – personal observation

Fibroma, oral – traumatic fibroma, oral polyp, focal intraoral fibrous dysplasia

Fibrosarcoma/spindle cell sarcoma

Fibrous hamartoma of infancy – skin tag-like papule *Ped Derm 16:65–67, 1999*

Follicular hamartoma with trichofolliculoma-like tumor with multiple trichogenic tumors *J Dermatol 18:465–471, 1991*

Folliculosebaceous cystic hamartoma – skin colored papule or nodule of central face or scalp; pedunculated or dome-shaped and umbilicated *BJD 157:833–835, 2007; Clin Exp Dermatol 31:68–79, 2006; AD 139:803–808, 2003; JAAD 34:77–81, 1996; Am J Dermatopathol 13:213–220, 1991; J Cutan Pathol 7:394–403, 1980;* skin tag-like papule *Ped Derm 16:65–67, 1999*

Giant folliculosebaceous cystic hamartoma – skin colored exophytic papules *BJD 160:454–456, 2009; AD 141:1035–1040, 2005; Am J Dermatopathol 13:213–220, 1991*

Granular cell tumor (granular cell myoblastoma), including granular cell tumor of the gingiva (congenital epulis) *Indian Dermatol Online J 7:390–392, 2016; Cutis 75:21,23–24, 2005; Ped Derm 15:318–320, 1998;* granular cell variant of epithelioid cell histiocytoma *Am J Dermatopathol 34:766–769, 2012*

Hair follicle nevus (hair follicle hamartoma) – pedunculated papule *Ped Derm 24:555–556, 2007; Cutis 32:79–82, 1983*

Kaposi's sarcoma *AD 141:1311–1316, 2005*

Leiomyoma of scrotum *SKINmed 9:323–325, 2011; Urology 39:376–379, 1992;* congenital leiomyoma of the heel *Ped Derm 3:158–160, 1986;* pedunculated congenital leiomyoma of tongue *Int J Pediatr Otorhinolaryngol 29:139–145, 1994*

Leiomyosarcoma – blue-black; also red, brown, yellow or hypopigmented *JAAD 46:477–490, 2002; J D Surg Oncol 9:283–287, 1983*

Lipofibroma *J Dermatol 27:288–290, 2000; JAAD 31:235–240, 1994*

Lymphoma – post-transplant primary cutaneous CD30 and CD56 ALCL polypoid scalp mass *Arch Pathol Lab Med 128:e96–99, 2004*

Median raphe cyst of the perineum – perianal polyp *Pathol 28:201–202, 1996*

Melanocytic nevus – compound nevi; congenital dermal melanocytic nevus *JAAD 49:732–735, 2003*

Melanoma *Derm Surg 26:127–129, 2002; Mayo Clin Proc 72:273–279, 1997; J Dermatol 22:527–529, 1995; Ann Plast Surg 5:432–435, 1980; Surg Gynecol Obstet 106:586–594, 1958;* amelanotic melanoma *AD 138:1245–1250, 2002;* vulvar melanoma – labia minora most common, then labia majora and clitoris; anorectal melanoma *JAAD 56:828–834, 2007;* congenital pigment synthesizing melanoma of the scalp (animal type melanoma); black, pedunculated, ulcerated scalp nodule *JAAD 71:366–375, 2014; JAAD 62:324–329, 2010;* acrochordon-like metastatic melanoma *AD 148:136–137, 2012;* polypoid lesion of anorectum, penis, sinonasal distribution *JAAD 71:366–375, 2014;* primary dermal melanoma – pedunculated pink papule, dark macule, blue pigmented nevus, dome-shaped hemorrhagic papule, changing pigmented nevus *JAAD 71:1083–1091, 2014;* ulcerated pedunculated *Am J Dermatopathol 39:593–598, 2017*

Melanotrichoblastoma – pedunculated pigmented papule *Cutis 100:243–246, 2017*

Merkel cell carcinoma – eyelid papule *Eyelid and Conjunctival Tumors, Shields JA and Shields CL, Lippincott Williams and Wilkins, 1999, p.101;* pedunculated telangiectatic *Indian J Dermatol 58:243, 2013*

Metastases – renal cell carcinoma; *Cancer 19:162–168, 1966;* clear cell type renal cell carcinoma *Cureus 11:e5021, 2019*

Mucinous nevus *BJD 148:1064–1066, 2003*

Cutaneous syncytial myoepithelioma *Am J Surg Pathol 37:710–718, 2013*

Myxoma – solitary cutaneous myxoma *JAAD 43:377–379, 2000*

Myxofibrosarcoma – presenting as large skin tag *Hautarzt 63:719–723, 22012*

Nasal glioma *J Postgrad Med 45:15–17, 1999*

Neuroblastoma *Dermatol Therapy 18:104–116, 2005*

Neurofibromas – including plexiform neurofibroma; neurofibromatosis *Eyelid and Conjunctival Tumors, Shields JA and Shields CL, Lippincott Williams and Wilkins, 1999, p.97;* nipple areolar complex neurofibromas *Case Rep Pathol Sept 6, 2018:6702561*

Nevus lipomatosis superficialis *Med J Armed Forces India 72:67–70, 2016;* pedunculated cerebriform nodule *Ped Derm 36:152–153, 2019;* skin tag-like papule *Ped Derm 16:65–67, 1999*

Nevus sebaceus – pink pedunculated nodule of scalp *Ped Derm 36:154–155, 2019; Ped Derm 25:355–358, 2008;* nevus sebaceous with hair collar sign -congenital pedunculated lesion of scalp with surrounding long dark hair *Ped Derm 27:525–526, 2010;* papillomatous pedunculated nevus sebaceus *BJD 176:204–208, 2017*

Olfactory neuroblastoma, pigmented – pigmented polypoid lesion of nasal cavity; confused with mucosal melanoma *AD 144:270–272, 2008*

Osseous choristoma of the tongue *Mol Clin Oncol 8:242–245, 2018; Br J Oral Surg 25:79–82, 1987*

Pilomatrixoma – polypoid lesion *Ped Derm 18:498–500, 2001;* giant pilomatrixoma *BJD 155:208–210, 2006; Ann Plast Surg 41:337–338, 1998*

Plantar fibromatosis *Foot Ankle Int 39:751–757, 2018*

Pleomorphic fibromas – polypoid *J Cutan Pathol 40:379–384, 2013*

Porocarcinoma *BJD 152:1051–1055, 2005*

Porokeratotic eccrine and ostial dermal duct nevus – linear, filiform, hyperkeratotic lesion *JAMA Derm 149:869–870, 2013*

Poroma *JAAD 44:48–52, 2001*

Primitive myxoid mesenchymal tumor of infancy – red pedunculated papules within a red plaque *Soc Ped Dermatol Annual Meeting, July, 2006; Am J Surg Pathol 30:388–394, 2006*

Pseudosarcomatous polyp, cutaneous *Ann Diagn Pathol 12:440–444, 2008; AD 139:93–98, 2003*

Rhabdomyomas – skin tag–like papule *Ped Derm 16:65–67, 1999*

Rhabdomyosarcoma – pedunculated tumor arising in a giant congenital melanocytic nevus *Ped Derm 31:584–587, 2014; Cutis 73:39–43, 2004*

Sebaceous adenoma *J Cutan Pathol 22:185–187, 1995;* pedunculated vascular nodule of dorsal penis *JAAD 57:S42–43, 2007*

Sebaceous carcinoma *JAAD 61:549–560, 2009; Dermatol Ther 21:459–466, 2008*

Seborrheic keratosis, including dermatosis papulosa nigra – polypoid, pedunculated *Indian J Sex Transm Dis AIDS 36:77–79, 2015; J Clin Aesthet Dermatol 13:17–19, 2020*

Soft fibroma *Dermatology 199:167–168, 1999*

Spitz nevus *J Cutan Pathol 38:747–752, 2011; BJD 142:128–132, 2000; Great Cases from the South; AAD Meeting; March 2000*

Squamous cell carcinoma – anal squamous cell carcinoma in situ – skin tag *J Clin Inf Dis 21:603–607, 1995;* squamous cell carcinoma *Curr Probl Cancer 4:1–44, 1980;* vulvar squamous cell carcinoma – papular and polypoid lesions; pedunculated red tumor of labia majora *BJD 171:7709–785, 2014;* verrucous white cobblestoned plaque *JAAD 66:867–880, 2012*

Stewart-Treves angiosarcoma – reddish-blue macules and/or nodules which become polypoid; pachydermatous changes, blue nodules, telangiectasias, palpable subcutaneous mass, ulcer *JAAD 67:1342–1348, 2012*

Syringocystadenoma papilliferum – pedunculated nodule of trunk, shoulders, axillae, or genitalia *AD 140:1393–1398, 2004; AD*

71:361–372, 1955; multiple nodules of legs associated with skin ulcers, burn scars, diabetic neuropathy, venous stasis

Trichoepithelioma *JAAD 37:881–883, 1997;* giant solitary trichoepithelioma *AD 120:797–798, 1984*

Undifferentiated sarcoma – giant pendulous cystic lesion of cheek *Soc Ped Derm Annual Meeting, July 2005*

Verrucifor xanthoma – pedunculated nodule *J Cutan Pathol 47:475–478, 2020*

Verrucous carcinoma of umbilicus *AD 141:779–784, 2005*

PARANEOPLASTIC DISORDERS

Eruptive skin tags associated with metastatic carcinoma – personal observation

Florid cutaneous papillomatosis – related to acanthosis nigricans and sign of Leser-Trelat

PRIMARY CUTANEOUS DISEASES

Ainhum *NY State Med J 81:1779–1781, 1981; J Am Podiatr Assoc 61:44–54, 1971*

Angiolymphoid hyperplasia with eosinophilia – personal observation

Infantile perianal pyramidal protrusion (anomalous anal papillae) – polypoid or filiform projections at the anus; almost exclusively in girls; in midline just anterior to anus; differential diagnosis includes hemorrhoids, rectal prolapse, skin tags, sexual abuse, sentinel tag of anal fissure, inflammatory bowel disease, perineal midline malformation, hemangioma *JAAD 54:1046–1049, 2006; Ped Derm 22:151–152, 2005; BJD 151:229, 2004; Ped Derm 19:15–18, 2002; J Pediatr 38:468–471, 1951;* vulvar pyramidal protrusion associated with lichen sclerosus *JAAD 56:S49–50, 2007*

Kerinokeratosis papulosa (waxy keratoses of childhood) *JAAD 50:S84–85, 2004; Clin Exp Dermatol 19:173–176, 1994*

Rudimentary polydactyly *BJD 66:402–408, 1954*

SYNDROMES

Adams-Oliver syndrome – autosomal dominant; terminal transverse limb anomalies, aplasia cutis congenita, cutis marmorata telangiectatica congenita, severe growth retardation, aplasia cutis congenita of knee, short palpebral fissures, dilated scalp veins, simple pinnae, skin tags on toes, hemangioma, undescended testes, supernumerary nipples, hypoplastic optic nerve, congenital heart defects *Ped Derm 24:651–653, 2007*

Amnion rupture malformation sequence (amniotic band syndrome) – congenital ring constrictions and intrauterine amputations; secondary syndactyly, polydactyly; distal lymphedema *JAAD 32:528–529, 1995; Am J Med Genet 42:470–479, 1992*

Cutis 44:64–66, 1989

Bannayan-Riley-Ruvalcaba syndrome (macrocephaly and subcutaneous hamartomas) (lipomas and hemangiomas) – autosomal dominant; multiple skin tags *JAAD 68:189–209, 2013; JAAD 53:639–643, 2005; AD 132:1214–1218, 1996; AD 128:1378–1386, 1992; Eur J Ped 148:122–125, 1988;* lipoangiomas (perigenital pigmented macules, macrocephaly) *AD 128:1378–1386, 1992;* lipomas in Ruvalcaba-Myhre-Smith syndrome *Ped Derm 5:28–32, 1988*

Basaloid follicular hamartoma syndrome – autosomal dominant; acrochordons, milia, comedone-like lesions, dermatosis papulosa nigra, skin tag-like lesions, hypotrichosis, multiple skin-colored, red, and hyperpigmented papules of the face in periorificial distribution, neck chest, back, proximal extremities, and eyelids; syndrome includes milia-like cysts, comedones, sparse scalp hair, palmar pits, and parallel bands of papules of the neck (zebra stripes); hypohidrosis *AD 144:933–938, 2008; Cutis 78:42–46, 2006; JAAD 49:698–705, 2003; BJD 146:1068–1070, 2002; JAAD 45:644–645, 2001; JAAD 43:189–206, 2000; JAAD 27:237–240, 1992*

Beare-Stevenson cutis gyrata syndrome – skin tags, localized redundant skin of scalp, forehead, face, neck, palms, and soles, acanthosis nigricans, craniofacial anomalies, anogenital anomalies, and large umbilical stump *Am J Med Genet 44:82–89, 1992*

Birt-Hogg-Dube syndrome – pedunculated lip papules on mucosal surface; thyroid nodules or cysts; mutation in *FLCN BJD 162:527–537, 2010*

Carney complex (NAME/LAMB syndrome) – autosomal dominant; pedunculated pink or skin colored myxomas, multiple lentigines of upper lips, genitalia, conjunctivae, inner and outer canthi, vulva, melanocytic nevi, small blue nevi, psammomatous schwannoma, cardiac myxomas, testicular Sertoli cell tumors, gynecomastia, myxoid breast fibroadenomas, pituitary adenomas, thyroid disease, Cushing's syndrome due to primary pigmented nodular adrenocortical disease; PRKAR1A (protein kinase A type-1 regulatory gene); lentigines fade with time *JAAD 59:801–810, 2008; Molec Genet Metab 78:83, 2003; J Clin Endocrinol 86:4041, 2001; Curr Prob in Derm VII:143–198, 1995; Medicine 64:270–283, 1985;* conjunctival lentigines *JAAD 42:145, 2000*; epithelioid blue nevus and psammomatous melanotic schwannoma *Semin Diagn Pathol 15:216–224, 1998; J Clin Invest 97:699–705, 1996; Dermatol Clin 13:19–25, 1995; JAAD 10:72–82, 1984*

Cowden's syndrome – acrochordons – personal observation

Costello syndrome – warty papules around nose and mouth, legs, perianal skin; loose skin of neck, hands, and feet, thick, redundant palmoplantar surfaces, hypoplastic nails, short stature, craniofacial abnormalities *Eur J Dermatol 11:453–457, 2001; Am J Med Genet 82:187–193, 1999; JAAD 32:904–907, 1995; Aust Paediat J 13:114–118, 1977*

Cutaneous segmental heterotopic meningeal tissue with multifocal neural and mesenchymal hamartomas – skin colored pedunculated papules of forehead, eyelids, scalp, ala nasi; hypertrichotic heterotopic meningeal nodule *BJD 156:1047–1050, 2007*

Delleman syndrome (oculocerebrocutaneous syndrome) – pedunculated facial papules and atrophic patches of neck; accessory tragi and aplasia cutis congenital; pedunculated typically hamartomatous or nodular skin appendages *Am J Med Genet C Semin Med Genet 178:414–422, 2018; AD 147:345–350, 2011; J Med Genet 25:773–778, 1988;* autosomal dominant with variable penetrance, multiple craniofacial skin tags, striated muscle hamartomas, orbital cysts (exophthalmia or microphthalmia), cerebral malformations, periorbital or postauricular appendages, focal dermal hypoplasia and aplasia (aplasia cutis congenita), rib defects, psychomotor retardation, seizures, skull defects; no ear abnormalities *Clin Genet 19:191–198, 1981*

Disorganization syndrome – filiform worm-like projections, syndactyly, popliteal pterygium, polydactyly, cleft lip/palate; ear abnormalities *Ped Derm 24:90–92, 2007; J Med Genet 26:417–420, 1989*

Encephalocraniocutaneous lipomatosis – polypoid and papular lesions of scalp and face; alopecia, scalp nodules, skin colored nodules, facial and eyelid papules – lipomas and lipofibromas; unilateral or bilateral skin colored or yellow domed papules or nodules of scalp (hairless plaque), head, and neck; ipsilateral cranial and facial asymmetry, cranial and ocular abnormalities, spasticity, mental retardation *JAAD 37:102–104, 1998; JAAD*

32:387–389, 1995; Ped Derm 10:164–168, 1993; Arch Neurol 22:144–155, 1970

Epidermal nevus syndrome – papillomatous epidermal nevi; linear arrays of pigmented papillomas *Curr Probl Pediatr 6:3–56, 1975;* pedunculated eyelid papules *JAAD 50:957–961, 2004*

Familial idiopathic fibroepithelial skin tags

Goldenhar syndrome (oculo-auricular-vertebral spectrum) *Syndromes of the Head and Neck, p.641–649, 1990*

Goltz's syndrome – raspberry-like papillomas; mutation in PORCN gene (encodes transmembrane endoplasmic reticulum proteins that target WNT signaling proteins

Infantile myofibromatosis – skin tag-like papule *Australas J Dermatol 41:156–161, 2000; Ped Derm 16:65–67, 1999;* giant necrotic pedunculated nodule *Ped Derm 27:29–33, 2010*

Juvenile hyaline fibromatosis – pearly white papules of face and neck; larger papules and nodules around nose, behind ears, on fingertips, multiple subcutaneous nodules of scalp, trunk, and extremities, papillomatous perianal papules; joint contractures, skeletal lesions, gingival hyperplasia, stunted growth

Muir-Torre syndrome – sebaceous adenoma, sebaceous epithelioma – personal observation

Multiple endocrine neoplasia syndrome (MEN I) – angiofibromas of vermilion border; facial angiofibromas, lipomas, abdominal collagenomas, cutis verticis gyrate, pedunculated skin tags, acanthosis nigricans, red gingival papules, confetti-like hypopigmented macules; café au lait macules; gingival papules; primary hyperparathyroidism with hypercalcemia, kidney stones, parathyroid, pituitary, pancreatic tumors; prolactinoma, gastrinoma, bilateral adrenal hyperplasia; mutation in menin, a nuclear protein involved in cell cycle regulation and proliferation *JAAD 61:319–324, 2009; J Clin Endocrinol Metab 89:5328–5336, 2004; AD 133:853–857, 1997;* pedunculated eruptive collagenomas *AD 148:1317–1322, 2012*

Neurofibromatosis –*JAAD 74:231–244, 2016; NEJM 365:2020, 2011*

Nevoid basal cell carcinoma syndrome – acrochordons (acrochordon-like basal cell carcinomas) *JAAD 60:857–861, 2009;* as presenting sign *JAAD 44:789–794, 2001*

Treacher-Collins syndrome – skin tags *Am J Med Genet 27:359–372,. 1987*

Tuberous sclerosis – pedunculated fibromas of the neck and axillae *JAAD 46:161–183, 2002*

Trisomy 13 – aplasia cutis congenita of scalp with holoprosencephaly, eye anomalies, cleft lip and/or palate, polydactyly, port wine stain of forehead *Am J Dis Child 112:502–517, 1966*

TRAUMA

Amputation neuroma *AD 108:223–225, 1973*

Frictional hypertrophy in bedridden patient – personal observation

VASCULAR DISEASES

Arteriovenous malformation *AD 143:1043–1045, 2007*

Hemangioma, proliferative

Hemangiopericytoma *J Cutan Pathol 35:748–751, 2008*

Mucocele of ventral surface of tongue (glands of Blandin-Nuhn) *Ped Derm 25:308–311, 2008*

PELVIS syndrome (may be part of urorectal septum malformation sequence) – macular telangiectatic patch; larger perineal hemangiomas, external genitalia malformations, lipomyelomeningocele, vesicorenal abnormalities, imperforate anus, and skin tags *AD 142:884–888, 2006*

Pyogenic granuloma – pedunculated nodule of scalp *Ped Derm 26:615–616, 2009;* periumbilical *Ped Derm 4:341–343, 1987;* congenital *J Cutan Pathol 46:691–697, 2019*

Verrucous localized lymphedema of penis, scrotum, vulva, pubis – polypoid, verrucous, cobblestoned lesions *JAAD 71:320–326, 2014*

PENILE EDEMA, ACUTE AND CHRONIC

AUTOIMMUNE DISORDERS

Allergic contact dermatitis

Angioedema *Clin Exp Dermatol 44:20–31, 2019;* "saxophone penis" *Indian Dermatol Online J 6:462–463, 2015*

Contact urticaria

Dermatomyositis *Acta Rheumatol Port 36:176–179, 2011*

Urticaria

CONGENITAL LESIONS

Congenital lymphedema (primary lymphedema) *Ped Derm 33:176, 2016*

DRUG REACTIONS

Topical imiquimod *JAMA Derm 150:1370–1371, 2014*

EXOGENOUS AGENTS

Etanercept *Cases J Nov 30, 2019*

Foreign body reaction

Silicone injection – foreign body reaction *J Dtsch Dermatol Ges 8:689–691, 2010*

INFECTIONS

Actinomycosis

Arachnidism *J Clin Aesthet Dermatol 2:40–43, 2009*

Cellulitis, erysipelas, recurrent

Chlamydia

Entomophthoromycosis (Basidiobolomycosis) *Indian J DV Leprol 81:616–618, 2015*

Filariasis (*Wuchereria bancrofti*) *Acta Trop 134:13–16, 2014*

Foreign body reaction

Gonorrhea *JAMA 241:157–158, 1979*

Granuloma inguinale

Herpes simplex infection

Lymphogranuloma venereum

Mycobacterial infections

Scabies

Summer penile syndrome – trombiculid (chigger) bites *Ped Derm 36:158–159, 2019; J Emerg Med 46:e21–22, 2014*

Syphilis – primary *Acta DV Croat 23:301–303, 2015;* secondary *Indian Dermatol Online J 28:585–586, 2019*

INFLAMMATORY DISORDERS

Balanoposthitis

Crohn's disease, metastatic – penile and scrotal swelling *JAMA Derm 156:334, 2020; Dermatol Online J Aug 15, 2018; Ped Derm 29:765–766, 2012;* anogenital granulomatosis *J Crohn's Colitis 11:454–459, 2017; Ped Derm 33:172–177, 2016*

Neutrophilic dermatoses

Peritonitis

Pyoderma gangrenosum

Sarcoidosis

METABOLIC DISEASES

Acute necrotizing pancreatitis *AD 137:1108–1110, 2001*

Fluid overload

Obesity *Human Pathol 44:277–281, 2012*

NEOPLASTIC DISORDERS

Pelvic neoplasms associated with pelvic obstruction, post-surgery, post-radiation

Penile metastases *Urol Case Rep April 5, 2020*

PRIMARY CUTANEOUS DISEASES

JAAD 64:993–994, 2011

Hidradenitis suppurativa

Idiopathic scrotal or penile edema

Inflammatory skin conditions

PSYCHOCUTANEOUS DISEASE

Self-mutilation *Scand J Urol 49:341–343, 2015*

SYNDROMES

Melkersson-Rosenthal syndrome *Ann Dermatol 28:232–236, 2010*

TRAUMA

Amputation of septic limb in diabetes *AD 127:1108–1110, 2001*

Child abuse

Compulsive masturbation *Arch Sex Behav 41:737–739, 2012*

Diagnostic paracentesis *Cureus 12:e7329, 2020*

Hair tourniquet *Urol Ann 7:1452–1453, 2019*

Penile fracture – "eggplant deformity" *Ann Emerg Med 69:374–380, 2017*

Penile ring entrapment *Urol Ann 12:15–18, 2020*

Zipper injury *Stat Pearls Dec 31, 2019*

VASCULAR DISORDERS

Acute hemorrhagic edema of infancy *Eur J Pediatr 170:1507–1511, 2011*

Henoch-Schonlein purpura *Arch Argent Pediatr 114:e249–251, 2016; Clin Case Rep 4:258–260, 2016;* mimicking child abuse *Clin Pediatr (Phila)52:988990, 2013*

Localized lymphedema, verrucous *JAAD 71:320–326, 2014; Hum Pathol 44:277–281, 2013*

Lymphatic obstruction

Lymphatic stasis in redundant skin after weight loss

Non-venereal sclerosing lymphangitis of the penis *BMJ Case Rep July 27, 2017*

Parenteral fluid overload

Venous thrombosis

PENILE LESIONS

AUTOIMMUNE DISEASES AND DISEASES OF IMMUNE DYSFUNCTION

Allergic contact dermatitis – poison ivy, antifungals, condoms *Contact Dermatitis 78:168–169, 2018;* benzocaine, textile dye *Indian Dermatol Online J 6:S24–26, 2015*

Angioedema *Dermatol Clin 3:85–95, 1985; JAAD 25:155–161, 1991*

Bullous pemphigoid

Cicatricial pemphigoid (mucous membrane pemphigoid) *Front Med (Lausanne) Jan 29, 2019; JAAD 46:S128–129, 2002; Oral Surg Oral Med Oral Pathol Oral Radiol Endod 88:56–68, 1999; BJD 118:209–217, 1988; Oral Surg 54:656–662, 1982*

IPEX syndrome – immune dysregulation (neonatal autoimmune enteropathy, food allergies), polyendocrinopathy (diabetes mellitus, thyroiditis), enteropathy (neonatal diarrhea), X-linked, rash (atopic dermatitis-like with exfoliative erythroderma and periorificial dermatitis; psoriasiform dermatitis, pemphigoid nodularis, painful fissured cheilitis, edema of lips and perioral area, urticaria secondary to foods); penile rash; thyroid dysfunction, diabetes mellitus, hepatitis, nephritis, onychodystrophy, alopecia universalis; mutations in *FOXP3* (forkhead box protein 3) gene – master control gene of T regulatory cells (Tregs); hyper IgE, eosinophilia *JAAD 73:355–364, 2015; BJD 160:645–651, 2009;* ichthyosiform eruptions *Blood 109:383–385, 2007; BJD 152:409–417, 2005; NEJM 344:1758–1762, 2001;* alopecia areata *AD 140:466–472, 2004*

Lupus erythematosus – discoid

Pemphigus vulgaris – balanitis – resembles Zoon's balanitis *Indian J DV 81:298–299, 2015; Acta DV 93:248–249, 2013; AD 137:756–758, 2001;*

Pemphigus vegetans – chronic balanitis *J Urol 137:289–291, 1987*

Rheumatoid nodule – penile nodule

Scleroderma *AD Syphilol 183:493, 1943*

Urticaria

CONGENITAL LESIONS

Congenital os penis *J Urol 91:663–664, 1964*

Congenital sinus or cyst of genitoperineal raphe (mucous cysts of the penile skin) *Cutis 34:495–496, 1984; AD 115:1084–1086, 1979*

Dermoid cysts *Dermatology 194:188–190, 1997*

Double penis (diphallia)

Foreskin cysts

True hermaphrodite

Median raphe canal of the ventral penis – with or without median raphe cysts; yellow cystic papules *Ped Derm 27:667–669, 2010; Am J Dermatopathol 23:320–324, 2001; Ped Derm 15:191–193, 1998; Genital Skin Disorders, Fischer and Margesson, CV Mosby, 1998, p. 80; Cutis 34:495–496, 1984, JAAD 26:273–274, 1992; AD 115:1084–1086, 1979;* differential diagnosis includes epidermoid or dermoid cysts, urethral diverticulosis, apocrine hidrocystoma

Median raphe cysts of the ventral penis – yellow cystic papules *Ped Derm 27:667–669, 2010;* differential diagnosis includes epidermoid or dermoid cysts, urethral diverticulosis, apocrine hidrocystoma

Urethral diverticulae

Urethral retention cyst – white papule at urethral opening of males

DRUG-INDUCED

Ashwagandha (*Withania sominifera*) (Indian herbal treatment) – fixed drug eruption; red plaque of penis *SKINmed 10:48–49, 2012*

BCG granuloma due to intravesical instillation – penile edema, ulcers, nodules *JAAD 55:328–331, 2006*

Corticosteroid atrophy – striae, dusky erythema, increased visibility of vessels *BJD 107:371–372, 1982*

Drug eruptions – bullous, morbilliform, fixed drug eruptions – red maculae, bullae *Cutis 45:242–244, 1990; Genitourin Med 62:56–58, 1986*

Coumarin necrosis *Pharmacotherapy 8:351–354, 1988*

Fixed drug eruption – tetracycline; finasteride *JAAD 60:168–169, 2009;* oxcarbazepine (Trileptal) – erosion of penis *AD 147:362–364, 2011;* propolis *SKINMed 17:306–309, 2019; Dermatitis 23:173–175, 2012*

Foscarnet – erosions/ulceration *Dermatol Reports 10:7749, June 20, 2018; JAAD 27:124–126, 1992*

Hydroxyurea – lichenoid eruption *AD 140:877–882, 2004*

Imiquimod – edema of penis *JAMA Derm 150:1370–1371, 2014*

Interferon-alpha2a-induced paraffin granulomas of penis *AD 147:1232–1233, 2011*

PUVA macules

Tegafur – pigmentation of glans penis *JAAD 71:203–214, 2014*

Vaginal use of triple sulfa vaginal cream *J Sex Med 9:758–760, 2012*

Vancomycin – linear IgA disease – personal observation

EXOGENOUS

Airborne contact dermatitis – penile dermatitis due to sawdust exposure in carpenters and cabinet makers

Condoms – chemical hypopigmentation

Diamond implants

Foreign body granuloma – penile nodule *JAAD 49:924–929, 2003*

Glass beads – penile nodules *Br J Urol 47:463, 1975*

High pressure injection injury – cellulitis *BJD 115:379–381, 1986*

Intracorporeal injection of vasoactive agents – fibrotic lesions *J Urol 140:615–617, 1988*

Irritant contact dermatitis *Australas J Dermatol 58:e68–72, 2017*

Occupational leukoderma

Paraffinoma (sclerosing lipogranuloma)- penile swelling *JAAD 64:1–34, 2011; BJD 105:451–456, 1981; Arch Pathol Lab Med 101:321–326, 1977;* mineral oil paraffinoma resulting in penile enlargement *JAAD 47:S251–253, 2002; JAAD 45:S222–224, 2001*

Penile implant *J Sex Med 15:1811–1817, 2018*

Penile ring – strangulation *Urol Ann 9:304, 2017;* painful swelling *J Coll Physicians Surg Pak 27:108–109, 2017;* streptococcal group A necrotizing cellulitis *Urology April 16, 2020*

Smooth beads – penile nodules *Cutis 89:237–239, 2012*

Tattoos – Koebner phenomenon in psoriasis *Biosci Rep 39:BSR 20193266.doi.10.1042/BSR 2019 3266 Dec 30, 2019; J Urol 186:498–503, 2011*

Terra firme *AD 146:679–680, 2010*

INFECTIONS AND INFESTATIONS

Abscess – edema of entire shaft of penis or nodule at base of penis

Actinomycosis – movable soft subcutaneous mass mimicking a "cyst" *Ann R Coll Surg Engl 94:e22–23, 2012*

African trypanosomiasis – penile edema

Amebiasis – *Entamoeba histolyticum* – balanitis *JAMA 120:827–828, 1942;* vegetating plaque of genitalia, perineum, and anus *Sex Transm Infect 88:585–588, 2012; Derm Clinics 17:151–185, 1999; Urology 48:151–154, 1996*

Arthropod bites – persistent nodular arthropod bite reactions (pseudolymphoma syndrome) *JAAD 38:877–905, 1998*

Aspergillosis – red penis *Ped Derm 19:439–444, 2002*

Bacillary angiomatosis

BCG-osis *BMJ Case Rep July 14, 2016*

Black widow spider bite – priapism *Cutis 69:257–258, 2002*

Candidal balanitis *JAAD 37:1–24, 1997;* penile involvement

Cellulitis – edematous penis and/or scrotum

Chancroid (*Haemophilus ducreyi*) *Cureus 2019 Dec 16;11 (12) e6397.doi:10.7759/Cureus 6397; Hum Pathol 27:1066–1070, 1996;* phagedenic chancroid

Chlamydia trachomatis – balanitis *Bull Soc Fr Dermatol Syphyligr 82:419–422, 1975*

Condylomata acuminate *JAAD 66:867–880, 2012*

Cryptococcosis – balanitis *Sex Transm Dis 39:792–793, 2012; Infect Urol 3:101–107, 1990*

Cytomegalovirus infection *NDT Plus 3:379–382, 2010*

Diphtheria *Rev Paul Med 39:371–373, 1951; An Bras Sifilogr 26:173–187, 1951; Acta DV 30:458–459, 1950*

Enterococcus – balanoposthitis

Epidemic typhus (*Rickettsia prowazekii*) (body louse) – pink macules on sides of trunk, spreads centrifugally; flushed face with injected conjunctivae; then rash becomes deeper red, then purpuric; gangrene of finger, toes, genitalia, nose *JAAD 2:359–373, 1980*

Erysipelas – edematous penis and/or scrotum with or without necrosis; may result in chronic lymphedema *Genital Skin Disorders, Fischer and Margesson, Mosby, 1998, p.20–23*

Escherichia coli – balanoposthitis

Filariasis – penile edema *Autops Case Rep 30:57–61, 2016; Int J Surg Case Rep 3:269–271, 2012*

Fournier's gangrene (necrotizing fasciitis) *J Coll Physicians Surg Pak 28:164–165, 2018; Transpl Infect Dis 13:392–396, 2011*

Furuncle

Fusarium *J Infect Chemother 24:660–663, 2018*

Gardnerella vaginalis – anaerobic balanitis *Br J Venerol Jis 58:243, 1982*

Giant condyloma of Buschke and Lowenstein – cerebriform, multilobulated giant tumor *Clin Case Rep 30:257–259, 2017; Chirurgia (Bucur)109:445–450, 2014; BJD 166:247–251, 2012*

Gonococcus – gonococcal nodule on one or both sides of frenum, abscess *Cutis 36:161–163, 1985;* pustule, furuncle, infected median raphe cyst in association with urethral gonococcal infection *Ann Emerg Med 9:314–315, 1980; Br J Infect Dis 49:364–367, 1973;* urethral gonorrhea – indurated nodule, penile edema

Granuloma inguinale – ulcers; penile edema *JAAD 11:43–47, 1984*

Haemophilus parainfluenza – balanoposthitis *JAAD 37:1–24, 1997*

Herpes simplex virus infection – perianal and genital verrucous papules and plaques *JAAD 57:737–763, 2007; Cutis 30:442–456, 1982;* crusted and/or verrucous *JAAD 37:1–24, 1997;* mimicking leukemia cutis *JAAD 21:367–371, 1989;* vegetative *Urology 87:e15–16, 2014*

Herpes zoster *Acta DV Croat 26:337–338, 2018; Braz J Infect Dis 15:599–600, 2011; JAAD 147:S177–179, 2002*

Histoplasmosis – balanitis *An Bras Dermatol 90:255–257, 2015; J Urol 149:848–850, 1993*

Bullous impetigo – personal observation

Klebsiella JAAD 37:1–24, 1997

Leishmaniasis *BJD 139:111–113, 1998; J Eur Acad Dermatol Venereol 10:226–228, 1998;* destruction of glans penis *JAAD 60:897–925, 2009;* postkala-azar dermal leishmaniasis – in India, hypopigmented macules; nodules develop after years; tongue, palate, genitalia *E Afr Med J 63:365–371, 1986*

Leprosy *Indian J Lepr 87:27–32, 2015; Lepr Rev 60:303–305, 1989*

Lymphogranuloma venereum – papulovesicle *Br J Vener Dis 49:193–202, 1973;* inguinal adenitis with abscess formation and draining chronic sinus tracts; rectal syndrome in women with pelvic adenopathy, periproctitis with rectal stricture and fistulae; esthiomene – scarring and fistulae of the buttocks and thighs with elephantiasic lymphedema of the vulva; lymphatics may develop abscesses which drain and form ulcers *Int J Dermatol 15:26–33, 1976*

Molluscum contagiosum *Cutis 86:230–236, 2010*

Morganella – balanoposthitis *JAAD 37:1–24, 1997*

Mucormycosis – penile necrosis *Clin Inf Dis 21:682–684, 1995*

Mycobacterium kansasii – papulonecrotic tuberculid *JAAD 36:497–499, 1997*

Mycobacterium tuberculosis – nodule of glans *Genital Skin Disorders, Fischer and Margesson, Mosby, 1998, p.31–32;* papulonecrotic tuberculid – dusky red crusted or ulcerated papules occur in crops on elbows, hands, feet, knees, legs; also ears, face, buttock, and penis; small ulcers *Dermatologica 174:151–152, 1987; JAAD 12:1104–1106, 1985;* with worm-eaten scarring *Genitourin Med 64:130–132, 1988;* primary tuberculosis of glans penis – periurethral red plaque *JAAD 26:1002–1003, 1992*

Myiasis – genital piercing *Sao Paolo Med J 136:594–596, 2018*

Phthirus pubis (pediculosis) *JAAD 82:551–569, 2020; JAMA Derm Sept 25, 2019; Med Clin NA 82:1081–1104, 1998*

Talaromyces marneffei – balanitis *Mycoses 34:245–249, 1991*

Proteus – balanoposthitis *JAAD 37:1–24, 1997*

Pseudomonas sepsis – penile gangrene *J Urol 124:431–432, 1980;* ecthyma gangrenosum *Pediatr Emerging Care 32:46–48, 2016*

Rhinosporidiosis – vascular nodules; may resemble condylomata *J Laryngol Otol 127:1020–1024, 2013; Trop Doct 42:174–175, 2012; Arch Otolaryngol 102:308–312, 1976*

Rhizopus oryzae (zygomycosis) – necrosis of distal penis *AD 142:1657–1658, 2006*

Scabies – burrows, papules and nodules *Genital Skin Disorders, Fischer and Margesson, Mosby, 1998, p.36–38; Dermatol Clinics 8:253–263, 1990;* crusted scabies – hyperkeratosis of penis *BJD 161:195–197, 2009*

Schistosomiasis – penile edema; penile papules *Ann DV 107:759–767, 1980; Br J Vener Dis 55:446–449, 1979*

Sporotrichosis – vegetative plaque of penis *AD 139:1647–1652, 2003*

Staphylococcus aureus – balanoposthitis *Br J Urol 63:196–197, 1989;* bullous impetigo

Streptococcal balanoposthitis – Group B beta-hemolytic strep *J Urol 135:1015, 1986;* Group B strep infection – circumferential erosion *AD 120:85–6, 1984;* penile edema *J Clin Inf Dis 24:516–517, 1997;* Group A beta-hemolytic strep *Pediatrics 88:154–156, 1991*

Summer penile syndrome – penile edema; trombiculid (chigger) bites *Ped Derm 36:158–159, 2019*

Syphilis – primary chancre; hard penile circumferential fold *JAAD 26:700–703, 1992;* primary – urethral irritation *Clin Inf Dis 68:1231–1234, 2019;* secondary – papules *Clin Dermatol 38:160–175, 2020;* exclusively peno-scrotal localization *G Ital DV 144:725–728, 2009;* multiple umbilicated papules of penis *Int J STD AIDS 30:707–709, 2019;* balanoposthitis and penile edema *Sex Transm Dis 42:524–525, 2015;* hard penile circumferential fold *JAAD 26:700703, 1992*

Tinea corporis (genitalis) *Med Glas (Zenica) 12:52–56, 2015; Mycosses 48:202–204, 2005; JAAD 44:864–867, 2001;* balanitis due to *Trichophyton rubrum* or *T. mentagrophytes Dermatologica 178:112–124, 1989*

Tinea versicolor *Acta DV Alp Pannonica Adriat 17:86–89, 2008; Trop Geogr Med 46:184–185, 1994*

Trichomonas – chancre or penile abscesses *Ann DV 108:731–738, 1981; Bull Soc Gr Dermatol Syphiligr 76:345, 1969;* chronic penile ulcers *Am J Trop Med Hyg 92:943–944, 2015*

Tuberculosis *Int J STD AIDS 28:1453–1455, 2017; J Clin Diagn Res 10:PD05–06, 2016; Scientifica (Cairo)2015; 2015:601624. doi.10.1155/2015/601624l; Arch Esp Urol 67:203–206, 2014*

Verrucae (condyloma acuminatum) – subclinical balanitis due to HPV *Genitourin Med 66:251–253, 1990; Acta DV 193:1–85, 1995*

Viper bite – severe penile edema; Levantine viper (*Macrovipera lebetina*) *NEJM 373:1059, 2015*

Yaws – secondary (daughter yaws, pianomas, framboesiomas) – small papules which ulcerate, become crusted; resemble raspberries; periorificial (around mouth, nose, penis, anus, vulva); extend peripherally (circinate yaws) *JAAD 29:519–535, 1993*

INFILTRATIVE LESIONS

Amyloidosis – primary cutaneous amyloidosis of the penis *JAMA Derm 151:910–911, 2015; BJD 171: 1245–1247, 2014; BJD 170:730–734, 2014; J Urol 140:830–831, 1988;* amyloid elastosis (primary systemic amyloid) – white cobblestoned plaque around urethral meatus *BJD 158:858–860, 2008*

Juvenile xanthogranuloma *Pediatr Radiol 39:176–179, 2009; J Urol 150:456–457, 1993*

Langerhans cell histiocytosis *Nippon Hinyokika Gakkai Zasshi 81:1904–1907, 1990;* chancre *AD 123:1274–1275, 1987;* eosinophilic granuloma *Bull Soc Fr Dermatol Syphiligr 82:44–45, 1975; BMC Urol 11:628, 2006; Urologe A38:42–45, 1999*

Verrucous xanthoma *Genital Skin Disorders, Fischer and Margesson, CV Mosby, 1998, p. 80; Br J Urol 70:574–575, 1992;*

Cutis 44:167–170, 1989; Urology 23:600–603, 1984; Arch Derm 117:516–518, 1981

Xanthogranuloma of penis – yellow papules *Ped Derm 34:603–604, 2017; JAAD 62:524, 2010; Actas Urol Esp 32:659–661, 2008; J Urol 150:456–457, 1993; Actas Urol Esp 14:210–213, 1990*

Zoon's balanitis – red plaque of glans penis *J Drugs Dermatol 16:285–287, 2017; Indian J Sex Transm Dis AIDS 37:129–138, 2016; J Drugs Dermatol 6:532–533, 2007; Am J Dermatopathol 24:459–467, 2002; J Urol 153:424–426, 1995; Dermatologica 10:51–57, 1952*

INFLAMMATORY LESIONS

Balanitis

    Amebic (*Entamoeba histolytica*) *Med J Aust 5:114–117, 1964*
    Aphthae
    Balanoposthitis – red patches and plaques *Int J STD AIDS 25:615–626, 2014*
    Candida *Int J STD AIDS 3:128–129, 1992; Clin Exp Dermatol 7:345–354, 1982*
    Chlamydial *Br J Hosp Med 29:6–11, 1983*
    Circinate – reactive arthritis *NEJM 276:157, 2017; J Cut Med Surg 17:180–188, 2013; J Clin Rheumatol 18:257–258, 2012*
    Gram negative bacteria
    Irritant; smegma, clothing, poor hygiene, detergent, water
    Erythroplasia of Queyrat
    Fixed drug eruption
    Lichen sclerosus (balanitis xerotica obliterans)
    Mixed infection – fusospirallary, bacterial, yeast
    Mycoplasma *NEJM 302:1063–1067, 1980; Bull Soc Fr Dermatol Syphilol 82:419–422, 1975*
    Plasma cell balanitis (Zoon's balanitis) *AD 149:440–445, 2013; J Urol 153:424–426, 1995; Genitourin Med 71:32–34, 1995; BJD 105:195–199, 1981;* red plaques *Dermatologica 105:1–7, 1952;* mucinous metaplasia in Zoon's balanitis – red plaque of glans penis *AD 147:735–740, 2011; JAAD 57:S6–7, 2007; Int J Dermatol 42:305–307, 2003*
    Porokeratosis of Mibelli
    Pseudoepitheliomatous keratotic and micaceous balanitis *Cutis 35:77–79, 1985*
    Relapsing chronic balanitis
    Streptococcal *Int J STD AIDS 3:128–129, 1992*
    Syphilitic balanitis (Follmann) *Br J Vener Dis 51:138–140, 1975*
    Titanium *Dermatologica 176:305–307, 1988*
    Traumatic – post-coital, zippers
    Trichomonal *Ann DV 108:731–738, 1981*
    Vincent's organism

Crohn's disease *Am J Dermatopathol 22:443–446, 2000; J Gastroenterol 32:817–821, 1997; Gut 27:329–333, 1986;* edema of prepuce and scrotum *JAAD:S182–183, 2003;* edema of penis and scrotum *JAAD 70:385, 2014; JAAD 65:449–450, 2011; Ped Derm 27:279–281, 2010;* granulomatous lymphangitis – penile and scrotal edema *Ped Derm 29:765–766, 2012*

Erythema multiforme – including Stevens-Johnson syndrome *BJD 174:1194–1227, 2016; Genital Skin Disorders, Fischer and Margesson, CV Mosby, 1998, p. 65*

Hidradenitis suppurativa – lymphedema of the penis *Cir 86:79–80, 2019*

Pyoderma gangrenosum *J Pak Med Assoc 68:1148–1150, 2018; Curr Urol 9:159–162, 2016; J Dermatol 40:840–843, 2013*

Sarcoid *J Cut Med Surg 4:202–204, 2000; JAAD 44:725–743, 2001; Urology 108:284–289, 1972*

Toxic epidermal necrolysis

Ulcerative colitis *Int J STD AIDS 5:72–73, 1994*

METABOLIC

Acrodermatitis enteropathica – penile dermatitis; mutation in SLC39A4 encodes ZIP4 zinc transporter *BJD 161:184–186, 2009*

Anasarca

Androgen excess – hyperpigmentation of areolae, axillae, external genitalia, perineum *Ghatan, Second Edition, 2002, p.165*

Calcific uremic arteriolopathy *Ann Afr Med 10:181–184, 2011*

Calcinosis cutis *Genital Skin Disorders, Fischer and Margesson, CV Mosby, 1998, p. 61;* idiopathic calcinosis cutis *JAAD 51:s118–119, 2004;* calcification of retained smegma

Calciphylaxis – penile necrosis *JAAD 82:799–816, 2020; Clin Exp Dermatol 43:645–647, 2018; J Emerg Med 52:e255–256, 2017; Am J Ther 19:e66–68, 2012; JAAD 54:736–737, 2006; AD 136:259–264, 2000; J Urol 160:764–767, 1998; AD 131:63–68, 1995;* biopsy contraindicated *J Sex Med 11:2611–2617, 2014;*

Cardiac failure – penile edema

Catastrophic antiphospholipid antibody syndrome – personal observation

Fabry's disease – angiokeratoma corporis diffusum (alpha galactosidase A) – X-linked recessive; of penis *BJD 157:331–337, 2007; AD 140:1440–1446, 2004; JAAD 46:161–183, 2002; JAAD 17:883–887, 1987; NEJM 276:1163–1167, 1967*

Fucosidosis – angiokeratomas *BJD 136:594–597, 1997*

Gout – tophus *AD 134:499–504, 1998*

Hypoproteinemia – penile edema

Male pseudohermaphroditism – ambiguous genitalia *Genital Skin Disorders, Fischer and Margesson, CV Mosby, 1998, p. 109*

Necrobiosis lipoidica diabeticorum – chronic balanitis

Dermatology 188:222–225, 1994

Pellagra

Renal failure – penile edema

NEOPLASTIC LESIONS

Abdominal cancer – edema of penis due to pelvic or abdominal cancer

Acrochordon – cerebriform nodule *JAAD 59:S35–37, 2008*

Angiokeratoma of Fordyce *Dermatol Ther (Heidelb) June 6, 2020; Aust Fam Physician 42:270–274, 2013*

Angiosarcoma *Int Urol Nephrol 44:1341–1343, 2012; Urology 51:130–131, 1998;* arising in Kaposi's sarcoma in AIDS – vascular penile nodule *JAAD 234:790–792, 1991; Cancer 15:1318–1324, 1981*

Apocrine cystadenoma *AD 113:1250–1251, 1977*

Atypical penile melanotic macules *AD 124:1267–1270, 1988*

Basal cell carcinoma *JAAD 20;1094–1097, 1989*

Benign penile lentigo *JAAD 42:640–644, 2000*

Blue nevus *J Cut Pathol 31:185–188, 2004; AD 139:1209–1214, 2003;* epithelioid blue nevus *BJD 145:496–501, 2001*

Bowen's disease *Genital Skin Disorders, Mosby, 1998, p.10;* red plaque *JAAD 66:867–880, 2012;* pigmented *Dermatol Onlin J April 16, 2014*

Bowenoid papulosis – irregular red papules of glans penis mimicking warts, psoriasis, or lichen planus *Cutis 86:278,295–296, 2010;* papules *AD 121:858–863, 1985;* hyperpigmented flat-topped papules *JAAD 81:1–21, 2019; Cutis 102:151–152,4, 2018; Ped Derm 2:297–301, 1985; Proc R Soc Med 68:345–346, 1975*

Cysts, calcified *J Dermatol 20:114–117, 1993*

Eccrine hidrocystoma – cystic papule of shaft of penis *SKINmed 13:331–333, 2015*

Eccrine poroma – pink papule of shaft of penis *SKINmed 13:331–333, 2015*

Eccrine syringofibroadenomatosis – balanitis *AD 130:933–934, 1994*

Epidermal nevus

Epidermoid cysts

Epithelioid sarcoma – penile nodule *J Sex Med 10:2871–1874, 2013; Ann Diagn Pathol 4:88–94, 2000; J Urol 147:1370–1372, 1992*

Erythroplasia of Queyrat – red plaque *AD 149:440–445, 2013; JID 115:396–401, 2000; Urology 8:311–315, 1976; Bull Soc Fr Dermatol Syphiligr 22:378–382, 1911*

Extramammary Paget's disease – red papule of penile shaft *AD 142:515–520, 2006;* red to brown scaly plaques; *JAAD 18:115–122, 1988;* red plaque of penis and pubis *AD 147:704–708, 2011;* red plaque of penis and scrotum and intertrigo *Cutis 94:35–38, 2014*

Fibroepithelioma of Pinkus *Cutis 31:519–521, 1983*

Fordyce spots (ectopic sebaceous glands) *Genital Skin Disorders, Fischer and Margesson, CV Mosby, 1998, p. 59;* of prepuce *Acta DV 70:344–345, 1990;* of glans penis

Glomus tumor *Curr Urol 9:113–118, 2016*

Granular cell tumor *Derm Surg 27:772–774, 2001*

Hidrocystoma *AD 142:1221–1226, 2006*

Histiocytoma – acquired mucosal indeterminate cell histiocytoma – red papule of glans penis *Ped Derm 24:253–256, 2007*

Horns *Acta DV Croat 20:30–33, 2012; Urology 30:156–158, 1987; JAAD 13:369–373, 1985*

Kaposi's sarcoma – penile lymphedema preceding appearance of Kaposi's sarcoma *JAAD 20:318–320, 2006; BJD 142:153–156, 2000; J Dermatol 26:240–243, 1999; J Med 27:211–220, 1996; JAAD 27:267–268, 1992; AD 102:461–462, 1970;* multilobulated nodules *JAAD 59:179–206, 2008;* skin colored nodule *BJD 142:153–156, 2000;* yellow-green penile plaques *Cutis 88:14–16, 2011*

Keloids *Ann Plast Surg 39:662–665, 1997*

Keratoacanthoma – ulcerated nodule *JAAD 15:1079–1082, 1986*

Leiomyoma *Scand J Urology 47:158–162, 2013; Diagn Pathol 7:140, 2012*

Leiomyosarcoma *Cancer 29:481–483, 1972*

Lentigines *JAAD 22:453–460, 1990; JAAD 20:567–570, 1989;* in the presence of lichen sclerosus *JAAD 50:690–694, 2004*

Leukemia – ulcerative balanoposthitis of the foreskin *Urology 56:669, 2000;* leukemia *Mediterr J Hematol Infect Dis 2013:5 (1):e2013008.doi:10.4084/MJHID.2013.008;* priapism *Int J Surg Case Rep 43:13–17, 2018*

Leukoplakia

Lipoma *Androlgia 51:e13289, 2019*

Lymphoma – infiltrative plaques with or without ulceration; B-cell, angiocentric T-cell lymphoma *JAAD 26:31–38, 1992;* cutaneous T-cell lymphoma; Hodgkin's disease; primary cutaneous CD30+ lymphoproliferative disorder (CD8+/CD4+) *JAAD 51:304–308, 2004;* diffuse large cell B-cell lymphoma, follicular lymphoma, extranodal NK/T-cell lymphoma, Burkitt's lymphoma, primitive T cell-rich B-cell lymphoma, ALK+ anaplastic large cell lymphoma, MALT lymphoma *Pathology 43:54–57, 2011*

Malignant tumors of the penis *JAAD 35:432–451, 1996; Urol Clin North Am 19:319–324, 1992*

Primary tumors

Soft tissue tumors

Angiosarcoma

Clear cell sarcoma

Epithelioid sarcoma

Fibrosarcoma

Hemangioendothelioma

Hemangiopericytoma

Kaposi's sarcoma

Leiomyosarcoma

Malignant Schwannoma

Melanoma *Eur J Dermatol 15:113–115, 2005; Urol Int 27:66–80, 1972;* melanoma in situ *JAAD 42:386–388, 2000*

Myxofibrosarcoma *Am J Surg Pathol 20:391–405, 1996*

Rhabdomyosarcoma

Undifferentiated sarcoma

Epithelial tumors

In situ carcinomas

Bowen's disease

Bowenoid papulosis

Erythroplasia of Queyrat

Extramammary Paget's disease

Invasive carcinomas

Squamous cell carcinomas *JAAD 69:73–81, 2013;–* preceded by erythroplasia, leukoplakia, or warty papule *Am J Surg Pathol 24:505–512, 2000; Urol Int 62:238–244, 1999; Ann Oncol 8:1089–1098, 1997*

Verrucous carcinoma – cutaneous horn *AD 126:1208–1210, 1990;* multinodular verrucous carcinoma *JAAD 29:321–324, 1993*

Melanoma *Eur J Surg Oncol 23:277–279, 1997; J Urol 139:813–816, 1988;* including desmoplastic melanoma – exophytic *JAAD 16:619–620, 1987;* amelanotic melanoma – red papule of penile shaft *AD 142:515–520, 2006*

Other tumors

Angiosarcoma *Cancer 47:1318–1324, 1981*

Dermatofibrosarcoma protuberans *Ann DV 105:267–274, 1978*

Leiomyosarcoma *Cancer 132:992–994, 1984; Ann DV 105:267–274, 1978*

Leukemia cutis *Mediterr J Hematol Infect Dis 2013:5 (1) e2013008.doi:4084/MJHID.2013.008; Eur J Dermatol 21:107–109, 2011;* penile ulcer *Am J Dermatopathol Jan 7, 2020;*

Recurrent Richter's transformation with penile ulcer *JAMA Derm 152:586–587, 2016*

Lymphomas *Hinyokika Kiyo 43:371–374, 1997;* anaplastic large cell lymphoma *World J Cases 26:3377–3383, 2019;* T-cell lymphoma *Int J Dermatol 51:973–975, 2012*

Malignant hemangioendothelioma

Neural tumors (Schwannomas)

Undifferentiated sarcoma

Secondary tumors

Metastases – nodules, often ulcerated *Int J Surg Pathol 19:597–606, 2011; J Urol 132:992–993, 1984;* metastatic male breast carcinoma – penile plaque with ulceration *JAAD 38:995–996, 1998;* transitional cell carcinoma of the bladder *J Natl Med Assoc 89:253–256, 1997;* presenting as penile and scrotal edema *JAAD 51:143–145, 2004;* lung cancer *South Med J 88:761–762, 1995;* supraglottic squamous cell carcinoma *J Urol 147:157–160, 1992;* prostate *AD 120:1604–1606, 1984;* rectal cancer *Br J Surg 62:77–79, 1975;* metastatic

gastric carcinoma – red swollen penis and scrotum *BJD 144:419–420, 2001*

Melanoma – lentiginous lesions of penis *AD 147:1181–1187, 2011; Mayo Clin Proceed 72:362–366, 1997*

Melanocytic nevus – genital nevi in children *JAAD 70:429–434, 2014;* in the presence of lichen sclerosus *JAAD 50:690–694, 2004;* divided nevus *BJD 143:1126–1127, 2000*

Melanotic macule (penile melanosis) *An Bras Dermatol 90:178–183, 2015*

Mucinous metaplasia – red plaques of glans penis *BJD 165:1263–1272, 2011*

Mucoid cysts *J Urol 115:397–400, 1976*

Myofibroma – skin colored to hyperpigmented nodules of hand, mouth, genitals, shoulders *JAAD 46:477–490, 2002*

Myointimoma – nodule of coronal sulcus *JAAD 53:1084–1086, 2005*

Neurinoma of the glans *Dermatologica 137:150–155, 1968*

Neurofibroma *Am J Med Genet 87:1–5, 1999*

Neuroma – solitary (palisaded) encapsulated neuroma *AD 140:1003–1008, 2004; BJD 142:1061–1062, 2000;* white penile papules – traumatic neuromas *JAAD 54:S54–55, 2006*

Nevus comedonicus *Acta DV (Stockh) 55:78–80, 1975*

Nodular hidradenoma (apocrine hidrocystoma) *Br J Urol 70:574–575, 1992*

Paget's disease *Dermatol Online J April 15, 2019; CMAJ 190:E1142, 2018; Ir Med J 111:772, 2018; JAMA Oncol 4:861–862, 2018; Plast Reconstr Surg 100:336–339, 1997; Ann Plast Surg 23:141–146, 1989*

Pearly penile papules (angiofibromas) *Int STD AIDS 10:726–727, 1999; AD 93:56–59, 1966; AD 90:166–167, 1964*

Penile horn – underlying benign epidermal hyperplasia, in situ carcinoma, verruca vulgaris, keratoacanthoma, hemangioma *JAAD 54:369–391, 2006*

Peyronie's disease – penile fibromatosis; thickened subcutaneous plaque *JAAD 41:106–108, 1999; J Clin Epidemiol 51:511–515, 1998*

Pilonidal cyst of penis *Arch Iran Med 21:131–133, 2018*

Plasmacytoma – red papule of glans penis *JAMA Derm 155:247–248, 2019*

Polyfibromatosis syndrome – Dupuytren's contracture, knuckle pads, Peyronie's disease, keloids, or plantar fibromatosis *Rook p. 2044, 1998, Sixth Edition;* stimulation by phenytoin *BJD 100:335–341, 1979*

Porokeratosis – of Mibelli *AD 142:1221–1226, 2006; BJD 144:643–644, 2001; Dermatology 196:256–259, 1998; JAAD 36:479–481, 1997; Clin Exp Dermatol 19:77–78, 1994;* linear porokeratosis *Ped Derm 26:216–217, 2009*

Pseudoepitheliomatous, micaceous, and keratotic balanitis *Dermatol Pract Concept Dec 31, 2019; Clin Exp Dermatol 42:424–426, 2017; J Clin Diagn Res 9:WD01–02, 2015; JAAD 54:369–391, 2006; JAAD 18:419–422, 1988; Cutis 35:77–79, 1985; Bull Soc Fr Dermatol Syphiligr 68:164–167, 1966*

Rhabdomyosarcoma, congenital *Clin Nucl Med 43:852–853, 2018;* embryonal *J Med Case Rep 20:353, 2016*

Sebaceous adenoma – pedunculated vascular nodule of dorsal penis *JAAD 57:S42–43, 2007*

Sebaceous hyperplasia – annular sebaceous hyperplasias of the penis *JAAD 48:149–150, 2003*

Seborrheic keratosis *J Sex Med 11:3119–3122, 2014; Urology 29:204–206, 1987*

Spitz nevi, eruptive – pigmented papules *BJD 164:873–877, 2011*

Squamous cell carcinoma – red or white plaque of penis *JAAD 69:73–81, 2013; JAAD 66:867–880, 2012; JAAD 62:284–290, 2010;* penile nodule *Genital Skin Disorders, Fischer and Margesson, CV Mosby, 1998, p. 83;* post PUVA; hyperkeratotic nodule of the penis *NEJM 374:164, 2016*

Syringomas – flesh-colored papules *JAAD 59:S46–47, 2008; Clin Exp Dermatol 18:384–385, 1993; Int J Derm 30:69, 1991; AD 123:1391–1396, 1987; AD 103:215–217, 1971;* eruptive syringomas *Ped Derm 32:145–146, 2015*

Trichofolliculomas *Dermatologica 181:68–70, 1990*

Verruciform xanthoma *J Urol (Paris) 93:41–42, 1987; AD 117:516–518, 1981*

Verrucous acanthoma

Verrucous carcinoma (giant condyloma of Buschke-Lowenstein) *AD 145:950–952, 2009; JAAD 32:1–21, 1995; AD 126:1208–1210, 1990; Int J Derm 18:608–622, 1979; JAAD 14:947–950, 1986*

PARANEOPLASTIC DISORDERS

Paraneoplastic pemphigus *BJD 176:1406–1408, 2017*

PRIMARY CUTANEOUS DISEASES

Acquired epidermodysplasia verruciformis – personal observation

Angiolymphoid hyperplasia with eosinophilia *JAAD 74:506–512, 2016*

Atopic dermatitis

Balanitis xerotica obliterans (lichen sclerosus of the glans) – non-bullous or bullous *World J Urol 18:382–387, 2000; AD 123:1391–1396, 1987;* white papules *JAMA Derm 149:23–24, 2013;* purpuric *Ped Derm 10:129–131, 1993*

Degos' disease (malignant atrophic papulosis) – penile lesions not rare *BJD 100:21–36, 1979; Ann Dermatol Venereol 79:410–417, 1954*

Ectopic hair of the glans *BJD 153:218–219, 2005*

Elastosis perforans serpiginosa *BJU Int 91:427, 2003*

Elephantiasis nostras verrucosa – penoscrotal *Int J Surg Case Rep 65:127–130, 2019*

Epidermolytic hyperkeratosis

Familial dyskeratotic comedones – shaft of penis *BJD 140:956–959, 1999; Eur J Dermatol 9:491–492, 1999; Arch Derm Research 282:103–107, 1990; JAAD 17:808–814, 1987*

Granuloma annulare *SKINMed 14:233–236, 2016; Ped Derm 25:260–262, 2008; JAAD 57:S45–46, 2007; J Pediatr Surg 40:1329–1331, 2005; Sex Transm Infect 75:186–187, 1999; J Cutan Pathol 17:101–104, 1997; Scand J Urol Nephrol 27:549–551, 1993; Genitourin Med 68:47–49, 1992; J Cutan Pathol 17:101–104, 1990*

Hailey-Hailey disease *J Cutan Pathol 21:27–32, 1994*

Lamellar ichthyosis

Lichen aureus – expression of Zoon's balanitis – purpuric eruption of the glans *JAAD 21:805–806, 1989*

Lichen nitidus *JAMA 308:1264–1265, 2012; Cutis 21:634–637, 1978; Urology 33:1–4, 1984*

Lichen planus – red plaques, papules, annular, erosive lesions *Sem Cut Med Surg 34:182–186, 2015*

Lichen sclerosus *BJD 174:687–689, 2016*

Lichen simplex chronicus

Mucha-Habermann syndrome *Genital Skin Disorders, Fischer and Margesson, Mosby, 1998, p. 53*

Necrobiotic granulomas *J Cutan Pathol 17:101–104, 1990*

Oid-oid disease – exudative discoid and lichenoid dermatitis

Papular acantholytic dyskeratosis of the penis *J Dermatol 36:427–429, 2009; Am J Dermatopathol 8:365–366, 1986*

Paraphimosis – penile edema

Pearly penile papules – angiofibromas *JAMA Derm 149:748–750, 2013*

Penile nodules *AD 12:1604–1606, 1984*

Pigmented purpuric eruption – personal observation

Pityriasis rosea *Genital Skin Disorders, Fischer and Margesson, Mosby, 1998, p. 52; JAAD 15:159–167, 1986*

Piebaldism

Pityriasis rosea – balanitis

Psoriasis *CMAJ 190:E747, 2018;* pustular psoriasis *Indian Dermatol Online J 9:96–100, 2018; J Eur Acad DV 18:742–743, 2004; Int J Dermatol 35:202–204, 1996*

Seborrheic dermatitis *Ann Dermatol 28:40–44, 2016; Urology 23:1–4, 1984*

Terra firme – verrucous plaque of distal shaft *Ped Derm 33:455–456, 2016*

Vitiligo *JAAD 38:647–666, 1998*

PSYCHOCUTANEOUS DISEASES

Factitial dermatitis *Int J STD AIDS 23:527–528, 2012; Acta DV Alp Pannonica Adriat 18:83–85, 2009*

Self-mutilation, self-inflicted, dermatitis artefacta *Int Med Case Rep 18:71–73, 2019*

SYNDROMES

Aarskog syndrome – hypoplastic penis with shawl-like scrotal folds covering the base of the penis *Atlas of Clinical Syndromes A Visual Aid to Diagnosis, 1992, pp.194–195; Birth Defects 11:25–29, 1975*

Ablepharon macrostomia – absent eyelids, ectropion, abnormal ears, rudimentary nipples, dry redundant skin, macrostomia, ambiguous genitalia *Hum Genet 97:532–536, 1996*

Anencephaly – hypoplastic penis *Syndromes of the Head and Neck, p. 565, 1990*

Bannayan-Riley-Ruvalcaba syndrome (Ruvalcaba-Myhre-Smith syndrome) (macrocephaly and subcutaneous hamartomas) (lipomas and hemangiomas) – autosomal dominant; hyperpigmented macules of glans and penile shaft, macrocephaly, hamartomatous intestinal polyps, lipid storage myopathy *JAAD 53:639–643, 2005; AD 132:1214–1218, 1996; AD 128:1378–1386, 1992; Ped Derm 5:28–32, 1988; Eur J Ped 148:122–125, 1988;* lipoangiomas (perigenital pigmented macules, macrocephaly) *AD 128:1378–1386, 1992*

Bazex syndrome – psoriasiform plaque of penis *JAMA Derm 150:1368–1370, 2014*

Behcet's disease – balanitis *JAAD 34:745–750, 1996;* ulcerations *Ugeskr Laeger 170:1440–1445, 2008;* dorsal vein thrombosis *Pan Afr Med J 24:17 May 2016*

Borjeson-Forssman-Lehmann syndrome – hypoplastic penis *Am J Med Genet 19:653–664, 1984*

Carney complex – pigmented epithelioid melanocytoma *J Dermatol 41:368–369, 2014; BJD 145:496–501, 2001*

Carpenter syndrome – hypoplastic penis *Am J Med Genet 28:311–324, 1987*

CHARGE syndrome – hypoplastic penis *Syndromes of the Head and Neck, p. 94, 1990*

Chromosomal abnormalities – hypospadias *NEJM 351;2319–2326, 2004*

del (9p) syndrome – hypoplastic penis *Pediatrics 73:670–675, 1984*

del (18p) syndrome – hypoplastic penis *Eur J Pediatr 123:59–66, 1976*

Down's syndrome – hypoplastic penis

Dubowitz syndrome – autosomal recessive, microcephaly, sloping forehead, telecanthus, erythema and scaling of face and extremities in infancy, sparse blond scalp and arched eyebrow hair, dysplastic low set ear pinnae, high pitched hoarse voice, delayed eruption of teeth, growth retardation, craniofacial abnormalities; syndactyly, cryptorchidism, hypospadias, developmental delay, transitory short stature, hyperactive behavior, blepharophimosis, ptosis of the eyelids, epicanthal folds, broad nose, palate anomalies, micrognathia, and severe atopic dermatitis *Ped Derm 22:480–481, 2005; Am J Med Genet 63:277–289, 1996; Clin Exp Dermatol 19:425–427, 1994; Am J Med Genet 47:959–964, 1993; Eur J Pediatr 144:574–578, 1986; Am J Med Genet 4:345–347, 1979; J Med Genet 2:12–17, 1965*

Femoral hypoplasia-unusual facies syndrome – hypoplastic penis *J Med Genet 21:331–340, 1984*

Floating-Harbor syndrome (unusual facies, short stature, hypoplastic penis) – hypoplastic penis *Birth Defects 11:305–309, 1975*

Glucagonoma syndrome – necrolytic migratory erythema, polymorphous, erosions and crusts of groin, perineum buttock, central face *AD 113:9=792–797, 1977;* stomatitis, angular cheilitis, elevated glucagon levels, weight loss, anemia, abnormal glucose tolerance *AD 113:749–754, 1977;* erythema of scrotum extending onto shaft of penis

Gorlin-Chaudhry-Moss syndrome – short and stocky with craniosynostosis, midface hypoplasia, hypertrichosis of the scalp, arms, legs, and back, anomalies of the eyes, digits, teeth, and heart, and genitalia hypoplasia *Am J Med Genet 44:518–522, 1992*

H syndrome (low height, heart, hallux valgus, hormonal, hypogonadism, hematologic) – autosomal recessive; micropenis; sclerodermoid changes of middle and lower body with overlying hyperpigmentation sparing the knees and buttocks; starts on feet and legs and progresses upward; hypertrichosis, short stature, facial telangiectasia, ichthyosiform changes, gynecomastia, varicose veins, skeletal deformities (camptodactyly of 5th fingers), scrotal masses with massively edematous scrotum obscuring the penis, hypogonadism, azoospermia, sensorineural hearing loss, dilated scleral vessels, exophthalmos, cardiac anomalies, hepatosplenomegaly, mental retardation; mutation in nucleoside transporter Hent3 *JAAD 70:80–88, 2014; BJD 162:1132–1134, 2010; Ped Derm 27:65–68, 2010; JAAD 59:79–85, 2008*

Hennekam syndrome – autosomal recessive; intestinal lymphangiectasia, lymphedema of legs and genitalia, gigantic scrotum and penis, multilobulated lymphatic ectasias, small mouth, narrow palate, gingival hypertrophy, tooth anomalies, thick lips, agenesis of ear, pre-auricular pits, wide flat nasal bridge, frontal upsweep, platybasia, hypertelorism, pterygia colli, bilateral single palmar crease, hirsutism, mild mental retardation, facial anomalies, growth retardation, pulmonary, cardiac, hypogammaglobulinemia *Ped Derm 23:239–242, 2006*

Hypereosinophilic syndrome – erosions *JAMA 247:1018–1020, 1982;* penile ulcers *Ceylon Med J 54:96–97, 2009*

IPEX syndrome – immune dysregulation (neonatal autoimmune enteropathy, food allergies), polyendocrinopathy (diabetes mellitus, thyroiditis), enteropathy (neonatal diarrhea), X-linked, rash (atopic dermatitis-like with exfoliative erythroderma and periorificial dermatitis; psoriasiform dermatitis, painful fissured cheilitis, edema of lips and perioral area, urticaria secondary to foods); penile rash; mutations in *FOXP3* gene – master control gene of T regulatory cells (Tregs); hyper IgE, eosinophilia *BJD 160:645–651, 2009;* ichthyosiform eruptions *Blood 109:383–385, 2007; NEJM 344:1758–1762, 2001;* alopecia areata *AD 140:466–472, 2004*

Johanson-Blizzard syndrome – hypoplastic penis *J Med Genet 19:302–303, 1981*

Klippel-Trenaunay-Weber syndrome – large penis *Mt Sinai J Med 49:66–70, 1982*

Laugier-Hunziker syndrome – genital pigmented macules *J Eur Acad Dermatol Venereol 15:574–577, 2001; Clin Exp Derm 15:111–114, 1990*

Lawrence-Seip syndrome (congenital generalized lipodystrophy) – lipoatrophic diabetes; enlarged penis *AD 91:326–334, 1965*

LEOPARD (Moynahan's) syndrome – CALMs, granular cell myoblastomas, steatocystoma multiplex, small penis, hyperelastic skin, low set ears, short webbed neck, short stature, syndactyly *JAAD 46:161–183, 2002; JAAD 40:877–890, 1999; J Dermatol 25:341–343, 1998; Am J Med 60:447–456, 1976; Am J Med 60:447–456, 1976; AD 107:259–261, 1973*

Leprechaunism (Donohue's syndrome) – decreased subcutaneous tissue and muscle mass, characteristic facies, severe intrauterine growth retardation, broad nose, low set ears, hypertrichosis of forehead and cheeks, loose folded skin at flexures, gyrate folds of skin of hands and feet; breasts, penis, clitoris hypertrophic *Endocrinologie 26:205–209, 1988*

Leschke's syndrome – growth retardation, mental retardation, diabetes mellitus, genital hypoplasia, hypothyroidism *Bolognia, p.859, 2003*

Meckel syndrome – hypoplastic penis *Birth Defects 18:145–160, 1982*

Neurofibromatosis – enlarged penis *J Urol 135:755–757, 1986; J Urol 130:1176–1179, 1983;* schwannoma *Clin Genitourin Cancer 14:198–202, 2016;* plexiform neurofibroma *Am J Med Genet 87:1–5, 1999*

Neu-Laxova syndrome – autosomal recessive; variable presentation; small genitalia; mild scaling to harlequin ichthyosis appearance; ichthyosiform scaling, increased subcutaneous fat and atrophic musculature, generalized edema and mildly edematous feet and hands, absent nails; microcephaly, intrauterine growth retardation, limb contractures, low set ears, sloping forehead, short neck; eyelid and lip closures, syndactyly, cleft lip and palate, micrognathia; uniformly fatal *Ped Derm 20:25–27,78–80, 2003; Curr Prob Derm 14:71–116, 2002; Clin Dysmorphol 6:323–328, 1997; Am J Med Genet 35:55–59, 1990*

Noonan syndrome – hypoplastic penis *J Med Genet 24:9–13, 1987*

Opitz G/BBB syndrome (hypertelorism-hypospadias syndrome) – X-linked and autosomal dominant forms; hypospadias; hypertelorism, upward-slanting palpebral fissures with epicanthal folds; broad flat nasal bridge, cleft lip +/- cleft palate; cryptorchidism, bifid scrotum, failure to thrive due to laryngotracheal clefts *NEJM 351;2319–2326, 2004*

Pallister-Hall syndrome – hypoplastic penis

Perlman syndrome – micropenis; nephroblastoma, renal hamartoma, facial dysmorphism, fetal gigantism *J Pediatr 83:414–418, 1973*

Peutz-Jegher's syndrome – hyperpigmented macules *Br J Ophthalmol 75:693–695, 1991*

Popliteal pterygium syndrome *J Med Genet 36:888–892, 1999; Int J Pediatr Otorhinolaryngol 15:17–22, 1988*

Prader-Willi syndrome – hypoplastic penis *Growth Genet Hormones 2:1–5, 1986*

Reactive arthritis – circinate balanitis; diffuse balanoposthitis *Genital Skin Disorders, Fischer and Margesson, Mosby, 1998, p. 51–52; Arthr Rheum 24:844–849, 1981; Semin Arthritis Rheum 3:253–286, 1974*

Robert's pseudothalidomide syndrome – enlarged penis *Hum Genet 61:372–374, 1982*

Robinow syndrome – hypoplastic penis *J Med Genet 23:350–354, 1986*

Rudiger syndrome – thick single palmar crease; somatic retardation, flexion contractures of hands, small fingers and nails, ureterovesical stenosis, micropenis, inguinal hernias, coarse facies, cleft soft palate *J Pediatr 79:977–981, 1971*

Russell-Silver syndrome – genital dysmorphia *JAAD 40:877–890, 1999; J Med Genet 36:837–842, 1999*

Sakati syndrome – hypoplastic penis *J Pediatr 79:104–109, 1971*

Short rib-polydacytyly syndromes – hypoplastic penis *J Med Genet 22:46–53, 1985*

Smith-Lemli-Opitz syndrome – autosomal recessive; hypospadias; failure to thrive, genital abnormalities in males, microcephaly, syndactyly of second and third toes, polydactyly; epicanthal folds, posteriorly rotated ears, ptosis, small pug nose, broad alveolar ridge, micrognathia; deficiency of 7-dehydrocholesterol reductase *NEJM 351;2319–2326, 2004; Am J Med Genet 66:378–398, 1996; Clin Pediatr 16:665–668, 1977*

Sweet's syndrome – in acute myelogenous leukemia *Urol Case Rep 2020 May 3:32:101235.doi:10.1016/j.eucr 2020.101235*

Triploidy syndromes – hypoplastic penis *Clin Genet 9:43–50, 1976*

49, XXXXY syndrome – hypoplastic penis *Clin Genet 33:429–434, 1988*

TOXINS

Chloracne – halogenated aromatic compounds; blackheads, cysts, pustules of cheeks, axillae, groin, post-auricular areas; dioxins, herbicides, Agent Orange *Stat Pearls April 24, 2020*

TRAUMA

Compression therapy of legs – edema of penis and scrotum

Compulsive masturbation – chronic penile lymphedema *Arch Sex Behav 41:737–739, 2012*

Concealed penis – complication of circumcision *Ped Derm 30:519–528, 2013*

Ecchymoses – tracking back along median raphe *Br J Vener Dis 49:467–468, 1972*

Epidermal inclusion cyst – complication of circumcision *Ped Derm 30:519–528, 2013*

Glandular adhesions – complication of circumcision *Ped Derm 30:519–528, 2013*

Hair coil strangulation (edema from accidentally wrapped hair around the penis) *Cutis 31:431–432, 1983*

Meatal stenosis – complication of circumcision *Ped Derm 30:519–528, 2013*

Mechanical trauma *Pediatr Emerg Care 14:95–98, 1998; Scand J Urol Nephrol 30:517–519, 1996*

Penile fracture – edema and purpura of penis *NEJM 372:1055, 2015; Br J Surg 67:680–681, 1980*

Penile skin bridge – complication of circumcision – penile nodules of shaft and rim of glans penis *Ped Derm 30:519–528, 2013*

Penile venereal edema *JAAD 38:645–646, 1998; JAMA 241:157–158, 1979; NEJM 289:108, 1973; AD 108:263, 1973*

Redundant foreskin – complication of circumcision *Ped Derm 30:519–528, 2013*

Rings

Squeezing of glans penis – petechiae *AD 112:121–122, 1976*

Traumatic urethral diverticulae – compressible nodulocystic lesions of the penile shaft *Br J Urol 37:560–568, 1969*

Urethrocutaneous fistuala – complication of circumcision *Ped Derm 30:519–528, 2013*

VASCULAR LESIONS

Acquired phlebectasia of penis *JAAD 13:824–826, 1985*

Acute hemorrhagic edema of infancy – purpura in cockade pattern of face, cheeks, eyelids, and ears; may form reticulate pattern; edema of penis and scrotum *JAAD 23:347–350, 1990*; necrotic lesions of the ears, urticarial lesions; oral petechiae *JAAD 23:347–350, 1990; Ann Pediatr 22:599–606, 1975*

Angiokeratoma corporis diffusum without metabolic abnormalities *AD 142:615–618, 2006*

Angiokeratoma of Fordyce *Genital Skin Disorders, Fischer and Margesson, CV Mosby, 1998, p. 78*; strawberry glans penis due to multiple angiokeratomas *BJD 142:1256–1257, 2000*

Angiolymphoid hyperplasia with eosinophilia – penile papule *JAAD 37:887–920, 1997; Cancer 47:944–949, 1981*; multiple violaceous papules of glans and corona *BJD 159:755–757, 2008*

Arteriosclerotic penile necrosis – personal observation

Arteriovenous malformation *J Pediatr Surg 35:1130–1131, 2000*

Calcemic uremic arteriopathy – in end stage renal disease – acral necrosis *The Ochsner Journal 14:380–385, 2014*

Dorsal vein thrombosis (Mondor's penile disease) *Case Rep Urol Aug 20, 2019; Urol Case Rep 19:34–35, 2018; Urology 67:587–588, 2006; Am J Emerg Med 15:67–69, 1997*

Elephantiasis nostras of penis *AD 137:1095–1100, 2001*

Eosinophilic granulomatosis with polyangiitis – penile papules *Ann DV 129:1049–1052, 2002*

Epithelioid hemangioma *Arch Pathol Lab Med 109:51–54, 1985*

Glomus tumor *Int J Urol 7:115–117, 2000*; glans penis *Derm Surg 21:895–899, 1995*

Granulomatosis with polyangiitis presenting as reactive arthritis – personal observation

Hemangioendothelioma

Hemangioma *Urology 56:153, 2000; J Urol 141:593–594, 1989*

Hemolymphangioma

Intravascular papillary endothelial hyperplasia (Masson's tumor) – blue subcutaneous nodule of penile shaft *Urol J 15:217–219, 2018; J Dermatol 20:657–659, 1993*

Lymphangioma – lymphangioma circumscriptum *Int J STD-AIDS 28:205–207, 2017; Plast Reconstr Surg 103:175–178, 1999; Cutis 28:642–643, 1981*; acquired lymphangioma *J Dermatol 21:358–362, 1994*; post-radiation *Acta DV Croat 26:53–57, 2018*

Lymphedema – due to penile strangulation *J Dermatol 23:648–651, 1996;* ambulatory peritoneal dialysis *Surg Gynecol Obstet 170:306–308, 1990;* amputation of limbs *Diabetes Res Clin Pract 21:197–200, 1993;* strangulation, thrombosis, acute necrotizing pancreatitis *J Ultrasound Med 15:247–248, 1996;* streptococcal disease *Clin Inf Dis 24:516–517, 1997*

Non-venereal sclerosing lymphangitis of the penis *Dermatol Online J July 15, 2014; Urology 127:987–988, 1982; BJD 104:607–695, 1981; Clin Exp Dermatol 2:65–67, 1977; AD 105:728–729, 1972*

Pyogenic granuloma *Ped Derm 19:39–41, 2002; Sex Transm Infect 76:217, 2000; Sex Transm Infect 74:221–222, 1998*

Retiform hemangioendothelioma *JAAD 38:143–175, 1998*

Spindle cell hemangioendotheliomas *Cutis 62:23–26, 1998*

Symmetric peripheral gangrene – penile necrosis and mummification

Varix

Vascular malformation *Aesthetic Surgery J 30:71–73, 2010*

Vasculitis – palpable purpura of shaft of penis; Henoch-Schonlein purpura *Iran J Pediatr 25:e2177, 2015; Genitourin Med 69:301–302, 1993*

Verrucous localized lymphedema of penis, scrotum, vulva, pubis – polypoid, verrucous, cobblestoned lesions *JAAD 71:320–326, 2014*

PENILE ULCERS

AUTOIMMUNE DISEASES AND DISEASES OF IMMUNE DYSFUNCTION

Cicatricial pemphigoid *J R Coll Surg Edinb 45:62–63, 2000;* anti-laminin 332 mucous membrane pemphigoid *BJD 165:815–822, 2011*

Dermatomyositis *J Clin Rheumatol 26:e7–8, 2020*

Lupus erythematosus *Clin Rheumatol 12:405–409, 1993*

Mixed connective tissue disease – orogenital ulcers *Am J Med 52:148–159, 1972*

Morphea

Pemphigus vulgaris

CONGENITAL LESIONS

Noma neonatorum – deep ulcers with bone loss, mutilation of nose, lips, intraorally, anus, genitalia; *Pseudomonas,* malnutrition, immunodeficiency

DEGENERATIVE DISEASES

Neurotrophic ulcer

DRUG-INDUCED

Anti-PD-1 therapy (nivolumab/pembrolizumab – lichenoid eruptions, vitiligo, dermatitis, red papules with scale, red papules and nodules, inflammation surrounding seborrheic keratosis, dyshidrosiform palmar lesions, penile erosions *JAMA Derm 152:1128–1136, 2016; JAAD 74:455–461, 2016*

BCG granuloma due to intravesical instillation – penile edema, ulcers, nodules *JAAD 55:328–331, 2006*

Corticosteroid (topical) abuse

Drug eruption

Fixed drug eruption; *Genitourin Med 62:56–58, 1986;* ornidazole *Indian J Dermatol 59:635, 2014*

Foscarnet – ulcers and/or erosions; *Dermatol Reports 10:7749, 2018; Int J Dermatol 32:519–520, 1993; JAAD 27:124–126, 1992*

HAART therapy – ritonavir and/or lamivudine *JAAD 61:164–165, 2009*

Hydralazine – induction of systemic lupus erythematosus *Postgrad Med J 57:378–379, 1981*

Mitomycin C – spillage; penile necrosis *JAAD 55:328–331, 2006*

Nicorandil *Scott Med J Aug 30, 2018*

Papaverine – self-induced injections *Urology 32:416–417, 1988*

EXOGENOUS AGENTS

Alkyl nitrites ("popper") – due contamination on the hands *JAMADerm153:233–224, 2017*

Dequalinium (quaternary ammonium antibacterial agent) – necrotizing ulcers of the penis *Trans St John's Hosp Dermatol Soc 51:46–48, 1965*

Nitrogen mustard (chemical warfare)

Paraffinoma (sclerosing lipogranuloma) *Eur Urol Focus 5:894–898, 2019; BJD 105:451–456, 1981; Arch Pathol Lab Med 101:321–326, 1977*

Silicone injections *Rev Med Interne 371:489–492, 2016*

Sodium hypochlorite – cleansing; ulcer at urethral meatus *NEJM 372:555, 2015*

INFECTIONS AND INFESTATIONS

Absidia corymbifera BJD 148:1286–1287, 2003

Actinomycosis

AIDS – acute HIV infection *Int J STD AIDS 22:766–767, 2011; AD 134:1279–1284, 1998;* aphthous ulcer of AIDS

Amebiasis – *Entameba histolytica* – solitary painful irregular ulcer *Cutis 90:310–314, 2012; Sex Transm Infect 85:585–588, 2012; Derm Clinics 17:151–185, 1999; Urology 48:151–154, 1996;* rupture of prepuce and erosion of shaft *Med J Aust 5:114–117, 1964*

Anaerobic erosive balanitis – ulcerative balanoposthitis – anaerobes and nontreponemal spirochetes *JAAD 37:1–24, 1997*

Candida – eroded or fissured candidal balanitis *Int J STD AIDS 3:128–129, 1992; Clin Exp Dermatol 7:345–354, 1982*

Chancriform pyoderma (*Staphylococcus aureus*) – ulcer with indurated base; eyelid, near mouth, genital *AD 87:736–739, 1963*

Chancroid (*Haemophilus ducreyi*), including phagedenic chancroid (deformity and mutilation) – round or oval ragged undermined ulcer with satellite ulcers; *Cureus 11:e6397, 2019; Int J STD AIDS 8:585–588, 1997; JAAD 19:330–337, 1988*

Chikungunya fever *Indian J Dermatol 54:128–131, 2009*

Chlamydia pneumonia – MIRM-like syndrome with cheilitis, penile erosions, morbilliform eruption *Ped Derm 34:465–472, 2017*

Cryptococcosis *Infect Urol 3:101–107, 1990; C. abidus* – ulcer of glans penis *BJD 143:632–634, 2000*

Cytomegalovirus *NDT plus 3:379–382, 2010; AD 145:931–936, 2009; Ann Int Med 119:1149, 1993*

Diphtheria, cutaneous (*Corynebacterium diphtheria*) – penile ulcers *Clin Inf Dis 57:iii, 2013; Indian J Dermatol Venereol Leprol 74:187, 2008;* black necrotic ulcers of penis and scrotum *Cutis 79:371–377, 2007*

Epstein-Barr virus *J Dtsch Dermatol Ges 16:1490–1492, 2018*

Fournier's gangrene *Niger J Clin Pract 19:426–430, 2016; Postgrad Med J 70:568–571, 1994*

Fusospirillary infections – deep ulcers with gangrene

Gonococcemia or gonococcal urethritis *Br J Inf Dis 49:364–367, 1973; Br J Vener Dis 46:336–337, 1970;* erosive balanitis; gonococcal penile ulcer *Br J Vener Dis 46:336–337, 1970*

Granuloma inguinale (*Klebsiella granulomatis*) *Dermatol Online J April 18, 2016; JAAD 11:43–47, 1984; JAAD 37:494–496, 1997*

Herpes simplex virus *NEJM 375:666–674, 2016; BJD 138:334–336, 1998; Br J Vener Dis 55:48–51, 1979;* recalcitrant pseudotumoral anogenital herpes simplex virus type 2 – ulcers and hypertrophic nodules *Clin Inf Dis 57:1648–1655, 2013*

Herpes zoster

Histoplasmosis – penile chancre *Aust N Z J Med 20:175–176, 1990; J Urol 57:781–787, 1947*

Infectious mononucleosis; *Can Med Assoc J 129:146–147, 1983*

Leishmaniasis *Indian D DV Leprol 80:247–249, 2014; Eur J Clin Microbiol Infect Dis 17:813–814, 1998; AD 130:1311–1316, 1994; Curr Opin Inf Dis 3:420–426, 1990;* denudation of penis and scrotum in AIDS; punched out ulcers of penis and scrotum *BJD 160:311–318, 2009*

Leprosy – erythema nodosum leprosum of glans penis *Int J Dermatol 54:1060–1063, 2015*

Lymphogranuloma venereum (*Chlamydia trachomatis*) *Int J STD AIDS 30:515–518, 2019; JAAD 37:1–24, 1997*

Mucormycosis

Mycobacterium avium-intracellulare Int J STD AIDS 9:56–57, 1998

Mycobacterium tuberculosis – tuberculosis cutis orificialis (acute tuberculous ulcer) – multiple, shallow, crusted ulcers *Ann DV 29:488–205, 1989;* primary tuberculosis *Australas J Dermatol 40:106–107, 1999; Urologica 34:171–175, 1973;* primary TB of glans penis *Tuber Lung Dis 75:319, 1994;* papulonecrotic tuberculid *Dermatologica 172:93–97, 1986; JAAD 12:1104–1106, 1985;* lupus vulgaris *Int J Dermatol 33:272–274, 1994;* penile ulcers *Indian J Sex Transm Dis AIDS 38:183–186, 2017*

*Mycobacterium ulcerans (*Buruli ulcer) *Prog Urol 15:736–738, 2005*

Mycoplasma-induced rash and mucositis (MIRM) – oral ulcers, lip ulcers, penile ulcers; erosive eyelid dermatitis, hemorrhagic erosive cheilitis, penile erosions *JAMA Derm 156:144–150, 2020*

JAMA 322, 2019

Mycoplasma hominis Sex Transm Dis 10:285–288, 1983

Myiasis – tumbu fly myiasis; *Diptera: Calliphoridae and Sarcophagidae Iran J Arthropod Borne Dis 4:72–76, 2010*

Necrotizing fasciitis – *Bacteroides spp.* in adults; streptococcal and staphylococcal in children

Noma

Penicillium marneffei Int J Derm 25:393–399, 1996; J Clin Inf Dis 23:125–130, 1996

Phagedenic ulcer *Genitourin Med 70:218–221, 1994*

Pseudomonas – ecthyma gangrenosum-like lesion *J Urol 24:431–432, 1980;* autoimmune neutropenia *Pediatr Emerg Care 32:46–48, 2016*

Scabies, with secondary infection

Schistosoma *haematobium Hum Pathol 17:333–345, 1986*

Sporotrichosis (*Sporothrix schenckii*) – irregular painful ulcerations of the glans penis *AD 139:1647–1652, 2003*

Staphylococcus aureus, methicillin resistant *Int J STD AIDS 23:524–526, 2012*

Streptococcal infection – Group A beta-hemolytic *South Med J 83:264, 1990;* Group B streptococcus – circumferential erosion *AD 120:85–86, 1984*

Syphilis (*Treponema pallidum*), primary – chancre *JAAD 82:1–14, 2020; AD 146:572, 2010;* condyloma lata – fissured and eroded; tertiary (gummas) *Genitourin Med 65:1–3, 1989;* reactivation of chancre in Jarisch-Herxheimer reaction *Acta DV 76:91–92, 1996;* herpetiform ulcers *Acta DV March 12, 2020*

Trichomonas – destructive lesion with sinus tract and fistula *Am J Trop Med Hyg 92:943–944, 2015; Br J Med 284:859–860, 1983*

Varicella/zoster

Yaws – ulcerated primary stage (mother yaw) – ulcerated nodule of glans

INFILTRATIVE DISORDERS

Amyloidosis, AL *Amyloid 23:203–204, 2016; J Cutan Pathol 41:791–796, 2014*

Langerhans cell histiocytosis – chancre *AD 123:1274–1275, 1987*

Zoon's balanitis (plasma cell balanitis) *JAAD 37:1–24, 1997*

INFLAMMATORY DISORDERS

Aphthosis – idiopathic; nonsexually acquired genital ulceration (Lipschutz ulcer) *J Eur Acad DV 33:1660–1666, 2019*

Balanoposthitis – ulcerative; poor hygiene; manifestation of chronic lymphocytic leukemia *Urology 56:669, 2000;* acute promyelomonocytic leukemia *J Urol 160:1430–1431, 1998*

Crohn's disease *J Eur Acad DV 30:e87–88, 2016; Cutis 72:432–437, 2003; J Eur Acad Dermatol Venereol 13:224–226, 1999; J Urol 159:506–507, 1998; J Gastroenterol 32:817–821, 1997; Genitourin Med 71:45–46, 1995; Int J STD AIDS 5:230–231, 1994; Gut 27:329–333, 1986; J R Soc Med 77:966–967, 1984; Urology 15:596–598, 1980; Gut 11:18–26, 1970*

Erythema multiforme *Medicine 68:133–140, 1989; JAAD 8:763–765, 1983;* Stevens-Johnson syndrome

Erythema of Jacquet *Ped Derm 15:46–47, 1998*

Hidradenitis suppurativa *Ann Int Med 97:520–525, 1982*

Pyoderma gangrenosum *J Dermatol 40:840–843, 2013; AD 141:1175–1176, 2005; Cutis 72:432–437, 2003; JAAD 32:912–914, 1995; J Urol 127:547–549, 1982; Int J Derm 9:293–300, 1970*

Ulcerative colitis *Nippon Shokakibyo Gakkai Zasshi 78:13030–1306, 1981*

METABOLIC DISEASES

Calciphylaxis – penile necrosis *CEN Case Report 7:204–207, 2018; JAAD 54:736–737, 2006*

Calcific uremic arteriolopathy *Dermatol Online J Feb15, 2019*

Multiple nutritional deficiencies – personal observation

Necrobiosis lipoidica diabeticorum *JAAD 49:921–924, 2003; BJD 135:154–155, 1996*

NEOPLASTIC DISEASES

Angiosarcoma *Int Urol Nephrol 44:1341–1343, 2012*

Basal cell carcinoma *Cutis 61:25–27, 1998*

Erythroplasia of Queyrat

Extramammary Paget's disease *Dermatol Online J Oct 15, 2008*

Kaposi's sarcoma *JAAD 27:267, 1992*

Keratoacanthoma – ulcerated nodule *JAAD 15:1079–1082, 1986*

Leukemia cutis – chronic eosinophilic leukemia *Am J Med 125:e5–6, 2012;* chronic lymphocytic leukemia *Clin Exp Dermatol 36:107–109, 2011;* acute myelomonocytic leukemia *Am J Dermatopathol Jan 7, 2020;* Richter's transformation *JAMA Derm 152:586–587, 2016;* chronic lymphocytic leukemia with ulcerative balanoposthitis of the foreskin *Urology 56:669, 2000;* HTLV-1 leukemia/lymphoma

Lymphoma – diffuse large B-cell lymphoma *Case Rep Pathol , 2012;* Richter transformation into diffuse large cell B-cell lymphoma *JAMA Derm 152:586–587, 2016;* primary anaplastic lymphoma *Genitourin Med 73:325, 1997; J Urol 153:1051–1052, 1995;* Hodgkin's disease primary CD30+ lymphoma *BJD 149:903–905, 2003;* T-cell lymphoma; plasmablastic lymphoma *Pathology 43:54–57, 2011;* follicular lymphoma, extranodal NK/T-cell lymphoma, Burkitt's lymphoma, chronic lymphocytic leukemia, primitive T-cell –rich B-cell lymphoma; ALK+ anaplastic large cell lymphoma, MALT lymphoma; primary penile lymphoma *J Urol 153:1051–1052, 1995*

Marjolin's ulcer *Tanzan J Health Res 14:288–292, 2012*

Metastatases – metastatic male breast carcinoma *JAAD 38:995–996, 1998;* adenocarcinoma of the lung *Med Oncol 26:228–232, 2009*

Mucoepidermoid carcinoma *Can Urol Assoc J 9:E27–29, 2015*

Penile intraepithelial neoplasia *Indian Dermatol Online J 11:120–122, 2020*

Porokeratosis of Mibelli – erosive balanitis *JAAD 36:479–481, 1997*

Squamous cell carcinoma *JAAD 37:1–24, 1997;* ulcerated nodule *NEJM 370:263–271, 2014; Urology 80:e9–10, 2012*

Waldenstrom's macroglobulinemia *An Bras Dermatol 91:236–238, 2016*

PRIMARY CUTANEOUS DISEASES

Acute parapsoriasis (pityriasis lichenoides et varioliformis acuta) (Mucha-Habermann disease) *AD 123:1335–1339, 1987; AD 118:478, 1982*

Balanitis xerotica obliterans *JAAD 37:1–24, 1997*

Erythema elevatum diutinum *Clin Dermatol 37:679–683, 2016*

Hailey-Hailey disease

Keratosis lichenoides chronica *JAAD 49:511–513, 2003*

Lichen planus – erosive lesions

Pilonidal sinus *BMJ Case Rep May 21, 2013; Scientific World J 4 (Suppl 1):258–259, 2004; J Cutan Pathol 26:155–158, 1999*

PSYCHOCUTANEOUS DISEASES

Factitial dermatitis *Acta DV Alp Pannonica Adryat 18:83–85, 2009*

Genital dermatillomania *Curr Urol 11:54–56, 2017*

SYNDROMES

Behcet's disease *NEJM 380:e7, 2019; JAAD 51:S83–87, 2004; Acta DV 54:299–301, 1974*

Degos' disease (malignant atrophic papulosis) *J Eur Acad DV 19:612–616, 2005; BJD 143:1320–1322, 2002*

Hypereosinophilic syndrome *JAMA 247:1018–1020, 1982*

MAGIC syndrome – combination of relapsing polychondritis and Behcet's syndrome *AD 126:940–944, 1990*

Reactive arthritis syndrome – moist red erosion in uncircumcised males *Cutis 71:198–200, 2003; Semin Arthritis Rheum 3:253–286, 1974*

TRAUMA

Condom catheter – gangrene of glans or shaft of penis *JAMA 244:1238, 1980*

Foreign body reaction *Int Marit Health 66:28–29, 2015*

Friction *Genital Skin Disorders, Fisher and Margesson, CV Mosby, 1998, p. 8*

Human bite *Int J STD AIDS 13:852–854, 2002; Sex Transm Dis 26:527–530, 1999;* orogenital traumatic contact *Dermatol Online J Aug 1, 2005*

Intravenous drug addiction (heroin ulcer) – dorsal vein of penis; *Cutis 29:62–72, 1981;* heroin ulcer *AD 107:121–122, 1973;* IVDA *Urol Int 73:302–304, 2004*

Longitudinal cleavage of the penis – catheter complication *Int Urol Nephrol 21:313–316, 1989*

Mechanical trauma including zipper trauma; penile metallic ring leading to strangulation *Hinyokika Kiyo 39:1179–1181, 1993*

Negative pressure device for erectile impotence *J Urol 146:1618–1619, 1991*

Persistent penile painful fissure

Physical trauma

Postoperative hyperemia of the glans penis with ulcers following revascularization surgery for vascular impotence *Dermatology 184:291–293, 1992*

Pressure necrosis *Int Wound J 11:696–700, 2014*

Radiation dermatitis

Zipper trauma – personal observation

VASCULAR DISEASES

Buerger's disease *Am J Clin Exp Urol 4:9–11, 2016*

Cholesterol emboli *BJD 150:1230–1232, 2004*

Granulomatosis with polyangiitis – necrotic penile ulcers *Urol J 17:210–212, 2020; Clin Rheumatol 17:239–241, 1998; JAAD 31:605–612, 1994; AD 130:1311–1316, 1994*

Non-venereal sclerosing lymphangitis of the penis

Polyarteritis nodosa *J Clin Rheumatol 11:167–169, 2005*

Prostatic artery embolization *Can Urol Assoc J Feb 4, 2020*

PERIANAL DERMATITIS AND HYPERTROPHIC PLAQUES

AUTOIMMUNE DISEASES AND DISEASES OF IMMUNE DYSFUNCTION

Allergic contact dermatitis – antipruritics, neomycin, caines, quinolones, lanolin, ethylenediamine *AD 144:749–755, 2008; Am J Contact Dermat 10:43–44, 1999; Contact Dermatitis 36:173–174,*

1997; Acta DV (Stockh) 60:245–249, 1980; or irritant contact dermatitis – liquid stools *J Wound Ostomy Continence Nurs 23:174–177, 1996;* vulvar or perianal dermatitis – allergic contact dermatitis to Cottonelle moist toilet paper (methylchloroisothiazolinone/methylisothiozolinone) *JAMA Derm 152:67–72, 2016; AD 146:886–890, 2010;* exogenous agents; textiles *Contact Dermatitis 81:66–67, 2019*

Cicatricial pemphigoid, drug-induced *BJD 102:715–718, 1980*

Dermatitis herpetiformis *Acta DV Alp Pannonica Adriat 15:52–54, 2006*

Dermatomyositis with epidermal necrosis

Linear IgA disease (chronic bullous disease of childhood) – intertriginous and perigenital *JAAD 51:95–98, 2004*

Lupus erythematosus – systemic lupus – perianal erythema *BJD 121:727–741, 1989;* discoid lupus erythematosus; perianal erythema *AD 118:55–56, 1982*

Pemphigoid vegetans – perianal hypertrophic plaques *Acta DV 64:450–452, 1984*

Pemphigus vegetans – perianal hypertrophic plaques *Int J Dermatol 38:29–35, 1999; Dermatol Clinics 11:429–452, 1993*

CONGENITAL LESIONS

Perineal groove – prominent wet sulcus from fourchette to anus *Ped Derm 27:626–627, 2010*

DRUG-INDUCED

Baboon syndrome (SDRIFE) *Clin Dermatol 33:462–465, 2015*

Etoposide/teniposide/amsacrine – perianal irritation *JAAD 71:203–214, 2014*

Fixed drug eruption

Imiquimod

Nicorandil *BJD 168:1136–1137, 2013*

Sorafenib (multikinase inhibitor) – hand-foot reactions; perianal dermatitis, facial seborrheic dermatitis, red plaques on sides of feet, hyperkeratotic plaque or blister of feet, red patches on pressure points, red swollen fingertips, gray blisters of fingerwebs, angular cheilitis *BJD 158:592–596, 2008*

Sulfonamide-induced acute lichen planus – personal observation

Sunitinib – multikinase inhibitor; bullous palmoplantar erythrodysesthesia, periungual erythema, perianal erythema, mucositis *AD 144:123–124, 2008*

EXOGENOUS AGENTS

Caffeine

Danthron (laxative) – irritant contact dermatitis; livedoid pattern *Clin Exp Dermatol 9:95–96, 1984*

Erythema of Jacquet – erosive diaper dermatitis; complication of adult urinary incontinence *Cutis 82:72–74, 2008;* perianal pseudoverrucous papules *J Pediatr 125:914–916, 1994; AD 128:240–242, 1992*

Poison ivy oral desensitization

INFECTIONS AND/OR INFESTATIONS

Actinomycosis – perianal hypertrophic plaques *Ann DV 109:789–790, 1982*

Amebic granuloma – perianal hypertrophic plaques; Entamoeba histolytica; protozoan; common sites are anus and buttocks, penis, and face; ulcer or granuloma; painful ulcer with raised thick borders and undermined edge with purulent exudate; diagnose by repeat stool examinations

Bacterial infection in immunosuppressed patients

Bejel – perianal hypertrophic plaques

Candidiasis *Int J Derm 38:618–622, 1999;* perianal hypertrophic plaques

Chancroid – perianal hypertrophic plaques; perianal fissuring; *Haemophilus ducreyi;* gram negative facultative anaerobe; incubation period is 3–7 days; soft papule with surrounding erythema progresses to pustular, eroded, ulcerative lesion with ragged and undermined edges; exudative; tender, painful, and multiple; bubo in 50% which may rupture; clinical variants: giant chancroid, large serpiginous ulcer, phagedenic chancroid, transient, follicular, papular (resembles condyloma latum)

Condylomata acuminata – perianal hypertrophic plaques *Ped Derm 20:440–442, 2003; BJD 128:575–577, 1993*

Coxsackie A – papular perianal dermatitis

Cryptococcosis – perianal hypertrophic plaques

Cutaneous larva migrans

Dermatophyte infection *AD 98:322–323, 1968*

Enterobiasis (*Enterobius vermicularis*) (pinworm) – anal and perineal pruritus and dermatitis *J Dermatol 21:527–528, 1994; Am Fam Phys 38:159–164, 1988;* perianal granuloma *J Pediatr 132:1055–1056, 1998*

Erythrasma

Filariasis – perianal hypertrophic plaques

Fournier's gangrene *Am J Med Jan 9, 2020; Am J Emerg Med 36:1719, Sept 2018; NEJM 376:1158, 2016*

Gonococcal infection – perianal fissuring; perianal hypertrophic plaques

Granuloma inguinale (*Calymmatobacterium granulomatis*) – ulcerated papule; perianal hypertrophic, sclerotic, or phagedenic plaques; intracellular gram negative rod; primary lesion is papule, nodule or ulcer; nodular variety ulcerates into red granulating surface; ulcerovegetative; hypertrophic, cicatricial; superinfection with fusospirochetes gives necrotic lesions with massive destruction; extragenital lesions around eye, axilla, oral mucosa, GI tract, and bone *JAAD 54:559–578, 2006*

Hand, foot, and mouth disease – personal observation

Herpes simplex virus – chronic; perianal hypertrophic verrucous papules and plaques *JAAD 57:737–763, 2007;* perianal vegetative tumid mass *JAMA Derm 156:453–454, 2020*

Herpes zoster *Acta DV (Stock)63:540–543, 1983; BJD 89:285–288, 1973*

Histoplasmosis – perianal hypertrophic plaques; perianal papule *Clin Inf Dis 62:361,397–398, 2016*

HIV disease – colonic and perianal ulceration, vacuolar interface dermatitis *Clin Case Rep 27:1478–1480 , 2019*

Bullous impetigo – personal observation

Insect bite – personal observation

Lymphogranuloma venereum (*Chlamydia trachomatis serovariant L1*) – perianal fissuring *Clin Inf Dis 20:576–581, 1995;* vegetating plaques

Malacoplakia – perianal hypertrophic plaques *JAAD 34:325–332, 1996*

Molluscum contagiosum – surrounding dermatitis

Mycetoma – perianal hypertrophic plaques

Mycobacterium tuberculosis – acid-fast, weakly gram positive non-motile rod; lupus vulgaris mimicking lichen simplex chronicus *Katmandu Univ Med J 1:238–241, 2014; J Dermatol 28:369–372, 2001;* tuberculosis verrucosa cutis – perianal fissuring; perianal hypertrophic plaques; solitary plaque

Orf – papules and plaques *JAAD 11:72–74, 1984*

Paracoccidioidomycosis – perianal red plaques *BJD 143:188–191, 2000*

Perianal hypertrophic plaques *Cutis 54:341–342, 1994*

Pinworm (oxyuriasis) (*Enterobius vermicularis*) – urticaria, erythema, pruritus *JAAD 57:371–392, 2007; J Dermatol 21:527–528, 1994*

Recurrent toxin-mediated perineal erythema – associated with *Staphylococcus aureus* or *Streptococcus pyogenes* pharyngitis *AD 144:239–243, 2008; AD 132:57–60, 1996; JAAD 39:383–398, 1998*

Rhinosporidiosis – perianal hypertrophic plaques

Scabies – personal observation

Scarlet fever

Schistosomal granuloma – perianal papules *JAAD 73:929–944, 2015; AD 138:1245–1250, 2002;* pruritic perianal papules *Br J Vener Dis 55:446–449, 1979;* perianal hypertrophic plaques; perianal fissuring; paragenital granulomas due to *S. haematobium;* communicating sinuses and fistulae *Br J Vener Dis 55:446–449, 1979*

Staphylococcus aureus – perianal dermatitis *Ped Derm 10:297–298, 1993;*

Staphylococcal scalded skin syndrome – personal observation

Streptococcus pyogenes – perianal erythema with ecthyma gangrenosum-like lesion (erythematous plaque with central black necrosis) in disseminated streptococcal disease *JAMA 311:957–958, 2014; Dis Colon Rectum 51:584–587, 2008;* perianal streptococcal dermatitis *Am J Clin Dermatol 4:555–560, 2003*

Strongyloidiasis – larva currens

Streptococcal perianal cellulitis – perianal erythema *JAMA 311:957–958, 2014; AD 141:790–792, 2005; Cutis 68:183–184, 2001; JAAD 42:885–887, 2000; Clin Pediatr (Phila) 39:500, 2000; NEJM 342:1877, 2000; Ped Derm 16:23–24, 1999;* perianal streptococcal dermatitis in children *AD 134:1147, 1150, 1998; Am J Dis Child 145:1058–1061, 1991; Ped Derm 7:97–100, 1990; AD 124:702–704, 1988;* in adults *BJD 135:796–798, 1996*

Syphilis – condylomata lata *Clin Inf Dis 55:1106,1164–1166, 2012; NEJM 352:708, 2005; ;* perianal hypertrophic plaques; annular verrucous perianal dermatitis in secondary syphilis *BJD 152:1343–1345, 2005*

Tinea cruris *JAMA Derm 152:486–487, 2016*

Vaccinia *Ann DV 105:339–341, 1979*

Varicella – "occult" *Pediatr Inf Dis 28:1073–1075, 2009*

Warts (human papilloma virus)

Yaws – perianal hypertrophic plaques

INFILTRATIVE

Amyloidosis – lichen amyloid *BJD 143:1266–1269, 2000;* pigmented macules and glossy hyperkeratotic lesions fanning out from anus *Jpn J Dermatol 91:398–443, 1981;* tumid amyloidosis – perianal hypertrophic plaques *AD 102:8–19, 1970;* perianal blistering purpuric dermatitis *JAMA Derm 151:1367–1368, 2015*

Langerhans cell histiocytosis *Curr Prob Derm VI Jan/Feb 1994; Clin Exp Derm 11:183–187, 1986; JAAD 13:481–496, 1985;* eosinophilic granuloma – dermatitis and/or perianal fissuring *Obstet Gynecol 67 (Suppl): 46s–49s, 1986;* in the adult – perianal plaque or dermatitis;

scrotal ulcer; solitary pink papule; red papules of trunk; ulceronecrotic plaque of scalp *BJD 167:1287–1294, 2012;* perianal ulcerated vegetative lesions *Am J Clin Dermatol 18:343–354, 2017; Clin Exp Dermatol 38: 203–204, 2013; Eur J Dermatol 23:551–552, 2013; Gastroenterol Clin Biol 34:95–97, 2010; JAAD 13:481–496, 1985*

Lipoid proteinosis – perianal hypertrophic plaques

Zoon's mucositis (plasma cell mucositis) – perianal moist red plaque *JAMA Derm 150:447–448, 2014*

INFLAMMATORY

Crohn's disease (contiguous extension) – dermatitis and/or perianal fissuring and fistulae, edema, inflammation, edematous skin tags; perianal hypertrophic plaques; non-specific cutaneous lesions include pyoderma gangrenosum, erythema nodosum, aphthous ulcers, signs of malnutrition, and pyostomatitis vegetans; specific lesions include metastatic granulomata, perianal papules or ulcers, sinus tracts *JAMA Derm 152:833–834, 2016; JAAD 68:189–209, 2013; Cutis 80:429–431, 2007; J R Soc Med 75:414–417, 1982; JAAD 5:689–695, 1981;* annular vegetative perianal plaque *JAAD 63:165–166, 2010*

Diverticulitis

Hidradenitis suppurativa – perianal red nodules *JAMA Derm 149:732–735, 2013*

Hirschsprung disease *Ann DV 123:549–551, 1996*

Sarcoidosis – perianal hypertrophic plaques *J Drugs Dermatol 16:1305–1306, 2017; Presse Med 45:146–147, 2016*

Ulcerative colitis – perianal hypertrophic plaques

METABOLIC DISEASES

Acrodermatitis enteropathica (zinc deficiency) – inherited or acquired *NEJM 371:67, 2014*

Biotinidase deficiency *BMJ Med Case Rep Sept 28, 2011*

Hyperhidrosis

Pellagra – perineal and scrotal erythema *BJD 164:1188–1200, 2011*

Short bowel syndrome – diaper dermatitis – personal observation

Verrucous xanthoma – anal nodule *Am J Proctol Gastroenterol Colon Rectal Surg 31:24–25, 1980*

Vitamin B6 deficiency *Clinics in Derm 17:457–461, 1999; JAAD 43:1–16, 2000*

NEOPLASTIC

Anorectal adenocarcinoma – abscess-like *Clin Colon Rectal surg 24:51–63, 2011*

Basal cell carcinoma *Case Rep Surg Nov 21, 2018:9021289; Case Rep Dermatol 21:25–28, 2015; Hautarzt 55:266–272, 2004*

Bowen's disease – perianal hypertrophic plaques *Clin Colon Rectal Surg 24:54–63, 2011; Ped Derm 27:166–169, 2010*

Bowenoid papulosis – HPV 16; perianal hypertrophic plaques *AD 125:651–654, 1989*

Epidermal nevi – perianal hypertrophic plaques

Extramammary Paget's disease *Int J Dermatol 58:871–879, 2019; JAAD 68:189–209, 2013; Br J Surg 75:1098–1092, 1988; JAAD 13:1009–1014, 1985; AD 115:706–708, 1979; Can Med Assoc J 118:161–162, 1978; BJD 85:476–480, 1971;* underlying adnexal carcinoma, adenocarcinoma of the rectum, cervix, or breast *AD 123:379–382, 1987*

ILVEN (inflammatory linear verrucous epidermal nevus) *Australas J Dermatol 50: 115–117, 2009*

Intraepithelial neoplasia, anal – perianal hyperpigmented patches, white and/or red plaques *JAAD 52:603–608, 2005*

Kaposi's sarcoma *Am J Surg 160:681–682, 1990*

Leukoplakia

Lymphoma – cutaneous T-cell lymphoma – personal observation; *Dermatology 190:313–316, 1995*

Melanocytic nevi *J Cutan Pathol 27:215–217, 2000*

Melanoma *Rum J Morphol Embryol 48:299–302, 2007; J Natl Med Assoc 97:726–731, 2005*

Rhabdomyomatous mesenchymal hamartoma – perianal papule *J Histol Histopathol 1:8, 2014*

Metastatic – anal carcinoma – personal observation

Porokeratosis – perianal inflammatory verrucous

porokeratosis (porokeratosis ptychotropica) – perianal papules *JAMA Derm 150:1007–1008, 2014; AD 146:911–916, 2010; JAAD 55:S120–122, 2006; BJD 140:553–555, 1999; BJD 132:150–151, 1995*

Seborrheic keratoses *Clin Colon Rectal Surg 32:394–402, 2019*

Squamous cell carcinoma – perianal hypertrophic plaques

anorectal carcinoma (abscess-like); perianal erythema – squamous cell carcinoma in situ *AD 137:14–16, 2001;* red plaque *Clin Colon Rectal Surg 24:54–63, 2011; Cutis 85:143–145, 2010*

Syringomas – milia-like syringomas *Dermatology 191:249–251, 1995*

Verrucous carcinoma (giant condylomata of Buschke and Lowenstein) – perianal hypertrophic plaques *JAAD 66:867:e1–14, 2012*

PARANEOPLASTIC

Acanthosis nigricans – perianal verrucous plaques *BJD 153:667–668, 2005*

Glucagonoma syndrome – alpha cell tumor of the pancreas; 50% of cases have metastasized by the time of diagnosis; periorificial dermatitis, including perianal dermatitis, angular stomatitis, cheilosis, beefy red glossitis, blepharitis, conjunctivitis, alopecia, crumbling nails; rarely, associated with MEN I or IIA syndromes *JAAD 54:745–762, 2006; AD 133:909–912, 1997; JAAD 12:1032–1039, 1985; Ann Int Med 91:213–215, 1979*

Nummular dermatitis – chronic and resistant to therapy

Paraneoplastic annular erythema – associated with colon cancer

PRIMARY CUTANEOUS DISEASE

Atopic dermatitis *JAAD 57:371–392, 2007*

Erythema of Jacquet – erosive diaper dermatitis *Ped Derm 15:46–47, 1998;* in adult *Cutis 82:72–74, 2008*

Fox-Fordyce disease

Genitoperineal papular acantholytic dyskeratosis – hypertrophic cobblestoned vulva; perianal hypertrophic dermatitis; mutation in *ATP2C1 BJD 166:210–212, 2012*

Granuloma gluteale infantum – perianal hypertrophic plaques; in adults due to incontinence *AD 114:382–383, 1978*

Infantile perianal pyramidal protrusion (anomalous anal papillae) – polypoid or filiform projections at the anus; almost exclusively in girls; in midline just anterior to anus; differential diagnosis includes hemorrhoids, rectal prolapse, skin tags, sexual abuse, sentinel tag of anal fissure, inflammatory bowel disease, perineal midline malformation, hemangioma *JAAD 54:1046–1049, 2006; Ped Derm*

22:151–152, 2005; BJD 151:229, 2004; Ped Derm 19:15–18, 2002; J Pediatr 38:468–471, 1951

Intertrigo

Lichen planus – perianal hypertrophic plaques *Dis Colon Rectum 41:111–114, 1998; Med Cutan Ibero Lat Am 12:339–344, 1984*

Lichen sclerosus et atrophicus *AD 134:1118–1120, 1998;* perianal hypertrophic plaques *J Cut Pathol 42:118–129, 2015; Mod Pathol 11:844–854, 1998*

Lichen simplex chronicus *Trans St John's Hosp Dermatol Soc 57:9–30, 1971;* perianal hypertrophic plaques

Malakoplakia – perianal nodules, vulvar nodules, skin-colored nodules, ulcerations, abscesses, red papules, masses *Arch Pathol Lab Med 132:113–117, 2008*

Papular acantholytic dermatosis – perianal papules; mutation in *ATP 2C1 BJD 179:1001–1002, 2018*

Perianal fissuring, idiopathic – acute, chronic *; Am Fam Physician 101:24–33, 2020; CMAJ 191:E737, 2019*

Perianal pseudoverrucous papules and nodules in children – perianal hypertrophic plaques; due to leakage of stool and/or urine *Cutis 67:335–338, 2001; J Pediatr 125:914–916, 1994; AD 128:240–242, 1992;* Hirschsprung's disease *Ped Derm 34:e343–344, 2017*

Perianal (infantile) pyramidal protrusion – manifestation of lichen sclerosus et atrophicus *AD 134:1118–1120, 1998*

Pruritus ani *Postgrad Med 77:56–59, 62, 65, 1985*

Psoriasis – dermatitis and/or perianal fissuring *Cutis 50:336–338, 1992;* perianal hypertrophic plaques; inverse psoriasis

Seborrheic dermatitis – dermatitis *JAAD 57:371–392, 2007;* and/or perianal fissuring; perianal hypertrophic plaques

Seborrhiasis (sebopsoriasis)

PSYCHOCUTANEOUS DISEASES

Factitial dermatitis

SYNDROMES

Baboon syndrome – generalized exanthem with accentuation of buttocks, anogenital area, flexures; systemic contact dermatitis to mercury precipitated often by inhalation of mercury vapor *Ped Derm 21:250–253, 2004*

Behcet's disease – perianal fissuring

Costello syndrome – perianal and vulvar papules; warty papules around nose and mouth, legs, perianal skin; loose skin of neck, hands, and feet; acanthosis nigricans; low set protuberant ears, thick palmoplantar surfaces with single palmar crease, gingival hyperplasia, hypoplastic nails, moderately short stature, craniofacial abnormalities, hyperextensible fingers, sparse curly hair, diffuse hyperpigmentation, generalized hypertrichosis, multiple nevi *Ped Derm 20:447–450, 2003; JAAD 32:904–907, 1995; Aust Paediat J 13:114–118, 1977*

Ectodermal dysplasia-skin fragility syndrome – autosomal recessive; plakophilin gene mutation (PKP1) – perianal erythema and erosions, follicular hyperkeratosis; widespread skin fragility, alopecia of scalp and eyebrows, focal palmoplantar keratoderma with painful fissures, hypohidrosis; skin peeling; generalized erythema and peeling at birth; perioral fissuring and cheilitis *JAAD 55:157–161, 2006; Acta DV 85:394–399, 2005; JID 122:1321–1324, 2004*

Hereditary mucoepithelial dysplasia (dyskeratosis) (Gap junction disease, Witkop disease) – autosomal dominant; non-scarring alopecia; dry rough skin; red eyes, non-scarring alopecia, follicular keratosis (keratosis pilaris), erythema of oral (hard palate, gingival, tongue) and nasal mucous membranes, cervix, vagina, and urethra; perineal and perigenital psoriasiform dermatitis (perineal erythema); hyperpigmented hyperkeratotic lesions of flexures (neck, antecubital and popliteal fossae); esophageal stenosis; keratitis (visual impairment) increased risk of infections, fibrocystic lung disease *Ped Derm 29:311–315, 2012; BJD 153:310–318, 2005; Ped Derm 11:133–138, 1994; Am J Med Genet 39:338–341, 1991; JAAD 21:351–357, 1989; Am J Hum Genet 31:414–427, 1979; Oral Surg Oral Med Oral Pathol 46:645–657, 1978*

Hermansky-Pudlak syndrome – perianal dermatitis with pilonidal cyst *Society of Pediatric Dermatology Annual Meeting, July, 2015*

Infantile systemic hyalinosis (juvenile hyaline fibromatosis) – perianal plaques; hyperpigmented papules; mimics atopic dermatitis; joint contractures, short stature, thickened skin and hyperpigmentation, pearly papules of face, perianal nodules, gingival hyperplasia, increased susceptibility to infection, osteopenia, protein losing enteropathy; mutation in *CMG2* (capillary morphogenesis protein 2) *Ped Derm 23:458–464, 2006; JAAD 58:303–307, 2008; Ped Derm 11:52–60, 1994; Dermatology 187:144–148, 1993; Pediatr Pathol 6:55–79, 1986;* perianal nodules; mutation of capillary morphogenesis protein 2 gene *BJD 157:1037–1039, 2007*

Kawasaki's disease – papular or papulovesicular perianal dermatitis, perianal erythema and desquamation *JAAD 69:501–510, 2013; JAAD 39:383–398, 1998; AD 124:1805–1810, 1988*

Keratitis-ichthyosis-deafness (KID) syndrome *Ped Derm 25:466–469, 2008*

KID syndrome with fissured lips – paronychial pustules, blepharitis without keratitis, perineal psoriasiform plaques, tongue erosions, honeycomb palmoplantar keratoderma; red gingivae; mutation in connexin 26 (*N14K*) *GJB2*

Olmsted syndrome – perianal hypertrophic plaques; palmoplantar and periorificial keratoderma of early childhood with alopecia universalis, tooth and nail defects, joint laxity, flexion contractures with constriction or autoamputation *BJD 122:245–252, 1990*

WILD syndrome – disseminated warts, diminished cell-mediated immunity, primary lymphedema, anogenital dysplasia; perianal hypertrophic plaque *AD 144:366–372, 2008*

TRAUMA

Child abuse *Pediatr Emerg Care 33:265–267, 2017*

Fecal incontinence

Sexual abuse *Arch Dis Child 87:262, 2002*

VASCULAR LESIONS

Hemorrhoids – surrounding dermatitis; erosions *Dermatitis 22:227–229, 2011; Dis Colon Rectum 43:561–563, 2000*

PERIANAL ULCERS, SINGLE OR MULTIPLE

AUTOIMMUNE DISEASES AND DISEASES OF IMMUNE DYSFUNCTION

Allergic contact dermatitis *Dermatitis 6:292–293, 2015*

Antineutrophil cytoplasmic antibody syndrome – purpuric vasculitis, orogenital ulceration, fingertip necrosis, pyoderma gangrenosum-like ulcers *BJD 134:924–928, 1996*

Bullous pemphigoid

Cicatricial pemphigoid; *BJD 118:209–217, 1988; Oral Surg 54:656–662, 1982*

Graft vs host disease *Clin Gastroenterol Hepatol 15:e53–54, 2017*

IgA pemphigus – oral and perianal ulcers *Cutis 80:218–220, 2007*

Leukocyte adhesion deficiency *BJD 178:335–349, 2018*

Mucous membrane pemphigoid – generalized bullae with perianal ulcers and esophageal ulcers; IgG and IgA antibodies to laminin 332 and type XVII collagen *BJD 166:1116–1120, 2012*

Pemphigus vulgaris

Pemphigus vegetans *JAAD 480–485, 1993*

Severe combined immunodeficiency in Athabascan American Indian children *AD 135:927–931, 1999*

CONGENITAL ANOMALIES

Congenital anorectal malformation (with polypoid lesions) *AD 123:1278–1279, 1987*

Congenital pemphigus vulgaris – perianal erosions *JAMA Derm 150:1223–1224, 2014*

Perineal groove (congenital malformation/wet sulcus (ulcer) – ulcer anterior to anus *Ped Derm 34:677–680, 2017; JAMA Derm 150:101–103, 2014; Pediatr Surg Int 19:554–556, 2003*

DRUG-INDUCED

Acetaminophen rectal suppositories – perianal necrosis (ergotism) *BJD 170:212–218, 2014*

All-trans retinoic acid induction chemotherapy in acute promyelocytic leukemia – fever, scrotal , vulvar, or perineal necrotic ulcers *JAMA Derm 153:1181–1182, 2017*

Analgesic suppositories *Australas J Dermatol 60:50–52, 2019*

Corticosteroids – topical corticosteroid atrophy with ulceration *Cutis 69:67–68, 2002*

Ergotism *Hautarzt 48:199–202, 1997; AD 128:1115–1120, 1992; Hautarzt 32:688–690, 1980*

Everolimus *Pediatr Transpl 22:doi:101111, Feb 2018*

Nicorandil (potassium channel activator) – large punched out perianal ulcers *Leuk and Lymph 53:334–335, 2012; BJD 156:394–396, 2007; JAAD 56:S116–117, 2007; BJD 155:494–496, 2006; BJD 152:1360–1361, 2005; BJD 152:809–810, 2005; BJD 150:394–396, 2004; Lancet 360:546–547, 2002;* peristomal ulcers, perianal ulcers; bowel perforation *BJD 167:1048–1052, 2012*

Sirolimus *BMT 51:132–133, 2016*

Sweet's syndrome – red plaques, nasal ulcers, perianal ulcers – celecoxib *JAAD 45:300–302, 2001*

EXOGENOUS AGENTS

Irritant contact dermatitis – anal fissures *JAAD 57:371–392, 2007*

Foreign body *AD 145:931–936, 2009*

Paraffinoma – injection for hemorrhoids; nodule, plaque, sinus *BJD 115:379–381, 1986*

Potassium permanganate bath *Hautarzt 61:535–538, 2010*

INFECTIONS AND INFESTATIONS

Actinomycosis *Ann DV 109:789–790, 1982*

Amebic ulcers (*Entamoeba histolytica*) – ulcers of vulva and perineum; often accompanied by diarrhea; serpiginous ulcer *Cutis 90:310–314, 2012; JAAD 60:897–925, 2009; AD 144:1369–1372, 2008; Ped Derm 23:231–234, 2006; Ped Derm 10:352–355, 1993; Pediatrics 71:595–598, 1983; Arch Dis Child 55:234–236, 1980; Mod Probl Paediatr 17:259–261, 1975; Am J Proctol 17:58–63, 1966*

Anorectal abscess

Bacteroides

Campylobacter jejuni

Candidiasis – erosive candidiasis

Cellulitis *AD 124:702–704, 1988;* streptococcal *JAAD 18:586–588, 1988*

Chancroid (*Hemophilus ducreyii*), including phagedenic chancroid (deformity and mutilation) – round or oval ragged undermined ulcer with satellite ulcers *Int J STD AIDS 8:585–588, 1997; JAAD 19:330–337, 1988*

Chikungunya fever *JAAD 75:1–16, 2016*

Chlamydia trachomatis lymphogranuloma venereum serovariant L1 – anal fissures *Clin Inf Dis 20:576–581, 1995*

Clostridial and non-clostridial gangrene *Surgery 86:655–662, 1979*

Cryptococcosis

Cytomegalovirus – in renal transplant patient *Clin Inf Dis 68:1747–1749, 2019; Gastroenterol 149:e11–12, 2015; AD 140:877–882, 2004; Cutis 67:43–46, 2001;* adult – *Am J Clin Path 47:124–128, 1967; JAAD 38:349–351, 1998;* perinatal CMV *JAAD 54:536–539, 2006;* pustules, ulcers, bullae, and vesicles in fatal CMV *AD 127:396–398, 1991;* livedo reticularis and perianal ulcers – CMV vasculopathy *JAAD 64:1216–1218, 2011*

Dermatophyte infection – deep dermatophytosis in inherited autosomal recessive CARD9 deficiency *NEJM 1704–1714, 2013*

Ecthyma gangrenosum *Am J Med 80:729–734, 1986;* due to *Citrobacter freundii JAAD 50:S114–117, 2004*

Entamoeba histolytica Ped Derm 23:231–234, 2006

Fournier's gangrene

Gonorrhea with rectal discharge – round or oval ulcers perianal fissuring *Sex Trans Dis 40:768–770, 2013; Ann Clin Lab Sci 6:184–192, 1976*

Granuloma inguinale (*Calymmatobacterium granulomatis*) – papule or nodule breaks down to form ulcer with overhanging edge; deep extension may occur; or serpiginous extension with vegetative hyperplasia; pubis, genitalia, perineum; extragenital lesions of nose and lips, or extremities *JAAD 32:153–154, 1995; JAAD 11:433–437, 1984*

Herpes simplex infection *NEJM 375:666–674, 2016; J Clin Microbiol 36:848–849, 1998;* chronic herpes simplex in HIV disease *JRSM Open July 7, 2015*

Herpes zoster *Acta DV (Stock) 63:540–543, 1983BJD 89:285–288, 1973*

Histoplasmosis *JAAD 77:197–218, 2017; J Cut Pathol 43:438–443, 2016; Mayo Clinic Proc 67:1089–1108, 1992*

HIV disease – idiopathic perianal ulcer *JRSM Open 6:2054270415593464, July, 2015; Ped Derm 23:43–48, 2006; Dis Colon Rectum 42:1598–1601, 1999*

Human papilloma virus infection

Klebsiella pneumoniae – necrotizing fasciitis *Indian J Pediatr 64:116–118, 1997*

Leishmaniasis *AD 141:1161–1166, 2005*

Lymphogranuloma venereum *Stat Pearls Nov 24, 2019*

Meleney's synergistic gangrene (synergistic necrotizing gangrene) *Surgery 86:655–662, 1979; Arch Surg 9:317–364, 1924*

Mycetoma *JAAD 53:931–951, 2005*

Mycobacterium kansasii JAAD 18:1146–1147, 1988

Mycobacterium tuberculosis – primary TB – indolent, irregular painful ulcers *Clin Dermatol 38:152–159, 2020; BJD 142:186–187, 2000;* fistulae, abscesses; lupus vulgaris, verrucous TB *Prensa Med Argent 56:622–623, 1969;* tuberculosis cutis orificialis (acute tuberculous ulcer) *Medicine (Balt) 97:e10836, June 2018; AD 145:931–936, 2009; DOJ 15:9, 2009; Dis Colon Rectum 42:110–112, 1999; J R Soc Med 89:584, 1996; Dis Colon Rectum 23:54–55, 1980*

Mycoplasma pneumonia (MIRM) – erosive eyelid dermatitis, hemorrhagic erosive cheilitis, penile erosions, perianal erosions *JAMA Derm 156:144–150, 2020*

Necrotizing anorectal and perineal infections – *Clostridium perfringens*, other clostridia, aerobic and anaerobic streptococci, *Pseudomonas* species *J Urol 124:431–432, 1980*

Orf *JAAD 11:72–74, 1984*

Paracoccidioidomycosis *J Clin Inf Dis 23:1026–1032, 1996*

Perirectal abscess

Pseudomonas sepsis in infants – perineal gangrenous changes (noma neonatorum) *Lancet 2:289–291, 1978*

Scabies – perianal ulcers *JAAD 57:371–392, 2007*

Schistosoma haematobium

Schistosoma mansoni – anal fissure with multilobulated giant anal polyp *AD 144:950–952, 2008*

Streptococcus – cellulitis; Group B streptococcal disease – decubitus ulcers *Clin Inf Dis 33:556–561, 2001;* chronic streptococcal carriage *Gastroenterology 155:1701–1702, 2018; JAAD 57:371–392, 2007*

Syphilis – primary chancre – ulcerated nodule, anal fissure *JAAD 82:1–14, 2020; ; Proc R Soc Med 49:629–631, 1966;* secondary syphilis – perianal fissures and proctitis *NEJM 375:666–674, 2016;* secondary (condyloma lata), endemic (bejel); congenital syphilis – diffuse perianal and perineal ulcers *Ped Derm 23:43–48, 2006;* perianal rhagades in congenital syphilis *Ped Derm 9:329–334, 1992;* tertiary (gummas) *Genitourin Med 65:1–3, 1989;* anal syphilis in men *Arch Pathol Lab Med 139:456–460, 2015*

Trichoderma JAAD 80:869–880, 2019

Yersinia enterocolitica Ann Surg 79:e271–272, 2013

INFILTRATIVE DISEASES

Langerhans cell histiocytosis – childhood *Int J Colorectal Dis 33:1501–1504, 2018; Eur J Dermatol 23:551–552, 2013; Ped Derm 23:43–48, 2006; Acta DV 80:49–51, 2000;* adult *BJD 160:213–215, 2009; Int J Colorectal Dis 22:1141–1142, 2007; AD 129:1261–1264, 1993; Dermatologica 155:283–291, 1977;* eosinophilic granuloma *AD 141:1161–1166, 2005*

Mastocytosis, systemic *Ped Derm 23:43–48, 2006*

INFLAMMATORY DISEASES

Crohn's disease – perianal ulcers, fissures, sinus tracts; rectal bleeding, perianal abscess, abdominal pain, perianal pustule, anal skin tags, scrotal swelling and erythema, labial erythema and edema, perianal erythema, granulomatous cheilitis *Ped Derm 35:566–574, 2018; Cutis 101:e8–10, 2018; Ped Derm 23:43–48, 2006; JAAD 10:33–38, 1984; J R Soc Med 75:414–417, 1982; JAAD 5:689–695, 1981;* anal fissures *JAAD 57:371–392, 2007*

Erythema multiforme, including Stevens-Johnson syndrome

Hidradenitis suppurativa *AD 145:931–936, 2009*

Malakoplakia *JAAD 34:325–332, 1996*

Perianal fissures, idiopathic

Pilonidal sinus tracts

Pyoderma fistulans sinifica (fox den disease) *Clin Inf Dis 21:162–170, 1995*

Pyoderma gangrenosum of adults or infants *JAMA Derm 154:1080–1081, 2018; Ped Derm 23:43–48, 2006; Ped Derm 11:10–17, 1994*

Sarcoidosis *AD 145:931–936, 2009*

Sterile abscesses

Toxic epidermal necrolysis

METABOLIC DISEASES

Acrodermatitis enteropathica; acquired zinc deficiency *Ped Derm 23:43–48, 2006*

Biotinidase deficiency

Constipation – anal fissures *JAAD 57:371–392, 2007*

Cystic fibrosis – diffuse perianal and perineal erosions *Ped Derm 23:43–48, 2006*

Essential fatty acid deficiency *Ped Derm 23:43–48, 2006*

Kwashiorkor – perianal erosions *Cutis 67:321–327, 2001*

Liver disease, chronic (cirrhosis) – zinc deficiency; generalized dermatitis of erythema craquele (crackled and reticulated dermatitis) with perianal and perigenital erosions and crusts; cheilitis, hair loss *Ann DV 114:39–53, 1987*

Necrolytic migratory erythema

Prolidase deficiency – autosomal recessive; peptidase D mutation (PEPD); increased urinary imidopeptides; leg ulcers, anogenital ulcers, short stature (mild), telangiectasias, recurrent infections (sinusitis, otitis); mental retardation; splenomegaly with enlarged abdomen, atrophic scarring, spongy fragile skin with annular pitting and scarring; dermatitis, hyperkeratosis of elbows and knees, lymphedema, purpura, low hairline, poliosis, canities, lymphedema, photosensitivity, hypertelorism, saddle nose deformity, frontal bossing, dull expression, mild ptosis, micrognathia, mandibular protrusion, exophthalmos, joint laxity, deafness, osteoporosis, high arched palate *JAAD 62:1031, 1034, 2010; Ped Derm 13:58–60, 1996; JAAD 29:819–821, 1993; AD 127:124–125, 1991; AD 123:493–497, 1987*

Riboflavin deficiency

NEOPLASTIC DISEASES

Bowenoid papulosis

Cloacogenic carcinoma – perianal nodule *JAAD 23:1005–1008, 1990*

Extramammary Paget's disease – perianal plaque *AD 123:379–382, 1987*

Kaposi's sarcoma

Leukemia – acute myelogenous leukemia *Proc R Soc Med 61:624–626, 1968*

Lymphoma – B-cell lymphoma *Ann R Coll Surg 92:W7–9, 2010;* angiocentric lymphoma *Dig Dis Sci 38:1162–1166, 1993*

Lymphomatoid papulosis *J R Soc Med 77 Suppl 14:9–11, 1984*

Marjolin's ulcer – from hidradenitis suppurativa *Plast Reconstr Surg Globe Open 7:e2054, 2019*

Metastatic squamous cell carcinoma in pilonidal cyst *JAAD 29:272–274, 1993*

Mucinous adenocarcinoma *Transl Gastroenterol Hepatol June 21, 2016*

Neuroendocrine small cell carcinoma *Am J Surg 84:e538–540, 2018*

Extramammary Paget's disease *Indian J Surg 79:380–382, 2017; Darier and Coulillaud, 1893*

Perianal polyps *Pathology 140:275–330, 1983*

Primary cutaneous plasmablastic lymphoma *Indian J Venereol Leprol 83:83–86, 2017*

Salivary ectopia – perianal skin tag *AD 123:1277–1278, 1987*

Squamous cell carcinoma, including anal squamous cell carcinoma in situ *J Clin Inf Dis 21:603–607, 1995*

Verrucous carcinoma (Buschke-Lowenstein tumor) *Dis Colon Rectum 37:950–957, 1994*

PRIMARY CUTANEOUS DISEASES

Behcet's disease

Complex aphthosis *J Cut Med Surg 23:105–107, 2019;* aphtha major perianalis *J Cut Med Surg 23:105–107, 2019*

Diaper dermatitis, erosive

Epidermolysis bullosa, recessive dystrophic – perianal ulcers resulting in anal stenosis *Epidermolysis Bullosa: Basic and Clinical Aspects. New York: Springer, 1992: 135–151*

Erythema of Jacquet – perineal punched out ulcers *Australas J Dermatol 43:1–6, 2002*

HAILEY-HAILEY DISEASE

Lichen planus *BJD 136:479, 1997*

Lichen sclerosus et atrophicus – anal fissures

Lichen simplex chronicus – anal fissures

Perianal pseudoverrucous papules and nodules in children *AD 128:240–242, 1992*

Psoriasis – anal fissures

Seborrheic dermatitis

PSYCHOCUTANEOUS DISEASES

Factitial dermatitis

SYNDROMES

Ankyloblepharon, ectrodactyly, cleft lip and palate syndrome (AEC syndrome) *Ped Derm 10:434–440, 1993*

Behcet's syndrome – inguinal fissures *JAAD 30:869–873, 1994;* fissures of anal margin *Br J Vener Dis 139:15–17, 1963*

Goltz's syndrome – perianal papillomas *JAAD 28:829–843, 1993*

Omenn's syndrome *Ped Derm 23:43–48, 2006*

Reactive arthritis syndrome – erosions with marginal erythema; circinate erosions *JAAD 59:113–121, 2008; NEJM 309:1606–1615, 1983; Semin Arthritis Rheum 3:253–286, 1974; Dtsch Med Wochenschr 42:1535–1536, 1916*

  Circinate balanitis – annular or serpiginous

  Asymptomatic oral mucosal erosions

  Keratoderma blenorrhagicum; soles, pretibial areas, dorsal toes, feet, fingers, hands, nails, scalp; may be associated with HIV disease *Ann Int Med 106:19–26, 1987; Semin Arthritis Rheum*

3:253–286, 1974; following gastroenteritis due to *Salmonella enteritidis, Shigella, Yersinia, Campylobacter species,* and Clostridium difficile *Clin Inf Dis 33:1010–1014, 2001*

Solitary rectal ulcer syndrome *Indian J Gastroenterol 38:173–177, 2019; GE Port J Gastroenterol 24:142–146, 2017*

Ulcerative vulvitis – red crusted plaques of vulva and perineum *JAAD 48:613–616, 2003; Arch Int Med 145:822–824, 1985*

TRAUMA

Anal fistulae, fissures, ulcerated hemorrhoids in homosexuals *Br J Surg 76:1064–1066, 1989*

Child abuse *JAAD 57:371–392, 2007*

Decubitus ulcers

Fissure *J Vasc Surg 152 (suppl2) S37–43, 2015*

Fistula

Mechanical trauma

Radiation dermatitis

Sadomasochism

Thermal burn

VASCULAR

Granulomatosis with polyangiitis – necrotic penile ulcers *Brit Med J Case Rep Jan 31, 2018; Clin Rheumatol 17:239–241, 1998; JAAD 31:605–612, 1994; AD 130:1311–1316, 1994*

Hemangioma, including infantile perianal hemangioma *JAAD 57:371–392, 2007; AD 138:126–127, 2002; AD 137:365–370, 2001; AD 106:382–383, 1972*

Hemorrhoids with perianal fissures

Ischemia *SKINMed 15:235–237, 2017*

PERIORBITAL EDEMA/ERYTHEMA (DERMATITIS)

AUTOIMMUNE DISEASES AND DISEASES OF IMMUNE DYSFUNCTION

Allergic contact dermatitis – cosmetics, aerosol sprays, matches, plants, occupational exposures, topical medicines, nickel *Surv Ophthalmol 24:57–88, 1989;* airborne allergic contact dermatitis; airborne allergen blepharitis *Clin Therap 17:800–810, 1995;* swimming goggles *JAAD 43:299–305, 2000;* epoxy resin in immersion oil *JAAD 47:954–955, 2002;* heliotrope – allergic contact dermatitis to phenylephrine drops *Ped Derm 30:975–977, 2019;* mango flesh *Int J Dermatol 43:195–196, 2004*

Angioedema *JAAD 53:373–388, 2005*

Dermatomyositis – periorbital edema as presenting sign *JAAD 48:617–619, 2003; Int J Dermatol 42:466–467, 2003; JAAD 47:755–765, 2002; Ped Derm 16:43–45, 1999; Curr Opin Rheum 11:475–482, 1999;* heliotrope *AD 148:1100–1101, 2012;* periorbital edema and arthralgias of dermatomyositis with anti-PL-12 autoantibodies (antisynthetase syndrome) *NEJM 367:2134–2146, 2012;* association with toxoplasmosis *Am J Med 75:313–320, 1983;* bleomycin *BJD 133:455–459, 1995;* associated with carcinomas of lung, breast, female genital tract, stomach, rectum, kidney, testis, nasopharyngeal carcinoma; lymphomas, thymoma, leukemias; Kaposi's sarcoma *AD 110:605–607, 1974;* myeloma, salivary pleomorphic adenoma *J R Soc Med*

76:787–788, 1983; dysgerminoma *Arthritis Rheum 26:572–573, 1983*

Graft vs. host reaction *AD 126:1324–1329, 1990;* including sclerodermatous graft vs. host reaction – periorbital papules *JAAD 26:49–55, 1992;* periorbital lichenoid graft vs. host reaction, chronic *AD 134:602–612, 1998;* periorbital edema *Am J Neuroradiol 18:730–732, 1997*

Lupus erythematosus – systemic *Lupus 12:866–869, 2003; BJD 143:679–680, 2000; BJD 134:601–602, 1996; J Rheumatol 20:2158–2160, 1993;* chronic cutaneous LE *JAAD 26:334–338, 1992;* periorbital mucinosis in SLE *JAAD 62:667–671, 2010;* DLE – acute periorbital mucinosis *JAAD 41:871–873, 1999;* DLE – periorbital edema *Dermatology 205:194–197, 2002;* eyelid plaques *AD 129:495, 1993;* bullous LE; lupus profundus *Hautarzt 50:889–892, 1999; JAAD 24:288–290, 1991; BJD 129:96–97, 1993; JAAD 24:288, 1991; Clin Exp Dermatol 13:406–407, 1988;* neonatal LE – periorbital erythema *Ped Derm 28:115–121, 2011; JAAD 40:675–681, 1999;* periorbital dermatitis – neonatal LE *Ped Derm 33:219–220, 2016;* tumid lupus erythematosus – periorbital red plaque *BJD 157:1081–083, 2007;* heliotrope *BJD 143:679–680, 2000*

Orbital myositis and giant cell myocarditis *JAAD 35:310–312, 1996; Ophthalmology 101:950–954, 1994*

Pemphigus – El-Bagre endemic pemphigus; facial scaling and crusting, conjunctival injection, eyelid erythema and edema, ectropion, meibomitis *JAAD 62:437–447, 2010*

Pemphigus vulgaris, erythematosus, foliaceus – erythema and erosions *JAAD 33:312–315, 1995*

Relapsing polychondritis *Respirology 8:99–103, 2003; JAAD 41:299–302, 1999*

Scleroderma – progressive systemic sclerosis and linear scleroderma resembling heliotrope *JAAD 7:541–544, 1982; Ann Int Med 80:273, 1974*

Sclerodermatomyositis – Gottron's papules, periorbital erythema, Raynaud's phenomenon, acrosteolysis, dysphagia, digital ulcers; high risk of interstitial lung disease *Arthr Research Therapy 16:R111, 2014; AD 144:1351–1359, 2008; Arthr Rheum 50:565–569, 2004; J Clin Immunol 4:40–44, 1984*

Serum sickness – personal observation

Sjogren's syndrome *Am J Dermpathol 21:129–137, 1999*

Still's disease (systemic onset juvenile idiopathic arthritis) – episodic fevers, polyarticular arthritis of both large and small joints; typical rash – evanescent salmon pink urticarial rash with fever on trunk, proximal extremities, pressure areas, face; atypical rash persistent eruption, periorbital edema, dermatomyositis-like rash; heliotrope *AD 148:947–952, 2012;* severe periorbital edema *Rheumatol Int 32:2233–2237, 2012; Ped Derm 21:580–588, 2004; Sem Hosp 59:1848–1851, 1983*

Urticaria – systemic, contact, physical *JAAD 47:755–765, 2002*

CONGENITAL DISORDERS

Congenital mucocoele

Dermoid cyst *Eyelid and Conjunctival Tumors, Shields JA and Shields CL, Lippincott Williams and Wilkins, 1999, p.159*

DEGENERATIVE DISORDERS

Blepharochalasis *Ann Plast Surg 45:538–540, 2000*

Loss of fenestration of the orbital septum

DRUG-INDUCED

Acitretin – conjunctival granulation tissue; swollen upper and lower eyelids *JAAD 58:S41–42, 2008*

Apixaban *J Gen Intern Med 33:232, 2018*

Aspirin – unilateral periorbital edema *Dent Update 34:3024, 2007; Ann Allergy Asthma Immunol 79:420–422, 1997; Allergy 48:366–369, 1993*

Atacurium

Augmentin – personal observation

Bleomycin, intrapleural – personal observation

BRAF inhibitors – eccrine hidradenitis *BJD 176:1645–1648, 2017*

Calcium channel blockers *JAAD 21:132–133, 1989*

Chemotherapy-induced eccrine neutrophilic hidradenitis – resembles periorbital cellulitis *JAAD 40:367–398, 1999*

Cisplatinum

Clozapine *Aust NZ J Psychiatry 45:1077–1078, 2011*

Contrast medium *Clin Radiol 40:108, 1989*

Corticosteroids – periorbital dermatitis and conjunctivitis *Eye 12:148–149, 1998;* methylprednisolone *AJ Ophth 113:588–590, 1992*

Diltiazem – periorbital edema *Arch Opthalmol 111:1027–1028, 1993*

Doxorubicin *Am J Ophthalmol 108:709–711, 1989*

Drug reaction with eosinophilia and systemic symptoms (DRESS) – morbilliform eruption, cheilitis (crusted hemorrhagic lips), diffuse desquamation, areolar erosion, periorbital dermatitis, vesicles, bullae, targetoid plaques, purpura, pustules, exfoliative erythroderma, facial edema, lymphadenopathy *JAAD 68:693–705, 2013;* Dilantin *AD 114:1350–1353, 1978*

Epidermal growth factor inhibitors – periorbital erythema *JAAD 70:821–838, 2014*

Erythropoietin

Ethosuximide *Curr Opin Ophthalmol 23:405–414, 2012*

5-fluorouracil – personal observation

Fixed drug eruption *Int J Derm 37:833–838, 1998*

Hyaluronidase *Australas J Dermatol 51:49–51, 2010; Eye (London)691–692, 2005*

Hydantoin *Arch Derm 114:1350, 1978*

Hydralazine

Irbesartan *J Drugs Dermatol 3:329–303, 2002*

Ibuprofen *J Dermatol 32:969–971, 2005; Am J Clin Dermatol 3:599–607, 2002*

Imatinib *Clin Ophthalmol 4:427–431, 2010; Arch Ophthalmol 125:985–986, 2007;* imatinib/dasatinib/nilotinib (tyrosine kinase inhibitors) – periorbital edema *JAAD 71:217–227, 2014*

Interferon beta – drug-induced dermatomyositis *AD 144:1341–1349, 2008*

Interleukin 4

Lamotrigine *Ann Pharmacother 33:557–550, 1997*

Mannitol

Metformin

Methotrexate-associated lymphoproliferative disorder – red papules and plaques of nose, cheeks, eyelids *JAAD 56:686–690, 2007*

Methuxsimide

Naproxen

Nifedipine *Am J Cardiol 55:1445, 1985*

Omeprazole – allergic contact dermatitis *Contact Dermatitis 15:36–51, 1986*

Oprelvekin

Pemetrexed *Indian J Pharmacol 48:741–742, 2016*

Piroxicam (Feldene) photodermatitis

Pioglitazone

Proton pump inhibitors – airborne contact dermatitis; red face and neck *Dermatitis 26:287–290, 2015*

Quinidine – photo-induced lichen planus

Resperidone *J Clin Psychopharm 25:709–710, 2008*

Rifampin *Arch Dis Child 62:1181, 1987*

Rosiglitazone

Sirolimus – eyelid edema *Transplantation 72:162–164, 2001*

Sorafenib *J Ocul Pharm Pract 25:2035–2037, 2019*

Sulfacetamide

Sulfafurazole

Sulfasalazine

Sunitinib *Arch Ophthalmol 125:985–986, 2007*

Thiazide diuretic – photoallergic dermatitis

Toxic epidermal necrolysis

Vaccination – post-influenza vaccination *Can Med Assoc J 116:724, 1977;* smallpox *Curr Opin Ophthalmol 23:405–414, 2012*

Verapamil

Yellow mercuric oxide *Contact Dermatitis 35:61, 1996*

Zoledronic acid

EXOGENOUS AGENTS

Artichoke injections (cosmetic surgery) – personal observation

Cocaine – nasolacrimal duct obstruction and orbital cellulitis due to chronic intranasal cocaine abuse *Arch Ophthalmol 117:1617–1622, 1999*

Epoxy resin

Hyaluronic acid and hydroxyapatite fillers (injections) – after administration of omalizumab for asthma; periorbital edema, erythema, and infiltration *J Cosmet Dermatol 19:824–826, 2020; Aesthet Surg J 38:NP109–113, 2018; BJD 166:1375–1376, 2012; J Dermatol 32:969–971, 2005*

Iododerma in chronic renal failure – edema of eyelids; pustulovesicular eruption, pustules, pseudovesicles, marked edema of face and eyelids, vegetative plaques *AD 140:1393–1398, 2004; JAAD 36:1014–1016, 1997; Clin Exp Dermatol 15:232–233, 1990; BJD 97:567–569, 1977*

Irritant contact dermatitis – eye shadow, eye shadow setting creams, eye-liners, mascaras, artificial eyelashes, eyebrow pencils, eye makeup removers *JAAD 47:755–765, 2002; The Clinical Management of Itching; Parthenon; p. 117, 2000*

Milk intolerance *Clin Pediatr (Phil) 34:265–267, 1995*

Food – rice *Allerg Immunopathol 20:171–172, 1992;* peanut allergy *Cutis 65:285–289, 2000*

Matches – recurrent facial eczema due to "strike anywhere" matches (phosphorus sesquisulphide) *BJD 106:477, 1982*

Ochronosis – exogenous ochronosis due to topical hydroquinone application

Paraffinoma – orbital and palpebral *Ophthal Plast Reconstr Surg 11:39–43, 1995; JAAD 26:833–835, 1992*

Silicone granulomas *JAAD 52:S53–56, 2005;* silicone breast implant – silicone granulomas, chronic eyelid edema *Ophthal Plast Reconstr Surg 14:182–188, 1998;* metastatic silicone granuloma –

eyelid papules, eyelid edema *AD 138:537–538, 2002;* silicone granulomas of the face *JAAD 52:53–56, 2005*

Sulfite hypersensitivity *J Korean Med Sci 11:356–357, 1996*

INFECTIONS AND INFESTATIONS

Surv Ophthalmol 52:422–433, 2007

Abscess – Pott's puffy tumor – sinusitis with frontal bone osteomyelitis and epidural abscess; swelling of upper eyelid *JAMA Derm 151:1261–1263, 2015; Am J Rhinol Allergy 26:e63–70, 2012; Eye (London)23:990–991, 2009; Postgrad Med 105:45–46, 1999*

Abscess, bacterial *Eyelid and Conjunctival Tumors, Shields JA and Shields CL, Lippincott Williams and Wilkins, 1999, p.171;* subgaleal abscess *Ann Emerg Med 18:785–787, 1989*

Acanthamebiasis – periorbital plaques *AD 147:857–862, 2011*

Acute hemorrhagic conjunctivitis

Acute sinusitis (acute maxillary sinusitis, acute ethmoiditis); chronic sinusitis *Ear Nose Throat J 93:E38–39, 2014*

Amebiasis *Am J Trop Med Hyg 35:69–71, 1986*

Anthrax (cutaneous palpebral anthrax) – *Bacillus anthracis;* swollen eyelids; malignant pustule; painless ulcer with vesicular lesions; face, neck, hands, fingers, arms, foot, knee; starts as painless erythema evolving into papule then into multiple vesicles or bulla on red base; then ulcer with hemorrhagic crust (eschar) with edema and erythema with small vesicles; edema of surrounding skin; takes six weeks to heal; edema of eyelids, lips, perioral area; slaughtering or milking of ill cows, sheep, or goats; handling of raw meat *Ped Derm 27:600–606, 2010; Ped Derm 18:456–457, 2001; Br J Opthalmol 76:753–754, 1992; J Trop Med Hyg 89:43–45, 1986; Bol Med Hosp Infant Mex 38:355–361, 1981*; preseptal cellulitis and cicatricial ectropion *Acta Ophthalmol Scand 79:208–209, 2001; Br J Opthalmol 76:753–754, 1992; Ophthalmic Physiol Opt 10:300–301, 1990*

Apical root dental abscess with unilateral periorbital edema *Oral Maxillofac Surg 21:271–279, 2017*

Ascariasis – unilateral eyelid edema *Klin Oczna 97:346–347, 1995 (Polish)*

Aspergillosis – orbital cellulitis *NEJM 341:265–273, 1999;* immunocompetent patients with chronic progressive proptosis, periorbital swelling, pain, visual impairment *Clin Inf Dis 59:iii, 2014;* retrobulbar; invasive sinusitis

Bacillus cereus BMJ 4:24, 1975

Bartonella henselae

Black widow spider *Wilderness Environ Med 31:116–118, 2020*

Bed bug infestation – erythema and edema of eyelids *Ped Derm 31:353–355, 2014;* unilateral edema *Ped Derm 29:695, 2012*

Blister beetle periorbital dermatitis and keratoconjunctivitis ("Nairobi eye") (rove beetle) *Eye 12:883–885, 1998;* due to skin contact with coelomic fluids (pederin); spp. *Paederi JAAD 56:685, 2007; J R Army Med Corps 139:17–19, 1993*

Brown recluse spider bite *Turk J Pediatr 53:87–90, 2011*

Cat scratch disease

Caterpillar dermatitis – urticarial papules surmounted by vesicles, urticaria, eyelid edema, bruising in children; conjunctivitis

Cavernous sinus thrombosis, septic *Arch Neurol 45:567–572, 1988*

Cellulitis, erysipelas – usually streptococcal, occasionally staphylococcal – eyelid erythema, edema *JAAD 48:617–1619, 2003;* association with sinusitis *J Eur Acad Dermatol Venereol 11:74–77, 1998;* periorbital cellulitis – erythema, induration, tenderness, warmth *JAAD 70:795–819, 2014;* orbital cellulitis – periorbital

findings and proptosis; limited ocular motility *JAAD 70:795–819, 2014*

Chagas' disease – American trypanosomiasis (*Trypanosoma cruzi*); Romana's sign – unilateral painless or painful bipalpebral edema of the eyelids, conjunctivitis, and inflammation of the lacrimal gland *NEJM 373:456–466, 2016; JAAD 60:897–925, 2009; JAAD 56:493, 2007;* megacolon, intestinal perforation; local lymphadenopathy, periorbital cellulitis, furuncular lesions (chagomas), panniculitis, cardiac involvement *JAAD 75:19–30, 2016; Plos Neglected Trop Dis 4:e711, 2010*

Chikungunya fever (Chikungunya virus) – Africa, Middle East, Europe, India, Southeast Asia; fever, arthralgias, morbilliform eruption; polyarthritis and tenosynovitis; hepatitis, myocarditis, hemorrhage, meningitis, encephalitis; palpebral edema; purpuric butterfly eruption of face; necrosis of skin of nose *Clin Inf Dis 62:78–81, 2016*

Chlamydia

Congestion of vessels of globe due to infection

Conidiobolus incongruus – cellulitis *Pharmacotherapy 21:351–354, 2001*

Cowpox – generalized cowpox in Darier's disease – crusted papules, pustules, and vesicles; cobblestoned appearance; with massive periorbital edema *BJD 164:1116–1118, 2011*

Cranial extradural empyema *Neurosurgery 44:748–753, 1999*

Cutaneous larva migrans

Cysticercosis (*Tenia solium*) – recurrent unilateral periorbital edema *JAMA Derm 154:734–735, 2018*

Dacryocystitis – lacrimal gland inflammation *J Craniofac Surg 30:e195–197, 2019; Eyelid and Conjunctival Tumors, Shields JA and Shields CL, Lippincott Williams and Wilkins, 1999, p.189*

Dengue fever

Dental abscess

Dermatophytosis, tinea faciei – personal observation

Dirofilariasis *JAAD 73:929–944 2015; Trop Parasitol 2:67–68, 2012*

Dracunculosis *JAAD 73:929–944, 2015*

Echinococcosis (hydatid cyst)

Ecthyma gangrenosum – in AIDS *Cutis 66:121–123, 2000*

Enterobacter cloacae – septic cerebral venous thrombosis; retroauricular pain, retrobulbar pain, putrid nasal discharge, chills, double vision, unilateral edema and erythema of right eyelid, red eye *NEJM 373:1553, 2015*

Epidemic keratoconjunctivitis – *Paederus spp.,* "Nairobi red eyes" *East Afr J Pub Health 7:242–245, 2010*

Chronic active Epstein-Barr virus – vulvitis, hemorrhagic cheilitis, necrotic ulcers, periorbital erythema and edema, maxillary sinusitis, hepatosplenomegaly *BJD 173:1266–1270, 2015*

Erysipelas – personal observation

Ethmoid sinusitis – personal observation

Filariasis *Eur J Ophthalmol 19:675–678, 2009*

Fusarium – of sinuses *JAAD 47:659–666, 2002*

Gnathostomiasis – migratory subcutaneous swellings; red and painful; upper body and periorbitally *Clin Inf Dis 16:33–50, 1993*

Gonorrheal conjunctivitis – profuse purulent discharge; swollen hemorrhagic eyelids *Am J Dis Child 144:5468, 1990*

Haemophilus influenzae periorbital cellulitis of children – violaceous erythema with edema *Pediatrics 62:492–493, 1978*

Hepatitis B prodrome – serum sickness, urticarial, angioedema *J Travel Med 18:224–225, 2011*

Herpes simplex infection, primary, recurrent; eczema herpeticum (Kaposi's varicelliform eruption) *Arch Dis Child 60:338–343, 1985*

Herpes zoster; herpes zoster with bacterial superinfection; post-herpes zoster dysesthesias – personal observation

Impetigo

Infectious mononucleosis – periorbital edema (Hoagland's sign) *Ped Derm 37:211–212, 2020; JAAD 72:1–19, 2015; Infection 41:1029–1030, 2013; Cutis 47:323–324, 1991; Pediatrics 75:1003–1010, 1985; J Pediatr 45:204–205, 1954; Am J Med 13:158–171, 1952*

Insect bites

Intraocular infections

Jellyfish envenomation

Lacrimal gland, chronic enlargement

Lassa fever *J Infect Dis 155:445–455, 1987*

Leishmaniasis – *L. aethiopica* – nasal infiltration with edema but no destruction *Trans R Soc Trop Med Hyg 63:708–737, 1969; Leishmania infantum* – periorbital granulomatous plaque *Dermatol Clin 33:579–593, 2015*

Lepidopterism

Leprosy *Lep Rev 84:316–321, 2013*

Leptospirosis *Eur J Case Rep Intern Med 3 (6)000447, Aug 26, 2016*

Loiasis – *Loa loa; Chrysops* (deer fly, horse fly, mangrove fly) – adult worms in conjunctiva with unilateral palpebral edema *JAAD 73:929–944, 2015; AD 108:835–836, 1973;* calabar swellings

Loxoscelism (brown recluse spider bite) - of eyelids *Cut Ocul Toxicol 30:302–305, 2011; Arch Ophthalmol 98:1997–1000, 1980*

Lyme disease *Ann Int Med 99:76–82, 1983;* dermatomyositis associated with Lyme disease *Clin Inf Dis 18:166–171, 1994;* conjunctivitis leading to blindness; keratitis, optic neuritis, periorbital edema; uveitis *JAAD 70:795–819, 2014; Br J Ophthalmol 107:581–587, 2000*

Lymphogranuloma venereum

Malaria

Measles

Millipede spray (*Polyconoceras spp.*) (*Saltpidobolus spp.*) – periorbital edema, periorbital mahogany hyperpigmentation, conjunctivitis, keratitis *JAAD 50:819–842, 2004*

Molluscum contagiosum, ruptured – personal observation

Moraxella species – preseptal cellulitis and facial erysipelas *Clin Exp Dermatol 19:321–323, 1994*

Mucormycosis (rhino-orbital) (zygomycosis) – ptosis with upper eyelid edema and necrosis *JAMA 309:2382–2383, 2013; Clin Inf Dis 40:990–996, 2005; NEJM 341:265–273, 1999; Sarcoidosis 12:143–146, 1995; AD 122:329–334, 1986;* invasive sinusitis

Myiasis – *Dermatobia hominis* – edema and erythema of eyelid *Ped Inf Dis 21:82–83, 2002*

Mycobacterium haemophilum BJD 149:200–202, 2003

Mycobacterium tuberculosis – tuberculous chancre – edema and irritation *Pakistan J Ophthalmol 4:37–40, 1988; Lancet i:1286–1289, 1955;* scrofula

Myiasis – *Hypoderma tarandi;* bumblebee-like fly of subarctic regions; eggs deposited on reindeer (caribou); larvae penetrate skin, hatch, and result in migratory swellings; ophthalmomyiasis may result in blindness *Euro Surveillance 22 (29)30576, July 20, 2017; NEJM 367:2456–2457, 2012;* ophthalmomyiasis due to sheep botfly (*Oestrus ovis*) *Optom Vis Sci 81:586–590, 2004*

Myospherulosis *Am J Rhinol 11:345–347, 1997*

Necrotizing fasciitis (streptococcal gangrene) *Graefes Arch Clin Exp Ophthalmol 244:268–270, 2006; AD 140:664–666, 2004; Eyelid and Conjunctival Tumors, Shields JA and Shields CL, Lippincott Williams and Wilkins, 1999, p.171; Eye 5:736–740, 1991; Ann Ophthalmol 19:426–427, 1987*

Neisseria meningitides – meningococcemia with orbital hemorrhage and DIC – periorbital edema and subconjunctival hemorrhage *Eye16:190–193, 2002*

Newcastle disease (fowlpox) – conjunctival inflammatory disease

Onchocerciasis

Ophthalmia neonatorum – conjunctival inflammatory disease

Orbital cellulitis (post-septal cellulitis) – emanating from infection of skin, teeth, nasolacrimal apparatus, paranasal sinuses (*Haemophilus influenzae, Streptococcus pneumoniae, Moraxella, catarrhalis Staphylococcus aureus, Streptococcus pyogenes, Strep. viridans Am J Otolaryngol 4:422–423, 1983*) *NEJM 341:265–273, 1999*

Orf *J Dermatol Treat 16:353–356, 2005*

Paederus beetle dermatitis – linear papular, vesicular, and pustular dermatitis *JAAD 57:297–300, 2007; Cutis 69:277–279, 2002*

Papular urticaria

Pasteurella multocida – periocular abscess and cellulitis *Am J Ophthalmol 128:514–515, 1999*

Periorbital cellulitis (pre-septal cellulitis) *Head Neck Surg 9:227–234, 1987*

Periorbital necrotizing fasciitis after minor trauma (streptococcal gangrene) *Case Rep Otolaryngol 2014:723408; Acta Ophthalmol 91:596–603, 2013; Graefes Arch Clin Exp Ophthalmol 244:268–270, 2006*

Phaeoacremonium inflatipes – fungemia in child with aplastic anemia; swelling and necrosis of lips, periorbital edema, neck swelling *Clin Inf Dis 40:1067–1068, 2005*

Pre-auricular cyst, infected

Preseptal cellulitis *NEJM 341:265–273, 1999*

Pythium insidiosum (pythiosis) (alga) (aquatic oocyte) – necrotizing hemorrhagic plaque; ascending gangrene of legs; Thailand; painful subcutaneous nodules, eyelid swelling and periorbital cellulitis, facial swelling, ulcer of arm or leg, pustules evolving into ulcers *BJD 175:394–397, 2016; J Infect Dis 159:274–280, 1989*

Rocky Mountain spotted fever – especially in children *Clin Dermatol 37:109–118, 2019; MMWR 65:1–44, May 13, 2016; Clin Pharm 7:109–116, 1988*

Roseola infantum (exanthem subitum) – human herpesvirus 6 – periorbital edema prior to onset of rash *Pediatrics 93:104–108, 1994; Ped 25:1034, 1960*

Ruptured frontal sinusitis

Russell's viper bite

Scabies

Scarlet fever

Schistosomiasis mansoni – purpura, urticaria, periorbital edema 4–6 weeks after penetration of the cercaria *Cutis 73:387–389, 2004; AD 112:1539–1542, 1976*

Septic thrombosis of the cavernous sinus *Arch Neurol 45:467–472, 1988*

Shewanella putrefaciens J Clin Inf Dis 25:225–229, 1997

Sparganosis (larvae of tapeworm) – *Spirometra mansonoides* – subcutaneous nodule, conjunctivitis, periorbital edema *JAMA Derm 152:831–832, 2016; Adv Parasitol 72:351–408, 2010; Derm Clinics 17:151–185, 1999*

Stye (hordeolum) – personal observation

Staphylococcal scalded skin syndrome

Subdural empyema

Subgaleal abscess *Ann Emerg Med 18:785–787, 1989*

Subperiosteal abscess – eyelid edema and erythema as sole sign *J Clin Neurosci 8:469–471, 2001; Br J Ophthalmol 73:576–578, 1989*

Syphilis – primary (chancre); secondary gumma with orbital cellulitis *NEJM 341:265–273, 1999*

Tarantula urticating hairs – generalized itchy rash, conjunctivitis and periorbital edema; tarantula flicks hundreds of hairs off its abdomen *Arch Dis Child 75:462–463, 1996*

Toxocariasis

Toxoplasmosis – heliotrope rash

Trichinosis (*Trichinella spiralis* or *T.britovi*) – periorbital edema, conjunctivitis; transient morbilliform eruption, splinter hemorrhages *JAAD 73:929–944, 2015; Can J Public Health 88:52–56, 1997; Postgrad Med 97:137–139, 143–144, 1995; South Med J 81:1056–1058, 1988*

Trypanosoma cruzi – Romana's sign

Tularemia – *Francisella tularensis*; skin, eye, respiratory, gastrointestinal portals of entry; ulceroglandular, oculoglandular, glandular types; toxemic stage heralds generalized morbilliform eruption, erythema multiforme-like rash, crops of red nodules on extremities *Cutis 54:279–286, 1994; Medicine 54:252–269, 1985*

Vaccinia – laboratory acquired vaccinia virus infection; painful inflamed ear and periorbital region; *MMWR 58:797–800, 2009;* ocular vaccinia *JAAD 50:495–528, 2004*

Verrucae planae (flat warts)

Wild boar meat *MMWR 58:1–7, 2009; Am J Trop Med Hyg 68:463–464, 2003; Can J Public Health 88:52–56, 1997*

Yellow fever *Lancet Inf Dis 19:750–758, 2019; Clin Dermatol 25:212–220, 2007*

INFILTRATIVE DISEASES

Amyloidosis – diffuse eyelid swelling *Ophthalmic Plast Reconstr Surg 29:e12–14, 2013; J Dermatol 19:113–118, 1992*

Colloid milium

Erdheim-Chester disease (non-Langerhans cell histiocytosis) – CD68+ and factor XIIIa+; negative for CD1a and S100; xanthoma and xanthelasma-like lesions; flat wart-like papules of face; bony lesions *AD 143:952–953, 2007; Hautarzt 52:510–517, 2001; Medicine (Baltimore) 75:157–169, 1996*

Primary and secondary intralymphatic histiocytosis – unilateral eyelid swelling *Am J Dermatopathol 31:140–151, 2009;* red patch of back; livedo reticularis *JAAD 70:927–933, 2014*

Intralymphatic histiocytosis – red patch overlying swollen knee; livedo reticularis, papules, nodules, urticaria, unilateral eyelid edema *AD 146:1037–1042, 2010*

Langerhans cell histiocytosis *Saudi J Ophthalmol 32:52–55, 2018; Ophthalmol Plast Reconstruct Surg 24:142–143, 2008*

Mast cell disease *Eye 17:788–790, 2003*

Mucinosis, cutaneous; in DLE *JAAD 41 (pt 2)871–873, 1999*

Orbital pseudotumor (eosinophilic or basophilic granulomas) (pseudotumor of orbit) *Ann Allergy 69:101–105, 1992*

Rosai-Dorfman disease – bilateral eyelid edema *Ped Derm 633–635, 2009*

Scleredema – periorbital edema *JAMA 315:1159–1160, 2016; Int J Dermatol 55:e100–102, 2016; Ped Derm 27:315–317, 2010; JAAD 52:S41–44, 2005*

Scleromyxedema *Hautarzt 65:454–457, 2014; JAAD 928–930, 1996*

Self-healing (papular) juvenile cutaneous mucinosis – juxta-articular painless nodules; also nodules of face, neck, scalp, abdomen, and thighs; arthralgias; white papules of head, neck, trunk, periarticular; deeper nodules of face and periarticular areas; periorbital edema *Am J Dermatopathol 34:699–705, 2012; Ped Derm 26:91–92, 2009; AD 145:211–212, 2009; JAAD 55:1036–1043, 2006; JAAD 50:S97–100, 2004; Ped Derm 20:35–39, 2003; JAAD 44:273–281, 2001; Ped Derm 14:460–462, 1997; AD 131:459–461, 1995; JAAD 11:327–332, 1984; Ann DV 107:51–57, 1980;* of adult *JAAD 50:121–123, 2004, BJD 143:650–651, 2000; Dermatology 192:268–270, 1996; Lyon Med 230:474–475, 1973*

Xanthogranuloma, adult *Eyelid and Conjunctival Tumors, Shields JA and Shields CL, Lippincott Williams and Wilkins, 1999, p.141;* periorbital xanthogranulomas (adult-onset asthma with periocular xanthogranulomas) – hyperpigmented indurated nodules of upper and lower eyelids (swollen eyelids); associated with asthma *AD 147:1230–1231, 2011; Arch Pathol Lab Med 133:1994–1997, 2009; Br J Ophthalmol 90:602–608, 2006; Trans Am Ophthalmol Soc 91:99–129, 1993*

Juvenile xanthogranuloma *JAAD 14:405–411, 1986*

Xanthoma disseminatum – periorbital papules *JAAD 15:433–436, 1991*

INFLAMMATORY DISEASES

Blepharitis granulomatosa – edema *AD 120:1141–1142, 1984*

Chronic dacryoadenitis *Jpn J Ophthalmol 43:109–112, 1999*

Cytophagic histiocytic panniculitis *Ped Derm 21:246–249, 2004*

Erythema multiforme, including Stevens-Johnson syndrome *J Korean Neurosurg Sci 58:163–166, 2015*

Juvenile xanthogranuloma, plaque-type – red plaques of face; swollen eyelids with periorbital edema *JAAD 59:S56–57, 2008*

Kikuchi's disease (histiocytic necrotizing lymphadenitis) – eyelid edema *Ped Derm 18:403–405, 2001; Ann DV 126:826–828, 1999; JAAD 36:342–346, 1997*

Neutrophilic eccrine hidradenitis – red/violaceous periorbital plaques *AD 139:531–536, 2003; JAAD 38:1–17,1998; AD 131:1141–1145, 1995; Arch Ophthalmol 112:1460–1463, 1994; JAAD 28:775, 1993*

Nodular fasciitis *Eyelid and Conjunctival Tumors, Shields JA and Shields CL, Lippincott Williams and Wilkins, 1999, p.147*

Orbital myositis *Rev Med Interne 22:189–193, 2001; Curr Opinion Rheumatol 9:504–512, 1997*

Orbital pseudotumor – eyelid swelling, proptosis, ophthalmoplegia *NEJM 341:265–273, 1999*

Orofacial granulomatosis – facial edema with swelling of lips, cheeks, eyelids, forehead, mucosal tags, mucosal cobblestoning, gingivitis, oral aphthae *BJD 143:1119–1121, 2000*

Periorbital cellulitis, myositis, vitiligo

Pruritic linear urticarial rash, fever, and systemic inflammatory disease of adolescents – urticaria, linear lesions, periorbital edema and erythema, and arthralgia *Ped Derm 21:580–588, 2004*

Rosai-Dorfman syndrome – eyelid edema, periorbital edema *BJD 145:323–326, 2001; Ophthalmic Plast Reconstr Surg 15:52–55, 1999*

Sarcoid *AD 118:356–357, 1982;* Parinaud's oculoglandular syndrome – conjunctival inflammatory disease; unilateral periorbital edema – facial nerve palsy and parotid gland enlargement *BJD 157:200–202, 2007*

Scleritis, episcleritis – in cutaneous lupus erythematosus *Clin Case Rep 14:1422–1425, 2019*

Whipple's disease – pseudotumor orbitae during therapy; macular and reticulated erythema; Addisonian hyperpigmentation; *Tropheryma whipplei JAAD 60:277–288, 2009*

METABOLIC DISEASES

Acrodermatitis enteropathica

Acromegaly – edematous thick eyelids *Hautarzt 60:502–504, 2009*

Carcinoid syndrome *JAAD 46:161–183, 2002*

Cardiac disease – congestive heart failure

Cushing's syndrome

Graves' disease – hyperthyroidism – unilateral eyelid edema *JAAD 48:617–619, 2003;* periorbital edema *NEJM 341:265–273, 1999; Med Clin NA 79:195–209, 1995*

Hepatic disease

Hypoalbuminemia *JAAD 48:617–619, 2003*

Hypothyroidism (myxedema) - puffy edema of the eyelids *NEJM 372;764, 2015; JAAD 26:885–902, 1992;* hyperthryroidism, Graves' disease (endocrine exopthhalmos), myxedema *Semin Neurol 20:43–54, 2000; Semin Ophthalmol 14:52–61, 1999;* congenital hypothyroidism *J Formosa Med Assoc 91:864–866, 1992*

Pellagra – eyelid edema *Cutis 69:96–98, 2002*

Pituitary apoplexy *ORL J Otorhinolaryngol Relat Spec 65:121–124, 2003*

Pregnancy – eyelid edema

Renal failure – glomerulonephritis, nephrotic syndrome *Practitioner 261:11–15, 2017* Hypothyroidism (myxedema) – puffy edema of eyelids *NEJM 372:764, 2015; JAAD 26:885–902, 1992;* hyperthyroidism, Graves' disease (endocrine exophthalmos), myxedema *Semin Neurol 20:43–54, 2000; Semin Ophthalmol 14:52–61, 1999;* congenital hypothyroidism *J Formosa Med Assoc 91:864–866, 1992*

Protein losing enteropathy *Lupus 15:102–104, 2006; Yohsei Med J 45:923–926, 2004; Z Gastroenterol 36:165–171, 1998; Clin Pediatr 134:265–267, 1995; Gut 25:1013–1015, 1984*

NEOPLASTIC DISEASES

Actinic keratosis

Aldosterone-producing tumors – heliotrope rash

Angiosarcoma of face and scalp (Wilson Jones angiosarcoma) – eyelid edema *AD 148:683–685, 2012; BJD 143:660–661, 2000; Hautarzt 51:419–422, 2000; JAAD 38:143–175, 1998; Am J Ophthalmol 125:870–871, 1998; Aust N Z J Ophthalmol 23:69–72, 1995;* eyelid edema *Hautarzt 51:419–422, 2000;* eyelid papule *Eyelid and Conjunctival Tumors, Shields JA and Shields CL, Lippincott Williams and Wilkins, 1999, p.125;* nodule *AD 121:549–550, 1985;* yellow plaques of eyelids *JAAD 34:308–310, 1996;* nodule *AD 121:549–550, 1985*

Atypical lymphoid hyperplasia *JAAD 37:839–842, 1997*

Basal cell carcinoma Benign and malignant ectodermal and mesodermal tumors (orbital tumors)

Blue nevus, cellular *Eyelid and Conjunctival Tumors, Shields JA and Shields CL, Lippincott Williams and Wilkins, 1999, p.90–91*

Bowen's disease

Chalazion

Dermoid cyst

Embryonal rhabdomyosarcoma – tumor of orbit, nasopharynx, nose; eyelid edema *AD 138:689–694, 2002*

Epidermal inclusion cyst

Eruptive hidradenoma – papules *Cutis 46:69–72, 1990*

Ethmoid sinus mucocele

Fibrosarcoma *Eyelid and Conjunctival Tumors, Shields JA and Shields CL, Lippincott Williams and Wilkins, 1999, p.148*

Fibrous histiocytoma *Eyelid and Conjunctival Tumors, Shields JA and Shields CL, Lippincott Williams and Wilkins, 1999, p.148*

Hidrocystoma

Hydroa vacciniforme-like cutaneous T-cell lymphoma (Epstein-Barr virus associated lymphoproliferative disorder), Epstein-Barr virus-related – edema, blisters, vesicles, ulcers, scarring, facial scars, swollen nose, lips, and periorbital edema, crusts with central hemorrhagic necrosis, facial dermatitis, photodermatitis, facial edema, facial papules and plaques, crusting of ears, pitted scars, fever *JAAD 81::534–540, 2019; JAAD 69:112–119, 2013; BJD 151:372–380, 2004*

Juvenile fibromatosis *Eyelid and Conjunctival Tumors, Shields JA and Shields CL, Lippincott Williams and Wilkins, 1999, p.14*

Kaposi's sarcoma *JAAD 59:179–206, 2008; NEJM 333:799–800, 1995; NEJM 332:1204, 1995 Cutis 56:104–106, 1995x*

Keratoacanthoma

Leiomyoma, retroperitoneal – periorbital and peripheral edema *Can J Surg 25:79–80, 1982*

Leukemia, including HTLV-1, acute myelogenous leukemia – papules *JAAD 40:966–978, 1999;* heliotrope as presentation of acute myelomonocytic leukemia *Leuk Lymphoma 25:393–398, 1997;* T-cell prolymphocytic leukemia *Ophthalmic Plast Reconstruct Surg 22:215–216, 2006*

Lymphoma – cutaneous T-cell or B-cell lymphoma *Eyelid and Conjunctival Tumors, Shields JA and Shields CL, Lippincott Williams and Wilkins, 1999, p.129;* CTCL mimicking facial erysipelas *BJD 152:1381–1383, 2005;* MALT (mucosa-associated lymphoid tissue) lymphoma *NEJM 372:363, 2015;* hydroa vacciniforme-like cutaneous T-cell lymphoma, Epstein-Barr virus-related – edema, blisters, vesicles, ulcers, scarring, facial scars, swollen nose, lips, and periorbital edema, crusts with central hemorrhagic necrosis, facial dermatitis, photodermatitis, facial edema, facial papules and plaques, crusting of ears, fever *JAAD 69:112–119, 2013;* Epstein-Barr virus-associated T-cell lymphoma – eyelid edema and intramuscular infiltration mimicking dermatomyositis; facial dermatitis and edema; lip edema *JAAD 72:2134, 2015; J Dermatol 41:29–39, 2014; BJD 147:1244–1248, 2002;* angiocentric lymphoma *Can J Ophthalmol 32:259–264, 1997;* B-cell lymphoma; nasal lymphoma *JAAD 38:310–313, 1998;* large cell B-cell lymphoma; midline granuloma presenting as orbital cellulitis *Graefes Arch Clin Exp Ophthalmol 234:137–139, 1996;* HTLV-1 lymphoma; CD4+ small to medium size pleomorphic T-cell lymphoma – red swollen eyelid with alopecia of eyebrow *Ped Derm 30:595–599, 2013; Cancer 73:2395–2399, 1994;* subcutaneous panniculitis-like T-cell lymphoma *Acta Med Iran 52:950–953, 2014*

Melanoma – primary orbital melanoma of infancy *Ped Derm 21:1–9, 2004;* congenital melanoma *Eyelid and Conjunctival Tumors, Shields JA and Shields CL, Lippincott Williams and Wilkins, 1999, p.93*

Merkel cell tumor

Metastases – breast cancer – periorbital edema and erythema *Cutis 70:291–293, 2002; BJD 146:919, 2002;* eyelid enlargement *JAAD*

37:362–364, 1997; also seen with gastrointestinal, lung, skin, and genitourinary tract malignancies; unilateral eyelid edema – metastatic breast cancer *Jpn J Ophthalmol 52:305–307, 2008;* mask-like metastases *Am J Dermatopathol 32:9–14, 2010*

Myeloma – cutaneous crystalline deposits *AD 130:484–488,1994*

Myxomas – periorbital cutaneous myxomas *JAAD 34:928–930, 1995*

Neuroblastoma, metastatic – lower lid edema *Ped Derm 37:29–39, 2020;* periorbital ecchymoses mimics child abuse; raccoon eyes *Ped Derm 26:473–474, 2009; Pediatr Radiol 25 (Suppl 1):S90–92, 1995*

Neuroendocrine carcinoma involving ethmoid and frontal sinuses *JAMA 309:605–606, 2013*

Neurofibroma, plexiform *Eyelid and Conjunctival Tumors, Shields JA and Shields CL, Lippincott Williams and Wilkins, 1999, p.97*

Orbital pseudotumor *Am J Emerg Med 18:83–85, 2000*

Orbital tumors *NEJM 341:265–273, 1999;* ethmoid sinus carcinoma

Phakomatous christoma *Eyelid and Conjunctival Tumors, Shields JA and Shields CL, Lippincott Williams and Wilkins, 1999, p.181*

Plasmacytoma – retrobulbar *NEJM 345:1917, 2001*

Rhabdomyosarcoma – rapid growth with explosive exophthalmos *Ped Derm 21:1–9, 2004; NEJM 350:494–502, 2004*

Sebaceous gland carcinoma

Seborrheic keratosis

Primary sweat gland carcinoma

Signet ring cell carcinoma, primary cutaneous *JAAD 54:532–536, 2006*

Squamous cell carcinoma *Eyelid and Conjunctival Tumors, Shields JA and Shields CL, Lippincott Williams and Wilkins, 1999, p.35*

Squamous cell carcinoma of the eyelid; of the lacrimal sac *Eyelid and Conjunctival Tumors, Shields JA and Shields CL, Lippincott Williams and Wilkins, 1999, p.185*

Syringomas

Transient myeloproliferative disorder associated with mosaicism for trisomy 21 – periorbital edema *Ped Derm 21:551–554, 2004*

Trichoepithelioma

Vellus hair cysts

PARANEOPLASTIC DISORDERS

Crystal-storing histiocytosis (composed of monoclonal immunoglobulins) – periorbital swelling *J Cut Pathol 42:136–143, 2015; Hum Pathol 27:84–87, 1996; AD 130:484–488, 1994;* fixed erythema of abdomen; paraneoplastic phenomenon in myeloma, lymphoplasmacytic lymphoma, B-cell lymphoma, or monoclonal gammopathy of uncertain significance (MGUS) *JAMA Derm 152:1159–1160, 2016*

Necrobiotic xanthogranuloma with paraproteinemia *Cutis 94:293–296, 2014; BJD 144:158–161, 2001*

Necrolytic migratory erythema (glucagonoma syndrome) – periorbital and perioral erythema; necrotic crusted plaques of legs *BJD 174:1092–1095, 2016*

Paraneoplastic pemphigus – erythema and erosions *JAAD 33:312–315, 1995*

PHOTODERMATITIS

Actinic granuloma (annular elastolytic giant cell granuloma) – periorbital *Graefes Arch Clin Exp Ophthalmol 236:646–651, 1998*

Chronic actinic dermatitis

Photoaging

Polymorphic light eruption

PRIMARY CUTANEOUS DISEASES

Acne rosacea *JAAD 37:346–348, 1997; AD 121:87, 1985;* rosacea lymphedema *AD 131:1069–1074, 1995;* periorbital chronic edema; *Arch Ophthalmol 108:561–563, 1990;*

Acne vulgaris – central forehead, periorbital skin, cheeks *Cutis 61:215–216, 1998; JAAD 22:129–130, 1990; AD 121:87–90, 1985;* ruptured acne cyst

Adult onset asthma with periocular xanthogranuloma *Ophthalmol Plast Reconstr Surg 29:104–108, 2013; AD 147:1230–1231, 2011; Br J Ophthalmol 90:602–608, 2006*

Alopecia mucinosa

Atopic dermatitis

Blepharitis granulomatosa *AD 120:1141, 1984*

Cutis laxa *Mymensingh Med 19:137–141, 2010*

Epidermolysis bullosa – junctional epidermolysis bullosa letalis (laminin 5 defect) – perioral and periorbital erosions

Granuloma annulare

Lichen planus of eyelids – heliotrope *JAAD 27:638, 1992*

Lichen sclerosus et atrophicus

Lichen simplex chronicus

Orbital fat herniation

Orofacial granulomatosis *Ophthalmic Plast Reconstr Surg 30:e151–155, 2014; J Oral Pathol Med 32:200–205, 2003*

Pityriasis rubra pilaris – personal observation

Psoriasis

Seborrheic dermatitis

Solid facial edema – rosacea lymphedema (Morbihan's disease) *An Bras Dermatol 91 (suppl 1)157–159, 2016; J Dermatol 27:214–216, 2000; AD 131:1069–1074, 1995, Cutis 61:321–324, 1998*

Chronic urticaria *Allergy Asthma Proc 40:437–440, 2019*

Vitiligo and sunburn

PSYCHOCUTANEOUS

Delusions of parasitosis

Factitial dermatitis mimicking dermatomyositis – personal observation

SYNDROMES

Anhidrotic ectodermal dysplasia

Ascher's syndrome – periorbital edema; edema of lips, double lip, blepharochalasis *AD 139:1075–1080, 2003; Klin Monatsbl Augenheilkd 65:86–97, 1920*

CANDLE syndrome (chronic atypical neutrophilic dermatosis with lipodystrophy and elevated temperature) – annular erythematous edematous plaques of face (periorbital erythema) and trunk which become purpuric and result in residual annular hyperpigmentation; urticarial papules; limitation of range of motion with plaques over interphalangeal joints; periorbital edema with violaceous swollen eyelids, edema of lips (thick lips), lipoatrophy of cheeks, nose, and arms, chondritis with progressive ear and saddle nose deformities, hypertrichosis of lateral forehead, gynecomastia, wide spaced nipples, nodular episcleritis and conjunctivitis, epididymitis, myositis, aseptic meningitis; short stature, anemia, abnormal liver functions, splenomegaly, protuberant abdomen; pleuritic chest pain; lymphadenopathy; arthralgia/oral ulcers *BJD 170:215–217, 2014; JAAD 68:834–853, 2013; Ped Derm 28:538–541, 2011; JAAD 62:487–495, 2010*

Ehlers-Danlos type VIIC (dermatosparaxis) – puffy around the eyes

Episodic angioedema associated with eosinophilia (Gleich syndrome) *Hematologica 100:300–307, 2015*

Fabry's disease (angiokeratoma corporis diffusum (alpha galactosidase A)) – X-linked recessive; upper eyelid edema *NEJM 276:1163–1167, 1967;* edema of hands, arms, eyelids *AD 140:1526–1527, 2004; Arch Ophthal 74:760, 1965*

Familial sea-blue histiocytosis – autosomal recessive; patchy gray pigmentation of face, upper chest, shoulders; eyelid edema, facial nodules *Dermatologica 174:39–44, 1987*

H syndrome – autosomal recessive; facial telangiectasias; sclerodermoid changes of middle and lower body with overlying hyperpigmentation sparing the knees and buttocks; hypertrichosis, short stature, facial telangiectasia, gynecomastia, camptodactyly of 5th fingers, scrotal masses with massively edematous scrotum obscuring the penis, hypogonadism, azospermia, sensorineural hearing loss, cardiac anomalies, hepatosplenomegaly; Arabic Palestinian population; gluteal lipoatrophy; hyperpigmentation, hearing loss, diabetes mellitus, lymphadenopathy, hypertrichosis, heart anomalies, micropenis, hallux valgus, hyperpigmentation induration and hypertrichosis of inner thighs and shins (sclerodermoid), chronic diarrhea, anemia, dilated lateral scleral vessels, episcleritis, exophthalmos, eyelid swelling, varicose veins, chronic rhinitis, renal abnormalities, bone lesions, arthritis, arthralgia; mutation in *SLC29A3 JAAD 70;80–88, 2014; JAAD 59:79–85, 2008*

Hemophagocytic lymphohistiocytosis syndrome – personal observation

Hypereosinophilic syndrome – personal observation

I-cell disease (mucolipidosis II) – puffy eyelids; small orbits, prominent eyes, fullness of lower cheeks; small telangiectasias; fish-mouth appearance, short neck; gingival hypertrophy *Birth Defects 5:174–185, 1969*

IgG4-related disease – cutaneous plasmacytosis (papulonodules); pseudolymphoma; angiolymphoid hyperplasia with eosinophilia; Mikulicz's disease – palpebral swelling, sicca syndrome (dry eyes and mouth), exophthalmos, fibroinflammatory changes including the pancreas, and enlarged salivary glands, lacrimal glands, submandibular glands, biliary tract, peritoneum, kidney, pituitary gland, thyroid gland, lung, prostate, testis, aorta, lymph nodes, orbital pseudotumors; psoriasiform dermatitis; morbilliform eruption; hypergammaglobulinemic purpura; urticarial vasculitis; ischemic digits; Raynaud's disease and digital gangrene; peritoneum (retroperitoneal fibrosis, sclerosing mesenteritis), kidney (tubulointerstitial nephritis), pituitary gland (autoimmune hypophysitis), thyroid gland (Riedel thyroiditis, Hashimoto thyroiditis), lung (interstitial pneumonia), prostate, testis (epididymo-orchitis), aorta (lymphoplasmacytic aortitis), lymph nodes (Rosai-Dorfman disease), orbital pseudotumors, sclerosing cholangitis *JAMA Derm 156:451, 2020; BJD 171:929,959–967, 2014*

   IgG4 disease
      Group 1 – pancreato-hepato-biliary disease
      Group 2 – retroperitoneal fibrosis and/or aortitis
      Group 3 – head and neck limited disease
      Group 4 – classic Mikulicz disease

Kawasaki's disease *Case Rep Ophthalmol 4:294–298, 2013; Heart Lung 39:164–172, 2010*

Lipoid proteinosis – moniliform blepharosis *Indian J Ophthalmol 63:793–795, 2015; BMJ Case Rep April 10, 2014*

Lymphedema-distichiasis syndrome – periorbital edema, vertebral abnormalities, spinal arachnoid cysts, congenital heart disease, thoracic duct abnormalities, hemangiomas, cleft palate, microphthalmia, strabismus, ptosis, short stature, webbed neck *Ped Derm 19:139–141, 2002*

Melkersson-Rosenthal syndrome – granulomatous blepharitis *Ophthalmic Plastic Reconstr Surg 21:243–245, 2005; J Eur Acad DV 19:107–111, 2005; BJD 149:222–224, 2003; AD 139:1075–1080, 2003; Dermatol Clin 14:371–379, 1996*

Multiple symmetric lipomatosis

NAME/LAMB syndromes

Neurofibromatosis – plexiform neuromas *Ped Derm 21:1–9, 2004*

Niemann-Pick disease, Type B *Metab Ped Syst Ophthal 15:16–20, 1992*

Noonan's syndrome – periorbital lymphedema *BJD 129:190–192, 1993*

Partial trisomy 16q24.1-qter *Am J Med Genet 113:339–345, 2002*

Schnitzler's syndrome – periorbital edema, chronic urticaria, monoclonal IgM gammopathy, bone lesions, recurrent fever, arthralgia, bone pain *BJD 156:1072–1074, 2007*

Sly syndrome

Sweet's syndrome *Eye 18:214, 2004; JAAD 24:140–141, 1991;* in acute myelogenous leukemia *JAAD 45:590–595, 2001*

Sybert syndrome – autosomal dominant; unknown mutation; thick hyperkeratotic; transgradiens, no nail changes nor hyperhidrosis; resembles Greither's PPK but more severe and widespread hyperkeratosis; lesions over elbows, knees, natal cleft, and groin; periorbital and perioral erythema; progressive; spontaneous amputations *Indian J Dermatol 55:297–299, 2010; Dermatol Online J 9:30, 2003; Prob Derm 14:71–116, 2002; JAAD 18:75–86, 1988*

Tumor necrosis factor (TNF) receptor 1-associated periodic fever syndromes (TRAPS) (same as familial hibernian fever, autosomal dominant periodic fever with amyloidosis, and benign autosomal dominant familial periodic fever) – erythematous patches, tender red plaques, fever, annular, serpiginous, polycyclic, reticulated, and migratory patches and plaques (migrating from proximal to distal), urticaria-like lesions, lesions resolving with ecchymoses, conjunctivitis, periorbital edema, myalgia, arthralgia, abdominal pain, headache; Irish and Scottish predominance; mutation in TNFRSF1A – gene encoding 55kDa TNF receptor *Frontiers in Immunology 10:1–24, 2019; Actas Dermosifiliogr Jan 17, 2013; AD 136:1487–1494, 2000; Mayo Clin Proc 72:806–817, 1997*

Wells' syndrome *AD 142:1157–1161, 2006*

Williams syndrome – puffy eyelids *Pediatrics 75:962–968, 1985*

Yellow nail syndrome

Zellweger (cerebrohepatorenal syndrome) syndrome – puffy eyelids *J Neurol Sci 69:9–25, 1985*

TOXINS

Arsenic poisoning – acute *BJD 149:757–762, 2003*

Alkali burn

Eosinophilia myalgia syndrome *J Rheumatol 17:1527–1533, 1990*

TRAUMA

Airbag injury

Carotid cavernous fistula – post traumatic; swelling, pain, decreased vision of eye *NEJM 371:1832, 2014*

Child abuse *Optom Clin 5:125–160, 1996*

Coma bullae – eyelid edema *Cutis 69:265–268, 2002*

Cryosurgery

Paranasal sinus fracture *J Oral Maxillofac Surg 63:1080–1087, 2005*

Physical trauma

Radiation blepharopathy – *Eyelid and Conjunctival Tumors, Shields JA and Shields CL, Lippincott Williams and Wilkins, 1999, p.21*

Subcutaneous emphysema *AD 134:557–559, 1998;* due to dental crown preparation resembling angioedema; trauma; head and neck surgery; general anesthesia; tooth extraction of mandibular 3rd molar *JAMA Derm 150:908, 2014;* of eyelid due to communication between paranasal space and eyelid

Subperiosteal hematomas *NEJM 341:265–273, 1999*

Surgery – after Mohs' surgery of nose – raccoon eyes; elephantiasis of the eyelids following repeated craniotomy *J Neurosurg 47:293–296, 1977;* post-rhinoplasty *Facial Plastic Surg 34:14–21, 2018;* blepharoplasty, halo fixation of cervical spine

Tape stripping – personal observation

VASCULAR DISEASES

Acute hemorrhagic edema of infancy – eyelid edema *Ped Derm30:e132–135, 2013; Cutis 68:127–128, 2001*

Angiolymphoid hyperplasia with eosinophilia *Ped Derm 15:91–96, 1998; Ann Allergy 69:101–105, 1992; Am J Ophthalmol 108:167–169, 1989*

Carotid-cavernous sinus fistula – eyelid edema *JAAD 48:617–619, 2003*

Cavernous sinus thrombosis *NEJM 341:265–273, 1999; Arch Neurol 45:567–572, 1988*

Congestive heart failure – eyelid edema *JAAD 48:617–619, 2003*

Disseminated intravascular coagulation *BJ Ophth 72:3417–379, 1988*

Dural arteriovenous malformation – eyelid edema *JAAD 48:617–619, 2003*

Elephantiasis

Eosinophilic granulomatosis with polyangiitis – non-pitting periorbital edema *Medicine 78:26–37, 1999*

Granulomatosis with polyangiitis *Eye 18:658–660, 2004;* pseudotumor orbiti; palatal ulcers and unilateral eyelid edema *Caspian J Intern Med 10:343–346, 2019*

Hemangiomas – subpalpebral skin colored mass *Ped Derm 37:40–1, 2020;* eyelid swelling *BJD 162:466–468, 2010;* rapid growth with explosive exophthalmos *Ped Derm 21:1–9, 2004; Int Med Case Rep J 10:255–259, 2017*

Henoch-Schonlein purpura (anaphylactoid purpura) *Arthritis Rheum 40:859–864, 1997;* hemorrhagic vesicles and bullae *Ped Derm 12:314–317, 1995;* C4 deficiency *JAAD 7:66–79, 1982;* eyelid and facial edema due to intracerebral hemorrhage *Brain and Development 24:115–117, 2002;* upper eyelid ecchymoses and edema *Arch Ophthalmol 117:842–843, 1999*

Kaposiform hemangioendothelioma of mediastinum and neck – periorbital edema and ecchymoses *Ped Derm 26:331–337, 2009*

Lemierre's syndrome – swollen red eyelid; due to *Fusobacterium necrophorum;* cavernous sinus thrombophlebitis, carotid artery thromboarteritis, abscess of parotid gland and subperiosteal orbit *NEJM 371:2018–2027, 2014*

Lymphatic malformation *Plast Reconstr Surg 115:22–30, 2005; Ped Derm 21:1–9, 2004*

Lymphedema *Mayo Clin Proc 92:1053–1060, 2017*

Microscopic polyangiitis *Klin Monatsbl Augenheilkd 221:964–969, 2004*

Neonatal hemangiomatosis

Nevus flammeus *Eyelid and Conjunctival Tumors, Shields JA and Shields CL, Lippincott Williams and Wilkins, 1999, p.116*

Polyarteritis nodosa *Clin Rheumatol 17:353–356, 1998*

Pyogenic granuloma

Recurrent cutaneous necrotizing eosinophilic vasculitis *AD 130:1159–1166, 1994*

Septic facial vein thrombosis (*Staphylococcus aureus*) *AD 145:1460–1461, 2009*

Sickle cell disease – orbital wall infarction *Am J Ophthalmol 146:595–601, 2008;* orbital compression syndrome *Acta Clin Belg 70:451–452, 2015; Eye 774–780, 2001; Ophthalmology 104:1610–1615, 1997*

Sturge-Weber syndrome

Superior vena cava syndrome *Cutis 79:362,367–368, 2007; Am Rev Respir Dis 141:1114–1118, 1990; JAAD 31:281–283, 1994*

Temporal arteritis *Acta Ophth 57:362–368, 1979*

Thrombotic thrombocytopenic purpura (TTP)

Valsalva maneuver – labor and delivery

Vascular malformations *Ped Derm 21:1–9, 2004*

Vein of Galen malformation – eyelid edema, telangiectatic patches of forehead and cheek, prominent superficial veins of forehead *JAMA Derm 149:249–251, 2013*

PERIORBITAL CONGENITAL NODULES, PEDIATRIC

Ped Derm 28:702, 2001

Dacryocystocele

Dermoid cyst

Encephalocele

Hemangioma, infantile

Nasal glioma

PERIOSTITIS

AUTOIMMUNE DISEASES AND DISORDERS OF IMMUNE DYSREGULATION

Interleukin-1 receptor antagonist deficiency – neutrophilic pustular dermatitis, periostitis, aseptic dermatitis, osteomyelitis, high acute phase reactants *J Med Case Rep June 23, 2015:9:145; Ped Derm 30:758–760, 2013*

DRUG REACTIONS

Interleukin-11 therapy – clavicle, long bones

Voriconazole *Semin Arth Rheumatol 49:319–323, 2019*

EXOGENOUS AGENTS

Skin popping – illicit drug use *Foot (Edinb)25:114–119, 2015*

INFECTIONS AND INFESTATIONS

Bacillary angiomatosis *Skeletal Radiology 23:569–571, 1994*

Bizarre parosteal osteochondromatous proliferation (Nora's tumor) – hands and feet

Cytomegalovirus infection, congenital

Leprosy *Indian J Leprosy 88:83–95, 2016*

Osteomyelitis – variable

Rubella, congenital

Subperiosteal abscess – eyelid edema and erythema as sole sign *Br J Ophthalmol 73:576–578, 1989*

Syphilis, congenital *Ped Derm 27:308–309, 2010; Turk J Ped 51:169–171, 2009*

Syphilis, secondary *Acta DV Croat 26:186–188, 2018; West J Med 140:35–42, 1984;* congenital syphilis – bone fractures, lytic bone lesions, periostitis *Turk J Ped 51:169–171, 2009;* pseudoparesis of Parrot *J Pediatr Nov 2017:190:282*

Systemic lupus erythematosus – variable

Yaws *Clin Orthop Relat Res 192:193–198, 1985*

INFILTRATIVE DISORDERS

Eosinophilic granuloma of bone (unifocal Langerhans cell histiocytosis) *J Manipulative Physiol Ther 28:274–277, 2005*

INFLAMMATORY DISORDERS

Crohn's disease *Gastroenterol Clin Biol 13:841–844, 1989; Gastroenterology 60:1106–1109, 1971*

Eosinophilic fasciitis *Z Rheumatol 39:236–250, 1980*

Facial infections – mandible, orbits

Erythema nodosum – ossifying granulomatous periostitis *Ital J Orthop Trauma 4:223–229, 1978*

Florid reactive periostitis – phalanges of hands and feet *Ped Radiol 20:186–189, 1990*

Hypertrophic osteoarthropathy – distal diaphysis of long bones and metacarpal joints

Ossifying fasciitis – variable

METABOLIC DISORDERS

Hyperparathyroidism *Radiographics 13:357–379, 1993*

Hypervitaminosis A *Ped Radiol 37:1264–1267, 2007*

Rickets, healing *Acad Forensic Pathol 7:240–262, 2017*

Thyroid acropachy (Graves' disease) *Orthopedics 31:98–100, 2008*

NEOPLASTIC DISORDERS

Chondrosarcoma – variable

Leukemia

Osteoblastoma – variable

PRIMARY CUTANEOUS DISEASES

Psoriatic onycho-pachydermoperiostitis – terminal phalanx

Psoriatic arthritis – phalanges of fingers and toes *Reumatismo 64:99–106, 2012; J Am Acad Orth Surg 20:28–37, 2012*

TRAUMA

Athletics – upper and lower extremities

Battered child syndrome

Chronic drug addiction (IVDA) – left forearm of right handed addicts and vice versa *Skeletal Radiology 15:209–212, 1986*

SYNDROMES

Menkes' syndrome

Pachydermoperiostosis (Touraine-Solente-Gole syndrome) – with hypertrophic osteoarthropathy; palmoplantar hyperhidrosis, arthritis, clubbing, cutis verticis gyrate, ptosis, seborrhea *Best Pract Res Clin Rheumatol April 11, 2020:101507; Indian J Nuc Med 27:201–204, 2012*

Periostitis ossificans (Garre's osteomyelitis) – variable; bony hard nontender swelling of mandible; young patients secondary to dental infection *OSOMOPOR Endodod 102:e14–19, 2006; Int J Ped Dent 16:59–64, 2006*

Reactive arthritis – phalanges of fingers and toes

SAPHO syndrome – variable *Eur J Ped 165:370–373, 2006;* bullhorn sign *Rheumatology (Oxford)42:1398–1403, 2003; Z Rheumatol 56:136–153, 1997*

VASCULAR DISORDERS

Cutaneous polyarteritis nodosa *Rev Med Interne 20:1132–1134, 1999*

Leg ulcers, chronic; chronic venous insufficiency – tibia *Sem Intervent Rad 22:162–168, 2005*

Cutaneous polyarteritis nodosa – lower extremities *Rev Med Interne 20:1132–1134, 1999*

Venous stasis dermatitis

PERIPHERAL EOSINOPHILIA

AUTOIMMUNE DISEASES AND DISORDERS OF IMMUNE DYSREGULATION

Asthma

Bullous pemphigoid *Acta DV 98:766–771, 2018; Acta DV 97:464–471, 2017;* pemphigoid nodularis *Exp Ther Med 17:1132–1138, 2019; BJD 179:1030, 2018*

Combined immunodeficiency with hypereosinophilia

Dermatomyositis

Dock 8 deficiency

Hyper IgE syndrome

IgG4 disease *Sci Rep 9:16483, Nov 11, 2019*

Non-episodic angioedema with eosinophilia *Case Rep Dermatol 9:164–168, 2017*

Rheumatoid arthritis *J Clin Rheumatol 14:211–213, 2008*

Scleroderma with skin ulcers *J Dermatol 46:334–337, 2019*

Sjogren's syndrome

DRUG REACTIONS

CD 30+ lymphomatoid angiocentric drug reactions *Am J Dermatopathol 39:508–517, 2017*

DRESS syndrome *Cureus June 27, 2019, 11 (6) e5015*

Drug hypersensitivity

IL-2 therapy

INFECTIONS AND INFESTATIONS

Aspergillosis – primary cutaneous, immunocompetent patient *Diagn Cytopathol 46:434–437, 2018*

Coccidioidomycosis *Human Pathol 45:153–159, 2014*

Histoplasmosis *Indian J Hematol Blood Transfus 33:130–132, 2017*

HIV disease *Am J Med 102:449–453, 1997*
    Leukopenia
    Reactions to medications
    Adrenal insufficiency
    Eosinophilic folliculitis

HTLV I and II

Katayama fever – exanthem, urticaria, fever, diarrhea *NEJM 374:469, 2016*

Parasites *BJD 176:212–215, 2017*
    Angiostrongyliasis costarincensis
    Ascara lumbricoides
    Enterobius vermicularis (pinworm) *Clin Pediatr (Phila)58:13–16, 2019*
    Filariasis – subcutaneous nodule *Trop Parasitol 8:121–123, 2018*
    Flukes – schistosomiasis, fascioliasis, clonorchiasis, paragonimiasis, fasciolopsiasis
    Gnathostomiasis
    Hookworm
    Onchocerciasis
    Strongyloides stercoralis
    Trichinella Ann Parasitol 65:177–189, 2019
    Tropical pulmonary eosinophilic loiasis
    Visceral larva migrans

Myiasis

Psittacosis *Resp Med Case Rep 23:138–142, 2018*

Scabies

INFILTRATIVE DISORDERS

Mastocytosis *Leukemia 34:1090–1101, 2020*

INFLAMMATORY DISORDERS

Eosinophilic esophagitis, gastritis, gastroenteritis, or colitis

Eosinophilic fasciitis – with prayer sign *Cureus Jan 7, 2020; e6581; Clin Dermatol 36:487–497, 2018*

Idiopathic eosinophilic synovitis

Loffler syndrome *Indian J Dermatol 61:190–192, 2016*

Pulmonary eosinophilia

Pyostomatitis vegetans *BJD 173:1556–1557, 2015; An Bras Dermatol 86:S137–140, 2011; Med Oral Patol Oral Cir Bucal 14:e114–117, 2009; Clin Exp Dermtol 29:1–7, 2004*

Sarcoidosis *Resp Med Case Rep Feb 16, 2013; Mayo Clin Proc 75:586–590, 2000*

METABOLIC DISORDERS

Adrenal insufficiency (Addison's disease) *J Am Coll Surg 183:589–596, 1996; Trop Geogr Med 40:241–243, 1988*

Monoclonal gammopathy *BJD 176:212–215, 2017*

NEOPLASTIC DISORDERS

Adenocarcinoma of the colon

Adenocarcinoma of the stomach

Adenocarcinoma of the uterus

Clonal eosinophilia, leukemia, myeloproliferative hypereosinophilic syndrome *BJD 176:212–215, 2017*

Large cell non-keratinizing cervical tumors

Large cell undifferentiated lung carcinomas

Lymphoma – cutaneous lymphoma *BJD 176:212–215, 2017;* cutaneous T-cell lymphoma, folliculotropic *SAGE Open Med Case Rep May 31, 2018;* Hodgkin's disease *Int Arch Allergy Immunol 110:244–251, 1996;* non-Hodgkin's lymphoma *Cutis 67:67–70, 2001;* peripheral T-cell lymphoma *J Fam Med Prim Care 6:427–430, 2017*

Lymphoproliferative disorders *BJD 176:212–215, 2017*

Malignancy
    Adenocarcinoma of the stomach, large bowel, or uterus
    Large cell non-keratinizing cervical tumors
    Large cell undifferentiated lung carcinomas

Metastases *BJD 176:212–215, 2017*

PARANEOPLASTIC DISORDERS

Pancreatic panniculitis as sign of pancreatic cancer *Acta Clin Belg 71:448–450, 2016*

PRIMARY CUTANEOUS DISEASES

Atopic dermatitis

Papuloerythroderma of Ofuji *Stat Pearls Nov 15, 2019 PMID 30969577*

SYNDROMES

Primary hypereosinophilic syndromes *BMJ Case Rep Oct 15, 2019; BJD 176:212–215, 2017*

Omenn syndrome

Allergic rhinitis syndrome

Wells' syndrome (eosinophilic cellulitis) *Dermatol Online J July 15, 2016*

TOXINS

Eosinophilic myalgia syndrome *Immunol Allergy Clin NA 35:453–476, 2015;* tryptophan *NEJM 322:874–881, 1990*

Toxic oil syndrome *Environ Health Perspect 110:457–464, 2002*

TRAUMA

Radiation exposure

VASCULAR LESIONS

Angiolymphoid hyperplasia with eosinophilia *Dermatol Online J Dec 15, 2019*

Atheroembolic disease (cholesterol emboli syndrome)

Cholesterol emboli *W V Med J 85:532–535, 1989*

Eosinophilic granulomatosis with polyangiitis *Oman Med J 34:345–349, 2019; Heart Asia June 5, 2019 vi (2) e011211*

Granulomatosis with polyangiitis

Kimura's disease – single or multiple nontender subcutaneous nodes of head and neck *Indian Dermatol Online J 9:282–283, 2010*

Thromboangiitis obliterans with eosinophilia of the temporal arteries

PERIPHERAL NEUROPATHY, CUTANEOUS MANIFESTATIONS

AUTOIMMUNE DISEASES AND DISORDERS OF IMMUNE DYSFUNCTION

Deficiency of adenosine deaminase – ADA 1 – autosomal recessive; severe combined immunodeficiency; ADA 2 – loss of function mutation in cat eye syndrome chromosome candidate 1 gene (*CECR1*); painless leg nodules with intermittent livedo reticularis, Raynaud's phenomenon, cutaneous ulcers, morbilliform rashes, Raynaud's phenomenon, digital gangrene, oral aphthae; vasculitis of small and medium arteries with necrosis, fever, early recurrent ischemic and hemorrhagic strokes, peripheral and cranial neuropathy, and gastrointestinal involvement (diarrhea); hepatosplenomegaly, systemic vasculopathy, stenosis of abdominal arteries *Ped Derm 37:199–201, 2020; NEJM 380:1582–1584, 2019; Ped Derm 33:602–614, 2016; NEJM 370:911–920, 2014; NEJM 370:921–931, 2014*

Dermatomyositis *Rev Med Interne 31:e13–15, 2010; Intern Med 42:1233–1239, 2003*

IgG4-related disease *Neurology 85:1400–1407, 2015; JAMA Neurology 70:502–505, 2013*

Lupus erythematosus, systemic *Clin Exp Rheumatol 37:146–155, 2019*

Mixed connective tissue disease *Medicine (Balt) 97: (31) e11360 Aug 2018*

Rheumatoid arthritis *Rheum Dis Clin NA 43:561–571, 2017*

Scleroderma *Semin Arthr Rheum 43:335–347, 2013*

Sjogren's syndrome-associated peripheral neuropathy *J Autoimmune 39:27–33, 2012; A Clinician's Pearls and Myths in Rheumatology pp.107–130; ed John Stone; Springer 2009; Neurology 43:1820–1823, 1993*

CONGENITAL DISORDERS

Syringomyelia – pseudoainhum *JAAD 44:381–384, 2001;* painless ulcer

DEGENERATIVE DISORDERS

Hereditary sensory neuropathy – primary; plantar ulcers *Int J Dermatol 23:664–668, 1984;* leg ulcers

Multiple sclerosis – secondary to anti-TNF therapy for psoriasis *J Dermatol Therapy 27:406–413, 2016*

Neuralgic amyotrophy – asymmetric atrophy of shoulder muscles *NEJM 362:2304, 2010*

Neuropathic ulcer (trophic ulcer) (mal perforans) (Charcot foot); including those associated with neuropathies – on metatarsal heads and heels with underlying sinus tract to joint or subfascial abscess
Trophic ulcers
Acrodystrophic neuropathy of Bureau and Barriere
Alcoholism
Amantadine-induced peripheral neuropathy
Autonomic trophic disorder of the cerebral hemispheres
Carpal tunnel syndrome
Cauda equina syndrome
Charcot-Marie-Tooth syndrome type 2A with neurotrophic foot ulcer
Compression syndrome
Cutaneous-mucous trophic disorder
Decubitus
Diabetes mellitus
Familial amyloid polyneuropathy type I
Giaccai syndrome
Gilbert's syndrome
Hereditary sensory and autonomic neuropathies (HSAN), four types *Clin Exp Derm 1:91–92, 1976*
Hereditary spastic paraplegia with sensory neuropathy
Leprosy
Lipomeningocele
Multiple sclerosis
Neuroacropathy
Paraplegias
Peripheral neuropathy
Poliomyelitis
Post-external fixation in quadriplegia
Post-retroperitoneoscopic lumbar sympathectomy
Post-spinal anesthesia
Post-surgery of trigeminal nerve
Reflex sympathetic dystrophy
Spina bifida
Split cord malformation with meningomyelocele (complex spina bifida)
Syringomyelia – trophic ulcer
Tabes dorsalis
Trigeminal trophic syndrome (Wallenberg's syndrome) – ulcers of nose and medial cheeks; scalp ulcers *Cutis 92:291–296, 2013; AD 144:984–986, 2008; J Dermatol 18:613–615, 1991*
Ulcerative-mutilating acropathy – inherited (Thavenard's syndrome) or acquired (Bureau-Barriere syndrome)
Werner's syndrome with torpid trophic ulcera cruris

Organic brain lesion

DRUGS

Bortezomib *Zhonghia Yi Xue Za Zhi 95:3297–3301, 2015*

Brentuximab – for cutaneous T-cell lymphoma including Sezary syndrome *J Neurooncol 132:439–446, 2017*

Chemotherapy-induced – cisplatin, vincristine, taxanes *J Natl Cancer Inst Feb 1, 2018 110 (2):doi:1011093*

Eribulin mesylate *Crit Rev Oncol Hematol 128:110–117, 2018*

Ganglion blocking and anticholinergic drugs

Levodopa *Musc Disord Clin Pract 6:96–103, 2018*

Reverse transcriptase inhibitor *Pharmacogenetics 10:623–637, 2009*

INFECTIONS AND INFESTATIONS

Acrodermatitis chronica atrophicans *Clin Inf Dis 59:866,903, 2014*

Diphtheria – bull neck due to lymphadenopathy, myocarditis, peripheral neuropathy, pharyngitis with membranes *Netter's Infectious Diseases pp.5–10, 2012; J Neurol Neurosurg Psychiatry 67:825–826, 1999;* cutaneous diphtheria *J R Soc Med 91:60, 1998*

Hepatitis B – mononeuritis multiplex and painful ulcerations *BMJ Case Rep May 2, 2013 pii:BCK2013009666*

Hepatitis C *World J Gastroenterol 21:2269–2280, 2015*

HTLV-1 *Handbook Clin Neurol 115:531–541, 2013; Semin Neurol 25:315–327, 2015*

Leprosy – including primary neural leprosy *Infect Dis Cases Aril 14, 2020:e00765; Clinics in Dermatol 33:8–18, 2015;* type 1 reaction demonstrates reappearance of resolved lesions, with erythema, edema, and paresthesias; acute peripheral neuritis, edema of hands, feet, arms, and face *JAAD 83:17–30, 2020; BJD 158:648–649, 2008; JAAD 57:914–917, 2007*

Lyme disease *Handbook Clin Neurol 145:453–474, 2017*

Varicella – congenital (fetal) varicella syndrome – infection between first and second trimester; dermatomal scars; low birth weight, localized absence of skin, papular lesions resembling connective tissue nevi, limb paresis, limb hypoplasia, malformed digits, ocular anomalies (chorioretinitis), central nervous system abnormalities *BJD 150:357–363, 2004*

Whipple's disease (*Tropheryma whipplie*) – non-palpable purpura, chronic leg edema, arthralgias; large dilated abdominal lymphatics; diarrhea, weight loss, abdominal pain, generalized hyperpigmentation, pulmonary hypertension, eye, cardiovascular, and neurologic disease *Clin Infect Dis 41:519–520,557–559, 2005*

Zika virus – ascending paralytic polyneuropathy; 20% are ill with mild viral syndrome; morbilliform eruption, arthralgias, non-purulent conjunctivitis, headache, retro-orbital pain *Clin Inf Dis 61:1445,1485–1486, 2015; NEJM 360:2536–2543, 2009*

INFILTRATIVE DISORDERS

Amyloidosis – subcutaneous nodular amyloidosis *Hum Pathol 32:346–348, 2001;* beta-2 microglobulin amyloidosis – shoulder pain, carpal tunnel syndrome, flexor tendon deposits of hands, lichenoid papules, hyperpigmentation, subcutaneous nodules (amyloidomas) *Int J Exp Clin Inves 4:187–211, 1997; South Med J 88:876–878, 1995; Arch Pathol Lab Med 118:651–653, 1994; J Clin Pathol 46:771–772, 1993; Nephron 55:312–315, 1990; Nephron 53:73–75, 1989;* dialysis-related beta-2 microglobulin amyloidosis of buttocks *BJD 149:400–404, 2003;* bilateral popliteal tumors *Am J Kidney dis 12:323–325, 1988;* familial amyloid polyneuropathy – atrophic scars *BJD 152:250–257, 2005;* familial amyloid polyneuropathy due to mutation in transthyretin – ulcers of knees *BJD 164:1398–1400, 2011*

Hereditary gelsolin amyloidosis (AGel amyloidosis) – cutis laxa, thin eyebrows, corneal lattice dystrophy, cranial and peripheral polyneuropathy *BJD 152:250–257, 2005*

Juvenile xanthogranuloma *Am J Surg Pathol 25:521–526, 2001*

INFLAMMATORY DISORDERS

Neuritis with onycholysis

Neurogenic muscle (pseudo)-hypertrophy – compensatory hypertrophy with swollen calf *Ned Tijdschr Geneeskd 147:2183–2186, 2003*

Radiculopathy – S1 radiculopathy – swollen calf *Lancet 365:1662, 2005; Arch Neurol 45:660–664, 1988*

Sarcoidosis *Handbook Clin Neurol 115:485–495, 2013; Chest 112:220–228, 1997*

METABOLIC DISORDERS

Angiokeratoma corporis diffusum (Fabry's disease (alpha galactosidase A) – X-linked recessive; skin dry or anhidrotic due to peripheral nervous system disease; lancinating shooting pain *Rev Neurol 173:650–657, 2017; JAAD 74:231–244, 2016; BJD 157:331–337, 2007; JAAD 46:161–183, 2002; Clin Auton Res 6:107–110, 1996; JAAD 17:883–887, 1987; NEJM 276:1163–1167, 1967*

Celiac disease *Acta Biomed 89 (9–5)22–32, 2018; Int J Environ Res Public Health July 14, 2017; Minerva Gastroenterol Dietol 62:197–206, 2016;* celiac neuropathy – pruritus ani *Neurology 60:1581–1585, 2003*

Cryoglobulinemia, mixed (non-hepatitis C) *Autoimmune Rev 18:778–785, 2019*

Diabetic neuropathy – hypohidrosis of legs with compensatory hyperhidrosis elsewhere *Mayo Clin Proc 64:617–628, 1989;* peripheral neuropathy with livedo reticularis *JAAD 52:1009–1019, 2005;* hemorrhagic callus

Hemochromatosis *J Neurol 257:1465–1472, 2010*

Hyperthermia

Idiopathic orthostatic hypotension

Pellagra – pain and dysesthesias of the legs, paresthesias of the toes and lower legs *NEJM 371:2218–2223, 2014*

Acute porphyria – acute intermittent porphyria, variegate porphyria, hepatoerythroporphyria *Br J Hematol 176:527–538, 2017*

Refsum's syndrome – phytanic acid oxidase deficiency – autosomal recessive; late onset (teens to 30's) mild ichthyosis vulgaris-like, some with lamellar type scale; retinitis pigmentosa, cataracts; deafness, anosmia, sensorimotor polyneuropathy, ataxia *Neurobiol Dis 18:110–118, 2005; Curr Prob Derm 14:71–116, 2002; J R Soc Med 84:559–560, 1991*

Vitamin B12 deficiency *J Assoc Physicians India 68:59, 2020; Rev Med Suisse 15:2152–2157, 2019; World J Gastroenterol 24:1343–1352, 2018*

NEOPLASTIC DISORDERS

Bronchial carcinoma – unilateral anhidrosis; with hyperhidrosis of opposite side *Eur J Dermatol 11:257–258, 2001*

Cervicothoracic syrinx and thoracic spinal cord tumor – dermatomal lichen simplex chronicus *Neurosurgery 30 (3):418–421, 1992*

Inflammation or tumors of hypothalamus

Light chain deposition disease – violaceous plaque of chin; involvement of kidneys (nephropathy), liver, heart, lungs, peripheral nerves *Hematol Oncol Clin NA 13:1235–1248, 1999*

Lymphoma – cutaneous T-cell lymphoma *Muscle Nerv 36:800–805, 2007;* granulomatous cutaneous T-cell lymphoma *J Med Assoc Thai 93:1321–1326, 2010*

Merkel cell carcinoma *JAMA Derm 156:597–598, 2020*

Monoclonal gammopathy *Rev Med Suisse 15:2152–2157, 2019*

Peripheral nerve lesion

PARANEOPLASTIC DISORDERS

Paraneoplastic peripheral neuropathies *Rev Neurol (Paris) 164:1068–1072, 2008;* anti-mu antibodies *Handbook Clin Neurol 115:713–726, 2013*

PRIMARY CUTANEOUS DISORDERS

Asteatotic dermatitis – in hypoesthetic skin *JAMA Derm 150:1088–1090, 2014*

Chronic idiopathic anhidrosis *Ann Neurol 18:344–348, 1985*

Congenital sensory neuropathy with anhidrosis – pseudoainhum *Ped Derm 11:231–236, 1994; JAAD 21:736–739, 1989*

Familial congenital anterior cervical hypertrichosis associated with peripheral sensory and motor neuropathy *J Pediatr Ophthalmol Strabismus 34:309–312, 1997*

Hereditary keratoderma, nail dystrophy, and hereditary motor and sensory neuropathy – autosomal dominant *J Med Genet 25:754–757, 1988*

Palmoplantar keratoderma, nail dystrophy, hereditary motor and sensory neuropathy

Partial lipodystrophy, complement abnormalities, vasculitis – macroglossia, polyarthralgia, mononeuritis, hypertrophy of subcutaneous tissue *Ann DV 114:1083–1091, 1987*

Xerosis – sympathetic nerve dystrophy – anhidrosis with xerosis

PSYCHOCUTANEOUS DISORDERS

Hysteria (conversion disorder) *Pain Res Manag 16:457–459, 2011*

SYNDROMES

Adie's syndrome – idiopathic, HIV, Lyme borreliosis, herpes simplex virus, parvovirus B19, syphilis *Neurol Sci 31:661–663, 2010*

Bannayan-Riley-Ruvalcaba syndrome – macrocephaly, genital lentiginosis, polyposis, multiple acrochordons *JAAD 53:639–643, 2005*

Bardet-Biedl syndrome – postaxial polydactyly (ulnar), retinal dystrophy, retinitis pigmentosa, obesity, neuropathy, mental disturbance *J Med Genet 36:599–603, 1999*

Begeer syndrome – cataracts, deafness, short stature, ataxia, polyneuropathy *Clin Dysmorphol 4:283–288, 1995*

Behcet's syndrome peripheral neuropathy is rare *Rev Med Interne 35:112–120, 2014;* peripheral facial paresis *Neurologist 14:77, 2008*

Brown-Crounse syndrome – 1–2 mm papules, plaques, and nodules, diffuse hypotrichosis resembling alopecia areata, basaloid follicular hamartomas, trichoepitheliomas, myasthenia gravis *AD 99:478–493, 1969*

Charcot Marie Tooth disease 2B – peripheral neuropathy, muscle weakness, recurrent foot ulcers *Int J Mol Sci Feb 4, 2017*

Chediak-Higashi syndrome – rare, autosomal recessive; partial albinism, recurrent infections, easy bruising, giant granules in many cells (leukocytes, platelets, hair shafts, melanocytes) *Muscle Nerve 55:359–365, 2017;* motor mononeuropathy *J Neurol Sci 344:203–207, 2017*

Cockayne's syndrome (cachectic dwarfism) – autosomal recessive; short stature, facial erythema in butterfly distribution leading to mottled pigmentation and atrophic scars, premature aged appearance with loss of subcutaneous fat and sunken eyes (enophthalmos with loss of periorbital fat), lipoatrophy of temples; canities, mental

deficiency, photosensitivity, disproportionately large hands, feet, and ears, ocular defects, demyelination *Ped Derm 20:538–540, 2003; J Med Genet 18:288–293, 1981*

Congenital insensitivity to pain – bruises, burns, lacerations, and fractures mimicking child abuse *Pediatr Emerg Care 12:116–121, 1996*

Congenital insensitivity to pain with anhidrosis – mutation in *NTRK1* gene encodes *TrkA* (receptor for nerve growth factor) *Ped Derm 30:754–756, 2013; BJD 166:888–891, 2012; Am J Med Genet 99:164–165, 2001; JID 112:810–814, 1999; Cutis 60:188–190, 1997;* congenital insensitivity to pain – bruises, burns, lacerations, and fractures mimicking child abuse *Pediatr Emerg Care 12:116–121, 1996;* self-mutilation *AD 124:564–566, 1988*

Cronkhite-Canada syndrome *Austral NZ J Med 21:379, 1991*

Familial dysautonomia (Riley-Day syndrome) (hereditary sensory and autonomic neuropathy type III) – Charcot joints *BMJ iv:277–278, 1967;* smooth tongue; absent fungiform papillae *Cesk Pediatrics 46:347–348, 1991;* congenital sensory neuropathy (Riley-Day syndrome) with anhidrosis *J Oral Maxillofac Surg 45:331–334, 1987*

Ectrodactyly-ectodermal dysplasia-cleft lip/palate syndrome (EEC syndrome) *Ped Derm 20:113–118, 2003*

Follicular keratotic papules with distal limb polyneuropathy *Am J Dermatopathol 39:e83–84, 2017; Am J Dermatopathol 39:549–550, 2017*

Guillain-Barre syndrome

Hereditary sensory and autonomic neuropathy type I – calluses over metatarsal heads which blister, necrose, and ulcerate

Hereditary sensory and autonomic neuropathy type II – acral whitlows and ulcers of fingers with mutilation

Hereditary sensory and autonomic neuropathy with phospholipid excretion *JAAD 21:736–739, 1989*

Hereditary sensory and autonomic neuropathy types II and IV – acral hypohidrosis (congenital insensitivity to pain with anhidrosis *Ped Derm 19:333–335, 2002*

Hereditary sensory and autonomic neuropathy type I–V (congenital insensitivity to pain) – ulcers with self-mutilation *Ped Derm 19:333–335, 2002*

Horner's syndrome – blepharoptosis, miosis, facial anhidrosis, iris hypochromia; medullary infarction, syringomyelia, multiple sclerosis, intraspinal tumors, aortic aneurysm, cervical lymphadenopathy, surgery, regional anesthesia, tumors – transient unilateral hyperhidrosis and vasoconstriction of the face with subsequent anhidrosis; Harlequin sign – hemifacial flushing and contralateral hypohidrosis in Horner's syndrome *Ped Derm 23:358–360, 2006*

Mobius syndrome – congenital bilateral facial paralysis; inability to abduct eyes *JAMA Derm 150:1019–1020, 2014*

Neurofibromatosis type 1 *Med Clin NA 103:1035–1054, 2019*

Oliver-McFarlane syndrome – autosomal recessive; trichomegaly, pigmentary degeneration of retina (retinitis pigmentosa), mental and growth retardation, peripheral neuropathy, anterior pituitary deficiencies *Br J Ophthalmol 87:119–120, 2003; Can J Ophthalmol 28:191–193, 1993; Genet Couns 2:115–118, 1991; Am J Med Genet 34:199–201, 1989; Am J Ophthalmol 101:490–491, 1986; Am J Dis Child 121:344–345, 1971; Arch Ophthalmol 74:169–171, 1965*

Pachyonychia congenita – neuropathic plantar pain *BJD 179:11–12, 2018; BJD 176:1144–1147, 2017*

POEMS syndrome (Takatsuki syndrome, Crowe-Fukase syndrome) – osteosclerotic bone lesions, peripheral polyneuropathy, hypothyroidism, and hypogonadism *Pract Neurol 18:278–290,*

2018; *JAAD 21:1061–1068, 1989; Cutis 61:329–334, 1998;* cicatricial alopecia with underlying plasmacytoma *JAAD 40:808–812, 1999*

Reflex sympathetic dystrophy (complex regional pain syndrome) *Cutis 68:179–182, 2001; JAAD 35:843–845, 1996; JAAD 22:513–520, 1990; Arch Neurol 44:555–561, 1987;* reticulated hyperpigmentation *Cutis 68:179–182, 2001*

Riga-Fede disease – white oral verrucous plaque of mucosal surface of lip, tongue, frenulum due to trauma; sign of infantile or natal teeth or sensory neuropathies *JAAD 47:445–447, 2002*

Ross' syndrome – progressive segmental anhidrosis with compensatory hyperhidrosis, Adie's pupils (tonic pupil), loss of reflexes, cholinergic supersensitivity *J Neurology 239:231–234, 1992; Neurology 32:1041–1042, 1982*

Schnitzler's syndrome – intracostal neuralgia *BJD 167:1392–1393, 2012*

Segmental hyperhidrosis with areflexia – diffuse loss of sweating *Neurophysiol Clin 23:363–369, 1993*

Speckled lentiginous nevus syndrome – speckled lentiginous nevus with ipsilateral sensory and motor neuropathy, hyperhidrosis, spinal muscle atrophy with fasciculations, dysesthesias, muscle weakness, muscle atrophy, nerve palsy *Ped Derm 26:298–301, 2009; Eur J Dermatol 12:133–135, 2002;* ipsilateral shortening of limb and vertebral malformations *Acta DV (Stockh)74:327–334, 1994*

TOXINS

Acrodynia (pink disease) – mercury poisoning; acral erythema and pain, hypertension, tachycardia, mental status changes *Arch Dis Child 86:453–2002; Ped Derm 21:254–259, 2004; Ann DV 121:309–314, 1994;* profuse sweating; red edematous hands and feet, hypertension, severe periumbilical pain, irritability *Ped Derm 29:199–201, 2012; Pediatr Nephrol 22:903–906, 2009; Arch Dis Child 62:293–295, 1987; Lancet 29:829–830, 1948; Arch Dermatol Syphilol 26:215–237, 1932; Rev Med Fr 3:51–74, 1830*

Alcoholic toxic polyneuropathy *Lancet ii:721–722, 1989; Z Hautkr 55:349–354, 1980*

Arsenic *Rev Environ Health 34:403–414, 2019*

Botulinum toxin injection – inhibits regional sweating *Clin Auton Res 6:123–124, 1996*

Thallium – anagen effluvium *JAMA Derm 152:724–726, 2016; Handbook Clin Neurol 131:253–296, 2015; JAAD 50:258–261, 2004;* nausea, vomiting, stomatitis, painful glossitis, diarrhea; severe dysesthesias and paresthesias in distal extremities, facial rashes of cheeks and perioral region, acneiform eruptions of face, hyperkeratosis of palms and soles, hair loss, Mees' lines *AD 143:93–98, 2007*

TRAUMA

Nerve injury, traumatic – surgical injury to lateral femoral cutaneous nerve with bulla and subsequent ulceration of lateral lower leg *Dermatol Wochenschri 136:971–973, 1957*

Sympathectomy

Sympathectomy-induced ichthyosis-like eruption *Int J Dermatol 39:146–151, 2000*

Quadriplegia

VASCULAR DISORDERS

Cutaneous polyarteritis nodosa *J Dermatol 41:266–267, 2014; Ann Vasc Dis 5:282–288, 2012; Arch Dermatol Res 301:117–121, 2009*

Eosinophilic granulomatosis with polyangiitis *Intern Med 56:3003–3008, 2017; JAAD 47:209–216, 2002; JAAD 37:199–203, 1997; JAAD 27:821–824, 1992; JID 17:349–359, 1951; Am J Pathol 25:817, 1949*

Giant cell arteritis – lower extremity ulcers *J Rheumatol 16:1366–1369, 1989; J Rheumatol 14:129–134, 1987; Postgrad Med J 60:670–671, 1984*

Granulomatosis with polyangiitis *Eur Neurol 73:197–204, 2015; Acta Rheumatol Port 39:96–97, 2014; Handbook Clin Neurol 115:463–483, 2013*

Henoch–Schonlein purpura *Handbook Clin Neurol 120:1101–1111, 2014; Ped Nephrol 16:1139–1141, 2001; Ped 75:687–692, 1985*

Hypocomplementemic urticarial vasculitis *J Neurol Sci 284:179–181, 2009*

Microscopic polyangiitis (ANCA+ vasculitis) *Curr Opinion Rheumatol 31:40–45, 2019; Rheum Dis Clin NA 43:633–639, 2017*

Polyarteritis nodosa – mononeuritis multiplex; peripheral neuropathy frequent and early symptom *Neurol Clin 37:345–357, 2019;* acrocyanosis and/or Raynaud's phenomenon; livedo reticularis with surrounding erythema; acrocyanosis, ulcers, papules *JAAD 74:247–270, 2016; JAAD 57:840–848, 2007; JAAD 52:1009–1019, 2005;* familial polyarteritis nodosa of Georgian Jewish, German, and Turkish ancestry – oral aphthae, livedo reticularis, leg ulcers, Raynaud's phenomenon, digital necrosis, nodules, purpura, erythema nodosum; systemic manifestations include fever, myalgias, arthralgias, gastrointestinal symptoms, renal disease, central and peripheral neurologic manifestations; mutation in adenosine deaminase 2 (*CECR1*) *NEJM 370:921–931, 2014*

PHAKOMATOSES

SYNDROMES

Aarskog syndrome (facio-digito-genital syndrome) – X-linked recessive – round face, hyperterlorism, ptosis, anteverted nostrils, long philtrum, broad nasal bridge; short broad hands with syndactyly, scrotal shawl (scrotal fold which surrounds the base of the penis); skeletal defects; delayed puberty; learning disabilities *J Clin Diagn Res 10:ZD09–11, 2016; Am J Med Genet 46:501–509, 1993; Am J Ophthalmol 109:450–456, 1990; Am J Med Genet 15:39–46, 1983; Hum Genet 42:129–135, 1978; J Pediatr 77:856–861, 1970*

Adams-Oliver syndrome – congenital scalp ACC and amniotic bands with reduction of terminal phalanges of fingers and toes (terminal transverse limb defects); occasionally severe bony defects with absent hands, feet, or lower legs; bony abnormalities of cranium; cutis marmorata telangiectatica congenita, severe growth retardation, aplasia cutis congenita of knee, short palpebral fissures, dilated scalp veins, simple pinnae, skin tags on toes, hemangioma, undescended testes, supernumerary nipples, hypoplastic optic nerve, central nervous system and congenital heart defects *Am J Med Genet A 173:790–800, 2017; Ped Derm 25:115–116, 2008; Ped Derm 24:651–653, 2007; BJD 157:836–837, 2007; Am J Med Genet 136A:269–274, 2005; Plast Reconstr Surg 100:1491–1496, 1997; Clin Genet 47:80–84, 1995; Int J Dermatol 32:52–53, 1993; Eur J Pediatr 126:289–295, 1977; JAAD 56:541–564, 2007*

Aicardi-Gutieres syndrome – autosomal recessive; type 1 interferonopathy; livedo reticularis, panniculitis, interstitial lung disease; chilblains, acrocyanosis, puffy hands and feet; blueberry muffin baby; intracranial calcification with enlarged ventricles; progressive encephalopathy; increased cerebrospinal fluid interferon alpha and lymphocytosis *Dermatol Clin 37:229–232, 2019; Ped Rheumatol Online J 14:35 June 4, 2016; Ped Derm 26:432–435, 2009; Am J Hum Genet 81:713–725, 2007; Ann Neurol 44:900–907, 1998*

Amelo-cerebro-hypohidrotic syndrome (Kohlschutter syndrome) – X-linked or autosomal recessive; hypohidrosis, hypoplastic yellow tooth enamel (amelogenesis imperfect), epilepsy, spasticity, mental retardation; *ROGD1* gene mutation *OSOMOPOR 125:e8–11, 2018; Helv Paediatr Acta 29:283–294, 1974*

Angelman syndrome – hypopigmentation, mental retardation; microcephaly, tongue protrusion, paroxysms of laughter; UBE3A mutation *Nat Rev Neurol 12:584–593, 2016; Am J Med Genet 40:454, 1991*

Ataxia telangiectasia – café au lait macules may be dermatomal; progeroid appearance with gray hair and skin atrophy; phosphatidylinositol 3-kinase *BJD 164:245–256, 2011; BJD 144:369–371, 2001; JAAD 42:939–969, 2000; JAMA 195:746–753, 1966;* autosomal recessive; telangiectasias of face, ocular telangiectasia, extensor surfaces of arms and bulbar conjunctiva; hypopigmented macules, melanocytic nevi, facial papulosquamous rash, hypertrichosis, bird-like facies; immunodeficiency, increased risk of leukemia, lymphoma; cerebellar ataxia with eye movement signs, mental retardation, and other neurologic defects; cafe au lait macules *JAAD 68:932–936, 2013; Ann Int Med 99:367–379, 1983*

Bafverstedt syndrome – linear horny excrescences of face and neck; mental retardation, seizures *Acta DV 22:207–212, 1941*

Bardet-Biedl syndrome – autosomal recessive; high arched palate, hearing loss, cardiac malformations, renal malformations leading to end stage renal disease; postaxial polydactyly (ulnar), retinal dystrophy, retinitis pigmentosa, obesity, neuropathy, mental disturbance *Adv Exp Med Biol 185:171–174, 2018 J Med Genet 36:599–603, 1999*

Berlin syndrome – ectodermal dysplasia; no vellus hairs; mottled pigmentation and leukoderma, flat saddle nose, thick lips, fine wrinkling around eyes and mouth (similar to Christ-Siemens ectodermal dysplasia); stunted growth, bird-like legs, mental retardation *Dermatologica 123:227–243, 1961*

Bowen-Armstrong syndrome (cleft lip-palate, ectodermal dysplasia, mental retardation) – ankyloblepharon; may be same as Hay-Wells syndrome *Iran J Ped 21:121–125, 2011; Clin Genet 9:35–42, 1976*

Braegger syndrome – proportionate short stature, IUGR, ischiadic hypoplasia, renal dysfunction, craniofacial anomalies, postaxial polydactyly, hypospadias, microcephaly, mental retardation *Am J Med Genet 66:378–398, 1996*

Brain tumors with pruritus – tumor invading floor of fourth ventricle – pruritus of nostrils; occasionally generalized pruritus *BJD 92:675–678, 1975;* brainstem glioma – unilateral facial pruritus *J Child Neurol 3:189–192, 1988;* cerebrovascular accidents – unilateral pruritus *AD 123:1527–1530, 1987; Ann Int Med 97:222–223, 1987*

Bregeat's syndrome (oculo-orbital-thalamoencephalic angiomatosis) – port wine stain of forehead and scalp with contralateral angiomatosis of the eye (subconjunctival masses around the limbus) and orbit (resulting in exophthalmos), and thalamoencephalic angiomatosis of the choroid plexus *Bull Soc Fr Ophthalmol 71:581–594, 1958*

C syndrome (Bohring-Opitz trigonocephaly syndrome) – glabellar and eyelid nevus flammeus; trigonocephaly, unusual facies with widely set eyes, wide alveolar ridges, multiple frenula, limb defects, visceral anomalies, redundant skin, mental retardation, hypotonia; striking posture seizures, minor cardiac anomalies, transient bradycardia; risk of Wilms' tumor *Gene Reviews Geb15, 2018; Am J Med Genet 9:147–163, 1981*

CADASIL (cerebral autosomal dominant arteriopathy with subcortical infarcts and leucencephalopathy) – petechiae and purpura; ischemic strokes, vascular dementia; skin biopsy for diagnosis; *NOTCH 3* mutation *Handbook Clin Neurol 148:733–743, 2018; Neurology 59:1134–1138, 2002; BJD 152:346–349, 2005*

Café au lait macules, temporal dysrhythmia, emotional instability *Int J Neuropsychiatry 2:179–187, 1966*

Carbohydrate deficient glycoprotein (CDG) syndrome type I – present at birth; lipodystrophic skin, sticky skin (peau d'orange), strabismus, psychomotor delay, floppy, failure to thrive, mental retardation, liver dysfunction, cerebellar ataxia, pericardial effusions *Ped Derm 22:75–78, 2005*

Caudal appendage, short terminal phalanges, deafness, cryptorchidism, and mental retardation *Clin Dysmorphol 3:340–346, 1994*

CDG-Ie (congenital disorder of glycosylation type Ie) – eyelid telangiectasia, hemangiomas, inverted nipples, microcephaly; neurologic abnormalities; dolichol-phosphate-mannose synthase *Mol Genet Metab 110:345–351, 2013; Ped Derm 22:457–460, 2005*

Cerebral cavernous malformations (cutaneous hyperkeratotic capillary-venous malformation associated with familial cerebral cavernous malformations) (familial cerebral cavernomas) type 1 – autosomal dominant; localized dark red hyperkeratotic plaques; violaceous to blue-black plaques (malformations); red blanchable patches; red hyperkeratotic plaques; deep blue nodules; cutaneous venous malformations; mutations in CCM-1 gene which encodes for Krev-1 interaction TRAP 1 protein (KRIT1) *Actas Dermosifiliogr 108:680–683, 2017; Ped Derm 26:666–667, 2009; JAAD 56:541–564, 2007; BJD 157:210–212, 2007; Hum Molec Genet 9:1351–1355, 2000; Ann Neurol 45:250–254, 1999; Lancet 352:1892–1897, 1998;* CCM2- malcaverin protein; CCM3 – PDCD10 protein

Cerebro-oculo-facial-skeletal syndrome – autosomal recessive; microcephaly, micrognathia, enlarged ears, bulbous nose, prominent nasal bridge, cataracts, blepharophimosis, short palpebral fissures, mental retardation, hyperkinesis, failure to thrive, orthopedic anomalies (kyphoscoliosis); mutation in *ERCC6 (CSB) Clin Genet 78:541–547, 2010; Ped Derm 26:97–99, 2009; JAMA Derm 149:1414–1418, 2013*

CHARGE syndrome – primary lymphedema, short stature, coloboma of the eye, heart anomalies, choanal atresia, somatic and mental retardation, genitourinary abnormalities, ear anomalies *Ped Derm 20:247–248, 2003;* immunodeficiency *Am J Med Genet C Semin Med Genet 175:516–523, 2017; Am J Med Genet C Semin Med Genet 175:397–406, 2017*

Chronic infantile neurological cutaneous articular syndrome (CINCA) (neonatal onset multisystem inflammatory disorder (NOMID)) – autosomal dominant; urticarial rash at birth, unique deforming arthropathy – bulging knees (premature patellar and long bone ossification), frontal bossing saddle nose, chronic aseptic meningitis; uveitis, mental retardation, short stature; mutation in *NLRP3 Orphanet J Rare Dis 11:167 Dec 7, 2016; Ped Derm 22:222–226, 2005; AD 136:431–433, 2000; Eur J Ped 156:624–626, 1997; J Pediatr 99:79–83, 1981;* IOMID – infantile-onset multisystem inflammatory disease – arthropathy, rash, and central nervous system involvement *AD 136:1487–1494, 2000*

Cleft lip-palate, posterior keratoconus, short stature, mental retardation, genitourinary anomalies *J Med Genet 19:332–336, 1982*

Cleft lip and palate, pili torti, malformed ears, partial syndactyly of fingers and toes, mental retardation *J Med Genet 24:291–293, 1987*

CLOVE syndrome – capillary, venous, and mixed vascular malformations, epidermal nevi, congenital lipomatous overgrowth; hemihypertrophy (milder than that of Proteus syndrome); ballooning of big toes, symmetrically overgrown feet; wrinkling of palms and soles; severe central nervous system involvement; *PIK5CA* mutation *Nature 558:540546, 2018; Clin Genet 91:14–21, 2017; JAAD 68:885–896, 2013; Am J Hum Genet 90:1108–1115, 2012; Ped Derm 27:311–312, 2010; Am J Med Genet 143A:2944–2958, 2007*

Cobb's syndrome (cutaneomeningospinal angiomatosis) – segmental port wine stain and vascular malformation of the spinal cord *AD 113:1587–1590, 1977; NEJM 281:1440–1444, 1969; Ann Surg 62:641–649, 1915*; port wine stain may be keratotic *Dermatologica 163:417–425, 1981;* segmental angiokeratoma-like lesions *Cutis 71:283–287, 2003;* paraplegia, quadriplegia *Surg Neurol Int 8:147 July 18, 2017*

Cockayne syndrome – autosomal recessive; xerosis with rough, dry skin, anhidrosis, erythema of hands, hypogonadism; short stature, facial erythema in butterfly distribution leading to mottled pigmentation and atrophic scars, premature aged appearance with loss of subcutaneous fat and sunken eyes, canities, mental deficiency, photosensitivity, disproportionately large hands, feet, and ears, ocular defects, demyelination *Stat Pearls May 2, 2019; JAAD 75:873–882, 2016; Ped Derm 20:538–540, 2003; Am J Hum Genet 50:677–689, 1992; J Med Genet 18:288–293, 1981*

Coffin-Lowry syndrome – X-linked inheritance; male patients with straight coarse hair, prominent forehead, prominent supraorbital ridges, hypertelorism, large nose with broad base, thick lips with mouth held open, large hands, tapering fingers, severe mental retardation; loose skin easily stretched, cutis marmorata, dependent acrocyanosis, varicose veins *Eur J Ped 161:179–187, 2002; Clin Genet 34:230–245, 1988; Am J Dis Child 112:205–213, 1966*

Congenital atrichia, palmoplantar keratoderma (Bazex-like), mental retardation, early loss of teeth *JAAD 30:893–898, 1994*

Congenital disorders of glycosylation (CDG-I/IIx or III) – depigmented macules, café au lait macules, neurologic abnormalities; phosphomannomutase-2; redundant excess fat; peau d'orange skin; facial dysmorphism, cerebellar hypoplasia, hypotonic neonate, strabismus *Ped Derm 22:457–460, 2005*

Congenital ichthyosis, alopecia, eclabion, ectropion, mental retardation – autosomal recessive; different from Sjogren Larsson syndrome *Clin Genet 31:102–108, 1987*

Congenital ichthyosis, retinitis pigmentosa, hypergonadotropic hypogonadism, small stature, mental retardation, cranial dysmorphism, abnormal electroencephalogram *Ophthalmic Genet 19:69–79, 1998*

Congenital insensitivity to pain with anhidrosis – autosomal recessive; recurrent episodic fevers, anhidrosis, absence of reaction to noxious stimuli, self-mutilation, mental retardation; type IV hereditary sensory and autonomic neuropathy *BJD 156:1084–1086, 2007; Arch Neurol 8:299–306, 1963;* secondary acquired generalized anhidrosis *BJD 150:589–593, 2004*

Cornelia de Lange (Brachmann-de Lange) syndrome – hypoplastic epidermal ridges of palms, soles, fingers, and toes; single palmar crease, hypoplastic nipples and umbilicus, umbilical hernia; generalized hypertrichosis, confluent eyebrows, low hairline, hairy forehead and ears, hair whorls of trunk, single palmar crease, cutis marmorata, psychomotor and growth retardation with short stature, specific facies, hypertrichosis of forehead, face, back, shoulders, and extremities, bushy arched eyebrows with synophrys; long delicate eyelashes, skin around eyes and nose with bluish tinge, small nose with depressed root, prominent philtrum, thin upper lip with crescent shaped mouth, widely spaced, sparse teeth, hypertrichosis of forehead, posterior neck, and arms, low set ears, arched palate, antimongoloid palpebrae; congenital eyelashes; xerosis, especially over hands and feet, nevi, facial cyanosis, lymphedema *Ped Derm 24:421–423, 2007; JAAD 56:541–564, 2007; JAAD 48:161–179, 2003; JAAD 37:295–297, 1997; Am J Med Genet 47:959–964, 1993*

Cross syndrome (Cross-McKusick-Breen syndrome (oculocerebral syndrome with hypopigmentation) – autosomal recessive; gingival fibromatosis, microphthalmia with cloudy opaque corneas, mental retardation, spasticity, growth retardation, athetosis, albino-like hypopigmentation, silvery gray hair, microphthalmos, post-natal growth retardation, nystagmus, spasticity *Ped Derm 18:534–536, 2001; Clin Genet 51:118–121, 1997; J Pediatr 70:398–406, 1967*

Cryopyrin-associated periodic syndrome (CAPS) – urticarial-like eruptions, fever, distal arthralgia, neurologic symptoms, eye disease, amyloidosis; mutation in *NLPR3* increases levels of interleukin-1 *J Clin Immunol 39:277–286, 2019; Ann Rheum Dis 76:942–947, 2017; JAAD 68:834–853, 2013*

Curry Jones syndrome – hypo- and hyperpigmented skin patches, along lines of Blaschko; streaks of atrophy with craniosynostosis, preaxial polysyndactyly, agenesis of the corpus callosum; gastrointestinal manifestations with severe constipation; mutation in *SMO BJD 182:212–217, 2020; Clin Dysmorphol 4:116–129, 1995*

Cutis laxa types IIA,B– autosomal recessive; facial dysmorphism with all the changes of wrinkly skin syndrome; pre and postnatal growth retardation, delayed motor development, delayed closure of large fontanelle, congenital hip dislocation, bone dysplasias, parallel strips of redundant skin of back *Int J Mol Sci 18:635 March 15, 2017; Ped Derm 23:225–230, 2006; Ped Derm 21:167–170, 2004*

Cutis marmorata telangiectatica congenita syndrome – body asymmetry, 2–3 toe syndactyly, hypotonia, developmental delay, midfacial vascular stains, joint laxity, loose skin; localized or generalized present at birth; red to purple vascular pattern admixed with telangiectasias *Orphanet J Rare Dis 14:283 Dec 4, 2019; Ped Derm 24:555–556, 2007*

Cutis tricolor parvimaculata (twin spotting – didymosis) – small café au lait macules and hypopigmented macules; ring chromosome 15 syndrome; low birth weight, failure to thrive, microcephaly, triangular face, clinodactyly, mental retardation *Ped Derm 35:e204–205, 2018; Quant Imaging Med Surg 6:525–534, 2016; Ped Derm 28:670–673, 2011; Dermatology 211:149–151, 2005*

Cutis verticis gyrata-mental deficiency syndrome *Am J Med Genet A173:638–646, 2017; Clin Dysmorphol 7:131–134, 1998*

De Barsy syndrome – autosomal recessive progeroid syndrome; cutis laxa-like wrinkled skin; cloudy corneas, mental retardation, pseudoathetoid movements, synophrys, pinched nose, thin skin, lack of subcutaneous tissue, sparse hair *Ped Anaesth 28:59–62, 2018; Clin Dysmorphol 25:190–191, 2016; Ped Derm 19:412–414, 2002; Eur J Pediatr 144:348–354, 1985*

Deletion of short arm of chromosome 4(4p(-) syndrome) (Wolf-Hirschorn syndrome) – typical facial appearance, "Greek warrior helmet" nose; mental retardation, deafness, seizures, ocular abnormalities *Genet Couns 25:299–303, 2014*

Deletion of short arm of chromosome 18 – mental and growth deficiency, microcephaly, ptosis; pectus excavatum, low ears, short neck *J Indian Soc Pedod Prev Dent 32:68–70, 2014; Am J Med Genet 66:378–398, 1996*

Delleman-Oorthuys syndrome – oculocerebrocutaneous syndrome – membranous aplasia cutis, eyelid tag, periorbital tags, facial tags, post-auricular crescent shaped lesion may be unique to this syndrome; orbital cysts, focal punched-out skin defects of the ala nasi, cerebral malformations, developmental delay *Am J Med Genet C Semin Med Genet 178:414–422, 2018; AD 147:345–350, 2010; Clin Dysmorphol 7:279–283, 1998; Clin Genetics 19:191–198, 1981;* pedunculated facial papules and atrophic patches of neck; accessory tragi and aplasia cutis congenita *AD 147:345–350, 2011; J Med Genet 25:773–778, 1988*

Depigmented hypertrichosis with dilated follicular pores, short stature, scoliosis, short broad feet, dysmorphic facies, supernumerary nipple, and mental retardation (cerebral-ocular malformations) *BJD 142:1204–1207, 2000*

DeSanctis-Cacchione syndrome – dwarfism, gonadal hypoplasia, mental deficiency, microcephaly, xeroderma pigmentosum *An Bras Dermatol 86:1029, 2011*

Didymosis aplasticosebacea – aplasia cutis congenita in a nevus sebaceus (Schimmelpenning syndrome); coloboma of eyelid *JAAD 63:25–30, 2010; Ped 24:514–516, 2007; Dermatology 202:246–248, 2001*

Diencephalic autonomic epilepsy (autonomic epilepsy) – paroxysmal flushing, tachycardia, hypertension due to catecholamine release; loss of consciousness or generalized seizures with olfactory or epigastric aura; due to acute distension of the third ventricle *JAAD 55:193–208, 2006*

Distal aphalangia, syndactyly, extra metatarsal, short stature, microcephaly, borderline intelligence – autosomal dominant *Ceylon Med J 50:33–34, 2005; Am J Med Genet 55:213–216, 1995*

Divry-van Bogaert syndrome (corticomeningeal angiomatosis) Divry-Van Bogaert syndrome – autosomal recessive; congenital livedo reticularis; diffuse leptomeningeal angiomatosis; rare cause of cerebral ischemic complications in young patients *J Neurol Sci 364:77–83, 2016; Ann Med Interne (Paris)146:280–283, 1995; J Neurol Sci 14:301–314, 1971*

Down's syndrome – idiopathic milia-like calcinosis cutis *Ped Derm 30:263–264, 2013; Ped Derm 19:271–273, 2002; JAAD 45:152–153, 2001; BJD 134:143–146, 1996; JAAD 32:129–130, 1995; AD 125:1586–1587, 1989;* atopic dermatitis, alopecia areata, elastosis perforans serpiginosa, skin infections *Cutis 66:420–424, 2000;* perforating milia-like calcinosis with syringomas in Down's syndrome *Ped Derm 11:258–260, 1994*

Dubowitz syndrome – autosomal recessive, microcephaly, sloping forehead, telecanthus, erythema and scaling of face and extremities in infancy, ichthyosiform eruption, sparse blond scalp and arched eyebrow hair, dysplastic low set ear pinnae, high pitched hoarse voice, delayed eruption of teeth, growth retardation, craniofacial abnormalities; syndactyly, cryptorchidism, hypospadias, developmental delay, transitory short stature, hyperactive behavior, blepharophimosis, ptosis of the eyelids, epicanthal folds, broad nose, palate anomalies, micrognathia, and severe atopic dermatitis; increased risk of malignancy *Am J Med Genet C Semin Med Genet 178:387–397, 2018; Ped Derm 22:480–481, 2005; Am J Med Genet 63:277–289, 1996; Clin Exp Dermatol 19:425–427, 1994; Am J Med Genet 47:959–964, 1993; Eur J Pediatr 144:574–578, 1986; Am J Med Genet 4:345–347, 1979; J Med Genet 2:12–17, 1965*

Dyggve-Melchior-Clausen syndrome – autosomal recessive; coarse facies, microcephaly; short trunk dwarfism and mental retardation; deficiency of dymeclin protein *Hum Mol Genet 24:2171–2183, 2015; Clin Dysmorphol 23:1–7, 2014; Clin Genet 14:24–30, 1978*

Elejalde syndrome (neuroectodermal lysosomal disease) – autosomal recessive; silvery hair, profound central nervous system dysfunction, normal immune function, bronze skin after sun exposure *Dermatol Onlin J Feb 22, 2015; Ped Derm 21:479–482, 2004; AD 135:182–186, 1999*

Encephalocraniocutaneous lipomatosis (Haberland syndrome) – alopecia, scalp nodules, skin-colored nodules, facial and eyelid papules – lipomas and lipofibromas; unilateral or bilateral skin-colored or yellow domed papules or nodules of scalp (hairless plaque) called nevus psiloliparus, head, and neck; ipsilateral cranial and facial asymmetry, cranial and ocular abnormalities, spasticity, mental retardation; mosaic *KRAS* mutation *Am J Med Genet A176:2253–2257, 2018; Am J Case Rep 18:1271–1275, 2017; Ped Derm 23:27–30, 2006; JAAD 37:102–104, 1998; JAAD 32:387–389, 1995; Ped Derm 10:164–168, 1993; Arch Neurol 22:144–155, 1970*

Epidermolysis bullosa simplex with or without neuromuscular diseases – autosomal recessive; muscular dystrophy, myasthenia gravis, spinal muscular atrophy; possible mental retardation; early death reported; plectin deficiency *J Dermatol Case Rep 30:39–48, 2016; BJD 168:808–814, 2013; AD 125:931–938, 1989*

Exudative retinopathy with bone marrow failure (Revesz syndrome) – intrauterine growth retardation, reticulate hyperpigmentation of trunk, palms, and soles; fine sparse hair, ataxia with cerebellar hypoplasia, hypertonia, progressive psychomotor retardation; variant of dyskeratosis congenital, retinal vasculopathy; *TINF2* mutation *Ophthalmic Genetic J 38:51–60, 2017; J Med Genet 29:673–675, 1992*

Familial eosinophilic cellulitis, short stature, dysmorphic habitus, and mental retardation – bullae, vesicles, and red plaques *JAAD 38:919–928, 1998*

Farber's disease (lipogranulomatosis) – lysosomal acid ceramidase deficiency (*N*-acylsphingosine amidohydrolase) (chromosome 8p22-21.2); deformed or stiff joints with painful limb contractures and red periarticular subcutaneous nodules (proximal and distal interphalangeal joints, wrist, elbow, knees, ankles, metatarsals), and progressive hoarseness; rarely nodules seen in conjunctivae, nostrils, ears, mouth; heart, liver, spleen, lung; progressive psychomotor retardation *Orphanet J Rare Dis 13:121 July 20, 2018; Ped Derm 26:44–46, 2009; Eur J Ped 157:515–516, 1998; AD 130:1350–1354, 1994*

FG syndrome (Opitz-Kaveggia syndrome) (MED12-related disorder)- macrocephaly, unusual facies, broad and flat thumbs, prominent forehead, ocular hypertelorism, corpus callosum deficient or absent; mental retardation, congenital hypotonia, imperforate anus; small ears *Am J Med Genet A 161A:2734–2740, 2013; Am J Med Genet 12:147–154, 1982*

Filippi syndrome – autosomal recessive; abnormal facies; polydactyly, syndactyly, microcephaly, growth retardation, and mental retardation; *CPKAP2L* mutation *Clin Dysmorphol 28:224–226, 2019; Clin Genet 93:1109–1110, 2018; Am J Med Genet 87:128–133, 1999*

Floating harbor syndrome – low hanging columella, short thumbs and broad fingertips, short stature

Focal dermal hypoplasia, morning glory anomaly, and polymicrogyria – swirling pattern of hypopigmentation, papular hypopigmented and herniated skin lesions of face, head, hands, and feet, basaloid follicular hamartomas, mild mental retardation, macrocephaly, microphthalmia, unilateral morning glory optic disc anomaly, palmar and lip pits, and polysyndactyly *Am J Med Genet 124A:202–208, 2004;* X-linked dominant; 90% females; *PORCN* pathogenic variant; fat nodules in the dermis; yellow-pink cutaneous nodules ; verrucoid papillomas of skin and mucous membranes *Gene Reviews July 21, 2016; Ped Derm 31:220–224, 2014*

Gangliosidosis (GM1-types 1,2,3) – X-linked; gingival hypertrophy, macroglossia, coarse facies, micrognathia, loose skin, inguinal hernia, delayed growth, hepatosplenomegaly, neonatal hypotonia, delayed motor development *Ped Derm 18:534–536, 2001*

Gingival fibromatosis, hypertrichosis, cherubism, mental and somatic retardation, and epilepsy (Ramon syndrome) *Am J Med Genet 25:433–442, 1986; (*gingival fibromatosis, hypertrichosis, epilepsy, mental retardation); swelling of jaw; hypertrichosis; homozygous mutation of *LMO2 Ann Maxillofac Surg 9:415–418, 2019; Clin Genet 93:703–706, 2018; Develop Med Child Neurol 31:538–542, 1989*

Glabellar port wine stain, mega cisterna magna, communicating hydrocephalus, posterior cerebellar vermis agenesis; autosomal dominant *J Neurosurg 51:862–865, 1979*

Happle-Tinschert syndrome – segmental basaloid follicular hamartomas; ipsilateral hypertrichosis; hypo- and hyperpigmentation along Blaschko's lines; linear atrophoderma; osseous, dental, and/or cerebral defects *BJD 182:212–217, 2020; BJD 169:1342–1345, 2013; Ped Derm 28:555–560, 2011; JAAD 65:e17–19, 2011; Dermatology 218:221–225, 2009; Acta DV 88:382–387, 2008*

Hennekam syndrome – autosomal recessive; intestinal lymphangiectasia, lymphedema of legs and genitalia, gigantic scrotum and penis, multilobulated lymphatic ectasias, small mouth, narrow palate, gingival hypertrophy, tooth anomalies, thick lips, agenesis of ear, pre-auricular pits, wide flat nasal bridge, frontal upsweep, platybasia, hypertelorism, pterygia colli, bilateral single palmar crease, hirsutism, mild mental retardation, facial anomalies, growth retardation, pulmonary, cardiac, hypogammaglobulinemia *BMC Med genet 16:28 April 30, 2015; Ped Derm 23:239–242, 2006*

Horner's syndrome, including congenital Horner's syndrome – ptosis, miosis, anhidrosis; contralateral unilateral facial flushing *ACS Chem Neurosci 9:177–186, 2018; JAAD 55:193–208, 2006; J Neurol Neurosurg Psychiatry 53:85–86;* Harlequin sign – hemifacial flushing and contralateral hypohidrosis in Horner's syndrome *Ped Derm 23:358–360, 2006*

Hunter's syndrome (mucopolysaccharidosis II) – X-linked recessive; scapular papules; cobblestoned skin colored papules also of posterior axillary lines, upper arms, forearms, chest, outer thighs; decreased sulfoiduronate sulfatase; skin colored papules overlying scapulae; linear and reticular patterns; also on shoulder, upper arms and chest, and lateral thighs; rough thickened skin, coarse straight bristly scalp hair, and hirsutism; coarse facies with frontal bossing, hypertelorism, and thick tongue; dysostosis multiplex; hunched shoulders and characteristic posturing; hepatosplenomegaly; upper respiratory infections due to laryngeal or tracheal stenosis; mental retardation; deafness; retinal degeneration and corneal clouding; umbilical and inguinal hernias; thickened heart valves lead to aortic regurgitation, stenosis, and congestive heart failure; iduronate-2-sulfatase deficiency *Ped Endocrinol Rev 12:Suppl 1:107–113, 2014BJD 159:249–250, 2008; BJD 148:1173–1178, 2003; Clin Exp Dermatol 24:179–182, 1999; AD 134:108–109, 1998; JAAD 39:1013–1015, 1998; Ped Derm 15:370–373, 1998; Am J Med Genet 47:456–457, 1993; Ped Derm 7:150–152, 1990*

Hoyeraal-Hreidarsson syndrome – reticulate

hyperpigmentation (severe form of dyskeratosis congenital with very short telomeres), growth retardation, microcephaly, mental retardation, cerebellar hypoplasia, progressive bone marrow failure, and mucocutaneous lesions *Br J Hem 170:457–471, 2015; Pediatr 136:390–393, 2000;* central nervous system calcifications *Ped Neurol 56:62–68, 2016*

Hurst syndrome – short stature, hypertonia, unusual facies, mental retardation, hemolytic anemia, delayed puberty *Am J Med Genet 29:107–115, 1988; Am J Med Genet 28:965–970, 1987*

Hypertensive diencephalic syndrome – hyperhidrosis and blotchy erythema of face and neck with salivation, tachycardia, and sustained hypertension
   Multiple sclerosis *JAAD 55:193–208, 2006*

Organic psychosis *Ann Int Med 98:30–34, 1983*
Lesions of pons, medulla, cortex
Tumors compressing the third ventricle
Increased intracranial pressure *J Neurosurg 92:1040–1044, 2000*
Parkinson's disease *JAAD 55:193–208, 2006*

Ichthyosis follicularis with atrichia and photophobia (IFAP) – X-linked recessive; atopic dermatitis; collodion membrane and erythema at birth; ichthyosis, spiny (keratotic) follicular papules (generalized follicular keratoses), non-scarring alopecia totalis, keratotic papules of elbows, knees, fingers, Achilles tendons; extensor surfaces, xerosis; punctate keratitis, photophobia with progressive corneal scarring; nail dystrophy, paronychia, psychomotor delay, short stature; enamel dysplasia, beefy red tongue and gingiva, angular stomatitis (angular cheilitis), lamellar scales, psoriasiform plaques, palmoplantar erythema; mutation of MBTPS2 (intramembrane zinc metalloproteinase needed for cholesterol homeostasis and endoplasmic reticulum stress response) *Mol Genomic Med 7:e812, 2019; JAAD 64:716–722, 2011; Ped Derm 26:427–431, 2009; Curr Prob Derm 14:71–116, 2002; JAAD 46:S156–158, 2002; BJD 142:157–162, 2000; AD 125:103–106, 1989; Ped Derm 12:195, 1995; Dermatologica 177:341–347, 1988; Am J Med Genet 85:365–368, 1999; BJD 21:165–189, 1909*

Ichthyosis, mental retardation, dwarfism, and renal impairment (ACD syndrome) – alopecia, contractures, dwarfism, mental retardation, ichthyosis *Eur J Ped 167:1057–1062, 2008 J Pediatr 92:766–768, 1978; Clin Genet 8:59–65, 1975*

Ichthyosis, mental retardation, asymptomatic spasticity *AD 126:1485–1490, 1990*

Ichthyosis with neurologic and eye abnormalities *AD 121:1149–1156, 1985*

   Keratosis-ichthyosis-deafness (KID) syndrome – autosomal dominant; reticulated severe diffuse hyperkeratosis of palms and soles, well marginated, serpiginous erythematous verrucous plaques, perioral furrows, leukoplakia, sensory deafness, photophobia with vascularizing keratitis, blindness; infectious and neoplastic complications; connexin 26 (*GJB2*) mutations *JAAD 69:127–134, 2013; BJD 156:1015–1019, 2007; JAAD 23:385–388, 1990; AD 123:777–782, 1987; AD 117:285–289, 1981;* KID syndrome with secondary dermatophytosis – cobblestoned palmoplantar keratoderma with ichthyosiform changes of face *AD 148:1199–1204, 2012*

   Netherton's syndrome – congenital ichthyosiform erythroderma or ichthyosis linearis circumflexa, hair shaft abnormalities (bamboo hair), and atopic diathesis (elevated IgE) *Cureus 10:e3070, 2018; SPINK5 mutation Mol Diagn Ther 21:137–152, 2017*

   Refsum's disease – autosomal recessive, childhood onset, deficiency of alpha phytanic acid hydroxylas, resembles ichthyosis vulgaris, cataracts, night blindness, polyneuritis, retinitis pigmentosa, ataxia; deafness, anosmia, short metacarpals and metatarsals, cardiomyopathy, arrhythmias *Gene Reviews June 11, 2015; AD 123:85–87, 1987*

   Sjogren-Larsson syndrome – autosomal recessive, lamellar ichthyosis, mental deficiency, macular degeneration of the retina, spastic paralysis, fatty alcohol oxidoreductase deficiency *Cutis 100:452–455, 2017; Curr Prob Derm 14:71–116, 2002*

   Trichothiodystrophy (Tay's syndrome) – BIDS – autosomal recessive; photosensitivity, recurrent infection, low sulfur or cysteine levels in hair; trichoschisis (transverse fracture through hair shaft), tiger tail under polarized light; brittle hair, intellectual impairment, decreased fertility, short stature

Dermatol Ther (Heidelb)9:421–448, 2019

Jaffe-Campanacci syndrome – coast of Maine CALMs, pigmented nevi, axillary freckling, non-ossifying fibromas in long bones and jaw, mental retardation, hypogonadism, cryptorchidism, precocious puberty, ocular anomalies, cardiovascular malformations and kyphoscoliosis *Hal J Ped May 11, 2020; Childs Nerv Syst 35:1051–1054, 2019; Curr Prob in Derm VII:143–198, 1995; Clin Orthop Rel Res 168:192–205, 1982*

Johanson-Blizzard syndrome – autosomal recessive; beaked nose with aplastic alae nasi, high forehead, prominent scalp veins; small stellate defects; membranous aplasia cutis; dwarfism, mental retardation, deafness, hypothyroidism, pancreatic insufficiency *Gene 570:153–155, 2015; Eur J Ped 170:179–183, 2011*

Kabuki makeup syndrome (Niikawa-Kuroki syndrome) – short stature, congenital heart defects, distinct expressionless face (frontal bossing, long palpebral fissures, eversion of the lower eyelids, sparse arched lateral eyebrows, epicanthus, telecanthus, prominent eyelashes, short flat nose with anteversion of the tip, short philtrum, large mouth with thick lips, high arched palate, cleft palate, dental malocclusion, micrognathia, large protuberant low set ears with thick helix), lowcut hairline, vitiligo, cutis laxa, hyperextensible joints, syndactyly of toes 2–3, brachydactyly, clinodactyly, fetal finger pads with abnormal dermatoglyphics, short great toes, blue sclerae, lower lip pits, cryptorchidism, mental retardation with microcephaly; preauricular dimple/fistula *Ped Derm 24:309–312, 2007; JAAD S247–251, 2005; Am J Med Genet 132A:260–262, 2005; Am J Med Genet 94:170–173, 2000;* pilomatrixoma *J Med Genet 56:89–95, 2019; Ped Derm 34:e26–27, 2017*

Keipert syndrome – broad thumbs/halluces, hearing loss, characteristic facial features including hypertelorism, prominent nose, wide mouth, broad forehead, prominent upper lip with Cupid's bow *Am J Hum Genet 104:914–924, 2019*

Keratoderma with mental retardation and spastic paraplegia – striate keratoderma of palms, diffuse keratoderma of the soles, pes cavus, X-linked *Am J Med Genet A 161A:1390–1393, 2013; Clin Genet 23:329–335, 1983*

Kotzot-Richter syndrome – autosomal recessive; tyrosinase-positive oculocutaneous albinism, granulocytopenia, thrombocytopenia, recurrent bacterial infections, microcephaly, mental retardation *Eur J Med Genet 56:570–576, 2013; Genet Couns 22:1–10, 2011; Am J Med Genet 66:378–398, 1996*

Krawinkel syndrome – lissencephaly, abnormal lymph nodes, spastic tetraplegia, transient arthritis, mental *Am J Med Genet 66:378–398, 1996*

Zimmermann-Laband syndrome (hereditary gingival fibromatosis) – soft, large floppy ears; bulbous soft nose, gingival fibromatosis; hypoplastic or absent nails; atrophic distal phalanges, hyperextensible joints, hepatosplenomegaly, hypertrichosis, mental retardation *Ped Derm 10:263–266, 1993; J Otol Pathol Med 19:385–387, 1990; Oral Surg Oral Med Oral Pathol 17:339–351, 1964*

Lennox-Gastaut syndrome (retardation with EEG abnormalities) – cutis verticis gyrate; several types of seizures, drop seizures characteristic *NEJM 378:1888–1897, 2018; Dev Med Child Neurol 16:196–200, 1974*

Leschke's syndrome – growth retardation, mental retardation, diabetes mellitus, genital hypoplasia, hyperthyroidism

Localized lipomatous hypertrophy with microcephaly, mental retardation, and deletion of short arm of chromosome 11 *AD 116:622, 1980; AD 115:978–979, 1979*

Lujan-Fryns syndrome – X-linked; hypernasal voice, large head and long narrow face; mental retardation with marfanoid habitus *Orphanet J Rare Dis July 10, 2006; Am J Med Genet 119A:363–366, 2003*

MC/MR syndrome with multiple circumferential skin creases – multiple congenital anomalies including high forehead, elongated face,

bitemporal sparseness of hair, broad eyebrows, blepharophimosis, bilateral microphthalmia and microcornea, epicanthic folds, telecanthus, broad nasal bridge, puffy cheeks, microstomia, cleft palate, enamel hypoplasia, micrognathia, microtia with stenotic ear canals, posteriorly angulated ears, short stature, hypotonia, pectus excavatum, inguinal and umbilical hernias, scoliosis, hypoplastic scrotum, long fingers, overlapping toes, severe psychomotor retardation, resembles Michelin tire baby syndrome *Am J Med Genet 62:23–25, 1996*

Macrocephaly-cutis marmorata telangiectatica congenita, macrocephalic neonatal hypotonia; midline facial nevus flammeus, congenital macrocephaly, macrosomia, segmental overgrowth, central nervous system malformations (hydrocephalus), connective tissue abnormalities, skin and joint hypermobility, toe syndactyly, frontal bossing, mental retardation *JAAD 56:541–564, 2007*

Alpha-mannosidosis – autosomal recessive; gingival hypertrophy, widely spaced teeth, macroglossia, coarse features, prognathism, thick eyebrows, low anterior hairline, deafness, lens opacities, hepatosplenomegaly, recurrent respiratory tract infections, muscular hypotonia, ataxia, bone disease, mental retardation *Int J Mol Sci 19:1500, May 17, 2018; Ped Derm 18:534–536, 2001*

Marden- Walker syndrome – autosomal recessive; mental retardation, failure to thrive, microcephaly, immobility of facial muscles with mask-like facies, blepharophimosis, congenital joint contractures, decreased muscular bulk, arachnodactyly, kyphoscoliosis, and transverse palmar creases; mutation in *PIE2O2 Indian J Hum Genet 18:256–258, 2012; J Child Neurol 16:150–153, 2001*

Marinesco-Sjogren syndrome – cataracts, mental retardation, microcephaly, short stature, hypogonadism, ataxia, hypotonia, myopathy, muscle weakness *Gene Reviews Nov 29, 2006; Clin Dysmorphol 4:283–288, 1995*

Megalencephaly-polymicrogyria-polydactyly-hydrocephalus syndrome – macrocephaly, face and limb asymmetry, craniofacial abnormalities, joint laxity or soft skin, distal limb malformation; developmental delay *Ped Derm 30:541–548, 2013;*

Nat Genet 44:934–940, 2012

MELAS syndrome – mitochondrial encephalomyopathy with lactic acidosis – reticulated hyperpigmentation; stroke-like episodes *Mol Genet Metab 116:4–12, 2015; JAAD 41:469–473, 1999;*

MEND – X-linked recessive; hypomorphic mutation of emopamil-binding protein (EBP); diffuse mild ichthyosis; telecanthus, prominent nasal bridge, low set ears, micrognathia, cleft palate large anterior fontanelle, polydactyly, 2-3 syndactyly, kyphosis, Dandy-Walker malformation, cerebellar hypoplasia, corpus callosal hypoplasia, hydrocephalus, hypotonia, developmental delay, seizures; bilateral cataracts, glaucoma, hypertelorism; cardiac valvular and septal defects, hypoplastic aortic arch; renal malformation, cryptorchidism, hypospadias *Mol Genet Genomic Med 7:e931, 2019; BJD 166:1309–1313, 2012*

Menkes' kinky hair syndrome – X-linked recessive; defective absorption of copper; polydactyly, syndactyly, fine hypopigmented easily plucked wiry hair, doughy skin, bone and connective tissue disturbances, progressive neurologic deterioration; tortuous intracranial vessels on angiography with intracranial hemorrhages *Cutis 90:183–185, 2012*

Mental retardation, X-linked, Snyder-Robinson type – marfanoid habitus *Clin Pediatr 8:669–674, 1969*

Mental retardation-enteropathy-deafness-neuropathy-ichthyosis-keratodermia (MEDNK) syndrome – defective copper metabolism, hypocupremia, hypoceruloplasminemia, liver overload; AP1S1 mutation *Brain 136 (pt 3)872–881, 2013; JAAD 63:607–641, 2010; Proc Natl Acad Sci USA 4:1–9, 2009*

Microcephalic osteodysplastic primordial dwarfism type II – autosomal recessive; craniofacial dysmorphism with slanting palpebral fissures, prominent nose, small mouth, micrognathia; fine sparse hair and thin eyebrows; café au lait macules; xerosis; mottling; dark pigmentation of neck and trunk; depigmentation (nevus depigmentosus); small pointed widely spaced teeth; low set ears missing lobule; widened metaphyses and relative shortening of distal limbs; cerebrovascular anomalies; insulin resistance, high pitched nasal voice, café au lait macules, thrombocytosis *Curr Osteoporosis Rep 15:61–69, 2017; Ped Derm 25:401–402, 2008*

MORFAN syndrome – mental retardation, prenatal and postnatal overgrowth, peculiar facies, diffuse and widespread acanthosis nigricans *Indian J Dermatol 64:231–234, 2019; Cutis 95:E20–21, 2015; JAAD 57:502–508, 2007; Am J Med Genet 45:525–528, 1993*

Mukamel syndrome – autosomal recessive; premature graying in infancy, lentigines, depigmented macules, mental retardation, spastic paraparesis, microcephaly, scoliosis *Am J Dis Child 139:1090–1092, 1985*

Mulvihill-Smith progeria-like syndrome (premature aging syndrome) – multiple congenital melanocytic nevi, freckles, blue nevi, short stature, unusual birdlike facies, lack of facial subcutaneous tissue, xerosis, telangiectasias, thin skin, fine silky hair, premature aging, low birth weight, , hypodontia, high-pitched voice, mental retardation, sensorineural hearing loss, hepatomegaly, microcephaly, immunodeficiency with chronic infections, progeroid, conjunctivitis, delayed puberty *Medicine (Balt)97:e0656, 2018; Am J Med Genet 69:56–64, 1997; J Med Genet 31:707–711, 1994; Am J Med Genet 45:597–600, 1993*

Nicolaides-Baraitser syndrome – congenital hypotrichosis, unusual facies (inverted triangular shaped face, low frontal hairline, mild facial hirsutism, deep set eyes, pointed nasal tip, thin nasal bridge, high arched palate, thick lower lip), interphalangeal swelling, short metacarpals ("drumstick fingers"), growth and mental retardation; *SMARCA2* mutation *Am J Med Genet A 173:195–199, 2017; JAAD 59:92–98, 2008*

Neurocutaneous melanosis *JAAD 35:529–538,1996; JAAD 24:747–755. 1991;* in association with large congenital nevi with satellite nevi; brain melanosis *Ped Derm 36:497–500, 2019; Ped Radiol 48:1786–1796, 2018; Ped Derm 26:79–82, 2009*

Neurofibromatosis type I (von Recklinghausen's syndrome) – café au lait macules, axillary/inguinal freckling, neurofibromas, increased generalized background pigmentation; juvenile xanthogranulomas, glomus tumors, blue-red macules, pseudoatrophic macules, nevus anemicus *Acta DV 100 (7):adv 00093;doi.10.2340/000115355-3249 March 25, 2020; AD 145:883–887, 2009; JAAD 61:1–14, 2009; Dermatol Clinics 13:105–111, 1995; Curr Prob Cancer 7:1–34, 1982; NEJM 305:1617–1627, 1981;* giant bathing trunk café au lait macule – type 2 segmental NF1 *JAAD 58:493–497, 2008*

Neurofibromatosis 1-like phenotype (Legius syndrome) – autosomal dominant; café au lait macules, axillary freckling, and macrocephaly; lipomas, Noonan-like facies; learning and behavioral disorders *SPRED1* gene; SPRED-1 protein negatively regulates Ras-mitogen activated protein kinase (MAPK) signaling (like neurofibromin) *JAAD 147:735–740, 2011; JAMA 302:2111–2118, 2009; Nat Genet 39:1120–1126, 2007*

Nevus comedonicus syndrome – preaxial polydactyly, skeletal defects, cerebral abnormalities, cataracts *Ped Derm 32:216–219, 2015; Indian J Dermatol 60 (4):421, July-Aug 2015; Ped Derm 15:304–306, 1998*

Nevus sebaceus syndrome (Schimmelpenning-Feuerstein-Mims syndrome) – cobblestoning of hard palate; trichilemmomas, sebaceomas, syringocystadenoma papilliferum, basal cell carcinoma and trichilemmal cysts *Int J Dermatol 57:599–604, 2018; G Ital DV 150:484–486, 2015; JAAD 52:S62–64, 2005; Am J Dis Child 104:675–679, 1962; Fortschr Roentgenstr 87:716–720, 1957;*

Nijmegen breakage syndrome – autosomal recessive; microcephaly, mental retardation, prenatal onset short stature, bird-like facies, café-au-lait macules; combined immunodeficiency predisposition to malignancy *Orphanet J Rare Dis Feb 28, 2012; Am J Med Genet 66:378–398, 1996*

NOMID – (neonatal onset multisystem inflammatory disease) – sporadic; generalized evanescent urticarial macules and papules (also includes CINCA (chronic infantile neurological cutaneous and articular syndrome) – cryopyrinopathy with mutation in *CIAS1* (encodes cryopyrin) (NLRP3); edematous papules and plaques, urticarial-like lesions in newborn, lesions, chronic aseptic meningitis, arthralgias of knees and ankles with disabling deforming arthropathy with epiphyseal bone formation (osseous overgrowth), deafness, hepatosplenomegaly, anterior uveitis, vitreitis, papilledema, corneal stromal keratopathy; blindness, mental retardation; high frequency hearing loss, developmental delay; recurrent fever and rash more severe in evening; headache, macrocephaly with frontal bossing, saddle back nose, large cephalic perimeter, cerebral atrophy; mutation in *NALP3 (CIAS 1)* which encodes cryopyrin *Orphanet J Rare Dis Dec 7, 2016; JAAD 68:834–853, 2013; AD 144:392–402, 2008; AD 142:1591–1597, 2006; NEJM 355:581–592, 2006; JAAD 54:319–321, 2006; Ped Derm 22:222–226, 2005; AD 141:248–263, 2005; Arthritis Rheum 52:1283–1286, 2005;*

NOVA syndrome – glabellar capillary malformation, communicating hydrocephalus, posterior fossa abnormalities, agenesis of the cerebellar vermis, Dandy-Walker malformation, mega cisterna magna, seizures *JAAD 56:541–564, 2007*

Oculocerebral syndrome with hypopigmentation of Cross-McKusick-Breen – generalized hypopigmentation of skin and hair with microphthalmia, corneal opacities; mental retardation and spasticity *Dermatology 223:306–310, 2011; Birth Defects 11:466–467,1975; J Pediatr 70:398–406, 1967*

Oculocerebral hypopigmentation syndrome of Preus – very short with thin build, ptosis, high arched palate, dental malocclusion, prominent central upper incisors, hair and skin hypopigmented, deafness, severe mental retardation with ataxia, decreased deep tendon reflexes, myopia, lens opacities, acetabular hypoplasia, and cerebral atrophy (especially occipital lobes) *Ped Derm 24:313–315, 2007; J Genet Hum 31:323–328, 1983*

Oculocerebrocutaneous syndrome (Delleman-Oorthuys syndrome) – membranous aplasia cutis; orbital cysts, cerebral malformations, facial skin tags, seizures, developmental delay *Am J Med Genet C Semin Genet 178:414–422, 2018; Ped Neurol 83:58–59, 2018*

Oliver-McFarlane syndrome – trichomegaly with mental retardation, dwarfism, and pigmentary degeneration of the retina; *PNPLA6* mutation *J Neurol Sci 15:391–392, 2018; JAAD 37:295–297, 1997; Can J Ophthalmol 28:191–193, 1993*

Oral-facial-digital syndrome type I ((13 forms) Papillon-League syndrome) – X-linked dominant; malformations or oral cavity, face, and extremities; short upper lip, hypoplastic ala nasi, hooked pug nose, hypertrophied labial frenulae, bifid or multilobed tongue with small tumors within clefts, clefting of hard and soft palate, teeth widely spaced, trident hand or brachydactyly, syndactyly, or postaxial (ulnar) polydactyly; hair dry and brittle, alopecic, numerous milia of face, ears, backs of hands, mental retardation *Ped Derm 9:52–56, 1992; Pediatrics 29:985–995, 1962; Rev Stomatol 55:209–227, 1954; J Ped Genet 7:92–96, 2018;* orofacial digital syndrome type VI – tongue hamartoma, multiple frenula, poly- syndactyly, molar tooth sign (MTS); hypoplasia of cerebellar vermis, partial ophthalmoplegia *Clin Genet 93:1205–1209, 2018; Orphanet J Rare Dis 7:4 Jan 11, 2012; J Med Genet 36:599–603, 1999*

Oral-facial-digital syndrome type III – lobulated hamartomatous tongue, mental retardation, eye abnormalities, dental abnormalities, bifid uvula, skeletal anomalies; malformation of cerebellar vermis, metronome eye movements *J Med Genet 30:870–872, 1993; Clin Genet 2:248–254, 1971*

Pallister-Killian (Killian-Teschler-Nicola syndrome) syndrome – short neck; Blaschko hyperpigmentation, streaks of hypo- and hyperpigmentation, mental retardation, coarse facies with prominent forehead fronto-parietal alopecia, short neck, hypertelorism, short nose with anteverted nostrils, flat nasal bridge, flat occiput, chubby cheeks, sparse eyebrows and eyelashes, long philtrum with thin upper lip (Pallister lip), bifid uvula; horizontal palpebral fissure, large low set ears with thick lobules, supernumerary nipples, Blaschko linear hypopigmented bands of face and shoulder; structural heart defects including atrial septal defect, ventricular septal defect, patent ductus arteriosus, patent foramen ovale, bicuspid aortic valve; i(12p) (tetrasomy 12p); tissue mosaicism; pigmentary mosaicism and localized alopecia *Clin Case Rep 5:774–777, 2017; Ped Derm 24:426–428, 2007; Ped Derm 23:382–385, 2006; Ped Derm 22:270–275, 2005; Ped Derm 17:151–153, 2000*

Patau's syndrome (non-mosaic trisomy 13) – phylloid hypomelanosis; parieto-occipital scalp defects, cleft lip/palate, abnormal helices, low set ears, loose skin of posterior neck, simian crease of hand, hyperconvex narrow nails, polydactyly, microcephaly, microphthalmia, severe central nervous system anomalies, congenital heart defects, holoprosencephaly; death in first year *Am J Med Genet A 167A2294–2299, 2015; Ped Derm 31:580–583, 2014; Am J Med Genet 143A:1739–1748, 2007; Ped Derm 22:270–275, 2005*

Patton syndrome – hypopigmentation, mental retardation, ataxia, myopia, occipital, cerebral atrophy, coxa valga, osteoporosis *J Med Genet 24:118–122, 1987*

PHACES syndrome – large facial hemangioma; Dandy-Walker malformation (posterior fossa cyst with hypoplasia of the cerebellar vermis; cystic dilatation of the fourth ventricle leading to hydrocephalus and increased head circumference) *Stat Pearls June 27, 2020; An Bras Dermatol 93:405–411, 2018; J Ped 178:24–33, 2016; Ped Derm 31:390–392, 2014; Ped Derm 26:730–734, 2009; Neuroradiology 16:82–84, 1978*

Phakomatosis pigmentokeratotica – hemiatrophy *BJD 155:225–226, 2006; AD 134:333–337, 1998;* coexistence of a Blaschko-esque organoid nevus (nevus sebaceous/epidermal nevus) and connective tissue nevus *SkinMed 11:125–128, 2013; Ped Derm 25:76–80, 2008; Ped Derm 22:44–47, 2005; AD 134:333–337, 1998*

Phakomatosis pigmentovascularis – port wine stain, oculocutaneous (dermal and scleral) melanosis, CNS manifestations; type I – PWS and linear epidermal nevus; type II – PWS and dermal melanocytosis; type III – PWS and nevus spilus; type IV – PWS, dermal melanocytosis, and nevus spilus; types II,III, and IV may also have nevus anemicus; type V – cutis marmorata telangiectatica congenita and dermal melanocytosis (cesiomarmorata type) *J Dermatol 46:843–848, 2019; JID 136:770–778, 2010; Ped Derm 21:642–645, 2004; J Dermatol 26:834–836, 1999; Ped Derm 15:321–323, 1998; Ped Derm 13:33–35, 1996; AD 121:651–653, 1985; Jpn J Dermatol 52:1–3, 1947*

PIBIDS (photosensitivity, ichthyosis, brittle hair, intellectual impairment, decreased fertility, short stature) – autosomal recessive; collodion baby, congenital erythroderma, sparse or absent eyelashes and eyebrows, sulfur deficient short brittle hair with tiger tail banding on polarized microscopy, trichomegaly, brittle soft nails with koilonychia, premature aging, very short stature, microcephaly, sexual immaturity, ichthyosis, photosensitivity, hypohidrosis, high arched palate, dysmyelination of white matter, bird-like facies, abnormal teeth with dental caries; trichothiodystrophy with ichthyosis, urologic malformations, hypercalciuria and mental and physical retardation; recurrent infections with neutropenia; ocular abnormalities, osteopenia; socially engaging personality; mutation in one of 3 DNA repair genes (XPB, XPA, TTDA, or TTDN1 *BMJ Case Rep Dec 22, 2018; JAAD 63:323–328, 2010; Curr Prob Derm 14:71–116, 2002; JAAD 44:891–920, 2001; Ped Derm 14:441–445, 1997; Pediatrics 87:571–574, 1991; Am J Med Genet 35:566–573, 1990; JAAD 16:940–947, 1987; Eur J Pediatr 141:147–152, 1984*

Prader-Willi syndrome – albinoid skin; almond-shaped eyes, narrow bifrontal diameter, thin upper lip with down-turned mouth, short stature, food seeking (hyperphagia) with excessive weight gain and central obesity, small hands and feet, mental retardation, hypogonadism, hypotonia at birth, excoriations, trichotillomania; temperature instability, hypersomnia, growth hormone, TSH deficiency, hypogonadism, central adrenal insufficiency *J Endocrinol Invest 38:1249–1263, 2015; Cutis 90;129–131, 2012; Growth Genet Hormones 2:1–5, 1986; Schweiz Med Wschr 86:1260–1261, 1956*

Premature aging syndrome with osteosarcoma, cataracts, diabetes mellitus, osteoporosis, erythroid macrocytosis, severe growth and developmental deficiency *Am J Med Genet 69:169–170, 1997*

Progressive spastic paraparesis, vitiligo, premature graying, and distinct facial appearance *Am J Med Genet 9:351–357, 1981*

Prolidase deficiency – autosomal recessive; peptidase D mutation (PEPD); increased urinary imidopeptides; leg ulcers, anogenital ulcers, short stature (mild), telangiectasias, recurrent infections (sinusitis, otitis); mental retardation; splenomegaly with enlarged abdomen, atrophic scarring, spongy fragile skin with annular pitting and scarring; dermatitis, hyperkeratosis of elbows and knees, lymphedema, purpura, low hairline, poliosis, canities, lymphedema, photosensitivity, hypertelorism, saddle nose deformity, frontal bossing, dull expression, mild ptosis, micrognathia, mandibular protrusion, exophthalmos, joint laxity, deafness, osteoporosis, high arched palate; extensive cystic changes of lungs *Ped Pulm 51:1229–1233, 2016; JAAD 62:1031, 1034, 2010; Ped Derm 13:58–60, 1996; JAAD 29:819–821, 1993; AD 127:124–125, 1991; AD 123:493–497, 1987*

Ramon syndrome – cherubism, gingival fibromatosis, epilepsy, cherubism, mental and somatic retardation, hypertrichosis, and stunted growth *Clin Genet 93:703–706, 2018; Develop Med Child Neurol 31:538–542, 1989; Am J Med Genet 25:433–442, 1986*

Richner-Hanhart syndrome (tyrosinemia type II) – autosomal recessive; tyrosine aminotransferase deficiency; chromosome 16q22-q24; painful palmoplantar keratoderma with circumscribed keratoses, linear hyperkeratotic plaques of soles; bullae may occur; dendritic (herpetiform) corneal ulcers, mental retardation; palmoplantar hyperhidrosis; signs include tearing, redness, pain and photophobia progressing to superficial and deep dendritic ulcers mental retardation; aggregated tonofibril bundles on electron microscopy; crystal structures *J Inherit Med Dis 40:461–462, 2017; Cutis 100:E20–22, 2017; Ped Derm 25:378–390, 2008; J Pediatr 126:266–269, 1995; AD 130:507–511, 1994; Ann DV 120:139–142, 1993; Dermatol 182:168–171, 1991; AD 126:1342–1346, 1990; JAAD 35:857–859, 1990*

Ring chromosome 11 – CALMs, microcephaly, short stature, microcephaly, growth delay, short broad neck; mental retardation *Mol Cytogenet 8:88 Nov 9, 2015; Am J Med Genet 30:911–916, 1988; JAAD 40:877–890, 1999*

Rubinstein-Taybi syndrome – mental deficiency, small head, broad thumbs and great toes, beaked nose, malformed low-set ears, capillary nevus of forehead, pilomatrixomas, obstructive sleep apnea, hypertrichosis of back and eyebrows, keloids, cardiac defects; mutation in *EP300 BMC Med Genet 19:36, March 5, 2018; Cutis 57:346–348, 1996; Am J Dis Child 105:588–608, 1963*

Rud's syndrome – autosomal recessive; sexual infantilism, macrocytic anemia, nerve deafness, pseudo-acanthosis nigricans;

ichthyosis with hypogonadism; congenital ichthyosis, hypogonadism, mental retardation, retinitis pigmentosa, hypertrophic polyneuropathy *Indian Dermatol Online J 5:173–175, 2014; Neuropediatrics 13:95–98, 1982*

Rutherfurd syndrome (gingival fibromatosis and corneal dystrophy) – autosomal dominant; gum hypertrophy, failure of tooth eruption, corneal opacities, mental retardation, aggressive behavior *Clin Dysmorphol 24:125–127, 2015; Ped Derm 18:534–536, 2001; Acta Paediatr Scand 55:233–238, 1966*

SADDAN syndrome – autosomal dominant; short stature, severe tibial bowing, severe achondroplasia with profound developmental delay and acanthosis nigricans; mutation in *FGFR3 J Ped Endocrinol Metab 24:851–852, 2011; BJD 147:1096–1011, 2002; Am J Med Genet 85:53–65, 1999*

SCALP syndrome – aplasia cutis congenita, pigmented nevus, nevus sebaceus; limbal dermoid, CNS malformations *JAAD 63:1–22, 2010;* sebaceous nevus syndrome, central nervous system malformations, aplasia cutis congenital, limbal dermoid, giant congenital melanocytic nevus with neurocutaneous melanosis *Am J Ophthalmol Case Rep 11:10–12, 2018; JAAD 58:884–888, 2008*

SCARF syndrome – ambiguous genitalia associated with skeletal abnormalities, cutis laxa, joint hyperextensibility, webbed neck, craniostenosis, psychomotor retardation, and facial abnormalities; multiple dislocations, face with premature aging, loose skin, umbilical and inguinal hernias *Clin Case Rep 2:74–76, 2014; Am J Med Genet 34:305–312, 1989*

Schinzel-Giedion syndrome – autosomal recessive; ectodermal dysplasia; prominent forehead, short upturned nose, midface retraction, hirsutism, telangiectasias of nose and cheeks, skeletal anomalies, mental retardation *Hum Genet 62:382, 1982; Am J Med Genet 1:361–375, 1978;* autosomal dominant form with *SETBP1* mutation; hydronephrosis, sclerotic skull base, broad ribs, increased cortical thickness *J Genet 97:35–46, 2018*

Short stature, characteristic facies, mental retardation, skeletal anomalies, and macrodontia (ring 14 syndrome) *Eur J Med Genet 55:374–380, 2012; Clin Genet 26:69–72, 1984*

Short stature, mental retardation, facial dysmorphism, short webbed neck, skin changes, congenital heart disease – xerosis, dermatitis, low set ears, umbilical hernia *Clin Dysmorphol 5:321–327, 1996*

Short stature, mental retardation, ocular abnormalities *Helv Paediat Acta 27:463–469, 1972*

Shprintzen-Goldberg syndrome – marfanoid features and craniostenosis (craniosynostosis), mental retardation; Hirschsprung disease, aortic root dilatation, dolichocephaly, low set ears , high arched palate, hypertelorism, proptosis, high prominent forehead *Pan Afr Med J 23:227 April 25, 2016; Am J Med Genet 76:202–212, 1998; J Craniofac Genet Dev Biol 2:65–74, 1982;* without mental retardation *Clin Dysmorphol 2:220–224, 1993*

Simpson-Golabi-Behmel syndrome – X-linked; males; increased growth, accessory nipples, coarse facies, polydactyly, midline defects, mental retardation; Wilms' and liver tumors, macrosomia, redundant furrowed skin over glabella, macroglossia, macrosomic multiple congenital anomalies *Gene Reviews Dec 19, 2000; Am J Med Genet 46:606–607, 1993*

Sjogren-Larsson syndrome – autosomal recessive; non-bullous congenital ichthyosiform erythroderma, ichthyosis with light peeling of trunk and lamellar-like ichthyosis of lower legs, yellow-brown hyperkeratosis around umbilicus, accentuated skin markings; mild to moderate mental retardation, spastic diplegia, short stature, kyphoscoliosis, retinal changes, yellow pigmentation, intertrigo – deficiency of fatty aldehyde dehydrogenase *Clin Genet 93:721–730, 2018; Cutis 78:61–65, 2006; Ped Derm 22:569–571, 2005; Curr Prob Derm 14:71–116, 2002; Chem Biol Interact 130–132:297–307, 2001;*

Am J Hum Genet 65:1547–1560, 1999; JAAD 35:678–684, 1996; Acta Psychiatr Scand 32:1–112, 1957

Smith-Fineman-Myers syndrome (unusual facies, short stature, and mental deficiency) *Am J Med Genet 46:727, 1993; Am J Med Genet 40:467–470, 1991; Am J Med Genet 22:301–304, 1985*

Smith-Lemli-Opitz syndrome – autosomal recessive; deficiency of 7-dehydrocholesterol-7-reductase (converts 7-DHC to cholesterol so have increased 7-DHC and decreased cholesterol) – sunburn with photosensitivity to UVA, polydactyly, syndactyly of 2nd and 3rd toes, growth and mental retardation, failure to thrive, dysmorphic facies, cleft palate, congenital heart disease, hypospadias *JAAD 67:1113–1127, 2012; AD 142:647–648, 2006; BJD 153:774–779, 2005; BJD 144:143–145, 2001; Photodermato Photoimmunol Photomed 15:217–218, 1999; BJD 141::406–414, 1999; JAAD 41:121–123, 1999; Am J Hum Genet 53:817–821, 1993; J Pediatr 64:210–217, 1964;* branchial midline defects *J Ped Endocrinol Metab 31:451–459, 2018*

Smith-Magenis syndrome – upper lip eversion (tented), brachycephaly, midface hypoplasia, short philtrum, prognathism, short broad hands with short fingers, clinodactyly of fifth fingers, fingertip pads, mental retardation; abnormal circadian rhythm of melatonin *Handbook Clin Neurol 111:295–296, 2013; Am J Med Genet 41:225–229, 1991*

Sparse hair, prominent nose, small mouth, micrognathia, cleft palate, crumpled upper helices, digit anomaly, mild developmental delay; limitation of flexion of DIP joints *Am J Med Genet 101:70–73, 2001*

Sturge-Weber syndrome (encephalofacial angiomatosis) – facial port wine stain almost invariably involving upper eyelid with homolateral leptomeningeal angiomatosis; somatic mutation of *GNAQ Ped Derm 35:30–42, 2018; NEJM 337:e11, 2017; NEJM 368:1971–1979, 2013; Pediatrics 76:48–51, 1985;* brain MRI, EEG *Ped Derm 35:575–581, 2018*

Tonoki syndrome – short stature, brachydactyly, nail dysplasia, mental retardation *Am J Med Genet 80:403–405, 1998*

Toriello syndrome – autosomal recessive; abnormally shaped ears, redundant anterior neck skin, midline structural abnormalities, with agenesis of corpus callosum, laryngeal anomalies, congenital heart defects, short hands; proportionate short stature, prenatal growth deficiency, delayed skeletal maturation, cataracts, enamel hypoplasia, neutropenia, microcephaly, mental retardation *Am J Med Genet A 170:2551–2558, 2016; Am J Med Genet 66:378–398, 1996*

Trichorrhexis nodosa with lip pits – autosomal dominant ectodermal dysplasia with central nervous system malformations *Am J Med Genet 71:226–228, 1997*

Trichothiodystrophy syndromes – BIDS, IBIDS, PIBIDS – facial hemiatrophy, lipoatrophy, sparse or absent eyelashes and eyebrows, brittle hair, premature aging, sexual immaturity, ichthyosis, dysmyelination, bird-like facies, dental caries; trichothiodystrophy with ichthyosis, urologic malformations, hypercalciuria and mental and physical retardation *Derm Ther (Heidelb)9:421–448, 2019; Ped Derm 14:441–445, 1997; JAAD 44:891–920, 2001*

Trisomy 9 – short stature, bulbous nose, marked palmar folds, low set ears, long philtrum, thin lips, low palpebral folds, cryptorchidism, mental retardation *Am J Med Genet A 155A:1033–1039, 2011; Ped Derm 26:482–484, 2009;* mosaic *Turk J Ped 60:729–734, 2018*

Trisomy D (13–15) – membranous aplasia cutis, holoprosencephaly, seizures, ocular abnormalities, deafness, neural tube defects

Trisomy 18 (Edward's syndrome) – posteriorly rotated low-set ears, redundant skin of back of neck, flat occiput, high-arched palate, flexed hands with overriding fingers, nail hypoplasia, and flexed elbows, short sternum, psychomotor retardation; major structural cardiac malformations *Am J Med Genet A 179:455–466, 2019; Orphanet J Rare Dis 7:81 Oct 23, 2012; Clin Genet 22:327–330, 1982*

Incomplete trisomy 22 (trisomy 22 mosaicism) – 46XX/47, XX + 22; complex congenital heart defect, membranous anal atresia without fistula, distal limb hypoplasia, partial cutaneous syndactyly of second and third toes, left preauricular pit; hypotonia, and delayed development *Am J Med Genet A 164A:181–193, 2014; Urology 40:259–261, 1992*

Tuberous sclerosis – adenoma sebaceum (angiofibromas) *Handbook Clin Neurol 148:813–822, 2018; BJD 165:912–916, 2011; AD 146:715–718, 2010; JAAD 57:189–202, 2007; JAAD 49:698–705, 2003; BJD 147:337–342, 2002; JAAD 45:731–735, 2001; Derm Surg 27:486–488, 2001; J Child Neurol 13:624–628, 1998; BJD 135:1–5, 1996; JAAD 32:915–935, 1995; J Clin Neurol 7:221–224, 1992; Ped Clin North Amer 38:991–1017, 1991; S Med J 75:227–228, 1982;* pulmonary manifestations *Am J Med Genet C Semin Med Genet 178:326–337, 2018;* renal manifestations *Am J Med Genet C Semin Med Genet 178:338–347, 2018*

Van den Bosch syndrome – X-linked recessive; acrokeratosis verruciformis with anhidrosis, skeletal deformities, mental deficiency and choroideremia *Am J Hum Genet 23:91–116, 1959*

Varadi syndrome (polydactyly, cleft lip/palate, lingual lump, cerebellar anomalies) – subtype of orofaciodigital syndrome that combines typical features with posterior fossa of Joubert syndrome *Am J Med Genet A 173:2439–2441, 2017; J Med Genet 17:119–122, 1980*

Von Hippel-Lindau disease – macular telangiectatic nevi, facial or occipitocervical; retinal angiomatosis, cerebellar or medullary or spinal hemangioblastoma, renal cell carcinoma. pheochromocytoma, café au lait macules *Arch Intern Med 136:769–777, 1976;* hemangioblastomas and endolymphatic sac tumors; autosomal dominant; mutation in *VHL* gene *JAMA Neurol 75:620–627, 2018;* hereditary renal tumors *JAAD 74:231–244, 2016; Cutis 81:41–48, 2008;* ocular findings *Ped Derm 2:98–117, 1984*

Watson's syndrome – café au lait macules, axillary and perianal freckling, pulmonic stenosis, low intelligence, short stature *JAAD 46:161–183, 2002; JAAD 40:877–890, 1999*

Weaver-Williams syndrome (cleft palate, microcephaly, mental retardation, musculoskeletal mass deficiency) – small mouth, prominent ears, long neck, clinodactyly of fingers *Birth Defects 13:69–84, 1977*

Wiedemann-Rautenstrauch syndrome (neonatal progeroid syndrome) – autosomal recessive; macrocephaly; aged facies at birth, frontal and biparietal bossing, scalp with sparse hair and prominent veins, retarded psychomotor development; death by age five; thin skin, rigid and thick joints *Am J Med Genet A 155A:1712–1715, 2011; Eur J Pediatr 136:245–248, 1981*

Wolf-Hirschhorn (4p deletion) syndrome (oculocerebrocutaneous syndrome) – growth and mental retardation (short stature) with seizures, microcephaly, hypospadias, cryptorchidism, facial and ear abnormalities, down-turned mouth with cleft lip and/or palate and short philtrum; hearing loss, abnormal tooth development, skeletal anomalies, heart lesions *Am J Med Genet C Semin Med Genet 169:216–223, 2015; Ped Derm 17:391–394, 2000*

Woodhouse-Sakati syndrome – autosomal recessive; triangular shaped face with prominent forehead, large low set ears, dystonia, hypotrichosis, with sparse eyebrows and eyelashes; alopecia, hypogonadism, diabetes mellitus, mental retardation, sensorineural deafness, extrapyramidal signs, low insulin-like growth factor 1; hypothyroidism with progressive childhood onset; facial hair absent in men; facial skin wrinkled causing progeroid appearance; must be differentiated from congenital hypotrichosis; mutation in *C2orf37 Gene Reviews Aug 4, 2016; Ped Derm 31:83–87, 2014; Am J Med Genet 143:149–160, 2007; J Med Genet 20:216–219, 1983*

Wrinkly skin syndrome – autosomal recessive *Clin Genet 38:307–313, 1990;* same as cutis laxa with growth and developmental delay; increased palmoplantar creases, prominent venous pattern over chest, mental retardation, microcephaly, hypotonia (joint laxity), musculoskeletal (decreased muscle mass, hip dislocation, winging of scapulae, vertebral deformities), short stature, craniofacial abnormalities, and connective tissue abnormalities *Ped Derm 23:225–230, 2006; Am J Med Genet 101:213–220, 2001; Ped Derm 6:113–117, 1999; Am J Med Genet 85:194, 1999; Clin Genet 4:186–192, 1973;* cutis laxa autosomal recessive type II or wrinkly skin syndrome *Indian Dermatol Online J 7:440–442, 2016; Gene Reviews March 19, 2009*

Wyburn-Mason (Bonnet-Duchaume-Blanc) syndrome – unilateral (trigeminal distribution, or midforehead, glabella, nose, upper lip) salmon patch with punctate telangiectasias or port wine stain; facial lesion may be arteriovenous malformation; unilateral retinal arteriovenous or vascular malformation, ipsilateral aneurysmal arteriovenous malformation of the midbrain *Stat Pearls July 2, 2020; Am J Ophthalmol 75:224–291, 1973; Brain 66:163–203, 1943; J Med Lyon 18:165–178, 1937;* red eyes *Ophthalmology 124:1763, 2017*

Xeroderma-talipes-enamel defect (Moynahan syndrome) – hypohidrosis, nail dystrophy, cleft palate, bilateral talipes, mental deficiency *Proc R Soc Med 63:447–448, 1970*

X-linked dysmorphic syndrome with mental retardation – sacral dimple; facial dysmorphism, clinodactyly, abnormal fundus of eye, subcortical cerebral atrophy *Clin Genet 32:326–334, 1987*

XLRI with mild mental retardation, chondrodysplasia punctata and short stature; steroid sulfatase deficiency *Eur J Med Genet 50:301–308, 2007; Am J Med Genet 41:184–187, 1991; Clin Genet 34:31–37, 1988*

Zlotogora-Ogur syndrome – ectodermal dysplasia, syndactyly, mental retardation, autosomal recessive; mutations in *PVRL1* the nectin-1 encoding gene *Am J Hum Genet 87:265–273, 2010; Am J Med Genet 70:211–215, 1997; J Med Genet 24:291–293, 1987*

Zunich neuroectodermal syndrome – migratory ichthyosiform dermatosis; craniofacial dysmorphism, bilateral colobomas of retina, sparse fine hair, hearing loss, ear anomalies, broad second toes *Ped Derm 13:363–371, 1996; AD 121:1149–1156, 1985*

PHARYNGITIS

NEJM 362:1993–2000, 2010

AUTOIMMUNE DISEASES

Juvenile rheumatoid arthritis (Adult onset Still's disease) – pharyngitis at presentation *Open Access Rheumatol 8:17–22, 2016; Clin Rheumatol 19:389–391, 2000; Med Chir Trans 80:47, 1897*

Hyper IgD syndrome *Expert Rev Clin Immunol 15:215–220, 2019; Scott Med J 64:103–107, 2019*

Leukocyte adhesion deficiency syndrome (congenital deficiency of leucocyte-adherence glycoproteins) (CD11a (LFA-1), CD11b, CD11c, CD18) (CD 18 beta2 subunit) – necrotic cutaneous abscesses, gingivitis, progressive periodontitis and oral infections, septicemia, ulcerative stomatitis, pharyngitis, otitis, pneumonia, peritonitis *JAAD 60:289–298, 2009;*

Dermatol Therapy 18:176–183, 2005; JAAD 31:316–9, 1994; Periodontol 6:26–36, 1994; Pediatr Pathol 12:119–130, 1992; BJD 123:395–401, 1990; Pediatr Dent 12:107–111, 1990

Mucous membrane pemphigoid *NEJM 369:265–274, 2013*

Pemphigus vulgaris *AD 127:887–888, 1991*

INFECTIONS AND INFESTATIONS

Acanthamebiasis in AIDS *AD 131:1291–1296, 1995*

Actinomycosis – ulcerated plaque of palate and gingiva *JAAD 65:1135–1136, 2011;* necrotic oral plaques *Ped Derm 29:519–520, 2012*

Adenovirus – pharyngoconjunctival fever, painful throat, modest lymphadenopathy *MMWR 66:1039–1042, 2017*

AIDS – human immunodeficiency virus – acute primary infection syndrome; acute retroviral syndrome – oral erythema with palatal and buccal erosions *AD 138:117–122, 2002; AD 134:1279–1284, 1998;* aphthae of AIDS – major aphthae *BJD 142:171–176, 2000;* HIV gingivitis/periodontitis *Oral Dis 3 Suppl 1:S141–148, 1997;* linear gingival erythema of HIV; necrotizing stomatitis

Anthrax – ingestion of contaminated meat *Clin Inf Dis 19:1009–1014, 1994*

Aspergillosis – invasive aspergillus stomatitis in acute leukemia (Aspergillus flavus); gingival ulcer with or without necrosis of the alveolar bone *Clin Inf Dis 33:1975–1980, 2001;* rhinocerebral aspergillus with palatal necrosis

Babesiosis *NEJM 366:2397–2407, 2012*

Bejel – primary chancre

Calymmatobacterium granulomatis (Donovanosis) *J Clin Inf Dis 25:24–32, 1997*

Cancrum oris (Noma) – *Fusobacterium necrophorum, Prevotella intermedium Am J Trop Med Hyg 60:150–156, 1999; Br J Plast Surg 45:193–198, 1992; Cutis 39:501–502, 1987;* S Afr Med J 46:392–394, 1972

Candidiasis – thrush

Capnocytophaga canimorsus Int J Infect Dis 82:104–105, 2019; Eur J Epidemiol 12:521–533, 1996

Cat scratch disease – indistinguishable from bacterial tonsillitis *Ann DV 140:614–618, 2013; J Laryngol Otol 115:826–828, 2001*

Chancroid *Sex Transm Infect 74:95–100, 1998*

Chlamydia pneumonia – bronchitis, pneumonia; acute or chronic pharyngitis *Kekkaku 81:581–588, 2006:* MIRM due to *Chlamydia pneumonia Ped Derm 34:465–472, 2017*

Chlamydia psittaci – psittacosis *AD 120:1227–1229, 1984*

Coccidioidomycosis *JAAD 55:929–942, 2006;* "a sore throat in the Southwest" *Am J Med 122:233–235, 2009; Ann Oto Rhino Laryngol 112:98–101, 2003*

Coronavirus – common cold

Corynebacterium diphtheria – tonsillar pseudomembrane, myocarditis; crusts around nose and mouth with faucial diphtheria; bull neck due to lymphadenopathy, myocarditis, peripheral neuropathy, pharyngitis with membranes; pharyngitis, rash, adenopathy, fever *Netter's Infectious Diseases pp.5–10, 2012; Ann Med Interne (Paris) 152:227–235, 2001; Schweiz Rundsch Med Prax 87:1188–1190, 1998; Postgrad Med J 72:619–620, 1996; Am J Epidemiol 102:179–184, 1975*

Corynebacterium haemolyticum – pharyngitis, scarlatiniform rash *Ann Int Med 105:867–872, 1986; J Infect Dis 154:1037–1040, 1986*

Covid-19 *Trans Rev April 15, 2020; J Dermatol Sci April 29, 2020; Cleve Clin J Med May 14, 2020; J Eur Acad DV April 15, 2020*

Coxsackie virus type A – herpangina, hand, foot, and mouth disease

Coxsackie B5 – fever, headache, pharyngitis, morbilliform rash sparing palms and soles; elevated ferritin *ID Cases 6:14–16, 2016*

Cryptococcosis *Oral Surg Oral Med Oral Pathol 64:449–453, 454–459, 1987;* stellate ulcerated plaque of hard palate *AD 144:1651–1656, 2008*

Cytomegalovirus *NEJM 371:358–366, 2014; Dermatology 200:189–195, 2000; J Oral Pathol Med 24:14–17, 1995; Oral Surg Oral Med Oral Pathol 77:248–253, 1994; JAAD 18:1333–1338, 1988; Oral Surg 64:183–189, 1987;* lip ulcer; mononucleosis-like syndrome

Dengue fever – fever, headache, myalgias, rash, pharyngitis *J Coll Physicians Surg Pak 18:8–12, 2008*

Ebola virus hemorrhagic fever (Filovirus) – dark red discoloration of soft palate, pharyngitis, oral ulcers, glossitis, gingivitis; morbilliform exanthem which becomes purpuric with desquamation of palms and soles; high fever, body aches, myalgia, arthralgias, prostration, abdominal pain, watery diarrhea; disseminated intravascular coagulation *Int J Dermatol 51:1037–1043, 2012; JAMA 287:2391–2002; Int J Dermatol 51:1037–1043, 2012; JAAD 65:1213–1218, 2011; MMWR 44, No.19, 382, 1995*

Echovirus (Boston exanthem) echovirus 18 pharyngitis and vesicular exanthem *Ped Inf Dis 30:259–260, 2011*

Enterobacter cloacae Cutis 59:281–283, 1997

Epiglottis

Epstein-Barr virus – infectious mononucleosis; Lipschutz ulcer (ulcus vulvae acutum) (genital ulcers in teenagers) – acute genital (vulvar) ulcer accompanying tonsillitis and fever with flu-like symptoms; Epstein-Barr virus in 1/3 of patients *Int J Dermatol April 28, 2020:doi;10.1111/ijd 14887; NEJM 371:358–366, 2014; Cutis 91:273–276, 2013; JAAD 63:44–51, 2010; AD 145:38–45, 2009; Ped Derm 25:113–115, 2008; Eur J Dermatol 13:297–298, 2003; J Pediatr 11:185, 1998; Obstet Gynecol 92:642, 1998; Sex Transm Infec 74:296–297, 1998; BJD 135:663–665, 1996; Archives of Dermatology Syphilol 20:363–396, 1912;* associated with upper respiratory infections, viral gastroenteritis, Epstein-Barr virus, cytomegalovirus, *Mycoplasma,* influenza A, streptococcal pharyngitis, mumps *JAAD 68:885–896, 2013;* oral aphthosis

Escherichia coli

Exanthem subitum – human herpesvirus 6 – uvulo-palatoglossal junctional ulcers *J Clin Virol 17:83–90, 2000; Med J Malaysia 54:32–36, 1999*

Fusobacterium necrophorum – Lemierre's syndrome (human necrobacillosis) – suppurative thrombophlebitis of tonsillar and peritonsillar veins and internal jugular vein; oropharyngeal pain, neck swelling, pulmonary symptoms, arthralgias *Clin Inf Dis 31:524–532, 2000*

Giardia lamblia infection – aphthous ulcer *B J Dent 166:457, 1989*

Hand, foot, and mouth disease (*Coxsackie A5,10,16*) – vesicular *NEJM 369:265–274, 2013; Oral Medicine/Oral Pathology Forum; AAD Annual Meeting, Feb 2002; BJD 79:309–317, 1967;* Enterovirus 71 *Clin Inf Dis 32:236–242, 2001;* Enterovirus 71 – myocarditis, encephalitis, aseptic meningitis, pulmonary edema *BJD 160:890–892, 2009; NEJM 341:929–935, 1999*

Herpangina – soft palatal ulcers *Oral Medicine/Oral Pathology Forum; AAD Annual Meeting, Feb 2002;* Coxsackie A1, A6, A10, A22, B1–5, Echovirus types 9, 11, 17 *J Infect Dis 15:191, 1987; Prog Med Virol 24:114–157, 1978*

Herpes simplex virus infection – primary herpetic gingivostomatitis *JAAD 57:737–763, 2007; Infection 25:310–312, 1997;* recurrent herpes simplex *JAAD 18:169–172, 1988; NEJM 314:686–691, 1986; NEJM 314:749–757, 1986*

Herpes zoster *Oral Medicine/Oral Pathology Forum; AAD Annual Meeting, Feb 2002;* sore throat and headache *J Emerg Med 50:e99–101, 2016*

Histoplasmosis *JAAD 56:871–873, 2007; AD 132:341–346, 1996;* in AIDS *JAAD 23:422–428, 1990*

Acute HIV infection – fever, rash , pharyngitis, mucosal ulcers *BJD 134:257–261, 1996; NEJM 371:358–366, 2014*

Influenza virus *BMC Infect Dis Jan 20, 2012*

Kikuchi's disease (histiocytic necrotizing lymphadenitis) (subacute necrotizing lymphadenitis) – morbilliform eruption, urticarial, and rubella-like exanthems; red papules of face, back, arms; red plaques; erythema and acneiform lesions of face; exanthem overlying involved lymph nodes; red or ulcerated pharynx; cervical adenopathy; associations with SLE, lymphoma, tuberculous adenitis, viral lymphadenitis, infectious mononucleosis, and drug eruptions *AD 142:641–646, 2006; Ped Derm 18:403–405, 2001; JAAD 22:909–912, 1990; Am J Surg Pathol 14:872–876, 1990;* rubella-like eruption, generalized erythema and papules *BJD 146:167–168, 2002*

Klebsiella pneumoniae Cutis 59:281–283, 1997; lip ulcer *Braz Dent J 11:161–165, 2000*

Kyasanur Forest disease (*Flavivirus*) – hemorrhagic fever in India (monkey fever); hemorrhagic exanthem, papulovesicular palatine lesions, conjunctival injection *Indian J Med Res 148:145–150, 2018*

Lassa fever – capillary leak syndrome with severe swelling of head and neck, oral ulcers, tonsillar patches *JAAD 65:1213–1218, 2011*

Leishmaniasis – espundia (mucocutaneous leishmaniasis) – ulcers of mouth and lips *Oral Surg 73:583–584, 1992; Int J Derm 21:291–303, 1982;* ulcer of hard palate in AIDS *BJD 160:311–318, 2009;* multiple ulcerated plaques – New World leishmaniasis *Ped Derm 24:657–658, 2007;* ulcerated nodule of buttock; *L. Mexicana, L. venezuelensis, L. amazonensis, L. braziliensis. L. peruviana, L. guyanensis, L. panamensis;* lip ulcers, crusted ulcer of face; ulcers of nasal septum, palate, lips, pharynx, larynx can develop months to years after initial infection

Leprosy *Indian Dermatol Online J 3:101–104, 2012*

Ludwig's angina – submandibular space infection

Measles *J Infect Chemother 14:291–295, 2008*

Mixed anaerobes – Vincent's angina (necrotizing gingivostomatitis

Monkeypox – exanthem indistinguishable from smallpox (papulovesiculopustular) (vesicles, umbilicated pustules, crusts) but is centrifugal; fever, chills, headache, back pain, sore throat, myalgias, diaphoresis, cough, nausea, vomiting, nasal congestion, blepharitis, oral ulcers, centrifugally clustered umbilicated papules and pustules, lymphadenopathy; heal with varioliform scarring *JAAD 55:478–481, 2006; JAAD 55:478–481, 2006; NEJM 355:962–963, 2006; CDC Health Advisory, June 7,2003; JAAD 44:1–14, 2001; J Infect Dis 156:293–298, 1987; Bull World Health Organ 46:593–597, 1972*

Mucormycosis *Oral Surg 68:624–627, 1989*

Mumps *Aust Fam Physician 26:978, 1997;* orchitis, meningitis, pancreatitis in post-vaccine era *Medicine (Balt)89:96–116, 2010*

Mycobacterium avium complex (MAC) JAAD 37:450–472, 1997

Mycobacterium chelonei Br J Oral Surg 13:278–281, 1976

Mycobacteria kansasii Ped Derm 18:131–134, 2001

Mycobacterium tuberculosis – tuberculosis cutis orificialis (acute tuberculous ulcer) – oral ulcers; lip ulcers, floor of mouth, soft palate, anterior tonsillar pillar, and uvula; *Clin Inf Dis 19:200–202, 1994; J Oral Surg 36:387–389, 1978;* tongue ulcer *Cutis 60:201–202, 1997;* lupus vulgaris

Mycoplasma pneumonia – bronchitis, pneumonia *Scand J Infect Dis 133:782–783, 2001;* MIRM mucositis *Clin Case Rep 6:551–552, 2018; Eur J Case Rep Intern Med Nov 28, 2015; JAAD 72:239–245, 2015*

Myospherulosis *Int J Oral Maxillofacial Surg 22:234–235, 1993*

Neisseria gonorrhoeae – pharyngitis, tonsillitis; gonococcal stomatitis *Pediatrics 84:623–625, 1989*

Neisseria meningitidis – pharyngitis, fever, headache, nausea and vomiting, neck stiffness and petechial rash *Infez Med 24:234–236, 2016*

North American blastomycosis *Oral Surg Oral Med Oral Pathol 47:157–160, 1979;* ulceration of the lip

Omsk hemorrhagic fever – papulovesicular eruption of soft palate *Lancet 376:2104–2113, 2010*

Orf – oral bullae and erosions as part of generalized severe blistering eruptions *JAAD 58:49–55, 2008*

Paecilomyces sinusitis – eroded hard palate *Clin Inf Dis 23:391–393, 1996*

Paracoccidioidomycosis (South American blastomycosis) (*Paracoccidioides brasiliensis*) – oral and perioral lesions; mulberry-like ulcerated swellings; – painful ulcerative stomatitis with punctuate vascular pattern over a granulomatous base (Aguiar-Pupo stomatitis) *JAAD 53:931–951, 2005; Cutis 40:214–216, 1987;* ulceration of the lip

Parainfluenza virus – cold, croup

Parvovirus B 19 – pharyngitis *G Ital DV 147:119–121, 2012; Med Pediatr Oncol 31:66–72, 1998;* including papular-purpuric "gloves and socks" syndrome – oral erosions *JAAD 41:793–796, 1999; AD 120:891–896, 1984;* bullous papular-purpuric gloves and socks syndrome with oral aphthae of tongue *JAAD 60691–695, 2009*

Periodontitis

Peritonsillar abscess

Proteus infections

Pseudomonas

Relapsing fever

Rhinovirus – common cold

Rickettsial pox *AD 139:1545–1552, 2003*

Australian rickettsiosis, Flinders Island spotted fever – fever, arthralgia, pharyngitis, morbilliform, petechial rash; *R honei, strain marmionis Emerging Infect Dis 13:566–573, 2007*

Rubella

Salmonella colitis *Am J Roent 158:918, 1992*

Schizophyllum – palatal ulcer *Sabouraudia 11:201–204, 1973*

Serratia

Smallpox *Otolaryngol Head Neck Surg 151:208–214,*

Sporotrichosis *Case Rep Dermatol 10:231–237, 2018; Oral Dis 7:134–136,2010*

Stenotrophomonas maltophilia – lip edema with ulcers *AD 149:495–497, 2013*

Group A streptococci – pharyngitis, scarlet fever; rheumatic fever with erythema marginatum, subcutaneous nodules *NEJM 376:1972, 2017;* guttate psoriasis *Cutis 104:248–249, 2019*

Group C and group G streptococci – pharyngitis

Streptococcal gingivostomatitis

Syphilis, primary – chancre *Rev Stomatol Chir Maxillofac 85:391–398, 1984;* ulcerated tonsil; secondary syphilis *NEJM 371:358–366, 2014; NEJM 368:561, 2013; AD 131:833, 1995; J Clin Inf Dis 21:1361–1371, 1995; Br J Dent 160:237–238, 1986;* gingival erosion *AD 147:869–870, 2011;* tertiary – gumma – ulcers of palate with palatal perforation; endemic (Bejel); congenital

Toxic shock syndrome *J Emerg Med 54:807–814, 2018*

Toxic streptococcal syndrome, Group A streptococcal pharyngitis, cellulit, followed by scarlatiniform rash and shock *Australas J Dermatol 38:158–160, 1997; J Microbiol Immunol Infect 42:276–279, 2009; J Microbiol Immunol Infect 41:351–354, 2008*

Toxoplasma gondii – small nontender lymphadenopathy; Amazonian toxoplasmosis – fever, lymphadenopathy, hepatosplenomegaly, morbilliform rash *Ped Infect Dis 38:e39–42, 2019*

Trichosporon beigelii

Tularemia (*Francisella tularensis*) – inhalational tularemia with pneumonia, tonsillitis, pharyngitis with cervical lymphadenopathy *Jpn J Infect Dis 67:295–299, 2014; MMWR 62:963–966, 2013; Turk J Pediatr 54:105–112, 2012*

Vaccinia

Varicella – pharyngitis, rash, pneumonia *Oral Medicine/Oral Pathology Forum; AAD Annual Meeting, Feb 2002; Int J Infect Dis 2:205–210, 1998*

Vesicular stomatitis virus – vesicles of fingers, gums, buccal, and pharyngeal mucosa *NEJM 277:989–994, 1967*

Vincent's disease (Vincent's angina) – acute necrotizing ulcerative infection of gingiva and tonsils *Otolaryngol Head and Neck Surg 161:1056–1057, 2019*

Yersinia enterocolitica – pharyngitis, enterocolitis

Yersinia pestis – plague *Adv Exp Med Biol 918:293–312, 2016; Emerging Infect Dis 11:1456–1457, 2005*

INFLAMMATORY DISORDERS

Acid reflux

Erythema multiforme, including Stevens-Johnson syndrome

PRIMARY CUTANEOUS DISEASES

Lichen planus *J Oral Pathol Med 37:582–586, 2008*

Periadenitis mucosa necrotica recurrens (Sutton's disease) *AD 133:1161–1166, 1997*

SYNDROMES

Behcet's disease *Dermatopathology (Basel)4:7–12, 2017*

FAPA – periodic fever, aphthosis, stomatitis, pharyngitis, adenitis; predominantly in young children *Ped Infect Dis 25:463–465, 2006; J Pediatr 146:283–285, 2005; JAAD 52:500–508, 2005*

Kawasaki's disease *Dermatol Online J 25 (7)13-3-/qt38c0f8gF July 15, 2019; NEJM 323:1189–1199, 1990*

Periodic fever, aphthous stomatitis, pharyngitis, and cervical adenopathy syndrome (PFAPA) *Ped Derm 28:290–294, 2011; J Pediatr 135:98–101, 1999; J Ped Hem Onc 25:212–218, 1996; Ped Inf Dis J 8:186–187, 1989; J Pediatr 110:43–46, 1987*

PHOTOERUPTION AND SEBORRHEIC DERMATITIS-LIKE ERUPTION

AUTOIMMUNE DISEASES AND DISEASES OF IMMUNE DYSFUNCTION

Allergic contact dermatitis – Vitamin E, poison ivy, mango; bufex-amac *Dermatology 197:183–186, 1998;* benzophenone *JAAD 49:S259–261, 2003;* oxybenzone – photoallergic contact dermatitis *BJD 131:124–129, 1994;* photoallergic contact dermatitis to plant and pesticide allergens *AD 135:67–70, 1999;* airborne allergic contact dermatitis to *Parthenium* resembling photodermatitis *Contact Derm 18:183–190, 2007;* allergic contact dermatitis to methylchloroisothiazolinone/methylisothiozolinone *BJD 173:1343–1344, 2015;* methylisothiazolinone *Contact Dermatitis 76:303–304, 2014;* benzydamine hydrochloride – photocontact dermatitis

Contact Dermatitis 23:125–126, 1990; cadmium reaction in tattoos – mercury-cadmium photoallergic reaction in red pigment *Ann Int Med 67:984–989, 1967;* yellow *South Med J 55:792–795, 1962; AD 88:267–271, 1963;* cobalt salts – photocontact dermatitis *Contact Dermatitis 8:383–388, 1982;* in a bricklayer *Contact Dermatitis 7:154–155, 1981;* diallyl disulfide – photoallergic contact dermatitis *Contact Dermatitis 45:179, 2001;* diaminodiphenylmeth-ane – occupational photosensitivity *Contact Dermatitis 9:488–490, 1983;* epoxy resin – persistent photosensitivity *AD 115:1307–1310, 1979;* fentichlor – photoallergic contact dermatitis *Contact Dermatitis 18:3180320, 1988;* fepradinol – photoallergic contact dermatitis *Contact Dermatitis 39:194–195, 1998;* flufenamic acid – photoallergic contact dermatitis *Contact Dermatitis 37:139–140, 1997;* fragrances – musk ambrette contact photoallergy *Australas J Dermatol 27:134–137, 1986; BJD 114:667–675, 1986;* pigmented photoallergic contact dermatitis *Contact Dermatitis 24:229–231, 1991; AD 117:432–434, 1981; Contact Dermatitis 5:251–260, 1979;* fungicide – mancozeb – photoallergic contact dermatitis *Contact Dermatitis 35:183, 1996;* Jadit *Arch Klin Exp Dermatol 233:287–295, 1966;* halogenated salicylanilides – photo-contact dermatitis *AD 113:1372–1374, 1977; JID 54:145–149, 1970; AD 97:136–244, 1968;* bath soaps *Am J Hosp Pharm 29:856–860, 1972; NEJM 278:81–84, 109, 1968; AD 94:255–262, 1966;* mercury-cadmium photoallergic reaction in red pigment of tattoos *Ann Int Med 67:984–989, 1967;* mineral oil – photoallergic contact dermatitis *Contact Dermatitis 20:291–294, 1989;* nonoxynol – anti-septic preparation; contact photosensitivity *Photodermatol Photoimmunol Photomed 10:198–201, 1994;* PABA – allergic contact photodermatitis *Contact Dermatitis 6:230–231, 1980; AD 114:1665–1666, 1978; Parthenium hysterophorus* – photocontact dermatitis *Dermatologica 157:206–209, 1978;* pesticides – maneb and fenitrothion – airborne photocontact dermatitis *Contact Dermatitis 40:222–223, 1999; Primula* photodermatitis *Contact Dermatitis 25:265–266, 1991;* rhubarb wine – photoallergic contact dermatitis *Photodermatol 1:43–44, 1984;* sandalwood oil – photoal-lergy *AD 96:62–63, 1967;* soaps and detergents – photoallergic contact dermatitis *Clin Dermatol 14:67–76, 1996;* sunscreen ingredients – UVA *Contact Dermatitis 37:221–232, 1997; Contact Dermatitis 13:473–481, 1995;* PABA derivatives, benzophenones – oxybenzone *Photodermatol Photoimmunol Photomed 10:144–147, 1994; BJD 131:124–129, 1994; AD 125:801–804, 1989;*

dibenzoylmethanes – Parsol 1789 (4-tert.butyl-4'-methoxy-dibenzoyl-methane *Contact Dermatitis 32:251–252, 1995; Contact Dermatitis 26:177–181, 1992; Contact Dermatitis 21:109–110, 1989; Photodermatol 3:140–147, 1986;* cinnamates – Parsol MCX (ethyl-hexyl-p-methoxycinnamate) *Contact Dermatitis 32:304–305, 1995;* 2-ethoxyethyl-p-methoxycinnamate *Contact Dermatitis 16:296, 1987; Contact Dermatitis 8:190–192, 1982;* camphor derivatives; benzocaine; thiourea – photocontact dermatitis *BJD 116:573–579, 1987;* osylamide/formaldehyde resin – contact dermatitis with photosensitivity *Contact Dermatitis 42:311–312, 2000;* ultraviolet-cured ink *AD 113:770–775, 1977;* Vitamin B6 – occupational and systemic contact dermatitis *Contact Dermatitis 44:184, 2001*

Bruton's hypogammaglobulinemia – dermatomyositis-like syndrome

Bullous pemphigoid – UV-A provoked *Acta DV 74:314–316, 1994;* seborrheic dermatitis-like *Clin Dermatol 5:6–12, 1987; Hautarzt 31:18–20, 1980;* photoexacerbation *BJD 126:91–92, 1992*

Complement deficiency-associated lupus erythematosus – homozy-gous C2 deficiency *J Clin Invest 58:853–861, 1976;* discoid lesions of lupus erythematosus *Arthritis Rheum 19:517–522, 1976;* C4 deficiency discoid LE-like lesions *Acta DV (Stockh) 64:552–554, 1984; JAAD 7:66–79, 1982;* C5, C6, C7, C8, and C9 – SLE, DLE *Medicine 63:243–273, 1984*

C1q deficiency – discoid LE-like lesions *BJD 142:521–524, 2000;*

Clin Exp Dermatol 48:353–358, 1982

C1 esterase inhibitor deficiency – angioedema with discoid LE-like lesions *Am J Med 56:406–411, 1974*

C3 deficiency – discoid LE-like lesions *BJD 121:809–812, 1989*

C4 deficiency

C5 deficiency – discoid LE-like lesions *JCI 57:1626–1634, 1976*

CD4+ lymphocytopenia – photoaccentuated erythroderma with CD 4+ T lymphocytopenia *JAAD 35:291–294, 1996*

Chronic granulomatous disease – seborrheic dermatitis-like *AD 130:105–110, 1994;* seborrheic dermatitis of scalp *Dermatol Therapy 18:176–183, 2005; AD 103:351–357, 1971;* DLE and LE-like skin lesions and stomatitis in female carriers of X-linked chronic granulomatous disease – photosensitivity, chilblain lupus of fingertips and toes, rosacea-like lesions of face, lupus profundus, red plaques, stomatitis *Ped Derm 3:376–379, 1986; BJD 104:495–505, 1981;* autosomal recessive *Clin Genet 30:184–190, 1986;* photoeruption *JAAD 70:576–580, 2014*

Common variable hypogammaglobulinemia with polymorphic light eruption *Clin Exp Dermatol 24:273–274, 1999*

Dermatomyositis *J of Autoimmunity 48–49:122–127, 2014; Dermatology 42:631–641, 2012; JAMA 305:183–190, 2011; JAAD 56:148–153, 2008; Curr Opin Rheum 11:475–482, 1999; BJD 139:1116–1118, 1998; BJD 131:205–208, 1994; JAAD 24:959–966, 1991;* juvenile dermatomyositis *Ped Derm 2:207–212, 1985;* amyopathic dermatomyositis *BJD 174:158–164, 2016;* seborrheic area erythema *Dermatology 217:374–377, 2008;* sunburn sign and suntan sign in Hispanic patients *J Eur Acad DV July 17, 2020*

DiGeorge's syndrome – seborrheic dermatitis

Epidermolysis bullosa acquisita – photoexacerbation *BJD 142:517–520, 2000*

Fogo selvagem *JAAD 20:657–659, 1989;* endemic pemphigus of El Bagre region of Colombia with photosensitivity resembling Senear-Usher syndrome *JAAD 49:599–608, 2003*

Graft vs. host reaction – seborrheic dermatitis-like eruption *Ped Derm 35:343–353, 2018; JAAD 66:515–532, 2012;* dermatomyositis-like *BJD 138:558–559, 1998;* systemic lupus erythematosus-like *JID 104:177–182, 1995*

Hyper IgE syndrome

Immunodeficiency and DNA repair defects *Clin Exp Immunol 121:1–7, 2000*

Lichen planus pemphigoides

Linear IgA disease *BJD 171:1578–1581, 2014*

Lupus erythematosus – systemic lupus erythematosus *Ped Derm 15:342–346, 1998; BJD 136:699–705, 1997; BJD 135:355–362, 1996; JID 100:58S–68S, 1993;* discoid lupus erythematosus; *NEJM 269:1155–1161, 1963;* DLE in children *Ped Derm 20:103–107, 2003;* subacute cutaneous lupus erythematosus – annular and polycyclic lesions of face, chest, arms *BJD 156:1321–1327, 2007; JAAD 38:405–412, 1998; Med Clin North Am 73:1073–1090, 1989; JAAD 19:1957–1062, 1988;* bullous, neonatal *Clin Exp Dermatol 26:105–106, 2001; Clin Exp Dermatol 26:184–191, 2001; Lupus 9:3–10, 2000; JAAD 40:675–681, 1999; Ped Derm 3:417–424, 1986; Medicine 63:362–378, 1984;* tumid lupus *JAAD 41:250–253, 1999;* drug-induced lupus erythematosus – various medications including hydralazine, procainamide, tiopronin *JAAD 31:665–667, 1994;* 6-demethyl-6-deoxy-4-dedimethylaminotetracycline (COL-3) *AD 137:471–474, 2001;* cutaneous lupus photosensitivity *JAAD 69:205–213, 2013*

　Systemic lupus-like lesions with primary immunodeficiency disorders *BJD 178:335–349, 2018*

　　C2 deficiency

　Also other complement disorders: C3, C4, C1q, C1r, C1s, C5, C1 esterase inhibitor deficiency

Chronic granulomatous disease *Ped Derm 33:e114–120, 2016; Arch Ped 21:1364–1366, 2014; Arthr Rheum 34:101–105, 1991*

Common variable immunodeficiency

IgA deficiency

Spondyloenchondro-dysplasia with immunodysregulation BJD 178:335–349, 2018

Mixed connective tissue disease – personal observation *J Assoc Physicians India 58:515–517, 2010; Am J Med 52:148–159, 1972*

Photoaggravated contact dermatitis (chronic actinic dermatitis) *BJD 162:1406–1408, 2010*

Pemphigus – El-Bagre endemic pemphigus; facial scaling and crusting (seborrheic dermatitis-like_, conjunctival injection, eyelid erythema and edema, ectropion, meibomitis *JAAD 62:437–447, 2010*

Pemphigus erythematosus – both photodistributed and seborrheic distribution *JAAD 10:215–222, 1984;* induced by penicillamine, propranolol, captopril, pyritinol, thioproline

Pemphigus foliaceus – starts in seborrheic distribution (scalp, face, chest, upper back) *AD 148:1173–1178, 2012; AD 83:52–70, 1961*

Pemphigus vulgaris – photoexacerbation *J Dermatol 23:559–563, 1996; J Cutan Pathol 7:429–430, 1980*

Sjogren's syndrome – annular urticarial-like erythema, localized cutaneous nodular amyloidosis (brown nodule), leukocytoclastic vasculitis, photosensitivity *JAAD 79:736–745, 2018;* annular erythema *BJD 147:1102–1108, 2002*

Severe combined immunodeficiency syndrome – desquamative erythematous, morbilliform or vesiculopapular eruption of newborn (3 weeks); erythroderma, seborrheic dermatitis-like eruption; morbilliform eruptions, lichen planus-like eruptions, dermatitis; mutations in cytokine common gamma chain, JAK3, RAG1 or RAG2, IL-7Rgamma, adenosine deaminase *JAAD 66:292–311, 2012; Ped Derm 26:213–214, 2009; AD 144:342–346, 2008; Dermatol Therapy 18:176–183, 2005; Ped Derm 17:91–96, 2000; AD 136:875–880, 2000; J Pediatr 123:564–572, 1993; Ped Derm 8:314–321, 1991; Birth Defects 19:65–72, 1983*

Urticaria, including solar urticaria

DEGENERATIVE DISORDERS

Dysuse hyperkeratosis of scalp – hyperkeratotic hypertrophic plaque of scalp *SKINmed 10:46–47, 2012*

DRUGS AND EXOGENOUS AGENTS

JAAD 33:551–573, 1995; Semin Dermatol 8:149–157, 1989

PHOTOALLERGIC DRUG ERUPTIONS

Aceclofenac – photoallergic contact dermatitis *Contact Dermatitis 45:170, 2001*

Acyclovir cream – photoallergic *Ann DV 128:184, 2001; Contact Dermatitis 41:54–55, 1999*

Amantadine – UVA *Contact Dermatitis 9:165, 1983*

Amiodarone – UVA *AD 144:92–96, 2008; Ann Pharmacother 34:1075, 2000; Circulation 92:1665, 1995; Acta DV 67:76–79, 1987; BJD 115:253–254, 1986; AD 120:1591–1594, 1984; BJD 110:451–456, 1984*

Amitriptyline *Am J Hematol 53:49–50, 1996*

Ampiroxicam *Dermatology 195:409–410, 1997; Contact 34:298–299, 1996*

Antidepressants

Antifungals (topical)

Azacitidine *J Oncol Pharm Pract 23:473–475, 2017*

Jadit *Med J Aust 1 (13):651–652, 1973; BJD 82:224–229, 1970*

Multifungin *AD 95:287–291, 1967*

Fentichlor *AD 95:287–291, 1967*

Arsenic

Azeperone – UVA

Azapropazone

Benadryl photoeruption – personal observation

Bendroflumethiazide – UVA

Benoxaprofen (NSAID) – UVA and UVB; persistent photosensitivity *BJD 121:551–562, 1989; BJD 115:515–516, 1986; JAAD 7:689–690, 1982;* photo-onycholysis *JAAD 7:678–680, 1982*

Benzydamine hydrochloride (NSAID) – UVA

Benzocaine – photocontact allergy *AD 117:77–79, 1981*

Benzodiazepines – UVB

Beta blockers

Bleomycin, intrapleural – personal observation

Capecitabine (Xeloda) *JAAD 47:453, 2002;* photolichenoid *BMC Cancer 17:866, Dec 19, 2017*

Carprofen – UVA

Chlordiazepoxide *AD 91:362–363, 1965*

Chlorpropamide *Dermatologica 146:25–29, 1973*

Chlorothiazide

Cinchocaine (dibucaine) – photocontact dermatitis *Contact Dermatitis 39:139–140, 1998*

Clinoril

Clioquinol

Clomipramine *Am J Psychiatry 146:552–553, 1989*

Clobazam – photo-induced TEN *BJD 135:999–1002, 1996*

Clozapine *J Clin Psychiatry 56:589, 1995*

Dapsone *Lepr Rev 78:401–404, 2007; Eur J Dermatol 11:50–53, 2001; Z Hautkr 63:53–54, 1988 (German); Lepr Rev 58:425–428, 1987*

Desoximetasone – UVA

Diazepam

Diphenhydramine – UVB *AD 110:249–252, 1974;* photoallergic contact dermatitis *Contact Dermatitis 38:282, 1998*

Doxepin cream *JAAD 34:143–144, 1996*

D-penicillamine *JAAD 35:147–169, 1996*

Dronedarone (novel anti-arrhythmic) *J Drugs Dermatol 12:946–947, 2013*

Droxicam *Int J Dermatol 36:318–320, 1997*

Efavirenz – in HIV disease *JAAD 49:159–160, 2003; AIDS 15:1085–1086, 2001*

Enoxacin *Photodermatol Photoimmunol Photomed 9:159–161, 1993;* photoallergy *Photodermatol 6:57–59, 1989*

Erbitux – personal observation

Fenofibrate *JAAD 35:775–777, 1996; Photodermatol Photoimmunol Photomed 7:136–137, 1990*

Fibric acid derivatives – UVA/UVB *JAAD 27:204–208, 1992*

Fleroxacin *Clin Exp Dermatol 21:46–47, 1996*

Fluorescein dye, IV *Retina 20:370–373, 2000; Photodermatol Photoimmunol Photomed 11:178–179, 1995*

Fluoroqinolones – lomafloxacin (UVA/?UVB) *AD 130:808–809, 1994;* ofloxacin *Int J Dermatol 32:413–416, 1993;* ciprofloxacin *BJD 123:9–20, 1990;* norfloxacin *J Dermatol Sci 18:1–10, 1998; Contact Derm 26:5–10, 1992; AD 130:261, 1994;* sparfloxacin *JAAD 38:945–949, 1998;*

5-fluorocytosine *JAAD 8:229–235, 1983*

Fluoxetine *J Clin Psychiatry 56:486, 1995*

Flutamide *Photodermatol Photoimmunol Photomed 12:216–218, 1996; Eur J Dermatol 8:427–429, 1998;* with residual vitiligo *Contact Dermatitis 38:68–70, 1998*

Fluvoxamine *Australas J Dermatol 37:62, 1996*

Gefitinib (epidermal growth factor receptor inhibitor) *JAAD 58:545–570, 2008*

Glyburide *Photodermatol 5:42–45, 1988*

Hydroxychloroquine *Ann DV 128:729–731, 2001*

Ibuprofen – UVA *JAAD 26:114–116, 1992*

Indomethacin, topical *BJD 90:91–93, 1974*

Interferon-alpha and ribavirin *BJD 147:1142–1146, 2002*

Ketoconazole *Clin Exp Dermatol 13:54, 1988*

Ketoprofen – UVA, photocontact dermatitis *Am J Contact Dermatitis 12:180–181, 2001; Contact Dermatitis 43:16–19, 2000;* prolonged photosensitivity *Dermatology 201:171–174, 2000*

Kit and BCR-ABL inhibitors – imatinib, nilotinib, dasatinib – facial edema morbilliform eruptions, pigmentary changes, lichenoid reactions, psoriasis, pityriasis rosea, pustular eruptions, DRESS, Stevens-Johnson syndrome, urticarial, neutrophilic dermatoses, photosensitivity, pseudolymphoma, porphyria cutanea tarda, small vessel vasculitis, panniculitis, perforating folliculitis, erythroderma *JAAD 72:203–218, 2015*

Melofenamic acid – UVA

6-mercaptopurine

Mesalazine *Am J Gastroenterol 94:3386–3387, 1999*

Methyldopa *AD 124:326–327, 1988*

Methylene blue *Pediatrics 97:717–721, 1996*

Minoxidil – UVA

Nicotinamide

Olaquindox – UVA and UVB

Oral contraceptives *Am Fam Physician 4:68–74, 1971; Med Ann Distr Columbia 40:501–503, 1971; Obstet Gynecol Surg 25:389–401, 1970; AD 101:181–186, 1970; BJD 81:946–949, 1969; JAMA 203:980–981, 1968*

Oxolinic acid *Photochem Photobiol 39:57–61, 1984*

Oxyphenbutazone – UVA

Phenothiazines

Phenylbutazone – UVA

Pembrolizumab – pruritus, hypopigmentation, morbilliform eruption, photosensitivity *JAMADerm151:1206–1212, 2015*

Pirfenidone (for idiopathic pulmonary fibrosis) *Eur J Dermatol 27:545–546, 2017; BJD 175:425–426, 2016*

Phenelzine *Photodermatol 5:101–102, 1988*

Phenothiazines (promethazine, chlorpromazine) – UVA *AD 111:1364–1365, 1975*

Piketoprofen *Contact Dermatitis 43:315, 2000*

Pilocarpine – UVA – photocontact dermatitis *Contact Dermatitis 25:133–134, 1991*

Plaquenil

Protriptyline

Pyrimethamine

Pyridoxine (Vitamin B6) *Dermatology 201:356–360, 2000; JAAD 35:304–305, 1996, JAAD 39:314–317, 1998; JAAD 35:304–305, 1996;* photoallergic *J Dermatol 23:708–709, 1996*

Quinapril *J Eur Acad DV 18:389–390, 2004*

RAF inhibitors (MAPK pathway) – vemurafenib and dabrafenib – exanthema warts and other hyperkeratotic lesions, keratoacanthomas, squamous cell carcinoma, melanocytic nevi, keratosis pilaris, seborrheic dermatitis, hyperkeratotic hand-foot reactions, photosensitivity, panniculitis with arthralgias, alopecia *JAAD 72:221–236, 2015*

Ranitidine *Dermatology 201:71–73, 2000; Clin Exp Dermatol 20:146–148, 1995;* drug-induced SCLE *J Cutan Pathol 26:95–99, 1999*

Ribavirin – photoallergic *Am J Gastroenterol 94:1686–1688, 1999*

Rilmenidine *Photodermatol Photoimmunol Photomed 14:132–133, 1998*

Risperidone *Postgrad Med J 74:252–253, 1998*

Saquinavir *Genitourin Med 73:323, 1997*

Simvastatin *Contact Dermatitis 33:274, 1995;* chronic actinic dermatitis *Contact Dermatitis 38:294–295, 1998*

Stilbenes

Sulfanilamides

Suprofen (NSAID) – UVA photocontact dermatitis *J Dermatol 21:352–357, 1994*

Tamsulosin *Singapore Med J 59:3367, 2018*

Tetrazapam *Dermatology 197:193–194, 1998*

Thiabendazole – photoaggravated allergic contact dermatitis *Contact Dermatitis 28:243–244, 1993*

Thiazide diuretics – photoallergic dermatitis *AD 125:1355–1358, 1989; BJD 116:749–760, 1987; AD 121:522–524, 1985; J Dermatol 7:293–296, 1980;* thioridazine – photoallergy *Contact Dermatitis 17:241, 1987*

Tiaprofenic acid (NSAID) – UVA – systemic or topical *Contact Dermatitis 20:270–273, 1989; Br J Rheumatol 22:239–242, 1983*

Tolbutamide *J Indian Med Assoc 82:289–291, 1984*

Triamterene *Contact Dermatitis 17:114–115, 1987*

Triflusal *J Eur Acad DV 14:219–221, 2000*

Trimethoprim *J Infect Dis 153:1001, 1986*

Valsartan *Pharmacotherapy 18:866–868, 1998*

Verteporfin *Arch Soc Esp Oftalmol 78:277–279, 2003*

Zyrtec photoeruption – personal observation

PHOTO-INDUCED HYPERPIGMENTATION

Afloqualone – photoleukomelanodermatitis (Kobori) *J Dermatol 21:430–433, 1994*

Argyria – slate-gray pigmentation of sun-exposed areas (forehead, nose, hands) *Am J Kidney Dis 37:1048–1051, 2001; BJD 104:19–26, 1981; AD 114:373–377, 1978*

Atabrine (mepacrine) – greenish–yellow pigmentation of face, hands, feet; then diffuse *Am J Med Sci 192:645–650, 1936*

Desipramine – blue–gray photo-pigmentation *AD 129:474–476, 1993*

Gold (chrysiasis) – slate-blue hyperpigmentation around the eyes and in sun-exposed areas *JAAD 39:524–525, 1998*; oral gold therapy with laser therapy *AD 131:1411–1414, 1995*

Diltiazem *JAAD 38:201–206, 1998;* reticulated, blue–gray, photodistributed hyperpigmentation *AD 142:206–210, 2006; AD 137:179–182, 2001;* drug-induced SCLE *Hum Pathol 28:67–73, 1997*

Imipramine – brown, slate-gray, or purple hyperpigmentation *JAAD 40:159–166, 1999; JAMA 254:357–358, 1985*

Tricyclic antidepressants – UVA/?UVB – dermal pigmentation *JAAD 40:290–293, 1999*

Vandetanib (kinase and growth factor receptor inhibitor) – photosensitivity, xerosis, and blue–gray perifollicular macules; also blue gray pigment within scars *JAAD 72:203–218, 2015; AD 48:1418–1420, 2012; AD 145:923–925, 2009*

PHOTO-RECALL REACTIONS

Ampicillin – ultraviolet recall manifested as erythema, bullae *JAAD 56:494–499, 2007*

Aspirin – UVA; aspirin and dialuminate – ultraviolet recall manifested as erythema, purpura *JAAD 56:494–499, 2007*

Bufferin *Eur J Dermatol 8:280–282, 1998*

Cefazolin – photo-recall reaction *Cutis 73:79–80, 2004;* cefazolin and gentamicin – ultraviolet recall manifested as morbilliform eruption *JAAD 56:494–499, 2007; Cutis 46:59–61, 1990*

Ceftazidime *Lancet 341 (8854):1221–1222, 1993*

Ciprofloxacin – photo-recall *JAAD 44:1054–1058, 2001*

Docetaxel *Photodermatol Photoimmunol Photomed 28:222–223, 2012*

Etoposide and cyclophosphamide – ultraviolet recall *Clin Exp Dermatol 18:452–453, 1993;* etoposide, methotrexate, and total body irradiation – ultraviolet recall manifested as edema, erythema, bullae, hemorrhagic crusting, macules, papules, ulceration, necrosis *JAAD 56:494–499, 2007*

Gemcitabine – ultraviolet recall manifested as erythema *JAAD 56:494–499, 2007*

Methotrexate photo-recall – ultraviolet recall manifested as edema, erythema, bullae, hemorrhagic crusting, macules, papules, ulceration, necrosis 1–5 days following sun exposure *Cutis 89:233–236, 2012; JAAD 56:494–499, 2007; Cutis 66:379–382, 2000; JAAD 40:367–398, 1999; Photodermatol Photoimmunol Photomed 11:55–56, 1995; AD 117:310–311, 1981; Arch Int Med 115:285–293, 1965*

Paclitaxel – ultraviolet recall manifested as erythema, bullae *JAAD 56:494–499, 2007*

Piperacillin, tobramycin, ciprofloxacin – ultraviolet recall manifested as morbilliform eruption *JAAD 56:494–499, 2007; JAAD 44:1054–1058, 2001*

Simvastatin – *Clin Oncol R Coll Radiol 7:325–326, 1995*

Sorafenib *Invest New Drug 29:1111–1113, 2011*

Suramin-induced sun exposed keratoses *AD 131:1147–1153, 1995;* ultraviolet recall manifested as urticarial eruptions or dermatitis *JAAD 56:494–499, 2007*

Taxotere photo-recall

Tobramycin – photo-recall *JAAD 44:1054–1058, 2001*

Trimethoprim-sulfamethoxazole – ultraviolet recall manifested erythema, bullae *JAAD 56:494–499, 2007*

PHOTOLICHENOID REACTIONS

JAAD 33:551–73, 1995

Chloroquine

Demeclocycline – phototoxic and photolichenoid eruptions *AD 109:97–98, 1974*

Diflunisal – UVA – lichenoid photoreactive epidermal necrosis *JAAD 20:850–851, 1989*

Enalapril – photolichenoid eruption *Dermatology 187:80, 1993*

Ethambutol *JAAD 33:675–676, 1995*

Hydrochlorothiazide – UVA

Hydroxychloroquine

Isoniazid – photo-lichenoid eruption *Photodermatol Photoimmunol Photomed 14:77–78, 1998;* pellagrous dermatitis *JAAD 46:597–599, 2002*

Fenofibrate – photolichenoid dermatitis *Photodermatol Photoimmunol Photomed 9:156–158, 1993*

Pyrazinamide – lichenoid photodermatitis *JAAD 40:645–646, 1999*

Quinidine *Cutis 17:72–74, 1976; AD 1221:525–528, 1985; AD 119:39–43, 1983;* photo-induced lichen planus *Cutis 29:595–597, 600, 1982;* photo-livedoid reticularis *JAAD 12:332–336, 1985; Dermatologica 148:371–376, 1974; AD 108:100–101, 1973*

Quinine dermatitis – UVA *Clin Exp Dermatol 19:246–248, 1994; Contact Dermatitis 26:1–4, 1992; BJD 117:631–640, 1987; AD 122:909–911, 1986;* persistent light reactivity *Photodermatol Photoimmunol Photomed 7:166–168, 1990;* lichenoid or eczematous photodermatitis *Dermatologica 174:285–289, 1987*

Sulfonamides

Sulfonylureas

Terazosin – photolichenoid dermatitis *BJD 158:426–427, 2008*

Tiopronin *JAAD 31:66–67, 1994*

Torsemide (loop diuretic) – photolichenoid reaction *Mayo Clin Proc 72:930–931, 1997*

PHOTOTOXIC REACTIONS

Alprazolam (Xanax) – phototoxic *JAAD 40:832–833, 1999; Dermatologica 181:75, 1990*

Amiodarone *Circulation 92:1665–1995*

Atovaquone/proguanil *J Dermatol 41:346–348, 2014*

Calcipotriene and UVB *AD 131:1305–1307, 1995;* bullous phototoxicity *JAAD 62:1081–1082, 2010*

Chloroquine *AD 118:290, 1982;* phototoxicity leading to vitiligo *J R Army Med Corps 144:163–165, 1998*

Chlorpromazine – phototoxicity and photoallergy *AD 98:354–363, 1968;* lichenoid dermatitis *Dermatologica 159:46–49, 1979;* immediate and delayed photoallergy *AD 111:1469–1471, 1975*

Ciprofloxacin *Photodermatol Photoimmunol Photomed 28:258–260, 2012*

Clorazepate dipotassium – photo-onycholysis *JAAD 21:1304–1305, 1989*

Dacarbazine – UVA/?UVB – phototoxicity *JAAD 50:783–785, 2004; JAAD 40:367–398, 1999; Photodermatol 6:140–141, 1989; JAAD 4:541–543, 1981*

Demeclocycline – phototoxic and photolichenoid eruptions *AD 109:97–98, 1974*

Disperse blue 35 – textile phototoxic dermatitis in factory workers *BJD 85:264–271, 1971;* bikini dermatitis *AD 112:1445–1447, 1976*

Doxycycline – crusted erosions *Indian J Med Res 150:103–104, 2019; JAAD 66:862–863, 2012; Contact Dermatitis 37:93–94, 1997; Clin Exp Dermatol 18:425–427, 1993;* papular photosensitivity *AD 108:837–838, 1973;* photo-onycholysis solar urticaria *J Drugs Dermatol 14:1358–1359, 2015*

Etretinate – UVA/?UVB

Farmorubicin – erythematobullous photoeruption *Contact Dermatitis 30:303–304, 1994*

5-fluorouracil, capecitabine, tegafur – photosensitivity; lupus erythematosus *JAAD 71:203–214, 2014*

5-fluorouracil – phototoxicity *JAAD 40:367–398, 1999; JAAD 25:905–908, 1991; Cutis 22:609–610, 1978;* photo-distributed hyperpigmentation *JAAD 71:203–214, 2014;* topical *JAAD 4:633–649, 1981*

Furosemide – phototoxic blisters *BJD 94:495–499, 1976*

Isotretinoin – UVA/?UVB *Am J Clin Dermatol 9:255–261, 2008*

Itraconazole – photodermatitis and retinoid-like dermatitis *J Eur Acad Dermatol Venereol 14:501–503, 2000; J Eur Acad DV 14:444, 2000*

Methylene blue phototoxicity – erythema of anterior neck *BJD 166:907–908, 2012*

Nalidixic acid – UVA *Photochem Photobiol 39:57–61, 1984;* bullous photoreaction *Am J Med 58:576–580, 1975; BJD 91:523–528, 1974*

Paraquat – due to percutaneous absorption *Contact Dermatitis 29:163–164, 1993*

Photodynamic therapy

Piroxicam (UVA) *JAAD 23:479–483, 1990; JAAD 20:706–707, 1989; Contact Dermatitis 17:73–79, 1987; JAAD 15:1237–1241, 1986*

Psoralens – UVA *JAAD 36:183–185, 1997; Curr Probl Dermatol 15:25–38, 1986;* bath PUVA *Acta DV 77:385–387, 1997*

Quinine derivatives – photo-onycholysis *Clin Exp Dermatol 14:335, 1989*

Retinoids *Pharmacol Ther 40:123–135, 1989; BJD 115:275–283, 1986*

Selective serotonin reuptake inhibitors – phototoxicity *JAAD 56:848–853, 2007; Am J Clin Dermatol 3:329–339, 2002; Am J Psychiatry 145:425–430, 1988*

Sulfonamides – UVB; sulfisoxazole ointment (phototoxic) *Arch Ophthalmol 100:1286–1287, 1982; Arch Ophthalmol 99:609–610, 1981*

Tars – coal tar smarting reaction *Curr Opinion in Pediatrics 9:377–387, 1997; JID 84:268–271, 1985; AD 113:592–595, 1977;* bitumen *Contact Dermatitis 35:188–189, 1996;* phototoxic keratoconjunctivitis from coal tar pitch volatiles *Science 198:841–842, 1977*

Tazarotene photosensitivity – personal observation

Tegafur (chemotherapy) – phototoxicity *JAAD 40:367–398, 1999*

Tetracycline – UVA; phototoxic sunburn; solar urticaria *Australas J Dermatol 41:181–184, 2000; BJD 132:316–317, 1995;* photo-onycholysis *J Am Pod Med Assoc 75:658–660, 1985; Acta DV 63:555–557, 1983; J Am Podiatry Assoc 68:172–177, 1978*

Textiles – phototoxic (bikini dermatitis) *AD 112:1445–1447, 1976*

Ultraviolet ink *J Burn Care Res 33:e213–215, 2012*

Vandetanib *Medicine 98:e16392, 2019; Cutis 103:E24–29, 2019*

Varenicline (Champix) – for smoking cessation; photosensitivity with burning and itching *JAAD 69:484, 2013*

Vemurafenib/dabrafenib – photosensitivity; cystic lesions of face, keratosis pilaris-like eruptions, hyperkeratotic plantar papules, squamous cell carcinoma; multiple nodules of cheeks; follicular plugging; exuberant seborrheic dermatitis-like hyperkeratosis of face; hand and foot reaction; diffuse spiny follicular hyperkeratosis; cobblestoning of forehead *JAMA Derm 151:1103–1109, 2015; JAAD 71:217–227, 2014; JAAD 67:1375–1379, 2012; AD 148:357–361, 2012*

Vinblastine – UVB phototoxicity *JAAD 40:367–398, 1999; AD 111:1168–1170, 1975*

Voriconazole – photodistributed erythema *BJD 168:179–185, 2013;* photodermatitis with acute and chronic changes of sun damage *AD 146:300–304, 2010; JAAD 62:31–37, 2010; Clin Med Res 6:83–85, 2008; JAAD 52:S81–85, 2005;* photodermatitis and retinoid-like dermatitis *Ped Derm 21:675–678, 2004; Pediatr Infect Dis J 21:240–248, 2002; Clin Exp Dermatol 26:648–653, 2001;* voriconazole photosensitivity with red plaques on cheeks in patient with chronic granulomatous disease *JAAD 70:576–580, 2014;* lupus erythematosus-like in chronic granulomatous disease *J Cutan Pathol 38:677–678, 2011; Ped Derm 27:105–106, 2010;* acral photo-distributed lentigines *JAMA Derm 150:334–335, 2014;* in children *JAAD 72:314–320, 2015*

DERMATOMYOSITIS-LIKE REACTIONS

Benzalkonium chloride – allergic reaction simulating dermatomyositis *Contact Dermatitis 31:50, 1994*

Capecitabine (Xeloda) *JAAD 47:453, 2002;* – dermatomyositis-like rash *JAMA Derm 156:103–104, 2020*

BCG *Scand J Rheumatol 8:187–191, 1979*

Carbamazepine *Br Med J ii:1434, 1966*

Cyclophosphamide and etoposide *Int J Dermatol 41:885–887, 2002*

Hydroxyurea – acral dermatomyositis lesions *JAAD 48:439–441, 2003; JAAD 21:797–799, 1989; JAAD 36:178–182, 1997;* hydroxyurea-associated squamous dysplasia – photodistributed red scaly patches *JAAD 51:293–300, 2004;* photodistributed squamous cell carcinoma *AD 146:305–310, 2010;* dermatomyositis-like eruptions *AD 146:305–310, 2010; Clin Exp Dermatol 30:191—192, 2005; JAAD 48:439–441, 2003; Clin Exp Dermatol 26:141–148, 2001; JAAD 36:178–182, 1997; BJD 134:1161–1163, 1996; BJD 133:455–459, 1995; JAAD 21:797–799, 1989*

Interferon beta – drug-induced dermatomyositis *AD 144:1341–1349, 2008*

Ipilimumab – monoclonal antibody to cytotoxic T-lymphocyte antigen 4; dermatomyositis eruption with cuticular hypertrophy, photosensitive rash with knuckle papules *JAMA Derm 151:195–199, 2015*

NSAIDS (niflumic acid and diclofenac) *Dermatologica 178:58–59, 1989*

Penicillamine *J Rheumatol 14:997–1001, 1987*

Omeprazole-induced dermatomyositis *BJD 154:557–558, 2006*

Simvastatin – amyopathic dermatomyositis *BJD 161:206–208, 2009*

Tumor necrosis factor inhibitors *AD 146:780–784, 2010*

LUPUS-LIKE REACTIONS

JAAD 31:665–667, 1994

ACE-inhibitors-induced SCLE *Hum Pathol 28:67–73, 1997*

Atenolol-induced lupus erythematosus *JAAD 37:298–299, 1997*

Captopril – including drug-induced SCLE *Lancet 345:398, 1995;* LE-like *Ann DV 115:167–169, 1988; Acta DV 65:447–448, 1985*

Capecitabine

Chrysotherapy – drug-induced SCLE *JAAD 35:147–169, 1996*

Cilazapril-induced SCLE *Lancet 345:398, 1995*

Cimetidine

Cinnarizine – drug-induced SCLE *Lupus 7:364–366, 1998*

COL-3 – non-antibiotic tetracycline derivative anti-cancer agent – drug-induced lupus erythematosus *AD 137:471–474, 2001*

5-fluorouracil – granulomatous septal panniculitis *JAAD 71:203–214, 2014;*

Griseofulvin *Photodermatol 5:272–274, 1988;* drug-induced SCLE *JAAD 21:343–346, 1989; J Dermatol 15:76–82, 1988;* exacerbation of lupus erythematosus *Cutis 17:361–363, 1976*

Hydralazine

Hydrochlorothiazide – drug-induced SCLE *Ann Int Med 103:49–51, 1985;* photoeruption – personal observation

Drug-induced lupus erythematosus – multiple drugs including nitrendipine, hydrochlorothiazide and triamterene, chlorothiazide, acebutolol, captopril, cilazapril, paclitaxel, tamoxifen, capecitabine, ranitidine, brompheniramine, cinnarizine and thiethylperazine, leflunomide, carbamazepine, pravastatin, efalizumab, lansoprazole, piroxicam, leuprorelin, PUVA, PUVA and UVB, bupropion, tiotropium, ticlopidine, hay with fertilizer, chlorpromazine, cotrimoxazole, phenytoin, ethosuximide, gold salts, isoniazide, lithium, methylthiouracil, minocin, naproxen *BJD 164:465–472, 2011; JAMA 268:51–52, 1992;* para-amino salicylic acid, penicillamine, phenylbutazone, phenylethylacetylurea, practolol, propylthiouracil, quinidine, reserpine, rifampin *Clin Exp Dermatol 26:260–262, 2001;* streptomycin, sulfasalazine *BJD 139:1132–1133, 1998;* tetracycline, trimethadone pravastatin, simvastatin, enalapril, lisinopril, diltiazem, nifedipine, interferon-alpha and beta, oxprenolol, procainamide, etanercept, infliximab *AD 139:45–49, 2003; Lancet 359:579–580, 2002*

Interferon beta – drug-induced SCLE *Lancet 352:1825–1826, 1998*

Methyldopa

Oral contraceptives

Oxyprenolol – drug-induced SCLE *JAAD 35:147–169, 1996*

Pazopanib (multikinase inhibitor) – subacute cutaneous lupus erythematosus *BJD 171:1559–1561, 2014*

Penicillins

Phenytoin

Piroxicam (NSAID) – drug-induced SCLE *JAAD 35:147–169, 1996*

Procainamide – drug-induced LE and drug-induced SCLE *JAAD 35:147–169, 1996*

Spironolactone – drug-induced SCLE *JAAD 35:147–169, 1996*

Drug-induced subacute cutaneous LE – photodistributed erythema, annular scaly lesions – alpha-methyl dopa, carbamazepine *AD 141:103–104, 2005;* anastrazole (aromatase inhibitor)-induced SCLE *BJD 158:628–629, 2008;* docetaxel *JAAD 58:545–570, 2008*

Sulfonamides

Sulfonylureas, including drug-induced SCLE *JAAD 35:147–169, 1996*

Tegafur – granulomatous septal panniculitis *JAAD 71:203–214, 2014*

Terbinafine – drug-induced SCLE *BJD 148:1056, 2003; JAAD 44:925–931, 2001; AD 137:1196–1198, 2001*

Tetracycline,

Thiazide-induced lupus erythematosus *J Toxicol Clin Toxicol 33:729–733, 1995; Ann Int Med 103:49–51, 1985*

Thiouracil

Tiopronin

Trimethadone

Verapamil – drug-induced SCLE *Hum Pathol 28:67–73, 1997*

Voriconazole – SLE-like photodermatitis *Ped Derm 27:105–106, 2010*

Yohimbine – lupus-like syndrome *JAAD 53:S105–107, 2005*

PELLAGROUS DERMATITIS

BJD 176:902–909, 2017; JAAD 67:1113–1127, 2012; JAAD 46:597–599, 2002; Semin Dermatol 10:282–292, 1991

Antidepressants

Azathioprine *JAAD 46:597–599, 2002*

Carbamazepine *JAAD 46:597–599, 2002*

Chloramphenicol – pellagrous dermatitis *JAAD 46:597–599, 2002*

Ethionamide – pellagrous dermatitis *JAAD 46:597–599, 2002*

Ethosuximide

5-fluorouracil

Hydantoin – pellagrous dermatitis *JAAD 46:597–599, 2002*

INH

Kombucha tea – pellagra *JAAD 53:S105–107, 2005*

6-mercaptopurine

Phenobarbital

Phenytoin

Protionamide – aphthous ulcers and fissured cheilitis *JAAD 46:597–599, 2002*

Pyrazinamide

Sulfapyridine

Sulfonamides

Valproic acid

PERIORAL DERMATITIS-LIKE REACTION

Corticosteroids – steroid perioral dermatitis

PHOTO-INDUCED TELANGIECTASIAS

Amlodipine – photo-induced telangiectasia *BJD 142:1255–1256, 2000; BJD 136:974–975, 1997*

Calcium channel blockers – felodipine, nifedipine, amlodipine, diltiazem – photodistributed telangiectasias *JAAD 45:323–324, 2001; BJD 136:974–975, 1997; J Allergy Clin Immunol 97:852–855, 1996*

Cefotaxime – photodistributed telangiectasia *BJD 143:674–675, 2000*

Felodipine-induced photodistributed facial telangiectasia *JAAD 45:323–324, 2001*

Nifedipine – UVB *JAAD 38:201–206, 1998;* photodistributed facial telangiectasia *BJD 129:630–633, 1993; Dermatologica 182:196–198, 1991;* drug-induced SCLE *Hum Pathol 28:67–73, 1997*

Venlaxifine – photodistributed eruptive telangiectasias of face, forearms, dorsal hands *BJD 157:822–824, 2007*

PORPHYRIA CUTANEA TARDA-LIKE REACTIONS

Chloracne – porphyria-like changes *Br J Ind Med 50:699–703, 1993*

Cyclophosphamide – porphyria cutanea tarda *JAAD 71:203–214, 2014*

Fluoroqinolones – drug-induced porphyria cutanea tarda *Dermatol Clinic 4:291–296, 1986*

Nabumetone – UVA; pseudo-PCT *J Rheumatol 27:1817–1818, 2000; JAAD 40:492–493, 1999*

Naproxen – UVA – pseudoporphyria *Scand J Rheumatol 24:108–111, 1995*; drug-induced SCLE *JAAD 35:147–169, 1996*

Oxaprozin – pseudoporphyria *AD 132:1519–1520, 1996*

Propionic acid derivatives (NSAIDS) – pseudo-PCT *J Cut Med Surg 3:162–166, 1999*

Tetracycline – porphyria cutanea tarda and erythropoietic protoporphyria-like changes *AD 112:661–666, 1976*

SEBORRHEIC DERMATITIS-LIKE ERUPTIONS

BJD 96:99–106, 1977

Alpha methyl dopa

Antidepressants

Azathioprine *JAAD 46:597–599, 2002*

Carbamazepine *JAAD 46:597–599, 2002*

Cetuximab (epidermal growth factor receptor inhibitor) – seborrheic dermatitis-like eruption *JAAD 58:545–570, 2008; JAAD 55:429–437, 2006; J Clin Oncol 18:904–914, 2000*

Chloramphenicol – pellagrous dermatitis *JAAD 46:597–599, 2002*

Chlorpromazine

Cimetidine – seborrheic dermatitis-like eruption *AD 117:65–66, 1981*

Erlotinib – seborrheic distribution of papules and pustules *JAAD 58:545–570, 2008; JAAD 55:429–437, 2006*

Ethionamide – pellagrous dermatitis *JAAD 46:597–599, 2002*

5-fluorouracil

Gold – seborrheic dermatitis-like eruption

Hydantoin – pellagrous dermatitis *JAAD 46:597–599, 2002*

INH

6-mercaptopurine

Phenobarbital

Phenytoin

Pyrazinamide

Sorafenib (multikinase inhibitor) – hand-foot reactions (hyperkeratosis with erythema); facial seborrheic dermatitis-like erythema, red plaques on sides of feet, hyperkeratotic plaque or blister of feet, red patches on pressure points, red swollen fingertips, gray blisters of fingerwebs, angular cheilitis, perianal dermatitis *JAAD 71:217–227, 2014; AD 144:886–892, 2008; BJD 158:592–596, 2008*

Sulfonamides

Sunitinib – hand/foot reaction; seborrheic dermatitis; alopecia; yellow coloration of face *JAAD 71:217–227, 2014; J Clin Oncol 24:5786–5788, 2006*

Vemurafenib/dabrafenib – photosensitivity; cystic lesions of face, keratosis pilaris-like eruptions, hyperkeratotic plantar papules, squamous cell carcinoma; multiple nodules of cheeks; follicular plugging; exuberant seborrheic dermatitis-like hyperkeratosis of face; hand and foot reaction; diffuse spiny follicular hyperkeratosis; cobblestoning of forehead *JAAD 71:217–227, 2014; JAAD 67:1375–1379, 2012; AD 148:357–361, 2012*

EXOGENEOUS AGENTS

PHYTOPHOTODERMATITIS (DERMATITIS BULLOSA STRIATA)

J Cutan Med Surg 3:263–279, 1999; Am J Contact Dermatol 10:89–93, 1999; Clin Dermatol 15:607–613, 1997; Clin Dermatol 4:102–121, 1986

Angelica *Photodermatol Photoimmunol Photomed 8:84–85, 1991*

Bergamot aromatherapy oil – bullous phototoxic reactions *JAAD 45:458–461, 2001*

Buttercup

Carrot extract containing sunscreen *Dermatol Online J Jan 15, 2018*

Celery *Int J Dermatol 33:116–118, 1994; AD 127:912–913, 1991; AD 126:1334–1336, 1990*

Celery soup *BJD 135:334, 1996*; celery diet *BJD 175:e133, 2016*

Chenopodium album (Lamb's quarters, white goosefoot) – red face with bullae *Dermatitis 25:140–146, 2014; Ped Derm 28:674–676, 2011*

Chlorella *Int J Dermatol 23:263–268, 1984*

Citrus hystrix BJD 140:737–738, 1999

Cyprus and geranium products – facial massage; contain furocoumarins *NEJM 371:559, 2014*

Dill

Fennel

Figs (*Ficus carica*) *Israel Med Assoc J 14:399–400, 2012; Dermatol Online J 14:9 Dec 15, 2008; Cutis 48:151–152, 1991*; "Florida water" or "Kananga water" – phytophotodermatitis due to oil of bergamot *Cutis 70:29–30, 2002*

Furocoumarins

Garden carrot

Gas plant (*Dictamnus albus*) *Can Med Assoc J 130:889–891, 1984; NEJM 276:1484–1486, 1967*

Lemon *Wounds 29:E118–124, 2017*

Lichens *Contact Dermatitis 3:213–214, 1977*

Lime and Persian lime *Med Clin (Barc)151:44, July 13, 2018; Med J Aus 207:328, 2017; NEJM 357:e1, 2007*

6-methyl coumarin (fragrance) – photocontact dermatitis *JAAD 2:124–127, 1980; Contact Dermatitis 4:283–288, 1978*

Meadow dermatitis (*Umbelliferae*); limes *Am J Epidemiol 125:509–514, 1987*

Mokihana fruits in Hawaiian lei *Contact Dermatitis 10:224–226, 1984*

Mustard

Parsley *Practitioner 229:673–675, 1985*

Parsnip – parsnip *J Accid Emerg Med 16:453–454, 1999; NEJM 276:1484–1486, 1967*; wild parsnip *Dermatol Online J Feb 15, 2018*

Psrolea corylifolia (babchi) *JAAD 53:S105–107, 2005*

Ruta graveolens (garden rue or common rue) *Contact Dermatitis 41:232, 1999; Ruta montana* – photocontact dermatitis *Dermatitis 18:52–55, 2007; Contact Dermatitis 33:284, 1995*

Seaweed *Pan Afr Med J 15:58m June 20, 2013*

St. John's wort (*Hypericum perforatum*) *Med J Aus 172:302, March 20, 2000*

Sweet oranges (exocarp) – photo-cheilitis *Contact Dermatitis 9:201–204, 1983*

Wild carrot

Zabon (citrus maxima) *JAAD 46: S146–147, 2002*

Acriflavine (dye) (acridine derivative)

Aloe vera *Int J Dermatol 31:372, 1992*

Anabolic steroid abuse – worsening seborrhea *Cutis 44:30–35, 1989*

Anthracene

Anthraquinone (dye) *Contact Dermatitis 18:171–172, 1988*

Argyria – homebrew silver solution *AD 145:1053–1058, 2009*

Benzocaine – erosive papulonodular vulvar dermatitis *JAAD 55:S74–80, 2006*

Bithionol *JAMA 199:89–92, 1967*

Bovine collagen, injectable – granulomatous allergic reaction; linear red plaques of nasolabial folds *JAAD 64:1–34, 2011*

Chromate and cobalt – contact allergy with immediate and delayed photoaggravation *Contact Dermatitis 33:282–284, 1995*

Chromium *BJD 97:411–416, 1977*

Compositae family *Acta DV Suppl (Stockh) 134:69–76, 1987; Contact Dermatitis 7:129–136, 1981; JAAD 2:417–424, 1980*

Creosote bush (Larrea) *JAAD 14:202–207, 1986*

Dioxins – hyperpigmentation in sun-exposed areas

Eosin

Ethylenediamine – photocontact dermatitis *Contact Dermatitis 15:305–306, 1986*

Etofenamate *Contact Dermatitis 37:139–140, 1997*

Fluorescent lamps *BJD 89:351–359, 1973; BJD 81:420–428, 1969*

Flupenthixol *Photodermatol Photoimmunol Photomed 13:159–161, 1997*

Food allergy – seborrheic dermatitis-like eruption

Halogen lamp *Dermatology 193:207–211, 1996*

Hexachlorophene – persistent light reaction *JAAD 24:333–334, 1991*

Oakmoss *Contact Dermatitis 18:240–242, 1988*

Occlusive dressings – photosensitivity following treatment of occlusive dressings *AD 102:276–279, 1970*

Persistent light reactions to photoallergens due to:
    Fragrances – musk ambrette, 6-methylcoumarin – UVA
    Halogenated salicylanilides – UVA/?UVB
    Sunscreens
    Optical whiteners

Peucedanum panculatum – endemic to Corsica *Contact Dermatitis 80:249–250, 2019; Clin Toxicol (Phila)57:68–69, 2019*

Phenothiazines – photocontact dermatitis in pharmacist *Tohoku J Exp Med 176:249–252, 1995*

Quinine and tonic water *BJD 1331:734–735, 1994*

Rivanol (dye) (acridine derivative)

Rose bengal

Saccharin *JAAD 8:565, 1983*

Shiitake mushroom toxicoderma – seborrheic dermatitis-like eruption *JAAD 24:64–66, 1991*

Sodium ferrous citrate *Contact Dermatitis 34:77, 1996*

Solar urticaria

St. John's wort (*Hypericum perforatum*) *Med J Aust 172:302, 2000*

Sulfite food derivatives – UVB

Weed trimming *AD 127:1419–1420, 1991*

Welders – polymorphic light eruption due to UVC *JAAD 62:150–152, 2010*

INFECTIONS AND INFESTATIONS

AIDS – seborrheic dermatitis photodermatitis, and/or hyperpigmentation, photolichenoid eruption of AIDS *The Southern African Journal of HIV Medicine, 2016; Clin Exp Dermatol 28:265–268, 2003; AD 130:609–613, 1994;* as presenting sign *AD 130:618–623,*

1994; photodistributed hypertrophic lichen planus *Cutis 55:109–111, 1995;* chronic actinic dermatitis *BJD 137:431–436, 1997;* butterfly rash *NEJM 311:189, 1984*

Candida – chronic mucocutaneous candidiasis – seborrheic dermatitis-like

Cellulitis *Dermatitis 25:322, 2014*

Chikungunya fever – morbilliform exanthem of trunk and limbs with islands of sparing; high fever, headache, photophobia, myalgia, arthralgias *JAMA Derm 151:257–258, 2015; Tyring, p.513, 2002*

Coxsackie virus – photodistributed exanthem *Tyring, p.460, 2002*

Dermatophyte infection – widespread dermatophyte infection mimicking photosensitivity *JAAD 23:855–857, 1990;* tinea faciei – photodistributed or mimicking seborrheic dermatitis *Ped Derm 22:243–244, 2005; NEJM 314:315–316, 1986;* corporis/capitis (seborrheic dermatitis-like) *Dermatologica 177:65–69, 1988; AD 114:250–252, 1978; Cutis 17:913–915, 1976; Cutis 17:913–915, 1976;* tinea corporis mimicking Casal's necklace; tinea incognito

Epstein-Barr virus – association with hydroa vacciniforme *BJD 140:715–721, 1999*

Erysipelas – mimics photosensitive eruption *Dermatitis 25:322, 2014; Am J Med 123:414–416, 2010; Postgrad Med 89:225–228, 233–234, 1991*

Favus – seborrheic dermatitis-like

Hepatitis A *Dermatology 200:266–269, 2000*

Herpes simplex – recurrent *Dermatitis 25:322, 2014; JID 65:341–346, 1975;* including eczema herpeticum

HIV-1 dermatitis – lichenoid photodermatitis *JAAD 28:167–173, 1993;* photosensitivity *AD 130:618–623, 1994*

Histoplasmosis – mimicking seborrheic dermatitis *JAAD 29:311–313, 1993*

Infectious eczematoid dermatitis with photodistributed absorption reaction

Leishmaniasis – in AIDS presenting with dermatomyositis-like eruption *JAAD 35:316–319, 1996*

Leprosy *Int J Lepr Other Mycobact Dis 45:67, 1977;* multibacillary leprosy mimicking malar rash of lupus *Lupus 24:1095–1102, 2015*

Lyme disease – malar erythema *NEJM 321:586–596, 1989; AD 120:1017–1021, 1984;* Borrelia lymphocytoma butterfly rash *Am J Dermatopathol 40:216–218, 2018;* photosensitivity *Cureus 11:e6509, Dec 30, 2019*

Lymphogranuloma venereum – photo-induced papular, urticarial and plaques in subacute stage of LGV *Int J Dermatol 15:26–33, 1976*

Measles *Dermatol Online J 16:March 15, 2010;* atypical *JAAD 22:1107–1109, 1990*

Mycobacterium tuberculosis Postgrad Med 89:225–228, 1991

Nocardia asteroides BJD 144:639–641, 2001

Parvovirus B19 – Parvovirus B19 – erythema infectiosum (fifth disease) *Hum Pathol 31:488–497, 2000; J Clin Inf Dis 21:1424–1430, 1995;* lupus-like rash *Hum Pathol 31:488–497, 2000;* dermatomyositis-like facial and upper extremity erythema *Hum Pathol 31:488–497, 2000*

Rubella – congenital rubella syndrome – seborrhea, cutis marmorata, hyperpigmentation *JAAD 46:161–183, 2002*

Scabies, crusted (Norwegian) – including seborrheic-like dermatitis of scalp; *Cutis 61:87–88, 1998;* crusted scabies in IPEX syndrome (immunodysregulation, polyendocrinopathy, enteropathy, X-linked inheritance) *JAAD 56:S48–49, 2007*

Strongyloides hyperinfection – with *Streptococcus bovis* meningitis; photophobia *NEJM 371:1051–1060, 2014*

Syphilis – secondary – mimicking seborrheic dermatitis over central face and along hairline (corona veneris) *Lupus 10:299–303, 2001*

Tinea capitis – seborrheic dermatitis-like eruption *Cutis 78:189–196, 2006*

Tinea faciei – mimicking lupus *Cutis 53:297–298, 1994*

Tinea imbricata – seborrheic dermatitis-like *Cutis 83:186–191, 2009*

Tinea versicolor – mimics seborrheic dermatitis *Semin Dermatol 4:173–184, 1985*

Toxoplasmosis – dermatomyositis-like eruption *JAAD 60:897–925, 2009; AD 115:736–737, 1979; BJD 101:589–591, 1979*

Tularemia *Photodermatol 2:122–123, 1985*

Varicella – photolocalized varicella *Ped Derm 31:609–610, 2014; BJD 170:1195–1196, 2014; BJD 142:584–585, 2000; Cutis 62:199–200, 1998; Pediatr Infect Dis J 15:921–922, 1996; JAAD 26:772–774, 1992; Ped Derm 3:215–218, 1986; Ped Derm 3:215–218, 1986; AD 107:628, 1973;* actinic varicella vaccine rash *Ped Inf Dis 30:1116–1118, 2011*

Viral exanthems – photodistributed *Pediatrics 59:484, 1977; Pediatrics 54:136–138, 1974*

INFILTRATIVE DISEASES

Colloid milium *Clin Exp Dermatol 18:347–350, 1993; BJD 125:80–81, 1991*

Jessner's lymphocytic infiltrate *AD 124:1091–1093, 1988*

Langerhans cell histiocytosis – seborrheic dermatitis-like papules, crops of red-brown or red-yellow papules, vesicopustules, erosions, scaling, and petechiae, purpura, solitary nodules, bronze pigmentation, lipid infiltration of the eyes, white plaques of the oral mucosa, onycholysis, and onychodystrophy *Clin Dermatol 38:223–234, 2020; Curr Prob Derm VI Jan/Feb 1994; Clin Exp Derm 11:183–187, 1986; JAAD 13:481–496, 1985;* adult Langerhans cell histiocytosis – papular eruption of central chest and submammary areas *JAAD 54:910–912, 2006;* Hand-Schuller-Christian disease – seborrheic dermatitis-like *JAAD 56:290–294, 2007; Clin Exp Dermatol 8:177–183, 1983*

Mastocytosis – telangiectasia macularis eruptiva perstans

Reticulated erythematous mucinosis *Dermatitis 25:322, 2014*

INFLAMMATORY DISEASES

Erythema multiforme *Photodermatol 4:52–54, 1987; Photodermatol 2:176–177, 1985; JAAD 9:419–423, 1983; AD 116:477, 1980*

Kikuchi's disease (histiocytic necrotizing lymphadenitis) – resembles lupus erythematosus or polymorphic light eruption *Ped Derm 18:403–405, 2001*

Lymphocytoma cutis; *Cancer 69:717–724, 1992; Acta DV (Stockh)62:119–124, 1982; BJD 84:25–31, 1971*

Neutrophilic sebaceous adenitis – annular erythematous indurated plaques of face and chest *JAAD 60:887–888, 2009;* persistent malar erythema with atrophy; annular without surface change, photodistributed *JAMA Derm 154:1215–1216, 2018; JAAD 36:845–846, 1997; AD 129:910–911, 1993*

Sarcoidosis – mimicking lupus erythematosus, polymorphic light eruption *JAAD 66:699–716, 2012; Photodermatol Photoimmunol Photomed 27:156–158, 2011; Clin Derm 4:35–46, 1986*

Sarcoidosis – lupus pernio *Postgrad Med 89:225–228, 233–234, 1991*

Whipple's disease (*Tropheryma whipplei*) – dermatomyositis-like eruption *JAAD 60:277–288, 2009*

METABOLIC DISEASES

Addison's disease – hyperpigmentation of face, often photo-accentuated *Ped Derm 25:215–218, 2008*

Biotinidase deficiency (juvenile form of multiple carboxylase deficiency) – seborrheic dermatitis-like rash *Ped Derm 21:231–235, 2004*

Central nervous system disorders – seizures, Parkinson's disease – seborrheic dermatitis

Chronic active hepatitis – lupus-like eruptions

Folic acid deficiency – gray–brown photo-hyperpigmentation *JAAD 12:914–917, 1985*

Hartnup's disease *Cutis 68:31–34, 2001; Ped Derm 16:95–102, 1999;* presenting in adulthood *Clin Exp Dermatol 19:407–408, 1994;* autosomal recessive; defective transport of neutral amino acids including tryptophan in small intestine and kidneys; pellagra-like photosensitive eruption; cerebellar ataxia; psoriasiform red scaly plaques, generalized alopecia, widespread edema; aminoaciduria *JAAD 67:1113–1127, 2012; Ped Derm 23:262–265, 2006*

Hemochromatosis – idiopathic (autosomal recessive) or secondary to chronic iron intoxication (Bantu hemochromatosis), chronic liver disease and iron overload, hepatic hemosiderosis in anemia with ineffective erythropoiesis, congenital transferrin deficiency – blue–gray, bronze, gray–brown hyperpigmentation especially of face, flexures, and exposed parts *J Drugs in Dermatol 9:719–722, 2010; Clev Clin J Med 76:599–606, 2009; AD 113:161–165, 1977; Medicine 34:381–430, 1955*

Holocarboxylase synthetase deficiency – autosomal recessive; scaly eyebrows, eyelashes, scalp *Ped Derm 23:142–144, 2006*

Hydroxykynureninuria

Kwashiorkor *Int J Dermatol 49:500–506, 2010*

Kynureninase deficiency (xanthurenicaciduria) – pellagrous dermatitis

Malabsorption

Mitochondrial disorders – erythematous photodistributed eruptions followed by mottled or reticulated hyperpigmentation; alopecia with or without hair shaft abnormalities including trichothiodystrophy, trichoschisis, tiger tail pattern, pili torti, longitudinal grooving, and trichorhexis nodosa *Pediatrics 103:428–433, 1999*

Multiple carboxylase deficiency – holocarboxylase deficiency; neonatal form; seborrheic rash of scalp, eyebrows, eyelashes, then spreads to periorificial areas *Ped Derm 21:231–235, 2004*

Necrolytic migratory erythema – recurrent seborrheic, serpiginous, annular papulosquamous eruptions; glucagonoma, chronic liver disease, inflammatory bowel disease, heroin abuse, pancreatitis, malabsorption syndromes *Int J Dermatol 49:24–29, 2010*

Neurologic disease – seborrheic dermatitis *Postgrad Med 117:43–44, 2005*

Panhypopituitarism

Pellagra (niacin deficiency) – red pigmented sharply marginated photodistributed rash; hyperpigmented scaly photodermatitis including drug-induced pellagra-like dermatitis – 6-mercaptopurine, 5-fluorouracil,INH (all of the above – also seb derm-like); resembles Hartnup disease *NEJM 371:2218–2223, 2014; BJD 164:1188–1200, 2011; Cutis 68:31–34, 2001; Ped Derm 16:95–102, 1999; BJD 125:71–72, 1991;* sebaceous gland hyperplasia and seborrhea of ala nasi, forehead, scalp, face, neck; associate with celiac disease *Yale J Biol Med 72:1518, 1999;* Hartnup disease – pellagrous dermatitis, cerebellar ataxia, psychosis *Lancet 2:421–428, 1956*; with anorexia nervosa *Dermatol 38:1037–1040, 2011*

Phenylketonuria – phenylalanine hydroxylase deficiency; fair skin and hair with light sensitivity

Porphyrias *Semin Cut Med Surg 18:285–292, 1999; Clin Dermatol 16:251–264, 1998; Ann Rev Med 41:457–469, 1990*

   Congenital erythropoietic porphyria – blisters, scarring, hyperpigmentation, mutilating ulcers, hypertrichosis, erythrodontia, corneal scarring, keratoconjunctivitis, cataracts; gingival recession; bullous photosensitivity, photomutilation, fixed flexion deformities, resorption of fingertips, blepharitis, ectropion, meibomian cysts, conjunctivitis, loss of eyebrows, erythrodontia (purple teeth), dental caries, overcrowding of teeth, facial hypertrichosis, scarring alopecia due to recurrent blistering, dyschromatosis; neonatal jaundice, hemolytic anemia, splenomegaly due to pancytopenia *BJD 167:988–900, 2012; JAAD 67:1093–1110, 2012; AD 141: 1575–1579, 2005; Semin Liver Dis 2:154–63, 1982*

   Erythropoietic porphyria *Dermatol Clin 4:291–296, 1986; Int J Biochem 9:921–926, 1978; BMJ 3 (5984):621–623, 1975*; congenital – photodistributed bullae, hypertrichosis of face and neck, depigmented scars, milia, sclerosis of hands; mutation of URO III synthase *Ped Derm 35:833–834, 2018*; or GATA1 *Eur J Haematol 94:491–497, 2015*

   Erythropoietic protoporphyria – photodistributed crusted erosions with weathered wrinkled appearance *BJD 171:412–414, 2014; Eur J Pediatr 159:719–725, 2000; J Inherit Metab Dis 20:258–269, 1997; BJD 131:751–766, 1994; Curr Probl Dermatol 20:123–134, 1991; Am J Med 60:8–22, 1976*; autosomal recessive EPP with decreased risk of liver disease *BJD 155:574–581, 2006*; X-linked dominant EPP with increased risk of liver disease *J Dermatol 43:44–48, 2016; Am J Med Genet 83:408–414, 2008*; red dorsal hands and feet *JAMA Derm 152:937–938, 2016*

   Hepatoerythropoietic porphyria – extreme photosensitivity, skin fragility in sun-exposed areas, hypertrichosis, erythrodontia, pink urine, sclerodermoid changes *AD 146:529–533, 2010;AD 138:957–960, 2002; JAAD 11:1103–1111, 1984; AD 116:307–311, 1980*

   Hereditary coproporphyria *BJD 96:549–554, 1977; Q J Med 46:229–241, 1977; BJD 84:301–310, 1971*

   Porphyria cutanea tarda – weather-beaten appearance; vesicles, bullae, crusts, skin fragility, atrophic scars, milia; associated with hepatic tumors *J Dermatol 9:131–137, 1982*; hepatitis *Clin Exp Dermatol 10:169–173, 1985*

   Sideroblastic anemia, abnormal porphyrins, and photosensitivity *JAAD 27:287–292, 1992*

   Transient neonatal porphyrinemia – phototherapy-induced blisters *Ped Derm 35:e272–275, 2018*

   Variegate porphyria – weather-beaten appearance *Skin Pharmacol Appl Skin Physiol 11:310–320, 1998; Postgrad Med J 69:781–786, 1993; AD 96:98–100, 1967*; homozygous variegate porphyria – erosions, photosensitivity, short stature *BJD 144:866–869, 2001*

Porphyria cutanea tarda-like dermatitis (pseudoporphyria) associated with:
   AIDS *Int J Derm 31:474–479, 1992; AD 130:630–633, 1994*
   Amiodarone *Photodermatol 5:146–147, 1988*
   Bumetanide
   Chlorthalidone
   Etretinate *Clin Exp Dermatol 14:437–438, 1989*
   Fluoroquinolone *Dermatologic Clinics 4:291–296, 1986*
   Furosemide
   Hemodialysis in chronic renal failure *NEJM 299:292–294, 1978*
   Isotretinoin

Nalidixic acid
Naproxen *J Pediatr 117:660–664, 1990; Arthritis Rheum 33:903–908, 1990*
Peritoneal dialysis and erythropoietin therapy *J Pediatr 121:749–752, 1992*
Status-post liver transplant *AD 130:614–617, 1994*
Sunbed use *Acta DV 70:354–356, 1990*
Tetracycline
Voriconazole *J Ped Infect Dis 4:e22–24, 2015*

Prolidase deficiency – autosomal recessive; peptidase D mutation (PEPD); increased urinary imidopeptides; leg ulcers, anogenital ulcers, short stature (mild), telangiectasias, recurrent infections (sinusitis, otitis); mental retardation; splenomegaly with enlarged abdomen, atrophic scarring, spongy fragile skin with annular pitting and scarring; dermatitis, hyperkeratosis of elbows and knees, lymphedema, purpura, low hairline, poliosis, canities, lymphedema, photosensitivity, hypertelorism, saddle nose deformity, frontal bossing, dull expression, mild ptosis, micrognathia, mandibular protrusion, exophthalmos, joint laxity, deafness, osteoporosis, high arched palate *JAAD 62:1031, 1034, 2010; Ped Derm 13:58–60, 1996; AD 127:124–125, 1991*

Sprue (celiac disease) – gluten sensitivity

Tuftsin deficiency – seborrheic dermatitis *Ped Derm 17:91–96, 2000*

Vitamin B1 deficiency *Clinics in Derm 17:457–461, 1999*

Vitamin B2 deficiency (riboflavin deficiency) – conjunctivitis and periorificial dermatitis; seborrheic dermatitis-like eruption; crusting of scrotum *JAAD 68:211–243, 2013; Ped Derm 16:95–102, 1999; Clinics in Derm 17:457–461, 1999; JAAD 21:1–30, 1989*

Vitamin B6 deficiency (pyridoxine deficiency) – periorificial dermatitis (seborrheic dermatitis-like) *JAAD 68:211–243, 2013; Ped Derm 16:95–102, 1999;JAAD 15:1263–1274, 1986*

Vitamin E deficiency *JAAD 43:1–16, 2000*

Zinc deficiency, chronic – seborrheic dermatitis-like changes *Cutis 81:314, 324–326, 2008; Acta DV 17:513–546, 1936*

NEOPLASTIC

Acanthomas – eruptive acanthomas following sunburn *BJD 133:493–494, 1995*

Actinic cheilitis *Dermatologica 135:465–471, 1967*

Actinic keratoses *JAAD 44:1052–1053, 2001*

Basal cell carcinomas

Bowen's disease – giant of face *Dermatol Ther 33:e13263, 2020; Open Access Macedonian J Med Sci 7:606–609, 2019*

Ephelides

Epstein-Barr virus associated lymphoproliferative lesions *BJD 151:372–380, 2004*

Keratoacanthomas *Oral Surg Oral Med Oral Pathol 38:918–927, 1974*; multiple self-healing keratoacanthomas of Ferguson-Smith *JAAD 49:741–746, 2003; BJD 46:267–272, 1934* Large cell acanthomas

Lichen planus-like keratoses simulating photodermatitis *JAAD 13:201–206, 1985*

Lymphoma – cutaneous T-cell lymphoma (plaque type) mimicking actinic reticuloid *BJD 113:497–500, 1985*; exfoliative CTCL mimicking chronic actinic dermatitis *BJD 160:698–703, 2009*; chronic actinic dermatitis with adult T-cell leukemia *JAAD 52:S38–40, 2005*; hydroa vacciniforme-like cutaneous T-cell lymphoma, Epstein-Barr virus-related – edema, blisters, vesicles, ulcers, scarring, facial scars, swollen nose, lips, and periorbital edema, crusts with central hemorrhagic necrosis, facial dermatitis, photodermatitis, facial edema, facial papules and plaques, crusting of ears, fever *JAAD 81:534–540, 2019; JAAD 69:112–119, 2013;*angiocentric CTCL of childhood (hydroa vacciniforme-like lymphoma) (atypical hydroa vacciniforme in childhood) – Latin America and Asia associated with Epstein- Barr virus *Clin Exp Dermatol 26:242–247, 2001; JAAD 40:283–284, 1999; AD 133:1081–1086, 1997; JAAD 38:574–579, 1998;* lymphomatoid granulomatosis (angiocentric lymphoma)

Lymphomatoid papulosis – hydroa vacciniforme-like *Case Rep Dermatol Med July 16, 2019:1765210; JAAD 32:378–381, 1995*

Melanocytic nevi *Dermatol Clin 13:595–603, 1995*

Melanoma

Metastases – gastric carcinoma – personal observation

Porokeratosis – disseminated superficial actinic porokeratosis *Cutis 67:286, 296–298, 2001; Australas J Dermatol 9:335–344, 1968;* actinic porokeratosis

Pseudo-cutaneous T-cell lymphoma in HIV disease *JAAD 41:722–727, 1999*

Squamous cell carcinoma

Syringomas *Cutis 77:33–36, 2006*

Tumors of the follicular infundibulum, multiple – papules in sun-exposed areas *JAAD 39:853–857, 1998*

PARANEOPLASTIC DISORDERS

Carcinoid syndrome – pellagrous dermatitis (skin fragility, erythema, and hyperpigmentation over knuckles), flushing, patchy cyanosis, hyperpigmentation, telangiectasia, pellagrous dermatitis, salivation, lacrimation, abdominal cramping, wheezing, diarrhea *BJD 152:71–75, 2005; AD 77:86–90, 1958; Am Heart J 47:795–817, 1954*

Glucagonoma syndrome (necrolytic migratory erythema) *Autops Case Rep 9:e2019129 Nov 27, 2019; Int J Dermatol 57:642–645, 2018;*

JAAD 12:1032–1039, 1985; AD 113:792–797, 1977

Renal cell carcinoma – discoid lupus erythematosus-like syndrome and hypercalcemia associated with renal cell carcinoma *Cutis 26:402–403, 1980*

PHOTODERMATOSES

Acquired brachioradial cutaneous dyschromatosis (dermatoheliosis) *JAAD 42:680–684, 2000*

Actinic cheilitis granulomatosa *J Dermatol 19:556–562, 1992*

Actinic comedones (Favre-Racouchot syndrome) *Cutis 60:145–146, 1997;* actinic comedonal plaque *Clin Exp Dermatol 18:156–158, 1993; JAAD 3:633–636, 1980*

Actinic prurigo – bullae of face and hands; cheilitis; conjunctivitis *SKINmed 13:287–295, 2015; The Dermatologist May, 2015,pp.47–48, 50, 2015; Dermatol Ther 16:40–44, 2003; JAAD 44:952–956, 2001; Australas J Dermatol 42:192–195, 2001; Photodermatol Photoimmunol Photomed 15:183–187, 1999; BJD 140:232–236, 1999; Int J Dermatol 34:380–384, 1995; JAAD 26:683–692, 1992; JAAD 5:183–190, 1981; Clin Exp Dermatol 2:365–372, 1977;* familial, in North American Indians *Int J Dermatol 10:107–114, 1971;* in Caucasians *BJD 144:194–196, 2001;* polymorphic light eruption of American Indians; occurrence in non-Indians *JAAD 34:612–617, 1996;* Southeast Asian*; Photodermatol Photoimmunol Photomed 9:225–228, 1992;* lower lip *Oral Surg Oral Med Oral Pathol 65:327–332, 1988*

Actinic reticuloid (chronic actinic dermatitis) – chronic photosensitivity disorder associated with CTCL; sensitive to UVB. *BJD 162:1406–1408, 2010; Ann Acad Med Singapore 30:664–667, 2001; BJD 137:431–436, 1997; Int J Dermatol 38:335–342, 1999; JAAD 38:877–905, 1998; Semin Diagn Pathol 8:109–116, 1991; JAAD 21:205–214, 1989; JAAD 21:1134–1137, 1989; AD 118:672–675, 1982; Sem Derm 161, Sept 1982; AD 115:1078–1083, 1979;* erythrodermic actinic reticuloid *AD 131:1298–1303, 1995; Arch Dermatol Res 277:159–166, 1985; AD 115:1078–1083, 1979*

Actinic superficial folliculitis *BJD 139:359–360, 1998; BJD 138:1070–1074, 1998; Clin Exp Dermatol 14:69–71, 1989; BJD 113:630–631, 1985*

Benign summer light eruption *JAAD 17:690–691, 1987*

Chronic actinic dermatitis – acute, subacute, or chronic dermatitis with lichenification, papules, plaques, erythroderma, stubby scalp and eyebrow hair *BJD 152:784–786, 2005; JAMA Derm 153:427–435, 2017; Photodermatol Photomed 20:312–314, 2004; Clin Exper Dermatol 28:265–268, 2003; Dermatologic Therapy 16:45–51, 2003; Yonsei Med J 41:190–194, 2000; AD 136:1215–1220, 2000; AD 130:1284–1289, 1994; JAAD 28:240–249, 1993; AD 126:317–323, 1990;* sensitization by sesquiterpene lactone mix *BJD 132:543–547, 1995;* associated with musk ambrette *Cutis 54:167–170, 1994; JAAD 3:384–393, 1980;* simvastatin *Contact Dermatitis 38:294–295, 1998*

Cutis rhomboidalis nuchae

Dermatoheliosis (solar elastosis) (sun damage – basophilic alteration of collagen)

Diffuse elastoma of Dubreuilh *Soc Ital Dermatol Sifilogr Sezioni Interprov Soc Ital Dermatol Sifilogrn 92:153–160, 1951*

Hydroa aestivale

Hydroa vacciniforme – red macules progress to tender papules or vesiculopapules, hemorrhagic vesicles or bullae, umbilication and crusting; pock-like scars, crusts of helices *Cutis 88:245–253, 2011; BJD 144:874–877, 2001; JAAD 42:208–213, 2000; Dermatology 189:428–429, 1994; JAAD 25:892–895, 1991; JAAD 25:401–403, 1991; BJD 118:101–108, 1988; BJD 118:101–108, 1988; AD 118:588–591, 1982;* familial *BJD 140:124–126, 1999; AD 114:1193–1196, 1978; AD 103:223–224, 1971;* late onset *BJD 144:874–877, 2001;* hydroa vacciniforme (Epstein-Barr virus-related) – red macules progress to tender papules or vesiculopapules, hemorrhagic vesicles or bullae, umbilication and crusting; pock-like scars; edema of cheeks, eyelids, ears, and lips *AD 142:587–595, 2006*

Juvenile spring eruption – vesicular eruption of helices, lips and cheeks due to Parvovirus B19 *JAMA Derm 154:1356–1357*

Melasma *Dermatol Online J Oct 15, 2019; Dermatol Ther (Heidelb)7:305–318, 2017; Ann DV 139:Suppl 4:S144–147, 2012*

Persistent light reactor – personal observation

Photo-onycholysis, spontaneous *BJD 113:605–610, 1985*

Poikiloderma of Civatte *Derm Surg 26:823–827, 2000*

Polymorphic light eruption – papules, plaques, and vesicles *BJD 144:446–447, 2001; JID 115:467–470, 2000; JAAD 42:199–207, 2000; Eur J Dermatol 8:554–559, 1998; Photodermatol Photoimmunol Photomed 13:89–90, 1997; Int J Dermatol 33:233–239, 1994; Photodermatol Photoimmunol Photomed 7:186–191, 1990; Dermatol Clin 4:243–251, 1986; JAAD 3:329–343, 1980;* papulovesicular variant *AD 121:1286–1288, 1985; Acta DV 62:237–240, 1982;* exacerbation with exposure to photocopier *AD 117:373–374, 1981;* pinhead papular eruption of the face *J Drugs in Dermatol 12:1285–1286, 2013*

Riehl's melanosis (pigmented contact dermatitis) *Stat Pearls May 30, 2020*

Solar pruritus *Acta DV 75:488–489, 1995*

Solar purpura – in PMLE *Photodermatol Photoimmunol Photomed 11:31–32, 1995;* in EPP *Dermatologica 167:220–222, 1983*

Solar urticaria *Am J Contact Dermat 11:89–94, 2000; BJD 142:32–38, 2000; Int J Dermatol 38:411–418, 1999; AD 134:71–74, 1998; JAAD 21:237–240, 1989;* PCT presenting as solar urticaria *BJD 141:590–591, 1999;* in an infant *BJD 136:105–107, 1997*

Spring and summer eruptions of the elbows – form of polymorphic light eruption; papules and plaques of elbows *JAAD 68:306–312, 2013*

PRIMARY CUTANEOUS DISEASES

Absorption reaction – personal observation

Acantholytic dyskeratotic epidermal nevus (unilateral Darier's disease) – induced by ultraviolet B radiation *JAAD 39:301–304, 1998*

Acne aestivalis (Mallorca acne) *Cutis 26:254–256, 1980; AD 111:891–892, 1975*

Acne rosacea *Dermatitis 25:322, 2014; AD 134:679–683, 1998; JID 88:56s–60s, 1987;* lupus miliaris disseminata faciei (granulomatous rosacea) *Int J Dermatol 9:173–176, 1970*

Acne vulgaris exacerbation of acne vulgaris by ultraviolet light *AD 114:221–223, 1978*

Actinic folliculitis *Clin Exp Dermatol 30:659–661, 2005; Clin Exp Dermatol 14:69–71, 1989; BJD 113:630–631, 1985*

Actinic granuloma – annular elastolytic giant cell granuloma *NEJM 376:475, 2017; AD 137:1647–1652, 2001; Cutis 62:181–187, 1998;* periorbital *Graefes Arch Clin Exp Ophthalmol 236:646–651, 1998*

Actinic rhinophyma *Cutis 57:389–392, 1996*

Albinism *Stat Pearls April 17, 2020; An Bras Dermatol 94:503–520, 2019*

Alopecia mucinosa

Annular atrophic plaques of the face *AD 100:703–716, 1969*

Atopic dermatitis – UV light as aggravating factor *Dermatology Online J 4:10, 1998;* with chronic actinic dermatitis *BJD 142:845, 2000*

Brachioradial pruritus *JAAD 41:656–658, 1999; Dermatology 195:414–415, 1997; BJD 135:486–487, 1996; BJD 115:177–180, 1986*

Confluent and reticulated papillomatosis *J Dermatol 36:251–253, 2009*

Darier's disease (keratosis follicularis) – seborrheic distribution; photoexacerbated *Ann DV 121:393–395, 1994; Clin Dermatol 19:193–205, 1994; JAAD 27:40–50, 1992; AD 120:1484–1487, 1984*

Dyshidrosis – photo-induced dyshidrosis *JAAD 50:55–60, 2004;* piroxicam photosensitivity and dyshidrosis *JAAD 15:1237–1241, 1986*

Elastotic nodules of ears

Eosinophilic pustular folliculitis of Ofuji – circinate and serpiginous plaques with overlying papules and pustules in seborrheic areas; pustules are follicular *Dermatology 208:229–230, 2004; J Dermatol 16:388–391, 1989; Acta DV 50:195–203, 1970*

Epidermolytic hyperkeratosis – persistent actinic epidermolytic hyperkeratosis *J Cutan Pathol 6:272–279, 1979*

Erythema elevatum diutinum *G Ital DV 117:31–34, 1982*

Erythromelanosis follicularis faciei *JAAD 32:863–866, 1995*

Erythrosis pigmentata faciei (erythrose peribuccale pigmentaire of Brocq)

Frictional lichenoid dermatitis of childhood (Sutton's summer prurigo) *Acta DV 58:549–61, 1978*

Granuloma annulare, photo-induced in AIDS with UVB photosensitivity *Am J Dermatopathol 39:625–627, 2017; Clin Exp Dermatol 34:e53–55, 2009; AD 126:830–831, 1990; AD 122:39–40, 1986*

Granuloma faciale

Grover's disease – transient or persistent acantholytic dermatosis *Z Hautkr 62:369–370, 375–378, 1987 (German); BJD 102:515–520, 1980*

Hailey-Hailey disease – seborrheic dermatitis-like *JAMA Derm 150:97–99, 2014; SkinMed 5:250–252, 2006; BJD 126:294–296, 1992*

Juvenile spring eruption *N Z Med J 109:389, 1996; BJD 125:402, 1991; BJD 124:375–378, 1991; Int J Dermatol 29:284–286, 1990; Clin Exp Dermatol 14:462–463, 1989*

Keratosis lichenoides chronica (Nekam's disease) – reticulated flat-topped keratotic papules, linear arrays, atrophy, comedo-like lesions, prominent telangiectasia; conjunctival injection, seborrheic dermatitis-like eruption; acral dermatitis over toes; punctate keratotic papules of palmar creases; scaly red papules of face; seborrheic dermatitis-like rash of face; nail dystrophy; oral and genital erosions, conjunctivitis *AD 147:1317–1322, 2011; Cutis 86:245–248, 2010; Ped Derm 26:615–616, 2009; AD 145:867–69, 2009; AD 144:405–410, 2008; Am J Dermatopathol 28:260–275, 2006; JAAD 49:511–513, 2003; Dermatology 201:261–264, 2000; JAAD 38:306–309, 1998; JAAD 37:263–264, 1997; Dermatopathol Pract Concept 3:310–312 1997; AD 131:609–614, 1995; Dermatology 191:188–192, 1995; AD 105:739–743, 1972; Presse Med 51:1000–1003, 1938; Arch Dermatol Syph (Berlin) 31:1–32, 1895;* in children *JAAD 56:S1–5, 2007*

Leiner's disease *Dermatol Therapy 18:176–183, 2005*

Lichen nitidus *Cutis 81:266–268, 2008; JAAD 54:S48–49, 2006; AD 134:1302–1303, 1998; Ped Derm 8:94–95, 1991; JAAD 4:404–411, 1981; Dermatologica 157:115–125, 1978*

Lichen planus, including actinic lichen planus (lichen planus actinicus) *Ped Derm 34:713–714, 2017; JAMA Derm 151:1121–1122, 2015; Cutis 72:377–381, 2003; JAAD 20:226–231, 1989; Clin Exp Dermatol 14:65–68, 1989; JAAD 4:404–411, 1981;* facial erythema of actinic lichen planus *BJD 1032–1034, 2002;* actinic lichen planus mimicking melasma *JAAD 18:275–278, 1988;* photopigmentation in lichen planus actinicus *BJD 163:662–663, 2010;* tropical lichen planus (lichenoid melanodermatitis) *BJD 101:651–658, 1979;* lichen planus/DLE overlap syndrome

Lichen simplex chronicus

Periorbital dermatitis (periorbital variant of perioral dermatitis) – idiopathic or topical corticosteroid–associated; distributed around nasolabial folds in seborrheic distribution; including facial Afro-Caribbean childhood eruption (FACE) *BJD 91:435–438, 1976*

Pityriasis rosea – mimicking seborrheic dermatitis

Pityriasis rubra pilaris –PRP type V – hyperkeratotic scaly patches of dorsal hands, annular brown macules, red patches; *CARD14* mutation (caspase recruitment domain family 14) *JAMA Derm 153:66–70, 2017;* seborrheic dermatitis-like eruption *Ped Derm 3:446–451, 1986;* seborrheic dermatitis in infants *BJD 157:202–204, 2007;* early or late may resemble severe explosive seborrheic dermatitis; photoexacerbated *Photodermatol Photoimmunol Photomed 10:42–45, 1994; AD 102:603–612, 1970*

Progressive symmetric erythrokeratoderma – personal observation

Psoriasis – photosensitive (photoexacerbated) psoriasis *Semin Dermatol 11:267–268, 1992; Photodermatol 6:241–243, 1989; Ann DV 115:47–50, 1988; JAAD 17:752–758, 1987; Acta DV Suppl (Stockh) 131:1–48, 1987; Photodermatol 3:317–326, 1986;* psoriasis in seborrheic distribution or mimicking seborrheic dermatitis (scalp, eyebrows, ears) photo-exacerbated; pustular psoriasis

Seborrheic dermatitis*; J Cutan Genitourin Dis 5:12, 1887;* severe seborrheic dermatitis in AIDS *Clin Dermatol 38:160–175, 2020*

    Blepharitis
    Cradle cap
    Dandruff
    Dermatitic plaques
    Erythrodermic
    Facial
    Flexural (intertrigo)
    Follicular
    Petaloid
    Pityriasiform

Vitiligo

PSYCHOCUTANEOUS DISORDERS

Factitial dermatitis intentionally mimicking dermatomyositis – personal observation *Ped Derm 21:205–211, 2004;* presenting as photodermatosis *Hautarzt 58:153–155, 2007*

SYNDROMES

Acrokeratosis marginalis

Alagille syndrome *Gastroenterology 99:831–835, 1990*

Apert's syndrome – seborrhea with severe acne; cutaneous and ocular hypopigmentation; craniosynostosis, midface malformation, syndactyly

Ataxia-telangiectasia – seborrheic dermatitis and photosensitivity *Dermatol Therapy 18:176–183, 2005; JAAD 10:431–438, 1984*

Bloom's syndrome (congenital telangiectatic erythema and stunted growth) – autosomal recessive; blisters of nose and cheeks; slender face, prominent nose; facial telangiectatic erythema and hyperpigmentation with involvement of eyelids, ear, hand and forearms; bulbar conjunctival telangiectasias; cheilitis of upper and lower lips; stunted growth; CALMs, clinodactyly, syndactyly, congenital heart disease, annular pancreas, high-pitched voice, testicular atrophy (hypogonadism); no neurologic deficits; DNA repair defect with chromosomal breaks, sister chromatid exchanges, and triradial and quadriradial chromosomes; *BLM* gene (Bloom helicase) encodes mutation in recQ DNA helicase (important in DNA repair) *BJD 178:335–349, 2018; JAAD 75:855–870, 2016; Ped Derm 27:174–177, 2010; Ped Derm 22:147–150, 2005; Curr Prob Derm 14:41–70, 2002; Ped Derm 14:120–124, 1997; JAAD 17:479–488, 1987; AD 114:755–760, 1978; Clin Genet 12:85–96, 1977; Am J Hum Genet 21:196–227, 1969; Am J Dis Child 116:409–413, 1968; AD 94:687–694, 1966; Am J Dis Child 88:754–758, 1954*

Bronze baby syndrome – gray–brown pigmentation after phototherapy for hyperbilirubinemia in neonates *JAAD 12:325–328, 1985*

Cardio-facio-cutaneous syndrome (Noonan-like short stature syndrome) (NS) – xerosis/ichthyosis, eczematous dermatitis, growth failure, hyperkeratotic papules, ulerythema ophryogenes, seborrheic dermatitis, CALMs, nevi, keratosis pilaris, autosomal dominant, patchy or widespread ichthyosiform eruption, sparse curly short scalp hair and eyebrows and lashes, hemangiomas, acanthosis nigricans, congenital lymphedema of the hands, redundant skin of the hands, short stature, abnormal facies, cardiac defects *JAAD*

46:161–183, 2002; Ped Derm 17:231–234, 2000; JAAD 28:815–819, 1993; AD 129:46–47, 1993; JAAD 22:920–922, 1990; port wine stain *Clin Genet 42:206–209, 1992*

Cerebro-oculo-facio-skeletal syndrome – autosomal recessive; UV-sensitivity; nucleotide excision repair defect *JAAD 67:1113–1127, 2012;* in aboriginal families – microcephaly, facies – micrognathia, small eyes, enlarged ears, bulbous nose, prominent nasal bridge, microphthalmia with poor vision, cataracts, blepharophimosis, short palpebral fissures, onychogryphosis, photosensitivity, mental retardation, hyperkinesis, failure to thrive, developmental delay, hypotonia, orthopedic anomalies (kyphoscoliosis), joint contractures; overhanging upper lip, small jaw *JAAD 75:873–882, 2016; Ped Derm 26:97–99, 2009; Atlas of Clinical Syndromes A Visual Aid to Diagnosis, 1992, pp.556; JAMA Derm 149:1414–1418, 2013*

Chanarin-Dorfman syndrome (neutral lipid storage disease) – erythrokeratoderma variabilis-like ichthyosis with seborrheic-like scaling along hairline *BJD 153:838–841, 2005*

Chediak-Higashi syndrome – photosensitivity *Allergo Immunopathol (Mads) 47:598–603, 2019*

Clouston's syndrome – photophobia, mild sensorineural hearing loss, alopecia, thick dystrophic nail plates, palmoplantar keratoderma; mutation in *GJB2* and *GJB6 JAMA Derm 149:1350–1351, 2013*

Cockayne syndrome – photosensitivity *Ped Derm 20:538–540, 2003; Hum Mutat 14:9–22, 1999; JAAD 39:565–570, 1998; JAAD 30:329–335, 1994; Am J Dermatopathol 7:387–392, 1985; J Med Genet 18:288–293, 1981; Pediatrics 60:135–139, 1977;* and xeroderma pigmentosum *Neurology 55:1442–1449, 2000; Am J Hum Genet 50:677–589, 1992*

Degos-Touraine syndrome – incontinentia pigmenti with poikiloderma in photodistribution, bullae of face, extremities; chronic erythroderma with subsequent hyperpigmentation *Soc Gr Dermatol Syph 68:6–10, 1961*

DeSanctis-Cacchione syndrome (variant of XP with neurologic manifestations) *Hum Mol Genet 9:1171–1175, 2000; Indian J Pediatr 64:269–272, 1997; AD 115:676, 1979; Neurol Psychiatr (Bucur) 16:47–51, 1978; AD 113:1561–1563, 1977; JID 63:392–396, 1974*

Down's syndrome – seborrheic dermatitis

Dubowitz's syndrome

Ectodermal dysplasia – ankyloblepharon, absent lower eyelashes, hypoplasia of upper lids, coloboma, seborrheic dermatitis, cribriform scrotal atrophy, ectropion, lacrimal duct hypoplasia, malaligned great toenails, gastroesophageal reflux, ear infections, laryngeal cleft, dental anomalies, scalp hair coarse and curly, sparse eyebrows, xerosis, hypohidrosis, short nose absent philtrum, flat upper lip *BJD 152:365–367, 2005*

Familial hemophagocytic lymphohistiocytosis – seborrheic dermatitis with purpura; ichthyosis-like *Ped Derm 28:494–501, 2011*

Elejalde syndrome – autosomal recessive; silvery hair, profound central nervous system dysfunction, normal immune function, photo-hyperpigmentation (bronze coloration) *Ped Derm 21:479–482, 2004*

Haber's syndrome – autosomal dominant; photo-aggravated rosacea-like rash of face; papules, pustules, scarring and telangiectasia; reticulate pigmented macules and keratotic plaques on trunk and extremities *Australas J Dermatol 38:82–84, 1997; BJD 77:1–8, 1965*

Hartnup's disease

Hereditary acrokeratotic poikiloderma of Weary-Kindler (Kindler's syndrome) *Ped Derm 6:91–101, 1989; AD 103:409–422, 1971*

Hereditary mucoepithelial dystrophy – autosomal dominant; angular cheilitis; red eyes, non-scarring alopecia, keratosis pilaris, erythema of oral (palate, gingiva) and nasal mucous membranes, cervix, vagina, and urethra; photophobia, keratosis pilaris, non-scarring alopecia, psoriasiform perineal plaques, angular cheilitis, nail deformity, increased risk of infections, fibrocystic lung disease *BJD 153:310–318, 2005; Ped Derm 12:195, 1995; JAAD 21:351–357, 1989; Am J Hum Genet 31:414–427, 1979; Oral Surg Oral Med Oral Pathol 46:645–657, 1978*

Hermansky-Pudlak syndrome *Ped Derm 34:638–646, 2017*

Hypereosinophilic syndrome – presenting as solar urticaria *Int J Dermatol 38:234, 1999*

Ichthyosis follicularis with atrichia and photophobia (IFAP) – X-linked recessive; linear plantar hyperkeratosis of heels; linear hairless scalp area in female carriers; ichthyosis, atopic dermatitis, alopecia, follicular papules, nail dystrophy, hyperextensible joints, photophobia, cheilitis, growth and psychomotor retardation, recurrent respiratory and skin infections, cryptorchidism, muscular hypotonia, skeletal abnormalities, inguinal hernia, congenital aganglionic megacolon, corneal vascularization and blindness; mutation in *MBTPS2* (membrane bound transcription factor protease, site 2) (zinc metalloprotease) *JAAD 64:716–722, 2011; Am J Med Genet 85:365–368, 1999; BJD 163:886–889, 2010; JAAD 46:S156–158, 2002*

Ichthyosis prematurity syndrome ("self-healing congenital verruciform hyperkeratosis") – autosomal recessive; erythrodermic infant with caseous vernix-like desquamation; fine scaling of scalp; evolves into generalized xerosis and mild flexural hyperkeratosis and of lower back; cutaneous cobblestoning; keratosis pilaris-like changes; fine desquamation of ankles; focal erythema, diffuse alopecia, red and white dermatographism; in utero polyhydramnios with premature birth, thick caseous desquamating skin (thick vernix caseosalike covering) (hyperkeratotic scalp) neonatal asphyxia; later in childhood, dry skin with follicular keratosis; mutation in fatty acid transporter protein 4 (FATP4) *JAAD 66:606–616, 2012; JAAD 63:607–641, 2010; JAAD 59:S71–74, 2008*

Keratosis follicularis spinulosa decalvans – conjunctivitis; keratosis pilaris, follicular atrophoderma, facial erythema, scarring alopecia, ulerythema oophyrogenes, photophobia *JAAD 58:499–502, 2008; Arch Dermatol Syphilol 151:384–387, 1926*

Kindler's syndrome – autosomal recessive; photosensitivity, cigarette paper atrophy, atrophied gingiva, poikiloderma, mucosal fragility, gingivitis, periodontitis; fermitin family homolog 1 mutation *JAAD 67:113–1127, 2012; BJD 160:233–242, 2009; Ped Derm 23:586–588, 2006; AD 142:1619–1624, 2006; AD 142:620–624, 2006; AD 140:939–944, 2004; BJD 144:1284–1286, 2001; AD 132:1487–1490, 1996; Ped Derm 13:397–402, 1996; Ped Derm 6:91–101, 1989; Ped Derm 6:82–90, 1989; BJD 66:104–111, 1954*

Lipoid proteinosis – severely scarred and photoaged skin *BJD 151:413–423, 2004; JID 120:345–350, 2003; Hum Molec Genet 11:833–840, 2002*

Mucoepithelial dysplasia – photophobia due to keratitis *Genetic Skin Disorders, Second Edition, 2010,pp.698–700*

Multicentric reticulohistiocytosis *JAAD 11:713–723, 1984;* mimicking dermatomyositis – macular photodistributed erythema *JAAD 48:S11–14, 2003; Br J Rheumatol 33:100–101, 1994*

Neutral lipid storage disease (Chanarin-Dorfman disease) – autosomal recessive; focal or diffuse alopecia; congenital non-bullous ichthyosiform erythroderma, collodion baby; seborrheic dermatitis-like rash of face and scalp; leukonychia; erythrokeratoderma variabilis-like presentation; mutation in ABHD5 which encodes protein of esterase/lipase/thioesterase subfamily *BJD 153:838–841, 2005*

Noonan's syndrome – extreme cradle cap

Pachydermoperiostosis – seborrhea *J Dermatol 27:106–109, 2000*

Pigmented xerodermoid – late onset; clinically resembles xeroderma pigmentosum *Bull Cancer 65:347–350, 1978*

Poikiloderma with neutropenia – autosomal recessive; Navajo Indians; erythematous rash of limbs, trunk, and face beginning in infancy; evolves into poikiloderma; recurrent infections; palmoplantar keratoderma; pachyonychia of great toenails, photosensitivity; growth retardation; dental caries; atrophic scars; mutation in *C16orf57 BJD 163:866–869, 2010; Am J Med Genet A 146A:2762–2769, 2008; Am J Hum Genet 86:72–76, 1991*

Pseudohypoaldosteronism type I – pustular miliaria, acneiform eruptions, extensive scaling of the scalp *Ped Derm 19:317–319, 2002*

Reactive arthritis syndrome

REM (reticular erythematous mucinosis) syndrome *JAAD 27:825–828, 1992; Ped Derm 7:1–10, 1990; Z Hautkr 63:986–998, 1988 (German); JAAD 19:859–868, 1988; AD 115:1340–1342, 1979; BJD 91:191–199, 1974; Z Hautkr 49:235–238, 1974*

Rothmund-Thomson syndrome – poikiloderma, photosensitivity (early erythema, edema, blistering of face); sparse hair, sparse eyebrows, small stature, palmoplantar keratoderma, skeletal anomalies, cataracts osteosarcoma in 30%; *JAAD 75:855–870, 2016; JAAD 67:1113–1127, 2012; Curr Prob Derm 14:41–70, 2002; BJD 139:1113–1115, 1998; Ped Derm 6:325–328, 1989; Ped Derm 6:321–324, 1989; JAAD 17:332–338, 1987;* mutations in DNA helicase gene *RECQL4 Nat Genet 22:82–84, 1999*

Schinzel-Giedion syndrome – widespread seborrheic rash *JAAD 48:161–179, 2003*

Sjogren's syndrome – erythema of nose and cheeks; photosensitivity *Stat Pearls July 4, 2020*

Smith-Lemli-Opitz syndrome – autosomal recessive; deficiency of 7-dehydrocholesterol-7-reductase (converts 7-DHC to cholesterol so have increased 7-DHC and decreased cholesterol) – sunburn with photosensitivity to UVA, polydactyly, syndactyly of 2nd and 3rd toes, growth and mental retardation, failure to thrive, dysmorphic facies, cleft palate, congenital heart disease, hypospadias *JAAD 67:1113–1127, 2012; AD 142:647–648, 2006; BJD 153:774–779, 2005; BJD 144:143–145, 2001; Photodermatol Photoimmunol Photomed 15:217–218, 1999; BJD 141::406–414, 1999; JAAD 41:121–123, 1999; Am J Hum Genet 53:817–821, 1993; J Pediatr 64:210–217, 1964*

Sweet's syndrome *BJD 149:675–678, 2003; AD 137:1106–1108, 2001; J Dermatol 12:191–194, 1985*

Trichothiodystrophy syndromes – BIDS, IBIDS, PIBIDS – photosensitivity, sparse or absent eyelashes and eyebrows, no freckling; brittle hair,; neuroectodermal defects, premature aging, sexual immaturity, ichthyosis, dysmyelination, bird-like facies, dental caries; trichothiodystrophy with ichthyosis, urologic malformations, hypercalciuria and mental and physical retardation; mutation in transcription/DNA repair factor IIH *Ped Derm 25:264–267, 2008; Trends Genet 17:279–286, 2001; Ped Derm 14:441–445, 1997; JAAD 44:891–920, 2001; Hum Mutat 14:9–22, 1999; JAAD 28:820–826, 1993; Ped Derm 9:369–370, 1992; JAAD 22:705–717, 1990; JAAD 13:683–686, 1985*

Turner's syndrome

Universal dyschromatosis with photosensitivity and neurosensory hearing defect *AD 126:1659–1660, 1990*

Unusual facies, vitiligo, canities, and progressive spastic paraplegia – hyperpigmentation of exposed areas *Am J Med Genet 9:351–357, 1981*

UV-sensitive syndrome – new syndrome with defective transcription-coupled DNA repair; acute sunburn, dryness, freckling, telangiectasias, no neurologic defects; pigmentary abnormalities *JAAD 75:873–882, 2016; JAAD 67:1113–1127, 2012; Am J Hum Genet 56:1267–1276, 1995*

X-linked reticulate pigmentary disorder with systemic manifestations (familial cutaneous amyloidosis) (Partington syndrome II) – X-linked; rare; Xp21–22; boys with generalized reticulated muddy brown reticulated pigmentation (dyschromatosis) with hypopigmented corneal dystrophy (dyskeratosis), coarse unruly hair, unswept eyebrows, silvery hair, hypohidrosis, recurrent sinus disease and pneumonia with chronic obstructive disease, clubbing; photophobia, failure to thrive, female carriers with linear macular nevoid Blaschko-esque hyperpigmentation; gastroenteritis, diarrhea; intronic mutation of *POLA1* gene *JAMA Derm 153:817–818, 2017; Ped Derm 32:871–872, 2015; Am J Med Genet 161:1414–1420, 2013; Eur J Dermatol 18:102–103, 2008; Ped Derm 22:122–126, 2005; Semin Cut Med Surg 16:72–80, 1997; Am J Med Genet 32:115–119, 1989; Am J Med Gen 10:65–75, 1981*

    Differential diagnosis includes:
        Dermatopathia pigmentosa reticularis – adermatoglyphia, palmoplantar keratoderma, non-scarring alopecia; mutation in *K14*
        Dowling-Degos syndrome – *K5* mutation
        Dyskeratosis congenital – mutation in *DKC1*
        Naegeli-Franceschetti-Jadassohn syndrome
        Myloidois cutis dyschromia
        Rothmund-Thomson syndrome
        Kindler's syndrome

Xeroderma pigmentosum – early acute sunburn, persistent erythema, freckling – initially discrete, then fuse to irregular patches of hyperpigmentation, dryness on sun-exposed areas; with time telangiectasias and small angiomas, atrophic white macules develop; vesiculobullous lesions, superficial ulcers lead to scarring, ectropion; multiple malignancies; photophobia, conjunctivitis, ectropion, symblepharon, neurologic abnormalities; short stature, conjunctivitis, photophobia, pyogenic granulomas in toddlers *JAAD 75:855–870, 2016; BJD 168:1109–1113, 2013; Adv Genet 43:71–102, 2001; Hum Mutat 14:9–22, 1999; Mol Med Today 5:86–94, 1999; Derm Surg 23:447–455, 1997; Dermatol Clin 13:169–209, 1995; Recent Results Cancer Res 128:275–297, 1993; AD 123:241–250, 1987; Ann Int Med 80:221–248, 1974;* XP variant *AD 128:1233–1237, 1992*

TOXINS

Mercury exposure – anorexia, weight loss, photosensitivity, sweaty palms *Lancet 336:1578–1579, 1990*

TRAUMA

Air bag dermatitis *AD 138:1383–1384, 2002*

Radiation therapy – radiation recall; ultraviolet recall manifested as edema, erythema, bullae, hemorrhagic crusting, macules, papules, ulceration, necrosis *JAAD 56:494–499, 2007;*

post-radiation activation of actinic keratoses

Spinal cord injury – development of seborrheic dermatitis *AD 83:379–385, 1961*

Sunburn

VASCULAR DISEASES

Acute hemorrhagic edema of infancy (Finkelstein's disease) *AD 139:531–536, 2003; Cutis 68:127–129, 2001; J Dermatol 28:279–281, 2001; Cutis 61:283–284, 1998; AD 130:1055–1060, 1994*

Emboli – from cardiac myxomas; red-violet malar flush *BJD 147:379–382, 2002*

Hereditary benign telangiectasia – autosomal dominant; lips, neck, trunk, arms, hands, and knees; photodistributed *JAAD 57:814–818, 2007; Ped Derm 6:194–197, 1989; Trans St.Johns Hosp Dermatol Soc 57:148–156, 1971*

Idiopathic systemic capillary leak syndrome – skin-colored or red papules of face, neck, abdomen, upper back, elbows, and hands; purpuric macules of lateral fingers, infiltrative edema of hands with sclerodermoid appearance, livedo reticularis of lower extremities; photodistributed eruption of face, neck, and arms *Dermatology 209:291–295, 2004*

Livedo reticularis, photosensitive *AD 108:100–101, 1973;* quinidine-induced photosensitive livedo reticularis *AD 125:417–418, 1989; JAAD 12:332–336, 1985*

Mitral stenosis – malar flush

Primary pulmonary hypertension

Superior vena cava obstruction – suffusion of face *Rev Med Interne 40:480–481, 2019; Emerg Med Clin NA 36:577–584, 2018; Clin Exp Dermatol 25:198–200, 2000*

Takayasu's arteritis

Temporal arteritis *BJD 76:299–308, 1964*

Vasculitis

PIGMENTARY RETINOPATHY OR CONE-ROD DYSTROPHY WITH DERMATOLOGIC MANIFESTATIONS

BJD 164:878–880, 2011

Alopecia areata – lens involvement, pigmentary clumping

Alstrom syndrome – acanthosis nigricans, alopecia, hirsutism; dilated cardiomyopathy, insulin resistance, short stature, hyperlipidemia, scoliosis, renal failure; mutation in *ALMS1*; subcapsular cataracts; cone-rod dystrophy, photophobia, nystagmus, blindness

CINCA syndrome (chronic infantile neurologic cutaneous and articular syndrome; NOMID) *JAAPOS 20:365–368, 2016*

Cone-rod congenital amaurosis – congenital hypertrichosis, hirsutism, cone-rod dystrophy

Edwards syndrome – acanthosis nigricans, pigmentary retinopathy, similar to ALMS but with mental retardation

HJDM (congenital hypotrichosis with juvenile macular dystrophy) – alopecia, congenital hypotrichosis, fusiform beading of hair shaft, pili torti; mutation in *CDH3* (gene encoding p-cadherin)

Hypotrichosis, cadherin 3 mutation *Doc Ophthalmol 138:153–160, 2019*

Jalili syndrome – autosomal recessive; cone-rod dystrophy and amelogenesis imperfect *PLoS One 8 (10);e78529.doi:10.1371/journa.pore 0078529*

Joubert syndrome – hirsutism, pigmentary retinopathy; mutation in *OFD* (ciliary protein disorder)

Lipodystrophy with congenital cataracts and neurodegeneration – acanthosis nigricans, pigmentary retinopathy, congenital cataracts, nystagmus, ocular dysmetria, juvenile macular (cone-rod) dystrophy

Mulibrey nanism (muscle, liver, brain, eye nanism) – acanthosis nigricans, cutaneous nevi on limbs, pigmentary retinopathy, macular changes, hypoplasia of choroid, astigmatism, strabismus

Mucopolysaccharidosis type IIIc (Sanfilippo syndrome) – hirsutism, coarse hair, pigmentary retinopathy; mutation in *HGSNAT*

Mutation CEP78 – hearing loss, ciliopathy *Am J Hum Genet 99:770–776, 2016*

Oliver-MacFarlane syndrome – frontal alopecia, trichomegaly, long eyebrows, pigmentary retinopathy, ring iris heterochromia, nystagmus

PITUITARY DISEASE, CUTANEOUS MANIFESTATIONS

AUTOIMMUNE DISEASES AND DISORDERS OF IMMUNE DYSREGULATION

Dermatomyositis and central diabetes insipidus *Endocrinol Diabetes Metab Case Rep Feb7, 2020 pii EDN 190070*

IgG4 disease – multisystem inflammatory disease with papules, plaques, and nodules; parotitis with parotid gland swelling, lacrimal gland swelling, dacryoadenitis, sialadenitis, proptosis; idiopathic pancreatitis, retroperitoneal fibrosis, aortitis; Mikuliczs syndrome, angio lymphadenopathy with eosinophilia, Riedel's thyroiditis, biliary tract disease, renal disease, meningeal disease, pituitary gland; Kuttner tumor, Rosai-Dorfman disease; elevated IgG4 with plasma cell dyscrasia, diffuse or localized swelling or masses; lymphocytic and plasma cell infiltrates with storiform fibrosis *Clin Rheumatol 37:1153–1159, 2018; NEJM 375:1469–1480, 2016; JAAD 75:177–185, 2016*

DRUG REACTIONS

Bromocriptine-induced bromoderma in a pituitary adenoma *J Dermatol 44:e95–99, 2017*

DRESS and syndrome of inappropriate ADH ((SIADH) *Intern Med 55:1393–1396, 2016; Clin Exp Dermatol 33:287–290, 2008*

Iatrogenic Cushing's syndrome – topical steroid abuse in psoriasis *Dermatol Ther May 6, 2020:e13514; Case Rep Endocrinol 2017:8320254 Nov 13, 2017; Indian J Dermatol 61:120, 2016*

Ipilimumab – hypophysitis (anterior and posterior pituitary), uveitis with metastatic melanoma *J Natl Compr Canc Netw 12:1077–1081, 2014*

INFECTIONS

Exanthem subitum and SIADH *Pediatr Infect Dis 16:532–533, 1997*

Herpes virus-6 infection – rash and SIADH *Pediatr Int 46:497–498, 2004*

Leprosy *Indian J Endocrinol Metab 19:369–372, 2015*

Tuberculosis *Intern Med 54:1247–1251, 2015*

INFILTRATIVE DISORDERS

Erdheim-Chester disease (non-Langerhans cell histiocytosis) – CD68+ and factor XIIIa+; negative for CD1a and S100; xanthoma and xanthelasma-like lesions (red-brown-yellow papules and plaques); flat wart-like papules of face; lesions occur in folds; skin becomes slack with atrophy of folds and face; also lesions of

eyelids, axillae, groin, neck; pretibial dermopathy, pigmented lesions of lips and buccal mucosa; long bone sclerosis; diabetes insipidus, painless exophthalmos, retroperitoneal fibrosis, renal (hairy kidneys), cerebellar syndrome, and pulmonary histiocytic infiltration; differential diagnosis includes Graves' disease, Hashimoto's thyroiditis, sarcoid *J Cutan Pathol 38:280–285, 2011; Int J Urol 15:455–456, 2008; Austral J Dermatol 44:194–198, 2003; JAAD 57:1031–1045, 2007; AD 143:952–953, 2007; Hautarzt 52:510–517, 2001; Medicine (Baltimore) 75:157–169, 1996; Virchow Arch Pathol Anat 279:541–542, 1930; diabetes insipidus BMJ Case Rep Oct 17, 2018*

Juvenile xanthogranuloma – central diabetes insipidus, growth hormone deficiency, panhypopituitarism *Pediatr Blood Cancer May 8, 2020:e28381*

Langerhans cell histiocytosis in adult *Praxis (Bern 1994)99:381–384, 2010;* fever, hyperprolactinemia *An Med Interna 22:535–537, 2005*

Xanthoma disseminatum – hypopituitarism *JAMA Derm 153:813–814, 2017;* rash, diabetes insipidus, laryngeal stenosis *NEJM 328:1138–1143, 1998*

INFLAMMATORY DISORDERS

Sarcoidosis *Pan Afr Med J June 7, 2019:33–92, doi:11604;* hypopituitarism *Pituitary 19:19–29, 2016;* neurosarcoidosis *J Neurol 264:1023–1028, 2017*

METABOLIC DISORDERS

Acromegaly *Clin Dermatol 38:79–85, 2020;* cutis verticis gyrate *NEJM 380:e31, 2019*

Cushing's syndrome *Clin Dermatol 38:79–85, 2020*

Delayed puberty – panhypopituitarism, developmental defects of the pituitary; tumors (craniopharyngioma, germinoma)

Fanconi's anemia – autosomal recessive; endocrine abnormalities with hypothyroidism, decreased growth hormone, diabetes mellitus, café au lait macules, diffuse hyperpigmented macules, guttate hypopigmented macules, intertriginous hyperpigmentation, skeletal anomalies (thumb hypoplasia, absent thumbs, radii, carpal bones), oral/genital erythroplasia with development of squamous cell carcinoma, hepatic tumors, microphthalmia, ectopic or horseshoe kidney, broad nose, epicanthal folds, micrognathia, bone marrow failure, acute myelogenous leukemia, solid organ malignancies (brain tumors, Wilms' tumor) *BJD 164:245–256, 2011; JAAD 54:1056–1059, 2006*

Generalized pruritus – diabetes insipidus

Growth hormone deficiency – short stature *NEJM 368:1220–1228, 2013*

Hemochromatosis – hypogonadotropic hypogonadism *Am J Case Rep April 24, 2020; 21:e923108*

Hyperprolactinemia – pituitary microadenoma *Arch Gynecol Obstet 264:90–92, 2000;* macroproprolactinoma *Minerva Endocrinol 21:67–71, 1996;* prolactinomas *Clin Endocrinol (Oxf) 30:131–140, 1989;* primary hypothyroidism *Curr Ther Endocrinol Metab 6:223–226, 1997*

Hypopituitarism – yellow tinge to skin with pallor; Sheehan's syndrome – yellow, dry skin diffuse loss of pigment

NEOPLASTIC DISORDERS

Carcinoid tumor of pituitary *Natl Med J India 29:209–211, 2016*

Hypothalamic-pituitary germinoma – presented as generalized hypohidrosis *Eur J Dermatol 17: 297–299, 2017*

Methotrexate associated lymphoproliferative disorder – multiple subcutaneous nodules and hypopituitarism *Endocrinol Diabetes Metab Case Rep Oct 12, 2019; pii: EDM 190082*

Rosai-Dorfman disease *Clin Endocrinol (Oxf) 50:133–137, 1999*

PARANEOPLASTIC DISORDERS

SIADH, T-cell lymphoma – pruritus and papular exanthem *Dtsch Med Wochenschr 140:997–1000, 2015*

SYNDROMES

Behcet's disease – lymphocytic hypophysitis *Neuro Endocrinol Lett 39:43–48, 2018*

Carney complex – pituitary adenoma *Exp Clin Endocrinol Diabetes 127:156–164, 2019; Clin Dermatol 24:299–316, 2006*

Cleft lip-palate and pituitary dysfunction *Syndromes of the Head and Neck p. 781, 1990*

Cowden's syndrome *QJM 111:735–736, 2018*

Fleisher syndrome – X-linked, proportionate short stature, hypo-gammaglobulinemia, isolated growth hormone deficiency *Am J Med Genet 66:378–398, 1996*

Maffucci's syndrome (enchondromatosis) – enchondromas and multiple venous malformations; spindle cell hemangioendothelioma; oral and intra-abdominal venous and lymphatic anomalies; short stature, shortened long bones with pathologic fractures; enchondromas undergo sarcomatous change in 30–40%; breast, ovarian, pancreatic, parathyroid, pituitary tumors *JAAD 56:541–564, 2007; Ped Derm 17:270–276, 2000; Ped Derm 12:55–58, 1995*

MEN I – most common pituitary tumors are prolactinoma, growth hormone producing, ACTH producing, gonadotrophin and non-functioning *Clin Dermatol 24:299–316, 2010*

Neurofibromatosis type I associated panhypopituitarism *BMJ Case Rep Nov 3, 2015*

Oliver-McFarlane syndrome – autosomal recessive; trichomegaly, pigmentary degeneration of retina (retinitis pigmentosa), mental and growth retardation, peripheral neuropathy, anterior pituitary deficiencies *Br J Ophthalmol 87:119–120, 2003; Can J Ophthalmol 28:191–193, 1993; Genet Couns 2:115–118, 1991; Am J Med Genet 34:199–201, 1989; Am J Ophthalmol 101:490–491, 1986; Am J Dis Child 121:344–345, 1971; Arch Ophthalmol 74:169–171, 1965*

Panhypopituitary dwarfism – short stature, excess subcutaneous fat, high pitched voice, soft, wrinkled skin, child-like facies *Birth Defects 12:15–29, 1976*

POEMS syndrome *J Clin Endocrinol Metab 104:2140–2146, 2019; BMC Endocr Disord March 22, 2019*

Sheehan's syndrome *BMJ Case Rep Feb 3, 2018*

VASCULAR DISORDERS

Granulomatosis with polyangiitis *Arthritis Rheum 71:1124, 2019; Rheumatol Int 39:1467–1476, 2019; Pituitary 20:594–601, 2017*

PHACES syndrome – hypopituitarism with growth hormone deficiency *J Pediatr Endocrinol Metab 32:1283–1286, 2019; Sem Cut Med Surg 35:108–116, 2016*

PITYRIASIS ROSEA-LIKE ERUPTIONS

AUTOIMMUNE DISEASES AND DISEASES OF IMMUNE DYSFUNCTION

Bone marrow transplant *JAAD 31:348–351, 1994*

Graft vs. host disease – inverse pityriasis rosea-like eruption *Ped Derm 35:343–353, 2018; JAAD 72:690–695, 2015; J Cut Med Surg 14:249–253, 2010*

Lupus erythematosus – subacute cutaneous lupus erythematosus *JAAD 35:147–169, 1996*

DRUG-INDUCED

Checkpoint inhibitors – pityriasis rosea-like eruptions *JAAD 80:990–997, 2019*

Influenza vaccine – widespread lichenoid eruption *J Drugs Dermatol 13:873–875, 2014*

Lichen planus-like drug eruption

Pityriasis rosea-like drug reactions *JAAD Case Rep 4:800–801, 2018; JAAD 61:303–318, 2009; JAAD 31:348–351, 1994; JAAD 15:159–167, 1986*
  Adalimumab *J Eur Acad DV 21:1294–1296, 2007*
  Allopurinol *Indian J Pharmacol 44:792–797, 2012*
    Arsenicals *JAAD 15:159–167, 1986*
  Asenapine *J Drugs Dermatol 12:1050–1051, 2013*
    Barbiturates *AD 118:186–187, 1982*
  BCG (bacillus Calmette-Guerin) therapy *Cutis 57:447–450, 1996; Isr J Med Sci 25:570–572, 1989;* intravesical *Ann Dermatol 24:360–362, 2012*
    Beta blockers, atenolol *Hum Exp Toxicol 35:229–231, 2016*
    Bismuth, including bismuth subsulfate *Cutis 77:166–168, 2006*
  Bupropion *Hum Exp Toxicol 33:1294–1296, 2014*
    Captopril *AD 118:186–187, 1982.*
  Chloroquine
  Clonidine
  Clozapine *Neuropsychiatr Dis Treat 11:2547–2549, 2015; Gen Hosp Psychiatry 34:703, 2012*
  Diphtheria toxoid *JAAD 5:475–476, 1981*
  Ergotamine tartrate *J Dermatol 32:407–409, 2005*
  Etanercept *Eur Rev Med Pharmacol Sci 13:383–387, 2009*
  Pooled gamma globulin
  Gold *Ann Rheum Dis 51:881–884, 1992*
  Graft vs. host disease
    Griseofulvin
  Hepatitis B vaccination *Clin Exp Rheumatol 18:81–85, 2000*
  Ibrutinib *JAAD Case Rep 4:55–57, 2017*
  Imatinib mesylate (multikinase inhibitor) *JAAD 58:545–570, 2008; JAAD 53:S240–243, 2005; AD 323 (suppl 3) S360–363, 201*
  Infliximab *J Dermatol 41:354–355, 2014*
  Isotretinoin dermatitis *Cutan Oculo Toxicol 37:100–102, 2018; Cutis 34:297–300, 1984*
    Ketotifen *Dermatologica 171:355–356, 1977 (1985)*
  Kit and BCR-ABL inhibitors – imatinib, nilotinib, dasatinib – facial edema morbilliform eruptions, pigmentary changes, lichenoid reactions, psoriasis, pityriasis rosea, pustular eruptions, DRESS, Stevens-Johnson syndrome, urticarial, neutrophilic dermatoses, photosensitivity, pseudolymphoma, porphyria cutanea tarda, small vessel vasculitis, panniculitis, perforating folliculitis, erythroderma *JAAD 72:203–218, 2015*
    Lamotrigine *JAAD 68:E180–181, 2013*
    Levamisole *JAAD 15:159–167, 1986*
    Lisinopril *J Eur Acad Dermatol Venereol 18:7435, 2004*

Lithium *Clin Drug Investig 24:493–393, 2004*

MEK inhibitors (selumetinib, cobimetinib, trametinib) – pityriasis rosea-like hypersensitivity reactions *JAMA Derm 151:78–81, 2015*

Methoxypromazine *JAAD 15:159–167, 1986*

Metronidazole *AD 113:1457–1458, 1977*

Nortriptyline *J Low Genit Tract Dis 17:226–229, 2013*

Ondansetron *Br J Clin Pharmacol 84:1077–1080, 2018*

Organic mercurials

NSAIDS

Omeprazole *BJD 135:660–661, 1996*

Penicillamine *JAAD 15:159–167, 1986*

Penicillin

Pneumococcal vaccine *J Dermatol 30:245–247, 2003*

Pyribenzamine

Quinidine

Ranitidine

Rituximab *J Dermatol 40:495–496, 2013*

Salvarson

Smallpox vaccination *JAAD 15:159–167, 1986*

Terbinafine *Indian J Pharmacol 47:680–681, 2015; BJD 138:529–532, 1998*

Thiazides

Tripelennamine *AD 118:186–187, 1982*

Tyrosine kinase inhibitors

Vaccines – diphtheria, smallpox, pneumococcal, hepatitis B, BCG *J Eur Acad DV 30:544–545, 2016*

Vasotec

EXOGENOUS AGENTS

Herbicides *JAAD 15:159–167, 1986*

Mustard oil (topical) *Indian J Dermatol Venereol Leprol 71:282–284, 2005*

INFECTIONS AND INFESTATIONS

Brucellosis *Cutis 63:25–27, 1999; AD 117:40–42, 1981*

Covid-19 infection – digitate papulosquamous eruption *JAMA Derm 156:819–820, 2020*

Gianotti-Crosti syndrome – mimics inverse papular PR *J R Coll Physicians Edinb 45:218–225, 2015*

HHV 6/HHV7 *Dermatology 230:23–26, 2015; JID 119:793–797, 2002*

HIV – pityriasis rosea-like exanthem *Mayo Clin Proc 67:1089–1108, 1992; JAAD 22 (pt 2)1270–1272, 1990*

Leishmaniasis

Leprosy *AD 147:345–350, 2011; Clin Inf Dis 35:1388–1389, 2002; JAAD 15:204–208, 1986;* borderline tuberculoid leprosy mimicking cutaneous T-cell lymphoma *SKINmed 11:379–381, 2013*

Pinworm infestation (*Enterobius vermicularis*) *Acta DV 70:526–529, 1990*

Scabies *Cureus 9:e1961, 2017*

Scrub typhus (*Orienta tsutsugamuchi*) – eschar and exanthem *NEJM 373:2455, 2015*

Syphilis, secondary – macular syphilids morbilliform or papular (copper red; *J Clin Inf Dis 21:1361–1371, 1995*

Tinea corporis – *Trichophyton rubrum, T. megninii, Epidermophyton floccosum Am Fam Physician 97:38–44, 2018; Mycoses 52:67–71, 2009; T. verrucosum* – extensive annular lesions of trunk and neck *AD 94:35–37, 1966*

Tinea versicolor *Semin Dermatol 4:173–184, 1985*

Varicella – personal observation

Viral exanthem

Yaws – secondary pianides

INFILTRATIVE DISEASES

Amyloid elastoidosis *AD 121:498, 1985*

Lymphocytoma cutis – personal observation

INFLAMMATORY DISEASES

Erythema multiforme

Lymphocytoma cutis

Sarcoid – personal observation

NEOPLASTIC DISEASES

Castleman's disease – widespread oval hyperpigmented patches *JAAD 65:430–432, 2011*

Familial cutaneous collagenoma *JAAD 40:255–257, 1999*

Kaposi's sarcoma *Clin in Dermatol 38:52–62, 2020; JAMA 313:514–515, 2015; Cutis 56:104–106, 1995; Cutis 31, 1982;* HIV associated Kaposi's sarcoma; in HIV disease with immune reconstitution syndrome *NEJM 369:1152–1161, 2013*

Leiomyomas, multiple (Reed syndrome) *The Dermatologist, July 2016, pp.47–49; JAAD 62:168–170, 2010; AD 120:1618–1620, 1984*

Leukemia cutis – myeloid dendritic cell leukemia *BJD 158:1129–1133, 2008;* acute myelogenous leukemia; relapse presenting as pityriasis rosea – personal observation

Lymphoma – acute lymphoblastic leukemia with T-cell lymphoma; cutaneous T-cell lymphoma *Cutis 100:56–58, 2018; JAAD 70:205–220, 2014; AD 133:649–654, 1997;* eruptive Hodgkin's disease – presenting as atypical pityriasis rosea *J Dermatol Case Rep 30:81–84, 2015; AD 133:649–654, 1997;* epidermotropic B-cell lymphoma *Am J Dermatopathol 38:105–112, 2016;* epidermotropic CXCR3 marginal zone lymphoma *Dermatol Online J 25:13030, July 15, 2019*

Lymphomatoid papulosis

Metastases, signet ring cancer of bladder *Cutis 49:324, 1992;* bronchogenic carcinoma *AD 133:649–654, 1997;* breast cancer – personal observation

Plasmacytomas – primary cutaneous plasmacytosis – brown–red macules; polyclonal hypergammaglobulinemia and lymphadenopathy *JAAD 56:S38–40, 2007; Dermatol 189:251, 1994; JAAD 31:897–900, 1994; AD 122:1314, 1986; Atlantic Derm Meeting, May 1994; Atlantic Derm Meeting, May 2000*

Seborrheic keratoses *J Dermatol 25:272–274, 1998*

PRIMARY CUTANEOUS DISEASES

Acute parapsoriasis (pityriasis lichenoides et varioliformis acuta) (Mucha-Habermann disease) *AD 123:1335–1339, 1987; AD 118:478, 1982*

Anetoderma of Jadassohn *AD 120:1032–1039, 1984*

Annular lichenoid dermatitis of youth *JAMA Derm 154:357–358, 2018; JAAD 49:1029–1036, 2003*

Digitate dermatosis (small plaque parapsoriasis) (persistent superficial dermatitis) *New England Dermatological Society Conference, Sept 15, 2007; Ann Dermatol Syph 3:433–468, 1902*

Erythema annulare centrifugum – personal observation

Erythema dyschromicum perstans *JAAD 44:351–353, 2001; Int J Dermatol 43:230–232, 2004; Acta Derm Ven 54:69*

Lichen planus

Nummular dermatitis *Am Fam Physician 97:38–44, 2018*

Parakeratosis variegata

Parapsoriasis en plaque *JAAD 5:373–395, 1981*

Generalized pigmented purpuric eruption – personal observation

Pityriasis alba

Pityriasis lichenoides chronica *The Dermatologist p.47, July, 2014; The Clinical Management of Itching; Parthenon; p. 137, 2000; Ped Derm 15:1–6, 1998*

Pityriasis rosea *JAAD 61:303–318, 2009; JAAD 15:159–167, 1986;* atypical pityriasis rosea; vesicular pityriasis rosea *Lancet 2:493, 1971;* purpuric *JAAD 28:1021, 1993;* purpuric PR with palatal petechiae *Dermatologica 160:142–144, 1980;* urticarial PR *JAMA 82:178–183, 1924;* papular PR *Cutis 70:51–55, 2002;* unilateral PR *JAMA 82:178–183, 1924; BJD 26:329, 1914*

Pityriasis rubra pilaris – personal observation

Post-inflammatory hyperpigmentation after pityriasis rosea

Psoriasis, guttate – personal observation

Seborrheic dermatitis

Sebo-psoriasis (seborrhiasis)

Surrounding nevi – Meyerson's phenomenon

Acute urticaria – personal observation

SYNDROMES

Epidermodysplasia verruciformis – pityriasis rosea-like appearance *BJD 145:669–670, 2001*

MEN2A – dermal hyperneury with pityriasis rosea-like papules *JAMA Derm 153:1298–1301, 2017*

Reed syndrome – leiomyomatosis *The Dermatologist July, 2016, pp47–49*

VASCULAR DISEASES

Purpura annularis telangiectoides – personal observation

PLANTAR ERYTHEMA

AUTOIMMUNE DISEASES AND DISEASES OF IMMUNE DYSFUNCTION

Allergic contact dermatitis

Angioedema

Bullous pemphigoid *Cureus Jan 11, 2020;12 (1) e6630*

Dermatomyositis *Indian J Dermatol 57:375–381, 2012;* anti-synthetase syndrome *BJM 111:329–330, 2018*

Graft vs. host reaction

Lupus erythematosus – systemic; neonatal lupus erythematosus – annular plaque of sole *AD 142:1351–1356, 2006*

Rheumatoid arthritis, including rheumatoid neutrophilic dermatitis

CONGENITAL ANOMALIES

Syringomyelia

DEGENERATIVE DISEASES

Acral localized acquired cutis laxa *JAAD 21:33–40, 1989*

Neurotrophic erythema

DRUG-INDUCED

Acral erythema of proximal nail fold and onychodermal band due to cyclophosphamide and vincristine *Cutis 52:43–44, 1993*

Bromocriptine ingestion mimicking erythromelalgia *Neurology 31:1368–1370, 1981*

Chemotherapy-induced acral dysesthesia syndrome (palmoplantar erythrodysesthesia syndrome) *Stat Pearls Oct 25, 2019–2020; JAAD 24:457–461, 1991; AD 122:1023–1027, 1986*

Chemotherapy-induced Raynaud's phenomenon

Dermatomyositis-like lesions associated with long term hydroxyurea administration *JAAD 21:797–799, 1989*

Drug eruption

DRESS syndrome

Nifedipine ingestion mimicking erythromelalgia *JAAD 21:797–799, 1989*

Nivolumab infusion reaction *Thoracic Cancer 8:706–709, 2017*

Oral contraceptives

EXOGENOUS AGENTS

Irritant contact dermatitis

INFECTIONS AND INFESTATIONS

Cellulitis

Clostridial sepsis

Covid-19 – Kawasaki-like illness in children

Endocarditis, including acute and subacute bacterial endocarditis

Erysipelas

Erythrasma

HIV – acute HIV infection – acral erythema *Cutis 40:171–175, 1987*

Human parechovirus *Virusu 65:17–26, 2015*

Japanese spotted fever *Emerging Infect Dis 24:1633–1641, 2018; Kansenshogaku Zasshi 85:638–643, 2011*

Leprosy – erythroderma *An Bras Dermatol 94:86–92, 2019*

Leptospirosis

Measles – atypical measles

Meningococcemia

Parvovirus B19 (erythema infectiosum) *Hum Pathol 31:488–497, 2000;* including papular pruritic petechial glove and sock syndrome *Cutis 54:335–340, 1994*

Pitted keratolysis – painful plaque-like pitted keratolysis *Ped Derm 9:251–254, 1992*

Pseudomonas hot-foot syndrome – 1–2 cm plantar nodules; spontaneous resolution in 14 days *NEJM 345:335–338, 2001*

Rat bite fever

Rocky Mountain spotted fever

Scabies

Syphilis – secondary

Tinea pedis

Toxic shock syndrome, either staphylococcal or streptococcal – erythema and edema of the palms and soles *JAAD 39:383–398, 1998*

Viral exanthem

INFILTRATIVE DISORDERS

Mastocytosis

INFLAMMATORY DERMATOSES

Erythema multiforme *Dermatology 207:386–389, 2003*

Erythema nodosum *Dermatology 199:190, 1999; JAAD 29:284, 1993; AD 129:1064–1065, 1993;* unilateral in sarcoid *Arthritis Rheumatol 70:297, 2018*

Goodpasture's syndrome – annular erythematous macule *AD 121:1442–1444, 1985*

Lipoatrophic panniculitis *AD 123:1662–1666, 1987*

Neutrophilic eccrine hidradenitis

METABOLIC DISEASES

Acrodermatitis enteropathica

Antiphospholipid antibody syndrome

Cold agglutinins

Cryofibrinogenemia

Cryoglobulinemia

Diabetes mellitus

Hyperestrogenic states – liver disease, exogenous estrogens

Hyperthyroidism

Polycythemia vera – acral ischemia with lividity

Pregnancy

Pseudoglucagonoma syndrome due to malnutrition *AD 141:914–916, 2005*

Thrombocythemia – acral ischemia with lividity, livedo reticularis, acrocyanosis, erythromelalgia, gangrene, pyoderma gangrenosum *Leuk Lymphoma 22 Suppl 1:47–56, 1996; Br J Haematol 36:553–564, 1977; AD 87:302–305, 1963*

NEOPLASTIC DISEASES

Angioimmunoblastic lymphadenopathy

Atrial myxoma *Br Heart J 36:839–840, 1974*

Eccrine angiomatous hamartoma (painful) *AD 125:1489–1490, 1989*

Leukemia – chronic myelogeous leukemia with leukostasis (livedo) *AD 123:921–924, 1987*

Lymphoma – angioimmunoblastic T- or B-cell lymphoma

Plantar fibromatosis *JAAD 12:212–214, 1985*

Waldenstrom's macroglobulinemia

PARANEOPLASTIC DISEASES

Bazex syndrome

Necrolytic migratory erythema (glucagonoma syndrome) *Biomedica 36:176–181, 2016*

Necrotizing eccrine squamous syringometaplasia *J Cutan Pathol 18:453–456, 1991*

PRIMARY CUTANEOUS DISEASES

Atopic foot dermatitis *Ped Derm 18:102–106, 2001*

Circumscribed palmar or plantar hypokeratosis – red atrophic patch *JAAD 51:319–321, 2004; JAAD 49:1197–1198, 2003; JAAD 47:21–27, 2002*

Epidermolytic hyperkeratosis

Erythroderma

Erythrokeratolysis hiemalis (Oudtshoorn disease) (keratolytic winter erythema) – palmoplantar erythema, cyclical and centrifugal peeling of affected sites, targetoid lesions of the hands and feet – seen in South African whites; precipitated by cold weather or fever *BJD 98:491–495, 1978*

Erythrokeratoderma variabilis

Follicular mucinosis, erythrodermic

Granuloma annulare, generalized *JAAD 20:39–47, 1989*

Greither's palmoplantar keratoderma (transgrediens et progrediens palmoplantar keratoderma) – red hands and feet; hyperkeratoses extending over Achilles tendon, backs of hands, elbows, knees; livid erythema at margins *Ped Derm 20:272–275, 2003; Cutis 65:141–145, 2000*

Hereditary palmo-plantar erythema (Lane's disease) *Ped Derm 34:590–594, 2017; JAAD 63;E46, 2010; Rev Med Suisse Romande 79:564–571, 1959*

Juvenile plantar dermatosis – glazed erythema and fissuring of forefoot *Clin Exp Dermatol 31:453–454, 2006*

Lamellar ichthyosis

Lichen planus

Mal de Meleda – autosomal dominant, autosomal recessive transgrediens with acral erythema in glove-like distribution *Dermatology 203:7–13, 2001; AD 136:1247–1252, 2000; J Dermatol 27:664–668, 2000; Dermatologica 171:30–37, 1985*

Palmoplantar pustulosis

Pityriasis rubra pilaris

Progressive symmetric erythrokeratoderma

Psoriasis

Symmetrical lividity of the soles *BJD 37:123–125 1985; BJD 37:123–125, 1925*

SYNDROMES

Eosinophilia myalgia syndrome *JAAD 23:1063–1069, 1990*

Familial Mediterranean fever (erysipelas-like lesions) *Acta Pediatr 20:382–385, 2013;* palmoplantar erythema *Frontiers in Immunology 10:1–24, 2019*

Hereditary lactate dehydrogenase M-subunit deficiency – annually recurring acroerythema *JAAD 27:262–263, 1992*

Ichthyosis follicularis with atrichia and photophobia (IFAP) – palmo-plantar erythema; collodion membrane and erythema at birth; ichthyosis, spiny (keratotic) follicular papules (generalized follicular keratoses), non-scarring alopecia, keratotic papules of elbows, knees, fingers, extensor surfaces, xerosis; punctate keratitis, photophobia; nail dystrophy, psychomotor delay, short stature; enamel dysplasia, beefy red tongue and gingiva, angular stomatitis, atopy, lamellar scales, psoriasiform plaques *Curr Prob Derm 14:71–116, 2002; JAAD 46:S156–158, 2002; BJD 142:157–162, 2000; Ped Derm 12:195, 1995; AD 125:103–106, 1989; Dermatologica 177:341–347, 1988; Am J Med Genet 85:365–368, 1999*

Kawasaki's disease *JAAD 39:383–398, 1998; Praxis (Bern 1994) 85:1211–1216, 1996*

Netherton's syndrome

Schopf-Schulz-Passarge syndrome – psoriasiform plantar dermatitis (palmoplantar keratoderma); eyelid cysts (apocrine hidrocystomas), hypotrichosis, decreased number of teeth, brittle and furrowed nails *AD 140:231–236, 2004; BJD 127:33–35, 1992; JAAD 10:922–925, 1984; Birth Defects XII:219–221, 1971*

Wells' syndrome – red plaques of soles *Cutis 72:209–212, 2003*

TOXINS

Infantile acrodynia ("pink disease") (erythema with or without exfoliation; hands and feet dusky pink along with nose: "puffy, pink, painful, paresthetic, perspiring and peeling" hands and feet *AD 124:107–109, 1988*

TRAUMA

Chilblains (perniosis) *JAAD 23:257–262, 1990*

Cold erythema *JAMA 180:639–42, 1962*

Delayed pressure urticaria

Frostbite, recovery phase

Heat exposure

Reflex sympathetic dystrophy (causalgia), Stage 1 *JAAD 50:456–460, 2004; JAAD 22:513–520, 1990*

Traumatic plantar urticaria (delayed pressure urticaria) *JAAD 18:144–146, 1988*

Vibratory urticaria

VASCULAR DISEASES

Acquired progressive lymphangioma – plantar red plaques *JAAD 49:S250–251, 2003*

Acrocyanosis

Acrocyanosis with atrophy *AD 124:263–268, 1988*

Angiodyskinesia – dependent erythema after prolonged exercise or idiopathic *Surgery 61:880–890, 1967*

Arteriosclerotic peripheral vascular disease – dependent erythema of the dorsum of the foot (Buerger's sign) *JAAD 50:456–460, 2004*

Emboli – cholesterol, septic, fat

Erythrocyanosis

Erythromelalgia – associations include essential thrombocythemia, polycythemia vera, diabetes mellitus, peripheral neuropathy, systemic lupus erythematosus, rheumatoid arthritis, hypertension, frostbite, colon cancer, gout, calcium channel blockers, bromocriptine *JAAD 50:456–460, 2004;* all types exacerbated by warmth; may affect one finger or toe; ischemic necrosis *JAAD 22:107–111, 1990;* primary (idiopathic) – lower legs, no ischemia *JAAD 21:1128–1130, 1989;* secondary to peripheral vascular disease *JAAD 43:841–847, 2000; AD 136:330–336, 2000;* following influenza vaccine *Clin Exp*

Rheumatol 15:111–113, 1997; erythromelalgia with thrombocythemia *JAAD 24:59–63, 1991*

Differential diagnosis of erythromelalgia *JAAD 23:166, 1990*
1. Arterial insufficiency (peripheral vascular disease, arteriosclerosis obliterans
2. Recovery phase of frostbite
3. Hyperperfusion phase of Raynaud's disease
4. Reflex sympathetic dystrophy
5. Neuropathy associated acral paresthesia and vasodilatation

Polyarteritis nodosa

Port wine stain

Raynaud's phenomenon

Thromboangiitis obliterans

Vasculitis – leukocytoclastic, other

Venous gangrene (erythema) *AD 123:933–936, 1987*

Venous stasis

PNEUMONIA AND PNEUMONIA-ASSOCIATED DISEASE, CUTANEOUS MANIFESTATIONS

AUTOIMMUNE DISEASES AND DISORDERS OF IMMUNED DYSREGULATION

Chronic granulomatous disease – autosomal recessive or X-linked recessive; defective oxidative burst in neutrophils and macrophages; *Staphylococcus aureus* and *Aspergillus spp.* Most common organisms; infection with *Burkholderia, Serratia,* or *Nocardia* warrant a screen for chronic granulomatous disease; hidradenitis suppurativa, cutaneous abscesses and pneumonia *Indian J Pediatr 83:345–353, 2016*

Common variable immunodeficiency – recurrent sinopulmonary infection, pneumonia, chronic lung disease bronchiectasis *Cureus 12 (1) e6711 Jan 20, 2020; Ped Derm 26:155–158, 2009; BJD 147:364–367, 2002; J Allergy Clin Immunol 109:581, 1999;* interstitial lung fibrosis and granulomatosis; necrotizing and sarcoidal granulomas of skin *Clin Exp Dermatol 40:379–382, 2015*

Complement deficiencies – C1q *Clin Exp Immunol 38:52–63, 1979;* pneumonia *Mol Immunol 48:1643–1655, 2011*

Dermatomyositis – anti-Jo1/anti-synthase syndrome; arthritis, Raynaud's, mechanic's hands interstitial lung disease; lung cancer; aspiration pneumonia; interstitial pneumonia , dermatomyositis, adenocarcinoma of the lung *Intern Med 57:849–853, 2018;* and thymic carcinoma *Thorac Cancer 10:2131–2034, 2019*; mechanics hands as sign of lung involvement *BMC Res Notes May 17, 2014*

Dock8 deficiency syndrome (dedicator of cytokinesis 8 gene) (autosomal recessive form of hyper IgE syndrome) – immunodeficiency; resembles Job's syndrome; decrease T and B cells; increased IgE, decreased IgM, increased eosinophilia; recurrent sinopulmonary infections, severe cutaneous viral infections and lymphopenia; warts, dermatitis, asthma, cutaneous staphylococcal abscesses; malignancies – aggressive T-cell lymphoma vulvar squamous cell carcinoma, diffuse large B-cell lymphoma; Job's syndrome may be differentiated by presence of pneumatoceles and bronchiectasis, rash at birth, osteoporosis, scoliosis, craniosynostosis, minimal trauma fractures, joint hyperextensibility; dominant negative STAT3 mutation *AD 148:79–84, 2012*

GATA2 deficiency (includes MOMOMAC syndrome, Emberger syndrome (lymphedema and myelodysplasia), familial acute leukemia and myelodysplasia) – disseminated mycobacterial infection, human papilloma virus and fungal infections, primary alveolar proteinosis, panniculitis, erythema nodosum-like lesions, primary lymphedema *BJD 170:1182–1186, 2014; Blood 123:809–821, 2014; JAAD 71:577–580, 2014*

Graft vs. host disease, chronic – rippled skin overlying deep sclerodermoid changes *JAAD 66:515–532, 2012; AD 138:924–934, 2002*

Hyper IgE syndrome (Job's, Buckley's, Quie-Hill syndromes (allergic rhinitis)) – autosomal dominant; dermatitis, recurrent cold abscesses of neck and trunk, coarse facial skin with broad nose; rough thickened skin with prominent follicular ostia; atrophoderma vermiculatum; retained primary dentition, bone abnormalities, cyst-forming pneumonia, elevated IgE levels; papular, pustular, excoriated dermatitis of scalp, buttocks, neck, axillae, groin; furunculosis; xerosis; folliculitis-like papular and papulopustular lesions; oral candida; chronic paronychia; growth failure; otitis media common; *STAT3* (transcription 3 gene activator and signal transducer) mutations (abnormality of JAK-STAT cytokine signaling pathway *Ped Derm 30:621–622, 2013; JAAD 65:1167–1172, 2011; NEJM 357:1608–1619, 2007; JAAD 54:855–865, 2006; Dermatol Therapy 18:176–183, 2005; AD 140:1119–1125, 2004; Pediatr 141:572–575, 2002; Curr Prob in Derm 10:41–92, 1998; Clin Exp Dermatol 11:403–408, 1986; Medicine 62:195–208, 1983;* pneumatoceles, recurrent pneumonia *Medicine (Baltimore) 97 (14) e2015 April 2018*

Hyper IgM syndrome – severe infections, recurrent pulmonary and diarrheal infections; mutation in gene encoding CD40 and CD40L ligand; bronchiectasis, skin infections, deep abscesses; lymphadenopathy *Clin Immunol 198:19–30, 2019*

IgG4-related disease – lung mass, pleural effusion *NEJM 373:1762–1772, 2015*

Leukocyte adhesion deficiency (beta-2 integrin deficiency) congenital deficiency of leukocyte-adherence glycoproteins (CD11a (LFA-1), CD11b, CD11c, CD18) – necrotic cutaneous abscesses, cellulitis, skin ulcerations, pyoderma gangrenosum; ulcerative stomatitis *BJD 139:1064–1067, 1998; J Pediatr 119:343–354, 1991; Ann Rev Med 38: 175–194, 1987; J Infect Dis 152:668–689, 1985;* congenital deficiency of leucocyte-adherence glycoproteins (CD11a (LFA-1), CD11b, CD11c, CD18) – necrotic cutaneous abscesses, psoriasiform dermatitis, gingivitis, periodontitis, septicemia, ulcerative stomatitis, pharyngitis, otitis, pneumonia, peritonitis *BJD 123:395–401, 1990*

leukocyte gingivitis,

Lupus erythematosus, systemic – pneumonitis *Am J Case Rep April 2020 e921299;* diffuse alveolar hemorrhage *J Clin Rheum 21:305–310, 2015*

Relapsing polychondritis – tracheal stenosis, tracheal collapse, pneumonia *Clin Rheumatol 32:1329–1335, 2013; Chest 116:1669–1675, 1999;* self-expandable stents

Rheumatoid arthritis – interstitial lung disease, nodules, unilateral pleural effusion, drug induced toxicity, Caplan syndrome (multiple peripheral pulmonary nodules in coal miners with RA) *Clin Chest Med 40:545–560, 2019*

SAVI-Sting associated vasculopathy with onset in infancy (type 1 interferonopathy) – progressive digital swelling, necrosis and amputation; red purpuric plaques over cold sensitive acral areas, nasal tip, ears, cheeks; nasal septal destruction; reticulate erythema of arms and legs; violaceous and telangiectatic malar plaques; severe interstitial lung disease *Ped Derm 33:602–614, 2016; JAAD 74:186–189, 2016; JAMA Derm 151:872–877, 2015; NEJM 371:507–518, 2014*

Scleroderma – diffuse and bilateral basilar reticulonodular infiltrates; multiple pulmonary nodules *Tuberk Toraks 60:370–374, 2012*

Sjogren's syndrome – chronic interstitial lung disease *Eur Respir Rev 25:110–123, 2016*

Still's disease – polyserositis *BMJ Case Rep April 25, 2019 12 (4) e228210;* chronic interstitial lung disease *JRSM Open Apr 2, 2020; (11)4;095440622091;* pleuritic, ARDS *Ann Rheum Dis 78:1722–1731, 2019*

Wiskott-Aldrich syndrome – X-linked congenital disease with "eczema", thrombocytopenia, and immune deficiency, recurrent pneumonia, mutation in *WASP J Clin Immunol 38:13–27, 2018*

WHIM syndrome – warts, hypoglobulinemia, infections, myelokathexis; mutation in *CXCR4 AD 146:931–932, 2010*

X-linked hypogammaglobulinemia *Medicine (Baltimore)85:193–202, 2006*

DRUG REACTIONS

All-trans-retinoic acid – Sweet's syndrome-like neutrophilic panniculitis; solitary red nodule *JAAD 56:690—693, 2007;* All-retinoic acid syndrome; fever, respiratory distress, weight gain, leg edema, pleural effusions, renal failure, pericardial effusions, hypotension, vasculitis, hypercalcemia, bone marrow necrosis and fibrosis, thromboembolic events, erythema nodosum *Leuk Lymphoma 44:547–548, 2003*

Amiodarone – blue skin and pulmonary nodules *Clin Case Rep 4:276–278, 2016*

DRESS syndrome – eosinophilic pneumonia *Respirol Case Rep Feb 20< 2020; 8 (3) e00541*

Methimazole-induced vasculitis – pulmonary hemorrhage; eschar-like leg ulcers *JAMA Derm 153:223–224, 2017*

Ustekinumab – non-infectious pneumonia *JAMA Derm 155:221–224, 2019*

EXOGENOUS AGENTS

Cocaine – pneumonitis ("crack lung") – fever, dyspnea, pleuritic chest pain, hemoptysis; pulmonary foreign body granulomas, pulmonary artery muscle hypertrophy, idiopathic pulmonary hypertension, pulmonary vascular granulomatosis *Rev Mal Respir 37:45–59, 2020; Clin Inf Dis 61:1840–1849, 2015;* crack lung – smoking crack cocaine

Intravenous drug abuse – contaminants, fillers (silica, cellulose, talc) crack lung, pulmonary foreign body granulomas, pulmonary artery muscle hypertrophy, idiopathic pulmonary hypertension, pulmonary vascular granulomatosis *Clin Inf Dis 61:1840–1849, 2015; Chem Biol Interact 206:444–451, 201*

INFECTIONS AND INFESTATIONS

Actinomycosis – sinus tracts or subcutaneous abscesses may develop adjacent to pleural abnormalities (effusions, thickening, empyema); may simulate lung cancer or tuberculosis *Semin Respir Infect 3:352–361, 1988*

Anaplasma phagocytophilum – tickborne; fever, headache, cervical lymphadenopathy, pulmonary infiltrates, macular eruption sparing the face *NEJM 373:2162–2172, 2015; NEJM 371:358–366, 2014*

Anthrax (malignant pustule) – *Bacillus anthracis;* painless ulcer with vesicular margin and surrounding edema; swollen eyelids; face, neck, hands, fingers, arms, foot, knee; starts as painless erythema evolving into papule then into multiple vesicles or bulla on red base; then ulcer with hemorrhagic crust (eschar) with edema and erythema with small vesicles; edema of surrounding skin; takes six weeks to heal; edema of eyelids, lips, perioral area; slaughtering or milking of ill cows, sheep, or goats; handling of raw meat; bioterrorism of 2001 *Ped Derm 27:600–606, 2010; Ped Derm 18:456–457, 2001; Br J Opthalmol 76:753–754, 1992; J Trop Med Hyg 89:43–45, 1986; Bol Med Hosp Infant Mex 38:355–361, 1981*; preseptal cellulitis and cicatricial ectropion *Acta Ophthalmol Scand 79:208–209, 2001; Br J Opthalmol 76:753–754, 1992; Ophthalmic Physiol Opt 10:300–301, 1990*

Ascariasis – Loeffler's-like pneumonia *JAAD 73:929–944 2015*

Aspergillosis – pneumonia with necrotic cutaneous lesion *SKINmed 13:329–330, 2015;* pulmonary cavitation, nodules with halo sign *Clin Microbiol Infect 24 (10):1105, e1–1105;* diffuse bilateral pulmonary infiltrates and nodules with hemorrhagic infarctions, *A. flavus Eur J Dermatol 12:93–98, 2002*

Babesiosis – pulmonary edema, fever, mottled skin, severe anemia *NEJM 370:753–762, 2014*

Bacillary angiomatosis – *Bartonella henselae B. quintana;* fleas and domestic cats, solitary or widespread lesions, angiomatous tumors with scaling collarette at base; friable, resembling pyogenic granulomas or skin-colored nodules *An Bras Dermatol 94:594–602, 2019*

Burkholderia pseudomallei (melioidosis) – Southeast Asia and Australia; pneumonia and cutaneous ulcers *MMWR 64:1–9 JULY 3, 2020;* deep seated abscesses, ulcers, pustules, nodules *J Clin Diagn Res 10:WD01–02, 2016;* cavitary lung lesions; lung mass and subcutaneous abscess *Am J Case Rep 16:272–275, 2015;* necrotizing pneumonia, acute suppurative parotitis *JAAD 75:1–16, 2013; Clin Inf Dis 60:243–250, 2015*

Candidiasis – congenital candidiasis – neonatal papules and vesicles; pneumonia *Cutis 93:229–232, 2014; J Perinatol 25:680–682, 2005*

Chikungunya fever – rash, fever, arthralgia, myalgia, and pneumonia *Am J Forensic Med Pathol 41:48–51, 2020*

Coccidioidomycosis – residence or travel to San Joaquin Valley, southern California or southwestern Texas, southern Arizona, New Mexico *Cutis 85:25–27, 2010; AD 144:933–938, 2008;* acute pneumonia, chronic progressive pneumonia, solitary pulmonary nodules pleural effusions, cavitary disease *Sem Resp Crit Care Med 32:754–763, 2011; ; An Circulo Med Argent 15:585–597, 1892*

Covid-19 – varicella like rash, reticulated purpura, Kawasaki-like illness in children, "covid toes"; dengue-like *JAAD 82:E177, May 2020*

Cryptococcosis – skin lesions, meningitis, and bronchopneumonia or lobar consolidation; cellulitis-like lesions *An Bras Dermatol 92 (suppl1) 69–72, 2017*

Cutaneous larva migrans – *Ancylostoma brasiliensis;* transient pulmonary infiltrates; CLM and eosinophilic pneumonia *Pneumonol Alergol Pol 79:365–370, 2011*

Cytomegalovirus – skin ulcer, purpuric morbilliform eruption, immunocompromised *Am J Clin Pathol 92:96–100, 1989*

Dengue virus – RNA Flavivirus; *Aedes aegypti, A. albopictus;* fever for 5–7 days, retro-orbital pain, red rash with islands of normal skin, flushed face, injected conjunctivae, hemorrhagic manifestations *NEJM 353:2522–2533, 2005*

Ebola virus – laboratory worker or traveler from endemic area in Africa; fever, severe headache, diarrhea, vomiting, alveolar hemorrhage, morbilliform rash of arms and trunk *NEJM 383:1382–1842, 2020*

Echinococcus granulosis (hydatid cyst) – necrotizing pneumonia, pleural effusion, cutaneous leukocytoclastic vasculitis *Turk Pediatr Ars 53:117–119, 2018*

Ehrlichiosis (*Ehrlichia chaffeensis*) – human monocytic ehrlichiosis; acute respiratory distress syndrome; fever, headache, myalgia, abdominal pain, petechial or morbilliform eruption or diffuse erythema *MMWR 65:1–44, 2016; Clin Inf Dis 34:1206–1212, 2002*

Enterovirus – hand, foot, and mouth disease with pneumonia; *Southeast Asian J Trop Med Public Health 46:449–459, 2015*

Epstein Barr virus *NEJM 373:2162–2172, 2015*

Fusarium *Clin Microbiol Infect 24 (10):1105e1–1105, 2018; Semin Respir Crit Care Med 36:706–714, 2015;* similar to aspergillus in lungs with alveolar infiltrates, nodules without halo sign, ground glass infiltrates, pleural effusions; disseminated papular and nodular skin lesions with central necrosis

Glanders – *Pseudomonas mallei* – cellulitis which ulcerates with purulent foul-smelling discharge, regional lymphatics become abscesses; nasal and palatal necrosis and destruction; metastatic papules, pustules, bullae over joints and face, then ulcerate; deep abscesses with sinus tracts occur; polyarthritis, meningitis, pneumonia

Hantavirus – exposure to rodent droppings, urine, saliva; pulmonary interstitial edema *Am J Emerg Med 31:978–982, 2013*

Herpes simplex – pneumonia in pregnancy *Obstet Med 10:58–60, 2017; Radiographics 22:S137–149, 2002*

Herpes zoster *Pediatr Int 61:1216–1220, 2019; BMJ Case Rep Sep 23, 2017; BMJ Case Rep March 20, 2013*

HHV-6 – pneumonia *Infect Drug Resist 11:701–705, 2018; J Infect 75:155–159, 2017;* HHV-6 reactivation fever and rash in immuno-compromised host; interstitial pneumonitis

H1N1 influenza – morbilliform exanthem of thighs, lower legs, and dorsal feet *AD 146:101–102, 2010*

Histoplasmosis, disseminated – crusted papulonodules *Ped Derm 27:549–551, 2010; AD 145:1447–1452, 2009; JAAD 23:422–429, 1990;* tongue nodules *Cutis 55:104–106, 1995;* facial papules, crusted papules muscle weakness, pulmonary infiltrates, morbilliform rash with scale *BJD 173:797–800, 2015*

Infective endocarditis – metastatic infection, *Staphylococcus aureus;* Austrian syndrome of meningitis, pneumonia, and endocarditis due to *Streptococcus pneumoniae Cureus April 17, 2019; 11 (4) e4486;* Olser's nodes (tips of fingers and toes, tender), splinter hemorrhages (distal third of nail), Janeway lesions (palms and soles, non-painful), Roth spots *Br J Hosp Med (London)74:C139–142, 2013; BMJ Case Rep Sep 6, 2013;* gram positive coccobacilli in the dermal abscess of Janeway lesion suggest septic microemboli are the cause *JAAD 22 (6pt1);1088–1090, 1990*

Kala azar

Legionnaire's disease (*Legionella pneumophila*) – exposure to contaminated aerosols (air coolers, hospital water supply); morbilliform, erythematous, petechial skin lesions; Legionella urine antigen testing or diagnosis *Resp Med Case Rep 15:95–100, 2015;* leg nodules *Transplant Inf Dis 16:307–314, 2014;* diffuse macular rash *Acta DV 85:343–344, 2005;* mimicking severe drug reaction *Clin Exp Dermatol 34e:72–74, 2009;* panniculitis *BMC Infect Dis 18:467, 2018;* painful non-pruritic erythematous macules, pretibial on day 5 *JAMA 245:1758–1981*

Lemierre's syndrome (human necrobacillosis) – Fusobacterium necrophorum; suppurative thrombophlebitis of tonsillar and peritonsillar veins and internal jugular vein; oropharyngeal pain, neck swelling, pulmonary symptoms, arthralgias *Clin Inf Dis 31:524–532, 2000*

Leptospirosis – exposure to wild rodents, dogs, cats, pigs, cattle, or horses or exposure to water contaminated with animal urine; outbreaks after heavy rain or flooding; chest x-ray non-specific, patchy or nodular infiltrates, lower lobes, uni- or bilateral, pulmonary hemorrhage *Respirology 23:28–35, 2018; Semin Respir Infect 12:44–49, 1997;* fever, myalgia, headache, conjunctival suffusion, pretibial macular erythema

Measles, including atypical measles *NEJM 371:358–366, 2014;* severe nodular pneumonia and atypical measles in adult *BMJ Case Rep Sep 23, 2015;* measles and pneumonia with respiratory failure *Acta Med Port 31:341–345, 2018; Clin Respir J 10:673–675, 2016*

Melioidosis – pneumonia and cutaneous ulcers *MMWR 64:1–9, July 3, 2015*

Meningococcemia, chronic – pneumonia *Clin Inf Dis 69:iii–iv, 2019*

Mycobacterium tuberculosis – scrofuloderma; bullous +PPD; – neck abscess *Cutis 85:85–89, 2010;* abscess *Ped Derm 30:7–16, 2013;* hot abscess; cold abscess (tuberculous gumma) *SKINmed 10:28–33, 2012;* tuberculous gumma (metastatic tuberculous ulcer) – firm subcutaneous nodule or fluctuant swelling breaks down to form undermined ulcer; bluish surrounding skin bound to the inflammatory mass; sporotrichoid lesions along draining lymphatics; extremities more than trunk *Am J Clin Dermatol 3:319–328, 2002; Tyring, p.327, 2002; BJD 142:387–388, 2000; Scand J Infect Dis 32:37–40, 2000; Scand J Inf Dis 35:149–152, 1993; JAAD 19:1067–1072, 1988; JAAD 6:101–106, 1982; Semin Hosp Paris 43:868–888, 1967;* of the neck *BJD 142:387–388, 2000;* paradoxical subcutaneous tuberculous abscess *J Clin Inf Dis 26:231–232, 1998; J Clin Inf Dis 24:734, 1997;* cutaneous metastatic tuberculous abscess *Ped Derm 19:90–91, 2002; Cutis 66:277–279, 2000;* nodules, lupus vulgaris; tuberculosis cutis miliaris acuta generalisita *Clin Inf Dis 57:1210–1201, 2013;* cavitary nodules, right upper lobe infiltrate, unilateral hilar adenopathy; erythema nodosum, erythema induratum, papulonecrotic tuberculid *NYS J Med 88:499–501, 1988;* lupus vulgaris turkey ear *BJD 157:816–818, 2007;* large tumors of earlobes *Cutis 67:311–314, 2001; Int J Dermatol 26:578–581, 1987;* extensive destruction *Cutis 15:499–509, 1975*

Mycobacterium haemophilum – tender erythematous papules or noodles that suppurate and ulcerate, usually on extremities; pulmonary infiltrates, nodules, cavitary lung disease *Clin Inf Dis 33:330–337, 2001;* cellulitis *JAAD 30:804–806, 1994*

Mycoplasma pneumoniae – diffuse pulmonary infiltrates, right lower lobe and apical segment of left lower lobe; mucositis; MIRM (mycoplasma-induced rash and mucositis) syndrome *J Eur Acad DV 29:595–598, 2015; JAAD 72:239–245, 2015;* morbilliform and urticarial eruptions *Dermatology 231:152–157, 2015*

Nocardia – long term immunosuppression, worsening pulmonary symptoms and relapsing pustular lesions *Case Rep Pulmon 2017:9567175; JAAD 20 (pt2)889–892, 1989;* several subcutaneous livid red nodules forearm and lung mass mimicked lung cancer *Eur J Dermatol 10:47–51, 2000*

North American blastomycosis (*Blastomyces dermatitidis*) – skin, bone, lungs and central nervous system *JAAD 21:1285–1293, 1989;* leg ulcer and pneumonia *Inf Dis Clin Pract 20:196–197, 2012;* bronchopneumonia or lobar consolidation; verrucous, warty or ulcerative plaques, misdiagnosed as keratoacanthoma, pyoderma gangrenosum *NEJM 373:955–961, 2015; NEJM 373; 1554–1564, 2015; Transpl Am Clin Climatol Assoc 125:188–202, 2014*

Paracoccidioidomycosis – Southern Mexico, parts of Central and South America; bronchopneumonia or lobar consolidation; superficial ulcer with granular appearance and hemorrhagic points (mulberry-like stomatitis), lips result in macrocheilia; gingiva, palate (sometimes palatal perforation), lips, buccal mucosa and tongue; contiguous spread to skin around mouth and nose *Clin Dermatol 30:610–615, 2012*

Paragonimus westermani – eating fresh water crabs or flesh of wild boars in East Asia; migrating subcutaneous mass with pruritus, reticulonodular lesions of right lung and pleural effusion of left lung,

eosinophilia *Intern Med 39:433–436, 2000;* cutaneous pruritic subcutaneous mass of abdomen, pleural effusion *Int J Dermatol 49:699–702, 2003;* pulmonary infiltrates *JAAD Case Reports 1:239–240, 2015*

Pasteurella multocida – skin and soft tissue infection from scratch or bite of infected dogs and cats; cellulitis *Medicine 63:133–154, 1984;* pneumonia, tracheobronchitis, empyema, lung abscess *Respir Med Case Rep 26:31–34, 2018*

Pneumocystis carinii (jirovecii) – classified as fungus (not protozoan); red or skin colored papules or nodules in ear or external auditory canal *JAAD 60:897–925, 2009;* red nodular infiltrated ear; polyps within external auditory canal *Am J Med 85:250–252, 1988;* bilateral hyperpigmented axillary nodules *Am J Med Sci 313:182–186, 1997*

Poxviridae (smallpox, generalized vaccinia) – aerosol CDC Category A bioterrorism agent, centrifugal spread of papules, then vesicles and classic pustules (pox) crusts by day 14 *Resp Care 53:40–53, 2008*

Psittacosis (*Chlamydia psittaci*) – exposure to birds (parrots, cockatoos, pigeons, turkeys) *Resp Med Case Rep 23:138–142, 2018;* peripheral ground glass opacities with consolidation in both lungs

Rat bite fever (*Streptobacillus moniliformis*) – Haverhill fever; hemorrhagic vesicles of hands and feet with petechiae *JAMA Derm 153:707–708, 2017; Clin Microbiol Rev 20:13–22, 2007;* interstitial pneumonia *Am J Clin Pathol 91:612–616, 1989;* finger pustules *NEJM 381:1762, 2019;* petechiae and acral hemorrhagic pustules and bullae with painful arthritis *Clin Inf Dis 54:1514–1515, 2012*

Rocky Mountain spotted fever *JAAD 49:363–392, 2003; Clin Inf Dis 16:629–634, 1993;* eschar at bite site; DIC *J Clin Inf Dis 21:429, 1995;* massive skin necrosis *South Med J 71:1337–1340, 1978; NEJM 373:2162–2172, 2015*

Scedosporium apiospermum – pneumonia and erythematous nodules chest, shoulders, and arms *J Cut Pathol 39:458–460, 2012*

Sporotrichosis – pulmonary cavitation *Mycopathologica 182:1119–1123, 2017; Clin Dermatol 30:437–443, 2012;* fixed and lymphocutaneous

Stenotrophomonas maltophilia – hemorrhagic pneumonia; cellulitis *J Cut Pathol 43:1017–1020, 2016;* infected mucocutaneous ulcers, metastatic cellulitis *Ann Acad Med Singapore 35:897–900, 2006*

Strongyloides hyperinfection – pneumonia *JAAD 73:929–944 2015;* thumb print purpura or periumbilical parasitic purpura *JAAD 23:324–326, 1990;* gram negative pneumonia *JAAD 73:929–944, 2015; Trop Med Infect Dis Feb 12, 2019*

Syphilis, secondary – lung abscess *Int J STD AIDS 29:1027–1032, 2018;* multiple pulmonary nodules *Korean J Intern Med 28:231–235, 2013; Chest 125:2322–2327, 2004;* "community acquired pneumonia" *Medicina (B Aires) 79:415–418, 2019;* congenital syphilis – pneumonia alba

Talaromyces (Penicillium) marneffei Emerg Microbes Inf March 9, 2016; Transplant Inf Dis 6:28–32, 2004; 14:434–439, 2012

Tropheryma whipplei (Whipples disease) *J Infect 69:103–112, 2014;* pneumonia, melanoderma, hyperpigmentation *J Infect 61:266–269, 2010*

Tularemia – exposure to infected animalas during trapping, hunting, or skinning (rabbits, hares, foxes, squirrels) or bites of infected flies, ticks *Resp Care 57:457–459, 2012;* cavitary pneumonia *Respir Care 57:457–459, 2012; Int J Dermatol 54:e33–37, 2015*

Varicella – oral vesicles, pneumonia *Arch Iran Med 21:223–225, 2018; QJM 111:827, 2018; J Clin Pathol 45:267–269, 1992*

West Nile virus – pneumonia *Transpl Ind Dis 20:800–803, 2007;* *Culex* mosquito; morbilliform eruption of trunk, encephalitis *Clin Dermatol 37:109–118, 2019*

Black death (pneumonic plague, *Yersinia pestis*) and kala azar

INFILTRATIVE DISEASES

Primary amyloidosis – pulmonary nodules, infiltrates, diffuse thin-walled cysts; peribronchovascular and subpleural *Korean J Radiol 20:1368–1380, 2019*

Erdheim-Chester disease (non-Langerhans cell histiocytosis) – CD68+ and factor XIIIa+; negative for CD1a and S100; xanthoma and xanthelasma-like lesions (red–brown–yellow papules and plaques); flat wart-like papules of face; lesions occur in folds; skin becomes slack with atrophy of folds skin and face; also lesions of eyelids, axillae, groin, neck; bony lesions; diabetes insipidus, painless exophthalmos, retroperitoneal, renal, and pulmonary histiocytic infiltration *NEJM 373:1762–1772, 2015; BJD 173:540–543, 2015; JAAD 57:1031–1045, 2007; AD 143:952–953, 2007; Hautarzt 52:510–517, 2001; Medicine (Baltimore) 75:157–169, 1996; Virchow Arch Pathol Anat 279:541–542, 1930*

Langerhans cell histiocytosis – erythematous plaques and papules of inframammary and inguinal skin *AD 144:649–653, 2008; Clin Chest Med 25:561–571, 2004; Eur J Med Res 9:510–514, 2004; NEJM 352:700–707, 2005;* self-regressive Langerhans cell histiocytosis (Hashimoto-Pritzker disease) – hypopigmented macules of trunk, solitary papules with necrosis, erosive and ulcerated papules, keratotic plantar papules *AD 146:149–156, 2010;* early pulmonary nodules, ulcerate or cavitate; later small nodules and cysts with bizarre and irregular shape, upper lung predominance, sparing costophrenic angles *Korean J Radiol 20:1368–1380, 2019*

INFLAMMATORY DISORDERS

Ankylosing spondylitis – chest wall constriction, apical fibrobullous disease, spontaneous pneumothorax, bronchiectasis *Clin Chest Med 31:547–554, 2010;* psoriasis, inflammatory bowel disease, aortic insufficiency, reactive arthritis

Pyoderma gangrenosum – nodules or interstitial lung disease; nodular lung lesions, some with cavitation and pneumonitis with multiple nodular lesions *Ped Derm 25:509–519, 2008; Presses Med 36 (10pt1):1395–1398, 2007*

Sarcoid – lupus pernio, erythema nodosum, Lofgren's syndrome, Darier-Roussy subcutaneous nodules; 1,2,3 sign of hilar lymphadenopathy, upper and midlung field micronodules, larger nodules or galaxy sign, pulmonary fibrosis with honeycombing, bullae and traction bronchiectasis *Semin Ultrasound CT MR 40:200–212, 2019;* fingertip nodules *JAAD 44:725–743, 2001; JAAD 11:713–723, 1984;* on palmar aspects of fingers *AD 132:459–464, 1996;* lupus pernio *JAAD 16:534–540, 1987; BJD 112:315–322, 1985*

Stevens-Johnson syndrome – acute sloughing of bronchial mucosa with respiratory failure requiring mechanical ventilation *Crit Care Med 42:118–128, 2014;* late bronchiolitis obliterans *Ped Radiol 26:22–25, 1996; Am J Case Rep 20:171–174, 2019;* bronchiectasis

Sweet's syndrome – fever, erythematous facial plaques and ground glass opacities of upper lung fields, bone marrow biopsy *MDS Aerugi 63:938–944, 2014;* cryptogenic organizing pneumonia and Sweet's syndrome *Clin Respir J 10:250–254, 2016;* bilateral pneumonia, pleural effusions and oral mucosal pustules, tender red plaques and multiple pustules of main bronchi *Eur J Respir J 11:978–980, 1998*

Toxic epidermal necrolysis – acute bronchopneumonia requiring mechanical ventilation, ARDS; chronic – bronchiolitis obliterans, bronchiectasis *Burns 42:20–27, 2016*

METABOLIC DISORDERS

Alpha-1 antitrypsin deficiency-associated panniculitis; painful ulcerative neutrophilic panniculitis *Int J Dermatol 57:952–958, 2018; JAAD 51:645–655, 2004; AD 123:1655–1661, 1987;* emphysema (severe hyperinflation)

Congenital neutropenia *Blood Rev 2:178–185, 1988; Am J Med 61:849–861, 1976*

Cyclic neutropenia *Ped Derm 18:426–432, 2001; Am J Med 61:849–861, 1976*

Cystic fibrosis – aquagenic wrinkling of hands in cystic fibrosis *Ped Derm 25:150–157, 2008; AD 141:621–624, 2005; Med Biol Immunol 25:205–210, 1975; Lancet 2:953, 1974;* cystic fibrosis – polycyclic psoriasiform dermatitis, resembling necrolytic migratory erythema *JAAD 58:S29–30, 2008;* chronic obstructive pulmonary disease, cystic bronchiectasis, pneumothorax

Mannosidosis – autosomal recessive; gingival hypertrophy, macroglossia, coarse features, prognathism, thick eyebrows, low anterior hairline, deafness, lens opacities, hepatosplenomegaly, recurrent respiratory tract infections , muscular hypotonia, mental retardation *Ped Derm 18:534–536, 2001*

NEOPLASTIC DISORDERS

Angiosarcoma – scalp of face of elderly; metastasize to lung; cystic lesions, solid lesions, pneumothorax or hemothorax *Derm J 22:167–168, 2018 PMID 30005733*

Atrial myxoma *Vrach Delo 9:70–72, 1979; J Lancet 85:328–330, 1965*

Blastic plasmacytoid dendritic cell neoplasm – solitary or multiple nodules; plaques of bruise-like infiltrates, may involve lungs, eyes, CNS *BJD 169:570586, 2013*

Carney complex *Clin Cardiol 34:83–86, 2011;* 6-month history intermittent painful, violaceous, blanching macules of fingers *Australasian J Dermatol 56:218–220, 2015;* purpuric patches palms and soles *Ann Dermatol 24:337–340, 2012*

Carcinoid syndrome – flushing and rosacea, scleroderma-like, pellagra-like, cutaneous metastases *JAAD 68:e1–21, 2013;* leonine facies *JAMA Derm 153:925–926, 2017; Radiologe 57:397–406, 2017;* cough, hemoptysis, obstructive pneumonia *Minerva Chir 57:403–423, 2002*

Cutaneous metastases from lung cancer – rare; alopecia neoplastica *Clin Case Rep 7:1796–1797, 2019;* radiotherapy-resistant upper limb edema; multiple immobile hard metastases to scalp from adenocarcinoma of lung *Oncol Targets Ther Sep 21, 2018; 11:6147–6151*

Kaposi sarcoma/HIV – primary pulmonary Kaposi sarcoma in HIV disease *ID Cases July 3,2018:e00420; Pneumocystis pneumonia;* pulmonary cavitation, pleural effusions, respiratory failure *J Community Hosp Intern Med Perspect 9:351–354, 2019;* pulmonary Kaposi's sarcoma after HIV disease *Lung 194:163–169, 2016;* immunosuppression, transplantation of lungs *J Heart Lung Transplant 37:798–799, 2018;* kidney transplantation *Cureus 12:e6719, Jan 2020*

Lymphoma, Hodgkin's disease – pulmonary cavitation; mimicking bronchiolitis obliterans organizing pneumonia *Pneumologia 64:4–45, 2015;* presenting as non-resolving pneumonia with endobronchial nodule; so in involvement rare, ulcers, plaques, nodules and papules *World J Clin Cases 7:2513–2518, 2019;* erythematous indurated papules and plaques *Am J Dermatopathol 37:499–502, 2015; JAAD 58:295–298, 2008;* cutaneous T-cell lymphoma *Cancer 109:1550–1555, 2007;* rarely involve lungs, most common radiologic pulmonary finding solitary nodule or multiple progressing nodules; diffuse involvement with angiocentric infiltration of tumor cells and distal pulmonary infarctions *Thoracic Imaging 17:157–159, 2002;* ground glass opacities of mid and upper lung fields *J Thoracic Imaging 22:366–368, 2007*

Lymphomatoid granulomatosis – Epstein-Barr virus+ B-cell lymphoproliferative disorder; papules, subcutaneous nodules, atrophic or indurated plaques, angiocentric angiodestructive infiltrates of atypical lymphocytes, alveolar or interstitial bilateral pulmonary infiltrates, lung nodules; morbilliform eruption *Ped Derm 17:369–372, 2000; JAAD Case Rep 1:234–237, 2015*

PARANEOPLASTIC DISORDERS

Primary leukocytoclastic vasculitis – initial presentation of myelodysplastic syndrome *Tuberc Respir Dis (Seoul)79:302–306, 2016;* presented as non-resolving pneumonia

Paraneoplastic pemphigus – necrosis of eyelids and oral mucosa; bronchiolitis obliterans *JAAD 80:1544–1549, 2019; Great Cases from the South, AAD Meeting, March 2000*

Tripe palms – associated with interstitial lung disease *JAAD Case Rep 2:59–62, 2016;* lung cancer *J Clin Oncol 7:669–678, 1989*

PRIMARY CUTANEOUS DISEASES

Atopic dermatitis – asthma

Cutis laxa – autosomal dominant, autosomal recessive, or X-linked; bloodhound appearance, redundant loose, sagging skin, eyelid ptosis; recurrent pneumonia; childhood onset pulmonary emphysema; *FBLN5*-related cutis laxa *Int J Mol Sci March 15, 2017*

Dahl's sign – symmetric slanting areas of hyperpigmentation of medial thighs (Thinker's sign) due to repeated pressure on thighs from COPD *NEJM 371:357, 2014*

Febrile ulceronecrotic Mucha- Habermann disease (pityriasis lichenoides et varioliformis acuta) *J Rheumatol 16:387–389, 1989;* crusted ulcerated red plaques; diarrhea, pulmonary involvement, abdominal pain, CNS symptoms, arthritis *Ped Derm 29:53–58, 2012*

Mal de Meleda *Cutis 93:193–198, 2014*

X-linked hypohidrotic ectodermal dysplasia – female carriers, mosaicism – V-shaped hypopigmented linear lesions, patchy hypotrichosis, abnormal teeth *Ped Derm 24:551–554, 2007*

X-linked reticulate pigmentary disorder with systemic manifestations (familial cutaneous amyloidosis) (Partington syndrome II) – X-linked; rare; Xp21–22; boys with generalized reticulated muddy brown pigmentation (dyschromatosis) with hypopigmented corneal dystrophy (dyskeratosis), photophobia, coarse unruly hair, unswept eyebrows, silvery hair, hypohidrosis, recurrent pneumonia with chronic obstructive disease, clubbing; diarrhea, hypospadias, failure to thrive, female carriers with linear macular nevoid Blaschko-esque hyperpigmentation *Ped Derm 32:871–872, 2015; Am J Med Genet 161:1414–1420, 2013; Eur J Dermatol 18:102–103, 2008; Ped Derm 22:122–126, 2005; Semin Cut Med Surg 16:72–80, 1997; Am J Med Gen 10:65:1981*

SYNDROMES

APLAID (autoinflammation and PLAID) – sinopulmonary infections, interstitial pneumonitis, eye inflammation, colitis, arthralgias; epidermolysis bullosa-like eruptions in infancy with vesiculopustular lesions and red plaques *JAAD 73:367–381, 2015*

Birt-Hogg-Dube syndrome – fibrofolliculomas, trichodiscomas, acrochordons, renal cancers; pulmonary cysts of lower peripheral lungs and along mediastinum, pneumothoraces recurrent *Respir Med Case Rep 18:90–92, 2016*

Dyskeratosis congenita – X-linked recessive; interstitial fibrosis *Thorax 56:891–894, 2001;* pulmonary fibrosis, pulmonary arteriovenous malformations *JAAD 1194–1196, 2017*

Epidermodysplasia verruciformis – molluscum contagiosum, bronchiectasis, lymphoma *JAAD 76:1161–1175, 2017*

Familial Mediterranean fever *Rheum Int 2=32:1801–1804, 2012;* erysipelas like erythema subsides 24–72 hours; *MEFV* mutation; IgA associated recurrent vasculitis, unusual locations (face and trunk), younger children *Rheumatol Int 55:1153–1158, 2016;* polyarteritis nodosa with elevated ASLO not hepatitis B antigen titer *Semin Arthritis Rheum 30:281–287, 2001*

Good syndrome – adult acquired primary immunodeficiency in context of past or current thymoma; sinopulmonary infections; lichen planus, oral lichen planus of tongue, gingivitis, oral erosions *BJD 172:774–777, 2015; Am J Med Genet 66:378–398, 1996*

Goodpasture's syndrome – annular erythematous macule *AD 121:1442–1444, 1985;*

Graft vs host disease – rippled skin overlying deep sclerodermoid changes *JAAD 66:515–532, 2012; AD 138:924–934, 2002*

Hereditary fibrosing poikiloderma of Weary – tendon contractures, myopathy, fibrosis, pulmonary fibrosis and alopecia *FAMiiiB* mutation *BJD 176:534–536, 2017*

Hereditary mucoepithelial dysplasia (dyskeratosis) (Gap junction disease, Witkop disease) – autosomal dominant; non-scarring alopecia; dry rough skin; red eyes, non-scarring alopecia, follicular keratosis (keratosis pilaris), erythema of oral (hard palate, gingival, tongue) and nasal mucous membranes, cervix, vagina, and urethra; perineal and perigenital psoriasiform dermatitis (perineal erythema); hyperpigmented hyperkeratotic lesions of flexures (neck, antecubital and popliteal fossae); esophageal stenosis; keratitis (visual impairment) increased risk of infections, fibrocystic lung disease *Ped Derm 29:311–315, 2012; BJD 153:310–318, 2005; Ped Derm 11:133–138, 1994; Am J Med Genet 39:338–341, 1991; JAAD 21:351–357, 1989; Am J Hum Genet 31:414–427, 1979; Oral Surg Oral Med Oral Pathol 46:645–657, 1978*

Hermansky-Pudlak syndrome – types 1–8; autosomal recessive; Arecibo, Puerto Rico; pigmentary dilution of skin, hair, eyes; ocular manifestations of albinism; bleeding tendency, platelet dysfunction (absent dense bodies), granulomatous colitis (ceroid deposits), interstitial pulmonary fibrosis *Ped Derm 34:638–646, 2017*

Kawasaki's disease – pulmonary involvement rare, pleural effusions>pneumonia, pulmonary nodules (days of fever, 4/5 cervical lymphadenopathy, bilateral non-purulent conjunctivitis, oropharyngeal mucosal changes (red or strawberry tongue), polymorphous rash, erythema of palms or soles and edema of hands or feet *J Med Case Rep 13:344, Nov 25, 2019*

Lipoid proteinosis – rare; autosomal recessive; *ECM1* mutation; hoarse voice PAS+ hyaline material deposited in skin, mucous membranes, and viscera *Ped Derm18:21–26, 2001;* Pox-like and acneiform scars, infiltration and thickening of skin and oral mucosa, eyelid margin beading (moniliform blepharosis) *Mol Syndromol 7:26–31, 2016*

Marfan's syndrome – fibrillin 1 gene mutation; aortic root dilatation and mitral valve prolapse; Morgagni hernia; pectus excavatum compression of lungs; increased density of right paracardiac lung fields mimic pulmonary infiltrate *Rontgenblatter 43:298–300, 1990*

Multicentric reticulohistiocytosis – interstitial fibrosis *AD 148:228–232, 2012;* multiple pulmonary nodules *Clin Exp Dermatol 34:183–185, 2009; JAAD 49:1125–1127, 2003*

Nijmegen breakage syndrome – autosomal recessive; chromosome instability syndrome; mutations in *NBS-1* gene which encodes bibirin (DNA damage repair); microcephaly, receding mandible, prominent midface, growth retardation, epicanthal folds, large ears, sparse hair, clinodactyly/syndactyly; freckling of face, café au lait macules, vitiligo, photosensitivity of the eyelids, telangiectasias; pigmented deposits of fundus; IgG, IgA deficiencies, agammaglobulinemia, decreased CD3 and CD4 T cells with recurrent respiratory and urinary tract infections *Ped Derm 26:106–108, 2009; DNA Repair 3:1207–1217, 2004; Arch Dis Child 82:400–406, 2000*

Osler-Weber-Rendu syndrome – telangiectatic macules, papules, clubbing, pulmonary arteriovenous fistulae (right to left shunt manifest as cyanosis, polycythemia, cold, and migraine, cerebrovascular accident, hemoptysis and spontaneous hemothorax *Actas Dermosifilogr 110:526–532, 2019*

Pachydermoperiostosis – clubbing, subperiosteal new bone formation (hypertrophic osteoarthropathy); primary and secondary; lung cancer or pleural mesothelioma and benign conditions including pulmonary infections, COPD *Medicine 96:e7985, Sep 2017*

Schwachman-Diamond syndrome – periodontal disease and caries; abscesses, short stature, delayed puberty, skeletal changes, pancreatic exocrine deficiency, pancytopenias, failure to thrive, hepatomegaly, pneumonia, otitis media, osteomyelitis *Ped Derm 28:568–569, 2011*

Sweet's syndrome – fever, erythematous facial plaques and ground glass opacities of upper lung fields *MDS Aerugi 63:938–944, 2014;* cryptogenic organizing pneumonia and Sweet's syndrome *Clin Respir J 10:250–254, 2016;* bilateral pneumonia, pleural effusions and oral mucosal pustules, tender red plaques and multiple pustules on mainstem bronchi *Eur J Respir Dis 11:978–980, 1998*

Superior vena cava syndrome – facial edema, swelling or discoloration of neck and upper extremities; garland sign; lung cancer, non-Hodgkin's lymphoma, and intravascular devices *Emerg Med Clin NA 36:577–584, 2018;* rare cause tertiary syphilitic aortic aneurysm *Clin Inf Dis 27:1331–1332, 1998; Am J Med 71:171–173, 1981*

Trichorhinophalangeal syndrome type I – autosomal dominant; slow growing short blond hair, receding frontotemporal hairline with high bossed forehead; thin nails, koilonychias, leukonychia, facial pallor, pear-shaped nose with bulbous nose tip, wide long philtrum, thin upper lip, triangular face, receding chin, tubercle of normal skin below the lower lip, protruding ears, distension and deviation with fusiform swelling of the PIP joints; hip malformation, brachydactyly, prognathism, fine brittle slow growing sparse hair, lateral eyebrows sparse and brittle, dense medially, bone deformities (hands short and stubby), joint hyperextensibility, cone-shaped epiphyses of bones of hand, lateral deviation of interphalangeal joints, flat feet, hip malformations, high arched palate, supernumerary teeth, dental malocclusion, mild short stature; hypotonia, hoarse deep voice, recurrent respiratory infections, hypoglycemia, diabetes mellitus, hypothyroidism, decreased growth hormone, renal and cardiac defects, mutation in zinc finger nuclear transcription factor (TRPS1 gene) *Cutis 89:56,73–74, 2012; Ped Derm 26:171–175, 2009; Ped Derm 25:557–558, 2008; BJD 157:1021–1024, 2007; AD 137:1429–1434, 2001; JAAD 31:331–336, 1994; Hum Genet 74:188–189, 1986; Helv Paediatr Acta 21:475–482, 1966*

Tuberous sclerosis – lymphangiomyomatosis, predominantly women with high morbidity and mortality; cough, dyspnea, hemoptysis, pneumothorax *Nat Rev Dis Primers 2016 May 26:2:16035; Eur J Radiol 83:39–46, 2014;* folliculocystic and collagen hamartoma – comedo-like openings, multilobulated cysts, scalp cysts and nodules *JAAD 66:617–621, 2012*

Urban-Rifkin-Davis syndrome – autosomal recessive; flattened midface; wide nasal bridge long philtrum, micrognathia, hypertelorism, periorbital fullness, receding forehead; severe pulmonary, gastrointestinal, and genitourinary abnormalities; mutation in *LTBP4 JAAD 66:842–851, 2012*

X-linked reticulate pigmentary disorder with systemic manifestations – rare; Xp21-22; boys with generalized reticulated muddy brown dyschromatosis, hypopigmented corneal dystrophy, photophobia, coars unruly hair, unswept eyebrows, silvery hair, hypohidrosis; clubbing; recurrent pneumonia with obstructive disease *Ped Derm 32:871–872, 2015; Am J Med Genetics 161:1414–1420, 2013*

Yellow nail syndrome – yellow slow growing thickened nails with a notable hump, lymphedema, pleural effusion, bronchiectasis, chronic sinusitis, recurrent pneumonia *Orphanet J Rare Dis 12:42 Feb 27, 2017; Ped Derm 27:533–534, 2010; JAAD 56:537–538, 2007; BJD 156:1230–1234, 2007; JAAD 28:792–794, 1993; JAAD 1:509–512, 1984*

TOXINS

Berylliosis *Toxicol Pathol 25:2–12, 1997; Environ Health Prev Med 12:161–164m 2007*

Eosinophilic myalgia syndrome – tryptophan-eosinophilic fasciitis associate disease *AD 127:217–220, 1991; Am J Med 88:542–546, 1990;* interstitial lung disease *Kans Med 94:175–177, 1993*

Mustard gas exposure *AD 128:775–780, 1992; JAAD 32:765–766, 1995, JAAD 39:187–190, 1998*

TRAUMA

Fat embolism syndrome- 24–48 hours following long bone fracture; petechiae of upper chest and face; confusion, respiratory distress, hypoxic ARDS *Spin J 14:e1–5, 2014; BMJ Case Rep July 5, 2013; Orthopedics 19:41–48, 1996*

Radiation therapy – radiation pneumonitis *Clin Chest Med 38:201–208, 2017*

VASCULAR DISORDERS

Eosinophilic granulomatosis with polyangiitis (EGPA) – palpable purpura, subcutaneous nodules (of scalp or bilateral extensor extremities) *Case Rep Dermatol 10:175–181, 2018;* elbow papules and nodules may become necrotic or ulcerative *JAAD 37 (pt1) 199–203, 1997;* asthma often precede by allergic rhinitis, eosinophilic pneumonia, migratory infiltrates, peripheral nodules, ground glass opacities *Autoimmune Rev 14:341–348, 2015*

Henoch-Schonlein purpura – alveolar hemorrhage *ID Cases 12:47–48, 2018; Semin Arthritis Rheum 42:391–400, 2013; Clin Rheumatol 20:293–296, 2001*

Hypersensitivity vasculitis – hypersensitivity pneumonia in pigeon breeder *Rom J Morphol Embryol 60:3325–331, 2019;* interstitial lung disease and ANCA-associated vasculitis *J Clin Rheumatol March 31, 2020*

Hypocomplementemic urticarial vasculitis *Ann DV 142:557–562, 2015;* hemoptysis, pleural effusion,

COPD *Dtsch Arztebl Int 106:656–663, 2009*

Microscopic polyangiitis – most MPO-ANCA+ small vessel vasculitis affecting lungs and kidneys; diffuse alveolar hemorrhage and pulmonary fibrosis *Clin Rheumatol 34:1273–1277, 2015; Clin Exp Nephrol 17:667–671, 2013;* organizing pneumonia *Respirol Case Rep 3:122–124, 2015*

Granulomatosis with polyangiitis – strawberry gums; vasculitis, pyoderma gangrenosum-like lesions, ulcerating acne, saddle nose deformity; asthma, pulmonary infiltrates, single or multiple nodules (frequently cavitated) and masses, resolving nodules C-ANCA: facial vegetative ulcers and peri-auricular lesions *Infect Disord Drug Targets Nov 14, 2019;* enlarging painful facial ulcers *Case Rep Rheumatol 2014;850364;* unilateral eyelid edema *Caspian J Intern Med 10:343–346, 2019;* pyoderma gangrenosum-like ulcers *Rheumatol Int 38:1139–1151, 2018*

POIKILODERMAS OF ADULTHOOD

AUTOIMMUNE DISEASES AND DISORDERS OF IMMUNE DYSREGULATION

Dermatitis herpetiformis *Clin Dermatol 24:486–492, 2006; JAAD 48:S11–14, 2003; Australas J Dermatol 43:136–139, 2002*

Dermatomyositis *J Med Case Rep March 24, 2018; BMJ Case Rep May 30, 2018*

Graft vs. host disease, chronic *JAAD 66:515–532, 2012; JAAD 38:369–392, 1998; AD 134:602–612, 1998*

Lupus erythematosus – SCLE – generalized poikiloderma *Clin Exp Dermatol 34:e859–861, 2009; Dermatology 207:285–290, 2003; JAAD 42:286–288, 2000*

Scleroderma (progressive systemic sclerosis)

DRUGS

Etanercept-induced dermatomyositis – eyelid erythema, poikiloderma, acral erythema, paronychial erythema *JAMA Derm 149:1204–1208, 2013*

Hydroxyurea – atrophic, scaling, poikilodermatous patches with erosions on the backs of the hands, sides of the feet (dermatomyositis-like) *Int J Dermatol 45:158–160, 2006; JAAD 45:321–322, 2001; JAAD 36:178–182, 1997*

INFECTIONS AND INFESTATIONS

Lyme borreliosis (*Borrelia burgdorferi*) – acrodermatitis chronica atrophicans – red to blue nodules or plaques; tissue-paper-like wrinkling; pigmented; poikilodermatous; hands, feet, elbows, knees *JAAD 72:683–689, 2015; BJD 121:263–269, 1989: Int J Derm 18:595–601, 1979*

INFILTRATIVE DISORDERS

Amyloidosis – poikiloderma-like cutaneous amyloidosis *J Dermatol 25:730–734, 1998;* macular amyloidosis – presenting as poikiloderma *J Dermatol 45:241–243, 2018; J Korean Med Sci 15:724–726, 2000; Int J Dermatol 31:277–278, 1992;* primary cutaneous amyloid *Dermatologica 155:301–309, 1977*

NEOPLASTIC DISORDERS

Granulomatous slack skin syndrome – cutaneous T-cell lymphoma *AD 133:231–236, 1997*

Lymphoma, including cutaneous T-cell lymphoma *JAMA Derm 155:958–959, 2019; Acta DV Croat 26:48–52, 2018; JAAD 65:313–319, 2011; BJD 157:1064–1066, 2007; Semin Cutan Med Surg 19:91–99, 2000; Clin Exp Dermatol 21:205–208, 1996;* syringotropic cutaneous T-cell lymphoma – punctate red papules; hyperkeratotic follicular papules, punctate red papules; anhidrosis; palmoplantar keratoderma; poikiloderma vasculare atrophicans *JAAD 71:926–934, 2014; Am J Surg Pathol 35:100–109, 2011; Eur J Dermatol 15:262–264, 2005;* CD8+ cutaneous T-cell lymphoma *BJD 161:826–830, 2009;* granulomatous cutaneous T-cell lymphoma *Clin Exp Dermatol 34:718–720, 2009*

PHOTODERMATOSES

Acquired brachial cutaneous dyschromatosis – a form of dermatoheliosis *JAAD 42:680–684, 2000*

Poikiloderma of Civatte, extracervical *An Bras Dermatol 89:655–656, 2014*

PRIMARY CUTANEOUS DISEASES

Atopic dermatitis – presenting as generalized poikiloderma *J Dermatol 41:230–231, 2014*

Poikiloderma vasculare atrophicans *AD 124:366–372, 1988; BJD 115:383–385, 1986; Cutis 17:938–941, 1976; BJD 87:405–411, 1972;* associated with cutaneous T-cell lymphoma *JAAD 52:706–708, 2005*

Parakeratosis variegata *Eur J Dermatol 26:300–302, 2016*

SYNDROMES

Blau syndrome – poikilodermatous dermatitis; granulomatous arthritis, synovial cysts, iritis, rash; autosomal dominant; resembles childhood sarcoid – red papules, uveitis; chromosome 16p12–q21 *JAAD 49:299–302, 2003*

COPS syndrome – poikiloderma, calcinosis cutis, osteoma cutis, skeletal abnormalities

Dyskeratosis congenita *BMJ Case Rep Nov 28, 2018:11 (1) p ii e226736*

Fascioscapular muscular dystrophy *AD 107:115–117, 1973*

Hereditary fibrosing poikiloderma – with tendon contractures, pulmonary fibrosis; *FAM IIIB* mutation *J Dermtol 46:1014–1018, 2019; Rev Mal Respir 35:968–973, 2018*

Hereditary sclerosing poikiloderma – with calcific aortic and mitral valvular stenosis *Cardiovasc Pathol 25:195–199, 2016*

Hereditary sclerosing poikiloderma of Weary *BJD 140:366–368, 1999*

Kindler's syndrome *Dermatol Online J March 15, 2018:24 (3) p ii 13030*

Multicentric reticulohistiocytosis – poikilodermatous patch *AD 144:1360–1366, 2008*

Rothmund-Thomson syndrome *JAAD 75:855–870, 2016; Ped Derm 19:312–316, 2002*

Werner's syndrome *SKINMed 8:184–186, 2010*

Xeroderma pigmentosum *JAAD 75:855–870, 2016*

TOXINS

Sulfur mustard gas *Cutan Ocul Toxicol 31:214–219, 2012*

TRAUMA

Heat and infrared radiation (erythema ab igne)

Radiation dermatitis, chronic *Cutan Ocul Toxicol 34:242–244, 2015; JAAD 54:28–46, 2006; Acta DV 49:64–71, 1969;* subacute radiodermatitis due to fluoroscopy *Cutis 91:230–232, 2013*

Sternal erythema, post- sternal thoracotomy *JAAD 53:893–896, 2005*

POIKILODERMAS OF CHILDHOOD

AUTOIMMUNE DISEASES AND DISORDERS OF IMMUNE DYSREGULATION

Dermatomyositis (poikilodermatomyositis) *JAAD 56:148–153, 2008; Lancet 355 (9197):53–57, 2000;* reticulate telangiectatic erythema in older lesions with hyper- and hypopigmentation

Graft vs. host disease, chronic *AD 138:924–934, 2002;*

JAAD 38:369–392, 1998; AD 134:602–612, 1998

Lupus erythematosus – subacute cutaneous lupus erythematosus *JAAD 42:286–288, 2000;* neonatal lupus erythematosus *Ped Derm 15:38–42, 1998*

METABOLIC DISORDERS

Fanconi's anemia

PHOTODERMATOSES

Poikiloderma of Civatte *Plast Reconstr Surg 107:1376–1381, 2001; J Cutan Laser Ther 1:45–48, 1999; AD 126:547–548, 1990*

PRIMARY CUTANEOUS DISEASES

Atopic dermatitis – poikiloderma-like lesions of the neck *J Dermatol 17:85–91, 1990*

Dermatopathia pigmentosa reticularis

Diffuse and macular atrophic dermatosis – generalized poikilodermatous prematurely aged (sun-damaged) appearance *Clin Exp Dermatol 5:57–60, 1980*

SYNDROMES

Acrogeria (Gottron's syndrome) – micrognathia, atrophy of tip of nose, atrophic skin of distal extremities with telangiectasia, easy bruising, mottled pigmentation or poikiloderma of extremities, dystrophic nails; acro-osteolysis, shortened fingers *BJD 151:497–501, 2004; BJD 103:213–223, 1980; Arch Dermatol Syphiligr 181:571–583, 1941*

AEC (ankyloblepharon, ectodermal defects, cleft lip and palate) syndrome (Hay-Wells syndrome) – poikilodermatous patches of trunk, shoulders, and upper back; similar to Rapp-Hodgkin with syndactyly, supernumerary nipple, lacrimal duct aplasia, scalp dermatitis, and recurrent scalp infections *Ped Derm 22:415–419, 2005*

Ataxia telangiectasia

Ballard-Gerold syndrome – poikiloderma, craniosynostosis, radial ray defects, patellar and palatal abnormalities, dislocated joints, diarrhea, short stature, slender nose, normal intellect *RECQL4* mutations *JAAD 75:855–870, 2016; Soc Ped Dermatol Annual Meeting, 2006*

Blau syndrome – poikilodermatous dermatitis; granulomatous arthritis, synovial cysts, iritis, rash; autosomal dominant; resembles childhood sarcoid – red papules, uveitis; chromosome 16p12–q21 *JAAD 49:299–302, 2003*

Bloom's syndrome *JAAD 75:855–870, 2016*

Cockayne's syndrome (cachectic dwarfism) – xerosis with rough, dry skin, anhidrosis, erythema of hands, hypogonadism; autosomal recessive; short stature, facial erythema in butterfly distribution leading to mottled pigmentation and atrophic scars, premature aged appearance with loss of subcutaneous fat and sunken eyes, canities, mental deficiency, photosensitivity, disproportionately large hands, feet, and ears, ocular defects, demyelination *Am J Hum Genet 50:677–689, 1992; J Med Genet 18:288–293, 1981*

Congenital poikiloderma with unusual hypopigmentation and acral blistering at birth *J Eur Acad Dermatol Venereol 12:54–58, 1999*

Congenital poikiloderma with verruciform hyperkeratoses (Dowling type) *Hautarzt 49:586–590, 1998*

COPS syndrome (calcinosis cutis, osteoma cutis, poikiloderma, with skeletal abnormalities) *Eur J Pediatr 150:343–346, 1991*

Degos-Touraine syndrome – incontinentia pigmenti with poikiloderma in photodistribution, bullae of face, extremities; chronic erythroderma with subsequent hyperpigmentation *Soc Gr Dermatol Syph 68:6–10, 1961*

Dyskeratosis congenita (Zinsser-Engman-Cole syndrome) *J Blood Med 5:157–167, 2014; Br J Haematol 145:164–172, 2009; Semin Cut Med Surg 16:72–80, 1997; Dermatol Clin 13:33–39, 1995; BJD 105:321–325, 1981*

Franceschetti-Jadassohn syndrome

Greither's syndrome – poikiloderma of face and extremities; warty keratoses over hands, feet, and legs; plantar keratoderma; normal nails and hair *Hautarzt 9:364–369, 1958*

Hallerman-Streiff syndrome

Hereditary (bullous) acrokeratotic poikiloderma of Weary (acrokeratotic poikiloderma) – autosomal dominant; vesiculopustular eruption of hands and feet in infancy and childhood; extensive dermatitis in childhood, persistent poikiloderma sparing face, scalp and ears, verrucous papules of hands, feet, elbows, and knees *AD 103:409–422, 1971;* pseudoainhum and sclerotic bands *Int J Dermatol 36:529–533, 1997*

Hereditary fibrosing poikiloderma with tendon contracture, myopathy, fibrosis, and alopecia; FAM IIIB mutation – mimics Rothmund-Thomson syndrome *Cases of the Year, Pre-AAD Pediatric Dermatology Meeting, 2016*
  Poikiloderma of cheeks
  Alopecia
  Myopathy – fatty infiltration of muscles
  Hypohidrosis
  Lymphedema of hands and legs
  Exocrine pancreatic insufficiency
  Extraocular muscle weakness
  Tendon contractures
  Pulmonary fibrosis

Hereditary sclerosing poikiloderma of Weary – autosomal dominant; generalized poikiloderma; sclerosis of palms and soles; linear hyperkeratotic and sclerotic bands in flexures of arms and legs *BJD*

140:366–368, 1999; Ann DV 122:618–620, 1995; AD 125:103–106, 1989; AD 100:413–422, 1969; AD 100:413–422, 1969

Huriez syndrome – autosomal dominant; palmoplantar keratoderma with sclerodactyly and scleroatrophy of distal extremities with nail changes (hypoplasia, longitudinal ridging, distal splitting); hypohidrosis, poikilodermatous changes of nose, flexion contractures of fingers *AD 146:1419–1424, 2010; TIG 13:229, 1997*

Kindler's syndrome – acral blistering at birth; progressive poikiloderma; cigarette paper atrophy of hands and feet (scleroatrophy), atrophied gingiva, photosensitivity; mutation in *FERMT1* (fermitin family homologue 1) gene *BJD 160:233–242, 2009; BJD 159:1192–1196, 2008; BJD 158:1375–1377, 2008; BJD 157:1252–1256, 2007; BJD 157:1281–1284, 2007; AD 142:1619–1624, 2006; AD 142:620–624, 2006; AD 140:939–944, 2004; BJD 144:1284–1286, 2001; AD 132:1487–1490, 1996; AD 133:1111–1117, 1997; Ped Derm 6:82–90, 1989; BJD 66:104–111, 1954*

Mandibulo acral dysplasia *JAAD 33:900–2, 1995*

Mendes de Costa syndrome (X-linked epidermolysis bullosa) – poikiloderma, retarded growth *Proc R Soc Med 66:234–236, 1973*

Mitochondrial DNA syndrome *JAAD 39:819–823, 1998*

Pangeria (Werner's syndrome)

Pearson's syndrome (mitochondrial syndrome) – exocrine pancreatic insufficiency, renal tubular dysfunction

Poikiloderma and megaloblastic anemia *AD 107:231–236, 1973*

Poikiloderma, alopecia, retrognathism, and cleft palate (PARC syndrome) *Dermatologica 181:142–144, 1990*

Poikiloderma with neutropenia – autosomal recessive; Navajo Indians; erythematous rash of limbs, trunk, and face beginning in infancy; evolves into poikiloderma; recurrent infections; palmoplantar keratoderma; pachyonychia of great toenails, photosensitivity; growth retardation; dental caries; atrophic scars; cryptorchidism; hepatosplenomegaly; mutation in *USB1* gene; mutation in *C16orf57* *BJD 168:665–666, 2013; Ped Derm 29:463–472, 2012; BJD 163:866–869, 2010; Am J Med Genet A 146A:2762–2769, 2008; Am J Hum Genet 86:72–76, 1991; Am J Hum Genet 49:A661, 1991*

Progeria (Hutchinson-Gilford syndrome) *AD 125:540–544, 1989*

Rothmund-Thomson syndrome (poikiloderma congenitale) – autosomal recessive *Am J Med Genet 22:102:11–17, 2001; Ped Derm 18:210212, 2001; Ped Derm 16:59–61, 1999; Dermatol Clin 13:143–150, 1995; JAAD 27:75–762, 1992; Arch Ophthalmol (German) 4:159, 1887*

Schopf-Schulz-Passarge – facial poikiloderma

Scleroatrophic syndrome of Huriez – poikiloderma of the nose, scleroatrophy of the hands *BJD 137:114–118, 1997; Ped Derm 15:207–209, 1998*

Trichothiodystrophy syndromes – BIDS, IBIDS, PIBIDS – poikiloderma, sparse or absent eyelashes and eyebrows, brittle hair, premature aging, sexual immaturity, ichthyosis, dysmyelination, bird-like facies, dental caries; trichothiodystrophy with ichthyosis, urologic malformations, hypercalciuria and mental and physical retardation (autism) *JAAD 44:891–920, 2001; Ped Derm 14:441–445, 1997*

Xeroderma pigmentosum

TRAUMA

Cold poikiloderma of the waistband – personal observation

Chronic radiation dermatitis – personal observation

VASCULAR LESIONS

Poikilodermatous plaque-like hemangioma *JAAD 81:1257–1270, 2019*

POLIOSIS, LOCALIZED OR GENERALIZED (CANITIES)

JAAD 69:625–633, 2013

AUTOIMMUNE DISORDERS

Graft vs host disease *Saudi J Ophthalmol 27:215–222m 2013*

CONGENITAL LESIONS

Congenital poliosis

DRUGS

Acitretin *JAAD 69:625–633, 2013; J Drugs Dermatol 11:247–239, 2012*

Bimatoprost, topical *AD 142:250–251, 2006*

Cetuximab *JAAD 69:625–633, 2013*

Chloramphenicol *JAAD 69:625–633, 2013*

Chloroquine *An Bras Dermatol 41:57–68, 1966*

Cituximab *Ophthalmology 125:294, 2018; J Clin Oncol 29:e532–533, 2011*

Cyclosporine *Med Clin (Barc) 97:39, 1991*

Imiquimod *JAAD 69:625–633, 2013; Dermatol Surg 34:844–845, 2008*

Ipilimumab *Med Clin (Barc)142:234, 2014*

Latanoprost – bilateral poliosis and granulomatous anterior uveitis *Actas Dermosifiliogr 106:74–75, 2015; Eye 15:347–349, 2001*

Prostaglandin analogs *JAAD 69:625–633, 2013*

Travoprost, topical *AD 142:250–251, 2006*

Tumor-infiltrating lymphocyte immunotherapy *JAAD 69:625–633, 2013*

EXOGENOUS AGENTS

Hair dyes in blacks – pseudo-white forelock *Cutis 52:273–279, 1993*

INFECTIONS AND INFESTATIONS

Post-herpetic (herpes zoster) *AD 142:250–251, 2006*

INFLAMMATORY DISORDERS

Blepharitis *JAAD 69:625–633, 2013*

Post-inflammatory

Sarcoid *AD 142:250–251, 2006; EYE 19:1015–1017, 2005*

Sympathetic ophthalmia *AD 142:250–251, 2006*

Uveitis, idiopathic *AD 142:250–251, 2006*

METABOLIC DISORDERS

Prolidase deficiency *AD 142:250–251, 2006*

NEOPLASTIC DISORDERS

Halo nevus *Ophthalmic Plast Reconstr Surg 32:e73–74, 2016; Korean J Ophthalmol 24:237–239, 2010*

Lymphoma – folliculotropic cutaneous T-cell lymphoma *Dermatol Online J 24 (12)13-30/qt5w68b51q Dec 15, 2018*

Melanocytic nevi – poliosis may be associated with congenital or acquired intradermal nevi *AD 129:1333, 1336, 1993*; halo nevi *AD 135:859–861, 1999*; scalp nevi *BJD 140:1182–1184, 1999*; giant congenital nevus *AD 135:859–861, 1999*

Melanoma *Am J Med 132:1417–1418, 2019; Arch Ophthalmol 129:1382–1383, 2011; Arch Ophthalmol 126:1006–1007, 2008; AD 131:618–619, 1995; AD 114:439–441, 1978*; scalp melanoma with associated poliosis *Clin Exp Dermatol 40:872–874, 2015*

Neurofibroma *AD 98:631–633, 1968*

Nevus comedonicus

Nevus depigmentosus *AD 142:250-251, 2006*

PRIMARY CUTANEOUS DISEASES

Alopecia areata *JAAD 69:625–633, 2013*

Isolated white forelock *JAAD 80:1776–1778, 2019*

Isolated occipital white lock (X-linked recessive)

Migratory poliosis *JAAD 42:1076–1077, 2000*

Piebaldism – autosomal dominant, hyperpigmented macule within amelanotic macule, medial eyebrows and eyelashes usually white, no other health associations, triangular or diamond shaped forehead macule, white forelock *Int J Dermatol 43:716–719, 2004; JAAD 44:288–292, 2001; AD 135:859–861, 1999*

Poliosis – deafness, unilateral tapetoretinal degeneration

Vitiligo *AD 142:250–251, 2006; JAAPOS 9:295–296, 2005*

SYNDROMES

Alezzandrini's syndrome – hearing loss, unilateral tapetoretinal degeneration, ipsilateral facial vitiligo, poliosis *Dermatology 222:8–9, 2011; JAAD 26:496–497, 1992*

Book's syndrome – autosomal dominant, bicuspid aplasia, hyperhidrosis, premature whitening of hair

Chediak-Higashi syndrome – silvery–gray hair

Fanconi's syndrome – fair hair

Fisch's syndrome – deafness, early graying of hair

Griscelli's syndrome – silvery–gray hair

Marfan's syndrome *Cutis 12:479–484, 1991*

Myotonia dystrophica – autosomal dominant, canities in 2nd or 3rd decade, cataracts, lugubrious physiognomy, myotonia, premature frontal balding, severe muscle wasting

Neurofibromatosis *Dermatol Online J 16:11, 2010; AD 135:859–861, 1999; AD 98:631–633, 1968*

Progeria – gray hair, sparse

Robert's syndrome – hypomelia-hypotrichosis-facial hemangioma syndrome – silvery blond hair

Rothmund-Thomson syndrome – autosomal dominant, cataracts, erythema, hypogonadism, photosensitivity, poikiloderma, premature canities, short stature, small skull

Rubenstein-Taybi syndrome *AD 142:250–251, 2006; Clin Exp Dermatol 19:170–172, 1994*

Seckel's syndrome – autosomal recessive, bird-head profile, hypodontia, pancytopenia, premature graying, skeletal defects, trident hands

Siccardi's syndrome – silver hair

Tietz's syndrome – autosomal dominant; congenital deafness and congenital hypopigmented patches of skin, no heterochromic irides *JAAD 69:625–633, 2013*

Trigeminal autonomic cephalalgia *JAAD 69:625–633, 2013; Australas J Dermatol 51:66–68, 2010*

Tuberous sclerosis – poliosis occurs and can be independent of hypomelanotic macule *Ped Derm 25:486–487, 2008; NEJM 355:1345–1346, 2006; JAAD 49 (CR) S164–166, 2003; AD 135:859–861, 1999*

Vogt-Koyanagi-Harada syndrome – alopecia, dysacusia, poliosis, uveitis, tinnitus, aseptic meningitis, vitiligo *Surv Ophthalmol 62:1–25, 2017; JAAD 44:129–131, 2001; Neurology 20:965–974, 1970*

Waardenburg's syndrome – autosomal dominant, congenital deafness, heterochromic irides, hypomelanotic macule, lateral displacement of the inner canthi and lacrimal punctae, prominence of nasal root and medial eyebrows, white forelock *AD 135:859–861, 1999*

Werner's Syndrome – autosomal recessive, graying hair by age of 20

White forelock with osteopathia striata (autosomal or X-linked dominant)

White forelock with multiple malformations (autosomal or X-linked recessive)

Woolf's Syndrome – autosomal recessive, piebaldism and deafness

Ziprkowski-Margolis Syndrome – deafness, heterochromic irides, piebald-like hypomelanosis skin and hair

TRAUMA

Post-traumatic

Repetitive plucking *J Cut Med Surg 14:193–194, 2010*

Other graying hair syndromes -
Chediak-Higashi syndrome
Down's syndrome
Hallerman-Streiff syndrome
Homocystinuria
Menkes' kinky hair syndrome
Oasthouse disease
Phenylketonuria
Pierre-Robin syndrome
Treacher-Collins syndrome
Tyrosinuria
Vitiligo

POLYDACTYLY (PPD, PAP, AND COMPLEX TYPES)

SYNDROMES

Acrocallosal syndrome (Greig cephalopolysyndactyly syndrome) – abnormal upper lids, frontonasal dysostosis, callosal agenesis, cleft lip/palate, redundant skin of neck, grooved chin, bifid thumbs, polydactyly, syndactyly; *G13* mutation *Dev Dyn 240:931–942, 2011; Orphanet J Rare Dis April 24, 2008; Am J Med Genet 43:938–941, 1992*

AKT serine/threonine kinase – megalencephaly-capillary malformation syndrome/megalencephaly-polymicrogyria-polydactyly-hydrocephalus syndrome – *AKT3, PIK3R2, PIK3CA JAAD 68:885–896, 2013*

Bardet-Biedl syndrome – postaxial polydactyly (ulnar), rod-cone dystrophy (retinal dystrophy), retinitis pigmentosa, obesity, neuropathy, mental disturbance, renal abnormalities, hypogonadism *Ped Derm 36:346–348, 2019; J Med Genet 36:599–603, 1999*

Bifid epiglottis syndrome – accessory auricles with preauricular sinus, polycystic kidney disease with intrahepatic biliary dilatation, endocardial cushion defect, polydactyly *Ped Int 52:723–728, 2010*

Braegger syndrome – proportionate short stature, IUGR, ischiadic hypoplasia, renal dysfunction, craniofacial anomalies, postaxial polydactyly, hypospadias, microcephaly, mental retardation *Am J Med Genet 66:378–398, 1996*

Cleft lip/palate, preaxial and postaxial polydactyly of hands and feet, congenital heart defect, and genitourinary anomalies *Syndromes of the Head and Neck, p. 751, 1990*

Cleft palate, absent tibiae, preaxial polydactyly of the feet, and congenital heart defect *Am J Dis Child 129:714–716, 1975*

Congenital dyserythropoietic anemia type I – small or absent nails; partial absence or shortening of fingers and toes, mesoaxial polydactyly, syndactyly of hands and feet; short stature, vertebral abnormalities and Madelung deformity; mutation in *CDAN1 Clin Exp Dermatol 515–517, 2020*

Dandy Walker syndrome *Am J Med Genet 85:183–184, 1999;* and postaxial polydactyly, Pierquin syndrome *Clin Dysmorphol 22:51–53, 2013*

Disorganization syndrome – filiform worm-like projections, syndactyly, popliteal pterygium, polydactyly, cleft lip/palate; ear abnormalities *Ped Derm 24:90–92, 2007; J Med Genet 26:417–420, 1989*

Ellis-van Creveld syndrome (chondroplastic dwarf with defective teeth and nails, and polydactyly) – autosomal recessive; chondrodysplasia, polydactyly, peg-shaped teeth or hypodontia, short upper lip bound down by multiple frenulae; nail dystrophy, hair may be normal or sparse and brittle; cardiac defects; ichthyosis, palmoplantar keratoderma; *EVC* mutation *Dev Dyn 240:931–942, 2011; Ped Derm 18:485–489, 2001; Ped Derm 18:68–70, 2001; J Med Genet 17:349–356, 1980; Arch Dis Child 15:65–84, 1940*

Epidermal (sebaceus) nevus syndrome

Fetal hydantoin syndrome *Clin Genet 51:343–345, 1997*

Filippi syndrome – polydactyly, syndactyly, microcephaly, growth retardation, and mental retardation *Am J Med Genet 87:128–133, 1999*

Goltz's syndrome (focal dermal hypoplasia) – linear alopecia *Cutis 53:309–312, 1994; J Dermatol 21:122–124, 1994;* asymmetric linear and reticulated streaks of atrophy and telangiectasia; yellow–red nodules; raspberry-like papillomas of lips, perineum, acrally, at perineum, buccal mucosa; xerosis; scalp and pubic hair sparse and brittle; short stature; asymmetric face; syndactyly, polydactyly; ocular, dental, and skeletal abnormalities with osteopathia striata of long bones *JAAD 25:879–881, 1991*

Kaufman-McKusick syndrome – hydrometrocolpos, hydronephrosis, postaxial polydactyly, congenital heart defect, vaginal atresia *J Med Genet 36:599–603, 1999; Eur J Pediatr 136:297–305, 1981*

Macrocephaly-CMTC (cutis marmorata telangiectatica congenita syndrome) – renamed "macrocephaly-capillary malformation syndrome" – macrocephalic neonatal hypotonia and developmental delay; frontal bossing, segmental overgrowth, syndactyly, asymmetry, distended linear and serpiginous abdominal wall veins, patchy reticulated vascular stain without atrophy; telangiectasias of face and ears; midline reticulated facial nevus flammeus (capillary malformation) (vascular stains), hydrocephalus, skin and joint hypermobility, hyperelastic skin, thickened subcutaneous tissue, polydactyly, 2–3 toe syndactyly, post-axial polydactyly, hydrocephalus, frontal bossing, hemihypertrophy with segmental overgrowth; neonatal hypotonia, developmental delay *Ped Derm 33:570–584, 2016; Ped Derm 29:384–386, 2012; JAAD 63:805–814, 2010; Ped Derm 26:342–346, 2009; AD 145:287–293, 2009; JAAD 58:697–702, 2008; Ped Derm 24:555–556, 2007; JAAD 56:541–564, 2007; Ped Derm 16:235–237, 1999; Genet Couns 9:245–253, 1998; Am J Med Genet 70:67–73, 1997; Clin Dysmorphol 6:291–302, 1997;*

(Note: Beckwith-Wiedemann syndrome demonstrates dysmorphic ears, macroglossia, body asymmetry, midfacial vascular stains, visceromegaly with omphalocele, neonatal hypoglycemia, BUT NO MACROCEPHALY)

Megalencephaly-polymicrogyria-polydactyly-hydrocephalus syndrome – macrocephaly, face and limb asymmetry, craniofacial abnormalities, joint laxity or soft skin, distal limb malformation; developmental delay, *Nat Genet 44:934–940, 2012; Ped Derm 30:541–548, 2013*

Meckel syndrome – microcephaly, microphthalmia, congenital heart defects, postaxial polydactyly, polycystic kidneys, cleft lip/palate *J Med Genet 8:285–290, 1971*

Menkes' kinky hair syndrome – X-linked recessive; polydactyly, syndactyly, fine hypopigmented wiry hair, doughy skin, bone and connective tissue disturbances, progressive neurologic deterioration; intracranial hemorrhages *Cutis 90:183–185, 2012*

Nevoid basal cell carcinoma syndrome (Gorlin's syndrome) – autosomal dominant; macrocephaly, frontal bossing, hypertelorism, cleft lip or palate, papules of the face, neck, and trunk, facial milia, lamellar calcification of the falx cerebri and tentorium cerebelli, cerebral cysts, calcifications of the brain, palmoplantar pits, mandibular keratocysts, skeletal anomalies, including enlarged mandibular coronoid, bifid ribs, kyphosis, spina bifida, polydactyly of the hands or feet, syndactyly; basal cell carcinomas; multiple eye anomalies – congenital cataract, microphthalmia, coloboma of the iris, choroid, and optic nerve; strabismus, nystagmus, keratin-filled cysts of the palpebral conjunctivae; also medulloblastomas, ovarian tumors (fibromas), mesenteric cysts, cardiac fibromas, fetal rhabdomyomas, astrocytomas, meningiomas, craniopharyngiomas, fibrosarcomas, ameloblastomas; renal anomalies; hypogonadotropic hypogonadism, *BJD 165:30–34, 2011; AD 146:17–19, 2010; JAAD 39:853–857, 1998; Dermatol Clin 13:113–125, 1995; JAAD 11:98–104, 1984; NEJM 262:908–912, 1960;* linear unilateral nevoid basal cell nevus syndrome *JAAD 50:489–494, 2004*

Nevus comedonicus syndrome – preaxial polydactyly, skeletal defects, cerebral abnormalities, cataracts *Ped Derm 15:304–306, 1998*

Onychoheterotopia – mimics polydactyly; nail tissue growing outside of classic nail unit; congenital or familial; seen in Pierre-Robin syndrome and abnormal long arm chromosome 6 *JAAD 64:161–166, 2011*

Oral-facial-digital syndrome type I (Papillon-League syndrome) – X-linked dominant; short upper lip, hypoplastic ala nasi, hooked pug nose, hypertrophied labial frenulae, bifid or multilobed tongue with small tumors within clefts, clefting of hard and soft palate, teeth widely spaced, trident hand or brachydactyly, syndactyly, or postaxial (ulnar) polydactyly; hair dry and brittle, alopecic, numerous milia of face, ears, backs of hands, mental retardation *Ped Derm 9:52–56, 1992; Pediatrics 29:985–995, 1962; Rev Stomatol 55:209–227, 1954;*

orofacial digital syndrome type VI – hypoplasia of cerebellar vermis, partial ophthalmoplegia *J Med Genet 36:599–603, 1999*

Pallister-Hall syndrome – *GL13* mutation

Patau's syndrome (trisomy 13) – polydactyly, simian crease of hand, loose skin of posterior neck, parieto-occipital

scalp defects, abnormal helices, low set ears, hyperconvex narrow nails *Ped Derm 22:270–275, 2005*

Polydactyly (preaxial) (radial) with radial and tibial dysplasia *Cutis 77:365–366, 2006;* thumb duplication *Curr Pediatr Rev 14:91–96, 2016*

Polydactyly (postaxial) (ulnar), hypoplastic nails, hypothalamic dysfunction; autosomal dominant *Sem Pediatr Neurol 6:238–242, 1999*

Polyonychia *Ann Dermatol 30:105–106, 2018; Dermatol Online J 18:10, 2015*

Popliteal pterygium (popliteal web) syndrome – autosomal dominant; bilateral popliteal pterygia, intercrural pterygium, hypoplastic digits, absence of labia majora, hypertrophied clitoris, cryptorchidism, bifid scrotum, valgus or varus foot deformities, syndactyly with or without polydactyly, cryptorchidism, umbilical or inguinal hernia, cleft scrotum, lower lip pits, cleft palate, mucous membrane bands (syngnathia) (fibrous bands connecting maxilla and mandible), eyelid adhesions (ankyloblepharon), hypertelorism, defect of alveolar ridge; mutation in *IRF6* (this mutation also seen in van der Woude syndrome) *Ped derm 28:333–334, 2011: J Med Genet 36:888–892, 1999; Int J Pediatr Otorhinolaryngol 15:17–22, 1988*

Postaxial polydactyly-dental-vertebral syndrome *J Pediatr 90:230–235, 1977*

Proteus syndrome *J Mol Diagn 19:487–497,613–624, 2017*

Rudimentary polydactyly (supernumerary digits) *Cutis 77:365–366, 2006; Ped Derm 20:108–112, 2003; Arch Pediatr Adolesc Med 149:1284, 1995*

Saldino–Noonan short rib polydactyly syndrome – autosomal recessive; mutations in *DYNC2H1 Clin Genet 92:158–165, 2017*

Smith-Lemli-Opitz syndrome – autosomal recessive; deficiency of 7-dehydrocholesterol-7-reductase (converts 7-DHC to cholesterol so have increased 7-DHC and decreased cholesterol) – sunburn with photosensitivity to UVA, polydactyly, syndactyly of 2nd and 3rd toes, growth and mental retardation, failure to thrive, dysmorphic facies, cleft palate, congenital heart disease, hypospadias *JAAD 67:1113–1127, 2012; AD 142:647–648, 2006; BJD 153:774–779, 2005; NEJM 351;2319–2326, 2004;BJD 144:143–145, 2001; Photodermato Photoimmunol Photomed 15:217–218, 1999; BJD 141::406–414, 1999; JAAD 41:121–123, 1999; Am J Med Genet 66:378–398, 1996 Am J Hum Genet 53:817–821, 1993; Clin Pediatr 16:665–668, 1977; J Pediatr 64:210–217, 1964*

Tibial aplasia with polydactyly and triphalangeal thumbs – autosomal dominant *J Hum Genet 59:467–470, 2014*

Townes-Brocks syndrome – preaxial polydactyly, external ear abnormalities, hearing loss, imperforate anus, renal malformations; autosomal dominant; chromosome 16q12.1 *Cutis 77:365–366, 2006*

Trisomy 2p syndrome – postaxial (ulnar) polydactyly *Am J Med Genet 87:45–48, 1999*

Trisomy 13 – total body milia; polydactyly, congenital cystic adenomatoid malformation, pulmonary hypertension, apnea, atrial septal defect, umbilical hernia, epilepsy, dislocated hip joint, ocular hypertelorism, microphthalmia, retinal hypoplasia, irideremia, small ears, deafness, broad flat nose, cleft palate, micrognathia, mental retardation *Ped Derm 27:657–658, 2010*

Ulnar-mammary syndrome – autosomal dominant; ulnar defects, nipple or apocrine gland hypoplasia; wide face, nasal base and tip, protruding chin; cardiac abnormalities *TXB3* mutation *Eplasty 27:14:ic35, e collection 2014, 2014 September*

Werner mesomelic syndrome – autosomal dominant

PORE

AD 125:827–832, 1989

AUTOIMMUNE DISEASES

Lupus erythematosus, discoid – personal observation

CONGENITAL ABNORMALITIES

Dermoid cyst of the nose

Preauricular fistula

Sacrococcygeal pore with underlying spinal defects (spinal dysraphism)

INFECTIONS AND INFESTATIONS

Dental sinus

Furunculoid myiasis (tumbu fly) – pore overlying furuncular lesion *JAMA Derm 154:737–738, 2018*

INFLAMMATORY DISORDERS

Post-inflammatory scar

NEOPLASTIC DISORDERS

Basal cell carcinoma (trichoid basal cell carcinoma) *JAAD 47:727–732, 2002;* within a dilated pore of Winer *Dermatol Surg 26:874–876, 2000*

Dilated pore nevus (variant of nevus comedonicus) *Am J Dermatopathol 15:169–171, 1993*

Epidermoid cyst

Nevus comedonicus *JAAD 43:927–929, 2000*

Pilar sheath acanthoma *JAAD 47:727–732, 2002; Yonsei Med J 30:392–395, 1989; Dermatologica 167:335–338, 1983; AD 114:1495–1497, 1978*

Sebaceous hyperplasia *JAAD 47:727–732, 2002*

Sebaceous trichofolliculoma *J Cut Pathol 7:394–403, 1980*

Trichoblastoma – with dilated pore *JAAD 54:357–358, 2006*

Trichofolliculoma *AD 125:827, 830, 1989; AD 81:922–930, 1960*

PRIMARY CUTANEOUS DISEASES

Aggregated dilated pores *J Dermatol 26:332–333, 1999*

Comedone

Dilated pore of Winer – infundibuloma *JAAD 47:727–732, 2002; Am J Dermatopathol 23:246–253, 2001; JID 23:181–188, 1954;* in external auditory canal *Auris Nasus Larynx 28:349–352, 2001*

Epidermolytic hyperkeratosis *J Dermatol 14:286–288, 1987*

Facial pore, enlarged – (1) high sebum secretion; (2) decreased elasticity around pore; (3) increased hair follicle volume *Dermatol Surg 42:277–285, 2016*

Fistula of dorsum of nose *AD 109:227–229, 1974*

Hair cortex comedo *Am J Dermatopathol 18:322–325, 1996*

Pilonidal sinus

Pits of lower lip – mucous secreting labial glands

SYNDROMES

Trichothiodystrophy syndromes – BIDS, IBIDS, PIBIDS – pre-auricular pits, poikiloderma, sparse or absent eyelashes and eyebrows, brittle hair, premature aging, sexual immaturity, ichthyosis, dysmyelination, bird-like facies, dental caries; trichothiodystrophy with ichthyosis, urologic malformations, hypercalciuria and mental and physical retardation *Ped Derm 14:441–445, 1997; JAAD 44:891–920, 2001*

TRAUMA

Piercing

Scars *JAAD 47:727–732, 2002*

PORT WINE STAIN

Ped Derm 14:466–469, 1997

DRUGS

Following administration of isotretinoin *Clin Exp Dermatol 30:587–588, 2005*

SYNDROMES

Beckwith-Wiedemann syndrome – nevus flammeus of central forehead and upper eyelids, macroglossia, macrosomia, omphalocele or other umbilical anomalies, linear grooves of the ear lobes *Syndromes of the Head and Neck 1990:323–328*

Bonnet-Dechaume-Blanc syndrome (Wyburn-Mason syndrome) – facial port wine stain, unilateral retinal arteriovenous malformation with ipsilateral intracranial arteriovenous malformation *Bibl Ophthalmol 76:124–128, 1968; Brain 66:163–203, 1943*

Bregea's syndrome – angiomatosis of the eye and orbit, port wine stain in scalp and contralateral forehead, and ipsilateral thalamencephalic angiomatosis

Cobb syndrome – segmental port wine stain or angiokeratoma of torso with a vascular malformation of the spinal cord *Dermatology 221:11–112, 2010; Ped Neurol 39:423–425, 2008; Ann Surg 62:641–649, 1915*

Cutis marmorata telangiectatica congenita *J Dermatol 35:471–472, 2008*

Klippel-Trenaunay syndrome – port wine stain, venous varicosities, hypertrophy of soft tissues *BMJ Case Rep 12:e230146 Aug 2019; Cutis 40:51–53, 1987*

Macrocephaly-CMTC (cutis marmorata telangiectatica congenita syndrome) – renamed "macrocephaly-capillary malformation syndrome" – macrocephalic neonatal hypotonia and developmental delay; frontal bossing, segmental overgrowth, syndactyly, asymmetry, distended linear and serpiginous abdominal wall veins, patchy reticulated vascular stain without atrophy; telangiectasias of face and ears; midline reticulated facial nevus flammeus (capillary malformation) (vascular stains), hydrocephalus, skin and joint hypermobility, hyperelastic skin, thickened subcutaneous tissue, polydactyly, 2–3 toe syndactyly, post-axial polydactyly, hydrocephalus, frontal bossing, hemihypertrophy with segmental overgrowth; neonatal hypotonia, developmental delay *Ped Derm 29:384–386, 2012; JAAD 63:805–814, 2010; Ped Derm 26:342–346, 2009; AD 145:287–293, 2009; JAAD 58:697–702, 2008; Ped Derm 24:555–556, 2007; JAAD 56:541–564, 2007; Ped Derm 16:235–237, 1999; Genet Couns 9:245–253, 1998; Am J Med Genet 70:67–73, 1997; Clin Dysmorphol 6:291–302, 1997;*

(Note: Beckwith-Wiedemann syndrome demonstrates dysmorphic ears, macroglossia, body asymmetry, midfacial vascular stains, visceromegaly with omphalocele, neonatal hypoglycemia, BUT NO MACROCEPHALY)

Nova syndrome – glabellar port wine stain, mega cisterna magna, communicating hydrocephalus, and posterior cerebellar vermis agenesis

Parkes-Weber syndrome – port wine stain and arteriovenous fistula, soft tissue and bony hypertrophy, congenital varicose veins

Phakomatosis pigmentovascularis – combinations of nevus flammeus with epidermal nevus (type I), aberrant Mongolian spots with or without nevus anemicus (type II), nevus silus with or without nevus anemicus (type III), and aberrant mongolian spots, nevus spilus, with or without nevus anemicus *J Dermatol 46:843–848, 2019; AD 102:640–645, 1970*

Proteus syndrome – hemihypertrophy, partial gigantism of the hands and/or feet, macrocephaly, subcutaneous hamartomatous tumors, epidermal nevi, visceral abnormalities, and early accelerated growth *Eur J Pediatr 140:5–12, 1983*

Robert's syndrome – hypomelia-hypotrichosis-facial hemangioma (pseudothalidomide) syndrome – mid forehead and midfacial port wine stain, cleft lip and/or palate, sparse silvery blonde hair, limb reduction defects, and marked growth retardation, hypoplastic ear lobules *Clin Genet 5:1–16, 1974*

Rubenstein-Taybi syndrome – forehead port wine stain

Short arm chromosome 4 deletion syndrome (Wolf-Hirschhorn syndrome)

Spinal dysraphism – associated port wine stain *Ped Derm 26:688–695, 2009*

Sturge-Weber syndrome (encephalotrigeminal angiomatosis) – unilateral port wine stain in trigeminal area, ipsilateral leptomeningeal venous malformation, atrophy and calcifications in cerebral cortex, neurologic, and ophthalmologic defects *Ped Derm 35:30–42, 2018*

TAR syndrome – thrombocytopenia-absent radii – port wine stain of head and neck

Thalidomide embryopathy – pronounced facial port wine stain

Turner's syndrome *Int J Dermatol 51:207–210, 2012*

Trisomy 13 syndrome – forehead port wine stain

Trisomy 18 syndrome – port wine stain

von Hippel-Lindau syndrome – facial or occipitocervical port wine stain, retinal angiomatosis, either cerebellar, medullary, or spinal hemangioblastomas, and renal cell carcinoma

XXYY syndrome

TRAUMA

Post traumatic port wine stain *AD 136:897–899, 2000*

VASCULAR DISORDERS

Diffuse phlebectasia (Brockenheimer's disease) *Ped Derm 17:100–104, 2000*

Inflammatory nuchal-occipital port wine stain – psoriasiform plaque *JAAD 35:811–813, 1996*

Butterfly-shaped mark – red-violet triangular or rhomboidal vascular mark on sacrum *Pediatrics 85:1069–1071, 1990*

Port wine stain – autosomal dominant *J Pediatr 73:755–757, 1968*

Port wine stain of the face and ocular defects – glaucoma, choroidal vascular anomalies, orbital lesions *Can J Ophthalmol 10:136–139, 1975*

Port wine stain with underlying spina bifida occulta or tethered cord or other anomalies of spinal dysraphism

Rorschach inkblot port wine stain

Salmon patch (nevus simplex) *Pediatr Clin North Am 30:465–482, 1983*

PREAURICULAR SINUSES (EAR PITS)

Ped Derm 21:191–196, 2004; Cutis 88:275–278–280, 2012

PRIMARY CUTANEOUS DISEASES

Sporadic *Cutis 88:275–278–280, 2012*

Familial – autosomal dominant

SYNDROMES

Bilateral defects, male transmission – bilateral cervical branchial sinuses, bilateral preauricular sinuses, bilateral malformed auricles, bilateral hearing impairment *Hum Genet 56:269–273, 1981*

Bifid epiglottis syndrome – accessory auricles with preauricular sinus, polycystic kidney disease with intrahepatic biliary dilatation, endocardial cushion defect, polydactyly *Ped Int 52:723–728, 2010*

Branchio-oto-renal syndrome (BOR) – autosomal dominant; mutation in EYA1 gene; conductive, sensorineural, mixed hearing loss; pre-auricular pits, structural defects of outer, middle, or inner ear; renal anomalies, renal failure, lateral cervical fistulae, cysts, or sinuses; nasolacrimal duct stenosis or fistulae *Am J Kidney Dis 37:505–509, 2001; Cutis 68:353–354, 2001*

Branchio-otic syndrome – autosomal dominant; branchial anomalies, preauricular pits, hearing loss, no renal dysplasia *J Med Genet 39:71–73, 2002*

Branchio-oto-ureteral syndrome – autosomal dominant; bilateral sensorineural hearing loss, preauricular pit or tag, duplication of ureters or bifid renal pelvises *J Dermatol 29:157–159, 2002*

Branchio-oto-costal syndrome – autosomal dominant; branchial arch anomalies, hearing loss, ear and commissural lip pits, and rib anomalies *Ear Nose Throat J 92:306–309, 2013; J Craniofac Genet Dev Biol 1 (suppl):287–295, 1985*

Branchio-oculo-facial syndrome – abnormal upper lip, malformed nose with broad nasal bridge and flattened tip, lacrimal duct obstruction, malformed ears, branchial cleft sinuses and/or linear skin lesions behind ears *Ann Otol Rhinol Laryngol 100:928–932, 1991*

Cat's eye syndrome – sporadic; *CECR2*; iris colobomas, imperforate anus with fistulae, down slanting palpebral fissures, congenital heart anomalies *Cutis 88:275–278–280, 2012*

Deafness, pre-auricular sinus, external ear anomaly, and commissural lip pit syndrome – autosomal dominant; pinna dysplasia, mixed or conductive hearing loss *Cutis 88:275–278–280, 2012*

Ectodermal dysplasia – preauricular pits, tetra-amelia, ectodermal dysplasia, hypoplastic lacrimal ducts and sacs opening toward exterior, peculiar facies, developmental retardation *Ann Genet 30:101–104, 1987*

Emanuel syndrome – microcephaly, preauricular tag of sinus, ear anomalies, cleft or high arched palate, micrognathia, congenital heart disease, structural brain abnormalities, genital anomalies in males *Genet Counsel 23:319–328, 2012*

Hemifacial microsomia syndrome – bilateral preauricular sinuses, facial steatocystoma multiplex associated with pilar cysts, sensorineural hearing loss, facial palsy, microtia or anotia, cervical appendages containing cartilage *Am J Med Genet 22:135–141, 1985*

Hennekam syndrome – autosomal recessive; intestinal lymphangiectasia, lymphedema of legs and genitalia, gigantic scrotum and penis, multilobulated lymphatic ectasias, small mouth, narrow palate, gingival hypertrophy, tooth anomalies, thick lips, agenesis of ear, pre-auricular pits, wide flat nasal bridge, frontal upsweep, platybasia, hypertelorism, pterygia colli, bilateral single palmar crease, hirsutism, mild mental retardation, facial anomalies, growth retardation, pulmonary, cardiac, hypogammaglobulinemia *Ped Derm 23:239–242, 2006*

Lip pits – preauricular sinuses, conductive deafness, commissural lip pits, external ear abnormalities *J Med Genet 24:609–612, 1987; preauricular pits, commissural lip pits, congenital conductive/mixed deafness Ann Otol Rhinol Larngol 100:928–932, 1991*

Rares syndrome of bilateral defects – male transmission to male; bilateral cervical sinus and branchial sinus; malformed ears; bilateral hearing impairment *Cutis 88:275–278–280, 2012*

Steatocystoma multiplex – pilar cysts and

Tetralogy of Fallot and clinodactyly – characteristic facies, preauricular pits, fifth finger clinodactyly, tetralogy of Fallot *Clin Pediatr (Phila)27:451–454, 1988*

Complete trisomy 22 – maternal origin of extra chromosome; primitive low-set ears, bilateral preauricular pit, broad nasal bridge, antimongoloid palpebral fissures, macroglossia, enlarged sublingual glands, cleft palate, micrognathia, clinodactyly of fifth fingers, hypoplastic fingernails, hypoplastic genitalia, short lower limbs, bilateral sandal gap, deep plantar furrows *Pediatrics 108:E32, 2001*

Incomplete trisomy 22 (trisomy 22 mosaicism) – 46XX/47, XX + 22; complex congenital heart defect, membranous anal atresia without fistula, distal limb hypoplasia, partial cutaneous syndactyly of second and third toes, left preauricular pit; hypotonia, and delayed development *Urology 40:259–261, 1992*

Waardenburg syndrome – bilateral preauricular sinuses *Acta Paediatr 86:17—172, 1997*

PREGNANCY, CUTANEOUS MANIFESTATIONS

J Drugs Dermatol 14:512–513, 2015

AUTOIMMUNE DISEASES

Pemphigoid gestationis (herpes gestationis) – urticaria-like lesions *JAAD 62:541–555, 2010; BJD 157:388–389, 2007; JAAD 55:823–828, 2006; JAAD 40:847–849, 1999; JAAD 17:539–536, 1987; Clin Exp Dermatol 7:65–73, 1982*

INFECTIONS EXACERBATED BY PREGNANCY

J Epidemiol Glob Health 7:63–70, 2017

Candidal vaginitis

Condylomata acuminatum

Herpes simplex *Clin Perinatol 46:235–236, 2019*

Leprosy reaction – reversal reaction and erythema nodosum leprosum

Pityrosporum folliculitis

Trichomonas vaginalis

Varicella, especially 3rd trimester *Clin Dermatol 34:368–377, 2016*

INFLAMMATORY DISORDERS

Sweet's syndrome, recurrent *JAAD 30 (PT 2)297–300, 1994; Ob Gyn Surg 48:584–587, 1993*

METABOLIC DISORDERS

Gigantomastia of pregnancy – ulceration of breast *Br J Surg 74:585–586, 1987*

Gingival hyperemia or hyperplasia (marginal gingivitis) *JAAD 52:491–499, 2005; J Int Med Res 30:353–355, 2002; J Am Dent Assoc 110:365–368, 1985*

Hirsutism

Hyperpigmentation of nipples, axillae, linea nigra, pseudoacanthosis nigricans, vulvar melanosis

Intrahepatic cholestasis of pregnancy – intense generalized pruritus beginning on palms and soles *J Drugs Dermatol 14:512–513, 2015; JAAD 6:977–998, 1982; Acta Med Scand 196:403–410, 1974*

Miliaria

Pigmentary demarcation lines of pregnancy *Cutis 38:263–266, 1986; JAAD 11:438–440, 1984*

Pruritic urticarial papules and plaques of pregnancy (polymorphic eruption of pregnancy) – zebra stripe dermatitis *JAAD 39:933–939, 1998; JAAD 10:473–480, 1984; Clin Exp Dermatol 7:65–73, 1982; JAMA 241:1696–1699, 1979;* post-partum PUPPP *Cutis 95:344–347, 2015*

Prurigo of Besnier (Nurse's early prurigo of pregnancy, papular dermatitis of Spangler) – widespread papular and urticarial eruption *JAAD 45:1–19, 2001*

Pruritus, generalized – cholestasis of pregnancy *JAAD 6:977–998, 1982; Acta Med Scand 196:403–410, 1974*

Subungual hyperkeratosis *J Drugs Dermatol 14:512–513, 2015*

NEOPLASTIC DISORDER IMPACTED BY PREGNANCY

Clin Dermatol 34:359–367, 2016

Acrochordon

Dermatofibroma *Dermatol Online J May 15, 2019*

Dermatofibrosarcoma protuberans

Glomangioma

Glomus tumor

Hemangioendothelioma

Hemangioma

Keloid

Leiomyoma *J Cut Med Surg 20:334–336, 2016*

Melanocytic nevus

Melanoma

Neurofibroma

Pyogenic granuloma

PRIMARY CUTANEOUS DISEASES

Acne vulgaris, exacerbation; rosacea fulminans *Open Access Maced J Med Sci 6:1438–1441, 2018*

Atopic eruption of pregnancy *J Drugs Dermatol 14:512–513, 2015*

Dyshidrosis

Hyperhidrosis

Impetigo herpetiformis – generalized pustular psoriasis *Int J Womens Health 10:109–115, 2018*

Postpartum telogen effluvium

Pruritic folliculitis of pregnancy *AD 117:20–22, 1981*

Striae distensae gravidarum (white or purple)

Urticaria

VASCULAR DISORDERS

Cutis marmorata of legs

Edema, non-pitting – eyelids, face, legs

Hemorrhoids

Palmar erythema

Port wine stains – marked enlargement and palpability

Spider telangiectasias (spider angioma, nevus araneus) *JAAD 6:977–998, 1982*

Unilateral nevoid telangiectasia *AD 146:1167–1172, 2010; Dermatology 209:215–217, 2004; JAAD 37:523–549, 1997; JAAD 8:468–477, 1983; Monatsschr Prakt Dermat 28:451, 1899*

Pyogenic granulomas

Varicosities

PREMATURE AGING SYNDROMES (PROGEROID SYNDROMES)

AUTOIMMUNE DISEASES

Lupus erythematosus, systemic – shortened telomere length in SLE *Expert Rev Clin Immunol 9:1193–1204, 2013; Arthritis Rheum 65:1319–1323, 2013*

EXOGENOUS AGENTS

Methamphetamine abuse *JAAD 69:135–142, 2013*

Smoker's face – linear wrinkling and atrophy *AD 128:255–262, 1992*

INFECTIONS

HIV disease *Clin Exp Immunol 187:44–52, 2017; Ann Rev Med 62:141–155, 2011*

INFILTRATIVE DISORDERS

Mastocytosis, systemic – premature aged facial appearance due to pruritus and rubbing *Ped Derm 19:184–185, 2002*

METABOLIC DISORDERS

Congenital erythropoietic porphyria *JAMA Derm 149:969–970, 2013*

Cystinosis – skin atrophy and telangiectasia mimicking premature aging; normal skin; subcutaneous plaques *JAAD 62:AB26, 2010; JAAD 68:e111–116, 2013*

Diabetic cheiroarthropathy – thickened immobile skin

Pituitary dwarfism

Porphyria – erythropoietic protoporphyria; premature aged appearance of hands *BJD 155:574–581, 2006*

Prolidase deficiency – fragile skin *FEBS J 285;3422–3441, 2018*

PHOTODERMATOSES

Actinic damage (photoaging)

Congenital photosensitivity syndromes
   Poikiloderma congenitale
   Xeroderma pigmentosum
   Cockayne's syndrome

Ultraviolet radiation – excess exposure to ultraviolet radiation (dermatoheliosis)

PRIMARY CUTANEOUS DISEASES

Blepharochalasis *Can J Ophthalmol 27:10–15, 1992; Cutis 45:91–94, 1990; Br J Ophthalmol 72:863–867, 1988; AD 115:479–481, 1979*

Congenital generalized lipodystrophy *Atlas of Clinical Syndromes A Visual Aid to Diagnosis, 1992, pp.280–281*

SYNDROMES

Acrogeria (Gottron's syndrome) – micrognathia, atrophy of tip of nose, atrophic skin of distal extremities with telangiectasia, easy bruising, mottled pigmentation or poikiloderma of extremities, dystrophic nails *BJD 103:213–223, 1980*

Acrometageria *Am J Med Genet 44:334–339, 1992*

Anhidrotic ectodermal dysplasia (Christ-Siemens-Touraine syndrome) *J Dermatol 26:44–47, 1999;* X-linked recessive – premature aged appearance with finely wrinkled skin, especially around eyes; absent or reduced sweating, hypotrichosis, and total or partial anodontia *J Med Genet 28:181–185, 1991;* autosomal recessive *Ped Derm 7:242, 1990*

Ataxia telangiectasia *Aging Res Rev 33:76–88, 2017; AD 134:1145–1150, 1998*

Atypical progeroid syndrome – diffuse mottled hyperpigmentation – mutations in *LMNA* gene *Ped Derm 36:913–917, 2019*

Baraitser syndrome (premature aging with short stature and pigmented nevi) – lack of facial subcutaneous fat, fine hair, hypospadius, dental abnormalities, hepatomegaly *J Med Genet 25:53–56, 1988*

Barber-Say syndrome – generalized hypertrichosis, dysmorphic facies (bilateral ectropion, hypertelorism, macrostomia, abnormal ears, bulbous nose, sparse eyebrows and eyelashes, hypoplasia of nipples with absence of mammary glands, transposition of scrotum, club feet, short neck, lax skin, premature aged appearance, cleft palate, conductive hearing loss *Ped Derm 23:183–184, 2006; Syndrome Ident 8:6–9, 1982*

Berardinelli-Seip syndrome – progeroid syndrome present at birth; lack of body fat, muscularity from birth, acanthosis nigricans, acromegaloid features, umbilical hernia, clitoromegaly, mild hypertrichosis, hyperinsulinemia, impaired glucose tolerance, hypertriglyceridemia *Ped Derm 22:75–78, 2005*

Bloom's syndrome – progeroid syndrome with predisposition to solid and hematologic malignancy; butterfly rash, telangiectasia, photosensitivity, atrophy, hypo- or hyperpigmentation, atrophy, CALMs, acanthosis nigricans, small testes *Curr Opinion Genet Dis 26:41–46, 2014*

Carbohydrate deficient glycoprotein (CDG) syndrome type I – present at birth; lipodystrophic skin, sticky skin (peau d'orange), strabismus, psychomotor delay, floppy, failure to thrive, mental retardation, liver dysfunction cerebellar ataxia, pericardial effusions *Ped Derm 22:75–78, 2005*

Cockayne syndrome – begins in early childhood, xerosis with rough, dry skin, anhidrosis, erythema of hands, hypogonadism; autosomal recessive; short stature with growth failure, microcephaly, facial erythema in butterfly distribution leading to mottled pigmentation and atrophic scars, premature aged appearance with loss of subcutaneous fat and sunken eyes, canities, ataxia, mental deficiency, photosensitivity, disproportionately large hands, feet, and ears, ocular defects, (optic atrophy, pigmentary demyelination), deafness, demyelination *Ped Derm 22:75–78, 2005; Ped Derm 20:538–540, 2003; Am J Hum Genet 50:677–689, 1992; J Med Genet 18:288–293, 1981*

Cutis laxa – congenital cutis laxa – autosomal recessive type 1 – premature aged appearance, diaphragmatic hernia, emphysema *Ped Derm 24:525–528, 2007;* inherited; acquired – with amyloidosis, myeloma, lupus erythematosus, hypersensitivity reaction, complement deficiency, penicillamine, inflammatory skin disease; generalized cutis laxa – autosomal dominant or autosomal recessive; bloodhound appearance of premature aging

Cutis laxa type IIIB – loose folds of wrinkled skin, progeroid facies, osteopenia, central nervous system abnormalities *JAMA Derm 155:257–259, 2019*

DeBarsy syndrome – autosomal recessive progeroid syndrome; present at birth, aged appearance, large helices, eye abnormalities (myopia, strabismus, and cataracts), lax joints, lax and wrinkled skin, neurologic abnormalities (hypotonia, development delay, athetoid movements), cloudy corneas, mental retardation, synophrys, pinched nose, thin skin, sparse hair *Ped Derm 22:75–78, 2005; Eur J Pediar 144:348–354, 1985*

Down's syndrome – trisomy 21 *NEJM 382:2344–2352, 2020; Dev Disabil Res Rev 18:51–67, 2013; Ped Derm 17:282–285, 2000; Pediatrics 16:43–54, 1955*

Dunnigan type familial partial lipodystrophy type 2 – loss of subcutaneous tissue from trunk and limbs; fat accumulation of neck and face; insulin resistant diabetes mellitus, premature atherosclerosis; mutation *LMNA Nucleus 9:249–260, 2018; Aging Cell 17:e12766, 2018*

Dwarfism, bilateral club feet, premature aging, progressive panhypogammaglobulinemia *J Rheumatol 21:961–963, 1994*

Dyskeratosis congenita – bone marrow failure syndrome; cancer predisposition syndrome; triad of oral leukoplakia, nail dystrophy, and reticulated hyperpigmentation; mutation in *DKC1* affecting telomeres *JCI 126:1621–1629, 2016; Mut Res 730:43–51, 2012*

Ehlers-Danlos syndrome type IV (acrogeric type) – acrogeric appearance (thinning and translucency of skin) *BJD 144:1086–1087, 2001;* type VIII – autosomal dominant; skin fragility, abnormal scarring, severe early periodontitis with loss of adult dentition by end of third decade; cigarette paper scars of shin; marfanoid habitus (tall, long limbs, arachnodactyly); triangular face, prominent eyes, thin nose, prematurely aged appearance, thin skin with prominent veins, no joint hypermobility, easy bruising, blue sclerae *JAAD 55:S41–45, 2006*

Familial mandibuloacral dysplasia (craniomandibular dermatodysostosis) – onset at age 3–5 years; atrophy of skin over hands and feet with club shaped terminal phalanges and acro-osteolysis, mandibular dysplasia, delayed cranial suture closure, short stature, dysplastic clavicles, prominent eyes and sharp nose, alopecia, sharp nose, loss of lower teeth, multiple Wormian bones, acro-osteolysis *Ped Derm 22:75–78, 2005; BJD 105:719–723, 1981; Birth Defects x:99–105, 1974*

GAPO syndrome – begins at 1–2 years, growth retardation, alopecia, pseudoanodontia, ocular manifestations (optic atrophy), aged appearance with coarse facial features including frontal bossing, wide anterior fontanelle, saddle nose, micrognathia, protruding thick lips, low set ears, antimongoloid slant, prominent scalp veins, loose skin, small hands, lax joints *Ped Derm 27:156–161, 2010; Ped Derm 22:75–78, 2005; Am J Med Genet 19:209–216, 1984; Odontol Tilster 55:484–493, 1947*

Geroderma osteodysplastica (Bamatter syndrome) (osteodysplastic geroderma) – autosomal recessive; short stature, cutis laxa-like changes with drooping eyelids and jowls (characteristic facies with hypoplastic midface), osteoporosis and skeletal abnormalities; lax wrinkled, atrophic skin, joint hyperextensibility, growth retardation *Ped Derm 23:467–472, 2006; Ped Derm 16:113–117, 1999; Am J Med Genet 3:389–395, 1979; Hum Genet 40:311–324, 1978; Ann Paediatr 174:126–127, 1950*

Hallermann-Streiff syndrome – present at birth, atrophic, thin, taut skin of face and scalp, telangiectasias, hypotrichosis of scalp, xerosis/ichthyosis, beaked pinched nose; brachycephaly, mandibular hypoplasia, ocular abnormalities (cataracts, microphthalmos, nystagmus), dental abnormalities *Ped Derm 22:75–78, 2005*

Hutchinson-Gilford syndrome (progeria) – premature aged appearance; age of onset is 1–2 years, short stature, weight low for height, loss of subcutaneous fat, plucked bird appearance, lax and wrinkled skin, prominent eyes, prominent scalp and leg veins, hyper- and hypomelanosis, alopecia of scalp, eyebrows, and eyelashes; mid-facial cyanosis around mouth and nasolabial folds, decreased sweating, sclerodermoid changes, cobblestoning of soft pebbly nodules, acro-osteolysis, widened metaphyses, and osteoporosis; mutation in lamin A *Aging Res Rev 33:18–29, 2017; Ped Derm 32:271–275, 2015; Ped Derm 22:75–78, 2005; Am J Med Genet 82:242–248, 1999*

Hypohidrotic ectodermal dysplasia

KID syndrome – keratosis, ichthyosis, deafness syndrome – fixed orange, symmetrical hyperkeratotic plaques of scalp, ears, and face with perioral rugae; aged or leonine facies; erythrokeratoderma-like; later hyperkeratotic nodules develop *Ped Derm 17:115–117, 2000; Ped Derm 13:105–113, 1996*

Kindler's syndrome *Orphanet J Rare Dis July 24, 2019*

Klinefelter's syndrome *Metabolism 86:135–144, 2018*

Leprechaunism – progeroid syndrome; present at birth, elfin-like facies, hyperglycemia, insulin resistance, failure to thrive, hypertrichosis, decreased subcutaneous fat, acanthosis nigricans, prominent nipples, enlarged genitalia, loose skin *Ped Derm 22:75–78, 2005*

Mandibuloacral dysplasia – autosomal recessive; progeroid facies; facial asymmetry, micrognathia, small nose, prominent eyes, large open fontanelles; congenital brown pigmentation of ankles progresses to mottled pigmentation; hypoplastic clavicles with acro-osteolysis; contractures of lower extremities; failure to thrive; progressive glomerulopathy; subcutaneous calcified nodules; mutation in *ZMPSTE24* (lamin) *JAMA Derm 151:561–562, 2015;*acral poikiloderma over hands and feet, subcutaneous atrophy *Biochem Soc Trans 39:1752–1757, 2011; Am J Med Genet 95:293–295, 2000; Clin Genet 26:133–138, 1984*

MDM 2-associated progeroid syndrome

Metageria – autosomal recessive; dry, atrophic, mottled skin, pinched face with beaked nose *Hautarzt 48:657–661, 1997; BJD 91:243–262, 1974*

Miescher syndrome

Myotonic dystrophy (Steinert syndrome) type 1 – autosomal dominant; muscular hypotonia, distal weakness of muscles, frontal alopecia, cataract, sensorineural hearing loss, dysarthria, dysphagia, diabetes mellitus, hypothyroidism, cardiac arrhythmias *Dtsch Arztebl Int 116:489–496, 2019; J Med Genet 19:341–348, 1982*

Nestor-Guillermo syndrome – secondary laminopathy; failure to thrive with onset at age 2; atrophic skin with senile shin spots, generalized lipoatrophy, prominent superficial vein, osteoporosis, scoliosis "chronic progeria", longer survival; mutation in *BANF1 Nucleus 9:249–260, 2018*

Premature aging syndrome (Mulvihill-Smith syndrome) – premature aging and immunodeficiency; multiple congenital melanocytic nevi, freckles, blue nevi, lack of facial subcutaneous tissue, xerosis, telangiectasias, thin skin, fine silky hair, premature aging, low birth weight, short stature, birdlike facies, hypodontia, high-pitched voice, mental retardation, sensorineural hearing loss, hepatomegaly *Am J Med Genet 69:56–64, 1997; J Med Genet 31:707–711, 1994; Am J Med Genet 45:597–600, 1993*

Osteodysplastic geroderma (Walt Disney dwarfism) – short stature, cutis laxa-like changes with drooping eyelids and jowls, osteoporosis and skeletal abnormalities *Am J Med Genet 3:389–395, 1979*

Partial or generalized lipodystrophy, insulin resistance

Penttinen syndrome – progeroid disorder with overgrowth; resembles mandibuloacral dysplasia (which has micrognathia); hypertelorism, malar hypoplasia, prognathia, narrow nose; open font, shallow orbits, lipoatrophy with thin translucent skin; scars overlying joints; acroosteolysis *Am J Med Genet A 161A:1786–1791, 2013; Am J Med Genet 69:182–187, 1997*

Premature aging syndrome with osteosarcoma, cataracts, diabetes mellitus, osteoporosis, erythroid macrocytosis, severe growth and developmental deficiency *Am J Med Genet 69:169–170, 1997*

PYCR1-related cutis laxa – hair loss, prominent scalp veins, triangular shaped face, microcephaly, short stature, hypermobility of joints, thin atrophic skin, wrinkled skin, muscle weakness, finger contractures *Dtsch Arztebl Intl 16:489–496, 2019*

Restrictive dermopathy – autosomal recessive, progeric appearance; erythroderma at birth, with extensive erosions and contractures; taut shiny skin; sparse or absent eyelashes, fetal akinesia, multiple joint contractures, dysmorphic facies with fixed open mouth, hypertelorism, pulmonary hypoplasia, bone deformities; uniformly fatal *Ped Derm 19:67–72, 2002; Ped Derm 16:151–153, 1999; AD 134:577–579, 1998; AD 128:228–231, 1992*

Rothmund-Thomson syndrome *Stat Pearls Jan 22, 2020; Genomics 61:268–276, 1999*

Ruijs-Aalfs syndrome – premature aging and cancer predisposition syndrome; facial and skeletal abnormalities; hepatoma in teenage years; triangular face, small deep set eyes, micrognathia ,small upper lip, bulbous nose; *SPRTN* gene *Nature Genet 46:1239–1244, 2014*

Setleis syndrome – aged leonine appearance, scar-like defects of the temples, absent or multiple rows of upper eyelashes, eyebrows slanted up and out, scar-like median furrow of chin *Pediatrics 32:540–548, 1963*

Short stature, premature aging, pigmented nevi *J Med Genet 25:53–56, 1988*

Sparse hair, prominent nose, small mouth, micrognathia, cleft palate, crumpled upper helices, digit anomaly, mild developmental delay *Am J Med Genet 101:70–73, 2001*

Storm syndrome – calcific cardiac valvular degeneration with premature aging; Werner-like syndrome *Am J Hum Genet 45 (suppl) A67, 1989*

Trichothiodystrophy syndromes – BIDS, IBIDS, PIBIDS – autosomal recessive; collodion baby, congenital erythroderma, sparse or absent eyelashes and eyebrows, sulfur deficient short brittle hair with tiger tail banding on polarized microscopy, trichomegaly, brittle soft nails with koilonychia, premature aging (progeria), very short stature, microcephaly, sexual immaturity, ichthyosis, photosensitivity, hypohidrosis, high arched palate, dysmyelination of white matter, osteoporosis, bird-like facies, abnormal teeth with dental caries; hearing loss, cataracts, trichothiodystrophy with ichthyosis, urologic malformations, hypercalciuria and mental and physical retardation; recurrent infections with neutropenia; ocular abnormalities, osteopenia; socially engaging personality; mutation in one of 3 DNA repair genes (XPB, XPA, TTDA, or TTDN1 *JAAD 75:873–882, 2016; JAAD 63:323–328, 2010; Curr Prob Derm 14:71–116, 2002; JAAD 44:891–920, 2001; Ped Derm 14:441–445, 1997*

Werner's syndrome (pangeria) – autosomal recessive; mutation of *WRN* manifesting in adulthood; gray thinning hair, sclerodermoid skin changes, regiona atrophy of subcutaneous fat, high pitch voice, cataracts, diabetes mellitus, skin ulcers, calcification of Achilles tendon, cancers *BJD 152:1030–1032, 2005; Ann N Y Acad Sci 908:167–179, 2000; Cancer 54:2580–2586, 1984; AD 118:106–108, 1982; Medicine 45:177–221, 1966*

Wiedemann-Rautenstrauch (neonatal progeroid syndrome) – autosomal recessive; present at birth, generalized lipoatrophy, macrocephaly, sparse hair, premature aging, wide open sutures, aged and triangular face with hypoplasia of facial bones, persistent fontanelles, prominent scalp veins, growth retardation, low set ears, beak shaped nose, neonatal teeth, slender limbs, large hands and feet with long fingers, joint contractures, large penis, pseudohydrocephalus, psychomotor retardation; osteosarcoma, thyroid carcinoma, melanoma; mutation in helicase *BJD 164:245–256, 2011; Ped Derm 22:75–78, 2005; J Med Genet 34:433–437, 1997; Am J Med Genet 35:91–94, 1990; Eur J Pediatr 130:65–70, 1979; Eur J Pediatr 124:101–111, 1977*

Wrinkly skin syndrome (possibly same as geroderma osteodysplastica) – autosomal recessive; aged appearance with wrinkled skin on abdomen and dorsal aspects of hands and feet, increase palmoplantar creases, prominent venous pattern on chest, intrauterine growth retardation, mental retardation, microcephaly, hypotonia, musculoskeletal abnormalities *Ped Derm 25:66–71, 2008; Ped Derm 23:467–472, 2006; Am J Med Genet 101:213–220, 2001; Ped Derm 16:113–117, 1999*

Xeroderma pigmentosum – multiple skin cancers *Acta DV 99L360–369, 2019*

PRIMARY IMMUNODEFICIENCIES WITH GRANULOMA FORMATION

JAAD 73:367–381, 2015

APLAID (autoinflammation and PLAID) – sinopulmonary infections, interstitial pneumonitis, eye inflammation, colitis, arthralgias; epidermolysis bullosa-like eruptions in infancy with vesiculopustular lesions and red plaques *JAAD 73:367–381, 2015*

Ataxia telangiectasia

Chronic granulomatous disease

Common variable immunodeficiency

Hypomorphic *RAG* mutation

Nijmegen breakage syndrome

PLAID (*PLCG2*-associated antibody deficiency and immune dysregulation) – evaporative cold urticaria; neonatal ulcers in cold sensitive areas; granulomatous lesions sparing flexures; blotchy pruritic red rash, spontaneous ulceration of nasal tip with eschar of nose; erosion of nasal cartilage, neonatal small papules and erosions of fingers and toes; brown granulomatous plaques with telangiectasia and skin atrophy of cheeks, forehead, ears, chin; atopy; recurrent sinopulmonary infections *JAAD 73:367–381, 2015; JAMA Derm 151:627–634, 2015*

Subacute combined immunodeficiency disease – mutations in IL-2R; hypomorphic *RAG* mutations; granulomatous skin disease and autoimmunity; with adenosine deaminase deficiency results in dermatofibrosarcoma protuberans *JAAD 73:367–381, 2015*
   X-linked recessive SCID – IL-2Rgamma mutation
   RAG mutation – OMENN syndrome (infantile erythroderma lymphadenopathy, hepatosplenomegaly, alopecia), autoimmunity, granulomas
   Hypomorphic *RAG1 or 2* mutations – destructive granulomas
   Adenosine deaminase deficiency – severe fungal, viral , bacterial infections in infancy; dermatofibrosarcoma protuberans

PROPTOSIS

JAMA 309:605–606, 2013

AUTOIMMUNE DISORDERS

CREST syndrome *Ophthalmic Plast Reconstr Surg 34:e43–45, 2018*

IgG4-related disease *BJD 171:957–967, 29014*

Relapsing polychondritis *Ophthalmology 93:681–689, 1986*

CONGENITAL DISORDERS

Dermoid cyst

Neonatal thyrotoxicosis *NEJM 370:1237, 2014*

INFECTIOUS DISEASES

Aspergillus – immunocompetent patients; chronic progressive proptosis, periorbital swelling, pain, visual impairment *Clin Inf Dis 59:iii, 2014*

Dacryoadenitis

Mucormycosis *Clin Inf Dis 54:S35–S43, 2012; Clin Microbiol Infect 15:Suppl 15:98–102, 2009*

Periorbital cellulitis – often unilateral *Stat Pearls Jan 21, 2020;PMID:29261970*

INFILTRATIVE DISEASES

Erdheim-Chester disease *Am J Med Sci 321:66–75, 2001*

Sarcoidosis *J Rheumatol 45:141–142, 2018; Arch Soc Esp Ofalpol 90:578–581, 2015*

INFLAMMATORY DISEASES

Idiopathic orbital inflammation

Orbital myositis

METABOLIC DISEASES

Cushing's syndrome – fat within the orbit

Graves' disease – often bilateral

NEOPLASTIC DISEASES

Metastases – to extraocular muscles *Clin Exp Ophthalmol 46:687–694, 2018*

Multiple malignancies

Myeloid sarcoma – may be seen as isolated finding or as part of myelodysplastic syndrome, myeloproliferative disease, or acute myelogenous leukemia *NEJM 369:2332, 2013*

Neuroblastoma

Neuroendocrine carcinoma (high grade) involving ethmoid and frontal sinuses *JAMA 309:605–606, 2013*

PRIMARY CUTANEOUS DISORDERS

Angiolymphoid hyperplasia with eosinophilia *JAMA Ophthalmology 132:633–636, 2014*

SYNDROMES

Hutchinson-Gilford progeria syndrome – mountain range rippling of skin; sclerodermoid changes; facies – mid-frontal bossing, protruding ears with small lobes, prominent eyes, glyphic nose (broad, mildly concave nasal ridge), mild micrognathia, vertical midline groove of chin, thin lips *BJD 163:1102–1115, 2010; AD 144:1351–1359, 2008; BJD 156:1308–1314, 2007*

Neurofibromatosis – pulsating exophthalmos *Neurosurg Focus 15:E2, 2006*

Orbital pseudotumor

Pfeiffer syndrome

TRAUMA

Orbital fracture – apex, floor, medial wall, zygomatic bone

Retrobulbar hemorrhage

VASCULAR DISORDERS

Aortic insufficiency – pulsatile proptosis

Arteriovenous malformation, post-traumatic

Blue rubber bleb nevus syndrome – with orbital varix thrombosis *Ophthalmic Plast Reconstr Surg 31:e82–86, 2015*

Bilateral multifocal hemangiomas of orbit *Ophthalmology 109:537–541, 2002*

Carotid-cavernous sinus fistula

Granulomatosis with polyangiitis *Exp Mol Pathol 99:271–278, 2015; Ped Derm 30:e37–42, 2013*

Hemangioma

High altitude cerebral edema

PRURITIC TUMORS

The Clinical Management of Itching; Parthenon; p. 150, 2000

Alveolar soft part sarcoma of the glabella *Int J Ped Otorhinolaryngol 68:569–571, 2004*

Angiolymphoid hyperplasia with eosinophilia *Open Access Maced J Med Sci 14:794–796, 2019; Ann Dermatol 22:358–361, 2010*

Angiokeratomas *J Dermatol 20:247–251, 1993; JAAD 12:51–53, 1985*

Dermatofibroma *J Drugs Dermatol 12:1483–1484, 2103; Int J Derm 30:507–508, 1991*

Eccrine poromas; malignant eccrine poroma *Dermatologica 167:243–249, 1983*

Eccrine spiradenoma

Epidermal nevi

Epithelial sheath neuroma *Clin Neuropathol May 8, 2020 doi:10.5414/NP301251*

Eruptive xanthomas

Follicular basal cell nevus with comedo-like lesions *Acta DV 63:77–79, 1983*

Granular cell tumor *AD 136:1165–1170, 2000*

Inflammatory linear verrucous epidermal nevus (ILVEN) *Cutis 102:111–114, 2018; Ann Plastic Surg 28:292–296, 1992*

Keloids *Clin Plast Surg 14:253–260, 1987*

Keratoacanthoma, generalized eruptive, of Grzybowski *Int J Dermatol 53:131–136, 2014; Int J Clin Oncol 15:413–415, 2010; BJD 142:800–803, 2000; JAAD 37:786–787, 1997*

Leiomyoma *Dermatol Onlin J 11 (1):20, March 1, 2005*

Leiomyosarcoma *J Med Life 15:270–273, 2014*

Leukemia – acute lymphoblastic leukemia with eosinophilia *Ped Derm 20:502–505, 2003*

Lymphoma – intravascular B-cell lymphoma; pruritic patches *JAAD 39:318–322, 1998*; adult T-cell leukemia/lymphoma *JAAD 13:213–219, 1985*; cutaneous T-cell lymphoma; primary cutaneous marginal zone lymphoma *Dermatol Online J 22 (12):13030/qt9r97c4fd Dec 15, 2016*

Lymphomatoid papulosis – in HIV positive man *AIDS Patient Care STDS 18:563–567, 2004*

Mastocytoma *J Cutan Pathol 45:176–179, 2018*

Melanocytic nevi

Melanoma *Clin Exp Dermatol 16:344–347, 1991;* Meyerson's phenomenon; melanoma in situ *Acta DV Croat 24:81–82, 2016*

Merkel cell tumor *Case Rep Dermatol 29:316–321, 2015*

Metastasis – uterine papillary serous carcinoma *Am J Dermatopathol 27:436–438, 2005*

Molluscum contagiosum *Dermatol Online J March 16, 2016q22 (3)13–30/qt8v2669cj*

Myelodysplastic syndrome – prurigo-nodularis-like lesions *JAAD 33:187–191, 1995*

Myofibroblastic tumor *Ped Dev Pathol 21:444–448, 2018*

Neurilemmomas – linear of the forehead *Clin Exp Dermatol 16:247–249, 1991*

Neurofibromas

Neuromas

Paget's disease of the vulva *Am J Obstet Gynecol 187:281–284, 2002 ; JAAPA 32:33–34, 2019;* ectopic extramammary Paget's disease – plaque of back *Cutis 101:422–424, 2018*

Plasmacytoma – thigh plaque *Am J Dermatopathol 34:537–540, 2012*

Eruptive papular pruritic porokeratosis *J Dermatol 19:109–112, 1992*

Seborrheic keratoses

Smooth muscle hamartoma, acquired *Dermatol Online J 15 (8):12 Aug 15, 2009*

Squamoid eccrine ductal carcinoma of the scalp *Australas J Dermatol 57:e117–119, 2016*

Squamous cell carcinoma with perineural invasion – localized pruritus without rash or tumor *Cutis 85:121–123, 2010*

Syringocystadenoma papilliferum *Dermatol Surg 30:468–471, 2004*

Syringomas *Ann DV 143:521–528, 2016*

Verrucous lymphangioma circumscriptum *Dermatol Online J 18 (12):9. Dec 15, 2012: J Cutan Pathol 26:150–154, 1999*

PRURITUS, ANAL

AUTOIMMUNE DISEASES AND DISEASES OF IMMUNE DYSFUNCTION

Allergic contact dermatitis *Acta DV (Stockh) 60:245–249, 1980;* adult wipes (methylchlorisothiazolinone/methylisothiazolinone) *Dermatitis 30:323, 2019;* systemic contact dermatitis to nickel *Dermatitis 22:50–55, 2011;* textile dye *Contact Dermatitis 81:66–67, 2019*

Atopic dermatitis *The Clinical Management of Itching; Parthenon; p. 115, 2000*

Dermatitis herpetiformis *Clin Exp Dermatol 44:728–731, 2019; Dermatol Clin 29:463–468, 2011;* celiac neuropathy *Neurology 60:1581–1585, 2003*

DRUGS

Antibiotic-induced proctitis (broad spectrum, tetracycline)

Colchicine

Drug eruptions

Gemcitabine *NEJM 340:655–656, 1999*

Hydrocortisone sodium phosphate, intravenous – perianal burning or itching *Clin Pharmacol Therapeutics 20:109–112, 1976*

Quinidine

EXOGENOUS AGENTS

Beer *Postgrad Med 82:76–80, 1987*

Chocolate *Postgrad Med 82:76–80, 1987*

Cinnamon

Citrus fruit *Postgrad Med 82:76–80, 1987*

Coffee *Postgrad Med 82:76–80, 1987*

Contact dermatitis, irritant

Food and drink – beer, colas, sine, Scotch, bourbon, gin, tea, coffee, decaffeinated coffee *Clin Colon Rectal Surg 29:38–42, 2016; Gastroenterol Clin NA 42:801–813, 2013; Cutis 40:421–422, 1987*

Irritant contact dermatitis – perfumes, cleansers, condoms, sweat, urine, feces, garments

Mineral oil

Poison ivy oral desensitization

Popcorn Pork *Postgrad Med 82:76–80, 1987*

Soda *Postgrad Med 82:76–80, 1987*

Spices *Postgrad Med 82:76–80, 1987*

Tea *Postgrad Med 82:76–80, 1987*

Tomatoes, tomato paste *Postgrad Med 82:76–80, 1987*

INFECTIONS AND INFESTATIONS

Candida

Condyloma acuminate *J Cutan Med Surg 17:Suppl 2:855–860, 2013*

Dermatophyte infection *Stat Pearls Feb 15, 2020*

Entamoeba histolytica

Enterobiasis (*Enterobius vermicularis*) (pinworm) – anal and perineal pruritus *NEJM 381:e1, July 4, 2019; Cutis 71:268–270, 2003 Am Fam Phys 38:159–164, 1988*

Erythrasma (*Corynebacterium minutissimum*) *Acta DV (Stockh)51:444–447, 1971*

Herpes simplex *The Clinical Management of Itching; Parthenon; p. 115, 2000*

Larva currens (*Strongyloides stercoralis*) *Case Rep Dermatol Med 2013:381583.doi:10.1155/2013/381583*

Larva migrans *Indian J DV 84:440, 2018*

Molluscum contagiosum

Oxyuriasis (pinworm)

Pediculosis

Streptococcus pyogenes – perianal streptococcal cellulitis *AD 141:790–792, 2005*

Strongyloides

Threadworms

Tinea cruris

Trichomonas vaginalis

Warts

INFILTRATIVE DISEASES

Amyloidosis, cutaneous – pigmented macules and glossy hyperkeratotic lesions fanning out from anus *Jpn J Dermatol 91:398–443, 1981*

Langerhans cell histiocytosis

Plasma cell (Zoon's) vulvitis *AD 141:789–790, 2005*

INFLAMMATORY LESIONS

Folliculitis

Hidradenitis suppurativa *Clin Colon Rectal Surg 24:71–80, 2011*

METABOLIC DISEASES

Diarrhea

NEOPLASTIC DISEASES

Basal cell carcinoma – anogenital pruritus *Am J Obstet Gynecol 121:173–174, 1975*

Bowen's disease *Dis Colon Rectum 30:782–785, 1987*

Bowenoid papulosis *BJD 129:648–649, 1993*

Cloacagenic carcinoma – anogenital pruritus *JAAD 23:1005–1008, 1990*

Extramammary Paget's disease *Medicine (Balt)97:e11638, 2018; Acta Chir Belg 116:187–192, 2016; Br J Surg 75:1089–1092, 1988*

Giant condylomata of Buschke and Lowenstein *SKINMed 12:114–115, 2011*

Kaposi's sarcoma *Case Rep Gastroenterol 5:416–421, 2011*

Lymphoma – cutaneous T-cell lymphoma

Squamous cell carcinoma – anogenital pruritus *Rev Clin Esp (Barc)214:87–93, 2014*

Syringomas, vulvar – pruritus vulvae *JAAD 48:735–739, 2003*

PRIMARY CUTANEOUS DISEASES

Anal fissure *Ann Int Med 101:837–846, 1984; Am Surgeon 59:666–668, 1993*

Dermatographism

Excessive hair

Fistulae

Hyperhidrosis

Intertrigo *The Clinical Management of Itching; Parthenon; p. 115, 2000*

Lichen planus

Lichen sclerosus et atrophicus *Ped Derm 35:198–201, 2018; Int J Womens Health 8:511–515, 2015*

Lichen simplex chronicus

Mucosal prolapse

Papular acantholytic dyskeratosis

Pruritus ani *Ann Int Med 101:837–846, 1984*

Psoriasis

Seborrheic dermatitis

Stricture

PSYCHOCUTANEOUS DISEASES

Psychiatric disease – depression, anxiety, phobias

SYNDROMES

Sjogren's syndrome

TRAUMA

Physical trauma

VASCULAR DISEASES

Hemorrhoids

PRURITUS, ERYTHEMATOUS PAPULES

AUTOIMMUNE DISEASES

Allergic contact dermatitis – prurigo nodularis-like lesions due to allergic contact dermatitis to para-phenylenediamine *Dermatitis 25:90–92, 2014*

Autoimmune estrogen dermatitis *JAAD 32:25–31, 1995*

Autoimmune progesterone dermatitis – papulovesicular dermatitis *Eur J Obstet Gynecol Reprod Biol 47:169–171, 1992; AD 113:426–430, 1977*

Bullous pemphigoid, urticarial phase, non-bullous *JAAD 78:989–995, 2018*

Dermatitis herpetiformis

Dermatomyositis – leukocytoclastic vasculitis as presenting feature *AD 147:1313–1316, 2011*

Fogo selvagem – prurigo nodularis-like lesions

Graft vs. host disease, acute *J Cutan Pathol 45:817–823, 2018*

Herpes (pemphigoid) gestationis *JAAD 40:847–849, 1999*

IgG4-related disease *Australas J Dermatol 55:132–136, 2014*

Still's disease *JAAD 73:294–303, 2015; J Dermatol 41:407–410, 2014; Int J Dermatol 23:120–122, 1984; AD 113:489–490, 1977*

DRUGS

Chemotherapy induced inflammation of actinic keratoses *SKINMed 14:473–474, 2016; Dermatol Online J 20:21246 Jan 15, 2014*

Drug eruptions, morbilliform, pustular, others

EXOGENOUS AGENTS

Fiberglass *AD 130:785, 788, 1994; J Dermatol 14:590–593, 1987*

Irritant contact dermatitis

Plants – stinging hairs of nettles, cactus ("Sabra dermatitis), barley awns

Red sea coral contact dermatitis *Int J Dermatol 30:271–273, 1991*

Sabra dermatitis – to prickly pear cactus *Cutis 68:183–184, 2001*

Shiitake mushroom dermatitis *Pharmacogn Rev 10:100–114, 2016; An Bras Dermatol 90:276–278, 2015*

INFECTIONS AND INFESTATIONS

AIDS – papular pruritic eruption *J Dermatol 22:428–433, 1995; Acta DV 74:219–220, 1994; AD 125:629–632, 1989;* prurigo nodularis-like lesions *AD 125:629–632, 1989;* pruritic papular eruption with HIV in Uganda *JAMA 292:2614–2621, 2004*

Avian mite *Clin Exp Dermatol 25:129–131, 2000;* pet gerbils *AD 157:167–170, 2001*

Bartonellosis (*Bartonella bacilliformis*) – 1–4 mm pruritic red papules *Clin Inf Dis 33:772–779, 2001*

Caterpillar dermatitis – urticarial papules surmounted by vesicles, urticaria, eyelid edema, bruising in children; conjunctivitis

Cat flea rickettsiosis (*Rickettsia felis*) – pruritic macules and papules of chest, abdomen and legs; eschar *JAAD 75:1–16, 2016*

Cat scratch disease – pruritic exanthem *Pediatrics 81:559–561, 1988*

Cercarial dermatitis – schistosomes; pruritic red papules; fresh water avian cercarial dermatitis (swimmer's itch) *Cutis 23:212–216, 1979; Cutis 19:461–467, 1977;* sea water avian cercarial dermatitis *Bull Mrine Sci Gulf Coast 2:346–348, 1952*; fresh water mammalian cercarial dermatitis *Trans R Soc Trop Med Hyg 66:21–24, 1972;* cercarial dermatitis from snail (*Lymnaea stagnalis*) in aquarium tank *BJD 145:638–640, 2001*

Cheyletiella mites – abdomen, thighs, chest, arms *JAAD 15:1130–1133, 1986; JAMA 251:2690, 1984; AD 116:435–437, 1980*

Chicken mite (*Dermanyssus gallinae*) *Clin Exp Dermatol 38:374–377, 2013*

Chiggers (grass mites) *Cutis 99:386–388, 2017*

Cimex lecutlaris/hemiptosus (bed bugs) *NEJM 382:2230–2237, 2020*

Cytomegalovirus infections – prurigo nodularis-like lesions *JAAD 24:346–352, 1991*

Demodex folliculorum J Am Optometric Assoc 61:637–639, 1990

Dermatophytids *J Dermatol 21:31–34, 1994*

Dogger bank itch (weed rash) – allergic contact dermatitis to microscopic marine organisms; *Alcyonidium gelatinosum, A. hirsutum, Electra pilosa*; seaweed – Sargassum muticum *Br Med J 5496:1142–1145, 1966; Proc Roy Soc Med 59:1119–1120, 1966*

Dracunculosis *JAAD 73:947–957, 2015; JAAD 73:929–941, 2015*

Ectopic schistosomiasis *An Bras Dermatol 89:646–648, 2014*

Enterobiasis *Acta DV Alp Pannonica Adriat 28:179–181, 2019*

Gamasoidosis – mite infestation *An Bras Dermatol 95:250–251, 2020*

Grain mites (*Aeroglyphus robustus*) *BJD 174:454–456, 2016*

Insect bite reaction; sandfly bites (urticaria multiformis endemica (harara)) – urticarial papules, papulovesicles, bullae; papules with overlying vesicle; bullae in children, associated with CLL *Acta DV (Stockh)57:81–92, 1977;* natural killer cell lymphocytosis *AD 126:362–368, 1990;* HIV disease *JAAD 29:269–272, 1993;* fleas, mosquitoes, gnats, midges, flies, mites, bugs; thrips (thunder flies), beetles, mites (copra itch, grocer's itch, barley itch, grain-shoveller's itch, grain itch, straw itch, cotton seed dermatitis); *Haematosiphoniasis* (Mexican chicken bug) – wheals, papules, vesicles, pustules, crusts

Leprosy, histiocytoid type 1 lepra reaction *Int J Dermatol 54:564–567, 2015*

Lone star tick larval bites *AD 142:491–494, 2006*

Mansonelliasis (filariasis) (*M. ozzardi*) – biting midges or black flies; angioedema, chronic pruritus with hyperpigmentation, papular eruption *JAAD 75:19–30, 2016*

Mites – birds, rodent, reptile mites – papules and papulovesicles; avian mites from pet gerbils *AD 137:167, 2001;* cheese mite (*Glyciphagus*) bites – papulovesicles and pustules *Dermatol Clin 8:265–275, 1990;* trombiculid mites – harvest mites – papules and papulovesicles *Int J Dermatol 22:75–91, 1983*

Monkeypox – varioliform rash with progression from papules to vesicles, umbilicated pustules, and crusting; prairie dogs infected in shipment with Gambian rat *AD 140:656, 2004*

Onchocerciasis – acute onchodermatitis; non-specific papular rash *BJD 121:187–198, 1989;* chronic papules *AD 133:381–386, 1997*

Oxyuriasis

Papular urticaria *Ped Derm 34:701–702, 2017; Cutis 68:89–91, 2001*

Pediculosis – head lice – pruritic papules of nape of neck; generalized pruritic eruption *NEJM 234:665–666, 1946;* pubic lice

Pigeon lice *An Bras Dermatol 93:285–287, 2019*

Pityrosporum folliculitis *J Dermatol 27:49–51, 2000; Int J Dermatol 38:453–456, 1999; JAAD 234:693–696, 1991; Ann Int Med 108:560–563, 1988; JAAD 12:56–61, 1985*

Pseudomonas folliculitis – swimming pool or hot tub *Harefuah 151:381–387, 2012*

Sarcoptic mange – chest, abdomen, thighs, forearms *JAAD 10:979–986, 1984*

Scabies – periaxillary, periareolar, abdomen, periumbilical, buttocks, thighs; animal scabies – camels, cats, cows, dogs, goats, pigs, sheep, water buffaloes, Arabian oryx, barbary sheep, elands, ferrets, mountain gazelles, Nubian oryxes

Seabather's eruption – *Linuche unguiculata* (thimble jellyfish); Edwardsiella lineata (sea anemone)

Sea urchin sting – red rash on knees and ankles *Dermatologica 180:99–101, 1990*

Sparganosis (*S. proliferum*) – subcutaneous nodules and pruritic papules *Am J Trop Med Hyg 30:625–637, 1981*

Stick tight flea *Cutis 100:40–49, 2017; Cutis 89:57–58, 2012; Cutis 68:250, 2001; Hautarzt 48:714–719, 1997*

Syphilis, secondary *Oxf Med Case Rep Feb 1, 2018*

Talaromyces marneffei Mycopathologia 184:129–139, 2019

Tanapox virus – few pruritic papules undergoing central necrosis, then evolving into ulcerated nodules, healing with scarring

Tarantula urticating hairs *Cutis 70:162–163, 2002*

Tick bites – papular urticaria

Trombiculiasis – larvae of *N. autumnalis* mite *Infez Med 26:77–80, 2018; Emerging Infect Dis 20:1059–1060, 2014*

Toxocariasis – prurigo nodularis *JAAD 75:19–30, 2016*

Trypanosoma brucei NEJM 375:2380, 2016; rhodesiense, gambiense; cruzii Dermatol Ther 32:e12665, July, 2019; Int J Dermatol 51:501–508, 2012

Viral exanthem

INFILTRATIVE DISEASES

Langerhans cell histiocytosis *Ped Ann 43:e9–12, 2014*

Lichen amyloidosis – papular pruritis syndrome *Dermatology 194:62–64, 1997*

Mastocytosis – urticaria pigmentosa; *Ped Derm 43:e13–15, 2014; Acta DV (Stockh) 42:433–439, 1962;* telangiectasia macularis eruptiva perstans

INFLAMMATORY DISEASES

Eosinophilic pustular folliculitis of HIV disease *BJD 145:514–515, 2001; J Dermatol 25:178–184, 1998*

Neutrophilic eccrine hidradenitis *SKINMed 15:297–299, 2017; BJD 147:797–800, 2002*

Sarcoidosis *Dermatology 234:220–225, 2018*

METABOLIC DISEASES

Intrahepatic cholestasis of pregnancy *AD 143:757–762, 2007*

Pruritic folliculitis of pregnancy – limbs and abdomen *An Bras Dermatol 91:suppl 1)66–68, 2016; JAAD 43:132–134, 2000; Semin Derm 8:23–25, 1989; AD 117:20–22, 1981*

Pruritic urticarial papules and plaques of pregnancy *Cutis 95:344–347, 2015; J Reprod Med 50:61–63, 2005; JAAD 10:473–480, 1984; Clin Exp Dermatol 7:65–73, 1982; JAMA 241:1696–1699, 1979*

Reactive perforating collagenosis *Stat Pearls Jan 24, 2020; Case Rep Dermatol 3:209–211, 2011*

NEOPLASTIC DISEASES

Eruptive papular pruritic porokeratosis *J Dermatol 19:109–112, 1992*

Keratoacanthoma, generalized eruptive, of Grzybowski *Int J Dermatol 53:131–136, 2014; BJD 142:800–803, 2000; JAAD 37:786–787, 1997*

Leukemia – acute lymphoblastic leukemia with eosinophilia *Ped Derm 20:502–505, 2003;* acute myelogenous leukemia with plasmacytoid dendritic cells *J Cutan Pathol 38:893–898, 2001;* chronic lymphocytic leukemia *Dermatol Online J 17:7, Sept 15, 2011*

Lymphoma – adult T-cell leukemia/lymphoma *JAAD 13:213–219, 1985;* cutaneous T-cell lymphoma; primary cutaneous marginal zone lymphoma *Dermatol Online J 22:13030/qtqr97c4fd:Dec 15, 2016;* pityriasis lichenoides-like T-cell lymphoma *Acta DV Croat 27:37–39, 2019*

Lymphomatoid papulosis *Dermatol Online J 21:13030/qt71j79320 Jan 15, 2015*

Myelodysplastic syndrome – prurigo-nodularis-like lesions *JAAD 33:187–191, 1995*

Waldenstrom's macroglobulinemia *Ann Dermatol 30:87–96, 2018*

PHOTODERMATOSES

Polymorphic light eruption – papules, plaques, and vesicles *BJD 144:446–447, 2001; JID 115:467–470, 2000; JAAD 42:199–207, 2000*

Porokeratosis – disseminated superficial actinic porokeratosis *J Dermatol 39:946–948, 2012*

PRIMARY CUTANEOUS DISEASES

Albopapuloid pretibial epidermolysis bullosa – prurigo nodularis-like lesions *JAAD 29:974–981, 1993*

Angiolymphoid hyperplasia with eosinophilia *Acta DV Croat 27:40–41, 2019*

Atopic dermatitis – papular variant

Dermatographism, including follicular dermographism *Cutis 32:244–245, 254, 260, 1983*

Epidermolysis bullosa pruriginosa – mild acral blistering at birth or early childhood; violaceous pruritic papular and nodular lesions in linear array on shins, forearms, trunk; lichenified hypertrophic and verrucous plaques in adults *BJD 172:778–781, 2015; BJD 130:617–625, 1994*

Granuloma annulare *Ann Dermatol 23:409–411, 2011*

Itchy red bump disease (papular prurigo, dermatitis herpetiformis-like dermatitis, subacute prurigo, papular dermatitis) *JAAD 38:929–933, 1998; JAAD 24:697–702, 1991; JAAD 4:723–729, 1981*

Kyrle's disease *Indian J Pathol Microbiol 61:414–417, 2018*

Lichen planus – lichen planopilaris of face *Skin Appendage Disorder 21:72–75, 2016*

Lichen sclerosus et atrophicus, extragenital *Indian J Dermatol 60:105, 2015*

Neutrophilic urticarial *SKINMed 15:471–472, 2017*

Papular eruption of black men

Pityriasis lichenoides et varioliformis acuta (acute parapsoriasis)

Prurigo pigmentosa – red papules or reticulate plaques with post-inflammatory hyperpigmentation *Am J Clin Dermatol 16:533–543, 2015; Dermatology 188:219–221, 1994; AD 129:365–370, 1993; BJD 120:705–708, 1989; AD 125:1551–1554, 1989*

Psoriasis

Transient or persistent acantholytic dermatosis (Grover's disease) *Acta DV Croat 27:192–194, 2019; Dermatol Online J 25:1030/qt2vm7509r March 15, 2019; JAAD 35:653–666, 1996;* folliculitis *JAAD 11:253–256, 1984; AD 101:426–434, 1970*Urticaria

SYNDROMES

Blau syndrome – granulomatous arthritis, synovial cysts, iritis, rash; autosomal dominant; resembles childhood sarcoid – red pruritic papules coalescing into plaques, uveitis; chromosome 16p12-q21 *JAAD 49:299–302, 2003; Am J Hum Genet 76:217–221, 1998; Am J Hum Genet 59:1097–1107, 1996*

Hypereosinophilic syndrome *Med Clin (Barc)106:304–306, 1996; AD 132:535–541, 1996*

TRAUMA

Chilblains – tender, pruritic red or purple digital papules; plantar nodule *Ped Derm 15:97–102, 1998*

Radiotherapy-induced polymorphic pruritic eruption *AD 135:804–810, 1999*

PRURITUS, GENERALIZED, WITHOUT PRIMARY SKIN LESIONS

NEJM 368:1625–1634, 2013; JAMA 309:2443–2450, 2013; JAAD 45:892–896, 2001; JAAD 14:375–392, 1986

AUTOIMMUNE DISEASES

Anaphylaxis *Mayo Clin Proc 69:16–23, 1994;* exercise-induced *Med Sci Sports Exerc 24:849–850, 1992; J Allergy Clin Immunol 75:479–484, 1985;* to bacitracin ointment *Cutis 83:127–129, 2009; Am J Emerg Med 25:95–96, 2007; J Allergy Clin Immunol 101:136–137, 1998; Am J Contact Derm 6:28–31, 1995; Am J Contact Derm 1:162–164, 1990; AD 120:909–911, 1984; AD 100:450–452, 1969*

Asthma, childhood – prodrome of pruritus *Lancet 2:154–155, 1984*

Autoimmune estrogen dermatitis *JAAD 32:25–31, 1995*

Autoimmune hepatitis – pruritus, fatigue, lethargy, anorexia, nausea, abdominal pain, and arthralgia *NEJM 354:54–66, 2006*

Autoimmune progesterone dermatitis *Eur J Obstet Gynecol Reprod Biol 47:169–171, 1992; AD 113:426–430, 1977*

Bullous pemphigoid *JAAD 81:355:363, 2019; JAMA Derm 149:950–953, 2013; JAMA 309:2443–2450, 2013; Int J Derm 37:508–514, 1998; BJD 109:237–239, 1983*

Dermatitis herpetiformis

Graft vs. host disease *JAAD 45:892–896, 2001*

Sjogren's syndrome *Dermatologica 137:74, 1968*

DEGENERATIVE DISEASES

Degenerative joint disease – dermatomal pruritus *J Dermatol 14:512–513, 1987;* degenerative cervical spine disease – scalp dysesthesia *JAMA Derm 149:200–203, 2013*

Meralgia paresthetica (Bernhard-Roth syndrome) (lateral femoral cutaneous nerve neuralgia) – pruritus or dysesthesia of lateral or antero-lateral upper thigh; association with diabetes *JAAD 74:215–228, 2016*

Multiple sclerosis – paroxysmal itch *J Neurol Neurosurg Psychiatry 44:19–22, 1981; BJD 95:555–558, 1976*

Senescence (senile pruritus) (generalized pruritus of the elderly) *BJD 161:306–312, 2009; JAAD 27:560–564, 1992; J Am Geriatr Soc 15:750–758, 1967*

Small fiber neuropathies *JAAD 72:328–332, 2015*

DRUG-INDUCED

Afatinib (epidermal growth factor receptor-tyrosine kinase inhibitors) – xerosis, paronychia, acneiform eruptions, pruritus *JAMA Derm 152:340–342, 2016*

Antimalarial drugs

Drug abuse (IVDA); heroin abuse – pruritus of face and genitalia, and at site of injection *JAAD 69:135–142, 2013*

Cancer immunotherapy – generalized pruritus *JAMA Derm 155:249–250, 2019*

Chloroquine pruritus in malaria *Trop Doct 28:210–211, 1998; Br J Clin Pharmacol 44:157–161, 1997; Afr J Med Med Sci 18:121–129, 1989; AD 120:80–82, 1984*

Cholestatic drugs – azathioprine, oral contraceptives, erythromycin estolate, chlorpromazine, penicillamine, promazine, sulfadiazine, testosterone, anabolic steroids, tolbutamide

Clonidine

Cocaine abuse – "coke bugs", "crack bugs", formication

Drug hypersensitivity without rash (subclinical drug hypersensitivity) – multiple drugs *JAMA 2443–2450, 2013*

Erlotinib (EGFR inhibitor) – pruritus, acneiform eruptions, xerosis, paronychia *JAMA Derm 152:340–342, 2016; JAAD 69:463–472, 2013; J Drugs Dermatol 9:1229–1234, 2010*

Gefitinib/erlotinib/cetuximab/panitumumab (epidermal growth factor receptor inhibitors) – pruritus *JAMA Derm 152:340–342, 2016; JAAD 71:217–227, 2014*

Gold salts

Hepatotoxic drugs – chloroform, valproic acid

Hydroxyethyl starch infusions – intravascular volume expander; pruritus begins 1–6 weeks after infusion and lasts 9–15 weeks *JAAD 59:151–153, 2008; BJD 152:1085–1086, 2005; BJD 152:3–12, 2005; Dermatology 192:222–226, 1996*

Interferon alpha *Semin Oncol 14:1–12, 1987*

Ipilimumab – generalized pruritus without rash, enterocolitis, uveitis, iridocyclitis *JAAD 71:161–169, 2014; JAAD 71:217–227, 2014*

Lithium

Morphine, including epidural morphine *Anesth Analg 61:490–495, 1982*

Naltrexone *Australas J Dermatol 38:196–198, 1997*

Neurologic mechanisms – butorphanol, codeine, cocaine, fentanyl, morphine, tramadol

Opiate hypersensitivity

Paroxetine (selective serotonin reuptake inhibitor) *JAAD 56:848–853, 2007; BJD 150:787–788, 2004*

PD-1 inhibitors – nivolumab, pembrolizumab *JAAD 72:221–236, 2015*

Pembrolizumab – pruritus, hypopigmentation, morbilliform eruption, photosensitivity *JAMA Derm 151:1206–1212, 2015*

Phenytoin-induced Hodgkin's disease *Int J Dermatol 24:54–55, 1985*

Polypharmacy in the elderly – thiazides, calcium channel blockers *Drugs Aging 32:201–205, 2015*

PUVA therapy

Sorafenib *JAAD 60:299–305, 2009*

Targeted anti-cancer therapies – pruritus and excoriations *JAAD 69:708–720, 2013*

Xerosis, drug-induced

EXOGENOUS AGENTS

Aquagenic pruritus *JAAD 13:91–96, 1985;* associated with acute lymphoblastic leukemia *BJD 129:346–349, 1993;* myelodysplastic syndrome *BJD 176:255–258, 2017; Clin Exp Dermatol 19:257–258, 1994;* myelofibrosis *BJD 176:255–258, 2017;* metastatic cervical carcinoma *Clin Exp Dermatol 19:257–258, 1994;* hypereosinophilic syndrome *BJD 176:255–258, 2017; BJD 122:103–106, 1990;* juvenile xanthogranuloma *Clin Exp Dermatol 18:253–255, 1993;* polycythemia vera *Dermatology 187:130–133, 1993;* hemochromatosis *Ann Int Med 98:1026, 1983;* Hodgkin's disease, mastocystosis, essential thrombocythemia; alcohol-induced pruritus with hot showers in sarcoidosis *BJD 176:255–258, 2017; Bolognia, p.100, 2004;* polycythemia vera *BJD 176:255–258, 2017; J Dtsch Dermatol Ges 8:797–804, 2010;* antimalarial therapy *Arthritis Rheum 41:744–745, 1998;* juvenile xanthogranuloma *BJD 176:255–258, 2017*

Atmokinesis – pruritus provoked by contact with air *Cutis 44:143–144, 1989*

Caffeine

Caterpillar – airborne disease due to oak processionary caterpillar *Ped Derm 23:64–66, 2006*

Ciguatera fish poisoning *Z Gastroenterol 35:327–330, 1997; Am Fam Physician 50:579–584, 1994; Revue Neurol 142:590–597, 1986;* pruritus of palms and soles *JAAD 20:510–511, 1989*

Cleansing agents – dishwashing liquids used in bathing *Ann Allergy 39:284, 1977*

Dialysis – either hemodialysis or peritoneal dialysis *Ann Int Med 93:446–448, 1980*

Drinking black tea – dermatomal pruritus *BJD 143:1355–1356, 2000*

External magnetic fields – used in therapy of multiple sclerosis *Int J Neuroscience 75:65–71, 1994*

Fiberglass exposure *AD 130:785, 788, 1994; J Dermatol 14:590–593, 1987*

Filariasis *Clin in Dermatol 37:644–656, 2019*

Helicobacter pyloris Clin in Dermatol 37:644–656, 2019

Itching powder – spicules of cowhage plant

Methamphetamine abuse *JAAD 69:135–142, 2013*

Nitrate intolerance *J Allergy Clin Immunol 104:1110–1111, 1999*

Peanut allergy *Cutis 65:285–289, 2000*

Vitamin A intoxication

INFECTIONS AND INFESTATIONS

AIDS/HIV *JAAD 70:659–664, 2014; Semin Cutan Med Surg 30:101–106, 2011; Am J Clin Dermatol 4:177–188, 2003; JAAD 45:892–896, 2001; JAAD 24:231–235, 1991*

Amebiasis – *Entamoeba histolytica Int J Derm 20:261, 1981*

Avian mite dermatitis/rat mite/pig mite

Ascariasis

Brain abscess *JAAD 45:892–896, 2001*

Candida – chronic mucocutaneous candidiasis

Chronic infection (bacterial, fungal, parasitic) *JAAD 45:892–896, 2001*

Creutzfeld-Jacob disease *Neurology 46:940–941, 1996*

Dengue fever *Kaohsiung J Med Sci 5:50–57, 1989*

Dipetalonemiasis

Dracunculosis – *Dracunculus medinensis* – initially fever, pruritus, urticaria, edema *Int J Zoonoses 12:147–149, 1985*

Echinococcosis

Filariasis *Int J Derm 26:171–173, 1987*

Giardiasis, acute *Ann Allergy 65:161, 1990*

Gnathostomiasis (nematode)

Hepatitis B *JAAD 8:539–548, 1983*

Hepatitis C *JAAD 45:892–896, 2001; AD 131:1185–1193, 1995*

Hookworm

Insect bites

Leptospirosis – Weil's disease

Malaria *Ann Emerg Med 18:207–210, 1989*

Mansonelliasis (filariasis) (*M. ozzardi*) – biting midges or black flies; angioedema, chronic pruritus with hyperpigmentation, papular eruption *JAAD 75:19–30, 2016*

Nocardia brain abscess – unilateral itching *Neurology 34:828–829, 1984*

Octopus bite – blue-ringed octopus *J Emerg Med 10:71–77, 1992*

Onchocerciasis – initial presentation of pruritus before appearance of dermatitis *Cutis 65:293–297, 2000; AD 120:505–507, 1984*

Pediculosis corporis

Scabies *Curr Opinion Infect Dis 23:111–118, 2010; JAMA 2443–2450, 2013*

Schistosomiasis

Streptocerciasis – *Mansonella streptocerca* – similar rash to onchocerciasis; acute or lichenified papules with widespread lichenification and hypopigmented macules; pruritus, lymphadenopathy *JAAD 73:929–944 2015; Derm Clinics 17:151–185, 1999*

Strongyloides stercoralis Cutis 71:22–24, 2003; Cesk Dermatol 52:121–123, 1977

Swimmer's itch (cercarial dermatitis) – schistosomes; pruritus initially then development of pruritic red papules; fresh water avian cercarial dermatitis (swimmer's itch) *Cutis 19:461–467, 1977;* sea

water avian cercarial dermatitis *Bull Mrine Sci Gulf Coast 2:346–348, 1952;* fresh water mammalian cercarial dermatitis *Trans R Soc Trop Med Hyg 66:21–24, 1972;* cercarial dermatitis from snail (*Lymnaea stagnalis*) in aquarium tank *BJD 145:638–640, 2001*

Syphilis – tabes dorsalis – unilateral itching

Thysanoptera (thrips) *AD 148:864–865, 2012*

Toxocariasis – (*T. canis, T. cati, T. leonensis*) visceral larva migrans *Clin in Dermatol 37:644–656, 2019; JAAD 59:1031–1042, 2008; Dermatologica 144:129–143, 1972*

Trichinosis

Trichuris (whipworm) *Dermatol Clin 7:275–290, 1989*

Trypanosomiasis *Am J Trop Med Hyg 22:473–476, 1973*

INFILTRATIVE

Amyloidosis – primary familial amyloidosis – pruritus in childhood *BJD 112:201–208, 1985*

Mastocytosis – mastocytoma, systemic mastocytosis *Dermatology 197:101–108, 1998; Arch Belg Dermatol 11:10–22, 1955*

INFLAMMATORY DISEASES

Guillain-Barre syndrome *Am J Clin Hypnosis 32:168–173, 1990*

Sarcoidosis – with elevation of IgA *Ann Allery Asthma Immunol 74:387–389, 1995*

METABOLIC DISEASES

Adrenergic pruritus *NEJM 368:1625–1634, 2013*

Anemia *Clin in Dermatol 37:644–656, 2019*

Asthma *Clin in Dermatol 37:644–656, 2019*

Biliary atresia *The Clinical Management of Itching; Parthenon; p. 28, 2000;* congenital biliary atresia *Ped Derm 25:403–404, 2008*

Choledocholithiasis *GE Port J Gastroenterol 22:65–69, 2015*

Cholinergic pruritus *BJD 121:235–237, 1989*

Congestive heart failure *Clin in Dermatol 37:644–656, 2019; BJD 172:1541–1546, 2015*

Diabetes insipidus

Diabetes mellitus – scalp, vulva *Diabetes Care 9:273–275, 1986;* truncal pruritus, diabetic polyneuropathy *Diabetes Care 33:150–155, 2010*

Dumping syndrome *BJD 107:70, 1982*

Extrahepatic biliary obstruction *JAAD 45:892–896, 2001*

Hemochromatosis – hyperferritinemia *Dermatol Online J Sept 17, 2015; BJD 112:629, 1985*

Hepatic disease, including intrahepatic biliary obstruction (cholestatic) *JAAD 81:1371–1378, 2019; JAAD 45:892–896, 2001;* obstructive biliary disease *AD 119:183–184, 1983;* primary biliary cirrhosis, cholestasis *JAAD 41:431–434, 1999; Am J Med 70:1011–1016, 1981;* primary ascending cholangitis; drug-induced cholestasis (chlorpromazine, birth control pills, testosterone) *Semin Dermatol 14:302–312, 1995;* primary biliary cirrhosis *JAAD 45:892–896, 2001*

Hepatitis B and C *JAAD 30:629–632, 1994*

Hypercalcemia

Hyperparathyroidism *Scand J Surg July 13, 2019; Nephrology (Carlton) March 2017; 22Suppl 2:47–50; Clin J Am Soc Nephrol 8:313–318, 2013; Iran J Kidney Dis 7:42–46, 2013*

Hyperphosphatemia *Nephrol Dial Transplant 28:2961–2968, 2013*

Hyperthyroidism, including thyrotoxicosis *BMJ Case Rep June 15, 2018 bcr 2018225347;doi:10.1136/bcr 2018–225347; JAAD 45:892–896, 2001; J Allergy Clin Immunol 48:73–81, 1971; South Med J 62:1127–1130, 1969*

Hypoparathyroidism

Hypothyroidism *JAAD 45:892–896, 2001*

Intrahepatic cholestasis of pregnancy *OB Gyn 124:120–133, 2014; AD 143:757–762, 2007; JAAD 6:977–998, 1982*

Iron deficiency with or without anemia *BJD 151 (Suppl 68):35, 2004; AD 119:630, 1983; JAMA 236:2319–2320, 1976; BJD 89 (Suppl 9):10, 1973*

Malabsorption

Miliaria

Porphyria – porphyria cutanea tarda *Ann DV 113:133–136, 1986;* erythropoietic protoporphyria – pruritus (without rash) in photodistribution *BJD 157:1030–1031, 2007*

Postmenopausal (perimenopausal) pruritus

Premenstrual pruritus – due to cholestasis *Trans St Johns Hosp Dermatol Soc 56:11–13, 1970*

Renal disease, chronic *NEJM 372:964–968, 2015; JAAD 49:842–846, 2003; JAAD 45:892–896, 2001; Clin Exp Dermatol 25:103–106, 2000; AD 118:154–160, 1982;* uremia

Starvation-associated pruritus *JAAD 27:118–120, 1992*

NEOPLASTIC AND PARANEOPLASTIC DISEASES

J Geriat Dermatol 3:172–181, 1995; JAAD 21:1317, 1989; JAAD 16:1179–1182, 1987

Angioimmunoblastic T-cell lymphoma *Asian Pac J Allergy Immunol 5:119–123, 1987;* mimicking chronic urticarial *Case Rep Med 2016:doi.10.1155/2016/8753235*

Brain tumors – tumor invading floor of fourth ventricle – pruritus of nostrils; occasionally generalized pruritus *BJD 92:675–678, 1975;* brainstem glioma – unilateral facial pruritus *J Child Neurol 3:189–192, 1988;* cerebrovascular accidents – unilateral pruritus *AD 123:1527–1530, 1987; Ann Int Med 97:222–223, 1987*

Breast carcinoma *Lancet 2:696, 1981*

Central pruritus *Pain 45:307–308, 1991*

Cervical spinal cord compression – lower extremity burning and itching *J Computed Tomography 6:57–60, 1982*

Cervicothoracic syrinx and thoracic spinal cord tumor *Neurosurgery 30:418–421, 1992*

Carcinoma – breast, stomach, lung, larynx *JAAD 45:892–896, 2001*

Ganglioma – cervical ganglioma of C6; localized pruritus of neck, shoulder, and arm *AD 149:446–449, 2013*

Gastrointestinal cancers – tongue, stomach, colon *Dermatologica 155:122–124, 1977*

Hematologic malignancy and cholangiocarcinoma *JAAD 70:651–658, 2014*

Kaposi's sarcoma

Leukemia *J Derm Surg Oncol 10:278–282, 1984;* chronic lymphocytic leukemia *JAAD 45:892–896, 2001;* HTLV-1 (acute T-cell leukemia) *JAAD 49:979–1000, 2003;* chronic myelomonocytic leukemia, myelodysplastic syndrome *BMJ Case Rep 12:e232480 Oct 23, 2019*

Lymphoma – cutaneous T-cell lymphoma ("invisible mycosis fungoides") *JAMA 2443–2450, 2013; JAAD 47:S168–171, 2002;* *JAAD 45:318–319, 2001; JAAD 42:324–328, 2000;* adnexotropic T-cell lymphoma *JAAD 38:493–497, 1998;* Sezary syndrome *JAAD 72:1003–1009, 2015; JAAD 33:678–680, 1995;* Hodgkin's disease – legs *JAMA 241:2598–2599, 1979;* especially with alcohol *Cancer 56:2874–2880, 1985;* Hodgkin's disease *Cutis 87:169–172, 2011*

Lung cancer *Clin Exp Dermatol 8:459–461, 1983; Arizona Med 37:831–833, 1980*

Mastocytoma, malignant

Metastastic disease *Dermatologica 155:122–124, 1977;* metastatic hepatocellular carcinoma *J Drugs Dermatol 13:1440, 2014*

Multiple myeloma *JAAD 45:892–896, 2001; Br Med J 2:1154, 1977*

Myelofibrosis *Clin in Dermatol 37:644–656, 2019*

Myeloproliferative disorders *Clin in Dermatol 37:644–656, 2019*

Pancreatic carcinoma – pruritus antedating obstructive jaundice – personal observation

Polycythemia vera – within minutes of water contact (aquagenic pruritus); *JAK2V617F* mutation *Clin Exp Dermatol 44:e33, 2019; Acta DV 98:185–190, 2018; Lancet 337:241, 1991; BJD 116:21–29, 1987; Blood 28:2319–2320, 1966*

Prostatic carcinoma

Spinal tumors – excoriations due to paresthesias; brachio-radial pruritus due to spinal cord ependyomoma of C4–C7 *JAAD 46:437–440, 2002*

Thyroid carcinoma

Uterine carcinoma

Waldenstrom's macroglobulinemia

PARANEOPLASTIC DISORDERS

Paraneoplastic pruritus, colon cancer *Dermatol Ther 23:590–596, 2010*

PHOTODISTRIBUTED DERMATOSES

Actinic prurigo – generalized pruritus and cheilitis *JAMA Derm 156:697–698, 2020*

Brachioradial pruritus *Cutis 81:37–40, 2008; Cutis 80:21,23–24, 2007; JAAD 52:142–145, 2005; BJD 150:786–787, 2004; JAAD 50:800–801, 2004; JAAD 48:825–828, 2003; JAAD 48:521–524, 2003; BJD 115:177–180, 1986;* generalized pruritus without rash *JAAD 68:870–873, 2013*

Photosensitive drug eruptions *JAMA 2443–2450, 2013*

Polymorphic light eruption sine eruption *BJD 118:73–76, 1988*

Sunburn

PRIMARY CUTANEOUS DISEASES

Anhidrosis – itching, burning, tingling skin due to small fiber neuropathy *BJD 172:412–418, 2015*

Atopic dermatitis *JAAD 45:892–896, 2001*

Epidermolysis bullosa pruriginosa (dystrophic epidermolysis bullosa) – hyperkeratosis of the nails, excoriations, lichenification of shins, white papules *JAMA Derm 149:727–731, 2013;* pruritus without rash *BJD 129:443–446, 1993*

Fox-Fordyce disease (apocrine miliaris) *Stat Pearls Aug 31, 2019 PMID 31424791;* of the nipple *J Eur Acad DV 29:7–13, 2015*

Grover's disease *JAMA 2443–2450, 2013*

Hereditary localized pruritus

Multilevel symmetric neuropathic pruritus *JAAD 75:774–781, 2016*

Notalgia paresthetica (localized) *Int J Dermatol 57:388–392, 2018; Cleve Clin J Med 80:550–552, 2013; JAAD 32:287–289, 1995*

Paroxysmal itching *JAAD 13:839–840, 1985*

Pruritus ani – nocturnal

Xerosis (dry skin itch, winter itch) *JAMA 2443–2450, 2013*

PSYCHOCUTANEOUS DISEASES

Anorexia nervosa *Am J Clin Dermatol 6:165–173, 2005; BJD 134:510–511, 1996*

Delusions of parasitosis *Dermatol Clin 14:429–438, 1996*

Emotional stress *Dermatol Clin 14:429–438, 1996*

Monosymptomatic hypochondriacal psychosis

Psychogenic pruritus – obsessive compulsive disorder *JAAD 76:779–791, 2017;* – perianal, vulvar

SYNDROMES

Alagille syndrome (arteriohepatic dysplasia) – paucity of interlobular hepatic ducts; autosomal dominant; pruritus and failure to thrive; wispy hair, triangular face, broad forehead, deep-set eyes, mild hypertelorism, straight nasal bridge with saddle nose, small pointed chin, ventricular hypertrophy, pulmonary artery stenosis; xanthomas; supernumerary digital flexion creases of middle phalanges; *JAG1* and *Notch2* mutations *JAAD 58:S9–11, 2008;* cutis laxa-like changes with resolution of xanthomas after liver transplantation *JAAD 58:S9–11, 2008; Atlas of Clinical Syndromes A Visual Aid to Diagnosis, 1992, pp.553; Ped Derm 15:199–202, 1998; Clin Exp Dermatol 8:657–661, 1983;* dysmorphic facies, follicular hyperkeratosis *BJD 138:150–154, 1998,* palmar linear plane xanthomas, porphyria cutanea tarda due to retained porphyrins

Carcinoid syndrome *Ann Int Med 58:989–993, 1963*

Hypereosinophilic syndrome – intractable pruritus, pulmonary infiltrates, eosinophilic gastroenteritis, endomyocardial fibrosis, thromboembolism *NEJM 380:1336–1346, 2019; AD 132:535–541, 1996; Med Clin (Barc)106:304–306, 1996*

Multicentric reticulohistiocytosis *Cutis 93:243–246, 2014*

Neurofibromatosis type I *JAAD 61:1–14, 2009; JAAD 43:958–961, 2000; Clin Exp Dermatol 10:590–591, 1985*

Trigeminal trophic syndrome

TOXINS

Eosinophilia myalgia syndrome *JAAD 23:1063–1069, 1990*

Mercury exposure – pruritus *Eur J Ped 17):747–750, 2011;* anorexia, weight loss, photosensitivity, sweaty palms *Lancet 336:1578–1579, 1990*

Mothball intoxication (paradichlorobenzene) – refractory pruritus of arms and hands; ichthyosis *AD 148:404–405, 2012*

Sulfur mustard – chronic pruritus *Cutan Oculo Toxicol 31:220–225, 2012*

VASCULAR

Aagenaes syndrome (hereditary cholestasis with lymphedema) – autosomal recessive; lymphedema of legs due to congenital lymphatic hypoplasia; pruritus, growth retardation

Intramedullary vascular malformation – segmental pruritus *Schweizer Archiv Neurol Psychiatrie 145:13–16, 1994*

Stroke – unilateral pruritus *JAAD 45:892–896, 2001*

Temporal arteritis – scalp dysesthesia *JAAD 74:215–228, 2016*

PRURITUS, VULVAR

AUTOIMMUNE DISEASES AND DISORDERS OF DYSREGULATION

Allergic contact dermatitis – methylisothiazolinone in wipes; textile dyes in underwear; fragrance in douche or antiperspirant; rubber accelerators in condoms, underwear adhesive in pads, panty liners, tampons, latex rubber; semen *Dermatitis 24:64–72, 2012; Am J Contact Derm 8:137–140, 1997*

Atopic dermatitis *Ob Gyn Clin NA 44:371–378, 2017; Australasian J Dermatol 42:225–236, 2001*

INFECTIONS AND INFESTATIONS

Candidiasis *Dtsch Arztebl Int 116:126–133, 2020*

Chlamydia

Condylomata acuminata

Cutaneous larva migrans

Gonorrhea

Haemophilus influenzae

Herpes simples

Molluscum contagiosum

Neisseria meningitides

Parasites

Pediculosis

Pinworm

Scabies *Drugs Aging 25:299–306, 2008; Am J Clin Dermatol 3:9–18, 2002*

Shigella

Staphylococcus aureus

Streptococcus pneumoniae

Streptococcus pyogenes

Tinea cruris

Trichomonas

Yersinia

INFILTRATIVE DISORDERS

Langerhans cell histiocytosis *Australas J Dermatol 52:e8–14, 2011*

Plasma cell vulvitis *Dermatology 230:113–118, 2015*

INFLAMMATORY DISORDERS

Sarcoidosis *J Cut Med Surg 17:287–290, 2013*

Folliculitis

NEOPLASTIC DISORDERS

Basal cell carcinoma *Singapore Med J 60:479–482, 2019; Dermatol Online J 17:8, Jan 2011*

Extramammary Paget's disease

Inflammatory linear verrucous epidermal nevus (ILVEN)

Invasive vulvar squamous cell carcinoma *Int J Gyn Ob 143:suppl 2;4–13, 2018;* in Turner's syndrome – lichen sclerosus, squamous cell carcinoma *Endocrinol Diabetes Mellitus Case Rep 2016:160016:doi:10.1530/EDM-16-0016*

Melanoma, amelanotic *Am J Dermatopathol 37:e75–77, 2015*

Merkel cell carcinoma *Gyn Oncol Res Pract Jan 25, 2017;4:2:doi;1186/s40661-017-1137*

Syringoma *J Clin Design Res 8:FD06, 2014*

Verrucous carcinoma *J Low Genit Tract Dis 20:114–118, 2016*

Vulvar intraepithelial neoplasia (squamous epithelial neoplasia)

PRIMARY CUTANEOUS DISEASES

Irritant contact dermatitis

Lichen planus *BJD 170:218–220, 2014; BJD 169:337–343, 2013; BJD 138:569–575, 1998*

Lichen sclerosus et atrophicus *JAAD 44:803–806, 2001*

Lichen simplex chronicus *Dermatol Clin 28:669–680, 2010*

Poor hygiene

Pruritus vulvae

Psoriasis *Acta DV 88:132–135, 2008*

Red vulva syndrome *JAMA Derm 154:731–733, 2018*

Seborrheic dermatitis, seborrhiasis

PSYCHOCUTANEOUS DISEASES

Psychogenic itch

Vulvodynia *Low Genit Tract Dis 19:248–252, 2015*

TRAUMA

Vaginal prolapse *Indian J Sex Transm Dis AIDS 38:15–21, 2017*

VASCULAR LESIONS

Angiokeratoma *Sur J Gyn Oncol 32:597–598, 2011*

Arteriovenous malformation of the vulva *J Low Genit Tract Dis 18:E12–15, 2014*

PSEUDOXANTHOMA ELASTICUM-LIKE CHANGES

AUTOIMMUNE DISORDERS

Dermatomyositis *J Dermatol 29:423–426, 2002*

DEGENERATIVE DISORDERS

Aging

DRUGS

Penicillamine *Ann Plast Surg 29:367–370, 1992; BJD 123:305–312, 1990; BJD 114:381–388, 1986; J R Soc Med 78:794–798, 1984*

Topical corticosteroids

EXOGENOUS AGENTS

Acquired pseudoxanthoma elasticum *BJD 151:242–244, 2004;* after liver transplantation *JAAD 64:873–878, 2011;* acquired pseudoxanthoma elasticum – farmers exposed to saltpeter (calcium-ammonium-nitrate salts); antecubital fossa; yellow macules and papules *JAAD 51:1–21, 2004; Acta DV 78:153–154, 1998; Acta DV 58:319–321, 1978*

Saltpetre ingestion – PXE-like lesions *Clinics Dermatol 23:23–32, 2005; JAAD 44:33–39, 2001*

INFECTIONS AND INFESTATIONS

Acrodermatitis chronica atrophicans

INFILTRATIVE DISORDERS

Amyloidosis *Clin Exp Dermatol 11:87–91;* primary cutaneous amyloidosis masquerading as pseudoxanthoma elasticum *JAMA Derm 150:1091–1094, 2014;*

Lichen myxedematosus – personal observation

INFLAMMATORY DISORDERS

Inflammatory skin disease in the absence of other signs of pseudoxanthoma elasticum *J Cutan Pathol 34:777–781, 2007*

Post-inflammatory elastolysis

METABOLIC DISEASES

Beta-thalassemia and sickle cell disease in Greeks *Clinics in Dermatol 23:23–32, 2005;* beta thalassemia *Hemoglobin 41:254–259, 2017; JAAD 44:33–39, 2001*

Calcinosis cutis – idiopathic, tumoral calcinosis, calciphylaxis; pseudoxanthoma elasticum-like lesions *JAAD 44:33–39, 2001*

Calciphylaxis – with PXE-like changes *Am J Dermatopathol Nov 26, 2019; J Cutan Pathol 45:118–121, 2018; J Cutan Pathol 44:1064–1069, 2017; Am J Dermatopathol `18:396–399, 1996*

Cutaneous laxity due to marked weight loss – wasting syndrome, marasmus

Cystic fibrosis *AD 145:1292–1295, 2009*

Hyperphosphatemia – pseudoxanthoma elasticum-like lesions *JAAD 44:33–39, 2001; Am J Med 83:1157–1162, 1987*

Porphyria – congenital erythropoietic porphyria *Eur J Dermatol 24:401–402, 2014*

Post-partum periumbilical pseudoxanthoma elasticum *Indian J DV Leprol 67:139–140, 2001;* perforating *JAAD 19:384–388, 1988*

Recovery from severe edema

Renal disease – end stage renal disease *Clinics in Dermatol 23:23–32, 2005*

Sickle cell anemia *Br J Haematol 148:342, 2010*

NEOPLASTIC DISORDERS

Collagenomas, disseminated

Granulomatous slack skin – CTCL *JID 89:183, 1987*

PHOTODERMATOSES

Dermatoheliosis

PRIMARY CUTANEOUS DISEASES

Anetoderma – primary, secondary

Cutis laxa, congenital *JAAD 44:33–39, 2001; AD 92:373, 1965*

Cutis laxa, acquired
  Myeloma *AD 112:853–855, 1976*
  Systemic lupus erythematosus *JAAD 8:869, 1983*
  Hypersensitivity reaction *AD 123:1211–1216, 1987*
  Complement deficiency, penicillamine therapy *Lancet ii:858, 1983*
  With osteoma cutis *Indian J DV 83:464–467, 2017; JAAD 43:337–339, 2000*
  With ossification *Int J Dermatol 43:375–378, 2004*
  With multiple coagulation factor deficiency *Ann DV 135:162–163, 2008; J Invest Dermatol 127:581–587, 2007; JAAD 21:1150–1152, 1989*

Elastoderma *JAAD 33:389, 1995*

Elastosis perforans serpiginosa with PXE

Focal dermal elastolysis – pseudoxanthoma elasticum-like lesions *JAAD 27:113–115, 1992;* late onset focal dermal elastosis *Am J Dermatopathol 39:e73–74, 2017; Cutis 85:195–197, 2010*

Linear focal elastolysis *AD 131:855, 1995*

Mid-dermal elastolysis (perifollicular atrophy) (wrinkled skin) *JAAD 48:846–851, 2003; Cutis 71:312–314, 2003; J Cut Med Surg 4:40–44, 2000; JAAD 26:490–492, 1992; JAAD 26:169–173, 1992; AD 125:950–951, 1989*

Papillary dermal elastolysis – side of neck, axilla; post-menopausal and elderly women *JAAD 67:128–135, 2012*

decreased oxytalan and elaunin elastic fibers *Int J Dermatol 58:93–97, 2019; J Cutan Pathol 36:1010–1013, 2009; J Eur Acad DV 22:368–369, 2008; J Dermatol 34:709–711, 2007; JAAD 51:958, 2004; JAAD 51:165–185, 2004; J Eur Acad Dermatol Venerol 51:175–178, 2004;* yellow papules of neck with coarse furrows or wrinkles *JAAD 51:165–185, 2004; AD 136:791–796, 2000; JAAD 26:648–650, 1992;* PXE-like papillary mid-dermal elastolysis – yellowish-white papules resembling PXE on neck and supraclavicular areas of elderly people (photoaging) *JAAD 47:S189–192, 2002; JAAD 28:938–942, 1993; JAAD 26:648–650, 1992*

Periumbilical perforating PXE *AD 132:224–225, 227–228, 1996; JAAD 19:384, 1989; JAAD 19:384–388, 1988; AD 121:1321, 1985*

Striae distensae

White fibrous papulosis of the neck (fibroelastolytic papulosis) – cobblestoning with 2–4 mm skin colored papules *JAAD 51:958–964, 2004; Int J Derm 35:720–722, 1996; JAAD 20:1073–1077, 1989*

SYNDROMES

Buschke-Ollendorff syndrome (dermatofibrosis lenticularis disseminate) *BJD 144:890–893, 2001*

De Barsky syndrome *Dermatology Foundation Vol. 4 12/96:1–15*

Ehlers-Danlos syndrome type IX – X-linked

Leprechaunism *AD 117:531, 1981*

Neurofibromatosis

Pseudoxanthoma elasticum – *ABCC6* mutation

Pseudoxanthoma elasticum with amyloid *Acta DV 93:204–205, 2013; BJD 158:858–860, 2008; BJD 148:154–159, 2003; JAAD 22:27–34, 1990; AD 121:498–502, 1985*

Pseudoxanthoma elasticum with generalized arterial calcification of infancy – missense mutation in *ENPP1* gene *BJD 166:1107–1111, 2012*

Trisomy 18 – redundant skin, rocker-bottom feet, clenched fist

Wrinkly skin syndrome

TOXINS

Eosinophilia myalgia syndrome *Clinics in Dermatol 23:23–32, 2005; JAAD 24:657–658, 1991; Dermatologica 183:57–61, 1991*

Hydrophilic polymer vasculopathy *J Cutan Pathol 44:393–386, 2017*

VASCULAR DISEASES

Moya-Moya disease – elastosis perforans serpiginosa with pseudoxanthoma elasticum-like changes in Moya-Moya disease (bilateral stenosis and occlusion of basa intracranial vessels and carotid arteries) *BJD 153:431–434, 2005*

PSORIASIFORM DERMATITIS

AUTOIMMUNE DISEASES AND DISEASES OF IMMUNE DYSFUNCTION

Anti-laminin-gamma-1 (anti-p200) pemphigoid – vesicles and bullae; autoantibody targeting laminin 311 of the lower lamina lucida; strong association with psoriasis *BJD 168:1367–1369, 2013; BJD 167:1179–1183, 2012; J Dermatol 34:1–8, 2007; JID 106:1333, 1996; Med J Rec 130:246–248, 1929*

Dermatomyositis – psoriasiform scalp dermatitis *JAAD 51:427–439, 2004;* dermatomyositis with anti-transcriptional intermediary factor-1gamma antibodies – hypopigmented and telangiectatic patches (red and white patches); palmar hyperkeratotic papules; psoriasiform plaques *JAAD 72:449–455, 2015*

Graft vs. host disease *Cutis 92:151–153, 2013; JAAD 66:515–532, 2012; Biol Blood Marrow Transplant 12:1101–1113, 2006*

ICF syndrome – immunodeficiency, centromere instability, facial anomaly syndrome *BJD 178:335–349, 2018*

IgA pemphigus – personal observation

IL 1OR defects – post-auricular and diaper psoriasiform dermatitis *BJD 178:335–349, 2018*

IPEX syndrome – immune dysregulation (neonatal autoimmune enteropathy, food allergies), polyendocrinopathy (diabetes mellitus, thyroiditis), enteropathy (neonatal diarrhea), X-linked, rash (atopic dermatitis-like with exfoliative erythroderma and periorificial dermatitis; psoriasiform dermatitis, pemphigoid nodularis, painful fissured cheilitis, edema of lips and perioral area, urticaria secondary to foods); penile rash; thyroid dysfunction, diabetes mellitus, hepatitis, nephritis, onychodystrophy, alopecia universalis; mutations in *FOXP3* (forkhead box protein 3) gene – master control gene of T regulatory cells (Tregs); hyper IgE, eosinophilia *JAAD 73:355–364, 2015; BJD 160:645–651, 2009;* ichthyosiform eruptions *Blood 109:383–385, 2007; BJD 152:409–417, 2005; NEJM 344:1758–1762, 2001;* alopecia areata *AD 140:466–472, 2004*

Leukocyte adhesion deficiency syndrome – congenital deficiency of leucocyte-adherence glycoproteins (CD11a (LFA-1), CD11b, CD11c, CD18) – necrotic cutaneous abscesses, psoriasiform dermatitis, gingivitis, periodontitis, septicemia, ulcerative stomatitis, pharyngitis, otitis, pneumonia, peritonitis *BJD 123:395–401, 1990*

LIG4 syndrome *BJD 178:335–349, 2018*

Linear IgA disease – annular psoriasiform, serpiginous red plaques of palms *JAAD 51:S112–117, 2004*

Lupus erythematosus including systemic lupus erythematosus, discoid lupus erythematosus, subacute cutaneous lupus erythematosus *Clinics in Derm 10:431–442, 1992*

Pemphigus foliaceus – personal observation

Pemphigus vulgaris – psoriasiform scalp dermatitis in pregnancy *Cutis 94:206–209, 2014*

SCID with microcephaly, growth retardation, and sensitivity to radiation syndrome *BJD 178:335–349, 2018*

Still's disease in the adult – brown coalescent scaly papules; persistent psoriasiform papular lesions *JAAD 52:1003–1008, 2005*

CONGENITAL LESIONS

Urachal sinus – presenting as periumbilical psoriasiform dermatitis *BJD 157:419–420, 2007*

DRUG-INDUCED

Acetazolamide – pustular psoriasis *J Dermatol 22:784–787, 1995*

Acral dysesthesia syndrome – personal observation

Adalimumab (TNF-inhibitor) – flare of psoriasis *J Drugs Dermtol 1152–1154, 2015; BJD 169:1141–1147, 2013;* pustular psoriasis; palmoplantar pustular psoriasis *JAAD 56:327–328, 2007*

Anakinra (IL-1 receptor antagonist) – psoriasiform drug eruption *BJD 158:1146–1148, 2008*

Atenolol – induces pustular psoriasis *AD 126:968–969, 1990; Clin Exp Derm 9:92–94, 1984*

Beta blocker-induced psoriasiform eruption *Int J Dermatol 27:619–627, 1988*

Botulinum A toxin, intramuscular *Cutis 50:415–416, 1992*

Bupropion (Zyban) – psoriatic erythroderma or pustular psoriasis *BJD 146:1061–1063, 2002*

Capecitabine (Xeloda) – acral dysesthesia syndrome

Checkpoint inhibitors – psoriasiform eruptions *JAAD 80:990–997, 2019*

Chloroquine

Drug-induced pseudolymphoma – allopurinol, amiloride, carbamazepine, cyclosporine, clomipramine, diltiazem, phenytoin *AD 132:1315–1321, 1996*

Efalizumab – intertriginous (flexural) papular psoriasis *AD 143:900–906, 2007*

Etanercept – pustular psoriasis; palmoplantar pustular psoriasis *JAAD 56:327–328, 2007; BJD 151:506–507, 2004*

Fluoxetine (selective serotonin reuptake inhibitor) – flare of psoriasis *JAAD 56:848–853, 2007; Am J Psychiatry 159:2113, 2002*

G-CSF – pustular psoriasis *AD 134:111–112, 1998*

Hepatitis B vaccine – necrolytic acral erythema; psoriasiform dermatitis, acral erythema and scale, cheilitis, verrucous papules of eyelids and around nose *BJD 171:1255–1256, 2014*

Infliximab – psoriasiform eruption *Cutis 80:231–237, 2007; Ann Pharmacother 38:54–57, 2004;* pustular psoriasis; palmoplantar pustular psoriasis *JAAD 56:327–328, 2007; BJD 151:506–507, 2004*

Interferon alpha *AD 130:890–893, 1994;* interferon beta *BJD 160:716–717, 2009*

Interleukin-2 *AD 124:1811–1815, 1988;* induction of reactive arthritis by IL-2 *JAAD 29:788–789, 1993*

Kit and BCR-ABL inhibitors – imatinib, nilotinib, dasatinib – facial edema morbilliform eruptions, pigmentary changes, lichenoid reactions, psoriasis, pityriasis rosea, pustular eruptions, DRESS, Stevens-Johnson syndrome, urticarial, neutrophilic dermatoses, photosensitivity, pseudolymphoma, porphyria cutanea tarda, small vessel vasculitis, panniculitis, perforating folliculitis, erythroderma *JAAD 72:203–218, 2015*

Lichenoid drug eruption – psoriasiform appearance – amiphenazole, captopril, gold *AD 109:372–376, 1974;* isoniazid, levamisole *J R Soc Med 73:208–211, 1980;* levopromazine, methyldopa, metropromazine, propranolol, exprenolol, labetalol (beta-blockers), chlorpropamide, enalapril, pyrimethamine *Clin Exp Dermatol 5:253–256, 1980;* antimalarials, penicillamine, thiazide diuretics, streptomycin, hydroxyurea, tiopronin, naproxen, carbamazepine, ethambutol, simvastatin, para-amino salicylic acid, pravastatin *JAAD 29:249–255, 1993; Cutis 61:98–100, 1998;* includes photo-LP (demeclocycline *AD 109:97–98, 1974*) oral LP, and contact LP; quinacrine – lichenoid dermatitis *JAAD 4:239–248, 1981;* quinine – lichenoid photodermatitis *Clin Exp Dermatol 19:246–248, 1994*

Lithium *Int J Dermatol 49:1351–1361, 2010; Am J Clin Dermatol 5:3–8, 2004; Am J Clin Dermatol 1:159–165, 2000*

Mitomycin C – intravesical administration *Arch Esp Urol 42:670–672, 1989*

Nifedipine *JAAD 38:201–206, 1998*

Nivolumab (PD-1 inhibitor) – psoriasiform eruption *JAMA Derm 151:797–798, 2015*

Paroxetine (selective serotonin reuptake inhibitor) – flare of psoriasis *JAAD 56:848–853, 2007; Ann Pharmacother 26:211–212, 1992*

Pembrolizumab (anti-PD-1) – fiery red eroded inguinal intertrigo (baboon syndrome) *JAMA Derm 152:590–592, 2016*

Penicillamine *J Rheumatol 8 (Suppl 7):149–154, 1981*

Ponitinib – pityriasis rubra pilaris-like changes, eyebrow thinning, ichthyosiform changes *BJD 173:574–577, 2015*

Propranolol *Lancet 1, 808, 1986; Cutis 24:95, 1979*

Rofecoxib (Vioxx) – exacerbation of psoriasis *AD 139:1223, 2003*

Secukinumab *JAMA Derm 153:1194–1195, 2017*

Sofosbuvir – pityriasis rubra pilaris-like eruption *J Drugs Dermtol 1161–1162, 2015*

Sorafenib *J Drugs Dermatol 9:169–171, 2010*

Terbinafine *JAAD 36:858–862, 1997*

TNF alpha blockers *BJD 178:281–283, 2018*

DRUGS EXACERBATING PSORIASIS

Acebutolol

Acetyl salicylic acid

Alprenolol

Atenolol

Beta blockers

Captopril

Calcium channel blockers

Chlorthalidone

Chloroquine

Cimetidine

Clomipramine

Clonidine

Clopidogrel – pustular psoriasis *BJD 155:630–631, 2006*

Cyclosporine

Dipyridamole

Fluoxetine

Gemfibrozil

Gold

Glyburide

Ibuprofen

IL-2 *JAMA 258:3120–3121, 1987*

Indomethacin

Interferon alpha *JAAD 37:118–120, 1997*

Labetalol

Lithium

Meclofenamate

Metaprolol

Nadolol

NSAIDS

Omeprazole

Oxprenelol

Oxyphenbutazone

Penicillamine

Penicillin

Phenylbutazone

Pindolol

Propranolol

Pyrazolone

Quinacrine

Quinidine

SARTANS – Orally active angiotensin II type I receptor antagonists *BJD 147:617–618, 2002*

Terbinafine *JAAD 36:858–862, 1997*

Terfenadine

Tetracycline

Timolol

Trazodone

Tumor necrosis factor inhibitors *BJD 161:1081–1088, 2009*

Vitamin K

EXOGENOUS AGENTS

Silicone – psoriasiform dermatitis of buttocks *AD 148:1212–1213, 2012*

INFECTIONS AND INFESTATIONS

AIDS-associated psoriasiform dermatitis *Int J Dermatol 35:484–488, 1996; AD 126:1457–1461, 1990;* exacerbation of psoriasis; Reiter's syndrome with or without zinc deficiency *Int J Derm 27:342–343, 1988*

Botryomycosis *Cutis 55:149–152, 1995*

Brucellosis *Cutis 63:25–27, 1999; AD 117:40–42, 1981*

Candidiasis

Generalized dermatophytosis personal observation

Epidermodysplasia verruciformis – autosomal recessive, X-linked recessive (one family); 17 HPV types isolated; HPV 3 and 10 most common with types 5 and 8 associated with malignant lesions; epidermodysplasia verruciformis HPV remain extrachromosomal in cutaneous tumors *AD 131:1312–1318, 1995; JAAD 22:547–566, 1990; Proc Nat Acad Sci USA 79:1634, 1982*

Erythrasma – personal observation

Gianotti-Crosti syndrome – personal observation

Hepatitis C infection – necrolytic acral erythema; red to hyperpigmented psoriasiform plaques with variable scale or erosions of feet or shins *JAAD 63:259–265, 2010; JAAD 53:247–251, 2005; Int J Derm 35:252–256, 1996*

Histoplasmosis, disseminated – *Histoplasma capsulatum*; mimicking psoriasis *JAAD 29:311–313, 1993;* dimorphic; 2–5 micron oval or budding yeast forms surrounded by halo within macrophages; cutaneous lesions in disseminated disease include macules and papules, plaques, punched-out ulcers, purpuric lesions, abscesses, dermatitis, subcutaneous nodules, cellulitis, exfoliative erythroderma, acneiform eruptions, transepidermal elimination papules, oral ulcers and tongue nodules *Diagnostic Challenges Vol V:77–79, 1994; AD 127:721–726, 1991*

Leishmaniasis – primary or leishmaniasis recidivans (lupoid leishmaniasis) – extensive psoriasiform dermatitis *Clin Dermatol 38:140–151, 2020*

Leprosy, borderline tuberculoid – personal observation

Mycobacterium tuberculosis – tuberculosis verrucosa cutis; usually solitary lesion resulting from exogenous inoculation of tubercle bacilli into individual with preexistent moderately high degree of immunity to TB; or from autoinoculation *AD 125:113–118, 1989;* lichen scrofulosorum – psoriasiform dermatitis with pustules *Ped Derm 28:532–534, 2011*

Pinta

Scabies, crusted (Norwegian scabies) – psoriasiform lesions of hands, hails, trunk, feet, ears, scalp *Cutis 92:193–198, 2013; Ped Derm 27:93–94, 2010; AD 127:1833, 1991; JAAD 17:434–436, 1987*

Scarlet fever

Staphylococcal scalded skin syndrome

Syphilis, secondary – *Treponema pallidum*; 8–14 regular rigid spirals; 3 main elements on electron microscopy 1) Protoplasmic cylinder (protoplast) 2) Axial filament 3) Outer envelope (cell wall); penicillin disrupts the synthesis of the outer envelope; psoriasiform dermatitis of scalp *JAAD 82:1–14, 2020; NEJM 371:2017, 2014; AD 148:1317–1322, 2012;* syphilitic keratoderma resembles reactive arthritis, psoriasis *AD 144:255–260, 2008*

Tinea corporis – *Trichophyton rubrum* including tinea corporis in HIV – *Microsporum gypseum AD 132:233–234, 1996;* tinea capitis; tinea pedis – mimics pustular psoriasis; tinea cruris; the three most common causes in the U.S. are *Trichophyton rubrum, Microsporum canis,* and *Trichophyton mentagrophytes; Trichophyton concentricum* (tinea imbricata) common in the Pacific Islands.

Tinea versicolor – personal observation

Yaws – secondary pianides

INFILTRATIVE DISEASES

Langerhans cell histiocytosis (Letterer-Siwe disease) *JAAD 56:302–316, 2007*

Lichen amyloidosis

Rosai-Dorfman disease – deep red plaques of lower back and buttocks *AD 145:571–574, 2009*

Waldenstrom's macroglobulinemia – psoriasiform plaques of knees *Annual AAD Meeting 2000*

INFLAMMATORY DISEASES

Erythema multiforme

Rosai-Dorfman disease (sinus histiocytosis with massive lymphadenopathy) – psoriasiform exfoliative dermatitis *JAAD 50:159–161, 2004; JAAD 41:335–337, 1999*

Sarcoidosis – psoriasiform dermatitis *JAAD 51:448–452, 2004; AD 106:896, 1972;* psoriasiform scalp dermatitis *AD 140:1003–1008, 2004*

Whipple's disease – psoriasiform dermatitis; macular and reticulated erythema; Addisonian hyperpigmentation; *Tropheryma whipplei JAAD 60:277–288, 2009*

METABOLIC

Acrodermatitis enteropathica or acquired zinc deficiency – autosomal recessive or acquired due to gastrointestinal disorders, dietary deficiencies, trauma, malignancy, renal disorders, parasitic infections; periorificial dermatitis, generalized dermatitis, vesicular, bullous, pustular, desquamative dermatitis, psoriasiform dermatitis, alopecia, paronychia, perleche *Ped Derm 27:395–396, 2010; JAAD 56:116–124, 2008; Ped Derm 25;56–59, 2008; Ped Derm 19:426–431, 2002; Ped Derm 19:426–431, 2002; AD 116:562–564, 1980; Acta DV (Stockh) 17:513–546, 1936*

Biotin-responsive multiple carboxylase deficiency – psoriasiform, periorificial intertriginous dermatitis; diarrhea, alopecia *Ped Derm 33:457–458, 2016; NEJM 304:820–823, 1981*

> Biotin is water soluble B complex vitamin.
> Pyruvate carboxylase, propionyl coenzyme A carboxylase , and beta methylcrotonyl Co-A carboxylase are all mitochondrial in location.
> Acetyl Co-A carboxylase is cytosolic.
> Late onset – deficiency of biotinidase.
> Early onset – holocarboxylase synthetase deficiency.

Cystic fibrosis – polycyclic psoriasiform dermatitis, resembling necrolytic migratory erythema *JAAD 58:S29–30, 2008*

Essential fatty acid deficiency – especially linoleic acid

Hartnup disease – autosomal recessive; defective transport of tryptophan in small intestine and kidneys; pellagra-like photosensitive eruption; cerebellar ataxia; psoriasiform red scaly plaques, generalized alopecia, widespread edema *Ped Derm 23:262–265, 2006*

Idiopathic hypoparathyroidism *Eur J Dermatol 9:574–576, 1999; Acta Med Scand (Suppl) 121:1–269, 1941*

Hereditary lactic dehydrogenase M-subunit deficiency – elbows and knees; circinate and psoriasiform lesions resembling circinate lesions of erythrokeratoderma variabilis, ichthyosis linearis circumflexa, necrolytic migratory erythema, pellagra, and zinc deficiency; isozymes of LDH are tetramers of 2 different polypeptides, M and H; isozyme LDH 5 contains four identical M chains and predominates in the epidermis *AD 122:1420–1424, 1986*

Methylmalonic acidemia – deficiency of methylmalonyl coenzyme A mutase or its cofactors adenosylcobalamin (vitamin B12) and methylcobalamin; affects metabolism of four amino acids (valine isoleucine, threonine, methionine); these patients fed low protein diets limited in branched chain amino acids *Ped Derm 24:455–456, 2007; Dermatol Pediatr Lat 1:46–48, 2003; Ped Derm 16:95–102, 1999; AD 133:1563–1566, 1997; J Pediatr 124:416–420, 1994; BJD 131:93–98, 1994*

Necrolytic acral erythema – cutaneous marker for hepatitis C infection; psoriasiform hyperpigmented, hyperkeratotic plaques of acral palmar, plantar, dorsal surfaces of hands and feet; darker, more velvety and verrucous than psoriasis; burning, pruritic dusky red plaques *Cutis 81:356–360, 2008; JAAD 55:S108–110, 2006; JAAD 53:247–251, 2005; AD 141:85–87, 2005; Int J Derm 44:916–921, 2005; JAAD 50:s121–124, 2004, Int J Derm 35:252–256, 1996*

Pellagra

Propionic aciduria – psoriasiform eruptions *Ped Derm 16:95–102, 1999*

Acquired zinc deficiency – personal observation

NEOPLASTIC

Eccrine syringofibroadenomatosis – varied clinical presentation including solitary nodules, psoriasiform dermatitis of palms and soles, dermatomal papules, vegetating hyperkeratotic nodule, pyogenic granuloma-like lesion, crusted papules, keratotic papules *JAAD 26:805–813, 1992*

Kaposi's sarcoma – personal observation

Keratoacanthomas – Grzybowski type

Lymphoma – cutaneous T-cell lymphoma – 2.8% of all lymphomas *JAAD 70:205–220, 2014; JAAD 52:393–402, 2005; JAAD 51:111–117, 2004; Curr Prob Derm Dec. 1991;* HTLV-1 lymphoma *JAAD 36:869–871, 1997;* cytotoxic T-cell lymphoma – psoriasiform dermatitis with widespread ulcerations *AD 145:801–808, 2009*

Lymphomatoid papulosis

Porokeratosis – disseminated superficial actinic porokeratosis – personal observation

PARANEOPLASTIC

Acrokeratosis paraneoplastica (Bazex syndrome) – associated with upper aerodigestive system malignancies; three stages – 1) fingers and toes, helices and nose; 2) palms and soles, face (violaceous plaques); 3) hands, elbows and knees, arms, forearms, thighs, legs and trunk *NEJM 373:2161, 2015; JAAD 55:1103–1105, 2006; JAAD 54:745–762, 2006; JAAD 52:711–712, 2005; AD 141: 389–394, 2005; Cutis 74:289–292, 2004; JAAD 40:822–825, 1999; AD 124:1852, 1855, 1988; JAAD 17:517–518, 1987; Bull Soc Fr Dermatol Syphilol 72:182–185 1965; Paris Med 43:234–237, 1922*

Necrolytic migratory erythema – glucagonoma syndrome *JAAD 49:325–328, 2003*

Paraneoplastic neutrophilic figurate erythema – arcuate psoriasiform plantar dermatitis *BJD 156:396–398, 2007*

PHOTODERMATOSES

Polymorphous light eruption, psoriasiform

Psoriasis, photosensitive

PRIMARY CUTANEOUS DISEASE

Acrodermatitis continua of Hallopeau *Ped Derm 34:715–716, 2017*

Acute parapsoriasis (pityriasis lichenoides et varioliformis acuta) (Mucha-Habermann disease) *AD 123:1335–1339, 1987; AD 118:478, 1982*

Annular epidermolytic hyperkeratosis – personal observation

Atopic dermatitis

Atypical epidermolytic hyperkeratosis with palmoplantar keratoderma with keratin 1 mutation – palmoplantar keratoderma with psoriasiform plaques of elbows and antecubital fossae *BJD 150:1129–1135, 2004*

Axillary granular parakeratosis *AD 140:1161–1166, 2004*

Circumscribed palmar hypokeratosis *JAMA Derm 153:609–611, 2017*

Dermatitis of the legs

Diaper dermatitis with rapid dissemination – expanding nummular dermatitis of trunk, and red scaly plaques of neck and axillae ("psoriasiform id") *BJD 78:289–296, 1966*

Dyshidrosis – personal observation

Epidermolysis bullosa, dominant dystrophic type; reduced numbers of anchoring fibrils; chondroitin 6-sulfate proteoglycan and KF-1 are reduced

Epidermolytic hyperkeratosis – polycyclic psoriasiform plaques; mutation in keratin 1 gene *Exp Dermatol 8:501–503, 1999*

Erythema annulare centrifugum – mimics recurrent circinate erythematous psoriasis of Bloch and Lapiere

Erythematous and keratotic components – differential diagnosis *Ped Derm 19:285–292, 2002*

    Erythrokeratoderma en cocardes
    Erythrokeratoderma variabilis
    Erythrokeratolysis heimalis (Oudtshoorn disease) – targetoid peeling with repeated cycles of hyperkeratosis and peeling
    Keratosis-ichthyosis-deafness (KID) syndrome – linear hyperkeratotic erythema; fine granular palmoplantar keratoderma
    Netherton's syndrome – flexural lichenification
    Non-bullous congenital ichthyosiform erythroderma
    Progressive symmetric erythrokeratoderma
    Loricrin keratoderma

Erythrokeratoderma progressiva symmetrica – plaques on medial buttocks, extremities, face, palms and soles; increased mitotic activity of cells with lipid vacuoles in stratum corneum cells

AD 122:434–440, 1986; Dermatologica 164:133–141, 1982

Erythrokeratoderma variabilis – psoriasiform plaques, urticarial plaques and palmoplantar keratoderma *BJD 173:309–311, 2015; Ped Derm 23:382–385, 2006; Clin in Dermatol 23:23–32, 2005; Ped Derm 12:351–354, 1995; Ann DV (Stockh) 6:225–258, 1925*

Granuloma annulare

Grover's disease (transient acantholytic dermatosis) *AD 113:431–435, 1977*

Hailey-Hailey disease – personal observation

Hyperkeratotic dermatitis of the palms *BJD 109:205–208, 1983; BJD 107:195–202, 1982*

Ichthyosis

Ichthyosis bullosa of Siemens – personal observation

Impetigo herpetiformis (pustular psoriasis) *Acta Obstet Gynecol Scand 74:229–232, 1995*

Infantile febrile psoriasiform dermatitis *Ped Derm 12:28–34, 1995*

Juvenile circumscribed pityriasis rubra pilaris *Ped Derm 25:125–126, 2008*

Juvenile plantar dermatosis – personal observation

Keratosis lichenoides chronica (Nekam's disease) – linear reticulate papular, nodular violaceous lesions

Lamellar ichthyosis – episodic psoriasiform pattern *Cutis 122:428–433, 1986*

Lichen planus – of palms or hypertrophic lichen planus

Lichen simplex chronicus – psoriasiform neurodermatitis

Lichen spinulosus *JAAD 22:261–264, 1990; Cutis 43:557–560, 1989*

Lichen striatus – personal observation

Necrolytic acral erythema – hyperpigmented psoriasiform serpiginous, verrucous plaques of dorsal aspects of hands, legs; associated with hepatitis C infection *JAAD 81:23–41, 2019; JAAD 50:S121–124, 2004; Int J Derm 35:252–256, 1996*

Palmoplantar keratoderma, epidermolytic hyperkeratosis – personal observation

Parakeratosis pustulosa – psoriasiform dermatitis of children; paronychial skin with thickening of nail edges *BJD 79:527–532, 1967*

Parapsoriasis en plaque – small plaque parapsoriasis *JAAD 59:474–482, 2008; Ann Dermatol Syphiligr (Paris)3:313–315, 1902*

Perioral dermatitis – personal observation

Pityriasis lichenoides chronica *BJD 172:372–379, 2015; JAAD 56:205–210, 2007; BJD 129:353–354, 1993; AD 119:378–380, 1983; Arch Dermatol Syphilol 50:359–374, 1899*

Pityriasis rosea

Pityriasis rotunda

Pityriasis rubra pilaris – psoriasiform patches of elbows and knees; seborrheic keratoses become more prominent if the erythroderma of PRP persists

    Adult – Classic (1), Atypical (2)
    Juvenile – Classic (3), Juvenile Circumscribed – psoriasiform dermatitis of knees and ankles with palmoplantar keratoderma *Ped Derm 31:138–145, 2014; (4), Atypical (5)* (early onset with chronic course) *JAAD 59:943–948, 2008; J Dermatol 27:174–177, 2000; JAAD 31:997–999, 1994; JAAD 20:801, 1989*

Poikiloderma vasculare atrophicans

Progressive symmetric erythrokeratoderma (Gottron's syndrome) – autosomal dominant; large fixed geographic symmetric scaly red–orange plaques; shoulders, cheeks, buttocks, ankles, wrists *Ped Derm 25:633–634, 2008; AD 122:434–440, 1986; Dermatologica 164:133–141, 1982*

Psoriasiform neurodermatitis (lichen simplex chronicus)

Psoriasis vulgaris *JAAD 65:137–174, 2011;* plantar psoriasis *BJD 168:1243–1251, 2013;* severe psoriasis in AIDS *Clin Dermatol 38:160–175, 2020*

RAG2-/-, I kappa B-alpha-/- chimeras *JID 115:1124–1133, 2000*

Seborrheic dermatitis

SYNDROMES

Activated STING in Vascular and Pulmonary syndrome – autoinflammatory disease; butterfly telangiectatic facies; acral violaceous psoriasiform, papulosquamous and atrophic vasculitis of hands; nodules of face, nose, and ears; fingertip ulcers with necrosis; nail dystrophy; nasal septal perforation; interstitial lung disease with fibrosis; polyarthritis; myositis *NEJM 371:507–518, 2014*

Arthropathy, rash, chronic meningitis, eye lesions, mental retardation *Jnl Ped 99:79, 1981*

Chanarin-Dorfman syndrome (neutral lipid storage disease) – erythrokeratoderma variabilis-like ichthyosis with keratotic plaques of elbows and knees and seborrheic-like scaling along hairline *BJD 153:838–841, 2005*

CHILD syndrome – linear demarcation of half-body psoriasiform dermatitis with hemidysplasia; mutation in NSDHL (NAD (P)H steroid dehydrogenase-like protein *BJD 159:1204–1206, 2008; Ped Derm 15:360–366, 1998*

Conradi-Hunermann syndrome (chondrodysplasia punctata – X-linked dominant) – ichthyotic and psoriasiform lesions *JAAD 33:356–360, 1995*

Craniosynostosis, anal anomalies, and porokeratosis (CAP/CDAGS) – autosomal recessive; craniosynostosis, clavicular hypoplasia, delayed fontanel closure, cranial defects (parietal foramina), deafness, imperforate anus or anterior placement of anus, genitourinary abnormalities (hypospadias and urethrorectal fistula), and skin eruption (porokeratosis-like lesions), mental retardation, scant hair, *Staphylococcus aureus* infections *JAAD 68:881–884, 2013; Am J Hum Genet 77:161–168, 2005; J Med Genet 35:763–766, 1998*

Erythrokeratoderma en cocarde

Familial pityriasis rubra pilaris – ichthyosiform scaling; psoriasiform dermatitis; gain of function mutation of *CARD14 BJD 171:420–422, 2014; Am J Hum Genet 91:163–170, 2012*

Haim-Munk syndrome – autosomal recessive; palmoplantar keratoderma, periodontitis, psoriasiform plaques of palms and soles, onychogryphosis, arachnodactyly, acro-osteolysis, flexion contractures; mutation of lysosomal protease cathepsin C *JAAD 58:339–344, 2008;* pes planus *BJD 77:42–54, 1965*

Hereditary focal transgressive palmoplantar keratoderma – autosomal recessive; hyperkeratotic lichenoid papules of elbows and knees, psoriasiform lesions of scalp and groin, spotty and reticulate hyperpigmentation of face, trunk, and extremities, alopecia of eyebrows and eyelashes *BJD 146:490–494, 2002*

Hereditary lactate dehydrogenase M subunit deficiency without IL-36 receptor antagonist mutation – pustular psoriasis-like eruption; erythematous skin lesions; psoriasiform dermatitis; annular desquamative plaques; fatigue, myalgia, myoglobinuria, increased creatine kinase *BJD 172:1674–1676, 2015; JAAD 27:262–263, 1992; JAAD 24:339–342, 1991; AD 122:1420–1424, 1986*

Hereditary mucoepithelial dysplasia (dyskeratosis) – red eyes, non-scarring alopecia, keratosis pilaris, erythema of oral (palate, gingiva) and nasal mucous membranes, cervix, vagina, and urethra; perineal and perigenital psoriasiform dermatitis; increased risk of infections, fibrocystic lung disease *BJD 153:310–318, 2005; Ped Derm 11:133–138, 1994; JAAD 21:351–357, 1989; Am J Hum Genet 31:414–427, 1979; Oral Surg Oral Med Oral Pathol 46:645–657, 1978*

HOPP syndrome – hypotrichosis, striate, reticulated pitted palmoplantar keratoderma, acro-osteolysis, psoriasiform plaques, lingua plicata, onychogryphosis, ventricular arrhythmias, periodontitis *BJD 150:1032–1033, 2004; BJD 147:575–581, 2002*

Ichthyosis follicularis with alopecia and photophobia (IFAP) – large psoriasiform plaques; knees; alopecia, photophobia, non-inflammatory spiny follicular projections, hyperkeratosis of dorsum of fingers, legs, knees, and elbows; to be differentiated from ulerythema ophryogenes, atrichia with papular lesions, atrophoderma vermiculata, keratosis pilaris rubra atrophicans facei, keratosis follicularis spinulosa decalvans, and KID syndrome *BJD 142:157–162, 2000; AD 121:1167–1174, 1985*

IgG4-related disease – cutaneous plasmacytosis (papulonodules); pseudolymphoma; angiolymphoid hyperplasia with eosinophilia; Mikulicz's disease; psoriasiform dermatitis; morbilliform eruption; hypergammaglobulinemic purpura; urticarial vasculitis; ischemic digits; Raynaud's disease and digital gangrene *BJD 171:929,959–967, 2014*

IPEX syndrome – X-linked; immune dysregulation, polyendocrinopathy (diabetes mellitus, thyroiditis), autoimmune enteropathy; mutation of FOXP3 gene encodes DNA-binding protein that suppresses transcription of multiple genes involved in cytokine production and T cell proliferation; atopic-like or nummular dermatitis, ichthyosiform dermatitis, urticaria, scaly psoriasiform plaques of trunk and extremities, penile rash, alopecia universalis, trachyo-

nychia, bullae; pemphigoid nodularis (bullae and prurigo nodularis), membranous glomerulonephritis, autoimmune thyroid disease, hepatitis, exocrine pancreatitis *NEJM 378:1132–1141, 2018; JAAD 55:143–148, 2006; AD 140:466–472, 2004; J Pediatr 100:731–737, 1982*

Kawasaki's syndrome – psoriasiform eruptions of face scalp and extremities *JAAD 75:69–76, 2016; Ped Derm 31:651–652, 2014; JAAD 69:501–510, 2013; Acta Paediatr 99:1102–1104, 2010; Ped Derm 24:336–337, 2007; J Pediatr 137:578–580, 2000*

Keratosis-ichthyosis-deafness (KID) syndrome (knees) – widespread erythrokeratotic lesions with grainy leatherlike appearance; reticulated and serpiginous hyperkeratotic plaques of the face; follicular keratosis, perioral wrinkling, loss of visual acuity, sensory impairment, susceptibility to bacterial and fungal infections *AD 123:777–782, 1987;* psoriasiform scalp dermatitis *BJD 148:649–653, 2003*

KID syndrome with fissured lips – paronychial pustules, blepharitis without keratitis, perineal psoriasiform plaques, tongue erosions, honeycomb palmoplantar keratoderma; red gingivae; mutation in connexin 26 (N14K) GJB2

Lipoid proteinosis – psoriasiform plaques *BJD 151:413–423, 2004; JID 120:345–350, 2003; BJD 148:180–182, 2003; Hum Molec Genet 11:833–840, 2002*

Mal de Meleda *AD 136:1247–1252, 2000*

Multicentric reticulohistiocytosis *AD 118:173, 1982*

Naxos syndrome – personal observation

Netherton's syndrome – presenting as congenital psoriasis *Ped Derm 14:473–476, 1997;* psoriasiform plaques of knees *Int J Dermatol 37:268–270, 1998;* generalized psoriasiform plaques *JAMA Derm 152:435–442, 2016*

Neutral lipid storage disease (Chanarin-Dorfman disease) – autosomal recessive; erythrokeratoderma variabilis-like presentation; focal or diffuse alopecia; congenital non-bullous ichthyosiform erythroderma, collodion baby; seborrheic dermatitis-like rash of face and scalp; leukonychia; mutation in ABHD5 which encodes protein of esterase/lipase/thioesterase subfamily *BJD 153:838–841, 2005*

Nijmegen breakage syndrome *BJD 178:335–349, 2018*

Papillon-Lefevre syndrome – autosomal recessive; diffuse transgradiens palmoplantar keratoderma and periodontopathy with loss of deciduous and permanent dentition ; psoriasiform plaques of elbows , knees, pretibial areas, and trunk; recurrent cutaneous and systemic pyodermas; mutation in cathepsin C gene *Cutis 93:193–198, 2014; Cutis 79:55–56, 2007; AD 141:779–784, 2005; JAAD 48:345–351, 2003; J Periodontol 66:413–420, 1995; Ped Derm 11:354–357, 1994; Ped Derm 6:222–225, 1989; AD 124:533–539, 1988*

Reactive arthritis – erosions with marginal erythema; circinate erosions *JAAD 59:113–121, 2008; NEJM 309:1606–1615, 1983; Semin Arthritis Rheum 3:253–286, 1974; Dtsch Med Wochenschr 42:1535–1536, 1916*

> Circinate balanitis – annular or serpiginous
> Asymptomatic oral mucosal erosions
> Keratoderma blenorrhagicum; soles, pretibial areas, dorsal toes, feet, fingers, hands, nails, scalp; may be associated with HIV disease *Ann Int Med 106:19–26, 1987; Semin Arthritis Rheum 3:253–286, 1974;* following gastroenteritis due to Salmonella enteritidis, *Shigella, Yersinia, Campylobacter species,* and *Clostridium difficile Clin Inf Dis 33:1010–1014, 2001*
> Pustular psoriasis
> Psoriasiform plaques
> Nail changes
> Geographic tongue

Aortic insufficiency

Cardiac conduction abnormalities

Conjunctivitis, uveitis, keratitis – sterile mucopurulent discharge

IgA nephropathy

Myelopathy

Palatal erosions, oral ulcers, glossitis

Seronegative non-suppurative arthritis – polyarticular knees, ankles, metatarsophalangeal, sacroiliac joints; relative sparing of hands and wrists; occasionally monoarticular; enthesitis

Spondylitis

Achilles tendonitis

Plantar fasciitis

Sausage digits – dactylitis

Urethritis

Ulcerative vulvitis – red crusted plaques of vulva and perineum

SAM syndrome (severe dermatitis, multiple allergies, metabolic wasting) – biallelic loss of function mutations in desmoglein1 (Dsg1); palmoplantar keratoderma, psoriasiform plaques, multiple allergies *BJD 172:257–261, 2015*

SAPHO syndrome – palmoplantar pustulosis with sternoclavicular hyperostosis; acne fulminans, acne conglobata, hidradenitis suppurativa, psoriasis, multifocal osteitis *Cutis 71:63–67, 2003; Cutis 62:75–76, 1998; Rev Rheum Mol Osteoarthritic 54:187–196, 1987; Ann Rev Rheum Dis 40:547–553, 1981*

Sweet's syndrome – personal observation

Transgradiens pachyonychia congenital – palmoplantar kerato-derma with psoriasiform plaques *BJD 166:124–128, 2012*

Turner's syndrome *JAAD 36:1002–1004, 1996*

PSORIASIFORM PLAQUE, FOCAL OR SOLITARY

AUTOIMMUNE DISEASES AND DISEASES OF IMMUNE DYSFUNCTION

Bullous pemphigoid

Dermatomyositis – personal observation

Lupus erythematosus – systemic lupus – psoriasiform plaques of palms and soles *BJD 81:186–190,1969;* discoid lupus erythemato-sus; *NEJM 269:1155–1161, 1963;* subacute cutaneous lupus erythematosus *Med Clin North Am 73:1073–1090, 1989; JAAD 19:1957–1062, 1988*

Pemphigus foliaceus

DRUGS

Chemotherapy-associated acral dysesthesia syndrome

Drug-induced pseudolymphoma *AD 132:1315–1321, 1996*

Erythropoietin-induced Sweet's syndrome – personal observation

Fixed drug eruption, chronic

Gamma interferon injection site *AD 126:351–355, 1990*

Tumor necrosis factor alpha antagonists – lichen planus-like eruptions; psoriasiform plaque of elbow *JAAD 61:104–111, 2009*

Vitamin K injection (Aquamephyton)

EXOGENOUS XOGENOUS AGENTS

Silica granulomas

INFECTIONS AND INFESTATIONS

African histoplasmosis (*Histoplasma capsulatum* var. *duboisii*) -exclusively in Central and West Africa and Madagascar *Clin Inf Dis 48:441, 493–494, 2009*

Alternaria chartarum – red, scaly plaque *BJD 142:1261–1262, 2000*

Chromomycosis *AD 113:1027–1032, 1997; Fonsecaea pedrosoi Clin Inf Dis 58:1734–1737, 2014*

Erythrasma, including disciform erythrasma

Impetigo – crusted red plaque *J Drugs in Dermatol 12:369–374, 2013*

Leishmaniasis – recidivans leishmaniasis *Clin Dermatol 38:140–151, 2020; JAAD 51:S125–128, 2004; JAAD 34:257, 1996*

Leprosy – type 1 reaction in borderline tuberculoid

Mycobacteria, non-tuberculous

Mycobacterium haemophilum Clin Inf Dis 33-330–337, 2001

Mycobacterium tuberculosis – lupus vulgaris; starts as red–brown plaque, enlarges with serpiginous margin or as discoid plaques; apple-jelly nodules; plaque form – psoriasiform, irregular scarring, serpiginous margins; head, neck, around nose, extremities, trunk *Int J Dermatol 26:578–581, 1987; Cutis 27:510, 1981; Acta Tuberc Scand 39 (Suppl 49):1–137, 1960;* tuberculosis verrucosa cutis (inoculation tuberculosis) *Cutis 78:309–316, 2006; JAAD 41:860–862, 1999; AD 125:113, 1989; BJD 66:444–448, 1954*

Nocardia *Clin Dermatol 38:152–159, 2020*

North American blastomycosis

Pinta *AD 135:685–688, 1999*

Scarlet fever

Sporotrichosis (fixed cutaneous sporotrichosis) *JAMA Derm 156:913–914, 2020; Derm Clinics 17:151–185, 1999*

Syphilis – secondary; tertiary

Tinea corporis – *Trichophyton rubrum;* including tinea corporis in HIV – *Microsporum gypseum AD 132:233–234, 1996;* Majocchi's granuloma; tinea cruris, pedis, capitis; tinea faciei *AD 114:250–252, 1978*

Trichosporon JAMA Derm 151:1139–1140, 2015

Warts – personal observation

INFILTRATIVE DISEASES

Amyloidosis – lichen amyloidosis

Erdheim-Chester disease, pediatric – facial plaques, psoriasiform plaques, papulosquamous lesions, annular lesions, central atrophic scarring; osteolysis and osteosclerosis *BJD 178:261–264, 2018*

Langerhans cell histiocytosis

Lymphoplasmacytic plaque of children – psoriasiform or red-brown plaque of ankle *Ped Derm 31:515–516, 2014; AD 146:95–96, 2010; AD 145:299–302, 2009*

INFLAMMATORY DISEASE

Erythema multiforme

Olecranon bursal sac inflammation – personal observation

Rosai-Dorfman disease *JAAD 41:335–337, 1999*

Sarcoidosis *JAAD 66:699–716, 2012; AD 133:882–888, 1997; AD 106:896–898, 1972*

METABOLIC DISEASES

Acrodermatitis enteropathica *Ped Derm 19:426–431, 2002*

Necrobiosis lipoidica diabeticorum

Necrolytic acral erythema – psoriasiform plaque with erosions at margins; hepatitis C *Cutis 83:309–314, 2009*

NEOPLASTIC DISEASES

Actinic keratosis

Basal cell carcinoma, including superficial basal cell carcinoma, basal cell carcinoma of the palm *JAAD 33:823–824, 1995*

Bowen's disease *JAAD 79:860–868, 2018*

Bowenoid papulosis – papules *AD 121:858–863, 1985;*

Clear cell acanthoma of nipple *JAAD 80:749–755, 2019*

Epidermal nevus

Erythroplasia of Queyrat

Extramammary Paget's disease – red psoriasiform plaque of pubic area *Cutis 95:132,135–136, 2015; Sem Cut Med Surg 21:159–165, 2002*

Inflammatory Becker's nevus – histopathology resembling ILVEN *Ped Derm 25:390–391, 2008*

Inflammatory linear verrucous epidermal nevus (ILVEN) – linear dermatitic and/or psoriasiform plaques; often on leg *AD 113:767–769, 1977; AD 104:385–389, 1971*

Kaposi's sarcoma

Leukemia cutis *AD 108:416–418, 1973*

Lymphoma – cutaneous T-cell lymphoma *JAAD 47:914–918, 2002;* of hands *Ped Derm 27:607–613, 2010;* CTCL with plantar psoriasiform plaques *AD 145:677–682, 2009;* gamma/delta T cell lymphoma *AD 136:1024–1032, 2000;* Woringer-Kolopp disease (pagetoid reticulosis) – annular hyperkeratotic psoriasiform plaque *JAMA Derm 156:585–586, 2020; Ann Dermatol Syphilol 67:945–958, 1939; JAAD 70:205–220, 2014; JAAD 14:898–901, 1986;* psoriasiform plaque of finger *JAAD 55:276–284, 2006;* post-transplant CTCL *Ped Derm 26:112–113, 2009;* CD8+ granulomatous cutaneous T-cell lymphoma associated with immunodeficiency – violaceous papules and nodules with psoriasiform scale; red plaques and tumors *JAAD 71:555–560, 2014*

Melanoma – amelanotic lentigo maligna; amelanotic acral melanoma – psoriasiform plaque of great toe *JAAD 69:700–707, 2013*

Paget's disease – nipple *Surg Gynecol Obstet 123:1010–1014, 1966*

Porokeratosis of Mibelli *JAAD 63:886–891, 2010; JAAD 57:665–668, 2007; Cutis 72:391–393, 2003;* giant verrucous porokeratosis of Mibelli *JAAD 57:665–668, 2007;* in gluteal cleft *BJD 132:150, 1995; Clin Exp Dermatol 9:509, 1984*

Squamous cell carcinoma, anal – psoriasiform perianal plaque *JAAD 54:189–206, 2006*

PARANEOPLASTIC DISEASES

Bazex syndrome – psoriasiform plaques and bullae of hands and feet *JAAD 40:822–825, 1999*

PHOTODERMATOSES

Phytophotodermatitis of the helix *AD 127:912–913, 1991*

PRIMARY CUTANEOUS DISEASES

Acanthosis nigricans *Ped Derm 19:12–14, 2002*

Acrodermatitis continua of Hallopeau

Alopecia mucinosa (follicular mucinosis) *Dermatology 197:178–180, 1998; AD 125:287–292, 1989; JAAD 10:760–768, 1984; AD 76:419–426, 1957*

Axillary granular parakeratosis *JAAD 37:789–790, 1997*

Circumscribed palmar or plantar hypokeratosis – red depressed or atrophic patch with ridged border *JAAD 51:319–321, 2004; JAAD 49:1197–1198, 2003; JAAD 47:21–27, 2002*

Epidermolysis bullosa – dominant dystrophic

Epidermolytic hyperkeratosis

Erythema elevatum diutinum *BJD 67:121–145, 1955*

Hailey-Hailey disease

Hyperkeratotic dermatitis of the palms *BJD 109:205–208, 1983; BJD 107:195–202, 1982*

Ichthyosis bullosa of Siemens

Lichen planus – ulcerative of soles – psoriasiform or lichenified plaque prior to ulceration; hypertrophic lichen planus

Lichen simplex chronicus; lichen simplex chronicus of posterior scalp (psoriasiform neurodermatitis)

Lichen striatus

Nummular dermatitis – personal observation

Pityriasis rubra pilaris

Progressive symmetric erythrokeratoderma

Psoriasis

Psoriasiform neurodermatitis – personal observation

Reactive perforating collagenosis

Tinea amientacea

SYNDROMES

Bazex syndrome – psoriasiform plaque of penis *JAMA Derm 150:1368–1370, 2014*

Epidermodysplasia verruciformis – psoriasiform plaques *Ped Derm 20:176–178, 2003;* psoriasiform groin intertrigo *AD 138:527–532, 2002*

Epidermolytic palmoplantar keratoderma, woolly hair, and dilated cardiomyopathy – striated palmoplantar keratoderma, follicular keratosis, clubbing, vesicles and bullae on trunk, psoriasiform keratoses on knees, legs, and feet *JAAD 39:418–421, 1998*

Hereditary mucoepithelial dysplasia (dyskeratosis) – autosomal dominant; red eyes, non-scarring alopecia, keratosis pilaris, erythema of oral (palate, gingiva) and nasal mucous membranes, cervix, vagina, and urethra; photophobia, keratosis pilaris, non-scarring alopecia, psoriasiform perineal plaques, angular cheilitis, nail deformity, increased risk of infections, fibrocystic lung disease *BJD 153:310–318, 2005; JAAD 21:351–357, 1989; Am J Hum Genet 31:414–427, 1979; Oral Surg Oral Med Oral Pathol 46:645–657, 1978*

Ichthyosis follicularis with atrichia and photophobia (IFAP) – psoriasiform plaques; collodion membrane and erythema at birth; ichthyosis, spiny (keratotic) follicular papules (generalized follicular keratoses), non-scarring alopecia, keratotic papules of elbows, knees, fingers, extensor surfaces, xerosis; punctate keratitis, photophobia; nail dystrophy, psychomotor delay, short stature; enamel dysplasia, beefy red tongue and gingiva, angular stomatitis, atopy, lamellar scales, palmoplantar erythema *Curr Prob Derm*

14:71–116, 2002; JAAD 46:S156–158, 2002; BJD 142:157–162, 2000; Am J Med Genet 85:365–368, 1999; AD 125:103–106, 1989; Ped Derm 12:195, 1995; Dermatologica 177:341–347, 1988

Lipoid proteinosis *BJD 151:413–423, 2004; JID 120:345–350, 2003; BJD 148:180–182, 2003; Hum Molec Genet 11:833–840, 2002*

Papillon-Lefevre syndrome – psoriasiform plaques of elbows *BJD 169:948–950, 2013; JAAD 49:S240–243, 2003; JAAD 48:345–351, 2003; JAAD 46:S8–10, 2002*

Reactive arthritis syndrome – balanitis circinata (sicca); keratoderma blenorrhagicum; soles, pretibial areas, dorsal toes, feet, fingers, hands, nails, scalp *Semin Arthritis Rheum 3:253–286, 1974*

Schopf-Schulz-Passarge syndrome – eyelid cysts (apocrine hidrocystomas), psoriasiform plantar dermatitis (palmoplantar keratoderma), hypotrichosis, decreased number of teeth, brittle and furrowed nails *AD 140:231–236, 2004; BJD 127:33–35, 1992; JAAD 10:922–925, 1984; Birth Defects XII:219–221, 1971*

Vohwinkel's syndrome – starfish hyperkeratotic plaque of the knees

TOXINS

Arsenic – Bowen's disease, single or multiple lesions; arsenic toxicity due to contaminated ground water consumption; especially in Bangladesh and West Bengal, India; also in India, Argentina, China, Chile, Thailand, and Mexico *SkinMed 11:211–216, 2013*

TRAUMA

Frictional dermatitis – palms and/or elbows

Occupational callosity; carpenter's calluses – personal observation

VASCULAR DISEASES

Inflammatory nuchal-occipital port wine stain *JAAD 35:811–813, 1996*

Lymphoangioendothelioma (acquired progressive lymphangioma) *JAAD 39:126–128, 1998*

PTERYGIUM (WEBBING)

SYNDROMES

Antecubital pterygia syndrome *Clin Genet 44:1–7, 1993*

Arthrogryposis multiplex congenita *Med Pregl 59:375–379, 2006*

Bartsocas/Papas lethal popliteal pterygium syndrome; cocoon syndrome *Ann Plast Surg 76:459–462, 2016; Am J Med Genet A 167A:545–552, 2015*

Bruck syndrome *Calcif Tissue Int 102:296–309, 2018; Endokrynol Pol 66:170–174, 2015; Am J Med Genet 70:28–31, 1997*

Craniocarpotarsal dysplasia (Whistling face syndrome) – pterygium colli *Birth Defects 11:161–168, 1975*

Disorganization syndrome – filiform worm-like projections, syndactyly, popliteal pterygium, polydactyly, cleft lip/palate; ear abnormalities *Ped Derm 24:90–92, 2007; J Med Genet 26:417–420, 1989*

Distichiasis and lymphedema – pterygia colli (webbed neck)

Haspleslagh syndrome *Clin Genet 47:332–334, 1995*

Hennekam syndrome – autosomal recessive; intestinal lymphangiectasia, lymphedema of legs and genitalia, gigantic scrotum and penis, multilobulated lymphatic ectasias, small mouth, narrow palate, gingival hypertrophy, tooth anomalies, thick lips, agenesis of ear, pre-auricular pits, wide flat nasal bridge, frontal upsweep, platybasia, hypertelorism, pterygia colli, bilateral single palmar crease, hirsutism, mild mental retardation, facial anomalies, growth retardation, pulmonary, cardiac, hypogammaglobulinemia *Ped Derm 23:239–242, 2006*

Hereditary onycho-osteodysplasia – pterygium of the elbow *Pathologica 83:365–372, 1991*

Klippel-Feil syndrome – pterygia colli (webbed neck) *Cleft Palate 17:65–88, 1980*

LEOPARD syndrome *Birth Defects 7:110–115, 1971*

Multiple lethal pterygium syndrome

Multiple pterygium syndrome (Escobar syndrome) *Am J Dis Child 142:794–798, 1988; Eur J Pediatr 147:550–552, 1988;* lethal *BMJ Case Rep 12:e229045, 2019*

Nail patella syndrome – antecubital pterygium *JAAD 49:1086–1087, 2003; J Formos Med 101:653–660, 2002; J Pediatr Orthop B 7:27–31, 1998; Am J Med Genet 38:9–12, 1991*

Noonan's syndrome – pterygia colli (webbed neck) *J Med Genet 24:9–13, 1987*

Pena-Shoker syndrome *Am J Med Genet 16:213–224, 1983*

Popliteal pterygium (popliteal web) syndrome – autosomal dominant; bilateral popliteal pterygia, intercrural pterygium, hypoplastic digits, absence of labia majora, hypertrophied clitoris, cryptorchidism, bifid scrotum, valgus or varus foot deformities, syndactyly with or without polydactyly, cryptorchidism, umbilical or inguinal hernia, cleft scrotum, lower lip pits, cleft palate, mucous membrane bands (syngnathia) (fibrous bands connecting maxilla and mandible), eyelid adhesions (ankyloblepharon), hypertelorism, defect of alveolar ridge; mutation in *IRF6* (this mutation also seen in van der Woude syndrome) *Ped Derm 28:333–334, 2011: J Med Genet 36:888–892, 1999; Int J Pediatr Otorhinolaryngol 15:17–22, 1988*

Turner's syndrome – pterygia colli (webbed neck) *Endocrinology 23:566–578, 1938*

PTERYGIUM OF THE NAIL

DORSAL PTERYGIUM

AUTOIMMUNE DISEASES AND DISORDERS OF IMMUNE DYSREGULATION

Bullous pemphigoid *Dermatol Clin 29:511–513, 20122*

Cicatricial pemphigoid *Clin Exp Dermatol 10:472–475, 1985*

CREST syndrome – personal observation

Dermatomyositis and scleroderma – personal observation

Graft vs. host disease, chronic *JAAD 66:515–532, 2012; BJD 122:841–843, 1990*

Lupus erythematosus, systemic – personal observation

Pemphigus foliaceus

CONGENITAL DISORDERS

Congenital pterygium

DRUGS

Taxotere – personal observation

INFECTIONS AND INFESTATIONS

Bacterial infection

Leprosy – type 2 reaction *Indian Dermatol Online J 11:195–201, 2020; Cutis 44:311–312, 1989*

INFLAMMATORY DISORDERS

Erythema multiforme

Sarcoid *AD 121:276–277, 1985*

Stevens-Johnson syndrome *BJD 177:924–935, 2017*

Toxic epidermal necrolysis

METABOLIC DISORDERS

Diabetic vasculopathy

NEOPLASTIC DISORDERS

Linear porokeratosis *Int J Dermatol 45:1077–179, 2006*

Onychomatricoma *JAAD 59:990–994, 2008: ACTA DV 86:369–370, 2006*

PRIMARY CUTANEOUS DISEASES

Epidermolysis bullosa dystrophica recessiva

GABEB – generalized atrophic benign epidermolysis bullosa

Idiopathic atrophy of the nail *Dermatology 190:116–118, 1995*

Lichen planus

Twenty nail dystrophy *Indian J DV Leprol 54:155–156, 1988*

PSYCHOCUTANEOUS DISORDERS

Onychotillomania

SYNDROMES

Ankyloblepharon-ectrodactyly-cleft lip/palate (AEC) syndrome – thin or absent nail plates, pterygia of the nails *AD 141:1591–1594, 2005*

Clouston syndrome *J Dermatol 46:e329–330, 2019*

Cronkhite-Canada syndrome – personal observation

Dyschromatosis universalis hereditaria *Clin Exp Dermatol 27:477–479, 2002*

Dyskeratosis congenita (Zinsser-Engman-Cole syndrome) – Xq28; oral bullae and erosions; distal ridging, splitting, pterygia *Ped Derm 14:411–413, 1997; J Med Genet 33:993–995, 1996; Dermatol Clin 13:33–39, 1995; BJD 105:321–325, 1981*

Keratosis lichenoides chronica *AD 120:1471–1474, 1984*

Marfan's syndrome *J Dermatol 29:164–167, 2002*

Nail-patella syndrome (hereditary onychodysplasia syndrome) (Hood syndrome)

TRAUMA

Burns

Nail biting

Radiation therapy

Physical trauma/injuries *Prim Care 42:677–691, 2015*

VASCULAR DISORDERS

Peripheral vascular disease

Raynaud's phenomenon – pterygium unguis inversum

VENTRAL PTERYGIUM (PTERYGIUM UNGUIS INVERSUM)

AUTOIMMUNE DISEASES AND DISORDERS OF IMMUNE DYSREGULATION

Acrylate allergic contact dermatitis *JAAD 58:S53–54, 2008*

Graft vs host disease – of lung *J Eur Acad DV 33:637–642, 2019; BMT 49:1521–1527, 2014*

Lupus erythematosus, systemic *AD 129:1307–1309, 1993; AD 108:817–818, 1973*

Scleroderma *JAAD 76:1115–1123, 2017; AD 129:1307–1309, 1993; AD 113:1429–1430, 1977*

CONGENITAL DISORDERS

Congenital *Ann Dermatol Venereol 107:83–86, 1980; Hautarzt 26:543–544, 1975; AD 110:89–90, 1974*

DEGENERATIVE DISORDERS

Hemiparesis

Paresis *Int J Dermatol 27:491–494, 1988*

EXOGENOUS AGENTS

Formaldehyde-containing nail hardeners *Semin Dermatol 10:29–33, 1991; Contact Dermatitis 15:256–257, 1986*

Gel polish *J Eur Acad DV 32:160–163, 2018*

INFECTIONS AND INFESTATIONS

Leprosy *Int J Dermatol 52:1621–1623, 2013; AD 126:1110, 1990; type 2 lepra reaction Cutis 44:311–312, 1989*

NEOPLASTIC DISORDERS

Porokeratosis of Mibelli – pterygium unguis inversus *BJD 156:1384–1385, 2007*

Subungual exostosis – mimics pterygium unguis inversum *Dermatology 193:354–355, 1996*

PRIMARY CUTANEOUS DISEASES

Familial pterygium unguis inversum *Ann DV 107:949–950, 1980*

Hyperkeratosis punctata of the palmar creases *Dermatologica 162:209–212, 1981*

Idiopathic *Clin Ped (Phila)49:394–395, 2010; AD 129:1307–1309, 1993*

Lenticular atrophy of the palmar creases *Dermatologica 162:209–212, 1981*

Unilateral *Int J Dermatol 27:491–494, 1988*

SYNDROMES

Neurofibromatosis *AD 113:1429–1430, 1977*

TRAUMA

Causalgia of the median nerve *Current Problems in Dermatol Basel, Switzerland: Karger-Basel 102–149, 1981*

Onychophagia *Case Rep Dermatol Med Jan 30, 2018*

Physical trauma

Scarring near the distal nail groove *AD 129:1307–1309, 1993; Clin Exp Dermatol 3:437–438, 1978*

VASCULAR DISORDERS

Peripheral vascular disease

Raynaud's phenomenon

Stroke – hemiparetic hand *JAAD 53:501–503, 2005; Int J Dermatol 27:491–494, 1988*

PUBERTY, DELAYED (HYPOGONADISM)

Ped Rev 22:309–315, 2001; Horm Res 51 (Suppl3):95–100, 1999

Constitutional delay of growth and puberty – most common cause of delayed puberty *NEJM 366:443–453, 2012*

Idiopathic

Pubertal delay due to chronic diseases
　Acrodermatitis enteropathica – hypogonadism, testicular atrophy *Ped Derm 19:426–431, 2002*
　Asthma
　Gastrointestinal diseases
　Hepatic diseases
　Renal failure
　Endocrine diseases
　Hematologic abnormalities
　Collagenosis
　Infections
　Undernutrition
　Intense exercise
　Cancer
　Anorexia nervosa
　Stress
　Drugs

Hypogonadism
　Aarskog syndrome *Birth Defects 11:25–29, 1975*
　Ablepharon macrostomia – absent eyelids, ectropion, abnormal ears, rudimentary nipples, dry redundant skin, macrostomia, ambiguous genitalia *Hum Genet 97:532–536, 1996*
　Acromegaly – amenorrhea and impotence
　Albright's hereditary osteodystrophy – pseudohypoparathyroidism, round face, short neck, osteomas of skin with overlying hyperpigmentation, short stature, hypogonadism, macrocephaly, psychomotor retardation, endocrinologic abnormalities; mutation in GNAS1 *Ped Derm 28:135–137, 2011; Endocrinology 30:922–932, 1942*
　Anencephaly *Syndromes of the Head and Neck, p. 565, 1990*
　Anorexia nervosa – hypogonadotropic hypogonadism *Psychosomatics 27:737–739, 1986*
　Asthma

Ataxia, dementia, hypogonadotropism – disordered ubiquitination; mutation in *RNF216 NEJM 368:1992–2003, 2013*
Ataxia telangiectasia *JAAD 10:431–438, 1978*
Autoimmune polyglandular endocrinopathy and anterior hypophysitis *J Pediatr Endocrinol Metab 14:909–914, 2001*
Bardet-Biedl syndrome – postaxial polydactyly (ulnar), rod-cone dystrophy (retinal dystrophy), retinitis pigmentosa, obesity, neuropathy, mental disturbance, renal abnormalities, hypogonadism *Ped Derm 36:346–348, 2019; J Med Genet 36:599–603, 1999*
Bloom's syndrome (congenital telangiectatic erythema and stunted growth) – autosomal recessive; blisters of nose and cheeks; slender face, prominent nose; facial telangiectatic erythema and hyperpigmentation with involvement of eyelids, ear, hand and forearms; bulbar conjunctival telangiectasias; cheilitis of upper and lower lips; stunted growth; CALMs, clinodactyly, syndactyly, congenital heart disease, annular pancreas, high-pitched voice, testicular atrophy (hypogonadism); no neurologic deficits; DNA repair defect with chromosomal breaks, sister chromatid exchanges, and triradial and quadriradial chromosomes; BLM gene encodes mutation in recQ DNA helicase (important in DNA repair) *Ped Derm 27:174–177, 2010; Ped Derm 22:147–150, 2005; Curr Prob Derm 14:41–70, 2002; Ped Derm 14:120–124, 1997; JAAD 17:479–488, 1987; AD 114:755–760, 1978; Clin Genet 12:85–96, 1977; Am J Hum Genet 21:196–227, 1969; Am J Dis Child 116:409–413, 1968; AD 94:687–694, 1966; Am J Dis Child 88:754–758, 1954*
Borjeson-Forssman-Lehman syndrome *Am J Med Genet 19:653–664, 1984*
Cancer
Carpenter syndrome (acrocephalosyndactyly) *Am J Med Genet 28:311–324, 1987*
CHARGE syndrome – coloboma, heart disease, atresia choanae, genital hypoplasia, low-set malformed small ears *JAAD 46:161–183, 2002; Perspect Pediatr Pathol 2:173–206, 1975*
Cockayne syndrome *Syndromes of the Head and Neck, p. 492, 1990*
Congenital cataracts, sensorineural deafness, hypogonadism, hypertrichosis, short stature *Clin Dysmorphol 4:283–288, 1995*
Congenital ichthyosis, hypogonadism, small stature, facial dysmorphism, scoliosis, and myogenic dystrophy *Ann Genet 42:45–50, 1999*
Congenital ichthyosis, retinitis pigmentosa, hypergonadotropic hypogonadism, small stature, mental retardation, cranial dysmorphism, abnormal electroencephalogram *Ophthalmic Genet 19:69–79, 1998*
Cornelia de Lange (Brachmann-de Lange) syndrome – hypoplastic genitalia, single palmar crease, hypoplastic epidermal ridges of palms, soles, fingers, and toes; hypoplastic nipples and umbilicus, umbilical hernia *Syndromes of the Head and Neck, p.303, 1990;* generalized hypertrichosis, confluent eyebrows, low hairline, hairy forehead and ears, hair whorls of trunk, single palmar crease, cutis marmorata, psychomotor and growth retardation with short stature, specific facies, hypertrichosis of forehead, face, back, shoulders, and extremities, bushy arched eyebrows with synophrys; long delicate eyelashes, skin around eyes and nose with bluish tinge, small nose with depressed root, prominent philtrum, thin upper lip with crescent shaped mouth, widely spaced, sparse teeth, hypertrichosis of forehead, posterior neck, and arms, low set ears, arched palate, antimongoloid palpebrae; congenital eyelashes; xerosis, especially over hands and feet, nevi, facial cyanosis, lymphedema *Ped Derm 24:421–423, 2007; JAAD 56:541–564, 2007; JAAD 48:161–179, 2003; Ped Derm 19:42–45, 2002; JAAD 37:295–297, 1997; Am J Med Genet 47:959–964, 1993; Am J Med Genet 20:453–459, 1985*

Cryptophthalmos syndrome *Syndromes of the Head and Neck, p. 817, 1990*

del (9p) syndrome *Syndromes of the Head and Neck, p. 84, 1990*

del (18p) syndrome *Syndromes of the Head and Neck, p. 52, 1990*

dup (3q) syndrome *Syndromes of the Head and Neck, p. 73, 1990*

dup (4p) syndrome *Syndromes of the Head and Neck, p. 73, 1990*

DeSanctis-Cacchione syndrome – dwarfism, gonadal hypoplasia, mental deficiency, microcephaly, xeroderma pigmentosum

Dyskeratosis congenita – hypogonadism *JAAD 77:1194–1196, 2017*

Emotional stress

Endocrine diseases

Estrogen receptor alpha variant – mutation in gene encoding *ESR1;* absent breast development *NEJM 369:164–171, 2013*

Fanconi's syndrome (pancytopenia with congenital defects) – generalized olive-brown hyperpigmentation, especially of lower trunk, flexures, and neck with depigmented macules; hypoplastic anemia, slender build, short broad thumbs, tapered fingers, microcephaly, hypogonadism *Semin Hematol 4:233–240, 1967*

Femoral hypoplasia-unusual facies syndrome *Syndromes of the Head and Neck, p. 731, 1990*

Floating-Harbor syndrome *Syndromes of the Head and Neck, p. 914, 1990*

Gastrointestinal diseases

Gorlin-Chaudhry-Moss syndrome – short and stocky with craniosynostosis, midface hypoplasia, hypertrichosis of the scalp, arms, legs, and back, anomalies of the eyes, digits, teeth, and heart, and genitalia hypoplasia *Am J Med Genet 44:518–522, 1992*

H syndrome – sclerodermoid changes of middle and lower body with overlying hyperpigmentation sparing the knees and buttocks; hypertrichosis, short stature, facial telangiectasia, gynecomastia, camptodactyly of 5th fingers, scrotal masses with massively edematous scrotum obscuring the penis, hypogonadism, azoospermia, sensorineural hearing loss, cardiac anomalies, hepatosplenomegaly *JAAD 59:79–85, 2008*

Hallerman-Streiff syndrome *Syndromes of the Head and Neck, p. 308, 1990*

Hematologic abnormalities

Hepatic diseases

Hurst syndrome – short stature, hypertonia, unusual facies, mental retardation, hemolytic anemia, delayed puberty *Am J Med Genet 29:107–115, 1988; Am J Med Genet 28:965–970, 1987*

Hypergonadotropic hypogonadism *Curr Ther Endocrinol Metab 6:223–226, 1997*

Hypogonadism *NEJM 368:1220–1228, 2013*

Hypogonadism with cleft lip-palate *Syndromes of the Head and Neck, p. 780, 1990*

Hypogonadotropic hypogonadism (eunuchoidism) (Kallmann's syndrome) *Int J Impot Res 12:269–271, 2000; J Pediatr Endocrinol Metab 11:631–638, 1998*

Infections

Intense exercise

Isolated gonadotrophin deficiency *Molec Genet Metab 68:191–199, 1999; J Pediatr 111:684–692, 1987*

Jaffe-Campanacci syndrome – coast of Maine CALMs, pigmented nevi and freckle-like macules, fibromas in long bones and jaw, mental retardation, hypogonadism, cryptorchidism, precocious puberty, ocular anomalies, cardiovascular malformations and kyphoscoliosis *Curr Prob in Derm VII:143–198, 1995; Clin Orthop Rel Res 168:192–205, 1982*

Johanson-Blizzard syndrome *Syndromes of the Head and Neck, p. 812, 1990*

Kabuki syndrome – vitiligo, developmental delay, short stature, congenital heart defects, skeletal defects, cleft palate, dental abnormalities, cryptorchidism, lip pits, prominent fingertip pads, autoimmune disorders, blue sclerae, prominent eyelashes, thinning of central eyebrows, protuberant ears *Amer J Med Genet 132A:260–262, 2005*

Klinefelter's syndrome *Syndromes of the Head and Neck, p. 58, 1990*

Langerhans cell histiocytosis – delayed puberty *Am J Med 60:457–463, 1976*

LEOPARD syndrome (multiple lentigines syndrome; Moynahan syndrome) – autosomal dominant; generalized lentiginosis, especially over neck and trunk; structural cardiac abnormalities, electrocardiographic abnormalities, genitourinary abnormalities (gonadal hypoplasia, hypospadias, delayed puberty), neurologic defects, cephalofacial dysmorphism, short stature or low birth weight, skeletal abnormalities *Curr Prob in Derm VII:143–198, 1995*

Leschke's syndrome – growth retardation, mental retardation, diabetes mellitus, genital hypoplasia, hypothyroidism

Malnutrition

Marinesco-Sjogren syndrome – cataracts, mental retardation, microcephaly, short stature, hypogonadism, ataxia, hypotonia *Clin Dysmorphol 4:283–288, 1995*

Martsolf syndrome – cataracts, facial dysmorphism, microcephaly, short stature, hypogonadism *Am J Med Genet 1:291–299, 1978; Syndromes of the Head and Neck, p. 906, 1990*

Meckel syndrome *Syndromes of the Head and Neck, p. 725, 1990*

MEND – X-linked recessive; hypomorphic mutation of emopamil-binding protein; diffuse mild ichthyosis; telecanthus, prominent nasal bridge, low set ears, micrognathia, cleft palate large anterior fontanelle, polydactyly, 2-3 syndactyly, kyphosis, Dandy-Walker malformation, cerebellar hypoplasia, corpus callosal hypoplasia, hydrocephalus, hypotonia, developmental delay, seizures; bilateral cataracts, glaucoma, hypertelorism; cardiac valvular and septal defects, hypoplastic aortic arch; renal malformation, cryptorchidism, hypospadias *BJD 166:1309–1313, 2012*

Michelin tire baby syndrome – either nevus lipomatosis or diffuse smooth muscle hamartoma; degenerative collagen, scarring; excessive folds of firm skin on extremities, especially ankles and wrists; generalized hypertrichosis, palmar cerebriform plaques; low set malformed ears with thickened helix and anti-helix; wide or depressed nasal bridge; epicantal folds, hypertelorism, cleft palate, micro-ophthalmia or deep set eyes, flat or hypoplastic midface, short neck, decreased hearing, hypoplastic malformed genitalia, micrognathia, histologically increased periadnexal fat and subcutaneous fat and smooth muscle hamartomas; mental retardation, tendinous hyperlaxity, seizures, mastocytosis, complex malformations syndrome (bilateral calcaneovalgus deformity, cleft palate, inguinal hernia, hip deformity, clefting of lateral mouth commissures, shawl scrotum, absent foreskin; developmental delay, microcephaly, mental retardation *Ped Derm 31:659–663, 2014JAAD 63:1110–1111, 2010; Ped Derm 27:79–81, 2010; Ped Derm 24:628–231, 2007; Ped Derm 22:245–249, 2005; Ped Derm 20:150–152, 2003; BJD 129:60–68,1993; JAAD 28:364–370, 1993; Atlas of Clinical Syndromes A Visual Aid to Diagnosis, 1992, pp.308–309; Ped Derm 6:329–331, 1989; Am J Med Genet 28:225–226, 1987; AD 115:978–979, 1979; diffuse lipomatous hypertrophy AD 100:320–323, 1969; generalized muscular nevus Ann DV 107:923–927, 1980*

Myotonic dystrophy *Syndromes of the Head and Neck, p. 587, 1990*

Phosphoglucomutase 1 deficiency – autosomal recessive; disorder of glycosylation with impaired glycoprotein production; liver dysfunction, bifid uvula, malignant hyperthermia, hypogonadotropic hypogonadism, growth retardation, hypoglycemia, myopathy, dilated cardiomyopathy, cardiac arrest *NEJM 370:533–542, 2014*

POEMS syndrome (Crowe-Fukase syndrome, Takatsuki syndrome) (PEP syndrome – plasma cell dyscrasia, endocrinopathy, polyneuropathy) – plethora, angiomas (cherry, globular, glomeruloid) presenting as red nodules of face, trunk, and extremities, diffuse hyperpigmentation, hypertrichosis, scleroderma-like changes, either generalized or localized (legs), hyperhidrosis, clubbing, leukonychia, papilledema, pleural effusion, peripheral edema, ascites, pulmonary hypertension, weight loss, fatigue, diarrhea, thrombocytosis, polycythemia, fever, renal disease, arthralgias; osteosclerotic myeloma (IgG or IgA lambda) bone lesions, progressive symmetric sensorimotor peripheral polyneuropathy, hypothyroidism, and hypogonadism; peripheral edema, thrombocytosis, cutaneous angiomas, blue dermal papules associated with Castleman's disease (benign reactive angioendotheliomatosis), maculopapular brown-violaceous lesions, purple nodules; papilledema *JAAD 58:671–675, 2008; JAAD 55:149–152, 2006; JAAD 44:324–329, 2001, JAAD 40:808–812, 1999; AD 124:695–698, 1988, Cutis 61:329–334, 1998; JAAD 21:1061–1068, 1989; JAAD 12:961–964, 1985; Nippon Shinson 26:2444–2456, 1968*

– hypogonadism with gynecomastia; insulin-dependent diabetes mellitus, primary hypothyroidism

Popliteal pterygium (popliteal web) syndrome – autosomal dominant; bilateral popliteal pterygia, intercrural pterygium, hypoplastic digits, absence of labia majora, hypertrophied clitoris, cryptorchidism, bifid scrotum, valgus or varus foot deformities, syndactyly with or without polydactyly, cryptorchidism, umbilical or inguinal hernia, cleft scrotum, lower lip pits, cleft palate, mucous membrane bands (syngnathia) (fibrous bands connecting maxilla and mandible), eyelid adhesions (ankyloblepharon), hypertelorism, defect of alveolar ridge; mutation in *IRF6* (this mutation also seen in van der Woude syndrome) *Ped Derm 28:333–334, 2011: J Med Genet 36:888–892, 1999; Int J Pediatr Otorhinolaryngol 15:17–22, 1988*

Prader-Willi syndrome – albinoid skin; almond-shaped eyes, narrow bifrontal diameter, thin upper lip, short stature, central obesity, small hands and feet, mental retardation, hypogonadism, hypotonia at birth, excoriations, trichotillomania *Cutis 90;129–131, 2012; Growth Genet Hormones 2:1–5, 1986; Schweiz Med Wschr 86:1260–1261, 1956*

Renal failure

Rubinstein-Taybi syndrome – multiple hemangiomas; hypogonadotropic hypogonadism; autosomal dominant; mutations or deletions of chromosome 16p13.3; human cAMP response element binding protein *Ped Derm 21:44–47, 2004; JAAD 46:161–183, 2002;JAAD 46:159, 2002*

Schwachman-Diamond syndrome – periodontal disease and caries; abscesses, short stature, delayed puberty, skeletal changes, pancreatic exocrine deficiency, pancytopenias, cyclic neutropenia, failure to thrive, hepatomegaly, pneumonia, otitis media, metaphyseal dysplasia, osteomyelitis *Ped Derm 28:568–569, 2011; Am J Med genet 66:378–398, 1996*

Multiple hormonal deficiency states

Emotional stress – growth hormone deficiency and delayed puberty *Am J Med 76:737–742, 1984*

Familial cytomegalic adrenocortical hypoplasia – X-linked; pubertal failure *Arch Dis Child 56:715–721, 1981*

Hemochromatosis *J Clin Endocrinol Metab 76:357–361, 1993*

Idiopathic

Langerhans cell histiocytosis

Nevoid basal cell carcinoma syndrome – hypogonadism in males *JAAD 11:98–104, 1984*

Radiation therapy *Med Pediatr Oncol 22:250–254, 1994*

Sarcoid

Tuberculosis

Tumors – Sertoli-Leydig cell tumor *Am J Obstet Gynecol 152:308–309, 1985*

Vascular disease

Zinc deficiency, endemic *Am J Clin Nutr 30:833–834, 1977; Arch Int Med 111:407–428, 1963*

Hyperprolactinemia – pituitary microadenoma *Arch Gynecol Obstet 264:90–92, 2000;* macroproprolactinoma *Minerva Endocrinol 21:67–71, 1996;* prolactinomas *Clin Endocrinol (Oxf) 30:131–140, 1989;* primary hypothyroidism *Curr Ther Endocrinol Metab 6:223–226, 1997*

Specific syndromes with hypogonadotropism

Bloom's syndrome – small testes

Cerebellar ataxia

Cohen's syndrome *J Med Genet 17:430–432, 1980*

Cockayne syndrome

Cutis laxa – generalized cutis laxa – autosomal dominant – lesions often preceded in infancy by episodes of edema; infantile genitalia; scant body hair; bloodhound appearance of premature aging

Down's syndrome *Syndromes of the Head and Neck, p. 33, 1990*

Hutchinson-Gilford syndrome (progeria) – absent sexual maturity *Am J Med Genet 82:242–248, 1999; J Pediatr 80:697–724, 1972*

Johnson-McMillin syndrome – autosomal dominant, facial nerve palsy, hearing loss, hyposmia, hypogonadism, microtia, alopecia

Laurence-Moon-Biedl syndrome

Multiple lentigines syndrome

Noonan's syndrome *Syndromes of the Head and Neck, p. 805, 1990*

Pallister-Hall syndrome *Syndromes of the Head and Neck, p. 903, 1990*

Popliteal pterygium syndrome *Syndromes of the Head and Neck, p. 629, 1990*

Prader-Willi syndrome *Eur J Pediatr 160:69–70, 2001*

Pseudohypothyroidism *Syndromes of the Head and Neck, p. 141, 1990*

Rothmund-Thomson syndrome (poikiloderma congenitale) – autosomal recessive; hypogonadism *Ped Derm 18:422–425, 2001; Ped Derm 18:210–212, 2001; Am J Med Genet 22:102:11–17, 2001; Ped Derm 16:59–61, 1999; Dermatol Clin 13:143–150, 1995; JAAD 27:75–762, 1992; BJD 122:821–829, 1990; Ped Derm 6:325–328, 1989; Ped Derm 6:321–324, 1989; JAAD 17:332–328, 1987; JAAD 17:332–338, 1987*

Rubinstein-Taybi syndrome – hypogonadotropic hypogonadism; autosomal dominant; mutations or deletions of chromosome 16p13.3; human cAMP response element binding protein *Ped Derm 21:44–47, 2004*

Rud's syndrome

Sakati syndrome *Syndromes of the Head and Neck, p. 558, 1990*

Sclerodactyly, non-epidermolytic palmoplantar keratoderma, multiple cutaneous squamous cell carcinomas, periodontal disease with loss of teeth, hypogenitalism with hypospadias, altered sex hormone levels, hypertriglyceridemia, 46XX *JAAD 53:S234–239, 2005*

Seckel syndrome *Syndromes of the Head and Neck, p. 313, 1990*

Short rib-polydactyly syndromes *Syndromes of the Head and Neck, p. 218–219, 1990*

Triploidy syndrome *Syndromes of the Head and Neck, p. 64, 1990*

Complete trisomy 22 – primitive low-set ears, bilateral preauricular pit, broad nasal bridge, antimongoloid palpebral fissures, macroglossia, enlarged sublingual glands, cleft palate, micrognathia, clinodactyly of fifth fingers, hypoplastic finger-nails, hypoplastic genitalia, short lower limbs, bilateral sandal gap, deep plantar furrows *Pediatrics 108:E32, 2001*

Turner's syndrome – gonadal dysgenesis *Curr Ther Endocrinol Metab 6:223–226, 1997; Syndromes of the Head and Neck, p. 54, 1990*

Walker-Warburg syndrome *Syndromes of the Head and Neck, p. 593, 1990*

Werner's syndrome

X-linked ichthyosis *Clin Exp Dermatol 22:201–204, 1997*

49,XXXXY syndrome *Syndromes of the Head and Neck, p. 59, 1990*

Systemic disease

AIDS *Trop Doct 31:233, 2001; J Acquir Immune Defic Syndr 21:333–337, 1999*

Alagille syndrome – xanthomas of palmar creases, extensor fingers, nape of neck; growth retardation, delayed puberty *Ped Derm 22:11–14, 2005*

Anorexia nervosa, unwarranted dieting *Nutr Rev 42:14–15, 1984*

Biliary atresia *J Pediatr Surg 25:808–811, 1990*

Chronic renal failure *Pediatr Nephrol 7:551–553, 1993;* congenital magnesium-losing kidney *Ann Clin Biochem 30:494–498, 1993*

Congenital heart disease

Cushing's disease *J Pediatr Endocrinol 6:201–204, 1993*

Cystic fibrosis *Clin Pediatr (Phila) 37:573–576, 1998; Pediatrics 99:29–34, 1997; Pediatrician 14:253–260, 1987*

Diabetes mellitus

Gaucher's disease type 1 *Isr Med Assoc J 2:80–81, 2000*

Gluten intolerance

Hypothyroidism

Inflammatory bowel disease

Sickle cell disease *West Indian Med J 44:20–23, 1995*

Thalassemia major *J Pediatr Endocrinol Metab 10:175–184, 1997; Eur J Pediatr 156:777–783, 1997*

Trichothiodystrophy, mental retardation, short stature, ataxia, and gonadal dysfunction *Am J Med Genet 35:566–573, 1990*

Trisomy 18 mosaicism *Am J Med Genet 50:94–95, 1994*

X-linked agammaglobulinemia with growth hormone deficiency and delayed growth and puberty *Acta Paediatr 83:99–102, 1994*

Zinc deficiency *Ann Rev Nutr 5:341–363, 1985*

Excessive exercise *Ann NY Scad Sci 709:55–76, 1994*

Low gonadotropins – pubertal failure

Congenital

Kallmann's syndrome

Luteinizing hormone deficiency

Follicle stimulating hormone deficiency

Marinesco-Sjogren syndrome – cataracts, mental retardation, microcephaly, short stature, hypogonadism, ataxia, hypotonia *Clin Dysmorphol 4:283–288, 1995*

Nevoid basal cell carcinoma syndrome (Gorlin's syndrome) – auto-somal dominant; macrocephaly, frontal bossing, hypertelorism, cleft lip or palate, papules of the face, neck, and trunk, facial milia, lamellar calcification of the falx cerebri and tentorium cerebelli, cerebral cysts, calcifications of the brain, palmoplantar pits, mandibular keratocysts, skeletal anomalies, including enlarged mandibular coronoid, bifid ribs, kyphosis, spina bifida, polydactyly of the hands or feet, syndactyly; basal cell carcinomas; multiple eye anomalies – congenital cataract, microphthalmia, coloboma of the iris, choroid, and optic nerve; strabismus, nystagmus, keratin-filled cysts of the palpebral conjunctivae; also medulloblastomas, ovarian tumors (fibromas), mesenteric cysts, cardiac fibromas, fetal rhabdomyomas, astrocytomas, meningiomas, craniopharyngiomas, fibrosarcomas, ameloblastomas; renal anomalies; hypogonadotropic hypogonadism, *BJD 165:30–34, 2011; AD 146:17–19, 2010; JAAD 53:S256–259, 2005; JAAD 39:853–857, 1998; Dermatol Clin 13:113–125, 1995; JAAD 11:98–104, 1984; NEJM 262:908–912, 1960;* linear unilateral nevoid basal cell nevus syndrome *JAAD 50:489–494, 2004*

Panhypopituitarism

Septo-optic dysplasia

Developmental defects of the pituitary

Prader-Willi syndrome

Laurence-Moon-Biedl syndrome

Acquired

Tumors (craniopharyngioma, germinoma)

Langerhans cell histiocytosis

Radiotherapy

Surgery

Head injury

Infections

Hypergonadotropic hypogonadism

Males

Anorchia and bilateral cryptorchidism (undescended testes)

Gonadal dysgenesis (XO/XY) or (XX)

Klinefelter's syndrome (XYY)

Hormonal abnormalities

Biosynthesis and androgen receptors

Females

Ullrich-Turner's syndrome (XO) *J Med Genet 29:547–551, 1992; Ped Clin North Am 37:1421–1440, 1990*

Gonadal dysgenesis (XO/XY) or (XX)

Androgen insensitivity (testicular feminization syndrome)

Both sexes

Polymalformation syndromes

Alstrom syndrome

Steiner's myotonic dystrophy

Down's syndrome

Irradiation and cytotoxic drugs

Myotonic dystrophy

Noonan's syndrome – scant pubic hair, short stature or normal height with broad short, webbed neck, lymphedema of feet and legs, orbital edema, leukokeratosis of lips and gingiva, low posterior hairline, hypertrichosis of cheeks or shoulders, ulerythema oophyrogenes *Arch Dis Child 84:440–443, 2001; JAAD 40:877–890, 1999*

Orchitis (mumps)

Polycystic ovarian disease

17-beta hydroxylase deficiency

Surgical accidents (during herniorrhaphy)

Testicular torsion

Acquired elevated gonadotropins

Males

Bilateral orchitis

Surgical or traumatic castration

Chemotherapy

Females

Surgical or traumatic castration

Premature idiopathic ovarian failure

Chemotherapy

Insensitivity to androgens

PUBERTY, PREMATURE

J Clin Endocrinol Metab 74:239–247, 1992; Pediatr Rev 11:229–237, 1990

Complete – true – Cyp21B gene point mutations *Clin Endocrinol (Oxf) 48:555–560, 1998*

Constitutional
 Sporadic
 Familial
Cerebral/neurogenic *Best Pract Res Clin Endocrinol Metab 33:101262, 2019*
 Tumors – hypothalamic hamartoma, astrocytoma, ependymoma, optic or hypothalamic glioma, pinealoma, neurofibroma, dysgerminoma, craniopharyngioma
 Developmental defects *Dev Med Child Neurol 41:392–395, 1999*
 Central nervous system infections – abscess, meningitis, tuberculosis, encephalitis
 Central nervous system trauma
  Sarcoidosis, radiation, asphyxia
  Cranial radiation – premature activation of gonadotropin-releasing hormone *Klin Padiatr 213:239–243, 2001; Horm Res 39:25–29, 1993*
 Central precocious puberty – activating mutations of *KISS1R, KISS1* genes; inactivating mutations of *MKRN3* (familial); chromosomal abnormalities *J Endocrin Soc 25:979–995, 2019*
 Congenital malformations *Arch Endocrinol Metab 60:163–172, 2016*
  Suprasellar cyst
  Arachnoid cyst
  Sept-optic dysplasia
  Hydrocephalus
  Spina bifida
  Vascular malformation
  Meningomyelocele
  Ectopic pituitary lobe
  Pituitary duplication
 Epidermal nevus syndrome with wooly hair nevus *JAAD 35:839–842, 1996*
 Hypothalamic hamartoma *Arch Pediatr 2:438–441, 1995; Am J Dis Child 144:225–228, 1990*
 Jaffe-Campanacci syndrome – coast of Maine CALMs, pigmented nevi and freckle-like macules, fibromas in long bones and jaw, mental retardation, hypogonadism, cryptorchidism, precocious puberty, ocular anomalies, cardiovascular malformations and kyphoscoliosis *Curr Prob in Derm VII:143–198, 1995; Clin Orthop Rel Res 168:192–205, 1982*
 McCune-Albright syndrome (polyostotic fibrous dysplasia) – giant café au lait macules; triad of fibrous dysplasia of bone (proximal femur and base of skull), café au lait macules and precocious puberty; associated hyperthyroidism, growth hormone excess, renal phosphate wasting with or without rickets, osteomalacia, Cushing's syndrome; mutation in *GNAS* (stimulatory G protein) *Ped Derm 31:80–82, 2014; Clin in Dermatol 23:56–67, 2005; Ped Derm 8:35–39, 1991; Dermatol Clin 5:193–203, 1987*
Peutz-Jeghers syndrome *Endocr Dev 29:230–239, 2016*
 Neurofibromatosis *Syndromes of the Head and Neck, p. 392, 1990*
 Tuberous sclerosis
 Rabson-Mendenhall syndrome – insulin-resistant diabetes mellitus, unusual facies, dental precocity, hypertrichosis, acanthosis nigricans, and premature sexual development
 Russell-Silver syndrome – large head, short stature, premature sexual development, CALMs, clinodactyly, syndactyly of toes, triangular face *Nat Rev Endocrinol 13:105–124, 2017; JAAD 40:877–890, 1999; J Med Genet 36:837–842, 1999*
 Hypothyroidism, childhood – sexual precocity
 Pineal lesions
Incomplete puberty

Premature thelarche
Premature pubarche
False – pseudopuberty
 Adrenal lesions
  Congenital adrenal hyperplasia *Pediatr Adolesc Gyn 30:520–534, 2017*
  Tumor
  Cushing's syndrome/hyperplasia
 Ovarian tumors
 Testicular tumors
 Iatrogenic (sex hormones)
Extrapituitary gonadotrophin-secreting tumors
 Teratoma
 Chorionepithelioma
 Hepatoblastoma
Other causes:

Angelman syndrome *Brain Dev 16:249–252, 1994*

Buschke-Ollendorf syndrome – with precocious puberty *Ped Derm 11:31–34, 1994; AD 106:208–214, 1972*

Estrogen exposure – estrogen or placenta-containing hair products *Clin Pediatr 134:82–89, 1999*

Hidradenitis suppurativa – presenting feature of premature adrenarche *BJD 129:447–448, 1993*

Hypophosphatemic Vitamin D-resistant rickets, precocious puberty, and epidermal nevus syndrome *AD 133:1557–1561, 1997*

Kabuki make-up syndrome – premature thelarche *Acta Paediatr Jpn 36:104–106, 1994*

Leprechaunism *Ann Genet 30:221–227, 1987*

Microphthalmia with linear skin defects (MIDAS syndrome) – Xp22.3 deletion *Ped Derm 20:153–157, 2003*

Peutz-Jeghers syndrome – autosomal dominant; ovarian tumors, precocious puberty with hormone secreting tumors *Gut 30:1588–1590, 1989*

Premature pubarche, ovarian hyperandrogenism, hyperinsulinism, and polycystic ovarian syndrome *J Endocrinol Invest 21:558–566, 1998*

Phenylketonuria *J Pediatr Endocrinol 7:361–363, 1994*

Rothmund-Thomson syndrome – hypogonadism *JAAD 75:855–870, 2016*

Rubinstein-Taybi syndrome *Am J Med Genet 23:365–366, 1999*

Sotos syndrome *Pediatr Med Chir 17:353–357, 1995*

Mutation in 3 beta-hydroxysteroid dehydrogenase type II *J Mol Endocrinol 12:119–122, 1994*

Mutation in 3 beta-hydroxysteroid dehydrogenase type II *J Mol Endocrinol 12:119–122, 1994*

Trichothiodystrophy – PIBIDS; cryptorchidism, delayed puberty *Ped Derm 32:865–866, 2015*

Woodhouse-Sakati syndrome – autosomal recessive; triangular shaped face with prominent forehead, large low set ears, dystonia, hypotrichosis, with sparse eyebrows and eyelashes; alopecia, hypogonadism, diabetes mellitus, mental retardation, sensorineural deafness, extrapyramidal signs, low insulin-like growth factor 1; must be differentiated from congenital hypotrichosis; mutation in *C2orf37 Ped Derm 31:83–87, 2014; Am J Med Genet 143:149–160, 2007; J Med Genet 20:216–219, 1983*

Xeroderma pigmentosum with DeSanctis-Cacchione syndrome – gonadal hypoplasia *JAAD 75:855–870, 2016*

X-linked adrenal hypoplasia congenita *J Clin Endocrinol Metab 86:4068–4071, 2001; Clin Endocrinol (Oxf) 53:249–255, 2000*

PULMONARY DISEASE ASSOCIATED WITH SKIN DISEASE

PULMONARY INTERSTITIAL LUNG DISEASE/ INFILTRATES/PNEUMONIA/ (CUTANEOUS MANIFESTATIONS OF PULMONARY DISEASE)

AUTOIMMUNE DISEASES AND DISORDERS OF IMMUNE DYSREGULATION

Dermatomyositis – anti-CADM-140 antibodies; anti-synthase antibodies; rapidly progressive interstitial lung disease *JAAD 78:776–785, 2018; JAMA 305:183–190, 2011*

DOCK2 deficiency – early onset invasive bacterial and viral infections *NEJM 372:2409–2422, 2015*

DOCK 8 deficiency syndrome – respiratory infections *Dermatol Clinics 35:11–19, 2017*

GATA2 deficiency (includes MONOMAC syndrome, DCML, Emberger syndrome (lymphedema and myelodysplasia) (familial acute leukemia and myelodysplasia) – monocytopenia, B-cell and natural killer cell lymphopenia, myeloid leukemias, disseminated mycobacterial infection, human papilloma virus infection, fungal infection; GATA2-transcription factor in early hematopoietic differentiation and lymphatic and vascular development; primary pulmonary alveolar proteinosis; panniculitis; erythema nodosum-like lesions; primary lymphedema *BJD 170:1182–1186, 2014*

Graft vs host disease

Hyper IgM syndrome – recurrent pulmonary and diarrheal infections; mutation in gene encoding CD40 ligand

IgG4 disease – lung mass, pleural effusion *NEJM 373:1762–1772, 2015*

Leukocyte adhesion deficiency (beta-2 integrin deficiency) congenital deficiency of leukocyte-adherence glycoproteins (CD11a (LFA-1), CD11b, CD11c, CD18) – necrotic cutaneous abscesses, cellulitis, skin ulcerations, pyoderma gangrenosum; ulcerative stomatitis *BJD 139:1064–1067, 1998; J Pediatr 119:343–354, 1991; Ann Rev Med 38: 175–194, 1987; J Infect Dis 152:668–689, 1985;* congenital deficiency of leucocyte-adherence glycoproteins (CD11a (LFA-1), CD11b, CD11c, CD18) – necrotic cutaneous abscesses, psoriasiform dermatitis, gingivitis, periodontitis, septicemia, ulcerative stomatitis, pharyngitis, otitis, pneumonia, peritonitis *BJD 123:395–401, 1990*

Lupus erythematosus *NEJM 373:1762–1772, 2015*

Relapsing polychondritis

Rheumatoid arthritis *NEJM 373:1762–1772, 2015*

Scleroderma – progressive systemic sclerosis with pulmonary fibrosis; silica dust – occupational scleroderma; digital ulcers, interstitial lung disease of lower lobes, myocardial dysfunction, cancer *JAAD 72:456–464, 2015*

Sclerodermatomyositis – Gottron's papules, periorbital erythema, Raynaud's phenomenon, acrosteolysis, dysphagia, digital ulcers; high risk of interstitial lung disease *Arthr Research Therapy 16:R111, 2014; AD 144:1351–1359, 2008; Arthr Rheum 50:565–569, 2004; J Clin Immunol 4:40–44, 1984*

Sjogren's syndrome *NEJM 374:74–81, 2016;* bronchiectasis; interstitial lung disease *A Clinician's Pearls and Myths in Rheumatology pp.107–130; ed John Stone; Springer 2009*

STING (stimulator of interferon genes)--associated vasculopathy with onset in infancy (SAVI) (type 1 interferonopathy) – autosomal dominant; progressive digital necrosis, swelling of fingers, amputation of several digits, violaceous and telangiectatic malar plaques, nasal septal destruction, chronic leg myalgias, atrophic skin over knees, red-purpuric plaques over cold-sensitive areas (acral areas) (cheeks, nasal tip, ears), red ears which ulcerate with necrosis; reticulate erythema of arms and legs *JAAD 74:186–189, 2016;* red plaques of face and hands; chilblain-like lesions; atrophic plaques of hands, telangiectasias of cheeks, nose, chin, lips, acral violaceous plaques and acral cyanosis (livedo reticularis of feet, cheeks, and knees), distal ulcerative lesions with infarcts (necrosis of cheeks and ears), gangrene of fingers or toes with ainhum, nasal septal perforation, nail loss and nail dystrophy ; small for gestational age; paratracheal adenopathy, abnormal pulmonary function tests; severe interstitial lung disease with fibrosis with ground glass and reticulate opacities; gain of function mutation in transmembrane protein 173 (STING) (*TMEM173*) (stimulator of interferon genes) leading to chronic activation of Type I interferon pathway; mimics granulomatosis with polyangiitis; *Ped Derm 33:602–614, 2016; JAMA Derm 151:872–877, 2015; NEJM 371:507–518, 2014*

> Interferonopathies – mutations in *PSMB8*
> > Aicardi-Goutieres syndrome
> > Familial chilblain lupus erythematosus
> > Spondyloench dysplasia

STK4 or Macrophage-stimulating 1 deficiency (MST1) – similar to DOCK 8 deficiency with viral, bacterial, fungal, respiratory infections; cardiac anomalies *Dermatol Clinics 35:11–19, 2017*

WHIM syndrome – warts, hypoglobulinemia, infections, myelokathexis; mutation in *CXCR4 AD 146:931–932, 2010*

X-linked hypogammaglobulinemia *Medicine (Baltimore)85:193–202, 2006*

DRUGS

DRESS syndrome

Methimazole-induced vasculitis – pulmonary hemorrhage; eschar-like leg ulcers *JAMA Derm 153:223–224, 2017; J Formos Med Assoc 100:772–775, 2000*

Ustekinumab – non-infectious pneumonia *JAMA Derm 155:221–224, 2019*

INFECTIONS AND INFESTATIONS

Anaplasma phagocytophilum (anaplasmosis) tickborne; fever, headache, cervical lymphadenopathy, pulmonary infiltrates; macular eruption sparing the face *NEJM 373:2162–2172, 2015; NEJM 371:358–366, 2014; Clin Microbiol Infect 8:763–772, 2002*

Aspergillosis

Babesiosis – pulmonary edema, fever, mottled skin, severe anemia *NEJM 370:753–762, 2014*

Candidiasis – congenital candidiasis – neonatal papules and vesicles; pneumonia *Cutis 93:229–232, 2014; J Perinatol 25:680–682, 2005*

Coccidioidomycosis – acute pulmonary coccidioidomycosis – macular, papular, urticarial, morbilliform, and targetoid lesions of exanthem *NEJM 363:2046–2054, 2010; JAAD 55:929, 942, 2006; AD 142:744–746, 2006;* macular red rash in 10% *Am Rev Resp Dis 117:559–585; 727–771, 1978;* morbilliform toxic erythema *Dermatol Clin 7:227–239, 1989;* hypersensitivity reaction in primary pulmonary coccidioidomycosis *JAAD 46:743–747, 2002*

Covid-19 – coronavirus; microthrombi with striking pulmonary infiltrates in severely ill patients; varicella-like rash, reticulated purpura, Kawasaki-like disease, chilblain-like lesions of toes

Cryptococcosis *NEJM 373:2162–2172, 2015*

Cytomegalovirus infection *NEJM 373:2162–2172, 2015*

Ehrlichiosis *NEJM 373:2162–2172, 2015; Ehrlichia chaffeensis* (human monocytic ehrlichiosis) – acute respiratory distress syndrome; fever, headache, malaise, myalgia; nausea, vomiting, diarrhea, abdominal pain; 1/3 with petechial or morbilliform eruption or diffuse erythema *MMWR 65:1–44, May 23, 2016; Clin Inf Dis 34:1206–1212, 2002; J Clin Gastroenterol 25:544–545, 1997*

Epidemic typhus (*Rickettsia prowazekii*) – morbilliform eruption becomes petechial exanthema; fever, nausea, diarrhea, delirium, respiratory failure, shock *JAAD 82:551–569, 2020*

Epstein-Barr virus *NEJM 373:2162–2172, 2015*

Glanders – *Pseudomonas mallei* – cellulitis which ulcerates with purulent foul-smelling discharge, regional lymphatics become abscesses; nasal and palatal necrosis and destruction; metastatic papules, pustules, bullae over joints and face, then ulcerate; deep abscesses with sinus tracts occur; polyarthritis, meningitis, pneumonia

H1N1 influenza A – morbilliform exanthema of thighs, lower legs, and dorsal feet *AD 146:101–102, 2010*

Herpes simplex virus – eczema herpeticum (Kaposi's varicelliform eruption) *Cutis 73:115–122, 2004; Arch Dis Child 60:338–343, 1985;* Kaposi's varicelliform eruption associated with Grover's disease *JAAD 49:914–915, 2003;* herpes simplex virus-associated exanthem following stem cell transplantation *AD 144:902–907, 2008*

Herpes virus 6 – interstitial pneumonitis, fever, rash

Herpes zoster – acute retinal necrosis, optic neuritis, acute glaucoma, episcleritis, scleritis, keratitis *NEJM 369;255–263, 2013; J Laryngol Otol 100:337–340, 1986*

Histoplasmosis (disseminated) in AIDS – facial papules, crusted papules, muscle weakness, pulmonary infiltrates; morbilliform rash with scale *BJD 173:797–800, 2015; Cutis 55:161–164, 1995; AD 121:1455–1460, 1985; Am J Med 64:923, 1978;* id reaction *JAAD 48:S5–6, 2003*

HIV disease *NEJM 373:2162–2172, 2015*

Kala azar

Legionella – painful non-pruritic erythematous macules; pretibial on day 5 *JAMA 245:1758, 1981*

Lyme disease *NEJM 373:2162–2172, 2015*

Malakoplakia (*Rhodococcus equi*) – pulmonary nodules, pneumonia, cavitation, abscesses *Clin Inf Dis 61:661–662, 2015*

Measles – pneumonia *Clin Respir J 10:673–675, 2016; Clin Microbiol Infect 20:O242–O244, 2014; NEJM 371:358–366, 2014*

Melioidosis (*Burkholderia pseudomallei*) – abscesses, abdominal pain, nausea, vomiting, cough, chest pain, fever, joint pain, necrotizing pneumonia, acute suppurative parotitis *JAAD 75:1–16, 2016; Clin Inf Dis 60:243–250, 2015*

Chronic meningococcemia – pneumonia *Clin Inf Dis 69:iii–iv, 2019*

Mycobacterium tuberculosis – lupus vulgaris – "turkey ear" *BJD 157:816–818, 2007;* – extensive destruction *Cutis 15:499–509, 1975;* starts as red-brown plaque, enlarges with serpiginous margin or as discoid plaques; apple-jelly nodules; myxomatous form with large tumors of the earlobes *Cutis 67:311–314, 2001; Int J Dermatol 26:578–581, 1987; Acta Tuberc Scand 39 (Suppl 49):1–137, 1960;* giant infiltrated ear lobe (lupus vulgaris) *AD 138:1607–1612, 2002;* papulonecrotic tuberculid – dusky red crusted or ulcerated papules occur in crops on elbows, hands, feet, knees, legs; also ears, face, buttock, and penis *Ped Derm 15:450–455, 1998; Int J Dermatol 30:487–490, 1991; Ped Derm 7:191–195, 1990;* multilobulated tumor of the earlobe *BJD 150:370–371, 2004;* tuberculosis verrucosa cutis; miliary tuberculosis

Mycoplasma pneumoniae

North American blastomycosis *NEJM 373:955–961, 2015; NEJM 373:1554–1564, 2015*

Paracoccidioidomycosis

Paragonimiasis (*Paragonimus westernani*) – eating raw crustaceans or raw meat; pulmonary infiltrates; edematous plaque of vulva *JAAD Case Reports 1:239–240, 2015*

Parvovirus *NEJM 373:2162–2172, 2015*

Proteus syndrome – pulmonary embolus with deep vein thrombosis *BJD 175:612–614, 2016*

Psittacosis – morbilliform rash *AD 120:1227, 1984*

Radiation therapy

Q fever (*Coxiella burnetii*) – pneumonia, high fever, headache, hepatitis, myocarditis *NEJM 376:869–874, 2017*

Rat bite fever – macular and petechial rash on palms and soles; acral hemorrhagic pustules; palpable purpura; arthritis, pustules; endocarditis, pericarditis, interstitial pneumonia, hepatitis, nephritis, septic arthritis, systemic vasculitis *JAMA Derm 152:723–724, 2016; J Clin Microbiol 51:1987–1989, 2013; AD 148:1411–1416, 2012; Clin Microbiol Rev 20:13–22, 2007; Clin Inf Dis 43:1585–1586, 1616–1617, 2006; JAAD 38:330–332, 1998*

Rocky Mountain spotted fever *NEJM 373:2162–2172, 2015*

Strongyloides hyperinfection

INFILTRATIVE DISORDERS

Erdheim-Chester disease (non-Langerhans cell histiocytosis) – CD68+ and factor XIIIa+; negative for CD1a and S100; xanthoma and xanthelasma-like lesions (red-brown-yellow papules and plaques); flat wart-like papules of face; lesions occur in folds; skin becomes slack with atrophy of folds and face; also lesions of eyelids, axillae, groin, neck; pretibial dermopathy, pigmented lesions of lips and buccal mucosa; long bone sclerosis; diabetes insipidus, painless exophthalmos, retroperitoneal fibrosis, renal (hairy kidneys), cerebellar syndrome, and pulmonary histiocytic infiltration; differential diagnosis includes Graves' disease, Hashimoto's thyroiditis, sarcoid *J Cutan Pathol 38:280–285, 2011; Int J Urol 15:455–456, 2008; Austral J Dermatol 44:194–198, 2003; JAAD 57:1031–1045, 2007; AD 143:952–953, 2007; Hautarzt 52:510–517, 2001; Medicine (Baltimore) 75:157–169, 1996; Virchow Arch Pathol Anat 279:541–542, 1930*

Langerhans cell histiocytosis – upper lobes

INFLAMMATORY DISORDERS

Ankylosing spondylitis – associated findings include psoriasis, anterior uveitis, inflammatory bowel disease, lung abnormalities, heart conduction defects, aortic insufficiency, renal abnormalities, osteoporosis, vertebral fractures *Euro J Intern Med 22:554–560, 2011; Int J Rheumatol 2011:1–10*

Erythema multiforme

Pyoderma gangrenosum *Ann DV 140:363–366, 2013; JAAD 59:S114–116, 2008*

Sarcoidosis *NEJM 373:1762–1772, 2015*

Stevens-Johnson syndrome/toxic epidermal necrolysis – impaired diffusion capacity of lungs *BJD 172:400–405, 2015*

Toxic epidermal necrolysis

METABOLIC DISORDERS

Congenital neutropenia *Blood Rev 2:178–185, 1988; Am J Med 61:849–861, 1976*

Cyclic neutropenia *Ped Derm 18:426–432, 2001; Am J Med 61:849–861, 1976*

Mannosidosis – autosomal recessive; gingival hypertrophy, macroglossia, coarse features, prognathism, thick eyebrows, low anterior hairline, deafness, lens opacities, hepatosplenomegaly, recurrent respiratory tract infections , muscular hypotonia, mental retardation *Ped Derm 18:534–536, 2001*

NEOPLASTIC DISORDERS

Atrial myxoma

Blastic plasmacytoid dendritic cell neoplasm – solitary or multiple nodules, plaques or bruise-like infiltrates; may involve lung, eyes, CNS *BJD 169:579–586, 2013; Arch Path Lab Med 134:1628–1638, 2010; Arch Path Lab Med 132:326–348, 2008*

Cancer *NEJM 373:2162–2172, 2015*

Kaposi's sarcoma

Leukemia cutis with pulmonary involvement

Light chain deposition disease – violaceous plaque of chin; involvement of kidneys (nephropathy), liver, heart, lungs, peripheral nerves *Hematol Oncol Clin NA 13:1235–1248, 1999*

Lymphoma – cutaneous T-cell lymphoma; non-Hodgkin's lymphoma

Lymphangitic metastases

Myelodysplastic syndrome

PARANEOPLASTIC DISORDERS

Paraneoplastic pemphigus – bronchiolitis obliterans *JAAD 80:1544–1549, 2019*

PRIMARY CUTANEOUS DISEASES

Dahl's sign – symmetric slanting areas of hyperpigmentation of the medial thighs ((Thinker's sign) due to repeated pressure on thighs from COPD *NEJM 371:357, 2014*

Febrile ulceronecrotic Mucha- Habermann disease (pityriasis lichenoides et varioliformis acuta) *J Rheumatol 16:387–389, 1989;* crusted ulcerated red plaques; diarrhea, pulmonary involvement, abdominal pain, CNS symptoms, arthritis *Ped Derm 29:53–58, 2012*

Mal de Meleda *Cutis 93:193–198, 2014*

X-linked hypohidrotic ectodermal dysplasia – female carriers, mosaicism – V-shaped hypopigmented linear lesions, patchy hypotrichosis, abnormal teeth *Ped Derm 24:551–554, 2007*

X-linked reticulate pigmentary disorder with systemic manifestations (familial cutaneous amyloidosis) (Partington syndrome II) – X-linked; rare; Xp21-22; boys with generalized reticulated muddy brown pigmentation (dyschromatosis) with hypopigmented corneal dystrophy (dyskeratosis), photophobia, coarse unruly hair, unswept eyebrows, silvery hair, hypohidrosis, recurrent pneumonia with chronic obstructive disease, clubbing; diarrhea, hypospadias, failure to thrive, female carriers with linear macular nevoid Blaschko-esque hyperpigmentation *Ped Derm 32:871–872, 2015; Am J Med Genet 161:1414–1420, 2013; Eur J Dermatol 18:102–103, 2008; Ped Derm 22:122–126, 2005; Semin Cut Med Surg 16:72–80, 1997; Am J Med Gen 10:65:1981*

SYNDROMES

APLAID (autoinflammation and PLAID) – sinopulmonary infections, interstitial pneumonitis, eye inflammation, colitis, arthralgias; epidermolysis bullosa-like eruptions in infancy with vesiculopustular lesions and red plaques *JAAD 73:367–381, 2015*

Blau or Jabs syndrome (familial juvenile systemic granulomatosis) – autosomal dominant; onset under 4 years of age; generalized micropapular rash of trunk and extremities infancy (ichthyosiform); translucent skin-colored papules (non-caseating granulomas) of trunk and extremities or dense lichenoid yellow to red-brown papules with grainy surface with anterior or panuveitis, synovitis, symmetric granulomatous polyarthritis; polyarteritis, multiple synovial cysts; red papular rash in early childhood; exanthem resolves with pitted scars; camptodactyly (flexion contractures of PIP joints); no involvement of lung or hilar nodes; sialadenitis, lymphadenopathy, erythema nodosum, leukocytoclastic vasculitis, transient neuropathies, interstitial lung disease, nephritis, arterial hypertension, pericarditis, pulmonary embolism, hepatic granulomas, chronic renal failure; activating mutations in NOD2 (nucleotide-binding oligomerization domain 2) (caspase recruitment domain family, member 15; *CARD* 15) *Ped Derm 34:216–218, 2017; Ped Derm 27:69–73, 2010; AD 143:386–391, 2007; Clin Exp Dermatol 21:445–448, 1996; J Pediatr 107:689–693, 1985*

Carcinoid syndrome

Dyskeratosis congenita – pulmonary fibrosis; pulmonary arteriovenous malformations *JAAD 77:1194–1196, 2017*

Epidermodysplasia verruciformis – *RHOH* deficient patients; bronchopulmonary disease and Burkitt's lymphoma *JAAD 76:1161–1175, 2017; CORO1A*-deficiency – molluscum contagiosum, bronchiectasis and lymphoma *JAAD 76:1161–1175, 2017*

Good syndrome – adult acquired primary immunodeficiency in context of past or current thymoma; sinopulmonary infections; lichen planus, oral lichen planus of tongue, gingivitis, oral erosions *BJD 172:774–777, 2015; Am J Med Genet 66:378–398, 1996*

Hereditary fibrosing poikiloderma with tendon contracture, myopathy, fibrosis, pulmonary fibrosis, and alopecia; FAM IIIB mutation – mimics Rothmund-Thomson syndrome; mutation in *FAMIIIB (POIKTMP) BJD 176:534–536, 2017; Cases of the Year, Pre-AAD Pediatric Dermatology Meeting, 2016*

> Papulovesicular facial eruption at birth
> Poikiloderma of cheeks
> Alopecia
> Cataracts
> Myopathy – fatty infiltration of muscles
> Gingivitis
> Poor dentition
> Hypohidrosis
> Lymphedema of hands and legs
> Exocrine pancreatic insufficiency
> Extraocular muscle weakness
> Tendon contractures
> Pulmonary fibrosis
> Palmoplantar keratoderma
> Red hands
> Sclerosis of fingers
> Photosensitivity

Hereditary mucoepithelial dysplasia (dyskeratosis) (Gap junction disease, Witkop disease) – autosomal dominant; non-scarring alopecia; dry rough skin; red eyes, non-scarring alopecia, follicular keratosis (keratosis pilaris), erythema of oral (hard palate, gingival, tongue) and nasal mucous membranes, cervix, vagina, and urethra; perineal and perigenital psoriasiform dermatitis (perineal erythema); hyperpigmented hyperkeratotic lesions of flexures (neck, antecubital and popliteal fossae); esophageal stenosis; keratitis (visual impairment) increased risk of infections, fibrocystic lung disease *Ped Derm*

29:311–315, 2012; BJD 153:310–318, 2005; Ped Derm 11:133–138, 1994; Am J Med Genet 39:338–341, 1991; JAAD 21:351–357, 1989; Am J Hum Genet 31:414–427, 1979; Oral Surg Oral Med Oral Pathol 46:645–657, 1978

Hermansky-Pudlak syndrome – oculocutaneous albinism, hemorrhage, ceroid-like material deposited in several organs; granulomatous colitis, pulmonary fibrosis, renal failure, cardiomyopathy, hypothyroidism *Ped Derm 34:638–646, 2017; SKINMed 12:313–315, 2014;* freckling in sun-exposed skin *JAAD 19:217–255, 1988*

Hunter syndrome (mucopolysaccharidosis type II) – accumulation of glycosaminoglycans; X-linked recessive; iduronate 2-sulfatase deficiency; recurrent otitis media, respiratory infections, hepatosplenomegaly, hernias, cardiomyopathy *Ped Derm 33:594–601, 2016*

Kawasaki's disease

Neurofibromatosis – lower lobes

Nijmegen breakage syndrome – autosomal recessive; chromosome instability syndrome; mutations in *NBS-1* gene which encodes bibirin (DNA damage repair); microcephaly, receding mandible, prominent midface, prenatal onset short stature, growth retardation, bird-like facies with epicanthal folds, large ears, sparse hair, clinodactyly/syndactyly; freckling of face, café au lait macules, vitiligo, photosensitivity of the eyelids, telangiectasias; pigmented deposits of fundus; IgG, IgA deficiencies, agammaglobulinemia, decreased CD3 and CD4 T cells with recurrent respiratory and urinary tract infections *Ped Derm 26:106–108, 2009; DNA Repair 3:1207–1217, 2004; Arch Dis Child 82:400–406, 2000; Am J Med Genet 66:378–398, 1996*

Multicentric reticulohistiocytosis

Nijmegen breakage syndrome – autosomal recessive; chromosome instability syndrome; mutations in *NBS-1* gene which encodes bibirin (DNA damage repair); microcephaly, receding mandible, prominent midface, growth retardation, epicanthal folds, large ears, sparse hair, clinodactyly/syndactyly; freckling of face, café au lait macules, vitiligo, photosensitivity of the eyelids, telangiectasias; pigmented deposits of fundus; IgG, IgA deficiencies, agammaglobulinemia, decreased CD3 and CD4 T cells with recurrent respiratory and urinary tract infections *Ped Derm 26:106–108, 2009; DNA Repair 3:1207–1217, 2004; Arch Dis Child 82:400–406, 2000*

Trichorhinophalangeal syndrome type I – autosomal dominant; slow growing short blond hair, receding frontotemporal hairline with high bossed forehead; thin nails, koilonychias, leukonychia, facial pallor, pear-shaped nose with bulbous nose tip, wide long philtrum, thin upper lip, triangular face, receding chin, tubercle of normal skin below the lower lip, protruding ears, distension and deviation with fusiform swelling of the PIP joints; hip malformation, brachydactyly, prognathism, fine brittle slow growing sparse hair, lateral eyebrows sparse and brittle, dense medially, bone deformities (hands short and stubby), joint hyperextensibility, cone-shaped epiphyses of bones of hand, lateral deviation of interphalangeal joints, flat feet, hip malformations, high arched palate, supernumerary teeth, dental malocclusion, mild short stature; hypotonia, hoarse deep voice, recurrent respiratory infections, hypoglycemia, diabetes mellitus, hypothyroidism, decreased growth hormone, renal and cardiac defects, mutation in zinc finger nuclear transcription factor (TRPS1 gene) *Cutis 89:56,73–74, 2012; Ped Derm 26:171–175, 2009; Ped Derm 25:557–558, 2008; BJD 157:1021–1024, 2007; AD 137:1429–1434, 2001; JAAD 31:331–336, 1994; Hum Genet 74:188–189, 1986; Helv Paediatr Acta 21:475–482, 1966*

Tuberous sclerosis – pulmonary lymphangioendotheliomatosis

X-linked reticulate pigmentary disorder – recurrent pneumonia, bronchiectasis, chronic diarrhea, failure to thrive, diffuse reticulated hyperpigmentation, hypohidrosis, corneal disease leading to

blindness; facies with unswept hair, flared eyebrows; female carriers display blaschko hyperpigmentation; *POLA1* gene *Ped Derm 33:602–614, 2016*

Yellow nail syndrome – pleural effusion, chronic bronchitis, bronchiectasis; lymphedema *J Dtsch Dermatol Ges 12:131–137, 2014; Case Rep Dermatol 3:251–258, 2011; Ped Derm 27:533–534, 2010; Chest 134:375–381, 2008; JAAD 56:537–538, 2007; BJD 156:1230–1234, 2007; JAAD 28:792–794, 1993*

TOXINS

Eosinophilia myalgia syndrome

Mustard gas exposure – flushing *JAAD 39:187–190, 1998; JAAD 32:765–766, 1995; AD 128:775–780, 1992*

Tear gas – exfoliative erythroderma

Trauma

Radiation injury

VASCULAR DISORDERS

Eosinophilic granulomatosis with polyangiitis – pulmonary infiltrates; mononeuritis multiplex; purpuric patches, stellate purpura; palpable purpura, hemorrhagic lesions *JAMA Derm 154:486–487, 2018; Autoimmunol Rev 14:341–348, 2015; JAAD 48:311–340, 2003; AD 141:873–878, 2005; AD 139:715–718, 2003; JAAD 48:311–340, 2003; JAAD 47:209–216, 2002; JAAD 47:209–216, 2002; JAAD 37:199–203, 1997; JAAD 27:821–824, 1992; JID 17:349–359, 1951; Am J Pathol 25:817, 1949; Mayo Clinic Proc 52:477–484, 1977;* purpura and petechiae of legs *JAAD 37:199–203, 1997;* acral purpura of finger and/or toe tips *Cutis 67:145–148, 2001;* necrotic purpura of scalp *Ann DV 122:94–96, 1995;* presenting as purpura fulminans *Clin Exp Dermatol 29:390–392, 2004*

Fat embolism syndrome – persistent somnolence, fever, tachycardia, respiratory symptoms, petechial eruption *NEJM 375:370–378, 2016*

Granulomatosis with polyangiitis – pleuritis, pulmonary nodules *NEJM 373:1762–1772, 2015*

Lymphomatoid granulomatosis (angiocentric lymphoma) – morbilliform eruption *Ped Derm 17:369–372, 2000*

Microscopic polyangiitis

Superior vena cava syndrome

PULMONARY NODULES

AUTOIMMUNE DISEASES AND DISORDERS OF IMMUNE DYSREGULATION

Dermatomyositis *NEJM 373:1762–1772, 2015;* pseudomediastinum *JAAD 78:776–785, 2018*

IgG4-related disease *NEJM 373:1762–1772, 2015*

Lupus erythematosus *NEJM 373:1762–1772, 2015*

Rheumatoid arthritis – Caplan syndrome *NEJM 373:1762–1772, 2015*

Scleroderma

DRUG REACTIONS

Amiodarone

Nivolumab – sarcoid-like parotid enlargement, pulmonary granulomas *BJD 176:1060–1063, 2017*

INFECTIONS AND INFESTATIONS

Coccidioidomycosis – acute pulmonary coccidioidomycosis – macular, papular, urticarial, morbilliform, and targetoid lesions of exanthem *NEJM 363:2046–2054, 2010; JAAD 55:929, 942, 2006; AD 142:744–746, 2006;* macular red rash in 10% *Am Rev Resp Dis 117:559–585; 727–771, 1978;* morbilliform toxic erythema *Dermatol Clin 7:227–239, 1989;* hypersensitivity reaction in primary pulmonary coccidioidomycosis *JAAD 46:743–747, 2002*

Cryptococcosis

Dirofilaria repens – red plaques (cellulitis-like) and pulmonary nodules *BJD 173:788–791, 2015*

Fusarium

Histoplasmosis (disseminated) in AIDS *Clin Inf Dis 70:1003–1010, 2020;* morbilliform rash with scale *Cutis 55:161–164, 1995; AD 121:1455–1460, 1985; Am J Med 64:923, 1978;* id reaction *JAAD 48:S5–6, 2003*

Katayama fever (acute schistosomiasis) – pulmonary nodules, red papular exanthem, fever, cough, urticarial eruption, fatigue *NEJM 374:469, 2016*

Malakoplakia (*Rhodococcus equi*) – pulmonary nodules, pneumonia, cavitation, abscesses *Clin Inf Dis 61:661–662, 2015*

Mycobacterium tuberculosis

Mycobacterium haemophilum

North American blastomycosis *NEJM 373:955–961, 2015*

Paragonimiasis – pulmonary nodule and brown chest nodule *Clin Inf Dis 60:1532,1582–1583, 2015*

Sporotrichosis

Strongyloides hyperinfection (*Strongyloides stercoralis*) *Clin Inf Dis 59:559,601–602, 2014*

Syphilis, secondary

Tularemia

Varicella

INFILTRATIVE DISORDERS

Primary amyloidosis

Erdheim-Chester disease (non-Langerhans cell histiocytosis) – multiple pink exophytic nodules – skin, pulmonary, vocal cord *NEJM 373:1762–1772, 2015; BJD 173:540–543, 2015; Virchows Arch Pathol Anat 173:561–602, 1930*

INFLAMMATORY DISORDERS

Pyoderma gangrenosum

Sarcoidosis *NEJM 373:1762–1772, 2015*

NEOPLASTIC DISORDERS

Cancer *NEJM 373:1762–1772, 2015*

Cylindromas *BJD 179:662–668, 2018; JAAD 19:397–400, 1988*

Kaposi's sarcoma – HIV disease

Lymphoma/leukemia – cutaneous T-cell lymphoma (Sezary syndrome) *JAAD 70:205–220, 2014; NEJM 369:559–569, 2013; Cutis 89:229–232,236, 2012; JAAD 27:427–433, 1992; JAAD 41:254–259, 1999; Semin Oncol 26:276–289, 1999;* exfoliative CTCL mimicking chronic actinic dermatitis *BJD 160:698–703, 2009;* adult T-cell leukemia/lymphoma *BJD 155:617–620, 2006;* presenting as papuloerythroderma *Clin Exp Dermatol 20:161–163, 1995; BJD 130:773–736, 1994;* syringotropic CTCL *BJD 148:349–352,*

2003; angioimmunoblastic lymphadenopathy with dysproteinemia (angioimmunoblastic T-cell lymphoma) *JAAD 38:992–994, 1998; JAAD 36:290–295, 1997; BJD 104:131–139, 1981;* HTLV-1 (adult T-cell leukemia) *JAAD 46:S137–141, 2002; JAAD 36:869–871, 1997; JAAD 27:846–849, 1992;* Hodgkin's disease, non–Hodgkin's lymphoma, leukemia, myelodysplasia; chronic T-cell lymphocytic leukemia *JAAD 8:874–878, 1983;* Ki-1 (CD30) positive anaplastic large cell lymphoma *JAAD 47:S201–204, 2002*

Lymphomatoid granulomatosis

Metastases – lung cancer associated dermatomyositis

Paraneoplastic Disorders

Lung cancer associated with dermatomyositis, pachydermoperiostosis

SYNDROMES

Eosinophilic granulomatosis with polyangiitis *JAAD 47:209–216, 2002; JAAD 37:199–203, 1997; JAAD 27:821–824, 1992; JID 17:349–359, 1951; Am J Pathol 25:817, 1949*

Gorlin's syndrome – metastatic basal cell carcinoma *JAMA Derm 150:877–879, 2014*

Multicentric reticulohistiocytosis

Osler-Weber-Rendu syndrome

Pachydermoperiostosis

Tuberous sclerosis/LAM *Eur J Radiol 83:39–46, 2014*

VASCULAR DISORDERS

Eosinophilic granulomatosis with vasculopathy

Granulomatosis with polyangiitis *NEJM 373:1762–1772, 2015*

Infantile hemangiomas *Pediatr Pulmonol 49:829–833, 2014; Ped Radiol 40:S63–67, 2010; J Clin Pathol 60:943–945, 2007; Pediatr Dev Pathol 5:283–292, 2002*

PLEURAL EFFUSIONS

AUTOIMMUNE DISORDERS

IgG4-related disease *NEJM 373:1762–1772, 2015*

Rheumatoid arthritis

Still's disease

Systemic lupus erythematosus

INFECTIONS AND INFESTATIONS

Actinomycosis

Coccidioidomycosis

Echinococcus (hydatid cyst)

Fusarium

Legionella

Mycoplasma pneumoniae dermatitis (MIRM)

Neisseria meningitides group y *Tidsskr Nor Laegeforen Nov 13, 2017*

North American blastomycosis *Can Report J 13:441–444, 2006*

Paracoccidioidomycosis

Paragonimiasis

Scrub typhus *Infect Chemother 51:161–170, 2019*

Tuberculosis

INFLAMMATORY DISORDERS

Acute pancreatitis

NEOPLASTIC DISORDERS

Angiosarcoma

Kaposi's sarcoma *J Community Hosp Intern Med Perspect 9:351–354, 2019*

Metastatic melanoma

PRIMARY CUTANEOUS DISEASE

Kawasaki's disease

SYNDROMES

Hereditary hemorrhagic telangiectasia

Hurler's syndrome (mucopolysaccharidosis type I-H)– disorder of glycosaminoglycans accumulation; autosomal recessive; coarse facies, macroglossia, short stature, macrocephaly, hepatospleno-megaly, hernias, corneal clouding, vision and hearing loss; cardiac anomalies; respiratory infections; alpha-I-iduronate deficiency *Ped Derm 33:594–601, 2016; Atlas of Clinical Syndromes A Visual Aid to Diagnosis, 1992, pp.118–119*

Hypereosinophilic syndrome – intractable pruritus, pulmonary infiltrates, eosinophilic gastroenteritis, endomyocardial fibrosis, thromboembolism *NEJM 380:1336–1346, 2019; AD 132:535–541, 1996; Med Clin (Barc)106:304–306, 1996*

Hypotrichosis-Lymphedema-Telangiectasia-Renal failure syn-drome – diffuse reticulated capillary malformation, hypertensive emergency with transient ischemic attack, dilatation or aortic root, pleural effusions, acute kidney injury, thin facies with telangiectasias of cheeks, livedo reticularis of trunk and extremities; mutation in *SOX18* gene *Cases of the Year, Pre-AAD Pediatric Dermatology Meeting, 2016*

Sweet's syndrome

X-linked reticulate pigmentary disorder with systemic manifestations (familial cutaneous amyloidosis) (Partington syndrome II) – X-linked; rare; Xp21-22; boys with generalized reticulated muddy brown reticulated pigmentation (dyschromatosis) with hypopigmented corneal dystrophy (dyskeratosis), coarse unruly hair, unswept eyebrows, silvery hair, hypohidrosis, recurrent sinus disease and pneumonia with chronic obstructive disease, clubbing; photophobia, failure to thrive, female carriers with linear macular nevoid Blaschko-esque hyperpigmentation; gastroenteritis, diarrhea; intronic mutation of *POLA1* gene *JAMA Derm 153:817–818, 2017; Ped Derm 32:871–872, 2015; Am J Med Genet 161:1414–1420, 2013; Eur J Dermatol 18:102–103, 2008; Ped Derm 22:122–126, 2005; Semin Cut Med Surg 16:72–80, 1997; Am J Med Genet 32:115–119, 1989; Am J Med Gen 10:65–75:1981*

Differential diagnosis includes:
Dermatopathia pigmentosa reticularis – adermatoglyphia, palmoplantar keratoderma, non-scarring alopecia; mutation in *K14*
Dowling-Degos syndrome – *K5* mutation
Dyskeratosis congenita – mutation in *DKC1*
Naegeli-Franceschetti-Jadassohn syndrome
Amyloidosis cutis dyschromia
Rothmune-Thomson syndrome
Kindler's syndrome

Yellow nail syndrome – pleural effusion, chronic bronchitis, bronchiectasis; lymphedema *J Dtsch Dermatol Ges 12:131–137, 2014; Case Rep Dermatol 3:251–258, 2011; Ped Derm 27:533–534,* 2010; *Chest 134:375–381, 2008; JAAD 56:537–538, 2007; BJD 156:1230–1234, 2007; JAAD 28:792–794, 1993*

VASCULAR DISORDERS

Diffuse capillary malformation and pleural effusions *Ped Derm 32:70–75, 2015*
Macrocephaly capillary malformation syndrome
CLOVES syndrome (congenital lipomatous overgrowth, vascular malformation, epidermal nevus, spinal/skeletal anomalies/scoliosis)

Hypocomplementemic urticarial vasculitis

PULMONARY INFARCTS/EMBOLI

Infective endocarditis

Lemierre syndrome (suppurative jugular thrombophlebitis)

Atrial myxoma

Cutaneous T-cell lymphoma *J Thorac Imaging 17:157–159, 2002*

Cocaine use

PULMONARY CYSTS

Birt-Hogg-Dube syndrome

Neurofibromatosis

Ehlers-Danlos syndrome

Sarcoidosis

Amyloidosis *Am J Respir Crit Care Med 192:17–29, 2015*

Light chain deposit disease

Sjogren's syndrome *Ann Am Thorac Soc 13:371–375, 2016*

Lymphangiomyomatosis

Langerhans cell histiocytosis

Angiosarcoma, metastatic

Coccidioidomycosis

Echinococcus (hydatid cyst)

Paragonimiasis

Pneumocystis jiroveci

Staphylococcal pneumonia

PNEUMOTHORAX

Birt-Hogg-Dube syndrome *BJ Cancer 105:1912–1919, 2011*

Tuberous sclerosis complex/LAM

Cystic fibrosis

Coccidioidomycosis *BMJ Case Rep July 30,2018*

Marfan's syndrome

Homocystinuria *Am J Respir Crit Care Med 199:1344–1347, 2019*

Cocaine use

Cutis laxa

Ehlers-Danlos type IV

Alpha-1-antitrypsin deficiency

ALVEOLAR HEMORRHAGE

Systemic lupus erythematosus *Medicine (Balt) 76:192–202, 1997*

Goodpasture's syndrome (anti-GBM)

Henoch-Schonlein purpura

Granulomatosis with polyangiitis

Microscopic polyangiitis

Celiac disease

Eosinophilic granulomatosis with polyangiitis

Rheumatoid arthritis

Behcet's syndrome

Primary antiphospholipid antibody syndrome

Scleroderma

Pneumocystis jirovecii

Stenotrophomonas maltophilia

Hepatitis C cryoglobulinemia

Hantavirus

Leptospirosis

CMV pneumonia

HSV pneumonia

Aspergillosis, invasive

Legionella

Mycoplasma

Kaposi's sarcoma

Cocaine – intravenous, inhaled cocaine or crack

Medications
  Amiodarone,
  Anticoagulants
  Retinoic acid
  Cytarabine
  Fludarabine
  Gemcitabine
  Mitomycin C
  Cyclosporine
  Methotrexate
  Sirolimus
  Rituximab

Methimazole-induced vasculitis

Fat embolism

Cholesterol embolism

Insect bite

PULSATILE PAPULES

NEOPLASTIC DISORDERS

Glomus tumor

Multiple myeloma, subcutaneous tumors

Osteosarcoma (egg shell crackling with pulsation) *Dermatologica 138:59–63, 1969*

Renal cell carcinoma, metastasis *Indian J Vascular and Endovascular Surg 4:214–216, 2017; Derm Surg 27:192–194, 2001; Mayo Clin Proc 72:935–941, 1997;* pulsatile cutaneous horn of nose *BMJ Case Rep 2017:bcr 2017220913*

Thyroid carcinoma, metastasis; follicular thyroid carcinoma *BMJ case Rep 2012:bcr 0920103354*

PRIMARY CUTANEOUS DISEASES

Angiolymphoid hyperplasia with eosinophilia *Indian J DV Leprol 82:413–415, 2016; G Ital Dermatol Venereol July 11, 2014*

VASCULAR DISORDERS

Aneurysm

Arteriovenous malformation

Arteriovenous fistulae – intracranial dural arteriovenous malformation; subcutaneous pulsatile nodule *AD 146:808–810, 2010;* congenital; red pulsating nodules with overlying telangiectasia – extremities, head, neck, trunk *Trauma Case Rep 17:43–47, 2018*

Arteriovenous shunt

Caliber persistent artery of the lip *Case Rep Dent 2015:747428; Australas J Dermatol 53:e18–19, 2012*

Facial vein pulsation – severe tricuspid regurgitation *The Lancet 393:1330, 2019*

Kasabach-Merritt syndrome

Pseudoaneurysm of face and forehead – pulsatile subcutaneous vascular nodule; hematoma with sinus tract communicating with lumen; following Mohs' surgery *JAMA Derm 150:546–549, 2014;* of wrist following transradial coronary angiography *NEJM 373:1361, 2015;* ulnar artery pseudoaneurysm *JAAPA 31:55–56, 2018*

Sinus pericranii – pulsatile scalp protrusion *JAAD 54:S50–52, 2006*

Temporal arteritis

Temporal artery aneurysm, pseudoaneurysm *Trauma Case Rep 17:43–47, 2018; BMJ March 24, 2015*

Thrombus in temporal artery aneurysm

Vascular malformation

Vascular tumor

PULSATILE PROPTOSIS

Absence sphenoid wing in neurofibromatosis type 1

Carotid-cavernous fistula

Orbital roof fractures

Arteriovenous malformation

PUNCTATE AND RETICULATE HYPERPIGMENTATION

AUTOIMMUNE DISEASES AND DISORDERS OF IMMUNE DYSREGULATION

Contact dermatitis – prurigo pigmentosa *Contact Dermatitis 44:289–292, 2001*

Scleroderma *J Med Case Rep 9:219, 2015; Clin Exp Dermatol 30:131–133, 2005*

DRUGS

Benzoyl peroxide *Acta DV 78:301–302, 1998*

Bleomycin *Dermatologica 180:255–257, 1990*

Chemotherapy *World J Clin Case 4:390–400, 2016*

Cyclophosphamide *Int J Clin Pharm 35:309–312, 2013*

Diltiazem *J Dermatol 37:807–811, 2010; AD 137:179–182, 2001*

5-fluorouracil – reticulate pigmentation *Int J Derm 34:219–220, 1995*

Hydroxychloroquine *J Cutan Pathol 35:1134–1137, 2008*

Paclitaxel *World J Clin Case 4:390–400, 2016*

INFILTRATIVE DISORDERS

Macular amyloid

METABOLIC DISORDERS

Fanconi's anemia *Br J Hematol 85:9–14, 1993*

Vitamin B12 deficiency *Ped Derm 35:796–799, 2018*

NEOPLASTIC DISEASES

Lymphoma (CTCL) *Int J Derm 30:658–659, 1991*

PRIMARY CUTANEOUS DISEASES

Acropigmentation symmetrica of Dohi (reticulate acropigmentation of Dohi) (dyschromatosis symmetrica hereditaria) – autosomal dominant or sporadic acral mottled pigmentation with depigmentation of dorsa of hands, feet, arms, and legs ((reticulate pattern becoming patches with hypopigmented macules of face, trunk, distal extremities); Asians with onset under 20 years of age; *JAAD 43:113–117, 2000; BJD 140:491–496, 1999; JAAD 37:884–886, 1997*

Anonychia with flexural pigmentation

Atopic dermatitis – "dirty neck"; reticulate pigmentation of the neck *Clin Exp Derm 12:1–4, 1987*

Confluent and reticulated papillomatosis (Gougerot-Carteaud syndrome) *Acta DV 93:493–494, 2013; Acta DV Suppl (Stockh)59:185–187, 1979*

Dermatopathia pigmentosa reticularis – autosomal dominant; reticulate pigmentation, alopecia, nail changes, palmoplantar hyperkeratosis, loss of dermatoglyphics *JAAD 75:379–382, 2019; Ped Derm 24:566–570, 2007; JAAD 26:298–301, 1992; AD 126:935–939, 1990*

Diffuse pigmentation with macular depigmentation of trunk with reticulate pigmentation of neck *Hautarzt 6:458–460, 1955*

Dyschromatosis ptychotropica *Eur J Ped 169:495–500, 2010*

Epidermolysis bullosa simplex with mottled pigmentation *Dermatology 189:173–178, 1994*

Erythromelanosis follicularis faciei et colli – with reticulated hyperpigmentation of the extremities *Clin Case Rep 5:1576–1579, 2017*

Familial pigmentary anomaly

Familial pigmentation – Becker

Familial progressive hyperpigmentation (Moon-Adams) *AD 103:581–598, 1971; Hautarzt 11:262–265, 1960*

Hidrotic ectodermal dysplasia – reticulate acropigmentation *JAAD 6:476–480, 1982*

Lichen planus pigmentosus *Dermatol Online J Dec 15, 2016; Indian J Dermatol 61:700, 2016*

Prurigo pigmentosa *Ped Derm 24:277–279, 2007; Am J Dermatopathol 25:117–129, 2003; Dermatology 188:219–221, 1994*

Reticulate hyperpigmentation in zosteriform fashion (progressive cribriform and zosteriform hyperpigmentation) (zosteriform reticulate hyperpigmentation) *BJD 121:280, 1989; in children BJD 117:503–17, 1987; AD 114:98–99, 1978*

Reticulate, patchy, and mottled pigmentation of the neck *Dermatology 197:291–296, 1998*

Terra firme *Acta DV 143:446–452, 2016; SkinMed 14:345–348, 2016*

SYNDROMES

Cantu's syndrome

Da Costa's syndrome *Ped Derm 6:91–101, 1989*

Dowling-Degos syndrome (reticulated pigmented anomaly of the flexures) – reticulated pigmentation of axillae, groin, and other intertrigenous areas, freckles of vulva, comedo-like lesions, pitted scars around mouth *JAAD 40:462–467, 1999; Clin Exp Dermatol 9:439–350, 1984;* hidradenitis suppurativa, mutation in *PSENEN BJD 178:502–508, 2018;* mutation in *POFUT4 BJD 173:584–586, 2015*

Down's syndrome – short stature, cutis marmorata, acrocyanosis, low-set, small ears *JAAD 46:161–183, 2002;*

Dyschromatosis universalis hereditaria – autosomal dominant; generalized with mucosal involvement; alopecia, onychodystrophy, hypopigmented macules, loss of dermatoglyphics, sweating disorders, plantar hyperkeratosis, acral non-scarring bullae *Clin Exp Dermatol 27:477–479, 2002*

Dyskeratosis congenita– X-linked recessive; reticulate hyperpigmentation (poikiloderma) of neck, chest, thighs; nail dystrophy, oral, ocular, and anal leukoplakia *J Med Genet 25:843–846, 1988*

Franceschetti-Jadassohn-Naegeli syndrome *Indian J Dermatol 64:3250328, 2019; JAAD 28:942–950, 1993*

Galli-Galli syndrome – Dowling-Degos disease with acantholysis – hyperkeratotic follicular papules *JAAD 56: S86–91, 2007; JAAD 45:760–763, 2001*

Goltz's syndrome

Haber's syndrome *JAAD 40:462–467, 1999*

Hereditary acrokeratotic poikiloderma of Weary – vesiculopustules of hands and feet at age 1–3 months which resolve; widespread atopic dermatitis-like dermatitis; diffuse poikiloderma with striate and reticulate atrophy; keratotic papules of hands and feet, elbows and knees; autosomal dominant *AD 103:409–422, 1971*

Hereditary sclerosing poikiloderma – involve entire body, but spares upper chest

Hoyeraal-Hreidarsson syndrome – reticulate

hyperpigmentation (resembles dyskeratosis congenita), growth retardation, microcephaly, mental retardation, cerebellar malformation, progressive bone marrow failure, and mucocutaneous lesions *J Pediatr 136:390–393, 2000*

Hypotrichosis, striate, reticulated pitted palmoplantar keratoderma, acro-osteolysis, psoriasiform plaques, lingua plicata, ventricular arrhythmias, periodontitis *BJD 147:575–581, 2002*

Incontinentia pigmenti (hypopigmentation) *AD 139:1163–1170, 2003; Ped Derm 7:174–178, 1990*

Keratosis-ichthyosis-deafness (KID) syndrome – reticulated severe diffuse hyperkeratosis of palms and soles, well marginated, serpiginous erythematous verrucous plaques, perioral furrows, leukoplakia, sensory deafness, photophobia with vascularizing keratitis, blindness *BJD 148:649–653, 2003; AD 117:285–289, 1981*

Kindler's syndrome – reticulated erythema precedes poikiloderma *JAAD 46:447–450, 2001*

Macrocephaly – cutis marmorata telangiectatica congenita syndrome (macrocephaly, cutis marmorata, hemangioma, and syndactyly syndrome) – macrocephaly, hypotonia, hemihypertrophy, hemangioma, cutis marmorata telangiectatica congenita, internal arterio-venous malformations, syndactyly, joint laxity, hyperelastic skin, thickened subcutaneous tissue, developmental delay, short stature, hydrocephalus *Ped Derm 16:235–237, 1999; Genet Couns 9:245–253, 1998; Am J Med Genet 70:67–73, 1997*

Microphthalmia with linear skin defects syndrome (MLS syndrome) *Am J Med Genet 49:229–234, 1994*

Navajo syndrome – pigmentation acral initially, then spreads to trunk

Phakomatosis pigmentovascularis type 5 – cutis marmorata telangiectatica congenital and Mongolian spot *BJD 148:148:342–345, 2003*

Pigmented reticularis faciei and colli with epithelial cystomatosis *Dermatologie Tokyo: University of Tokyo Press 89–90, 1982*

Pseudoxanthoma elasticum – linear and reticulated yellow papules and plaques *AD 124:1559, 1988; JAAD 42:324–328, 2000; Dermatology 199:3–7, 1999*; pseudoxanthoma elasticum resembling reticulated pigmented disorders *BJD 134:1157–1159, 1996*; penicillamine-induced pseudoxanthoma elasticum *JAAD 30:103–107, 1994; Dermatology 184:12–18, 1992;* saltpetre-induced pseudoxanthoma elasticum *Acta DV 58:323–327, 1978*

Reflex sympathetic dystrophy – reticulated hyperpigmentation *Cutis 68:179–182, 2001*

Reticular pigmented genodermatosis with milia (Naegeli-Franceschetti-Jadassohn syndrome?) *Clin Exp Dermatol 20:331–335, 1995*

Reticulate acropigmentation of Kitamura – autosomal dominant; freckle-like pigmentation of dorsae of hands, palmar pits *AD 139:657–662, 2003; J Dermatol 27:745–747, 2000; JAAD 40:462–467, 1999; BJD 109:105–110, 1983; ADAM 10* mutation *Clin Exp Dermatol 44:700–703, 2019*

Reticulate hyperpigmentation of Iijima, Naito, and Uyeno *Acta DV 71:248–250, 1991*

Reticulolinear aplasia cutis congenita of the face and neck – Xp deletion syndrome, MIDAS (microphthalmia, dermal aplasia, sclerocornea), MLS (microphthalmia and linear skin defects), and Gazali-Temple syndrome; lethal in males; residual facial scarring in females, short stature, organ malformations *BJD 138:1046–1052, 1998*

Revesz syndrome

Rothmund-Thompson syndrome – photodistributed erythema followed by mottled pigmentation

Speckled pigmentation, palmoplantar punctate keratoses, childhood blistering *BJD 105:579–585, 1981*

Trisomy 13 mosaicism *Ped Derm 31:580–583, 2014*

Trisomy 14 mosaicism syndrome – patchy reticulated hyperpigmentation resembling that of incontinentia pigmenti *Syndromes of the Head and Neck, p.89, 1990*

Trisomy 18 – reticulate vascular nevus or port wine stain *J Pediatr 72:862–863, 1968*

Tumor necrosis factor (TNF) receptor 1-associated periodic fever syndromes (TRAPS) (same as familial hibernian fever, autosomal dominant periodic fever with amyloidosis, and benign autosomal dominant familial periodic fever) – erythematous patches, tender red plaques, fever, annular, serpiginous, polycyclic, reticulated, and migratory patches and plaques (migrating from proximal to distal), urticaria-like lesions, lesions resolving with ecchymoses, conjunctivitis, periorbital edema, myalgia, arthralgia, abdominal pain, headache; Irish and Scottish predominance; mutation in TNFRSF1A – gene encoding 55kDa TNF receptor *AD 136:1487–1494, 2000*

X-linked reticulate pigmentary disorder (formerly familial or X-linked cutaneous amyloidosis) *BJD 177:e200–201, 2017; Am J Med Genet A 161A:1414–1420, 2013; Am J Med Genet 52:75–78, 1994; Am J Med Genet 10:67–75, 1981*

Xp microdeletion syndrome – linear skin defects of head and neck (congenital smooth muscle hamartomas) (MIDAS syndrome – microphthalmia, dermal aplasia, sclerocornea) *Ped Derm 14:26–30, 1997*

TOXINS

Heavy metal poisoning

VASCULAR DISORDERS

Erythema ab igne – heating pad; "toasted skin syndrome" *Acta DV 94:365–367, 2014*

Laptop computer-induced hyperpigmentation *Dermatol Online J Dec 15< 2018; An Bras Dermatol 91:79–80, 2016*

PURPURA

AUTOIMMUNE DISEASES AND DISEASES OF IMMUNE DYSFUNCTION

Allergic contact dermatitis to azo textile dyes and resins – purpuric *J Eur Acad Dermatol Venereol 14:101–105, 2000;* purpuric patch tests due to azo dyes *Contact Dermatitis 42:23–26, 2000;* disperse blue 106 and 124, cobalt, epoxy resin, methylmethacrylate, EMLA, n-phenyl n'isopropyl para-phenylenediamine *JAAD 45:456–458, 2001;* p-phenylene diamine, Balsam of Peru *Contact Dermatitis 11:207–209, 1984;* rubber in clothing *Trans St John's Hosp Dermatol Soc 54:73–78, 1968;* optical whiteners *BJD 83:296–301, 1970;* benzoyl peroxide *JAAD 22:358–361, 1990;* ethyleneurea melamineformaldehyde, dimethylol dihydroxyethyleneurea, tetramethylol acetylenediurea, urea formaldehyde, melamine formaldehyde, Disperse Red 17 *JEADV 14:101–105, 2000;* splinter hemorrhage; methyl methacrylate allergic contact dermatitis in dentist – fingertip purpura *JAMA Derm 150:784–785, 2014;* purpuric allergic contact dermatitis to textile dyes, formaldehyde, epoxy resins *J Eur Acad Dermatol Venereol 14:101–105, 2000;* purpuric contact dermatitis – Balsam of Peru, benzoyl peroxide, Disperse Blue 85, elastic in underwear, EMLA, nitrodisc purpura, proflavine, unprocessed wool, woolen garments *Contact Dermatitis 36:11–13, 1997; JAAD 22:359–361, 1990; Contact Dermatitis 34:213–215, 1996*

Antineutrophil cytoplasmic antibody syndrome – purpuric vasculitis, orogenital ulceration, fingertip necrosis, pyoderma gangrenosum-like ulcers *BJD 134:924–928, 1996*

Autoimmune lymphoproliferative syndrome – petechiae and purpura; germline *FAS* mutation *NEJM 369:853–863, 2013*

Autoimmune progesterone dermatitis *S Afr Med J 106:48–50, 2016;* palpable pinpoint purpura *Cutis 98:E12–13, 2016*

Autosensitivity to DNA – painful pruritic ecchymoses *Am J Med Sci 251:145–147, 1966*

Bowel-associated dermatitis-arthritis syndrome *AD 135:1409–1414, 1999; JAAD 14:792–796, 1986; Mayo Clin Proc 59:43–46, 1984; AD 115:837–839, 1979*

Bullous pemphigoid

CANDLE syndrome (chronic atypical neutrophilic dermatosis with lipodystrophy and elevated temperature) – recurrent annular red or violaceous plaques of face and trunk which evolve to purpura then annular hyperpigmentation, purple swollen eyelids and lips (thick lips), limitation of range of motion with plaques over interphalangeal joints; arthralgia without arthritis, panniculitis, lipoatrophy of cheeks and arms, myositis, aseptic meningitis, nodular episcleritis, lymphadenopathy, ear and nose chondritis with saddle nose deformity, epididymitis, cold-induced pernio-like lesions of hands and feet, delayed physical development with short stature, splenomegaly, protuberant abdomen, nodular episcleritis and conjunctivitis *Ped Derm 33:602–614, 2016; JAAD 62:489–495, 2010*

C2 deficiency – Henoch-Schonlein purpura-like lesions *BJD 178:335–349, 2018*

C4 deficiency – Henoch-Schonlein purpura-like lesions *BJD 178:335–349, 2018*

Chediak-Higashi syndrome – photophobia, nystagmus, decreased pigmentation of iris *BJD 178:335–349, 2018*

Common variable immunodeficiency *BJD 178:335–349, 2018*

Connective tissue disease – vasculitis; retiform purpura *JAAD 82:783–796, 2020*

Dermatitis herpetiformis – palmar or plantar purpura, especially in children *JAMA Derm 156:695, 2020; JAMA Derm 150:1353–1354, 2014; Dermatology 227:1–4, 2013; JAAD 64:1017–1024, 2011; Cutis 70:217–223, 2002; Ped Derm 14:319–322, 1994; JAAD 19:577, 1988; JAAD 16:1274–1276, 1987; Cutis 37:184–187, 1986;* oral petechiae *Oral Surg 62:77–80, 1986;* digital petechiae *JAMA Derm 150:1353–1354, 2014; Ped Derm 29:209–212, 2012; BJD 84:386–388, 1971; BJD 85:314–319, 1971; AnnDV 110:121–126, 1983;* purpura of fingers with red patches and pustules – leukocytoclastic vasculitis as presentation of dermatitis herpetiformis *AD 137:1313–1316, 2011;* purpura of fingertips *JAMA Derm 150:1353–1354, 2014;* linear petechiae of fingertips *Dermatology 227:1–4, 2013*

Dermatomyositis

Epidermolysis bullosa acquisita, including buccal mucosa *JAAD 11:820–832, 1984*

Graft vs. host reaction – petechiae *AD 125:1685–1688, 1989;* oral purpura *Postgrad Med 66:187–193, 1979*

Hepatic venoocclusive disease with immunodeficiency *BJD 178:335–349, 2018*

IgG4-related disease – small purpuric papules *NEJM 376:775–786, 2017;* Raynaud's phenomenon, digital gangrene, and hyperglobulinemic purpura *BJD 165:1364–1366, 2011*

IKAROS defect *BJD 178:335–349, 2018*

Linear IgA disease *JAAD 22:362–365, 1990*

Lupus erythematosus – systemic lupus erythematosus with thrombocytopenia or vasculitis *JAAD 48:311–340, 2003;* purpuric macules, purpuric urticaria, palpable purpura *BJD 135:355–362, 1996;* with antiphospholipid antibodies – purpura fulminans *Haematologica 76:426–428, 1991;* splinter hemorrhages with vasculitis *Arch Int Med 116:55–66, 1965;* systemic lupus erythematosus – lesions of palate, buccal mucosa, gums; red or purpuric areas with red haloes break down to form shallow ulcers *BJD 135:355–362, 1996; BJD 121:727–741, 1989;* neonatal lupus *JAAD 40:675–681, 1999; Clin Exp Rheumatol 6:169–172, 1988;* follicular petechiae in SLE *BJD 147:157–158, 2002*

Morphea

Pemphigus vulgaris – subungual hematoma *Hautarzt 38:477–478, 1987*

Perforating neutrophilic and granulomatous dermatitis of the newborn – cutaneous eruption of immunodeficiency; papules, plaques, vesicles, crusts, ulcers; boggy pustular masses; purpuric lesions; prominent involvement of palms and soles; sparing of trunk *Ped Derm 24:211–215, 2007*

Periodic fever, immunodeficiency, and thrombocytopenia – severe oral ulcers leading to scarring and microstomy; fever, poor growth, infections, thrombocytopenia *Ped Derm 33:602–614, 2016*

Rheumatoid arthritis – vasculitis – palpable purpura, petechiae *JAAD 53:191–209, 2005; JAAD 48:311–340, 2003; BJD 147:905–913, 2002;* purpuric infarcts of paronychial areas and digital pads (Bywater's lesions) purpuric papules *Cutis 71:462, 464, 2003; BJD 77:207–210, 1965;* bullae of fingertips and toetips with or without

purpura *BJD 77:207–210, 1965;* large hemorrhagic lesions, gangrene with necrotizing arteritis

Rheumatoid neutrophilic dermatosis – edematous plaque, purpuric papules *JAAD 79:1009–1022, 2018*

RNASAEH2 (A-C) deficiency (AGS2-4) *BJD 178:335–349, 2018*

SAMHD1 deficiency (AGS5) *BJD 178:335–349, 2018*

Schwachman-Bodian-Diamond syndrome *BJD 178:335–349, 2018*

Serum sickness *J Invest Allergol Clin Immunol 9:190–192, 1999; Medicine (Balt) 67:40–57, 1988*

Sjogren's syndrome – palpable purpura – vasculitis *NEJM 378:931–939, 2018; A Clinician's Pearls and Myths in Rheumatology pp.107–130; ed John Stone; Springer 2009;* ecchymoses of legs *JAAD 48:311–340, 2003;* cryoglobulinemia, hyperglobulinemic purpura

TREX1 deficiency (Aicardi-Goutieres syndrome) *BJD 178:335–349, 2018*

WIP deficiency, WAS phenotype *BJD 178:335–349, 2018*

Urticaria – purpura due to rubbing

CONGENITAL DISEASES

Injury

Neonatal purpura – deficiency of clotting factors, protein C or protein S deficiency (neonatal purpura fulminans) *Semin Thromb Hemost 16:299–309, 1990;* thrombocytopenia due to maternal ITP or SLE, Rh factor antibodies *Lancet i:137–138, 1989*

Neonatal rubella

Volkmann ischemic contracture, congenital (neonatal compartment syndrome) – upper extremity circumferential contracture from wrist to elbow; necrosis, cyanosis, edema, eschar, bullae, purpura; irregular border with central white ischemic tissue with formation of bullae, edema, or spotted bluish color with necrosis, a reticulated eschar or whorled pattern with contracture of arm; differentiate from necrotizing fasciitis, congenital varicella, neonatal gangrene, aplasia cutis congenital, amniotic band syndrome, subcutaneous fat necrosis, epidermolysis bullosa *BJD 150:357–363, 2004*

Wiskott-Aldrich syndrome

DEGENERATIVE DISORDERS

Digital myxoid cyst – personal observation

Reflex sympathetic dystrophy *JAAD 35:843–845, 1996*

DRUG-INDUCED

Amlodipine *J Postgrad Med 57:341–342, 2011*

Amoxicillin – personal observation

Arthus reaction – erythema, edema, hemorrhage, occasional necrosis

Aspirin

Azathioprine hypersensitivity reaction – occurs within first four weeks of treatment; fever, malaise, arthralgias, myalgias, nausea, vomiting, diarrhea; morbilliform eruption, leukocytoclastic vasculitis, acute generalized exanthematous pustulosis, erythema nodosum, Sweet's syndrome; red papulonodules with pustules *JAAD 65:184–191, 2011*

Axitinib (VEGF inhibitor) – purpuric livedoid vasculopathy of feet *JAMA Derm 152:222–223, 2016*

BCG vaccination – morbilliform or purpuric eruptions with arthralgia, abdominal pain *BJD 75:181–192, 1963*

Bendamustine *Int J Hematol 95:311–314, 2012*

Cabozantinib – VEGFR2 inhibitor; c-met; RET multitargets; tyrosine kinase inhibitor; hand foot skin reactions with bullae, hyperkeratosis, acral erythema; skin and hair depigmentation, splinter hemorrhages, xerosis, red scrotum *JAMA Derm 151:170–177, 2015*

Calcium gluconate extravasation – hematoma *AD 138:405–410, 2002*

Carbamazepine

Chemotherapy-induced eccrine neutrophilic hidradenitis *JAAD 40:367–398, 1999*

Chlorpromazine

Chlorzoxazone – leukocytoclastic vasculitis *BJD 150:153, 2004*

Clindamycin – leukocytoclastic vasculitis – personal observation

Cocaine – levamisole-adulterated; *J Clin Rheumatol 25:e16–26, 2019;* reversible retiform purpura *CMAJ 183:E597–600, 2011;* thrombotic vasculopathy *Am J Med Sci 342:524–526, 2011;* levamisol vasculopathy *Semin Arth Rheum 48:921–926, 2019; Cutis 102:169,170,175, 176, 2018*

Corticosteroid purpura – systemic, inhaled, topical – hands, forearms, and legs *JAAD 54:1–15, 2006*

Coumarin necrosis – acral purpura *JAAD 14:797–802, 1986; Plast Reconstr Surg 48:160–166, 1971;* hemorrhagic plaques of breast, buttock, thighs *JAAD 82:783–796, 2020; JAAD 60:1–20, 2009;* begins as paresthesia, then progresses to edema, petechiae, ecchymosis, hemorrhagic bulla, and necrosis; preferential sites are abdomen, buttocks, thighs, legs, breasts; may occur acrally; associated with protein C deficiency (autosomal dominant); begins 3–5 days after commencing coumarin therapy; also associated with priapism, hepatitis, alopecia, morbilliform eruption *JAAD 61:325–332, 2009; JAAD 60:1–20, 2009; Acta Med Scand 148:453–462, 1954; NYS J Med 43:1121, 1943; Am J Physiol 41:250–257, 1916*

Coumarin purple toe syndrome

Cytarabine – purpuric intertriginous plaques, scalp involvement, papules coalesce into papular purpuric violaceous generalized exanthema, red knee, red feet *JAAD 73:821–828, 2015*

Diclofenac – thrombotic thrombocytopenic purpura *J Med Case Rep 23:190 June 23, 2019*

Dilantin hypersensitivity syndrome

DPT vaccination site – embolia cutis medicamentosa (Nicolau syndrome) *Actas Dermosifiliogr 95:133–134, 2004*

Drug reaction with eosinophilia and systemic symptoms (DRESS) – morbilliform eruption, cheilitis (crusted hemorrhagic lips), diffuse desquamation, areolar erosion, periorbital dermatitis, vesicles, bullae, targetoid plaques, purpura, pustules, exfoliative erythroderma, facial edema, lymphadenopathy *JAAD 68:693–705, 2013; Pharmacotherapy 31:332, 2011;* purpura of legs *AD 146:1373–1379, 2010*

Drug-induced vasculitis – retiform purpura *JAAD 82:783–796, 2020*

EMLA cream *Ped Derm 22:566–568, 2005*

Epidermal growth factor inhibitors – purpura with pustules *JAMA Derm 153:906–910, 2017*

Gold

Griseofulvin

Heparin – heparin-induced thrombocytopenia *JAAD 82:799–816, 2020; Thrombosis Res 100:115–125, 2000;* heparin necrosis with thrombocytopenia and thrombosis *Br J Haematol 111:992, 2000; Ann R Coll Surg Engl 81:266–269, 1999; JAAD 37:854–858, 1997;*

NEJM 336:588–589, 1997; Nephron 68:133–137, 1994; Dermatol 18:138–141, 1993; Clin Exp Dermatol 18:138–141, 1993; low molecular weight heparin *Ann Haematol 77:127–130, 1998;* at injection site *Dermatology 196:264–265, 1998; Thromb Haemost 78:785–790, 1997; Australas J Dermatol 36:201–203, 1995;* bullous hemorrhagic dermatitis *AD 145:603–605, 2009;* heparin, low molecular weight – intraepidermal bullous hemorrhage *BJD 161:191–193, 2009*

Indomethacin

Infliximab – eczematid-like purpura of Doucas and Kapetenakis *JAAD 49:157–158, 2003*

Interferon alfa – as treatment for hepatitis C – pigmented purpuric eruption *JAAD 43:937–938, 2000*

Iodides

IVIG – thrombotic vasculitis *JAAD 55:S112–113, 2006*

Lenalidomide – neutrophilic dermatosis; crusted hemorrhagic ulcerated nodules *JAAD 61:709–710, 2009;* polycyclic pigmented purpuric eruption *JAAD 65:654–656, 2011*

Leukocytoclastic vasculitis, drug-induced *AD 142:155–161, 2006*

Lithium intoxication *Chin Med J (Engl)128:284 Jan 20, 2015*

Meprobamate – pigmented purpuric eruption *JAAD 41:827–829, 1999*

Montelukast – Churg-Strauss syndrome induced by montelukast *BJD 147:618–619, 2002*

Morbilliform drug eruption

Nitroglycerin – pigmented purpuric eruption *JAAD 41:827–829, 1999*

NSAIDs (non-steroidal anti-inflammatory drugs)

Orlistat (pancreatic lipase inhibitor) *Cutis 91:148–149, 2013*

Panitumumab – purpuric drug eruption *J Dermatol 46:e221–222, 2019*

Penicillamine dermatopathy *AD 125:92–97, 1989*

Phenylbutazone

Pigmented purpuric eruptions – drug-induced
    Acetaminophen *JAAD 27:123–124, 1992*
    Ampicillin
    Apremilast *JAMA Derm 153:1197–1198, 2017*
    Aspirin
    Barbiturates
    Bezafibrate
    Carbromal *JAAD 41:827–829, 1999*
    Chlordiazepoxide *JAAD 41:827–829, 1999*
    Cola drink and apple cherry fruit spritzer
    Creatine/hydroxymethylbutyrate
    Dipyridamol
    Energy drink
    5-fluorouracil, topical *JAAD 41:827–829, 1999*
    Furosemide *JAAD 41:827–829, 1999*
    Gefitinib (EGFR inhibitor) – reticulated purpuric eruption *AD 144:269–270, 2008*
    Glipizide *JAAD 41:827–829, 1999*
    Glybuzole
    Herbal medicine *SkinMed 17:138–139, 2019; Explore (NY)14:152–160, 2018*
    Hydralazide
    Hydrochlorthiazide
    Interferon-alpha
    Isotretinoin *JAMA Derm 150:182–184, 2014*
    Medroxyprogesterone acetate
    Meprobamate
    NSAIDS

Nitroglycerin

Phenobarbital

Pseudoephedrine

Reserpine-hydralazine

Sildenafil *Cutan Oculo Toxicol 32:91–92, 2013*

Trichlormethiazide *JAAD 41:827–829, 1999*

Vitamin B1 *JAAD 41:827–829, 1999*

Zomepirac

Propylthiouracil – thrombotic vasculitis – facial and ear purpura *JAAD 41:757–764, 1999;* ANCA+ leukocytoclastic vasculitis *AD 142:879–880, 2006*

Prostacyclin (epoprostenol) – diffuse erythema with or without mottling, exfoliation, or palpable purpura *JAAD 51:98–102, 2004*

PUVA – subungual hemorrhage

Quinidine-induced photosensitive purpuric livedo reticularis *Blood 67:1377–1381, 1986; JAAD 12:332–336, 1985*

Quinine *J Exp Med 107:665–690, 1958;* "cocktail purpura" – immune thrombocytopenia *Am J Kidney Dis 33:133–137, 1999*

Ranitidine (Zantac)

Sedormid *Am J Med 14:605–632, 1953*

Selective serotonin reuptake inhibitors – petechiae, ecchymoses, leukocytoclastic vasculitis *JAAD 56:848–853, 2007*

Sorafenib – splinter hemorrhages *JAAD 60:299–305, 2009;* erythema marginatum hemorrhagicum – annular scalloped hemorrhagic macules *JAAD 64:1194–1196, 2011;* annular leukocytoclastic vasculitis *J Drugs in Dermatol 9:697–698, 2010*

Staphylococcal protein A column immunoadsorption therapy – leukocytoclastic vasculitis *Cutis 64:250–252, 1999*

Sulfonamides

Sunitinib – splinter hemorrhages *BJD 161:1045–1051, 2009;* purpura simplex *Int J Dermatol 58:e153–155, 2019*

Thrombocytopenia, drug-induced – oral hemorrhagic bullae *Cutis 62:193–195, 1998*

Tissue plasminogen activator – painful purpura following tissue plasminogen activator *AD 126:690–691, 1990*

Ustekinumab – leukocytoclastic vasculitis – purpuric necrotic targetoid bullae *J Drugs Dermatol 15:358–361, 2016*

Vancomycin – purpuric drug eruption *Asian Pac J Allergy Immunol 38:47–51, 2020*

Vascular endothelial growth factor receptor (VEGFR) inhibitors – bevacizumab, ranibizumab – mucocutaneous hemorrhage, disturbed wound healing *JAAD 72:203–218, 2015*

EXOGENOUS AGENTS

Agave americana (century plant) dermatitis – palpable purpuric agave dermatitis; linear purpura *Cutis 72:188–190, 2003; Cutis 66:287–288, 2000; JAAD 40:350–355, 1999*

Catheter-related thrombus (sterile) – periungual purpura, splinter hemorrhages, Janeway lesions and Osler's nodes *AD 141:1049, 2005*

Cheut sah – Chinese coin rubbing *JAAD 64:811–824, 2011*

Cocaine abuse – leukocytoclastic vasculitis *Clin Inf Dis 61:1840–1849, 2015; JAAD 59:483–487, 2008;* levamisole contaminating cocaine – retiform purpura; necrotic purpura, purpura of ears, cheeks, and nose; stellate livedo racemosa *JAAD 65:722–725, 2011; JAAD 63:530–535, 2010; J Cutan Pathol 37:1212–1219, 2010;* levamisole with cocaine ANCA+ autoimmune disease with agranulocytosis *JAAD 69:954–959, 2013*

Coral dermatitis *JAMA Derm 155:107, 2019; J Emerg Med 53:e111–113, 2017*

Drug abuse – intra-arterial injection with vasculitis *Int J Dermatol 27:512–513, 1988*

Endovascular devices – microemboli from hydrophilic polymer from endovascular devices – purpuric livedo racemosa *JAAD 73:666–675, 2015*

Foreign body emboli – following cardiac catheterization – purpuric macules of palm *AD 142:1077–1078, 2006*

Intra-arterial injection of polidocanol – retiform purpura *Acta DV 85:372–373, 2005*

Mountain climbers – petechiae *Br Med J 296:822–824, 1992*

Rhus – ingestion of Rhus as folk medicine remedy *BJD 142:937–942, 2000*

Toxic purpura due to capillary damage – arsenic, atropine, bismuth, barbiturates, chloramphenicol, chlorothiazide, chlorpromazine, diethylstilbestrol, gold, hair dye, INH, iodides, menthol, meprobamate, paraaminosalicylic acid, piperazine, quinidine, quinine, reserpine, snake venoms, sodium salicylate, sulfonamides, tartrazine and other food additives *AD 109:49–52, 1974;* thiouracil, tolbutamide, glyceryl trinitrate

Transfusion – post-transfusion purpura; 2–14 days following transfusion; thrombocytopenia due to platelet alloantibodies *Thrombosis Res 100:115–125, 2000*

Weed wacker dermatitis *AD 127:1419–1420, 1991*

INFECTIONS AND INFESTATIONS

Acanthamoeba species *Am J Dermatopath 15:146–149, 1993*

Aeromonas hydrophilia – purpura fulminans *Southeast Asian J Trop Med Public Health 16:532–533, 1985*

African tick bite fever (*Rickettsia africae*) – hemorrhagic pustule, purpuric papules; transmitted by *Amblyomma hebraeum or A variegatum* ticks – high fever, arthralgia, myalgia, fatigue, rash in 2–3 days, with eschar, maculopapules, vesicles, and pustules *AD 148:247–252, 2012; JAAD 48:S18–19, 2003*

AIDS – palatal petechiae

Alternariosis *Cutis 56:145–150, 1995*

Arboviral hemorrhagic fevers

Arenaviruses (hemorrhagic fevers) – Lassa fever (rats and mice) (West Africa), Junin virus (Argentine pampas), Machupo virus (Bolivian savannas), Guanarito virus (Venezuela), Sabia virus (Southeast Brazil), Whitewater virus (California, New Mexico), Tacaribe virus complex (mice) – swelling of face and neck, oral hemorrhagic bullae, red eyes *JAAD 49:979–1000, 2003*

Argentinian hemorrhagic fever

Arthropod bite

Aspergillosis, primary cutaneous – hemorrhagic vesicles, pustules, and nodules *JAAD 12:313–318, 1985;* necrotic purpura *JAAD 53:213–219, 2005; Aspergillus fumigatus* – necrotic purpura with ulcers; verrucous crusted black giant plaque of back *Ped Derm 27:403–404, 2010; Aspergillus fumigatus* – painful, purpuric necrotic papules and pustules in tattoo *BJD 170:1373–1375, 2014*

Avian mite dermatitis – large bruise *Cutis 23:680–682, 1979*

Babesiosis – purpura and ecchymoses due to thrombocytopenia *JAAD 49:363–392, 2003*

Bites – snake, spider, insect, human

Borrelia recurrentis – relapsing fever; louse-borne; tick-borne (*B. duttoni, B hermsi*) – fever and petechial or purpuric rash *J Infect Dis*

140:665–675, 1979; Trans R Soc Trop Med Hyg 65:776–781, 1971; Q J Med 39:129–170, 1970; Medicine 48:129–149, 1969

Boutonneuse fever – *Rickettsia conorii* – petechial, purpuric, or hemorrhagic; Marseilles fever, South African tick fever, Kenya tick typhus, Israel tick typhus, and Indian tick typhus *JAAD 49:363–392, 2003*

Brazilian purpuric fever – *Haemophilus influenzae biogroup aegyptius* strains *J Infect Dis 171:209–212, 1995; Pediatr Infect Dis J 8:239–241, 1989*

Brown recluse spider bite – blister of finger with purpuric base *Clin Inf Dis 32:595,636–637, 2001;* purpuric morbilliform eruption in children at 24–48 hours *JAAD 44:561–573, 2001;* purpuric plaque *Int J Dermatol 39:287–289, 2000;* ecchymosis, ischemic pallor and erythema, livedoid necrosis, eschar *JAMA Derm 150:1205–1208, 2014*

Brucellosis *Cutis 63:25–27, 1999; Ann Trop Paediatr 15:189–192, 1995; Dermatologica 171:126–128, 1985; AD 117:40–42, 1981;* with thrombocytopenic purpura *Clin Inf Dis 31:904–909, 2000*

Bunyavirus hemorrhagic fever (Crimean Congo hemorrhagic fever, Rift Valley fever, Hantavirus) – ticks (Hyalomma genus) petechial eruption orally and on upper trunk *JAAD 49:979–1000, 2003*

Campylobacter jejuni Scand J Urol Nephrol 28:179–181, 1994

Candidiasis – disseminated *Am J Med 80:679–684, 1986;* palpable purpura *JAAD 53:544–546, 2005; Candida krusei AD 131:275–277, 1995;* Candida tropicalis – purpuric papules *Cutis 71:466–468, 2003; C. parapsilosis* emboli *J Dermatol 43:216–217, 2016*

Capnocytophaga canimorsus sepsis – dog and cat bites or scratch; necrosis with eschar; cellulitis, macular and morbilliform eruptions, petechiae, purpura fulminans, symmetrical peripheral gangrene *Cutis 60:95–97, 1997; Eur J. Epidemiology 12 (5)521–533, 1996; JAAD 33:1019–1029, 1995*

Cat scratch disease (*Bartonella henselae*) – petechial exanthem *Ann DV 125:894–896, 1998;* thrombocytopenia *Clin Pediatr (Phila) 41:117–118, 2002*

Caterpillars (*Lonomia*) – fatal hemorrhagic syndrome (disseminated intravascular coagulation); colonies of caterpillars in fruit trees *JAAD 67:331–344, 2012*

Caterpillar dermatitis (*Euproctis crysorrhoea*) – bruising in children *Clin Exp Dermatol 5:261, 1980;* puss caterpillar (larval stage of flannel moth, *Megalopyge opercularis*) – hemorrhagic papulovesicles or bullae *JAAD 62:1–10, 2010; Cutis 71:445–448, 2003;* parallel purpuric linear patches *Cutis 32:114–119, 1990; Lonomia* – hemorrhagic diathesis *JAAD 62:1–10, 2010*

Cellulitis – personal observation

Chikungunya fever – purpura in children *Ped Derm 33:238–240, 2016*

Chromobacterium violaceum JAAD 54:S224–228, 2006

Coccidioidomycosis – hemorrhagic papules or nodules in AIDS *Clin Microbiol Rev 8:440–450, 1995*

Colorado tick fever – *Orbivirus;* macules, papules, petechiae *JAAD 49:363–392, 2003*

Corynebacterium jeikeium endocarditis – palpable purpura *AD 127:1071–1072, 1991*

Covid-19 – retiform purpura *Transl Res 220:1–13, 2020;* autoimmune thrombotic thrombocytopenic purpura *Ann Hematol 99:1673–1674, 2020; J Eur Acad DV April 27, 2020, June 3, 2020; JAAD July2, 2020; Covid Registry;* pediatric inflammatory multisystem syndrome (Kawasaki-like) *JAMA June 8, 2020*

Cowpox – hemorrhagic pustules *JAAD 44:1–14, 2001*

Coxsackie *virus A5,A9,B4,B5,B6* – leukocytoclastic vasculitis – personal observation; Coxsackie A6 – generalized vesicular exanthema

with flexural vesicles; acral purpuric macules of palms and soles *Ped Derm 33:429–437, 2016*

Crimean-Congo hemorrhagic fever (*Bunyavirus*) – fine petechiae of back, then widespread purpura and palatal petechiae *Cutis 87:165–167, 2011*

Cryptococcosis *BMJ Case Rep July 21, 2015; Arch Int Med 138:1412–1413, 1978*

Cytomegalovirus – palpable purpura *AD 126:1497–1502, 1990; JAAD 13:845–852, 1985; JAAD 24:860–867, 1991;* purpura in neonate

AD 130:243–248, 1994; petechiae in neonate due to thrombocytopenia; petechial lesions

Dengue fever (flavivirus) – mosquito vector (Aedes aegypti and Haemogogus species) *JAAD 75:1–16, 2016; JAAD 49:979–1000, 2003; Ann DV 124:237–241,477–478, 1997;* dengue hemorrhagic fever *JAAD 49:979–1000, 2003;* palmar petechiae *JAAD 46:430–433, 2002*

Dysgonic fermenter type 2 sepsis – purpura fulminans *AD 125:1380–1382, 1989*

Ebola virus hemorrhagic fever (Filovirus) – morbilliform exanthem which becomes purpuric with desquamation of palms and soles; ecchymoses, petechiae, high fever, body aches, myalgia, arthralgias, prostration, abdominal pain, watery diarrhea; disseminated intravascular coagulation *JAAD 75:1–16, 2016; Int J Dermatol 51:1037–1043, 2012; JAMA 287:2391–2002; Int J Dermatol 51:1037–1043, 2012; JAAD 65:1213–1218, 2011; MMWR 44, No.19, 382, 1995*

Echovirus 11,19 – petechial rash *Arch Dis Child 57:22–29, 1982;* echovirus 3,4,9,25 *JAAD 49:363–392, 2003*

Ecthyma gangrenosum

Ehrlichiosis – human monocytic ehrlichiosis and leukocytoclastic vasculitis (palpable purpura) *J Int Med 247:674–678, 2000;* human granulocytic ehrlichiosis with acute renal failure mimicking TTP; petechial and purpuric rash of human monocytic ehrlichiosis *Am J Nephrol 19:677–681, 1999; Skin and Allergy News, Oct. 2000, p.40; Ann Int Med 120:736–743, 1994; Ehrlichia chaffeensis* – diffusely erythematous or morbilliform, scattered petechiae or macules *Clin Inf Dis 33:1586–1594, 2001*

Endocarditis – acute or subacute bacterial endocarditis – acral purpura *J Pediatr 120:998–1000, 1992;* splinter hemorrhages *Br Med J ii:1496–1498, 1963*

Enterobacter cloacae sepsis

Epidemic typhus (*Rickettsia prowazeki*) (body louse) – pink macules on sides of trunk, spreads centrifugally; flushed face with injected conjunctivae; then rash becomes deeper red, then purpuric; gangrene of finger, toes, genitalia, nose *JAAD 2:359–373, 1980*

Epstein-Barr virus – flexural purpura *Int J Dermatol 37:130–132, 1998;* infectious mononucleosis (*Epstein-Barr virus*) – petechiae at the junction of the hard and soft palate on the second or third day of fever *JAAD 72:1–19, 2015;* petechial or purpuric exanthems; papular-purpuric gloves and socks syndrome

Escherichia coli – purpura in neonate *J Appl Microbiol 88 Suppl:24S–30S, 2000; AD 130:243–248, 1994; Ann Int Med 109:705–712, 1988*

Exanthem subitum (*HHV-6*) – cutaneous and palatal petechiae *J Ped Hem Onc 24:211–214, 2002*

Filoviruses – Marburg and Ebola virus; transient morbilliform rashes, purpura, red eyes *JAAD 49:979–1000, 2003*

Fire ant stings

Fusarium, disseminated – purpuric papules *JAAD 47:659–666, 2002;* palpable purpura with myositis *JAAD 23:393–398, 1990;*

JAAD 16:260–263, 1987; purpuric eschar; purpuric paronychia *AD 147:1317–1322, 2011;*

Gianotti-Crosti syndrome – papular acrodermatitis of childhood, hemorrhagic variant *Clin Exp Derm 22:301–302, 1997; Ped Derm 8:169–171, 1991*

Gnathostomiasis – including urticarial migratory lesions; intermittent migratory swellings and nodules; subcutaneous hemorrhages along tracks of migration; abdominal pain, nausea and vomiting, diarrhea; South East Asia *JAAD 73:929–944, 2015; JAAD 73:929–944, 2015; JAAD 11:738–740, 1984; AD 120:508–510, 1984*

Gonococcemia (*Neisseria gonorrhea*) – hemorrhagic pustules with halo of erythema *AD 107:403–406, 1973; Arch Int Med 112:731–737, 1963;* gonorrheal conjunctivitis – profuse purulent discharge; swollen hemorrhagic eyelids

Grass mite bites – personal observation

Haemophilus influenzae – sepsis-associated purpura fulminans *N C Med J 46:516–517, 1985*

Hand, foot, and mouth disease – purpura of palms and soles; onycholysis with splinter hemorrhages *BJD 170:748–749, 2014*

Hantavirus hemorrhagic fever – Sin nombre virus, Black Creek Canal virus, Bayou virus, New York virus, Hantaan virus, Seoul virus, Puumala virus, Dobrava virus, Khabarovsk virus – petechial axillary rash, facial flushing, generalized purpura *JAAD 49:979–1000, 2003*

Hepatitis A, B, and C – vasculitis; hepatitis C-associated mixed cryoglobulinemia *AD 131:1185–1193, 1995;* hepatitis C – autoimmune thrombocytopenic purpura *AD 131:1185–1193, 1995;* splinter hemorrhage

Herpes simplex – purpura in neonate *AD 130:243–248, 1994*

Herpes zoster – purpuric, umbilicated, necrotic bullae of leg *Neth J Med 70:189, 195, 2012; Lancet 278:1324 Oct 8, 2011; AD 147:235–240, 2011*

HHV6 and protein S deficiency (anti-protein S antibodies) – disseminated intravascular coagulation *BJD 161:181–183, 2009*

Histoplasmosis *Postgraduate Med 49:226–230, 1971*

HIV – neonatal purpura *JAAD 37:673–705, 1997;* splinter hemorrhage; TTP-like syndrome *Thromb J 16:35 Dec 13, 2018*

Influenza A virus – acute rash, fever, and petechiae *Clin Infect Dis 29:453–454, 1999*

Israel spotted fever – purpura fulminans *Emerging Infect Dis 24:835–840, 2018*

Janeway lesion – faint red macular lesions of thenar and hypothenar eminences *Br J Hosp Med (London)74:139–142, 2013; BMJ Case Rep Sept 6, 2013; AD 137:957–962, 2001; NEJM 295:1500–1505, 1976;* hemorrhagic lesions *Med News 75:257–262, 1899*

Kenya tick typhus – R. conorii

Klebsiella species

Kyasanur Forest disease (*Flavivirus*) – hemorrhagic exanthem, papulovesicular palatine lesions

Lassa fever (*arenavirus*) – morbilliform or petechial rash with conjunctivitis *J Infect Dis 155:445–455, 1985*

Legionella species – DIC *Respir Med Case Rep 19:95–100, 2015*

Leishmaniasis – post kala-azar leishmaniasis

Leprosy – Lucio's phenomenon – hemorrhagic stellate patches *AD 114:1023–1028, 1978;* erythema nodosum leprosum (vasculitis) *AD 111:1575–1580, 1975*

Leptospirosis (Weil's disease) – purpura and jaundice *Medicine 39:117–134, 1960;* Haverhill fever

Listeria monocytogenes – neonatal purpuric, bluish papules of trunk and legs, pustular and morbilliform eruptions *AD 130:245,248,*

1994; painful red papules with central pustulation in veterinarians of arms and hands *Hautarzt 11:201–204, 1960*

Louse-borne relapsing fever (*Borrelia recurrentis*) – high fever, headache, dizziness, myalgias, fatigue, hemorrhage, liver disease, renal failure; relapse ever 7–19 days *JAAD 82:551–569, 2020*

Lyme disease (*Borrelia burgdorferi*) – central purpura or hemorrhagic bulla

Marseilles fever – *Rickettsia conorii*

Marburg virus (filovirus) – maculopapular-vesicular eruption progressing to purpura *S Afr Med J 60:751–753, 1981*

Measles – during prodrome *Can Med Assoc J 8:49, 1918; J Ped 36:35–38, 1950;* atypical measles *BMJ Case Rep Sept 23, 2015; Ann Int Med 90:877–881, 1979*

Mediterranean spotted fever – *Rickettsia conorii*; morbilliform exanthem, spares the face, involves the palms and soles; petechial conjunctival lesions *Ann NY Acad Sci 1166:167–171, 2009; Int J Med Sci 6:126–127, 2009;* petechiae *JAAD 49:363–392, 2003*

Meningococcemia – meningococcal meningitis – scattered petechiae and purpura *NEJM 372:1454–1462, 2015;* acute or chronic (petechial); acute; initially ecchymoses, purpuric papules and plaques with surrounding erythema, vesicles, bullae, hemorrhagic necrosis, purpura fulminans; or chronic (petechial) *Pediatr Infect Dis J 8:224–227, 1989; Rev Infect Dis 8:1–11, 1986;* splinter hemorrhage; purpuric plaque in chronic meningococcemia *BJD 153:669–671, 2005;* meningococcal purpura fulminans *BMC Infect Dis 19:252 March 12, 2019*

Mucormycosis *Semin Resp Crit Care Med 41:99–114, 2020; JAAD 80:869–880, 2019; JAMA Derm 150:79–81, 2014*

Morganella morganii – septic emboli; stellate purpura *JAMA Derm 151:1125–1126, 2015;* retiform purpura *BMJ Case Rep 12:e233344.doi:10.1136/bcr-2019-233344*

Murine typhus (*Rickettsia typhi*) – petechial rash *MMWR 52:1224–1226, 2003;* retiform purpura *Clin Exp Dermatol 42:928–930, 2017*

Mycobacterium tuberculosis – acute miliary *J Clin Inf Dis 23:706–710, 1996;* pulmonary TB with cutaneous leukocytoclastic vasculitis *Infection 28:55–57, 2000;* large crops of blue papules, vesicles, pustules, hemorrhagic papules; red nodules; vesicles become necrotic to form ulcers *Practitioner 222:390–393, 1979; Am J Med 56:459–505, 1974; AD 99:64–69, 1969;* erythema induratum; associated leukocytoclastic vasculitis *Rheum Int 26:1154–1157, 2006*

Mycoplasma pneumoniae – purpura and necrosis *Clin Exp Immunol 14:531–539, 1973*

Necator americanus (hookworm) *Scand J Hematol 30:174–176, 1983*

Necrotizing fasciitis – bruise or purpuric plaque with bullae *AD 138:893–898, 2002; AD 126:815–820, 1990; Surg Gynecol Obstet 154:92–102, 1982;* periorbital edema and ecchymosis *AD 140:664–666, 2004*

North Asian tick-borne typhus – *F. siberica*

Octopus tentacles – curvilinear lesions due to suction purpura; *Int J Dermatol 53:e174–175, 2014; JAAD 61:733–750, 2009*

Omsk hemorrhagic fever (*Flavivirus*) – western Siberia; muskrat hunting

Orf

Oriental spotted fever – R. japonica

Oroya fever – *Bartonella bacilliformis*; petechial or ecchymotic eruption *Ann Rev Microbiol 35:325–338, 1981*

Paecilomyces lilacinus – purpuric macules, hemorrhagic vesicles, hemorrhagic papules *JAAD 39:401–409, 1998*

Papular purpuric gloves and socks syndrome – hepatitis B *BJD 145:515–516, 2001;* also parvovirus B19, measles *JAAD 30:291–292, 1994;*, Coxsackie B6 *AD 134:242–244, 1998;* cytomegalovirus *Dermatology 191:269–270, 1995; Epstein-Barr virus, HHV-6 AD 134:242–244, 1998;* HHV-7, rubella *JAAD 47:749–754, 2002; Arcanobacterium haemolyticum, hepatitis B Oral Dis 10:118–122, 2004;* Parvovirus B19 bullous papular-purpuric gloves and socks syndrome *JAAD 60:691–695, 2009*

Parvovirus B19 – including papular purpuric petechial gloves and socks syndrome *Hum Pathol 31:488–497, 2000; Diagn Microbiol Infect Dis 36:209–210, 2000; JAAD 41:793–796, 1999; Ped Derm 15:35–37, 1998; Clin Infect Dis 27:164–168, 1998; JAAD 27:835–838, 1992; JAAD 25:341–342, 1991;* annular purpura of palms and feet *JAAD 54:896–899, 2006;* generalized petechial exanthem *Pediatrics 125:e787, 2010;* neonatal purpura *JAAD 37:673–705, 1997;* syndrome resembling thrombotic thrombocytopenic purpura *Clin Inf Dis 32:311–312, 2001;* generalized petechial eruption *Clin Pediatr 45:275–280, 2006 JAAD 52:S109–113, 2005;* petechial exanthema in male bathing trunk area *Ped Derm 22:430–433, 2005;* bullous papular-purpuric gloves and socks syndrome *JAAD 60:691–695, 2009*

Phaeohyphomycosis

Plague (*Yersinia pestis*) – purpura, DIC in septicemic plague *JAAD 54:559–578, 2006;* symmetrical peripheral gangrene *AD 135:311–322, 1999*

Pneumococcal cellulitis – hemorrhagic bullae *AD 132:81–86, 1996*

Portuguese man-o'-war (*Physalia physalis*) stings *An Bras Dermatol 87:644–645, 2012; J Emerg Med 10:71–77, 1992*

Proteus mirabilis

Providencia stuartii – septic vasculitis *JAAD Case Rep 6:422–425, 2020*

Pseudomonas aeruginosa – ecthyma gangrenosum in Pseudomonas sepsis *JAAD 11:781–787, 1984; Arch Int Med 128:591–595, 1971;* purpura in neonate *AD 130:243–248, 1994*

Psittacosis – disseminated intravascular coagulation *AD 120:1227–1229, 1984;* splinter hemorrhage

Purpura fulminans (disseminated intravascular coagulation) *JAAD 69:450–462, 2013; AD 124:1387–1391, 1988*
  Candida sepsis
  Capnocytophaga canimorsus Scand J Infect Dis 44:635–639, 2012
  Enterobacter cloacae Int Med 54:2425–2426, 2015
  Escherichia coli Cutis 96:E3–4, 2015; J Clin Microbiol 52:4404–4406, 2014
  Hemophilus influenza NC Med J 46:516–517, 1985
  Indian tick typhus *Indian J Dermatol 62:1–6, 2017*
  Klebsiella oxytoca Intern Med 58:1801–1802, 2019
  Legionella pneumophilia
  Leptospirosis
  Malaria *Braz J Infect Dis 17:712–713, 2013;*

Indian J DV 77:110, 2011
  Meningococcemia *QJM 110:755–756, 2017; Mil Med 181:e1702–1705, 2016*
  Pasteurella multocida *BMJ Case Rep Feb 19, 2014*
  Rocky Mountain spotted fever
  Roseola
  Rubella
  Scarlet fever
  Staphylococcal sepsis *Clin Inf Dis 40:941–947, 2005;* MRSA *Am J Dermatopathol 37:643–646, 2015; Am J Emerg Med 30:1013 July 2012;*
  Streptococcus pneumonia BMJ Case Rep Oct 20, 2017; Actas Dermosifiliogr 104:623–627, 2013; CJEM 16:339–342, 2014

Streptococcus pyogenes, group A, B-hemolytic *Ann Clin Microbiol Antimicrob 17:31 July 9, 2018; Eur J Ped 170:657–660, 2011*
  Streptococcal sepsis Groups A, B, C
  Varicella *Ped Emerg Care 26:932–934, 2010*
  Vibrio parahemolyticus
  West Nile virus, acute *J Clin Virol 75:1–4, 2010*

Puss caterpillar sting – hemorrhagic papules, papulovesicles *Cutis 60:125–126, 1997;* train track purpura *Cutis 71:445–448, 2003*

Q fever – generalized petechiae *Pediatr Infect Dis J 19:358, 2000*

Queensland tick typhus – *Rickettsia australis*

Rat bite fever (*Streptobacillus moniliformis*) – acral hemorrhagic pustules; petechial exanthem *Clin Inf Dis 43:1585–1586;1616–1617, 2006; JAAD 38:330–332, 1998;* palpable purpura *JAMA Derm 152:723–724, 2016*

Reduviid bugs (assassin bugs, kissing bugs) (*Triatominae hemiptera*) – hemorrhagic nodules

Respiratory syncytial virus *Ped Infec Dis J 32:e186–191, 2013; Clin Ped (Phila)32:355–356, 1993*

Rheumatic fever – petechiae; splinter hemorrhage

Rhizopus (zygomycosis) – necrotic purpuric plaque of arm *Ped Derm 31:249–250, 2014*

Rickettsia conorii – purpura fulminans *J Med Case Rep 12:145, May 2018*

Rickettsia parkeri rickettsiosis – Gulf coast tick (*Amblyomma maculatum*); eschar with surrounding petechiae, fever, fatigue, headache, myalgia, arthralgia, morbilliform or vesiculopapular rash of trunk and extremities, palms and soles, and occasionally the face; some lesions with small vesicle or pustule *Clin Inf Dis 47:1188–1196, 2008*

Rift Valley fever

Rocky Mountain spotted fever (*Rickettsia rickettsii*) – initially blanching pink macules, or morbilliform eruption of wrists and ankles; soon spreads to face, trunk, and extremities; palms and soles involved; becomes purpuric with acral gangrene *ASM News 71:65–70, 2005; JAAD 2:359–373, 1980; South Med J 71:1337–1340, 1978*

Rubella – Forscheimer's spots – red macules and petechiae on soft palate *NEJM 369:558, 2013;* congenital rubella – purpuric exanthem

Salmonella – purpura in neonate *AD 130:243–248, 1994;* meningitis with purpura fulminans; typhoid fever presenting as ITP *S Afr Med J 51:3, 1977*

Scarlet fever – Pastia's lines; purpura fulminans; idiopathic thrombocytopenic purpura

Scedosporium – bullous necrotic purpura *Ann DV 125:711–714, 1998; S. apiospermum* – stellate purpura *Cutis 84:275–278, 2009*

Schistosomiasis (*S. japonicum*) – Katayama fever – purpura, arthralgia, systemic symptoms *Dermatol Clin 7:291–300, 1989; S. mansoni* – purpura, urticaria, periorbital edema 4–6 weeks after penetration of the cercaria *Cutis 73:387–389, 2004*

Scrub typhus – *Rickettsia tsutsugamuchi* – fever, headache, myalgia, rash and eschar *Trans R Soc Trop Med Hyg 11:43–54, 2017*

Sea anemone sting

Sepsis – septic vasculitis – retiform purpura *JAAD 82:783–796, 2020;* multiple organisms – neonatal purpura *JAAD 37:673–705, 1997;* purpura of proximal nail folds *Dermatol Clin 33:207–241, 2015;* acral purpura; splinter hemorrhage *J Ped 131:398–404, 1997; Ped 84:1051–1055, 1989*

Septic emboli – with pseudoaneurysms due to *Staphylococcus aureus* following percutaneous transluminal coronary angioplasty;

palpable purpura, petechiae, and livedo reticularis *Cutis 66:447–452, 2000; JAMA Derm 151:1125–1126, 2015;* unilateral stellate purpura of ankle due to *Streptococcus viridans* endocarditis *Cureus 11:e4635, 2019;* aortofemoral bypass graft infection *AD 117:430–431, 1981*

Severe fever with thrombocytopenia (STS bunyavirus) – fever, nausea and vomiting, abdominal pain, myalgia, lymphadenopathy, confusion, headache, conjunctival congestion, and cough *NEJM 364:1523–1532, 2011*

Shigellosis

Smallpox – purpura of palms and soles *Cutis 71:319–321, 2003;*

Snake bites – edema, erythema, pain, and ecchymosis (within 3–6 hours of bite), necrosis *NEJM 347:347–356, 2002*

Solenopsis fugax bites – generalized papular purpuric eruption *An Bras Dermatol 93:570–572, 2018*

South American Arenaviruses (Junin, Machupo, Sabia, Guanarito)

Spider bite – brown recluse spider *J Cutan Med Surg 21:425–437, 2027*

Staphylococcus aureus sepsis *Am J Med 83:801–803, 1987; Staphylococcus aureus* purpura fulminans and toxic shock syndrome *Clin Inf Dis 40:941–947, 2005;* neonatal purpura fulminans due to MRSA *Ped Derm 30:266–267, 2013*

Stenotrophomonas maltophilia Cut Pathol 43:1017–1020, 2016; purpura fulminans *J Dermatol 18:225–229, 1991*

Stingray bite *BJD 143:1074–1077, 2000; Cutis 58:208–210, 1996*

Streptococcus pyogenes group A beta hemolytic toxic shock-like syndrome – hemorrhagic bullae *J Ped Surg 48:e1–3, 2013; AD 131:73–77, 1995;* petechiae; *Group B streptococcus* – purpura in neonate, purpura fulminans *Am J Case Rep 14:315–317, 2013; Ped Hem Onc 27:620–625, 2010*

Streptococcus pneumoniae

Streptococcus suis – meningitis (sensorineural hearing loss) and sepsis; petechiae, ecchymoses, hemorrhagic cutaneous necrosis *Clin Inf Dis 48:617–625, 2009*

Streptococcus viridans, S. mitis, S. bovis

Strongyloides stercoralis – hyperinfection *Clin Inf Dis 59:559,601–602, 2014; JAAD 63:896–902, 2010; AD 146:191–196, 2010; Braz J Inf Dis 9:419–424, 2005; JAAD 49:S157–160, 2003;* periumbilical thumb print parasitic purpura acquired from cadaveric renal transplant *Transplant Inf Dis 13:58–62, 2011; JAAD 31:255–259, 1994;* anasarca, renal failure, serpiginous abdominal purpura *Clin Inf Dis 59:559, 601–602, 2014;* dermoscopy *Int J Dermatol 57:e30–31, 2018*

Subacute bacterial endocarditis – Henoch-Schonlein purpura with SBE *Cutis 69:269–273, 2002;* leukocytoclastic vasculitis *Am J Clin Dermatol 9:71–92, 2008; Clin Dermatol 24:414–429, 2006; JAAD 48:311–340, 2003;* splinter hemorrhage; *S. Bovis* ANCA + vasculitis *Clin Nephrol 62:144–148, 2004*

Tacaribe viruses – Argentinian, Bolivian, and Venezuelan hemorrhagic fevers – erythema of face, neck, and thorax with petechiae *JAMA 273:194–196, 1994; Lancet 338:1033–1036, 1991*

Tick bite – Argasid tick *Centr Afr J Med 26:212–213, 1980;* purpura from tick bite *Am J Med 130:e131–132, 2017*

Tick typhus (Boutonneuse fever, Kenya tick typhus, African and Indian tick typhus) (ixodid ticks) – small ulcer at site of tick bite (tache noire) – black necrotic center with red halo; pink morbilliform eruption of forearms, then generalizes, involving face, palms, and soles; may be hemorrhagic; recovery uneventful *JAAD 2:359–373, 1980*

Tinea corporis – *Trichophyton rubrum* – Majocchi's granuloma (nodular folliculitis) may be hemorrhagic *AD 81:779–785, 1960; AD 64:258–277, 1954;* invasive dermatophyte CARD9 deficiency *NEJM*

369:1704–1714, 2013; STAT3 BJD 179:567–568, 2018; hemorrhagic purpuric leg nodules in transplant patient – invasive *T. rubrum AD 149:475–480, 2013*

Toxic shock syndrome – petechiae and fever Stat Pearls June 28, 2020; Lancet Infect Dis 19:e313–321, 2019

Toxoplasmosis – purpuric nodules *JAAD 14:600–605, 1986;* congenital toxoplasmosis – oval purpuric macules *JAAD 60:897–925, 2009; JAAD 12:697–706, 1985;* petechial eruption

Trichinosis – periorbital edema, conjunctivitis; transient morbilliform eruption, splinter hemorrhages *Can J Public Health 88:52–56, 1997; Postgrad Med 97:137–139, 143–144, 1995; South Med J 81:1056–1058, 1988*

Trichophyton verrucosum (cattle ringworm) – tinea profunda; purpuric plaque of pubis *Ped Derm 33:673–674, 2016*

Trichosporon beigelii, disseminated – purpuric papules and nodules *AD 129:1020–1030, 1993*

Trypanosomiasis – African; edema of face, hands, feet with transient red macular, morbilliform, petechial or urticarial dermatitis; circinate, annular of trunk *AD 131:1178–1182, 1995*

Tularemia *Cutis 54:279–286, 1994*

Varicella, hemorrhagic – varicella with anti-protein S antibodies, protein S deficiency and DIC *J Thromb Haemost 3:1243–1249, 2005; Am J Emerg Med 11:633–638, 1993*

Vasculitis, infectious (not embolic)

Vibrio vulnificus sepsis *BJD 142:386–387, 2000; JAAD 24:397–403, 1991; Am J Gastroenterol 80:706–708, 1985;* edema, erythema, and purpura of ankles *BJD 145:280–284, 2001;* acral purpura and bullae *Arch Int Med 148:1825–1827, 1988*

Viral exanthem, including measles

Viral insect borne and hemorrhagic fevers
   Togavirus – maculopapular/petechial
      Sindbis fever
      Chikungunya fever
      Japanese encephalitis
      O'nyong nyong fever
      Ross river fever *Pathology 47:171–173, 2015*
      Barmah forest fever
   Flavivirus *J Leukoc Biol 106:695–70 1, 2019*
      Dengue fever *Postgrad Med 95:676 Dec 2019; JAAD 58:308–316, 2008*
      West Nile fever
      Kunjin fever
      Usutu – fever, rash, hepatitis *J Neurovirol 26:149–154, 2020*
      Yellow fever
      Zika virus
   Arena virus – maculopapular-petechial
      Guanarito fever
      Lassa fever
      Junin fever
      Machupo fever
      Sabia fever
   Filovirus
      Marburg fever
      Ebola fever
   Bunyavirus
      Bwamba fever
      Rift valley fever
      Crimean/Congo fever
      Hanta virus

Yersinia pseudotuberculosis, enterocolitica

Zika virus – pinpoint red papules coalescing into exanthema; arthralgias, arthritis, conjunctivitis, petechiae of hard palate, headache, lethargy; incubation 3–12 days *Can J Microbiol 66:87–*

98, 2020; JAMA Derm 152:691–693, 2016; Dermatol Online J July 15, 2016

Zygomycosis – purpuric plaque *JAAD 20:989–1003, 1989*

INFILTRATIVE DISEASES

Amyloidosis – primary systemic – petechiae, purpura, ecchymoses in body folds, eyelids, sides of neck, axillae, umbilicus, oral, anogenital areas; periorbital pinch purpura; perianal post-procto-scopic purpura; purpuric halos around cherry angiomas; purpuric papules of eyelids, lips, and nose *JAMA Derm 153:593–594, 2017; NEJM 374:264–274, 2016; JAMA Derm 152:207–208, 2016; AD 148:247–252, 2012; NEJM 349:583–596, 2003; Cutis 48:141–143, 1991; BJD 112:209–211, 1985; Gewebelehre. Berlin: A. Hirschwald: 1858;* easy bruising *JAMA Derm 150:1357–1358, 2014;* nodular tumefactive amyloid; oral hemorrhagic bullae in primary systemic amyloidosis *Oral Surg Oral Med Oral Pathol Oral Radiol Endod 101:734–740, 2006;* hereditary gelsolin amyloidosis (AGel amyloidosis) – cutis laxa with easy bruisability, petechiae, purpura, corneal lattice dystrophy, cranial and peripheral polyneuropathy *BJD 152:250–257, 2005;* secondary systemic (AA amyloidosis) – occasional purpura, easy bruisability *BJD 152:250–257, 2005;* hereditary apolipoprotein A1 amyloidosis – yellow papules, petechiae, purpura *BJD 152:250–257, 2005;* diffuse hemorrhage *Clin Exp Dermatol 33:94–96, 2008;* pinch purpura *Int J Dermatol 98:e195–196, 2019*

Colloid milium – stroke induced purpura *Cutis 56:109–113, 1995;* juvenile colloid milium *JAAD 49:1185–1188, 2003*

Eosinophilic endomyocarditis – Janeway lesions and splinter hemorrhages *JAMA Derm 151:907–908, 2015*

Langerhans cell histiocytosis – crops of red-brown or red-yellow papules, vesicopustules, erosions, scaling, and seborrheic dermatitis-like papules, petechiae, purpura, solitary nodules, bronze pigmentation, lipid infiltration of the eyes, white plaques of the oral mucosa, onycholysis, and onychodystrophy *JAAD 78:1047–1056, 2018; Curr Prob Derm VI Jan/Feb 1994; Clin Exp Derm 11:183–187, 1986; JAAD 13:481–496, 1985;* purpuric papules in the neonate; petechial eruptions *Clin Dermatol 38:223–234, 2020;* masquerading as lichen aureus *Ped Derm 8:213–216, 1991;* Letterer-Siwe disease *JAAD 18:646–654, 1988;* purpuric vesicles *JAAD 37:314–317, 1997;* in adults *Clin Exp Dermatol 30:603–604, 2005;* adult multisystem Langerhans cell histiocytosis – purpuric intertrigo *AD 144:649–653, 2008;* splinter hemorrhages; purpuric nail striae with paronychia *Ped Derm 37:18–183, 2020*

Mastocytosis – urticaria pigmentosa; ecchymoses *Eur J Dermatol 5:237–239, 1995*

Self-healing reticulohistiocytosis – purpuric papules in the neonate

Xanthoma disseminatum – intertriginous violaceous-yellow purpuric papules, confluent xanthomatous plaques in axillae, groin, other folds; face, eyelids, chest upper back, globe of eyeball *AD 147:459–464, 2011*

INFLAMMATORY DISEASES

Acute generalized exanthematous pustulosis – pustules, purpura, fever and rash – etiologies include multiple drugs, mercury, enterovirus, adenovirus, Epstein-Barr virus, cytomegalovirus, hepatitis B virus, *Mycoplasma pneumoniae Ped Derm 17:399–402, 2000*

Cullen's sign – periumbilical hemorrhage with hemorrhagic pancreatitis *Gastroenterology 115:253, 2018; QJM 170:315, 2017; Int J Surg Case Rep 3:143–146, 2012; Am J Obstet Disorders in Women and Child 78:457, 1918*

Endometriosis, cutaneous – of umbilicus (Villar's nodule_ *Int J Women's Dermatol 6:214–215, 2020*

Eosinophilic panniculitis *JAAD 12:161–164, 1985*

Erythema multiforme *Medicine 68:133–140, 1989; JAAD 8:763–765, 1983*

Erythema nodosum, late – bruised appearance (erythema nodosum contusiforme) – personal observation;

Grey-Turner sign – purpura of flank associated with retroperitoneal hemorrhage (hemorrhagic pancreatitis) *Stat Pearls Jan 13, 2019; Intern Emerg Med 10:387–388, 2015; Br J Surg 7:394–395, 1920*

Histiocytic cytophagic panniculitis – ecchymotic nodules with or without ulceration *JAAD 20:177–185, 1989*

Lipophagic granulomatous panniculitis – mimics purpura *Clin Exp Rheumatol 20:432, 2002*

Neutrophilic eccrine hidradenitis – purpuric nodules *JAAD 38:1–17, 1998; JAAD 26:793–794, 1992; JAAD 23:1110–1113, 1990*

Pyoderma gangrenosum *Br J Plast Surg 53:441–443, 2000; JAAD 18:559–568, 1988;* may resemble purpura fulminans

Rosai-Dorfman disease – vasculitis-like lesions *JAAD 46:775–778, 2002*

Sarcoid – splinter hemorrhages; pigmented purpuric-like *J Dermatol 4:629–631, 2015; Eur J Dermatol 21:110–111, 20122*

Subcutaneous fat necrosis of newborn

Urticaria multiforme – wheals, fever, arcuate, annular, polycyclic lesions; ecchymotic center or central pallor; edema of hands and feet; aged 4 months to 4 years *Cutis 89:260:262–264, 2012; Pediatrics 119:e1177–1183, 2007*

METABOLIC DISEASES

Alpha-1 antitrypsin deficiency – ecchymotic panniculitis – personal observation; *BJD 174L753, 762, 2010; JAAD 33:913–916, 1995*

Angiokeratoma corporis diffusum – Fabry's disease – purpura –like appearance (alpha galactosidase A) – angiokeratomas mimicking purpura *Ped Derm 19:85–87, 2002; NEJM 276:1163–1167, 1967;* petechia-like *Arch Dermatol Syphil 43:187, 1898;* fucosidosis (alpha-I-fucosidase) *AD 107:754–757, 1973;* Kanzaki's disease (alpha-N-acetylgalactosidase) *AD 129:460–465, 1993;* aspartylgly-cosaminuria (aspartylglycosaminidase) *Paediatr Acta 36:179–189, 1991;* adult-onset GM1 gangliosidosis (beta galactosidase) *Clin Genet 17:21–26, 1980;* galactosialidosis (combined beta-galactosi-dase and sialidase) *AD 120:1344–1346, 1984;* no enzyme deficiency

Antithrombin III deficiency *JAAD 82:799–816, 2020*

Blueberry muffin baby – widespread blue, purple, or red macules papules or nodules of trunk, head, and neck; may develop pete-chiae on surface
   Dermal erythropoiesis (erythroblastosis fetalis)
      Congenital infections (TORCH)
         Rubella
         Cytomegalovirus
         Coxsackie B2
         Syphilis
         Toxoplasmosis
         Herpes simplex
        Hereditary spherocytosis
      Rh incompatibility
        ABO blood-group incompatibility
        Twin-twin transfusion syndrome
      Neoplastic infiltrates
        Congenital leukemia
        Neuroblastoma

Congenital rhabdomyosarcoma
Other disorders
Neonatal lupus erythematosus

Calciphylaxis – retiform purpura; livedo racemosa; calciphylaxis with stellate necrosis and retiform purpura unassociated with renal disease; associated with hypoalbuminemia, malignancy, systemic corticosteroid therapy, coumarin, chemotherapy, systemic inflammation, cirrhosis, protein C or S deficiency, obesity, rapid weight loss, infection *JAAD 82:783–796, 2020; JAMA Derm 149:946–949, 2013; AD 145:451–458, 2009*

Chronic renal failure – ecchymoses *Lancet ii:1205–1208, 1988;* splinter hemorrhage

Coagulopathy – coagulation defects usually present with large ecchymoses without petechiae

Cold agglutinins *JAAD 82:799–816, 2020*

Congenital disorders of glycosylation (CDG-Ix) – nuchal skin folds, facial dysmorphism, inverted nipples, hypoplastic nails, petechiae and ecchymoses, edema; neurologic, gastrointestinal and genitourinary abnormalities, pericardial effusion, ascites, oligohydramnios *Ped Derm 22:457–460, 2005*

Cryofibrinogenemia *JAAD 82:799–816, 2020; AD 144:405–410, 2008; Am J Med 116:332–337, 2004*

Cryoglobulinemia – retiform purpura *JAAD 82:799–816, 2020;* ecchymoses, palpable purpura *JAAD 48:311–340, 2003; JAAD 13:636–644, 1985;* pustules and purpura of feet – pustular cryoglobulinemic vasculitis *AD 147:235–240, 2011*

Cushing's syndrome *Ped Derm 15:253–258, 1998*

Factor V Leiden *JAAD 82:783–796, 799–816, 2020*

Interstitial cryoglobulinosis – non-palpable petechial purpura, necrotic ulcers, hemorrhagic bullae; renal failure *JAAD 77:1145–1158, 2017*

Cystic fibrosis-associated episodic arthritis – pink macules, urticarial papules, arthritis, purpura of legs, erythema nodosum, cutaneous vasculitis *JAMA Derm 155:375–376, 2019; Respir Med 88:567–570, 1994; Am J Dis Child 143:1030–1032, 1989; Ann Rheum Dis 47:218–223, 1988; Arch Dis Child 59:377–379, 1984*

cystic fibrosis – leukocytoclastic vasculitis – personal observation; splinter hemorrhages

Diabetes mellitus – hemorrhagic plantar callus

Dysproteinemias
Cryofibrinogenemia
Cryoglobulinemia – mixed cryoglobulinemia *NEJM 374:74–81, 2016*
Hypergammaglobulinemic purpura of Waldenstrom *JAAD 23:669–676, 1990; Acta Med Scand 266 (Suppl):931–946, 1952*
Hyperglobulinemia (polyclonal) due to sarcoid, lupus erythematosus, Sjogren's syndrome, myeloma
Lambda light chain vasculopathy; kappa light chains and IgA vasculitis *Clin Lymphoma Myeloma Leuk 11:373–374, 2011*

Essential thrombocythemia *JAAD 82:799–816, 2020*

Ethyl malonic aciduria and normal fatty acid oxidation – petechiae *J Ped 124:79–86, 1994*

Fanconi's anemia – skeletal abnormalities *BJD 178:335–349, 2018*

Fucosidosis – red papules, purpura, short stature *Ped Derm 24:442–443, 2007*

Galactosialidosis – autosomal recessive; combined deficiency of beta-galactosidase and neuraminidase; due to defect of lysosomal protein (prospective protein); angiokeratoma corporis diffusum; macular cherry red dots and petechia; conjunctival telangiectasia, telangiectasias of joints, Mongolian-like spots, café au lait macules, skin hyperextensibility, nevus of Ito *BJD 149:405–409, 2003*

Gamma heavy chain disease – vascular nodules *JAAD 23:988–991, 1990*

Gray platelets, idiopathic purpura (acquired platelet dysfunction with eosinophilia)- *NBEAL2* mutation *J Ped Hematol Oncol 41:47–50, 2019; Platelets 29:632–635, 2018*

Hemochromatosis – splinter hemorrhages

Hemolytic uremic syndrome *JAAD 82:799–816, 2020*

Hemophilia

Hemorrhagic disease of the newborn *JAAD 37:673–705, 1997*

Hereditary clotting factor deficiencies *JAAD 37:673–705, 1997*

Hypercoagulable state *JAAD 82:783–796, 799–816, 2020*

Hyperhomocysteinemia *JAAD 783–796, 799–816, 2020*

Hypothyroidism – purpura and ecchymoses *JAAD 26:885–902, 1992*

Hypothrombinemia (vitamin K deficiency)

Idiopathic thrombocytopenic purpura

Kwashiorkor

Liver disease, acute or chronic; splinter hemorrhage; chronic active hepatitis – allergic capillaritis

Mitral stenosis – splinter hemorrhages

Monoclonal gammopathy – leukocytoclastic vasculitis *J Dermatol 45:1009–1012, 2018; JAAD 43:955–957, 2000*

Multiple sclerosis – splinter hemorrhages

Myxedema – pancytopenia *Case Rep Med July 14, 2019*

Neonatal purpura fulminans – ecchymoses of limbs at sites of pressure in first day of life; enlarge rapidly, hemorrhagic bullae with central necrosis; homozygous protein C or protein S deficiency *Semin Thromb Hemost 16:299–309, 1990*

Oxalosis – retiform purpura *JAAD 82:783–796, 2020*

Paroxysmal nocturnal hemoglobinuria – petechiae, ecchymoses, red plaques which become hemorrhagic bullae with necrosis; lesions occur on scalp, legs, abdomen, chest, nose, and ears; fever; acute edema of head and face *JAAD 82:799–816, 2020; AD 148:660–662, 2012; JAAD 53:1090–1092, 2005; AD 138:831–836, 2002;* livedo racemosa, painful ecchymoses, purpura, hemorrhagic bullae, ulcers; mutation *PIGA* gene which encodes glycosylphosphatidylinositol-anchored proteins (decrease in GPI proteins in cell membranes); complement-induced intravascular hemolysis; increased thrombosis *BJD 171:908–910, 2014;* purpura fulminans *Eur J Dermatol 26:397–398, 2016*

Platelet abnormalities – immune platelet destruction – post-transfusion, antilymphocyte globulin, ITP, marrow transplant, alloimmune neonatal thrombocytopenia, maternal autoimmune thrombocytopenia (ITP, lupus), drug-related immune thrombocytopenia; primary platelet production/function defects – bone marrow aplasia, thrombocytopenia with absent radii syndrome, Wiskott-Aldrich syndrome, Fanconi syndrome, congenital amegakaryocytic thrombocytopenia, giant platelet syndromes (Bernard-Soulier, May-Hegglin), trisomy 13 or 18, Alport syndrome variants, gray platelet syndrome, Glanzmann thrombasthenia, Hermansky-Pudlak syndrome – all are causes of neonatal purpura *JAAD 82:799–816, 2020; JAAD 37:673–705, 1997;* thrombocytopenia – bone marrow aplasia, uremia, alcohol, drugs, leukemia, lymphoma, myeloma, myelofibrosis; consumption – hemolytic-uremic syndrome, thrombotic thrombocytopenic purpura; hypersplenism; abnormal platelet function; thrombocytopenia – usually demonstrates petechiae; thrombopathia, thrombasthenia, von Willebrand's disease, severe anemia, fibrinogen; thrombocythemia – livedo reticularis, acrocyanosis, erythromelalgia, gangrene, pyoderma gangrenosum

Porphyria – itching purpura-like dermatitis *Arch Klin Exp Derm 223:128–135, 1965;* erythropoietic protoporphyria – petechiae and ecchymoses *BJD 155:574–581, 2006; Eur J Pediatr 159:719–725, 2000; J Inherit Metab Dis 20:258–269, 1997; BJD 131:751–766, 1994; Curr Probl Dermatol 20:123–134, 1991; Am J Med 60:8–22, 1976;* splinter hemorrhages

Prolidase deficiency – autosomal recessive; skin spongy and fragile with annular pitting and scarring; leg ulcers; photosensitivity, telangiectasia, purpura, premature graying, lymphedema *Ped Derm 13:58–60, 1996; JAAD 29:819–821, 1993; AD 127:124–125, 1991; AD 123:493–497, 1987*

Protein C deficiency with purpura fulminans – necrotic purpura in neonatal protein C deficiency *Pediatr Hematol Oncol 18 (7):453–458, 2001; AD 124:1387–1391, 1988;* purpuric plaque with thrombotic vasculopathy *JAAD 82:799–816, 2020; Neonatology Netw 30:153–159, 2011; Ped Derm 24:57–60, 2007*

Protein S deficiency – purpura at IV site *JAAD 82:799–816, 2020;* retiform purpura *Actas Dermosifiliogr 107:430, 2016*

Prothrombin III mutation *JAAD 783–796, 799–816, 2020*

Pulmonary disease – splinter hemorrhages

Red blood cell occlusion – sickle cell disease, thalassemia, hereditary spherocytosis, severe malaria *JAAD 82:799–816, 2020*

Ruptured ectopic pregnancy – periumbilical hemorrhage and pigmentation *JAAD 72:1066–1073, 2015; Can Med Assoc J 85:1003–1004, 1961*

Scurvy – large ecchymoses and fresh hemorrhage; perifollicular hemorrhage with hemosiderin staining of legs; hemorrhagic gingivitis, stomatitis, epistaxis *NEJM 379:282–289, 2018; JAAD 76:S52–54, 2017; NEJM 374:1369–1374, 2016; AD 148:1073–1078, 2012; Ped Derm 28:444–446, 2011; AD 146:1167–1172, 2010; Cutis 86:205–207, 2010; AD 145:195–200, 2009; JAAD 59:901–903, 2008; NEJM 357:392–400, 2007; Int J Dermatol 45:909–913, 2006; AD 142:658, 2006; Oral Surg Oral Med Oral Pathol Oral Radiol Oral Endodontol 100:688–692, 2005; Am J Hematol 74:85–87, 2003; Ann DV 127:510–512, 2000; Cutis 66:39–44, 2000; JAAD 41:895–906, 1999; AD 120:1212, 1984; NEJM 314:892–902, 1986;* palpable purpura *AD 139:1363–1368, 2003;* purpura of legs *JAMA 1911–1912, 2011;* upper eyelid ecchymoses *Arch Ophthalmol 117:842–843, 1999;* splinter hemorrhages ; corkscrew hairs in 10 year old boy *Ped Derm 28:444–446, 2011*

Splenomegaly – platelet sequestration

Thrombocytopenia – congenital; idiopathic thrombocytopenic purpura; drug hypersensitivity, post-transfusion, DIC, Kasabach-Merritt syndrome, prosthetic heart valves, thrombotic thrombocytopenic purpura, uremia; aplastic anemia, bone marrow suppression; functional platelet disorders (Bernard-Soulier syndrome, Glanzmann's disease, storage pool disease, von Willebrand's disease)

Thrombotic thrombocytopenic purpura – ADAMTS13 *JAAD 82:799–816, 2020; Blood Adv 26:1510–1516, 2018*

Uremia – purpura, ecchymoses

Vitamin A intoxication – ecchymoses *NEJM 315:1250–1254, 1986*

Waldenstrom's hyperglobulinemic purpura *J Neurol Sci 367:275–277. 2016' JAAD 72:374–376, 2015; Indian J DV Leprol 77:205–208, 2011*

NEOPLASTIC DISEASES

Angioimmunoblastic T-cell lymphoma *JAAD 38:992–994, 1998; JAAD 36:290–295, 1997; Dermatol Clin 3:759–768, 1985;* acral petechiae *JAAD 46:325–357, 2002;* purpura fulminans *Cutis 95:113–115, 2015;* morbilliform eruption; arthralgias, purpura,

petechiae, urticaria, nodules *JAAD 65:855–862, 2011; NEJM 361:900–911, 2009; BJD 144:878–884, 2001; JAAD 36:290–295, 1997; JAAD 1:227–32, 1979;*

Angiosarcoma *JAAD 34:308–310, 1996;* of face and scalp – bruise-like *Cutis 76:313–317, 2005; JAAD 50:867–874, 2004; Sem Cut Med Surg 21:159–165, 2002; JAAD 38:143–175, 1998; JAAD 38:310–313, 1998;JAAD 38:837–840, 1998; BJD 76:21–39, 1964;* Stewart-Treves angiosarcoma – bruise-like (purple plaque) *JAMA Derm 151:1226–1229, 2015; Cutis 89:129–132, 2012; JAAD 38:837–840, 1998;* hemorrhage ulcerated nodule in chronic lymphedema *AD 146:337–342, 2010;* multilobulated large tumor *Cutis 83:91–94, 2009*

Atrial myxoma – palpable purpura, splinter hemorrhages, petechiae of hands and feet *Cutis 62:275–280, 1998; JAAD 32:881–883, 1995*

Blastic plasmacytoid dendritic cell neoplasm – purpuric plaque; ecchymotic-like lesion *BJD 169:579–586, 2013;* violaceous nodule with golden contusiform rim *JAMA Derm 150:73–76, 2014;* bruising of face and shoulder *JAMA Derm 150:1109–110, 2014*

Cytophagic histiocytic panniculitis – manifestation of hemophago-cytic syndrome; purpuric red tender nodules; may evolve into T-cell lymphoma, B-cell lymphoma, histiocytic lymphoma, sinus histiocyto-sis with massive lymphadenopathy (Rosai-Dorfman disease) *JAAD 4:181–194, 1981; Arch Int Med 140:1460–1463, 1980*

Dermatofibrosarcoma protuberans – bruise-like nodule of buttocks in infancy *Ped Derm 25:317–325, 2008*

Eccrine pilar angiomatous nevi – bruise-like (ecchymotic) hairy nodules *Cutis 71:449–455, 2003; Ped Derm 13:139–142, 1996; JAAD 29:274–275, 1993; Am J Dermatopathol 14:161–164, 1992; NY State J Med 68:2803–2806, 1968; AD 96:552–553, 1967; Dermatologica 127:9–16, 1963*

Essential thrombocythemia *JAAD 24:59–63, 1992*

Extramedullary hematopoiesis in chronic myelogenous leukemia – bruises or myelofibrosis with central nodule *Ann Int Med 735–738, 1979*

Hemophagocytic lymphohistiocytosis (hemophagocytic syndrome) – erythroderma and edema *J Dermatol 33:628–631, 2006; AD 138:1208–1212, 2002; J Pediatr 130:352–357, 1997; AD 128:193–200, 1992*

Intravascular lymphomatosis (malignant angioendotheliomatosis) – purpuric papules, plaques, and nodules with overlying telangiecta-sias *AD 128:255, 258, 2003; JAAD 18:407–412, 1988*

Intravascular B-cell lymphoma *JAAD 67:e238–240, 2012; Am J Dermatopathol 30:295–299, 2008*

Kaposi's sarcoma – mimicking a bruise *Dermatol Clin 24:509–520, 2006; JAAD 38:143–175, 1998;* periorbital edema with ecchymosis-like appearance *JAAD 59:179–206, 2008*

Leukemia cutis –*BJD 143:773–779, 2000;* congenital leukemia (AML) (purpuric papules or nodules in the neonate) *JAAD 54:S22–27, 2006;* acute myelogenous leukemia with leukemic vasculitis – purpuric plaque of scalp *JAMA Derm 152:571–572, 2016;* acute lymphocytic leukemia – widespread purpura *Cutis 93:228,241–242, 2014;* adult T-cell leukemia *BJD 152:350–352, 2005; JAAD 13:213–219, 1985;* T-cell prolymphocytic leukemia – facial purpuric plaques; petechial periorbital eruption *JAAD 55:467–477, 2006;* acute leukemia in children (viral-induced purpura) *AD 134:319–323, 1998;* congenital monocytic leukemia *Ped Derm 6:306–311, 1989;* gingival hemorrhage *Oral Surg 55:572–578, 1983;* splinter hemorrhages natural killer cell CD 56- large granular lymphocytic leukemia – purpuric ulcerated plaques *JAAD 62:496–501, 2010;* purpuric and ulcerated nodules – aleukemic leukemia cutis with T-cell acute lymphoblastic leukemia *Ped Derm 28:535–537, 2011*

Leukemic vasculitis – retiform purpura *JAAD 82:783–796, 2020*

Lymphoma – pigmented purpuric eruption *Cutis 94:297–300, 2014; JAAD 19:25–31, 1988;* lichen aureus-like CTCL *JAAD 60:359–375, 2009; BJD 142:564–567, 2000; BJD 62:177–178, 1950;* lichenoid pigmented purpuric eruption of Gougerot-Blum *Dermatology 205:191–193, 2002;* pigmented purpuric eruption-like *Ped Derm 23:350–354, 2006; JAAD 19:25–31, 1988;* CTCL with malignancy of FOXP3 regulatory cells – erosive and ulcerative hemorrhagic pyoderma gangrenosum-like lesions *JAAD 61:348–355, 2009;* primary cutaneous peripheral T-cell lymphoma – purpuric plaques *BJD 164:677–679, 2011;* HTLV-1 leukemia/lymphoma – purpura *Blood 117:3961–3967, 2011; JAAD 36:869–871, 1997;* intravascular large cell lymphoma – purpuric patches *JAAD 39:318–321, 1998;* angiotropic large cell lymphoma presenting as TTP *Cancer 75:1167–1170, 1995;* cutaneous T-cell lymphoma (CTCL) *JAAD 46:325–357, 2002; JAAD 19:25–31, 1988;* CTCL presenting as pigmented purpuric eruption *Dermatology 207:246–247, 2003; J Eur Acad Dermatol Venereol 15:62–64, 2001; JAAD 39:858–863, 1998; Am J Dermatopathol 19:108–118, 1997; JAAD 8:417, 1983;* angiotropic B cell lymphoma (malignant angioendotheliomatosis) – hemorrhagic papules, nodules, and plaques; natural killer T-cell (CD 56+) lymphoma – bruise like circumscribed swelling (contusiform lesions) (purpuric plaque) *BJD 144:432–434, 2001; BJD 142:1021–1025, 2000; Am J Surg Pathol 20:202–210, 1996;* lymphomatoid granulomatosis (angiocentric lymphoma) – red, brown, or violaceous plaques with epidermal atrophy and purpura *JAAD 20:571–578, 1989; AD 124:571–576, 1988;* CD56+ natural killer cell lymphoma – contusiform lesions *AD 132:550–553, 1996;* adult T-cell lymphoma/leukemia *JAAD 46:S137–141, 2002;* splinter hemorrhages in CTCL; blastic NK-lymphoma associated with myelodysplastic syndrome – ecchymotic lesions of skin and tongue *BJD 149:869–876, 2003;* hematodermic/plasmacytoid dendritic cell CD4+ CD56+ lymphoma – bruise-like lesions *JAAD 58:480–484, 2008; Blood 99:1556–1563, 2002;* MALT lymphoma – purpuric papules *AD 145:955–958, 2009;* intravascular B-cell lymphoma – white blood cell occlusion *JAAD 82:799–816, 2020; Am J Dermatopathol 30:295–299, 2008;* primary cutaneous epidermotropic CD8+ T-cell lymphoma – mixture of patches, plaques, papulonodules with central ulceration, necrosis, and hemorrhage *JAAD 62:300–307, 2010;* primary cutaneous anaplastic large cell lymphoma – ulcerated purpuric nodule of nasal tip *Ped Derm 28:570–575, 2011;* disseminated mantle cell lymphoma – petechial morbilliform eruption *JAMA Derm 150:94–96, 2014; ;* autoimmune lymphoproliferative syndrome due to germline *FAS* mutation – petechiae *NEJM 369:853–863, 2013;* CD8+ cutaneous T-cell lymphoma – pigmented purpuric eruption-like patches *JAAD 77:489–496, 2017*

Melanocytic nevus, traumatized

Melanoma – hematoma-like melanoma metastases *JAAD 55:1106–1107, 2006; JAAD 49:912–913, 2003;* subcutaneous metastatic melanoma with overlying ecchymoses *AD 144:561–562, 2008; Br J Plast Surg 56:76, 2003; ;* primary dermal melanoma – pedunculated pink papule, dark macule, blue pigmented nevus, dome-shaped hemorrhagic papule, changing pigmented nevus *JAAD 71:1083–1091, 2014*

Merkel cell tumor

Metastases – telangiectatic metastatic breast carcinoma – purpuric plaque *Cancer 59:1184–1186, 1987;* malignant mesothelioma of testis *AD 131:483–488, 1995;* carcinoma telangiectatica – purpuric plaques

Multiple myeloma – ecchymosis *AD 127:69–74, 1991*

Myelodysplastic syndromes *JAAD 33:187–191, 1995;* granuloma annulare in myelodysplastic syndrome *JAAD 38:106–108, 1998*

Squamous cell carcinoma of cervix – post-coital bleeding *NEJM 370:2031, 2014*

Waldenstrom's macroglobulinemia – reticulate purpura and bullae *Clin Exp Dermatol 26:513–517, 2001;* acral purpura or mucosal bleeding due to hyperviscosity *JAAD 45:S202–206, 2001;* cryoglobulin-associated purpura, leukocytoclastic vasculitis *JAAD 45:S202–206, 2001;* petechiae *Int J Dermatol 55:e361–362, 2016*

Waldenstrom's IgM storage papules – skin colored translucent papules on extensor extremities, buttocks, trunk; may be hemorrhagic, crusted, or umbilicated *JAAD 45:S202–206, 2001*

PARANEOPLASTIC DISEASES

Chilblains in chronic lymphocytic leukemia – personal observation

Eosinophilic dermatosis of myeloproliferative disease – face, scalp; scaly red nodules; trunk – red nodules; extremities – red nodules and hemorrhagic papules *AD 137:1378–1380, 2001*

Paraneoplastic pemphigus – hemorrhagic bullae *JAAD 27:547–553, 1992*

Paraneoplastic vasculitis – leukocytoclastic vasculitis – palpable purpura, petechiae *J Rheumatol 18:721–727, 1991; Medicine 67:220–230, 1988;* paraneoplastic Henoch-Schonlein purpura *Cutis 81:131–137, 2008; JAAD 55:S65–70, 2006;* granulomatous vasculitis with lymphoma, chronic myelogenous leukemia, or preleukemia *JAAD 14:492–501, 1986;* in chronic myelogenous leukemia *Am J Med 80:1027–1030, 1986*

PHOTODERMATOSES

Actinic purpura – Bateman's purpura – hands, forearms, and legs *J Eur Acad DV 32:e383–384, 2018; J Drugs in Dermatol 10:718–722, 2011; Dermatol Clin 5:109–1121, 1987*

Hydroa vacciniforme – purpuric blisters *Ped Derm 18:71–73, 2001*

Photodermatitis (phototoxic)

Phototherapy-induced purpura in transfused neonates due to transient pophyrinemia *Ped Derm 31:e152–153, 2014; J Drugs Dermatol 10:306–307, 2011; Pediatrics 100:360–364, 1997*

Purple nails – phototoxicity, numerous causes

Sunburn purpura

Solar purpura *AD 124:24–25, 1988;* mimics leukocytoclastic vasculitis *Pathology 45:484–488, 2013*

Sunlight *J R Soc Med 79:423–424, 1986*

PRIMARY CUTANEOUS DISEASES

Angina bullosa hemorrhagica (blood blisters) *Br Dent J 180:24–25, 1996; JAAD 31:316–319, 1994*

Atopic dermatitis

Cutis laxa, acquired

Darier's disease – hemorrhagic stellate macules with blistering on palms *JAAD 27:40–50, 1992; Hautarzt 51:857–861, 2000; AD 89:523–527, 1964;* splinter hemorrhages

Dermatosparaxis – easy bruisability *AD 129:1310–1315, 1993*

Dyshidrosis – hemorrhagic dyshidrosis *Clin Exp Derm 13:342–343, 1988*

Epidermolysis bullosa simplex, Ogna variant – autosomal dominant; plectin abnormality; seasonal blistering of hands and feet, bruising, hemorrhagic bullae, onychogryphotic first toenails *Hum Hered 23:189–196, 1973;* may mimic child abuse

Erythema annulare centrifugum – purpura, rarely

Erythema craquele – linear hemorrhage or purpura; personal observation

Erythema elevatum diutinum *BJD 67:121–145, 1955*

Febrile ulceronecrotic pityriasis lichenoides et varioliformis acuta *Ped Derm 22:360–365, 2005*

Granuloma annulare – resembling septic emboli in myelodysplastic syndrome *JAAD 38:106–108, 1998*

Hematidrosis – spontaneous bleeding of skin *AD 148:960–961, 2012*

Keratosis lichenoides chronica – facial purpuric lesions in children *JAAD 56:S1–5, 2007*

Lichen nitidus *AD 105:430–431, 1972; Acta DV 238–246, 1959;* purpuric palmar lichen nitidus *Acta DV 91:108–109, 2011; Clin Exp Dermatol 13:347–349, 1988;* oral purpuric papules *Acta DV (Stockh)39:238–246, 1959*

Lichen planus,- hemorrhagic nails in bullous lichen planus *JAMA Derm 151:674–675, 2015;* resolving lichen planus; lichen planus pigmentosus inversus *JAAD 60:359–375, 2009*

Lichen sclerosus et atrophicus – vulvar purpura *Ped Derm 31:95–98, 2014; Ped Derm 10:129–131, 1993*

Nummular dermatitis

Perioral dermatitis

Pigmented purpuric eruptions *Dermatologica 140:45–53, 1970*
  Associated with dental abscesses *JAAD 46:942–944, 2002*
  Cutaneous T-cell lymphoma – presenting as pigmented purpuric eruption *Cutis 94:297–300, 2014; Eur J Dermatol 21:272–273, 2011*
  Eczematoid-like pigmented purpuric eruption of Doukas and Kapetanakis *Ped Derm 32:291–292, 2015*
  Familial pigmented purpuric eruptions (Schamberg's or purpura annularis telangiectoides *Dermatologica 132:400–408, 1966*
  Gougerot and Blum (lichenoid PPE) *AD 144:405–410, 2008; Bull Soc Fr Deratol Syphiligr 32:161, 1925*
  Granulomatous pigmented purpuric eruption *An Bras Dermatol 94:582–585, 2019; Cutis 100:256–258, 2017;* Blaschkoid distribution *Clin Exp Dermatol 40:387–390, 2015; Am J Dermatopathol 3:146–148, 2012*
  Gravitational purpura (acroangiodermatitis) – minute purpuric macules coalescing into plaques of lower legs and feet *AD 92:515–518, 1965*
  Itching purpura of Doucas and Kapetenakis *Cutis 25:147–151, 1980; AD 91:351–356, 1965*
  Lichen aureus – resembles a bruise; red-brown papules *AD 144:1169–1173, 2008; JAAD 8: 417–420, 1983;* Blaschko distribution *Ped Derm 33:351–352, 2016*
  Majocchi's purpura – purpura annularis telangiectoides *Eur J Dermatol 29:546–547, 2019; G Ital J Cutan Dis 33:129–141, 1915; Mal Vener Pelle 31:263–264, 1896;* variant is purpura telangiectatic arciformis of Touraine *Z Haut-u Geschlkrankh 17:331–336, 1957*
  Meprobamate, carbromal, phenacetin, hydrochlorothiazide Schamberg's disease *An Bras Dermatol 92:246–248, 2017; JAMA Derm 149:223–228, 2013; BJD 13:1–5, 1901*
  Palmoplantar purpura in pigmented purpuric eruptions *Cutis 40:109–113, 1987*
  Zosteriform pigmented purpura (lichen aureus-like) *Int J Dermatol 30:654–655, 1991; Dermatologica 180:93–95, 1990; Hautarzt 40:373–375, 1989;* associated with deep vein thrombosis *Int J Dermatol 53:e87–88, 2014*

Pigmented purpuric stomatitis *Oral Surg 74:780–782, 1992*

Pityriasis lichenoides et varioliformis acuta – personal observation

Pityriasis rosea, purpuric *Indian J DV Leprol 80:551–553, 2014; JAAD 28:1021, 1993;* purpuric PR with palatal petechiae *Dermatologica 160:142–144, 1980*

Purpura simplex (female easy bruising syndrome) – thighs of women

Relapsing annular erythema (neutrophilic figurate erythema of infancy) – facial, polycyclic borders; may be bullous, purpuric, or targetoid *Ped Derm 37:209–210, 2020;* recurrent annular erythema with purpura – leukocytoclastic vasculitis *BJD 135:972–975, 1996; Ann DV 192:457, 2002*

Splinter hemorrhages *JAAD 50:289–292, 2004*

Spontaneous atrophic patches in extremely premature infants *AD 132:671–674, 1996*

Striae atrophicae

PSYCHOCUTANEOUS DISEASES

Anorexia nervosa – thrombocytopenia *Am J Clin Dermatol 6:165–173, 2005;* diffuse reticulate purpura (malnutrition associated capillary hyperpermeability and supporting tissue fragility) *Intern Med 58:2417, 2019; CMAJ 187:E514, 2015; Dermatol Sinica 21:68–74, 2003*

Factitial purpura *Ped Derm 21:205–211, 2004; Clin Exp Dermatol 17:238–239, 1992;* suction purpura of chin from drinking glass *AD 106:238–241, 1972; Clin Pediatr 10:183–184, 1971*

Factitial traumatic panniculitis *JAAD 13:988–994, 1985;* factitial dermatitis *Ped Derm 32:604–608, 2015; Ped Derm 26:597–600, 2009*

Psychogenic purpura *Clin Paediatr 21:700–704, 1985*

SYNDROMES

Achenbach's syndrome – paroxysmal hematoma of the finger – mimics bruising or steroid atrophy *BJD 132:319, 1995; Medizinische 52:2138–2140, 1958*

Acrogeria – thin skin *Dermatol Clin 5:109–1121, 1987*

Antiphospholipid antibody syndrome – petechiae, purpura, ecchymoses, splinter hemorrhages *JAAD 82:799–816, 2020; NEJM 346:752–763, 2002; Semin Arthritis Rheum 31:127–132, 2001; JAAD 36:149–168, 1997; JAAD 36:970–982, 1997; BJD 120:419–429, 1989*

Baboon syndrome – intertriginous follicular purpura *BJD 150:788–789, 2004*

Behcet's disease – palpable purpura *BJD 147:331–336, 2002; JAAD 40:1–18, 1999; JAAD 41:540–545, 1999; NEJM 341:1284–1290, 1999; JAAD 36:689–696, 1997;* bullous necrotizing vasculitis *JAAD 21:327–330, 1989;* splinter hemorrhages

CADASIL (cerebral autosomal dominant arteriopathy with subcortical infarcts and leucencephalopathy) – petechiae and purpura *BJD 152:346–349, 2005*

Congenital insensitivity to pain – bruises, burns, lacerations, and fractures mimicking child abuse *Pediatr Emerg Care 12:116–121, 1996*

Dercum's disease (adiposis dolorosa) – painful peri-articular lipomas and ecchymoses *JAAD 44:132–136, 2001*

Dyskeratosis congenita – pancytopenia *BJD 178:335–349, 2018*

Ehlers-Danlos syndrome – types I, II – easy bruising *JAAD 19:656–666, 1988;* type IV (ecchymotic type); type V *Rook p.2032–2038, 1998, Sixth Edition;* type VI – blue sclerae, scleral fragility, joint hypermobility, skin hyperextensibility, easy bruising, atrophic scarring, marfanoid habitus, scoliosis, neonatal hypotonia, arterial dissection; type VIII – autosomal dominant; skin fragility, abnormal scarring, severe early periodontitis with loss of adult dentition by end of third decade; cigarette paper scars of shin;

marfanoid habitus (tall, long limbs, arachnodactyly); triangular face, prominent eyes, thin nose, prematurely aged appearance, thin skin with prominent veins, no joint hypermobility, easy bruising, blue sclerae *JAAD 55:S41–45, 2006; Ped Derm 18:156–158, 2001; Heritable Disorders of Connective Tissue, 4th Ed, St. Louis: Mosby 1972;* simulating child abuse *AD 120:97–101, 1984;* periodontal EDS – type VIII; periodontitis, marked skin fragility, over shins, pretibial bruising, cigarette paper scars, atrophy, wrinkling, skin thin and translucent with visible venous pattern, marfanoid habitus with triangular face, long nose, thin philtrum; decrease types III and I collagen *BJD 158:825–830, 2008; Ped Derm 24:189–191, 2007; Clin Pediatr 34:552–555, 1995; Clin Oral Investig 4:66–69, 2000; Birth Defects 13:85–93, 1983; JAAD 5:297–303, 1981*

Familial cold urticaria

Familial Mediterranean fever – purpuric lesions of face, trunk, extremities; lesions of Henoch-Schonlein purpura *Acta Paediatr 89:177–182, 2000; AD 134:929–931, 1998; J Rheumatol 24:323–327, 1997; Eur J Pediatr 155:540–544, 1996; J Rheumatol Suppl 35:1–9, 1992; Am J Med 43:227–253, 1967;* neutrophilic lobular panniculitis – subcutaneous red nodules of extremities with contusiform changes *JAMA Derm 150:213–214, 2014*

Gardner-Diamond syndrome (painful bruising syndrome) (auto-erythrocyte sensitization) – arms and legs *J Clin and Aesthet Dermatol 12:44–46, 2019; J Cutan Med Surg 22:607, 2018; JAAD 27:829–832, 1992; Ann Med Interne (Paris)125:323–332, 1974; Blood 10:675–690, 1955;* autosensitization to DNA *Ann Int Med 60:886–891, 1964;* zebra stripe and annular purpura *BJD 164:672–673, 2011*

Hemophagocytic syndrome (hemophagocytic lymphohistiocytosis) (familial hemophagocytic syndrome) – morbilliform eruptions, purpuric macules, acral blanching red macules, erythroderma and edema *JAAD 56:302–316, 2007; AD 138:1208–1212, 2002;AD 128:193–200, 1992;* fever, pancytopenia, lymphadenopathy, hepatomegaly, splenomegaly, neurologic, joint, purpura, morbilliform eruption, kidney, and cardiac involvement, central nervous system dysfunction *Eur Rev Med Pharmacol Sci, 16:1414–1424, 2012; Genes Immunol 13:289–298, 2012;* familial hemophagocytic lymphohistiocytosis – seborrheic dermatitis with purpura; ichthyosis-like *Ped Derm 28:494–501, 2011*

   Familial HLH – known genetic defects (perforin)
   Immune deficiencies
      Chediak-Higashi syndrome
      Griscelli syndrome
      X-linked lymphoproliferative syndrome
   Acquired
      Infections
      Endogenous products
      Rheumatic diseases
      Neoplasms

Hermansky-Pudlak syndrome – platelet defects with oculocutaneous albinism *Orphanet J Rare Dis Feb 21, 2019; BJD 178:335–349, 2018; Platelets 29:91–94, 2018; Ped Derm 34:638–646, 2017;*

Histiophagocytic syndrome – ecchymoses, purpura, palpable purpura *Am J Med 93:177–180, 1992; AD 128:193–200, 1992*

Hutchinson-Gilford syndrome (progeria) – easy bruisability; bruising due to loss of subcutaneous tissue *JAMA Derm 150:197–198, 2014; Am J Med Genet 82:242–248, 1999; J Pediatr 80:697–724, 1972*

Hypereosinophilic syndrome associated with T-cell lymphoma – splinter hemorrhages *JAAD 46:S133–136, 2002*

Hyper-IgD syndrome – autosomal recessive; red macules or papules, urticaria, red nodules, urticaria, combinations of periodic fever, arthritis, arthralgias, and rash, annular erythema, and pustules, abdominal pain with vomiting and diarrhea, lymphade-

nopathy; elevated IgD and IgA – mevalonate kinase deficiency *Ped Derm 22:138–141, 2005; AD 136:1487–1494, 2000; AD 130:59–65, 1994; Medicine 73:133–144, 1994; Lancet 1:1084–1090, 1984*

IgG4-related disease – cutaneous plasmacytosis (papulonodules); pseudolymphoma; angiolymphoid hyperplasia with eosinophilia; Mikulicz's disease; psoriasiform dermatitis; morbilliform eruption; hypergammaglobulinemic purpura; urticarial vasculitis; ischemic digits; Raynaud's disease and digital gangrene *BJD 171:929,959–967, 2014*

Kabuki syndrome – idiopathic thrombocytopenic purpura, vitiligo, developmental delay, short stature, congenital heart defects, skeletal defects, cleft palate, dental abnormalities, cryptorchidism, lip pits, prominent fingertip pads, autoimmune disorders, blue sclerae, prominent eyelashes, thinning of central eyebrows, protuberant ears *Amer J Med Genet 132A:260–262, 2005*

Kasabach-Merritt syndrome – thrombocytopenia and purpura associated with Kaposiform hemangioendothelioma or tufted angioma; enlargement, tenderness, induration, and ecchymosis occur within the vascular lesion; consumptive coagulopathy with hemorrhage *Ped Derm 11:79–81, 1994; Am J Dis Child 59:1063–1070, 1940*

Kawasaki's disease *Ped Derm 36:274–282, 2019*

Marfan's syndrome

MELAS syndrome *J Neurol Sci 103:37–41, 1991; J Dermatol 18:295–301, 1991*

Neutrophilic dermatosis (pustular vasculitis) of the dorsal hands – variant of Sweet's syndrome – hemorrhagic pustular nodules *AD 138:361–365, 2002*

Neurofibromatosis – purpura in plexiform neurofibromas in NF-1 *AD 137:233–234, 2001*

Niemann-Pick disease – autosomal recessive; sphingomyelinase deficiency; purpuric lesions *Medicine 37:1–95, 1958*

Noonan's syndrome – easy bruising *Ped Derm 20:447–450, 2003*

Osteogenesis imperfecta *Postgrad Med J 76:743–749, 2000*

Partial lipodystrophy, complement abnormalities, vasculitis – macroglossia, polyarthralgia, mononeuritis, hypertrophy of subcutaneous tissue *Ann DV 114:1083–1091, 1987*

POEMS syndrome *JAAD 37:887–920, 1997; JAAD 40:808–812, 1999*

Premature aging syndromes – hands, forearms, and legs

Progeria – thin skin *Dermatol Clin 5:109–1121, 1987*

Pseudoxanthoma elasticum

Relapsing polychondritis – palpable purpura *Clin Exp Rheumatol 20:89–91, 2002;* purpura *Medicine 80:173–179, 2000*

Shulman's syndrome – eosinophilic fasciitis; hemorrhage *JAAD 1:221–226, 1979; Ann Rheum Dis 36:354–359, 1977*

Sjogren's syndrome – splinter hemorrhages; dependent purpura; annular purpura *J Korean Med Sci 15:115–118, 2000;* macular and palpable purpura *Seminars Arthr Rheum 29:296–304, 2000*

Sneddon's syndrome – retiform purpura; occlusive non-vasculitic vasculopathy *Am J Dermatopathol 39:637–662, 2017; Hemato Oncol Clin NA 22:67–77, 2008; JAAD 36:970–982, 1997; BJD 122:115–116, 1990*

Sweet's syndrome – chronic recurrent Sweet's syndrome of myelodysplasia – purpuric plaques *AD 142:1170–1176, 2006;* giant cellulitis-like; bullae and purpura *JAMA Derm 149:79–83, 2013*

Tumor necrosis factor (TNF) receptor 1-associated periodic fever syndromes (TRAPS) (same as familial hibernian fever, autosomal dominant periodic fever with amyloidosis, and benign autosomal dominant familial periodic fever) – erythematous patches, tender red plaques, fever, annular, serpiginous, polycyclic, reticulated, and migratory patches and plaques (migrating from proximal to distal), urticaria-like lesions, lesions resolving with ecchymoses, conjunctivitis, periorbital edema, myalgia, arthralgia, abdominal pain, headache; Irish and Scottish predominance; mutation in TNFRSF1A – gene encoding 55kDa TNF receptor *AD 136:1487–1494, 2000; Mayo Clin Proc 72:806–817, 1997*

Wells' syndrome – blaschkolinear purpura *J Drugs Dermatol 16:1036–1038, 2017*

Werner's syndrome – thin skin *Dermatol Clin 5:109–1121, 1987*

Whipple's disease (*Tropheryma whipplie*) – non-palpable purpura, chronic leg edema, arthralgias; large dilated abdominal lymphatics; diarrhea, weight loss, abdominal pain, generalized hyperpigmentation, pulmonary hypertension, eye, cardiovascular, and neurologic disease *Clin Infect Dis 41:519–520,557–559, 2005*

Wiskott-Aldrich syndrome – dermatitis of scalp, face, flexures, napkin area with petechiae and purpura; Xp11.22–11.23; WASP gene – actin polymerization *BJD 178:335–349, 2018; Ped Derm 24:417–418, 2007; Cell Mol Life Sci 61:2361–2385, 2004; Semin Hematol 35:332–345, 1998; J Pediatr 125:876–885, 1994; Int J Dermatol 24:77–81, 1985*

TOXINS

Chemicals

TRAUMA

Accidental bruising – mimicking child abuse

Air emboli *JAAD 82:783–796, 2020*

Altitude injury – petechiae and hemorrhagic bullae of external auditory canal in pilots descending from high altitudes *Laryngoscope 56:225–236, 1946*

Asphyxia – facial congestion, facial edema, cyanosis, periorbital or conjunctival petechiae *JAAD 64811–824, 2011*

Bathtub suction purpura *Ped Derm 21:146–149, 2004*

Bite marks – human bite marks; annular erythema with central bruising *JAAD 64:811–824, 2011*

Black dot heel (talon noir) *JAAD 55:290–301, 2006*

Bungee jumping *Unfauchirurg 98:447–448, 1995*

Callus, hemorrhagic

Cephalohematoma

Chilblains, resolving

Child abuse – bruising of protected sites (upper arms, axillae, medial and posterior thighs, hands, palms or soles, inner wrists, trunk, cheeks, earlobes, ears, neck, genitalia, dorsal feet, buttocks, and oral mucosa); child under 9 months of age; bruising away from bony prominences; multiple bruises in clusters; bruises in defined pattern or with imprint of an implement; cutaneous and physical injuries other than bruises *JAAD 57:371–392, 2007; Child Abuse and Neglect 30:549–555, 2006; Arch Pathol Lab Med 130:1290–1296, 2006; Arch Dis Child 90:182–186, 2005;* petechiae; erythema and petechia of ear due to head slap *Ped Derm 23:311–320, 2006;* traumatic asphyxia *JAAD 23:972–974, 1990;* oral petechiae at junction of hard and soft palate *Ped Derm 23:311–320, 2006;* linear and arcuate purpura – human bites *Ped Derm 33:223–224, 2016*

Chin purpura *Arch Ped 25:280–282, 2018*

Coin rubbing ("cao gio") (Southeast Asia); "cheut sah" (Chinese) – intercostal spaces, glabella, elbow and knee flexures *JAAD 64:811–824, 2011; Am J Forensic Med Pathol 15:257–260, 1994*

Coma blisters – stellate purpura or hemorrhagic bullae *JAAD 27:269–270, 1992*

Crack fingers, crack cocaine hands – fingertip burns *An Bras Dermatol 88:850–852, 2013; Cutis 50:193–194, 1992*

Cupping *JAAD 57:371–392, 2007; Aust J Dermatol 12:89–96, 1971*

Deep dissecting hematoma in dermatoporosis *AD 144:1303–1308, 2008*

Doughnut

Ecchymoses of median raphe of penis *Br J Vener Dis 49:467–468, 1972*

Exercise-induced leukocytoclastic vasculitis of the legs – palpable purpura *Cutis 83:319–322, 2009; AD 145:601–602, 2009*

Exercise-induced purpura *Ped 2019 April 143(4) e20182797. doi:10.1542/peds.2018–2797;* periorbital exercise-induced purpura *Ped 215:277, 2019*

Fat embolism syndrome – persistent somnolence, fever, tachycardia, respiratory symptoms, petechial eruption *JAAD 82:783–796, 2020; NEJM 375:370–378, 2016*

Flip-flop vasculitis – exercise induced; purpuric papules of dorsal feet *JAMA Derm 149:751–756, 2013*

Frostbite

GAGA ball purpura – waffle-like purpuric patches *Ped Derm 35:406–407, 2018*

Golfer's purpura *J Eur Acad DV 30:1403–1404, 2016*

Hemiscrotal ecchymosis – torsion of spermatic cord with testicular infarction of neonate; high venous pressure during delivery *Br Med J 298:1492–1493, 1989*

Hypothermia – platelet sequestration

Ice pack dermatosis – red plaque, retiform purpura with purpuric papules and ulcers *JAMA Derm 149:1314–1318, 2013*

Increased transmural pressure gradient
    Acute – Valsalva, coughing, vomiting, childbirth, weight lifting, suction purpura *G Ital DV 151:570–571, 2016*
    Chronic – venous stasis

Irritant contact dermatitis – linear purpura of legs due to laser waxing and depilatory *Ped Derm 37:190–191, 2020*

Kidney biopsy – periumbilical purpura

Laser hair removal *J Med Case Rep 12:60 Feb 27, 2018*

Loom band purpura – purpura of fingers *Ped Derm 33:667–668, 2016*

Mechanical trauma

Physical injuries

Paintball purpura *JAAD 53:901–902, 2005; Cutis 75:157–158, 2005*

Passion marks

Penile fracture – edema and purpura of penis *NEJM 372:1055, 2015;* hematoma of entire shaft of penis *Genital Skin Disorders, Mosby, 1998, p.9*

Penile purpura – rough sex

Physical trauma to vessels

Piano glissando purpura *J Eur Acad DV 30:683, 2016*

Press stroking (gua sha) *Int J Dermatol 52:892–893, 2013; Complement Ther Med 20:340–344, 2012*

Opera glove

Powerlifter's purpura – neck purpura *Cutis 70:93–94, 2002*

Rubbing or scratching any dermatosis (urticaria/atopic)

Seizures *Seizure 7:337–339, 1998*

Sports related injuries – black dot heel, black palm, petechia of ankles in long distance runners, hardball injury (ping-pong patch), annular purpura of legs with aerobics, tennis or jogger's toe (subungual purpura), splinter hemorrhages

Suction cup – forehead ecchymosis *Cutis 18:216, 1976*

Suction pump injuries *Forensic Sci Med Pathol 11:626–628, 2015*

Traumatic asphyxia *JAAD 23:972–974, 1990*

Vacuum extraction during child birth

Valsalva purpura

Vibex (linear purpura)

Video game playing with thrombocytopenia – purpura of palmar aspects of first phalanges *Cutis 97:35–38, 2016*

VASCULAR DISEASES

Acquired progressive lymphangioma (benign lymphangioendothelioma) – abdomen, thigh, calf; bruise or bruise-like plaque *JAAD 37:656–657, 1997; JAAD 23:229–235, 1990; JAAD 31:362–368, 1994; J Cutan Pathol 19:502–505, 1992; JAAD 24:813–815, 1991; AD 124:699–701, 1988*

Acral pseudolymphomatous angiokeratoma – cobblestoned pink and purpuric plaque of heel *JAAD 76:S25—27, 2017*

Acroangiodermatitis (gravitational purpura) *AD 92:515–518, 1965*

Acute hemorrhagic edema of infancy (Finkelstein's disease) (Seidlmayer's purpura) – purpura in cockade pattern of face, cheeks, eyelids, and ears; may form reticulate pattern; edema of penis and scrotum *Ped Derm 36:274–282, 2019; Cutis 102:359–362, 2018; Clin Inf Dis 61:1553,1624–1625, 2015; JAMA 309:2159–2160, 2013; JAAD 59:684–695, 2008; Ped Int 45:697–700, 2003; Cutis 68:127–129, 2001; J Dermatol 28:279–281, 2001; Cutis 61:283–284, 1998; AD 130:1055–1060, 1994; JAAD 23:347–350, 1990; JAMA 61:18–19, 1913;* annular purpura *AD 146:1037–1042, 2010;* necrotic lesions of the ears, urticarial lesions; oral petechiae *JAAD 23:347–350, 1990; Ann Pediatr 22:599–606, 1975;* edema of limbs and face *Cutis 68:127–129, 2001*

ANCA vasculitis = retiform purpura *JAAD 82:783–796, 2020*

Angiokeratoma circumscriptum – petechial appearance *Ped Derm 23:192–193, 2006*

Angioma serpiginosum – petechial appearance *Postgrad Med J 67:1065–1066, 1991; AD 92:613–620, 1965*

Arterial catheterization – unilateral splinter hemorrhages

Atherosclerosis – acral purpura

Benign lymphangioendothelioma – slow growing red or bruise-like plaque *Histopathology 35:319–327, 1999; Am J Surg Pathol 26:328–327, 2002*

Capillary fragility

Capillary leak syndrome – large ecchymoses *BJD 150:150–152, 2004*

Cholesterol emboli – livedo racemosa of flank *JAMA Derm 151:97–98, 2015;* acral purpura *JAAD 82:783–796, 2020 ;JAAD 55:786–793, 2006; BJD 146:511–517, 2002; Medicine 74:350–358, 1995; Angiology 38:769–784, 1987; AD 122:1194–1198, 1986;* splinter hemorrhages

Dependent purpura

Diffuse dermal angiomatosis (benign reactive angioendotheliomatosis) – red-brown or violaceous nodules or plaques with petechiae or ecchymoses on face, arms, or legs *JAAD 40:257–259, 1999; JAAD 38:143–175, 1998;* with arteriosclerotic peripheral vascular disease *AD 138:456–458, 2002*

Disseminated intravascular coagulation, including purpura fulminans, symmetrical peripheral gangrene) – obstetric complications, extensive tissue damage, gram-negative septicemias, immune reactions, malignancy, snake bites, angiomas, protein S or protein C deficiency *JAAD 82:783–796, 2020; Br Med J 312:683–687, 1996; BJD 88:221–229, 1973*

Elder abuse *JAAD 68:533–542, 2013*

Emboli – septic, fat, air, cholesterol, marantic; retiform purpura *JAAD 82:783–796, 2020;* atheromatous (cholesterol crystal emboli); fat emboli – petechiae of upper trunk 2 days after major trauma *Lancet 1:284–285, 1976; Lancet ii:825–828, 1960;* infectious organisms – septic emboli from infected pseudoaneurysms following coronary angioplasty *Cutis 66:447–452, 2000;* cardiac myxomas – petechiae, splinter hemorrhages *BJD 147:379–382, 2002;* tumor emboli, traumatic aneurysm; septic emboli *JAMA Derm 151:1125–1126, 2015;* unilateral palpable purpura – septic emboli infected aortofemoral bypass graft *AD 117:430–431, 1981*

Eosinophilic granulomatosis with polyangiitis – purpuric patches, stellate purpura; palpable purpura, hemorrhagic lesions *JAMA Derm 154:486–487, 2018; Autoimmunol Rev 14:341–348, 2015; JAAD 48:311–340, 2003; AD 141:873–878, 2005; AD 139:715–718, 2003; JAAD 48:311–340, 2003; JAAD 47:209–216, 2002; JAAD 47:209–216, 2002; JAAD 37:199–203, 1997; JAAD 27:821–824, 1992; JID 17:349–359, 1951; Am J Pathol 25:817, 1949; Mayo Clinic Proc 52:477–484, 1977;* purpura and petechiae of legs *JAAD 37:199–203, 1997;* acral purpura of finger and/or toe tips *Cutis 67:145–148, 2001;* necrotic purpura of scalp *Ann DV 122:94–96, 1995;* presenting as purpura fulminans *Clin Exp Dermatol 29:390–392, 2004;* with ischemic strokes *J Stroke Cerebrovasc Dis 21:911, 2012*

Eosinophilic vasculitis syndrome *Sem Derm 14:106–110, 1995;* eosinophilic vasculitis in connective tissue disease *JAAD 35:173–182, 1996;* recurrent cutaneous necrotizing eosinophilic vasculitis – palpable purpura; necrosis *BJD 149:901–902, 2003; Acta DV 80:394–395, 2000;* with angioedema *AD 130:1159–1166, 1994*

Equestrian perniosis – annular, arcuate, concentric purpuric plaques of lateral thighs *JAMA Derm 153:83–84, 2017*

Eruptive capillary angiomas

Glomeruloid angioendotheliomatosis – red purpuric patches and acral necrosis – associated with cold agglutinins *JAAD 49:887–896, 2003*

Granulomatosis with polyangiitis – purpuric papules *NEJM 382:1750–1758, 2020;* acneiform facial and truncal lesions with crusted necrotic papules, ulcers; palpable purpura *JAAD 72:859–867, 2015;* petechiae, palpable purpura, facial purpuric plaque *JAAD 48:311–340, 2003; AD 130:861–867, 1994; JAAD 10:341–346, 1984;* splinter hemorrhages *Eur J Ped 173:1685–1689, 2014*

Hemangioma – infantile hemangioma with pseudoecchymotic stain *JAAD 50:875–882, 2004;* acquired elastotic hemangioma *JAAD 47:371–376, 2002*

Henoch-Schonlein purpura (anaphylactoid purpura) *NEJM 369:1843, 2013; Curr Opin Rheumatol 22:598–602, 2010; Int J Dermatol 48:1157–1165, 2009; JAAD 48:311–340, 2003; Semin Arthritis Rheum 32:149–156, 2002; Arthritis Rheum 40:859–864, 1997;* hemorrhagic vesicles and bullae *Ped Derm 12:314–317, 1995; Berl Klin Wochenschr 11:641–643, 1874;* C4 deficiency *JAAD 7:66–79, 1982;* upper eyelid ecchymoses and edema *Acta DV 97:1160–1166, 2017; Arch Ophthalmol 117:842–843, 1999*

Hypersensitivity vasculitis – fever and petechiae

Hypocomplementemic urticarial vasculitis

Idiopathic thrombocytopenic purpura *Hem Am Soc Hem Educ Program 2019:561–567, 2018*

IgA vasculitis – retiform purpura *JAAD 82:783–796, 2020*

Infantile hemangiomas with minimal or arrested growth – bruise-like appearance; telangiectatic patch; red plaques; more often on lower body *AD 146:971–976, 2010*

Intravascular microemboli from polymer coats of intravascular device – hemorrhagic panniculitis presenting as ecchymosis; nodules of buttocks, arms, and trunk *JAMA Derm 151:204–207, 2015*

Kaposiform hemangioendothelioma – red-blue tumid swelling; red plaque or nodule with ecchymotic or purpuric border *Ped Derm 19:388–393, 2002; JAAD 38:799–802, 1998; AD 133:1573–1578, 1997;* purpuric macules *JAAD 38:799–802, 1998; Am J Surg Pathol 17:321–328, 1993;* kaposiform hemangioendothelioma of mediastinum and neck – periorbital edema and ecchymoses *Ped Derm 26:331–337, 2009;* Kaposiform hemangioendothelioma with Kasabach-Merritt syndrome – livedoid enlarging bruise of back *JAMA Derm 149:1337–1338, 2013; AJDC 59:1063–1070, 1940*

Kasabach-Meritt syndrome – purpura with edema; associated with tufted angioma *Ped Derm 35:635–638, 2018; Ped Derm 26:347–348, 2009;* associated with hemangiopericytoma *Br J Plast Surg 48:240–242, 1995;* associated with angiosarcoma *Acta DV 88:193–194, 2008;* giant congenital hemangioma of scalp *Eur J Pediatr 166:619–620, 2007; AJDC 59:1063–1070, 1940*

Livedoid vasculopathy (atrophie blanche en plaque; atrophie blanche with summer ulceration) – painful purpuric papules and plaques; leg and ankle ulcers; atrophic white scars; livedo reticularis *JAAD 69:1033–1042, 2013;* petechiae early *JAAD 8:792–798, 1993; AD 119:963–969, 1983*

Livedoid purpura *JAMA Derm 151:659–660, 2015*
  Lucio's phenomenon
  Purpura fulminans
  Anti-phospholipid antibodies
  Cholesterol emboli
  Levamisole
  Perniosis

Lymphatic malformation

Lymphangioma; lymphangiomatous malformation with overlying bruises *AD 122:1065–1070, 1986; JAAD 5:663–667, 1983*

Acquired progressive lymphangioma (benign lymphangioendothelioma) – red plaque with bruise-like appearance at borders *Ped Derm 35:486–489, 2018*

Lymphangiosarcoma (Stewart-Treves tumor) – red-brown or ecchymotic patch, nodules, plaques in lymphedematous limb; bruising in lymphedematous extremity *Arch Surg 94:223–230, 1967; Cancer 1:64–81, 1948*

Macular arteritis – reticulated purpuric macules mimicking pigmented purpuric eruption *Ped Derm 26:93–95, 2009;* asymptomatic hyperpigmented macules of legs in black patients *JAAD 52:364–366, 2005; JAAD 49:519–522, 2003*

Marantic emboli *JAAD 82:783–796, 2020*

Microscopic polyangiitis *AD 133:4474–477, 1997*

Petechial cherry angiomas – personal observation

Polyarteritis nodosa – palpable purpura, livedo, nodules, urticaria, skin necrosis with ulcers *BJD 159:615–620, 2008; JAAD 48:311–340, 2003;* petechiae or gross hemorrhage *JAAD 31:561–566, 1994;* cutaneous infarcts presenting as purpuric plaques; microscopic polyarteritis nodosa (polyangiitis) – arthralgias, leg ulcers, fever, livedo, nodules, urticaria, palpable purpura, petechiae, ecchymoses, acral bullae, plantar red plaque *BJD 159:615–620, 2008; JAAD 57:840–848, 2007; Eur J Dermatol 14:255–258, 2004;* microscopic polyarteritis nodosa – hemorrhagic papules (palpable purpura) *JAAD 48:311–340, 2003; AD 128:1223–1228, 1992;* oral purpura *Oral Surg 56:597–601, 1983;* cutaneous (livedo with nodules) – purpura; painful or asymptomatic red or skin colored

multiple nodules with livedo reticularis of feet, legs, forearms face, scalp, shoulders, trunk *BJD 146:694–699, 2002;* splinter hemorrhages; familial polyarteritis nodosa of Georgian Jewish, German, and Turkish ancestry – oral aphthae, livedo reticularis, leg ulcers, Raynaud's phenomenon, digital necrosis, nodules, purpura, erythema nodosum; systemic manifestations include fever, myalgias, arthralgias, gastrointestinal symptoms, renal disease, central and peripheral neurologic manifestations; mutation in adenosine deaminase 2 (*CECR1*) *NEJM 370:921–931, 2014*

Postcardiotomy syndrome

Pseudo-Kaposi's sarcoma (Stewart-Bluefarb syndrome) *Cutis 103:336–339, 2019; Wounds 30:E105–107, 2018*

Purpura simplex

Purpura fulminans – symmetric peripheral gangrene; meningococcemia, staphylococcal sepsis, *Capnocytophaga canimorsus JAAD 57:944, 956, 2007; Br Med J 2:8–9, 1891*

Reactive angioendotheliomatosis (proliferating angioendotheliomatosis) – red purple-purpuric patches and plaques; bruised appearance; includes acroangiomatosis, diffuse dermal angiomatosis, intravascular hitiocytosis, glomeruloid angioendotheliomatosis, angiopericatomatosis (angiomatosis with cryoproteins) *JAAD 49:887–896, 2003; JAAD 42:903–906, 2000; AD 122:314–319, 1986*

Recurrent annular erythema with purpura – variant of leukocytoclastic vasculitis *BJD 135:972–975, 1996*

Retiform purpura – ANCA+ vasculitis; antiphospholipid antibodies, mixed cryoglobulins (types I, II, and III), DIC, heparin-induced thrombocytopenia, septic vasculitis, coumarin necrosis, lupus anticoagulant *JAAD 63:530–535, 2010*

Sickle cell disease *Am J Dermatopathol 21:384–386, 1999*

Superficial lymphatic malformation (formerly targetoid hemosiderotic hemangioma/ hobnail hemangioma) – purpuric plaque *AD 138:117–122, 2002;* brown to violaceous papule or nodule with ecchymotic halo; violaceous papule with ecchymotic or brown ring *JAAD 66:112–115, 2012; int J Dermatol 47:991–992, 2008; AD 142:1351–1356, 2006; Cutis 72:51–52, 2003; AD 138:117–122, 2002; AD 136:1571–1572, 2000; J Cutan Pathol 26:279–286, 1999; JAAD 41:215–224, 1999; JAAD 32:282–284, 1995; J Cutan Pathol 17:233–235, 1990; JAAD 19:550–558, 1988*

Temporal arteritis – resembling Henoch-Schonlein purpura *BJD 76:299–308, 1964;* reticulated purpura of frontal scalp *Dermatol Online J June 15, 2012*

Thrombotic thrombocytopenic purpura (Moschcowitz syndrome) *NEJM 380:e23, 2019; Expert Rev Hematol 12:383–395, 2019; Eur J Hematol 101:425–434, 2018; Ann Hematol 79:66–72, 2000; Cor Vasa 30:60–72, 1988*

Thrombotic vasculitis (venous thrombosis) – retiform purpura *JAAD 82:783–796, 2020; AD 133:1051–1052, 1997*
  Disseminated intravascular coagulation
  Essential thrombocythemia
  Hemolytic uremic syndrome
  Heparin-induced thrombocytopenia
  Hypercoagulable state
    Anti-phospholipid antibody syndrome
    Factor V Leiden mutation
    Protein C deficiency
    Protein S deficiency
    Prothrombin III mutation
    Anti-thrombin III deficiency
    Hyperhomocystinemia
  Paroxysmal nocturnal hemoglobinuria
  Platelet diathesis
  Red blood cell occlusion – thalassemia, sickle cell disease, hereditary spherocytosis, severe malaria

Activated protein C resistance

Temperature-related – cryoglobulins, type I, cryofibrinogenemia, cold agglutinins

Thrombotic thrombocytopenic purpura

Warfarin necrosis

White blood cell occlusion – intravascular B-cell lymphoma

Tufted angioma – purpuric plaque *JAAD 20:214–225, 1989*

Urticarial vasculitis, including urticarial vasculitis associated with mixed cryoglobulins, hepatitis B or C infection, IgA multiple myeloma, infectious mononucleosis, monoclonal IgM gammopathy (Schnitzler's syndrome), fluoxetine ingestion, metastatic testicular teratoma, serum sickness, Sjogren's syndrome, systemic lupus erythematous *Clin Rev Allergy Immunol 23:201–216, 2002; JAAD 38:899–905, 1998; Medicine 74:24–41, 1995; JAAD 26:441–448, 1992*

Vasculitis – palpable purpura; splinter hemorrhages; urticarial vasculitis – painful purpuric plaques on edematous hands *AD 141:1457–1462, 2005;* livedoid purpura – septic vasculitis secondary to catheterization and pseudoaneurysm of femoral artery *AD 142:936–938, 2006*

Venous stasis – stasis purpura (orthostatic purpura); acute or chronic; stasis dermatitis

PURPURA, NEONATAL

AUTOIMMUNE DISEASES

Alloimmune neonatal thrombocytopenia *Int J Dermatol 76:suppl 1:361–363, 2002*

Maternal autoimmune thrombocytopenia (ITP, LE) *Singapore Med J 59:390393, 2018*

DRUGS

Drug-related immune thrombocytopenia

INFECTIONS AND INFESTATIONS

Aspergillus fumigatus – necrotic purpura with ulcers; verrucous crusted black giant plaque of back *Ped Derm 27:403–404, 2010*

HIV infection

Infections, multiple organisms – *Neisseria meningitidis*

Parvovirus B19

Purpura fulminans (DIC) *J Ped Hem Oncol 40:625–627, 2019*

Sepsis

TORCH syndrome

INFILTRATIVE DISORDERS

Langerhans cell histiocytosis *JAAD 78:1035–1044, 1047–1056, 2018;* blueberry muffin baby *JAAD 53 (suppl 2) S143–146, 2005*

METABOLIC DISORDERS

Congenital megakaryocytic thrombocytopenia *J Indian Med Assoc 50:209–211, 1968*

Extramedullary hematopoiesis (blueberry muffin baby) *Dermatol Online J 14:8, 2008*

Fanconi's anemia *Front Ped 3:50, 2015*

Hemophagocytic lymphohistiocytosis *J Dermatol 33:628–631, 2006*

Hemorrhagic disease of the newborn

Hereditary clotting factor deficiencies

Hereditary thrombocytopenias

Primary platelet production/function defects

Protein C deficiency *Neonatal Netw 30:153–159, 2011*

Protein S deficiency

Thrombotic thrombocytopenic purpura (Upshaw-Schulman syndrome) *J Matern Fetal Neonatal Med 29:1977–1979, 2016; Arch Ped 23:78–81, 2016*

NEOPLASTIC DISEASES

Neuroblastoma, metastatic – periocular ecchymoses (raccoon eyes) *Ped Derm 26:473–474, 2009;* blueberry muffin baby *JAAD 64:1197–1198, 2011*

PHOTODERMATOSES

Purpuric phototherapy-induced eruption – with transient porphyrinemia *J Drugs Dermatol 10:306–307, 2011*

SYNDROMES

Acardi-Goutieres syndrome – blueberry muffin baby *Ped Derm 26:432–435, 2009*

Alport syndrome variants – myosin heavy chain-related disorders *Clin Kidney J 6:516–518, 2013*

Giant platelet syndromes (Bernard-Soulier, May-Hegglin)

Hemorrhagic disease of the newborn

Glanzmann's thrombasthenia

Gray platelet syndrome *Br J Hem 173:662, 2016*

Hermansky-Pudlak syndrome

Thrombocytopenia with absent radii syndrome *Ann Hematol 78:401–407, 1999*

Trisomy 13

Trisomy 18 *Ped Int 62:240–242, 2020*

Volkmann ischemic contracture, congenital (neonatal compartment syndrome) – upper extremity circumferential contracture from wrist to elbow; necrosis, cyanosis, edema, eschar, bullae, purpura; irregular border with central white ischemic tissue with formation of bullae, edema, or spotted bluish color with necrosis, a reticulated eschar or whorled pattern with contracture of arm; differentiate from necrotizing fasciitis, congenital varicella, neonatal gangrene, aplasia cutis congenita, amniotic band syndrome, subcutaneous fat necrosis, epidermolysis bullosa *BJD 150:357–363, 2004*

Wiskott-Aldrich syndrome *J Ped Hem Oncol 40:240–242, 2018*

X-linked recessive thrombocytopenia

TRAUMA

Bryant's sign – scrotal ecchymosis due to retroperitoneal hemorrhage from traumatic delivery (perinatal liver laceration) *NEJM 365:1824, 2011*

Physical trauma

Stabler's sign – inguinal ecchymosis due to retroperitoneal hemorrhage from traumatic delivery (perinatal liver laceration) *NEJM 365:1824, 2011*

VASCULAR DISORDERS

Extramedullary hematopoiesis (blueberry muffin baby) *JAAD 37:673–705, 1997*

Granulomatosis with polyangiitis – herpetiform necrotic purpuric papules over joints (ankles, elbows) *AD 148:849–854, 2012*

Kaposiform hemangioendothelioma of infancy – red-blue tumid swelling; red plaque or nodule with ecchymotic or purpuric border *Ped Derm 19:388–393, 2002; JAAD 38:799–802, 1998; AD 133:1573–1578, 1997; Am J Surg Pathol 17:321–328, 1993*

Kasabach-Meritt syndrome *Br J Heme 112:851–862, 2001*

Vasculitis, cutaneous
  Collagen vascular diseases
  Cutaneous small vessel vasculitis – ulcerated purpuric necrotic plaques *AD 148:887–888, 2012*
  Henoch-Schonlein purpura *Ped Derm 15:357–359, 1998; Ped Derm 12:314–317, 1995; Am J Dis Child 99:833–854, 1960* associated with *Mycoplasma pneumoniae* infection *Cutis 87:273–276, 2011*
  Infectious vasculitis (not embolic)
  Paraneoplastic vasculitis
  Systemic vasculitis

PURPURIC RASH AND FEVER

JAAD 37:673–705, 1997

AUTOIMMUNE DISEASES AND DISEASES IMMUNE DYSFUNCTION

Allergic contact dermatitis – Nigella Sativa oil *JAMA Derm 154:1062–1065, 2018*

Antineutrophil cytoplasmic antibody syndrome – purpuric vasculitis, orogenital ulceration, fingertip necrosis, pyoderma gangrenosum-like ulcers *BJD 134:924–928, 1996*

Autoimmune lymphoproliferative syndrome – petechiae and purpura; germline *FAS* mutation *NEJM 369:853–863, 2013*

Bowel-associated dermatitis-arthritis syndrome *AD 135:1409–1414, 1999; JAAD 14:792–796, 1986; Mayo Clin Proc 59:43–46, 1984; AD 115:837–839, 1979*

CANDLE syndrome (chronic atypical neutrophilic dermatosis with lipodystrophy and elevated temperature) – recurrent annular red or violaceous plaques which evolve to purpura then hyperpigmentation, purple swollen eyelids and lips, arthralgia without arthritis, panniculitis, lipoatrophy, aseptic meningitis, nodular episcleritis, lymphadenopathy, ear and nose chondritis, epididymitis, cold-induced pernio-like lesions of hands and feet, delayed physical development, splenomegaly, conjunctivitis *Ped Derm 33:602–614, 2016*

Graft vs. host reaction – petechiae *AD 125:1685–1688, 1989;* oral purpura *Postgrad Med 66:187–193, 1979*

Lupus erythematosus – systemic lupus erythematosus with thrombocytopenia or vasculitis *JAAD 48:311–340, 2003; Arch Fam Med 9:553–556, 2000;* purpuric macules, purpuric urticaria, palpable *BJD 135:355–362, 1996;* with antiphospholipid antibodies – purpura fulminans *Haematologica 76:426–428, 1991;* splinter hemorrhages with vasculitis *Arch Int Med 116:55–66, 1965;*

systemic lupus erythematosus – lesions of palate, buccal mucosa, gums; red or purpuric areas with red haloes break down to form shallow ulcers *BJD 135:355–362, 1996; BJD 121:727–741, 1989;* neonatal lupus *JAAD 40:675–681, 1999; Clin Exp Rheumatol 6:169–172, 1988;* follicular petechiae in SLE *BJD 147:157–158, 2002;* splinter hemorrhages

Rheumatoid arthritis – vasculitis – palpable purpura, petechiae *JAAD 53:191–209, 2005; JAAD 48:311–340, 2003; BJD 147:905–913, 2002;* purpuric infarcts of paronychial areas and digital pads (Bywater's lesions) purpuric papules *Cutis 71:462, 464, 2003; BJD 77:207–210, 1965;* bullae of fingertips and toetips with or without purpura *BJD 77:207–210, 1965;* large hemorrhagic lesions, gangrene with necrotizing arteritis; splinter hemorrhages

Serum sickness *J Invest Allergol Clin Immunol 9:190–192, 1999; Medicine (Balt) 67:40–57, 1988*

Still's disease – mimicking acute bacterial endocarditis *Eur Heart J 16:1448–1450, 1995*

Wiskott-Aldrich syndrome – personal observation

DRUG-INDUCED

Dilantin hypersensitivity syndrome

Drug hypersensitivity

Drug reaction with eosinophilia and systemic symptoms (DRESS) – morbilliform eruption, cheilitis (crusted hemorrhagic lips), diffuse desquamation, areolar erosion, periorbital dermatitis, vesicles, bullae, targetoid plaques, purpura, pustules, exfoliative erythroderma, facial edema, lymphadenopathy *JAAD 68:693–705, 2013;* purpura of legs *AD 146:1373–1379, 2010*

Drug-induced vasculitis – livedo racemosa *JAAD 82:783–796, 2020*

EXOGENOUS AGENTS

Cocaine-induced vasculitis *Curr Rheum Rep 14:532–538, 2012;* levamisole tainted cocaine *J Burn Care Res 38:e638–646, 2017; Cutis 98:E15–19, 2010*

INFECTIONS AND INFESTATIONS

Acanthamoeba species *Am J Dermatopath 15:146–149, 1993*

Aeromonas hydrophilia

African tick bite fever – *Rickettsia africae; Amblyomma hebraeum or A variegatum;* petechiae, purpura, fever, leg edema *AD 148:247–252, 2012*

AIDS – palatal petechiae

Alternariosis *Cutis 56:145–150, 1995*

Angioinvasive fungi – retiform purpura *JAAD 82:783–796, 2020*

Arboviral hemorrhagic fevers

Arcanabacterium haemolyticum AD 132:61–64, 1996

Arenaviruses (hemorrhagic fevers) – Lassa fever (rats and mice) (West Africa), Junin virus (Argentine pampas), Machupo virus (Bolivian savannas), Guanarito virus (Venezuela), Sabia virus (Southeast Brazil), Whitewater virus (California, New Mexico), Tacaribe virus complex (mice) – swelling of face and neck, oral hemorrhagic bullae, red eyes *JAAD 49:979–1000, 2003*

Arthropod bite

Arthropod vectors – Zika virus, dengue fever, Eastern equine encephalitis, West Nile virus, Chikungunya fever, Rift valley fever

Aspergillosis, primary cutaneous – hemorrhagic vesicles, pustules, and nodules *JAAD 82:783–796, 2020; JAAD 12:313–318, 1985;*

Aspergillus fumigatus – necrotic purpura with ulcers in neonate; verrucous crusted black giant plaque of back *Ped Derm 27:403–404, 2010*

Avian mite dermatitis – large bruise *Cutis 23:680–682, 1979*

Babesiosis (*Babesia microti*) – purpura and ecchymoses due to thrombocytopenia *JAAD 49:363–392, 2003*

Bacterial endocarditis, acute – *Staphylococcus aureus;* livedo reticularis of trunk, purpuric eruption of hands; fever, confusion, thrombocytopenia, renal failure *NEJM 370:651–660, 2014*

Bites – snake, spider, insect, human, etc.

Borrelia recurrentis – relapsing fever; fever and petechiae *J Infect Dis 140:665–675, 1979; Trans R Soc Trop Med Hyg 65:776–781, 1971*

Brazilian purpuric fever – *Haemophilus influenzae biogroup aegyptius* strains *J Infect Dis 171:209–212, 1995; Pediatr Infect Dis J 8:239–241, 1989*

Brown recluse spider bite – purpuric morbilliform eruption in children at 24–48 hours *JAAD 44:561–573, 2001*

Brucellosis *Case Rep Infect Dis Sept 23, 2018; Dermatologica 171:126–128, 1985; Cutis 63:25–27, 1999; Ann Trop Paediatr 15:189–192, 1995; AD 117:40–42, 1981;* with thrombocytopenic purpura *Clin Inf Dis 31:904–909, 2000*

Bubonic plague – *Yersinia pestis; Xenopsylla cheopis* (Oriental rat flea); 2–6 day incubation period; fever, painful lymphadenitis, buboes; septicemia with disseminated intravascular coagulation *Cutis 86:282–284, 2010*

Bunyavirus hemorrhagic fever (Crimean Congo hemorrhagic fever, Rift Valley fever, Hantavirus) – ticks (Hyalomma genus) petechial eruption orally and on upper trunk *JAAD 49:979–1000, 2003*

Campylobacter jejuni Scand J Urol Nephrol 28:179–181, 1994

Candidiasis – disseminated *Am J Med 80:679–684, 1986;* palpable purpura *JAAD 53:544–546, 2005;* Candida krusei *AD 131:275–277, 1995; NEJM 23:1650, 1994; JAAD 26:295–297, 1992*

Capnocytophaga canimorsus sepsis – dog and cat bites or scratch; necrosis with eschar; cellulitis, macular and morbilliform eruptions, petechiae, purpura fulminans, symmetrical peripheral gangrene *NEJM 369:1238–1248, 2014; Cutis 60:95–97, 1997; Eur J. Epidemiology 12 (5)521–533, 1996; JAAD 33:1019–1029, 1995*

Cat scratch disease *Ann DV 125:894–896, 1998;* petechiae *JAAD 31:535–536, 1994*

Cellulitis – hemorrhagic bullae

Chagas' disease – reactivation; fever purpuric plaque after heart transplant for Chagasic cardiomyopathy *Int J Dermatol 51:829–834, 2012*

Chikungunya fever – purpuric rashes *Ped Derm 35:408–409, 2018; Ped Derm 31:392–396, 2018*

Colorado tick fever – Orbivirus; macules, papules, petechiae *JAAD 58:308–316, 2008; JAAD 49:363–392, 2003*

Corynebacterium jeikeium endocarditis – palpable purpura *AD 127:1071–1072, 1991*

Covid 19 chilblain-like lesions *BJD June 25, 2020;* generalized petechial eruption *JAMA Derm 156:821–822, 2020*

Cowpox – hemorrhagic pustules *JAAD 44:1–14, 2001*

Coxsackie virus A6 (atypical hand, foot, and mouth disease) – red papulovesicles of fingers, palmar erythema, red papules of ears, red papules of antecubital fossa, perioral papulovesicles, vesicles of posterior pharynx; crusted papules of scalp, ears, and face; purpuric targetoid painful vesicular lesions of hands and feet, arthritis, fissured scrotum, headache *JAMA Derm 153:219–220, 2017; Ped Derm 33:429–437, 2016; J Clin Virol 60:381–386, 2014; J Clin Virol*

59:201–203, 2014; JAMA Derm 149:1419–1421, 2013; JAAD 69:736–741, 2013; MMWR 61:213–214, 2012

Coxsackie virus A9 *JAAD 49:363–392, 2003;* Coxsackie B4 exanthem

Crimean-Congo hemorrhagic fever – fine petechiae of back, then widespread purpura and palatal petechiae; conjunctivitis *Cutis 87:165–167, 2011; JAAD 58:308–316, 2008;*

Cryptococcosis *Arch Int Med 138:1412–1413, 1978*

Cytomegalovirus – vasculitis; palpable purpura *AD 126:1497–1502, 1990; JAAD 13:845–852, 1985; JAAD 24:860–867, 1991;* purpura in neonate *AD 130:243–248, 1994*

Dengue hemorrhagic fever – petechiae and thrombocytopenia *JAAD 75:1–16, 2016; Dermatol Clinics 29:33–38, 2011; JAAD 58:308–316, 2008;* hyperpigmentation of nose (chik sign); transient flushing, purpuric lesions, scleral injection, morbilliform exanthema with circular islands of sparing, aphthous ulcers, lichenoid papules, flagellated pigmentation, urticarial lesions, erythema multiforme-like *Ped Derm 36:737–739, 2019; Indian Dermatol Online J 8:336–342, 2017; Indian J DV Leprol 76:671–676, 2010*Diphtheria

Dysgonic fermenter type 2 sepsis – purpura fulminans *AD 125:1380–1382, 1989*

Ebola virus hemorrhagic fever (Filovirus) – exanthem which becomes purpuric with desquamation of palms and soles; ecchymoses, petechiae, high fever, body aches, myalgia, arthralgias, prostration, abdominal pain, watery diarrhea; disseminated intravascular coagulation *JAAD 75:1–16, 2016; Int J Dermatol 51:1037–1043, 2012; JAMA 287:2391–2002; Int J Dermatol 51:1037–1043, 2012; JAAD 65:1213–1218, 2011; MMWR 44, No.19, 382, 1995*

Echovirus 9; Echovirus 11,19 – petechial rash *Arch Dis Child 57:22–29, 1982*

Ecthyma gangrenosum – retiform purpura *JAAD 82:783–796, 2020; JAAD 82:783–796, 2020*

Ehrlichiosis – human granulocytic ehrlichiosis with acute renal failure mimicking TTP; petechial and purpuric rash of human monocytic ehrlichiosis *JAAD 75:1–16, 2016; Am J Nephrol 19:677–681, 1999; Skin and Allergy News, Oct. 2000, p.40; Ann Int Med 120:736–743, 1994*

Ehrlichia chaffeensis – diffusely erythematous or morbilliform, scattered petechiae or macules *Clin Inf Dis 33:1586–1594, 2001*

Endocarditis -; bacterial endocarditis – splinter hemorrhages *Br Med J ii:1496–1498, 1963;* acute bacterial endocarditis (*Staphylococcus aureus*) – purpuric emboli; acute, subacute; acral purpura *JAAD 22:1088–1090, 1990;* infective endocarditis and aortitis due to *Staphylococcus aureus;* livedo reticularis of trunk, purpuric eruption of hands, fever, confusion, thrombocytopenia, renal failure *J Card Surg June 19, 2020; NEJM 370:651–660, 2014;* subacute bacterial endocarditis – personal observation; Janeway lesion – hemorrhagic lesions *Med News 75:257–262, 1899*

Enterobacter cloacae sepsis – Enterobacter species *Cutis 41:361–363, 1988*

Enterovirus
  Coxsackie virus B4
  Echo 9

Epidemic typhus (*Rickettsia prowazekii*) – morbilliform eruption becomes petechial exanthem; fever, nausea, diarrhea, delirium, respiratory failure, shock *JAAD 82:551–569, 2020*

Epstein-Barr virus – flexural purpura *Int J Dermatol 37:130–132, 1998;* infectious mononucleosis (Epstein-Barr virus) – petechiae at the junction of the hard and soft palate on the second or third day of fever petechial or purpuric exanthems *Clin Inf Dis 59:95, 136–137, 2014;* papular-purpuric gloves and socks syndrome; infectious mononucleosis (Epstein-Barr virus) – purpuric exanthema, pharyngitis, cervical lymphadenopathy *Clin Inf dis 59:95, 136–137, 2014*

Escherichia coli – purpura in neonate *J Appl Microbiol 88 Suppl:24S–30S, 2000; AD 130:243–248, 1994; Ann Int Med 109:705–712, 1988; Cutis 41:361–363, 1988*

Exanthem subitum (HHV-6) (roseola infantum) – cutaneous and palatal petechiae *J Ped Hem Onc 24:211–214, 2002*

Fire ant stings

Fusarium – palpable purpura with myositis *JAAD 82:783–796, 2020; JAAD 23:393–398, 1990; JAAD 16:260–263, 198*

Gianotti-Crosti syndrome – papular acrodermatitis of childhood, hemorrhagic variant *Ped Derm 8:169–171, 1991*

Gonococcal sepsis (gonococcemia) (*Neisseria gonorrhea*) – hemorrhagic pustules, petechiae, purpuric lesions *Dermatol Online J 2017 Jan 15, 23:1 (13030)/qt33b2.4006 Arch Fam Med 9:553–556, 2000; Arch Int Med 112:731–737, 1963*

Group B streptococcus – purpura in neonate

Guanarito virus (Venezuela) *JAAD 49:979–1000, 2003*

H1N1 virus pandemic of 2009 *J Med Case Rep April 11, 2011; Ped Int 53:426–430, 2011*

Haemophilus influenzae – sepsis-associated purpura fulminans *N C Med J 46:516–517, 1985*

Hand, foot, and mouth disease – palmoplantar purpuric macules *Ped Derm 33:428–437, 2016*

Hantavirus hemorrhagic fever – infected rodent waste; flulike prodrome; nausea, vomiting, shock, extensive ecchymoses; oliguria, pulmonary edema, coagulopathy *JAAD 58:308–316, 2008; AD 140:656, 2004*

Hemorrhagic fever – Puumala virus *Clin Inf Dis 20:255–258, 1995*

Hepatitis A, B, and C *Arch Fam Med 9:553–556, 2000*

Herpes simplex – purpura in neonate *AD 130:243–248, 1994*

Herpes zoster

Histoplasmosis *Postgraduate Med 49:226–230, 1971*

HIV – neonatal purpura *JAAD 37:673–705, 1997*

Influenza A virus – acute rash, fever, and petechiae *Clin Infect Dis 29:453–454, 1999*

Junin virus (Argentine pampas) *JAAD 49:979–1000, 2003*

Kyasanur forest disease *JAAD 58:308–316, 2008*

Klebsiella sepsis *Diagn Microbiol Infect Dis 37:275–277, 2000*

Lassa fever – rats and mice *JAAD 58:308–316, 2008; JAAD 49:979–1000, 2003*

Legionella species

Leprosy – Lucio's phenomenon – retiform purpura *JAAD 82:783–796, 2020*; hemorrhagic stellate patches *AD 114:1023–1028, 1978*; erythema nodosum leprosum

Leptospirosis – Haverhill fever (*Listeria monocytogenes*) – neonatal purpuric, pustular and morbilliform eruptions *JAAD 58:308–316, 2008; AD 130:245,248, 1994*

Machupo virus (Bolivian savannahs) *JAAD 49:979–1000, 2003*

Malaria *JAAD 58:308–316, 2008*

Marburg virus (Filovirus) – exanthem which becomes purpuric with desquamation of palms and soles *JAAD 65:1213–1218, 2011; JAAD 58:308–316, 2008*

Measles, including atypical measles *BMJ Case Rep Se[t 23, 2015*

Mediterranean spotted fever – *Rickettsia conorii*; petechiae *JAAD 49:363–392, 2003*

Meningococcemia – retiform purpura *JAAD 82:783–796, 2020; JAAD 82:783–796, 2020;* acute or chronic (petechial); acute; initially ecchymoses, purpuric papules, nodules, and plaques with surrounding erythema, vesicles, bullae, hemorrhagic necrosis, purpura fulminans; fever and arthralgias *Clin Exp Rheumatol 20:553–554, 2002;* or chronic (petechial) *Pediatr Infect Dis J 8:224–227, 1989; Rev Infect Dis 8:1–11, 1986;* purpuric plaque in chronic meningococcemia *BJD 153:669–671, 2005;* widespread purpuric macules in chronic meningococcemia *Ped Derm 33:559–560, 2016;* splinter hemorrhage

Morganella morganii

Mucormycosis (rhino-orbito-cerebral mucormycosis) – central facial destruction, hematoma, and ecchymosis *JAAD 82:783–796, 2020; Dermatol Online J March 15, 2017; JAAD 65:241–243, 2011; AD 141:1035–1040, 2005; JAAD 50:549–552, 2004*

Murine typhus

Mycobacterium tuberculosis – acute miliary tuberculosis; large crops of blue papules, vesicles, pustules, hemorrhagic papules; red nodules; vesicles become necrotic to form ulcers *J Clin Inf Dis 23:706–710, 1996; Practitioner 222:390–393, 1979; Am J Med 56:459–505; AD 99:64–69, 1969;* pulmonary TB with cutaneous leukocytoclastic vasculitis *Infection 28:55–57, 2000;* erythema induratum

Mycoplasma pneumoniae

Necator americanus (hookworm)

Necrotizing fasciitis – bruise or purpuric plaque with bullae *AD 126:815–820, 1990; Surg Gynecol Obstet 154:92–102, 1982*

North Asian tick-borne typhus – *Forcipomyia siberica*

Omsk hemorrhagic fever *JAAD 58:308–316, 2008*

Orf

Paecilomyces lilacinus – purpuric macules, hemorrhagic vesicles, hemorrhagic papules *JAAD 39:401–409, 1998*

Paracoccidioidomycosis, disseminated (*Paracoccidioides brasiliensis*) – disseminated purpuric ulcerated nodules in HIV disease *Clin Inf Dis 58:1431–1432,2014*

Parvovirus B19 – petechial gloves and socks syndrome *Diagn Microbiol Infect Dis 36:209–210, 2000; JAAD 41:793–796, 1999; Ped Derm 15:35–37, 1998; Clin Infect Dis 27:164–168, 1998; JAAD 27:835, 1992;* generalized petechial and purpuric eruption *Clin Pediatr 45:275–280, 2006;* purpuric eruption and Koplik spots *JAAD 27:466, 1992;* neonatal purpura *JAAD 37:673–705, 1997;* mimicking measles; bullous papular-purpuric gloves and socks syndrome *JAAD 60:691–695, 2009;* periflexural purpuric eruption (baboon-like syndrome) *JAAD Case Rep 6:63–65, 2019; JAAD 71:62–69, 2014*

Phaeohyphomycosis

Proteus mirabilis – sepsis-associated purpura fulminans *JAAD 37:673–705, 1997*

Pseudomonas aeruginosa sepsis – including purpura in neonate *AD 130:243–248, 1994*

Post kala-azar leishmaniasis

Purpura fulminans (DIC) *Stat Pearls Jan 23, 2020*
  Candida sepsis
  Hemophilus influenza NC Med J 46:516–517, 1985
  Klebsiella pneumonia
  Leptospirosis
  Meningococcemia *Indian J Pathol Microbiol 61:284–286, 2018*
  Pneumococcal sepsis
  Rickettsia conorii J Med Case Rep 12:145, 2018
  Rocky Mountain spotted fever
  Roseola
  Rubella

Scarlet fever

Staphylococcal sepsis

Streptococcus pneumonia BMJ Case Rep Oct 20, 2017

Streptococcal sepsis *JAAD 47:496, 2002*

Varicella

Vibrio parahemolyticus

Puss caterpillar sting – hemorrhagic papules, papulovesicles *Cutis 60:125–126, 1997*

Q fever (*Coxiella burnetti*) *Pediatr Infect Dis J 19:358, 2000; Q J Med 45:193–217, 1976*

Rat bite fever – hemorrhagic vesicles of hands and feet with petechiae *JAMA Derm 153:707–708, 2017; Clin Microbiol Rev 20:13–22, 2007;* macular and petechial rash on palms and soles; acral hemorrhagic pustules; palpable purpura; arthritis, pustules; endocarditis, pericarditis, interstitial pneumonia, hepatitis, nephritis, septic arthritis, systemic vasculitis *JAMA Derm 152:723–724, 2016; J Clin Microbiol 51:1987–1989, 2013; AD 148:1411–1416, 2012; Clin Microbiol Rev 20:13–22, 2007; Clin Inf Dis 43:1585–1586, 1616–1617, 2006; JAAD 38:330–332, 1998*

Relapsing fever (tick-borne relapsing fever) – Ornithodoros soft ticks transmitting *Borrelia hermsii, B.turicata,* or *B. parkeri*; 1–2 cm rose-colored macules, papules, petechiae, purpura, facial flushing; arthralgias, iritis, myalgia *JAAD 49:363–392, 2003;* diffuse macular rash

Respiratory syncytial virus

Rheumatic fever – petechiae

Rickettsial diseases

    African tick bite fever (*R. africae*) – hemorrhagic pustule, purpuric papules; transmitted by Amblyomma ticks) – high fever, arthralgia, myalgia, fatigue, rash in 2–3 days, with eschar, maculopapules, vesicles, and pustules *JAAD 48:S18–19, 2003*

    Boutonneuse fever – *Rickettsia conori* – Marseilles fever, South African tick fever, Kenya tick typhus, Israel tick typhus, and Indian tick typhus

    Epidemic typhus *Rickettsia prowazekii*

    Kenya tick typhus – *R. conorii*

    Louse-borne typhus

    Marseilles fever – *R. conorii*

    Mediterranean spotted fever *Trop Geogr Med 42:78–82, 1990*

    Oriental spotted fever – *R. japonica*

    Queensland tick typhus – *R. australis*

    Rickettsia parkeri rickettsiosis – Gulf coast tick (*Amblyomma maculatum*); eschar with surrounding petechiae, fever, fatigue, headache, myalgia, arthralgia, morbilliform or vesiculopapular rash of trunk and extremities, palms and soles, and occasionally the face; some lesions with small vesicle or pustule *Clin Inf Dis 47:1188–1196, 2008*

    Rocky Mountain spotted fever – massive skin necrosis *Ped Derm 36:119–123, 2017; J Cutan Pathol 24:604–610, 1997; South Med J 71:1337–1340, 1978*

    Scrub typhus – *Rickettsia tsutsugamuchi*

Rotavirus

Rubella – Forscheimer's spots (red macules and petechiae on soft palate)

Sabia virus (Southeast Brazil) *JAAD 49:979–1000, 2003*

Salmonella species – purpura in neonate *AD 130:243–248, 1994;* meningitis with purpura fulminans; typhoid fever presenting as ITP *S Afr Med J 51:3, 1977*

*Saprochaeta clavata (*formerly *Geotrichum clavatum)* sepsis – purpuric macules and papules *Ped Derm 36:990–991, 2019*

Scedosporium – bullous necrotic purpura *Ann DV 125:711–714, 1998*

Schistosomiasis (*S. japonicum*) – Katayama fever – purpura, arthralgia, systemic symptoms *Dermatol Clin 7:291–300, 1989*

Sea anemone sting

Sepsis – multiple organisms – neonatal purpura *JAAD 37:673–705, 1997*

Septic emboli *JAAD 82:783–796, 2020*

Septic vasculitis *JAAD 82:783–796, 2020*

Severe fever with thrombocytopenia (STS bunyavirus) – fever, nausea and vomiting, abdominal pain, myalgia, lymphadenopathy, confusion, headache, conjunctival congestion, and cough *NEJM 364:1523–1532, 2011*

Shigellosis

Small pox – macular and papular exanthem of face and extremities develop vesicles, pustules, and umbilicated crusts; hemorrhagic smallpox more severe *JAAD 65:1213–1218, 2011*

South American Arenaviruses (Junin, Machupo, Sabia, Guanarito)

Staphylococcus aureus – retiform purpura *JAAD 82:783–796, 2020;* purpura fulminans and toxic shock syndrome *Clin Inf Dis 40:941–947, 2005; Staphylococcus aureus* in AIDS; Staphylococcus aureus sepsis *Am J Med 83:801–803, 1987;* abscess in acute myelogenous leukemia – personal observation

Stingray bite *Cutis 58:208–210, 1996*

Streptococcus dysgalactiae – septic embolic from infected pseudoaneurysm of femoral artery; purpuric macules and papules of foot and toes *JAMA Derm 156:452, 2020*

Streptococcus pyogenes – scarlet fever; retiform purpura; Pastia's lines *JAAD 82:783–796, 2020*

Streptococcus pyogenes toxic shock-like syndrome – hemorrhagic bullae *Ped Int Child Health 38:223–226, 2018; AD 131:73–77, 1995*

Streptococcus pneumoniae – pneumococcal cellulitis – bilateral hemorrhagic bullae *AD 132:81–86, 1996;* peripheral symmetric gangrene – personal observation

Streptococcus suis – meningitis (sensorineural hearing loss) and sepsis; petechiae, ecchymoses, hemorrhagic cutaneous necrosis *Clin Inf Dis 48:617–625, 2009*

Streptococcus viridans

Strongyloides stercoralis – retiform purpura *JAAD 82:783–796, 2020;* hyperinfection; thumb-print purpura *JAMA Derm 155:957, 2019; Clin Inf Dis 59:559,601–602, 2014; AD 146:191–196, 2010; Braz J Inf Dis 9:419–424, 2005; JAAD 49:S157–160, 2003; JAAD 31:255–259, 1994; JAAD 21:1123, 1989;* thumbprint sign *JAAD 23:324–326, 1990;* periumbilical purpura *Transplant Inf Dis 13:58–62, 2011; JAMA 256:1170–1171, 1986;* anasarca, renal failure, serpiginous abdominal purpura *Clin Inf Dis 59:559, 601–602, 2014*

Tacaribe viruses – Argentinian, Bolivian, and Venezuelan hemorrhagic fevers – erythema and edema of face, neck, and thorax with petechiae; oral hemorrhagic bullae *JAAD 49:979–1000, 2003; Lancet 338:1033–1036, 1991; JAMA 273:194–196, 1994*

TORCH syndrome – neonatal purpura; blueberry muffin baby (extramedullary hematopoiesis)

Toxic shock syndrome

Toxoplasmosis – purpuric nodules *JAAD 14:600–605, 1986;* congenital toxoplasmosis *JAAD 12:697–706, 1985*

Trichinosis – subungual petechiae

Trichosporon beigelii, disseminated – purpuric papules and nodules *Mycoses 39:195–199, 1996; AD 129:1020–1030, 1993*

Trypanosomiasis, African *AD 131:1178–1182, 1995*

Tularemia *Cutis 54:279–286, 1994*

Varicella-zoster virus – herpes zoster, disseminated herpes zoster, varicella

Vasculitis, infectious (not embolic)

Vibrio vulnificus sepsis – hemorrhagic bullae *JAAD 61:733–750, 2009; BJD 142:386–387, 2000; JAAD 24:397–403, 1991; Am J Gastroenterol 80:706–708, 1985*

Viral exanthem, including measles – personal observation

Viral hemorrhagic fevers – including Argentine hemorrhagic fever, Bolivian hemorrhagic fever, Lassa fever, Venezuelan hemorrhagic fever, Kyasanur Forest disease, Omsk hemorrhagic fever, yellow fever and

Viral insect borne and hemorrhagic fevers *Dermatol Clinics 17:29–40, 1999*
  Togavirus
    Sindbis fever
    Chikungunya fever
    O'nyong nyong fever
    Ross river fever
    Barmah forest fever
  Flavivirus
    Dengue fever (flavivirus) – morbilliform or scarlatiniform eruption on day 3–4, then becomes petechial; joint and bone pain with severe backache *Ann DV 124:237–241, 1997; Bull Soc Pathol Exot 86:7–11, 1993*
    West Nile fever
    Kunjin fever
    Kyasanur Forest disease
    Omsk hemorrhagic fever *AD 140:656, 2004*
  Arena virus
    Lassa fever
    Junin fever
    Machupo fever
  Filovirus
    Marburg virus – maculopapular-vesicular *S Afr Med J 60:751–753, 1981*
    Ebola viral hemorrhagic fever – morbilliform rash *MMWR 44:468–469, 1995*
  Bunyavirus
    Bwamba fever
    Rift valley fever
    Crimea/Congo fever
    Hanta virus (hemorrhagic fever with renal syndrome (Hanta virus))

Whitewater virus (California, New Mexico) *JAAD 49:979–1000, 2003*

Xanthomonas maltophilia – purpura fulminans *J Dermatol 18:225–229, 1991*

Yellow fever *Dermatol Clinics 29:33–38, 2011*

Yersinia- *Yersinia pestis* (plague) – purpura, including symmetrical peripheral gangrene *AD 135:311–322, 1999*

Zygomycosis – purpuric plaque *JAAD 20:989–1003, 1989;* bulls-eye cutaneous infarct *JAAD 51:996, 2004*

INFLAMMATORY DISORDERS

Acute generalized exanthematous pustulosis – pustules, purpura, fever and rash – etiologies include multiple drugs, mercury, enterovirus, adenovirus, Epstein-Barr virus, cytomegalovirus, hepatitis B virus, *Mycoplasma pneumoniae Ped Derm 17:399–402, 2000*

METABOLIC DISEASES

Cryofibrinogenemia *Am J Med 116:332–337, 2004*

Cryoglobulinemia *Saudi J Kidney Dis Transpl 30:663–669, 2019*

Disseminated intravascular coagulation, purpura fulminans – personal observation

Paroxysmal nocturnal hemoglobinuria *AD 114:560, 1978*

Purpura fulminans *JAAD 47:493–496, 2002*
  Neisseria meningitides
  Streptococcus pneumoniae
  Group A streptococcus
  Group B streptococcus
  Streptococcus suis
  Staphylococcus albus
  Haemophilus influenzae
  Haemophilus aegyptius
  Rickettsia reckettsii
  Klebsiella pneumoniae
  Escherichia coli
  Neisseria cararrhalis
  Proteus mirabilis
  Proteus mirabilis
  Proteus vulgaris
  Enterobacter sp
  Pseudomonas sp
  Salmonella paratyphi
  Pasteurella multocida
  Capnocytophaga canimorsus
  Acinetobacter calcoaceticus anitratus
  Vibrio sp
  Xanthomonas maltophilia
  Mycobacterium tuberculosis

NEOPLASTIC DISEASES

Atrial myxoma – purpuric macules of palms and soles *BMC Ped 18:373, 2018; Ann Dermatol 24:337–340, 2012*

Leukemia/lymphoma *Arch Fam Med 9:553–556, 2000;* autoimmune lymphoproliferative syndrome due to germline *FAS* mutation – petechiae *NEJM 369:853–863, 2013*

Myelodysplastic syndrome *Adian Pac J Cancer Prev 17:1535–1537, 2016*

PRIMARY CUTANEOUS DISORDERS

Febrile purpuric pityriasis rosea – personal observation

SYNDROMES

Familial Mediterranean fever – purpuric lesions of face, trunk, extremities; lesions of Henoch-Schonlein purpura *Eur J Pediatr 155:540–544, 1996; J Rheumatol Suppl 35:1–9, 1992; Q J Med 75:607–616, 1990; Am J Med 43:227–253, 1967*

Hemophagocytic lymphohistiocytosis syndrome – criteria include – fever, pancytopenia, lymphadenopathy, hepatomegaly, hypertriglyceridemia, or hypofibrinogenemia, hemophagocytosis, low or absent NK cell activity, elevated CD 25 (IL-2 receptor alpha domain), ferritin >5000, splenomegaly also observe joint, purpura, morbilliform eruption, kidney, and cardiac involvement, central nervous system dysfunction *Arch Dis Child 102:279–284, 2017; Eur Rev Med Pharmacol Sci, 16:1414–1424, 2012; Genes Immunol 13:289–298, 2012*

Familial HLH – known genetic defects (perforin)
Immune deficiencies
   Chediak-Higashi syndrome
   Griscelli syndrome
   X-linked lymphoproliferative syndrome
Acquired
   Infections
   Endogenous products
   Rheumatic diseases
   Neoplasms

Sweet's syndrome *BMJ Case Rep June 11, 2020*

Tumor necrosis factor (TNF) receptor 1-associated periodic fever syndromes (TRAPS) (same as familial hibernian fever, autosomal dominant periodic fever with amyloidosis, and benign autosomal dominant familial periodic fever) – erythematous patches, tender red plaques, fever, annular, serpiginous, polycyclic, reticulated, and migratory patches and plaques (migrating from proximal to distal), urticaria-like lesions, lesions resolving with ecchymoses, conjunctivitis, periorbital edema, myalgia, arthralgia, abdominal pain, headache; Irish and Scottish predominance; mutation in TNFRSF1A – gene encoding 55kDa TNF receptor *AD 136:1487–1494, 2000*

Wells' syndrome – serpiginous purpura *J Drugs Dermatol 16:1036–1038, 2017*

TRAUMA

Fat embolism syndrome – persistent somnolence, fever, tachycardia, respiratory symptoms, petechial eruption *NEJM 375:370–378, 2016; Am J Gastroenterol 68:476–480, 1977*

VASCULAR DISEASES

Acute hemorrhagic edema of infancy (Seidlmayer's purpura, Finkelstein's syndrome) *Ped Int 45:697–700, 2003; JAMA 61:18–19, 1913*

ANCA-negative vessel vasculitis *Intern Med 54:2759–2763, 2015*

Cholesterol embolism syndrome *Am J Dermatopathol 29:44–55, 2007; Kyobu Geka 57:477–48-2004*

Granulomatosis with polyangiitis – hemorrhagic bullae *JAAD 82:783–796, 2020; J Adv Res 24:311–315, 2020; Mymensingh Med J 22:196–199, 2013; Am J Kidney Dis 37:E5, 2001; Arch Fam Med 9:553–556, 2000*

Henoch-Schonlein purpura *NEJM 369:1843, 2013; Arch Fam Med 9:553–556, 2000*

IgA vasculitis *JAAD 82:783–796, 2020; Intern Med 57:3141–3147, 2018*

Microscopic polyangiitis *BJD 134:542–547, 1996*

Polyarteritis nodosa *Arch Fam Med 9:553–556, 2000;* familial polyarteritis nodosa of Georgian Jewish, German, and Turkish ancestry – oral aphthae, livedo reticularis, purpura, leg ulcers, Raynaud's phenomenon, digital necrosis, nodules, purpura, erythema nodosum; systemic manifestations include fever, myalgias, arthralgias, gastrointestinal symptoms, renal disease, central and peripheral neurologic manifestations; mutation in adenosine deaminase 2 (*CECR1*) *NEJM 370:921–931, 2014*

Vasculitis, hypersensitivity vasculitis *Arch Fam Med 9:553–556, 2000*

PUSTULAR AND VESICOPUSTULAR ERUPTIONS IN THE NEWBORN

AUTOIMMUNE DISEASES AND DISORDERS OF IMMUNE DYSREGULATION

Bullous pemphigoid *Ped Derm 33:367–374, 2016*

Chronic granulomatous disease – neonatal pustules *Arch Dis Child 65:942–945, 1990*; vesiculopustular eruptions *JAAD 36:899–907, 1997;* scalp folliculitis *AD 103:351–357, 1971*

DIRA (IL-1 receptor deficiency) – loss of function mutation of *IL1RN*; infantile pustulosis and exfoliative erythroderma *AD 148:747–752, 2012; Ped Radiol 42:495–498, 2012; NEJM 360:2426–2437, 2009*

Hyper IgE syndrome – papulopustular eruption of face and scalp (newborn vesiculopustular eosinophilic eruption *J Cut Med Surg 20:340–342, 2016; JAAD 54:855–865, 2006*

IgA pemphigus – neonatal vesicopustules in a one-month old *JAAD 48:S22–24, 2003*

IL-36 receptor antagonist deficiency – generalized pustular psoriasis *Ped 132:e1043–1047, 2013; NEJM 365:620–628, 2011*

Linear IgA disease *Curr Opinion Pediatr 28:500–506, 2016*

Maternal bullous disease

Pemphigoid gestations *Dermatologica 176:143–147, 1988*

Pemphigus vulgaris *Ped Derm 33:367–374, 2016*

STAT1 gain of function mutation – congenital candidiasis; most common cause of chronic mucocutaneous candidiasis; demodicidosis with facial papulopustular eruptions, blepharitis, chalazion, dermatitis of the neck, nail dystrophy *Ped Derm 37:159–161, 2020*

INFECTIONS AND INFESTATIONS

Acinetobacter sepsis *Indian Pediatr 30:1413–1416, 1993*

Aspergillus infection *Ped Derm 19:439–444, 2002; BJD 103:681–684, 1980*

Candidiasis – neonatal – oral *Candida* with or without diaper *Candida*; may be generalized, including palmar pustules; *Clin Inf Dis 32:1579,1637–1638, 2001; Ped Derm 6:206–209, 1989;* congenital cutaneous candidiasis – from ascending maternal chorioamnionitis; on face and chest then spreads; progression from pink to red macules, papules, vesicles, pustular, bullous lesions; no oral involvement *Ped Derm 29:507–510, 2012; Ann DV 113:125–130, 1986; JAAD 6:926–928, 1982; Arch Dis Child 57:528–535, 1982*

Chlamydia trachomatis Ped Derm 21:667–669, 2004

Citrobacter sepsis *Indian J Pediatr 57:781–784, 1990*

Cytomegalovirus *Ped Derm 19:210–215, 2002*

Ecthyma gangrenosum *Ped Derm 19:210–215, 2002*

Epstein-Barr syndrome, congenital

Escherichia coli

Haemophilus influenzae

Herpes simplex infection – neonatal or intrauterine *Clin Ob Gyn 61:157–176, 2018; Curr Opinion Ped 29:240–248, 2017; Semin Perinatol 22:64–71, 1998; Neonatal Neurol 15:11–15, 1996*

Herpes zoster *Nepal Med Coll J 9:281–283, 2007; Ginecol Obstet Mex 72:63–67, 2004; Acta Pediatr Jpn 33:57–60, 1991*

Impetigo neonatorum *Ped Derm 31:609, 2014*

Klebsiella pneumoniae

Listeria monocytogenes – disseminated petechial pustular lesions of the newborn *AD 130:245,248, 1994*

Malassezia furfura pustulosis – a form of neonatal acne; red papulopustular lesions of face and scalp of neonates *AD 132:190–193, 1996*

Post-scabietic syndrome

Post-streptococcal pustulosis of palms and soles *JAMA Derm 345–346, 2015*

Pseudomonas aeruginosa

Scabies *Ped Derm 11:264–266, 1994; Am J Dis Child 133:1031–1034, 1979*

Sepsis

Staphylococcus aureus – pyoderma, impetigo neonatorum *World J Clin Cases 4:191–194, 2016; Ped Derm 31:609–610, 2014;* scalded skin syndrome, folliculitis, ecthyma *Alaska Med 28:99–103, 1986;* pustular eruption *Ann Emerg Med 65:464–469, 2015*

Streptococcus, including beta-hemolytic Group A and Group B

Tinea faciei, capitis *Pediatr Ann 43:e16–18, 2014*

Trichophyton verrucosum Mycoses 32:411–415, 1989

Syphilis *Med J Austral 165:382–385, 1996*

Varicella, neonatal *Lancet 2:371–373, 1989;* congenital *Arch Dis Child Fetal Neonatal Ed 96:F296–297, 2011*

INFILTRATIVE DISEASES

Congenital self-healing histiocytosis (Hashimoto-Pritzker disease) *Dermatol Online J Aug 15, 2019; JAAD 56:290–294, 2007*

Langerhans cell histiocytosis *AJP Rep 3:63–66, 2013; Ped Derm 19:210–215, 2002*

Mastocytosis, bullous, diffuse cutaneous

INFLAMMATORY DISORDERS

Erosive pustular dermatosis of the scalp

Erythema multiforme *Ped Derm 19:210–215, 2002*

Miliaria pustulosa *Ped Derm 19:210–215, 2002;* miliaria crystallina *Cutis 47:103–106, 1991;* rubra *Ann DV 134:253–256, 2007*

METABOLIC DISORDERS

Acrodermatitis enteropathica *J Drugs Dermatol 13:1153–1154, 2014; Ann Dermatol 23:S326–328, 2011*

Erythropoietic protoporphyria

Protein C deficiency

Toxic epidermal necrolysis

NEOPLASTIC DISORDERS

Transient myeloproliferative disorder in trisomy 21 or normal patients – small papules, vesicles, and pustules; pancytopenia, hepatosplenomegaly, immature circulating leukocytes; mutation in globin transcription factor 1 (*GATA 1*) *JAAD 60:869–871, 2009; AD 141:1053–1054, 2005;* transient myeloproliferative disorder associated with trisomy 21 *Cutis 85:286–288, 2010; BJD 156:1373–1374, 2007; JAAD 54:562–564, 2006; AD 141:1053–1054, 2005;*

Ped Derm 21:551–554, 2004; AD 137:760–763, 2001; Ped Derm 20:232–237, 2001; associated with mosaicism for trisomy 21 – pustular, papulovesicular, vesiculopustular rash, facial dermatitis *Cutis 83:234–236, 2009; JAAD 54:S62–64, 2006; NEJM 348:2557–2566, 2003;* periorbital vesiculopustules, red papules, crusted papules, and ulcers; with periorbital edema *Ped Derm 21:551–554, 2004;* vesiculopustular eruptions in neonates with Down's syndrome and myeloproliferative disorders (leukemoid reaction) *AD 137:760–763, 2001*

PRIMARY CUTANEOUS DISEASES

Absent dermatoglyphics and transient facial milia (vesicles) *JAAD 32:315–8, 1995*

Acne, neonatal, infantile (benign cephalic pustulosis); *Malassezia furfura* pustulosis – a form of neonatal acne; red papulopustular lesions of face and scalp of neonates *AD 134:995–998, 1998; AD 132:190–193, 1996; Malassezia sympodialis*

Acropustulosis of infancy *BJD 115:735–739, 1986; Cutis 36:49–51, 1985; AD 115:834–836, 1979*

Aplasia cutis congenita – blister-like

Bullous ichthyosiform erythroderma

Diaper dermatitis *Ped Derm 19:210–215, 2002*

Ectodermal dysplasias

Eosinophilic pustular folliculitis of infancy *Clin Exp Dermatol 26:251–255, 2001; Ped Derm 16:118–120, 1999*

Epidermolysis bullosa *Ped Derm 19:210–215, 2002*

Epidermolytic hyperkeratosis

Erosive and vesicular dermatosis

Erythema toxicum neonatorum *Eur J Dermatol 21:271–272, 2011; Ped Derm 23:301–302, 2006; Ped Derm 16:137–141, 1999*

Irritant contact dermatitis *Ped Derm 19:210–215, 2002*

Pustular bacterid

Pustular psoriasis *Ped Derm 10:277–282, 1993*

Seborrheic dermatitis *Ped Derm 19:210–215, 2002*

Subcorneal pustular dermatosis *AD 109:73–77, 1974*

Toxic erythema of the newborn *Pediatr Med Chir 27:22–25, 2005;Dermatology 185:18–22, 1992*

Transient neonatal pustular melanosis *Int J Derm 18:636–638, 1979; J Pediatr 88:831–835, 1976*

SYNDROMES

Behcet's syndrome, neonatal *BMJ Case Rep Feb 6, 2013*

Down's syndrome (trisomy 21) – clue to transient myeloproliferative disorder (leukemoid reactions) – neonatal pustules, vesicles, papulovesicles, vesicopustules *Ped Derm 36:702–706, 2019; Cutis 85:286–288, 2010; Ped Derm 20:232–237, 2003; AD 137:760–763, 2001*

Incontinentia pigmenti *Hautarzt 68:149–152, 2017; JAAD 47:169–187, 2002; Cutis 54:161–166, 1994*

Sweet's syndrome *Ped Derm 29:38–44, 2012*

TRAUMA

Sucking blisters

VASCULAR LESIONS

Rapidly involuting hemangioma with pustules *Ped Derm 31:398–400, 2014*

PUSTULES AND PUSTULAR ERUPTIONS OF THE PALMS AND SOLES

Sorld J Surg Oncol 14:145, 2016; Adv Exp Med Biol 755:307–310, 2013; AD 130:861–867, 1994

Acrodermatitis continua of Hallopeau – osteolysis of tuft of distal phalanx *JAMA Derm 154:1346–1347, 2018; AD 148:297–299, 2012; AD 118:434–437, 1982;* tapered sclerodermoid changes

Acropustulosis of infancy – acral plantar pustules *JAAD 62:906–908, 2010; Hautarzt 39:1–4, 1988*

Acute palmoplantar pustulosis

Adalimumab (TNF-inhibitor) – pustular psoriasis; palmoplantar pustular psoriasis *J Drugs Dermatol 12:16–17, 2013; AD 147:1228–1230, 2011; JAAD 56:327–328, 2007*

Adult Still's disease – palmoplantar vesiculopustular eruption with fixed facial papules *J Korean Med Sci 17:852–855, 2002*

Allergic contact dermatitis

Blistering distal dactylitis

Bullous pemphigoid *J UOEH 33:183–187, 2011*

Candidiasis, congenital cutaneous *Clin Inf Dis 32:1579, 1637–1638, 2001*

Chronic recalcitrant pustular eruptions of the palms and soles *BJD 168:1243, 2013; Clin Exp Dermatol 34:219, 2010;*

Cutis 68:216–218, 2001

Contact dermatitis *Contact Derm 39:108–111, 1998*

CRMO – chronic recurrent multifocal osteomyelitis and synovitis; acne, pustulosis, hyperostosis, osteitis; palmoplantar pustules, Sweet's syndrome, pyoderma gangrenosum *JAAD 70:767–773, 2014*

Cryoglobulinemia – pustules and purpura of feet – pustular cryoglobulinemic vasculitis *AD 147:235–240, 2011*

Drug eruption

Dyshidrotic dermatitis *J Dermatol 46:399–408, 2019*

Endocarditis – acute bacterial endocarditis, MRSA – personal observation

Eosinophilic pustular folliculitis *Cutis 74:107–110, 2004; Dermatology 185:276–280, 1992; Dermatologica 149:1240–1247, 1974*

Etanercept – pustular psoriasis; palmoplantar pustular psoriasis *AD 147:1228–1230, 2011; Ann Dermatol 22:212–215, 2010; JAAD 56:327–328, 2007*

Gonococcemia – personal observation

Gouty tophi *J Med Assoc Thai 92:979–982, 2009*

Hereditary acrokeratotic poikiloderma – vesicopustules of hands and feet at 1–3 months of age; widespread dermatitis; keratotic papules of hands, feet, elbows, and knees *AD 103:409–422, 1971*

Herpes simplex *Dermatol Online J Sept 16, 2014*

Histoplasmosis, disseminated *Braz J Infect Dis 4:255–261, 2000*

Hot tub folliculitis *JAAD 57:596–600, 2007*

Hypothyroidism – palmoplantar pustulosis *BJD 121:487–491, 1989*

IgA pemphigus – personal observation

Impetigo herpetiformis (pustular psoriasis of pregnancy) *Dermatology 198:61–64, 1999*

Incontinentia pigmenti

Infliximab – pustular psoriasis; palmoplantar pustular psoriasis *JAAD 56:327–328, 2007; AD 143:1449, 2007*

Intravenous gammaglobulin (IVIG)

Kawasaki's disease *Int J Dermatol 45:1080–1082, 2006*

Langerhans cell histiocytosis – plantar papulopustules *BJD 142:1234–1235, 2000*

Lymphoma – cutaneous T-cell lymphoma mimicking palmoplantar pustulosis *JAAD 51:139–141, 2004; JAAD 47:914–918, 2002; JAAD 23:758–759, 1990*

Milker's nodule

Monkeypox

Mycobacterium abscessus – acquired in swimming pools; pustules of palms, soles, and arms *Ped Derm 31:292–297, 2014*

Orf

Palmoplantar pustulosis *Am J Clin Dermatol 21:355–370, 2020; J Eur Acad DV 31:38–44, 2017; AD 145:1224–1226, 2009*

Pustular bacterid of Andrews *J Gen Fam Med 19:32–33, 2017; Lancet Infect Dis 13:655–656, 2013; Hautarzt 44:221–224, 1993; Am J Dermatopathol 7:200, 1985; Arch Dermatol Syphilol 32:837–847, 1935*

Pustular idiopathic recurrent palmoplantar hidradenitis *JAAD 47:S263–265, 2002*

Pustular psoriasis of palms and soles *BJD 171:646–649, 2014; BJD 168:820–824, 2013; Eur J Dermatol 2:311–314, 1992; Dermatol Clin 2:455–470, 1984;* pustular psoriasis due to beta blocker *Cutis 94:153–155, 2014*

Rat bite fever – palmoplantar papulopustules, fever, arthralgias *NEJM 381:1762, 2019; Ned Tijdschr Geneeskd 142:2006–2009, 1998*

Recurrent self-healing cutaneous mucinosis – red papules of palms and fingertips with pustules and vesicles *BJD 143:650–652, 2000*

Reactive arthritis – personal observation

Rituximab – palmoplantar pustular psoriasis *BJD 171:S1546–1549, 2014*

SAPHO syndrome – palmoplantar pustulosis with sternoclavicular hyperostosis; non-palmoplantar pustulosis, acne fulminans, acne conglobata, hidradenitis suppurativa, psoriasis, multifocal osteitis *BJD 179:959–962, 2018; JAAD 72:550–553, 2015; AD 149:475–480, 2013; JAAD 68:834–853, 2013; Cutis 71:63–67, 2003; Cutis 62:75–76, 1998; Rev Rheum Mol Osteoarthritic 54:187–196, 1987; Ann Rev Rheum Dis 40:547–553, 1981;* with neutrophilic dermatosis (bullous Sweet's syndrome) *AD 143:275–276, 2007*

Scabies *Ped Derm 11:264–266, 1994; Am J Dis Child 133:1031–1034, 1979*

Secondarily infected hand or foot dermatitis

Stevens-Johnson syndrome – peplomycin *J Dermatol 31:802–805, 2004*

Sweet's syndrome *J Med Assoc Thai 94:S119–122, 2011; JAAD 42:332–334, 2000*

Syphilis, secondary *Sex Transm Dis 5:115–118, 1978*

Terbinafine *Ann DV 127:279–281, 2000*

Tularemia

Tumor necrosis factor inhibitors *BJD 161:1081–1088, 2009*

Whirlpool dermatitis *Dtsch Med Wochenschr 139:1459–1461, 2014*

PUSTULES AND PUSTULAR ERUPTIONS

AUTOIMMUNE DISEASES AND DISEASES OF IMMUNE DYSFUNCTION

Allergic contact dermatitis – isoconazole nitrate *Am J Contact Dermat 8:229–230, 1997; Contact Derm 32:309–310, 1995; Cutis 27:630–631, 1981;* 5-fluorouracil – pustular contact hypersensitivity *AD 121:240–242, 1985*

Amicrobial pustulosis associated with autoimmune disease treated with zinc *BJD 143:1306–1310, 2000;* exudative erythema, erosions, pustules of scalp, axillae, ears, thighs *JAAD 57:523–526, 2007; BJD 154:568–569, 2006*

Bowel-associated dermatitis-arthritis syndrome – vesicopustules, red papules, erythema nodosum-like lesions *JAAD 79:1009–1022, 2018; Ped Derm 25:509–519, 2008; AD 138:973–978, 2002; BJD 142:373–374, 2000; AD 135:1409–1414, 1999; JAAD 14:792–796, 1986; Mayo Clin Proc 59:43–46, 1984; AD 115:837–839, 1979*

Bowel bypass syndrome *AD 115:837–839, 1979;* jejunal ileal bypass *QJ Med 51:445–460, 1982*

Bullous pemphigoid – eosinophilic pustules *J IOSH 33:183–187, 2011; BJD 136:641–642, 1997*

Chronic granulomatous disease – neonatal pustules *Arch Dis Child 65:942–945, 1990;* vesiculopustular eruptions *JAAD 36:899–907, 1997;* scalp folliculitis *Dermatol Therapy 18:176–183, 2005; AD 103:351–357, 1971*

Dermatitis herpetiformis – vesiculopustular facial eruption; purpura of fingers with red patches and pustules – leukocytoclastic vasculitis as presentation of dermatitis herpetiformis *AD 137:1313–1316, 2011*

Dermatomyositis – papules and pustules of the elbows and knees in Asian children *Ped Derm 17:37–40, 2000*

Deficiency of interleukin-1 receptor antagonist (DIRA) (IL-1 receptor deficiency) –autosomal recessive; loss of function mutation of *IL1RN;* neutrophilic pustular dermatosis with confluent pustules and lakes of pus; infantile pustulosis and exfoliative erythroderma; oral ulcers, joint swelling; periostitis, aseptic multifocal osteomyelitis; failure to thrive; increased acute phase reactants *JAAD 70:767–773, 2014; Ped Derm 30:758–760, 2013; AD 148:747–752, 2012; Arthritis Rheum 63:4018–4022, 2011; Arthritis Rheum 63:4007–4017, 2011*

Deficiency of IL-36 receptor antagonist (DITRA) – familial severe pustular psoriasis *JAMA Derm 153:473–475, 2017; JAMA Derm 153:106–108, 2017; BJD 172:302–304, 2015;* erythrodermic pustular psoriasis *BJD 174:417–420, 2016*

Fogo selvagem *JAAD 20:657, 1989*

HyperIgD syndrome – cephalic pustulosis; pink plaques and nodules, recurrent fevers, cervical adenopathy, oral aphthae, abdominal pain, vomiting, diarrhea, myalgia, arthralgia; mevalonate kinase deficiency *Ped Derm 35:482–485, 2018*

Hyper IgE syndrome – papular, pustular, excoriated dermatitis of scalp, buttocks, neck, axillae, groin; papulopustules of face and scalp in first year of life; mimics atopic dermatitis; furunculosis; growth failure; neonatal acne-like eruption; resembles eosinophilic pustular folliculitis of infancy; monomorphic folliculitis of back *JAAD 65:1167–1172, 2011; AD 140:1119–1125, 2004; J Pediatr 141:572–575, 2002; Clin Exp Dermatol 11:403–408, 1986; Ped Derm 1:202–206, 1984; Medicine 62:195–208, 1983*

Id reaction *Niger Med J 55:274–275, 2014; Dermatitis 21:E11–15, 2010*

IgA pemphigus (intraepidermal (subcorneal) IgA pemphigus) – annular flaccid pustules *JAMA Derm 153:921–922, 2017;* pustular eruption *BJD 171:650–656, 2014; BJD 168:224–226, 2013; Eur J Dermatol 11:41–44, 2001; JAAD 43:546–549, 2000;* vesiculopustules *JAAD 82:1386–1392, 2020; JAAD 43:923–926, 2000; JAAD 32:352–357, 1995; JAAD 31:502–504, 1994; JAAD 24:993, 1992;* intercellular IgA dermatosis resembling subcorneal pustular dermatosis *AD 123:1062–1065, 1987;* with autoantibodies to desmocollin-1 *BJD 143:144–148, 2000*

Juvenile rheumatoid arthritis – Still's disease; evanescent rash; persistent pruritic papules and plaques; urticarial and urticarial-like rash, vesiculopustular eruptions, edema of the eyelids, widespread non-pruritic persistent erythema *Medicine 96:e6318, 2017*

Linear IgA dermatosis – pustules, vesicles, and erosions *AD 129:897–898, 900–901, 1993*

Lupus erythematosus – amicrobial pustulosis of the folds *J Cutan Pathol 44:367–372, 2019; Ann DV 144:169–175, 2017; Lupus 6:514–520, 1997*

Mixed connective tissue disease – personal observation

Neutrophilic IgA dermatosis *JAAD 31:502–504, 1994*

Pemphigoid gestationis – erythematopustulous rash in newborn *Dermatologica 176:143–147, 1988;* pustular pemphigoid gestationes *AD 119:91–93, 1983*

Pemphigoid vegetans – rare intertriginous variant of bullous pemphigoid *J Cutan Pathol 35:1144–1147, 2008; JAAD 28:331–335, 1993*

Pemphigus – vulgaris, pemphigus vegetans (pustular) *AD 123:609–614, 1987; Dermatol Clinics 1:171–177, 1983; Ann DV 109:549–555, 1982; AD 114:627–628, 1978;* pemphigus vulgaris mimicking pustular psoriasis of hands and feet *Cutis 86:138–140, 2010;* acute pemphigus foliaceus *BJD 145:132–136, 2001;* pemphigus herpetiformis *JAAD 48:117–122, 2003;* IgA pemphigus – neonatal vesicopustules in a one-month old *JAAD 48:S22–24, 2003;* endemic pemphigus of El Bagre region of Colombia *JAAD 49:599–608, 2003*

Pyrin-associated autoinflammatory neutrophilic disease (PAAND) – autosomal dominant; facial pustules, pyoderma gangrenosum lesions; mutation in *MEFV Ped Derm 33:602–614, 2016*

Rheumatoid arthritis – erosive pustular dermatitis of the scalp *J Dermatol 45:198–201, 2018; Int J Dermatol 34:148, 1995;* rheumatoid neutrophilic dermatosis

Eur J Dermatol 18:347–349, 1998

Still's disease – adult onset Still's disease – vesicopustules of hands and feet *JAAD 52:1003–1008, 2005; J Eur Acad Dermatol Venereol 19:360–363, 2005;* palmoplantar vesiculopustular eruption *J Korean Med Sci 17:852–855, 2002*

X-linked agammaglobulinemia *Pediatr Anna 16:414–411, 1987*

CONGENITAL LESIONS

Cephalic pustulosis (neonatal acne) *AD 134:995–998, 1998*

Erythema toxicum neonatorum (toxic erythema of the newborn) – blotchy macular erythema (one to several hundred lesions); surmounted by pustules; including scrotal pustules *Arch Pediatr Adolesc Med 150:649–650, 1996; Dermatology 185:18–22, 1992*

Impetigo – widespread pustules in neonate *Ped Derm 31:609–610, 2014;* streptococcal impetigo *J Dermatol Sci 17:45–53, 1998;* staphylococcus *Cutis 81:115–122, 2008; Acta DV 72:58–60, 1992*

Transient myeloproliferative disorder – small papules, vesicles, and pustules; mutation in transcription factor *GATA 1 JAAD 60:869–871, 2009; AD 141:1053–1054, 2005;* transient myeloproliferative disorder associated with mosaicism for trisomy 21 – pustular, papulovesicular, vesiculopustular rash, facial dermatitis *JAAD 54:S62–64, 2006; NEJM 348:2557–2566, 2003*; periorbital vesiculopustules, red papules, crusted papules, and ulcers; with periorbital edema *Ped Derm 21:551–554, 2004*

Transient neonatal pustular melanosis – flaccid, superficial fragile pustules; chin, neck, forehead, back, buttocks *Int J Dermatol 18:636–638, 1979; J Pediatr 88:831–835, 1976;*

DRUG-INDUCED

BJD 130:514–519, 1994

Acetaminophen *AD 139:1181–1183, 2003*

Acetylsalicylic acid *Schweiz Med Wochenschr 123:542–546, 1993*

Acute generalized exanthematous pustulosis (pustular drug eruptions) – multiple drugs *NEJM 375:471–475, 2016; JAAD 73:843–848, 2015; BJD 169:1223–1232, 2013; Cutis 83:291–298, 2009; AD 142:1080–1081, 2006; Semin Cutan Med Surg 15:244–249, 1996; AD 127:1333–1338, 1991;* pustules and hemorrhagic bullae *AD 147:697–670, 2011;* plaquenil – tongue pustules; widespread pustular exanthema including palms and soles *NEJM 372:161, 2015*

Adalimumab (TNF-inhibitor) – pustular psoriasis; palmoplantar pustular psoriasis *JAAD 56:327–328, 2007*

Allopurinol *Clin Exp Dermatol 19:243–245, 1994*

Amoxicillin *Dermatitis 30:274–275, 2019; Hautarzt 42:713–716, 1991*

Amoxicillin/clavulanate – AGEP *Ped Derm 26:623–625, 2009*

Ampicillin *AD 130:787, 790, 1994*

Azathioprine – multiple pustules on large red plaque covering lower legs in patients with inflammatory bowel disease *AD 143:744–748, 2007;* azathioprine hypersensitivity reaction – occurs within first four weeks of treatment; fever, malaise, arthralgias, myalgias, nausea, vomiting, diarrhea; morbilliform eruption, leukocytoclastic vasculitis, acute generalized exanthematous pustulosis, erythema nodosum, Sweet's syndrome; red papulonodules with pustules *JAAD 65:184–191, 2011*

Baboon syndrome – cetuximab (EGFR inhibitor); intertrigo with pustules *AD 144:272–274, 2008*

Bacampicillin *J Dermatol 25:612–615, 1998*

BCG vaccination – lichenoid and red papules and papulopustules *Ped Derm 13:451–454, 1996*

Bromoderma – single or multiple papillomatous nodules or plaques studded with pustules on face or extremities *Ped Derm 18:336–338, 2001; AD 115:1334–1335, 1979;* iodides, bromides – intertriginous pustular plaques *AD 123:393–398, 1987;* pustular red plaque with pustules at margins to distinguish it from pyoderma gangrenosum *JAAD 58:682–684, 2008*

Captopril *Cutis 56:276–278, 1995*

Carbamazepine *AD 124:178–9, 1988;* eosinophilic pustular folliculitis (Ofuji's disease) *JAAD 38:641–643, 1998*

Cefaclor acetazolamide *AD 139:1181–1183, 2003*

Cefazolin *JAAD 19:571, 1988; JAAD 16:1051–1052, 1987*

Ceftriaxone – AGEP *Ped Derm 36:514–516, 2019*

Cephalexin *Dermatologica 177:292–294, 1988*

Cephadrine *Cutis 38:58–60, 1986*

Cetuximab (epidermal growth factor receptor inhibitor) – follicular papules and pustules *JAAD 58:545–570, 2008; AD 138:129–131, 2002*

Chemotherapy-induced eccrine neutrophilic hidradenitis *JAAD 40:367–398, 1999*

Chloroquine *Int J Dermatol 37:713–714, 1998*

Chloramphenicol *Dermatologica 146:285–291, 1973*

Chlorpromazine *BMJ 309:97, 1994*

Cimetidine

Clemastine *Clin Exp Dermatol 21:293–295, 1996*

Clopidogrel – pustular psoriasis *BJD 155:630–631, 2006;* AGEP *BJD 162:1402–1403, 2010*

Co-trimoxazole *Br Med J 293:1279–1280, 1986*

Corticosteroid acne *Int J Derm 37:772–777, 1998*

Corticosteroids, systemic – withdrawal of steroids resulting in acute pustular psoriasis *BJD 161:964–966, 2009*

Cyclosporine – withdrawal of cyclosporine *Clin Exp Dermatol 24:10–13, 1999; BJD 136:132–133, 1997*

Dactinomycin

Dapsone *JAAD 35:346–349, 1996*

Dexamethasone – injections *Dermatology 193:56–58, 1996*

Dihydrocodone phosphate – pustular drug eruption in *IL36RN* mutation *JAMA Derm 151:311–315, 2015*

Diltiazem *JAAD 38:201–206, 1998; Clin Exp Dermatol 20:341–344, 1995*

Dithranol ointment *Hautarzt 49:781–783, 1998*

Doxorubicin *Acta DV 81:224, 2001*

Doxycycline *Dermatology 186:75–78, 1993*

Drug reaction with eosinophilia and systemic symptoms (DRESS) – morbilliform eruption, cheilitis (crusted hemorrhagic lips), diffuse desquamation, areolar erosion, periorbital dermatitis, vesicles, bullae, targetoid plaques, purpura, pustules, exfoliative erythroderma, facial edema, lymphadenopathy *JAAD 68:693–705, 2013*

Enalapril *Clin Exp Dermatol 21:54–55, 1996*

Epidermal growth factor inhibitors (chemotherapy) – purpura with pustules *JAMA Derm 153:906–910, 2017; JAAD 55:657–670, 2006*

Eprazinone *Hautarzt 35:200–203, 1984*

Erlotinib (epidermal growth factor receptor inhibitor) – papulopustular eruption; painful annular pustular eruption; targetoid lesions *Clin in Dermatol 29:587–601, 2011; Cutis 88:281–283, 2012; JAAD 58:545–570, 2008;* pustules of neck *JAAD 147:735–740, 2011*

Erythromycin

Etanercept – pustular psoriasis; palmoplantar pustular psoriasis *JAAD 56:327–328, 2007*

Ferrous fumarate *Dermatology 192:294–295, 1996*

Flucloxacillin – AGEP *BJD 171:1539–1545, 2014*

5-fluorouracil *JAAD 25:905–908, 1991;* pustular contact hypersensitivity *AD 121:240–242, 1985*

Furosemide *Dermatologica 146:285–291, 1973*

Gefitinib/erlotinib/cetuximab/panitumumab (epidermal growth factor receptor inhibitor) – papulopustular eruption *JAAD 71:217–227, 2014; JAAD 58:545–570, 2008;* sea of pustules covering entire scalp *JAMA 310:1068–1069, 2013*

Gentamycin *AD 139:1181–1183, 2003*

GM-CSF – subcorneal pustular eruption at injection site *JAAD 30:787–789, 1994; Ann Hematol 63:326–327, 1991*

Hydroxychloroquine *Acta DV 70:250–251, 1990*

Hydroxyzine – AGEP *BJD 157:1296–1297, 2007*

Icodextrin – palmoplantar pustulosis, erythroderma, generalized exanthematous pustulosis *AD 137:309–310, 2001*

Imatinib mesylate (Gleevec) (multikinase inhibitor) – AGEP *JAAD 58:545–570, 2008*

Imipenem *Ann DV 116:407–409, 1989*

Immune checkpoint inhibitors – CTLA-4, PD-1/PD-L1 inhibitors – pustular psoriasis *Clin in Dermatol 38:94–104, 2020*

Infliximab – pustular psoriasis; palmoplantar pustular psoriasis *JAAD 56:327–328, 2007*

INH *BJD 112:504–505, 1985*

Iododerma – after intravenous pyelogram *Dermatologica 171:463–468, 1985;* in chronic renal failure – 2–5 days, fever, edema of eyelids; pustulovesicular eruption, pustules, pseudovesicles, marked edema of face and eyelids, vegetative plaques *AD 140:1393–1398, 2004; JAAD 36:1014–1016, 1997; Clin Exp Dermatol 15:232–233, 1990; BJD 97:567–569, 1977;* pustules on a plaque *JAAD 36:1014–1016, 1997; JAAD 31:344–347, 1994;* radioactive iodine for thyroid ablation – acneiform and generalized pustular eruption *J Drugs in Dermatol 9:1070–1071, 2011;* papulopustular eruptions *Australas J Dermatol 28:119–122, 1987*

Iohexol and iodixanol – iodinated radiocontrast material; AGEP *Am J Roentgenol 187:W198–201, 2006; J Dermatol 30:723–726, 2003*

Iopamidol – AGEP *Ann DV 131:831–832, 2004*

Ioversol – non-ionic, non-iodinated radiocontrast material; AGEP *AD 145:683–687, 2009*

Kit and BCR-ABL inhibitors – imatinib, nilotinib, dasatinib – facial edema morbilliform eruptions, pigmentary changes, lichenoid reactions, psoriasis, pityriasis rosea, pustular eruptions, DRESS, Stevens-Johnson syndrome, urticarial, neutrophilic dermatoses, photosensitivity, pseudolymphoma, porphyria cutanea tarda, small vessel vasculitis, panniculitis, perforating folliculitis, erythroderma *JAAD 72:203–218, 2015*

Levofloxacin – localized exanthematous pustulosis of forehead *BJD 152:1076–1077, 2005*

Lithium *Clin Exp Derm 21:296–298, 1996*

MEK inhibitors – C1-1040, selumetinib, trametinib – morbilliform eruption, papulopustular eruptions, xerosis, paronychia *JAAD 72:221–236, 2015*

Mesalazine *JAAD 45:S220–221, 2001*

Methylphenidate hydrochloride (Ritalin) – AGEP *AD 147:872–873, 2011*

Metronidazole *AD 139:1181–1183, 2003*

Mexiletine *Eur J Dermatol 11:469–471, 2001*

Minocycline *Acta DV 77:168–169, 1997; AD 131:490–491, 1995*

Minoxidil – pustular contact dermatitis *Contact Dermatitis 38:283–284, 1998*

Naproxen *Dermatologica 179:57–58, 1989*

Nitrazepam

Norfloxacin – subcorneal pustular eruption *Cutis 42:24–27, 1988*

Nystatin *Hautarzt 49:492–495, 1998*

Ofloxacin *Acta DV 73:382–384, 1993*

Olanzapine *JAAD 41:851–853, 1999*

Oxytetracycline

Paclitaxel *Int J Dermatol 36:559–560, 1997*

Panitumumab – epidermal growth factor receptor inhibitor *AD 146:926–927, 2010*

Paracetamol *Dermatology 193:56–58, 1996*

Penicillin *Cutis 54:194–196, 1994*

Phenobarbital *AD 139:1181–1183, 2003*

Phenytoin hypersensitivity eruption *JAAD 18:721–741, 1988; AD 127:1361–1364, 1991*

Piperazine ethionamate *Dermatologica 146:285–291, 1973*

Piperacillin

Pneumococcal vaccine *Dermatology 187:217, 1993*

Prednisolone *Dermatol Monatsschr 174:221–225, 1988*

Proguanil

Pustular drug eruptions – personal observation

PUVA *AD 139:1181–1183, 2003*

Pyrimethamine *Dermatologica 146:285–291, 1973*

Resprim *AD 139:1181–1183, 2003*

Ritodrine *J Eur Acad DV 11:91–93, 1998*

Roxithromycin *AD 139:1181–1183, 2003*

Secukinumab – AGEP *JAMA Derm 152:482–483, 2016*

Sorafenib – pustular drug eruption (AGEP) *JAMA Derm 130:664–666, 2014;* localized pustular eruption *BJD 165:443–445, 2011*

Spiramycin

Streptomycin *AD 117:444–445, 1981*

Sulfasalazine

Tacrolimus ointment – rosacea-like dermatosis with overgrowth of Demodex folliculorum *AD 140:457–460, 2004*

Terbinafine *JAAD 49:158–159, 2003; Australas 41:42–45, 2000; JAAD 37:653–655, 1997, JAAD 39:115–117, 1998*

Tetracycline *AD 139:1181–1183, 2003*

Thalidomide – toxic pustuloderma *Clin Exp Dermatol 22:297–299, 1997*

Ticlopidine *AD 139:1181–1183, 2003*

Trimethoprim-sulfamethoxazole *AD 139:1181–1183, 2003*

Vemurafenib/dabrafenib – papulopustular facial rash *JAAD 71:217–227, 2014*

Vitamin B12 *DICP 23:1033–1044, 1989*

EXOGENOUS AGENTS

Antimony melting workers *J Occup Med 35:39–45, 1993*

Aromatic polycyclic hydrocarbons *G Ital Med Lav Ergon 19:152–163, 1997*

Chloracne *Stat Pearls April 24, 2020*

Clam digger's itch (cercarial dermatitis)

Fiberglass dermatitis *Int J Dermatol 58:1107–1111, 2019*

Irritant contact dermatitis – *Malva neglecta* Wallr *Dermatitis 25:140–146, 2014*

Mineral oils – folliculitis

Occlusion folliculitis

Oil folliculitis

Patch tests – acute generalized exanthematous pustulosis due to patch test to acetaminophen *AD 139:1181–1183, 2003*

Potassium iodide patch-test reactions *Arch Dermatol Forsch 242:137–152, 1972*

Rhus – ingestion of *Rhus* lacquer from Japanese lacquer tree as folk medicine remedy; AGEP *JAAD 63:166–168, 2010;* pustules *BJD 142:937–942, 2000*

Tar folliculitis – occupational *Int J Dermatol 54:868–869, 2015;* coal tar *J Dermatol Treat 18:329–334, 2007;* Goeckerman regimen *Ped Derm 27:518–524, 2010*

INFECTIONS AND INFESTATIONS

Acanthamoeba in AIDS *JAAD 42:351–354, 2000; AD 131:1291–1296, 1995; JAAD 26:352–355, 1992;* in lung transplant patient – personal observation

Acinetobacter calcoaceticus var anitratus – pustules *J Hosp Infect 1:125–131, 1980*

Actinomycosis

Actinomycetoma – due to *Nocardia brasiliensis;* pustules, scarring, sinus tracts, multilobulated nodules, grains *JAAD 62:239–246, 2010*

Aeromonas hydrophila folliculitis – mimicking hot tub folliculitis *Ped Derm 26:601–603, 2009;* due to inflatable swimming pool *Australas J Dermatol 49:39–41, 2008*

African tick bite fever (*Rickettsia africae*) – hemorrhagic pustule, purpuric papules; transmitted by Amblyomma ticks) – high fever, arthralgia, myalgia, fatigue, rash in 2–3 days, with eschar, maculo-papules, vesicles, and pustules *Clin Inf Dis 39:700–701, 741–742, 2004; JAAD 48:S18–19, 2003*

AIDS-associated eosinophilic pustular folliculitis – face, trunk, and extremities *NEJM 318:1183–1186, 1988; Sex Transm Infec 4 (3):229–230, 1987;* acute HIV infection – vesicopustular eruptions *AD 138:117–122, 2002*

Alternariosis *BJD 145:484–486, 2001; J Formos Med Assoc 91:462–466, 1992*

Ancylostoma caninum larvae *AD 127:247–250, 1991*

Anthrax – *Bacillus anthracis;* malignant pustule; face, neck, hands, arms; starts as papule then evolves into bulla on red base; then hemorrhagic crust with edema and erythema with small vesicles; edema of surrounding skin *Br J Ophthalmol 76:753–754, 1992; J Trop Med Hyg 89:43–45, 1986; Bol Med Hosp Infant Mex 38:355–361, 1981; Arch Intern Med 1955:387–396, 1956*

Aspergillosis – pustules *JAAD 80:869–880, 2019;* primary cutaneous aspergillosis – pustules and erythema under tape *Ped Derm 31:609–610, 2014; JAAD 31:344–347, 1994;* in neonates *Clin Inf Dis 22:1102–1104, 1996;* red plaque with pustules – *Aspergillus ustus JAAD 38:797–798, 1998;* disseminated – morbilliform rash which becomes pustular *Ped Derm 19:439–444, 2002; Aspergillus fumigatus* – red plaque with pustules *Ped Derm 26:592–596, 2009;* pustular violaceous plaque from hospital arm board *Ped Derm 26:493–495, 2009; Aspergillus fumigatus* – painful, purpuric necrotic papules and pustules in tattoo *BJD 170:1373–1375, 2014*

Bacillus cereus – cutaneous infection begins with vesicle and/or pustule and becomes cellulitis; then a non-healing ulcer with a black eschar *Cutis 79:371–377, 2007; Lancet Mar 18;1 (8638):601–603, 1989*

Disseminated BCG infection – in patient with severe combined immunodeficiency disease – abscesses, nodules, papules and pustules *Ped Derm 36:672–676, 2019*

Blastomycosis-like pyoderma *Australas J Dermatol 58:139–141, 2017; J Clin Diagn Res 10:W 003–004, 2016; AD 142:1643–1648, 2006; AD 115:170–173, 1979*

Blister beetle (Rove beetle) – pustular dermatitis *Mil Med 169:57–60, 2004*

Bockhart's impetigo (staphylococcal folliculitis)

Botryomycosis – plaques with pustules and crusts *J Drugs Dermatol 13:976–978, 2014; J Dermatol 36:551–554, 2009; AD 139:93–98, 2003; Cutis 55:149–152, 1995;* disseminated botryomy-cosis – due to *Staphylococcus aureus;* disseminated pustules of nose, papules of eyelids, eschars of extremities *J Drugs Dermatol 13:976–78, 2014*

Brown recluse spider bite *Hautarzt 41:218–219, 1990;* AGEP *Ped Derm 28:685–688, 2011*

Candidiasis – flexural candidiasis with satellite pustules *Clin Obstet Gynecol 24:407–438, 1981;* disseminated candidiasis, congenital cutaneous candidiasis – papulopustular eruption of newborn *Ped Derm 35:683–684, 2018; Pediatrics 105:438–444, 2000; AJDC 135:273–275, 1981;* necrotic pustules *JAAD 37:817–823, 1997;* mimicking tinea barbae *Int J Derm 36:295–297, 1997;* candidiasis, systemic in drug addicts – purulent nodules of scalp and follicular pustules of beard, axilla, and pubis *Br Med J 287:861–862, 1983; Candida kefyr* – unilateral red nodules of leg, bullae, pustules; arterial thrombus of left iliac artery *Cutis 91:137–140, 2013*

Carbuncle *Stat Pearls May 2, 2020*

Cat scratch disease – inoculation pustule, papule, or vesicle *JAAD 18:239–259, 1988; Ped Derm 5:1–9, 1988*

Cellulitis with overlying pustules – personal observation

Cheyletiella mite infestation – papulovesicles, pustules, necrosis *JAAD 50:819–842, 2004; AD 116:435–437, 1980*

Chromobacterium violaceum Ped Infect Dis 11:583–586, 1992

Clostridium perfringens Clin Inf Dis 26:501–502, 1998

Clostridium welchii

Coccidioidomycosis – papulopustules *JAAD 55:929–942, 2006; JAAD 26:79–85, 1992;* red plaque with pustules *JAAD 46:743–747, 2002*

Cowpox (feline orthopoxvirus) – papule progresses to vesicle to hemorrhagic vesicle to umbilicated pustule, then eschar with ulcer; tongue ulcer, targetoid and umbilicated indurated papules, vesicles, pustules with central necrosis; exposure to pet rat *Clin Inf Dis 68:1063–1064, 2019; JAAD 49:513–518, 2003; JAAD 44:1–14, 2001; BJD 1331:598–607, 1994;* generalized cowpox in Darier's disease – crusted papules, pustules, and vesicles; cobblestoned appearance; with massive periorbital edema *BJD 164:1116–1118, 2011*

Coxsackie A6 – hand, foot, and mouth disease; intertrigo, acral pustules and vesicopustules *Cutis 102:353–356, 2018; Coxsackie A9, B4* – AGEP *AD 139:1181–1183, 2003; Coxsackie A16* – hand, foot, and mouth disease; blisters and vesicopustules; perioral dermatitis *Cutis 102:353–356, 2018*

Cryptococcosis *BMJ Case Rep July 21, 2015; Med Mycol 48:785–791, 2010; Clin Exp Dermatol 34:e751–753, 2009; JAAD 37:116–117, 1997*

Cytomegalovirus infection – AGEP *AD 139:1181–1183, 2003;* pustules, ulcers, bullae, and vesicles in fatal CMV *JAMA Derm 151:1380–1381, 2015; AD 127:396–398, 1991*

Dematiacious fungal infections in organ transplant recipients – all lesions on extremities
  Alternaria Transpl Infect Dis 12:242–250, 2010
  Bipolaris hawaiiensis
  Exophiala jeanselmei, E. spinifera, E. pesciphera, E. castellani, E. pisciphila Rev Infect Dis 13:379–382, 1991
  Exserohilum rostratum
  Fonsacaea pedrosoi
  Phialophora parasitica

Demodex folliculitis *Hautarzt 50:491–494, 1999; Clin Exp Dermatol 21:148–150, 1996; JAAD 15:1159, 1986;* of scalp – demodex-associated papulopustular folliculitis *BJD 170:1219–1225, 2014; Am J Dermatopathol 18:589–591, 1996; Cutis 76:321–324, 2005;* mimicking favus; hyperkeratotic patchy alopecia, papules, vesicles, pustules *JAAD 57:S19–21, 2007;*

papular facial dermatitis in children with acute lymphoblastic leukemia *Ped Derm 22:407–411, 2005;* pustules of nose *Ped Derm 24:417–418, 2007*

Dermatophilus congolensis – due to contact with infected animals *BJD 145:170–171, 2001; JAAD 29:351–354, 1993*

Diphtheria, cutaneous – painful vesicle evolving into pustule then anesthetic shallow punched out ulcer with gray-black membrane *Cutis 79:371–377, 2007*

Echinococcosis – cystic echinococcosis of the liver with acute generalized exanthematous pustulosis *BJD 148:1245–1249, 2003*

Echovirus 6, 30, 11

Ecthyma

Ecthyma gangrenosum *Am J Med 70:1133–1135, 1981;* disseminated *Candida; Chromobacterium violaceum JAAD 54:S224–228, 2006*

Eczema herpeticum (Kaposi's varicelliform eruption) *Stat Pearls Jan 10, 2020; Cutis 75:33–36, 2005; Hautarzt 55:646–652, 2004; JAAD 49:198–205, 2003;* in Darier's disease *JAAD 72:481–484, 2015*

Eczema vaccinatum *Am J Health Syst Pharm 60:749–756, 2003*

Ehrlichiosis – human granulocytic ehrlichiosis *JAAD 49:363–392, 2003*

Enterovirus infection – acral pustular eruption *Tyring, p.460, 2002*

Epstein-Barr virus – AGEP *AD 139:1181–1183, 2003*

Erysipelas – personal observation

Erysipeloid

Favus – follicular pustules

Felon

Fire ant stings (*Solenopsis invicta*) – clusters of vesicles evolve into umbilicated pustules on red swollen base; crusting, heal with scars; urticaria; pustule formation due to piperidine (alkaloids) *NEJM 370:1432–1439, 2014; JAAD 67:331–344, 2012; Cutis 83:17–20, 2009; Cutis 75:85–89, 2005; JAMA 284:2162–2163, 2000; J S C Med Assoc 95:231–235, 1999; Ann Allergy Asthma Immunol 77:87–95, 1996; Allergy 50:535–544, 1995; Ped Derm 9:44–48, 1992;* reached United States from Brazil through port of Mobile, Alabama in 1930s *Ann Rev Entomol 20:1–30, 1975; Solenopsis invicta* – red imported fire ant; *S. xyloni* – native southern fire ant; *S. richteri* – black imported fire ant; *S aurea* – desert fire ant; *S. geminate* – tropical fire ant; *Pogonomyrmex rugosus* – rough harvester ant; *P. Maricopa* – Maricopa harvester ant; *P. barbatus* – red harvester ant; *P. ejectus* – twig or oak ant; *Hypoponera punctatissima; Pachycondyla chinensis–* Asian needle ant *Cutis 83:17–20, 2009*

Folliculitis – multiple organisms; follicular pustules of neck *J Drugs in Dermatol 12:369–374, 2013*

Fusarium, disseminated *JAAD 47:659–666, 2002; Ped Derm 13:118–121, 1996;* with myositis *Ped Derm 13:118–121, 1996; Ped Derm 9:62–65, 1992; Dermatology 186:232–235, 1993; JAAD 23:393–398, 1990; F. falciforme* – red plaques, vesicles, pustules, necrosis *BJD 157:407–409, 2007*

Glanders (farcy) – *Burkholderia (Pseudomonas) mallei* – cellulitis which ulcerates with purulent foul-smelling discharge, regional lymphatics become abscesses; nasal and palatal necrosis and destruction; metastatic papules, pustules, bullae over joints and face, then ulcerate; deep abscesses with sinus tracts occur; polyarthritis, meningitis, pneumonia *JAAD 54:559–578, 2006*

Gonorrhea – penile pustules of coronal sulcus; gonococcemia – hemorrhagic pustules with halo of erythema *Dermatol Online J Jan 15:23 (1)13030/qt33624006; NEJM 380:1565, 2019; Int J Dermatol 42:208–209, 2003AD 107:403–406, 1973*

Gram negative folliculitis *NEJM 352:1463–1472, 2005; Int J Dermatol 38:270–274, 1999; Fortschr Med 115:42–44, 1997*

Haematosiphoniasis (Mexican chicken bug) – wheals, papules, vesicles, pustules, crusts

Hand foot and mouth disease – *Coxsackie A16, A5, A7, A9, A10, B2, B3, B5, Enterovirus 71;* vesicular *BJD 160:890–892, 2009; Ped*

Derm 20:52–56, 2003; BJD 79:309–317, 1967; Enterovirus 71 – myocarditis, encephalitis, aseptic meningitis, pulmonary edema *BJD 160:890–892, 2009; NEJM 341:929–935, 1999*

Hepatitis B infection – AGEP *AD 139:1181–1183, 2003*

Herpes simplex – papules and pustules *BJD 172:278–280, 2015;* pustules of chest wall with disseminated herpes simplex *Clin Inf Dis 56:559,613–614, 2013; AD 113:983–986, 1997;* herpetic whitlow *Case Rep Orthop 2014:906487.doi:10.1155/2014/906487.Epub Nov 4*

Herpes zoster *AD 113:983–986, 1997*

Histoplasmosis, disseminated *Clin Dermatol 30:592–598, 2012; AD 143:255–260, 2007; AD 132:341–346, 1996; JAAD 25:418–422, 1991; JAAD 23:422–428, 1990*

Hookworm folliculitis – ancylostoma *AD 127:547, 1991*

Hot tub folliculitis *Ped Derm 28:590–591, 2011; JAAD 57:596–600, 2007*

Impetigo contagiosa *Ped Derm 31:609–610, 2014;* pregnancy *Dermatol Onlin J April 18, 2016*

Insect bites – sandflies (*Phlebotomus, Lutzomyia*) – harara, urticaria multiformis endemica in Middle East; vesicopustules *The Clinical Management of Itching; Parthenon; p. 64, 2000*

Kerion – pustular plaque of scalp *Ped Derm 27:361–363, 2010*

Leclaria adecarboxylata – cellulitis with necrotic pustules in acute lymphoblastic leukemia *Ped Derm 28:162–164, 2011*

Leprosy – erythema nodosum leprosum *J Eur Acad DV 31:705–711, 2017; JAAD 51:416–426, 2004; AD 111:1575–1580, 1975;* erythema nodosum leprosum *Lepr Rev 85:322–327, 2014*

Listeriosis, congenital – grey–white papules or pustules with red margins; predilection for the back *J Natl Med Assoc 57:290–296, 1965;* purpura, morbilliform rashes *Am J Dis Child 131:405–408, 1977; J Cutan Pathol 18:474–476, 1991;* contact listeriosis – localized vesicles or pustules *JAAD 48:759, 2003;* septic vasculitis *Rev Chilena Infectol 31:764–769, 2014*

Lobomycosis (*Lacazia loboi*) – earliest lesion is a small pustule or papule *JAAD 53:931–951, 2006; J Clin Microbiol 38:1283–1285, 2000*

Lyme disease – annular lesion with central papulopustule *QJM Nov 4, 2019; JAAD 49:363–392, 2003*

Majocchi's granuloma – crusted papules and pustules of leg *JAMA Derm 153:205–206, 2017*

Meleney's synergistic gangrene

Melioidosis – *Burkholderia pseudomallei* – pustules *JAAD 75:1–16, 2016; JAAD 54:559–578, 2006; Clin Inf Dis 33:29–34, 2001; Med J Malaysia 48:248–249, 1993*

Meningococcemia – acute, chronic *Rev Infect Dis 8:1–11, 1986;* septic vasculopathy *Int J Dermatol 52:1071–1080, 2013*

Microsporum gypseum – plaque with multiple nodules and pustules *BJD 146:311–313, 2002*

Milker's nodule – vesiculopustules of dorsal hand *JAMA Derm 156:93, 2020; JAAD 49:910–911, 2003;* chronic *Ped Derm 13:483–487, 1991*

Mites – cheese mite (Glyciphagus) bites – papulovesicles and pustules *Dermatol Clin 8:265–275, 1990*

Molluscum contagiosum *AD 133:983–986, 1997*

Monkeypox – exanthem indistinguishable from smallpox (papulovesiculopustular) (vesicles, umbilicated pustules, crusts) except for presence of adenopathy – prairie dogs infected by Gambian rat *JAAD 49:979–1000, 2003; CDC Health Advisory, June 7,2003; JAAD 44:1–14, 2001; J Infect Dis 156:293–298, 1987;* cervical, maxillary, and inguinal adenopathy; headache, fatigue; rash begins on face and moves downward; begins as macular eruption then papular, vesicular, pustular *Clin Inf Dis 58:260–267, 2014*

Moraxella osloensis – gonococcemia-like infection *Cutis 21:657–659, 1978*

Mucormycosis – red plaque with pustules *JAAD 59:542–544, 2008;* pustules – *Mucor, Rhizopus oryzi, Rhizomucor, Lichtheimia, Saksenaea, Cunninhghamella, Apophysomyces* pink papules *JAAD 80:869–880, 2019; Mycopatholgia 173:187–192, 2012*

Mycetoma *JAAD 32:311–315, 1995; Cutis 49:107–110, 1992; Australas J Dermatol 31:33–36, 1990; JAAD 6:107–111, 1982; Sabouraudia 18:91–95, 1980; AD 99:215–225, 1969*

Mycobacterium abscessus – acquired in swimming pools; pustules of palms, soles, and arms *Ped Derm 31:292–297, 2014*

Mycobacterium avium intracellulare – resembles lupus vulgaris *J Cut Med Surg 272–274, 2016; BJD 136:264–266, 1997;* disseminated infection in AIDS – pustules *BJD 130:785–790, 1994*

Mycobacterium bollettii – leg plaques and abscesses due to foot baths for pedicures *AD 147:454–458, 2011*

Mycobacterium bovis JAAD 28:264–266, 1993

Mycobacterium chelonae BJD 171:79–89, 2014; Clin Exp Dermatol 29:254–257, 2004; Rev Clin Exp 196:606–609, 1996; with pustules *JAAD 24:867–870, 1991;* hemorrhagic pustules of face and neck ; mimicking *Demodex* folliculitis *Clin Exp Dermatol 45:469–470, 2020*

Mycobacterium fortuitum

Mycobacterium hemophilum BJD 149:200–202, 2003; Ann Int Med 120:118–125, 1994; JAAD 28:264–266, 1993;

Mycobacterium kansasii – pustules *JAAD 40:359–363, 1999;* papulopustules *JAAD 41:854–856, 1999; JAAD 36:497–499, 1997*

Mycobacterium marinum – disseminated pustular eruption resembling varicella in subacute combined immune deficiency *Clin Inf Dis 21:1325–1327, 1995*

Mycobacterium malliliense – leg plaques, pustules, and abscesses due to foot baths for pedicures *AD 147:454–458, 2011*

Mycobacterium tuberculosis – acute miliary tuberculosis – multiple pustules *Clin Inf Dis 57:1162–1163,1210–1211, 2013; JAAD 50:S110–113, 2004; J Clin Inf Dis 23:706–710, 1996;* papulopustular eruption *Ped Derm 3:464–467, 1986;* large crops of blue papules, vesicles, pustules, hemorrhagic papules; red nodules; vesicles become necrotic to form ulcers *Practitioner 222:390–393, 1979; Am J Med 56:459–505, 1974; AD 99:64–69, 1969;* lichen scrofulosorum – yellow to red-brown flat-topped papules, slightly scaly, surmounted with minute pustule; trunk scrofulosorum *Ped Derm 17:373–376, 2000; AD 124:1421–1426, 1988; Clin Exp Dermatol 1:391–394, 1976;* acne scrofulosorum – follicular papules heal with scarring; domed papulopustular follicular lesions *Clin Exp Dermatol 6:339–344, 1981; BJD 7:341–351, 1895;* lichen scrofulosorum – psoriasiform dermatitis with pustules *Ped Derm 28:532–534, 2011;* papulonecrotic tuberculid – papulopustules; dusky red crusted or ulcerated papules occur in crops on elbows, hands, feet, knees, legs; also ears, face, buttock, and penis; may evolve into pustules *NEJM 380:275–283, 2019; Dermatol Therapy 21:154–161, 2008; JAAD 14:815, 1986; Ped Derm 15:450–455, 1998;* disseminated lupus vulgaris presenting as granulomatous folliculitis *Int J Dermatol 28:388–392, 1989*

Mycobacterium ulcerans Clin Inf Dis 21:1325–1327, 1995

Mycoplasma pneumoniae – AGEP *AD 139:1181–1183, 2003*

Myiasis, including tumbu fly myiasis; furuncular myiasis *Med Sant Trop 28:375–377, 2018; AD 131:951, 1995; Dermatobia hominis Acta DV Croat 26:267–269, 2018;*

Necrotizing fasciitis – streptococcal *Ann DV 128:376–381, 2001; AD 130:1150–1158, 1994;* methicillin-resistant *Staphylococcus aureus NEJM 352:1445–1453, 2005; Serratia marcescens Clin Inf Dis 23:648–649, 1996; JAAD 20:774–778, 1989; Bacteroides spp.* in penile necrotizing fasciitis *JAAD 37:1–24, 1997;* neonatal *Pediatrics 103:e53, 1999;* in infancy *Ped Derm 2:55–63, 1984;* Clostridial cellulitis (gangrene); progressive synergistic gangrene; gangrenous cellulitis (*Pseudomonas*); Fournier's gangrene

Nocardia asteroides Cureus 11:e5860, 2019; J Dermatol Case Rep 7:52–55, 2013; JAAD 41:338–340, 1999; JAAD 20:889–892, 1989; AD 121:898–900, 1985; Rev Infect Dis 6:164–180, 1984; JAMA 242:333–336, 1979; lymphocutaneous nocardiosis – crusted verrucous plaques with sporotrichoid nodules, abscesses, and pustules *Cutis 85:73–76, 2010*

North American blastomycosis – pustulonodular infiltration of nose *JAMA 312:2564–2565, 2014; AD 138:1371–1376, 2002; Cutis 50:422–424, 1992; Int J Dermatol 16:277–280, 1977;* disseminated – papulopustules *JAAD 61:355–358, 2009; NEJM 356:1456–1462, 2007; Cutis 30:199–202l 1982; Int J Dermatol 16:277–278, 1977;* red plaque with pustules *JAAD 53:740–741, 2005;* disseminated blastomycosis – red plaque with pustules *Ped Derm 23:541–545, 2006*

Onchocerciasis (*Onchocerca volvulus*) – acute papular onchodermatitis – papules, vesicles, pustules *JAAD 73:929–944, 2015*

Orf – vesiculo-pustules of four fingers *Cutis 100:148, 158, 2017;* pustular nodule *The Dermatologist March 2015, pp 47–50;* hemorrhagic pustule *AD 145:321–326, 2009; Ann DV 113:1065–1076, 1986*

Paecilomyces lilacinus (cutaneous hyalohyphomycosis) – folliculitis *JAAD 35:779–781, 1996; JAAD 37:270–271, 1997; P. variotii Transp Infect Dis 20:e12871, 2018*

Paederus beetle dermatitis – linear papular, vesicular, and pustular dermatitis *JAAD 57:297–300, 2007; Cutis 69:277–279, 2002*

Parvovirus B19 *Am J Med 84:968–972, 1988;* including vesicopustules of the hard and soft palate (papular-purpuric "gloves and socks" syndrome) *JAAD 41:793–796, 1999;* AGEP *AD 139:1181–1183, 2003*

Pasteurella multocida – vesicopustules of palms *Cutis 89:269–272, 2012*

Peloderma strongyloides (nematode larvae) – exanthem of papules and pustules *JAAD 51:S181–184, 2004; JAAD 51:S109–112, 2004; Cutis 48:123–126, 1991*

Penicillium marneffei JAAD 37:450–472, 1997; J Clin Inf Dis 23:125–130, 1996

Phaeohyphomycosis – nodule with pustules; *Exophiala J Clin Inf Dis 19:339–341, 1994;* diffuse infiltrated pigmented plaques; subcutaneous cysts, abscesses, ulcerated plaques, hemorrhagic pustules, necrotic papulonodules, cellulitis *JAAD 75:19–30, 2016; JAAD 40:364–366, 1999; JAAD 28:34–44, 1993; AD 127:721–726, 1991; JAAD 19:478–481, 1988; AD 123:1346–1350, 1987*

Pityrosporum folliculitis – upper trunk and upper arms *JAAD 52:528, 2005; J Dermatol 27:49–51, 2000; Int J Derm 38:453–456, 1999; Int J Derm 37:772–777, 1998; JAAD 24:693–696, 1991; Ann Int Med 108:560–563, 1988; JAAD 12:56–61, 1985; AD 107:388–391, 1973;* Splendore-Hoeppli phenomenon in pityrosporum folliculitis *J Cutan Pathol 18:293–297, 1991*

Plague (*Yersinia pestis*) – umbilicated vesicles or pustules *J Infect Dis 129:S78–84, 1974*

Novel poxvirus (related to Yoka virus) – vesicopustule *Clin Inf Dis 61:1543–1548, 2015*

Protothecosis – red plaque with pustules and ulcers *BJD 146:688–693, 2002*

Pseudomonas – ecthyma gangrenosum *Cureus Aug 31, 2019;* periumbilical pustules with necrotic ulcers; extensive necrosis in neutropenic patients *JAAD 11:781–786, 1984; AD 97:312–318, 1968;* diving suit folliculitis *JAAD 31:1055–1056, 1994;* hot tub folliculitis; swimming pool *Ped Derm 28:590–591, 2011; Public*

Health Rep 96:246–249, 1981; AD 120:1304–1307, 1984; following depilation Ann Derm Venereol 123:268–270, 1996; Rev Infect Dis 5:1–8, 1983; wet suit Pseudomonas dermatitis – pustules and papules Ped Derm 458–459, 2003

Pustular bacterid J Gen Fam Med 19:32–33, 2017; Lancet Infect Dis 13:655–656, 2013; Am J Dermatopathol 7:200, 1985

Pythium insidiosum (pythiosis) (alga) (aquatic oocyte) – necrotizing hemorrhagic plaque; ascending gangrene of legs; Thailand; painful subcutaneous nodules, eyelid swelling and periorbital cellulitis, facial swelling, ulcer of arm or leg, pustules evolving into ulcers BJD 175:394–397, 2016; J Infect Dis 159:274–280, 1989

Rat bite fever (Streptobacillus moniliformis) – fever, arthritis, exanthema; papules and papulopustules of face and hand; hand and foot swellings Ped Derm 29:767–768, 2012; acral hemorrhagic pustules; petechial exanthem abscesses NEJM 381:1762, 2019; JAMA 321:1930–1931, 2019; AD 148:1411–1416, 2012; Clin Inf Dis 43:1585–1586;1616–1617, 2006; JAAD 38:330–332, 1998

Rhinoscleroma

Rickettsia parkeri rickettsiosis – Southeastern United States; Gulf coast tick (Amblomma maculatum); eschar with surrounding petechiae, fever, lethargy, fatigue, headache, myalgia, arthralgia, morbilliform or vesiculopapular or papulopustular rash of trunk and extremities, palms and soles, and occasionally the face 0.5 to 4 days after fever; some lesions with small vesicle or pustule; morbilliform eruptions, discrete round macules and papules AD 146:641–648, 2010; Clin Inf Dis 47:1188–1196, 2008

Rickettsial pox Ann NY Acad Sci 990:36–44, 2003

Salmonella – veterinarians with nodules with central pustulation Rook p.1143, 1998, Sixth Edition; toxic shock syndrome – personal observation

Scabies Cutis 101:169, 178, 2018; Am J Dis Child 133:1031–1034, 1979

Scedosporium (asexual form of Pseudallescheria boydii) – eumyce-toma; red swollen arm with numerous pustules AD 148:1199–1204, 2012

Schistosoma haematobium Am J Dermatopathol 16:442–446, 1994

Serratia – eccrine hidradenitis (pustule) JAAD 22:1119–1120, 1990; S. marcescens – papular eruption with pustules AIDS 10:1179–1180, 1996

Smallpox (variola) – macular and papular exanthem of face and extremities develop vesicles, pustules, and umbilicated crusts; hemorrhagic smallpox more severe JAAD 65:1213–1218, 2011; Am J Health Syst Pharm 60:749–456, 2003; JAAD 44:1–14, 2001

Smallpox vaccination Clin Inf Dis 37:241–250, 2003; generalized vaccinia – umbilicated vesicopustules Clin Inf Dis 37:251–271, 2003

Sparganosis – linear migratory erythema with or without pustules

Spider bite (brown recluse spider) – acute generalized exanthema-tous pustulosis JAAD 55:525–529, 2006

Sporotrichosis Stat Pearls Nov 27, 2019; ID cases 12:99–100, 2018; JAMA 242:333–336, 1979

Staphylococcal abscesses (furuncle), folliculitis; periporitis of neonate AD Syphilol 69:543–553, 1954; chronic folliculitis of the legs of Indian males Indian J DV 39:35–39, 1973

Streptococcal disease – pustulosa acuta generalisata JAAD 58:1056–1058, 2008; Ped Derm 24:272–276, 2007; BJD 133:135–139, 1995; streptococcal pyoderma; group A pustulosis Ped Derm 36:995–996, 2019; streptococcal impetigo; infectious eczematoid dermatitis D Eur Acad DV 29:203–208, 2015

Streptococcal gangrene (necrotizing fasciitis), streptococcal pyoderma

Swimmer's itch (cercarial dermatitis) – fresh water Environ Health 17:73, 2018; Cutis 19:461–465, 1977

Sycosis barbae – deep staphylococcal folliculitis Dermatol Wochenschr 152:153–167, 1966

Syphilis – secondary; miliary pustular syphilis J Clin Inf Dis 21:1361–1371, 1995; Cutis 34:556–558, 1984; noduloulcerative secondary syphilis AD 113:1027–1032, 1997; Sex Transm Dis 5:115–118, 1978; congenital; malignant lues Indian J Dermatol 62:524–527, 2017; Infection 43:231–236, 2015; frambesiform Br J Vener Dis 53:195–199, 1977

Tinea – tinea corporis; tinea barbae – Trichophyton verrucosum Clin Infect Dis 23:1308–1310, 1996; tinea capitis Int J Derm 33:255–257, 1994; tinea capitis of adult females – pustular eruptions JAAD 49:S177–179, 2003; kerion Mycoses 42:581–585, 1999; tinea pedis JAAD 42:132–133, 2000; Trichophyton rubrum tinea pedis – plantar pustules JAAD 42:132–133, 2000

Tick larvae J Dermatol 8:157–159, 1981

Tinea faciei – Trichophyton mentagrophytes – red plaque of eyelid with pustules Ped Derm 34:711–712, 2017

Toxic shock syndrome, either streptococcal or staphylococcal – widespread macular erythema, scarlatiniform, and papulopustular eruptions; occasional vesicles and bullae; edema of hands and feet; mucosal erythema; second week morbilliform or urticarial eruption occurs with desquamation at 10–21 days JAAD 39:383–398, 1998; Rev Infect Dis 11 (Suppl 1):S1–7, 1989; JAAD 8:343–347, 1983

Toxoplasma gondii AD 136:791–796, 2000

Trichophyton erinacei – pustules and erosion of dorsal hand; pet hedgehog JAMA Derm 154:967–968, 2018

Trichosporon beigelii – disseminated – papulopustular AD 129:1020–1023, 1993

Tsukamurella paurometabolum New Microbes New Infection 22:6–12, 2018; J Clin Inf Dis 23:839–840, 1996

Tufted folliculitis BJD 138:799–805, 1998

Tularemia – Francisella tularensis (non-encapsulated gram-nega-tive coccobacillus); transmitted in tick feces; skin, eye, respiratory, gastrointestinal portals of entry; ulceroglandular, oculoglandular, glandular types; typhoidal, pneumonic, oropharyngeal, and gastrointestinal types; toxemic stage heralds macular, generalized morbilliform eruption, vesicular, pustular, nodular or plaque-like secondary eruption; erythema multiforme-like rash, crops of red nodules on extremities; ulceroglandular tularemia – starts as papule, then pustule, then ulcer, then lymph node; fever, head-ache, chills, body aches, coryza, sore throat JAAD 65:1213–1218, 2011; JAAD 49:363–392, 2003; Cutis 54:279–286, 1994; Medicine 54:252–269, 1985; vesiculopapular lesions of trunk and extremi-ties Cutis 54:279–286, 1994; Photodermatology 2:122–123, 1985; pustule of toe; lymphangitis of foot Ped Derm 35:478–481, 2018

Tungiasis – pustules of hand JAAD 82:551–569, 2020; JAMA Derm Aug 14, 2019; NEJM 380:e19, 2019; J Public Health Afr 2:e21, 2011; Emerging Infect Dis 9:949–955, 2003; Acta Dermatovenereol (Stockh)76:495, 1996; Cutis 56:206–207, 1995

Vaccinia – sycosis vaccinatum – folliculocentric pustules of bearded region JAMA Derm 151:799–800, 2015; JAAD 44:1–14, 2001

Varicella – reinfection varicella Clin Inf Dis 52:907–909, 2011

Viral syndrome

Yersinia enterocolitica Medicine (Balt)95:e3988, 2016

Zygomycosis – red plaque with pustules JAAD 30:904–908, 1994

INFILTRATIVE DISORDERS

Congenital self-healing histiocytosis (Hashimoto-Pritzker disease) – congenital crusted red or blue nodules, pustules *Ped Derm 18:41–44, 2001*

Langerhans cell histiocytosis – children; adults – follicular pustules in scalp and groin *Dermatol Online J Aug 15, 2019; JAAD 78:1047–1056, 2018; J Drugs Dermatol 13:1153–1154, 2014; J Eur Acad DV 14:212–215, 2000; JAAD 29:166–170, 1993;* vesicopustules *Curr Prob Derm 14:41–70, 2002; JAAD 13:481–496, 1985;* pustules, ulcers *Obstet Gynecol 67:46–49, 1986;* umbilicated blisters and pustules *Hematol Oncol Clin North Amer 12:269–286, 1998*

INFLAMMATORY DISORDERS

Acute generalized exanthematous pustulosis – pustules, purpura, fever and rash – etiologies include multiple drugs, mercury, enterovirus, adenovirus, Epstein-Barr virus, cytomegalovirus, hepatitis B virus, mycoplasma pneumoniae *Semin Immunopathol 38:75–86, 2016; JAAD 73:843–848, 2015; AD 140:1172–1173, 2004; Ped Derm 17:399–402, 2000;* loxoscelism *BJD 161:208–209, 2009*

Chronic recurrent multifocal osteomyelitis (CRMO) – seen with varied neutrophilic dermatoses including SAPHO syndrome, pyoderma gangrenosum, acne fulminans, pustular psoriasis, Sweet's syndrome *Ped Derm 26:497–505, 2009*

Crohn's disease – perianal pustule *Ped Derm 35:566–574, 2018;* vesiculopustular lesions; palmoplantar pustulosis *JAAD 36:697–704, 1997;* pustular eruption *Ped Derm 13:127–130, 1996;* neutrophilic dermatosis – vesiculopustules of face and trunk *Ped Derm 30:619–620, 2013*

Deficiency of interleukin-1 receptor antagonist (DIRA) – autosomal recessive; life threatening systemic inflammation with bone and skin involvement; anonychia; chronic cutaneous pustulosis resembling pustular psoriasis; bone lesions include lytic bone lesions, periostitis, osteopenia, long bone epiphyseal ballooning and erosions, widening of clavicle and anterior rib ends, periosteal elevation, heterotopic ossification; vascular occlusions, interstitial pulmonary fibrosis; red eyes *Front Immunol 10:2448, 2019; AD 148:301–304, 2012; NEJM 360:2426–2437, 2009*

Dissecting cellulitis of the scalp (perifolliculitis capitis abscessus et suffodiens) *Minn Med 34:319–325, 1951; AD 23:503–518, 1931; BJD 174:916–918, 2016; JAAD 53:1–37, 2005;* perifollicular pustules *Dermatol Online J 20:22092, 2014*

Eosinophilic pustular folliculitis – annular pustular eruption in butterfly distribution *JAMA Derm 155:481–482, 2019; JAAD 55:285–289, 2006;* infantile eosinophilic pustular folliculitis – pustules of scalp, face, trunk, and limbs *Ped Derm 26:195–196, 2009; AD 144:105–110, 2008; Ped Derm 25:52–55, 2008; JAAD 55:285–289, 2006;* pustules of scalp and extremities *Ped Derm 30:621–622, 2013;* HIV-associated *JAAD 55:285–289, 2006;* 2–3 months following stem-cell transplantation *Ped Derm 34:326–330, 2017*

Erythema multiforme with subcorneal pustules *J Eur Acad DV 20:1353–1355, 2006; Ped Derm 17:202–204, 2000; BJD 88:605–607, 1973*

Folliculitis decalvans *Cutis 78:162–164, 2006; JAAD 53:1–37, 2005; J Dermatol 28:329–331, 2001; JAAD 39:891–893, 1998*

Folliculitis spinulosa decalvans – pustules, keratotic papules of scalp, scarring alopecia *Cutis 98:175–178, 2016; Ped Derm 23:255–258, 2006*

Hidradenitis suppurativa *An Bras Dermatol 95:203–206, 2020; BMJ Case Rep Feb 10, 2017; AD 133:967–970, 1997*

Interleukin 36 receptor antagonist deficiency (IL36RN) – pustular psoriasis *NEJM 365:620–628, 2011; Am J Hum Genet 89:432–437, 2011*

Kikuchi's disease (histiocytic necrotizing lymphadenitis) (subacute necrotizing lymphadenitis) – papulopustules, morbilliform eruption, urticarial, and rubella-like exanthems; red papules of face, back, arms; red plaques; erythema and acneform lesions of face; exanthem overlying involved lymph nodes; red or ulcerated pharynx; cervical adenopathy; associations with SLE, lymphoma, tuberculous adenitis, viral lymphadenitis, infectious mononucleosis, and drug eruptions *AD 142:641–646, 2006; Ped Derm 18:403–405, 2001; JAAD 22:909–912, 1990; Am J Surg Pathol 14:872–876, 1990;* rubella-like eruption, generalized erythema and papules *BJD 146:167–168, 2002*

Malignant pyoderma – head and neck variant of pyoderma gangrenosum *Eur J Dermatol 11:595–596, 2001; AD 122:295–302, 1986;* papulopustules, skin ulcers, violaceous nodules with central necrosis, tongue, pharyngeal, and nasal ulcers *AD 146:102–104, 2010; AD 98:561–576, 1968*

Meibomitis with ocular rosacea – personal observation

Miliaria pustulosa *Int J Dermatol 58:86–90, 2019; JAMA 148:1097–1100, 1952*

Neutrophilic dermatosis of the dorsal hands (variant of Sweet's syndrome) – ulcerated pustules of dorsal hands *JAMA Derm 150:897–898, 2014; AD 142:57–63, 2006*

Neutrophilic eccrine hidradenitis *Ped Derm 6:33–38, 1989; AD 131:1141–1145, 1995; JAAD 38:1–17, 1998*

Pustulotic arthro-osteitis *Semin Musculoskelet Radiol 5:89–93, 2001;* pustular vasculitis with sternoclavicular hyperostosis *Dermatology 186:213–216, 1993*

Pyoderma gangrenosum – pustular pyoderma gangrenosum *JAAD 79:1009–1022, 2018;* solitary pustule *JAAD 18:359–368, 1988;* triplet of pustules *BJD 157:1235–1239, 2007;* pustular pyoderma gangrenosum with colitis in children *JAAD 15:608–614, 1986;* pyoderma gangrenosum, palmoplantar pustulosis, and chronic recurrent multifocal osteomyelitis *Ped Derm 15:435–438, 1998;* pustular pyoderma gangrenosum *Clin Rev Allergy Immunol 45:202–210, 2013; Inflamm Bowel Dis 2013, Oct 13; SKINmed 9:196–198, 2011; AD 114:1061–1064, 1978;* pustular pyoderma gangrenosum in pregnancy *Cutis 81:255–258, 2008;* in children *Ped Derm 25:509–519, 2008;* peristomal pyoderma gangrenosum *BJD 161:1206–1207, 2009*

Pyoderma fistulans sinifica (fox den disease) *Wounds 27:170–173, 2015; Dermatology Online J June 15, 2013; J Clin Inf Dis 21:162–170, 1995*

Pyoderma vegetans – crusted hyperplastic vegetative plaques, mimic blastomycosis; ulceration mimicking pyoderma gangrenosum; crusted red plaques with pustules; may be intertriginous; association with ulcerative colitis *JAAD 75:578–584, 2016; J Cutan Med Surg 5:223–227, 2001; BJD 144:1224–1227, 2001; J Derm 19:61–63, 1992; JAAD 20:691–693, 1989; J Derm Surg Onc 12:271–273, 1986;* with pyostomatitis vegetans *JAAD 46:107–110, 2002;* pustules on a plaque *JAAD 31:336–341, 1994*

Pyostomatitis vegetans – gingival pustules; *JAAD 50:785–788, 2004; Oral Surg Oral Med Oral Pathol 75:220–224, 1993; Gastroenterology 103:668–674, 1992; JAAD 21:381–387, 1989; AD 121:94–98, 1985;* erosive yellow crusted plaques of lips with lip ulcers; lip swelling with cobblestoning, micropustules *JAMA Derm 156:335, 2020; JAAD 75:578–584, 2016; NEJM 368:1918, 2013*

Relapsing polychondritis – aseptic pustules *Medicine 80:173–179, 2001*

Rosai-Dorfman disease (sinus histiocytosis with massive lymphadenopathy) – red plaque with pustules *JAAD 41:335–337, 1999;* pustules *BJD 154:277–286, 2006; JAAD 50:159–161, 2004*

Sarcoidosis – pustular folliculitis *AD 133:882–888, 1997*

Stevens-Johnson syndrome *Ped Derm 17:202–204, 2000*

Superficial granulomatous pyoderma *BJD 153:684–686, 2005; JAAD 18:511–521, 1988*

Trichodysplasia spinulosa – immunosuppression; eyebrow alopecia, acneiform eruptions, follicular spicules, inflammatory papules and pustules *Ped Derm 27:509–513, 2010; JID Symp Proc 4:268–271, 1999; Hautarzt 46:841–846, 1995;* trichodysplasia spinulosa–associated polyoma virus *Transpl Infect Dis 31:e13342, 2020; Ped Derm 36:723–724, 2019; J Med Virol 91:1896–1900, 2019; JAAD Case Rep 24:23–25, 2019*

Ulcerative colitis – pustular vasculitis *Cutis 56:297–300, 1995;* vesicopustular eruption *AD 119:91–93, 1983; AD 114:1061–1064, 1978*

Vulvar pustulosis – associated with plantar pustulosis *Clin Exp Dermatol 13:344–346, 1988*

METABOLIC

Acrodermatitis enteropathica

Cryoglobulinemia – pustules and purpura of feet – pustular cryoglobulinemic vasculitis *AD 147:235–240, 2011*

Hepatobiliary disease – vesiculopustular eruption *Int J Dermatol 36:837–844, 1997*

Impetigo herpetiformis (pustular psoriasis of pregnancy); symmetrical and grouped lesions starting in flexures (inguinocrural areas) *Stat Pearls April 29, 2020; Ind J Womens Health 10:109–115, 2018; Dermatol Res Pract April 4, 2018; AD 136:1055–1060, 2000; AD 127:91–95, 1996; Acta Ob Gyn Scand 74:229–232, 1995; AD 118:103–105, 1982*

Miliaria pustulosa

Myeloperoxidase deficiency – pustular candidal dermatitis *J Clin Inf Dis 24:258–260, 1997*

Prolidase deficiency – papulopustular dermatitis, chronic ulcers, dermatitis with crusting of face and extremities, telangiectasias, photosensitivity, chronic otitis media, sinusitis, splenomegaly *Biology (Basel)9:108, 2020; J Ped 11:242, 1971*

Pruritic folliculitis of pregnancy *Am Fam Physician 39:189–193, 1989*

Vitamin A deficiency *JAAD 29:447–461, 1993*

Vitamin C deficiency *JAAD 29:447–461, 1993*

Zinc deficiency – bullous pustular dermatosis *JAAD 69:616–624, 2013;* papulopustular acneiform eruption

NEOPLASTIC DISEASES

Epstein-Barr virus associated lymphoproliferative lesions – papulopustules *BJD 151:372–380, 2004*

Glucagonoma *Indian J DV Leprol Aug 1, 2019; Am J Dermatopathol 41:e29–32, 2019; Int J Dermatol 57:642–645, 2018; JAAD 19:377, 1988*

IgA intraepidermal pustulosis with IgA myeloma *Dermatologica 181:261–263, 1990*

Leukemia – chronic lymphocytic leukemia – transient annular erythema with pustular folliculitis *BJD 150:1129–1135, 2004*

Leukemoid eruption, congenital *JAAD 35:330–333, 1996*

Lymphoma – cutaneous T-cell lymphoma *JAAD 46:325–357, 2002; Cutis 54:202–204, 1994; AD 93:221, 1966;* generalized pustular

eruption *JAAD 61:908–909, 2009;* CD 30+ anaplastic large cell lymphoma *J Drugs Dermatol 15:1132–1135, 2016; Am J Surg Pathol 23:244–246, 1999;* palmoplantar pustulosis *JAAD 23:758–759, 1990;* vesiculopustular palmoplantar keratoderma *AD 131:1052–1056, 1995;* lymphomatoid granulomatosis *AD 127:1693–1698, 1991;* erythrodermic CTCL with pustulosis *BJD 144:1073–1079, 2001*

Lymphomatoid papulosis *J Dtsch Dermatol Ges 18:199–205, 2020; JAAD 68:809–816, 2013; JAAD 27:627, 1992;* papulopustules *JAAD 38:877–905, 1998*

Nevus comedonicus, inflammatory – papulopustules *JAAD 38:834–836, 1998*

Polycythemia vera – disseminated pustular dermatosis *JAAD 18:1212, 1988*

Squamous syringometaplasia of the eccrine glands *AD 123:1202–1204, 1987*

Transient myeloproliferative disorder associated with mosaicism for trisomy 21 – vesiculopustular rash

in trisomy 21 or normal patients; periorbital vesiculopustules, red papules, crusted papules, and ulcers *Ped Derm 36:702–706, 2019; Ped Derm 28:189–190, 2011; NEJM 348:2557–2566, 2003;* with periorbital edema *Ped Derm 21:551–554, 2004*

PARANEOPLASTIC DISORDERS

Eosinophilic dermatosis of hematologic malignancy *Am J Clin Dermatol May 11, 2020; JAAD 81:74–75, 2019*

Eosinophilic pustular folliculitis associated with mantle cell lymphoma – papulopustular eruption of face *Cutis 101:454–457, 2018*

Neutrophilic dermatosis associated with cutaneous T-cell lymphoma *AD 141:353–356, 2005*

Paraneoplastic IgA pemphigus – tense bullae, vesicopustules *JAAD 56:S73–76, 2007*

Solid pseudopapillary tumor of pancreas – produced GCSF; pustules of legs, palms and soles; evolve into crusted plaques *BJD 177:1122–1126, 2017*

PHOTODERMATITIS

Acne aestivalis (Mallorca acne) *Clin Exp Dermatol 30:659–661, 2005*

Actinic superficial folliculitis *BJD 138:1070–1074, 1998; Clin Exp Dermatol 14:69–71, 1989; BJD 113:630–631, 1985*

Hydroa vacciniforme – pustules *Ped Derm 18:71–73, 2001*

PRIMARY CUTANEOUS DISEASES

Acne keloidalis nuchae *JAAD 39:661, 1998; Dermatol Clin 6:387–395, 1988*

Acne necrotica miliaris *Australas J Dermatol 59:e53–58, 2018; AD 132:1367–1370, 1996*

Acne neonatorum – neonatal Malassezia furfur pustulosis *AD 132:190–193, 1996*

Acne rosacea *AD 134:679–683, 1998*

Acne vulgaris, pyoderma faciale, acne conglobata *J Derm 19:61–63, 1992*

Acrodermatitis continua of Hallopeau (dermatitis repens) – palms and soles *JAAD 60:532–535, 2009; BJD 135:644–646, 1996; JAAD 11:755–62, 1984*

Acropustulosis of infancy (infantile acropustulosis) – vesicopustules on palms, soles, sides of feet, dorsal aspects of hands, feet, fingers *Ped Derm 15:337–341, 1998; AD 132:1365–1366, 1368–1369, 1996; AD 122:1155–1160, 1986; Dermatologica 165:615–619, 1982; AD 115:831–833, 1979; AD 115:834–836, 1979*

Acute palmoplantar pustulosis

Acute parapsoriasis (Mucha-Habermann disease) – mimicking varicella

Alopecia mucinosa *Derm 197:178–180, 1998*

Amicrobial pustulosis – exudative erythema, erosions, pustules, diffuse alopecia with dermatitis; associated with systemic autoimmune disorders; scalp, axillae, ears, thighs JAAD 57:523–526, 2007; BJD 154:568–569, 2006; Communication no.11. Journees Dermatologiques de Paris, March 1991.

Atopic dermatitis Acta Derm Vener suppl 171:1–37, 1992; thick-walled pustules with heavy crusting; periorbital crusting in atopic dermatitis due to group A beta hemolytic streptococcus; herpetiform lesions Ped Derm 28:230–234, 2011

Chronic recalcitrant pustular eruptions of the palms and soles *Cutis 68:216–218, 2001*

Darier's disease *J Derm 25:469–475, 1998*

Dermatitis repens

Disseminated and recurrent infundibulofolliculitis – occasional pustules *J Derm 25:51–53, 1998; AD 105:580–583, 1972*

Dyshidrosis with secondary infection

Elastosis perforans serpiginosa *J Derm 20:329–340, 1993*

Eosinophilic pustular dermatitis of infancy – acneiform pustules of chin and feet *BJD 167:1189–1191, 2012*

Eosinophilic pustular folliculitis – red plaque with pustules *JAAD 51:S71–73, 2004; JAAD 46:S153–155, 2002;* sterile papules, pustules, and plaques of face, trunk, arms, palms, soles *JAAD 23:1012–1014, 1990; JAAD 14:469–474, 1986;* palmar pustulosis *Dermatology 185:276–280, 1992; AD 121:917–920, 1985;* eosinophilic pustular folliculitis of childhood – may see pustules on scalp, limbs, genitals, behind ears *JAAD 27:55–60, 1992; Ped Derm 8:189–193, 1991;* of infancy – mostly of scalp *Ped Derm 16:118–120, 1999; BJD 132:296–299, 1995;* eosinophilic pustular folliculitis of infancy – pustules of scalp; papules and pustules of trunk and extremities *JAAD 68:150–155, 2013*

Erosive pustular dermatosis of the scalp – in elderly; erosions, sterile pustules, scarring alopecia; sign of chronic actinic damage; chronic atrophic erosive dermatosis of the scalp and extremities *JAAD 57:421–427, 2007;* in child following craniofacial surgery *Ped Derm 36:697–701, 2019*

Familial pustular psoriasis – mutation in IL-36 receptor antagonist *NEJM 365:620–628, 2011*

Febrile ulceronecrotic Mucha-Habermann disease (acute parapsoriasis) *JAAD 55:557–572, 2006; NJAAD 54:1113–1114, 2006; Ped Derm 22:360–365, 2005; BJD 152:794–799, 2005; JAAD 49:1142–1148, 2003; BJD 147:1249–1253, 2002; Ped Derm 8:51–57, 1991; AD 100:200–206, 1969; Ann DV 93:481–496, 1966*

Granuloma annulare – follicular, pustular granuloma annulare *BJD 138:1075–1078, 1998;* pustular generalized granuloma annulare *BJD 149:866–868, 2003*

Hailey-Hailey disease *Dermatol Ther 32:e12945, 2019; Australas J Dermatol 37:196–198, 1996; BJD 126:275–282, 1992; Arch Dermatol Syphilol 39:679–685, 1939*

Ichthyosiform erythroderma with generalized pustulosis *BJD 138:502–505, 1998*

Ichthyosis bullosa of Siemens

Keratosis pilaris *Ann Derm Vener 118:69–75, 1991*

Kyrle's disease *J Derm 20:329–340, 1993*

Lichen nitidus *Cutis 62:247–248, 1998*

Lichen planopilaris *JAAD 27:935–942, 1992*

Lichen spinulosus *Int J Derm 34:670–671, 1985*

Miliaria, including congenital miliaria crystallina *Cutis 47:103–106, 1991*

Ofuji's disease – pustulosis of the palms *Cutis 44:407–409, 1989*

Perioral dermatitis *Derm 195:235–238, 1997*

Pityriasis rosea *The Clinical Management of Itching; Parthenon; p. 137, 2000*

Pityriasis rubra pilaris *BJD 133:990–993, 1995*

Pseudofolliculitis – barbae *Derm Surg 26:737–742, 2000; J Emerg Med 4:283–286, 1986;* pubis; of scalp *AD 113:328–329, 1977;* of nasal hairs *AD 117:368–369, 1981*

Psoriasis – pustular psoriasis (von Zumbusch) *BJD 173:239–241, 2015; NEJM 365:620–628, 2011; Ped Derm 13:45–46, 1996; Dermatol Clin 13:757–770, 1995; Dermatol Clin 2:455–470, 1984;* pustular psoriasis with IL36RN mutations *BJD 170:202–204, 2014;* generalized pustular psoriasis in children *Ped Derm 31:575–579, 2014;* psoriasis with pustules; acropustulosis with destructive pustulation of nail unit; annular pustular psoriasis *Ped Derm 19:19–25, 2002*; palmoplantar pustular psoriasis; psoriasis with pustules; pustular psoriasis in children *Ped Derm 24:401–404, 2007;* intertriginous pustular psoriasis of childhood *JAAD 60:679–683, 2009*

Pustulosis acuta generalisata – pustular eruption of palms, trunk; scattered sterile pustules with red inflammatory haloes; arthropathy; post-streptococcal *JAAD 58:1056–1058, 2008; Ped Derm 24:272–276, 2007*

Pustulosis vegetans *AD 120;1355–1359, 1984*

Rosacea fulminans – acute pustular eruption of face; pustules; red eyes *BJD 163:877–879, 2010; Dermatology 188:251–254, 1994; AD 41:451–462, 1940*

Scleredema of Buschke (pseudoscleroderma) – in diabetics, preceded by erythema or pustules *Clin Exp Dermatol 14:385–386, 1989*

Subcorneal pustular dermatosis of Sneddon-Wilkinson – pustules which expand to annular and serpiginous lesions with scaly edge; heal with hyperpigmentation *BJD 176:1341–1344, 2017;*

JAAD 73:809–820, 2015; Clin Exp Dermatol 33:229–233, 2008; Am J Clin Dermatol 3:389–400, 2002; BJD 144:1224–1227, 2001; Clin Dermtol 18:301–313, 2000; J Dermatol 27:669–672, 2000; Cutis 61:203–208, 1998; BJD 68:385–394, 1956; subcorneal pustular dermatosis associated with IgA paraproteinemia *JAAD 24:325–8, 1991*

Transient acantholytic dermatosis (Grover's disease) – pustular or vesiculopustular *Am J Dermatopathol 40:445–448, 2018; JAAD 35:653–666, 1996*

SYNDROMES

Behcet's disease – papulopustules seen more frequently in patients with arthritis *BJD 157:901–906, 2007; BJD 147:331–336, 2002; Ann Rheum Dis 60:1074–1076, 2001; JAAD 40:1–18, 1999; JAAD 41:540–545, 1999; NEJM 341:1284–1290, 1999; JAAD 19:767–779, 1988; JAAD 36:689–696, 1997;*

CARD14 – gain of function mutation in caspase recruitment domain family member – pustular eruptions *JAAD 70:767–773, 2014*

CRMO – chronic recurrent multifocal osteomyelitis and synovitis; acne, pustulosis, hyperostosis, osteitis; palmoplantar pustules, Sweet's syndrome, pyoderma gangrenosum *JAAD 70:767–773, 2014*

Deficiency of the interleukin-1 receptor antagonist (DIRA) – autosomal recessive; widespread neonatal onset cutaneous pustulosis with recurrent oral ulcers, sterile multifocal osteomyelitis and periostitis, hepatosplenomegaly *JAAD 68:834–853, 2013; NEJM 360:2426–2437, 2009*

Down's syndrome – with transient myeloproliferative disorder (leukemoid reactions) – neonatal pustules, vesicles, papulovesicles *Ped Derm 20:232–237, 2003*

Familial Mediterranean fever

Hereditary acrokeratotic poikiloderma (Kindler's syndrome)– vesiculopustules of hands and feet at age 1–3 months which resolve *AD 103:409–422, 1971*

Hereditary lactate dehydrogenase M subunit deficiency without IL-36 receptor antagonist mutation – pustular psoriasis-like eruption; erythematous skin lesions; psoriasiform dermatitis; annular desquamative plaques; fatigue, myalgia, myoglobinuria, increased creatine kinase *BJD 172:1674–1676, 2015; JAAD 27:262–263, 1992; JAAD 24:339–342, 1991; AD 122:1420–1424, 1986*

Incontinentia pigmenti *JAAD 47:169–187, 2002; Clin Exp Immunol 127:470–480, 2001*

Jung's syndrome – atopic dermatitis, pyoderma, folliculitis, blepharitis *Lancet ii:185–187, 1983*

Kawasaki's disease – micropustular eruption, macular, morbilliform, urticarial, scarlatiniform, erythema multiforme-like, erythema marginatum-like exanthems *Ped Derm 32:547–548, 2015; JAAD 69:501–510, 2013; Cutis 72:354–356, 2003; JAAD 39:383–398, 1998; Am J Dermatopathol 10:218–223, 1988; Hifubyo Shinryo (Japan) 2:956–961, 1980*

Keratosis follicularis spinulosa decalvans – X-linked dominant and autosomal dominant; alopecia, xerosis, thickened nails, photophobia, spiny follicular papules (keratosis pilaris), scalp pustules, palmoplantar keratoderma *JAAD 53:1–37, 2005; Ped Derm 22:170–174, 2005*

Keratosis-ichthyosis-deafness (KID) syndrome – autosomal recessive; paronychial pustules; dotted waxy, fine granular, stippled, or reticulated surface pattern of severe diffuse hyperkeratosis of palms and soles (palmoplantar keratoderma), ichthyosis with well marginated, serpiginous erythematous verrucous plaques, hyperkeratotic elbows and knees, perioral furrows, leukoplakia, bilateral sensorineural deafness, photophobia with vascularizing keratitis, blindness, hypotrichosis of scalp, eyebrows, and eyelashes, dystrophic nails, chronic mucocutaneous candidiasis, otitis externa, abscesses, blepharitis; connexin 26 mutation *Ped Derm 23:81–83, 2006; JAAD 51:377–382, 2004; BJD 148:649–653, 2003; Cutis 72:229–230, 2003; Ped Derm 19:285–292, 2002; Ped Derm 15:219–221, 1998; Ped Derm 13:105–113, 1996; BJD 122:689–697, 1990; JAAD 23:385–388, 1990; JAAD 19:1124–1126, 1988; AD 123:777–782, 1987; AD 117:285–289, 1981; J Cutaneous Dis 33:255–260, 1915*

hyperkeratotic papules and plaques of face, scalp, trunk, extremities; exaggerated diaper dermatitis

Lipoid proteinosis – vesiculopustular periorbital eruption *JAAD 39:149–171, 1998; Ped Derm 14:22–25, 1997; extrafacial pustules BJD 151:413–423, 2004; JID 120:345–350, 2003; Hum Molec Genet 11:833–840, 2002*

Majeed syndrome (autoinflammatory syndrome) – autosomal recessive; chronic recurrent multifocal osteomyelitis; congenital dyserythropoietic anemia and neutrophilic dermatosis; periodic fevers; Sweet's syndrome; chronic pustulosis; mutation in *LPIN2* (lipin 2 gene) *JAAD 70:767–773, 2014; J Clin Immunol 28 (Suppl 1) S73–83, 2008; J Med Genet 4:551–557, 2005; Eur J Pediatr 160:705–710, 2001*

Netherton's syndrome – recurrent pustular eruptions *Ped Derm 32:147–148, 2015*

Neutrophilic dermatosis (pustular vasculitis) of the dorsal hands – variant of Sweet's syndrome – hemorrhagic pustular nodules *AD 138:361–365, 2002; JAAD 43:870–874, 2000; JAAD 32:192–198, 1995*

Pseudohypoaldosteronism type I – pustular miliaria, acneiform eruptions, extensive scaling of the scalp *Ped Derm 19:317–319, 2002*

Reactive arthritis syndrome – keratoderma blenorrhagicum; soles, pretibial areas, dorsal toes, feet, fingers, hands, nails, scalp *Semin Arthritis Rheum 3:253–286, 1974*

SAPHO syndrome – pustulosis palmaris et plantaris with chronic recurrent multifocal osteomyelitis *JAAD 12:927–930, 1985; palmoplantar pustulosis with sternoclavicular hyperostosis; chronic synchondrosis, osteosclerosis, hypertrophic osteitis, synovitis JAAD 68:834–853, 2013; Dtsch Med Wochenschr 124:114–118, 1999; Cutis 62:75–76, 1998; J Pediatr 93:227–231, 1978*

SAVI – (STING (stimulator of interferon genes)-associated vasculopathy) – progressive digital necrosis, swelling of fingers, amputation of several digits, violaceous and telangiectatic malar plaques, nasal septal destruction, chronic leg myalgias, atrophic skin over knees, red-purpuric plaques over cold-sensitive areas (acral areas) (cheeks, nasal tip, ears), reticulate erythema of arms and legs *JAAD 74:186–189, 2016*

Sweet's syndrome – pustules and/or pustular plaques; red plaque with central pustule *AD 145:608–609, 2009; papules with supervening pustules Ped Derm 22:525–529, 2005; Hautarzt 46:283–284, 1995; JAAD 16:458–462, 1987; AD 123:519–524, 1987; BJD 76:349–356, 1964; chronic recurrent Sweet's syndrome of myelodysplasia – pustules, plaques, and papules AD 142:1170–1176, 2006; neutrophilic pustulosis with CML – a unique form of Sweet's syndrome Acta Haematol 88:154–157, 1992; pediatric Sweet's syndrome and immunodeficiency Ped Derm 22:530–535, 2005; necrotizing Sweet's syndrome – edematous red plaque studded with pustules JAAD 67:945–954, 2012*

Trichothiodystrophy syndromes – BIDS, IBIDS, PIBIDS – palmar pustules, poikiloderma, sparse or absent eyelashes and eyebrows, brittle hair, premature aging, sexual immaturity, ichthyosis, dysmyelination, bird-like facies, dental caries; trichothiodystrophy with ichthyosis, urologic malformations, hypercalciuria and mental and physical retardation *JAAD 44:891–920, 2001; Ped Derm 14:441–445, 1997*

Wells' syndrome – with subcorneal pustules *Indian J DV 81:301–303, 2015*

TOXINS

Arsenic – acute arsenic intoxication; initially morbilliform eruption with development of vesicles, pustules on red background; followed by generalized desquamation and palmoplantar lamellar desquamation *BJD 141:1106–1109, 1999*

Mercury intoxication – acute generalized exanthematous pustulosis *AD 139:1181–1183, 2003; JAAD 37:653–655, 1997; Contact Dermatitis 9:411–417, 1983; pustular eruption JAAD 43:81–90, 2000*

Potato poisoning – rash of lower abdomen and medial thighs consisting of red papules which progress to pustules and crusted lesions; facial and abdominal edema; headache, vomiting, diarrhea *J R Coll Physicians Edinb 36:336–339, 2007*

TRAUMA

Chilblains – pustular chilblains (acrodermatitis pustulosa hiemalis) *Cases J 2:6500, 2009; Covid-19 BJD April 29, 2020*

Erosive pustular dermatosis of face – following cosmetic resurfacing *JAMA Derm 153:1021–1025, 2017*

Occlusion folliculitis – beneath adhesive dressings or plasters

Physical or chemical trauma – folliculitis

Traction folliculitis – papules and pustules *Cutis 79:26–26–30, 2007*

Waxing folliculitis with secondary staphylococcal infection – personal observation

VASCULAR DISEASES

Degos' disease – ulceropustular lesions *Ann DV 79:410–417, 1954*

Henoch-Schonlein purpura – personal observation

Levamisole tainted cocaine-induced vasculitis *J Wound Ostom Continence Nurs 47:182–189, 2020*

Primary idiopathic cutaneous pustular vasculitis *JAAD 14:939–944, 1986*

RICH (rapidly involuting congenital hemangioma) with pustules *Ped Derm 31:398–400, 2014*

Vasculitis – including leukocytoclastic vasculitis *AD 134:309–315, 1998;* pustular vasculitis – annular pustular plaques with central necrosis; acral vesiculopustular lesions

Venous insufficiency – erosive pustular dermatosis of the legs – in setting of chronic venous insufficiency *BJD 147:765–769, 2002*

Polyangiitis with granulomatosis *JAAD 10:341–346, 1984*

RED CHEST

AUTOIMMUNE DISEASES AND DISORDERS OF IMMUNE DYSREGULATION

Allergic contact dermatitis

Dermatomyositis *JAAD 79:77–83, 2018*

Lupus erythematosus

Pansclerotic morphea *Nat Rev Rheumatol 5:513–516, 2009*

Scleroderma – acute edematous phase; cellulitis-like

DRUGS

Acetaminophen – exanthem of breasts *Cutis 89:284–286, 2012*

DRESS

Drug hypersensitivity reaction

EXOGENOUS AGENTS

Reticular telangiectatic erythema associated with implantable cardioverter defibrillator *Cutis 78:329–331, 2006; AD 137:1239–1241, 2001*

INFECTIONS AND INFESTATIONS

Cellulitis

Dermatophytosis

Herpes zoster

Lyme disease – erythema chronicum migrans

Nocardiosis *JAAD 23:399–400, 1990; JAAD 13:125–133, 1985; Nocardia asteroides* – cellulitis *BJD 144:639–641, 2001; AD 121:898–900, 1985; N. brasiliensis* cellulitis of legs, arms, trunk, and face *J Inf Dis 134(3):286–289, 1976; Nocardia nova* – red plaque of hand *BJD 145:154–156, 2001*

Nontuberculous mycobacterial infection following surreptitious breast augmentation

Osteomyelitis of medial clavicle; osteomyelitis of sternum *BMJ Case Rep Oct 30, 2012*

Tinea versicolor

Unilateral laterothoracic exanthem *JAAD 34:979–984, 1996*

INFILTRATIVE DISORDERS

Reticular erythematous mucinosis syndrome

INFLAMMATORY DISORDERS

Costochondritis – overlying erythema

Erythema multiforme

Interstitial granulomatous dermatitis - annular erythematous plaques of medial thighs, lateral chest, abdomen *JAMA Derm 149:626–627, 2013; AD 140:353–358, 2004*

Periductal mastitis – cellulitis-like *JAAD 43:733–751, 2000*

METABOLIC DISORDERS

Paroxysmal nocturnal hemoglobinuria – petechiae, ecchymoses, hemorrhagic bullae; ulcers; red plaques which become hemorrhagic bullae with necrosis; lesions occur on legs, abdomen, chest, nose, and ears; fever; deficiency of enzymes – decay-accelerating factor (DAF) and membrane inhibitor of reactive lysis (MIRL) *AD 148:660–662, 2012; AD 138:831–836, 2002; AD 122:1325–1330, 1986; AD 114:560–563, 1978*

NEOPLASTIC DISORDERS

Carcinoid syndrome

Carcinoma erysipelatoides - mimicking infectious cellulitis *JAAD 67:177–185, 2012; Ann Int Med 142:47–55, 2005; J R Soc Med 78:Suppl 11:43–45, 1985; AD 113:69–70, 1977*

Lymphoma – angioimmunoblastic T- or B-cell lymphoma

peripheral T-cell lymphoma *Cutis 81:33–36, 2008*

Melanoma - red patch of upper central chest – signet ring melanoma metastases of cervical lymph nodes *JAAD 65:444–446, 2011*

Metastatic melanoma – erythematous annular plaques of trunk *AD 148:531–536, 2012*

PHOTODERMATOSES

Allergic photocontact dermatitis

Dermatoheliosis

Polymorphic light eruption

PRIMARY CUTANEOUS DISEASES

Generalized granuloma annulare

Ichthyosis en confetti (congenital reticulated ichthyosiform erythroderma)(CRIE) – reticulated erythroderma with guttate hypopigmentation, palmoplantar keratoderma; loss of dermatoglyphics; temporary hypertrichosis of normal skin *BJD 166:434–439, 2012; JAAD 63:607–641, 2010*

Poikiloderma vasculare atrophicans

Seborrheic dermatitis

Urticaria

SYNDROMES

Aesop syndrome(adenopathy and extensive skin patch overlying plasmacytoma) – extensive asymptomatic red-violaceous skin patch or plaque of chest overlying a solitary bone plasmacytoma with regional adenopathy; dermal mucin and vascular hyperplasia (mucinous angiomatosis) *JAAD 55:909–910, 2006*

NOD 2 mutations(nucleotide-binding oligomerization domain 2) – dermatitis, weight loss with gastrointestinal symptoms, episodic self-limiting fever, polyarthritis, polyarthralgia, red plaques of face and forehead, urticarial plaques of legs, patchy erythema of chest, pink macules of arms and back *JAAD 68:624–631, 2013*

REM(reticular erythematous mucinosis) syndrome *AD 148:768–769, 2012; JAAD 27:825–828, 1992; Ped Derm 7:1–10, 1990; Z Hautkr*

63:986–998, 1988(German); JAAD 19:859–868, 1988; AD 115:1340–1342, 1979; BJD 91:191–199, 1974; Z Hautkr 49:235–238, 1974

SAPPHO syndrome *Rheum Clinic 11:108–111, 2015*

Wells' syndrome(eosinophilic cellulitis) – red plaques resembling urticaria or cellulitis *Cutis 89:191–194, 2012; AD 142:1157–1161, 2006; Ann Int Med 142:47–55, 2005; JAAD 52:187–189, 2005; NEJM 350:904–912, 2004; AD 139:933–938, 2003; Ped Derm 20:276–278, 2003; BJD 140:127–130, 1999; JAAD 18:105–114, 1988; Trans St. Johns Hosp Dermatol Soc 51:46–56, 1971;* bullous Wells' syndrome – red plaque with bullae *Ped Derm 29:762–764, 2012*

TOXINS

Scombroid fish poisoning

TRAUMA

Cutaneous radiation-associated angiosarcoma of the breast – livedoid violaceous plaques with nodules of the breast *JAMA Derm 149:973–974, 2013*

Lightning strike – Lichtenberg figures; frond-like (ferning pattern) transient non-blanching pink-red erythema beginning 20 minutes to 3 ½ hours after the strike and lasting up to 48 hours *Cutis 80:141–143, 2007; Arch Neurol 61:977, 2005; Injury 34:367–371, 2003; Burns Incl Thermal Inj 13:141–146, 1987; Proc IEE 123:1163–1180, 1976; Memoirs Med Soc London 2:493–507, 1794*

Postirradiation pseudosclerodermatous panniculitis *Ann Int Med 142:47–55, 2005; Am J Dermatopathol 23:283–287, 2001; Mayo Clin Proc 68:122–127, 1993*

Radiation dermatitis, acute – erythema *JAAD 54:28–46, 2006; Acta DV 49:64–71, 1969;* fluoroscopy-induced radiation injury; post-radiation vascular proliferations of breast (atypical vascular lesions of the breast) – erythema; erythema with underlying induration or ulceration, telangiectasias, papules, plaques, nodules, *JAAD 57:126–133, 2007*

Radiation recall – erythema, vesiculation, erosions, hyperpigmentation; red hyperpigmented patch *Cutis 91:17–18, 2013;* dactinomycin and doxorubicin *Radiother Oncol 59:237–245, 2001; Mayo Clin Proc 55:711–715, 1980;* edatrexate, melphalan, etoposide, vinblastine, bleomycin, fluorouracil, hydroxyurea, methotrexate *Rook p. 3469, 1998, Sixth Edition*

Subcutaneous emphysema – extensive erythema of upper chest *AD 147:254–255, 2011*

VASCULAR DISEASES

Diffuse dermal angiomatosis (reactive angioendotheliomatosis), including diffuse dermal angiomatosis of the breast; reticulated ulcerations of breasts *AD 144:693–694, 2008; AD 142:343–347, 2006*

Flushing syndromes

Superior vena cava syndrome

RED ELBOW

AUTOIMMUNE DISEASES AND DISEASES OF IMMUNE DYSFUNCTION

Allergic contact dermatitis – poison ivy; allergic contact dermatitis (dermal hypersensitivity) to titanium elbow implant

Dermatomyositis *JAAD 79:77–83, 2018; JAAD 49:295–298, 2003;* red knees *BJD 156:1390–1392, 2007;* amyopathic dermatomyositis *BJD 174:158–164, 2016*

Dermatitis herpetiformis

Linear scleroderma

Lupus erythematosus – systemic, discoid lupus erythematosus *NEJM 269:1155–1161, 1963*

Pemphigus foliaceus

Rheumatoid arthritis - intravascular or intralymphatic histiocytosis in rheumatoid arthritis; confluent papules over swollen elbows *JAAD 50:585–590, 2004*

Scleroderma – CREST syndrome with calcinosis cutis of elbows

Still's disease (juvenile rheumatoid arthritis)

DRUG

Capecitabine reaction mimicking dermatomyositis - personal observation

Drug eruption

Sorafenib - personal observation

EXOGENOUS AGENTS

Foreign body reaction (granuloma) – orthopedic implants mimicking infectious cellulitis *Ann Int Med 142:47–55, 2005; Ann DV 123:686–690, 1996*

INFECTIONS AND INFESTATIONS

AIDS – popular mucinosis of AIDS - personal observation

Erysipelas/cellulitis, including "transplant elbow"

Gianotti-Crosti syndrome *Cutis 89:169–172, 2012*

Helicobacter cinaedi - multifocal cellulitis *Clin Inf Dis 70:531,533–534, 2020*

Herpes simplex virus infection, disseminated

Human herpesvirus 8 – relapsing inflammatory syndrome; fever, lymphadenopathy, splenomegaly, edema, arthrosynovitis, exanthem of hands, wrists, and elbows *NEJM 353:156–163, 2005*

Leprosy – tuberculoid, erythema nodosum leprosum *JAAD 51:416–426, 2004*

Lyme disease – erythema chronicum migrans

Meningococcus - periarticular erythema of chronic meningococcemia; with arthritis *AD 102:97–101, 1970*

Mycobacterium haemophilum cellulitis

Mycobacterium marinum

Olecranon bursitis – staphylococcal, sterile; *Scedosporium apiospermium* (asexual state of *Pseudallescheria boydii*) *Clin Inf Dis 34:398–399, 2002;* transplant elbow (*Staphylococcus aureus* bursitis)

Parvovirus B19

Scabies

Septic arthritis

Streptococcal suppurative panniculitis - personal observation

Suppurative panniculitis

Tinea corporis

Toxoplasmosis

"Transplant elbow" – *Cutaneous Signs of Infection in the Immunocompromised Host; Grossman, et al 2ⁿᵈ Edition, Springer 2012*

INFILTRATIVE DISORDERS

Langerhans cell histiocytosis *Int J Dermatol 57:911–912, 2018*

INFLAMMATORY DISEASES

Erythema nodosum

Erythema multiforme

Erythema nodosum

Olecranon bursitis with or without psoriasis

Sarcoid

METABOLIC DISEASES

Alpha 1 antitrypsin panniculitis - personal observation

Calcinosis cutis, metastatic, perforating *SKINMed 11:314–315, 2013*

Chronic obstructive pulmonary disease - frictional erythema of elbow

Congenital heart disease – livedo reticularis - personal observation

Gouty tophi - personal observation

Necrolytic migratory erythema

Pruritic urticarial papules and plaques of pregnancy (PUPPP)

Zinc deficiency, acquired

PHOTODERMATITIS

Actinic granuloma

NEOPLASTIC DISEASE

Ruptured epidermoid cyst

Waldenstrom's macroglobulinemia - IgM storage papule

PRIMARY CUTANEOUS DISEASES

Dyshidrosis

Dermatitis herpetiformis-like dermatitis – personal observation

Epidermolysis bullosa – dominant dystrophic

Erythema elevatum diutinum *Stat Pearls Dec 20, 2019; Cutis 34:41–43, 1984*

Granuloma annulare

Generalized essential telangiectasia

Lichen myxedematosus - personal observation

Necrolytic migratory erythema without glucagonoma - personal observation

Papular prurigo (itchy red bump disease)(subacute prurigo)

Pityriasis rubra pilaris

Pruritic urticarial papules and plaques of pregnancy

Psoriasis

SYNDROMES

Haim-Munk syndrome – autosomal recessive; mutation in cathepsin C gene (like Papillon-Lefevre syndrome); palmoplantar keratoderma, scaly red patches on elbows, knees, forearms, shins, atrophic nails, gingivitis with destruction of periodontium, onychogryphosis, arachnodactyly, recurrent pyogenic infections *BJD 152:353–356, 2005*

Keratosis linearis with ichthyosis congenita and sclerosing keratoderma (KLICK syndrome) *BJD 153:461, 2005; Acta DV (Stockh) 77:225–227, 1997; AD 125:103–106, 1989*

Lipoid proteinosis

Multicentric reticulohistiocytosis

Rothmund-Thomson syndrome

TRAUMA

Frictional lichenoid dermatitis

Pressure

VASCULAR

Cholesterol emboli

Lymphangiosarcoma in lymphedematous extremity

Granulomatosis with polyangiitis - palisaded neutrophilic and granulomatous dermatitis *Cutis 70:37–38, 2002*

Rapidly involuting congenital hemangioma (RICH) – red mass of elbow with white halo *Ped Derm 37:40–1, 2020*

RED FACE

Clinics in Dermatology 11:189–328, 1993; See Erythrodermas

AUTOIMMUNE DISEASES AND DISEASES OF IMMUNE DYSFUNCTION

Allergic contact dermatitis – poison ivy; multiple causes; facial cosmetics *JAAD 49:S259–261, 2003; Clin Dermatol 11:289–295, 1993;* mango ingestion; allergic granulomatous reaction to microneedle therapy with Vita C serum for skin rejuvenation *JAMA Derm 150:68–72, 2014;* nickel allergy with orthodontic appliance *Angle Orthod 79:1194–1196, 2009*

Anaphylaxis

Cholinergic urticaria

Dermatomyositis *AD 140:723–727, 2004; Clin Dermatol 11:261–273, 1993;* dusky red face *Clin Rev Allergy Immunol 5:293–302, 2016*

Graft vs. host disease, chronic – begins with facial erythema, then becomes lichenoid

Lupus erythematosus - systemic, SCLE, tumid, discoid lupus erythematosus *JAAD 65:54–64, 2011; NEJM 269:1155–1161, 1963;* edematous, neonatal *Int J Dermatol 35:44–44, 1996; Clin Dermatol 11:253–260, 1993;* neonatal lupus *Ped Derm 22:240–242, 2005;* neonatal lupus – red patch of entire forehead *Ped Derm 25:253–254, 2008*

Morphea – linear erythema of forehead as early presentation of en coup de sabre *Clin Exp Dermatol 45:470–471, 2020*

Pemphigus erythematosus

Pemphigus foliaceus

Pemphigus vulgaris *AD 143:1033–1038, 2007; AD 141:680–682, 2005*

Scleroderma - progressive systemic sclerosis and linear scleroderma resembling heliotrope *JAAD 7:541–544, 1982; Ann Int Med 80:273, 1974*

Still's disease, adult onset – evanescent rash, persistent papules and plaques *Clin Rheumatol 35:1377–1382, 2016*

CONGENITAL DISORDERS

Neonatal lupus erythematosus *NEJM 370:958, 2014*

Rubor – transient neonatal rubor due to vasodilatation and hyperemia, especially of the head *JAAD 60:669–675, 2009*

DRUG-INDUCED

Cimetidine - seborrheic dermatitis-like eruption

Cisplatin - lighting up of actinic keratoses *JAAD 17:192–197, 1987*

Corticosteroid (topical) atrophy; steroid (topical) rosacea - personal observation

Corticosteroid abuse and withdrawal *JAAD 41:435–442, 1999*

Cyclosporine, intravenous

Dactinomycin-dacarbazine-vincristine sulfate – lighting up of actinic keratoses *JAAD 17:192–197, 1987*

Deoxycoformycin - lighting up of actinic keratoses *JAAD 17:192–197, 1987*

Disulfiram

Dupilumab *Biologics 13:79–82, 2019; JAAD Case Rep 5:888–891, 2019*

Doxorubicin - lighting up of actinic keratoses *JAAD 17:192–197, 1987*

Drug reaction with eosinophilia and systemic symptoms (DRESS) *AD 146:1373–1379, 2010; AD 145:63–66, 2009*

EMLA

Erlotinib – facial swelling and erythema *Cut Ocul Toxicol 37:96–99, 2018*

Everolimus – mTOR inhibitor; broad red patches of face, scalp, upper trunk; also widespread dermatitis, acneiform eruptions *The Dermatologist July 2015;pp.47–48*

5-fluorouracil - topical or systemic *JAAD 17:192–197, 1987*

Fludarabine - lighting up of actinic keratoses *JAAD 17:192–197, 1987*

Hydroxyurea *JAAD 49:339–341, 2003*

Iododerma – due to computed tomography scans; red papules and plaques *J Drugs in Dermatol 12:574–576, 2013*

Isotretinoin (Accutane) – acute facial erythema and edema *Ped Derm 23:518–519, 2006*

Itraconazole - photodermatitis and retinoid-like dermatitis *J Eur Acad Dermatol Venereol 14:501–503, 2000*

Methyldopa - seborrheic dermatitis-like eruption

Palifermin exanthema - personal observation

Penicillamine - seborrheic dermatitis-like eruption

Phosphodiesterase 5 inhibitors (sildenafil, vardenafil, tadalafil) – facial erythema and rosacea *BJD 160:719–720, 2009*

Phototoxic drug eruption

Prostacycline – for primary pulmonary hypertension

Proton pump inhibitors – airborne contact dermatitis; red face and neck *Dermatitis 26:287–290, 2015*

Retinoids - topical, systemic

Rifampin overdosage in children

Sorafenib – seborrheic dermatitis-like facial erythema *BJD 161:1045–1051, 2009; JAAD 60:299–305, 2009; AD 144:886–892, 2008*

Sunitinib – facial erythema *BJD 161:1045–1051, 2009*

Vancomycin - red man syndrome *Pediatrics 86:572–580, 1990*

Vandetanib (kinase and growth factor receptor inhibitor) – photosensitivity and blue-gray perifollicular macules; also blue gray pigment within scars *AD 48:1418–1420, 2012; AD 145:923–925, 2009*

Vemurafenib - erythema and edema of face and neck *J Eur Acad DV 29:61–68, 2015; BJD 169:934–938, 2013*

Voriconazole – photodermatitis and retinoid-like dermatitis *Ped Derm 21:675–678, 2004; Pediatr Infect Dis J 21:240–248, 2002; Clin Exp Dermatol 26:648–653, 2001*

EXOGENOUS AGENTS

Alcohol-induced flushing, especially in Asians

Contact dermatitis - airborne, irritant, allergic

Sorbic acid - immediate nonallergic facial erythema from cosmetics - *Cutis 61:17, 1998; Cutis 40:395–397, 1987*

Tacrolimus and alcohol ingestion – facial flushing

INFECTIONS

Anaplasmosis - personal observation

Candidiasis – rosacea-like eruption *AD 142:945–946, 2006;* candidal infection after ablative laser therapy – weeping bright red erythematous plaques *JAAD 73:15–24, 2015*

Chikungunya fever – flushed face *Ped Derm 35:408–409, 2018;*

Crimean-Congo hemorrhagic fever – flushing and edema of face and neck

Demodicidosis(*Demodex folliculorum*) – demodex folliculitis; acneiform eruption with conjunctivitis and red face *JAMA Derm 150:61–63, 2014;* erythema of face and neck mimicking acute graft vs. host reaction *BJD 170:1219–1225, 2014; JAMA Derm 149:1407–1409, 2013; Bone Marrow Transplant 37:711–712, 2006*

Dengue hemorrhagic fever – facial flushing; circumoral cyanosis *JAAD 75:1–16, 2016*

Epidemic typhus(*Rickettsia prowazeki*)(body louse) - pink macules on sides of trunk, spreads centrifugally; flushed face with injected conjunctivae; then rash becomes deeper red, then purpuric; gangrene of finger, toes, genitalia, nose *JAAD 2:359–373, 1980*

Epstein-Barr virus – swollen erythema of face *BJD 143:1351–1353, 2000*

Erysipelas *Clin Dermatol 11:307–313, 1993*

Fusarium – of sinuses; malar erythema *JAAD 47:659–666, 2002*

Haemophilus influenza – buccal cellulitis - personal observation

Herpes simplex – eczema herpeticum

Herpes zoster

HIV primary infection *J Dermatol 32:137–142, 2005*

Leprosy - autoaggressive Hansen's disease *JAAD 17:1042–1046, 1987*

Lyme disease – malar erythema *NEJM 321:586–596, 1989; AD 120:1017–1021, 1984;* acrodermatitis chronica atrophicans *Dermatology 189:430–431, 1994*

Measles *JAMA 311:345–346, 2014*

Mucormycosis – unilateral localized facial edema with slight erythema; within days goes on to necrosis *JAAD 66:975–984, 2012;* ptosis with upper eyelid edema and necrosis *JAMA 309:2382–2383, 2013*

Mycobacterium tuberculosis – lupus vulgaris; starts as red-brown plaque, enlarges with serpiginous margin or as discoid plaques; apple-jelly nodules; plaque form – psoriasiform, irregular scarring, serpiginous margins *Int J Dermatol 26:578–581, 1987; Acta Tuberc Scand 39(Suppl 49):1–137, 1960*

Necrotizing fasciitis

Noma

Omsk hemorrhagic fever – hyperemia of face, upper body, and mucous membranes

Parvovirus B19 infection - erythema *Hum Pathol 31:488–497, 2000; J Clin Inf Dis 21:1424–1430, 1995*

Rift Valley fever – flushed face

Rubella

Scabies, crusted (Norwegian scabies) *Dermatology 197:306–308, 1998; AD 124:121–126, 1988*

Scarlet fever – *Streptococcus pyogenes*; scarlatiniform (sandpaper) rash, red face with perioral pallor; erythema marginatum *JAAD 39:383–398, 1998*

Staphylococcal scalded skin syndrome - personal observation

Staphylococcal toxic shock syndrome - personal observation

Streptococcus, Group B – facial cellulitis

Tacaribe viruses – Argentinian, Bolivian, and Venezuelan hemorrhagic fevers – erythema of face, neck, and thorax with petechiae *Lancet 338:1033–1036, 1991; JAMA 273:194–196, 1994*

Tinea faciei *Clin Dermatol 32:734–738, 2014; JAAD 29:119–120, 1993;* tinea incognito *J Dermatol 22:706–707, 1995*

Varicella

Viral exanthems

INFILTRATIVE DISEASES

Lymphocytoma cutis

Mastocytosis *Clin Derm 32:800–808, 2014*

INFLAMMATORY DISEASES

Erythema multiforme - personal observation

Kikuchi's disease (histiocytic necrotizing lymphadenitis) – facial erythema, multiple red to red-brown papules of face, scalp, chest, back, arms; red plaques; erythema and acneiform lesions of face; morbilliform, urticarial, and rubella-like exanthems; red or ulcerated pharynx; cervical adenopathy; associations with SLE, lymphoma, tuberculous adenitis, viral lymphadenitis, infectious mononucleosis, and drug eruptions *AD 142:641–646, 2006; BJD 144:885–889, 2001; JAAD 36:342–346, 1997;Am J Surg Pathol 14:872–876, 1990*

Diffuse cutaneous reticulohistiocytosis - personal observation

Orofacial granulomatosis *Dermatol Clin 33:509–630, 2015*

Rosai-Dorfman disease – granulomatous rosacea-like *Chin Med J (Eng)124:793–794, 2011; BJD 149:672–674, 2003*

Scleredema – secondary to paraproteinemia *JAMADerm 150:788–789, 2014*

Sarcoid, erythrodermic

Stevens-Johnson syndrome

Toxic epidermal necrolysis

METABOLIC DISEASES

Cryoglobulinemia - personal observation

Cushing's syndrome – tumor, iatrogenic; bilateral macronodular adrenal hyperplasia *NEJM 369:2115–2125, 2013; NEJM 369:2105–2114, 2013*

Diabetes mellitus - diabetic rubor *Dermatol Clin 7:531–546, 1989*

Exercise-induced erythema

Flushing (see chapter on flushing, p. 223)

Hyperthyroidism – flushing of face *JAAD 26:885–902, 1992*

Miliaria rubra

Polycythemia vera

Porphyria - congenital erythropoietic porphyria (Gunther's disease), erythropoietic protoporphyria

Zinc deficiency, acquired - personal observation

NEOPLASTIC DISEASES

Angiosarcoma – rosacea-like angiosarcoma *JAMADerm 156:587–588, 2020; AD 148:683–685, 2012; AD 143:75–77, 2007; JAAD 38:837–840, 1998*

Atrial myxoma - malar flush with erythema and cyanosis of digit *Br M J 36:839–840, 1974*

Breast cancer – metastatic telangiectatic breast carcinoma *JAAD 48:635–636, 2003*

Carcinoid syndrome – persistent erythema with or without telangiectasia; rosacea; flushing, thick skin with venous telangiectasias, purplish vascular lesions of face; chronic facial erythema *JAAD 68:189–209, 2013*

Field cancerization (multiple actinic keratosis) *BJD 166:150–159, 2012*

Hemophagocytic lymphohistiocytosis(hemophagocytic syndrome) – red face and proximal extremity rash; erythroderma and edema *J Dermatol 33:628–631, 2006; AD 138:1208–1212, 2002; J Pediatr 130:352–357, 1997; AD 128:193–200, 1992*

Keratoacanthomas of Grzybowski - personal observation

Intranasal carcinoma - mimics rosacea

Leukemia – mimicking viral exanthem *J Dermatol 26:216–219, 1999;* juvenile chronic myelogenous leukemia - eczematous dermatitis *JAAD 26:620–628, 1992*

Lymphoma - cutaneous T-cell, B-cell, HTLV-1 lymphoma *Clin Dermatol 11:319–328, 1993;* folliculotropic cutaneous T-cell lymphoma *JAAD 70:205e1–e16, 2014; AD 144:738–746, 2008;* primary and secondary cutaneous follicle center lymphoma - red macules of face and scalp *JAAD 75:1000–1006, 2016;* anaplastic large cell lymphoma *Acta Clin Belg 67:127–129, 2012;* Sezary syndrome

Melanoma – amelanotic lentigo maligna - red patch of cheek *JAAD 50:792–796, 2004*

Metastases – intravascular metastatic breast carcinoma – carcinoma telangiectoides *JAAD 60:633–638, 2009;* metcervical carcinoma; erythema, edema, and telangiectasia of entire central face *JAAD 56:S26–28, 2007*

Pancreatic tumor with ectopic secretion of luteinizing hormone *J Endocrinol Invest 27:361–365, 2004;* VIPoma *Clin Dermatol 32:800–808, 2014*

Pheochromocytoma *Clin Derm 32:800–808, 2014*

PARANEOPLASTIC DISORDERS

Brenner's sign – erythema of face in patient with malignant melanoma *AD 143:1001–1004, 2007*

Sweet's syndrome, bullous

PHOTOSENSITIVITY DISORDERS

Actinic prurigo - eczematous dermatitis *JAAD 26:683–692, 1992*

Chronic actinic dermatitis, including actinic reticuloid *Clin Dermatol 11:297–305, 1993*

Dermatoheliosis

Hydroa vacciniforme – initial erythema and edema *Ped Derm 18:71–73, 2001*

Neonatal sunburn *AD 145:1285–1291, 2009*
  Cockayne syndrome
  Congenital erythropoietic porphyria
  Neonatal lupus erythematosus
  Trichothiodystrophy
  Xeroderma pigmentosum

Photocontact dermatitis *Clin Dermatol 11:289–295, 1993*

Polymorphic light eruption

PUVA burn from tanning salon - personal observation

PRIMARY CUTANEOUS DISEASES

Acne rosacea – erythematotelangiectatic rosacea *JAAD 72:49–58, 2015; Cutis 92:234–240, 2013; AD 147:1258–1260, 2011*

Acne vulgaris

Atopic dermatitis

CARD 14-associated papulosquamous eruption – features of psoriasis, pityriasis rubra pilaris, atopic dermatitis *JAAD 79:487–494, 2018*

Dowling-Degos disease

Eosinophilic pustular folliculitis *AD 121:917–920, 1985*

Epidermolysis bullosa, generalized junctional (Herlitz type) *The Dermatologist, October 2016, pp17–18*

Erythrokeratoderma variabilis *BJD 152:1143–1148, 2005*

Erythromelanosis follicularis faciei et colli – red-brown granular appearance *JAAD 67:320–321, 2012; Cutis 79:459–461, 2007; Cutis 51:91–92, 1992; JAAD 5:533–534, 1981*

Erythrose peribuccale pigmentaire

Granulosis rubra nasi

Keratosis pilaria – unilateral generalized keratosis pilaris *Cutis 94:203–205, 2014*

Keratosis pilaris faciei including ulerythema ophryogenes (keratosis pilaris atrophicans)

Keratosis rubra pilaris (keratosis pilaris rubra faciei) *Ped Derm 33:443–446, 2016; AD 142:1611–1616, 2006; BJD 147:822–824, 2002*

Lamellar ichthyosis - personal observation

Lichen myxedematosus - personal observation

Lichen planus - facial erythema of actinic lichen planus *BJD 1032–1034, 2002*

Lichen planus pigmentosus – annular pigmented macules on background of erythema *JAMADerm 154:717–718, 2018*

Papuloerythroderma of Ofuji

Pityriasis folliculorum - red patch *JAAD 21:81–84, 1989*

Pityriasis rubra pilaris *AD 143:1597–1599, 2007*

Progressive symmetric erythrokeratoderma - personal observation

Pseudochromhidrosis *BJD 142:1219–1220, 2000*

Psoriasis

Seborrheic dermatitis

Solid facial edema

Symmetric progressive erythrokeratoderma(Gottron's syndrome) – autosomal dominant; large fixed geographic symmetric scaly red-orange plaques; shoulders, cheeks, buttocks, ankles, wrists *AD 122:434–440, 1986; Dermatologica 164:133–141, 1982*

Seborrheic dermatitis *Am J Clin Dermatol 1:75–80, 2000*

PSYCHOCUTANEOUS DISEASES

Factitial dermatitis

Hematohidrosis – linear dripping blood tinged discharge from eyes, ears, axilla, mouth, rectum, vagina, urethra, scalp, neck, trunk, extremities *Indian J Dermatol 58:478–480, 2013; Indian Pediatr 50, 2013; Am J Clin Dermatol 11:440–443, 2010; Am J Dermatopathol 30:135–139, 2008; Ophthalmic Plastic Reconstr Surg 20:442–447, 2004*

SYNDROMES

Amyoplasia congenita disruptive sequence – midfacial macular telangiectatic nevi *Am J Med Genet 15:571–590, 1983*

Auriculotemporal syndrome(von Frey's syndrome) – damage to auriculotemporal nerve due to injury, abscess, after parotitis, surgery in parotid area; linear flush and/or sweating on cheek, over parotid region, neck, and temporal scalp after eating *Ped Derm 26:302–305, 2009; Ann Plast Surg 57:581–584, 2006; Ped Derm 17:415–416, 2000; AD 133:1143–1145, 1997; Rev Neurol 2:97–104, 1923;* after facial trauma *J Oral Maxillofac Surg 55:1485–1490, 1997;* parotidectomy *Laryngoscope 107:1496–1501, 1997;* after thyroidectomy *BJD 79:519–526, 1967*

Beckwith-Wiedemann syndrome (Exomphalos-Macroglossia-Gigantism)(EMG) syndrome – autosomal dominant; zosteriform rash at birth, exomphalos, macroglossia, visceromegaly, facial salmon patch of forehead, upper eyelids, nose, and upper lip and gigantism; linear earlobe grooves, circular depressions of helices; increased risk of Wilms' tumor, adrenal carcinoma, hepatoblastoma, and rhabdomyosarcoma *JAAD 74:231–244, 2016; JAAD 37:523–549, 1997; Am J Dis Child 122:515–519, 1971*

Bregeat's syndrome(oculo-orbital-thalamoencephalic angiomatosis) – port wine stain of forehead and scalp with contralateral angiomatosis of the eye (subconjunctival masses around the limbus) and orbit (resulting in exophthalmos), and thalamoencephalic angiomatosis of the choroid plexus *Bull Soc Fr Ophthalmol 71:581–594, 1958*

Bloom's syndrome *JAAD 17:479–488, 1987*

Cardiofaciocutaneous syndrome - personal observation

dsCoats' disease – cutaneous telangiectasia or unilateral macular telangiectatic nevus with retinal telangiectasia *AD 108:413–415, 1973*

Glabellar port wine stain, mega cisterna magna, communicating hydrocephalus, posterior cerebellar vermis agenesis; autosomal dominant *J Neurosurg 51:862–865, 1979*

Haber's syndrome *JAAD 40:462–467, 1999*

Harlequin syndrome – damage to sympathetic innervation of one side of face; decreased sweating and flushing on one side of face; compensatory increased sweating and flushing on normal side of face *BJD 169:954–956, 2013*

Hereditary neurocutaneous angioma – autosomal dominant; port wine stains with localized CNS vascular malformations *J Med Genet 16:443–447, 1979*

Hermansky-Pudlak syndrome – mucocutaneous granulomatous disease in Hermansky-Pudlak syndrome; butterfly red plaques of face; linear ulcers of groin and vulva; pink plaques of thighs; swollen vulva; indurated nodules of vulva; axillary ulcers, red face *JAMADerm 150:1083–1087, 2014*

Histiophagocytic syndrome – parvovirus B19-induced histiophago-cytic syndrome – bilateral facial rash and generalized morbilliform eruption *J Infect Dis 58:149–151, 2005;* in systemic lupus erythe-matosus *JAAD 57:S111–114, 2007*

Ichthyosis follicularis with atrichia and photophobia (IFAP) – X-linked; mild collodion membrane and erythema at birth; red cheeks; ichthyosis, spiny (keratotic) follicular papules (generalized follicular keratoses), congenital atrichia, non-scarring alopecia, keratotic papules of elbows, knees, fingers, extensor surfaces, xerosis; punctate keratitis, photopho-bia; nail dystrophy, psychomotor delay, short stature; enamel dysplasia, beefy red tongue and gingiva, angular stomatitis, atopy, lamellar scales, psoriasiform plaques, palmoplantar erythema; skeletal abnormalities, inguinal hernias, cryptorchidism, seizures, atopy, respiratory and cutaneous infections; mutation in *MBTPS2* (membrane-bound transcription factor peptidase sete 2) *BJD 163:886–889, 2010; JAAD 63:607–641, 2010; Curr Prob Derm 14:71–116, 2002; JAAD 46:S156–158, 2002; BJD 142:157–162, 2000; AD 125:103–106, 1989; Ped Derm 12:195, 1995; Dermatologica 177:341–347, 1988; Am J Med Genet 85:365–368, 1999*

Incontinentia pigmenti – facial erythema preceding blisters in Blaschko distribution *AD 139:1163–1170, 2003*

Kawasaki's disease

Keratitis, ichthyosis, deafness (KID) syndrome – neonatal facial erythema *Ped Derm 23:81–83, 2006;* symmetric hyperkeratotic red plaques of face *Clin in Dermatol 23:23–32, 2005*

Keratosis follicularis spinulosa decalvans – conjunctivitis; keratosis pilaris, follicular atrophoderma, facial erythema, scarring alopecia, ulerythema ophryogenes, photophobia *JAAD 58:499–502, 2008; Arch Dermatol Syphilol 151:384–387, 1926*

Kikuchi's disease (histiocytic necrotizing lymphadenitis) – red papules of face, back, arms; red plaques; erythema and acneiform lesions of face; morbilliform, urticarial, and rubella–like exanthems; red or ulcerated pharynx; cervical adenopathy; associations with SLE, lymphoma, tuberculous adenitis, viral lymphadenitis, infectious mononucleosis, and drug eruptions *Ped Derm 18:403–405, 2001; BJD 144:885–889, 2001; JAAD 36:342–346, 1997; Am J Surg Pathol 14:872–876, 1990; JAAD 59:130–136, 2008;* morbilliform eruption *Ped Derm 24:459–460, 2007*

Kindler's syndrome *BJD 157:1281–1284, 2007*

Lethal multiple pterygium syndrome - midfacial macular telangiec-tatic nevi *Am J Med Genet 12:377–409, 1982*

Macrocephaly-CMTC(cutis marmorata telangiectatica congenita syndrome) – macrocephalic neonatal hypotonia and developmental delay; distended linear and serpiginous abdominal wall veins, patchy reticulated vascular stain without atrophy; telangiectasias of face and ears; midline reticulated facial nevus flammeus (capillary malforma-tion), hydrocephalus, skin and joint hypermobility, hyperelastic skin, thickened subcutaneous tissue, polydactyly, 2–3 toe syndactyly,

hydrocephalus, frontal bossing, hemihypertrophy with segmental overgrowth; neonatal hypotonia, developmental delay *AD 145:287–293, 2009; JAAD 58:697–702, 2008; Ped Derm 24:555–556, 2007; JAAD 56:541–564, 2007; Ped Derm 16:235–237, 1999; Genet Couns 9:245–253, 1998; Am J Med Genet 70:67–73, 1997*

(Note: Beckwith-Wiedemann syndrome demonstrates dysmorphic ears, macroglossia, body asymmetry, midfacial vascular stains, visceromegaly with omphalocele, neonatal hypoglycemia, BUT NO MACROCEPHALY)

MARSH syndrome *Clin Exp Dermatol 24:42–47, 1999*

Mast cell activation syndrome

Netherton's syndrome *AD 140:1275–1280, 2004;* facial erythema (especially perioral) and peeling *AD 122:1420–1424, 1986*

Phakomatosis pigmentovascularis – port wine stain, oculocutaneous (dermal and scleral) melanosis, CNS manifestations; type I – PWS and linear epidermal nevus; type II – PWS and dermal melanocytosis; type III – PWS and nevus spilus; type IV – PWS, dermal melanocytosis, and nevus spilus *J Dermatol 26:834–836, 1999; AD 121:651–653, 1985*

POEMS syndrome (Crow-Fukasi syndrome, Takatsuki syndrome) – plethora, angiomas (cherry, globular, glomeruloid) presenting as red nodules of face, trunk, and extremities, diffuse hyperpigmentation, hypertrichosis, scleroderma-like changes, hyperhidrosis, clubbing, leukonychia, papilledema, sclerotic bone lesions, pleural effusion, peripheral edema, ascites, pulmonary hypertension, weight loss, fatigue, diarrhea, thrombocytosis, polycythemia, fever, renal disease, arthralgias *JAAD 55:149–152, 2006*

Prader-Willi syndrome *Lancet 345:1590, 1995*

Proteus syndrome – port wine stains, subcutaneous hemangiomas and lymphangiomas, lymphangioma circumscriptum, hemihypertro-phy of the face, limbs, trunk; macrodactyly, cerebriform hypertrophy of palmar and/or plantar surfaces, macrocephaly; verrucous epidermal nevi, sebaceous nevi with hyper- or hypopigmentation *Am J Med Genet 27:99–117, 1987;* vascular nevi, soft subcutane-ous masses; lipodystrophy, café au lait macules, linear and whorled macular pigmentation *Am J Med Genet 27:87–97, 1987; Pediatrics 76:984–989, 1985; Eur J Pediatr 140:5–12, 1983*

Reactive arthritis

Robert's syndrome(hypomelia-hypotrichosis-facial hemangioma syndrome) – autosomal recessive; midfacial port wine stain extending from forehead to nose and philtrum, cleft lip +/– cleft palate, sparse silver-blond hair, limb reduction malformation, characteristic facies, malformed ears with hypoplastic lobules, marked growth retardation *Clin Genet 31:170–177, 1987; Clin Genet 5:1–16, 1974*

Rombo syndrome – autosomal dominant; acral erythema, cyanotic redness of hands and lips, follicular atrophy (atrophoderma vermiculata), milia-like papules and cysts of the face and trunk, telangiectasias, red face with perioral cyanotic erythema, red ears with telangiectasia, thin eyebrows, sparse beard hair, basal cell carcinomas, trichoepitheliomas, short stature with short trunk *Ped Derm 23:149–151, 2006; BJD 144:1215–1218, 2001; JAAD 39:853–857, 1998; Acta DV 61:497–503, 1981*

Rothmund Thompson syndrome *JAAD 27:750–762, 1992*

Rubinstein-Taybi syndrome – port wine stain of forehead

SAVI – (STING (stimulator of interferon genes)-associated vasculopathy) – facial erythema and telangiectasia, progressive digital necrosis, swelling of fingers, amputation of several digits, violaceous and telangiectatic malar plaques, nasal septal destruc-tion, chronic leg myalgias, atrophic skin over knees, red-purpuric plaques over cold-sensitive areas (acral areas)(cheeks, nasal tip, ears), reticulate erythema of arms and legs; painful ulcers, eschars *JAAD 74:186–189, 2016*

   Overlaps with:
      Familial chilblain lupus (interferonopathy)
      Aicardi-Goutieres syndrome

Sturge-Weber syndrome (encephalofacial angiomatosis) – facial port wine stain with homolateral leptomeningeal angiomatosis *Ped Der 25:452–454, 2008; Pediatrics 76:48–51, 1985*

Sweet's syndrome

Trisomy 13 – ACC of scalp with holoprosencephaly, eye anomalies, cleft lip and/or palate, polydactyly, port wine stain of forehead *J Med Genet 5:227–252, 1968; Am J Dis Child 112:502–517, 1966*

Thrombocytopenia-absent radii (TAR) syndrome – congenital thrombocytopenia, bilateral absent or hypoplastic radii, port wine stain of head and neck *AD 126:1520–1521, 1990; Am J Pediatr Hematol Oncol 10:51–64, 1988*

Wyburn-Mason(Bonnet-Duchaume-Blanc) syndrome – unilateral (trigeminal distribution, or midforehead, glabella, nose, upper lip) salmon patch with punctate telangiectasias or port wine stain; facial lesion may be arteriovenous malformation; unilateral retinal arteriovenous or vascular malformation, ipsilateral aneurysmal arteriovenous malformation of the midbrain *Am J Ophthalmol 75:224–291, 1973; Brain 66:163–203, 1943; J Med Lyon 18:165–178, 1937*

Xeroderma pigmentosum – presenting in infancy with sunburn *AD 145:1285–1291, 2009*

TOXINS

Acrodynia (pink disease) – mercury poisoning; red cheeks and nose *Ped Derm 21:254–259, 2004; AD 124:107–109, 1988*

Dioxin exposure - *JAAD 19:812–819, 1988*

Mustard gas exposure - sunburn-like erythema *JAAD 19:529–536, 1988*

Scombroid fish poisoning

Self-defense sprays *Ann DV 114:1211–1216, 1987*

TRAUMA

Airbag dermatitis – bizarre shapes of erythema, resembling factitial dermatitis *JAAD 33:824–825, 1995*

Asphyxia – facial congestion, facial edema, cyanosis, periorbital or conjunctival petechiae *JAAD 64811–824, 2011*

Burns - thermal, ultraviolet, X-ray, laser

Changes in temperature

Cold panniculitis in children *Burns Incl Therm Inj 14:51–52, 1988*

Dermabrasion

Erythema ab igne

Erythromelalgia, pediatric – mutation in *SCN9A*; encodes sodium channel protein Na(v)1.7 subunit – red feet, red hands, red legs (cellulitis-like), red face, ears, nose; purple hue, cool, painful *JAAD 66:416–423, 2012*

Frostbite

Neonatal cold injury – facial erythema or cyanosis; firm pitting edema of extremities spreads centrally; skin is cold; mortality of 25% *Br Med J 1:303–309, 1960*

Physical trauma

Popsicle panniculitis

Sunburn

VASCULAR DISEASES

Capillary malformation(port wine stain, salmon patch, angel's kiss, stork bite, nevus simplex, vascular stain) *JAAD 56:353–370, 2007*

Capillary malformations, hereditary, without arteriovenous malformation; autosomal dominant; port wine stain with multifocal <1–3 cm round or oval pink macules of face, trunk, or extremities; 50% with blanched halo; arteriovenous malformations of brain, spine, skin, bone, muscle; inactivating mutations of *RASA1 Ped Derm 30:409–415, 2013; BJD 158:1035–1040, 2008; JAAD 56:541–564, 2007; Am J Hum Genet 73:1240–1249, 2003*

Cutis marmorata telangiectatica congenita – hyperemic face *BJD 137:119–122, 1997; JAAD 20:1098–1104, 1989; AD 118:895–899, 1982; Am J Dis Child 112:72–75, 1966*

Nevus simplex (salmon patch ("stork bite")) – pink macules with fine telangiectasias of the nape of the neck, glabella, forehead upper eyelids, tip of nose, upper lip, midline lumbosacral area *Ped Derm 6:185–187, 1989; Ped Derm 73:31–33, 1983*; extensive nevus simplex of scalp, nose, upper and lower lip mimicking port wine stain *JAAD 68:885–896, 2013*

PHACES syndrome *BJD 169:20–30, 2013; Ped Derm 29:316–319, 2012*

Port wine stain (true capillary-venular malformations of the superficial vascular plexus) *JAMADerm 155:435–441, 2019; JAAD 74:527–535, 2016; BJD 172:684–691, 2015; JAMADerm 150:1336–1340, 2014; BJD 167:1215–1233, 2012; JAAD 60:669–675, 2009;* bilateral port wine stain *AD 142:994–998, 2006*

Septic facial vein thrombosis (*Staphylococcus aureus*) *AD 145:1460–1461, 2009*

Sturge-Weber syndrome – red face *Ped Derm 36:524–527, 2019;* red patch of face *BJD 171:861–867, 2014;* central facial mosaic port wine stain in the midline crossing the nose and temporal area incurs highest risk for Sturge-Weber syndrome *JAAD 72:473–480, 2015; BJD 171:861–867, 2014; NEJM 368:1971–1979, 2013; Pediatrics 87:323–327, 1991*

Superior vena cava syndrome – ruddy complexion *Cutis 79:362, 367–368, 2007; Am Rev Respir Dis 141:1114–1118, 1990*

Tufted angioma - personal observation

RED FEET

AUTOIMMUNE DISEASES AND DISEASES OF IMMUNE DYSFUNCTION

Allergic contact dermatitis – plantar foot dermatitis due to dialkylurea *Ped Derm 36:514–516, 2019*

Bullous pemphigoid

Dermatomyositis

Goodpasture's syndrome (annular erythematous macules) *AD 121:1442–1444, 1985*

Graft vs. host reaction - plantar erythema, TEN-like erosions, flat-topped papules *Ped Derm 30:335–341, 2013*

Lupus erythematosus – systemic; reticulated telangiectatic erythema of thenar and hypothenar eminences, finger pulps, toes, lateral feet, and heels; bluish red with small white scars discoid lupus erythematosus *JAAD 45:142–144, 2001*

Pemphigus erythematosus

Rheumatoid arthritis

Rheumatoid neutrophilic dermatitis

Serum sickness

CONGENITAL ANOMALIES

Acrocyanosis

Syringomyelia

DEGENERATIVE DISEASES

Neurotrophic erythema

Thermally induced cutaneous vasodilatation in aging *J Gerontol 48:M53–57, 1993*

DRUG-INDUCED

Capecitabine (Xeloda) – acral dysesthesia syndrome

Cyclophosphamide and vincristine - acral erythema of proximal nail fold and onychodermal band *Cutis 52:43–44, 1993*

Bromocriptine ingestion mimicking erythromelalgia *Neurology 31:1368–1370, 1981*

Chemotherapy-induced hand-foot syndrome(acral dysesthesia syndrome)(palmoplantar erythrodysesthesia syndrome) – pegylated liposomal doxorubicin, capecitabine, 5-fluorouracil, cytarabine, docatael, sorafenib, sunitinib, axitinib, pazopanib, regorafenib, vemurafenib *JAAD 71:787–794, 2014; AD 131:202–206, 1995; JAAD 24:457–461, 1991; AD 122:1023–1027, 1986*

Chemotherapy-induced Raynaud's phenomenon *Ann Int Med 95:288–292, 1981*

Coumadin purple toe syndrome

Cytarabine – purpuric intertriginous plaques, scalp involvement, papules coalesce into papular purpuric violaceous generalized exanthema, red knee, red feet *JAAD 73:821–828, 2015*

Dilantin hypersensitivity syndrome

Docataxel

Pegylated liposomal doxorubicin – red hands and feet (acral erythrodysesthesia); follicular exanthem, intertrigo, alopecia, nail changes, stomatitis *BJD 176:507–509, 2017*

Erythromelalgia, drug-induced – erythema and edema of feet; nifedipine, pergolide, bromocriptine, felodipine, nicardipine *Cutis 75:37–40, 2005*

Etoposide/teniposide/amsacrine – hand/foot syndrome *JAAD 71:203–214, 2014*

Felodipine - erythromelalgia *Cutis 75:37–40, 2005*

5-fluorouracil, capecitabine, tegafur – hand/foot syndrome *JAAD 71:203–214, 2014*

Hydroxyurea – dermatomyositis-like lesions associated with long-term hydroxyurea administration *JAAD 21:797–799, 1989*

Morbilliform or scarlatiniform drug eruptions

Necrotizing eccrine squamous syringometaplasia *J Cut Pathol 18:453–456, 1991*

Nicardipine - erythromelalgia *Cutis 75:37–40, 2005*

Nifedipine - erythromelalgia *Cutis 75:37–40, 2005*

Paclitaxel – acral erythema of chemotherapy *AD 148:1333–1334, 2012*

Pergolide – erythromelalgia *Cutis 75:37–40, 2005*

6-mercaptopurine and mesalamine – erythrodysesthesia; red and eroded palms and soles *AD 144:1079–1080, 2008*

Sorafenib – acral erythema of chemotherapy *JAAD 71:217–227, 2014; Clin in Dermatol 29:587–601, 2011*

Sunitinib – acral erythema of chemotherapy *JAAD 71:217–227, 2014; Clin in Dermatol 29:587–601, 2011*

Toxic erythema of chemotherapy – erythema of hands and feet with giant bullae *Clin in Dermatol 29:587–601, 2011*

   Cytosine arabinoside

   Doxorubicin and other anthracyclines

   5-fluorouracil

   Capecitabine

   Docataxel and other taxanes

   Methotrexate

Tyrosine kinase inhibitor-induced hand-foot syndrome *AD 148:546–547, 2012*

Vandetanib – erythema of palms and soles *AD 148:1418–1420, 2012*

Vemurafenib – cystic lesions of face, keratosis pilaris-like eruptions, hyperkeratotic plantar papules, squamous cell carcinoma; multiple nodules of cheeks; follicular plugging; exuberant seborrheic dermatitis-like hyperkertosis of face; hand and foot reaction; diffuse spiny follicular hyperkeratosis; cobblestoning of forehead *JAAD 67:1375–1379, 2012;*

AD 148:357–361, 2012

Verapamil - erythromelalgia *BJD 127:292–294, 1992*

Vincristine/vinblastine/vinorelbine – hand/foot syndrome *JAAD 71:203–214, 2014*

EXOGENOUS AGENTS

Irritant contact dermatitis

Sea urchin spine injury *Harefuah 118:639–640, 1990*

INFECTIONS AND INFESTATIONS

AIDS - acute HIV infection - acral erythema *Cutis 40:171–175, 1987*

Cutaneous borreliosis – acrodermatitis chronica atrophicans, cutis laxa-like changes, red patches, erythema migrans, erythema and edema of foot, poikilodermatous changes, red macules and telangiectasias *JAAD 72:683–689, 2015; acrodermatitis chronica atrophicans mimicking peripheral vascular disease Acta Med Scand 220:485–488, 1980; red blue foot BMJ Case Rep June 22, 2016*

Cellulitis

Endocarditis

Erysipelas – bullous erysipelas

Leprosy

Lyme disease

Mycobacterium marinum NEJM 373:1761, 2015

Painful plaque-like pitted keratolysis *Ped Derm 9251–254, 1992*

Parvovirus B19 infection - papular-purpuric gloves and socks syndrome (Parvovirus B19) *JAAD 71:62–69, 2014; bullous papular-purpuric gloves and socks syndrome JAAD 60691–695, 2009*

Human Parechovirus type 3 infection – generalized morbilliform eruption with bright red feet *Ped Derm 31:258–259, 2014*

Scopulariopsis Dermatology 193:149–151, 1996

Septic emboli

Syphilis – secondary

Tinea pedis, moccasin type

Vibrio vulnificus - edema, erythema, and purpura of ankles *BJD 145:280–284, 2001*

INFILTRATIVE DISORDERS

Mastocytosis – diffuse infiltrative mastocytosis (xanthelasmoidea)

INFLAMMATORY DISEASES

Angioedema

Erythema multiforme

Erythema nodosum *JAAD 29:284, 1993; AD 129:1064–1065, 1993*

Hashimoto-Pritzker Langerhans cell histiocytosis – urticating lesions *Ped Derm 18:41–44, 2001*

Inflammatory lymphedema and inflammatory vasculitis – red feet and edema of legs in Air Force basic trainees *JAMADerm 151:395–400, 2015*

Interstitial granulomatous dermatitis – red plaques of feet *Cutis 90:30–32, 2012*

Lipoatrophic panniculitis *AD 123:1662–1666, 1987*

Neutrophilic eccrine hidradenitis, including recurrent palmoplantar hidradenitis in children *AD 131:817–820, 1995*

METABOLIC DISEASES

Cold agglutinins

Cryofibrinogenemia

Cryoglobulinemia

Diabetes mellitus – erysipelas-like erythema of legs or feet *Acta Med Scand 196:333–342, 1974*

Gout - mimicking infectious cellulitis *Ann Int Med 142:47–55, 2005*

Hyperestrogenic states - liver disease, exogenous estrogens

Hyperthyroidism

Neuropathy-associated acral paresthesia and vasodilatation

Nutritional melalgia – nutritional deficiency associated with anorexia nervosa *AD 140:521–524, 2004*

Pellagra *Int J Dermatol 37:599, 1998*

Porphyria - congenital erythropoietic porphyria; erythropoietic protoporphyria *JAMADerm 152:937–938, 2016*

Waldenstrom's macroglobulinemia

NEOPLASTIC DISEASES

Atrial myxoma *Br Heart J 36:839–840, 1974*

Eccrine angiomatous hamartoma – vascular nodule; macule, red plaque, acral nodule of infants or neonates; painful, red, purple, blue, yellow, brown, skin-colored *JAAD 47:429–435, 2002; Ped Derm 13:139–142, 1996; JAAD 37:523–549, 1997*

Essential thrombocythemia - acral ischemia with lividity

Inflammatory carcinoma *JAAD 31:689–690, 1994*

Kaposi's sarcoma

Leukemia - acral livedo with leukostasis in chronic myelogenous leukemia *AD 123:921–924, 1987*

Plantar fibromatosis *JAAD 12:212–214, 1985*

Polycythemia vera - acral ischemia with lividity; acral erythema

PARANEOPLASTIC DISEASES

Acrokeratosis paraneoplastica (Bazex syndrome) *Hautarzt 43:496–499, 1992*

Erythromelalgia associated with thrombocythemia *JAAD 24:59–63, 1991*

PRIMARY CUTANEOUS DISEASES

Acrodermatitis continua of Hallopeau *Dtsch Med Wochenschr 123:386–390, 1998*

Atopic hand and foot dermatitis

Cutis laxa - acral localized acquired cutis laxa *JAAD 21:33–40, 1989*

Epidermolytic hyperkeratosis - personal observation

Erythema elevatum diutinum

Erythroderma

Erythrokeratoderma variabilis

Erythrokeratolysis hiemalis(Oudsthoorn disease)(keratolytic winter erythema) – palmoplantar erythema, cyclical and centrifugal peeling of affected sites, targetoid lesions of the hands and feet – seen in South African whites; precipitated by cold weather or fever *BJD 98:491–495, 1978*

Familial acral erythema *AD 95:483–486, 1967*

Greither's palmoplantar keratoderma(transgrediens et progrediens palmoplantar keratoderma) – red hands and feet; hyperkeratoses extending over Achilles tendon, backs of hands, elbows, knees; livid erythema at margins *Ped Derm 20:272–275, 2003; Cutis 65:141–145, 2000*

Follicular mucinosis, erythrodermic

Granuloma annulare, generalized *JAAD 20:39–47, 1989*

Infectious eczematoid dermatitis - personal observation

Juvenile plantar dermatosis *Clin Exp Dermatol 11:529–534, 1986; Semin Dermatol 1:67–75, 1982; Clin Exp Dermatol 1:253–260, 1976*

Lamellar ichthyosis

Lichen planus *Dermatol J Online Dec 16, 2014* Mal de Meleda – autosomal dominant, autosomal recessive transgrediens with acral erythema in glove-like distribution *Dermatology 203:7–13, 2001; AD 136:1247–1252, 2000; J Dermatol 27:664–668, 2000; Dermatologica 171:30–37, 1985*

Pityriasis rosea - personal observation

Pityriasis rubra pilaris - personal observation

Progressive symmetric erythrokeratoderma

Psoriasis, including pustular psoriasis

Symmetrical lividity of the soles *Int J Dermatol 17:739–744, 1978; BJD 37:123–125, 1925*

SYNDROMES

Acrogeria *J Dermatol 20:572–576, 1993*

Antiphospholipid antibody syndrome

Familial Mediterranean fever - mimicking infectious cellulitis *Ann Int Med 142:47–55, 2005; Isr Med Assoc J 1:31–36, 1999; Q J Med 75:607–616, 1990*

Goodpasture's syndrome - annular erythematous macules on instep *AD 121:1442–4, 1985*

Hereditary lactatate dehydrogenase M-subunit deficiency – annually recurring acroerythema *JAAD 27:262–263, 1992*

Hypereosinophilic syndrome – palmoplantar erythema *JAAD 46:s133–136, 2002*

Ichthyosis follicularis with atrichia and photophobia (IFAP) – palmoplantar erythema; collodion membrane and erythema at birth; ichthyosis, spiny (keratotic) follicular papules (generalized follicular keratoses), non-scarring alopecia, keratotic papules of elbows, knees, fingers, extensor surfaces, xerosis; punctate keratitis, photophobia; nail dystrophy, psychomotor delay, short stature; enamel dysplasia, beefy red tongue and gingiva, angular stomatitis, atopy, lamellar scales, psoriasiform plaques *Curr Prob Derm 14:71–116, 2002; JAAD 46:S156–158, 2002; BJD 142:157–162, 2000; Ped Derm 12:195, 1995; AD 125:103–106, 1989; Dermatologica 177:341–347, 1988; Am J Med Genet 85:365–368, 1999*

Kawasaki's disease

Klippel-Trenaunay-Weber

Netherton's syndrome - personal observation

Red ear syndrome – may be manifestation of erythromelalgia; irritation of third cervical root; temporomandibular joint dysfunction, thalamic syndrome, headache, antiphospholipid antibody syndrome, neuropsychiatric lupus erythematosus, idiopathic; red hands and feet *Ped Derm 36:686–689, 2019; Lupus 9:301–303, 2000; Neurology 47:617, 620, 1996;* rare migraine variant

Schamberg's disease *JAMA Derm 149:223–228, 2013; BJD 13:1–5, 1901*

Schopf-Schulz-Passarge syndrome – psoriasiform plantar dermatitis (palmoplantar keratoderma); eyelid cysts (apocrine hidrocystomas), hypotrichosis, decreased number of teeth, brittle and furrowed nails *AD 140:231–236, 2004; BJD 127:33–35, 1992; JAAD 10:922–925, 1984; Birth Defects XII:219–221, 1971*

Scleroatrophic syndrome of Huriez - red hands and feet early in disease *Ped Derm 15:207–209, 1998*

Sweet's syndrome

Wells' syndrome – red plaques of soles *Cutis 72:209–212, 2003*

TOXINS

Ciguatera fish poisoning *Dtsch Med Wochenschr 126:812–814, 2001*

Eosinophilia myalgia syndrome *JAAD 23:1063–1069, 1990*

Mercury - infantile acrodynia (erythema with or without exfoliation) *Arch Dis Child 86:453, 2002; AD 124:107–109, 1988*

TRAUMA

Chilblains *JAAD 23:257–262, 1990; AD 117:26–28, 1981*

Delayed pressure urticaria

Frostbite, recovery phase

Heat exposure

Long distance running

Reflex sympathetic dystrophy (causalgia)(complex regional pain syndrome), Stage 1 *JAAD 22:513–520, 1990*

Thermal burn

Traumatic plantar urticaria (delayed pressure urticaria) *JAAD 18:144–146, 1988*

Vibratory urticaria

VASCULAR

Acquired port wine stain - personal observation

Acquired progressive lymphangioma – plantar red plaques *JAAD 49:S250–251, 2003*

Acral ischemia with lividity in polycythemia vera or essential thrombocythemia

Acroangiodermatitis of Mali (pseudo-Kaposi's sarcoma) *Indian J DV Leprol 76:553–556, 2010*

Acrocyanosis with atrophy *AD 124:263–268, 1988*

Acute venous congestion - personal observation

Angiodyskinesia – dependent erythema after prolonged exercise or idiopathic *Surgery 61:880–890, 1967*

Arteriosclerotic peripheral vascular disease (arterial insufficiency, arteriosclerosis obliterans) – dependent erythema of the dorsum of the foot (Buerger's sign) *JAAD 50:456–460, 2004*

Cholesterol emboli - personal observation

Erythrocyanosis

Erythromelalgia *BJD 172:412–418, 2015; SKINmed 12:271–275, 2014; AD 147:309–314, 2011; AD 144:320–324, 2008; AD 142:1583–1588, 2006; AD 142:283–286, 2006; BJD 153:174–177, 2005; AD 139:1337–1343, 2003; JAAD 43:841–847, 2000; AD 136:330–336, 2000;* pediatric erythromelalgia – mutation in *SCN9A;* encodes sodium channel protein Na(v)1.7 subunit – red feet, red hands, red legs (cellulitis-like), red face, ears, nose; purple hue, cool, painful *JAAD 66:416–423, 2012*

Fat emboli

Generalized essential telangiectasia

Granulation tissue - personal observation

Granulomatosis with polyangiitis *AD 130:861–867, 1994*

Hemangiomatosis *Acta DV 66:449–451, 1986*

Infantile hemangiomas of the extremities – zosteriform or segmental; red hand or red foot *JAAD 75:556–563, 2016*

Klippel-Trenaunay syndrome - personal observation

Parkes-Weber syndrome – arteriovenous malformation with multiple arteriovenous fistulae along extremity with limb (usually leg) overgrowth; arteriovenous shunting; cutaneous red stain; lymphedema; high output congestive heart failure, hypertrophied digits with severe deformity; red foot *JAAD 56:541–564, 2007;*

Curr Prob in Dermatol 13:249–300, 2002; BJD 19:231–235, 1907

Polyarteritis nodosa *AD 130:884–889, 1994*

Progressive ascending telangiectasia - personal observation

Raynaud's disease or phenomenon – hyperperfusion phase

Thromboangiitis obliterans

Vascular malformation - nevus flammeus

Vasculitis, leukocytoclastic

Venous congestion, acute

Venous gangrene - erythema *AD 123:933–936, 1987*

Venous stasis

RED NOSE

AUTOIMMUNE DISEASES AND DISEASES OF IMMUNE DYSFUNCTION

Allergic contact dermatitis

Dermatomyositis

Lupus erythematosus - discoid lupus erythematosus *NEJM 269:1155–1161, 1963;* subacute cutaneous LE, systemic lupus – facial erythema and telangiectasia; nasal chondritis *Clin Exp Rheumatol 5:349–353, 1987*

Pemphigus, multiple types *JAAD 47:875–880, 2002*

Relapsing polychondritis

Urticaria

CONGENITAL DISEASES

Nevus simplex (capillary ectasias) – glabella, eyelids, nose, upper lip, nape of neck

Salmon patch (nevus simplex)("stork bite") – pink macules with fine telangiectasias of the nape of the neck, glabella, forehead, upper eyelids, tip of nose, upper lip, midline lumbosacral area *Ped Derm 73:31–33, 1983*

DRUG-INDUCED

Corticosteroids - topical corticosteroid-induced telangiectasia and atrophy

Tetracycline and doxycycline photosensitivity

EXOGENOUS AGENTS

Irritant contact dermatitis

INFECTIONS AND INFESTATIONS

Actinomycosis - indurated red nose *JAAD 38:310–313, 1998*

AIDS - seborrheic dermatitis

Aspergillosis *Oral Surg Oral Med Oral Pathol 59:499–504, 1985*

Candidiasis - chronic mucocutaneous candidiasis

Cat scratch disease

Chikungunya fever *Ped Derm 35:408–409, 2018*

Cryptococcosis - indurated red nose *JAAD 38:310–313, 1998*

Erysipelas/cellulitis

Fusarium – of sinuses; nasal erythema with conjunctivitis *JAAD 47:659–666, 2002*

Herpes simplex virus infection - personal observation

Herpes zoster

Histoplasmosis - indurated red nose *JAAD 38:310–313, 1998*

Bullous impetigo - personal observation

Leishmaniasis - indurated red nose *JAAD 38:310–313, 1998;* nasal erythema and crusting *JAMA 312:1250–1251, 2014*

Leprosy - indeterminate – red macules lepromatous leprosy*;* indurated red nose *JAAD 38:310–313, 1998*

Mycobacterium tuberculosis - lupus vulgaris with indurated red nose *JAAD 38:310–313, 1998;* lupus vulgaris erythematoides *Dermatol Online J May 15, 2013*

North American blastomycosis - indurated red nose *JAAD 38:310–313, 1998;* red plaque with pustules *JAAD 53:740–741, 2005*

Paracoccidioidomycosis - indurated red nose *JAAD 38:310–313, 1998*

Rhinoscleroma - indurated red nose *JAAD 38:310–313, 1998; Cutis 40:101–103, 1987*

Sporotrichosis - indurated red nose *JAAD 38:310–313, 1998*

Staphylococcus aureus - nasal carriage with intranasal folliculitis or vestibulitis

Syphilis - indurated red nose *JAAD 38:310–313, 1998*

Tinea faciei – *Microsporum gypseum Ped Derm 22:536–538, 2005;* tinea incognito, treated with topical corticosteroids

Varicella – with or without secondary Staphylococcal infection

INFILTRATIVE DISEASES

Amyloidosis, including nodular amyloidosis *J Cut Med Surg 5:101–104, 2001*

Hereditary progressive mucinous histiocytosis *JAAD 35:298–303, 1996*

Histiocytosis - non-Langerhans cell histiocytosis *JAAD 30:367–370, 1994*

Jessner's lymphocytic infiltrate

Lichen myxedematosus

Lymphocytoma cutis

INFLAMMATORY DISEASES

Rosai-Dorfman disease (sinus histiocytosis with lymphadenopathy) *BJD 134:749–753, 1996*

Sarcoidosis - lupus pernio - indurated red nose *AD 149:493–494, 2013; Rheum Dis Clin North Amer 39:277–297, 2013; JAAD 38:310–313, 1998;* angiolupoid sarcoid – red and telangiectatic nose *JAAD 66:699–716, 2012*

METABOLIC DISEASES

Flushing

Porphyria - porphyria cutanea tarda, erythropoietic protoporphyria, congenital erythropoietic porphyria, variegate porphyria

Pregnancy

NEOPLASTIC DISEASES

Aggressive intranasal carcinoma - edema and erythema *Cutis 42:288–293, 1988*

Angiofibroma

Angiosarcoma - indurated red nose *JAAD 54:883–885, 2006; JAAD 38:310–313, 1998; JAAD 38:837–840, 1998*

Basal cell carcinoma mimicking rhinophyma - indurated red nose *JAAD 38:310–313, 1998*

Carcinoid syndrome

Epithelioid sarcoma *J Cutan Pathol 27:186-190, 2000*

Kaposi's sarcoma

Keratoacanthoma

Leukemia cutis – chronic lymphocytic leukemia – red infiltrated nose with necrosis *Cutis 80:208–210, 2007*

Lymphoma - indurated red nose *JAAD 38:310–313, 1998;* malignant lymphoma of the nasal cavity *Acta Pathol Jpn 42:333–338, 1992;* cutaneous T-cell lymphoma; nasal lymphoma *JAAD 38:310–313, 1998;* B–cell lymphoma *Leuk Lymph 34:682–684, 2010*

Merkel cell tumor

Metastatic carcinoma – cervical carcinoma *Dermatology 199:171–173, 1999;* indurated red nose *JAAD 38:310–313, 1998*

Nasal septal carcinoma – mimicking rosacea *J Derm Surg 13:1021–1024, 1987*

Sebaceous carcinoma - indurated red nose *JAAD 38:310–313, 1998*

Squamous cell carcinoma - indurated red nose *JAAD 38:310–313, 1998;* clown nose *BMJ Case Rep Jan 31, 2014*

PARANEOPLASTIC DISORDERS

Bazex syndrome (acrokeratosis paraneoplastica) *AD 141: 389–394, 2005*

.

PHOTODERMATOSES

Actinic prurigo

Chronic actinic damage

Chronic actinic dermatitis

Polymorphic light eruption

PRIMARY CUTANEOUS DISEASES

Acne vulgaris

Acne rosacea, including granulomatous rosacea - indurated red nose *JAAD 38:310–313, 1998*

Granuloma faciale

Granulosis rubra nasi *Ann DV 123:106–108, 1996; G Ital DV 125:275–276, 1990; Derm Z 71:79–84, 1935*

Lichen simplex chronicus

Perioral dermatitis

Psoriasis

Rhinophyma - indurated red nose *JAAD 38:310–313, 1998*

Seborrheic dermatitis

PSYCHOCUTANEOUS DISORDERS

Factitial dermatitis - personal observation

SYNDROMES

Amyoplasia congenita disruptive sequence – midfacial macular telangiectatic nevi *Am J Med Genet 15:571–590, 1983*

Beckwith-Wiedemann syndrome (Exomphalos-Macroglossia-Gigantism)(EMG) syndrome – autosomal dominant; zosteriform rash at birth, exomphalos, macroglossia, visceromegaly, facial salmon patch of forehead, upper eyelids, nose, and upper lip and gigantism; linear earlobe grooves, circular depressions of helices; increased risk of Wilms' tumor, adrenal carcinoma, hepatoblastoma, and rhabdomyosarcoma *JAAD 37:523–549, 1997; Am J Dis Child 122:515–519, 1971*

Bloom's syndrome *J Dermatol Case Rep 6:29–33, 2012*

Bonnet-Dechaume-Blanc syndrome – midfacial arteriovenous malformation *Textbook of Neonatal Dermatology, p. 329, 2001*

Cornelia de Lange syndrome – specific facies, hypertrichosis of forehead, face, back, shoulders, and extremities, synophrys; long delicate eyelashes, cutis marmorata, skin around eyes and nose with bluish tinge, red nose *Ped Derm 19:42–45, 2002; JAAD 37:295–297, 1997*

Familial chilblain lupus - interferonopathy *Orphan Diseases Online J Aug 26, 2017*

Lethal multiple pterygium syndrome - midfacial macular telangiectatic nevi *Am J Med Genet 12:377–409, 1982*

Lipoid proteinosis *Ped Derm 9:264–267, 1992*

Multicentric reticulohistiocytosis

Robert's syndrome (hypomelia-hypotrichosis-facial hemangioma syndrome) – autosomal recessive; midfacial port wine stain extending from forehead to nose and philtrum, cleft lip +/– cleft palate, sparse silver-blond hair, limb reduction malformation, characteristic facies, malformed ears with hypoplastic lobules, marked growth retardation *Clin Genet 5:1–16, 1974; Clin Genet 31:170–177, 1987*

Sjogren's syndrome – erythema of nose and cheeks

Sphenopalatine syndrome – chronic and intermittent edema of face with unilateral lacrimation, rhinitis, erythema of the bridge of the nose

Trichorhinophalangeal syndrome (bulbous nose) *Ped Derm 10:385–387, 1993*

Tuberous sclerosis – adenoma sebaceum *Plast Reconstruct Surg 70:91–93, 1981*

Wyburn-Mason (Bonnet-Duchaume-Blanc) syndrome – unilateral (trigeminal distribution, or midforehead, glabella, nose, upper lip) salmon patch with punctate telangiectasias or port wine stain; facial lesion may be arteriovenous malformation; unilateral retinal arteriovenous or vascular malformation, ipsilateral aneurysmal arteriovenous malformation of the midbrain *Am J Ophthalmol 75:224–291, 1973; Brain 66:163–203, 1943; J Med Lyon 18:165–178, 1937*

TOXIC

Acrodynia (mercury) *AD 124:107–109, 1988*

TRAUMA

Cold-induced injury - indurated red nose *JAAD 38:310–313, 1998*

Nostril piercing – persistent telangiectatic erythema following nostril piercing *Int J Dermatol 53:e145–151, 2014*

Post-rhinoplasty *Plast Recontr Surg 67:661–664, 1981*

Pseudorhinophyma – eyeglass frames restricting superficial venous and lymphatic drainage from nose *Skin and Allergy News, November 2001, p. 42*

VASCULAR

Angioendotheliosarcoma *Acta DV64:88–90, 1984*

Angiomatous nevus

Arteriovenous and cavernous angioma *Dtsch Med Wochenschr 116:416–420, 1991*

Erythromelalgia, pediatric – mutation in *SCN9A*; encodes sodium channel protein Na(v)1.7 subunit – red feet, red hands, red legs (cellulitis-like), red face, ears, nose; purple hue, cool, painful *JAAD 66:416–423, 2012*

Granulomatosis with polyangiitis - indurated red nose *JAAD 38:310–313, 1998*

Hemangioma

Nevus flammeus - personal observation

Progressive ascending telangiectasia

Sturge-Weber syndrome

Symmetric peripheral gangrene (disseminated intravascular coagulation)

Vascular malformation

RED PATCH

AUTOIMMUNE DISEASES AND DISEASES OF IMMUNE DYSFUNCTION

Allergic contact dermatitis - mimicking infectious cellulitis *Ann Int Med 142:47–55, 2005;* painful oral erythema due to 2-hydroxyethyl methacrylate *Australas J Dermatol 42:203–206, 2001*

Arthus reaction – erythema, edema, hemorrhage, occasional necrosis

Dermatomyositis – over scalp, face, arms, thighs, trunk *AD 142:65–69, 2006;* oval palatal erythematous patch in dermatomyositis with anti-TIF1 gamma (p155) antibody *JAMADerm 152:1049–1054, 2016*

Flavorings (cinnamic aldehyde) – oral erythema *QJM 93:507–511, 2000*

Food additives (benzoic acid) – oral erythema *QJM 93:507–511, 2000*

Graft vs. host disease – acute – oral erythema chronic - erythema red macules or folliculocentric papules of face, ears, palms and soles, periungual areas, upper back and neck *AD 143:67–71, 2007*

Juvenile rheumatoid arthritis - Still's disease; evanescent rash; persistent pruritic papules and plaques; urticarial and urticarial-like rash, vesiculopustular eruptions, edema of the eyelids, widespread non-pruritic persistent erythema *Medicine 96:e6318, 2017*

Lupus erythematosus - systemic lupus erythematosus *BJD 135:355–362, 1996;* mimicking infectious cellulitis *Ann Int Med 142:47–55, 2005;* intraoral red patch of hard palate; red oral mucosa *BJD 144:1219–1223, 2001; Int J Oral Surg 13:101–147, 1984;* follicular erythema and petechiae of SLE *BJD 147:157–159, 2002;* lupus profundus *Ann Int Med 142:47–55, 2005*

Morphea, early *Ann Int Med 142:47–55, 2005;* early morphea resembles macular vascular nevus or acquired port wine stain *Ped Derm 31:591–594, 2014; JAAD 64:779–782, 2011;* superficial morphea *JAAD 51:S84–86, 2004*

Pemphigoid gestations *JAAD 55:823–828, 2006*

Pemphigus foliaceus of children *JAAD 46:419–422, 2002; Ped Derm 3:459–463, 1986*

Still's disease – salmon-pink urticaria-like macular lesions *JAAD 50:813–814, 2004*

Urticaria; mimicking infectious cellulitis *Ann Int Med 142:47–55, 2005*

CONGENITAL DISEASES

Blueberry muffin baby - personal observation

Erythema toxicum neonatorum

Harlequin color change - neonatal vasomotor instability; occurs days 2–5 lasting 30 seconds to 20 minutes; increased prostaglandin E1 *Ped Derm 21:573–576, 2004; Lancet 263:1005–1007, 1952*

Nevus simplex (capillary ectasias)(true capillary malformation) (salmon patches) – glabella, eyelids, nose, upper lip, nape of neck *JAAD 60:669–675, 2009*

Rubor – transient neonatal rubor due to vasodilatation and hyperemia, especially of the head *JAAD 60:669–675, 2009*

Self-limited neonatal periumbilical erythema *Ped Derm 34:730–731, 2017*

Spinal dysraphism with overlying port wine stain *AD 114:573–577, 1978; AD 112:1724–1728, 1976*

DEGENERATIVE DISEASES

Sympathetic nerve dystrophy – erythema

DRUGS

Azathioprine – neutrophilic dermatosis (azathioprine hypersensitivity syndrome) – palpebral conjunctival erythema, pink macules, pink or red plaques *JAMA Derm 149:592–597, 2013*

Cabozantinib – VEGFR2 inhibitor; c-met; RET multitargets; tyrosine kinase inhibitor; hand foot skin reactions with bullae, hyperkeratosis, acral erythema; skin and hair depigmentation, splinter hemorrhages, xerosis, red scrotum *JAMADerm 151:170–177, 2015*

Colchicine *BJD 150:581–588, 2004*

Cyclophosphamide – radiation recall *JAAD 71:203–214, 2014*

Dimethyl fumarate (therapy for multiple sclerosis) – eosinophilic fasciitis-like disorder *J Drugs Dermatol 13:1144–1147, 2014*

Docataxel radiation recall reaction *BJD 153:674–675, 2005*

Doxorubicin, pegylated - periaxillary erythema *JAAD 58:S44–46, 2008;* doxorubicin/daunorubicin – radiation recall *JAAD 71:203–214, 2014*

Everolimus – mTOR inhibitor; broad red patches of face, scalp, upper trunk; also widespread dermatitis, acneiform eruptions *The Dermatologist July 2015;pp.47–48*

Fixed drug eruption – mimicking cellulitis *NEJM 350:904–912, 2004*

Gemcitabine – radiation recall *JAAD 71:203–214, 2014*

Injection site reactions *JAAD 49:826–831, 2003*

Lanreotide – radiation recall; erythema of abdomen *BJD 157:1061–1063, 2007*

Methotrexate – photorecall; administration of methotrexate after occurrence of sunburn *JAAD 58:903–905, 2008*

Mogamulizumab granulomatous drug eruption – red macules and patches, scaly red plaques *JAMADerm 155:968–971, 2019*

Pemetrexed – radiation recall; confluent erythema *JAAD 58:545–570, 2008;* painful red patches *JAAD 65:241–243, 2011*

Prostacyclin (epoprostenol) – diffuse erythema with or without mottling, exfoliation, or palpable purpura *JAAD 51:98–102, 2004*

Radiation recall – chemotherapy, antituberculous drugs, antibiotics, simvastatin, interferon, codeine, tamoxifen *Cancer Treat Rev 31:555–570, 2005;* pemetrexed *JAAD 58:545–570, 2008;* capecitabine, doxorubicin, taxanes, gemcitabine; erythema and desquamation; edema; vesicles and papules; ulceration and skin necrosis *The Oncologist 15:1227–1237, 2010*

Retinoid dermatitis

Voriconazole – in immunosuppressed patients; chronic phototoxicity with aggressive squamous cell carcinomas; sunburn-like erythema, multiple lentigines, multiple actinic keratoses, cheilitis, exfoliative dermatitis, pseudo-porphyria cutanea tarda, telangiectasias *JAAD 62:31–37, 2010*

EXOGENOUS AGENTS

Foreign body reaction (granuloma) – orthopedic implants mimicking infectious cellulitis *Ann Int Med 142:47–55, 2005; Ann DV 123:686–690, 1996*

Injection of ricin – infectious and toxic cellulitis *BJD 150:154, 2004*

Irritant contact dermatitis

Marlex graft infection, intermittent cellulitis; geometric red patches overlying Marlex graft - personal observation

Reticular telangiectatic erythema associated with implantable cardioverter defibrillator, pacemakers, knee prostheses, spinal cord stimulators, infusion pumps *Dermatitis 25:98–99, 2014; Mayo Clinic Proc 88:117–119, 2013; Contact Dermatitis 64:280–288, 2011; Cutis 78:329–331, 2006; AD 137:1239–1241, 2001;* overlying intrathecal pump *Soc Ped Derm Annual Meeting, July 2005; AD 141:106–107, 2005;* overlying a pacemaker *Hautarzt 32:651–654, 1981*

INFECTIONS AND INFESTATIONS

Acanthamebiasis in AIDS *AD 131:1291–1296, 1995*

Acinetobacter calcoaceticus – cellulitis *Medicine 56:79–97, 1977*

Aeromonas hydrophila – cellulitis complicating injuries in fresh water or soil *NEJM 350:904–912, 2004; Clin Inf Dis 19:77–83, 1994; Clin Inf Dis 16:79–84, 1993*

Anaerobic myonecrosis – gas gangrene; *Clostridium perfringens, septicum NEJM 350:904–912, 2004*

Anthrax – cellulitis in intravenous drug abuse *Clin Inf Dis 61:1840–1849, 2015;* confused with cellulitis *NEJM 350:904–912, 2004*

Aspergillosis – red patch *JAAD 80:869–880, 2019;* primary cutaneous aspergillosis in premature infants; red patch with pustules *Ped Derm 19:439–444, 2002*

Bacillary angiomatosis – intraoral red patch

Black widow spider bite *Semin Cutan Med Surg 26:168–179, 2007*

Brown recluse spider bite *Semin Cutan Med Surg 26:168–179, 2007*

Cutaneous borreliosis – acrodermatitis chronica atrophicans, cutis laxa-like changes, red patches, erythema migrans, erythema and edema of foot, poikilodermatous changes, red macules and telangiectasias *JAAD 72:683–689, 2015*

Buruli ulcer – diffuse erythema, edema, and necrosis of dorsal hand *JAMADerm 130:669–671, 2014*

Candidiasis - intraoral red patch

Caterpillar envenomation – pain, erythema, and edema; saddleback caterpillar (*Acharia stimulea*), Io moth (*Automeris io*), hag moth (*Phobetron pithecium*), buck moth (*Hemileuca maia*) *Cutis 80:110–112, 2007;* puss caterpillar (*Megalopyge opercularis*) – severe sting with edema, erythema, and hemorrhagic papular eruptions; systemic reactions *JAAD 62:1–10, 2010*

Cellulitis *NEJM 350:904–912, 2004*
    Periorbital cellulitis – *Staphylococcus aureus, pneumococcus, Group A streptococcus*
    Buccal cellulitis – *Haemophilus influenzae*
    Cellulitis complicating body piercing – *Staphylococcus aureus, Group A streptococcus*
    Mastectomy – *non-group A hemolytic streptococcus*
    Lumpectomy - *non-group A hemolytic streptococcus*
    Harvest of saphenous vein for coronary artery bypass - Group A or non-group A hemolytic streptococcus
    Liposuction - *Group A streptococcus, peptostreptococcus*
    Postoperative (very early) wound infection - *Group A streptococcus*
    Injection drug user - *Staphylococcus aureus, streptococci (groups A, C, F, G), Enterococcus faecalis, viridans-group streptococci, coagulase negative staphylococci, anaerobic bacteria (bacteroides, clostridium), Enterobacteriaceae*
    Perianal cellulitis - *Group A streptococcus*

Crepitant cellulitis – gas gangrene; *Clostridium perfringens, septicum*
Gangrenous cellulitis
Erythema migrans – *Borrelia burgdorferi*
Paraplegia
Dog or cat bite – *Pasteurella multocida, Staph aureus, S. intermedius, Neisseria canis, Haemophilus felix, Capnocytophaga canimorsus,* anaerobes
    Human bites – *Bacteroides species, peptostreptococci, Eikenella corrodens, viridans streptococci, Staphylococcus aureus*

Centipede bite – cellulitis-like *Semin Cutan Med Surg 26:168–179, 2007*

Chagas disease (reactivation posttransplant) *Cutis 48:37–40, 1991*

Chrysaora plocamia ("true jellyfish") – widespread erythema with bullae *JAAD 61:733–750, 2009*

Citrobacter diversus - cellulitis *Cutis 61:158–159, 1998*

Citrobacter freundii – cellulitis, ecthyma, ulcers, red plaque with central ulceration and caseation *AD 143:124–125, 2007*

Clostridium botulinum, sordelli, novyi – cellulitis in intravenous drug abuse *Clin Inf Dis 61:1840–1849, 2015*

Contiguous spread of subcutaneous infections *Semin Cutan Med Surg 26:168–179, 2007*

Corals (true corals)(Anthozoa) – erythema, bullae, ulcers *JAAD 61:733–750, 2009*

Corynebacterium diphtheriae – respiratory diphtheria; pharyngeal erythema with purulent posterior pharyngeal exudate; swollen neck *NEJM 369:1544, 2013*

Cryptococcosis – cellulitis *Cutis 72:320–322;2003; J Dermatol 30:405–410, 2003; Clin Inf Dis 33:700–705, 2001; Australas J Dermatol 38:29–32, 1997; JAAD 32:844–850, 1995; Scand J Infect Dis 26:623–626, 1994; Clin Inf Dis 16:826–827, 1993; Clin Inf Dis 14:666–672, 1992; Int J Dermatol 29:41–44, 1990; JAAD 17:329–332, 1987; Cutis 34:359–361, 1984*

Dematiaceous fungal infections in organ transplant recipients
    Alternaria
    Bipolaris hawaiiensis
    Exophiala jeanselmei, E. spinifera, E. pisciphera, E. castellani
    Exserohilum rostratum
    Fonsacaea pedrosoi
    Phialophora parasitica

Demodicidosis (*Demodex folliculorum*) – red patch of cheeks *JAAD 60:453–462, 2009*

Dental sinus or abscess *Semin Cutan Med Surg 26:168–179, 2007*

Dermatophytosis – cellulitis-like *Semin Cutan Med Surg 26:168–179, 2007*

Dirofilaria repens – red plaques (cellulitis-like) and pulmonary nodules *BJD 173:788–791, 2015*

Dracuncula medinensis (dracunculosis)(Guinea worm) – stagnant water with copepods; painful popular lesions, nausea and vomiting, fever, syncope, urticarial, red papulonodular lesions which become vesiculobullous, cellulitis lesions *JAAD 73:929–944, 2015*

Echovirus 25,32 – cherry spots

Ehrlichia chaffeensis – diffusely erythematous or morbilliform, scattered petechiae or macules *Clin Inf Dis 33:1586–1594, 2001*

Eikenella corrodens – cellulitis *Clin Infect Dis 33:54–61, 2001*

Erysipeloid - *Erysipelothrix insidiosa NEJM 350:904–912, 2004*

Erythrasma - personal observation

Escherichia coli sepsis – rose spots

Fish stings – venomous fish; lesser weever fish, spiny dogfish, stingray, scorpion fish, catfish, rabbit fish, stone fish, stargazers, toadfish – erythema, edema mimicking cellulitis

Fusarium – sepsis; red-gray macules *JAAD 47:659–666, 2002; Fusarium solani* – digital cellulitis

Glanders – *Burkholderia mallei* – cellulitis which ulcerates with purulent foul-smelling discharge, regional lymphatics become abscesses; nasal and palatal necrosis and destruction; metastatic papules, pustules, bullae over joints and face, then ulcerate; deep abscesses with sinus tracts occur; polyarthritis, meningitis, pneumonia

Gnathostomiasis/paragonimus - migratory cellulitis-like plaques *JAAD 33:825–828, 1995; JAAD 13:835–836, 1985; AD 120:508–510, 1984*

Haemophilus influenzae – facial cellulitis in children *Am J Med 63:449, 1977*

Helicobacter cinaedi - cellulitis *Ann Int Med 121:90–93, 1994; J Clin Inf Dis 20:564–570, 1995*

Herpes simplex – red patch with erosions – Kaposi's varicelliform eruption in Darier's disease *JAAD 72:481–484, 2015*

Herpes zoster – pre-vesicular stage with red dermatomal patches *Semin Cutan Med Surg 26:168–179, 2007*

Histoplasmosis - in AIDS *JAAD 23:422–8, 1990;* cellulitis *AD 118:3–4, 1982; S Med J 74:635–637, 1981; AD 95:345–350, 1967*

Hydrozoa (medusa) – red patch *JAAD 61:733–750, 2009*

Insect bites *NEJM 350:904–912, 2004; The Clinical Management of Itching; Parthenon; p. 60, 2000;* mimicking infectious cellulitis *Ann Int Med 142:47–55, 2005*

Janeway lesion – faint red macular lesions of thenar and hypothenar eminences *NEJM 295:1500–1505, 1976*

JC virus annular erythema - personal observation

Klebsiella pneumoniae - cellulitis *JAAD 51:836, 2004*

Legionella micdadei - cellulitis *Am J Med 92:104–106, 1992*

Leishmaniasis - Kala azar – red patches

Leprosy – indeterminate – red macules of face, arms, buttocks, trunk; lepromatous leprosy; reversal reaction in leprosy – periarticular erythema and edema of hand with edema of red plaques of trunk; existing lesions become red and tumid with edema of the hands, neuritis, sensory and motor loss with foot drop, wrist drop, facial palsy, lagophthalmos, keratitis and blindness *JAAD 71:795–803, 2014*

Listeria monocytogenes – red macules progressing to pustules

Lyme disease - acrodermatitis chronica atrophicans – annular erythematous slightly atrophic patches of ankles and feet; violaceous patches *JAAD 74:685–692, 2016; Clin Inf Dis 57:1751,1782–1783, 2013*

Millipede envenomation – erythema, hyperpigmentation, blindness *JAAD 67:347–354, 2012*

Mites and ticks – erythema, edema, papules *JAAD 67:347–354, 2012*

Morganella morganii

Mucormycosis – ptosis with eyelid edema and necrosis *JAMA 309:2382–2383, 2013*

Mycobacterium abscessus – erythematous patch *AD 142:1287–1292, 2006; Am J Respir Crit Care Med 156(pt 2):S1–S25, 1997; Clin Inf Dis 19:263–273, 1994; Rev Infect Dis 5:657–679, 1983;* cellulitis *J Clin Inf Dis 24:1147–1153, 1997;* breast implants adulterated with *Mycobacterium abscessus*

Mycobacterium avium intracellulare JAAD 33:528–531, 1995; JAAD 21:574–576, 1989

Mycobacterium bovis AD 126:123–124, 1990

Mycobacterium chelonae - erythematous patch *AD 142:1287–1292, 2006; Am J Respir Crit Care Med 156(pt 2):S1–S25, 1997; Clin Inf Dis 19:263–273, 1994; Rev Infect Dis 5:657–679, 1983;* cellulitis *J Infect Dis 166:405–412,1992*

Mycobacterium fortuitum - erythematous patch *AD 142:1287–1292, 2006; Am J Respir Crit Care Med 156(pt 2):S1–S25, 1997; Clin Inf Dis 19:263–273, 1994; Rev Infect Dis 5:657–679, 1983;* panniculitis *JAAD 39:650–653, 1998;* cellulitis *Dermatol Surg 26:588–590, 2000*

Mycobacterium hemophilum Am J Transplant 2:476–479, 2002; BJD 149:200–202, 2003; JAAD 40:804–806, 1994

Mycobacterium kansasii Semin Cutan Med Surg 26:168–179, 2007

Mycobacterium szulgai – diffuse cellulitis, nodules, and sinuses *Am Rev Respir Dis 115:695–698, 1977*

Mycobacterium tuberculosis *Clin Exp Dermatol 25:222–223, 2000*

Myiasis - palpebral myiasis presenting as preseptal cellulitis *Arch Ophthalmol 116:684, 1998*

Necrotizing fasciitis *NEJM 350:904–912, 2004; Streptococcus pyogenes Ann DV 128:376–381, 2001; AD 130:1150–1158, 1994; Pseudomonas aeruginosa, Escherichia coli, Klebsiella species, Peptostreptococcus, Bacteroides fragilis Clin Inf Dis 33:6–15, 2001;* Streptococcus pneumoniae – due to intramuscular injection *Clin Inf Dis 33:740–744, 2001; Serratia marcescens Clin Inf Dis 23:648–649, 1996; JAAD 20:774–778, 1989; Bacteroides spp.* in penile necrotizing fasciitis *JAAD 37:1–24, 1997;* neonatal *Pediatrics 103:e53, 1999;* in infancy *Ped Derm 2:55–63, 1984;* Clostridial cellulitis (gangrene); progressive synergistic gangrene; gangrenous cellulitis (Pseudomonas); Fournier's gangrene; necrotizing fasciitis associated with injection drug abuse – gram-positive aerobes - *Staphylococcus aureus, viridans group streptococci, Streptococcus pyogenes, coagulase-negative Staphylococcus species, Enterococcus species;* gram-negatives - *Pseudomonas aeruginosa, Enterococcus species; Clostridium perfringens, Clostridium species Clin Inf Dis 33:6–15, 2001*

Neisseria meningitidis – meningococcal endocarditis presenting as cellulitis *Clin Inf Dis 21:1023–1025, 1995;* periarticular erythema of chronic meningococcemia; red macules around knees *BJD 163:218–219, 2010; Ped Derm 13:483–487, 1996; Calif Med 103:87–90, 1965*

Nocardiosis *JAAD 23:399–400, 1990; JAAD 13: 125–133, 1985; Nocardia asteroides AD 121:898–900, 1985*

Onchocerciasis (erysipelas de la costa) *Semin Cutan Med Surg 26:168–179, 2007*

Osteomyelitis – acute osteomyelitis in children; red patch of upper arm – osteomyelitis of humerus *NEJM 370:352–360, 2014*

Paecilomyces lilacinus (cutaneous hyalohyphomycosis) – red macules with fine scale *JAAD 39:401–409, 1998*

Parvovirus B19 *Semin Cutan Med Surg 26:168–179, 2007*

Periductal mastitis - cellulitis-like *JAAD 43:733–751, 2000*

Phaeohyphomycosis *JAAD 18:1023–1030, 1988*

Phlegmon *Semin Cutan Med Surg 26:168–179, 2007*

Pinta – primary *AD 135:685–688, 1999*

Plague – *Yersinia pestis;* flea bite; cellulitic plaque becomes bullous and crusted like anthrax *West J Med 142:641–646, 1985*

Prevotella species J Clin Inf Dis (Suppl 2):S88–93, 1997

Protothecosis *JAAD 31:920–924, 1994; AD 125:1249–1252, 1989;* cellulitis *Cutis 63:185–188, 1999; JAAD 32:758, 1995; BJD 146:688–693, 2002*

Pseudallescheria boydii JAAD 21:167–179, 1989

Pseudomonas aeruginosa JAMA 248:2156, 1982; ecthyma gangrenosum in Pseudomonas sepsis *Arch Int Med 128:591–595, 1971*

Psittacosis – Horder spots (pink macules resembling rose spots) *JAAD 54:559–578, 2006; AD 120:1227–9, 1984*

Pyomyositis – faint erythema overlying edema of muscle *JAAD 51:308–314, 2004*

Recurrent toxin-mediated perineal erythema – associated with pharyngitis due to *Staphylococcus aureus* or *Streptococcus pyogenes AD 144:2390243, 2008; AD 132:57060, 1996*

Rheumatic fever

Rhizopus Arch Surg 111:532, 1976

Sea anemones – erythema, bullae, ulcers *JAAD 61:733–750, 2009*

Serratia marcescens - cellulitis *JAAD 49:S193–194, 2003; JAMA 250:2348, 1983*

Shewanella putrefaciens - cellulitis *J Clin Inf Dis 25:225–229, 1997*

Snake bites – edema, erythema, pain, and necrosis *NEJM 347:347–356, 2002*

Spider bites – cellulitis-like; black widow spider (*Latrodectus mactans*) – punctum with erythema and edema *AD 123:41–43, 1987;* brown recluse spider (*Loxosceles reclusa*) – erythema, edema, central bulla; targetoid lesion with central blue/purple, ischemic halo, outer rim of erythema; at 3–4 days central necrosis, eschar, ulcer, scar *South Med J 69:887–891, 1976;* wolf spider (*Lycosa*) – erythema and edema *Cutis 39:113–114, 1987*

Sporotrichosis *JAAD 40:272–274, 1999*

Staphylococcus aureus Ped 18:249, 1956; staphylococcal scalded skin syndrome *JAAD 59:342–346, 2008*

Staphylococcus epidermidis *AD 120:1099, 1984*

Streptococcus - Group B streptococcal disease – cellulitis *Clin Inf Dis 33:556–561, 2001;* neonatal group B Streptococcal cellulitis *Ped Derm 10:58–60, 1993;* Group G streptococcus *Arch Derm 118:934, 1982;* Streptococcus zooepidemicus (Lancefield Group C) - cellulitis *Aust NZ Med 20:177–178, 1990*

Streptococcus dysgalactiae – figurate red patches covering entire chest *JAAD 55:S91–92, 2006*

Streptococcus iniae NEJM 337:589–594, 1997

Streptococcus pneumoniae Am J Med 59:293, 1975

Streptococcus pyogenes – intravenous drug abuse *Clin Inf Dis 61:1840–1849, 2015;* perianal cellulitis *JAMA 311:957–958, 2014*

Group G streptococcus *AD 118:934, 1982*

Streptococcus zooepidemicus Aust NZ J Med 20:177–178, 1990

Syphilis – secondary; macular syphilid; red macules of hard palate (secondary syphilis) *JAAD 54:S59–60, 2006;*

Tinea versicolor

Trench fever – red macules, 1 cm or less; fever, malaise, chills, conjunctivitis, myalgias, arthralgias *Clinics in Dermatol 28:483–488, 2010*

Trichophyton rubrum – Majocchi's granuloma; invasive *Trichophyton rubrum Cutis 67:457–462, 2001*

Trichosporon cutaneum AD 129:1020–1023, 1993

Trypanosomiasis brucei rhodesiense (African trypanosomiasis) – annular red patch *NEJM 342:1254, 2000*

Typhoid fever – rose spots *Clin Inf Dis 48:615–616,683–684, 2009; NEJM 346:752–763, 2002*

Vaccinations – postvaccination; vaccinia (preseptal cellulitis); *Haemophilus influenza B* (periorbital and orbital cellulitis)

Vaccinia – vaccination site *NEJM 350:904–912, 2004;* progressive vaccinia - cellulitis with bullae *J Clin Inf Dis 25:911–914, 1997*

Vibrio alginolyticus – cellulitis *Acta DV 63:559–560, 1983*

Vibrio vulnificus sepsis – cellulitis *JAAD 24:397–403, 1991; J Infect Dis 149:558–564, 1984;* edema, erythema, and purpura of ankles *BJD 145:280–284, 2001*

Viral exanthem

Yaws *JAAD 54:559–578, 2006*

Yersinia enterocolitica – cellulitis *J Infect Dis 165:740–743, 1992*

Xanthomonas maltophilia AD 128:702, 1992

Zygomycosis *Ped Inf Dis J 4:672–676, 1985;* red plaque with central eschar *AD 131:833–834, 836–837, 1995*

INFILTRATIVE DISEASES

Crystal storage histiocytossis – intralysosomal crystals of immuno-globulin (primary and secondary intralymphatic histiocytosis) – red and pigmented patches of back and abdomen; livedo reticularis; facial swelling; associated with B-cell lymphomas and plasma cell dyscrasias *JAAD 77:1145–1158, 2017;*

JAAD 70:927–933, 2014

Intravascular or intralymphatic histiocytosis in rheumatoid arthritis *JAAD 50:585–590, 2004;* red patch overlying swollen knee; livedo reticularis *AD 146:1037–1042, 2010*

Mastocytosis, systemic – small pink patches, with flushing and diarrhea *NEJM 363:72–78, 2010; Leuk Res 25:519–528, 2001;* red macules in adults *Eur J Cancer 39:2341–2348, 2003;* telangiectasia macularis eruptive perstans – red macules *JAAD 74:885–891, 2016*

Rosai-Dorfman disease(non-Langerhans cell histiocytosis)(sinus histiocytosis with massive lymphadenopathy) – macular erythema; cervical lymphadenopathy; also axillary, inguinal, and mediastinal adenopathy *Am J Dermatopathol 17:384–388, 1995; Cancer 30:1174–1188, 1972;* red patches and plaques of back and upper extremities *AD 143:736–740, 2007; BJD 154:277–286, 2006*

INFLAMMATORY DISEASES

Arthritis - personal observation

Dissecting cellulitis of the scalp - mimicking infectious cellulitis *Ann Int Med 142:47–55, 2005*

Erythema nodosum – cellulitis-like

Erythema overlying infection or inflammation of underlying structure (erythema of flank overlying area of bowel perforation)

Hidradenitis suppurativa - mimicking infectious cellulitis *Ann Int Med 142:47–55, 2005*

Interstitial granulomatous dermatitis – red plaque with papules *Ped Derm 34:191–192, 2017*

Neutrophilic eccrine hidradenitis - personal observation

Panniculitis – Weber-Christian disease, cytophagic histiocytic panniculitis, post-steroid panniculitis all mimicking cellulitis *Ann Int Med 142:47–55, 2005;* pancreatic panniculitis *Ann Int Med 142:47–55, 2005*

Pyoderma gangrenosum mimicking cellulitis *NEJM 350:904–912, 2004*

Sarcoid – mimicking infectious cellulitis *Ann Int Med 142:47–55, 2005; Am Fam Physician 65:1581–1584, 2002*

Subcutaneous fat necrosis of the newborn – cellulitis-like *AD 117:36–37, 1981; AD 134:425–426, 1998*

Toxic epidermal necrolysis *BJD 68:355–361, 1956*

Whipple's disease – macular and reticulated erythema; Addisonian hyperpigmentation; *Tropheryma whipplei JAAD 60:277–288, 2009*

METABOLIC DISEASES

Alpha-1 antitrypsin deficiency panniculitis – trunk and proximal extremities *JAAD 51:645–655, 2004; JAAD 45:325–361, 2001;* cellulitis-like *JAAD 18:684–692, 1988*

Biotinidase deficiency – facial red patches *AD 141:1457–1462, 2005*

Cystic fibrosis-associated episodic arthritis – pink macules, urticarial papules, arthritis, purpura of legs, erythema nodosum, cutaneous vasculitis *JAMADerm 155:375–376, 2019; Respir Med 88:567–570, 1994; Am J Dis Child 143:1030–1032, 1989; Ann Rheum Dis 47:218–223, 1988; Arch Dis Child 59:377–379, 1984*

Metastatic calcification - personal observation

Calciphylaxis – early erythema mimicking cellulitis *Ann Int Med 142:47–55, 2005; Kidney Int 61:2210–2217, 2002*

Cholinergic erythema *BJD 109:343–348, 1983*

Crohn's disease – perianal erythema, perianal ulcers, fissures, sinus tracts; rectal bleeding, perianal abscess, abdominal pain, perianal pustule, anal skin tags, scrotal swelling and erythema, labial erythema and edema, granulomatous cheilitis *Ped Derm 35:566–574, 2018*

Congenital disorders of glycosylation (CDG-IIa) – N-acetylglucosaminyltransferase II; midfrontal capillary hemangioma, widespaced nipples; facial dysmorphism, neurologic and gastrointestinal abnormalities *Ped Derm 22:457–460, 2005*

Diabetes mellitus – erysipelas-like erythema of legs or feet *Acta Med Scand 196:333–342, 1974;* diabetic rubor of cheeks *Diabetes 14:201–208, 1965;* erythema, edema and atrophy of skin of legs

Gout - mimicking infectious cellulitis *Ann Int Med 142:47–55, 2005; NEJM 350:904–912, 2004*

Kwashiorkor - xerosis; begin as red-purple-brown patches which heal as flaky paint scaling *Cutis 67:321–327, 2001; JAAD 21:1–30, 1989*

Methylmalonic acidemia – erosive erythema; newborn and early infancy

Osteoma cutis – congenital plate-like osteoma cutis; oval red patch *Ped Derm 26:479–481, 2009*

Pellagra – sunburn *BJD 164:1188–1200, 2011*

Porphyria – erythropoietic protoporphyria photo-induced erythema in operating room - personal observation

Persistent cholinergic erythema

NEOPLASTIC DISEASES

Proliferative actinic keratosis – red patch with erosions *Derm Surg 26:65–69, 2000*

Acquired progressive lymphangioma *JAAD 24:813–5, 1991*

Atypical vascular lesions of breast following radiation therapy – red macule *JAAD 63:337–340, 2010*

Burkitt's lymphoma, disseminated – red macules and papules *BJD 174:184–186, 2016*

Carcinoma of the breast (primary)

Carcinoma erysipelatoides - mimicking infectious cellulitis *Ann Int Med 142:47–55, 2005; J R Soc Med 78:Suppl 11:43–45, 1985; AD 113:69–70, 1977*

Congenital smooth muscle hamartoma with livedo appearance – resembles cutis marmorata telangiectatica congenita with fibrotic appearance; serpiginous border *Ped Derm 37:204–206, 2020*

Dermal dendrocyte hamartoma – medallion-like; annular brown or red congenital lesion of central chest with slightly atrophic wrinkled surface *JAAD 51:359–363, 2004*

Dermatofibrosarcoma protuberans, congenital – annular red plaque, pink alopecic plaque, red macule, blue plaque, hypopigmented plaque *AD 143:203–210, 2007*

Eccrine angiomatous hamartoma – vascular nodule; macule, red plaque, acral nodule of infants or neonates; painful, red, purple, blue, yellow, brown, skin colored *JAAD 47:429–435, 2002; Ped Derm 13:139–142, 1996; JAAD 37:523–549, 1997;* hyperpigmented plaque and violaceous patches *Ped Derm 26:662–663, 2009*

Erythroplasia, oral – underside of tongue, floor of mouth, soft palate *J Oral Pathol 12:11–29, 1983*

Kaposi's sarcoma – intraoral red macule *JAAD 41:860–862, 1999; JAAD 38:143–175, 1998; Dermatology 190:324–326, 1995*

Leukemia cutis – monocytic leukemia – red, brown, violaceous patch or nodule *AD 123:225–231, 1971;* T-cell prolymphocytic leukemia – mimicking cellulitis *Ann Int Med 142:47–55, 2005;* B-cell chronic lymphocytic leukemia – violaceous telangiectatic circumferential patches of legs *JAAD 60:772–780, 2009*

Lymphangiosarcoma (Stewart-Treves tumor) – red-brown or ecchymotic patch, nodules, plaques in lymphedematous limb *Cancer 1:64–81, 1948*

Lymphoma – cutaneous T-cell lymphoma *JAAD 70:205–220, 2014;* pilotropic (follicular) CTCL – erythema of forehead *AD 138:191–198, 2002;* nasal NK/T-cell lymphoma *JAAD 46:451–456, 2002;* peripheral T-cell/NK- cell lymphoma - erysipelas-like erythema with violaceous nodule *Cutis 81:33–36, 2008;* angiocentric lymphoma *J Dermatol 24:165–169, 1997; Am J Med Sci 301:178–181, 1991;* intravascular B-cell lymphoma – red patch of thigh *BJD 178:215–221, 2018;* painful gray-brown, red, blue-livid patches, plaques, nodules, with telangiectasia and underlying induration; 40% of patients with intravascular lymphoma present with cutaneous lesions *BJD 157:16–25, 2007;* intravascular cytotoxic T-cell lymphoma *JAAD 58:290–294, 2008;* red patch overlying multiple subcutaneous nodules *JAAD 61:885–888, 2009;* angioimmunoblastic T-cell lymphoma *BJD 173:134–145, 2015;* primary skeletal muscle lymphoma – mimicking cellulitis *Ann Int Med 142:47–55, 2005; Cutis 68:223–226, 2001;* HTLV-1 leukemia/lymphoma (ATLL) – red brown annular patches, red papules and nodules *JAAD 72:293–301, 2015; BJD 152:76–81, 2005;* primary cutaneous diffuse large cell B-cell lymphoma, leg type – large red annular patches or thin plaques *JAAD 72:1016–1020, 2015;* primary cutaneous epidermotropic CD8+ T-cell lymphoma – mixture of patches, plaques, papulonodules with central ulceration, necrosis, and hemorrhage *JAAD 62:300–307, 2010;* HTLV-1 leukemia/lymphoma *Blood 117:3961–3967, 2011;* primary and secondary cutaneous follicle center lymphoma - red macules of face and scalp *JAAD 75:1000–1006, 2016;* CD8+ cutaneous T-cell lymphoma *JAAD 77:489–496, 2017*

Lymphomatoid papulosis in children – red scaly macules *BJD 171:138–146, 2014*

Melanoma – amelanotic melanoma *JAAD 61:230–241, 2009; AD 137:923–929, 2001;* amelanotic lentigo maligna; red patch of cheek *JAAD 50:792–796, 2004*

Metastases *JAAD 29:228–236, 1993;* carcinoma erysipelatoides - includes metastases from breast, lung, melanoma, ovary, stomach, tonsils, pancreas, kidney, rectum, colon, parotid, uterus *NEJM 350:904–912, 2004; JAAD 39:876–878, 1998; JAAD 30:304–307, 1994; JAAD 31:877–880, 1994;* larynx *Eur J Dermatol 11:124–126, 2001*

Mucinous syringometaplasia *JAAD 11:503–8, 1984*

Multinucleate cell angiohistiocytoma – women over 50 years old; thighs, knees, dorsal hands and fingers – violaceous macules or red-purple papules *JAMA Derm 149:357–362, 2013; J Cut Med Surg 14:178–180, 2010; New England Dermatological Society Conference, Sept 15, 2007; JAAD 38:143–175, 1998; AD 132:703–708, 1996; JAAD 30:417–422, 1994; BJD 121:113–121, 1989; BJD 113:15, 1985*

Nevus psiloliparus (mesodermal nevus of lipoma) – alopecia with pink nodule of scalp; when associated with aplasia cutis congenita (aplasticopsillipara), it is associated with encephalocraniocutaneous lipomatosis *Ped Derm 31:746–748, 2014*

Plasmacytomas – primary cutaneous plasmacytosis - brown-red macules; polyclonal hypergammaglobulinemia and lymphadenopathy *JAAD 56:S38–40, 2007; Dermatol 189:251, 1994; JAAD 31:897–900, 1994; AD 122:1314, 1986; Atlantic Derm Meeting, May 1994; Atlantic Derm Meeting, May 2000*

Porokeratotic adnexal ostial nevus(conifying porokeratotic eccrine ostial and dermal duct nevus) with porokeratotic eccrine and hair follicle nevus – linear, hyperkeratotic lesions with comedones; presents as red patch with red and atrophic linear and curvilinear erosions; unilateral breast hypoplasia and multifocal squamous cell carcinomas *JAAD 61:1060–1069, 2009; BJD 103:435–441, 1980; BJD 101:717–722, 1979*

Posttransplant lymphoproliferative disorder – violaceous macules and facial nodules *Ped Derm 36:681–685, 2019*

Squamous cell carcinoma – red patch of finger *JAAD 55:1092–1094, 2006;* intraoral red patch *Oral Oncol 31B:16–26, 1995;* diffuse epidermal and periadnexal squamous cell carcinoma in situ – diffuse erythema and hyperkeratosis of face, neck, and scalp *JAAD 53:623–627, 2005*

PARANEOPLASTIC DISORDERS

Brenner's sign – erythema of face or surrounding the tumor in patients with malignant melanoma *AD 143:1001–1004, 2007; J Eur Acad DV 19:514–515, 2005;* red patch of upper central chest – signet ring melanoma metastases of cervical lymph nodes *JAAD 65:444–446, 2011*

Crystal-storing histiocytosis (composed of monoclonal immunoglobulins) – fixed erythema of abdomen; paraneoplastic phenomenon in myeloma, lymphoplasmacytic lymphoma, B-cell lymphoma, or monoclonal gammopathy of uncertain significance (MGUS) *JAMADerm 152:1159–1160, 2016*

Generalized eruptive histiocytosis associated with acute myelogenous leukemia *JAAD 49:S233–236, 2003*

Glucagonoma syndrome – erythema mimicking cellulitis *JAAD 49:325–328, 2003*

PHOTODERMATOSES

Ultraviolet recall manifested as edema, erythema, bullae, hemorrhagic crusting, macules, papules, ulceration, necrosis *JAAD 56:494–499, 2007*

PRIMARY CUTANEOUS DISEASES

Circumscribed palmar or plantar acral hypokeratosis – pink macule or red atrophic patch of medial or lateral hand *JAMADerm 153:609–611, 2017; JAAD 76:S43–45, 2017; Cutis 93:97–101, 2014; BJD 166:221–222, 2012; AD 148:1427–1428, 2012; BJD 164:211–213,* 2011*; JAAD 61:1090–1091, 2009; AD 145:195–200, 2009; BJD 157:804–806, 2007; JAAD 51:319–321, 2004; JAAD 49:1197–1198, 2003; JAAD 47:21–27, 2002*

Erythromelanosis faciei - personal observation

Granuloma annulare – patch-type granuloma annulare *JAAD 51:39–44, 2004; JAAD 46:426–429, 2002*

Intertrigo

Necrolytic migratory erythema without glucagonoma - personal observation

Non-episodic angioedema with eosinophilia – erythema, livedo reticularis, edema of legs, urticaria *Cutis 93:33–37, 2014*

Pityriasis rubra pilaris – PRP type V – hyperkeratotic scaly patches of dorsal hands, annular brown macules, red patches; *CARD14* mutation (caspase recruitment domain family 14) *JAMADerm 153:66–70, 2017*

Progressive symmetric erythrokeratoderma (Gottron syndrome) *Ped Derm 19:285–292, 2002; AD 136:665, 668, 2000; AD 122:434–440, 1986*

Red scrotum syndrome *J Drugs Dermatol 6:935–936, 2007; Genital Skin Disorders, Fischer and Margesson, Mosby, 1998, p. 53*

Scleredema of Buschke (pseudoscleroderma) – in diabetics, preceded by erythema *Clin Exp Dermatol 14:385–386, 1989*

PSYCHOCUTANEOUS DISORDERS

Factitial dermatitis - personal observation

SYNDROMES

Acute anterior tibial compartment syndrome – cellulitis-like *Ann Int Med 142:47–55, 2005; JAAD 34:521–522, 1996*

Aesop syndrome (adenopathy and extensive skin patch overlying plasmacytoma) – extensive asymptomatic red-violaceous skin patch or plaque of chest overlying a solitary bone plasmacytoma with regional adenopathy; dermal mucin and vascular hyperplasia (mucinous angiomatosis) *JAAD 55:909–910, 2006*

AKT serine/threonine kinase – megalencephaly-capillary malformation syndrome/megalencephaly-polymicrogyria-polydactyly-hydrocephalus syndrome – *AKT3, PIK3R2, PIK3CA JAAD 68:885–896, 2013*

Amyoplasia congenita disruptive sequence – midfacial macular telangiectatic nevi *Am J Med Genet 15:571–590, 1983*

Angiokeratoma corporis diffusum

Bannayan-Riley-Ruvalcaba-Zonana syndrome (PTEN phosphatase and tensin homolog hamartoma) – dolicocephaly, frontal bossing, macrocephaly, ocular hypertelorism, long philtrum, thin upper lip, broad mouth, relative micrognathia, lipomas, penile or vulvar lentigines, café au lait macules, facial verruca-like or acanthosis nigricans-like papules, multiple acrochordons, angiokeratomas, transverse palmar crease, accessory nipple, syndactyly, brachydactyly, port wine stain (capillary (vascular) malformations), arteriovenous malformations, lymphangiokeratoma, subcutaneous and visceral lipomas, goiter, hamartomatous intestinal polyposis *JAAD 56:541–564, 2007; JAAD 53:639–643, 2005*

Beckwith-Wiedemann syndrome (Exomphalos-Macroglossia-Gigantism)(EMG) syndrome – autosomal dominant; zosteriform rash at birth, exomphalos, macrosomia, macroglossia, visceromegaly, facial salmon patch of forehead, upper eyelids, nose, and upper lip and gigantism; linear earlobe grooves, circular depressions of helices; increased risk of Wilms' tumor, adrenal carcinoma, hepatoblastoma, and rhabdomyosarcoma; neonatal hypoglycemia; uniparental disomy *JAAD 74:231–244, 2016; JAAD 65:893–906, 2011; JAAD 56:541–564, 2007; Ped Derm 22:482–487, 2005; Curr Prob in Dermatol 13:249–300, 2002; Am J Med Genet 79:268–273, 1998; JAAD 37:523–549, 1997; Am J Dis Child 122:515–519, 1971; Clin Genet 46:168–174, 1994*

Bloom's syndrome – telangiectatic erythema *JAAD 75:855–870, 2016*

Bowel-associated dermatitis-arthritis syndrome – red annular or oval macules, red papules, vesicles evolving into pustules *AD 138:973–978, 2002*

Cardiofaciocutaneous syndrome – port wine stain, hypotonia, mental retardation, atrial septal defect, pulmonary stenosis, dermatitis, hypotrichosis, characteristic facies *Clin Genet 42:206–209, 1992*

Carcinoid syndrome – persistent erythema with or without telangiectasia

C syndrome (Opitz trigonocephaly syndrome) – nevus flammeus; trigonocephaly, unusual facies with wide alveolar ridges, multiple frenula, limb defects, visceral anomalies, redundant skin, mental retardation, hypotonia *Am J Med Genet 9:147–163, 1981*

CLOVES syndrome – capillary, venous, and mixed vascular malformations, epidermal nevi, congenital lipomatous overgrowth; hemihypertrophy (milder than that of Proteus syndrome); epidermal nevi, spinal and skeletal abnormalities; ballooning of big toes, symmetrically overgrown feet; wrinkling of palms and soles; severe central nervous system involvement *JAAD 65:893–906, 2011; Ped Derm 27:311–312, 2010; Am J Med Genet 143A:2944–2958, 2007*

Coats' disease – cutaneous telangiectasia or unilateral macular telangiectatic nevus with retinal telangiectasia *AD 108:413–415, 1973*

Cobb's syndrome (cutaneomeningospinal angiomatosis) – segmental port wine stain and vascular malformation of the spinal cord *JAAD 56:541–564, 2007; AD 113:1587–1590, 1977; NEJM 281:1440–1444, 1969; Ann Surg 62:641–649, 1915*; PWS may be keratotic *Dermatologica 163:417–425, 1981*

Compartment syndrome – often of anterior tibial compartment; erythema mimicking cellulitis *Ann Int Med 142:47–55, 2005*

Cutis marmorata telangiectatica congenita syndrome – body asymmetry, 2–3 toe syndactyly, hypotonia, developmental delay, midfacial vascular stains, joint laxity, loose skin *Ped Derm 24:555–556, 2007*

Didymosis aplasticosebacea – aplasia cutis congenita in a nevus sebaceous (Schimmelpenning syndrome); coloboma of eyelid *Ped 24:514–516, 2007*

Familial dysautonomia (Riley-Day syndrome)(hereditary sensory and autonomic neuropathy type III) – blotchy erythema in infancy with 2–5 cm red macules on trunk and extremities *AD 89:190–195, 1964*

Familial Hibernian fever – mimicking infectious cellulitis *Ann Int Med 142:47–55, 2005; QJMed 51:469–480, 1982*

Familial Mediterranean fever - mimicking infectious cellulitis *Ann Int Med 142:47–55, 2005; NEJM 350:904–912, 2004; Isr Med Assoc J 1:31–36, 1999; Q J Med 75:607–616, 1990;* red patch with pale areas *AD 143:1080–1081, 2007*

Fegeler syndrome – acquired port wine stain following trauma *Ped Derm 21:131–133, 2004*

Goodpasture's syndrome - annular erythematous macules on instep - *AD 121:1442–4, 1985*

Gorham-Stout disease (disappearing bone disease) – vascular malformations, intraosseous vascular malformations, osteolysis (venous malformations) *JAAD 56:541–564, 2007*

Hemihyperplasia-Multiple Lipomatosis syndrome – hemihyperplasia at birth, moderate overgrowth, extensive congenital vascular stain (superficial capillary malformation), compressible blue nodule, multiple subcutaneous nodules, hemihypertrophy, hemifacial atrophy, café au lait macules; syndactyly, thickened but not cerebriform soles, dermatomyofibroma *Ped Derm 31:507–510, 2014; JAAD 56:541–564, 2007; Soc Ped Derm Annual Meeting, July 2005; Am J Med Genet 130A-111-122, 2004; Am J Med Genet 79:311–318, 1998*

Hemophagocytic syndrome (hemophagocytic lymphohistiocytosis) (familial hemophagocytic syndrome) – morbilliform eruptions, purpuric macules, acral blanching red macules, erythroderma and edema *JAAD 56:302–316, 2007; AD 138:1208–1212, 2002; AD 128:193–200, 1992*

Hereditary hemorrhagic telangiectasia – arteriovenous malformation; pulmonary arteriovenous malformations; mutation in ENG (endoglin)(a transforming growth factor beta protein) or ALK1 gene (product is activin-like tyrosine kinase1); both encode membrane glycoprotein on vascular endothelial cells as surface receptor for TGFR beta superfamily which mediates vascular remodeling effects on extracellular matrix production *JAAD 56:541–564, 2007; BJD 145:641–645, 2001*

Hereditary mucoepithelial dysplasia (dyskeratosis) – autosomal dominant; red eyes, non-scarring alopecia, keratosis pilaris, erythema of oral (palate, gingiva) and nasal mucous membranes, cervix, vagina, and urethra; photophobia, keratosis pilaris, non-scarring alopecia, psoriasiform perineal plaques, angular cheilitis, nail deformity, increased risk of infections, fibrocystic lung disease *BJD 153:310–318, 2005; JAAD 21:351–357, 1989; Am J Hum Genet 31:414–427, 1979; Oral Surg Oral Med Oral Pathol 46:645–657, 1978*

Hereditary neurocutaneous angioma – autosomal dominant; port wine stains with localized CNS vascular malformations *J Med Genet 16:443–447, 1979*

Hypereosinophilic syndrome – necrotizing eosinophilic vasculitis *BJD 143:641–644, 2000;* red macules, red papules, plaques, and nodules, urticaria, angioedema *AD 142:1215–1218, 2006; Am J Hematol 80:148–157, 2005; Allergy 59:673–689, 2004; AD 132:535–541, 1996; AD 114:531–535, 1978; Medicine 54:1–27, 1975; BJD 143:641–644, 2000; BJD 144:639, 2001; AD 132:583–585, 1996; Blood 83:2759–2779, 1994; AD 114:531–535, 1978;* urticaria and/or angioedema *Med Clin (Barc)106:304–306, 1996; AD 132:535–541, 1996; Sem Derm 14:122–128, 1995; Blood 83:2759–2779, 1994;* multiple large round and oval red patches of trunk; *FIP1L1-PDGFRA* fusion gene *BJD 157:1284–1287, 2007*

Hyper IgD syndrome - autosomal recessive; red macules or papules, urticaria, red nodules, urticaria, combinations of periodic fever, arthritis, arthralgias, and rash, annular erythema, and pustules, abdominal pain with vomiting and diarrhea, lymphadenopathy; elevated IgD and IgA - mevalonate kinase deficiency *JAAD 68:834–853, 2013; Ped Derm 22:138–141, 2005; AD 136:1487–1494, 2000; AD 130:59–65, 1994; Medicine 73:133–144, 1994; Lancet 1:1084–1090, 1984*

IRAK-4 deficiency (homozygous mutations of IL-receptor-associated kinase 4 gene) – cutaneous infections with *Staphylococcus aureus;* abscesses, cellulitis, impetigo *JAAD 54:951–983, 2006*

Kawasaki's disease – mimicking periorbital cellulitis *NEJM 350:904–912, 2004;* oral erythema *Oral Surg 67:569–572, 1989;* perianal erythema and desquamation *AD 124:1805–1810, 1988*

Klinefelter variants - macular telangiectatic vascular nevi *J Urol 119:103–106, 1978;* erythema, crusting, or necrosis of BCG inoculation sites *JAAD 69:501–510, 2013*

Kikuchi-Fujimoto disease – young Asians; fever, often painful lymphadenopathy, respiratory symptoms, arthralgias and myalgias; macules, patches, ulcers, red plaques, and papules, facial erythema, red macules and patches; scattered indurated nodules, photoeruptions; leukocytoclastic vasculitis; pruritus, conjunctival injection, pharyngitis with oral ulcers *JAAD 72:1–19, 2015; NEJM 369:2333–2343, 2013; Int J Dermatol 51:564–567, 2012; Indian J Otolaryngol Head Neck Surg 63:Suppl 1:110–112, 2011; Arch Pathol Lab Med 134:289–293, 2010; JAAD 59:130–136, 2008; Clin Rheumatol 26:50–54, 2007; BJD 144:885–889, 2001; JAAD 36:342–346, 1997*

Lethal multiple pterygium syndrome - midfacial macular telangiectatic nevi *Am J Med Genet 12:377–409, 1982*

Macrocephaly-CMTC (cutis marmorata telangiectatica congenita syndrome) – renamed "macrocephaly-capillary malformation syndrome" now renamed "megalencephaly capillary malformation syndrome - macrocephalic neonatal hypotonia and developmental delay; frontal bossing, segmental overgrowth, syndactyly, asymmetry, distended linear and serpiginous abdominal wall veins, patchy reticulated or telangiectatic port wine stain (vascular stain) without atrophy; fading of port wine stain in first year; telangiectasias of face and ears; midline reticulated facial nevus flammeus (capillary malformation)(vascular stains), central facial salmon patches; hydrocephalus, skin and joint hypermobility, hyperelastic skin, thickened subcutaneous tissue, polydactyly, 2–3 toe syndactyly, postaxial polydactyly, hydrocephalus, frontal bossing, hemihypertrophy with segmental overgrowth; enlarged hand (macrmano); connective tissue defects; *PIK3CA* mutations *BJD 175:810–814, 2016; JAAD 65:893–906, 2011; Ped Derm 26:342–346, 2009; AD 145:287–293, 2009; JAAD 58:697–702, 2008; Ped Derm 24:555–556, 2007; JAAD 56:541–564, 2007; Ped Derm 16:235–237, 1999; Genet Couns 9:245–253, 1998; Am J Med Genet 70:67–73, 1997; Clin Dysmorphol 6:291–302, 1997;*

(Note: Beckwith-Wiedemann syndrome demonstrates dysmorphic ears, macroglossia, body asymmetry, midfacial vascular stains, visceromegaly with omphalocele, neonatal hypoglycemia, BUT NO MACROCEPHALY)

Maffucci's syndrome – vascular malformation, enchondromas *Ped Derm 25:205–209, 2008; J Larygol Otol 115:845–847, 2001*

Muckle-Wells syndrome – autosomal dominant; macular erythema, urticaria, deafness, amyloidosis *JAAD 39:290–291, 1998*

Mulibrey nanism – nevus flammeus, muscle hypotonia, triangular face, thinness *JAAD 46:161–183, 2002; Birth Defects 11:3–17, 1975*

NOD 2 mutations (nucleotide-binding oligomerization domain 2) – dermatitis, weight loss with gastrointestinal symptoms, episodic self-limiting fever, polyarthritis, polyarthralgia, red plaques of face and forehead, urticarial plaques of legs, patchy erythema of chest, pink macules of arms and back *JAAD 68:624–631, 2013*

NOMID – neonatal onset multisystem inflammatory disease – generalized evanescent urticarial macules and papules

NOVA syndrome – autosomal dominant: glabellar capillary malformation, communicating hydrocephalus, posterior fossa abnormalities, agenesis of the cerebellar vermis, Dandy-Walker malformation, mega cisterna magna, seizures *JAAD 56:541–564, 2007; JAAD 63:805–814, 2010*

Peeling skin syndrome – red macules, erosions, desquamation, xerosis; mutation in corneodesmosin *JAMADerm 151:225–226, 2015*

Phakomatosis pigmentovascularis – cutis marmorata telangiectatica congenital and Mongolian spots *JAAD 66:341–342, 2012;* port wine stain (capillary malformation)(may be widespread), oculocutaneous (dermal and scleral) melanosis, CNS manifestations; type I – PWS and linear epidermal nevus; type II – PWS and dermal melanocytosis *Ped Derm 27:303–304, 2010;* type III – PWS and nevus spilus; type IV – PWS, dermal melanocytosis, and nevus spilus; types II,III, and IV may also have nevus anemicus *JAAD 58:88–93, 2008; JAAD 56:541–564, 2007; Ped Derm 21:642–645, 2004; Curr Prob in Dermatol 13:249–300, 2002; J Dermatol 26:834–836, 1999; AD 121:651–653, 1985; Jpn J Dermatol 52:1–3, 1947;* extensive Mongolian spot, nevus flammeus, cutis marmorata telangiectatica *BJD 156:1068–1071, 2007;* phakomatosis cesioflammea – Mongolian spots or dermal melanocytosis with one or more port wine stains *AD 141:385–388, 2005*

PIK3CA/AKT/mTOR-related overgrowth syndromes – reticulated port wine stain; hemihypertrophy *GeneReviews.http://ncbi.nlm.nih.gov/pubmed/23946963; Am J Med Genet 167:287–295, 2015; JAAD 69:589–594, 2013; Nature Genetics 44:934–940, 2012*

> CLOVES syndrome
> Macrocephaly capillary malformation syndrome (macrocephaly cutis marmorata telangiectatica congenita)(megalencephaly capillary malformation syndrome)
> Proteus syndrome

Proteus syndrome – extensive truncal and extremity port wine stains, subcutaneous hemangiomas and lymphangiomas, lymphangioma circumscriptum, hemihypertrophy of the face, limbs, trunk; macrodactyly, cerebriform hypertrophy of palmar and/or plantar surfaces, macrocephaly; verrucous epidermal nevi, sebaceous nevi with hyper- or hypopigmentation *JAAD 52:834–838, 2005 Clin Exp Dermatol 29:222–230, 2004;Curr Prob in Dermatol 13:249–300, 2002; Am J Med Genet 27:99–117, 1987; Eur J Pediatr 140:5–12, 1983; Birth Defects 15:291–296, 1979;* vascular nevi, soft subcutaneous masses; lipodystrophy, café au lait macules, linear and whorled macular pigmentation *Pediatrics 76:984–989, 1985; Am J Med Genet 27:87–97, 1987; Eur J Pediatr 140:5–12, 1983*

Relapsing eosinophilic perimyositis – fever, fatigue, and episodic muscle swelling; erythema over swollen muscles *BJD 133:109–114, 1995*

Relapsing polychondritis - mimicking infectious cellulitis *Ann Int Med 142:47–55, 2005; Semin Arthr Rheum 31:384–395, 2002*

REM (reticular erythematous mucinosis) syndrome *JAAD 27:825–828, 1992; Ped Derm 7:1–10, 1990; Z Hautkr 63:986–998, 1988(German); JAAD 19:859–868, 1988; AD 115:1340–1342, 1979; BJD 91:191–199, 1974; Z Hautkr 49:235–238, 1974*

Robert's pseudothalidomide syndrome (hypomelia-hypotrichosis-facial hemangioma syndrome)(Roberts/SC phocomelia syndrome) – autosomal recessive; midfacial port wine stain extending from forehead to nose and philtrum, cleft lip +/– cleft palate, sparse silver-blond hair, limb reduction malformation, characteristic facies, malformed ears with hypoplastic lobules, marked growth retardation *JAAD 56:541–564, 2007; Clin Genet 31:170–177, 1987; Clin Genet 5:1–16, 1974*

Rubenstein-Taybi syndrome – arciform keloids, hypertrichosis, long eyelashes, thick eyebrows, keratosis pilaris or ulerythema ophryogenes, low set ears, very short stature, broad terminal phalanges of thumbs and great toes, hemangiomas, nevus flammeus, café au lait macules, pilomatrixomas, cardiac anomalies, mental retardation *Ped Derm 19:177–179, 2002; Am J Dis Child 105:588–608, 1963;* port wine stain of forehead

Short arm 4 deletion syndrome – macular telangiectatic vascular nevi *Am J Dis Child 122:421–425, 1971*

TAR syndrome (thrombocytopenia-absent radii syndrome) – congenital thrombocytopenia, anemia, eosinophilia, leukemoid reactions, leg abnormalities, bilateral absent or hypoplastic radii; foreshortened forearms, port wine stain of forehead and neck *JAAD 56:541–564, 2007; AD 126:1520–1521, 1990; Am J Pediatr Hematol Oncol 10:51–64, 1988*

Trisomy 13 – port wine stain of forehead *J Med Genet 5:227–252, 1968*

Trisomy 18 – reticulate vascular nevus or port wine stain *J Pediatr 72:862–863, 1968*

Tumor necrosis factor (TNF) receptor 1-associated periodic fever syndromes (TRAPS)(same as familial hibernian fever and familial periodic fever) – autosomal dominant; prolonged periodic fevers (7–21 days); red patches evolve into serpiginous tender red plaques, fever, polycyclic, reticulated, and migratory patches and plaques, conjunctivitis, periorbital edema, myalgia, abdominal pain, headache; Irish and Scottish predominance; mutations in *TNFRSF1A JAAD 68:834–853, 2013; AD 136:1487–1494, 2000; Pre–AAD Pediatric Dermatology Meeting, March 2000; Mayo Clin Proc 72:806–817, 1997*

Von Hippel-Lindau disease – macular telangiectatic nevi, facial or occipitocervical; retinal angiomatosis, cerebellar or medullary or spinal hemangioblastoma, renal cell carcinoma, pheochromocytoma, café au lait macules *Arch Intern Med 136:769–777, 1976*

Wells' syndrome *JAAD 52:187–189, 2005; NEJM 350:904–912, 2004; Trans St. Johns Hosp Dermatol Soc 57:46–56, 1971*

Wyburn-Mason (Bonnet-Duchaume-Blanc) syndrome – unilateral (trigeminal distribution, or midforehead, glabella, nose, upper lip) salmon patch with punctate telangiectasias or port wine stain; facial lesion may be arteriovenous malformation; unilateral retinal arteriovenous or vascular malformation, ipsilateral aneurysmal arteriovenous malformation of the midbrain *Am J Ophthalmol 75:224–291, 1973; Brain 66:163–203, 1943; J Med Lyon 18:165–178, 1937*

XXYY syndrome - macular telangiectatic vascular nevi *AD 94:695–698, 1966*

TOXINS

L-tryptophan-induced eosinophilic myalgia syndrome – cellulitis-like

TRAUMA

Acquired cold-contact urticaria – painful erythema *JAMA 180:639-642, 1962*

Airbag dermatitis – bizarre shapes of erythema, resembling factitial dermatitis *JAAD 33:824–825, 1995*

Burns, first degree – erythema *Cutis 86:249–257, 2010*

Cold panniculitis – red patch of abdomen in febrile infant *Ped Derm 29:658–659, 2012; JAAD 45:325–361, 2001;* of neonate and children (Haxthausen's disease) *JAAD 33:383–385, 1995; Burns Incl Therm Inj 14:51–52, 1988; AD 94:720–721, 1966; BJD 53:83–89, 1941;* popsicle panniculitis – cellulitis-like *Pediatr Emerg Care 8:91–93, 1992*

Coma-induced sweat gland necrosis – pressure bulla; cellulitis-like *Ann Dermato Syphiligr 98:421–428, 1971*

Denture-induced stomatitis *J Oral Pathol 10:65–80, 1981*

Fegeler syndrome – acquired port wine stain following trauma *Arch Dermatol Syphilol 188:421–422, 1949*

Lightning strike – Lichtenberg figures; frond-like (ferning pattern) transient non-blanching pink-red erythema beginning 20 minutes to 3 ½ hours after the strike and lasting up to 48 hours *Cutis 80:141–143, 2007; Arch Neurol 61:977, 2005; Injury 34:367–371, 2003; Burns Incl Thermal Inj 13:141–146, 1987; Proc IEE 123:1163–1180, 1976; Memoirs Med Soc London 2:493–507, 1794*

Perniosis *AD 117:26–28, 1981*

Postirradiation pseudosclerodermatous panniculitis *Ann Int Med 142:47–55, 2005; Am J Dermatopathol 23:283–287, 2001; Mayo Clin Proc 68:122–127, 1993*

Postsurgical sternal erythema (post-traumatic reflex dystrophy following coronary artery bypass grafting) – red patch around sternotomy wound; with telangiectasia; poikiloderma *JAAD 53:893–896, 2005*

Radiation dermatitis, acute – erythema *JAAD 54:28–46, 2006; Acta DV 49:64–71, 1969;* fluoroscopy-induced radiation injury – red telangiectatic patch with ulceration of upper back or axilla *AD 143:637–640, 2007;* postradiation vascular proliferations of breast (atypical vascular lesions of the breast) – erythema; erythema with underlying induration or ulceration, telangiectasias, papules, plaques, nodules, *JAAD 57:126–133, 2007;* chlorambucil-induced radiation recall *SKINmed 13:317–319, 2015*

Radiation recall – erythema, vesiculation, erosions, hyperpigmentation; red hyperpigmented patch *Cutis 91:17–18, 2013;* dactinomycin and doxorubicin *Radiother Oncol 59:237–245, 2001; Mayo Clin Proc 55:711–715, 1980;* edatrexate, melphalan, etoposide, vinblastine, bleomycin, fluorouracil, hydroxyurea, methotrexate; rapamycin inhibitors, epidermal growth factor inhibitors, histone deacetylase inhibitors, BRAF inhibitor (vemurafenib) *Eur J Cancer 49:1662–1668, 2013*

Reflex sympathetic dystrophy (complex regional pain syndrome) – erythema and edema; muscle wasting *JAMADerm 150:640–642, 2014;* geometric marginated erythema *Cutis 68:179–182, 2001*

Reticular telangiectatic erythema – after placement of cardiac pacemakers, carioverter defibrillators, and morphine pumps *Contact Dermatitis 64:280–288, 2011*

Subcutaneous emphysema – extensive erythema of upper chest *AD 147:254–255, 2011*

VASCULAR DISEASES

Acquired digital arteriovenous malformation – red macule, purple macule *BJD 142:362–365, 2000*

Acquired port wine stain - personal observation

Acquired progressive lymphangioma – red plaque or patch *Clin Exp Dermatol 21:159–162, 1996;*

Acute venous congestion - personal observation

Angioma serpiginosum *JAAD 65:462–463, 2011*

Angiosarcoma *JAAD 50:867–874, 2004*

Arteriovenous malformations (fistulae) – congenital or acquired; may have appearance of port wine stain or involuting hemangioma; overlying port wine stain; extremities, head, neck, trunk including Wyburn-Mason, Bennet Dechaume-Blanc and Bregeat syndromes *JAAD 56:353–370, 2007;* of scalp – faint pink or blue macule *JAAD 46:934–941, 2002;* pink patch *Ped Derm 31:103–104, 2014*

Bier's spots – red or white spots in midst of cyanotic congestion after application of a tourniquet *JAAD 14:411–419, 1986*

Capillary malformation (port wine stain, salmon patch, angel's kiss, stork bite, nevus simplex, vascular stain) – glabella , forehead, nape of neck, upper eyelids, eyelids, scalp, upper and lower lip, upper back, lumbosacral region; GNAQ mutations *Ped Derm 33:570–584, 2016; JAAD 63:805–814, 2010; JAAD 56:353–370, 2007; Ped Derm 6:185–187, 1989; Ped Derm 1:58–68, 1983; Pediatrics 58:218–222, 1976; Arch Dermatol Syphilol 67:302–305, 1953*

Differential diagnosis of capillary malformations: *Ped Derm 33:570–584, 2016*

Angiokeratoma circumscriptum

Arteriovenous malformations
Congenital plaque-type glomuvenous malformation
Infantile hemangiomas
Linear morphea
Multifocal lymphangioendotheliomatosis with thrombocytopenia

Capillary malformations, hereditary, without arteriovenous malformation; autosomal dominant; port wine stain with multifocal <1–3 cm round or oval pink macules of face, trunk, or extremities; 50% with blanched halo; arteriovenous malformations of brain, spine, skin, bone, muscle; inactivating mutations of *RASA1 Ped Derm 33:570–584, 2016; Ped Derm 30:409–415, 2013; BJD 158:1035–1040, 2008; JAAD 56:541–564, 2007; Am J Hum Genet 73:1240–1249, 2003*

Capillary malformation-arteriovenous malformation syndrome (CM-AVM syndrome) – white halo surrounding red patch; *RASA1* mutation; vascular stains and cardiac failure; multiple capillary malformations, Parkes-Weber syndrome, pink stain overlying arteriovenous malformation; multiple infantile hemangiomas, pink patches; red patch of eyelid with white halo; mutation in *RASA1* or *EPHB4 Ped Derm 37:342–344, 2020; Ped Derm 37:64–68, 2020; JAMADerm 155:733, 2019; Ped Derm 32:128–131, 2015; Ped Derm 32:76–84, 2015; Am J Hum Genet 6:1240–1249, 2003; Acta DV 3:202–211, 1922*

Capillary malformations with bone and soft tissue overgrowth – reticulated capillary malformations *Ped Derm 33:570–584, 2016*

Capillary malformations, branchial clefts, lip pseudoclefts, and unusual facies *JAAD 56:541–564, 2007; J Laryngol Otol 71:597–603, 1957*

Cerebral cavernous malformations (cutaneous hyperkeratotic capillary-venous malformation associated with familial cerebral cavernous malformations)(familial cerebral cavernomas) type 1 – autosomal dominant; localized dark red hyperkeratotic plaques; violaceous to blue-black plaques (malformations); red blanchable patches; red hyperkeratotic plaques; deep blue nodules; cutaneous venous malformations; mutations in CCM-1 gene which encodes for Krev-1 interaction TRAP 1 protein (KRIT1) *Ped Derm 26:666–667, 2009; JAAD 56:541–564, 2007; BJD 157:210–212, 2007; Hum Molec Genet 9:1351–1355, 2000; Ann Neurol 45:250–254, 1999; Lancet 352:1892–1897, 1998;* CCM2- malcaverin protein; CCM3 – PDCD10 protein

Eosinophilic granulomatosis with polyangiitis *JAAD 47:209–216, 2002*

Congenital plaque-type glomuvenous malformations – glomulin gene on 1p21; loss of function mutation; atrophic at birth; livedoid plaques, blue plaques, vascular nodules, red patches, cerebriform, targetoid *AD 142:892–896, 2006*

Cutaneous angiomatosis following implanted osteosynthesis nail *BJD 142:1056–1057, 2000*

Cutis marmorata-arteriovenous malformation syndrome – *RASA1* mutation *JAAD 65:893–906, 2011*

Cutis marmorata telangiectatica congenita – reticulated capillary malformation with telangiectasias; ulcerated over elbows and knees; atrophy; limb hypoplasia or hypertrophy; associated with port wine stain or distant to it *JAAD 65:893–906, 2011; JAAD 56:541–564, 2007*

Deep venous thrombosis - mimicking infectious cellulitis *Ann Int Med 142:47–55, 2005; NEJM 350:904–912, 2004*

Dependent rubor – as sign of peripheral vascular disease *JAAD 67:177–185, 2012*

Diffuse capillary malformation with overgrowth – reticulated red patch with hypertrophy *Ped Derm 33:570–584, 2016; JAAD 69:589–594, 2013*

Erythromelalgia - mimicking infectious cellulitis *Ann Int Med 142:47–55, 2005; Am J Med 91:416–422, 1991*

Generalized acquired telangiectasia – cellulitis-like

Geographic capillary malformations *Ped Derm 33:570–584, 2016*
    Klippel-Trenaunay (capillary-lymphatic-venous malformations)
    Proteus syndrome
    CLOVES syndrome
    CLAPO syndrome – capillary malformation of lower lip, lymphatic malformation of face and neck, partial or generalized overgrowth *Am J Med Genet A 146:2583–2588, 2008*

Glomeruloid angioendotheliomatosis – red purpuric patches and acral necrosis – associated with cold agglutinins *JAAD 49:887–896, 2003*

Glabellar port wine stain, mega cisterna magna, communicating hydrocephalus, posterior cerebellar vermis agenesis; autosomal dominant *J Neurosurg 51:862–865, 1979*

Glomuvenous malformation - congenital plaque-type glomuvenous malformation – may resemble capillary malformation (red patch), venous malformation, or blue nevus *JAAD 56:353–370, 2007*

Granulomatosis with polyangiitis – presenting as reactive arthritis - personal observation

Hemangioma of infancy
    Differential diagnosis of hemangioma of infancy *JAAD 48:477–493, 2003*

        Capillary malformation
        Venous malformation
        Lymphatic malformation

        Arteriovenous malformation
        Non-involuting congenital hemangioma
        Rapidly involuting congenital hemangioma
        Pyogenic granuloma
        Tufted angioma
        Spindle cell hemangioendothelioma
        Kaposiform hemangioendothelioma
        Fibrosarcoma
        Rhabdomyosarcoma
        Myofibromatosis
        Nasal glioma
        Encephalocele
        Lipoblastoma
        Dermatofibrosarcoma protuberans
        Giant cell fibroblastoma
        Neurofibroma

Hemangioma - abortive or minimal growth infantile hemangiomas – reticulated red patch with telangiectasias *JAAD 58:685–690, 2008*

Henoch-Schonlein purpura – starts as red macules *Ped Derm 15:357–359, 1998; Ped Derm 12:314–317, 1995; Am J Dis Child 99:833–854, 1960;* in the adult *AD 125:53–56, 1989*

Klippel-Trenaunay syndrome(capillary-lymphatic-venous malformation) – geographic capillary malformation stains; slow flow with capillary, lymphatic, and venous elements *Ped Derm 30:541–548, 2013*; venous malformation, arteriovenous fistula, or mixed venous lymphatic malformation; hemihypertrophy; varicose veins *Ped Derm 33:570–584, 2016; JAAD 65:893–906, 2011; BJD 162:350–356, 2010; JAAD 56:541–564, 2007; JAAD 56:242–249, 2007; Curr Prob in Dermatol 13:249–300, 2002; Mayo Clin Proc 73:28–36, 1998; Br J Surg 72:232–236, 1985; Arch Gen Med (Paris) 3:641–672, 1900*

Lipodermatosclerosis – chronic venous insufficiency with hyperpigmentation, induration, inflammation *Ann Int Med 142:47–55, 2005; Lancet ii:243–245, 1982*

Lymphangioma – erythematous depressed patch of upper back as sign of underlying systemic lymphangiomatosis; history of chylothorax *BJD 163:875–877, 2010*

Lymphangitis - chemical, thermal, infectious

Lymphedema - mimicking infectious cellulitis *Ann Int Med 142:47–55, 2005*

Macrocephaly-capillary malformation (previously CTMC) syndrome – nevus simplex of philtrum and/or glabella; rare; widespread reticulated capillary malformations; somatic overgrowth, facial and limb asymmetry (hypoplasia more common); macrocephalic neonatal hypotonia; midline facial nevus flammeus (port wine stain of philtrum), congenital macrocephaly, macrosomia, segmental overgrowth, central nervous system malformations (hydrocephalus), connective tissue abnormalities, skin and joint hypermobility, toe syndactyly or polydactyly, frontal bossing, mental retardation, developmental delay *Ped Derm 35:724, 2018; JAAD 63:805–814, 2010; JAAD 56:541–564, 2007; Curr Prob in Dermatol 13:249–300, 2002*

Megalencephaly-capillary malformation polymicrogyria (MCAP) – reticulated capillary malformation *Ped Derm 33:570–584, 2016*

Microcephaly-capillary malformation syndrome (MICCAP) – reticulated capillary malformation *Ped Derm 33:570–584, 2016*

Multifocal lymphangioendotheliomatosis with thrombocytopenia – multiple congenital red-brown macules and blue nodules; gastrointestinal bleeding *Ped Derm 27:395–396, 2010; AD 140:599–606, 2004; JAAD 54:S214–217, 2006*

Nevus simplex *Ped Derm 26:661–662, 2009; Ped Derm 41:172–174, 2000*

Nevus roseus – phakomatosis spilorosea *BJD 159:489–491, 2008*

Nevus simplex – also known as salmon patch, angel's kiss, stork bite, fading macular stain, nevus roseus *Ped Derm 33:570–584, 2016*

  Seen in:

    Beckwith-Wiedemann syndrome *Clin Genet 46:168–174, 1994*
    Nova syndrome - familial communicating hydrocephalus, posterior cerebellar agenesis, mega cisterna magna *J Neurosurg 51:862–865, 1979*
    Odontodysplasia *Oral surg 46:675–684, 1978*
    Roberts-SC syndrome (Phocomelia syndrome) *clin Genet 45:107–108, 1994*

Nevus simplex with odontodysplasia – defects in dentin pulp, enamel, and dental follicle; failure of full eruption of affected teeth *JAAD 63:805–814, 2010;* extensive nevus simplex of scalp, nose, upper and lower lip mimicking port wine stain *JAAD 68:885–896, 2013*

Non-involuting capillary hemangioma (NICH) – red patch; blue patch; red nodules *JAAD 70:899–903, 2014*

Parkes-Weber syndrome – fast flow; capillary and arteriovenous shunts *Ped Derm 30:541–548, 2013;* combined vascular malformation like Klippel-Trenaunay syndrome with arteriovenous malformation with multiple arteriovenous fistulae along extremity with limb (usually leg) overgrowth; arteriovenous shunting; cutaneous red stain; lymphedema; high output congestive heart failure, hypertrophied digits with severe deformity; red foot *JAAD 65:893–906, 2011; JAAD 56:541–564, 2007; Curr Prob in Dermatol 13:249–300, 2002; BJD 19:231–235, 1907*

Phlebitis, superficial – cellulitis-like

Pigmented purpuric eruptions - lichen aureus *JAAD 8:722–724, 1983*

Popliteal artery occlusion - personal observation

Polyarteritis nodosa, infantile systemic – red patch heralding cutaneous infarction *J Pediatr 120:206–209, 1992;* oral erythema *Oral Surg 56:597–601, 1983*

Port wine stain *JAAD 74:527–535, 2016; BJD 172:684–691, 2015; BJD 167:1215–1233, 2012; Curr Prob in Dermatol 13:249–300, 2002;* segmental port wine stain in PHACES syndrome *Ped Derm 28:180–184, 2011; Neuroradiology 31:544–546, 1990;* somatic mutation in GNAQ *NEJM 368:1971–1979, 2013;* acquired port wine stain – red patches of neck, upper back, lower leg, posterior thigh *Ped Derm 37:93–97, 2020*

Acquired port wine stain – following penetrating trauma *Cutis 96:391–394, 2015; JAAD 65:462–463, 2011; AD 136:897–899, 2000; AD 122:1415–1416, 1986; Arch Dermatol Syphilol 188:416–422, 1949*

Port wine stains *JAAD 52:555–557, 2005*
  Beckwith-Wiedemann syndrome
  Coat's disease
  Cobb syndrome
  Phakomatosis pigmentovascularis
  Proteus syndrome
  Roberts syndrome
  Rubenstein-Taybi syndrome
  Sturge-Weber syndrome
  TAR syndrome
  Von Hippel-Lindau disease

Port wine stain with gingival hypertrophy and dental abnormalities *Ped Derm 33:570–584, 2016; J Craniofac surg 20:1629–1630, 2009*

Progressive ascending telangiectasia

Proteus syndrome – vascular malformations *AD 140:947–953, 2004*

Reticular infantile hemangioma with minimal or arrested growth associated with lipoatrophy *JAAD 72:828–833, 2015*

Roberts – SC phocomelia syndrome (pseudo-thalidomide syndrome) – symmetric limb defects, craniofacial abnormalities, prenatal and postnatal growth retardation and mental retardation *JAAD 63:805–814, 2010*

Salmon patch (nevus simplex)("stork bite") – pink macules with fine telangiectasias of the nape of the neck, glabella, forehead upper eyelids, tip of nose, upper lip, midline lumbosacral area *Ped Derm 73:31–33, 1983*

Servelle-Martorell syndrome – association of capillary stains and dysplastic veins with undergrowth of affected limb *Curr Prob in Dermatol 13:249–300, 2002*

Sinus pericranii – vertical red patch on midforehead to nasal root *Ped Derm 31:655, 2014*

Stewart-Bluefarb syndrome – arteriovenous malformation of leg with multiple fistulae and port wine stain-like purplish lesions (Mali's acroangiodermatitis/pseudo-Kaposi's sarcoma) – brown macules, purple nodules and plaques, edema, varicose veins, hypertrichosis, cutaneous ulcers, enlarged limb *JAAD 65:893–906, 2011*

Sturge-Weber syndrome – high risk port wine stains – hemifacial, median, forehead; capillary malformation of V1; choroidal and leptomeningeal involvement *Ped Derm 35:575–581, 2018; Ped Derm 33:570–584, 2016; BJD 171:861–867, 2014; Ped Derm 29:32–37, 2012; JAAD 56:541–564, 2007; Curr Prob in Dermatol 13:249–300, 2002: Pediatrics 87:323–327, 1991; Clin Soc Trans 12:162–167, 1879;* somatic mutation in GNAQ *NEJM 368:1971–1979, 2013;* central facial mosaic port wine stain in the midline crossing the nose and temporal area incurs highest risk for Strurge-Weber syndrome *JAAD 72:473–480, 2015*

Superficial thrombophlebitis – mimicking infectious cellulitis *Ann Int Med 142:47–55, 2005*

Temporal arteritis - personal observation

Tufted angioma (angioblastoma) - red stain; patchy dull red , purple, or red-brown patch and/or plaque; associated with erythema, edema, and hypertrichosis *BJD 171:474–484, 2014; Ped Derm 30:124–127, 2013; AD 144:1217–1222, 2008; Ped Derm 18:456–457, 2001;* overlying a port wine stain *AD 142:745–751, 2006*

Venous thrombosis – cellulitis-like; protein C deficiency, protein S deficiency, anti-thrombin III deficiency, hyperhomocystinemia, activated protein C resistance *AD 133:1027–1032, 1997*

Venous stasis – cellulitis-like

RED PLAQUE

AUTOIMMUNE DISEASES AND DISEASES OF IMMUNE DYSFUNCTION

Allergic contact dermatitis, including allergic contact dermatitis to metal joint replacements; cobalt – cellulitis-like *Ann Int Med 142:47–55, 2005;* mimicking infectious cellulitis *Ann Int Med 142:47–55, 2005;* dimethyl fumarate – epidemic of furniture-related dermatitis; extensive red plaques of back and buttocks *BJD 162:108–116, 2010*

Angioedema – lips, eyelids, genitalia *Ann Int Med 142:47–55, 2005; JAAD 25:155–161, 1991*

Autoimmune-related granulomatous dermatitis – confluent widespread red plaques; annular red plaques; autoimmune thyroid disease; autoimmune hepatitis *Case Rep Dermatol Med 2013; Case Rep Dermatol 4:80–84, 2012*

Bare lymphocyte syndrome *JAAD 17:895–902, 1987*

Bullous pemphigoid *JAAD 29:293–299, 1993;* anti-lamin gamma 1 pemphigoid antibodies (200kDa protein) – pruritic red brown plaques with blisters developing within plaques *BJD 163:1134–1136, 2010; J Dermatol 34:1–8, 2007;*

Chronic granulomatous disease - X-linked chronic granulomatous disease - discoid lupus-like lesions of face and hands in female carriers of X-linked chronic granulomatous disease *BJD 104:495–505, 1981*

Cicatricial pemphigoid – localized red plaque is site of recurrent blisters near mucosal surfaces *BJD 118:209–217, 1988; Oral Surg 54:656–662, 1982*

Combined immunodeficiency in children *JAAD 25:761–766, 1991*

Common variable immunodeficiency – granulomatous dermatitis with annular atrophic scarred and scaly plaques *J Clin Immunol 33:84–95, 2013; Dermatovenereol 18:107–113, 2010; J Clin Immunol 117:878–882, 2006; BJD 147:364–367, 2002; Mt Sinai Med J 68:326–330, 2001*

Congenital neutropenia

Cyclic neutropenia – cellulitis *Ped Derm 18:426–432, 2001; Am J Med 61:849–861, 1976*

Dermatitis herpetiformis – elbows, knees, buttocks, face *JAAD 64:1017–1024, 2011*

Dermatomyositis – small plaques over knees, elbows, knuckles, backs of finger joints, around fingernails; of the scalp; panniculitis - nodules and plaques on arms, thighs, buttocks, abdomen with lipoatrophy *AD 127:1846–1847, 1991; JAAD 23:127–128, 1990;* calcinosis cutis with cellulitis-like lesions due to extrusion of calcium cutaneous mucinosis *JAAD 48:S41–42, 2003*

Graft vs. host reaction, acute - red plaque with follicular papules *AD 142:1237–1238, 2006;* chronic – cellulitis-like *AD 134:602–612, 1998;* palmoplantar plaque *JAAD 33:711–717, 1975*

Cutaneous granulomas *Curr Opin Pediatr 25:492–497, 2013; Dermatology 223:13–19, 2011*
  Common variable immunodeficiency
  Inflammatory bowel disease
  Severe combined immunodeficiency
  Chronic granulomatous disease
  Ataxia telangiectasia

HyperIgD syndrome – recurrent transient and fixed pink plaques and nodules of face and extremities; cephalic pustulosis; mevalonate kinase deficiency *Ped Derm 35:482–485, 2018*

IgA pemphigus – red plaque with desquamation *BJD 171:650–656, 2014*

Juvenile rheumatoid arthritis - Still's disease; evanescent rash; persistent pruritic papules and plaques; urticarial and urticarial-like rash, vesiculopustular eruptions, edema of the eyelids, widespread non-pruritic persistent erythema *Medicine 96:e6318, 2017; AD 130:59–65, 1994*

IL-1 receptor-associated kinase 4 gene (IRAK-4) mutations – cellulitis, abscesses, impetigo *JAAD 54:951–983, 2006; Science 299:2076–2079, 2003*

Leukocyte adhesion deficiency

Linear IgA disease

Lupus erythematosus – discoid lupus of eyelid *JAMADerm 154:957–958, 2018;* mimicking infectious cellulitis *Ann Int Med 142:47–55, 2005;* subacute cutaneous LE; tumid lupus *JAAD 41:250–253, 1999;* lupus profundus *Ann Int Med 142:47–55, 2005;* lupus panniculitis - plaque with bullae *Fitzpatrick J of Clin Derm 2:32–34, 1994;* chilblain lupus - purple plaque *JAAD 19:909–910, 1988;* tumid lupus *AD 145:244–248, 2009;* non-bullous histiocytoid neutrophilic dermatosis; crusted red plaques *AD 144:1495–1498, 2008;* lupus mastitis - red plaque of breast (mimicking carcinoma erysipelatoides) *JAAD 60:1074–1076, 2009;* urticarial vasculitis - personal observation

Mendelian susceptibility to mycobacterial disease (MSMD) – *Mycobacterium bovis,* nontuberculous mycobacteria, *Salmonella* – mutations in IL-12, interferon gamma, IFNGR1, IFNGR2, STAT1, IL-12B, aIL-12RB1, IKBKG *Ped Derm 31:236–240, 2014*

Morphea, generalized; morphea profunda – red plaque of arm *Cutis 95:32–36, 2015; Ann Int Med 142:47–55, 2005; Ped Derm 8:292–295, 1991*

Pemphigoid gestationis *BJD 157:388–389, 2007*

Pemphigus foliaceus - face

Pemphigus herpetiformis – annular arcuate red plaques with edematous borders with erosions and vesicles; IgG to DSC1/3 and LAD-1 red plaque with vesicles, circinate desquamation, erosions, urticarial lesions *Ped Derm 34:342–346, 2017; BJD 169:719–721, 2013; AD 148:531–536, 2012*

Pemphigus vulgaris

Perforating neutrophilic and granulomatous dermatitis of the newborn – cutaneous eruption of immunodeficiency; papules, plaques, vesicles, crusts, ulcers; prominent involvement of palms and soles; sparing of trunk *Ped Derm 24:211–215, 2007*

Rheumatoid arthritis – rheumatoid neutrophilic dermatosis; edematous plaque, purpuric papules *JAAD 79:1009–1022, 2018; JAAD 45:596–600, 2001; J Dermatol 27:782–787, 2000;* intravascular or intralymphatic histiocytosis in rheumatoid arthritis; red livedoid plaques *JAAD 50:585–590, 2004*

Scleroderma – acute edematous phase; cellulitis-like

Still's disease – adult onset Still's disease - persistent plaques and linear pigmentation; flagellate erythema, erythema of eyelids, erythema of knuckles, red plaques of legs *JAAD 79:969–971, 2018;*

JAMA Derm 149:1425–1426, 2013; J Eur Acad Dermatol Venereol 19:360–363, 2005; Dermatology 188:241–242, 1994

STING-associated vasculopathy with onset in infancy (SAVI)(type 1 interferonopathy) – red plaques of face and hands; chilblain-like lesions; atrophic plaques of hands, telangiectasias of cheeks, nose, chin, lips, acral violaceous plaques and acral cyanosis (livedo reticularis of feet, cheeks, and knees), distal ulcerative lesions with infarcts (necrosis of cheeks and ears), gangrene of fingers or toes with ainhum, nasal septal perforation, nail dystrophy; small for gestational age; paratracheal adenopathy, abnormal pulmonary function tests; interstitial lung disease with fibrosis with ground glass and reticulate opacities; gain of function mutation in *TMEM173* (stimulator of interferon genes); mimics granulomatosis with polyangiitis *JAMADerm 151:872–877, 2015; NEJM 371:507–518, 2014; JAAD 74:186–189, 2016*

Systemic contact dermatitis to corticosteroids – red plaques with bullae *BJD 172:300–302, 2015*

Urticaria - mimicking infectious cellulitis *Ann Int Med 142:47–55, 2005*

X-linked agammaglobulinemia – cellulitis *Medicine (Baltimore)85:193–202, 2006*

CONGENITAL LESIONS

Choristia, periumbilical – intestinal mucosal cells; crusted, red perimbilical plaques *Ann DV 105:601–606, 1978*

Congenital mucinous eccrine nevi – red-brown hyperkeratotic plaques over ankle, foot, and toes *AD 148:140–142, 2012*

Congenital dermatofibrosarcoma protuberans – zosteriform red plaques *Cutis 90:285–288, 2012*

Mastocytoma *Cutis 99:261, 264, 2017*

Neonatal erythema of infancy – recurrent annular diffuse red plaques *JAMADerm 150:565–566, 2014; AD 117:145–148, 1981*
   Differential diagnosis:
      Urticaria
      Neonatal lupus erythematosus
      Erythema gryatum atrophicans transient neonatale
      Erythema annulare centrifugum
      Familial annular erythema
      Erythema gyratum perstans

Ectopic respiratory epithelium - red plaque of the neck *BJD 136:933–934, 1997*

Sclerema neonatorum - indurated violaceous plaques of back and legs *Cutis 92:83–87, 2013*

Subcutaneous fat necrosis of the newborn *Ped Derm 26:217–219, 2009; Ped Derm 20:257–261, 2003; JAAD 45:325–361, 2001;* due to therapeutic hypothermia *Ped Derm 29:59–63, 2012;* neutrophil-rich subcutaneous fat necrosis of the newborn – red papules and plaques *JAAD 75:177–185, 2016*

DRUG-INDUCED

Acral dysesthesia syndrome(chemotherapy-induced acral erythema)(toxic erythema of chemotherapy) – intertriginous eroded plaques and acral erythema; multiple chemotherapeutic agents including cytarabine, 5-fluorouracil, taxanes, anthracyclines, methotrexate *JAAD 63:175–177, 2010*

Adalibumab– eosinophilic cellulitis-like reaction *AD 142:218–220, 2006*

Alemtuzumab (CD52 monoclonal antibody) – red indurated plaque at injection site; localized cutaneous hemophagocytosis *JAMADerm 150:1021–1023, 2014*

Anakinra – lichenoid drug reaction *BJD 174:1417–1418, 2016*

Azathioprine – neutrophilic dermatosis (azathioprine hypersensitivity syndrome) – palpebral conjunctival erythema, pink macules, pink or red plaques *JAMA Derm 149:592–597, 2013*

BCGitis – red plaques in patient with transient hypogammaglobulinemia of infancy *Ped Derm 31:750–751, 2014*

BCG granuloma *AD 129:231–236, 1993*

Bleomycin (violaceous) - hyperkeratotic *JAAD 33:851–852, 1995*

Bortezomib – histiocytoid Sweet's syndrome; multiple red plaques of trunk *JAAD 71:217–227, 2014; JAAD 60:496–497, 2009*

BRAF inhibitors – eccrine hidradenitis *BJD 176:1645–1648, 2017*

Calcium gluconate extravasation – cellulitis-like *AD 138:405–410, 2002; AD 134:97–102, 1998*

Chemotherapy-related eccrine squamous syringometaplasia – red plaques of neck, axillae, and groin; lower eyelids; doxorubicin; bone marrow transplant regimen (cyclophosphamide, thiotepa, carboplatin) *JAAD 64:1092–1103, 2011; AD 133:873–878, 1997*

Chlorambucil – cellulitis-like *AD 122:1358, 1986*

Clopidogrel bisulfate *Mayo Clin Proc 78:618–620, 2003*

Corticosteroids – post-steroid panniculitis *JAAD 45:325–361, 2001; Ped Derm 5:92–93, 1988; J Cutan Pathol 12:366–380, 1985*

Coumadin necrosis (early) – cellulitis-like *JAAD 60:1–20, 2009*

Docataxel – acral dysesthesia syndrome – dusky red plaque *BJD 142:808–811, 2000;* extravasation *AD 146:1190–1191, 2010*

Doxorubicin – pegylated liposomal doxorubicin resulting in eccrine squamous syringometaplasia; red plaque with desquamation *AD 144:1402–1403, 2008*

Etanercept – eosinophilic cellulitis-like reaction *AD 142:218–220, 2006*

Fixed drug eruption – cellulitis-like *Ann Int Med 142:47–55, 2005; NEJM 350:904–912, 2004;* non-pigmenting *AD 134:929–931, 1999; JAAD 23:379, 1990;* pseudoephedrine *JAAD 48:628–630, 2003;* non-pigmenting fixed drug eruptions to pseudoephedrine and tetrahydrozoline *JAAD 17:403–407, 1987; JAAD 31:291–292, 1994;* to arsphenamine, acetaminophen; eperisine hydrochloride *BJD 144:1288–1289, 2001;* procarbazine *Med Pediatr Oncol 16:378–380, 1988;* piroxicam *JAAD 21:1300, 1989;* thiopental *Anesth Analg 70:216–217, 1990;* iothalamate (radiocontrast medium) *JAAD 23:379–381, 1990;* diflunisal *JAAD 24:1021–1022, 1991;* betahistine *Dermatology 193:248–250, 1996;* cimetidine *Dermatology 197:402–403, 1998;* paracetamol *J Invest Allergol Clin Immunol 9:399–400, 1999;* cotrimoxazole *Eur J Dermatol 10:288–291, 2000;* topotecan *J Eur Acad Dermatol Venereol 16:414–416, 2002*

Furosemide – cellulitis-like drug eruption

Gadolidium *JAMADerm 151:316–319, 2015*

Gemcitabine – erysipelas-like red plaques *JAAD 58:545–570, 2008*

GM-CSF-producing tumor cell vaccine *JAMADerm 153:332–334, 2017*

Heparin - local reaction *JAAD 21:703–707, 1989*

Hyaluronic acid filler – delayed hypersensitivity reaction

IL-2 therapy – cellulitis-like *JAAD 28:66–70, 1993*

Imatinib-associated Sweet's syndrome *AD 141:368–370, 2005*

Interferon alpha – sarcoidal papules *BJD 146:320–324, 2002;* granulomatous indurated erythema at injection site *JAAD 46:611–616, 2002*

Interferon beta-1b *JAAD 37:553–558, 1997*

Iohexol (intravenous contrast material) – annular plaque of breast *J Drugs in Dermtol 10:802–804, 2011*

Isotretinoin – granulations tissue as red plaques *Ped Derm 35:257–258, 2018*

L-asparaginase pseudocellulitis

Methotrexate photorecall

Nadroparin-calcium injections – calcifying panniculitis; crusted red plaques *BJD 153:657–660, 2005*

Nivolumab – lichen planus pemphigoides; bullae, erosions, red plaques *Cutis 103:224–226, 2019*

Non-pigmenting fixed drug eruption - personal observation

Pegfilgrastim - Sweet's syndrome due to pegfilgrastim (pegylated G-CSF) *JAAD 52:901–905, 2005*

Propranolol – annular telangiectatic perivascular angiomatosis – red to violaceous hyperpigmented annular plaques with central clearing and radial telangiectasia *BJD 169:1369–1371, 2013*

Pseudolymphoma secondary to drugs - antihistamines, allopurinol, amiloride, carbamazepine, cyclosporine, clomipramine, diltiazem phenytoin *JAAD 38:877–905, 1998; JAAD 32:419–428, 1995, AD 132:1315–1321, 1996;* anticonvulsants captopril, enalapril *J Clin Pathol 39:902–907, 1986;* atenolol *Clin Exp Dermatol 115:119–120, 1990;* ACE inhibitors , amitryptiline *Curr Probl Dermatol 19:176–182, 1990*

Quinidine photolichenoid dermatitis

Ramucirumab – angioma *JAMADerm 151:1240–1243, 2015*

Simvastatin – urticarial vasculitis *Dermatitis 21:223–224, 2010*

Sorafenib (multikinase inhibitor) – hand-foot reactions; facial seborrheic dermatitis, red plaques on sides of feet, hyperkeratotic plaque or blister of feet, red patches on pressure points, red swollen fingertips, gray blisters of fingerwebs, angular cheilitis, perianal dermatitis *BJD 158:592–596, 2008;* red scaly plaque with follicular papules (pityriasis rubra pilaris-like) *JAAD 65:452–453, 2011;* interstitial granulomatous dermatitis; red papules, nodules, and plaques of palms *AD 147:1118–1119, 2011*

Sweet's syndrome – red plaques, nasal ulcers, perianal ulcers - celecoxib, G-CSF, all-trans retinoic acid *JAAD 45:300–302, 2001*

Vaccination reaction

Vemurafenib – red plaque of cutaneous T-cell lymphoma *BJD 173:1024–1031, 2015*

Vitamin K allergy – cellulitis-like red plaque, typically lateral upper arm 1–2 weeks after injection *JAAD 28(PT2)345–347, 1993*

EXOGENOUS AGENTS

Cold urticaria - ice cube test

Bromoderma – vegetating bromoderma; pustular red plaque with pustules at margins to distinguish it from pyoderma gangrenosum *JAAD 58:682–684, 2008*

Foreign body reaction (granuloma) – orthopedic implants mimicking infectious cellulitis *Ann Int Med 142:47–55, 2005; Ann DV 123:686–690, 1996*

Irritant contact dermatitis – cellulitis-like *JAAD 67:177–185, 2012; Onopordum acanthium; Mandragora autumnalis Dermatitis 25:140–146, 2014*

Mercury exanthema *Contact Dermatitis 36:277–278, 1997*

Milk injections – cellulitis

Paraffinoma – grease gun injury; nodule, plaque, sinus of hand *BJD 115:379–381, 1986;* sclerosing lipogranuloma *JAAD 9:103–110, 1983*

Postvaccination *Semin Pediatr Infect Dis 14:196–198, 2003*

Radiocontrast material (meglumine ioxitalamate) – Sweet's syndrome *JAAD 58:488–489, 2008*

Silicone reaction/granuloma – recurrent cellulitis; red plaques of buttocks *AD 141:13–15, 2005; Derm Surg 27:198–200, 2001*

Squaric acid dibutyl ester – red plaque of arm; cutaneous lymphoid hyperplasia *JAAD 65:230–232, 2011*

INFECTIONS AND INFESTATIONS

Acanthamebiasis(*Balamuthia mandrillaris, Naegleria fowleri, Acanthamoeba spp, Sappinia pedata*) – cellulitis *AD 147:857–862, 2011;* centrofacial Balamuthiasis *J Cut Pathol 43:892–897, 2016; Adv Dermatol 23:335–350, 2007; JAAD 42:351–354, 2000; JAAD 42:351–354, 2000;* cellulitis *Ann DV 128:1237–1240, 2001 ;* balamuthiasis– amoebic infection of soft tissues and central nervous system; edematous erythematous infiltrated plaque of face, abdomen, extremities - red plaque with central necrosis; transmitted by organ transplant *Clin Inf Dis 63:878–888, 2016*

Acinetobacter calcoaceticus – cellulitis *Medicine 56:79–97, 1977; A. baumannii* – edematous cellulitis with small vesicles and hemorrhagic bullae after war trauma *JAAD 75:1–16, 2016; Clin Infect Dis 47:444–449, 2008;* cellulitis with overlying vesicles progress to necrotizing fasciitis with bullae *Surg Infect (Larchmt)11:49–57, 2010*

Aeromonas hydrophila – cellulitis complicating injuries in fresh water or soil *JAAD 61:733–750, 2009; Clin Inf Dis 19:77–83, 1994; Clin Inf Dis 16:79–84, 1993*

African histoplasmosis

AIDS - cutaneous CD8+ T-cell infiltrates in advanced HIV disease *JAAD 41:722–727, 1999 ;* AIDS-associated eosinophilic pustular folliculitis – red plaques with papulovesicular borders *JAAD 14:1020–1022, 1986*

Alternariosis (*A. alternata*) *JAAD 52:653–659, 2005; AD 124:1822–1825, 1988;* Alternaria chartarum – red, scaly plaque *BJD 142:1261–1262, 2000*

Anaerobic clostridial myositis

Anthrax *Int J Dermatol 20:203–206, 1981*

Aspergillosis, primary cutaneous *AD 136:1165–1170, 2000; JAAD 12:313–318, 1985; JAAD 31:344–347, 1994;* primary cutaneous aspergillosis in premature infants; red patch with pustules *Ped Derm 19:439–444, 2002;* primary cutaneous aspergillosis (*Aspergillus fumigatus*) at IV site in patient with mitochondrial disorder complex I (NADH dehydrogenase deficiency) *Cutis 92:219, 223–224, 2013; Aspergillus fumigatus* – red plaque with pustules *Ped Derm 26:592–596, 2009*

Bacillary angiomatosis - plaque with hyperkeratotic center *BJD 126:535–541, 1992*

Bacillus cereus – cutaneous infection begins with vesicle and/or pustule and becomes cellulitis; then a nonhealing ulcer with a black eschar *Cutis 79:371–377, 2007; Lancet Mar 18;1(8638):601–603, 1989*

Bacillus species - cellulitis *JAAD 39:285–287, 1998; Medicine 66:218–223, 1987;* plaque with hyperkeratotic center *BJD 126:535–541, 1992*

Bacterial panniculitis – extensive red plaque of upper chest with sandpaper texture *AD 147:499–504, 2011*

Bacteroides fragilis – cellulitis *J Hosp Infect 3303–304, 1982*

BCG granuloma

BCG vaccination – lupus vulgaris *Ped Derm 21:660–663, 2004*

Bilophila wadsworthia - cellulitis *J Clin Inf Dis (Suppl 2):S88–93, 1997*

Blastomycosis-like pyoderma *AD 142:1643–1648, 2006; AD 115:170–173, 1979*

Botryomycosis - granulomatous plaque *JAAD 24:393–396, 1991; AD 126:815–820, 1990*

Breast abscess – cellulitis-like *JAAD 43:733–751, 2000*

Brown recluse spider bite (loxoscelism) *Adv Hematol 2019:4091278*

Brucellosis - panniculitis *JAAD 35:339–341, 1996;* erysipelas-like *Cutis 63:25–27, 1999; AD 117:40–42, 1981*

Buruli ulcer (*Mycobacteria ulcerans subspecies shinshuense*) – ulcerated red plaque of face *JAMA Derm 150:64–67, 2014*

Campylobacter jejuni - erysipelas-like lesions in patient with hypogammaglobulinemia *Eur J Clin Microbiol Infect Dis 11:842–847, 1992; Campylobacter species* - red, annular, and serpiginous plaques of lower leg in HIV+ patient *AD 142:1240–1241, 2006*

Candidiasis – flexural candidiasis; invasive systemic candidiasis in premature neonate (C. albicans); erosive and crusted red plaques *Ped Derm 21:260–261, 2004;* chronic mucocutaneous candidiasis – crusted red plaques *Ped Derm 29:519–520, 2012; C. tropicalis –* cellulitis-like plaque *Cutis 93:204–206, 2014*

Capnocytophaga canimorsus sepsis – dog and cat bites; necrosis with eschar; cellulitis *Cutis 60:95–97, 1997; JAAD 33:1019–1029, 1995*

Cat scratch disease – red plaque *JAAD 48:474–476, 2003;* red plaque with pseudovesicular border (Sweet's-like) *JAAD 41:833–836, 1999*

Cellulitis/erysipelas – streptococcal; Groups A, B (infants under 3 months) *J Drugs in Dermatol 12:369–374, 2013; JAAD 67:163–174, 2012; Ped Derm 27:528–530, 2010; Am J Dis Child 136:631–633, 1982;* pelvic postoperative erysipelas *AD 120:85–86, 1994),* C, and G *AD 130:1150–1158, 1994; Haemophilus influenzae –* facial cellulitis in children; *Streptococcus pneumoniae Clin Inf Dis 14:247–250, 1992; Pseudomonas aeruginosa JAMA 248:2156–2157, 1982; Campylobacter jejuni Eur J Clin Microbiol Infect Dis 11:842–847, 1988;* congenital neutropenia *Blood Rev 2:178–185, 1988; Am J Med 61:849–861, 1976;* in leukocyte adhesion deficiency (beta 2 integrin deficiency) – abscesses, cellulitis, skin ulcerations, ulcerative stomatitis *BJD 139:1064–1067, 1998; J Pediatr 119:343–354, 1991; Ann Rev Med 38: 175–194, 1987; J Infect Dis 152:668–689, 1985; Paecilomyces marquandii, Paecilomyces lilacinus BJD 143:647–649, 2000*

Centipede bite – two legs/segment; not millipede; cellulitis-like *Int J Dermatol 153:869–872, 2014*

Chagas' disease - reactivation posttransplant; cellulitis *Dermatol Clinics 29:53–62, 2011; JAAD 58:529–530, 2008;* cellulitis *Cutis 48:37–40, 1991;* panniculitis; megacolon, intestinal perforation; unilateral painful bipalpebral edema, conjunctivitis, local lymphadenopathy, periorbital cellulitis, furuncular lesions (chagomas), cardiac involvement *JAAD 75:19–30, 2016*

Chromobacterium violaceum – nodules with cellulitis *JAAD 54:S224–228, 2006;* cellulitis following boating accident *Cutis 81:269–272, 2008*

Chromomycosis *JAAD 57:912–914, 2007*

Citrobacter diversus - cellulitis *Cutis 61:158–159, 1998*

Clostridium botulinum – wound botulism in drug addicts; cellulitis *Clin Inf Dis 31:1018–1024, 2000*

Clostridium cellulitis (gas gangrene)(*C. perfringens, C. oedematicus, C.septicum, C. histolyticum*) – crepitant, painful, swollen plaque with serous discharge; bullae, necrosis develop

JAAD 67:177–185, 2012; Br J Surg 64:104–112, 1977; NEJM 289:1129–1136, 1973

Coccidioidomycosis (granulomatous plaque) *JAAD 26:79–85, 1992;* red plaque with pustules *JAAD 46:743–747, 2002;* primary cutaneous coccidioidomycosis – ulcerated plaque *JAAD 49:944–949, 2003*

Corynebacterium jeikeium BJD 133:801–804, 1995

Coxsackie A16 - Sweet's-like red plaques

Cryptococcosis (*Cryptococcous neoformans*) – cellulitis *Clin Inf Dis 59:688, 745–746, 2014; JAMA 309:1632–1633, 2013; Cutis 72:320–322;2003; J Dermatol 30:405–410, 2003; Clin Inf Dis 33:700–705, 2001; Australas J Dermatol 38:29–32, 1997; JAAD 32:844–850, 1995; Scand J Infect Dis 26:623–626, 1994; Clin Inf Dis 16:826–827, 1993; Clin Inf Dis 14:666–672, 1992; Int J Dermatol 29:41–44, 1990; JAAD 17:329–332, 1987; Cutis 34:359–361, 1984;* crusted plaque of neck *AD 142:921–926, 2006;* panniculitis *Cutis 85:303–306, 2010;* edematous erythema with subcutaneous plaques of legs *JAMA 309:1632–1633, 2013*

Curvularia – cellulitis *Cutis 89:65–68, 2012*

Cytomegalovirus Medicina B Aires 62:572–574, 2002

Dematiacious fungal infections in organ transplant recipients - all lesions on extremities
  Alternaria
  Bipolaris hawaiiensis
  Exophiala jeanselmei, E. spinifera, E. pesciphera, E. castellani
  Exserohilum rostratum
  Fonsacaea pedrosoi
  Phialophora parasitica

Dermatophytosis *Ophthal Plast Reconstr Surg 19:244–246, 2003*

Dirofilaria repens – red plaques (cellulitis-like) and pulmonary nodules *BJD 173:788–791, 2015*

Dysgonic fermenters – gram-negative bacillus *Rev Infect Dis 9:884–890, 1987*

Eikenella corrodens – human bite wound; IV drug abuse *J Drugs in Dermatol 12:369–374, 2013; AD 125:849–850, 1989*

Erysipeloid - *Erysipelothrix insidiosa (rhusiopathiae)* - seal finger, blubber finger; red plaque of hand *JAAD 61:733–750, 2009; Clin Microbiol Rev 2:354–359, 1989; JAAD 9:116–123, 1983;* red plaque of thumb *AD 147:1456–1458, 2011*

Fish stings – venomous fish; lesser weever fish, spiny dogfish, stingray, scorpion fish, catfish, rabbit fish, stone fish, stargazers, toadfish – erythema, edema mimicking cellulitis

Flavimonas oryzihabitans Clin Inf Dis 18:808–809, 1994

Flavobacterium odoratum Clin Inf Dis 22:1112–1113, 1996

Fusarium solani – cellulitis *JAAD 56:873–877, 2007; AD 127:1735–1737, 1991;* digital cellulitis; localized fusariosis (*F. solani*) – red plaque of arm with eschar *AD 141:794–795, 2005;* cellulitis (*F. oxysporum*) *Acta DV 81:51–53, 2001;* cellulitis with necrosis *Am J Clin Pathol 75:304–311,1981; J Pediatr 84:561–564, 1974*

Gianotti-Crosti syndrome – lichenoid dermatitis *Am J Dermatopathol 22:162–165, 2000;* pink papules coalescing into plaques *Ped Derm 30:137–138, 2013*

Glanders – *Pseudomonas mallei* – cellulitis which ulcerates with purulent foul-smelling discharge, regional lymphatics become abscesses; nasal and palatal necrosis and destruction; metastatic papules, pustules, bullae over joints and face, then ulcerate; deep abscesses with sinus tracts occur; polyarthritis, meningitis, pneumonia

Gnathostomiasis/paragonimus - migratory tender red nodules or cellulitis-like plaques *JAAD 68:301–305, 2013; JAAD 33:825–828, 1995; JAAD 13:835–836, 1985*

Haemophilus influenzae – facial cellulitis in children *Am J Med 63:449, 1977*

Helicobacter cinaedi (formerly *Campylobacter cinaedi*) - cellulitis *BJD 175:62–68, 2016; Ann Int Med 121:90–93, 1994; J Clin Inf Dis 20:564–570, 1995;* multifocal cellulitis *Clin Inf Dis 70:531,533–534, 2020*

Hepatitis C infection - necrolytic acral erythema; red to hyperpigmented psoriasiform plaques with variable scale or erosions of feet or shins *JAAD 53:247–251, 2005; Int J Derm 35:252–256, 1996*

Herpes zoster

Histoplasmosis - panniculitis *JAAD 25:912–914, 1991; AD 132:341–346, 1996; JAAD 25:418–422, 1991; Medicine 60:361–373, 1990;* cellulitis *Clin Inf Dis 69:373–375, 2019; AD 118:3–4, 1982; S Med J 74:635–637, 1981; AD 95:345–350, 1967;* erysipelas-like *Trans Proc 37:4313–4314, 2005*

Hyalohyphomycosis – cellulitis *JAAD 80:869–880, 2019; Acute Med 15:88–91, 2016*

Impetigo – crusted red plaque *J Drugs in Dermatol 12:369–374, 2013*

Infected marlex mesh graft inserted during abdominal surgery

Insect bite reaction – mimicking infectious cellulitis *Ann Int Med 142:47–55, 2005*

Klebsiella pneumoniae - cellulitis *JAAD 51:836, 2004*

Leclaria adecarboxylata – cellulitis with necrotic pustules in acute lymphoblastic leukemia *Ped Derm 28:162–164, 2011*

Legionella micdadei - cellulitis *Am J Med 92:104–106, 1992*

Leishmaniasis - acute cutaneous leishmaniasis *AD 122:329–334, 1986; L. tropica* (dry, urban type) – brown nodule extends to plaque with central ulceration red plaque of neck – mucocutaneous leishmaniasis *JAMA 312:1250–1251, 2014;* multiple red plaques of trunk in AIDS *BJD 160:311–318, 2009;* Old World leishmaniasis – ulcerated red plaque *Ped Derm 35:384–387, 2018;* leishmaniasis recidivans (lupoid leishmaniasis) – brown-red or brown-yellow papules close to scar of previously healed lesion; resemble lupus vulgaris; may ulcerate or form concentric rings; keloidal form, verrucous form of legs, extensive psoriasiform dermatitis; red crusted plaque *Cutis 77:25–28, 2006; Ped Derm 23:78–80, 2006; JAAD 47:614–616, 2002;* localized cutaneous leishmaniasis – *L. viannia panamensis; Lutzomyia trapidoi* (vector) *AD 139:1075–1080, 2003; L. panamensis Clin Inf Dis 61:1314,1342–1343, 2015*

Leprosy – borderline – red or coppery-brown plaque *JAAD 54:559–578, 2006;* borderline lepromatous leprosy *Clin Inf Dis 50:1015–1016,1068–1069, 2010;* borderline tuberculoid leprosy *JAMADerm 150:643–644, 2014;* borderline tuberculoid leprosy mimicking cutaneous T-cell lymphoma *SKINmed 11:379–381, 2013;* acute borderline leprosy in immune reconstitution syndrome in AIDS – tender, red plaque of leg *Cutis 100:327–329, 2017;* indurated translucent red plaques *NEJM 356:1549–1551, 2011;* lepromatous – wine red plaques *J Drugs in Dermatol 13:210–215, 2014;* tuberculoid – well-defined edge, red, copper or purple colored plaque with hypopigmented center; hairless *AD 144:1051–1056, 2008;* erythema nodosum leprosum *JAAD 51:416–426, 2004;* Lucio's phenomenon - firm subcutaneous plaque *AD 114:1023–1028, 1978;* borderline; reversal reaction in leprosy – periarticular erythema and edema of hand with edema of red plaques of trunk; existing lesions become red and tumid with edema of the hands, neuritis, sensory and motor loss with foot drop, wrist drop, facial palsy, lagophthalmos, keratitis, and blindness *JAAD 71:795–803, 2014;* type 1 reaction demonstrates reappearance of resolved lesions, with erythema, edema, and paresthesias; acute peripheral neuritis, edema of hands, feet, arms, and face *BJD 158:648–649, 2008; JAAD 57:914–917, 2007;* type 1 reversal reaction – oval pink plaque *Cutis 95:222–226, 2015;* type 1 reaction in borderline leprosy; immune reconstitution inflammatory syndrome (IRIS) in HIV disease – ulcerated plaque *AD 140:997–1000, 2004*

Listeria monocytogenes

Lobomycosis *Emerging Inf Dis 25:65–660, 2019*

Lupus vulgaris – crusted hyperkeratotic plaque with nodules and scarring; due to BCG inoculation *BJD 144:444–445, 2001*

Lyme disease – annular red plaque *BJD 171:528–543, 2014*

Mastitis - infectious *JAAD 43:733–751, 2000;* periductal cellulitis-like *JAAD 43:733–751, 2000*

Microsporum gypseum – plaque with multiple nodules and pustules *BJD 146:311–313, 2002*

Moraxella species - preseptal cellulitis and facial erysipelas *Clin Exp Dermatol 19:321–323, 1994*

Mucormycosis – *Mucor, Rhizopus oryzi, Rhizomucor, Lichtheimia, Saksenaea, Cunninhghamella, Apophysomyces* cellulitis *JAAD 80:869–880, 2019; Clin Inf Dis 54(Suppl 1)523–534, 2012; AD 113:1075–1076, 1977;Ped Derm 20:411–415, 2003;* red plaque with pustules *JAAD 59:542–544, 2008;* red plaque of neck *Cutis 89:167–168, 2012;* red plaque with central eschar *AD 131:833–834,836–837, 1995; Ped Inf Dis J 4:672–676, 1985;* violaceous necrotic and crusted plaques; *Rhizopus spp. AD 143:417–422, 2007*

Mycobacterium abscessus - multinodular plaque *J Drugs Dermatol 13:1495–1497, 2014;* cellulitis *AD 142:1287–1292, 2006; Am J Respir Crit Care Med 156(pt 2):S1–S25, 1997; Clin Inf Dis 24:1147–1153, 1997; Clin Inf Dis 19:263–273, 1994; AD 129:1190–1191, 1193, 1993; Rev Infect Dis 5:657–679, 1983*

Mycobacterium avium-intracellulare JAAD 21:574–576, 1989; JAAD 33:528–531, 1995; red indurated plaque of scalp, ear, and lateral face *J Drugs in Dermatol 1:490–491, 2013*

Mycobacterium bollettii – leg plaques and abscesses due to foot baths for pedicures *AD 147:454–458, 2011*

Mycobacterium bovis AD 126:123–124, 1990

Mycobacterium chelonae – multinodular plaque *J Drugs Dermatol 13:1495–1497, 2014;* with pustules *BJD 171:79–89, 2014; JAAD 24:867–870, 1991;* cellulitis *Dermatol Clin 33:563–577, 2015; AD 142:1287–1292, 2006; Am J Respir Crit Care Med 156(pt 2):S1–S25, 1997; Clin Inf Dis 24:1147–1153, 1997; Clin Inf Dis 19:263–273, 1994; AD 129:1190–1191, 1193, 1993; J Infect Dis 166:405–412,1992; Rev Infect Dis 5:657–679, 1983*

Mycobacterium fortuitum panniculitis *JAAD 39:650–653, 1998;* cellulitis *AD 142:1287–1292, 2006; Dermatol Surg 26:588–590, 2000; Am J Respir Crit Care Med 156(pt 2):S1–S25, 1997; Clin Inf Dis 24:1147–1153, 1997; Clin Inf Dis 19:263–273, 1994; AD 129:1190–1191, 1193, 1993; Rev Infect Dis 5:657–679, 1983;* mimicking lupus vulgaris *BJD 147:170–173, 2002;* red plaque *Ped Derm 33:264–274, 2016*

Mycobacterium hemophilum Am J Transplant 2:476–479, 2002; BJD 149:200–202, 2003; JAAD 40:804–806, 1994; ulcerated red plaque *AD 141:897–902, 2005*

Mycobacterium kansasii - red plaque (cellulitis-like) *JAAD 41:854–856, 1999; JAAD 40:359–363, 1999; Am Rev Resp Dis 112:125,1979; JAAD 36:497–499, 1997; Cutis 31:87–89, 1983*

Mycobacterium marinum

Mycobacterium massiliense – leg plaques and abscesses due to foot baths for pedicures *AD 147:454–458, 2011*

Mycobacterium szulgai – diffuse cellulitis, nodules, and sinuses *Am Rev Respir Dis 115:695–698, 1977*

Mycobacterium thermoresistible – violaceous indurated plaque *Clin Inf Dis 31:816–817, 2000*

Mycobacterium tuberculosis – tuberculous cellulitis *JAAD 65:450–452, 2011;* lupus vulgaris - red plaque with papules and central atrophy *SKINmed 10:28–33, 2012;* lupus vulgaris simulating a port wine stain *BJD 119:127–128, 1988*; ulcerated plaque of buttocks (lupus vulgaris) *BJD 146:525–527, 2002*; starts as red-brown plaque, enlarges with serpiginous margin or as discoid plaques; apple-jelly nodules; plaque form – psoriasiform, irregular scarring, serpiginous margins; ulcerative and mutilating forms, vegetating forms – ulcerate, areas of necrosis, invasion of mucous membranes with destruction of cartilage (lupus vorax); tumor-like forms – deeply infiltrative; soft smooth nodules or red-yellow hypertrophic plaque; myxomatous form with large tumors of the earlobes; lymphedema prominent; papular and nodular forms; nasal, buccal, and conjunctival involvement with friable nodules which ulcerate; vegetative and ulcerative lesions of buccal mucosa, palate, gingiva, oropharynx; head, neck, around nose, extremities, trunk *Int J Dermatol 26:578–581, 1987; Acta Tuberc Scand 39(Suppl 49):1–137, 1960*; erythema induratum

Morganella morganii

Myiasis, subcutaneous (*Dermatobia hominis*) *Z Hautkr 61:958–962, 1986*

Necrotizing fasciitis – *Streptococcus pyogenes JAAD 67:177–185, 2012; Ann DV 128:376–381, 2001; AD 130:1150–1158, 1994; Pseudomonas aeruginosa, Escherichia coli, Klebsiella species, Peptostreptococcus, Bacteroides fragilis Clin Inf Dis 33:6–15, 2001; Streptococcus pneumoniae* – due to intramuscular injection *Clin Inf Dis 33:740–744, 2001; Serratia marcescens Clin Inf Dis 23:648–649, 1996; JAAD 20:774–778, 1989; Bacteroides spp.* in penile necrotizing fasciitis *JAAD 37:1–24, 1997*; neonatal *Pediatrics 103:e53, 1999*; in infancy *Ped Derm 2:55–63, 1984*; Clostridial cellulitis (gangrene); progressive synergistic gangrene; gangrenous cellulitis (*Pseudomonas*); Fournier's gangrene; necrotizing fasciitis associated with injection drug abuse – gram-positive aerobes - *Staphylococcus aureus, viridans group streptococci, Streptococcus pyogenes, coagulase-negative Staphylococcus species, Enterococcus species*; gram-negatives - *Pseudomonas aeruginosa, Enterococcus species; Clostridium perfringens, Clostridium species Clin Inf Dis 33:6–15, 2001*

Neisseria meningitidis - cellulitis *Clin Inf Dis 21:1023–1025, 1995*; periarticular erythema of chronic meningococcemia

Nocardiosis *JAAD 23:399–400, 1990; JAAD 13:125–133, 1985; Nocardia asteroides* – cellulitis *BJD 144:639–641, 2001; AD 121:898–900, 1985; N. brasiliensis* cellulitis of legs, arms, trunk, and face *J Inf Dis 134(3):286–289, 1976; N. brasiliensis* – ulcerated plaque, eschar, cellulitis, sporotrichoid pattern *JAMADerm 151:895–896, 2015; Nocardia nova* – red plaque of hand *BJD 145:154–156, 2001*

North American blastomycosis - disseminated blastomycosis – red plaque with pustules *Ped Derm 23:541–545, 2006*

Onchocerciasis - erysipelas–like acute lesions - erysipela de la Costa; eosinophilic cellulitis *J R Soc Med 78 Suppl 11:21–22, 1985*

Paecilomyces marquandii, P. lilacinus, variotii - cellulitis *BJD 143:647–649, 2000; JAAD 39:401–409, 1998; AD 122:1169, 1986; P. lilacinus* - crusted red plaque of leg *JAAD 55:S63–64, 2006*

Paracoccidioidomycosis - near mouth, anus, or genitalia *JAAD 53:931–951, 2005*

Parvovirus B19 infection – red/violaceous plaques resembling Sweet's syndrome *Hum Pathol 31:488–497, 2000*; erysipelas-like red plaque *Rev Med Interne 24:317–319, 2003*

Pasteurella multocida (P. haemolytica, pneumotropica, and *ureae)* – cellulitis with ulceration with hemorrhagic purulent discharge with sinus tracts; dog or cat bite *J Drugs in Dermatol 12:369–374, 2013; JAAD 33:1019–1029, 1995; Medicine 63:133–154, 1984*

Phaeohyphomycosis *JAAD 18:1023–1030, 1988*; diffuse infiltrated pigmented plaques; subcutaneous cysts, abscesses, ulcerated plaques, hemorrhagic pustules, necrotic papulonodules, cellulitis *JAAD 75:19–30, 2016; JAAD 40:364–366, 1999; JAAD 28:34–44, 1993; AD 127:721–726, 1991; JAAD 19:478–481, 1988; AD 123:1346–1350, 1987*

Phlegmon – cellulitis-like

Pinta – primary lesion with satellite papules *AD 135:685–688, 1999*; primary pinta - red scaly plaque *JAAD 54:559–578, 2006*

Plague – *Yersinia pestis*; flea bite; cellulitic plaque becomes bullous and crusted like anthrax *West J Med 142:641–646, 1985*

Pott's puffy tumor - nontender bogginess of forehead - underlying osteomyelitis

Prevotella species J Clin Inf Dis (Suppl 2):S88–93, 1997

Prototothecosis (*Prototheca wickerhamii*) – green alga *AD 142:921–926, 2006; JAAD 32:758–764, 1995; JAAD 31:920–924, 1994; AD 125:1249–1252, 1989*; cellulitis *Cutis 63:185–188, 1999; BJD 146:688–693, 2002; Am J Clin Pathol 61:10–19, 1974*; red plaque with focal ulcers covering entire arm *Clin Inf Dis 56:271, 307, 2013*

Pseudallescheria boydii JAAD 21:167–179, 1989

Pseudomonas aeruginosa JAMA 248;2156, 1982

Pyomyositis *Hawaii J Med Public Health 74:260–266, 2015; Pediatr Int 57:1053–1054, 2015; JAAD 51:308–314, 2004*

Pythiosis (*Pythium insidiosum*)(alga) – cellulitis, infarcts, ulcers *JAAD 52:1062–1068, 2005*

Rhizopus – violaceous targetoid plaque of thigh *Ped Derm 24:560–561, 2007; JAAD 51:996–1001, 2004; Mycoses 45(Suppl 1):27–30, 2002; A Surg 111:532, 1976*

Salmonella species – reptile exposure *J Drugs in Dermatol 12:369–374, 2013*

Scedosporium (asexual form of *Pseudallescheria boydii*) – eumycetoma; red swollen arm with numerous pustules *AD 148:1199–1204, 2012*

Schistosomiasis – ectopic cutaneous granuloma – skin-colored papule, 2–3 mm; group to form mamillated plaques *Dermatol Clin 7:291–300, 1989; BJD 114:597–602, 1986*

Serratia marcescens – moist red plaque *JAAD 55:357–358, 2006; JAMA 250:2348, 1983*; cellulitis *JAAD 49:S193–194, 2003*

Shewanella putrefaciens - cellulitis *J Clin Inf Dis 25:225–229, 1997*

Sparganosis – subcutaneous sparganosis (*Spirometra*/tapeworm) - (infective larvae of pseudophyllidean tapeworm of genus Spirometra) - urticaria-like lesions *BJD 170:741–743, 2014; BJD 148:369–370, 2003*

Spider bites – cellulitis-like; black widow spider (Latrodectus mactans) – punctum with erythema and edema *AD 123:41–43, 1987*; brown recluse spider (*Loxosceles reclusa*) – erythema, edema, central bulla; targetoid lesion with central blue/purple, ischemic halo, outer rim of erythema; at 3–4 days central necrosis, eschar, ulcer, scar *South Med J 69:887–891, 1976*; wolf spider (Lycosa) – erythema and edema *Cutis 39:113–114, 1987*

Sporotrichosis – cellulitis (erysipeloid-like) *JAAD 40:272–274, 1999*; fixed cutaneous sporotrichosis *Derm Clinics 17:151–185, 1999*; disseminated

Staphylococcus aureus Ped 18:249, 1956; staphylococcal

Staphylococcus epidermidis – cellulitis *Arch Derm 120:1099, 1984*

Stenotrophomonas maltophilia (formerly *Pseudomonas maltophilia*) – cellulitis, nodules, ecthyma gangrenosum lesions *Eur J Clin Microbiol Infect Dis 28:719–730, 2009l J Eur Acad Dermatol Venereol 21:1298–1300, 2007; Ann Pharmacother 36:63–66, 2002; Can J Infect Dis 7:383–385, 1996*

Stink bugs (*Pentatomidae*) – red plaques and vesicles *JAAD 67:331–344, 2012*

Streptococcus - Group B streptococcal disease – cellulitis *Clin Inf Dis 33:556–561, 2001;* neonatal group B Streptococcal cellulitis *Ped Derm 10:58–60, 1993;* Group G streptococcus *Arch Derm 118:934, 1982; Streptococcus zooepidemicus* (Lancefield Group C) - cellulitis *Aust NZ Med 20:177–178, 1990;* Group C streptococcal cellulitis (*S. dysgalactiae*) – pneumonia with chest cellulitis *JAAD 55:S91–92, 2006*

Streptococcus pneumoniae Am J Med 59:293, 1975; Clin Inf Dis 19:149–151, 1994

Streptococcal toxic shock syndrome – painful localized edema and erythema; progression to vesicles and bullae

Subcutaneous phycomycosis (*Basidiobolus haptosporus*) *Ped Derm 5:33–36, 1988; Basidiobolus ranarum* – violaceous indurated plaque of buttocks *Ped Derm 29:121–123, 2012*

Sycosis – deep staphylococcal folliculitis; red plaque studded with pustules *Dermatol Wochenschr 152:153–167, 1966*

Syphilis – secondary – red plaques of soles *JAAD 69:640–642, 2013;* tertiary

Tinea corporis, including *Trichophyton rubrum*, invasive *Cutis 67:457–462, 2001;* neonatal tinea corporis

Tinea capitis – kerion

Tinea faciei – *Trichophyton mentagrophytes* – red plaque of eyelid with pustules *Ped Derm 34:711–712, 2017*

Trichosporon – hyperpigmented and red annular plaque with surface change *JAMADerm 151:1139–1141, 2015*

Trichosporon beigelii AD 129:1020–1023, 1993; neonatal – cellulitis evolving into necrotic ulcer

Vaccinia - progressive vaccinia - cellulitis with bullae *J Clin Inf Dis 25:911–914, 1997*

Vibrio alginolyticus – cellulitis *Acta DV 63:559–560, 1983*

Vibrio vulnificus sepsis – history of travel with water contact; initially begins as cellulitis *Clin Inf Dis 40:718,754–755, 2005; JAAD 24:397–403, 1991; J Infect Dis 149:558–564, 1984*

Viral exanthem

Wasp sting – cellulitis-like plaque *Cutis 105:17–18, 2020*

Whipple's disease – septal panniculitis associated with Whipple's disease *BJD 151:907–911, 2004*

Xanthomonas maltophilia AD 128:702, 1992

Yersinia enterocolitica – cellulitis *J Infect Dis 165:740–743, 1992*

INFILTRATIVE DISORDERS

Amyloidosis – nodular localized primary cutaneous amyloidosis *BJD 145:105–109, 2001;* red plaque of nose – primary cutaneous amyloidosis *AD 143:535–540, 2007;* red plaque of glans penis – nodular amyloidosis *BJD 171:1245–1247, 2014;* lichen amyloidosis

Chronic neutrophilic plaques - hands *Acta DV (Stockh)69:415–418, 1989*

Erdheim-Chester disease – annular erythematous plaques *BJD 182:405–409, 2020*

Generalized eruptive histiocytosis – ameboid pink plaques of legs *The Dermatologist Dec 2015:pp39–42*

Jessner's lymphocytic infiltrate

Langerhans cell histiocytosis – in adult – eroded submammary bright red plaques – adult Langerhans cell histiocytosis *JAMADerm 150:1105–1106, 2014;* ulcerated red plaque of groin; eosinophilic granuloma

Lichen myxedematosus (papular mucinosis)

Lymphocytoma cutis - personal observation

Lymphoplasmacytic plaque of children – red-brown plaque of ankle *Ped Derm 31:515–516, 2014; AD 146:95–96, 2010; AD 145:299–302, 2009*

Mastocytoma

Mucinosis - plaque-like erythema with milia: a noninfectious dermal mucinosis mimicking cryptococcal cellulitis in a renal transplant recipient *JAAD 39:334–337, 1998;* follicular mucinosis (alopecia mucinosa) *JAAD 62:139–141, 2010; Dermatology 197:178–180, 1998; AD 125:287–292, 1989; JAAD 10:760–768, 1984*

Myxedema, localized pretibial; red, pink, or purple plaques *AD 145:1053–1058, 2009; Am J Clin Dermatol 6:295–309, 2005*

New England Dermatological Society Conference, Sept 15, 2007; J Clin Endocrinol Metab 87:438–461, 2002

Nodular eosinophilic infiltration *JAAD 24:352–355, 1991*

Plasma cell (Zoon's) balanitis – red plaque of glans penis *J Drugs Dermatol 6:532–533, 2007; J Urol 153:424–426, 1995;* plasma cell vulvitis – red plaque *JAAD 19:947–950, 1988;* Zoon's mucositis – perianal moist red plaque *JAMADerm 150:447–448, 2014* Zoon's mucositis

Plasmacytosis, primary cutaneous – red-brown to violaceous macules and plaques of extremities; associated with polyclonal hypergammaglobulinemia *Cutis 86:143–147, 2010*

Pretibial lymphoplasmacytic plaque – irregular reddish-brown plaque of children *AD 46:95–96, 2010;* aka benign primary cutaneous plasmacytosis *AD 145:299–302, 2009*

Rosai-Dorfman disease (non-Langerhans cell histiocytosis)(sinus histiocytosis with massive lymphadenopathy) – violaceous, red plaques; cervical lymphadenopathy; also axillary, inguinal, and mediastinal adenopathy *JAMADerm 150:177-18, 2014; AD 145:571–574, 2009; JAAD 41:335–337, 1999; Am J Dermatopathol 17:384–388, 1995; Cancer 30:1174–1188, 1972;* red patches and plaques of back and upper extremities *AD 143:736–740, 2007;* red plaque with multinodular areas *JAAD 65:890–892, 2011; JAAD 49:139–143, 2003*

Verruciform xanthoma *Ped Derm 37:355–357, 2020*

INFLAMMATORY DISEASE

Annular atrophic panniculitis of the ankles (lipophagic panniculitis of childhood) – nodules, plaques, and atrophy of the ankles; lobular panniculitis *Ped Derm 28:146–148, 2011; AD 146:877–881, 2010;* annular atrophy of the ankles or dorsal foot) – red nodules and red plaques of extremities

Atypical lymphocytic lobular panniculitis (T-cell dyscrasia) – spontaneously resolves; red plaques and nodules of arms and legs with associated edema; identical presentation as subcutaneous panniculitis-like T-cell lymphoma with hemophagocytosis *JAAD 61:875–881, 2009; J Cutan Pthol 31:300–306, 2004*

Crohn's disease - metastatic Crohn's disease – red papules and plaques with overlying scale/crust; red scaly plaque with shallow ulcer; red plaques and nodules; abscess-like lesions *JAAD 71:804–813, 2014; J Eur Acad Dermatol Venereol 15:343–345, 2001; J Eur Acad Dermatol Venereol 12:65–66, 1999; AD 132:928–932, 1996; JAAD 36:986–988, 1996; JAAD 10:33–38, 1984;* perianal red plaque *JAAD 41:476–479, 1999*

Cryoglobulinemia – with vasculitis *Dtsch Med Wochennschr 119:1239–1242, 1994*

Dissecting cellulitis of the scalp - mimicking infectious cellulitis *Ann Int Med 142:47–55, 2005*

Eosinophilic cellulitis - mimicking infectious cellulitis *Ann Int Med 142:47–55, 2005; Int J Dermatol 42:62–67, 2003; Int J*

Dermatol40:148–152, 2001; red plaques of breast *AD 148:990–992, 2012*

Eosinophilic cellulitis-like lesions associated with eosinophilic myositis *AD 133:203–206, 1997;* annular plaque with pustules *JAAD 51:S71–73, 2004*

Eosinophilic panniculitis – cellulitis-like *JAAD 34:229–234, 1996*

Eosinophilic pustular folliculitis – red plaque with pustules *JAAD 46:S153–155, 2002*

Erythema multiforme

Erythema nodosum – cellulitis-like *Ann Int Med 142:47–55, 2005*

Folliculitis decalvans

Hidradenitis suppurativa - mimicking infectious cellulitis *Ann Int Med 142:47–55, 2005*

IgG4 disease – multisystem inflammatory disease with papules, plaques, and nodules; parotitis with parotid gland swelling, lacrimal gland swelling, dacryoadenitis, sialadenitis, proptosis; idiopathic pancreatitis, retroperitoneal fibrosis, aortitis; Mikuliczs syndrome, angiolymphadenopathy with eosinophilia, Riedel's thyroiditis, biliary tract disease, renal disease, meningeal disease, pituitary gland; Kuttner tumor, Rosai-Dorfman disease; elevated IgG4 with plasma cell dyscrasia, diffuse or localized swelling or masses; lymphocytic and plasma cell infiltrates with storiform fibrosis *JAAD 75:177–185, 2016; JAAD 75:197–202, 2016*

Interstitial granulomatous dermatitis with arthritis – plaques (aka linear rheumatoid nodule, railway track dermatitis, linear granuloma annulare) – red, linear plaques with arthritis

JAAD 46:892–899, 2002; annular erythematous plaques of medial thighs, lateral chest, abdomen *JAMA Derm 149:626–627, 2013;*

AD 140:353–358, 2004

Kikuchi's disease (histiocytic necrotizing lymphadenitis) – red papules of face, back, arms; red plaques; erythema and acneiform lesions of face; morbilliform, urticarial, and rubella-like exanthems; red or ulcerated pharynx; cervical adenopathy; associations with SLE, lymphoma, tuberculous adenitis, viral lymphadenitis, infectious mononucleosis, and drug eruptions *AD 142:641-646, 2006; BJD 144:885–889, 2001; JAAD 36:342–346, 1997; Surg Pathol 14:872–876, 1990*

Lymphocytoma cutis

Lymphomatoid granulomatosis – pink plaques *AD 139:803–808, 2003*

Midline granuloma - presenting as orbital cellulitis *Graefes Arch Clin Exp Ophthalmol 234:137–139, 1996*

Neutrophilic dermatosis of the dorsal hands (variant of Sweet's syndrome) – ulcerative violaceous plaques *AD 142:57–63, 2006*

Neutrophilic eccrine hidradenitis - Ara-C, doxorubicin, erythro, cyclophosphamide *JAAD 28:775–776, 1993; AD 129:791–792, 1993; JAAD 35:819–822, 1996; JAAD 38:1–17, 1998; JAAD 11:584, 1984; AD 118:263–266, 1982;* childhood variant – plantar red plaque

Neutrophilic sebaceous adenitis – annular expanding red plaques of face and back with fever, lymphadenopathy *JAMADerm 150:1225–1226, AD 129:910–911, 1993*

Panniculitis – Weber-Christian disease, cytophagic histiocytic panniculitis, post-steroid panniculitis all mimicking cellulitis *Ann Int Med 142:47–55, 2005;* various types; cellulitis-like red plaque; pancreatic panniculitis *Ann Int Med 142:47–55, 2005; JAAD 45:325–361, 2001; JAAD 31:379–383, 1994*

Panniculitis, granulomatous – in Sjogren's syndrome; red nodules and plaques *AD 144:815–816, 2008*

Plasma cell granuloma (cutaneous inflammatory pseudotumor) *BJD 144:1271–1273, 2001*

Pseudolymphoma – CD 8+ pseudolymphoma in HIV disease *JAAD 49:139–141, 2003*

Pyoderma gangrenosum *NEJM 350:904–912, 2004*

Sarcoid – red pretibial plaques with atrophic scars, telangiectasias, venous prominence *JAMADerm 154:955–956, 2018*; mimicking infectious cellulitis *Ann Int Med 142:47–55, 2005; Am Fam Physician 65:1581–1584, 2002;* red plaques of scalp with scarring alopecia *JAAD 59:143–145, 2008*

Subacute migratory nodular panniculitis (Villanova)(erythema nodosum migrans) – red leg plaque *AD 128:1643–1648, 1992; Cutis 54:383–385, 1994; Acta DV (Stockh) 53:313–317, 1973; AD 89:170–179, 1964*

Subcutaneous fat necrosis of the newborn – cellulitis-like *AD 117:36–37, 1981; AD 134:425–426, 1998;* erythematous nodular plaque of back *BJD 160:423–425, 2009*

METABOLIC

Alpha-1 antitrypsin deficiency panniculitis – red plaque, ulcerated nodule; trunk and proximal extremities *BJD 174:753–762, 2016; Cutis 93:303–306, 2014; JAAD 51:645–655, 2004; JAAD 45:325–361, 2001;* cellulitis-like *JAAD 18:684–692, 1988*

Alpha heavy chain disease *AD 122:1243–1244, 1986*

Calciphylaxis – early erythema mimicking cellulitis *Ann Int Med 142:47–55, 2005; Kidney Int 61:2210–2217, 2002; AD 131:638–638, 1995*

Carbamyl phosphate synthetase deficiency

Citrullinemia - moist red scaly plaques on genitalia, abdomen, buttocks, and perioral skin

Congenital disorders of glycosylation (CDG-IIc)(Rambam-Hasharon syndrome) – GDP-L-fucose AKA leukocyte adhesion deficiency type 2 (LAD 2); localized cellulitis, neurologic abnormalities, distinctive facies, short stature *Ped Derm 22:457–460, 2005*

Cryoglobulinemia

Diabetes mellitus – erysipelas-like erythema of legs or feet *Acta Med Scand 196:333–342, 1974;* diabetic muscle infarction – swelling of thigh *AD 143:1456–1457, 2007; Diabetalogica 1:39–42, 1965*

Extramedullary hematopoiesis *QJMed 6:253–270, 1937*

Gamma heavy chain disease *AD 124:1538–1540, 1988*

Gouty arthritis – cellulitis-like *Ann Int Med 142:47–55, 2005*

Necrobiosis lipoidica diabeticorum – starts as red plaque *JAMA 311:2328, 2014; Int J Derm 33:605–617, 1994; JAAD 18:530–537, 1988*

Nephrogenic systemic fibrosis *JAAD 48:55–60, 2003*

Paroxysmal nocturnal hemoglobinuria – petechiae, ecchymoses, red plaques which become hemorrhagic bullae with necrosis; lesions occur on legs, abdomen, chest, nose, and ears; deficiency of enzymes – decay-accelerating factor (DAF) and membrane inhibitor of reactive lysis (MIRL) *AD 138:831–836, 2002*

Porokeratosis of Mibelli – pink plaque of forearm *AD 145:91–92, 2009*

Pruritic urticarial papules and plaques of pregnancy

Sickle cell disease *Oral Dis 7:306–309, 2001*

Spherocytosis – pseudoerysipelas due to recurrent hemolysis *JAAD 51:1019–1023, 2004*

Waldenstrom's macroglobulinemia – red-brown to violaceous plaques *JAAD 45:S202–206, 2001*

NEOPLASTIC DISEASES

Actinic reticuloid

Adenosquamous carcinoma of the skin – red keratotic papule or plaque of head, neck, or shoulder; extensive local invasion *AD 145:1152–1158, 2009*

Aggressive intranasal carcinoma *Cutis 42:288–293, 1988*

Anal intraepithelial neoplasia – perianal hyperpigmented patches, white and/or red plaques *JAAD 52:603–608, 2005*

Angiosarcoma - indurated red plaque of cheek and nose *JAAD 54:883–885, 2006;* red plaques of face and scalp *BJD 169:204–206, 2013;* cutaneous radiation-associated angiosarcoma of the breast – livedoid violaceous plaques with nodules of the breast *JAMA Derm 149:973–974, 2013;* ulcerated red plaque with eschar *JAMA 314:1169–1170, 2015; AD 143:75–77, 2007; J Eur Acad Dermatol Venereol 17:594–595, 2003; AD 138:831–836, 2002; JAAD 38:837–840, 1998; AD 133:1303–1308, 1997; JAAD 34:308–310, 1996; AD 128:1115, 1992;* of face and scalp - bruise-like *Sem Cut Med Surg 21:159–165, 2002; JAAD 38:143–175, 1998; JAAD 34:308–310, 1996; AD 128:115–120, 1990;* of face and scalp *JAAD 38:143–175, 1998;* angiosarcoma secondary to radiation of hemangioma - violaceous *JAAD 33:865–870, 1995;* erysipelas-like *Cancer 77:2400–2406, 1996;* congenital fatal angiosarcoma – violaceous *Soc Ped Derm Annual Meeting, July 2005*

Apocrine carcinoma - carcinoma erysipelatoides (red plaque of head and neck) *AD 147:1335–1337, 2011;* metastatic apocrine adenocarcinoma – red plaque of axilla *JAMADerm 152:111–113, 2016*

Apocrine hamartoma *Ped Derm 12:248–251, 1995*

Atypical granular cell schwannoma – oval red ulcerated plaque *Ped Derm 31:729–731, 2014*

Basaloid squamous cell carcinoma of the skin – ulcerated plaque of inguinal crease; necrotic linear ulcer of inguinal crease *JAAD 64:144–151, 2011*

Blastic plasmacytoid dendritic cell neoplasm – confluent brown-red plaques of trunk *BJD 169:579–586, 2013;* red plaques of temple *Ped Derm 32:283–284, 2015; Am J Surg Pathol 34:75–87, 2010*

Bowen's disease *JAAD 54:369–391, 2006;* perianal Bowen's disease *Ped Derm 27:166–169, 2010;* Bowen's disease of the penis – red plaque *JAAD 66:867–880, 2012*

Bowenoid papulosis - personal observation

Carcinoma erysipelatoides - mimicking infectious cellulitis *JAAD 67:177–185, 2012; Ann Int Med 142:47–55, 2005; J R Soc Med 78:Suppl 11:43–45, 1985; AD 113:69–70, 1977;* metastases *JAAD 29:228–236, 1993;* carcinoma erysipelatoides - includes metastases from breast, lung, melanoma *AD 147:1215–1220, 2011; NEJM 350:904–912, 2004; Forum Clin Oncol 1:76–79, 2002; Ann DV 120:831–833, 1993;* carcinoma erysipelatoides – violaceous plaques of neck and upper chest *AD 147:345–350, 2011;* ovary, stomach, tonsils, pancreas, kidney, rectum, colon, parotid, uterus *JAAD 43:733–751, 2000; JAAD 39:876–878, 1998; JAAD 33:161–182, 1995; JAAD 30:304–307, 1994; JAAD 31:877–880, 1994;* larynx *Eur J Dermatol 11:124–126, 2001;* prostate carcinoma *Cutis 65:215–216, 2000;* squamous cell carcinoma *Br J Plast surg 44:622–623, 1991;* gastric adenocarcinoma *Cutis 76:194–196, 2005;* prostate *JAAD 53:744–745, 2005;* peristomal red plaque with ulcers – metastatic adenocarcinoma of the rectum *AD 142:1372–1373, 2006;* adenocarcinoma presenting as cellulitis *Cutis 85:72, 2010;* hemangioma-like metastatic adenocarcinoma of the lung *AD 148:1317–1322, 2012*

Carcinosarcoma – ulcerated nodule or red plaque of scalp *Cutis 92:247–249, 2013*

Castleman's disease, including multicentric Castleman's disease *JAMADerm 153:449–452, 2017*

CD4+/CD56+ hematodermic neoplasm ("blastic natural killer cell lymphoma"; blastic plasmacytoid dendritic cell neoplasm) – red-brown facial plaque *AD 146:1167–1172, 2010*

CD 30+ lymphoproliferative disorders – red tumors, red plaques with or without necrosis, giant tumor *JAAD 72:508–515, 2015*

Clear cell acanthoma (velvety plaque) *JAAD 21:313–315, 1989*

Connective tissue nevus; purplish verrucous plantar plaque *BJD 146:164–165, 2002;* familial cutaneous collagenomas; mutations in *LEMD3* – pink oval plaques *BJD 156:375–377, 2007*

Cutaneous epithelioid sarcoma-like hemangioendothelioma – red plaque of foot *AD 149:459–465, 2013*

Dermatofibroma – congenital multiple clustered dermatofibroma - red plaque and papules *BJD 142:1040–1043, 2000; Ann DV 111:163–164, 1984*

Dermal dendritic hamartoma - personal observation

Dermatofibrosarcoma protuberans *JAAD 53:76–83, 2005;* congenital – annular red plaque, pink alopecic plaque, red macule, blue plaque, hypopigmented plaque *Ped Derm 25:317–325, 2008; AD 143:203–210, 2007;* Bednar tumor (pigmented dermatofibrosarcoma protuberans) – brown plaque *JAAD 40:315–317, 1999*

Dermatomyofibroma – red or tan nodule or plaque *Ped Derm 34:347–351, 2017; JAAD 46:477–490, 2002; Ped Derm 16:154–156, 1999*

Eccrine angiomatous hamartoma *AD 142:1351–1356, 2006;* red plaque of palm *Ped Derm 27:548–549, 2010;* congenital red plaques and papules of arm *Ped Derm 32:285–286, 2015;* congenital red-brown papules and plaques *Ped Derm 36:909–912, 2019*

Eccrine porocarcinoma – cobblestoned red plaque *JAAD 76:S73–75, 2017; Dermatol Ther 21:433–438, 2008; JAAD 35:860–864, 1996*

Eccrine syringofibroadenomas

Epidermoid cyst, ruptured - personal observation

Erythroplasia, oral – underside of tongue, floor of mouth, soft palate *J Oral Pathol 12:11–29, 1983*

Erythroplasia of Queyrat *JAAD 54:369–391, 2006; JID 115:396–401, 2000; Urology 8:311–315, 1976; Bull Soc Fr Dermatol Syphiligr 22:378–382, 1911*

Extramammary Paget's disease – underpants-pattern erythema *Sem Cut Med Surg 21:159–165, 2002; JAAD 40:966–978, 1999; JAAD 13:84–90, 1985;* of inguinal crease and scrotum *BJD 153:676–677, 2005;* red plaque of scrotum or vulva *JAMADerm 153:689–693, 2017; JAAD 67:327–328, 2012; JAAD 65:656–657, 2011; JAAD 57:S43–45, 2007;* red plaque of penis and pubis *AD 147:704–708, 2011;* red plaque of penis and scrotum and intertrigo *Cutis 94:35–38, 2014;* red plaque of pubis *Cutis 95:109–112, 2015;* red psoriasiform plaque of pubic area *Cutis 95:132,135–136, 2015*

Extramedullary hematopoiesis in chronic idiopathic myelofibrosis with myelodysplasia – ulcerated red plaque *JAAD 55:S28–31, 2006*

Fat-storing hamartoma of dermal dendrocytes – red-brown plaque of papules and nodules of lumbosacral area *AD 126:794–796, 1990*

Fibroepithelioma of Pinkus - personal observation

Fibrous hamartoma of infancy – red plaque of buttock *JAMA Derm 149:629–630, 2013*

Hyperkeratotic lichen planus-like reactions combined with infundibulocystic hyperplasia *AD 140:1262–1267, 2004*

Infantile myofibromatosis *Ped Derm 5:37–46, 1988; AD 134:625–630, 1998*

Kaposi's sarcoma *JAAD 59:179–206, 2008;* eruptive Kaposi's sarcoma *Cutis 87:34–38, 2011*

Keloid

Keratoacanthoma – Grzybowski type

Langerhans cell histiocytosis with leukemia

Large cell acanthoma

Leukemia cutis – violaceous plaques of skin and oral mucosa *Cutis 104:326–330, 2019; JAAD 44:365–369, 2001; Acta DV 78:198–200, 1998;* B-cell leukemia cutis *JAAD 33:341–345, 1995;* carcinoma erysipelatoides *JAAD 40:966–978, 1999;* leukemic infiltrates of breast *JAAD 43:733–751, 2000;* acute myelogenous leukemia – red-brown plaques of lower legs *JAAD 49:128–129, 2003;* acute promyelocytic leukemia – necrotic red plaques *AD 143:1220–1221, 2007;* eosinophilic leukemia *AD 140:584–588, 2004;* T-cell prolymphocytic leukemia – mimicking cellulitis *Ann Int Med 142:47–55, 2005;* HTLV-1 (acute T-cell leukemia) *JAAD 49:979–1000, 2003;* neonatal aleukemic leukemia cutis; natural killer cell CD 56- large granular lymphocytic leukemia – purpuric ulcerated plaques *JAAD 62:496–501, 2010;* leukemia/lymphoma – adult T-cell leukemia/ lymphoma – large red plaques of buttocks *BJD 165:437–439, 2011;* cutaneous precursor B-cell acute lymphoblastic leukemia – painful swollen red cheek *JAMA Derm 149:609–614, 2013;* plasma cell leukemia *J Drugs Dermatol 13:994–995, 2014*

Lymphangiosarcoma (Stewart-Treves tumor) – red-brown or ecchymotic patch, nodules, plaques in lymphedematous limb; edematous arm within violaceous plaque with nodules *NEJM 359:950, 2008; Cancer 1:64–81, 1948*

Lymphoma – cutaneous T-cell lymphoma, including folliculotropic CTCL *JAAD 70:205–220, 2014;* syringotropic cutaneous T-cell lymphoma – red plaques, leg ulcers, comedo-like lesions, palmoplantar hyperkeratosis *JAAD 71:926–934, 2014; JAAD 61:133–138, 2009;* primary cutaneous peripheral T-cell lymphoma – purpuric plaques *BJD 164:677–679, 2011;* granulomatous cutaneous T-cell lymphoma – violaceous plaques *JAAD 69:366–374, 2013; AD 144:1609–1617, 2008;* palmoplantar CTCL *AD 143109–114, 2007; AD 131:1052–1056, 1995; ;* CD8+ granulomatous cutaneous T-cell lymphoma associated with immunodeficiency – violaceous papules and nodules with psoriasiform scale; red plaques and tumors *JAAD 71:555–560, 2014;* subcutaneous panniculitic T-cell lymphoma – red plaques and nodules of arms and legs with edema of legs *The Dermatologist October 2014; pp.42–44; BJD 171:891–894, 2014; The Dermatologist, October 2014, pp.42–44; JAAD 61:875–881, 2009; BJD 149:542–553, 2003; JAAD 45:325–361, 2001;* red plaque of trunk *JAAD 72:21–34, 2015;* primary cutaneous epidermotropic CD8+ T-cell lymphoma – mixture of patches, plaques, papulonodules with central ulceration, necrosis, and hemorrhage *JAAD 62:300–307, 2010;* primary cutaneous follicle center lymphoma with diffuse CD30 expression – papules, plaques, nodules, multilobulated scalp tumor *JAAD 71:548–554, 2014;* angiotrophic lymphoma (violaceous) *JAAD 26:101–104, 1992; JAAD 21:727–733, 1989;* primary CD30+ anaplastic large cell lymphoma – solitary red plaque/nodule of back *AD 143:417–422, 2007;* folliculotropic CTCL – red plaques of head and neck; periauricular lesions; comedo-like, acneiform, cystic lesions, keratotic follicular papules *JAAD 62:418–426, 2010;* B-cell lymphoma; granulomatous slack skin syndrome (CTCL); HTLV-1 leukemia/lymphoma – nodulotumoral lesions, nodules, ulcerated nodules, multipapular lesions, red plaques, red patches, erythroderma *JAAD 72:293–301, 2015; Blood 117:3961–3967, 2011; BJD 128:483–492, 1993; Am J Med 84:919–928, 1988;* large cell lymphoma *JAAD 25: 912–915, 1991;* CD30+ anaplastic large cell lymphoma – ulcerated red plaque *BJD 157:1291–1293, 2007;*

lymphomatoid granulomatosis - red, brown, or violaceous plaques with epidermal atrophy and purpura *JAAD 20:571–578, 1989; AD 124:571–576, 1988* primary cutaneous B-cell lymphoma *JAAD 62:173–176, 2010;* immunocytoma (low grade B-cell lymphoma) – reddish-brown papules, red nodules, plaques and/or tumors on the extremities *JAAD 44:324–329, 2001;* B-cell lymphoma overlying acrodermatitis chronica atrophicans associated with *Borrelia burgdorferi* infection *JAAD 24:584–590, 1991;* primary skeletal muscle lymphoma with cellulitis-like appearance *Ann Int Med 142:47–55, 2005; Cutis 68:233–236, 2001;* NK/T-cell lymphoma *Ped Derm Meeting of AAD, March, 2000;* blastoid nasal T/natural killer-cell lymphoma *BJD 146:700–703, 2002;* primary cutaneous blastic NK-cell lymphoma of forehead – violaceous pearly edematous plaque with pseudovesicular appearance *JAAD 53:742–743, 2005;* peripheral T-cell/NK-cell lymphoma - erysipelas-like erythema with violaceous nodule *Cutis 81:33–36, 2008;* intravascular B-cell lymphoma (malignant angioendotheliomatosis) – purple plaques; red plaques with telangiectasias; painful gray-brown, red, blue-livid patches, plaques, nodules, with telangiectasia and underlying induration; 40% of patients with intravascular lymphoma present with cutaneous lesions *BJD 157:16–25, 2007; Cutis 72:137–140, 2003; Cancer 3:1738–1745, 1994;* intravascular cytotoxic T-cell lymphoma – painful gray-brown, red, blue-livid patches, plaques, nodules, with telangiectasia and underlying induration; 40% of patients with intravascular lymphoma present with cutaneous lesions *Cutis 82:267–272, 2008; BJD 157:16–25, 2007; Dermatology, February 2016; Cutis 82:267–272, 2008; JAAD 58:290–294, 2008; BJD 157:16–25, 2007;* Burkitt's lymphoma *JAAD 54:1111–1113, 2006;* plasmablastic lymphoma (HIV and EBV-associated) *BJD 149:889–891, 2003;* Woringer-Kolopp disease (localized pagetoid reticulosis) – red scaly plaques of buttocks *JAAD 61:120–123, 2009; JAAD 58:679–681, 2008; Ann Derm Syphilol 67:945–958, 1939;* red plaque of foot *Cutis 99:311,354–355, 2017; AD 120:1045–1051, 1984;* CD 20+ primary CTCL *BJD 160:894–896, 2009;* annular hyperkeratotic plaques of hands and feet *BJD 163:651–653, 2010;* primary cutaneous marginal B-cell lymphoma – violaceous plaques *JAAD 69:329–340, 2013;* in children *BJD 161:140–147, 2009;* anetodermic primary cutaneous B-cell lymphoma – associated with antiphospholipid antibodies *AD 146:175–182, 2010; Arthritis Rheum 36:133–134, 2010; Clin Exp Dermatol 31:130–131, 2006; Actas Dermosifiligr 94:243–246, 2003; Am J Dermatopathol 23:124–132, 2001; BJD 143:165–170, 2000;* secondary cutaneous marginal zone lymphoma *JAAD 63:142–145, 2010;* CD4+/CD56+ TdT+ haematodermic neoplasm (formerly blastic natural killer cell lymphoma); derived from plasmacytoid dendritic cells *BJD 162:1395–1397, 2010;* gamma-delta T-cell lymphoma – presenting as facial palsy *BJD 164:205–207, 2011;* primary cutaneous follicle center lymphoma, diffuse type (Crosti lymphoma) *JAAD 65:991–1000, 2011;* primary cutaneous follicle center lymphoma *JAAD 69:343–354, 2013;* primary cutaneous follicular helper cell lymphoma - red papules, red plaques, scalp nodule, facial plaques *AD 148:832–839, 2012;* primary cutaneous epidermotropic aggressive CD8+ T-cell lymphoma – red plaques with central necrosis (targetoid); ulcerated nodule *JAAD 67:748–759, 2012;* primary aggressive CD8+ CTCL *JAMADerm 150:320–322, 2014;* cutaneous extranodal natural killer/T-cell lymphoma – black nasal papules; edematous cheek; red plaques of arms *JAAD 70:716–723, 2014;* cutaneous extranodal natural killer T-cell lymphoma – multiple violaceous or red nodules of extremities, subcutaneous nodules, cellulitis, abscess-like lesions *JAAD 70:1002–1009, 2014;* Richter transformation – transformation of chronic lymphocytic leukemia to high grade lymphoma – red nodules and plaques of arm with generalized lymphadenopathy *BJD 172:513–521, 2015;* angioimmunoblastic T-cell lymphoma – red plaque of neck *Cutis 102:179–182, 2018*

Lymphomatoid granulomatosis – Epstein-Barr-related angiocentric T-cell-rich B-cell lymphoproliferative disorder; presents as urticarial dermatitis; papules and dermal nodules with or without ulceration, folliculitis-like lesions, maculopapules, indurated plaques, ulcers *BJD 157:426–429, 2007; JAAD 54:657–663, 2006*

Malignant histiocytosis – multiple erythematous plaques with depigmentation *Am J Dermatopathol 19:299–302, 1997*

Malignant nodular hidradenoma – ulcerated red plaque of back *Cutis 68:273–278, 2001*

Medallion-like dermal dendrocyte hamartoma – red plaque of neck; wrinkled pliable pink-yellow atrophic patch with plucked chicken appearance of lateral neck *Ped Derm 27:638–642, 2010*

Melanocytic nevus - congenital melanocytic nevus *AAD 1997, Ped Derm Section*; giant bathing trunk nevus; brown plaque *BJD 157:99–601, 2007*; congenital nevus - red, white, and blue plaque on flank of newborn mimicking a vascular tumor *Ped Derm 30:749–750, 2013*

Melanoma, amelanotic melanoma *JAAD 62:857–860, 2010; JAAD 27:464–465, 1992*; melanoma erysipelatoides (inflammatory melanoma) *BJD 143:904–906, 2000; JAAD 10:52–55, 1984*; acral lentiginous melanoma; metastatic melanoma – erythematous annular plaques of trunk *AD 148:531–536, 2012*

Merkel cell carcinoma *Cutis 100:103–104,124, 2017*;

mimicking angiosarcoma *AD 123:1368–1370, 1987*

Milia en plaque - face, eyelid, ears, and ear lobes *Ped Derm 15:282–284, 1998*

Mucinous eccrine nevus – red plaque in fold of wrist *Ped Derm 25:573–574, 2008*

Mucinous metaplasia – red plaques of glans penis *BJD 165:1263–1272, 2011*

Multiple myeloma *AD 139:475–486, 2003*; cutaneous crystalline deposits in myeloma *AD 130:484–488, 1994*; face with cellulitis-like appearance

Neurilemmomatosis (multiple neurilemmomatosis) *JAAD 10:744–754, 1984*

Nevus marginatus – red plaque with surrounding hyperpigmented serpiginous verrucous margin; *HRAS* mutation *BJD 168:892–894, 2013*

Nevus sebaceous

Paget's disease - nipple *Ann Int Med 142:47–55, 2005 Surg Gynecol Obstet 123:1010–1014, 1966*; extramammary - perianal *BJD 85:476-480, 1971*; vulvar *Cancer 46:590-594, 1980; Am J Clin Pathol 27:559–566, 1957*

Plantar fibromatosis

Plaque-like myofibroblastic tumor – red to violaceous plaque of back; ulcerated plaque *Ped Derm 34:176–179, 2017; Ped Derm 30:600–607, 2013*

  Differential diagnosis of fibrous tumors
    Dermatofibroma
    Dermatomyofibroma – 1–2 cm red-brown plaques or nodules of neck, arms, upper trunk
    Infantile myofibroma or myofibromatosis – skin-colored to vascular-appearing rubbery nodules of head, neck, trunk, and arms
    Fibrous hamartoma of infancy – 2–5 cm nodule of axilla, shoulders, upper chest
    Infantile digital fibromatosis – pink nodule of dorsal digit
    Desmoid-type fibromatosis – deep-seated nodule of head, neck, extremities, trunk
      Dermatofibrosarcoma protuberans – blue-red nodule of trunk or proximal extremities

Giant cell fibroblastoma – skin-colored nodule or subcutaneous nodules of back or legs

Plasmacytoid dendritic cell neoplasm – purple macules, violaceous papules, nodules, tumefactions; highly pigmented dark red, purpuric, necrotic lesions of face, neck *JAAD 66:278–291, 2012*

Plasmacytosis, cutaneous – multiple red-brown infiltrated plaques and flat tumors; anemia, fever, hypergammaglobulinemia, lymphadenopathy *JAAD 68:978–985, 2013; JAAD 36:876–880, 1997*; pruritic red plaque of arm *Ped Derm 31:387–388, 2014*

Plexiform fibrohistiocytic tumor *Ped Derm 23:71–12, 2006*

Porokeratosis (porokeratosis ptychotropica) *JAAD 60:501–503, 2009; JAAD 55:S120–122, 2006; Cutis 72:391–393, 2003; Clin Exp Dermatol 28:450–452, 2003; BJD 140:553–555, 1999; BJD 132:150–151, 1995*

Porokeratosis of Mibelli – pink-white plaque *AD 145:91–92, 2009; Cutis 79:22,53–54, 2007; JAAD 52:553–555, 2005; Gior Ital d Mal Ven 28:313–355, 1893*

Posttransplant Epstein-Barr virus-associated lymphoproliferative disorder – ulcerated plaques *JAAD 51:778–780, 2004; AD 140:1140–1164, 2004*

Primitive myxoid mesenchymal tumor of infancy – red pedunculated papules within a red plaque *Soc Ped Dermatol Annual Meeting, July, 2006; Am J Surg Pathol 30:388–394, 2006*

Recurrent, self-healing monoclonal plasmablastic infiltrates in HIV *BJD 153:828–832, 2005*

Reticulohistiocytoma of the dorsum (Crosti's syndrome) - B-cell lymphoma

Alveolar rhabdomyosarcoma, metastatic – red multinodular ulcerated plaque *Ped Derm 33:225–226, 2016*

Seborrheic keratosis

Squamous cell carcinoma *JAAD 54:369–391, 2006*; of penis *JAAD 66:867–880, 2012; JAAD 62:284–290, 2010*; squamous cell carcinoma of stump in recessive dystrophic epidermolysis bullosa *BJD 169:208–210, 2013*; squamous cell carcinoma associated with lichen planus – multilobulated, ulcerated, red nodule and plaque *JAAD 71:698–707, 2014*; oral squamous cell carcinoma – white to red oral plaques *JAAD 81:59–71, 2019*

Syringocystadenoma papilliferum

Trichilemmal carcinoma *JAAD 36:107–109, 1997*

Verrucous acanthoma

Verrucous carcinoma – genital red plaque

Waldenstrom's macroglobulinemia (macroglobulinosis) – red-brown to violaceous plaques, macules, or papulonodules; neoplastic B-cell infiltration *Ann DV 129:53–55, 2002; JAAD 45:S202–206, 2001; AD 124:1851–1856, 1988; Ann DV 112:509–516, 1985; BJD 106:217–222, 1982*; macroglobulinosis – ulcerated nodules and plaques with central necrosis; skin-colored papules of dorsal hands with central crusts *AD 146:165–169, 2010*

PARANEOPLASTIC DISEASES

Eosinophilic dermatosis of myeloproliferative disease – red papules, face, scalp; scaly red nodules; trunk – red nodules; extremities – red nodules and hemorrhagic papules *JAAD 81:246–249, 2019; AD 137:1378–1380, 2001*

Insect bite-like reactions associated with hematologic malignancies *AD 135:1503–1507, 1999*

Interstitial granulomatous dermatitis – annular red-brown plaque of back; associated with myeloma *Trichosporon* – hyperpigmented and red annular plaque with surface change *JAMADerm 151:1141–1142, 2015*

Necrobiotic xanthogranuloma with paraproteinemia *Medicine (Baltimore) 65:376–388, 1986*

Necrolytic migratory erythema (glucagonoma syndrome) – necrotic crusted plaques of legs *BJD 174:1092–1095, 2016*

Neutrophilic dermatosis associated with cutaneous T-cell lymphoma *AD 141:353–356, 2005*

Neutrophilic panniculitis associated with myelodysplastic syndrome *JAAD 50:280–285, 2004*

Paraneoplastic pemphigus

Superficial migratory thrombophlebitis – "pseudocellulitis"; red plaques of legs; paraneoplastic *J Clin Aesth Dermatol 10:49–51, 2017*

Wells' syndrome – associated with lung cancer *BJD 145:678–679, 2001;* anal squamous cell carcinoma *Acta DV (Stockh)66:213–219, 1986;* nasopharyngeal carcinoma *Ann DV 111:777–778, 1984*

PHOTODERMATOSES

Actinic granuloma

Actinic prurigo - red plaques on arms

Actinic reticuloid *JAAD 38:877–905, 1998*

Polymorphic light eruption

Solar elastotic bands – red plaques of forearms *JAAD 49:1193–1195, 2003*

Spring and summer eruptions of the elbows – form of polymorphic light eruption; papules and plaques of elbows *JAAD 68:306–312, 2013*

PRIMARY CUTANEOUS DISEASE

Acne rosacea

Axillary (intertrigenous) granular hyperkeratosis *JAAD 39:495–496, 1998*

Circumscribed palmar hypokeratosis – atrophic pink patches and plaques of palms *JAAD 57:285–291, 2007; JAAD 47:21–27, 2002*

Digitate dermatosis - personal observation

Eosinophilic fasciitis

Eosinophilic pustular folliculitis (Ofuji's disease) – sterile papules, pustules, and plaques of face, trunk, arms, palms, soles *JAAD 23:1012–1014, 1990; JAAD 14:469–474, 1986*

Epidermolysis bullosa pruriginosa (DDEB) – atrophic skin with erosions, hypertrophic scarring, hypopigmentation, and linear scars *JAAD 56:S77–81, 2007*

Erythema elevatum diutinum – red or violaceous plaques over lower legs *JAMADerm 152:331–332, 2016; BJD 159:733–735, 2008; Hautarzt 48:113–117, 1997; JAAD 26:38–44, 1992; Medicine (Baltimore) 56:443–455, 1977;* in AIDS *Cutis 68:41–42, 55, 2001;* mimicking Kaposi's sarcoma in AIDS *AD 127:1819–1822, 1991;* red-brown plaques of fingers and knees *JAAD 65:469–471, 2011*

Erythrokeratoderma variabilis (Mendes da Costa syndrome) – autosomal dominant – dark red fixed plaques with transient polycyclic red macules with fine scale *Ped Derm 23:382–385, 2006; JID 113:1119–1122, 1999; Ped Derm 12:351–354, 1995*

Febrile ulceronecrotic Mucha-Habermann disease – dusky plaque with bullae *Ped Derm 29:135–140, 2012;* crusted ulcerated red

plaques; diarrhea, pulmonary involvement, abdominal pain, CNS symptoms, arthritis *Ped Derm 29:53–58, 2012*

Granuloma annulare, generalized *JAAD 20:39–47, 1989*

Granuloma faciale - red, brown, violaceous, yellowish *JAAD 53:1002–1009, 2005;* extrafacial *BJD 145:360–362, 2001*

Granuloma multiforme – upper trunk and arms; papules evolving into annular plaques with geographical, polycyclic borders; heal centrally with depigmented macules; Central Africa

Hailey-Hailey disease - personal observation

Lichen myxedematosus - personal observation

Lichen planus – lichen planus actinicus – violaeous plaques of dorsal hands *JAMADerm 151:1121–1122, 2015;* annular lichen planus *Cutis 100:199, 2017*

Lichen planus follicularis tumidus – brown-violaceous acral plaques, cysts, milia, comedonal openings *Clin Exp Dermatol 45:638–641, 2020*

Lichen sclerosus et atrophicus

Lichen simplex chronicus

Malakoplakia *JAAD 30:834–836, 1994;* granulomatous plaque *JAAD 23:947–948, 1990*

Miescher's granuloma

Necrolytic acral erythema – acral hyperkeratotic hyperpigmented plaques with red to violaceous centers *Ped Derm 28:701–706, 2011*

Neutrophilic dermatosis of the dorsal hands *AD 142:57–63, 2006*

Nummular dermatitis

Parapsoriasis en plaque *JAAD 5:373–395, 1981*

Pityriasis rosea *JAAD 15:159–167, 1986*

Pityriasis rubra pilaris

Poikiloderma vasculare atrophicans

Prurigo pigmentosa – urticarial red pruritic papules, papulovesicles, vesicles, and plaques with reticulated hyperpigmentation *JAAD 55:131–136, 2006; Cutis 63:99–102, 1999; BJD 120:705–708, 1989; AD 125:1551–1554, 1989; JAAD 12:165–169, 1985*

Psoriasis *JAAD 65:137–174, 2011*

Pyoderma vegetans

Seborrheic dermatitis – scalp; genitalia

Scleredema of Buschke (pseudoscleroderma) – in diabetics, preceded by erythema; cellulitis-like *Clin Exp Dermatol 14:385–386, 1989*

Superficial granulomatous pyoderma

Symmetrical lividity of the palms and soles *Int J Dermatol 17:739–744, 1978*

Syringolymphoid hyperplasia *JAAD 49:1177–1180, 2003*

PSYCHOCUTANEOUS DISEASES

Factitial panniculitis *JAAD 45:325–361, 2001;* factitial dermatitis – red facial plaque *Ped Derm 24:327–329, 2007*

SYNDROMES

Acute anterior tibial compartment syndrome – cellulitis-like *JAAD 34:521–522, 1996*

Aesop syndrome – extensive red violaceous skin patch or plaque of chest overlying a solitary bone plasmacytoma with regional adenopathy; dermal mucin and vascular hyperplasia (mucinous angiomatosis) *JAAD 55:909–910, 2006; Medicine 82:51–59, 2003;*

JAAD 40:808–812, 1999; JAAD 21:1061–1068, 1989; J Neurol Neurosurgery Psychiatry 41:177–184, 1978; Br J Dis Chest 68:65–70, 1974; due to malignant blue cell tumor *AD 148:1431-1437, 2012*

Albright's hereditary osteodystrophy (pseudohypoparathyroidism) - osteomas

Ataxia telangiectasia – cutaneous granulomas present as papules or nodules, red plaques with atrophy or ulceration; telangiectasias of bulbar conjunctivae, tip of nose, ears, antecubital and popliteal fossae, dorsal hands and feet; atrophy with mottled hypo- and hyperpigmentation, dermatomal CALMs, photosensitivity, canities, acanthosis nigricans, dermatitis *JAAD 56:541–564, 2007; Clin in Dermatol 23:68–77, 2005; AD 134:1145–1150, 1998; JAAD 10:431–438, 1984*

Buschke-Ollendorff syndrome

Blau or Jabs syndrome (familial juvenile systemic granulomatosis) – autosomal dominant; translucent skin-colored papules (noncaseating granulomas) of trunk and extremities with uveitis, synovitis, symmetric polyarthritis; polyarteritis, multiple synovial cysts; red papular rash in early childhood; camptodactyly (flexion contractures of PIP joints); uveitis, iritis, vitritis, closed-angle glaucoma; mutations in NOD2 (nucleotide-binding oligomerization domain 2)(caspase recruitment domain family, member 15; *CARD* 15) *JAAD 68:834–853, 2013; AD 143:386–391, 2007; Clin Exp Dermatol 21:445–448, 1996;* chromosome 16p12-q21 *JAAD 49:299–302, 2003; Am J Hum Genet 76:217–221, 1998; Am J Hum Genet 59:1097–1107, 1996*

CANDLE syndrome (chronic atypical neutrophilic dermatitis with lipodystrophy and elevated temperature) – early onset periodic fevers, generalized annular erythematous or violaceous plaques, edema of eyelids, progressive facial lipodystrophy, arthralgia, delayed physical development; mutations in *PSMB8* (proteasome subunit beta type 8) *JAAD 68:834–853, 2013; JAAD 62:489–495, 2010*

Epidermodysplasia verruciformis *AD 131:1312–1318, 1995*

Farber's disease (disseminated lipogranulomatosis) – red papules and nodules of joints and tendons of hands and feet; deforming arthritis; papules, plaques, and nodules of ears, back of scalp and trunk *Am J Dis Child 84:449–500, 1952*

Familial eosinophilic cellulitis, short stature, dysmorphic habitus, and mental retardation - bullae, vesicles, and red plaques *JAAD 38:919–928, 1998*

Familial Hibernian fever – mimicking infectious cellulitis *Ann Int Med 142:47–55, 2005; QJMed 51:469–480, 1982*

Familial Mediterranean fever - autosomal recessive; erysipelas-like erythema - mutation in pyrin/marenostrin *JAAD 67:177–185, 2012; JAAD 42:791–795, 2000; AD 136:1487–1494, 2000;* mimicking infectious cellulitis *Ann Int Med 142:47–55, 2005; Isr Med Assoc J 1:31–36, 1999; Q J Med 75:607–616, 1990;* annular recurrent plaque of buttocks *Clin Inf Dis 58:1273–1338, 2014*

Fanconi's anemia – autosomal recessive; endocrine abnormalities with hypothyroidism, decreased growth hormone, diabetes mellitus, café au lait macules, diffuse hyperpigmented macules, guttate hypopigmented macules, intertriginous hyperpigmentation, skeletal anomalies (thumb hypoplasia, absent thumbs, radii, carpal bones), oral/genital erythroplasia with development of squamous cell carcinoma, hepatic tumors, microphthalmia, ectopic or horseshoe kidney, broad nose, epicanthal folds, micrognathia, bone marrow failure, acute myelogenous leukemia, solid organ malignancies *JAAD 54:1056–1059, 2006*

Glucagonoma syndrome – cellulitis-like *Ann Int Med 142:47–55, 2005*

Goltz's syndrome

Hermansky-Pudlak syndrome – mucocutaneous granulomatous disease in Hermansky-Pudlak syndrome; butterfly red plaques of face; linear ulcers of groin and vulva; pink plaques of thighs; swollen vulva; indurated nodules of vulva; axillary ulcers, red face *JAMADerm 150:1083–1087, 2014*

Histiophagocytic syndrome – parvovirus B19-induced histiophagocytic syndrome in systemic lupus erythematosus; violaceous plaques and erythema of scalp, face, and back with erosions and erosive cheilitis *JAAD 57:S111–114, 2007*

Hypereosinophilic syndrome, idiopathic; red macules, red papules, plaques, and nodules, urticaria, angioedema *AD 142:1215–1218, 2006; Allergy 59:673–689, 2004; Am J Hematol 80:148–157, 2005; AD 132:535–541, 1996; Medicine 54:1–27, 1975; BJD 143:641–644, 2000; BJD 144:639, 2001; AD 132:583–585, 1996; Blood 83:2759–2779, 1994; AD 114:531–535, 1978;* urticaria and/or angioedema *Med Clin (Barc)106:304–306, 1996; AD 132:535–541, 1996; Sem Derm 14:122–128, 1995; Blood 83:2759–2779, 1994*

Infantile systemic hyalinosis – autosomal recessive; dusky red plaques of buttocks, synophrys, thickened skin, perianal nodules, gingival hypertrophy, joint contractures, juxta-articular nodules (knuckle pads), osteopenia, growth failure, diarrhea, frequent infections, facial red papules *JAAD 50:S61–64, 2004*

IRAK-4 deficiency (homozygous mutations of IL-receptor-associated kinase 4 gene) – cutaneous infections with *Staphylococcus aureus;* abscesses, cellulitis, impetigo *JAAD 54:951–983, 2006*

Kawasaki's disease – mimicking periorbital cellulitis *NEJM 350:904–912, 2004*

KID syndrome – keratosis, ichthyosis, deafness syndrome – fixed orange, symmetrical hyperkeratotic plaques of scalp, ears, face, and extremities with perioral rugae; aged or leonine facies; erythrokeratoderma-like; later hyperkeratotic nodules develop *Ped Derm 17:115–117, 2000; Ped Derm 13:105–113, 1996*

Majeed syndrome – autosomal recessive; Sweet's syndrome-like lesions; LPIN2 mutations; chronic recurrent multifocal osteomyelitis, congenital dyserythropoietic anemia, fever, onset before 2 years *Arthr Rheum 56:960–964, 2007; J Med Genet 42:551–557, 2005*

Muckle-Wells syndrome

Multicentric reticulohistiocytosis

Multifocal idiopathic fibrosclerosis (hyper IgG4 syndrome) – sclerodermoid red plaque of breast; fibrosis of thyroid, mediastinum, retroperitoneum, orbits, pancreas, gallbladder *AD 148:1335–1336, 2012*

Neutrophilic dermatosis (pustular vasculitis) of the dorsal hands – variant of Sweet's syndrome *AD 138:361–365, 2002*

Nevoid basal cell carcinoma syndrome - personal observation

Nakajo syndrome - nodular erythema with digital changes

POEMS syndrome (hyperpigmented plaque) *JAAD 21:1061–1068, 1989*

Reactive arthritis syndrome – circinate balanitis (red plaque of penis)

Reflex sympathetic dystrophy – red plaque *JAAD 35:843–845, 1996; JAAD 28:29–32, 1993*

Relapsing polychondritis – initial inflammatory phase mimics cellulitis *Ann Int Med 142:47–55, 2005; Medicine 55:193–216, 1976*

Reticular erythematous mucinosis (REM) syndrome – red plaques in midline of back *Cutis 93:294–296, 2014;* red chest *AD 148:768–769, 2012*

Schopf syndrome – syringofibroadenomas – flat and fissured red plaques *JAAD 40:259–262, 1999*

Sweet's syndrome - red plaque (cellulitis-like) with or without bullae or pustules *NEJM 382:1543, 2020; Ped Derm 29:38–44, 2012; AD 145:608–609, 2009; Ann Int Med 142:47–55, 2005; NEJM 350:904–912, 2004; Cutis 71:469–472, 2003; JAAD 40:838–841, 1999; AD 134:625–630, 1998; JAAD 31:535–536, 1994; Int J Dermatol 31:598–599, 1992; BJD 76:349–356, 1964;* red plaque of neck *JAAD 69:557–564, 2013;* giant cellulitis-like Sweet's syndrome *JAMADerm 150:457–459, 2014;* bullae and purpura *JAMA Derm 149:79–83, 2013;* associated with myeloproliferative disorders *Cancer 51:1518–1526, 1983;* red annular targetoid plaques *AD 148:969–970, 2012;* histiocytoid Sweet's syndrome – red plaques of face and trunk *JAAD 61:882–884, 2009;* histiocytoid Sweet's of hands *JAMADerm 153:651–659, 2017;* zosteriform red plaques in acute myelogenous leukemia *AD 142:235–240, 2006;* chronic recurrent Sweet's syndrome of myelodysplasia - pustules, plaques, and papules *AD 142:1170–1176, 2006;* induced by or associated with granulocyte colony-stimulating factor, trimethoprim-sulfamethoxazole, minocycline, nitrofurantoin, anti-seizure medications, hydralazine, oral contraceptives, retinoids (all-trans retinoic acid) *AD 145:215–216, 2009; Ann Pharmacother 41:802–811, 2007; Cutis 71:469–472, 2003;* red breast *JAAD 49:907–909, 2003;* in children *Ped Derm 26:452–457, 2009;* subcutaneous Sweet's syndrome *Australas J Dermatol 32:61–64, 1991; Dermatologica 183:255–264, 1991;* associated with primary or secondary immunodeficiency *Ped Derm 26:452–457, 2009;* necrotizing Sweet's syndrome – red plaque mimicking necrotizing fasciitis *JAAD 67:945–954, 2012;* necrotizing Sweet's syndrome - edematous red plaque studded with pustules *JAAD 67:945–954, 2012;* histiocytoid Sweet's syndrome – multiple deep purple plaques of trunk and extremities *JAAD 72:131–139, 2015;* histiocytic Sweet's syndrome (leukemia cutis?) – red plaques of dorsal fingers *JAAD 70:1021–1027, 2014*

Tuberous sclerosis – shagreen patch; pink, yellow, or skin-colored plaque *JAAD 57:189–202, 2007;* fibrous cephalic plaque of face *Ped Derm 32:563–570, 2015*

Tumor necrosis factor (TNF) receptor 1-associated periodic fever syndromes (TRAPS)(same as familial hibernian fever, autosomal dominant periodic fever with amyloidosis, and benign autosomal dominant familial periodic fever) - erythematous patches, tender red plaques, fever, annular, serpiginous, polycyclic, reticulated, and migratory patches and plaques (migrating from proximal to distal), urticaria-like lesions, lesions resolving with ecchymoses, conjunctivitis, periorbital edema, myalgia, arthralgia, abdominal pain, headache; Irish and Scottish predominance; mutation in TNFRSF1A - gene encoding 55kDa TNF receptor *JAAD 67:177–185, 2012; AD 136:1487–1494, 2000; Mayo Clin Proc 72:806–817, 1997*

Vogt-Koyanagi-Harada syndrome - inflammatory vitiligo presenting as a red plaque around preexistent vitiliginous patches *JAAD 44:129–131, 2001*

Wells' syndrome (eosinophilic cellulitis) – red plaques resembling urticaria or cellulitis *JAMA 315:79–80, 2016; Cutis 89:191–194, 2012; AD 142:1157–1161, 2006; Ann Int Med 142:47–55, 2005; JAAD 52:187–189, 2005; NEJM 350:904–912, 2004; AD 139:933–938, 2003; Ped Derm 20:276–278, 2003; BJD 140:127–130, 1999; JAAD 18:105–114, 1988; Trans St. Johns Hosp Dermatol Soc 51:46–56, 1971;* bullous Wells' syndrome – red plaque with bullae *Ped Derm 29:762–764, 2012;* violaceous plaque of hand *JAMADerm 155:617–618, 2019*

WILD syndrome – disseminated warts, diminished cell-mediated immunity, primary lymphedema, anogenital dysplasia; perianal hypertrophic plaque *AD 144:366–372, 2008*

TOXINS

Arsenical keratoses; multiple Bowenoid keratoses in arsenical poisoning *AD 123:251–256, 1987*

L-tryptophan-induced eosinophilic myalgia syndrome – cellulitis-like

TRAUMA

Cardioversion (defibrillation) – hypopigmented, atrophic, telangiectatic, crusted erythematous plaque of back with rim of hyperpigmentation; delayed onset of years *AD 145:1411–1414, 2009*

Chemical scalp burn – hair highlighting with persulfate and hydrogen peroxide; red plaque with granulation tissue *Ped Derm 27:74–78, 2010*

Chilblains (perniosis) *AD 117:26–28, 1981*

Cold panniculitis *JAAD 45:325–361, 2001;* of neonate and children (Haxthausen's disease) *JAAD 33:383–385, 1995; Burns Incl Therm Inj 14:51–52, 1988; AD 94:720–721, 1966; BJD 53:83–89, 1941;* popsicle panniculitis – cellulitis-like *Pediatr Emerg Care 8:91–93, 1992;* red plaque on back following ice therapy for supraventricular tachycardia *Ped Derm 28:192–194, 2011*

Coma-induced sweat gland necrosis – pressure bulla; cellulitis-like *Ann Dermato Syphiligr 98:421–428, 1971*

Equestrian cold panniculitis – red plaques on hips *AD 116:1025–1027, 1980*

Ice pack dermatosis – red plaque, retiform purpura with purpuric papules and ulcers *JAMA Derm 149:1314–1318, 2013*

Postirradiation pseudosclerodermatous panniculitis *Ann Int Med 142:47–55, 2005; Am J Dermatopathol 23:283–287, 2001; Mayo Clin Proc 68:122–127, 1993*

Radiation therapy – acute and chronic fluoroscopy-induced radiation dermatitis *JAMA 314:1390–1391, 2015;* post-irrradiation pseudosclerodermatous panniculitis *JAAD 45:325–361, 2001;* cellulitis-like lesions of the breast *JAAD 54:28–46, 2006;* postradiation vascular proliferations of breast (atypical vascular lesions of the breast) – erythema; erythema with underlying induration or ulceration, telangiectasias, papules, plaques, nodules, *JAAD 57:126–133, 2007;* acnegenic radiation dermatitis – red plaque with acneiform lesions *AD 146:439–444, 2010; Br J Radiol 75:478–481, 2002;* acute and chronic fluoroscopy-induced radiation dermatitis *JAMA 314:1390–1391, 2015*

Salt-ice challenge of teenagers

Scar *JAMADerm 150:187–193, 2014*

VASCULAR

Acquired agminated acral angioma *AD 141:646–647, 2005*

Acquired elastotic hemangioma – red plaque with vascular appearance *JAAD 47:371–376, 2002*

Acquired progressive lymphangioma (benign lymphangioendothelioma) – abdomen, thigh calf; bruise or bruise-like plaque; red plaque or patch *JAAD 49:S250–251, 2003; JAAD 37:656–657, 1997; Clin Exp Dermatol 21:159–162, 1996; JAAD 23:229–235, 1990; JAAD 31:362–368, 1994; J Cutan Pathol 19:502–505, 1992; JAAD 24:813–815, 1991; AD 124:699–701, 1988*

Acral pseudolymphomatous angiokeratoma of children (APACHE) - unilateral multiple persistent vascular papules on hands and feet; may have keratotic surface or collar *Ped Derm 20:457–458, 2003*

Acroangiodermatitis of Mali - pseudo-Kaposi's sarcoma; chronic venous insufficiency, congenital or acquired arteriovenous malformations, hemodialysis arteriovenous shunts, paralysis, amputation stumps, minor trauma – dorsum of foot, tops of first and second toes; red-brown plaque *Cutis 86:239–240, 2010; JAAD 49:887–896, 2003; Eur J Vasc Endovasc Surg 24:558–560, 2002; Acta DV (Stockh) 75:475–478, 1995; Int J Dermatol 33:179–183, 1994; AD 92:515, 518, 1965;* red plaque of above-knee amputation stump *AD 145:1447–1452, 2009;* giant red plaque of calf *Cutis 103:336–339, 2019*

Acute hemorrhagic edema of infancy *Ped Derm 36:274–282, 2019*

Arteriovenous malformation – red plaque overlying large subcutaneous nodule *JAMADerm 155:256–257, 2019; JAAD 56:353–370, 2007*

Benign (reactive) angioendotheliomatosis (benign lymphangioendothelioma, acquired progressive lymphangioma, multifocal lymphangioendotheliomatosis) – present at birth; red-brown or violaceous nodules or plaques on face, arms, legs with petechiae, ecchymoses, and small areas of necrosis *AD 140:599–606, 2004; Am J Surg Pathol 26:328–327, 2002; Histopathology 35:319–327, 1999; JAAD 38:143–175, 1998; AD 114:1512, 1978*

Capillary lymphatic venous malformation *Ped Derm 37:272–277, 2020*

Cerebral cavernous malformation (familial cerebral cavernomas) – red hyperkeratotic plaques; cutaneous venous malformations *Lancet 352:1892–1897, 1998*

Churg-Strauss granuloma *AD 137:136, 2001;* necrotic eschar within red plaque; red papules of forehead and scalp *JAAD 65:244–246, 2011*

Congenital self-healing tufted angioma – annular red plaque *AD 142:749–751,2006*

CRMO – chronic recurrent multifocal osteomyelitis and synovitis; acne, pustulosis, hyperostosis, osteitis; palmoplantar pustules, Sweet's syndrome, pyoderma gangrenosum *JAAD 70:767–773, 2014*

Cutaneous epithelioid angiomatous nodule *AD 146:439–444, 2010; Am J Dermatopathol 26:14–21, 2004*

Cutaneous polyarteritis nodosa – inflammatory red plaque with peripheral nodules *JAAD 60:320–325, 2009*

Diffuse dermal angiomatosis (reactive angioendotheliomatosis) *JAAD 40:257–259, 1999;* ulcerated violaceous plaques *JAAD 45:462–465, 2001;* associated with peripheral vascular disease *JAAD 49:887–896, 2003;* diffuse dermal angiomatosis of the breast *AD 142:343–347, 2006;* associated with cutis marmorata telangiectatica congenita – crusted plaque *AD 146:1311–1312, 2010*

Eosinophilic vasculitis *AD 130:1159–1166, 1994*

Epithelioid angiosarcoma *JAAD 38:143–175, 1998*

Epithelioid hemangioendothelioma *JAAD 42:897–899, 2000*

Erythromelalgia – cellulitis-like *JAAD 67:177–185, 2012; Ann Int Med 142:47–55, 2005*

Generalized acquired telangiectasia – cellulitis-like

Glomeruloid angioendotheliomatosis – red purpuric patches and acral necrosis – associated with cold agglutinins *JAAD 49:887–896, 2003*

Glomus tumors (vascular plaque) *AD 126:1203–1207, 1990*

Hemangiopericytoma – solitary violaceous congenital lesion of plantar aspect *Ped Derm 23:84–86, 2006*

Hyperkeratotic capillary-venous malformations (dark red irregularly shaped) associated with cerebral cavernous malformation – KRIT1 mutations *Ped Derm 23:208–215, 2006*

Infantile hemangioma *JAAD 60:669–675, 2009;* red plaque of lower back – hemangioma with retroperitoneal hemangioma *Ped Derm 36:830–834, 2019;* zosteriform infantile hemangioma of face *Ped Derm 30:151–154, 2013;* hemangioma of lower lateral cheek

associated with airway obstruction; large facial hemangiomas of PHACES syndrome; sacral hemangiomas associated with spinal dysraphism *JAAD 48:477–493, 2003;* periocular hemangioma – red facial plaque *JAAD 55:614–619, 2006;* biker glove pattern of segmental infantile hemangioma – high risk of ulceration *JAAD 71:542–547, 2014*

Infantile hemangiomas with minimal or arrested growth – red plaques; more often on lower body *Ped Derm 34:64–71, 2017; AD 146:971–976, 2010*

IgG4 disease (sclerosing mesenteritis) - IgG4 disease – papules, plaques, nodules, parotid gland swelling (parotitis), lacrimal gland swelling, dacryoadenitis, sialadenitis, proptosis, idiopathic pancreatitis, sclerosing mesenteritis (retroperitoneal fibrosis), aortitis *JAAD 75:197–202, 2016*

Kaposiform hemangioendothelioma - red to purple plaque *JAAD 52:616–622, 2005; JAAD 38:799–802, 1998;* large violaceous plaque of abdomen in newborn with Kasabach-Merritt syndrome *AD 142:641–646, 2006;* of back with KMS *Ped Derm 26:365–366, 2009*

Klippel-Trenaunay-Weber syndrome – purple plaque of leg; hemihypertrophy *JAAD 66:71–77, 2012*

Lichen aureus *JAAD 8:722–724, 1983*

Lipodermatosclerosis – chronic venous insufficiency with hyperpigmentation, induration, inflammation *JAAD 67:177–185, 2012; Lancet ii:243–245, 1982;* cellulitis-like *Ann Int Med 142:47–55, 2005; JAAD 45:325–361, 2001*

LUMBAR syndrome (PELVIS syndrome) – cutaneous infantile hemangiomas of lower body; myelopathy, cutaneous defects, urogenital abnormalities, bony deformities, anorectal abnormalities, arterial anomalies, renal anomalies *JAAD 68:885–896, 2013; Ped Derm 27:588, 2010; J Pediatr 157:795–801, 2010; AD 42:884–888, 2006; Dermatology 214:40–45, 2007*

Acquired progressive lymphangioma (benign lymphangioendothelioma) – red plaque with bruise-like appearance at borders *Ped Derm 35:486–489, 2018*

Lymphangioma circumscriptum - personal observation

Lymphatic malformation – red-brown plaque of lumbosacral area; invasive lymphatic malformation (Gorham-Stout syndrome) (vanishing bone syndrome)(benign progressive acquired lymphangioma) of pelvis; progressive massive osteolysis *Ped Derm 30:374–378, 2013*

Lymphedema - mimicking infectious cellulitis *JAAD 67:177–185, 2012; Ann Int Med 142:47–55, 2005;* with lymphangiectasias – cellulitis-like

Malignant angioendotheliomatosis – scalp; livedoid red plaque of thigh with woody induration *JAAD 18:407–412, 1988*

Microvenular hemangioma – red-blue plaque *Ped Derm 20:266–267, 2003; AD 131:483–488, 1995*

Multifocal lymphangioendotheliomatosis – congenital appearance of hundreds of flat red-brown vascular papules and plaques associated with gastrointestinal bleeding, thrombocytopenia with bone and joint involvement; spontaneous resolution *JAAD 67:898–903, 2012; JAAD 54:S214–217, 2006; J Pediatr Orthop 24:87–91, 2004*

Non-involuting congenital hemangioma – thin red plaque *Ped Derm 36:466–470, 2019;* round to ovoid pink to purple papule or plaque with central or peripheral pallor, coarse telangiectasias *JAAD 50:875–882, 2004*

Thrombophlebitis, superficial – cellulitis-like *Ann Int Med 142:47–55, 2005*

Papillary intralymphatic angioendothelioma/retiform hemangioendothelioma spectrum – subcutaneous purple nodules or deep red plaques *BJD 171:474–484, 2014; Cancer 24:503–510, 1969*

PELVIS syndrome (may be part of urorectal septum malformation sequence)(also termed SACRAL – spinal dysraphism, anogenital, cutaneous, renal, urogenital anomalies, angioma of lumbosacral location) – macular telangiectatic patch; larger perineal hemangiomas, external genitalia malformations, lipomyelomeningocele, vesicorenal abnormalities, imperforate anus, and skin tags *Ped Derm 26:381–398, 2009; AD 142:884–888, 2006*

PHACES syndrome – large facial infantile hemangioma; posterior fossa malformations, cervicofacial hemangiomas, often segmental, arterial anomalies, cardiac defects, eye anomalies, and sternal clefting or supraumbilical raphe; Dandy-Walker malformation (posterior fossa cyst with hypoplasia of the cerebellar vermis; cystic dilatation of the fourth ventricle leading to hydrocephalus and increased head circumference) *Ped Derm 26:381–398, 2009; Pediatrics 124:1447–1456, 2009; Ped Derm 26:730–734, 2009; Ped Derm 23:476–480, 2006; JAAD 58:81–87, 2008; JAAD 55:1072–1074, 2006; Ped Derm 23:476–480, 2006; Clin Pediatr 44:747, 2005Neuroradiology 16:82–84, 1978;* association with hearing loss *AD 146:1391–1396, 2010;* ventral linear midline blanching with segmental infantile hemangioma *Ped Derm 32:180–187, 2015;* small red plaque *Ped Derm 35:622–627, 2018*

Poikilodermatous plaque-like hemangioma *JAAD 81:1257–1270, 2019*

Differential diagnosis:
Acrodermatitis chronica atrophicans
Cutaneous T-cell lymphoma
Fixed drug eruption
Hobnail hemangioma
Microvascular hemangioma
Pigmented purpuric eruption

Polyangiitis with granulomatosis *JAAD 28:710–718, 1993;* palisaded neutrophilic and granulomatous dermatitis *Cutis 70:37–38, 2002*

Polyarteritis nodosa – mimicking infectious cellulitis *Ann Int Med 142:47–55, 2005;* cutaneous polyarteritis nodosa - acrocyanosis and/or Raynaud's phenomenon; livedo reticularis with surrounding erythema; acrocyanosis, ulcers, peripheral gangrene, red plaques and peripheral nodules, papules, myalgias *JAAD 73:1013–1020, 2015*

Reactive angioendotheliomatosis – red purple-purpuric patches and plaques; includes acroangiomatosis, diffuse dermal angiomatosis, intravascular hitiocytosis, glomeruloid angioendotheliomatosis, angioperictomatosis (angiomatosis with cryoproteins) *JAAD 49:887–896, 2003*

Retiform hemangioendothelioma - *JAAD 42:290–292, 2000;* red plaque of scalp, arms, legs, and penis *JAAD 38:143–175, 1998*

Spindle cell hemangioma – purple plaque of sole *BJD 171:466–473, 2014*

Stasis dermatitis – solitary red plaque *JAAD 61:1028–1033, 2009*

Stewart-Bluefarb syndrome – arteriovenous malformation of leg with multiple fistulae and port wine stain-like purplish lesions (Mali's acroangiodermatitis/pseudo-Kaposi's sarcoma) – brown macules, purple nodules and plaques, edema, varicose veins, hypertrichosis, cutaneous ulcers, enlarged limb *JAAD 65:893–906, 2011;* violaceous plaques of feet *JAAD 59:179–1206, 2008;* ulcerated purple plaque *Ped Derm 18:325–327, 2001; AD 121:1038–1040, 1985*

Superficial migratory thrombophlebitis – "pseudocellulitis"; red plaques of legs; paraneoplastic *J Clin Aesth Dermatol 10:49–51, 2017*

Takayasu's arteritis - erythema induratum-like lesions; Sweet's syndrome associated with aortitis *Ped Derm 29:645–650, 2012*

Tufted angioma (angioblastoma of Nakagawa) - patchy dull red , purple, or red-brown patch and/or plaque; associated with ery-thema, edema, and hypertrichosis *Ped Derm 35:808–816, 2018; Int J Dermatol 53:1165–1176, 2014; Head and Neck Pathol 7:291–294, 2013; Ped Derm 30:124–127, 2013; AD 146:758–763, 2010; AD 145:847–848, 2009; AD 144:1217–1222, 2008; Ped Derm 24:397–400, 2007; JAAD 49:887–896, 2003; Ped Derm 19:388–393, 2002; Ped Derm 12:184–186, 1995; JAAD 20:214–225, 1989; JAAD 31:307–311, 1994; JAAD 33:124–126, 1995;* red plaque of lower leg of neonate *Ped Derm 26:347–348, 2009;* violaceous plaque *Ped Derm 36:963–964, 2019*

Urticarial vasculitis *JAAD 26:441–448, 1992*

Vasculitis - granulomatous, leukocytoclastic; Cutaneous small vessel vasculitis – ulcerated purpuric necrotic plaques *AD 148:887–888, 2012*

Venous congestion *JAAD 67:177–185, 2012*

Venous thrombosis, deep – cellulitis-like *Ann Int Med 142:47–55, 2005;* protein C deficiency, protein S deficiency, antithrombin III deficiency, hyperhomocystinemia, activated protein C resistance *AD 133:1027–1032, 1997*

Venous stasis – cellulitis-like

Verrucous hemangioma – red or red-brown hyperkeratotic plaque; behaves like vascular malformation *Ped Derm 23:208–215, 2006*

RED SCROTUM

AUTOIMMUNE DISORDERS AND DISEASES OF IMMUNE DYSFUNCTION

Allergic contact dermatitis *Semin Ped Surg 16:58–63, 2007*

DEGENERATIVE DISORDERS

Hernia of hydrocele *Semin Ped Surg 16:58–63, 2007*

Hernia sac torsion of peritoneum *Urology 89:126–128, 2016*

Hydrocoele *Case Rep Med Feb 8, 2018; 2862514*

Inguinal hernia *Semin Ped Surg 16:58–63, 2007*

Torsion of rudimentary vestigial appendages of testicle or epididy-mis – prepubertal boys *Semin Ped Surg 16:58–63, 2007*

DRUG REACTIONS

Capecitabine *AD 147:1123–1124, 2011*

Corticosteroid atrophy/addiction *Sex Health 10:452–455, 2013*

Fixed drug reaction

EXOGENOUS AGENTS

Irritant contact dermatitis

INFECTIONS AND INFESTATIONS

Bacterial epididymitis – gonococcal, chlamydial, *E.coli,* mycoplasma

Candidiasis – "red bag"

Cellulitis

Erythrasma – coral red fluorescence *NEJM 364:e25, 2011*

Fournier's gangrene *Medicine 97:e0140, 2018; Case Rep Urol May 9, 2018:5135616;* following vasectomy *J Urol 147:1613–1614, 1992*

Insect bite

Lyme disease

Mumps orchitis

Viral epididymitis – adenovirus, enterovirus, influenza, parainfluenza *JAAD Case Rep 3:464–465, 2017*

INFILTRATIVE DISORDERS

Eruptive xanthogranulomas *J Cut Pathol 44:385–387, 2017*

INFLAMMATORY DISORDERS

Acute idiopathic scrotal edema *Semin Ped Surg 16:58–63, 2007*

Appendicitis – perforated retrocecal appendix; hemiscrotal erythema *J Med Case Rep 5:27, 2011; CMAJ 166:1695, 2002;* acute appendicitis in neonate *J Afr Med J 62:1003–1005, 1982*

Crohn's disease *J Pediatric Child Health 50:158–160, 2014*

Epididymitis

Orchitis *Semin Ped Surg 16:58–63, 2007*

Testicular torsion (torsion of the spermatic cord) – in newborns and adolescents; "bell clapper" deformity *Semin Ped Surg 16:58–63, 2007*

METABOLIC DISORDERS

Vitamin B2 deficiency *Cutis 105:296–302, 2020*

NEOPLASTIC DISORDERS

Bowen's disease *Open Access Maced J Med Sci 5:545–546, 2017*

Epidermolytic acanthomas *Ann DV 144:295–300, 2017*

Extramammary Paget's disease *J Drugs Dermatol 5:652–654, 2006; Ned Tijdschr Geneeskd 138:914–916, 1994*

Giant angiofibroma of child *Urology 93:e15–16, 2016*

Lymphoma – B-cell lymphoma

Mucosal angiokeratoma *Indian J Dermatol 57:228–229, 2012*

Porokeratosis, genitocrural *J Cut Pathol 39:72–74, 2012*

Sseminoma – intrascrotal tumor; acute scrotum *Nihon Hinyokika Gakkai Zasshi 99:698–702, 2008*

Teratoma with hemorrhage – acute scrotum *Hinyookika Kiyo 35:1243–1245, 1989*

PRIMARY CUTANEOUS DISEASES

Angiolymphoid hyperplasia with eosinophilia *J Dermatol 37:355–359, 2010*

Red scrotum syndrome *Int J Dermatol 58:e162–263, 2019; Dermatologic Ther July 29, 2016; 244–248*

SYNDROMES

Hennekam syndrome – severe scrotal edema; intestinal lymphangiectasia, lymphedema of limbs and genitalia, mild mental retardation, facial anomalies *Ped Derm 23:239–242, 2006*

TRAUMA

Cardiac catheterization – hematoma *BMJ Case Rep May 5, 2017*

Hematoma – following vasectomy *BMJ Case Rep Jan 6, 2014*

Intraperitoneal hemorrhage from hernia repair *BMJ Case Rep 11:226676, 2018*

Physical trauma

Sexual abuse

VASCULAR DISORDERS

Acute hemorrhagic edema of infancy *Eur J Pediatr 170:1507–1511, 2011*

Angiokeratoma circumscriptum *Stat Pearls Oct 20, 2019*

Henoch–Schonlein purpura *Clin Rev Allergy Immunol 53:439–451, 2017; Semin Ped Surg 16:58–63, 2007*

Neonatal testicular hemangiolymphangioma *Arch Iran Med 18:386–388, 2015*

Testicular capillary hemangioma *Indian J Pathol Microbiol 55:557–559, 2012*

Vascular malformation

REDUNDANT SKIN

AUTOIMMUNE DISEASES AND DISEASES OF IMMUNE DYSFUNCTION

Severe combined immune deficiency

CONGENITAL LESIONS

Congenital erosive and vesicular dermatosis with reticulate supple scarring – widespread erosions, low set ears, syndactyly *JAAD 69:909–915, 2013; Ped Derm 24:384–386, 2007; Ped Derm 22:55–59, 2005; JAAD 45:946–948,2001; Ped Derm 15:214–218, 1998; Dermatol 194:278–280, 1997; JAAD 32:873–877, 1995; AD 126:544–546, 1990; JAAD 17:369–376, 1987; AD 121:361–367, 1985*

Infantile perineal protrusion *Dermatology 201:316–320, 2000*

Megaprepuce, congenital – redundant prepuce *Andrologia April 2018; BJU Int 86:519–522, 2000*

Smooth muscle hamartoma – generalized congenital smooth muscle hamartoma – inguinal and sacral redundancy with hypertrichosis *Ped Derm 25:236–239, 2008*

DRUGS

Dilantin – hypertrophy of retro-auricular folds *Cutis 30:207–209, 1982*

Penicillamine – pseudoxanthoma elasticum-like skin changes *Dermatology 184:12–18, 1992;* cutis laxa *Cutis 76:49–53, 2005*

Rofecoxib – aquagenic wrinkling of the palms *Ped Derm 19:353–355, 2002*

EXOGENOUS AGENTS

Aquagenic wrinkling of palms *Ped Derm 21:180, 2004*

Nephrogenic systemic fibrosis – late stage anetoderma (cutaneous wrinkling); due to gadolinium *AD 145:183–187, 2009*

Paraffinoma; *Plast Reconstr Surg 65:517–524, 1980*

INFECTIONS

Leprosy, lepromatous – redundant facial skin *Int J Lepr Other Mycobact Dis 42:297–302, 1974*

Onchocerciasis (*Onchocerca volvulus*) – hanging groin; redundant stretched abdominal skin *JAAD 73:929–944, 2015*

INFILTRATIVE DISEASES

Amyloidosis – elastolytic skin lesions of fingertips *AD 126:657–660, 1990;* primary systemic amyloidosis - cutis verticis gyrata lesions

Erdheim-Chester disease (non-Langerhans cell histiocytosis) – CD68+ and factor XIIIa+; negative for CD1a and S100; xanthoma and xanthelasma-like lesions (red-brown-yellow papules and plaques); flat wart-like papules of face; lesions occur in folds; skin becomes slack with atrophy of folds and face; also lesions of eyelids, axillae, groin, neck; bony lesions; diabetes insipidus, painless exophthalmos, retroperitoneal, renal, and pulmonary histiocytic infiltration *NEJM 374:470–477, 2016; JAAD 57:1031–1045, 2007; AD 143:952–953, 2007; Hautarzt 52:510–517, 2001; Medicine (Baltimore) 75:157–169, 1996; Virchow Arch Pathol Anat 279:541–542, 1930*

Lichen myxedematosus

Mastocytosis - diffuse cutaneous mastocytosis (xanthelasmoidea) (pseudoxanthomatous mastocytosis) – pachydermatous change to skin *BJD 65:296–297, 1963*

Scleromyxedema – facial and truncal redundant skin *JAAD 74:1194–1200, 2016*

INFLAMMATORY DISEASES

Hidradenitis suppurativa – redundant scars *JAAD 77:118–122, 2017; BJD 161:831–839, 2009*

METABOLIC DISEASES

Acromegaly

ACTH overproduction in infants

Congenital disorders of glycosylation (CDG-Ia) – phosphomanno-mutase-2; redundant excess fat; peau d'orange skin; facial dysmorphism, cerebellar hypoplasia, hypotonic neonate, strabismus *Ped Derm 22:457–460, 2005*

Congenital disorders of glycosylation (CDG-Ix) – nuchal skin folds, facial dysmorphism, inverted nipples, hypoplastic nails, petechiae and ecchymoses, edema; neurologic, gastrointestinal, and genitourinary abnormalities, pericardial effusion, ascites, oligohy-dramnios *Ped Derm 22:457–460, 2005*

Cushing's syndrome, infancy *NEJM 352:1047–1048, 2005*

Cystic fibrosis – aquagenic wrinkling of the palms *NEJM 369:2362–2363, 2013; AD 141:621–624, 2005*

Marasmus – malnutrition without edema *Stat Pearls March 21, 2020*

Massive weight loss *JAAD 81:1059–1069, 2019*

Obesity *JAAD 81:1059–1069, 2019*

Pretibial myxedema *Int J Low Extrem Wounds 13:152–154, 2014; Indian J Med Res 137:568, 2013; NEJM 352:918, 2005*

NEOPLASTIC DISEASES

Lymphoma - granulomatous slack skin syndrome *JAAD 70:205–220, 2014; Ped Derm 24:640–645, 2007; AD 141:1178–1179, 2005; AD 107:271–274, 1973;* cutaneous T-cell lymphoma; edematous

redundant eyelid skin – folliculotropic cutaneous T-cell lymphoma *JAMADerm 156:811–812, 2020*

Melanocytic nevi, including cerebriform nevi

Stewart-Treves angiosarcoma – reddish-blue macules and/or nodules which become polypoid; pachydermatous changes, blue nodules, telangiectasias, palpable subcutaneous mass, ulcer *JAAD 67:1342–1348, 2012*

PARANEOPLASTIC DISEASES

Tripe palms - rippled skin *J Clin Oncol 7:669–678, 1989*

PRIMARY CUTANEOUS DISEASES

Benign enlargement of the labia minora *Eur J Obstet Gynecol Reprod Biol 8:61–64, 1978*

Blepharochalasis *Br J Ophthalmol 72:863–867, 1988; AD 115:479–481, 1979*

Cutis laxa, acquired – with amyloidosis, myeloma, lupus erythema-tosus, hypersensitivity reaction, complement deficiency, penicilla-mine, inflammatory skin disease *Rook p. 2019, 1998, Sixth Edition;* acrolocalized acquired cutis laxa *BJD 134:973–976, 1996*

Cutis verticis gyrata – autosomal dominant *Ped Derm 15:18–22, 1998; AD 125:434–435, 1989*
   associated with: *Cutis 73:254–256, 2004*
      acanthosis nigricans
      acromegaly *AD Syphilol 42:1092–1099, 1940*
      amyloidosis
      chronic traction (trauma)
      cylindroma
      Darier's disease
      dermatofibroma
      Ehlers-Danlos syndrome
      fallopian tube carcinoma
      hamartoma
      histiocytofibroma
      Lennox-Gastart syndrome (retardation with EEG abnormalities) *Dev Med Child Neurol 16:196–200, 1974*
      leukemia
      lymphangioma
      melanocytic nevi (cerebriform) *Cutis 73:254–256, 2004; Dermatology 186:294–297, 1993*
      mental retardation *Am J Med Genet 38:249–250, 1991;*
Scott Med J 12:450–456, 1967
      mucinosis
      myxedema
      neurofibromas, fibromas *Ann Surg 118:154–158, 1943*
      nevus lipomatosis
      nevus sebaceous
      Noonan's syndrome *Ped Derm 22:142–146, 2005*
      pachydermoperiostosis
      paraneoplastic *AD 125:434–435, 1989*
      syphilis
      tuberous sclerosis
      Turner's syndrome *Ped Derm 22:142–146, 2005*

Dermatochalasis

Double lip – usually upper lip *Ann Plast Surg 28:180–182, 1992;* Ascher's syndrome – associated with blepharochalasis and goiter

Elastoderma - cutis laxa-like changes *JAAD 33:389–392, 1995*

Gynecomastia, massive

Lipedema - personal observation

Webbed neck

SYNDROMES

Ablepharon macrostomia – absent eyelids, ectropion, abnormal ears, rudimentary nipples, dry redundant skin, macrostomia, ambiguous genitalia *Hum Genet 97:532–536, 1996*

Apert's syndrome – excess skin wrinkling of forehead *Cutis 52:205–208, 1993*

Beare-Stevenson cutis gyrata syndrome – localized redundant skin of scalp, forehead, face, neck, palms, and soles, acanthosis nigricans, craniofacial anomalies, anogenital anomalies, skin tags, and large umbilical stump *Am J Med Genet 44:82–89, 1992*

C syndrome (Opitz trigonocephaly syndrome) – nevus flammeus; trigonocephaly, unusual facies with wide alveolar ridges, multiple frenula, limb defects, visceral anomalies, redundant skin, mental retardation, hypotonia *Am J Med Genet 9:147–163, 1981*

Cardiofaciocutaneous syndrome – autosomal dominant, xerosis/ichthyosis, eczematous dermatitis, alopecia, growth failure, hyperkeratotic papules, ulerythema ophryogenes (decreased or absent eyebrows), seborrheic dermatitis, CALMs, nevi, hemangiomas, keratosis pilaris, patchy or widespread ichthyosiform eruption, sparse curly scalp hair and sparse eyebrows and lashes, congenital lymphedema of the hands, redundant skin of the hands, short stature, abnormal facies with macrocephaly, broad forehead, bitemporal narrowing, hypoplasia of supraorbital ridges, short nose with depressed nasal bridge, high arched palate, low set posteriorly rotated ears with prominent helices, cardiac defects; gain of function sporadic missense mutations in *BRAF, KRAS, MEK1,* or *MEK2, MAP2K1/MAP2K2 BJD 163:881–884, 2010; Ped Derm 27:274–278, 2010; Ped Derm 17:231–234, 2000; JAAD 28:815–819, 1993; AD 129:46–47, 1993; JAAD 22:920–922, 1990;* port wine stain *Clin Genet 42:206–209, 1992*

Congenital fascial dystrophy - rippled skin *JAAD 21:943–950, 1989*

Costello syndrome - warty papules around nose and mouth, legs, perianal skin; loose thick skin of neck, hands, and feet, thick, redundant palmoplantar surfaces, hypoplastic nails, short stature, craniofacial abnormalities; linear papillomatous papules of upper lip *Ped Derm 30:665–673, 2013; BJD 168:903–904, 2013; Am J Med Genet 117:42–48, 2003; Eur J Dermatol 11:453–457, 2001; Am J Med Genet 82:187–193, 1999; JAAD 32:904–907, 1995; Am J Med Genet 47:176–183, 1993; Aust Paediat J 13:114–118, 1977*Cutis laxa (dermatochalasis connata) – autosomal dominant; mild disease of late onset *Ped Derm 21:167–170, 2004;* bloodhound appearance of premature aging *Ped Derm 19:412–414, 2002; JAAD 29:846–848, 1993; Clin Genet 39:321–329, 1991; Ped Derm 2:282–288, 1985*

Cutis laxa type I – autosomal recessive; diaphragmatic hernia, gastrointestinal and genitourinary diverticulae, pulmonary emphysema, cardiac abnormalities *Ped Derm 21:167–170, 2004*

Cutis laxa type II – autosomal recessive; pre and postnatal growth retardation, delayed motor development, delayed closure of large fontanelle, congenital hip dislocation, bone dysplasias, parallel strips of redundant skin of back *Ped Derm 21:167–170, 2004*

Cutis laxa type III – autosomal recessive; severe mental retardation, corneal clouding *Ped Derm 21:167–170, 2004*

Cutis laxa – X-linked recessive (occipital horn syndrome; formerly Ehlers-Danlos type IX) – lysyl oxidase deficiency, skeletal dysplasias, joint hypermobility, chronic diarrhea, obstructive uropathy *Ped Derm 21:167–170, 2004*

Cutis verticis gyrate-mental deficiency syndrome *Am J Med Genet 38:249–250, 1991*

Donohue syndrome (leprechaunism) – congenital insulin resistance; dwarfism; elfin-like face, large eyes, thick lips, low set ears, less

subcutaneous fat, excessive folding of skin *Pediatr 83:18, 1994; AD 117:531–535, 1981*

Ehlers-Danlos syndrome – atrophic scars over knees; redundant skin on palms and soles; redundant folds around eyes

GAPO syndrome - growth retardation, alopecia, pseudoanodontia, and progressive optic atrophy; midface hypoplasia; frontal bossing, wide anterior fontanelle, saddle nose, protruding thick lips, low set ears, anti-Mongoloid slant, diffuse scalp hypotrichosis, prominent scalp veins, sparse eyebrows and eyelashes, absent teeth, slightly redundant skin, impacted teeth *Ped Derm 27156–161, 2010; Ped Derm 19:226, 2002; J Craniofac Genet Dev Biol 19:189–200, 1999; Birth Defects 24:205–207, 1988; Am J Med Genet 19:209–216, 1984; Syndr Ident 8:14–16, 1982; Odont Tilster 55:484–493, 1947*

Geroderma osteodysplastica (Bamatter syndrome)(osteodysplastic geroderma) – autosomal recessive; short stature, cutis laxa-like changes with redundant abdominal skin, drooping eyelids and jowls (characteristic facies with hypoplastic midface), osteoporosis and skeletal abnormalities; lax wrinkled, atrophic skin, joint hyperextensibility, growth retardation *Ped Derm 23:467–472, 2006; Ped Derm 16:113–117, 1999; Am J Med Genet 3:389–395, 1979; Hum Genet 40:311–324, 1978; Ann Paediatr 174:126–127, 1950*

Gingival fibromatosis-hypertrichosis syndrome(Byars-Jurkiewicz syndrome) – autosomal dominant; fibroadenomas of breast; hypertrichosis of face, upper extremities, midback; redundant skin *Ped Derm 18:534–536, 2001; J Pediatr 67:499–502, 1965*

Hypomelanosis of Ito – excess skin folds *J Med Genet 25:809–818, 1988*

Laron dwarfism

Leprechaunism (Donohue's syndrome) – decreased subcutaneous tissue and muscle mass, characteristic facies, severe intrauterine growth retardation, broad nose, low set ears, hypertrichosis of forehead and cheeks, loose folded skin at flexures, gyrate folds of skin of hands and feet; breasts, penis, clitoris hypertrophic *Endocrinologie 26:205–209, 1988*

Lipoid proteinosis – rugose forehead *BJD 151:413–423, 2004; JID 120:345–350, 2003; BJD 148:180–182, 2003; Hum Molec Genet 11:833–840, 2002*

Localized familial redundant scalp *Clin Exp Dermatol 17:349–350, 1992*

Localized lipomatous hypertrophy with microcephaly, mental retardation, and deletion of short arm of chromosome 11 *AD 116:622, 1980; AD 115:978–979, 1979*

Michelin tire baby syndrome – either nevus lipomatosis or diffuse smooth muscle hamartoma; excessive folds of firm skin on extremities, especially ankles and wrists; generalized hypertrichosis, palmar cerebriform plaques; low set ears with thickened helix and antihelix; wide nasal bridge; histologically increased periadnexal fat and subcutaneous fat and smooth muscle hamartomas; mental retardation, tendinous hyperlaxity, seizures, mastocytosis, complex malformations syndrome (bilateral calcaneovalgus deformity, cleft palate, inguinal hernia, hip deformity, clefting of lateral mouth commissures, shawl scrotum, absent foreskin *JAAD 63:1110–1111, 2010; Ped Derm 27:79–81, 2010; Ped Derm 24:628–231, 2007; Ped Derm 22:245–249, 2005; Ped Derm 20:150–152, 2003; BJD 129:60–68,1993; JAAD 28:364–370, 1993; Atlas of Clinical Syndromes A Visual Aid to Diagnosis, 1992, pp.308–309; Ped Derm 6:329–331, 1989; Am J Med Genet 28:225–226, 1987; AD 115:978–979, 1979;* diffuse lipomatous hypertrophy *AD 100:320–323, 1969;* generalized muscular nevus *Ann DV 107:923–927, 1980*

Mucopolysaccharidoses (Hurler, Hurler-Schei, Sanfilippo, Morquio, Maroteaux-Lamy, Sly syndromes) - personal observation

Neurofibromatosis – rugose and plexiform neurofibromas *JAAD 52:191–195, 2005*

Noonan's syndrome – cutis verticis gyrata *Ped Derm 22:142–146, 2005*

Pachydermoperiostosis (Touraine-Solente-Gole syndrome) *JAAD 63: 1036–1041, 2010*

Patterson-David syndrome – redundant skin, hypertrichosis *Birth Defects 5:117–121, 1969*

Patau's syndrome (trisomy 13) – loose skin of posterior neck, parieto-occipital scalp defects, abnormal helices, low set ears, simian crease of hand, hyperconvex narrow nails, polydactyly *Ped Derm 22:270–275, 2005*

Proteus syndrome

Pseudoxanthoma elasticum – linear and reticulated cobblestoned yellow papules and plaques *AD 124:1559, 1988; JAAD 42:324–328, 2000; Dermatology 199:3–7, 1999*; PXE and acrosclerosis *Proc Roy Soc Med 70:567–570, 1977*; penicillamine-induced pseudoxanthoma elasticum *JAAD 30:103–107, 1994; Dermatology 184:12–18, 1992*; saltpeter-induced pseudoxanthoma elasticum *Acta DV 58:323–327, 1978*

RINZ syndrome – rare, autosomal recessive connective tissue disorder; soft redundant and /or hyperextensible skin *Am J Med Genetics A 170:2408–2415, 2016*

Soto's syndrome

Turner's syndrome – neonatal cutis verticis gyrata *Ped Derm 15:18–22, 1998*

Weaver syndrome - generalized somatic overgrowth; macrocephaly, broad forehead, flattened occiput, large low set ears, hypertelorism; soft loose skin, redundant nuchal skin folds; umbilical hernia; thin deep set nails *J Ped Genet 4:136–143, 2015; Cutis 83:255–261, 2009*

Williams' syndrome – premature laxity of skin, congenital heart disease (supravalvular aortic stenosis), baggy eyes, full cheeks, prominent lips, dental malocclusion, delayed motor skills, cocktail party personality *J Pediatr 113:318–326, 1988*

TRAUMA

Immersion foot - rippled skin

VASCULAR DISEASES

Glomerulovenous malformation – atrophic patch with redundant skin *Soc Ped Derm Annual Meeting, July 2005*

Hemangiomas, resolved – atrophy, telangiectasia, redundant skin *JAAD 48:477–493, 2003*; resolved rapidly involuting congenital hemangioma *BJD 158:1363–1370, 2008*

RENAL FAILURE, CUTANEOUS MANIFESTATIONS

AUTOIMMUNE DISEASES AND DISORDERS OF IMMUNE DYSREGULATION

Behcet's disease *Semin Arthr Rheum 38:241–248, 2008*

C1q deficiency – atrophic fingers and toes, hypopigmentation, finger tapering, butterfly rash, discoid lupus lesions, Raynaud's phenomenon; renal disease – segmental mesangiopathic glomerulonephritis; increased interferon 1 levels *Ped Derm 33:602–614, 2016*

IgG4 disease – multisystem inflammatory disease with papules, plaques, and nodules; parotitis with parotid gland swelling, lacrimal gland swelling, dacryoadenitis, sialadenitis, proptosis; idiopathic pancreatitis, retroperitoneal fibrosis, aortitis; Mikuliczs syndrome, angiolymphadenopathy with eosinophilia, Riedel's thyroiditis, biliary tract disease, renal disease, meningeal disease, pituitary gland; Kuttner tumor, Rosai-Dorfman disease; elevated IgG4 with plasma cell dyscrasia, diffuse or localized swelling or masses; lymphocytic and plasma cell infiltrates with storiform fibrosis *JAAD 75:177–185, 2016*

Lupus erythematosus – systemic lupus erythematosus *JAAD 65:54–64, 2011; Lupus 9:301–303, 2000; Clin Exp Rheum 5:349–353, 1987*; auricular chondritis with red ear *Clin Exp Rheumatol 5:349–353, 1987*; chilblain lupus *BJD 98:497–506, 1978*; perforation of pinna *Cutis 32:554–557, 1983*; neuropsychiatric lupus *Lupus 9:301–303, 2000*; discoid lupus erythematosus *NEJM 269:1155–1161, 1963*

Relapsing polychondritis *Rheumatol Int 31:707–713, 2011*; IgA nephropathy *Pathology 20:85–89, 1988*

Scleroderma *JAAD 74:231–244, 2016*

Tumor necrosis factor (TNF) receptor 1-associated periodic fever syndromes (TRAPS)(same as familial Hibernian fever, autosomal dominant periodic fever with amyloidosis, and benign autosomal dominant familial periodic fever) – painful erythematous patches, tender red plaques, fever for 7–21 days, annular, serpiginous, polycyclic, reticulated, and migratory patches and plaques (migrating from proximal to distal), urticaria-like lesions, purpuric lesions resembling Henoch-Schonlein purpura; lesions resolving with ecchymoses, conjunctivitis, periorbital edema, localized myalgia which may be migratory resulting in muscle stiffness, arthralgia, abdominal pain, headache; Irish and Scottish predominance; upper extremities most commonly involved; skin lesions and myalgias move proximal to distal; renal and hepatic involvement; mutation in *TNFRSF1A* - gene encoding 55kDa TNF receptor *JAAD 68:834–853, 2013; AD 144:392–402, 2008; AD 136:1487–1494, 2000*

DRUGS

All-trans retinoic acid – Sweet's syndrome-like neutrophilic panniculitis; solitary red nodule *JAAD 56:690—693, 2007*; All-retinoic acid syndrome; fever, respiratory distress, weight gain, leg edema, pleural effusions, renal failure, pericardial effusions, hypotension, vasculitis, hypercalcemia, bone marrow necrosis and fibrosis, thromboembolic events, erythema nodosum *Leuk Lymphoma 44:547–548, 2003*

Drug reaction with eosinophilia and systemic symptoms (DRESS) – acute interstitial nephritis *Cutis 102:322–326, 2018*; morbilliform eruption, cheilitis (crusted hemorrhagic lips), diffuse desquamation, areolar erosion, periorbital dermatitis, vesicles, bullae, targetoid plaques, purpura, pustules, exfoliative erythroderma, urticarial papular-confluent; facial edema, lymphadenopathy *JAAD 82:573–574, 2020; JAMADerm 152:1254–1257, 2016; BJD 170:866–873, 2014; JAAD 68:E1–14BJD 169:1071–1080, 2013; BJD 168:391–401, 2013; Am J Med 124:588–597, 2011; Ped Derm 28:741–743, 2011; JAAD 68:693–705, 2013; AD 146:1373–1379, 2010; NEJM 242:897–898, 1950*

Levamisole-contaminated cocaine – snorting, injection, smoking *Clin Inf Dis 61:1840–1849, 2015*

Ecchymoses, bullae, stellate lesions with red borders and necrotic center; especially on ears and cheeks; fixed drug eruptions; lichen planus, ulceration, morbilliform exanthem, hemorrhagic bullae, acute kidney failure

Vemurafenib – vemurafenib-induced Fanconi's syndrome with acute renal failure *JAMADerm 151:453–454, 2015*

EXOGENOUS AGENTS

Bullous dermatosis of hemodialysis *JAAD 21:1049–1051, 1989*

Intravenous drug abuse – MDMA; serotonin syndrome – tachycardia, hypothermia; *Ecstasy or Molly*; rhabdomyolysis with acute kidney injury; acute swollen leg *Clin Inf Dis 61:1840–1849, 2015; BMJ 309:1361–1362, 1994*

INFECTIONS AND INFESTATIONS

Bacterial endocarditis, acute – *Staphylococcus aureus;* livedo reticularis of trunk, purpuric eruption of hands; fever, confusion, thrombocytopenia, renal failure *NEJM 370:651–660, 2014;* immune complex glomerulonephritis, renal infarction, septic emboli, renal cortical necrosis, drug-induced acute interstitial nephritis

Ebola virus hemorrhagic fever (Filovirus) – proteinuria with hematuria, oliguria and azotemia; dark red discoloration of soft palate, pharyngitis, oral ulcers, glossitis, gingivitis; morbilliform exanthem which becomes purpuric with desquamation of palms and soles; high fever, body aches, myalgia, arthralgias, prostration, abdominal pain, watery diarrhea; disseminated intravascular coagulation *Int J Dermatol 51:1037–1043, 2012; JAMA 287:2391–2002; Int J Dermatol 51:1037–1043, 2012; JAAD 65:1213–1218, 2011; MMWR 44, No.19, 382, 1995*

Ehrlichiosis (*Ehrlichia chaffeensis*) – human monocytic ehrlichiosis and leukocytoclastic vasculitis (palpable purpura); fever, headache, malaise, myalgia; nausea, vomiting, diarrhea, abdominal pain; 1/3 with petechial or morbilliform eruption or diffuse erythema *MMWR 65:1–44, May 23, 2016; Clin Inf Dis 34:1206–1212, 2002; J Clin Gastroenterol 25:544–545, 1997; J Int Med 247:674–678, 2000;* human granulocytic ehrlichiosis with acute renal failure mimicking TTP; petechial and purpuric rash of human monocytic ehrlichiosis *Am J Nephrol 19:677–681, 1999; Skin and Allergy News, Oct. 2000, p.40; Ann Int Med 120:736–743, 1994; Ehrlichia chaffeensis* – diffusely erythematous or morbilliform, scattered petechiae or macules *Clin Inf Dis 33:1586–1594, 2001*

Influenza – myocarditis, myositis, acute renal failure *Netter's Infectious Diseases pp.34–37, 2012*

Leishmaniasis, visceral (kala azar) – acute renal failure, nephrotic syndrome, glomerulonephritis, interstitial nephritis

Leptospirosis – Weil's disease; hepatic renal dysfunction, fever, scleral injection (red eyes)

Leprosy - erythema nodosum leprosum with glomerulonephritis, painful facial nodules, fever, arthralgias, dactylitis, iridocyclitis, uveitis, orchitis, adenitis, edema, and hyperemia resulting in painful red eye, tibial periostitis *JAAD 83:17–30, 2020; JAAD 71:795–803, 2014; JAAD 51:416–426, 2004; AD 138:1607–1612, 2002*

Louse-borne relapsing fever (*Borrelia recurrentis*) – high fever, headache, dizziness, myalgias, fatigue, hemorrhage, liver disease, renal failure; relapse ever 7–19 days *JAAD 82:551–569, 2020*

Rocky Mountain spotted fever – acute renal failure *MMWR 65:1–44, May 13, 2016*

Scabies complicated by streptococcal infection *JAAD 82:533–548, 2020*

Schistosoma haematobium – chronic renal failure *NEJM 381:2493–2495, 2019*

Syphilis – nephrotic syndrome

Toxic shock syndrome *JAAD 10:267–272, 1984*

INFILTRATIVE DISORDERS

Amyloidosis – primary systemic; papules *JAAD 77:1145–1158, 2017; JAAD 74:247–270, 2016; Cutis 80:193–200, 2007;* Eyelid and Conjunctival Tumors, Shields JA and Shields CL, Lippincott Williams and Wilkins, 1999, p.175; Postgrad Med J 64:696–698, 1988; Clin Exp Dermatol 4:517–536, 1979; diffuse eyelid swelling *J Dermatol 19:113–118, 1992;* conjunctival amyloidosis with unilateral upper and lower eyelid edema *Korean J Ophthalmol 15:38–40, 2001*

Interstitial cryoglobulinosis – non-palpable petechial purpura, necrotic ulcers, hemorrhagic bullae; renal failure *JAAD 77:1145–1158, 2017*

Erdheim-Chester disease (non-Langerhans cell histiocytosis) – CD68+ and factor XIIIa+; negative for CD1a and S100; xanthoma and xanthelasma-like lesions (red-brown-yellow papules and plaques); flat wart-like papules of face; lesions occur in folds; skin becomes slack with atrophy of folds and face; also lesions of eyelids, axillae, groin, neck; bony lesions; diabetes insipidus, painless exophthalmos, retroperitoneal, renal, and pulmonary histiocytic infiltration *NEJM 374:470–477, 2016; JAAD 57:1031–1045, 2007; AD 143:952–953, 2007; Hautarzt 52:510–517, 2001; Medicine (Baltimore) 75:157–169, 1996; Virchow Arch Pathol Anat 279:541–542, 1930*

INFLAMMATORY DISEASES

Ankylosing spondylitis – associated findings include psoriasis, anterior uveitis, inflammatory bowel disease, lung abnormalities, heart conduction defects, aortic insufficiency, renal abnormalities, osteoporosis, vertebral fractures; renal amyloid most common type of renal disease *Saudi J Kidney Dis Transpl 29:386–391, 2018; Euro J Intern Med 2011:1–7; Int J Rheumatol 2011:1–10*

Sarcoid – *JAAD 74:231–244, 2016;* with hypercalcemia *NEJM 373:864–873, 2015;* fingertip nodules *JAAD 44:725–743, 2001; JAAD 11:713–723, 1984;* on palmar aspects of fingers *AD 132:459–464, 1996;* lupus pernio *JAAD 16:534–540, 1987; BJD 112:315–322, 1985;* renal manifestations *Int Braz J Urol 46:15–25, 2020*

METABOLIC DISORDERS

Calciphylaxis (vascular calcification cutaneous necrosis syndrome) (cutaneous calcinosis in end-stage renal disease) – necrotic cutaneous ulcers, livedo racemosa (livedoid necrosis), hemorrhagic patches, indurated plaques, hemorrhagic bullae *JAAD 56:569–579, 2007;* (chronic renal failure and hyperparathyroidism) *JAAD 74:247–270, 2016; JAMA Derm 149:946–949, 2013; JAMA Derm 149:163–167, 2013; JAAD 58:458–471, 2008; AD 143:152–154, 2007; Ped Derm 23:266–272, 2006; JAAD 40:979–987, 1999; JAAD 33:53–58, 1995; JAAD 33:954–962, 1995;J Dermatol 28:27–31, 2001; Br J Plast Surg 53:253–255, 2000; J Cutan Med Surg 2:245–248, 1998; JAAD 33:954–962, 1995; AD 131:786, 1995; AD 127:225–230, 1991; Arch Int Med 136:1273–1280, 1976;* acute reversible renal failure; associated with hepatitis C infection *JAAD 50:S125–128, 2004;* calciphylaxis with stellate necrosis and retiform purpura unassociated with renal disease; associated with hypoalbuminemia, malignancy, systemic corticosteroid therapy, coumarin, chemotherapy, systemic inflammation, cirrhosis, protein C or S deficiency, obesity, rapid weight loss, infection *AD 145:451–458, 2009*

Calcific uremic arteriolopathy *Clin J Am Soc Nephrol 9:201–218, 2014*

Cholesterol emboli – blue toes, livedo reticularis, gangrene, purpura, nail fold infarcts, ulcerations; post-intravascular catheterization; acute, subacute, chronic renal failure *Int J Mol Sci 18:1120, 2017*

Cryoglobulinemia *JAAD 74:231–244, 2016;* renal involvement *Clin Exp Med 18:466–471, 2018*

Cystinosis – white facial papules; renal failure, ocular, pancreatic, hepatic, muscular, dental, gonadal, and neurologic involvement, hypothyroidism *Ped Nephrol Feb 2020; JAMADerm 152:108–109, 2016*

Delayed puberty – chronic renal failure *Pediatr Nephrol 7:551–553, 1993;* congenital magnesium-losing kidney *Ann Clin Biochem 30:494–498, 1993*

Fabry's disease - angiokeratoma corporis diffusum (Fabry's disease (alpha galactosidase A) – X-linked recessive); initially, telangiectatic macules; perioral telangiectasias *Nephron 143:274–281, 2018; JAAD 74:231–244, 2016;; NEJM 276:1163–1167, 1967*

Fanconi's anemia – autosomal recessive; ectopic or horseshoe kidney; endocrine abnormalities with hypothyroidism, decreased growth hormone, diabetes mellitus, café au lait macules, diffuse hyperpigmented macules, guttate hypopigmented macules, intertriginous hyperpigmentation, skeletal anomalies (thumb hypoplasia, absent thumbs, radii, carpal bones), oral/genital erythroplasia with development of squamous cell carcinoma, hepatic tumors, microphthalmia, broad nose, epicanthal folds, micrognathia, bone marrow failure, acute myelogenous leukemia, solid organ malignancies (brain tumors, Wilms' tumor) *BJD 164:245–256, 2011; JAAD 54:1056–1059, 2006;Ped Derm 16:77–83, 1999*

Metastatic calcification

Nephrotic syndrome – yellow skin *JAAD 57:1051–1058, 2007*

Osteitis fibrosa (renal osteodystrophy) – nodule of hard palate *NEJM 359:74, 2008*

Oxalosis - acral necrosis with livedo; primary oxalosis (hyperoxaluria) – type 1 - alanine glyoxalate aminotransferase (transaminase) deficiency; chromosome 2q36-37; type 2 (rare) – D-glyceric acid dehydrogenase deficiency *AD 137:957–962, 2001; JAAD 22:952–956, 1990; AD 131:821–823, 1995;* primary hyperoxaluria; necrosis with limb gangrene *JAAD 49:725–728, 2003;* livedo reticularis, ulcers, and peripheral gangrene *AD 136:1272–1274, 2000;* autosomal recessive; livedo reticularis, acrocyanosis, peripheral gangrene, ulcerations, sclerodermoid changes (woody induration of extremities), eschar of hand (calcium oxalate); acral and/or facial papules or nodules; end-stage renal disease; primary hyperoxalosis – deficiency of alanine:glyoxylate aminotransferase; primary hyperoxalosis – deficiency of D-glycerate dehydrogenase/glyoxylate reductase *AD 147:1277–1282, 2011*

Post-reperfusion syndrome – massive edema of muscles; may lead to amputation; peripheral cyanosis, livedo reticularis, edema of foot; myocardial injury, renal failure *Int Wound J March 3, 2014; Semin Vasc Surg 22:52–57, 2009; Plast Reconstr Surg 117:1024–1033, 2006*

White tongue (leukoplakia) – chronic renal failure; xerostomia, uremic feter (ammoniacal odor), angular cheilitis

NEOPLASTIC DISORDERS

Light chain deposition disease – violaceous plaque of chin; involvement of kidneys (nephropathy), liver, heart, lungs, peripheral nerves *Hematol Oncol Clin NA 13:1235–1248, 1999*

PRIMARY CUTANEOUS DISEASES

Acquired perforating dermatosis of chronic renal disease *Int J Derm 32:874–876, 1993; Int J Dermatol 31:117–118, 1992; AD 125:1074–1078, 1989;* reactive perforating collagenosis *JAAD 75:247–270, 2016*

Epidermolysis bullosa, autosomal recessive – blisters and erosions, mild skin fragility, fatal interstitial lung disease, nephrotic syndrome,

sparse fine hair, large dystrophic toenails with distal onycholysis; integrin alpha-6 beta-4 mutation *NEJM 366:1508–1514, 2012*

Epidermolysis bullosa with pyloric atresia – alpha-6 beta-4 mutation; focal segmental glomerulosclerosis

Gingival hyperplasia - chronic renal failure *Pediatr Nephrol 18:39–45, 2003*

Hypopigmentation - hypopigmented hair transverse white nail bands half and half nails (Lindsay's nails); generalized pallor

Mee's lines (white transverse bands) seen with arsenic poisoning, pellagra, malnutrition, typhoid fever, Hodgkin's disease, renal failure, renal allograft rejection, and myocardial infarction *Dermatol Clin 6:305–313, 1988*

Perforating disorders *JAAD 74:247–270, 2016*

Periorbital edema - glomerulonephritis, nephrotic syndrome

Pruritus without primary dermatitis; chronic renal disease *JAAD 74:247–270, 2016; JAAD 45:892–896, 2001; Clin Exp Dermatol 25:103–106, 2000; AD 118:154–160, 1982;* uremia *JAAD 49:842–846, 2003*

Pseudoporphyria

Spiny keratoderma (multiple minute palmar-plantar digitate hyperkeratoses)(music box keratoderma)(punctuate/spiny keratoderma) – spiny, filiform, spiked, minute aggregate *JAAD 58:344–348, 2008; Cutis 54:389–394, 1994; BJD 121:239–242, 1989; JAAD 18:431–436, 1988; AD 104:682–683, 1971;* autosomal dominant; may remit with topical 5-fluorouracil; may be associated with autosomal dominant polycystic kidney disease *JAAD 34:935–936, 1996; JAAD 26:879–881, 1992;* questionable paraneoplastic associations *Dermatology 201:379–380, 2000;* digestive adenocarcinoma *Ann DV 124:707–709, 1997;* breast cancer *Ann DV 117:834–836, 1990*

Uremia – yellow skin

Uremic follicular hyperkeratosis *JAAD 26:782–783, 1992*

Uremic frost

Uremic glossitis – red tongue

Urticaria *Semin Dermatol 14:297–301, 1995*

Xerosis - chronic renal failure *Nephrol Dial Transplant 10:2269–2273, 1995*

SYNDROMES

Arthrogryposis, renal tubular dysfunction, and cholestasis (ARC) syndrome – ichthyosis, scarring alopecia, ectropion, arthrogryphosis of wrist, knee, and hip *Ped Derm 22:539–542, 2005*

Bardet-Biedl syndrome – postaxial polydactyly (ulnar), rod-cone dystrophy (retinal dystrophy), retinitis pigmentosa, obesity, neuropathy, mental disturbance, renal abnormalities, hypogonadism *Ped Derm 36:346–348, 2019; J Med Genet 36:599–603, 1999*

Beckwith-Wiedemann syndrome – nephrolithiasis, hydronephrosis, calyceal diverticula *JAAD 74:231–244, 2016*

Bifid epiglottis syndrome – accessory auricles with preauricular sinus, polycystic kidney disease with intrahepatic biliary dilatation, endocardial cushion defect, polydactyly *Ped Int 52:723–728, 2010*

Birt-Hogg-Dube syndrome – fibrofolliculomas, trichodiscomas, acrochordon, renal tumors, spontaneous pneumothoraces; mutation in folliculin gene

Blau or Jabs syndrome (familial juvenile systemic granulomatosis) – autosomal dominant; onset under 4 years of age; generalized micropapular rash of trunk and extremities infancy (ichthyosiform); translucent skin-colored papules (noncaseating granulomas) of trunk and extremities or dense lichenoid yellow to red-brown papules with grainy surface with anterior or panuveitis, synovitis, symmetric granulomatous polyarthritis; polyarteritis, multiple synovial cysts; red papular rash in early childhood; exanthema resolves with pitted scars; camptodactyly (flexion contractures of PIP joints); no involvement of lung or hilar nodes; sialadenoitis, lymphadenopathy, erythema nodosum, leukocytoclastic vasculitis, transeient neuropathies, interstitial lung disease, nephritis, arterial hypertension, pericarditis, pulmonary embolism, hepatic granulomas, chronic renal failure; activating mutations in NOD2 (nucleotide-binding oligomerization domain 2)(caspase recruitment domain family, member 15; *CARD* 15) *Ped Derm 34:216–218, 2017; Ped Derm 27:69–73, 2010; AD 143:386–391, 2007; Clin Exp Dermatol 21:445–448, 1996; J Pediatr 107:689–693, 1985*

Braegger syndrome – proportionate short stature, IUGR, ischiadic hypoplasia, renal dysfunction, craniofacial anomalies, postaxial polydactyly, hypospadias, microcephaly, mental retardation *Am J Med Genet 66:378–398, 1996*

Branchio-oto-renal syndrome (BOR) – autosomal dominant; mutation in EYA1 gene; conductive, sensorineural, mixed hearing loss; preauricular pits, structural defects of outer, middle, or inner ear; renal anomalies, renal failure, lateral cervical fistulae, cysts, or sinuses; nasolacrimal duct stenosis or fistulae *Am J Kidney Dis 37:505–509, 2001; Cutis 68:353–354, 2001*

Cowden's syndrome (PTEN hamartoma-tumor syndrome) – sclerotic fibromas; glomerulosclerosis, megalencephaly (macrocephaly), dysplastic gangliocytoma of the cerebellum (Lhermite-Duclos disease), hamartomatous intestinal polyposis *AD 142:625–632, 2006; J Cut Pathol 19:346–351, 1992;* type 2 segmental Cowden's disease – keratinocytic soft, thick papillomatous nevus, connective tissue nevi, vascular nevi (including cutis marmorata), angiomas, varicosities, lymphatic hamartomas, lipomas, lipoblastomatosis, hydrocephalus, seizures, hemihypertrophy of limbs, ballooning of toes, bowel polyps, macrocephaly *BJD 156:1089–1090, 2007; Eur J Dermatol 17:133–136, 2007*

Chanarin-Dorfman disease – coarse facies, ichthyosis with fine scaling of trunk, renal disease *BJD 176:545–548, 2017*

Familial Mediterranean fever – fever for 6–72 hours; monoarticular arthritis, severe abdominal pain, pleurisy, leukocytoclastic vasculitis resembling HSP and polyarteritis nodosa, scrotal pain and edema, AA amyloid *JAAD 68:834–853, 2013; AD 144:392–402, 2008; Medicine 77:268–297, 1998; AD 134:929–931, 1998; QJMed 75:607–616, 1990;* autosomal recessive; erysipelas-like erythema - mutation in MEFV/pyrin/marenostrin *JAAD 68:834–853, 2013; JAAD 42:791–795, 2000; AD 136:1487–1494, 2000;* mimicking infectious cellulitis *Ann Int Med 142:47–55, 2005; NEJM 350:904–912, 2004; Isr Med Assoc J 1:31–36, 1999; Q J Med 75:607–616, 1990;* red patch with pale areas *AD 143:1080–1081, 2007;* edema with or without erythema of the foot *AD 134:929–931, 1998*

H syndrome – autosomal recessive; facial telangiectasias; sclerodermoid changes of middle and lower body with overlying hyperpigmentation sparing the knees and buttocks; hypertrichosis, short stature, facial telangiectasia, gynecomastia, camptodactyly of 5th fingers, scrotal masses with massively edematous scrotum obscuring the penis, hypogonadism, azospermia, sensorineural hearing loss, cardiac anomalies, hepatosplenomegaly; Arabic Palestinian population; gluteal lipoatrophy; hyperpigmentation, hearing loss, diabetes mellitus, lymphadenopathy, hypertrichosis, heart anomalies, micropenis, hallus valgus, hyperpigmentation induration and hypertrichosis of inner thighs and shins (sclerodermoid), chronic diarrhea, anemia, dilated lateral scleral vessels, episcleritis, exophthalmos, eyelid swelling, varicose veins, chronic rhinitis, renal abnormalities, bone lesions, arthritis, arhthralgia; mutation in *SLC29A3 JAAD 70;80–88, 2014; JAAD 59:79–85, 2008*

Hemophagocytic lymphohistiocytosis syndrome – fever, pancytopenia, lymphadenopathy, hepatomegaly, splenomegaly, neurologic, joint, purpura, kidney, and cardiac involvement, central nervous system dysfunction *Eur Rev Med Pharmacol Sci, 16:1414–1424, 2012; Genes Immunol 13:289–298, 2012*

   Familial HLH – known genetic defects (perforin)
   Immune deficiencies
      Chediak-Higash syndrome
      Griscelli syndrome
      X-linked lymphoproliferative syndrome
   Acquired
      Infections
      Endogenous products
      Rheumatic diseases
      Neoplasms

Hermansky-Pudlak syndrome – oculocutaneous albinism, hemorrhage, ceroid-like material deposited in several organs; granulomatous colitis, pulmonary fibrosis, renal failure, cardiomyopathy, hypothyroidism *Ped Derm 34:638–646, 2017; SKINMed 12:313–315, 2014*

Hypotrichosis-Lymphedema-Telangiectasia-Renal failure syndrome – diffuse reticulated capillary malformation, hypertensive emergency with transient ischemic attack, dilatation or aortic root, pleural effusions, acute kidney injury, thin facies with telangiectasias of cheeks, livedo reticularis of trunk and extremities; mutation in *SOX18* gene *Cases of the Year, Pre-AAD Pediatric Dermatology Meeting, 2016*

Kaufman-McKusick syndrome – hydrometrocolpos, hydronephrosis, postaxial polydactyly, congenital heart defect, vaginal atresia *J Med Genet 36:599–603, 1999; Eur J Pediatr 136:297–305, 1981*

Mandibuloacral dysplasia – autosomal recessive; progeroid facies; facial asymmetry, micrognathia, small nose, prominent eyes, large open fontanelles; congenital brown pigmentation of ankles progresses to mottled pigmentation; hypoplastic clavicles; contractures of lower extremities; failure to thrive; progressive glomerulopathy; subcutaneous calcified nodules; mutation in *ZMPSTE24* (lamin) *JAMADerm 151:561–562, 2015*

Meckel syndrome – microcephaly, microphthalmia, congenital heart defects, postaxial polydactyly, polycystic kidneys, cleft lip/palate *J Med Genet 8:285–290, 1971*

MEND – X-linked recessive; hypomorphic mutation of emopamil-binding protein; diffuse mild ichthyosis; telecanthus, prominent nasal bridge, low set ears, micrognathia, cleft palate large anterior fontanelle, polydactyly, 2–3 syndactyly, kyphosis, Dandy-Walker malformation, cerebellar hypoplasia, corpus callosal hypoplasia, hydrocephalus, hypotonia, developmental delay, seizures; bilateral cataracts, glaucoma, hypertelorism; cardiac valvular and septal defects, hypoplastic aortic arch; renal malformation, cryptorchidism, hypospadias *BJD 166:1309–1313, 2012*

Muckle-Wells syndrome – autosomal dominant; macular erythema (evanescent red macules), urticaria (cold air urticaria), deafness, extremity pain, arthralgias of knees and ankles with arthritis; nephropathy, AA amyloidosis with neuropathy; fever and rash more severe in evening; mutation in gene encoding NALP3 (cryopyrin) *SkinMed 11:80–83, 2013; AD 142:1591–1597, 2006; BJD 151:99–104, 2004; JAAD 39:290–291, 1998; BJD 100:87–92, 1979; QJMed 31:235–248, 1962*

Nail patella syndrome – autosomal dominant; glomerulonephritis and end-stage renal disease; hyperextensible joints; absence of distal interphalangeal creases; webbing between digits; hypoplastic nails, triangular lunulae, absent or hypolastic patellae; iliac horns; mutation in *LMX1B Cutis 101:126–129, 2018; JAAD 74:231–244, 2016; Ped Derm 27:93–94, 2010; Dermatology 213:153–155, 2006*

Neurofibromatosis - renal artery stenosis, Wilms' tumor, angiomyolipoma *JAAD 74:231–244, 2016*

Noonan syndrome – renal abnormalities *Cutis 93:83–87, 2014;*

Oral-facial-digital syndrome type 1 (Papillon-Leage-Psaume syndrome) – X-linked dominant; congenital facial milia which resolve with pitted scars; milia of face, scalp, pinnae, and dorsal hands; short stature, hypotrichosis with dry and brittle hair, short upper lip, hypoplastic ala nasi and lower jaw, pseudoclefting of upper lip, hooked pug nose, hypertrophied labial frenulae, bifid or multilobed tongue with small white tumors within clefts, ankyloglossia, multiple soft hamartomas of oral cavity, clefting of hard and soft palate, teeth widely spaced with dental caries, trident hand or brachydactyly, syndactyly, clinodactyly, ulnar deviation of index finger, or polydactyly; hair dry and brittle, alopecic, numerous milia of face, ears, backs of hands, mental retardation with multiple central nervous system abnormalities, frontal bossing, hypertelorism, telecanthus, broad depressed nasal bridge; polycystic renal disease; combination of polycystic renal disease, milia, and hypotrichosis is highly suggestive of OFD 1 *Ped Derm 27:669–670, 2010; JAAD 59:1050–1063, 2008; Ped Derm 25:474–476, 2008; Ped Derm 9:52–56, 1992; Am J Med Genet 86:269–273, 1999; JAAD 31:157–190, 1994; Ped Derm 9:52–56, 1992; Pediatrics 29:985–995, 1962; Rev Stomatol 55:209–227, 1954*

Perlman syndrome – micropenis; nephroblastoma, renal hamartoma, facial dysmorphism, fetal gigantism *J Pediatr 83:414–418, 1973*

POEMS syndrome (Crow-Fukasi syndrome, Takatsuki syndrome) (PEP syndrome – plasma cell dyscrasia, endocrinopathy, polyneuropathy) – plethora, angiomas (cherry, globular, glomeruloid) presenting as red nodules of face, trunk, and extremities, diffuse hyperpigmentation, hypertrichosis, scleroderma-like changes, either generalized or localized (legs), hyperhidrosis, clubbing, leukonychia, papilledema, pleural effusion, peripheral edema, ascites, pulmonary hypertension, weight loss, fatigue, diarrhea, thrombocytosis, polycythemia, fever, renal disease, arthralgias; osteosclerotic myeloma (IgG or IgA lambda) bone lesions, progressive symmetric sensorimotor peripheral polyneuropathy, hypothyroidism, and hypogonadism;, blue dermal papules associated with Castleman's disease (benign reactive angioendotheliomatosis), maculopapular brown-violaceous lesions, purple nodules; *JAAD 58:671–675, 2008; JAAD 55:149–152, 2006; JAAD 44:324–329, 2001, JAAD 40:808–812, 1999; AD 124:695–698, 1988, Cutis 61:329–334, 1998; JAAD 21:1061–1068, 1989; JAAD 12:961–964, 1985; Nippon Shinson 26:2444–2456, 1968*

Reactive arthritis syndrome - erosions with marginal erythema; circinate erosions *JAAD 59:113–121, 2008; NEJM 309:1606–1615, 1983; Semin Arthritis Rheum 3:253–286, 1974; Dtsch Med Wochenschr 42:1535–1536, 1916*

Schimke immunoosseous dysplasia – disproportionate short stature, spondyloepiphyseal dysplasia, progressive nephropathy, episodic lymphopenia, pigmentary skin changes *Am J Med Genet 66:378–398, 1996*

Activated STING in Vascular and Pulmonary syndrome – autoinflammatory disease; butterfly telangiectatic facies; acral violaceous psoriasiform, papulosquamous and atrophic plaques of vasculitis of hands; nodules of face, nose, and ears; fingertip ulcers with necrosis; nail dystrophy; nasal septal perforation; interstitial lung disease with fibrosis; polyarthritis; myositis *NEJM 371:507–518, 2014*

Turner's syndrome – horseshoe kidney, urinary collecting system abnormalities, decreased renal blood flow *JAAD 74:231–244, 2016*

VACTERL syndrome (vertebral anomalies, anorectal malformations, cardiac defects, tracheoesophageal fistulae, renal or radial anomalies, limb malformations) – sporadic *J Pediatr 93:270–273, 1978*

TOXINS

Boric acid ingestion – "boiled lobster" erythema with subsequent desquamation; cardiogenic shock, seizures, renal failure *Clinical Toxicology 47:432, 2009; Inf Dis in ObGyn 6:191–194, 1998*

Nephrogenic systemic fibrosis (nephrogenic fibrosing dermopathy) (scleromyxedema-like illness of renal disease) - associated with chronic renal failure with or without hemodialysis; patterned cobblestoned rippled red to violaceous thin fixed plaques with polygonal, reticular, or ameboid patterns; sclerodermoid changes; edema of fingers, wrists, toes, ankles; decreased range of motion; induced by gadolinium *JAAD 65:1095–1106, 2011; BJD 165:828–836, 2011; JAAD 61:868–874, 2009; AD 145:1164–1169, 2009; AD 145:183–187, 2009; BJD 158:1358–1362, 2008; JAAD 56:21–26, 2007; Semin Dialysis 19:191–194, 2006; JAAD 54:S31–34, 2006; Semin Arthritis Rheum 35:238–249, 2006; Semin Arthritis Rheum 35:208–210, 2006; Curr Opin Rheumatol 18:614–617, 2006; BJD 152:531–536, 2005; Arthritis Rheum 50:2660–2666, 2004; JAAD 48:55–60, 2003; JAAD 48:42–47, 2003; Am J Med 114:563–572, 2003; AD 139:903–906, 2003; Am J Dermatopathol 25:358, 2003; Am J Dermatopathol 23:383–393, 2001; Lancet 356:1000–1001, 2000*

VASCULAR DISORDERS

Arteriosclerosis obliterans in patients with chronic renal failure *JAAD 57:322–326, 200*

Dialysis shunt-associated steal syndrome *Ann Dermatol Venereol 133:264–267, 2006; Curr Surg 63:130–136, 2006; AD 138:1296–1298, 2002*

Granulomatosis with polyangiitis – suppurative otitis *Laryngoscope 92:713–717, 1982;* destruction of ear *JAAD 74:231–244, 2016*

Henoch-Schonlein purpura – scalp and facial edema preceding HSP *Ped Derm 9:311, 1992;* eyelid and facial edema due to intracerebral hemorrhage *Brain and Development 24:115–117, 2002; JAAD 74:231–244, 2016; JAAD 48:311–340, 2003; Ped Derm 15:357–359, 1998; Ped Derm 12:314–317, 1995; Am J Dis Child 99:833–854, 1960;* HSP with renal impairment *JAAD 82:1393–1399, 2020*

Hypersensitivity angiitis *AD 138:1296–1298, 2002*

LUMBAR syndrome (PELVIS syndrome) – cutaneous infantile hemangiomas of lower body; myelopathy, cutaneous defects, urogenital abnormalities, bony deformities, anorectal abnormalities, arterial anomalies, renal anomalies *JAAD 68:885–896, 2013; Ped Derm 27:588, 2010; J Pediatr 157:795–801, 2010; AD 42:884–888, 2006; Dermatology 214:40–45, 2007*

Polyarteritis nodosa - acrocyanosis and/or Raynaud's phenomenon; livedo reticularis with surrounding erythema; acrocyanosis, ulcers, papules *JAAD 74:231–244, 2016; JAAD 57:840–848, 2007; JAAD 52:1009–1019, 2005;* familial polyarteritis nodosa of Georgian Jewish, German, and Turkish ancestry – oral aphthae, livedo reticularis, leg ulcers, Raynaud's phenomenon, digital necrosis, nodules, purpura, erythema nodosum; systemic manifestations include fever, myalgias, arthralgias, gastrointestinal symptoms, renal disease, central and peripheral neurologic manifestations; mutation in adenosine deaminase 2(*CECR1*) *NEJM 370:921–931, 2014*

Purpura fulminans – multiorgan failure

ACUTE RENAL FAILURE

Prerenal
   Volume depletion
      Adrenal insufficiency

Diuretics
Gastrointestinal losses
Renal salt wasting
Toxic shock syndrome, either streptococcal or staphylococcal – widespread macular erythema, scarlatiniform, and papulopustular eruptions; occasional vesicles and bullae; edema of hands and feet; mucosal erythema; second week morbilliform or urticarial eruption occurs with desquamation at 10–21 days *Clin Inf Dis 32:1470–1479, 2001; JAAD 39:383–398, 1998; Rev Infect Dis 11(Suppl 1):S1–7, 1989; JAAD 8:343–347, 1983*
Congestive heart failure
Adrenal insufficiency
Cardiogenic
Hemorrhagic
Inferior vena cava obstruction or stenosis *Am J Med 113:580–586, 2002; Eur J Med Research 1:334–338, 1996*
Septic - bacterial endocarditis, acute – *Staphylococcus aureus*; livedo reticularis of trunk, purpuric eruption of hands; fever, confusion, thrombocytopenia, renal failure *NEJM 370:651–660, 2014*; Rocky Mountain spotted fever – acute renal failure *MMWR 65:1–44, May 13, 2016*
Third spacing
Cirrhosis
Nephrosis
Renal artery stenosis
Renal
Glomerular
Anti-GBM antibody disease
ANCA-associated vasculitis
Granulomatosis with polyangiitis
Microscopic polyangiitis
Eosinophilic granulomatosis with polyangiitis
Immune complex glomerulonephritis
Cryoglobulinemia
Henoch-Schonlein purpura
IgA nephropathy
Membranoproliferative glomerulonephritis
Post-streptococcal glomerulonephritis
Subacute bacterial endocarditis
Systemic lupus erythematosus
Tubulointerstitial
Acute interstitial nephritis
Allergic interstitial nephritis
Infections
Sarcoidosis
TINU syndrome
Acute kidney injury
Crystalluria
Ischemia
Myeloma kidney
Nephrotoxicity
Pigment-induced
Tumor lysis syndrome
Vascular
Acute arterial embolus or thrombus
Antiphospholipid antibody syndrome
Cholesterol emboli
Cortical necrosis
Eclampsia
Hemolytic uremic syndrome
Malignant hypertension
Polyarteritis nodosa
Scleroderma renal crisis
Thrombotic thrombocytopenic purpura – altered mental status, renal injury, fever, livedo reticularis, purpura *NEJM 370651-660, 2014*

Postrenal
Bilateral ureteral obstruction or ureteral obstruction of single functioning kidney
Clot
Extrinsic compression by tumor
Papillary necrosis
Retroperitoneal fibrosis
Stone
Tumor
Obstruction of the bladder outlet
Bladder or prostate cancer
Clot
Neurogenic bladder
Obstructed Foley catheter
Stone disease

Ehrlichiosis – human monocytic ehrlichiosis and leukocytoclastic vasculitis (palpable purpura) *J Int Med 247:674–678, 2000;* human granulocytic ehrlichiosis with acute renal failure mimicking TTP; petechial and purpuric rash of human monocytic ehrlichiosis *Am J Nephrol 19:677–681, 1999; Skin and Allergy News, Oct. 2000, p.40; Ann Int Med 120:736–743, 1994; Ehrlichia chaffeensis* – diffusely erythematous or morbilliform, scattered petechiae or macules *Clin Inf Dis 33:1586–1594, 2001*

Henoch-Schonlein purpura – scalp and facial edema preceding HSP *Ped Derm 9:311, 1992;* eyelid and facial edema due to intracerebral hemorrhage *Brain and Development 24:115–117, 2002*

Hypersensitivity angiitis *AD 138:1296–1298, 2002*

Iododerma in chronic renal failure – marked facial edema and edema of eyelids; pustulovesicular eruption, pustules, pseudovesicles, vegetative plaques *AD 140:1393–1398, 2004; JAAD 36:1014–1016, 1997; Clin Exp Dermatol 15:232–233, 1990; BJD 97:567–569, 1977*

Leprosy - erythema nodosum leprosum with glomerulonephritis; iridocyclitis, uveitis, edema, and hyperemia resulting in painful red eye *JAAD 83:17–30, 2020; JAAD 71:795–803, 2014; JAAD 51:416–426, 2004; AD 138:1607–1612, 2002*

Rhabdomyolysis – acute swollen legs *BMJ 309:1361–1362, 1994*

Syphilis, secondary

Uremic frost

RENAL TUMOR, CUTANEOUS MANIFESTATIONS

AUTOIMMUNE DISEASES AND DISORDERS OF IMMUNE DYSREGULATION

Discoid lupus erythematosus-like syndrome and hypercalcemia associated with renal cell carcinoma *Cutis 26:402–403, 1980*

INFLAMMATORY DISORDERS

Bullous pyoderma gangrenosum; associations with solid tumors – gastric, renal, oral, parotid, hypopharynx, breast, colon *JAAD 64:1208–1211, 2011*

NEOPLASTIC DISORDERS

Metastases, cutaneous – vascular appearance of metastasis *Dermatol Online J May 2012;* alopecia neoplastica *J Eur Acad DV 33:1020–1028, 2019; Urology 63:1021, 1026, 2004; J Derm Surg Oncology 9:815–818, 1983;* metastatic renal cell carcinoma presenting as cutaneous horn *Cutis 64:111–112, 1999*

SYNDROMES

BAP1 mutant disease – clear cell renal cell carcinoma; melanoma, uveal melanoma, epithelioid atypical Spitz tumors *Adv Chronic Kid Dis 21:81–90, 2014*

Beckwith-Wiedemann syndrome – Wilms' tumor, renal cysts *JAAD 74:231–244, 2016*

Birt-Hogg-Dube syndrome - fibrofolliculomas – autosomal dominant; renal cell carcinoma (papillary variant) white or yellow facial and nose papules; comedo-like white papules, pedunculated lip papules of mucosal surface, thyroid nodules or cysts; pulmonary cysts, spontaneous pneumothoraces; mutation in *FLCN* (folliculin) gene *Am J Clin Dermatol 19:87–101, 2018; JAAD 74:231–244, 2016; AD 147:499–504, 2011; AD 146:1316–1318, 2010; BJD 162:527–537, 2010; JAAD 50:810–812, 2004; JAAD 49:698–705, 2003;* renal and colonic neoplasms *Cancer Epidemiol Biomarkers Prev 11:393–400, 2002; AD 135:1195–1202, 1999;* facial angiofibromas *JAAD 53:S108–111, 2005*

Cowden's syndrome/PTEN tumor hamartoma syndrome *J Urol 190:1990–1998, 2013*

Neurofibromatosis - Wilms' tumor, angiomyolipoma *JAAD 74:231–244, 2016*

New Multiple Neoplasm Disorder – case report of patient with family history of multiple cancers, lipomatosis; testicular seminoma, multiple colonic polyps, hyperpigmented skin lesions, renal cancer, pituitary adenoma; negative for *PTEN J Med Case Reports 1:9, 2007*

Reed's syndrome (familial leiomyomatosis cutis et utero) – renal cell cancer (papillary, tubulopapillary, and collecting duct variants) *The Dermatologist July, 2016, pp 47–49; JAAD 74:231–244, 2016; Cutis 81:41–48, 2008*

Tuberous sclerosis – renal cysts, renal cell carcinoma, angioleiomyolipomas *JAAD 74:231–244, 2016; Int Urol Nephrol 46:1685–1690, 2014*

VASCULAR DISORDERS

Urticarial vasculitis and renal carcinoma *Prog Urol 13:495–497, 2003*

Vasculitis *Arch Int Med 154:334–340, 1994*

Von Hippel-Lindau disease – clear cell renal cell carcinoma, macular telangiectatic nevi, facial or occipitocervical; retinal angiomatosis, cerebellar or medullary or spinal hemangioblastoma, renal cell carcinoma (clear cell variant), renal cysts, pheochromocytoma, café au lait macules *JAAD 74:231–244, 2016; NEJM 353:2477–2490, 2005; Arch Intern Med 136:769–777, 1976*

RETICULATED ERUPTIONS

AUTOIMMUNE DISEASES AND DISEASES OF IMMUNE DYSFUNCTION

Common variable immunodeficiency – reticulated eruption consisting of cutaneous granulomas *BJD 153:194–199, 2005*

Dermatomyositis – reticulate telangiectatic erythema in older lesions with hyper- and hypopigmentation DOCK8 hypereosinophilic syndrome – reticulated exanthem *Dermatology News August, 2015, p.39*

Graft vs. host disease, chronic; erythema craquele-like changes *JAAD 72:690–695, 2015;* acute oral changes of GVH *AD 120:1461–1465, 1984*

Hereditary angioedema – reticulated erythema may be prodrome *BJD 101:549–552, 1979; J Allergy Clin Immunol 53:352–355, 1974*

Morphea/scleroderma

Lupus erythematosus – neonatal LE (cutis marmorata telangiectatica congenita-like dermatosis) – reticulated erythema *Ped Derm 30:495–497, 2013; JAAD 40:675–681, 1999;* plate-like calcinosis cutis, in SLE *AD 126:1057–1059, 1990;* nodules and atrophy *AD 126:544–546, 1990;* reticulated telangiectatic erythema of thenar and hypothenar eminences, finger pulps, toes, lateral feet, and heels; bluish red with small white scars; tumid lupus – reticulated telangiectasias *JAAD 41:250–253, 1999*

Pemphigus foliaceus – resolved lesions

Serum sickness - vasculitis

Still's disease, adult onset – reticulated erythematous scaly eruption *JAAD 73:294–303, 2015*

CONGENITAL DISORDERS

Congenital diffuse mottling of the skin

Congenital erosive and vesicular dermatosis with reticulated scarring – vesicles of trunk and extremities, erosions, ulcers, erythroderma, collodion baby, ectropion, reticulated soft scarring, scarring alopecia, absent eyebrows, hypohidrosis with compensatory hyperhidrosis *JAAD 69:909–915, 2013; Ped Derm 29:756–758, 2012; JAAD 45:946–948, 2001; Ped Derm 15:214–218, 1998; JAAD 32:873–877, 1995; AD 121:361–367, 1985*

Cutis marmorata telangiectatica congenita (CMTC) *JAAD 48:950–954, 2003; BJD 142:366–369, 2000; BJD 137:119–122, 1997; JAAD 20:1098–1104, 1989; AD 118:895–899, 1982;* reticulate erosions

Pigmentary lines of the newborn *JAAD 28:942–950, 1993; JAAD 28:893–894, 1993*

Reticulolinear aplasia cutis congenita of the face and neck – syndromes linked to Xp22 *BJD 138:1046–1052, 1998*

DEGENERATIVE DISEASES

Reflex sympathetic dystrophy (complex regional pain syndrome) - reticulate hyperpigmentation *AD 127:1541–1544, 1991; J Drugs Dermatol 17:532–536, 2018*

DRUG-INDUCED

Benzoyl peroxide – reticulate hyperpigmentation *Acta DV 78:301–302, 1998*

Bleomycin *Dermatologica 180:255–257, 1990*

Cyclophosphamide *Int J Clin Pharm 35:309–312, 2013*

Cytarabine *Dermatology 231:312–318, 2015*

Diltiazem *Dermatol Online J July 2011*

5-fluorouracil *Actas Dermosifillogr 99:573–582, 2008*

Gefitinib (EGFR inhibitor) – reticulated purpuric eruption *AD 144:269–270, 2008*

Interferon injection - personal observation

Levetiracetam *J Drugs Dermatol 9:409–410, 2010*

Lichenoid drug reaction

Loncastuximab tesirine – blanching reticulated telangiectatic patches of upper and lower extremities *JAMADerm 156:601–603, 2020*

Mefenamic acid – reticulated multifocal fixed drug eruption *J Coll Physicians Surg Pak 15:562–563, 2005*

Paclitaxel *Dermatology 231:312–318, 2015*

Rovalpituzumab teserine - blanching reticulated telangiectatic patches of upper and lower extremities *JAMADerm 156:601–603, 2020*

EXOGENOUS AGENTS

Danthron (laxative) – irritant contact dermatitis; livedoid pattern *Clin Exp Dermatol 9:95–96, 1984*

Diode laser-assisted hair removal – reticulate erythema (probably a form of erythema ab igne) *JAAD 51:774–777, 2004*

Irritant contact dermatitis - personal observation

Reticular telangiectatic erythema associated with implantable cardioverter defibrillator, pacemakers, knee prostheses, spinal cord stimulators, infusion pumps *Dermatitis 25:98–99, 2014; Mayo Clinic Proc 88:117–119, 2013; Contact Dermatitis 64:280–288, 2011; Cutis 78:329–331, 2006; AD 137:1239–1241, 2001;* overlying intrathecal pump *Soc Ped Derm Annual Meeting, July 2005; AD 141:106–107, 2005;* overlying a pacemaker *Hautarzt 32:651–654, 1981; Cutis 78:329–331, 2006; AD 137:1239–1241, 2001;* overlying intrathecal pump *Soc Ped Derm Annual Meeting, July 2005; AD 141:106–107, 2005;* overlying a pacemaker *Hautarzt 32:651–654, 1981*

Transarterial chemoembolization with drug-eluting (doxorubicin) microspheres – retiform papules of trunk *JAMADerm 150:1118–1120, 2014*

INFECTIONS

Brown recluse spider bites *JAAD 67:347–354, 2012*

Coxsackie B4 hemorrhagic dermatitis

Hepatitis B - serum sickness - reticulated fine red blanching erythema; fever, myalgias, arthritis *NEJM 368:1239–1245, 2013*

Klebsiella sepsis - personal observation

Parvovirus B19 infection - erythema infectiosum *Hum Pathol 31:488–497, 2000; J Clin Inf Dis 21:1424–1430, 1995*

Pitted keratolysis and symmetric lividity of the soles - personal observation

Rheumatic fever - erythema marginatum; reticulated pattern *JAAD 8:724–728, 1983; Ann Int Med 11:2223–2272, 1937–1938*

Rocky Mountain spotted fever

Rubella - congenital rubella - reticulated erythema *JAAD 12:697–706, 1985*

Tinea corporis

Tinea versicolor

INFILTRATIVE DISEASES

Amyloidosis - familial or X-linked cutaneous amyloidosis (X-linked reticulate pigmentary disorder with systemic manifestations) *Am J Med Genet 52:75–78, 1994; Ped Derm 10:344–351, 1993; Am J Med Genet 10:67–75, 1981;;* macular amyloid in incontinentia pigmenti–like pattern *BJD 142:371–373, 2000*

Benign cephalic histiocytosis *Ped Derm 11:164–177, 1994*

Intravascular histiocytosis with hemophagocytosis – symmetric reticulated erythema of the breasts *Histopathology 69:1077–1081, 2016*

Mastocytosis (urticaria pigmentosa) – flexural hyperpigmented reticulated plaques *AD 139:381–386, 2003*

Xanthoma disseminatum

INFLAMMATORY DISORDERS

Erythema multiforme

Kawasaki's disease *Dermatol Online J July 2019*

Post-inflammatory hyperpigmentation with band-like mucin deposition *Int J Dermatol 37:829–832, 1998*

Sarcoid – reticulate yellow stippling with resolution of erythrodermic sarcoid

Whipple's disease – macular and reticulated erythema; Addisonian hyperpigmentation; *Tropheryma whipplei JAAD 60:277–288, 2009*

METABOLIC DISEASES

Calcinosis cutis – yellow reticulated plaques *JAAD 49:1131–1136, 2003*

Calciphylaxis;- retiform purpura; calciphylaxis with stellate necrosis and retiform purpura unassociated with renal disease (non-uremic calciphylaxis) – stellate necrosis beginning as mottled purpuric reticulated patches; associated with hyperparathyroidism, malignancy, alcoholic liver disease, connective tissue disease, diabetes mellitus, chemotherapy-induced protein C or S deficiency *JAAD 82:783–796, 2020; JAMA 310:1281–1282, 2013*

Cryoglobulinemia – reticulate (retiform) purpura and livedo reticularis *AD 139:803–808, 2003; BJD 129:319–323, 1993*

Homocystinuria *JAAD 56:541–564, 2007; JAAD 40:279–281, 1999*

Hunter's syndrome – reticulated 2–10 mm skin-colored papules over scapulae, chest, neck, arms; X-linked recessive; MPS type II; iduronate-2 sulfatase deficiency; lysosomal accumulation of heparin sulfate and dermatan sulfate; short stature, full lips, coarse facies, macroglossia, clear corneas (unlike Hurler syndrome), progressive neurodegeneration, communicating hydrocephalus, valvular and ischemic heart disease, lower respiratory tract infections, adenotonsillar hypertrophy, otitis media, obstructive sleep apnea, diarrhea, hepatosplenomegaly, skeletal deformities (dysostosis multiplex), widely spaced teeth, dolichocephaly, deafness, retinal degeneration, inguinal and umbilical hernias *Ped Derm 21:679–681, 2004*

Hypergammaglobulinemic purpura of Waldenstrom – reticulate purpura *Clin Exp Dermatol 24:469–472, 1999*

Kwashiorkor – reticulated scaly eruption *AD 137:630–636, 2001*

Methylmalonic acidemia with cobalamin F type - reticulate hyperpigmentation *Am J Human Genet 15A:353, 1992*

Mitochondrial disorders – erythematous photodistributed eruptions followed by mottled or reticulated hyperpigmentation; alopecia with or without hair shaft abnormalities including trichothiodystrophy, trichoschisis, tiger tail pattern, pili torti, longitudinal grooving, and trichorhexis nodosa *Pediatrics 103:428–433, 1999*

Nephrogenic fibrosing dermopathy (nephrogenic systemic fibrosis) – reticulate hyperpigmentation JAAD 48:42–47, 2003

Primary biliary cirrhosis – disseminated reticulate hypomelanosis *Dermatology 195:382–383, 1997*

Prolidase deficiency - reticulated erythema *AD 127:124–125, 1991*

Propionic acidemia – propionyl-CoA carboxylase deficiency; low isoleucine, valine, methionine, threonine *Ped Derm 24:508–510, 2007*

Vitamin B12 and/or folate deficiency - reticulated pigmentation of the palms *AD 107:231–236, 1973*

Zinc deficiency, chronic liver disease (cirrhosis) – zinc deficiency; generalized dermatitis of erythema craquele (crackled and reticulated dermatitis) with perianal and perigenital erosions and crusts; cheilitis, hair loss *Ann DV 114:39–53, 1987;* reticulated non-pruritic scaly dermatitis of trunk in alcoholics *AD 114:937–939, 1978*

NEOPLASTIC DISEASES

Bowen's disease

Chronic NK cell lymphocytosis – retiform purpura; activating mutations in *STAT3 Int J Dermatol 41:852–857, 2002; BJD 106:960–966, 1999*

Inflammatory linear verrucous epidermal nevus (ILVEN)

Infundibulomas, eruptive infundibulomas - papules

Ink spot lentigo (reticulated black solar lentigo) *AD 128:934–940, 1992*

Juvenile xanthogranulomas - reticulated maculopapular eruption *AD 105:99–102, 1972*

Lymphoma - cutaneous T-cell lymphoma; reticulate pigmentation in CTCL *Int J Derm 30:658–659, 1991;* reticulated petechial patches of elbows and knees; chronic facial edema; hydroa vacciniforme-like cutaneous T-cell lymphoma, Epstein-Barr virus-related – edema, blisters, vesicles, ulcers, scarring, facial scars, swollen nose, lips, and periorbital edema, crusts with central hemorrhagic necrosis, facial dermatitis, photodermatitis, facial edema, facial papules and plaques, crusting of ears, fever *JAAAD 72:21–34, 2015; J Dermatol 41:29–39, 2014; JAAD 69:112–119, 2013;*

Metastases – carcinoma telangiectoides from gallbladder cancer - personal observation

Nevus comedonicus – cribriform plaques *Ped Derm 21:84–86, 2004*

Porokeratosis of Mibelli - cribriform changes *AD 122:585–590, 1986*

Porokeratosis *Clin Exp Dermatol 17:178–181, 1992; AD 121:1542–3, 1985;* reticular erythema with ostial porokeratosis *JAAD 22:913–916, 1990*

Posttransplantation lymphoproliferative disorder – red reticulated indurated plaque *AD 140:1140–1164, 2004*

Syringomas - resembling confluent and reticulated papillomatosis *Cutis 61:227–228, 1998*

Waldenstrom's macroglobulinemia – reticulate purpura and bullae *Clin Exp Dermatol 26:513–517, 2001*

PARANEOPLASTIC DISORDERS

Lymphoma – reticulated plaques due to cutaneous granulomas associated with systemic lymphoma *JAAD 51:600–605, 2004*

Palmar fasciitis and polyarthritis syndrome - indurated reticulate palmar erythema *Australas J Dermatol 50:198–201, 2009*

PHOTOSENSITIVITY DISORDERS

Actinic lichen planus *JAAD 20:226–231, 1989*

Disseminated superficial actinic porokeratosis

Stellate pseudoscars *AD 105:551–554,1972; Acta DV 52:51–54, 1972*

PRIMARY CUTANEOUS DISEASES

Acquired epidermodysplasia verruciformis - personal observation

Atopic dermatitis – reticulate and poikiloderma-like lesions of the neck*; J Dermatol 17:85–91, 1990;* "dirty neck"

Atrophoderma vermiculatum - reticulated scarring *JAAD 18:538–542, 1988*

Atrophoderma, reticulated

Atrophoderma of Moulin - reticulated, atrophic, Blaschko lesions *Ped Derm 31:373–377, 2014*

Bullous prurigo pigmentosa – pruritic reticulated bullous eruption of neck and trunk *JAMADerm 150:1005–1006, 2014; Dermatologica sinica 27:103–110, 2009*

Confluent and reticulated papillomatosis of Gougerot and Carteaud *Cutis 93:199–203, 2014; AD 145:1325–1330, 2009; Cutis 78:239–240, 2006; JAAD 49:1182–1184, 2003; BJD 142:1252–1253, 2000; AD 132:1400–1401, 1996; BJD 129:351–353, 1993; Bull Soc Fr Dermatol Syphilol 34:719–721, 1927*

Dowling-Degos syndrome (reticulated pigmented anomaly of the flexures); mutation in *KRT5/JPOFUT1* (protein-O-fucosyl transferase)/*POGLUT1 BJD 173:584–586, 2015; JAAD 40:462–467, 1999; AD 114:1150–1157, 1978;*

Epidermolysis bullosa, Dowling-Meara epidermolysis bullosa with mottled, reticulate dyspigmentation *AD 122:900–908, 1986*

Epidermolysis bullosa simplex, Mendes de Costa variant - reticulate hyperpigmentation and atrophy *JAAD 21:425–432, 1989; Ped Derm 6:91–101, 1989*

Erythema craquele (asteatotic dermatitis) – following acute edema/distension *J Dermatol 43:709–710, 2016*

Erythrokeratoderma variabilis

Erythromelalgia and webbed neck - personal observation

Folliculitis ulerythematosa reticulata - scarring and honeycomb atrophy; associated with Noonan's syndrome *AD 124:1101–1106, 1988*

Frontal fibrosing alopecia - facial lesions - skin-colored facial papules, follicular red dots, perifollicular and diffuse erythema with reticulated pattern, pigmented macules *JAAD 73:987–990, 2015*

Galli-Gallli disease – reticulate, hyper- and hypopigmented macules and papules; intertrigo; mutation in keratin 5 *BJD 170:1362–1365, 2014*

Granular parakeratosis (axillary granular parakeratosis) *JAAD 59:177–178, 2008; JAAD 52:863–867, 2005; Ped Derm 20:215–220, 2003*

Granuloma annulare, generalized *Curr Prob in Derm 8:137–188, 1996*

Ichthyosis en confetti (congenital reticulated ichthyosiform erythroderma)(CRIE) – reticulated erythroderma with guttate hypopigmentation, palmoplantar keratoderma; loss of dermatoglyphics; temporary hypertrichosis of normal skin *BJD 166:434–439, 2012; JAAD 63:607–641, 2010*

Infantile febrile psoriasiform dermatitis *Ped Derm 12:28–34, 1995*

Keratosis lichenoides chronica(Nekam's disease) – reticulated flat-topped keratotic papules and hyperpigmented plaques, linear arrays, atrophy, comedo-like lesions, prominent telangiectasia; conjunctival injection, seborrheic dermatitis-like eruption; acral dermatitis over toes; punctate keratotic papules of palmar creases; scaly red papules of face; seborrheic dermatitis-like rash of face; nail dystrophy; oral and genital erosions, conjunctivitis *AD 147:1317–1322, 2011; Cutis 86:245–248, 2010; Ped Derm 26:615–616, 2009; AD 145:867–69, 2009; AD 144:405–410, 2008; Am J Dermatopathol 28:260–275, 2006; JAAD 49:511–513, 2003; Dermatology 201:261–264, 2000; JAAD 38:306–309, 1998; JAAD*

37:263–264, 1997; Dermatopathol Pract Concept 3:310–312 1997; AD 131:609–614, 1995; Dermatology 191:188–192, 1995; AD 105:739–743, 1972; Presse Med 51:1000–1003, 1938; Arch Dermatol Syph (Berlin) 31:1–32, 1895; in children *JAAD 56:S1–5, 2007*

Lichen planus of tongue/buccal mucosa *J Oral Pathol 14:431–458, 1985*

Linear reticulated pigmented purpuric eruption - personal observation

Lichen sclerosus et atrophicus, oral – bluish-white plaques; may mimic lichen planus*; BJD 131:118–123, 1994; Br J Oral Maxillofac Surg 89:64–65, 1991*

Mid-dermal elastophagocytosis – reticulate erythema *Australas J Dermatol 42:50–54, 2001*

Parakeratosis variegata – reticulated and atrophic *New England Dermatological Society Conference, Sept 15, 2007; Dermatology 201:54–57, 2000; BJD 137:983–987, 1997; Dermatology 190:124–127, 1995; Ann Dermatol Syph 3:433–468, 1902*

Periumbilical perforating pseudoxanthoma elasticum - plaque *AD 126:1639–1644, 1990; Arch Pathol Lab Med 100:544–546, 1976*

Pigmentatio reticularis faciei and colli with epithelial cystomatosis *JAAD 37:884–886, 1997; Dermatoligae Tokyo: University of Tokyo Press 89–90, 1982*

Poikiloderma vasculare atrophicans *AD 125:1265–70, 1989*

Prurigo pigmentosa – red papules with vesiculation and crusting arranged in reticulated pattern or reticulate plaques in young women; heals with reticulated hyperpigmentation; urticarial red pruritic papules, papulovesicles, vesicles, crusted papules, and plaques with reticulated hyperpigmentation *Ped Derm 35:239–241, 2018; JAMADerm 151:796–797, 2015; J Eur Acad Dermatol Venereol 26:1149–1153, 2012; Ped Derm 24:277–279, 2007; JAAD 55:131–136, 2006; Am J Dermatopathol 25:117–129, 2003; Cutis 63:99–102, 1999; JAAD 34:509–11, 1996; AD 130:507–12, 1994; BJD 120:705–708, 1989; AD 125:1551–1554, 1989; JAAD 12:165–169, 1985; J Dermatol 5:61–67, 1978; Jpn J Dermatol 81:78–91, 1971;* zosteriform reticulated crusted papules *Ped Derm 31:523–525, 2014*

Psoriasis

Ulceronecrotic Mucha Habermann disease - generalized reticulate necrotic lesions

Unilateral laterothoracic exanthem *JAAD 34:979–984, 1996*

Vermiculate atrophoderma – honeycomb atrophy

Zosteriform reticulate hyperpigmentation *BJD 121:280, 1989; BJD 117:503–510, 1987*

SYNDROMES

Acropigmentation symmetrica of Dohi – autosomal dominant, sporadic; Asians with onset under 20 years of age; acral hyperpigmentation (reticulate pattern becoming patches with hypopigmented macules of face, trunk, distal extremities) *JAAD 43:113, 2000*

Adams-Oliver syndrome – autosomal dominant, lack of digits, syndactyly, brachydactyly, congenital cardiac malformations, microcephaly; 10% with cutis marmorata telangiectatica congenita *JAAD 65:893–906, 2011; JAAD 58:697–702, 2008; Dermatology 187:205–208, 1993*

Ataxia telangiectasia

Beckwith-Wiedemann syndrome – exomphalos, neonatal macroglossia, gigantism, organomegaly, Wilms' tumor; cutis marmorata telangiectatica congenital *JAAD 58:697–702, 2008*

Cantu's syndrome – autosomal dominant, onset in early adolescence with 1 mm brown macules which become confluent over face,

feet, forearms; hyperkeratotic papules of palms and soles *Clin Genet 14:165, 1978*

Cardiofaciocutaneous syndrome - personal observation

Chanarin-Dorfman syndrome – ichthyosiform erythroderma; Jordan's anomaly (leukocyte vacuolization) *Clin Exp Dermatol 42:699–701, 2017*

CLOVE (congenital lipomatous overgrowth, vascular malformations and epidermal nevi) syndrome – capillary, venous, and mixed vascular malformations, epidermal nevi, lipomas; hemihypertrophy (milder than that of Proteus syndrome) *Am J Med Genet 143A:2944–2958, 2007*

Coffin-Lowry syndrome – X-linked inheritance; straight coarse hair, prominent forehead, prominent supraorbital ridges, hypertelorism, large nose with broad base, thick lips with mouth held open, large hands, tapering fingers, severe mental retardation; loose skin easily stretched, cutis marmorata, dependent acrocyanosis, varicose veins *Clin Genet 34:230–245, 1988; Am J Dis Child 112:205–213, 1966*

Congenital reticular ichthyosiform erythroderma (ichthyosis variegata) *BJD 139:893–896, 1998;* ichthyosis 'en confettis *Dermatology 188:40–45, 1994*

Cornelia de Lange (Brachmann-de Lange) syndrome – persistent cutis marmorata *AD 93:702–707, 1966;* generalized hypertrichosis, confluent eyebrows, low hairline, hairy forehead and ears, hair whorls of trunk, single palmar crease, cutis marmorata, psychomotor and growth retardation with short stature, specific facies, hypertrichosis of forehead, face, back, shoulders, and extremities, bushy arched eyebrows with synophrys; long delicate eyelashes, skin around eyes and nose with bluish tinge, small nose with depressed root, prominent philtrum, thin upper lip with crescent-shaped mouth, widely spaced, sparse teeth, hypertrichosis of forehead, posterior neck, and arms, low set ears, arched palate, antimongoloid palpebrae; congenital eyelashes; xerosis, especially over hands and feet, nevi, facial cyanosis, lymphedema *Ped Derm 24:421–423, 2007; JAAD 56:541–564, 2007; JAAD 48:161–179, 2003; JAAD 37:295–297, 1997; Am J Med Genet 47:959–964, 1993*

CRIE syndrome - congenital reticulated ichthyosiform erythroderma (ichthyosis variegata) *BJD 139:893–896, 1998; Dermatology 188:40–45, 1994*

Cutis marmorata-phacomatosis cesiomarmorata (CMTC with aberrant mongolian spots) *Ped Derm 24:555–556, 2007*

Cutis marmorata telangiectatica congenita syndrome – body asymmetry, 2–3 toe syndactyly, hypotonia, developmental delay, midfacial vascular stains, joint laxity, loose skin *Ped Derm 24:555–556, 2007*

Dermatopathia pigmentosa reticularis (dermatopathia pigmentosa reticularis hyperkeratosis et mutilans) – autosomal dominant; reticulate pigmentation, alopecia, nail changes, palmoplantar hyperkeratosis (punctate palmoplantar keratoderma), loss of dermatoglyphics; infantile bullae, reticular hyperpigmentation of flexures, ainhum-like contraction, periodontopathy *JAAD 26:298–301, 1992;AD 126:935–939, 1990*

Divry-Van Bogaert syndrome – autosomal recessive; congenital livedo reticularis; diffuse leptomeningeal angiomatosis *J Neurol Sci 14:301–314, 1971*

Down's syndrome – persistent cutis marmorata *AD 112:1397–1399, 1976*

Dyschromatosis universalis hereditaria *BJD 177:945959, 2017; Ped Derm 17:70–72, 2000*

Dyskeratosis congenita (Zinsser-Engman-Cole syndrome) – Xq28 *J Med Genet 33:993–995, 1996; Dermatol Clin 13:33–39, 1995; BJD 105:321–325, 1981*

Epidermolysis bullosa pruriginosa – reticulated linear hypopigmented plaques; bullae; scars; zebra stripe appearance; dyschromatosis *Ped Derm 32:549–550, 2015*; reticulate scarring, dermatitis with lichenified plaques, violaceous linear scars, albopapuloid lesions of the trunk, prurigo nodularis-like lesions, milia *BJD 152:1332–1334, 2005*

Extensive reticular hyperpigmentation and milia *Ped Derm 16:108–110, 1999*

Familial multiple follicular hamartoma *JAAD 37:884–886, 1997; Dermatologica 159:316–324, 1979*

Goltz's syndrome (focal dermal hypoplasia) – asymmetric linear and reticulated streaks of atrophy and telangiectasia; yellow-red nodules; raspberry-like papillomas of lips, perineum, acrally, at perineum, buccal mucosa; xerosis; scalp and pubic hair sparse and brittle; short stature; asymmetric face; syndactyly, polydactyly; ocular, dental, and skeletal abnormalities with osteopathia striata of long bones *JAAD 25:879–881, 1991*

Haber's syndrome - reticulate keratotic plaques on trunk and limbs; rosacea-like eruption of face *BJD 77:1–8, 1965*

Hereditary angioneurotic edema - reticulate erythema in prodromal stage *BJD 101:549–552, 1979*

Hereditary sclerosing poikiloderma *AD 100:413–422, 1969*

Hoyeraal-Hreidarrson syndrome – severe variant of dyskeratosis congenita *BJ Hematol 170:457–471, 2015*

Hunter's syndrome (mucopolysaccharidosis type II) – fleshy ivory white papules and nodules (pebbling) in ridging or reticular pattern, symmetric, involving area between the angle of the scapula and anterior axillary line; coarse facial features, bony abnormalities, recurrent umbilical and inguinal hernias; recurrent otitis media and pneumonia; developmental delay; coarse straight scalp hair; hypertrichosis of body and face; slate grey nevi; bilateral knee pain; decreased sulfoiduronate sulfatase (L-iduronate-2-sulfatase) resulting in buildup of dermatan sulfate and heparin sulfate *Ped Derm 37:369–370, 2020; Ped Derm 15:370–373, 1998*

Hutchinson-Gilford progeria syndrome – reticulated hyperpigmentation interspersed with hypopigmentation *NEJM 592–604, 2008*

Incontinentia pigmenti - hyper or hypopigmentation *Ped Derm 7:174–178, 1990*; reticulate hypohidrotic lines of posterior calves in stage IV *Clin Exp Dermatol 30:474–480, 2005*

Jackli syndrome – generalized reticulated hyperpigmentation with alopecia, microdontia, and childhood cataracts

Keratosis-ichthyosis-deafness (KID) syndrome – autosomal recessive; dotted waxy, fine granular, stippled, or reticulated surface pattern of severe diffuse hyperkeratosis of palms and soles (palmoplantar keratoderma), ichthyosis with well-marginated, serpiginous erythematous verrucous plaques, hyperkeratotic elbows and knees, perioral furrows, leukoplakia, follicular occlusion triad, scalp cysts, nodules (trichilemmal tumors, squamous cell carcinoma), bilateral sensorineural deafness, photophobia with vascularizing keratitis, blindness, hypotrichosis of scalp, eyebrows, and eyelashes, dystrophic nails, chronic mucocutaneous candidiasis, otitis externa, abscesses, blepharitis; connexin 26 mutation *JAAD 69:127–134, 2013; Ped Derm 27:651–652, 2010; Ped Derm 23:81–83, 2006; JAAD 51:377–382, 2004; BJD 148:649–653, 2003; Cutis 72:229–230, 2003; Ped Derm 19:285–292, 2002; Ped Derm 15:219–221, 1998; Ped Derm 13:105–113, 1996; JAAD 19:1124–1126, 1988; AD 123:777–782, 1987; AD 117:285–289, 1981; J Cutaneous Dis 33:255–260, 1915*

Kindler's syndrome - reticulate erythema *AD 133:1111–1117, 1997; Ped Derm 13:397–402, 1996*

Koraxitrachitic syndrome – self-healing collodion baby; heals with mottled reticulated atrophy; alopecia, absent eyelashes and eyebrows, conjunctival pannus, hypertelorism, prominent nasal root,

large mouth, micrognathia, brachydactyly, syndactyly of interdigital spaces *Am J Med Genet 86:454–458, 1999*

Macrocephaly-CMTC (cutis marmorata telangiectatica congenita syndrome) – macrocephalic neonatal hypotonia and developmental delay; distended linear and serpiginous abdominal wall veins, patchy reticulated vascular stain without atrophy; telangiectasias of face and ears; midline reticulated facial nevus flammeus (capillary malformation), hydrocephalus, skin and joint hypermobility, hyperelastic skin, thickened subcutaneous tissue, polydactyly, 2–3 toe syndactyly, hydrocephalus, frontal bossing, hemihypertrophy with segmental overgrowth; neonatal hypotonia, developmental delay *Ped Derm 33:570–584, 2016; AD 145:287–293, 2009; JAAD 58:697–702, 2008; Ped Derm 24:555–556, 2007; JAAD 56:541–564, 2007; Ped Derm 16:235–237, 1999; Genet Couns 9:245–253, 1998; Am J Med Genet 70:67–73, 1997* (Note: Beckwith-Wiedemann syndrome demonstrates dysmorphic ears, macroglossia, body asymmetry, midfacial vascular stains, visceromegaly with omphalocele, neonatal hypoglycemia, BUT NO MACROCEPHALY) *Ped Derm 16:235–237, 1999*

Megalencephaly-capillary malformation polymicrogyria (MCAP) syndrome – reticulated capillary malformation *Ped Derm 33:570–584, 2016*

MELAS syndrome - mitochondrial encephalomyopathy with lactic acidosis - reticulated hyperpigmentation *JAAD 41:469–473, 1999*

Mendes da Costa syndrome - hereditary bullous dystrophy, macular type; similar skin changes as Kindler's syndrome (Da Costa's) syndrome *Ped Derm 6:91–101, 1989*

Micrcephaly-capillary malformation syndrome (MICCAP) – reticulated capillary malformations – reticulated capillary malformations *Ped Derm 33:570–584, 2016*

Microphthalmia with linear skin defects (MIDAS syndrome)(MLS syndrome, Xp deletion syndrome, Xp 22.3 microdeletion syndrome) – Xp22.3 deletion – X-linked dominant; linear jagged skin defects of scalp, face, neck, and occasionally upper trunk, Blaschko-esque depressed patches of face, linear red atrophic patches (aplasia cutis-like), hyperpigmented Blascko thin facial patches, reticulate skin defects of head and neck, preauricular ear pit, severe short stature, congenital heart defects, agenesis of the corpus callosum, ambiguous genitalia, nail dystrophy, microphthalmia, sclerocornea; mutation in holocytochrome c synthase *Ped Derm 29:217–218, 2012; Ped Derm 25:548–552, 2008; Ped Derm 20:153–157, 2003; JAAD 44: 612–615, 2001; Am J Med Genet 49:229–234, 1994*

Mitochondrial disease - reticulated hyperpigmentation *Pediatrics 103:428–433, 1999*

Naegeli- Franceschetti-Jadassohn syndrome – autosomal dominant, reticulate gray to brown pigmentation of neck, upper trunk and flexures, punctate or diffuse palmoplantar keratoderma, hypohidrosis with heat intolerance, onycholysis, subungual hyperkeratosis, yellow tooth enamel *JAAD 28:942–950, 1993*

Naegeli-Franceschetti-Jadassohn syndrome variant – reticulate pigmentary dermatosis with hypohidrosis and short stature *Int J Dermatol 34:30–31, 1995*

Neurofibromatosis - nevus anemicus in neurofibromatosis type 1 *JAAD 69:768–775, 2013*

Nicolau syndrome - embolia cutis medicamentosa; sulfonamides, benzathine penicillin, gentamicin, phenobarbital, camphor-quinine, triflupromazine, chlorpromazine, interferon alpha *Ped Derm 12:187–190, 1995*

Odonto-onycho-dermal dyplasia – oligodontia with small widely spaced conical peg-shaped teeth, hypodontia, absence of secondary teeth; palmoplantar keratoderma, hyperhidrosis, dystrophic nails, erythematous telangiectatic, reticulated atrophic malar and ala nasal patches with vermiculate scarring *JAAD 57:732–733, 2007; Am J Med Genet 14:335–346, 1983*

Pachyonychia congenita with cutaneous amyloidosis and hyperpigmentation *JAAD 16 (pt 1)935–940, 1987*

Partington syndrome

Phakomatosis pigmentovascularis type V - extensive Mongolian spot, nevus flammeus, cutis marmorata telangiectatica *Ped Derm 25:198–200, 2008; BJD 156:1068–1071, 2007*

PIK3CA/AKT/mTOR-related overgrowth syndromes – reticulated port wine stain; hemihypertrophy *GeneReviews.http://ncbi.nlm.nih. gov/pubmed/23946963; Am J Med Genet 167:287–295, 2015; JAAD 69:589–594, 2013; Nature Genetics 44:934–940, 2012*
> CLOVES syndrome
> Macrocephaly capillary malformation syndrome(macrocephaly cutis marmorata telangiectatica congenita)(megalencephaly capillary malformation syndrome)
> Proteus syndrome

Reticulate acropigmentation of Dohi - dyschromatosis symmetrica hereditaria *Clin Exp Derm 20:477, 1995;* autosomal recessive *JAAD 43:113–117, 2000*

Reticulate acropigmentation of Kitamura *Dermatology 200:57–58, 2000; Dermatology 195:337–343, 1997; JAAD 37:884–886, 1997; Int J Dermatol 32:726–727, 1993; BJD 109:105–110, 1983; BJD 95:437–443, 1976*

Reticular erythematous mucinosis (REM syndrome) - red reticulated plaques of breasts and central back; asymptomatic, photosensitivity of middle-aged women *BJD 169:1207–1211, 2013; AD 147:710–715, 2011; BJD 161:583–590, 2009; BJD 150: 173–174, 2004; AD 140:660–662, 2004; JAAD 19:859–868, 1988; BJD 91:191–199, 1974; AD 82:980–985, 1960*

Reticulate hyperpigmentation of Iijima, Naito, and Uyeno *Acta DV 71:248–250, 1991*

Rothmund-Thomson syndrome – face spreading to buttocks and extremities, chronic reticulated hypo- and hyperpigmentation, punctate atrophy, and telangiectasias; poikiloderma *Gene Reviews Oct 6, 1999*

Schopf-Schulz-Passarge syndrome (congenital ectodermal dysplasia) – acral papules of syringocystadenoma papilliferum and syringofibroadenoma; reticulated palmoplantar keratoderma, hypodontia, hypotrichosis, nail dystrophy, multiple eyelid apocrine hidrocystomas, no dermatoglyphics of fingertips; mutation in WNT10A *JAAD 65:1066–169, 2011*

Trisomy 18 – persistent cutis marmorata *AD 145:287–293, 2009*

Trisomy 21 - congenital livedo reticularis *JAAD 56:541–564, 2007*

Tumor necrosis factor (TNF) receptor 1-associated periodic fever syndromes (TRAPS)(same as familial hibernian fever and familial periodic fever) - tender red plaques, fever, polycyclic, reticulated, and migratory patches and plaques, conjunctivitis, periorbital edema, myalgia, abdominal pain, headache; Irish and Scottish predominance *Pre-AAD Pediatric Dermatology Meeting, March 2000*

Weary's syndrome - hereditary and bullous acrokeratotic poikiloderma of Weary and Kindler *BJD 140:366–368, 1999*

Werner's syndrome

Woolly hair, alopecia, premature loss of teeth, nail dystrophy, reticulate acral hyperkeratosis, facial abnormalities *BJD 145:157–161, 2001*

Ziprkowski-Margolis syndrome

TOXINS

Acrodynia

Heavy metal poisoning

Ice pack dermatosis – red plaque, retiform purpura with purpuric papules and ulcers *JAMA Derm 149:1314–1318, 2013*

TRAUMA

Erythema ab igne *Cutis 88:290–292, 2012; JAAD 18:1003–1019, 1988;* car heater *Cutis 59:81–82, 1997;* heated car seat *AD 148:265–266, 2012*

Hysterosalpingogram - reticulated purpura with contrast medium after hysterosalpingogram *BJD 138:919–920, 1998*

Radiodermatitis, chronic *BJD 141:150–153, 1999*

VASCULAR DISEASES

Acute hemorrhagic edema of infancy – purpura in cockade pattern of face, cheeks, eyelids, and ears; may form reticulate pattern; edema of penis and scrotum *JAAD 23:347–350, 1990;* necrotic lesions of the ears, urticarial lesions; oral petechiae *JAAD 23:347–350, 1990; Ann Pediatr 22:599–606, 1975*

Atrophie blanche (livedoid vasculopathy)

Angioma serpiginosum

Bockenheimer's syndrome - diffuse generalized phlebactasia *Ped Derm 17:100–104, 2000; JAAD 40:257–259, 1999;*

Capillary malformations *Ped Derm 33:570–584, 2016; JAAD 56:541–564, 2007;* generalized

Capillary malformations with bone and soft tissue overgrowth *Ped Derm 33:570–584, 2016*

Cholesterol emboli- livedo racemosa *JAMADerm 151:97–98, 2015; AD 122:1194–1198, 1986*

Chronic NK cell lymphocytosis – retiform purpura; activating mutations in *STAT3 Int J Dermatol 41:852–857, 2002; BJD 106:960–966, 1999*

CLAPO syndrome – capillary malformation of lower lip; lymphatic malformation of face and neck; swollen lip, prominent veins of neck, jaw, and scalp, asymmetry of face and limbs, partial or generalized overgrowth reticulate erythema of neck ; *PIK3CA* mutation *Ped Derm 35:681–682, 2018*

Cutaneous polyarteritis nodosa – atrophie blanche lesions, acrocyanosis, Raynaud's phenomenon, peripheral gangrene, red plaques and peripheral nodules, myalgias; macular lymphocytic arteritis – red or hyperpigmented reticulated patches of legs *JAAD 73:1013–1020, 2015*

Cutis marmorata – physiologic vascular marbling
> Athyrotic (congenital) hypothyroidism
> Cornelia de Lange syndrome
> Adams-Oliver syndrome
> Trisomy 18
> Trisomy 21
> Homocystinuria
> Divry-Van Bogaert syndrome
> Neonatal vasomotor instability

Cutis marmorata telangiectatica congenita (Lohuizon syndrome) – reticulated capillary malformation with telangiectasias; ulcerated over elbows and knees; atrophy; limb hypoplasia *JAAD 56:541–564, 2007; JAAD 48:950–954, 2003; BJD 142:366–369, 2000*

Cutis marmorata telangiectatica congenita, congenital macrocephaly, macrosomia, segmental overgrowth, central nervous system malformations, connective tissue abnormalities, mental retardation *JAAD 56:541–564, 2007; Ped Derm 19:506–509, 2002*

Diffuse capillary malformation with overgrowth – reticulated red patch with hypertrophy *JAAD 69:589–594, 2013*

Diffuse dermal angiomatosis (reactive angioendotheliomatosis), including diffuse dermal angiomatosis of the breast; reticulated erythema with ulcerations of breasts; seen in patients with breast reduction or pendulous breasts *Int J Dermatol 55:e103–104, 2016; JAAD 71:1212–1217, 2014; AD 144:693–694, 2008; AD 142:343–347, 2006*

Eosinophilic granulomatosis with polyangiitis – reticulated purpura *AD 141:873–878, 2005;* pink reticulated plaques, purpuric patches, stellate purpura *JAMADerm 154:4867–487, 2018; Clin Rheumatol 30:573–580, 2010*

Generalized essential telangiectasia - familial or acquired *JAAD 37:321–325, 1997; JAMA 185:909–913, 1963*

Hemangioma - abortive or minimal growth infantile hemangiomas – reticulated red patch with telangiectasias *JAAD 58:685–690, 2008*

Henoch-Schonlein purpura in adults - reticulate purpura *AD 125:53–56, 1989*

Hereditary hemorrhagic telangiectasia

Klippel-Trenaunay-Weber syndrome – capillary-lymphatic-venous malformation with limb overgrowth *Ped Derm 24:356–362, 2007; Br J Surg 72:232–236, 1985; Arch Gen Med 3:641–672, 1900*

Lymphocytic thrombophilic arteritis – painless non-ulcerating livedo reticularis, reticulated hyperpigmentation, red nodules *AD 144:1175–1182, 2008*

Lymphedema – with reticulate vascular anomaly *BJD 135:92–97, 1996*

Macular arteritis – reticulated purpuric macules mimicking pigmented purpuric eruption *Ped Derm 26:93–95, 2009;* asymptomatic hyperpigmented macules of legs in black patients *JAAD 52:364–366, 2005; JAAD 49:519–522, 2003*

Net-like superficial vascular malformation (lymphatic malformation); deep red, purple, or red-brown *BJD 175:191–193, 2016*

Polyarteritis nodosa – reticulated lilac erythema

Port wine stain

Reticulate purpura *Indian J Derm 59:3–14, 2014*

Reticular infantile hemangioma – refractory punctuate and scattered ulcerations of buttocks, and/or perineum, involve legs of females, enlarged foot and limb; associated with ventral-caudal anomalies such as omphalocele, femoral artery hypoplasia, imperforate anus, solitary or duplicate kidney, tethered cord; congestive heart failure *Ped Derm 24:356–362, 2007*

Reticular infantile hemangioma with minimal or arrested growth associated with lipoatrophy *JAAD 72:828–833, 2015*

Sturge-Weber syndrome

Tufted angioma – reticulated solitary red-brown to violaceous plaque *Int J Dermatol 53:1165–1176, 2014; Head and Neck Pathol 7:291–294, 2013*

Unilateral dermatomal telangiectasia *JAAD 8:468–477, 1983*

Congenital Volkmann ischemic contracture(neonatal compartment syndrome) – upper extremity circumferential contracture from wrist to elbow; necrosis, cyanosis, edema, eschar, bullae, purpura; irregular border with central white ischemic tissue with formation of bullae, edema, or spotted bluish color with necrosis, a reticulated eschar or whorled pattern with contracture of arm; differentiate from necrotizing fasciitis, congenital varicella, neonatal gangrene, aplasia cutis congenita, amniotic band syndrome, subcutaneous fat necrosis, epidermolysis bullosa *BJD 150:357–363, 2004*

RETICULATED HYPERPIGMENTATION

Clin Exp Dermatol 9:439–450, 1984

AUTOIMMUNE DISEASES AND DISEASES OF IMMUNE DYSREGULATION

Graft vs. host disease, chronic *Dermatol Online J 19:20710, 2013*

X-linked reticulate pigmentary disorder – recurrent pneumonia, bronchiectasis, chronic diarrhea, failure to thrive, diffuse reticulated hyperpigmentation, hypohidrosis, corneal disease leading to blindness; facies with unswept hair, flared eyebrows; female carriers display blaschko hyperpigmentation; *POLA1* gene *Ped Derm 33:602–614, 2016*

DRUGS

Bleomycin *Dermatologica 180:255–257, 1990*

Cyclophosphamide *Int J Clin Pharm 35:309–312, 2013*

Diltiazem – reticulated photopigmentation *Dermatol Online jJ 17:142011; AD 142:206–210, 2006*

EXOGENOUS AGENTS

Tar melanosis *Contact Derm 3:249, 1977*

INFILTRATIVE DISORDERS

Amyloidosis, familial *BJD 161:1217–1224, 2009*

Amyloidosis, macular – intensive reticulated pigmented patches *BJD 161:1217–1224, 2009; Dermatology 207:65–67, 2003*

INFLAMMATORY DISORDERS

Post-inflammatory hyperpigmentation - secondary to allergic contact dermatitis to benzoyl peroxides

METABOLIC DISORDERS

Calcinosis cutis – hyperpigmented reticulated plaques *BJD 142:820–822, 2000*

Cryoglobulinemia – hepatitis C, vasculitis, lower leg reticulated pigmentation due to resolved livedo reticularis

Fanconi's syndrome *BJD 178:335–349, 2018; AD 103:581, 1971*

Vitamin B12 deficiency – sparse thin scalp hairs, generalized hyperpigmentation, hyperpigmentation over dorsal hands and feet, reticulate hyperpigmentation, glossitis, cheilitis *Ped Derm 35:796–799, 2018*

NEOPLASTIC DISORDERS

Acquired dermal melanocytosis *BJD 124:96, 1991*

Lymphoma - cutaneous T-cell lymphoma *Int J Derm 30:658, 1991*

Myeloma with reticulated pigmentation - personal observation

PHOTODERMATOSES

Poikiloderma of Civatte *Ann Dermatol Syphilol 9:381–420, 1938*

PRIMARY CUTANEOUS DISEASES

Atopic dirty neck

Atrophoderma of Moulin *JAAD Case Rep 2:10–12, 2016*

Confluent and reticulated papillomatosis of Gougerot and Carteaud *JAAD 56:896–898, 2007; Cutis 80:184, 201–202, 2007; Cutis 78:239–240, 2006; JAAD 49:1182–1184, 2003; BJD 142:1252–1253, 2000; AD 132:1400–1401, 1996; BJD 129:351–353, 1993; JAAD 2:401–410, 1980; Bull Soc Fr Dermatol Syphilol 34:719–721, 1927*

Congenital diffuse mottling of the skin – mottled pigmentation, café au lait macules, facial lentigines *Ped Derm 24:566–570, 2007*

Dermatitis *Clin Exp Derm 15:380–381, 1990*

Dyschromatosis symmetrica hereditaria (reticulate acropigmentation of Dohi)(acropigmentation symmetrica of Dohi) – involves extremities and face *BJD 177:945–959, 2017; BJD 153:342–345, 2005; BJD 150:633–639, 2004; BJD 144:162–168, 2001; JAAD 45:760–763, 2001; JAAD 43:113–117, 2000;* sun-exposed areas only *JAAD 10:1–16, 1984*

Dyschromatosis universalis hereditaria – mottled hyperpigmentation, small stature, high tone deafness *BJD 177:945–959, 2017; Ped Derm 24:566–570, 2007; Semin Cut Med Surg 16:72–80, 1997; Clin Exp Derm 2:45, 1977*

Ectodermal dysplasia *JAAD 6:476–480, 1982*

Ectodermal dysplasia and clefting – alopecia, tooth abnormalities, reticulated hyperpigmentation *Ped Derm 28:707–710, 2011*

Epidermolysis bullosa herpetiformis (Dowling-Meara) *Ped Derm 13:306–309, 1996*

Epidermolysis bullosa, autosomal recessive – diffuse palmoplantar keratoderma with pitting, pitted palmaar keratoderma, dystrophic toenails, blistering, generalized reticulated hyperpigmentation; dental caries with squamous cell carcinoma of tongue; keratin 14 mutation; must be differentiated from EBS with mottled pigmentation (keratin 5 mutation), Kindler's syndrome, Naegeli syndrome – inflammatory blisters and hypohidrosis (keratin 14 mutation), and dyskeratosis congenita (telomerase mutation) *BJD 162:880–882, 2010*

Epidermolysis bullosa simplex with mottled pigmentation – wart-like hyperkeratotic papules of axillae, wrists, dorsae of hands, palms and soles; P25L mutation of keratin 5 *JAAD 52:172–173, 2005;* non-scarring alopecia *BJD 177:945–959, 2017; BJD 174:633–635, 2016*

Familial pigmentation with dystrophy of the nails *AD 71:591–598, 1955*

Familial progressive hyperpigmentation *AD 103:581, 1971*

Galli-Galli disease – autosomal dominant; reticulated hyperpigmentated scaly plaques, red-brown macules, crusted papules, perioral pitted scars, comedones; suprabasal acantholysis, reticulate hyperpigmentation like Dowling-Degos disease; mutation in *KRT5* and *POFUT-1 (*protein O-fucotransferase 1) and *POGLUT-1* (protein o-glucosyltransferase-1) *BJD 177:945–959, 2017; BJD 176:270–274, 2017; JAMADerm 152:461–462, 2016*

Hereditary focal transgressive palmoplantar keratoderma – autosomal recessive; hyperkeratotic lichenoid papules of elbows and knees, psoriasiform lesions of scalp and groin, spotty and reticulate hyperpigmentation of face, trunk, and extremities, alopecia of eyebrows and eyelashes *BJD 146:490–494, 2002*

Keratosis lichenoides chronica - in children *JAAD 56:S1–5, 2007; Arch Dermatol Syph (Berlin) 31:1–32, 1895*

Lichen planus – generalized reticulated hyperpigmentation *Clin Exp Dermatol 34:e63–69, 2009*

Melanosis universalis hereditaria *AD 125:1442, 1989*

Pigmentatio reticularis faciei et colli with multiple epithelial cysts *AD 121:109, 1985*

Prurigo pigmentosa – red papules with vesiculation and crusting arranged in reticulated pattern or reticulate plaques in young women; heals with reticulated hyperpigmentation; urticarial red pruritic papules, papulovesicles, vesicles, and plaques with reticulated hyperpigmentation *JAMADerm 155:377–378, 2019; JAMADerm 154:353–354, 2018; JAMADerm 153:353–354, 2017; JAMADerm 151:796–797, 2015; J Eur Acad Dermatol Venereol 26:1149–1153, 2012; Ped Derm 24:277–279, 2007; JAAD 55:131–136, 2006; Am J Dermatopathol 25:117–129, 2003; Cutis 63:99–102, 1999; JAAD 34:509–11, 1996; AD 130:507–12, 1994; BJD 120:705–708, 1989; AD 125:1551–1554, 1989; JAAD 12:165–169, 1985; Jpn J Dermatol 81:78–91, 1971*

Reticulate acropigmentation of Kitamura – reticulate pigmentation of dorsal hands and feet with palmoplantar pits; differs from acropigmentation symmetrica of Dohi by the absence of hypopigmented macules *BJD 177:945–959, 2017; BJD 144:162–168, 2001; Semin Cut Med Surg 16:72–80, 1997; AD 115:760, 1979; BJD 95:437–443, 1976; Rinsho No Hifu Hitsunyo 1943:201*

Reticulate hyperpigmentation of Iijima, Naito, Vyeno *Arch Derm Vener 71:248–250, 1991*

Reticulate nonmelanocytic hyperpigmented anomaly *Int J Derm 30:39–42, 1991*

Riehl's melanosis – rapid onset of gray-brown reticulated hyperpigmentation of the face *J Drugs Dermatol 13:356–358, 2014*

SASH1-related lentigines, hyper- and hypopigmentation, alopecia, nail dystrophy, palmoplantar keratoderma, skin cancer *BJD 177:945–959, 2017*

Unilateral dermatomal pigmentary dermatosis *Semin Cut Med Surg 16:72–80, 1997*

X-linked reticulated pigmentary disorder – amyloid-associated *BJD 177:945–959, 2017*

Zosteriform reticulate hyperpigmentation *BJD 121:280, 1989; BJD 117:503–510, 1987*

SYNDROMES

Basaloid follicular hamartoma syndrome – reticulated hyperpigmentation of palms and soles - personal observation

Cantu's syndrome – reticulated hyperpigmentation of face, forearms, feet with palmoplantar keratoderma *Clin Genet 14:165, 1978*

Dermatopathia pigmentosa reticularis – autosomal dominant; localized mottled pigmentation *BJD 177:945–959, 2017*

reticulate pigmentation of trunk, neck, and proximal extremities, alopecia, nail changes (mild onychodystrophy), palmoplantar keratoderma, loss of dermatoglyphics, non-scarring alopecia; hyperpigmented tongue, hypo- or hyperhidrosis, non-scarring blisters of dorsal hands and feet, dark areolae, thin eyebrows; mutation in K14 *Ped Derm 24:566–570, 2007; J Dermatol 24:266-269, 1997; Semin Cut Med Surg 16:72–80, 1997; JAAD 26:298–301, 1992; AD 126:935–939, 1990; Hautarzt 6:262, 1960; Dermatol Wochenschr 138:1337, 1958*

Dowling-Degos disease (reticulated pigmented anomaly of the flexures)- autosomal dominant; reticulated hyperpigmentated scaly papules, plaques, red-brown macules, crusted papules,, perioral pitted scars, comedones; mutation in *KRT5* and *POFUT-1 (*protein O-fucotransferase 1)) and *POGLUT-1 (*protein o-glucosyltransferase-1) *BJD 177:945–959, 2017; BJD 176:270–274, 2017; JAMADerm 152:461–462, 2016; Semin Cut Med Surg 16:72–80, 1997; AD 114:1150, 1978;* acantholytic variant (Galli-Galli disease) *JAAD 178:502–508, 2018; JAAD 45:760–763, 2001; JAAD 24:888–892, 1991; Hautarzt 33:378–383, 1982; AD 114:1150–1157, 1978;* reticulated pigmentation of the vulva and perianal skin; pitted perioral scars; comedo-like lesions *AD 148:113–118, 2012*

Dyskeratosis congenita(Hoyeraal-Hreidarsson syndrome) – reticulated hyperpigmentation, dystrophic nails and oral leukoplakia; progressive bone marrow failure, myelodysplastic syndrome or acute myelogenous leukemia *BJD 178:335–349, 2018; JAAD 77:1194–1196, 2017; BJD 177:945–959, 2017; BJD 176:270–274, 2017; J Blood Med 5:157–167, 2014; Br J Haematol 145:164–172, 2009; Semin Cut Med Surg 16:72–80, 1997*

Exudative retinopathy with bone marrow failure (Revesz syndrome) – intrauterine growth retardation, reticulate hyperpigmentation of trunk, palms, and soles; fine sparse hair, ataxia with cerebellar hypoplasia, hypertonia, progressive psychomotor retardation *J Med Genet 29:673–675, 1992*

Franceschetti-Jadassohn-Naegeli syndrome – autosomal dominant; brown-gray reticulated hyperpigmentation fading after teens, hypohidrosis; palmoplantar hyperkeratosis; dental abnormalities, nail dystrophy, bleeding tendencies *Ped Derm 22:122–126, 2005; JAAD 10:1–16, 1984; Dematologica 108:1–28, 1954; Schweiz Med Wschr 8:48, 1927*

Galli-Galli disease –acantholytic variation of Dowling-Degos disease; reticulated hyperpigmentation with red macules, papules, and papulovesicles *BJD 163:197–200, 2010; JAAD 58:299–302, 2008; BJD 150:350–352, 2004; JAAD 45:760–763, 2001; Akt Dermatol 12:41–46, 1986; Hautarzt 33:378–383, 1982*

Generalized anhidrosis, diffuse reticular hyperpigmentation, syndactyly *J Dermatol 46:e154–155, 2019*

Griscelli's syndrome type 2 *BJD 178:335–349, 2018*

Haber's syndrome – autosomal dominant; photo-aggravated rosacea-like rash of face; papules, pustules, scarring and telangiectasia; reticulate pigmented macules and keratotic plaques on trunk and extremities *Australas J Dermatol 38:82–84, 1997; AD 117:321, 1981; BJD 77:1–8, 1965*

Incontinentia pigmenti - reticulated linear hyperpigmented patches *JAAD 64:508–515, 2011; Ped Derm 24:566–570, 2007*

Kindler's syndrome (hereditary bullous acrokeratotic poikiloderma of Weary-Kindler) *Ped Derm 23:586–588, 2006; AD 142:1619–1624, 2006; AD 142:620–624, 2006; AD 140:939–944, 2004; Int J Dermatol 36:529–533, 1997; AD 1487–1490, 1996; BJD 66:104–111, 1954*

Mendes da Costa syndrome (dystrophia bullosa, typus maculatus) – X-linked recessive; tense bullae, alopecia, coarse reticulated hyperpigmentation of face and extremities with atrophy, mental retardation *Acta DV (Stockh) 18:265, 1937*

Mitochondrial disorders – reticulate hyperpigmentation of cheeks, dorsal hands and forearms; hypertrichosis, hair shaft abnormalities, acrocyanosis

Mononeuritis multiplex, lividity, and purpura - personal observation

Naegeli-Franceschetti-Jadassohn syndrome – absent dermatoglyphics, reticulated hyperpigmentation, palmoplantar keratoderma, dental abnormalities, abnormal sweating SASH1-related lentigines, hyper- and hypopigmentation, alopecia, nail dystrophy, palmoplantar keratoderma, skin cancer *BJD 177:945–959, 2017*

Reticulate hyperpigmentation with alopecia, nail changes, and growth retardation with or without blisters *Schweiz Med Wochenschr 100:228–233, 1970; Monatsschr Kinderheilkd 78:773–781, 1939*

Revesz syndrome – fatal disease; fine sparse hair, fine reticulate hyperpigmentation, ataxia, cerebellar hypoplasia, cerebral calcifications; exudative retinopathy; bone marrow failure *J Med Genet 29:673–675, 1992*

X-linked reticulate pigmentary disorder with systemic manifestations (familial cutaneous amyloidosis)(Partington syndrome II) – X-linked; rare; Xp21-22; boys with generalized reticulated muddy brown reticulated pigmentation (dyschromatosis) (incontinenti pigmenti-like pigmentation) with hypopigmented corneal dystrophy (dyskeratosis), coarse unruly hair, unswept eyebrows, silvery hair, hypohidrosis, recurrent sinus disease and pneumonia with chronic obstructive disease, clubbing; photophobia, failure to thrive, female carriers with linear macular nevoid Blascko-esque hyperpigmentation; gastroenteritis, diarrhea; intronic mutation of *POLA1* gene *BJD 177:945–959, 2017; JAMADerm 153:817–818, 2017; Ped Derm 32:871–872, 2015; Am J Med Genet 161:1414–1420, 2013; Eur J Dermatol 18:102–103, 2008; Ped Derm 22:122–126, 2005; Semin Cut Med Surg 16:72–80, 1997; Am J Med Genet 32:115–119, 1989; Am J Med Gen 10:65–75:1981*

TOXINS

Arsenic intoxication

TRAUMA

Erythema ab igne; due to a laptop computer *Cutis 80:319–320 2007; Cutis 79:59–60, 2007; Dermatology 212:392–393, 2006; JAAD 50:973–974, 2004; Contact Dermatitis 50:105, 2004;* with pancreatic cancer *Am J Gastroenterol 67:77–79, 1977;* associated with cancer-related pain *Pain 87:107–108, 2000*

VASCULAR DISORDERS

Cutaneous arteritis – round, linear, reticulated hyperpigmentation *JAAD 49:519–522, 2003*

Cutaneous polyarteritis nodosa (livedo with nodules) – arthritis; arthralgias; painful or asymptomatic red or skin-colored multiple nodules with livedo reticularis of feet, legs, forearms face, scalp, shoulders, trunk; leg ulcers, atrophie blanche-like lesions; reticulate hyperpigmentation *JAMADerm 151:549–550, 2015; JAAD 63:602–606, 2010; JAAD 57:840–848, 2007; BJD 146:694–699, 2002;* anti-phosphatidylserine-prothrombin complex *JAAD 63:602–606, 2010;* macular lymphocytic arteritis – red or hyperpigmented reticulated patches of legs *JAAD 73:1013–1020, 2015*

Lymphocytic thrombophilic arteritis – painless non-ulcerating livedo reticularis, reticulated hyperpigmentation, red nodules *AD 144:1175–1182, 2008*

Superficial migratory thrombophlebitis – reticulated hyperpigmented patches with red subcutaneous nodules *Cutis 101:322,325–326, 2018*

DIFFUSE FRECKLE-LIKE OR RETICULATE HYPERPIGMENTATION OF DORSAL ASPECTS OF HANDS AND FEET, EXTREMITIES OR FLEXURES

Acromelanosis progressive

Hereditary symmetric dyschromatosis of Dohi

Reticulate acropigmentation of Kitamura

Heterochromia extremitarum

Dowling Degos disease

RETICULATED HYPERPIGMENTATION AND PUNCTATE KERATODERMA

Cantu syndrome (hyperkeratosis-hyperpigmentation syndrome)

Dermatopathia reticularis

Naegelli-Franceschetti-Jadassohn syndrome

RHINOPHYMATOUS ERUPTIONS

Acne rosacea *Am Fam Physician 50:1691–1697, 1994*

Actinic rhinophyma *Cutis 57:389–392, 1996*

Angioma *J Derm Surg Oncol 19:206–212, 1993*

Angiosarcoma *JAAD 49:530–531, 2001*

Basal cell carcinoma *AD 95:250–254, 1967*

Basosquamous carcinoma *AD 113:847–848, 1977*

Benign symmetric lipomatosis *Clin Exp Dermatol 19:531–533, 1994*

Cryptococcosis *Acta Haematol 84:101–103, 1990*

Cylindroma *Plast Reconstr Surg 59:582–587, 1977*

Granuloma faciale *Acta DV 80:144, 2000*

Leishmaniasis – post-kala-azar dermal leishmaniasis *Acta DV 79:330–331, 1999*

Lymphoma – cutaneous B-cell lymphoma *Australas J Dermatol 45:110–113, 2004;* systemic lymphoma *BJD 107:45–46, 1982;* diffuse large cell B-cell lymphoma *Cureus 10:e2536, 2018*

Metastases – squamous cell carcinoma of the lung *Cutis 57:33–36, 1997*

Microcystic adnexal carcinoma *Laryngorhinootologie 83:113–116, 2004*

Mycobacterium kansasii Otolaryngol Head Neck Surg 107:792–795, 1992

Paraneoplastic rhinophyma (retroperitoneal malignant hemangio-pericytoma) *Clin Exp Dermatol 14:253–255, 1989*

Phenytoin *Br J Plast Surg 53:521–522, 2000*

Rhinoscleroma *Ned Tijdschr Geneeskd 114:374–378, 1970*

Sarcoid *J Drugs Dermatol 3:333–334, 2003; Ann Otol Rhinol Laryngol 107:514-518, 1998*

Sebaceous adenoma *AD 95:250–254, 1967*

Sebaceous carcinoma *BJD 124:283–284, 1991*

Squamous cell carcinoma *Derm Surg 27:201–202, 2001;* adenoid squamaus cell carcinoma *AD 95:250–254, 1967;* intranasal squamous cell carcinoma *J Laryngol Oncol 87:1137–1141, 1973*

Tuberous sclerosis *Otolaryngology 86:ORL 904–908, 1978*

Vasculitis - localized chronic fibrosing vasculitis *Cutis 78:325–328, 2006*

Rhinophyma-like venous malformation *BJD 171:195–197, 2014*

RIPPLING OF SKIN

Aquagenic syringeal acrokeratoderma *The Dermatologist January, 2015, pp. 47–49, 2015; BJD 167:575–582, 2012; JAAD 59:S112–113, 2008; Ped Derm 24:197–198, 2007; Ped Derm 23:39–42, 2006; Cutis 78:317–318, 2006; JAAD 44:696–699, 2001*

Breast implant rippling *Aesthetic Plastic Surg 42:980–985, 2018*

Cellulite – association with obesity *JAAD 81:1037–1057, 2019*

Eosinophilic fasciitis (Shulman's syndrome) *Clin Dermatol 38:235–249, 2020*

Excess water exposure to palms and soles

Graft vs. host disease, chronic – sclerosis with subcutaneous involvement and fasciitis and rippling of skin *JAMADerm 151:635–637, 2015; JAAD 59:1070–1074, 2008;* calcinosis cutis in GVHD – umbilicated nodules, leg ulcers, rippled appearance *JAMADerm 156:814–817, 2020*

Hunter's syndrome – papules overlying scapulae with rippled appearance

Hutchinson-Gilford progeria syndrome – mountain range rippling of skin; sclerodermoid changes; facies – midfrontal bossing, protruding ears with small lobes, prominent eyes, glyphic nose (broad, mildly concave nasal ridge), mild micrognathia, vertical midline groove of chin, thin lips *BJD 156:1308–1314, 2007*

Infantile transient smooth muscle contraction of skin *JAAD 69:498–500, 2013*

Nevus of striated muscle – atrophic plaque with rippled surface on palmar surface *Ped Derm 31:254–256, 2014*

Phenylketonuria – autosomal recessive; deficiency of pheylalanine hydroxylase; sclerodermoid changes of thighs and buttocks in first year of life with rippled appearance of skin; contractures of legs; morphea-like lesions in older children, hypopigmentation, photosensitivity *Ped Derm 23:136–138, 2006; JAAD 26:329–333, 1992*

Plexiform neurofibroma – brown patch of back with appearance of bag of worms *Society of Pediatric Dermatology Annual Meeting, July, 2015*

Prune belly syndrome – hypoplastic abdominal musculature, cryptorchidism, urinary tract abnormalities *JAAD 72:1066–1073, 2015*

Tripe palms – metastatic squamous cell carcinoma of the tongue *NEJM 370:558, 2014*

Venous malformation – enlarged hand, hemihypertrophy, mountain range changes *BJD 157:558–562, 2007*

ROSETTE LESIONS

AUTOIMMUNE DISEASES

Bullous pemphigoid - personal observation

Dermatitis herpetiformis - personal observation

IgA mediated epidermolysis bullosa acquisita *JAAD 54:734–736, 2006*

IgA pemphigus – intraepidermal neutrophilic dermatosis *JAAD 82:1386–1392, 2020*

Intraepidermal neutrophilic IgA dermatosis *JAAD 22:917–919, 1990*

Linear IgA disease (chronic bullous disease of childhood) – string of pearls *Ped Derm 27:197–198, 2010; Ped Derm 26:28–33, 2009*

Pemphigoid en cocarde *JAAD 20:1125, 1989*

Pemphigoid gestationis – bullae in rosettes *JAAD 55:823–828, 2006*

Pemphigus herpetiformis – annular erythematous patches with hyperpigmentation with or without vesicles; rosette lesions *Ped Derm 27:488–491, 2010;* pemphigus herpetiformis and bullous pemphigoid *AD 149:502–504, 2013*

Pemphigus vulgaris – anti-desmoglein 1 antibody dominant *JAAD 52:839–845, 2005*

DRUG REACTIONS

Acute generalized exanthematous putulosis *Eur J Dermatol 12:475–478, 2002*

INFECTIONS AND INFESTATIONS

Fire ant stings *Cutis 75:85–89, 2005*

Smallpox vaccination – inadvertent inoculation *Clin Inf Dis 37:251–271, 2003*

Staphylococcal sepsis with widespread pustular exanthema

Syphilis, secondary – corymbose syphilis; explosion-like floral lesions with peripheral satellites *JAAD 82:1–14, 2020; JAMADerm 153:1317–1318, 2017;* congenital syphilis – string of pearl blisters *Ped Derm 36:735–736, 2019*

Chronic varicella-zoster in HIV disease - personal observation

Verrucae vulgaris – rosettes after cryotherapy or cantharadin

METABOLIC DISORDERS

Calcinosis cutis following liver transplantation *Ped Derm 20:225–228, 2003*

PRIMARY CUTANEOUS DISEASES

Epidermolysis bullosa - Dowling-Meara type

Erythrokeratoderma variabilis without mutations in connexin 31 *BJD 143:1283–1287, 2000*

Interstitial granulomatous dermatitis *Clin Exp Dermatol 33:712–714, 2008*

VASCULAR DISEASES

Acute hemorrhagic edema of infancy *Pediatr Ann 43:e4–8, 2014*

Henoch-Schonlein purpura - children or adults *AD 125:53–56, 1989*

SADDLE NOSE DEFORMITY

AUTOIMMUNE DISEASES

ANCA-associated vasculitis *APMIS SUPPL 1 27:32–36, 2009*

Relapsing polychondritis – saddle nose deformity, red ears, and airway collapse *NEJM 352:609–615, 2005; Chest 91:268–270, 1987; Medicine 55:193–216, 1976*

Rheumatoid arthritis *Arthritis Rheum 22:101–102, 1979*

EXOGENOUS AGENTS

Cocaine abuse *Autoimmune Rev 12:496–500, 2013; Ned Tijdschr Gmoeskd 157:A6035, 2013;* cocaine induced midline destructive lesions (CIMDL) *Rhinology 52:104–111, 2014*

INFECTIONS AND INFESTATIONS

Abscess of nasal septum *Eur Arch Otorhinolaryngology 276:417–420, 2019*

Fusarium Clin Infec Dis 68:705–709, 2019

Leishmaniasis *Acta Biomed 85:3–7, 2014*

Leprosy – lepromatous leprosy – misshapen nose with collapse of nose and saddle nose deformity *NEJM 352:609–615, 2005;* primary diffuse lepromatous leprosy (la lepra bonita) *JAAD 51:416–426, 2004;* leprous trigeminal neuritis–nasopharyngeal mutilation

Mycobacterium tuberculosis – lupus vulgaris; vegetating forms – ulcerate, areas of necrosis, invasion of mucous membranes with destruction of cartilage (lupus vorax); saddle nose deformity; nasal involvement with friable nodules which ulcerate *NEJM 352:609–615, 2005; Int J Dermatol 26:578–581, 1987; Acta Tuberc Scand 39(Suppl 49):1–137, 1960*

Rhinoscleroma–nasopharyngeal mutilation *NEJM 352:609–615, 2005; Ped Derm 21:134–138, 2004; Acta Otolaryngol 105:494–499, 1988; Cutis 40:101–103, 1987; Wien Med Wochenschr 20:1–5, 1870*

Syphilis – congenital – destruction of nasal septum; tertiary (gumma) *Dermatol Clin 24:497–507, 2006; NEJM 352:609–615, 2005;* endemic (bejel)–nasopharyngeal mutilation

INFLAMMATORY DISORDERS

Crohn's disease *J Craniomaxillofac Surg 40:17–19, 2012; Dig Dis Sci 52:1285–1287, 2007*

Pyoderma gangrenosum *J Laryngol Otol 112:870–871, 1998*

Sarcoidosis *Med Rheum 28:1053–1057, 2018*

METABOLIC DISORDERS

Prolidase deficiency – autosomal recessive; peptidase D mutation (PEPD); increased urinary imidopeptides; leg ulcers, anogenital ulcers, short stature (mild), telangiectasias, recurrent infections (sinusitis, otitis); mental retardation; splenomegaly with enlarged abdomen, atrophic scarring, spongy fragile skin with annular pitting and scarring; dermatitis, xerosis, hyperkeratosis of elbows and knees, lymphedema, purpura, low hairline, poliosis, canities, lymphedema, photosensitivity, hypertelorism, saddle nose deformity, frontal bossing, dull expression, mild ptosis, micrognathia, mandibular protrusion, exophthalmos, joint laxity, deafness, osteoporosis,

high arched palate *JAAD 62:1031, 1034, 2010; BJD 144:635–636, 2001; Ped Derm 13:58–60, 1996; JAAD 29:819–821, 1993; AD 127:124–125, 1991; AD 123:493–497, 1987*

NEOPLASTIC DISORDERS

Squamous cell carcinoma of the nasal septum *BMJ Case Rep Aug 5, 2014*

PRIMARY CUTANEOUS DISEASES

Anhidrotic ectodermal dysplasia – saddle-nose deformity *Ear Nose Throat J 91:E28–33, 2012*

Eosinophilic angiocentric fibrosis (variant of granuloma faciale) – red facial plaque with saddle nose deformity *BJD 152:574–576, 2005; Histopathology 9:1217–1225, 1985*

Hydroa vacciniforme – saddle nose deformity *Ped Derm 21:555–557, 2004*

SYNDROMES

CANDLE syndrome (chronic atypical neutrophilic dermatosis with lipodystrophy and elevated temperature) – annular erythematous edematous plaques of face and trunk which become purpuric and result in residual annular hyperpigmentation; limitation of range of motion with plaques over interphalangeal joints; periorbital edema with violaceous swollen eyelids, edema of lips (thick lips), lipoatrophy of cheeks, nose, and arms, chondritis with progressive ear and saddle nose deformities, hypertrichosis of lateral forehead, gynecomastia, wide spaced nipples, nodular episcleritis and conjunctivitis, epididymitis, myositis, aseptic meningitis; short stature, anemia, abnormal liver functions, splenomegaly, protuberant abdomen *Ped Derm 28:538–541, 2011; JAAD 62:487–495, 2010*

Hurler's syndrome–saddle-nose deformity

Mowat-Wilson syndrome *Orphanet J Rare Dis 2:42, 2007*

Robinow syndrome *Genet Counseling 16:297–300, 2005*

Takayasu's arteritis *J Laryngol Otol 120:59–62, 2006*

TRAUMA

Status/post nasal septoplasty *J Craniofac Surg 31:e62–65, 2020;* polydioxanone foil use in nasal surgery *Facial Plastic Surg 34:312–317, 2018*

VASCULAR DISEASES

Granulomatosis with polyangiitis *NEJM 352:609–615, 2005; NEJM 352:392, 2005; AD 130:861–867, 1993*

SCALP CYSTS

CONGENITAL ANOMALIES

Aplasia cutis congenita

Cephalocele – includes meningocele (rudimentary meningocele), meningoencephalocele, meningomyelocele; blue nodule with overlying hypertrichosis *JAAD 46:934–941, 2002; AD 137:45–50, 2001;* sequestrated meningocele *Ped Derm 11:315–318, 1994*

Congenital atrichia with papular lesions *Skin Appendage Disorders 4:129:130, 2018; JID 118:887–890 2002*

Congenital inclusion cysts of the subgaleal space *Surg Neurol 21:61–66, 1984; J Neurosurg 56:540–544, 1982*

Dermoid cyst and sinus *JAAD 46:934–941, 2002; Curr Prob in Dermatol 13:249–300, 2002; Neurosurg Clin N Am 6:359–366, 1995; Acta Neurochir (Wien) 128:115–121, 1994; AD 107:237–239, 1973*

Encephalocele

Epidermal inclusion cyst of anterior fontanel *Ped Derm 23:56–60, 2006; Surg Neurol 56:400–405, 2001*

Folliculocystic and collagen hamartoma *Ann Dermatol 27:593–596, 2015;* presenting as tuberous sclerosis *BJD 178:e276, 2018*

Heterotopic brain tissue (heterotopic meningeal nodules) – blue-red cystic mass with overlying alopecia *JAAD 46:934–941, 2002;* bald cyst of scalp with surrounding hypertrichosis *AD 131:731, 1995; JAAD 28:1015, 1993; BJD 129:183–185, 1993; AD 125:1253–1256, 1989*

Sinus pericranii – pulsatile scalp protrusion *Ned Tijdschr Geneeskd 159:A8007, 2015; JAAD 54:S50–52, 2006*

INFECTIONS AND INFESTATIONS

Molluscum contagiosum – occurring in an epidermoid cyst *Am J Dermatopathol 17:414–416, 1995; Cutis 26:180, 184, 1980*

Myiasis–Dermatobia hominis–scalp cyst in a child *Ped Derm 15:116–118, 1998*

INFILTRATIVE DISEASES

Eosinophilic granuloma, transcranial – subcutaneous scalp mass *J Derm Surg Oncol 19:631–634, 1993*

INFLAMMATORY DISEASES

Dissecting cellulitis of the scalp *BJD 159:506–507, 2008*

NEOPLASTIC DISEASES

Cutaneous ciliated cyst of the scalp *Am J Dermatopathol 16:76–79, 1994*

Cutaneous ectopic meningioma (psammoma)

Cystic panfolliculoma *Indian J Pathol Microbiol 56:437–439, 2013*

Epidermoid cyst *World Neurosurg 12:119–124, 2018; AD 125:1253–1256, 1989*

Hybrid cyst – combined epidermoid and pilar cyst *J Eur Acad Dermatol Venereol 17:83–86, 2003; JAAD 9:872–875, 1983*

Leiomyoma, vascular *Ped Derm 30:e27–29, 2013*

Lymphoma – cutaneous T-cell lymphoma with underlying epidermoid cysts *AD 115:622, 1979*

Malignant proliferating trichilemmal tumor *Am J Clin Oncol 24:351–353, 2001; JAAD 32:870–873, 1995*

Metaplastic synovial cyst *Am J Dermatopathol 10:531–535, 1988*

Metastasis – adenocarcinoma of the lung *JAAD 54:916–917, 2006;* mimicking epidermoid cyst *AD 104;301–303, 1971;* salivary gland adenocarcinoma mimicking kerion

Microcystic adnexal carcinoma *J Derm Surg Oncol 15:768–771, 1989*

Pilar cyst (trichilemmal cyst) *JAAD 46:934–941, 2002*

Pilomatrixoma

Proliferating trichilemmal cyst *AD 131:721, 724, 1995*

Squamous cell carcinoma arising in an epidermoid cyst *AD 117:683, 1981*

Steatocystoma multiplex suppurativa – giant cysts of neck and scalp *Case Rep Dermatol 19:71–76, 2019*

Steatocystoma simplex *Mymensingh Med J 669–671, 2018*

Teratoid cysts *Radiol Med 124:1049–1061, 2019*

Trichilemmal cysts *Anticancer Res 39:4253–4258, 2019*

PRIMARY CUTANEOUS DISEASES

Cutaneous ciliated cyst *Case Rep Med 2015:589831; Am J Dermatopathol 36:679–682, 2014*

Lichen planopilaris with cysts and comedones *Clin Exp Dermatol 17:346–348, 1992;* lichen planus follicularis tumidus– recurrent retroauricular cystic nodules *Dermatol Online J Oct 15, 2018*

Pseudocyst of the scalp – alopecic aseptic nodules of scalp *Dermatology 232:165–170, 2016' Dermatology 210:333–335, 2005*

SYNDROMES

Atrichia with keratin cysts – face, neck, scalp; then trunk and extremities *Ann DV 121:802–804, 1994*

Gardner's syndrome – epidermoid cysts *Imaging Sci Dent 46:267–272, 2016; Br J Dent 193:383–384, 2002*

Oral-facial-digital syndrome – milia of the scalp *Ped Derm 9:52–56, 1992*

Pachyonychia congenita *Skin Med 3:233–235, 2004*

Steatocystoma multiplex *Int J Dermatol 34:429–430, 1995; J Dermatol 22:438–440, 1995;* eruptive steatocystoma *J Dermatol 18:537–539, 1991*

Tuberous sclerosis – folliculocystic and collagen hamartoma – comedo-like openings, multilobulated cysts, scalp cysts and nodules *JAAD 66:617–621, 2012*

TRAUMA

Cephalohematoma

Cerebrospinal fluid cyst – post-operative *Br J Plast Surg 32:241–244, 1979*

Leptomeningeal cyst (traumatic) (growing fracture) – skull fracture with laceration of underlying dura *Ped Clin North Amer 6:1151–1160, 1993;* with brain herniation *JAAD 46:934–941, 2002*

VASCULAR DISORDERS

Angiolymphoid hyperplasia – mimicking a pilar cyst *J Derm Surg Oncol 6:935–937, 1980*

Cystic hygroma (lymphatic malformation)

Lymphangioma

Subepicranial hygromas *JAAD 46:934–941, 2002*

SCALP DERMATITIS

AUTOIMMUNE DISEASES AND DISEASES OF IMMUNE DYSFUNCTION

Allergic contact dermatitis *Contact Dermatitis 44:178, 2001; Contact Dermatitis 40:335, 1999; Contact Dermatitis 23:124–125, 1990;* preservatives, surfactants, hair dyes, nickel cobalt, balsam of Peru, fragrance mix, carba mix propylene glycol *Skin Appendage Disorders 3:7014, 2017*

Amicrobial pustulosis associated with autoimmune disease treated with zinc *BJD 143:1306–1310, 2000*

Bullous pemphigoid

Chronic granulomatous disease – scalp folliculitis *Dermatol Therapy 18:176–183, 2005; Ped Derm 21:646–651, 2004*

Cicatricial pemphigoid, Brunsting-Perry type *BJD 159:984–986, 2008; AD 75:489–501, 1957;* mimicking DLE *JAAD 65:886–887, 2011*

Dermatitis herpetiformis – elbows, knees, buttocks, shoulders, trunk, face, and scalp, oral lesions

Dermatomyositis *JAMA 272:1939–1941, 1994;* juvenile form *JAAD 45:28–34, 2001;* erythema of scalp with diffuse alopecia; poikilodermatomyositis of scalp

DiGeorge's syndrome–personal observation

Graft vs. host disease *Ann DV 126:51–53, 1999*

Hyper IgE syndrome – papulopustular dermatitis of scalp *J Cut Med Surg 20:340–342, 2016*

Immunodeficiency disorders – hypercupremia and decreased intracellular killing – blepharitis and pyoderma of the scalp *Ped Derm 1:134–142, 1983*

Linear IgA disease (chronic bullous disease of childhood) – scalp, annular polycyclic bullae *Ped Derm 15:108–111, 1998*

Lupus erythematosus; neonatal lupus erythematosus *JAAD 40:675–681, 1999*

Pemphigoid vegetans *AD 115:446–448, 1979*

Pemphigus foliaceus – starts in seborrheic distribution (scalp, face, chest, upper back) *JAAD 71:669–675, 2014; Ped Derm 3:459–463, 1986; AD 83:52–70, 1961;* endemic pemphigus of El Bagre region of Colombia *JAAD 49:599–608, 2003*

Pemphigus vulgaris – psoriasiform scalp dermatitis in pregnancy *Cutis 94:206–209, 2014;* scalp erosions *BJD 173:1557–1559, 2015; JAAD 55:S98–99, 2006; Ped Derm 3:459–463, 1986; AD 110:862–865, 1974*

Rheumatoid arthritis – erosive pustular dermatitis of the scalp *Int J Dermatol 34:148, 1995;* neutrophilic dermatitis *Ann DV 141:603–606, 2014*

Wiskott-Aldrich syndrome–personal observation

CONGENITAL DISEASES

Congenital erosive dermatosis with reticulated supple scarring *AD 126:544–546, 1990*

DRUGS

Cimetidine–seborrheic dermatitis-like eruption *Clin Dermatol 11:243–251, 1993*

Drug rash *Cutis 35:148–149, 1985*

Chemotherapy–inflammation of actinic keratoses from systemic chemotherapy *JAAD 17:192–197, 1987*

Cytarabine – purpuric intertriginous plaques, scalp involvement, papules coalesce into papular purpuric violaceous generalized exanthema, red knee, red feet *Am J Ther 26:e653–655, 2019; JAAD 73:821–828, 2015*

Dasatinib – seborrheic dermatitis-like eruption *J Clin Aesthet Dermatol 10:23–27, 2017*

Erlotinib folliculopathy–personal observation

Imatinib – psoriasiform eruption *Am J Hematol 93:467–468, 2018*

Methyldopa–seborrheic dermatitis-like eruption *Clin Dermatol 11:243–251, 1993*

Penicillamine–seborrheic dermatitis-like eruption *Clin Dermatol 11:243–251, 1993*

EXOGENOUS AGENTS

Contact dermatitis, irritant; *AD 108:102–103, 1973*

Fiberglass dermatitis

Iatrogenic–topical immunotherapy

INFECTIONS AND INFESTATIONS

AIDS – seborrheic dermatitis; photodermatitis of AIDS, including photo-lichenoid dermatitis

Book lice (Liposcelis mendax) *BJD 125:400–401, 1991*

Candidiasis – mucocutaneous candidiasis with candidal granuloma *BJD 86(Suppl.8):88–102, 1972*

Cladosporium – tinea capitis *SKINmed 10:393–394, 2012*

Coccidioidomycosis *Diagn Microbiol Infect Dis 89:218–221, 2017*

Coxsackie virus A6 (atypical hand, foot, and mouth disease) – crusted papules of scalp; red papulovesicles of fingers, palmar erythema, red papules of ears, red papules of antecubital fossa, perioral papulovesicles, vesicles of posterior pharynx; crusted papules of ears, and face; purpuric targetoid painful vesicular lesions of hands and feet, arthritis, fissured scrotum *JAMADerm 149:1419–1421, 2013; JAAD 69:736–741, 2013*

Cryptococcosis – mimicking kerion – personal observation

Demodicidosis – papular eruption in HIV patients of head and neck, trunk, and arms *JAAD 20:306–307, 1989; JAAD 20:197–201, 1989;* mimicking favus; hyperkeratotic patchy alopecia, papules, vesicles, pustules *JAAD 57:S19–21, 2007;* demodex-associated papulopustular folliculitis *Am J Dermatopathol 18:589–591, 1996;* demodex eosinophilic folliculitis *Clin Exp Dermatol 40:413–415, 2015*

Herpes simplex, neonatal

Herpes zoster – giant lichenification following herpes zoster *Clin Exp Dermatol 28:57–59, 2003;* lichen simplex chronicus as complication *BJD 138:921–922, 1998*

Human T-lymphotropic virus type 1-associated infective dermatitis – chronic relapsing dermatitis; severe red and exudative dermatitis with scaling and crusting of scalp, forehead, eyelids, paranasal area, neck, retroauricular, external ear, axillae, groin; chronic watery nasal discharge, crusting of anterior nares, blepharoconjunctivitis; generalized fine papular rash with lymph nodes; onset of rash at age 2 years; most common form of transmission is breast feeding; harbinger of development of adult T-cell lymphotropic leukemia and HTLV-1 associated myelopathy (HAM)/tropical spastic paralysis (TSP); Jamaica, Senegal, Brazil (endemic areas) *Semin Diagn Pathol 37:92–97, 2020; JAAD 64:152–160, 2011;*

Impetigo

Infectious eczematoid dermatitis

Insect bites

Kerion–personal observation
   Differential diagnosis includes:
      Psoriasis
      Seborrheic dermatitis
      Folliculitis decalvans
      Dissecting cellulitis
      Acne keloidalis
      Pseudolymphoma
      Abscess

Larva migrans *An Bras Dermatol 89:332–333, 2014; Rev Soc Bras Med Trop 32:187–189, 1999*

Leprosy – erythema nodosum leprosum of scalp *Indian J Lepr 87:23–26, 2015*

Mite infestation *Arch Int Med 147:2185–2187, 1987*

Mycobacterium tuberculosis

Myiasis *Int J Dermatol 58:336–342, 2019; Dermatol Online J Nov 18, 2015*

Pediculosis; *Dermatol Online J March 16, 2016; Dermatol Clin 8:219–228, 1990*

Scabies – scaly dermatitic scalp *JAAD 82:533–548, 2020; Infez Med 27:332–335, 2019; Ped Derm 27:525–526, 2010; Acta DV 61:360–362, 1981;* crusted (Norwegian) *Cutis 61:87–88, 1998;* immunocompromised patients *Ped Derm 10:136–138, 1993;* IPEX syndrome (immunodysregulation, polyendocrinopathy, enteropathy, X-linked inheritance) – Norwegian scabies *JAAD 56:S48–49, 2007*

Staphylococcal pyoderma

Sycosis – deep staphylococcal folliculitis *Dermatol Wochenschr 152:153–167, 1966*

Syphilis, secondary *J Med Case Rep 13:360, 2019; AD 128:530–534, 1992*

Tinea capitis – Trichophyton tonsurans; favus *Dermatol Clin 4:137–149, 1986;* in adults *Int J Dermatol 30:206–208, 1991; Cutis 41:284, 1988;* tinea incognito; tinea capitis of adult females – pustular eruptions *JAAD 49:S177–179, 2003;* in adults *Dermatol Online J March 16, 2016*

Tufted folliculitis

INFILTRATIVE LESIONS

Langerhans cell histiocytosis – crusted papules *JAMADerm 154:607–608, 2018; JAAD 10:968–969, 1984;* red-brown papules *AD 143:1067–1072, 2007;* red papules and erosions *AD 144:105–110, 2008*

INFLAMMATORY DISEASES

Dissecting cellulitis of the scalp

Eosinophilic pustular folliculitis of infancy – dermatitis with or without pustules *Ped Derm 26:195–196, 2009; Ped Derm 21:615–616, 2004; Ped Derm 16:118–120, 1999; Ped Derm 1:202–206, 1984*

Folliculitis

Folliculitis decalvans–personal observation

Folliculitis spinulosa decalvans – pustules, keratotic papules of scalp, scarring alopecia *Ped Derm 23:255–258, 2006*

Malignant pyoderma–pustular scalp dermatitis *AD 122:295–302, 1986*

Perforating folliculitis *Dermatologica 168:131–137, 1984*

Pyoderma gangrenosum *AD 125:1239–1242, 1989*

METABOLIC DISEASES

Acrodermatitis enteropathica *Ped Derm 16:95–102, 1999*

Biotin deficiency *J Pediatr 106:762–769, 1985*

Essential fatty acid deficiency *AD 113:939–941, 1977*

Holocarboxylase synthetase deficiency – autosomal recessive; scaly eyebrows, eyelashes, scalp *Ped Derm 23:142–144, 2006*

Porphyria–congenital erythropoietic porphyria *BJD 148:160–164, 2003*

Zinc deficiency, acquired *JAAD 69:616–624, 2013; Hautarzt 28:578–582, 1977*

NEOPLASTIC DISEASES

Basal cell carcinoma– personal observation

Bowen's disease

Epidermal nevus–verrucous scalp *AD 120:227–230, 1984*

Leukemia cutis *Clin Pediatr (Phila) 35:531–534, 1996;* HTLV-1 leukemia/lymphoma (acute T-cell leukemia)–HTLV-1 infective dermatitis–dermatitis of scalp, around ears and nose *JAAD 81:23–41, 2019; JAAD 49:979–1000, 2003; Braz J Infect Dis 4:100–102, 2000; AD 134:439–444, 1998;* violaceous dermatitis of scalp (AMML M5) *JAAD 64:1003–1004, 2011;* chronic lymphocytic leukemia *BMJ Case Rep Sept 21, 2015*

Leukemid in chronic lymphocytic leukemia– personal observation

Lymphoma – cutaneous T-cell lymphoma; anaplastic large cell T-cell lymphoma *BJD 99:99–106, 1978*

Melanocytic nevus – congenital nevus– personal observation

Squamous cell carcinoma in situ – in sclerodermatous graft vs host disease and voriconazole *Ped Derm 35:e165–169, 2018*

PARANEOPLASTIC DISORDERS

Paraneoplastic dermatitis, non-Hodgkin's lymphoma–personal observation

PHOTODERMATOSES

Chronic actinic dermatitis – acute, subacute, or chronic dermatitis with lichenification, papules, plaques, erythroderma, stubby scalp and eyebrow hair *AD 136:1215–1220, 2000; AD 130:1284–1289, 1994; JAAD 28:240–249, 1993; AD 126:317–323, 1990;* sensitization by sesquiterpene lactone mix *BJD 132:543–547, 1995;* associated with musk ambrette *Cutis 54:167–170, 1994; JAAD 3:384–393, 1980*

Giant actinic porokeratosis *BJD 149:654, 2003*

PRIMARY CUTANEOUS DISEASES

Acne necrotica miliaris

Alopecia mucinosa *Clin Exp Derm 14:382–384, 1989*

Amicrobial pustulosis – exudative erythema, erosions, pustules, diffuse alopecia with dermatitis; associated with systemic autoimmune disorders; scalp, axillae, ears, thighs *JAAD 57:523–526,*

2007; BJD 154:568–569, 2006; Communication no.11. Journees Dermatologiques de Paris, March 1991.

Atopic dermatitis Ped Derm 13:10–13, 1996

Darier's disease (keratosis follicularis) – seborrheic distribution; photoexacerbated Ann DV 121:393–395, 1994; Clin Dermatol 19:193–205, 1994; JAAD 27:40–50, 1992; AD 120:1484–1487, 1984

Dissecting cellulitis of the scalp BJD 177:e160, 2018

Epidermolysis bullosa–Herlitz junctional EB and junctional EB mitis–scalp erosions

Erosive pustular dermatosis of the scalp (chronic atrophic erosive dermatosis of the scalp and extremities)–in elderly; hyperkeratotic crusting, pustules, erosions, atrophy, scarring alopecia JAMADerm 152:694–697, 2016; JAAD 66:680–686, 2012; AD 145:1340–1341, 2009; JAAD 60:521–522, 2009; AD 144:795–800, 2008; JAAD 57:421–427, 2007; JAAD 57:S11–14, 2007; Ped Derm 23:533–536, 2006; AD 139:712–714, 2003; BJD 148:593–595, 2003; Dermatol Surg 27:766–767, 2001; JAAD 28:96–98, 1993; Hautarzt 43:576–579, 1992; Ann DV 118:899–901, 1991; BJD 118:441–444, 1988(S); BJD 100:559–566, 1979; BJD 97(Suppl):67, 1977; after perinatal scalp injury Ped Derm 23:533–36, 2006; following craniofacial surgery Ped Derm 36:697–701, 2019

Exfoliative erythroderma, multiple causes

Hailey-Hailey disease BJD 126:294–296, 1992

Ichthyosis – multiple types

Leiner's disease Pediatrics 49:225–232, 1972

Lichen planopilaris

Lichen simplex chronicus–psoriasiform neurodermatitis An Bras Dermatol 93:108–110, 2018; BJD 138:921–922, 1998

Lipedematous alopecia – boggy scalp with diffuse alopecia JAAD 52:152–156, 2005; AD Syphilol 32:688, 1935

Non-bullous congenital ichthyosiform erythroderma – personal observation

Pityriasis rubra pilaris – explosive seborrheic dermatitis in children and teenagers J Dermatol 27:174–177, 2000; JAAD 31:997–999, 1994; childhood form Ped Derm 4:21–23, 1987

Pityriasis capitis (dandruff)

Plica neuropathica – complete matting of scalp hair Clin Exp Dermatol 31:790–792, 2006

Psoriasis BJD 161:159–166, 2009; AD 98:248–259, 1968; tinea amiantacea Clin Exp Dermatol 2:137–143, 1977

Seborrheic dermatitis Dermatology 201:146–147, 2001; tinea amiantacea Cutis 63:169–170, 1999; Hautarzt 25:134–139, 1974

Terra firme

Tinea amiantacea (pityriasis amiantacea) Niger Postgrad Med 21:196–198, 2014; Clin Exp Dermatol 2:137–144, 1977
  Atopic dermatitis Int J Dermatol 42:260–264, 2003; Clin Exp Dermatol 2:137–143, 1977
  Adalimumab, rituximab Hautarzt 68:1007–1010, 2017; Clin Exp Dermatol 37:639–641, 2012
  Bacterial infection Clin Exp Dermatol 2:137–143, 1977
  Darier's disease Clin Exp Dermatol 34:554–556, 2009
  Dermatophyte infection (tinea capitis) AD 20:45–53, 1929
  Lichen planus Int J Dermatol 42:260–264, 2003
  Lichen simplex chronicus Int J Dermatol 42:260–264, 2003
  Melphalan Cutis 103:46–50, 2019
  Pityriasis rubra pilaris Dermatologica 166:314–315, 1983; Dermatologica 159:245–250, 1979
  Psoriasis
  Seborrheic dermatitis
  Vemurafenib Cut Oncol Toxicol 35:329–331, 2016

X-linked ichthyosis–personal observation

PSYCHOCUTANEOUS DISEASES

Factitial dermatitis – with underlying osteomyelitis of the scalp Int J Trichology 8:26–28, 2016; Acta Neurochir (Wien) 143:737–738, 2001; with resultant cerebral abscess Postgrad Med J 64:976–977, 1988; skull erosion and intracranial infection Acta Neurochir (Wien) 157:2227–2228, 2015

Neurotic excoriations

SYNDROMES

Andogsky syndrome – atopic dermatitis and unilateral cataracts Ped Derm 20:419–420, 2003; Klin Monatsbl Augenheilkd 52:824–831, 1914

Ankyloblepharon, ectodermal dysplasia, and cleft lip and palate syndrome (AEC syndrome) (Hay-Wells syndrome) – hair sparse or absent, dystrophic nails, dystrophic widely spaced pointed teeth are shed early, chronic scalp erosions (erosive scalp dermatitis) in early childhood; papular and pustular scalp dermatitis Ped Derm 28:313–317, 2011; Ped Derm 28:15–19, 2011; BJD 94:287–289, 1976; Ped Derm 14:149–150, 1997

CEDNIK syndrome (cerebral dysgenesis-neuropathy-ichthyosis-keratoderma) – microcephaly; dysmorphic face with small anterior fontanelles; pointed prominent nasal tip, small chin, inverted nipples and long toes, high palate, thick gingivae, cradle cap, sparse brittle coarse hair, scarring alopecia, fixed flexion posture; decreased SNAP 29 protein; mutation in SNARE proteins mediating vesicle trafficking; mutation in ABCA12 gene BJD 164:610–616, 2011; AD 144:334–340, 2008

Ectodermal dysplasias with clefting–scalp dermatitis JAAD 27:249–256, 1992

Ectrodactyly-ectodermal dysplasia-cleft lip/palate (EEC) syndrome Dermatology 194:191–194, 1997; BJD 132:621–625, 1995; JAAD 29:505–506, 1993

Happle syndrome (X-linked chondrodysplasia punctata) – scalp dermatitis at birth; Blaschko hyperkeratosis, follicular atrophoderma, cicatricial alopecia Ped Derm 18:442–444, 2001

Hay-Wells syndrome (ankyloblepharon-ectrodactyly-cleft lip/palate) syndrome (AEC syndrome)- scalp erosions and pustules AD 141:1591–1594, 2005; Ped Derm 10:334–340, 1993; AD 128:1378–1386, 1992; JAAD 12:810–815, 1985

Hyper IgE syndrome (Job's syndrome) (Buckley's syndrome) – papular, pustular, excoriated dermatitis of face, behind ears, scalp, axillae, and groin; recurrent bacterial infections of skin with cold abscesses, contact urticaria, infections of nasal sinuses and respiratory tract; growth failure AD 140:1119–1125, 2004; J Pediatr 141:572–575, 2002; NEJM 340:692–702, 1999; Curr Prob in Derm 10:41–92, 1998; Clin Exp Dermatol 11:403–408, 1986; Medicine 62:195–208, 1983; Pediatrics 49:59–70, 1972; Lancet 1:1013–1015, 1966

Hypoplastic enamel-onycholysis-hypohidrosis (Witkop-Brearley-Gentry syndrome) – marked facial hypohidrosis, dry skin with keratosis pilaris, scaling and crusting of the scalp, onycholysis and subungual hyperkeratosis, hypoplastic enamel of teeth Oral Surg 39:71–86, 1975

Ichthyosis follicularis with atrichia and photophobia (IFAP) – atopic dermatitis; collodion membrane and erythema at birth; ichthyosis, spiny (keratotic) follicular papules (generalized follicular keratoses), non-scarring alopecia, keratotic papules of elbows, knees, fingers, extensor surfaces, xerosis; punctate keratitis, photophobia; nail dystrophy, psychomotor delay, short stature; enamel dysplasia, beefy red tongue and gingiva, angular stomatitis, lamellar scales, psoriasiform plaques, palmoplantar erythema Curr Prob Derm

14:71–116, 2002; JAAD 46:S156–158, 2002; BJD 142:157–162, 2000; AD 125:103–106, 1989; Ped Derm 12:195, 1995; Dermatologica 177:341–347, 1988; Am J Med Genet 85:365–368, 1999

Keratosis-ichthyosis-deafness (KID) syndrome – autosomal recessive; dotted waxy, fine granular, stippled, or reticulated surface pattern of severe diffuse hyperkeratosis of palms and soles (palmoplantar keratoderma), ichthyosis with well marginated, serpiginous erythematous verrucous plaques, hyperkeratotic elbows and knees, perioral furrows, leukoplakia, bilateral sensorineural deafness, photophobia with vascularizing keratitis, blindness, hypotrichosis of scalp, eyebrows, and eyelashes, dystrophic nails, chronic mucocutaneous candidiasis, otitis externa, abscesses, blepharitis; connexin 26 mutation Ped Derm 27:651–652, 2010; Ped Derm 23:81–83, 2006; JAAD 51:377–382, 2004; BJD 148:649–653, 2003; Cutis 72:229–230, 2003; Ped Derm 19:285–292, 2002; Ped Derm 15:219–221, 1998; Ped Derm 13:105–113, 1996; BJD 122:689–697, 1990; JAAD 23:385–388, 1990; JAAD 19:1124–1126, 1988; AD 123:777–782, 1987; AD 117:285–289, 1981; J Cutaneous Dis 33:255–260, 1915; hyperkeratotic papules and plaques of face, scalp, trunk, extremities; exaggerated diaper dermatitis Ped Derm 13:105–113, 1996; BJD 122:689–697, 1990; psoriasiform scalp dermatitis BJD 148:649–653, 2003

Netherton's syndrome – flexural lichenification; trichorrhexis invaginata Ped Derm 19:285–292, 2002; AD 135:823–832, 1999; BJD 141:1097–1100, 1999; Curr Prob in Derm 10:41–92, 1998; Ped Derm 14:473–476, 1997; Ped Derm 13:183–199, 1996; BJD 131:615–619, 1994

Omenn's syndrome Acta Derm 782:71, 1988; presents in neonatal period with atopic-like dermatitis

Rapp-Hodgkin hypohidrotic ectodermal dysplasia–autosomal dominant; alopecia of wide area of scalp in frontal to crown area, short eyebrows and eyelashes, coarse wiry sparse hypopigmented scalp hair, sparse body hair, scalp dermatitis, ankyloblepharon, syndactyly, nipple anomalies, cleft lip and/or palate; nails narrow and dystrophic, small stature, hypospadias, conical teeth and anodontia or hypodontia; distinctive facies, short stature JAAD 53:729–735, 2005; Ped Derm 14:149–150, 1997;

Ped Derm 7:126–131, 1990; J Med Genet 15:269–272, 1968;

Red scalp syndrome Dermatology 219:179–181, 2009

Schwachman's syndrome – neutropenia, malabsorption, failure to thrive; generalized xerosis, follicular hyperkeratosis, widespread dermatitis, palmoplantar hyperkeratosis Ped Derm 9:57–61, 1992; Arch Dis Child 55:531–547, 1980; J Pediatr 65:645–663, 1964

Trichothiodystrophy syndromes–BIDS, IBIDS, PIBIDS – dermatitis, sparse or absent eyelashes and eyebrows, brittle hair, premature aging, sexual immaturity, ichthyosis, dysmyelination, bird-like facies, dental caries; trichothiodystrophy with ichthyosis, urologic malformations, hypercalciuria and mental and physical retardation JAAD 44:891–920, 2001; Ped Derm 14:441–445, 1997

Wiskott-Aldrich syndrome – dermatitis, thrombocytopenia, malignant lymphoma, leukemia Curr Prob Derm 14:41–70, 2002; Int J Dermatol 24:77–81, 1985

X-linked ectodermal dysplasia with immunodeficiency – NEMO mutation; erythroderma, alopecia, red scaly scalp, frontal bossing, periorbital wrinkling, intertrigo, thick everted lower lip AD 144:342–346, 2008

TOXINS

Selenium toxicity – transverse white nail bands; exfoliative scalp dermatitis with hair loss, dizziness, fatigue, amenorrhea, nausea and vomiting, joint pain; "Total Body Formula" dietary supplement JAAD 63:168–169, 2010

TRAUMA

Erosive pustular dermatitis of the scalp – following craniofacial surgery Ped Derm 36:697–701, 2019

Intrapartum internal fetal monitoring – infectious dermatitis Pediatrics 74:81–85, 1984

Radiation dermatitis Neurosurgery 34:1105, 1994; BJD 138:799–805, 1998

Radiation recall dermatitis Cureus 9:e1671, 2017

Video-EEG monitoring Neurodiagn J 56:139–150, 2016

SCALP NODULES

JAAD 46:934–941, 2002; JAAD 25:819–830, 1991

INFANTS

DEVELOPMENTAL DISORDERS

Branchial cleft cyst Ped Derm 27:204–206, 2010

Cephalocele – includes encephalocele, meningocele (rudimentary meningocele), meningoencephalocele, meningomyelocele; blue nodule with overlying hypertrichosis JAAD 46:934–941, 2002; AD 137:45–50, 2001

Congenital fibroblastic connective tissue nevi – red nodule Ped Derm 35:644–650, 2018

Dermal sinus tumor Cutis 76:377–382, 2005

Dermatofibrosarcoma protuberans – congenital AD 139:207–211, 2003

Dermoid cyst (cranial dermoids) – midline overlying anterior or posterior fontanelle or over occipito-parietal suture Ped Derm 30:706–711, 2013; Ped Derm 28:577–578, 2011; Dermatol Therapy 18:104–116, 2005; Ped Clin North Amer 6:1151–1160, 1993; midline lobulated scalp nodule Ped Derm 30:706–711, 2013
   Midline violaceous soft nodule of scalp
      Abscess
      Cephalohematoma
      Dermoid cyst
      Encephalocele
      Epidermoid cyst
      Infantile hemangioma
      Lipoma
      Lymphatic malformation
      Subgaleal hematoma

Desmoplastic trichoepithelioma, congenital – firm skin colored scalp nodule Ped Derm 34:189–190, 2017

Encephalocoele (hair collar sign) Dermatol Therapy 18:104–116, 2005

Heterotopic brain tissue (heterotopic meningeal nodules) – blue-red cystic mass with overlying alopecia BJD 156:1047–1050, 2007;

Dermatol Therapy 18:104–116, 2005; JAAD 46:934–941, 2002; bald cyst of scalp with surrounding hypertrichosis *AD 131:731, 1995; JAAD 28:1015, 1993; BJD 129:183–185, 1993; AD 125:1253–1256, 1989;* cyst with collar of hair (heterotopic meningeal nodules) *JAAD 28:1015–1017, 1993; AD 123:1253–1256, 1989*

Infantile hemangioma *Ped Derm 15:307–308, 1998*

Melanocytic nevus – mimicking RICH *Ped Derm 30:e164–165, 2013*

Rudimentary meningocele (primary cutaneous meningioma) – scalp or paraspinal region of children and teenagers; yellow plaque of scalp *AD 137:45–50, 2001; Ped Derm 15:388–389, 1998;* nodule with overlying alopecia or hypertrichosis *JAAD 46:934–941, 2002; AD 130:775–777, 1994; Cancer 34:728–744, 1974*

Meningoencephalocoele

Sinus pericranii – alopecic red nodule of scalp *JAAD 46:934–941, 2002*

Congenital xanthogranulomas *Ped Derm 35:582–587, 2018*
   Atrophic patch with yellow macules and papules

INFECTIONS AND INFESTATIONS

Abscesses *JAAD 46:934–941, 2002*

Bacille-Calmette-Guerin (BCG) infection, disseminated – nodules of scalp, back, and legs *Ped Derm 36:672–676, 2019*

Gonorrhea – newborn with gonococcal scalp abscess *South Med J 73:396–397, 1980; Am J Obstet Gynecol 127:437–438, 1977*

Mycoplasma hominis – neonatal scalp abscess *Ped Inf Dis 12:1171–1172, 2002*

Myiasis – cuterebrid myiasis *Ped Derm 21:515–516, 2004*

Scabies *Semin Dermatol 12:3–8, 1993*

INFILTRATIVE DISORDERS

Juvenile hyaline fibromatosis (infantile systemic hyalinosis) – limb contractures, sclerodermoid changes; gigantic lip fibromas, giant fibrous nodules of scalp and ears; giant nodules of frontal scalp and face; periarticular nodules of knees; gingival hypertrophy, bone deformities; mutation in gene encoding capillary morphogenesis protein 2 (*ANTRX2(CMG2)*) *Ped Derm 23:458–464, 2006; JAAD 55:1036–143, 2006; Ped Derm 21:154–159, 2004; Ped Derm 18:400–402, 2001; Ped Derm 11:52–60, 1994; Pediatrics 87:228–234, 1991;*

Juvenile xanthogranuloma *Ped Derm 27:666–667, 2010*

Langerhans cell histiocytosis – scalp papules and nodules *AD 137:1241–1246, 2001;* congenital self-healing variant

Self-healing Hashimoto-Pritzker histiocytosis *Ann DV 128:238–240, 2001; Arch Pediatr 7:629–632, 2000; Am J Dermatopathol 13:481–487, 1991*

INFLAMMATORY DISORDERS

Congenital cranial fasciitis – giant skin colored nodule *Ped Derm 24:263–266, 2007;*

mobile red subcutaneous mass *Ped Derm 16:232–234, 1999*

Eosinophilic granuloma – yellow to brown papule with hemorrhagic center *JAAD 46:934–941, 2002*

NEOPLASTIC DISORDERS

Adenoid cystic carcinoma–personal observation; primary cutaneous of scalp *Clin in Dermatol 37:468–486, 2019*

Infantile choriocarcinoma *JAAD 14:918–927, 1986*

Infantile myofibromatosis – red scalp nodule *Ped Derm 27:29–33, 2010;* purple *Ann Pathol 24:427–431, 2004; AD 123:1392–1393, 1395–1396, 1987*

Connective tissue nevus – associated with cardiomyopathy and hypogonadism *Ann Int Med 93:813–817, 1980*

Cylindromas *JAAD 81:1300–1307, 2019*

Dermatofibrosarcoma protuberans, subcutaneous *JAAD 77:503–511, 2017*

Epidermoid cyst *Cutis 76:377–382, 2005*

Fibrosarcoma

Giant cell fibroblastoma *JAAD 46:934–941, 2002*

Hamartoma with ectopic meningothelial elements – simulates angiosarcoma *Am J Surg Pathol 14:1–11, 1990*

Infantile myofibromatosis–red to violaceous nodules *JAAD 49:S148–150, 2003; AD 123:1391–1396, 1987*

Intracranial neoplasms with extension through the skull *JAAD 46:934–941, 2002*

Leukemia *Pediatr Ann 43:e25–27, 2014;* acute lymphoblastic B-cell leukemia *Cutis 103:E16–18, 2019; Ann Plast Surg 64:251–153, 2010;* acute myelogenous leukemia *SkinMed 8:305–306, 2010*

Leptomeningeal cyst (traumatic) (growing fracture) – skull fracture with laceration of underlying dura *Ped Clin North Amer 6:1151–1160, 1993;* with brain herniation *JAAD 46:934–941, 2002*

Lipoma *JAAD 46:934–941, 2002;* congenital frontal lipoma associated with agenesis of corpus callosum *Ped Derm 29:490–494, 2012*

Lymphoma *JAAD 46:934–941, 2002;* primary cutaneous follicle center B-cell lymphoma *JAAD 69:343–354, 2013*

Melanocytic nevus

Melanoma – congenital pigment synthesizing melanoma of the scalp (animal type melanoma); black, pedunculated, ulcerated scalp nodule *JAAD 62:324–329, 2010*

Meningioma *Cutis 76:377–382, 2005*

Meningothelial hamartoma (rudimentary meningocele) – alopecic fibrotic blue-purple plaque of scalp; may be tan-gray, red, or skin colored; nodular *Ped Derm 28:677–680, 2011;*

Zentralbl Pathol 138:355–361, 1992

Metastases *Cutis 76:377–382, 2005; JAAD 46:934–941, 2002;* neuroblastoma *Indian J Pathol Microbiol 52:374–376, 2009*

Mucoepidermoid carcinoma – skin colored nodule *Soc Ped Dermatol Annual Meeting, July, 2006*

Myofibromatosis – spontaneous regression of crusted nodule; lesions in heart, lung, gastrointestinal tract *JAMADerm 151:663–664, 2015; Cancer 48:1807–1818, 1981*
   Differential diagnosis includes:
      Fibrous tumors
      Xanthogranulomas
      Nasal gliomas
      Vascular or lymphatic tumors
      Dermoid cysts
      Neurofibromas
      Sarcomas *J Perinatol 28:160–162, 2008*
      Encephaloceles
      Meningiomas
      Lipomas
      Teratomas

Nevus sebaceous–large papillomatous, pedunculated, pink nodule *Ped Derm 25:355–358, 2008*

Pigment synthesizing melanocytic neoplasm with protein kinase C alpha (*PRKCA*) fusion – ATPase calcium transporting plasma membrane4 (ATp2B4)-protein kinase C-alpha (PRKCA) fusion transcript *JAMADerm 152:318–322, 2016*

Sarcoma *JAAD 46:934–941, 2002*

Teratoma *J Craniofac Surg 7:148–150, 1996*

PRIMARY CUTANEOUS DISEASES

Aplasia cutis congenita *Cutis 76:377–382, 2005*

Granuloma annulare *Ped Derm 35:e72–73, 2018; Cutis 76:377–382, 2005*

SYNDROMES

Fibrodysplasia ossificans progressiva – fibrous scalp nodules *JAAD 64:97–101, 2011; Clev Clin Q 51:549–552, 1984*

Lumpy scalp syndrome *Clin Exp Derm 15:240, 1989*

Congenital Wells' syndrome *Ped Derm 14:312–315, 1997*

TRAUMA

Cephalohematoma (Cephalohematoma deformans) – blood between outer table of skull and periosteum; fixed *Ped Clin North Amer 6:1151–1160, 1993;* cephalohematoma with secondary infection with Gardnerella vaginalis *Pediatr Inf Dis J 23:276–277, 2004* Subcutaneous fat necrosis of the newborn *J Eur Acad DV 12:254–257, 1999*

VASCULAR DISORDERS

Arteriovenous malformation *JAAD 46:934–941, 2002*

Hemangiomas *JAAD 46:934–941, 2002*

Hematoma *J Craniofac Surg 7:148–150, 1996*

Kaposiform hemangioendothelioma *Am J Surg Pathol 17:321–328, 1993*

Subepicranial hygromas *JAAD 46:934–941, 2002*

Venous cavernoma (venous malformation) *JAAD 46:934–941, 2002; Zentralbl Neurochir 59:274–277, 1998*

Subepidermal varix *JAAD 46:934–941, 2002*

Subgaleal scalp hematoma *Ped Clin North Amer 6:1151–1160, 1993*

CHILDREN

AUTOIMMUNE DISEASES

Benign rheumatoid nodules – healthy children; pretibial areas, feet, scalp *Aust NZ J Med 9:697–701, 1979*

Chronic granulomatous disease–crusted scalp nodule in infant *AD 130:105–110, 1994*

DEVELOPMENTAL DEFECTS

Aplasia cutis congenita with or without hair collar or port wine stain

Atretic encephalocele or meningocele

Branchial cleft sinuses–linear lesion; retroauricular tumor *Ped Derm 2:318–321, 1985*

Cephalocele – includes meningocele (rudimentary meningocele), meningoencephalocele, meningomyelocele; blue nodule with overlying hypertrichosis *JAAD 46:934–941, 2002; AD 137:45–50, 2001*

Encephalocoele

Heterotopic brain tissue (heterotopic meningeal nodules) – blue-red cystic mass with overlying alopecia *JAAD 46:934–941, 2002; AD 131:731, 1995; JAAD 28:1015, 1993*

Meningocele–classic meningocele; sequestrated meningocele–juicy nodule in parieto-occipital scalp *Ped Derm 14:315–318, 1994; rudimentary meningocele Ped Derm 18:368–381, 1998*

Sinus pericranii *JAAD 46:934–941, 2002*

DRUGS

Anti-tumor necrosis factor agents – erythematous boggy crusted alopecic plaque of scalp *Ped Derm 29:454–459, 2012*

Methotrexate-associated B-cell lymphoproliferative disease *JAMADerm 154:490–492, 2018*

INFECTIONS AND INFESTATIONS

Abscesses *JAAD 46:934–941, 2002*

Cryptococcosis in hyper IgM syndrome – mimicking kerion *Cases of the Year, Pre-AAD Pediatric Dermatology Meeting*

Filariasis (*Brugia*) – multiple nodules of forehead and scalp *Ped Derm 25:230–232, 2008*

Kerion *Ped Derm 29:479–482, 2012*

Mycetoma – due to *Microsporum canis* (pseudomycetoma) *Cutis 78:473–475, 2006; M. canis and Trichophyton mentagrophytes Mycopathologia 81: 41–48, 1983*

Myiasis, furuncular–*Dermatobia hominis*–human botflies *Clin Inf Dis 37:542, 591–592, 2003;* scalp cyst in a child *Ped Derm 15:116–118, 1998;* mimicking ruptured epidermoid cyst *Can J Surg 33:145–146, 1990;* house fly *BJD 76:218–222, 1964;* New World screw worm (Cochliomyia), Old World screw worm (Chrysomya), Tumbu fly (Cordylobia) *BJD 85:226–231, 1971;* black blowflies (Phormia) *J Med Entomol 23:578–579, 1986;* greenbottle (Lucilia), bluebottle (Calliphora), flesh flies (Sarcophaga, Wohlfartia) *Cutis 82:396–398, 2008; Neurosurgery 18:361–362, 1986;* rodent botflies (Cuterebra) *JAAD 21:763–772, 1989;* human botflies (Dermatobia hominis) *AD 126:199–202, 1990; AD 121:1195–1196, 1985*

Orf – scalp nodules with necrosis *AD 145:1053–1058, 2009*

Rheumatic fever – nodules of occiput

Scabies *Semin Dermatol 12:3–8, 1993*

Tinea capitis (Trichophyton verrucosum, T. mentagrophtes) – kerion *AD 114:371–372, 1978;* tinea capitis mimicking dissecting cellulitis – alopecia and inflammatory nodules of scalp *Ped Derm 30:753–754, 2013*

Wart

INFILTRATIVE DISORDERS

Eosinophilic granuloma – yellow to brown papule with hemorrhagic center *JAAD 46:934–941, 2002; J Derm Surg Oncol 19:631–634, 1993*

Hashimoto-Pritzker self-healing histiocytosis *Arch Pediatr 7:629–632, 2000*

Juvenile xanthogranuloma *Ped Dev Pathol 21:489–493, 2018; JAAD 36:355–367, 1997; Am J Surg Pathol 15:150–159, 1991*

Hereditary progressive mucinous histiocytosis – infantile dermal nodules of scalp, trunk, and extremities *Ped Derm 32:e273–276, 2015; Dermatology 36:958–960, 1997*

Langerhans cell histiocytosis *Head Neck Pathol 12:431–439, 2018*

Self-healing juvenile cutaneous mucinosis – red nodules of face, scalp, hand; macrodactyly (enlarged thumbs); periarticular papules and nodules, painful polyarthritis; linear ivory white papules, multiple subcutaneous nodules, indurated edema of periorbital and zygomatic areas *JAAD 55:1036–1043, 2006; Ped Derm 20:35–39, 2003; AD 131:459–461, 1995; Clin Exp Dermatol 19:90–93, 1994; Ann DV 107:51–57, 1980; Lyon Med 230:470–474, 1973*

INFLAMMATORY DISORDERS

Cranial fasciitis of childhood *Ped Derm 16:232–234, 1999*

Dissecting cellulitis – abscess-like scalp nodule *JAMADerm 152:1280–1281, 2016; Cutis 67:37–40, 2000*

Eosinophilic panniculitis *Ped Derm 12:35–38, 1995*

Sarcoid

METABOLIC DISORDERS

Alopecia an aseptic nodule of scalp *Ped Derm 34:697–700, 2017*

Progressive osseous heteroplasia

NEOPLASTIC DISORDERS

Apocrine poroma – red nodule of scalp *JAMADerm 151:553–554, 2015*

Basal cell carcinoma arising in nevus sebaceous *Ped Derm 28:138–141, 2011*

Cylindroma; malignant cylindroma *Dermatology 201:255–257, 2000*

Dermal sinus tumors

Dermatofibrosarcoma protuberans, metastasis *Am J Dermatopathol 38:e40–43, 2016; J Surg Res 170:69–72, 2011; JAAD 61:130–132, 2009*

Dermoid and epidermoid cysts *Australas J Dermatol 33:135–140, 1992*

Encephalocutaneous cranial lipomatosis *J Paediatr Child Health 36:603–605, 2000; Am J Med Genet 91:261–266, 2000; Ann DV 124:549–551, 1997*

Epidermoid cysts *JAAD 46:934–941, 2002*

Giant cell fibroblastoma *JAAD 46:934–941, 2002*

Granulocytic sarcoma *BJD 147:609–611, 2002*

Intracranial neoplasms with extension through the skull *JAAD 46:934–941, 2002*

Juvenile hyaline fibromatosis *Pathologica 106:70–72, 2014; Dermatology 198:18–25, 1999*

Keratoacanthomas–multiple self-healing keratoacanthomas of Ferguson-Smith – cluster around ears, nose, scalp; red nodule becomes ulcerated, resolve with crenellated scar; develop singly or in crops *Cancer 5:539–550, 1952;* one reported unilateral case *AD 97:615–623, 1968*

Leptomeningeal cyst (traumatic) (growing fracture) – skull fracture with laceration of underlying dura *Ped Clin North Amer 6:1151–1160, 1993;* with brain herniation *JAAD 46:934–941, 2002*

Leukemia cutis – acute myelogenous leukemia in children *SkinMed 8:305–306, 2010;* red scalp nodule *Ped Derm 36:658–663, 2019;* acute lymphoblastic leukemia *Pediatr Ann 43:e25–27, 2014; Ann Plast Surg 64:251–253, 2010*

Lipoma *JAAD 46:934–941, 2002; J Derm Surg Oncol 11:981–984, 1985*

Lipomatous mixed tumor *BJD 146:899–903, 2002*

Lymphoma–*JAAD 46:934–941, 2002;* cutaneous T-cell lymphoma (CTCL)

Lymphomatoid papulosis *Arch Pediatr 2:984–987, 1995*

Melanocytic nevus–atypical proliferative nodules in congenital melanocytic nevi *BJD 165:1138–1142, 2011*

Meningioma–nodule with overlying alopecia or hypertrichosis *JAAD 46:934–941, 2002; Eur J Pediatr Surg 10:387–389, 2000;* primary cutaneous meningioma *Asian J Neurosurg 13:110–112, 2018; J Cutan Pathol 21:549–556, 1994*

Merkel cell carcinoma *Cutis 103:261,280–282, 2019*

Metastases *JAAD 46:934–941, 2002;* lung cancer with emboli in pulmonary venous circulation; nodules of trunk and scalp *Cancer 19:162–168, 1966;* osteosarcoma – red scalp nodule *JAAD 49:124–127, 2003;* leiomyosarcoma *JAAD 72:910–912, 2015;* renal cell carcinoma – red-blue nodule *Cutis 99:14,25–26, 2017*

Multiple myeloma *AD 139:475–486, 2003*

Myofibromatosis *AD 123:1392–1395, 1987*

Myxoid neurothekeoma – skin colored scalp nodules *Ped Derm 28:333–334, 2011*

Myxoinflammatory fibroblastic sarcoma *Pediatr Dev Pathol 15:254–258, 2012*

Neurocristic cutaneous hamartoma *Am J Dermatopathol 37:e87–92, 2015; Mod Pathol 11:573–578, 1998*

Neurofibroma

Neurothekeoma

Nevus sebaceus–nodule with surrounding hypertrichosis *Ped Derm 89:84–86, 1991*

Osteogenic sarcoma

Osteoma *Cutis 76:377–382, 2005*

Pilomatrixoma *Arch Otolaryngol Head Neck Surg 124:1239–1242, 1998; JAAD 3:180–185, 1980;*

Porocarcinoma *AD 136:1409–1414, 2000*

Porokeratosis of Mibelli

Undifferentiated pleomorphic sarcoma (malignant fibrous histiocytoma) *BJD 163:431–433, 2010; Cancer 17:1445–1455, 1964*

PRIMARY CUTANEOUS DISEASES

Granuloma annulare, subcutaneous *Cutis 104:E15–17, 2019; Ped Derm 19:276–277, 2002; Curr Prob Derm 14:41–70, 2002; Pediatrics 107:E42, 2001; Pediatr Dev Pathol 1:300–308, 1998; Pediatrics 100:965–967, 1997; Curr Prob in Derm 8:137–188, 1996*

Subcutaneous necrobiotic granulomas of the scalp

SYNDROMES

Wells' syndrome *Ped Derm 14:312–315, 1997*

TRAUMA

Traumatic granuloma *Cutis 76:377–382, 2005*

VASCULAR DISORDERS

Arteriovenous malformation *JAAD 46:934–941, 2002*

Cephalohematoma deformans

Hemangiomas *JAAD 46:934–941, 2002*

Subepicranial hygromas *JAAD 46:934–941, 2002*

Subepidermal varix *JAAD 46:934–941, 2002*

Venous cavernoma (venous malformation) *JAAD 46:934–941, 2002*

ADULTS

AUTOIMMUNE DISEASES AND DISEASES OF IMMUNE DYSFUNCTION

Lupus erythematosus – discoid lupus erythematosus – calcinosis cutis of scalp – white papulonodules *JAMA Derm 149:246–248, 2013;* lupus profundus/panniculitis *Med Clin (Barc)151:444–449, 2018; Lupus 21:662–665, 2012*

Rheumatoid nodulosis *Arthritis Rheum 40:175–178, 1997*

DRUGS

Anti-retroviral agents *NEJM 352:63, 2005*

EXOGENOUS AGENTS

Iododerma *Australas J Dermatol 29:179–180, 1988*

Paraffinomas–lumpy scalp *AD 121:382–385, 1985*

INFECTIONS

Abscesses *JAAD 46:934–941, 2002*

Bacillary angiomatosis *Dermatol Online J 18:8, Aug 15, 2012*

Candidiasis, systemic in drug addicts – purulent nodules of scalp and follicular pustules *BJD 150:1–10, 2004; Clin Infect Dis 15:910–923, 1992; J Infect Dis 152:577–591, 1985; Br Med J 287:861–862, 1983*

Carbuncle

Folliculitis decalvans–personal observation

Herpes simplex folliculitis–violaceous nodules *Am J Dermatopathol 13:234–240, 1991*

Deep mycoses

Dirofilaria repens – self–limiting parasite of dogs *Ann DV 138:50–53, 2011*

Leprosy – rarely involves scalp *An Bras Dermatol 91:69–70, 2016*

Molluscum contagiosum *Ann Dermatol 25:109–110, 2013;* HIV and giant Mollusca *Int J Infect Dis 38:153–155, 2015*

Mycobacterium abscessus *Clin Exp Dermatol 41:768–770*

Mycobacterium haemophilum AD 138:229–230, 2002

Mycobacterium tuberculosis–scrofuloderma *J Dermatol 21:42–45, 1994*

Myiasis – *Dermatobia hominis Int J Dermatol 57:227–230, 2018BJD 151:1270, 2004;* cuterebrid myiasis *Ped Derm 21:515–516, 2004;* furunculoid myiasis; migratory myiasis–*Gasterophilus intestinalis, Hypoderma spp. JAAD 58:907–926, 2008*

New Jersey polyoma viremia

Nocardia Cutis 104:226–229, 2019; N. nova South Med J 103;1269–1271, 2010

Onchocercoma

Pott's puffy tumor – fluctuant nodule over frontal region in patients with chronic sinusitis *JAAD 46:934–941, 2002*

Pseudomycetoma of scalp – multiple scalp nodules; Trichophyton schoenleinii *BJD 145:151–153, 2001*

Scabies – single scalp nodule *G Ital DV 148:546–547, 2013; Acta DV (Stockh)61:360–362, 1981*

Syphilis – secondary *Int J Dermatol 58:e203–204, 2019; J Dermatol 44:1401–1403, 2017;* tertiary *Ann DV 121:146–151, 1994*

Tick bite – alopecia and nodule at site of tick attachment to scalp *Cutis 98:88–90, 2016*

Tinea capitis, kerion; presenting as acne keloidalis *JAAD 56:699–701, 2007;* masquerading as basal cell carcinoma *SkinMed 16:269–271, 2018*

Trichosporon beigelii, disseminated *JAAD 129:1020–1023, 1993*

Tufted folliculitis *BJD 174:e22, 2016*

Wart, mimicking keratoacanthoma–personal observation

Yaws *Infect Dis Poverty 9:1 Jan 30, 2020*

INFILTRATIVE DISORDERS

Amyloidosis–nodular primary cutaneous amyloidosis *Dermatol Pract Concept 31:184–187, 2018; JAAD 14:1058–1062, 1986*

Angioplasmocellular hyperplasia – red nodule with red rim, ulcerated nodule, vascular nodule of face, scalp, neck, trunk, and leg *JAAD 64:542–547, 2011*

Eosinophilic granuloma (Langerhans cell histiocytosis) *AD 143:1083–1084, 2007*

Erdheim-Chester disease *Ann Dermatol 22:439–443, 2010*

IgG4-related skin disease – plasma cells and fibrosis; FoxP3+ cells *G Ital DV 151:296–299, 2016; JAMA Derm 149:742747, 2013*

Indeterminate cell histiocytosis – widespread erythematous papulonodular eruption *BJD 158:838–840, 2008*

Lymphocytoma cutis *Cancer 69:717–724, 1992; Acta DV (Stockh)62:119–124, 1982; Cancer 24:487–502, 1969*

Mastocytoma – subcutaneous scalp nodule *JAAD 65:683–684, 2011*

Rosai-Dorfman disease – orange nodules of scalp *Cutis 100:157, 159–160, 2017*

Xanthogranuloma *AD 112:43–44, 1976;* polypoid lesion of scalp *Am J Dermatopathol 39:773–775, 2017*

Xanthoma disseminatum *Ann Dermatol 22:353–357, 2010*

INFLAMMATORY DISORDERS

Alopecia and aseptic nodules of the scalp *Indian J Dermatol 62:515–518, 2017; Dermatology 232:165–170, 2016*

Cranial fasciitis (nodular fasciitis) *Ped Derm 24:463, 2007; AD 125:674–678, 1989*

Dissecting cellulitis of the scalp (perifolliculitis capitis abscedens et suffodiens) – cerebriform scalp nodules *Ped Derm 34:e210–211, 2017; BJD 174:916–918, 2016; BJD 174:421–423, 2016; BJD 159:506–507, 2008; BJD 152:777–779, 2005; Cutis 67:37–40, 2001; AD 128:1115–1120, 1992; Minn Med 34:319–325, 1951; AD 23:503–518, 1931*

Fibroblastic rheumatism *JAAD 66:959–965, 2012*

Kikuchi's histiocytic necrotizing lymphadenitis *BJD 144:885–889, 2001*

Lymphocytoma cutis

Pseudolymphomatous folliculitis

Sarcoid *JAAD 44:725–743,2001*

METABOLIC DISORDERS

Metastatic Crohn's disease–personal observation

Osteoma cutis – platelet osteoma cutis presenting as cutis verticis gyrata *JAAD 64:613–615, 2011*

Pancreatic panniculitis *Eur J Case Rep Intern Med April 27, 2017*

Tuberous xanthoma *Indian J Dermatol 60:425, 2015*

NEOPLASTIC DISORDERS

Actinic keratosis

Adenoid cystic carcinoma, primary cutaneous – scalp papules or nodules *Cutis 81:243–246, 2008; JAAD 58:636–641, 2008; Cutis 77:157–160, 2006; JAAD 40:640–642, 1999*

Angiomyxoma, superficial – exophytic nodule of scalp *JAMA Derm 149:751–756, 2013*

Apocrine carcinoma *Cancer 71:375–381, 1993*

Apocrine epithelioma–retroauricular tumor *JAAD 13:355–363, 1985*

Apocrine nevus *Am J Dermatopathol 34:205–209, 2012; Ann Dermatol Syphiligr 101:251–261, 1974*

Atypical fibroxanthoma *Am J Dermatopathol 141:e79–79, 2019; Sem Cut Med Surg 21:159–165, 2002; Head Neck 23:399–403, 2001;* hemorrhagic scalp nodule *AD 143:653–658, 2007;* multilobulated, ulcerated, scalp nodule *JAAD 67:1091–1092, 2012*

Basal cell carcinoma *JAAD 56:448–452, 2007; Acta Pathol Microbiol Scand 88A:5–9, 1980; J Surg Oncol 5:431–463, 1975;* post-irradiation *Lancet i:509, 1974;* with cerebral invasion *Eur J Surg Oncol 27:510–511, 2001*

Benign chondroblastoma cutis–retroauricular tumor *AD 123:24–26, 1987*

Blastic plasmacytoid dendritic cell neoplasm (blastic natural killer cell lymphoma) – skin colored nodule of scalp *JAMA Derm 149:971–972, 2013; Indian J Dermatol 57:45–47, 2012*

Bowen's disease

Brooke-Spiegler syndrome *SkinMed 13:325–328, 2015*

Carcinoid–primary cutaneous carcinoid *Cancer 36:1016–1020, 1975*

Carcinosarcoma *JAAD 52:S124–126, 2005*

Cellular blue nevus *J Surg Oncol 74:278–281, 2000; Br J Plast Surg 51:410–411, 1998;* giant alopecic nodule *BJD 126:375–377, 1992*

Ceruminoma–retroauricular tumor *AD 98:344–348, 1968*

Chondroblastoma *JAAD 40:325–327, 1999*

Chondroid syringoma *Ear Nose Throat J 90:190–191; Cutis 71:49–55, 2003;* malignant *Indian Dermatol Online J 4:236–238, 2013*

Chondroma *Pan Afr Med J 21:64, 2015*

Chondromyxoid fibroma

Clear cell acanthoma *Cutis 67:149–151, 2001*

Clear cell hidradenoma (eccrine acrospiroma) – pink nodule of scalp *Cutis 94:268,271–272, 2014; AD 128:547–552, 1992; AD 125:985–990, 1989*

Congenital smooth muscle hamartoma *Ped Derm 11:431–433, 1996*

Connective tissue nevus–rare *Int J Trichology 5:88–90, 2015;* fibrous cephalic plaque in tuberous sclerosis *JAAD 78:721–724, 2018*

Cylindroma *Dermatol Online J 16:12, April 15, 2010; AD 145:1277–1284, 2009; BJD 155:182–186, 2006; NEJM 351:2530, 2004; JAAD 46:934–941, 2002; Am J Dermatopathol 17:260–265, 1995;* malignant cylindroma *Int J Surg Case Rep 4:587–592, 2013*

Deep penetrating nevus – black or darkly pigmented nevus of head, neck, and scalp *JAAD 71:1234–1240, 2014*

Dermatofibroma

Dermatofibrosarcoma protuberans *JAAD 56:448–452, 2007; JAAD 21:278–283, 1989;* multilobulated scalp nodule *JAAD 67:861–866, 2012*

Eccrine epithelioma–ulcerated nodule *JAAD 6:514–518, 1982*

Eccrine sweat gland carcinoma–clear reticulated cytoplasm; face, scalp, palm *J Cutan Pathol 14:65–86, 1987; JAAD 13:497–500, 1985; AD 120:768–769, 1984;* squamoid eccrine ductal carcinoma *Australas J Dermatol 57:e111–119, 2016*

Eccrine hidradenoma – dermal nodule with or without ulceration; face, scalp, anterior trunk *AD 97:651–661, 1968*

Eccrine porocarcinoma (malignant eccrine poroma) – red nodule *Am J Case Rep 20:179–183, 2019; Cutis 93:43–46, 2014*

Eccrine poroma – pigmented scalp nodule *BJD 146:523, 2002*

Eccrine spiradenoma *J Cutan Pathol 15:226–229, 1988;* malignant eccrine spiradenoma of scalp *Derm Surg 25:45–48, 1999;* zosteriform *Ann Chir Plast Ethet 61:65–68, 2016*

Eosinophilic dermatosis of myeloproliferative disease – face, scalp; scaly red nodules; trunk – red nodules; extremities – red nodules and hemorrhagic papules *AD 137:1378–1380, 2001*

Epidermoid cysts *JAAD 46:934–941, 2002;* ruptured epidermoid cysts *Jpn J Clin Dermatol 46:9–16, 1992*

Epithelial nevi and tumors

Extraskeletal Ewing's sarcoma *Ped Derm 5:123–126, 1988*

Fibrodysplasia ossificans progressiva – fibrous scalp nodules *Cleve Clin Q 51:549–552, 1984*

Fibrous dysplasia

Fibrosarcoma

Folliculosebaceous cystic hamartoma – skin colored papule or nodule of central face or scalp; pedunculated or dome-shaped and umbilicated *BJD 157:833–835, 2007; Clin Exp Dermatol 31:68–79, 2006; Am J Dermatopathol 13:213–220, 1991; J Cutan Pathol 7:394–403, 1980*

Giant cell angiofibroma *Surg Neurol Int Sept 30, 2013; Case Rep Pathol 2012:408575:doi.101155/408575*

Giant cell fibroblastoma *JAAD 46:934–941, 2002*

Giant folliculosebaceous cystic hamartoma *AD 141:1035–1040, 2005*

Granular cell tumor *Case Rep Pathol 2016:8043183:doi.10.1155/2016/8043183*

Hair follicle hamartoma–personal observation

Heterotopic meningeal nodules, familial cutaneous *JAAD 28:1015, 1017, 1993;* neuroglial heterotopia *Pathologica 108:42–44, 2016*

Hibernoma

Hidradenocarcinoma, metastases – red nodules of face and scalp *Indian J Dermatol 60:421, 2015; AD 147:998–999, 2011;* poroid hidradenoma *J Surg Case Rep May 9, 2019*

Hidradenoma papilliferum *JAAD 41:115–118, 1999; JAAD 19:133–135, 1988;* tubopapillary hidradenoma *J Cytol 30:142–144, 2013*

Cutaneous histiocytic sarcoma *Am J Dermatopathol 42:286–291, 2020*

Intracranial neoplasms with extension through the skull *JAAD 46:934–941, 2002*

Intravascular papillary endothelial hyperplasia (Masson tumor) *J Korean Neurosurg Soc 52:52–54, 2012*

Juvenile aponeurotic fibroma – rare on head/neck *Ear Nose Throat J 90:E14–16, 2011*

Juvenile hyaline fibromatosis (systemic hyalinosis) – translucent papules or nodules of scalp, face, neck, trunk, gingival hypertrophy, flexion contractures of large and small joints *JAAD 16:881–883, 1987*

Kaposi's sarcoma *Med J Malaysia 68:383–384, 2011*

Keloids

Keratoacanthoma–personal observation

Leukemia cutis *JAAD 34:375–378, 1996;* chronic myelogenous leukemia blast crisis *Indian J Dermatol 51:265–267, 2010*

Lipoma *JAAD 46:934–941, 2002;* sclerotic lipoma *J Cutan Pathol 47:286–290, 2020*

Liposarcoma, pleomorphic – metastatic to scalp *J Cutan Pathol 43:526–530, 2016*

Lymphoepithelioma-like carcinoma of the skin *AD 134:1627–1632, 1998*

Lymphoma *JAAD 46:934–941, 2002;* follicular-center B-cell lymphoma – nodules of face, scalp, trunk, extremities *BJD 144:1239–1243, 2001; AD 132:1376–1377, 1996;* primary cutaneous B-cell lymphoma *BJD 153:167–173, 2005;* cutaneous B-cell lymphoblastic lymphoma *JAAD 66:51–57, 2012;* primary cutaneous follicle center lymphoma *JAAD 69:343–354, 2013; AD 143:1520–1526, 2007; BJD 157:1205–1211, 2007;* primary cutaneous follicle center lymphoma with diffuse CD 30 expression – papules, plaques, nodules, multilobulated scalp tumor *JAAD 71:548–554, 2014;* plasmacytoid dendritic cell neoplasm (lymphoblastoid natural killer-cell lymphoma) – purple nodule of leg; nodule of face or scalp *BJD 162:74–79, 2010; AD 144:1155–1162, 2008;* primary cutaneous marginal zone lymphoma *JAAD 69:329–340, 2013;* post-transplant lymphoma *JAAD 81:600–602, 2019;* post-transplant primary cutaneous CD30 and CD56 acute large cell lymphoma–polypoid scalp mass *Arch Pathol Lab Med 128:e96–99, 2004;* cutaneous T-cell lymphoma–fungating ulcerative mass *AD 124:409–413, 1988;* Hodgkin's disease – ulcerated papules, plaques, and nodules of the scalp and face *AD 127:405, 408, 1991;* spindle cell B-cell lymphoma *BJD 145:313–317, 2001;* blastic natural killer-cell lymphoma *BJD 150:174–176, 2004;* others; cutaneous Richter syndrome (CLL rapidly developing into large cell lymphoma) *Am J Med 68:539–548, 1980;* primary cutaneous CD30+ anaplastic large cell lymphoma – arciform lesions *Ped Derm 26:721–724, 2009;* CD4+ small,/medium pleomorphic T-cell lymphoma – skin colored nodule of face, red nodule of scalp, red plaque of neck *JAAD 65:739–748, 2011;* primary cutaneous follicular helper T-cell lymphoma – red papules, red plaques, scalp nodule, facial plaques *AD 148:832–839, 2012;* precursor B-cell lymphoblastic lymphoma – scalp nodule of 4 year old *Ped Derm 30:135–136, 2013;* lymphoblastic lymphoma – red scalp nodule *JAAD 70:318–325, 2014;* primary cutaneous anaplastic large cell lymphoma *JAAD 74:1135–1143, 2016*

Lymphomatoid papulosis – scalp papules *BJD 171:1590–1592, 2014*

Malignant blue nevus *Int J Dermatol 37:126–127, 1998; Cutis 58:40–42, 1996*

Malignant eccrine spiradenoma *Derm Surg 25:45–48, 1999; Am J Dermatopathol 14:381–390, 1992*

Malignant fibrous histiocytoma, angiomatoid *J Clin Pathol 67:210–215, 2014*

Malignant peripheral nerve sheath tumors (neurofibrosarcoma) *AD 137:908–913, 2001*

Melanocytic nevi *ad 146:506–511, 2010;* including giant congenital melanocytic nevus, of scalp and cranium *Br J Plast Surg 50:20–25, 1997*

Melanoma *JAAD 56:448–452, 2007;* primary dermal melanoma – blue scalp nodule *AD 144:49–56, 2008;* red nodule *JAMADerm 150:1048–1055, 2014;* primary amelanotic rhabdoid melanoma – red scalp nodule *BJD 174:1156–1158, 2016;* amelanotic melanoma; desmoplastic *Am Surg Pathol 38:864–870, 2014*

Meningioma–intracranial malignant meningioma *JAAD 34:306–307, 1996;* osteolytic meningioma *JAAD 35:641, 1996;* metastatic meningioma – skin colored nodule of scalp *Cutis 101:386–389, 2018;* intracranial anaplastic meningioma *Dermatol Online J 18:6, Sept 15, 2012*

Merkel cell tumor *JAAD 31:271–2, 1994;* multilobulated red nodules of scalp *AD 145:494–495, 2009*

Metastases *JAAD 56:448–452, 2007; JAAD 46:934–941, 2002; JAAD 36:531–537, 1997;* cystic lesion–metastatic lung adenocarcinoma *JAAD 36:644–646, 1997;* prostate *AD 104:301–303, 1971;* lung and kidney in men; breast in women; also ovaries, uterus, gallbladder, testis, gastrointestinal tract, melanoma, leukemia, lymphoma *JAAD 31:319–321, 1994;* renal cell carcinoma *Cutis 98:376,383–384, 2016; AD 140:1393–1398, 2004; Derm Surg 27:192–194, 2001;* paraganglioma – painful *JAAD 44:321–323, 2001;* glioblastoma multiforme *JAAD 46:297–300, 2002;* salivary gland adenocarcinoma mimicking kerion; osteosarcoma *JAAD 49:757–760, 2003;* cholangiocarcinoma *JAAD 56:S58–60, 2007; JAAD 51:S108–111, 2004;* malignant mixed Mullerian tumor *BJD 151:943–945, 2004;* esophageal carcinoma *Cutis 70:230–232, 2002;* metastatic rhabdomyosarcoma *JAAD 58:S118–120, 2008;* red nodule–malignant fibrous histiocytoma of bone *JAAD 59:S88–91, 2008;* bladder carcinoma *AD 145:213–215, 2009;* alveolar soft part sarcoma *JAAD 61:117–120, 2009;* renal cell *Cases J 2:7948, 2009*

Microcystic adnexal carcinoma – skin colored plaque *JAAD 41:225–231, 1999;* skin colored or yellow nodule or plaque *JAAD 52:295–300, 2005; Derm Surg 27:979–984, 2001; Derm Surg 27:678–680, 2001; JAAD 45:283–285, 2001*

Mucinous carcinoma of skin (primary cutaneous mucinous carcinoma) *AD 148:849–854, 2012; JAAD 52:S76–80, 2005; JAAD 49:941–943, 2003; JAAD 36:323–326, 1997; Clin Exp Dermatol 18:375–377, 1993;* eyelid and scalp *Am J Surg Pathol 29:764–782, 2005*

Mucoepidermoid carcinoma – scalp nodule *Ped Derm 24:452–453, 2007; Derm Surg 27:1046–1048, 2001*

Myeloma – plasmacytoma *Int J Surg Case Rep 21:52–54, 2016*

Myoepithelioma *Ped Derm 29:345–348, 2012*

Myofibroma – giant tumor of scalp with surface telangiectasias *Ped Derm 27:525–526, 2010;* giant infantile myofibroma – large exophytic mass of scalp of newborn *Ped Derm 32:281–282, 2015; Australas J Dermatol 41:156–161, 2000; Cancer 7:973–978, 1054*

Cutaneous myopericytoma *Dermatopathol (Bazel)2:9–14, 2015*

Neurocristic cutaneous hamartoma – a dermal melanocytosis *Mod Pathol 11:573–578, 1998*

Neuroendocrine carcinoma of the skin *J Cutan Pathol 44:978–981, 2017*

Neurofibroma

Neurothekeoma – skin colored scalp nodule *Brain Tumor Res Treat 4:17–20, 2016; BJD 144:1273–1274, 2001*

Nevus lipomatosis superficialis *Cutis 43:143–144, 1989*

Nevus psiloliparus) (mesodermal nevus of lipoma) – alopecia with pink nodule of scalp; when associated with aplasia cutis congenita (aplasticopsillipara) it is associated with encephalocraniocutaneous lipomatosis *Ped Derm 31:746–748, 2014*

Nevus sebaceus, exophytic *Pediatr Neurosurg 44:144–147, 2008; Ped Derm 25:366–358, 2008; Ped Derm 8:84–86, 1991;* pink pedunculated nodule of scalp *Ped Derm 36:154–155, 2019*

Nuchal type fibroma of scalp *Ann Dermatol 27:194–196, 2015*

Osteogenic sarcoma *BMJ Case Rep May 18, 2018*

Osteoma

Pacinian collagenoma *J Cutan Pathol 47:291–294, 2020*

Paraganglioma, primary cutaneous – scalp papule, red nodule *JAAD 54:S220–223, 2006*

Parotid gland tumors–retroauricular tumor

Pilar cyst *JAAD 46:934–941, 2002;* proliferating pilar cyst – multi-lobulated scalp nodule *JAAD 69:849–850, 2013;*

Pilomatrixomas, also seen with myotonic dystrophy *Ped Derm 28:74–76, 2011; Arch Otolaryngol Head Neck Surg 124:1239–1242, 1998; JAAD 37:268–269, 1997;* tent sign, skin crease sign *Aust J Gen Pract 48:294–297, 2019*

Pilomatrix carcinoma *JAAD 44:358–361, 2001;* multiple of head and neck *Otolaryngol Head Neck Surg 109:543–547, 1993; JAAD 23:985–988, 1990*

Plasmacytosis, nodular cutaneous *Clin Exp Dermatol 21:360–364, 1996*

Pleomorphic fibroma *Dermatology 191:245–248, 1995*

Plexiform fibrohistiocytic tumor *Ped Derm 23:71–12, 2006*

Porocarcinoma *Dermatol Online J July 15, 2018:24 (7):13030/ qts307797*

Poroid hidradenoma – painful deep red nodule of arm, scalp, face, or trunk *AD 146:557–562, 2010*

Porokeratosis of Mibelli

Poroma (apocrine origin)–red, pink, purple *JAAD 44:48–52, 2001*

Post-auricular pilonidal sinus *Case Rep Surg 2017:5791972 doi.10.1155/2017/5791972*

Primary cutaneous primitive neuroectodermal tumor *JAAD 65:440–441, 2011*

Primary trichilemmal tumor of the scalp – ulcerated nodule *BJD 159:483–485, 2008*

Proliferating trichilemmal tumor *J Dermatol 27:687–688, 2000; Ann Plast Surg 43:574–575, 1999; Mund Kiefer Gesechtschir 2:216–219, 1998; AD 124:935–940, 1988; Cancer 48:1207–1214, 1981*

Pseudocyst of the scalp *Ann Dermatol 23:5267–5269, 2011*

Rhabdomyosarcoma – paraspinal alveolar rhabdomyosarcoma *Cutis 87:186–188, 2011*

Schwannoma – benign glandular schwannoma *BJD 145:834–837, 2001*

Sebaceous adenoma *J Cutan Pathol 11:396–414, 1984;* yellow nodule *Int J Trichol 3:123–124, 2011*

Sebaceous carcinoma *Br J Ophthalmol 82:1049–1055, 1998; Br J Plast Surg 48:93–96, 1995; JAAD 25:685–690, 1991; J Derm Surg Oncol 11:260–264, 1985*

Sebaceoma, giant *J Dermatol 21:367–369, 1994*

Seborrheic keratosis–personal observation

Solitary fibrous tumor of the skin – facial, scalp, posterior neck nodule *AD 142:921–926, 2006; JAAD 46:S37–40, 2002*

Spindle cell lipoma

Spiradenomas *Dermatol Online J Dec 15, 2012*

Spiradenocarcinoma – vascular scalp nodule *Cutis 69:455–458, 2002*

Spitz nevus

Squamous cell carcinoma *Am J Case Rep Aug 3, 2019; AD 143:889–892, 2007; JAAD 56:448–452, 2007;* squamous cell carcinoma arising in cyst with pilar differentiation–red nodule

Steatocystoma multiplex *Ann Dermatol 23:S258–260, 2011*

Sweat gland carcinoma–personal observation

Syringocystadenoma papilliferum *Dermatol Pract Concept 8:48–50, 2018*

Trichilemmal cyst *BMJ Case Re Nov 2011:bcr0720114492. doi.10.1136/bcr.07.2011.4492; Dermatol Surg 33:1102–1108, 2007;* ossifying, giant; proliferating

Trichoblastoma – pink or skin colored scalp nodule; umbilicated scalp nodule with central follicular plug *BJD 144:1090–1092, 2001; AD 135:707–712, 1999; J Cutan Pathol 26:490–496, 1999;* giant trichoblastoma *Am J Dermatopathol 15:497–502, 1993;* trichoblastic carcinoma *Dermatol Online J Sept 15, 2018*

Trichoepithelioma *Acta DV Croat 26162–165, 2018; AD 120:227–230, 1984*

Tubular apocrine adenoma *JAAD 11:639–642, 1984; AD 105:869–879, 1972*

Verrucous carcinoma *JAAD 56:506–507, 2007; Derm Surg 31:1363–1365, 2005*

Warty dyskeratoma *Iran J Public Health 43:1145–1147, 2014*

Wiener's nevus – red scalp nodule

PARANEOPLASTIC DISORDERS

Necrobiotic xanthogranuloma with paraproteinemia – scalp plaque *JAAD 57:1026–1030, 2007*

PRIMARY CUTANEOUS DISEASES

Acne keloidalis *BJD 157:981–988, 2007; Cutis 75:317–321, 2005*

Alopecic and aseptic nodule of scalp *Ped Derm 34:697–700, 2017; Nouv Dermatol 17:181, 1998; Jpn J Clin Dermatol 46:9–16, 1992*

Central centrifugal cicatricial alopecia – papules of scalp *Ped Derm 34:133–137, 2017*

Comedone

Cutis verticis gyrata–paraneoplastica *AD 125:434–435, 1989;* pachydermoperiostosis *AD 124:1831–1824, 1988;* neuropathic disease, tumors, cerebriform nevi, neurofibromas, fibromas, associated with acromegaly, myxedema, leukemia, syphilis, acanthosis nigricans, tuberous sclerosis, Apert's syndrome, amyloidosis; secondary cutis verticis gyrata- inflammatory disorders of the scalp–eczema, psoriasis, folliculitis, erysipelas, pemphigus

Granuloma annulare – forehead, scalp, and lower leg nodules in children *JAAD 75:457–465, 2016; BJD 70:179–181, 1958*

Granuloma faciale *JAAD 51:269–273, 2004*

Lichen planus follicularis tumidus – recurrent retroauricular cystic nodules *Dermatol Online J Oct 15, 2018*

Prurigo nodularis

Subcutaneous necrobiotic granulomas of the scalp *JAAD 3:180–185, 1980*

SYNDROMES

Birt-Hogg-Dube syndrome – trichoblastoma; multilobulated scalp nodule *BJD 160:1350–1353, 2009*

Brooke-Spiegler syndrome–trichoepitheliomas and cylindromas (face, scalp, and upper trunk) *Dermatol Surg 26:877–882, 2000*

Cowden's disease (multiple hamartoma syndrome) *JAAD 17:342–346, 1987*

Emcephalocranial lipomatosis (Haberlenn's syndrome) *J Dermatol Case Rep 7:46–48, 2013*

Farber's disease (disseminated lipogranulomatosis) – red papules and nodules of joints and tendons of hands and feet; deforming arthritis; papules, plaques, and nodules of ears, back of scalp

and trunk *Am J Dis Child 84:449–500, 1952*

Fibroblastic rheumatism – symmetrical polyarthritis, nodules over joints and on palms, elbows, knees, ears, neck, Raynaud's phenomenon, sclerodactyly; joint contractures, thick palmar fascia; scalp nodules, red tender swelling of toe tips, periarticular nodule; skin lesions resolve spontaneously *JAAD 66:959–965, 2012; Ped Derm 19:532–535, 2002; AD 131:710–712, 1995*

Fibrodysplasia ossificans progressiva – fibrous scalp nodules; heterotopic bone formation within soft tissues; multiple neonatal scalp nodules associated with malformation of the great toes (hallux valgus); hypoplastic great toes; development of tumors is cranial to caudal, dorsal to ventral and proximal to distal; ossification after infections or trauma; scalp nodules large, firm, and immobile; mutation in *ACVR1* gene *JAAD 64:97–101, 2011; Clev Clin Q 51:549–552, 1984*

Gardner's syndrome – red scalp nodules; metastatic pilomatrix carcinoma – personal observation

Giant congenital hemangioma of scalp associated with Kassabach-Merritt syndrome *Eur J Pediatr 166:619–620, 2007*

Hypereosinophilic syndrome *Case Rep Med Nov 18, 2019*

Juvenile hyaline fibromatosis – pearly white papules of face and neck; larger papules and nodules around nose, behind ears, on fingertips, multiple subcutaneous nodules of scalp, trunk, and extremities, papillomatous perianal papules; joint contractures, skeletal lesions, gingival hyperplasia, stunted growth; mutation of capillary morphogenesis protein 2 gene *JAAD 61:695–700, 2009; BJD 157:1037–1039, 2007*

Keratosis-ichthyosis-deafness (KID) syndrome – autosomal dominant; sporadic; inflammatory nodules of scalp; reticulated severe diffuse hyperkeratosis of palms and soles (grainy leather-like surface), well marginated, serpiginous erythematous verrucous plaques, perioral furrows, leukoplakia, sensory deafness, photophobia with vascularizing keratitis, blindness; connexin 26 (*GJB2*) mutations *BJD 156:1015–1019, 2007*

Lipoid proteinosis – yellow-brown nodules with alopecia *Int J Derm 39:203–204, 2000; Acta Paediatr 85:1003–1005, 1996; JAAD 27:293–297, 1992*

Lumpy scalp syndrome – autosomal dominant; irregular scalp nodules, deformed pinnae, rudimentary nipples *Int J Dermatol 29:657–658, 1990; Clin Exp Dermatol 15:240, 1989; BJD 99:423–430, 1978*

Multicentric reticulohistiocytosis – digital papule; knuckle pads; yellow papules and plaques *AD 126:251–252, 1990; Oral Surg Oral Med Oral Pathol 65:721–725, 1988; Pathology 17:601–608, 1985; JAAD 11:713–723, 1984; AD 97:543–547, 1968*

Multiple endocrine neoplasia syndrome (MEN I) – angiofibromas of vermilion border; facial angiofibromas, lipomas, abdominal collagenomas, cutis verticis gyrate, pedunculated skin tags, acanthosis nigricans, red gingival papules, confetti-like hypopigmented macules; primary hyperparathyroidism with hypercalcemia, kidney stones, prolactinoma, gastrinoma, bilateral adrenal hyperplasia; mutation in menin, a nuclear protein involved in cell cycle regulation and proliferation *JAAD 61:319–324, 2009; J Clin Endocrinol Metab 89:5328–5336, 2004; AD 133:853–857, 1997*

Muir-Torre syndrome – sebaceous carcinoma *Am J Dermatopathol 38:618–622, 2016; Int J Dermatol 45:311–312, 2006*

Neurofibromatosis *JAAD 23:866–869, 1990*

Oculo-ectodermal syndrome – macrocephaly, cutis aplasia, abnormal pigmentation, scalp nodules, corneal epibulbar dermoid cysts *BJD 151:953–960, 2004*

Proteus syndrome – multilobulated cerebriform scalp nodule (connective tissue nevus) *JAAD 67:890–897, 2012*

Tuberous sclerosis – folliculocystic and collagen hamartoma – comedo-like openings, multilobulated cysts, scalp cysts and nodules *JAAD 66:617–621, 2012;* fibrous cephalic plaques *JAAD 78:717–724, 2018*

Xeroderma pigmentosum – squamous cell carcinoma *BJD 152:545–551, 2005*

TRAUMA

Cephalohematoma

VASCULAR DISORDERS

Agminated eruptive pyogenic granuloma-like lesions over congenital vascular stains (capillary malformations) *Ped Derm 29:186–190, 2012*

Angiolymphoid hyperplasia with eosinophilia – red or pink papules or nodules *SkinMed 16:71–72, 2018; Cutis 88:122–128, 2011; AD 146:911–916, 2010;* retroauricular nodule *Dermatol Online J Oct 15, 2017;* (Kimuura's disease) *BJD 151:1103–1104, 2004; AD 137:863–865, 2001; AD 137:821–822, 2001; BJD 143:214–215, 2000;* retroauricular tumor *Ped Derm 1:210–214, 1984;* mimicking a pilar cyst *J Derm Surg Oncol 6:935–937, 1980;*

Angiosarcoma (Wilson-Jones angiosarcoma)–nodule or plaque *BJD 172:1156–1158, 2015; AD 148:683–685, 2012; BJD 162:697–699, 2010; BJD 160:456–458, 2009; JAAD 56:448–452, 2007; JAAD 40:872–876, 1999; Int J Dermatol 38:697–699, 1999; JAAD 38:143–175, 1998; BJD 136:752–756, 1997; Cancer 59:1046–1057, 1987;* multiple nodules *BJD 144:380–383, 2001;* mimicking epidermoid cyst *Dermatol Online J 14:13, June 15, 2008;* masquerading as squamous cell carcinoma *J Cut Med Surg 16:187–190, 2012*

Arteriovenous fistulae – intracranial dural arteriovenous malformation; subcutaneous pulsatile nodule *AD 146:808–810, 2010*

Cerebellar hemangioblastoma *JAMA 308:182–183, 2012*

Cutaneous epithelioid angiomatous nodules (CEAN) *Dermatol Online J 18:8, Aug 15, 2012*

Eosinophilic granulomatosis with polyangiitis – scalp nodules *JAAD 48:311–340, 2003; Medicine 78:26–37, 1999;* umbilicated nodules with central necrosis of scalp *BJD 127:199–204, 1992;* red papules of forehead and scalp *JAAD 65:244–246, 2011*

Extramedullary hematopoiesis – with myelofibrosis *J Dermatol 26:379–384, 1999*

Giant cell arteritis *Ann DV 127:304, 2000*

Hemangioma, congenital; intracranial hemangiomas; giant hemangiomas of scalp *Ped Derm 34:473–475, 2017; S Afr Med J 55:47–49, 1979*

Polyarteritis nodosa, systemic; cutaneous (livedo with nodules) – painful or asymptomatic red or skin colored multiple nodules with livedo reticularis of feet, legs, forearms face, scalp, shoulders, trunk *Ped Derm 15:103–107, 1998; AD 130:884–889, 1994; JAAD 31:561–566, 1994; JAAD 31:493–495, 1994*

Pyogenic granuloma

Rapidly involuting congenital hemangioma – large violaceous gray-blue nodule of scalp with overlying telangiectasia *Soc Ped Derm Annual Meeting, 2005*

Retiform hemangioendothelioma *JAAD 38:143–175, 1998;* composite hemangioendothelioma *JAAD 69:e98–99, 2013*

Subepicranial hygromas *JAAD 46:934–941, 2002*

Temporal arteritis – nodules over occipital artery *Ann DV 141:518–522, 2014; BJD 76:299–308, 1964*

Thrombus in temporal artery aneurysm

Vascular nevi

Venous malformation *JAAD 46:934–941, 2002*

SCALP POLIOSIS

Scalp poliosis
  Inflammatory or autoimmune
    Alopecia areata
    Alezzandrini syndrome
    Post-inflammatory hypopigmentation (DLE, trauma)
    Halo nevus
    Vitiligo
    Vogt-Koyanagi-Harada syndrome
  Inherited
    Isolated white forelock (possible form fruste of piebaldism)
    Isolated occipital white lock–X-linked
    Piebaldism (primarily midline frontal)
    Tuberous sclerosis
    Waardenburg's syndrome (primarily midline frontal)
    White forelock with multiple malformations–autosomal or X-linked recessive
    White forelock with osteopathia striata–autosomal or X-linked recessive
  Nevoid
    Associated with nevus comedonicus
    Congenital pigmented nevus *AD 129:1331–1336, 1993*
  Idiopathic

SCALP, RED PLAQUES

AUTOIMMUNE DISEASES AND DISORDERS OF IMMUNE DYSREGULATION

Contact dermatitis–allergic or irritant

Dermatomyositis

Lupus erythematosus–discoid lupus erythematosus *Acta DV Croat 22:150–159, 2014; NEJM 269:1155–1161, 1963;* cutaneous mucinosis *J Dermatol 16:374–378, 1989;* lupus profundus *Lupus 14:403–405, 2005;* neonatal lupus *Int J Dermatol 35:42–44, 1996*

DRUGS

Cytarabine *JAAD 73:821–828, 2015*

INFECTIONS AND INFESTATIONS

Herpes simplex

Herpes zoster

Kerion *SKINmed 10:14–16, 2012*

Molluscum contagiosum *New England Dermatological Society Conference, Sept 15, 2007*

Mycobacterium avium-intracellulare – red indurated plaque of scalp, ear, and lateral face *J Drugs in Dermatol 1:490–491, 2013*

Mycobacterium tuberculosis – lupus vulgaris *North Clin Istanb 1:53–56, 2014*

Tinea capitis (T. verrucosum, T. mentagrophtes) – including kerion *AD 114:371–372, 1978*

Tufted folliculitis *J Dermatol 29:427–430, 2002*

INFILTRATIVE DISEASES

Amyloid

Langerhans cell histiocytosis in the adult – ulceronecrotic plaque of scalp; scrotal ulcer; solitary pink papule; red papules of trunk; perianal plaque; perianal dermatitis *BJD 167:1287–1294, 2012; BJD 133:444–448, 1995*

Miescher's granuloma

Verrucous (verruciform) xanthoma–normolipemic; most commonly on mucosal surfaces, especially the oral mucosa; also nose, axilla, neck, and scalp *AD 143:1067–1072, 2007*

INFLAMMATORY DISORDERS

Dissecting cellulitis of the scalp–mimicking infectious cellulitis *Ann Int Med 142:47–55, 2005*

Erosive pustular dermatitis of the scalp *Australas J Dermatol 60:e322–326, 2019*

Erythema multiforme–personal observation

Folliculitis decalvans

Kikuchi's histiocytic necrotizing lymphadenitis *BJD 144:885–889, 2001*

Sarcoid – psoriasiform plaques and dermatitis *Dermatol Online J April 16, 2015; AD 140:1003–1008, 2004;* red plaques *JAAD 59:143–145, 2008;* yellow-red plaque of face and scalp *BJD 175:1111–1112, 2016* Subcutaneous fat necrosis of infancy *AD 136:1559–1564, 2000*

METABOLIC DISORDERS

Calcinosis cutis

Necrobiosis lipoidica diabeticorum *Dermatologica 135:11–26, 1967*

Platelike osteoma cutis – red oval patches and plaques *Ped Derm 26:479–481, 2009; AD 143:109–114, 2007*

Pretibial myxedema *JAAD 46:723–726, 2002*

NEOPLASTIC DISORDERS

Basal cell carcinoma

Carcinosarcoma – ulcerated nodule or red plaque of scalp *Cutis 92:247–249, 2013*

Eccrine angiomatous hamartoma – blue-red plaque of scalp *Ped Derm 26:316–319, 2009; Virchow Arch Pathol Anat 16:160, 1859*

Ectopic meningothelial hamartoma – white linear plaque of occipital scalp; congenital red plaque becomes orange-yellow then white *Ped Derm 34:99–100, 2017; Ped Derm 31:208–211, 2014; Ped Derm 28:677–680, 2011; Am J Surg Pathol 14:1–11, 1980*
  Differential diagnosis:
    Angiosarcoma
    Aplasia cutis congenital, membranous

Atretic meningocele

Epithelioid hemangioma

Giant cell fibroblastoma

Hypertrophic scar

Intravascular papillary endothelial hyperplasia

Spindle cell hemangioendothelioma

Hair follicle hamartoma – papules and plaques of scalp *BJD 143:1103–1105, 2000*

Leukemia cutis including chronic myelogenous leukemia; hairy cell leukemia cutis–violaceous plaques *JAAD 11:788–797, 1984*

Lymphocytoma cutis *Cancer 69:717–724, 1992; Acta DV (Stockh)62:119–124, 1982; Cancer 24:487–502, 1969*

Lymphoma–B-cell *JAAD 53:479–484, 2005;* cutaneous B-cell lymphoma *SKINmed 12:244–248, 2014;* annular red plaque of scalp with scarring alopecia – primary cutaneous follicle center B-cell lymphoma *BJD 165:204–208, 2011;* cutaneous T-cell lymphoma mimicking dissecting cellulitis of the scalp *JAAD 47:914–918, 2002; J Cutan Pathol 24:169–175, 1997;* primary cutaneous anaplastic large cell lymphoma *AD 143:255–260, 2007; ;* primary cutaneous follicle center cell lymphoma – multilobulated nodules, red plaques of scalp, nodules of head and neck, papules of head and neck *JAAD 70:1010–1020, 2014*

Lymphomatoid granulomatosis *AD 132:1464–1470, 1996*

Malignant angioendotheliomatosis *J Derm Surg Oncol 7:130–136, 1981*

Meningothelial hamartoma (rudimentary meningocele) – alopecic fibrotic blue-purple plaque of scalp *Ped Derm 28:677–680, 2011*

Merkel cell carcinoma – mimicking angiosarcoma *AD 123:1368–1370, 1987*

Metastases – gastric adenocarcinoma *Cutis 76:194–196, 2005*

Microcystic adnexal carcinoma *JAAD 41:225–231, 1999*

Nevus sebaceus – large red exophytic scalp mass *Case Rep Dermatol 17:298–302, 2015*

Porokeratosis of Mibelli of the scalp *Dermatologica 134:269–272, 1967*

Squamous cell carcinoma

Syringocystadenoma papilliferum

PRIMARY CUTANEOUS DISEASES

Alopecia mucinosa (follicular mucinosis) *Derm 197:178–180, 1998; JAAD 10:760–768, 1984; AD 76:419–426, 1957*

Granuloma faciale – red-brown plaques *JAMADerm 154:1312–1315, 2018; JAAD 53:1002–1009, 2005; Cutis 72:213–219, 2003*

Lichen planopilaris

Lichen simplex chronicus – psoriasiform neurodermatitis

Prurigo nodularis

Psoriasis *AD 98:248–259, 1968*

Seborrheic dermatitis

Tinea amiantacea

PSYCHOCUTANEOUS DISORDERS

Neurotic excoriation

SYNDROMES

Farber's disease (disseminated lipogranulomatosis) – red papules and nodules of joints and tendons of hands and feet; deforming arthritis; papules, plaques, and nodules of ears, back of scalp and trunk *Am J Dis Child 84:449–500, 1952*

Folliculocystic and collagen hamartoma of tuberous sclerosis – pink plaque of scalp with comedones *Ped Derm 31:249–250, 2014*

Histiophagocytic syndrome – parvovirus B19-induced histiophago-cytic syndrome in systemic lupus erythematosus; violaceous plaques and erythema of scalp, face, and back with erosions and erosive cheilitis *JAAD 57:S111–114, 2007*

Sweet's syndrome *Hautarzt 41:398–401, 1990*

VASCULAR DISORDERS

Angiosarcoma *BJD 172:1156–1158, 2015; AD 148:683–685, 2012; BJD 162:697–699, 2010Cancer 77:2400–2406, 1996;* linear red plaque of scalp *JAAD 62:538–539, 2010*

Klippel-Trenaunay-Weber syndrome

Retiform hemangioendothelioma–red plaque of scalp, arms, legs, and penis *JAAD 38:143–175, 1998*

SCARRING OF NECK

AUTOIMMUNE DISEASES

Bullous pemphigoid–localized Brunsting-Perry type *Hautarzt 44:110–113, 1993; Clin Dermatol 5:43–51, 1987; BJD 95:531–534, 1976*

Lupus erythematosus *Am J Clin Dermatol 10:365–381, 2009*

DEVELOPMENTAL DISORDERS

Branchial cleft sinus

DRUG REACTIONS

Stevens-Johnson syndrome

Toxic epidermal necrolysis

INFECTIONS AND INFESTATIONS

Actinomycosis

Anthrax

Dental sinus

Eczema herpeticum

Herpes zoster *Am J Clin Dermatol 17:893–897, 2018*

Leishmaniasis

Mycetoma

Mycobacterium tuberculosis–scrofuloderma *Dermatol Clin 33:541–562, 2015; Ped Derm 30:7–16, 2013*

Non-tuberculous mycobacterial infections in childhood *Br J Oral Maxillofac Surg 36:119–122, 1998*

Osteomyelitis

Smallpox

Spider bite

Syphilitic gumma

Varicella – including congenital varicella

INFLAMMATORY DISORDERS

Folliculitis decalvans *J Dermatol 28:329–331, 2001*

Pyoderma gangrenosum *J Dermatol 44:e244–245, 2017*

METABOLIC DISORDERS

Porphyria cutanea tarda *Ann Dermatol 140:589–597, 2013*

NEOPLASTIC DISORDERS

Basal cell carcinoma

Desmoplastic trichoepithelioma *Clin Exp Dermatol 32:522–524, 2007*

Squamous cell carcinoma arising in scarifying mucocutaneous disorders *Adv Dermatol 2:19–46, 1987; Head Neck 20:515–521, 1998*

PHOTODERMATOSES

Poikiloderma of Civatte with pseudoscars

PRIMARY CUTANEOUS DISEASES

Acne keloidalis nuchae *J Derm Surg Oncol 15:642–647, 1989*

Atrophoderma vermiculata *Clin Exp Dermatol 41:159–161, 2016*

Epidermolysis bullosa dystrophica inversa *Ped Derm 7:116–121, 1990*

Pseudoxanthoma elasticum *J Dermatol 43:454–456, 2016*

Reticulolinear aplasia cutis congenita of the face and neck – syndromes linked to Xp22 *BJD 138:1046–1052, 1998*

PSYCHOCUTANEOUS DISORDERS

Factititial dermatitis

TRAUMA

Burns

CO_2 laser resurfacing *J Cosmet Laser Ther 18:352–354, 2016; Lasers Surg Med 41:185–188, 2009*

Fiddler's neck *Ear Nose Throat J 96:76–79, 2017; BJD 98:669–674, 1978*

Surgical scars; thyroidectomy

Tracheotomy

Trauma

VASCULAR DISORDERS

Hemangioma, resolved

SCARS, LESIONS IN SCARS

AUTOIMMUNE DISEASES AND DISORDERS OF IMMUNE DYSREGULATION

Allergic contact dermatitis – to 2-octylcyanoacrylate

Bullous pemphigoid – in surgical wounds *Cutis 75:169–170, 2005; BJD 145:670–672, 2001*

Cicatricial pemphigoid (mucous membrane pemphigoid) *Dermatitis 27:75–76, 2016; Cutis 94:183–186, 2014*

Graft vs host disease–lichenoid reaction – at vaccination site *BJD 173:1050–1053, 2015*

Leukocyte adhesion deficiency with pyoderma gangrenosum *Ped Derm 28:156–161, 2011*

Lupus erythematosus, discoid *Lupus 19:1020–1028, 2010; BJD 161:1052–1058, 2009; JAAD 48:S54–55, 2003;* systemic LE – thrombotic vasculopathy *Am J Clin Dermatol 19:679–694, 2018*

Morphea – Addisonian keloid *Ped Derm 29:111–112, 2012; Int J Dermatol 31:422–423, 1992; Med Chir Trans 37:27–47, 1854*

CONGENITAL DISORDERS

Congenital erosive and vesicular dermatosis with reticulated scarring – vesicles of trunk and extremities, erosions, ulcers, erythroderma, collodion baby, ectropion, reticulated soft scarring, scarring alopecia, absent eyebrows, hypohidrosis with compensatory hyperhidrosis *Ped Derm 29:756–758, 2012; JAAD 45:946–948, 2001; Ped Derm 15:214–218, 1998;*

JAAD 32:873–877, 1995; AD 121:361–367, 1985
    Differential diagnosis:
        Aplasia cutis congenita
        Amniotic adhesions
        Cutaneous trauma
        Epidermolysis bullosa
        Focal dermal hypoplasia
        Intrauterine infection
        Intrauterine or perinatal trauma

DEVELOPMENTAL DISORDERS

Aplasia cutis congenita; autosomal dominant *Ped Derm 22:213–217, 2005;* Adams-Oliver syndrome – aplasia cutis congenita, cutis marmorata telangiectatica congenital, transverse limb defects *Ped Derm 22:206–209, 2005;* non-membranous aplasia cutis congenital – thickened hypertrophic scars *Ped Dem 26:362–363, 2009;* aplasia cutis congenita associated with fetus papyraceus – cutaneous ulcers, linear atrophic scars, atrophic scars of scalp, dystrophic nails *Ped Derm 32:858–861, 2015*

DRUGS

Argyria – secondary to silver sulfadiazine *JAAD 49:730–732, 2003*

Drug-induced leukocytoclastic vasculitis – vancomycin

Interleukin-2 reaction–erosions in surgical scar *JAMA 258:1624–1629, 1987*

Minocycline hyperpigmentation

Vandetanib (kinase and growth factor receptor inhibitor) – photosensitivity and blue-gray perifollicular macules; also blue gray pigment within scars *AD 145:923–925, 2009*

EXOGENOUS AGENTS

IVDA skin popping, stigmata – track marks, puffy hand syndrome, sooting tattoos *JAAD 69:135–142, 2013*

Silicone, injected – scarring, contractures, deformity *AD 141:13–15, 2005; Derm Surg 27:198–200, 2001*

INFECTIONS AND INFESTATIONS

Actinomycetoma–due to *Nocardia brasiliensis;* pustules, scarring, sinus tracts, multilobulated nodules, grains *JAAD 62:239–246, 2010*

Chromomycosis *Arq Bras Oftalmol 80:46–48, 2017*

Herpes simplex, recurrent – pock-like facial scars – personal observation

Herpes zoster *Am J Clin Dermatol 19:893–897, 2018*

Leishmaniasis recidivans (chronic relapsing leishmaniasis) – circinate papules at periphery of old scars *PLOS One 12:e89906, Dec 20, 2017; JAAD 73:897–908, 2015; Clin Inf Dis 33:1076–1079, 2001; JAAD 34:257–72, 1996;* discoid lupus like lesions *Clin Dermatol 38:140–151, 2020*

Lobomycosis (*Lacazia loboi*) *An Bras Dermatol 93:279–281, 2018*

Lymphogranuloma venereum – *Chlamydia trachomatis;* Jersild syndrome – perirectal abscesses, fistulae, sclerosis *JAAD 54:559–578, 2006*

Mycobacterium tuberculosis–scrofuloderma – abscess, ulcers, scars *JAMADerm 150:909–910, 2014; Dermatol Clin 33:541–562, 2015; Ped Derm 30:7–16, 2013;* papulonecrotic tuberculid – punctate depressed or varioliform scarring *Clin Exp Dermatol 45:238–240, 2020*

Mycobacterium ulcerans (Buruli ulcer) *Dermatol Clin 33:563–577, 2015*

Spider bite (*Loxosceles reclusa*) *BMJ Case Rep 2016:bcr 2016215832*

Varicella – post- varicella pock-like scarring

Verrucae *Actas Dermosifiliogr 105:96–97, 2014*

INFILTRATIVE DISORDERS

Amyloidosis

INFLAMMATORY DISORDERS

Crohn's disease

Dissecting cellulitis of the scalp *Curr Prob Dermatol 47:76–86, 2015*

Erythema multiforme *JAAD 48:S54–55, 2003*

Hidradenitis suppurativa – bridged scars *Dermatol Online J Jan 15, 2012; BJD 162:195–197, 2010; JAAD 62:205–217, 2010; BJD 158:370–374, 2008;* hypertrophic scars *JAMA Derm 149:1192–1194, 2013*

Pyoderma gangrenosum *JAMADerm 154:4616, 2018; NEJM 347:1419, 2002*

Sarcoidosis – scars become inflamed and infiltrated; in pre-existent scars, biopsy scars, BCG, tuberculin test sites, tribal scarification *JAMA Derm 149:1097–1098, 2013; JAAD 66:699–716, 2012; Cutis 87:234–236, 2011;* at venipuncture sites *Cutis 24:52–53, 1979;* subcutaneous sarcoid in melanoma surgical scar *Cutis 87:234–236, 2011*

Stevens-Johnson syndrome, sequela – macular white scarring; adhesions of labia *Dermatol Res Pract Jan 30, 2019:4917024; BJD 177:924–935, 2017;* hypertrophic scarring *Ped Derm 31:527–528, 2014;* gingival synechiae *AD 145:1332–1333, 2009*

Superficial vegetating pyoderma–personal observation

METABOLIC DISORDERS

Addison's disease – darkening of scars *Clin Dermatol 29:511–522, 2011*

Anasarca–personal observation

Congenital erythropoietic porphyria–sclerodactyly with crusted papules on dorsal hands; atrophic scars, erythrodontia *BJD 166:697–699, 2012*

Endometriosis, primary cutaneous – in C-section scars *J Plast Reconstr Aesthet Surg 66:e111–113, 2013; AD 145:605–606, 2009; Gynecol Endocrinol 22:284–285, 2006; Lancet 364:388, 2004; Obstet Gynaecol 22:553–554, 2002*

Erythropoietic protoporphyria *Ped Derm 24:E5–9, 2007*

Extramedullary hematopoiesis *JAAD 32:805–807, 1995*

Graves' disease – thyroid dermopathy (pretibial myxedema) in smallpox scar *Clin Exp Dermatol 25:132–134, 2000*

Osteoma cutis in prostatectomy scars or other postoperative scars *AD 117:797–801, 1981*

Porphyria – acute intermittent porphyria – surgical scars due to misdiagnosis *BMC Res Notes 11;552, 2018*

Porphyria cutanea tarda *Dermatol Clin 4:297–309, 1986; Med Clin NA 64:807–827, 1980*

Variegate porphyria *JAAD 2:36–43, 1980*

Xanthoma – erythropoietic protoporphyria scars in Alagille syndrome *Int J Dermatol 53:e112–114, 2014*

NEOPLASTIC DISORDERS

Angiosarcoma *BJD 149:1273–1275, 2003*

Basal cell carcinoma, morpheaform *Derm Surg 27:195–197, 2001; Derm Surg 25:965–968, 1999; JAAD 38:488–490, 1998;* in breast augmentation scar *Aesthetic Plast Surg 41:318–320, 2017*

Dermatofibroma *JAAD 48:S54–55, 2003*

Dermatofibrosarcoma protuberans – within smallpox scar *JAAD 48:S54–55, 2003;* injection site scar *Cutis 90:233–234, 2012*

Desmoid tumors – in Gardner's syndrome; arise in incisional scars of abdomen *Cancer 36:2327–2333, 1975; AD 90:20–30, 1964*

Desmoplastic trichoepithelioma–often mistaken for chicken pox scar *Acta DV Croat 27:282–284, 2019*

Eccrine poroma and eccrine porocarcinoma *BJD 150:1232–1233, 2004*

Epidermal inclusion cyst

Lymphoma–hydroa vacciniforme-like cutaneous T-cell lymphoma (Epstein-Barr virus associated lymphoproliferative disorder) – pitted scars, edema, blisters, vesicles, ulcers, scarring, facial scars, swollen nose, lips, and periorbital edema, crusts with central hemorrhagic necrosis, facial dermatitis, photodermatitis, facial edema, facial papules and plaques, crusting of ears, fever *JAAD 81::534–540, 2019; JAAD 69:112–119, 2013; BJD 151:372–380, 2004*

Kaposi's sarcoma *JAAD 59:179–206, 2008*

Keloids, spontaneous

Keratoacanthoma *Ped Derm 23:448–450, 2006; J Drugs Dermatol 3:193–194, 2004*

Leiomyosarcoma – in burn scar *Burns 24:68–71, 1998;* in smallpox scar *World J Surg Oncol July 16, 2012*

Liposarcoma *Burns 22:497–499, 1996*

Lymphoma – Burkitt's lymphoma; seeding of tumor after inguinal lymph node biopsy *JAAD 54:1111–1113, 2006;* hydroa vaccin-iforme-like cutaneous T-cell lymphoma, Epstein-Barr virus-related – edema, blisters, vesicles, ulcers, scarring, facial scars, swollen nose, lips, and periorbital edema, crusts with central hemorrhagic necrosis, facial dermatitis, photodermatitis, facial edema, facial papules and plaques, crusting of ears, fever *JAAD 69:112–119, 2013;* cutaneous T-cell lymphoma – scarring alopecia *Int J Dermatol 55:e40–41, 2016*

Bullous macroglobulinosis – bullae, scars, erosions, papules of dorsal hands *JAAD 77:1145–1158, 2017*

Malignant fibrous histiocytoma *Burns 26:305–310, 2000; Postgrad Med J 63:1097–1098, 1987*

Melanoma – recurrent melanoma in surgical scar *JAAD 48:S54–55, 2003; Ann Plast Surg 46:59–61, 2001; BJD 137:793–798, 1997;* desmoplastic melanoma *JAAD 68:825–833, 2013;* in burn scar *BMJ Case Rep 11:e227295, 2018*

Merkel cell tumor *Hum Pathol 32:680–689, 2001; Am J Dermatopathol 4:537–548, 1982*

Metastatic renal cell cancer in nephrectomy scar *BMC Cancer 18:266, 2018; Arch Pathol 76:339–46, 1963;* metastatic pancreatic carcinoma with seeding at time of surgery–personal observation

Infantile myofibromatosis–recurrent infantile myofibromatosis *SkinMed 11:371–373, 2013*

Nevus comedonicus–personal observation

Pseudoangiomatous stromal hyperplasia in breast cancer surgical scar *BMJ Case Rep Aug 11, 2011*

Squamous cell carcinoma *Derm Surg 25:965–968, 1999; JAAD 38:488–490, 1998;* in lesions of epidermolysis bullosa acquisita *BJD 152:588–590, 2005;* cutaneous horn *BJD 164:673–675, 2011;* Marjolin's ulcer *J Burn Care Res 39:636–639, 2018;* in Buruli ulcer scar *Pan Afr Med J July 23, 2019*

Synovial cyst – cutaneous metaplastic synovial cyst *JAAD 41:330–332, 1999*

Trichoepithelioma – in facial scar *J Craniofac Surg 24:e292–294, 2013*

PARANEOPLASTIC DISORDERS

Necrobiotic xanthogranuloma with paraproteinemia – yellow linear plaques within scars *Acta DV Croat 25:167–169, 2017; Int J Derm 43:293–295, 2004* (burn scar)*; Orbit 27:191–194, 2008; Mayo Clin Proc 72:1028–1033, 1997; AD 128:94–100, 1992* (surgical scars)

PHOTODERMATOSES

Annular elastolytic granuloma *Cutis 103:e5–7, 2019*

Hydroa vacciniforme *JAAD 78:637–642, 2018*

Stellate pseudoscars – at sites of chronic sun damage; due to application of topical corticosteroids *JAAD 54:1–15, 2006*

PRIMARY CUTANEOUS DISEASES

Acne vulgaris *Am J Clin Dermatol 19:139–144, 2018*

Acne keloidalis

Atrophia maculosa varioliformis cutis *Ped Derm 37:156–158, 2020; JAMADerm 155:245–246, 2019*

Atrophoderma vermiculata

Darier's disease–comedonal Darier's disease; nodules, cysts, ice pick scars *BJD 162:687–689, 2010*

Degos' disease *JAMADerm 153:1183–1184, 2017; J Eur Acad DV 31:e435–438, 2017; AD 145:321–326, 2009*

Epidermolysis bullosa pruriginosa – autosomal dominant or autosomal recessive; vesicles, erosions, crusting, linear violaceous hypertrophic scars; dystrophic form of epidermolysis bullosa; mutation in COL7A1 *Ped Derm 32:549–550, 2015; Ped Derm 29:725–731, 2012; AD 147:956–960, 2011;* flagellate scars *Clin Exp Dermatol 45:e5–6, 2019*

Excoriations–personal observation

Frontal fibrosing alopecia *J Cut Med Surg 27:182–189, 2018;* in men *JAAD 77:683–690, 2017*

Galli-Galli disease – autosomal dominant; reticulated hyperpigmen-tation, perioral pitted scars, comedones *JAMADerm 152:461–462, 2016*

Granuloma annulare–linear in scar *JAAD 50:S34–37, 2004*

Granuloma faciale *JAAD 53:1002–1009, 2005*

Idiopathic hypopigmented scarring of the chest and back–personal observation

Keratosis pilaris atrophicans

Lichen planus–Graham-Little syndrome *JAAD 75:1081–1099, 2016;* lichen planopilaris *Curr Prob Dermatol 47:76–86, 2015;* nail scarring *Ann DV 142:21–25, 2015;* erosive lichen planus–stricture of vulva *JAAD 82:1287–1298, 2020*

Lichen sclerosus et atrophicus *JAAD 32:393–416, 1995;*

JAAD 31:671–3, 1994

Milia – in scars of bullous diseases *J Dermatol 41:1003–1005, 2014*

Pityriasis rubra pilaris

Psoriasis, koebnerized in scar

PSYCHOCUTANEOUS DISORDERS

Delusions of parasitosis – white atrophic scars with erosions and ulcers *NEJM 371:2115–2123, 2014*

Factitial scarring (dermatitis artefacta) *Clin Dermatol 36:719–722, 2018; JAAD 76:779–791, 2017; Int J STD AIDS 23:527–528, 2012; Psychiatr Danub 23:73–75, 2011*

Skin picking – linear hypopigmented scars *JAAD 76:779–791, 2017*

SYNDROMES

Behcet's disease *Ann Bras Dermatol 92:452–464, 2017; Ped Derma 32:476–480, 2015*

Blau or Jabs syndrome (familial juvenile systemic granulomatosis) – autosomal dominant; onset under 4 years of age; generalized papular rash of infancy; translucent skin-colored papules (non-case-ating granulomas) of trunk and extremities or dense lichenoid yellow to red-brown papules with grainy surface with anterior or panuveitis, synovitis, symmetric polyarthritis; polyarteritis, multiple synovial cysts; red papular rash in early childhood; exanthema resolves with pitted scars; camptodactyly (flexion contractures of PIP joints); generalized poikiloderma; no involvement of lung or hilar nodes; activating mutations in NOD2 (nucleotide-binding oligomerization domain 2) (caspase recruitment domain family, member 15; *CARD*

15) *Ped Derm 27:69–73, 2010; AD 143:386–391, 2007; Clin Exp Dermatol 21:445–448, 1996; J Pediatr 107:689–693, 1985*

Cowden's syndrome (PTEN hamartoma tumor syndrome) – thyroidectomy scar; breast biopsy

Crouzon syndrome with acanthosis nigricans (CAN) – white hypopigmented scars; onset of acanthosis nigricans during childhood, dark melanocytic nevi, craniosynostosis, ocular proptosis, midface hypoplasia, choanal atresia, hypertelorism, anti-Mongoloid slant, posteriorly placed ears, hydrocephalus; mutation in *FGFR3 JAMA Derm 149:737–741, 2013; Ped Derm 27:43–47, 2010; Am J Med Genet 84:74, 1999*

Dowling-Degos syndrome – pitted acne scars, reticulate papules and pigmentation; mutation in *PSENEV BJD 178:502–508, 2018;* hidradenitis suppurativa scars *Dermatol Online J 19:18558 June 15, 2013*

Ehlers-Danlos syndrome – fish-mouthed scars; type IV – keloids *BJD 171:615–621, 2014;* type VIII – autosomal dominant; skin fragility, abnormal scarring, severe early periodontitis with loss of adult dentition by end of third decade; cigarette paper scars of shin; marfanoid habitus (tall, long limbs, arachnodactyly); triangular face, prominent eyes, thin nose, prematurely aged appearance, thin skin with prominent veins, no joint hypermobility, easy bruising, blue sclerae *JAAD 55:S41–45, 2006*

Goeminne syndrome – keloids; congenital torticollis, nevi, and varicosities *BJD 171:615–621, 2014*

Kindler's syndrome *Hum Mutation 32:1204–1212, 2011*

Lipoid proteinosis – crusted erosions leading to linear pitted and cribriform scars *Ped Derm 26:91–92, 2009; Ped Derm 18:21–26, 2001; Virchows Arch Pathol Anat 273:286–319, 1929*

Osteogenesis imperfecta

PIK3CA-related overgrowth syndromes – scars *JAMADerm 154:452–455, 2018*

Rubenstein-Taybi syndrome – multiple keloids; characteristic facies; broad thumbs; mutation in *CREBBP* and *EP300 BJD 171:615–621, 2014*

SCALP syndrome – aplasia cutis congenita, pigmented nevus, nevus sebaceus; limbal dermoid, CNS malformations *JAAD 63:1–22, 2010*

TRAUMA

Amputation stump neuroma

Linear scarring – pulse dye laser *Cutis 94:83–85, 2014*

Survivors of torture *D Eur Acad DV 33:1232–1240, 2019*

VASCULAR DISORDERS

Atrophie blanche en plaque (livedoid vasculopathy) – porcelain white scars *Int J Dermatol 57:732–741, 2018*

Benign lymphangiomatous papules of the skin *JAAD 52:912–913, 2005*

Cutis marmorata telangiectatica congenita

Granulomatosis with polyangiitis *Acta DV 45:288–95, 1965*

Hemangioma *Bol Med Hosp Infant Mex 76:167–175, 2019*

Lymphangiomas – benign lymphangiomatous papules (BLAP) often seen post radiation therapy or post-surgically *JAAD 52:912–913, 2005; Am J Surg Pathol 26:328–337, 2002; Histopathology 35:319–327, 1999*

Symmetrical peripheral gangrene – splenectomy scars; propensity for gram + sepsis and disseminated intravascular coagulation

Temporal arteritis biopsy site

SCLERODERMOID CHANGES

AUTOIMMUNE DISEASES AND DISEASES OF IMMUNE DYSFUNCTION

Dermatomyositis – sclerosis of skin; acrosclerosis

Graft vs. host disease, chronic – deep sclerosis and fasciitis; prayer sign *JAAD 66:515–532, 2012; Ped Derm 28:172–175, 2011; JAAD 59:1070–174, 2008; AD 144:1106–1109, 2008; Ped Derm 25:240–244, 2008; BJD 156:1032–1038, 2007; Am J Clin Dermatol 5:403–416, 2004; Blood 100:406–414, 2002; BJD 142:529–532, 2000; JAAD 38:369–392, 1998; NEJM 324:667–674, 1991; Clin Exp Dermatol 8:531–538, 1983;* sclerotic GVHD at sites of skin injury *AD 147:1081–1086, 2011;* bullous sclerodermoid changes *BJD 171:63–68, 2014; AD 121:1189–1192, 1985;* morphea-like lesions *JAAD 66:515–532, 2012; Clin Exp Dermatol 8:531–538, 1983;* sclerodermoid changes with ripply appearance *AD 138:924–934, 2002;* eosinophilic fasciitis *JAAD 53:591–601, 2005;* linear and curvilinear morphea-like chronic GVHD *AD 144:1229–1231, 2008*

Lupus erythematosus – systemic lupus – bound-down skin of face and limbs; discoid lupus with annular atrophic plaques of face, neck, behind ears *AD 112:1143–1145, 1976;* lupus mastitis–sclerosis of the breast *JAAD 29:343–346, 1993;* lupus panniculitis – morphea-like lesions *Clin Exp Dermatol 19:79–82, 1994;* neonatal lupus with morphea-like lesions *BJD 115:85–90, 1986;* acrosclerosis; papulonodular mucinosis in LE *JAAD 32:199–205, 1995*

Lupus erythematosus/dermatomyositis overlap

Mixed connective tissue disease–personal observation; *Am J Med 52:148–159, 1972*

Morphea *BJD 171:1243–1245, 2014; JAAD 64:217–228, 2011; JAAD 64:231–242, 2011; AD 147:1148–1150, 2011; JAAD 59:385–396, 2008;* linear morphea *Semin Cutan Med Surg 18:210–225, 1999; Semin Cutan Med Surg 17:27–33, 1998; Int J Derm 35:330–336, 1996;* en coup de sabre *JAAD 56;257–263, 2013;* morphea profunda with overlying hyper- or hypopigmentation *Ped Derm 8:292–295, 1991;* deep morphea (morphea profunda) *JAMADerm 152:1170–1172, 2016; AD 146:1009–1013, 2010;* following vaccination *Ped Derm 23:484–487, 2006;* morphea following hepatitis B vaccination *Presse Med 29:1046, 2000;* following BCG vaccination *Med Cutan Ibero Lat Am 11:329–332, 1983;* pansclerotic morphea – mutilating form of morphea *Ped Derm 26:59–61, 2009; JAAD 53:S115–119, 2005; AD 116:169–173, 1980;* generalized deep morphea *Semin Cutan Med Surg 26:90–95, 2007; Clin Dermatol 24:374–392, 2006; Mayo Clin Proc 70:1068–1076, 1995;* generalized morphea; *Borrelia*-associated early onset morphea *JAAD 60:248–255, 2009*

Rheumatoid arthritis – pseudoscleroderma

Scleroderma (progressive systemic sclerosis)–diffuse cutaneous form; CREST syndrome *NEJM 372:1056–1067, 2015;* en coup de sabre *JAAD 56:257–263, 2007;* linear scleroderma of the leg *BJD 156:1363–1365, 2007*

Sclerodermatomyositis – Gottron's papules, periorbital erythema, Raynaud's phenomenon, acrosteolysis, dysphagia, digital ulcers; high risk of interstitial lung disease *Arthr Research Therapy 16:R111, 2014; AD 144:1351–1359, 2008; Arthr Rheum 50:565–569, 2004;*

J Clin Immunol 4:40–44, 1984
Sjogren's syndrome

CONGENITAL LESIONS

Sclerema neonatorum – indurated violaceous plaques of back and legs *Cutis 92:83–87, 2013; JAAD 45:325–361, 2001; Ped Derm 10:271–276, 1993; Ped Derm 4:112–122, 1987*

Smooth muscle hamartoma *Ped Derm 13:222–225, 1996*

DEGENERATIVE DISORDERS

Limb immobilization

DRUG-INDUCED LESIONS

Appetite suppressants–amphetamine, diethylpropion *J Rheumatol 11:254–255, 1984*

Balicatib – drug-induced morphea *JAAD 59:125–129, 2008*

Bisoprolol–drug-induced morphea *Eur J Dermatol 3:108–109, 1993*

Bleomycin – sclerodermatous changes of hands *JAAD 71:203–214, 2014; Clin Rheumatol 18:422–424, 1999; J Korean Med Sci 11:454=456, 1996; JAAD 33:851–852, 1995; J Rheumatol 19:294–296, 1992; Hautarzt 34:10–12, 1983; AD 107:553–555, 1973*

Bromocriptine – morphea *Int J Dermatol 28:177–179, 1989*

Capecitabine – sclerodermoid changes *JAAD 71:203–214, 2014*

Carbidopa *NEJM 303:782–787, 1980*

Diltiazem – thickened skin of the feet *Int J Cardiol 35:115, 1992*

Dimethyl fumarate (therapy for multiple sclerosis) – eosinophilic fasciitis-like disorder *J Drugs Dermatol 13:1144–1147, 2014*

Docetaxel *JAAD 58:545–570, 2008; BJD 156:363–367, 2007; BJD 147:619–621, 2002; Cancer 88:1078–1081, 2000; Cancer 76:110–115, 1995*

Ergot

Ethosuximide

Gemcitabine – edema of legs with subsequent sclerodermoid changes *JAAD 51:S73–76, 2004*

Heparin, injected *Ann DV 112:245–247, 1985*

5-hydroxytryptophan with carbidopa – eosinophilia-myalgia-like lesions *NEJM 303:782–787, 1980*

Interferon alpha-induced eosinophilic fasciitis *JAAD 37:118–120, 1997*

Interferon beta 1b *JAAD 37:553–558, 1997*

Isoniazid

Meperidine – ulcer and fibrosis of forearm *JAMADerm 151:331–332, 2015*

Methysergide *BJD 153:224–225, 2005*

Paclitaxel *JAAD 58:545–570, 2008; BJD 156:363–367, 2007; JAAD 48:279–281, 2003; BJD 147:619–621, 2002;* edematous sclero-derma *BJD 164:1393–1395, 2011*

Peplomycin (derivative of bleomycin)-induced scleroderma *BJD 1213–1214, 2004*

D-penicillamine *BJD 116:95–100, 1987;* morphea-like reaction *Ann Rheum Dis 48:963–964, 1989; Ann Rheum Dis 40:42–44, 1981*

Pentazocine (Talwin), injected–woody induration with overlying ulceration *AD 132:1366–1369, 1996; AD 127:1591–1592, 1991; JAAD 22:694–695, 1990*

Sodium valproate *AD 116:621, 1980*

Taxane-induced scleroderma *BJD 173:1054–1058, 2015*

Uracil-tegafur (UFT) *JAAD 42:519–520, 2000*

Vitamin K (fat soluble) (phytonadione) injection (Texier's syndrome)–sclerodermiform atrophic plaques *AD 137:957–962, 2001; JAAD 38:322–324, 1998; Cutis 61:81–83, 1998; Int J Dermatol 34:201–202, 1995; Contact Derm 31:45–46, 1994; Cutis 43:364–368, 1989; AD 121:1421–1423, 1985*

Vitamin B12–drug-induced morphea *Derm Surg 30:152–1255, 2004*

EXOGENOUS AGENTS

Betel chewing–oral submucous fibrosis *JAAD 37:81–88, 1998*

Chlorethylene

Cocaine abuse *JAAD 10:525, 1984*

DPT vaccination – morphea secondary to DPT vaccination *Ped Derm 29:525–526, 2012*

Epoxy resin-associated fibrosis with arthralgia *Dermatologica 161:33–44, 1980*

Paraffin–paraffinoma

Pesticides–weed sprayer with sclerodactyly of fingers and toes with hyperkeratosis of palms and chloracne *Clin Exp Dermatol 19:264–267, 1994*

Plastics
    Epoxy resin-associated fibrosis *Dermatologica 161:33–44, 1980*
    Urea formaldehyde foam
    Vinyl chloride – thick skin of hands, face, and trunk *AD 106:219–223, 1972*

Polyvinyl chloride – acro-osteolysis, cutaneous sclerosis, Raynaud's phenomenon *Br Med J i:936–938, 1976*

Silica dust – occupational; digital ulcers, interstitial lung disease, myocardial dysfunction, cancer *JAAD 72:456–464, 2015; JAAD 22:444–448, 1990; Ann Int Med 66:323–334, 1967;* silica dust in gold mining–acro-osteolysis, cutaneous sclerosis, Raynaud's phenomenon *Br J Ind Med 42:838–843, 1985;* silica-associated systemic sclerosis in coal miners *BJD 123:725–734, 1990*

Silicone breast implant associated scarring dystrophy of arm *AD 131:54–56, 1995;* indurated inflammatory subcutaneous masses due to silicone bag-gel rupture

Subcutaneous silicone injections

Solvents *Acta DV (Stockh) 69:533–536, 1989; Clin Exp Dermatol 2:17–22, 1977*
    Aromatic hydrocarbons
    Aliphatic hydrocarbons
    Chlorinated hydrocarbons
    Ethylacetate *Arthritis Rheum 34:631–633, 1991*
    Hexachloroethane
    Isopropyl alcohol *Arthritis Rheum 34:631–633, 1991*
    Meta-phenyl diamine *Am J Med 85:114–116, 1988*
    Naphthalene *Arthritis Rheum 34:631–633, 1991*
    Perchlorethylene – like vinyl chloride disease *Schweiz Med Wochenschr 125:2433–2437, 1995; Clin Exp Dermatol 2:17–22, 1977*
    Toluene
    Trichloroethane *Acta DV (Stockh)67:263–264, 1987*
    Trichloroethylene *Acta DV (Stockh)67:263–264, 1987*
    Trimethylbenzene *Arthritis Rheum 34:631–633, 1991*
    Terpene derivatives *Arthritis Rheum 34:631–633, 1991*

INFECTIONS OR INFESTATIONS

Brucellosis *Int J Derm 33:57–59, 1994*

Filariasis

HIV-related porphyria cutanea tarda *J Acquir Immune Defic Syndr 4:1112–1117, 1991*

Leprosy – lepromatous; Lucio's phenomenon – gradual loss of eyebrow, eyelash, and body hair with generalized sclerodermoid thickening of skin

Lobomycosis (lacaziosis) (*Lacazia loboi*) – sclerodermiform plaques *Mycoses 55:298–309, 2012*

Lyme borreliosis–morphea-like changes *JAAD 48:376–384, 2003*; acrodermatitis chronica atrophicans – sclerodermiform with sclerosis of lower legs with ulceration *BJD 121:263–269, 1989: Int J Derm 18:595–601, 1979*

Lymphogranuloma venereum

Mycetoma – hyperpigmented firm, indurated subcutaneous swellings or papules *JAAD 53:931–951, 2005*

Mycobacterium tuberculosis – tuberculosis verrucosa cutis; deep papillomatous and sclerotic forms causing deformity of the extremities *Clin Exp Dermatol 13:211–220, 1988*

Syphilis–secondary in AIDS *AD 128:530–534, 1992*

Trichodysplasia spinulosa – DNA polyoma virus in renal transplant patient; alopecia, particulate matter, follicular papules, thickened skin, eyebrow alopecia, leonine facies *AD 148:726–733, 2012; AD 146:871–874, 2010; JAAD 60:169–172, 2009; J Cutan Pathol 34:721–725, 2007; AD 142:1643–1648, 2006; JAAD 50:310–315, 2004; J Invest Dermatol Symp Proc 4:268–271, 1999; Hautarzt 46:871–874, 1995*

Yaws–tertiary–cicatricial changes

INFILTRATIVE DISORDERS

Amyloidosis (pseudoscleroderma) – primary systemic *J Clin Rheumatol 14:161–165, 2008; Postgrad Med J 64:696–698, 1988; Clin Exp Dermatol 4:517–536, 1979; Can Med Assoc J 83:263–265, 1960*; amyloid elastosis *JAAD 22:27–34, 1990*; beta-2 microglobulin amyloidosis – subcutaneous masses of shoulders, wrists, and palms *JAAD 65:1095–1106, 2011*

Juvenile hyaline fibromatosis (infantile systemic hyalinosis) – limb contractures, sclerodermoid changes; gigantic lip fibromas, giant fibrous nodules of scalp and ears; giant nodules of frontal scalp and face; periarticular nodules of knees; gingival hypertrophy, bone deformities; mutation in gene encoding capillary morphogenesis protein 2 (*ANTRX2 (CMG2)*) *Ped Derm 23:458–464, 2006; JAAD 55:1036–143, 2006; Ped Derm 11:52–60, 1994; Pediatrics 87:228–234, 1991*

Mastocytosis – diffuse infiltrative mastocytosis

Scleredema – secondary to paraproteinemia *JAMADerm 150:788–789, 2014;* associated with diabetes *JAMA 315:1159–1160, 2016*

Scleromyxedema (lichen myxedematosus) (pseudoscleroderma)– linear papules, leonine facies, arthritis and rash, sclerodermoid changes *JAAD 69:66–72, 2013; Int J Derm 42:31–35, 2003; JAAD 44:273–281, 2001; JAAD 38:289–294, 1998; JAAD 33:37–43, 1995; JAAD 14:1–18, 1986; Arch Dermatol Syphilol 7:569–570, 1906*

Xanthosiderohistiocytosis – variant of xanthoma disseminatum; diffuse infiltration of skin, subcutis, and muscle *AD 82:171–174, 1960*

INFLAMMATORY DISORDERS

Connective tissue panniculitis – nodules, atrophic linear plaques of face, upper trunk, or extremities *AD 116:291–294, 1980*

Encephalitis with sclerodermoid changes–personal observation

Eosinophilic fasciitis (Shulman's syndrome) *Clin Dermatol 38:235–249, 2020; Curr Rheum Reports 4:113, 2002; Rheum Dis Clin North Am 21:231, 1995; Assoc Am Physicians 88:70, 1985; JAAD 1:221–226, 1979; Ann Rheum Dis 36:354–359, 1977; J Rheumatol 1(Suppl 1):46, 1974*

IgG4 related disease – indurated nodules of neck, cheek, temporal region, periauricular; lymphadenopathy *Adv Anat Pathol 20:10–16, 2013; Eur J Dermatol 23:241–245, 2013; JAMADerm 149:742–747, 2013;* sclerosing mesenteritis (retractile mesenteritis) – sclerodermoid changes with subcutaneous nodules *AD 146:1009–1013, 2010*

Sarcoid–morphea-like lesions *Dermatol Clin 33:509–630, 2015; JAAD 44:725–743, 2001; JAAD 39:345–348, 1998; Clin Exp Rheumatol 8:171–175, 1990;* mimicking lipodermatosclerosis *Cutis 75:322–324, 2005*

Subacute nodular migratory panniculitis *AD 128:1643–1648, 1992*

Subcutaneous fat necrosis of the newborn – red to bluish-red firm nodules and/or plaques; buttocks, thighs, shoulders, back, cheeks, and arms; associated with hypercalcemia *JAAD 16:435–439, 1987; Ped Derm 4:112–122, 1987; Clin Pediatr 20:748–750, 1981*

METABOLIC DISORDERS

Acromegaly

Bisalbuminemia – cold, blue hands; inability to extend fingers *BJD 95(Suppl.14):54–55, 1977*

Calcification–subcutaneous calcification (post-phlebitic subcutaneous calcification) – chronic venous insufficiency; non-healing ulcers; fibrosis *Radiology 74:279–281, 1960*

Congenital erythropoietic porphyria – sclerodactyly with crusted papules on dorsal hands; atrophic scars, erythrodontia *BJD 166:697–699, 2012*

Diabetes mellitus–diabetic hands (diabetic cheiroarthropathy) (prayer sign) (waxy hands)–limited joint mobility *JAAD 49:109–111, 2003; Ped Derm 11:310–314, 1994; J Rheumatol 10:797–800, 1983; Arthritis Rheum 25:1357–1361, 1982;* diabetic thick skin *JAAD 16:546–553, 1987;* with finger pebbling *JAAD 14:612–619, 1986;* scleredema *Dermatologica 146:193–198, 1973;* pigmented hypertrichotic indurated plaques of thighs *Ped Derm 24:101–107, 2007*

Hashimoto's thyroiditis

Hepatoerythropoietic porphyria – extreme photosensitivity, skin fragility in sun-exposed areas, hypertrichosis, erythrodontia, pink urine, sclerodermoid changes *AD 146:529–533, 2010*

Hunter's syndrome – decreased sulfoiduronate sulfatase – sclerodermoid changes of the hands *Ped Derm 15:370–373, 1998*

Hyaluronan metabolic abnormality–peau d'orange bound skin, generalized lax and cerebriform redundant skin *J Pediatr 136:62–68, 2000*

Hyperoxalosis – primary type I hyperoxalosis; glyoxylate aminotransferase deficiency; sclerodermoid changes of legs *BJD 151:1104–1107, 2004*

Hypopituitarism – post-partum; scleroderma-like

Hypothyroidism (myxedema) – edematous and indurated skin

Immunoglobulin G4-related sclerosing disorders *AD 146:1009–1013, 2010*

Mucolipidosis type II

Mucopolysaccharidoses (Hunter's and Hurler's syndromes)–acrosclerosis; Hurler–focal pebbly thickening of skin

Muscle glycogenosis – proximal extremities with contractures *Acta DV (Stockh)52:379–385, 1972*

Necrobiosis lipoidica diabeticorum *Int J Derm 33:605–617, 1994; JAAD 18:530–537, 1988*

Nephrogenic systemic fibrosis (nephrogenic fibrosing dermopathy) (scleromyxedema-like cutaneous fibrosing disorder)–associated with chronic renal failure with or without hemodialysis; patterned cobblestoned rippled red to violaceous thin fixed plaques with polygonal, reticular, or ameboid patterns; sclerodermoid changes; edema of fingers, wrists, toes, ankles; decreased range of motion; induced by gadolinium-containing contrast medium *BJD 165:828–836, 2011; JAAD 61:868–874, 2009; AD 145:1164–1169, 2009; AD 145:183–187, 2009; BJD 158:1358–1362, 2008; JAAD 56:21–26, 2007; Semin Dialysis 19:191–194, 2006; JAAD 54:S31–34, 2006; Semin Arthritis Rheum 35:238–249, 2006; Semin Arthritis Rheum 35:208–210, 2006; Curr Opin Rheumatol 18:614–617, 2006; BJD 152:531–536, 2005; Arthritis Rheum 50:2660–2666, 2004; JAAD 48:55–60, 2003; JAAD 48:42–47, 2003; Am J Med 114:563–572, 2003; AD 139:903–906, 2003; Am J Dermatopathol 25:358, 2003; Am J Dermatopathol 23:383–393, 2001; Lancet 356:1000–1001, 2000*

Niemann-Pick disease

Oxalosis (primary oxalosis) – autosomal recessive; livedo reticularis, acrocyanosis, peripheral gangrene, ulcerations, sclerodermoid changes (woody induration of extremities), eschar of hand (calcium oxalate); acral and/or facial papules or nodules; end stage renal disease; primary hyperoxalosis – deficiency of alanine: glyoxylate aminotransferase; primary hyperoxalosis – deficiency of D-glycerate dehydrogenase/glyoxylate reductase *AD 147:1277–1282, 2011*

Paraproteinemia

Phenylketonuria – autosomal recessive; deficiency of pheylalanine hydroxylase; sclerodermoid changes of thighs and buttocks in first year of life with rippled appearance of skin; contractures of legs; morphea-like lesions in older children, hypopigmentation, photosensitivity *Ped Derm 23:136–138, 2006; JAAD 26:329–333, 1992;* morphea resulting in atrophoderma of Pasini and Pierini with subcutaneous atrophy *JAAD 49:S190–192, 2003*

Porphyria–porphyria cutanea tarda *Clin Dermatol 38:235–249, 2020; AD 148:1317–1322, 2012; BJD 129:455–457, 1993; Dermatol Clinics 4:297–309, 1986;* variegate porphyria – pseudosclerodermatous changes of hands and fingers; hepatoerythropoietic porphyria *JAAD 67:1093–1110, 2012; JAAD 11:1103–1111, 1984; AD 116:307–313, 1980; BJD 96:663–668, 1977;* erythropoietic protoporphyria–"pseudoscleroderma" *Sybert's Genetic Skin Disorders, p.536, Oxford University Press, 1997;* Gunther's disease–congenital erythropoietic porphyria – sclerosis of hands *JAMA Derm 149:969–970, 2013; Ped Derm 20:498–501, 2003; Clin Exp Dermatol 12:61–65, 1987*

Scurvy – chronic *Nature 202:708–709, 1964*

Spherocytosis – pseudoerysipelas due to recurrent hemolysis with underlying sclerodermoid changes *JAAD 51:1019–1023, 2004*

Thyroid dermopathy – indurated arms *JAAD 64:1219–1220, 2011*

NEOPLASTIC DISEASES

Angiosarcoma in radiation site – late skin thickening and induration, edema, and dyspigmentation *JAAD 49:532–538, 2003*

Basal cell carcinoma, morpheaform *Acta Pathol Mibrobiol Scand 88A:5–9, 1980; Am J Surg 116:499–505, 1968*

Collagenoma–eruptive, familial, isolated

Dermatofibrosarcoma protuberans – indurated depressed blue-gray plaque in infancy *Ped Derm 25:317–325, 2008*

Desmoid tumors – extra-abdominal desmoids tumor *JAAD 34:352–356, 1996*

Desmoplastic hairless hypopigmented nevus (variant of giant congenital melanocytic nevus) *BJD 148:1253–1257, 2003*

Hair follicle hamartoma – sclerotic facial changes *BJD 143:1103–1105, 2000*

Hypertrophic scars

Keloids

Keratoacanthomas – Grzybowski eruptive keratoacanthomas; mask-like face *BJD 147:793–796, 2002*

Lymphoma – Hodgkin's disease presenting as generalized sclerodermoid changes *In J Derm 33:217–218, 1994;* CD30+ anaplastic large cell lymphoma – morphea-like plaques *Am J Dermatopathol 18:221–235, 1996;* lymphoma en cuirasse *JAAD 14:1096–1098, 1986;* Sezary syndrome; intravascular B-cell lymphoma – indurated hyperpigmented sclerodermoid plaques of thighs *AD 148:247–252, 2012;* angioimmunoblastic T-cell lymphoma mimicking morphea–personal observation

Lymphomatoid granulomatosis–morphea-like plaque *JAAD 20:571–578, 1989*

Malignant mesothelioma–hourglass abdominal induration *JAAD 21:1068–1073, 1989*

Melanocytic nevus, congenital–congenital giant melanocytic nevus with progressive sclerodermoid reaction *Ped Derm 18:320–324, 2001;* desmoplastic giant congenital nevus *JAAD 56:S10–14, 2007*

Melanoma–desmoplastic melanoma; metastatic *J Derm Surg Oncol 6:112–114, 1980*

Metastases–morphea-like changes in metastatic lesions–breast, lung, gut, kidney, lacrimal gland *JAAD 33:161–182, 1995;* sclerodermoid hyperpigmented plaques of breasts – metastatic renal cell carcinoma *AD 147:1215–1220, 2011;*

carcinoma en cuirasse (metastatic breast carcinoma, gastric, lung, cutaneous squamous cell carcinoma, penile squamous cell carcinoma) – scattered lenticular papulonodules, diffuse morphea-like indurated skin, red-blue discoloration, keloidal appearance *An Bras Dermatol 88:608–610, 2013; Dermatol Ther 23:581–589, 2012; Am J Dermatopathol 34:347–392, 2012; Indian J Pathol Microbiol 53:351–358, 2010;* metastatic male breast carcinoma – sclerodermoid ichthyosiform plaque of chest wall *AD 139:1497–1502, 2003*

Microcystic adnexal tumor – sclerodermoid plaque above eyebrow *Derm Surg 27:979–984, 2001*

Multiple myeloma *Dermatologica 144:257–269, 1972*

Neurofibroma–diffuse neurofibroma *BJD 121(suppl 34):24, 1989*

Paraproteinemia *AD 123:226–229, 1987*

Rhabdomyomatous mesenchymal hamartoma – indurated plaque of chin *Ped Derm 32:256–262, 2015*

Sebaceous carcinoma–morpheic plaque of eyelid *Am J Surg Pathol 8:597–606, 1984*

Trichilemmal carcinoma – indurated plaque *Dermatol Surg 28:284–286, 2002*

PARANEOPLASTIC DISEASES

Malignancy-associated scleroderma or CREST syndrome (lung, thyroid, ovary, cervix, brain esophagus, stomach, breast, lymphoma, leukemia, hepatoblastoma) *Act Rheum Port 39:87–90, 2014; Rheum Dis Clin North Am 39:905–920, 2013; Arthritis Rheum 65:1913–1921, 2013; Curr Opin Rheumatol 23:530–535, 2011; Clin Exp Rhrumatol 19:221–223, 2001; Medicine 58:182–207, 1979; AD 115:950–955, 1979; Nebraska Med J 58:186–188, 1973;* with fasciitis/panniculitis *Cancer 73:231–235, 1994*

Metastatic malignant melanoma – sclerodermoid changes *J Derm Surg 6:112–114, 1980*

Panniculitis-fasciitis syndrome with hairy cell leukemia–personal observation

Scleredema associated with paraproteinemia or myeloma *Arch Dermatol Forsch 248:379, 1974;* malignant insulinoma *BJD 126:527–528, 1992*

Xanthomatosis resembling scleroderma in multiple myeloma *Arch Pathol Lab Med 102:567–571, 1978*

PRIMARY CUTANEOUS DISEASES

Acrodermatitis chronica atrophicans – morphea-like lesions

Cold flexed fingers (bowed fingers) *J Rheumatol 8:266–272, 1981*

Eosinophilic fasciitis (Shulman's syndrome) *Rheum Dis Clin North Am 21:231–246, 1995; Clin Dermatol 12:449–455, 1994; JAAD 1:221–226, 1979; JAMA 240:451–453, 1978*

Idiopathic acro-osteolysis

Lamellar ichthyosis – limitation of joint movement, flexion contractures, digital sclerodactyly *Rook p.1500, 1998, Sixth Edition*

Lichen sclerosus et atrophicus *JAAD 65:1095–1106, 2011;* lichen sclerosus and morphea *AD 148:24–28, 2012*

Palmar fibromatosis–Dupuytren's contracture *JAAD 65:1095–1106, 2011*

Pityriasis rubra pilaris – sclerodermoid changes of hands in type V PRP *Clin Exp Dermatol 5:105–112, 1980*

Scleredema of Buschke (pseudoscleroderma) *Clin Dermatol 38:235–249, 2020; Clin Rheumatol 25:3–15, 2005; J Postgrad Med 46:91–93, 2000; JAAD 11:128–134, 1984;* associated with rheumatoid arthritis and Sjogren's syndrome *BJD 121:517–520, 1989;* with primary hyperparathyroidism *Int J Derm 27:647–649, 1988;* with anaphylactoid purpura *Acta DV (Stockh) 77:159–161, 1997*

Sclerema neonatorum – severely ill child; starts on legs then generalizes, diffuse yellow-white woody induration with immobility of limbs; mortality 50% *AD 97:372–380, 1968*

Sclerema edematosum

Sclerotic panatrophy – may follow morphea or occur spontaneously; linear or annular or circumferential bands around limbs

SYNDROMES

Acrogeria

Ataxia telangiectasia

Carcinoid syndrome–sclerodermoid changes *JAAD 68:189–209, 2013;* sclerosis of the legs *BJD 152:71–75, 2005; BJD 129:222–223, 1993;* scleroderma-like lesions *Arch Int Med 131:550–553, 1973*

Cataracts, alopecia, and sclerodactyly – ectodermal dysplasia syndrome on the island of Rodrigues *Am J Med Genet 32:500–532, 1989*

Cervical rib syndrome – indurated edema

Cockayne's syndrome

Congenital ichthyosiform dermatosis with linear keratotic flexural papules and sclerosing palmoplantar keratoderma *AD 125:103–106, 1989*

Congenital fascial dystrophy (stiff skin syndrome) (Parana hard skin syndrome) – autosomal recessive; hirsutism, limited joint mobility, localized areas of stony hard skin of buttocks and legs *Ped Derm 20:339–341, 2003; Ped Derm 19:67–72, 2002; JAAD 43:797–802, 2000; JAAD 21:943–50, 1989; Ped Derm 3:48–53, 1985; Ped Derm 2:87–97, 1984*

Congenital generalized fibromatosis

Dento-oculo-cutaneous syndrome – pigmented and indurated interphalangeal joints, thick and wide philtrum, ectropion, dental abnormalities, dystrophic fingernails *Int J Dermatol 12:285–289, 1973*

Dermochondrocorneal dystrophy–Francois' syndrome–hands *AD 124:424–428, 1988*

Diffuse lipomatosis–autosomal dominant *Proc Greenwood Genet Center 3:56–64, 1984*

Familial histiocytic dermoarthritis of Zayd

Familial scleroderma-like fingers (familial sclerodactyly) *JAAD 33:302–304, 1995*

Farber's lipogranulomatosis – lysosomal storage disease *AD 144:1351–1359, 2008*

Fibroblastic rheumatism – symmetrical polyarthritis, nodules over joints and on palms, elbows, knees, ears, neck, Raynaud's phenomenon, sclerodactyly; joint contractures, thick palmar fascia; scalp nodules, red tender swelling of toe tips, periarticular nodule; skin lesions resolve spontaneously *JAAD 66:959–965, 2012; AD 139:657–662, 2003; Ped Derm 19:532–535, 2002; AD 139:657–662, 2003; AD 131:710–712, 1995; Clin Exp Dermatol 19:268–270, 1994; AD 131:710–712, 1995; Clin Exp Dermatol 19:268–270, 1994; JAAD 14:1086–1088, 1986; Rev Rheum Ed Fr 47:345–351, 1980;* periungual papules *Ped Derm 19:532–535, 2002*

Flynn-Aird syndrome–progressive sensorineural deafness, neurologic signs and symptoms, sclerodermoid changes

Geleophysic dysplasia *Ann DV 125(suppl 1):1S 31–32, 1998; Am J Med Genet 72:85–90, 1997; Am J Med Genet 63:50–54, 1996; J Pediatr 117:227–232, 1990; Am J Med Genet 19:487–499, 1984; Lancet 2 (7715)97–98, 1971*

GEMSS syndrome–autosomal dominant; glaucoma, lens ectopia, microspherophakia, stiff joints, shortness, gingival hypertrophy, flexion contractures of joints, osteolytic defects, stunted growth, stocky pseudoathletic build, sclerosis of upper back and extremities *AD 131:1170–1174, 1995*

H syndrome (low height, heart, hallus valgus, hormonal, hypogo-nadism, hematologic) – sclerodermoid changes of middle and lower body with overlying hyperpigmentation sparing the knees and buttocks; starts on feet and legs and progresses upward; hypertri-chosis, short stature, facial telangiectasia, ichthyosiform changes, gynecomastia, varicose veins, skeletal deformities (camptodactyly of 5th fingers), scrotal masses with massively edematous scrotum obscuring the penis, hypogonadism, micropenis, azoospermia, sensorineural hearing loss, dilated scleral vessels, exophthalmos, cardiac anomalies, hepatosplenomegaly, mental retardation; mutation in nucleoside transporter hENT3 *Ped Derm 32:731–732, 2015; JAAD 70:80–88, 2014; Ped Derm 27:65–68, 2010; JAAD 59:79–85, 2008*

> Differential diagnostic considerations include:
> > Winchester syndrome – arthropathy, coarse facies, no hearing loss
> > POEMS syndrome–paraproteinemia

Hallermann-Streiff syndrome–taut, thin, atrophic skin, telangiecta-sias, hypotrichosis of scalp, xerosis/ichthyosis, pinched nose

Hereditary bullous acrokeratosis poikiloderma (Weary) – Kindler's syndrome? – pseudoainhum and sclerotic bands *Int J Dermatol 36:529–533, 1997*

Hereditary sclerosing poikiloderma – generalized poikiloderma; sclerosis of palms and soles; linear hyperkeratotic and sclerotic bands in flexures of arms and legs *AD 100:413–422, 1969*

Hunter's syndrome – (Mucopolysaccharidosis type II) – X-linked recessive, generalized skin thickening, ivory papules of scapulae, hypertrichosis, coarse facial features, dysostosis, dwarfism, hepatosplenomegaly, cardiovascular disease, deafness

Ped Derm 33:594–601, 2016; Adv Pediatr 33:269–302, 1986

Hurler's syndrome – thickening of digits resembling acrosclerosis *Ped Derm 33:594–601, 2016; Curr Rheumatol Reports 16:399, 2014; Adv Pediatr 33:269–302, 1986; AD 85:455–471, 1962*

Hutchinson-Gilford progeria syndrome – neonatal appearance of sclerodermoid changes of abdomen, trunk and thighs; mountain range rippling of skin; facies – mid-frontal bossing, protruding ears with small lobes, prominent eyes, glyphic nose (broad, mildly concave nasal ridge), mild micrognathia, vertical midline groove of chin, thin lips; prominent superficial veins; dyspigmentation, alopecia; mutation in *LMNA Ped Derm 32:271–275, 2015; Ped Derm 31:387–388, 2014; Ped Derm 31:196–202, 2014; JAMADerm 150:197–198, 2014; BJD 163:1102–1115, 2010; AD 144:1351–1359, 2008; BJD 156:1308–1314, 2007*

Ichthyosis cerebriformis – keratotic plugs, depressions, thick skin, palmoplantar keratoderma *JAAD 58:505–507, 2008*

IgG4 disease (retractile mesenteritis)–personal observation

Infantile myofibromatosis – subcutaneous induration with hypertri-chosis *Ped Derm 27:34–38, 2010*

Infantile restrictive dermopathy – autosomal recessive; taut shiny skin with flexion of joints *Eur J Ped 155:987–989, 1996; Am J Med Genet 24:631–648, 1986*

Infantile systemic hyalinosis – large subcutaneous nodules; hyperpigmented plaques over joints, diarrhea, recurrent infections; death by age 2 *JAAD 61:629–638, 2009; AD 144:1351–1359, 2008*

IgG4 disease (sclerosing mesenteritis, sclerodermoid cutaneous changes) – aortitis *NEJM 367:2335–2346, 2012*

Juvenile hyaline fibromatosis (infantile systemic hyalinosis) (Murray-Puretic-Drescher syndrome) – autosomal recessive; gingival fibromatosis with hypertrophy, focal skin nodularity with multiple subcutaneous tumors (nodular perianal lesions, facial red or pearly papules (paranasal, periauricular), dusky red plaques of buttocks, ears, lips), synophrys, thickened skin with sclerodermiform

atrophy, osteolytic (osteoporotic) skeletal lesions, stiff muscles with massive stiffness, flexural joint contractures, hyperpigmentation, flexion contractures of joints, juxta-articular nodules (knuckle pads), nodules of ears, diarrhea, recurrent suppurative infections failure to thrive with stunted growth (growth failure) and death in infancy; CMG2 (capillary morphogenesis protein 2) (transmembrane protein); deposition of collagen type VI (bound to laminin and collagen 4) mutation (chromosome 4q21) *JAAD 61:629–638, 2009; Ped Derm 25:557–558, 2008; JAAD 58:303–307, 2008; Ped Derm 21:154–159, 2004; JAAD 50:S61–64, 2004; Ped Derm 19:67–72, 2002; Ped Derm 18:534–536, 2001; Ped Derm 18:400–402, 2001; Dermatology 198:18–25, 1999; Int J Paediatr Dent 6:39–43, 1996; J Periodontol 67:451–453, 1996; Dermatology 190:148–151, 1995; Ped Derm 11:52–60, 1994; Ped Derm 6:68–75, 1989; Oral Surg 63:71–77, 1987; Arch Fr Pediatr 35:1063–1074, 1978*

> Differential diagnosis of infantile systemic hyalinosis
> > Winchester syndrome – autosomal recessive, patches of thick leathery skin, coarse facies, gingival hypertrophy, joint contractures
> > Lipoid proteinosis (Urbach-Wiethe disease) – autosomal recessive, vesiculopustulosis, ice-pick scars
> > Mucopolysaccharidosis type II (Hunter's syndrome) – X-linked recessive, generalized skin thickening, ivory papules of scapulae, hypertrichosis, coarse facial features, dysostosis, dwarfism, hepatosplenomegaly, cardiovascular disease, deafness

Klinefelter's syndrome – stasis changes–personal observation

Lipoid proteinosis–"pseudoscleroderma" *Ped Derm 18:21–26, 2001*

Macrocephaly with cutis marmorata, hemangioma, and syndactyly syndrome – macrocephaly, hypotonia, hemihypertrophy, heman-gioma, cutis marmorata telangiectatica congenita, internal arterio-venous malformations, syndactyly, joint laxity, hyperelastic skin, thickened subcutaneous tissue, developmental delay, short stature, hydrocephalus *Ped Derm 16:235–237, 1999*

Mandibuloacral dysplasia *JAAD 33:900–902, 1995*

Melorheostosis – cutaneous lesions resemble linear morphea overlying bony lesions (endosteal bony densities resembling candle wax) *Mayo Clin Proc 70:1068–1076, 1995; BJD 86:297–301, 1972*

Moore-Federman syndrome–short stature, stiffness of joints, characteristic facies *J Med Gen 26:320–325, 1989*

Muckle-Wells syndrome (possibly H syndrome) – hyperpigmented, hypertrichotic, sclerodermoid plaques *JAAD 61:725–727, 2009*

Multicentric reticulohistiocytosis–sclerosing lesion of leg *JAAD 20:329–335, 1989*

Multifocal idiopathic fibrosclerosis (hyper IgG4 syndrome) – sclero-dermoid red plaque of breast; fibrosis of thyroid, mediastinum, retroperitoneum, orbits, pancreas, gallbladder *AD 148:1335–1336, 2012*

Myhre syndrome – low birth weight, short stature, muscular build, limited joint mobility, cardiac defects, deafness, skeletal abnormali-ties, facial dysmorphism, thick skin, keratosis pilaris, coarse facies

Neonatal mucolipidosis II (I-cell disease) – lysosomal storage disease; mutation in n-acetylglucosamine-1 phosphotransferase; alpha/beta subunits precursor gene *AD 144:1351–1359, 2008*

Neu-Laxova syndrome – microcephaly; harlequin fetus-like changes; resembles restrictive dermopathy *Am J Med Genet 15:153–156, 1983*

Niemann-Pick disease – autosomal recessive; sphingomyelinase deficiency; waxy induration with transient xanthomas overlying enlarged cervical lymph nodes *Medicine 37:1–95, 1958*

Nijmegen breakage syndrome – autosomal recessive; microcephaly, growth retardation, chromosomal instability, and combined immunodeficiency; pink to red-brown firm papules and plaques with sclerosis and atrophy, clinodactyly, syndactyly, vitiligo, café au lait macules *Ped Derm 27:285–289, 2010*

Novel fibrosing disorder – subcutaneous fibrotic nodules, progressive distal joint contractures, marfanoid stature, forehead nodules, skin tightening (sclerodermoid changes), palmoplantar nodules, nodules of elbows and knees, linear arrays of nodules later in course; differentiate from Marfan's syndrome, congenital contractural arachnodactyly, Winchester syndrome, multicentric osteolysis nodulosis and arthropathy (MONA) syndrome *BJD 163:1102–1115, 2010*

Olmsted syndrome

Palmar fasciitis and polyarthritis syndrome – painful swelling over palmar PIP joints – indurated palmar skin; flexion contractures; may be paraneoplastic (transitional cell carcinoma of the bladder) *JAAD 64:1159–1163, 2011; Ann Int Med 96:424–431, 1982*

Panniculitis-fasciitis syndrome – associated with hairy cell leukemia – personal observation

Parana hard skin syndrome – frozen joints secondary to skin tightening *BJD 163:1102–1115, 2010; Lancet 1:215–216, 1974*

Parry-Romberg syndrome *JAAD 56:257–263, 2007*

POEMS syndrome (Takatsuki syndrome, Crow-Fukase syndrome) (PEP syndrome – plasma cell dyscrasia, endocrinopathy, polyneuropathy)–osteosclerotic myeloma (IgG or IgA lambda) bone lesions, progressive symmetric sensorimotor peripheral polyneuropathy, hypothyroidism, and hypogonadism; peripheral edema, sclerodermoid changes (thickening of skin), either generalized or localized (legs), pleural effusions, thrombocytosis, cutaneous angiomas, blue dermal papules associated with Castleman's disease (benign reactive angioendotheliomatosis), diffuse hyperpigmentation, maculopapular brown-violaceous lesions, purple nodules; papilledema *AD 146:615–623, 2010; JAAD 58:671–675, 2008; JAAD 55:149–152, 2006; JAAD 44:324–329, 2001, JAAD 40:808–812, 1999; AD 124:695–698, 1988, Cutis 61:329–334, 1998; JAAD 21:1061–1068, 1989; JAAD 12:961–964, 1985; Nippon Shinson 26:2444–2456, 1968*; AESOP syndrome – adenopathy, extensive skin patch thickening overlying a plasmacytoma seen in POEMS syndrome *Medicine (Baltimore)82:51–59, 2003*

Progeria (Hutchinson-Gilford syndrome) *Ped Derm 17:282–285, 2000; AD 125:540–544, 1989*

Pseudoxanthoma elasticum – with scleroderma *Dermatologica 140:54–59, 1970*

Reflex sympathetic dystrophy – area becomes indurated after initial edema; glossy edematous, sclerodermatous skin, taut fingers, alopecia *JAAD 58:320–322, 2008; Cutis 68:179–182, 2001; JAAD 35:843–845, 1996; AD 127:1541–1544, 1991; JAAD 22:513–520, 1990; Arch Neurol 44:555–561, 1987*

Restrictive dermopathy–autosomal recessive, erythroderma at birth with tight, taut, translucent skin, prominent superficial vasculature, extensive erosions and contractures; taut shiny skin; fetal akinesia, multiple joint contractures, dysmorphic facies with fixed open mouth, microstomia, micrognathia, hypertelorism, pulmonary hypoplasia, bone deformities; uniformly fatal in neonatal period; intrauterine growth retardation *AD 141:611–613, 2005; Ped Derm 19:67–72, 2002; Ped Derm 16:151–153, 1999; AD 134:577–579, 1998; AD 128:228–231, 1992; Am J Med Genet 24:631–648, 1986; Am J Med Genet 15:153–156, 1983; Eur J Obstet Gynecol Reprod Biol 10:381–388, 1980*

Rothmund-Thomson syndrome

Scalenus anticus syndrome – indurated edema

Scheie syndrome – mucopolysaccharidosis *Adv Pediatr 33:269–302, 1986*

Scleroatrophic syndrome of Huriez (familial scleroatrophic syndrome) – autosomal dominant; triad of diffuse scleroatrophy of the hands, ridging or hypoplasia of the nails, and lamellar palmoplantar keratoderma; development of aggressive squamous cell carcinoma of involved skin *BJD 143:1091–1096, 2000; BJD 137:114–118, 1997; Fr Dermatol Syphilol 70:743–744, 1963*

Sclerodactyly, non-epidermolytic palmoplantar keratoderma, multiple cutaneous squamous cell carcinomas, periodontal disease with loss of teeth, hypogenitalism with hypospadias, altered sex hormone levels, hypertriglyceridemia, 46XX *JAAD 53:S234–239, 2005*

Shoulder-hand syndrome – sclerodactyly, mild Raynaud's phenomenon, abnormal sweating

Stiff skin syndrome (congenital fascial dystrophy) – autosomal dominant; early age at onset; rock hard sclerodermoid changes of pelvic (buttocks and thighs) or shoulder girdle, limited joint mobility, mild overlying hypertrichosis, especially over lumbosacral area (contractures of knees and hips) and pelvic girdle; sharp demarcation at inguinal crease *JAAD 65:1095–1106, 2011; Rheumatology 48:849–852, 2009; AD 144:1351–1359, 2008; Ped Derm 20:339–341, 2003; Ped Derm 19:67–72, 2002; Dermatology 190:148–151, 1995; Ped Derm 2:87–97, 1984; Pediatrics 47:360–369, 1971*; unilateral (segmental) *JAAD 75:163–168, 2016*

Storm syndrome–calcific cardiac valvular degeneration with premature aging–Werner-like syndrome *Am J Hum Genet 45(suppl) A67, 1989*

Tricho rhino digital syndrome

Tuberous sclerosis–collagenoma–dermal fibrosis

Vohwinkel's syndrome–spindle-shaped fingers

Wells' syndrome–resolving lesions *JAAD 18:105–114, 1988; morphea-like lesions JAAD 52:187–189, 2005; Trans St. Johns Hosp Dermatol Soc 57:46–56, 1971*

Werner's syndrome (pangeria) – sclerodactyly with acral gangrene *Medicine 45:177–221, 1966*; atypical Werner's syndrome – sclerodermatous skin, premature aging, thin arms and legs *BJD 163:1102–1115, 2010*

Whistling face syndrome (craniocarpotarsal dysplasia syndrome) *Birth Defects 11:161–168, 1975*

Winchester syndrome (hereditary contractures with sclerodermoid changes of skin) – scleredema-like skin changes, joint contractures, gingival hyperplasia, dwarfism, arthritis of small joints, corneal opacities *JAAD 55:1036–1043, 2006; JAAD 50:S53–56, 2004; J Med Genet 26:772–775, 1989; Am J Med Genet 26:123–131, 1987; AD 111:230–236, 1975; J Pediatr 84:701–709, 1974; Pediatrics 47:360–369, 1971*

TOXINS

Eosinophilia myalgia syndrome (l-tryptophan related) – erythematous and edematous rashes, peripheral edema, morphea, urticaria, papular lesions; arthralgia *BJD 127:138–146, 1992; Int J Dermatol 31:223–228, 1992; Mayo Clin Proc 66:457–463, 1991; Ann Int Med 112:758–762, 1990; JAMA 264:213–217, 1990*

Mustard gas (Yperite) *Eur J Dermatol 15:140–145, 2005*

Spanish toxic oil syndrome – rapeseed oil denatured with aniline; early see pruritic morbilliform exanthem then white, yellow or brown papules; finally scleroderma-like syndrome *JAAD 18:313–324, 1988; JAAD 9:159–160, 1983*

TRAUMA

Burns

Mechanical trauma–jackhammer, chain saw

Post-vein stripping sclerodermiform dermatitis *AD 135:1387–1391, 1999*

Radiation exposure (radiation port scleroderma)–chronic radiation dermatitis; supervoltage external beam radiation *JAAD 35:923–927, 1996;* post-radiation morphea–chronic *JAAD 76:19–21, 2017; BJD 120:831–835, 1989;* postirradiation pseudosclerodermatous panniculitis *Ann Int Med 142:47–55, 2005; JAAD 45:325–361, 2001; Am J Dermatopathol 23:283–287, 2001; Mayo Clin Proc 68:122–127, 1993;* radiation fibrosis *JAAD 49:417–423, 2003*

Spinal injury–dermal fibrosis

Surgical trauma

VASCULAR DISORDERS

Angiosarcoma of the breast post-irradiation for breast cancer – late thickening, edema, or induration of the breast *JAAD 49:532–538, 2003*

Erythrocyanosis – may have ulceration, erythema, keratosis pilaris, desquamation, nodular lesions, edema, and fibrosis

Idiopathic systemic capillary leak syndrome – skin-colored or red papules of face, neck, abdomen, upper back, elbows, and hands; purpuric macules of lateral fingers, infiltrative edema of hands with sclerodermoid appearance, livedo reticularis of lower extremities; photodistributed eruption of face, neck, and arms *Dermatology 209:291–295, 2004*

Lipodermatosclerosis (hypodermatitis sclerodermiformis; sclerosing panniculitis) – chronic venous insufficiency with hyperpigmentation, induration, inflammation; champagne bottle legs *JAAD 62:1005–1012, 2010; JAAD 46:187–192, 2002; Lancet ii:243–245, 1982*

Lymphedema, chronic – pseudo-scleroderma; Kaposi-Stemmer sign; failure to pick up fold of skin

Malignant angioendotheliomatosis – scalp; livedoid red plaque of thigh with woody induration *JAAD 18:407–412, 1988*

SCROTAL NODULES WITH EROSIONS

AUTOIMMUNE DISEASES AND DISEASES OF IMMUNE DYSFUNCTION

Chronic granulomatous disease

Pemphigus vegetans

DRUG-INDUCED

5-fluorouracil therapy *JAAD 19:929–931, 1988*

INFECTIONS AND INFESTATIONS

Amebiasis – scrotal abscess *Trop Biomed 32:494–496, 2015*

Bacillary angiomatosis *JAAD 32:510–512, 1995*

Candida–candida granuloma; chronic mucocutaneous candidiasis

Chancroid, including phagedenic chancroid *JAAD 19:330–337, 1988*

Coccidioidomycosis

Condylomata acuminata

Cryptococcosis

Cytomegalovirus

Granuloma inguinale *Dermatol Online J 12:14, 2006*

Group B beta hemolytic streptococcal infection

Herpes simplex *Case Rep Infect Dis 2017:1509356; Clin Inf Dis 57:1648–1655, 2013*

Histoplasmosis

Orf *JAAD 11:72–74, 1985*

Scabies

Schistosomal granulomas (Schistosoma haematobium) *J Dtsch Dermatol G 13:165–167, 2015*

Syphilis – chancre; Jarisch-Herxheimer reaction *JAMADerm 149:1429–1430, 2013*

Talaromyces marneffei Indian J DV Leprol 76:45–48, 2010

Verruga peruana

Yaws, including secondary yaws (exudative lesion)

INFILTRATIVE DISEASES

Langerhans cell histiocytosis–Letterer-Siwe disease

Lymphocytoma cutis

Verruciform xanthoma *AD 120:1378–1379, 1984*

INFLAMMATORY DISEASES

Crohn's disease

Malacoplakia *JAAD 34:325–332, 1996*

METABOLIC DISEASES

Acrodermatitis enteropathica

NEOPLASTIC DISEASES

Extramammary Paget's disease *JAAD 17:497–505, 1987*

Kaposi's sarcoma

Leiomyoma *AD 125:417–422, 1989*

Leiomyosarcomas *JAAD 20:290–292, 1989*

Leukemia–acute myelogenous leukemia *JAAD 21:410–413, 1989*

Lymphoma–primary cutaneous epidermotropic CD8+ T-cell lymphoma – mixture of patches, plaques, papulonodules with central ulceration, necrosis, and hemorrhage *JAAD 62:300–307, 2010*

Malignant mesothelioma–thick scrotum *J Cut Pathol 10:213–216, 1983*

Malignant papillary mesothelioma of the testis *JAAD 17:887–890, 1987*

Melanoma – primary scrotal melanoma *AD 145:1071–1072, 2009;* amelanotic melanoma metastases

Metastases–renal cell, thyroid (Hurthle cell carcinoma of the thyroid), colonic, prostatic, gastric carcinomas *Am J Dermatopathol 32;392–394, 2010*

Multinucleate cell angiohistiocytoma–red to brown nodules *JAAD 30:417–422, 1994*

Squamous cell carcinoma, including mule spinner's disease; squamous cell carcinoma in cotton textile workers *AD 121:370–372, 1985*

Verrucous carcinoma (giant condylomata of Buschke and Lowenstein) *JAAD 23:723–727, 1990; Z Hautkr 58:1325–1327, 1983*

PARANEOPLASTIC DISORDERS

Multicentric reticulohistiocytosis *Clin Exp Dermatol 3:183–185, 2009*

PRIMARY CUTANEOUS DISEASES

Atopic dermatitis

Darier's disease

Erythema of Jacquet *Cutis 82:72–74, 2008*

Granuloma gluteale infantum *J Dermatol 40:1038–1041, 2013*

Lichen planus

Lichen simplex chronicus

SYNDROMES

Behcet's syndrome

TOXINS

Dioxin exposure *JAAD 19:812–819, 1988*

Mustard gas exposure *JAAD 19:529–536, 1988*

TRAUMA

Child abuse

VASCULAR DISEASES

Angiokeratoma

Angiosarcoma *Clin Exp Dermatol 31:706–707, 2006*

Arteriovenous malformation *J Emerg Med 42:e133–135, 2012*

Cutaneous chylous scrotum (weeping scrotum)

Hemangiomas

Pyogenic granulomas *Cutis 62:282, 1998*

SCROTAL PAPULES AND NODULES

AUTOIMMUNE DISEASES AND DISEASES OF IMMUNE DYSFUNCTION

Chronic granulomatous disease

Cicatricial pemphigoid

Pemphigus vegetans

CONGENITAL ANOMALY

Dermoid cyst *Curr Prob in Dern 8:137–188, 1996*

Fibrous hamartoma of infancy *JAAD 41:857–859, 1999*

Median raphe cyst of the scrotum and perineum *JAAD 55:S114–115, 2006*

Transient neonatal pustular melanosis – brown papules of scrotum *Ped Derm 35:845–846, 2018*

DRUG-INDUCED

Cyclosporine

EXOGENOUS AGENTS

Foreign body granuloma

Sclerosing lipogranuloma of penis and scrotum due to paraffin or mineral oil injection

Hydrocarbon (tar) keratosis – flat-topped papules of face and hands; keratoacanthoma-like lesions on scrotum *JAAD 35:223–242, 1996*

INFECTIONS AND INFESTATIONS

Abscess–parasitic (tumbu fly, guinea worm, filariasis, bacterial)

Amblyomma americacum (turkey mite infestation) – scrotal papules *Cutis 93:64–66, 2014*

Amebiasis

Bacillary angiomatosis

Blastomycosis-like pyoderma–scrotal plaque *JAAD 36:633–634, 1997*

Candida, including candida granuloma

Chancroid

Coccidioidomycosis

Condylomata acuminata

Cytomegalovirus

Dirofilariasis, subcutaneous (migratory nodules) – eyelid, scrotum, breast, arm, leg, conjunctiva *JAAD 73:929–944, 2015; JAAD 35:260–262, 1996*

Filariasis – Wuchereria bancrofti – calcified scrotal nodules

Furuncle

Granuloma inguinale *SKINMed 15:73–75, 2017*

Herpes simplex virus – scarring; chronic herpes simplex–vegetative nodule *JAMA Derm 149:881–883, 2013*

Histoplasmosis

Leishmania *India J DV Leprol 64:243–244, 1998*

Lymphocytoma cutis of Lyme borreliosis (Borrelia burgdorferi) *JAAD 47:530–534, 2002; Cutis 66:243–246, 2000; JAAD 38:877–905, 1998*

Lymphogranuloma venereum–remnant of chancre

Myiasis – *Dermatobia hominis JAMADerm 151:1389–1390, 2015*

Mycobacterium tuberculosis Trop Doct 48:240–242, 2018

Onchocerciasis with calcified encysted nodules *Zentralbl Bakteriol 289:371–379, 1999; BJD 74:136–140, 1962*

Orf *East Afr Med J 76:635–638, 1999; JAAD 11:72–74, 1985*

Paracoccidioidomycosis – red plaques of scrotum *BJD 143:188–191, 2000*

Paragonimiasis *Medicine (Baltimore)97:e328, 2018*

Phaeohyphomycosis–flat papules

Scabies, nodular *J Parasit Dis 39:581–583, 2015; J Cutan Pathol 19:124–127, 1992*

Schistosomal granulomas (S. mansoni) *AD 115:869–870, 1979;* S. haematobium *JAAD 49:961–962, 2003;* nodule *J Dtsch Dermatol Ges 13:165–167, 2015*

Staphylococcus aureus – abscesses

Syphilis – chancre; condylomata lata; Jarisch-Herxheimer reaction; periorificial nodules – malignant secondary syphilis *JAMADerm 152:829–830, 2016; AD 99:70–73, 1969; BJD 9:11–26, 1897;* lichenoid plaque *Indian Dermatol Online J 28:585–586, 2019;* weeping papules *Am Fam Physician 94:140–142, 2016*

Talaromyces marneffei Indian J DV Leprol 76:45–48, 2010

Tinea genitalis – lichenified plaques, favus-like scutula-like, pseudomembranous-like, white dot *Indian J Dermatol 160:422, 2015*

INFILTRATIVE DISEASES

Langerhans cell histiocytosis *JAAD 25:1044–1053, 1991*

Lymphocytoma cutis *Acta DV (Stockh)42:3–10, 1962*

Verruciform xanthoma – pink nodule *Dermatol J Online Aug 15, 2015; Cutis 94:139–141, 2014; BJD 150:161–163, 2004; AD 138:689–694, 2002; AD 120:1378–1379, 1984;* cauliflower-like appearance *J Dermatol 16:397–401, 1989*

Xanthoma disseminatum – perioral papules; eyelid papules; scrotal papules; intertrigo *BJD 170:1177–1181, 2014*

INFLAMMATORY DISEASES

Crohn's disease

Hidradenitis suppurativa *Int J Dermatol 57:1471–1480, 2018*

Malakoplakia *JAAD 34 (pt 2)) 325–332, 1996*

Meconium periorchitis *J Ultrasound Med 13:491–494, 1994*

Rosai-Dorfman disease *Semin Diagn Pathol 7:19–73, 1990*

Sarcoid *J Cut Med Surg 4:202–204, 2000;* scrotal edema and papules *Cutis 83:133–137, 2009*

Sclerosing lipogranuloma *Acta Cytol 42:1181–1183, 1998*

METABOLIC

Calcinosis – idiopathic calcinosis of the scrotum *NEJM 369:965, 2013; NEJM 365:647, 2011; JAAD 51:S97–101, 2004; Genital Skin Disorders, Fischer and Margesson, CV Mosby, 1998, p. 76; Br J Plast Surg 42:324–327, 1989; Int J Derm 20:134–136, 1981; AD 114:957, 1978;* dystrophic calcinosis of benign epithelial cyst *BJD 144:146–150, 2001*

Fabry's disease – after years may develop blue-violaceous nodules *Stat Pearls Oct 19, 2019*

Fucosidosis–angiokeratomas *BJD 136:594–597, 1997*

Gout – tophi *Rein Foie 2:143–145, 1961*

Verrucous xanthoma *Acta DV 99:466–467, 2019; J Dermatol 16:397–401, 1989; J Dermatol 12:443–448, 1985; AD 120:1378–1379, 1984*

Xanthomas

NEOPLASTIC

Angiomyxoma *Pediatr Dev Pathol 6:187–191, 2003;* pink polypoid scrotal mass; may be associated with Carney complex *Ped Derm 28:200–201, 2011*

Angiomyofibroblastoma *Am J Surg Pathol 16:373–382, 1992*

Basal cell carcinoma *Dermatol Surg 38:783–790, 2012; Cutis 59:116–117, 1997; JAAD 26:574–578, 1992*

Bowen's disease *J Eur Acad DV 19:232–235, 2005*

Bowenoid papulosis *J Dermatol Surg Oncol 12:1114–1115, 1986*

Clear cell acanthoma, polypoid *J Dermatol 31:236–238, 2004*

Cutaneous horn

Dermatofibroma, atypical fibrous histiocytoma *Ann Diagn Pathol 7:370–373, 2003*

Epidermal nevus

Erythroplasia of Queyrat *Urol Clin NA 19:139–142, 1992*

HPV high grade dysplasia – hyperpigmented hyperkeratotic plaque of scrotum *JAMADerm 153:1332–1334, 2017*

Isolated epidermolytic acanthoma *AD 101:220–223, 1970*

Epidermoid cyst *Hinyokika Kiyo 44:683–685, 1998*

Extramammary Paget's disease – red plaque of scrotum *JAMADerm 153:689–693, 2017; JAAD 67:327–328, 2012; JAAD 65:656–657, 2011; JAAD 57:S43–45, 2007;* perigenital red nodules of scrotum and pubic region *Cutis 94:276–278, 2014*

Fibroma, including pendulous fibromas

Fibrosarcoma

Fibrous hamartoma of infancy *Ped Derm 15:326, 1998*

Folliculosebaceous cystic hamartoma – cobblestoned umbilicated nodules covering half of scrotum *BJD 157:833–835, 2007*

Giant cell fibroblastoma *Tumori 379:367–369, 1993*

Granular cell Schwannomas (multiple) – skin colored nodule *Ped Derm 25:341–343, 2008; Dermatol Online J 11:25, 2005; Arch Esp Urol 54:374–375, 2001; Arch Esp Urol 52:169–170, 1999; Cutis 63:77–80, 1999; Urol 45:332–334, 1995*

Kaposi's sarcoma *Int J Surg Case Rep 5:1986–1087, 2014*

Leiomyoma – pedunculated nodule *SKINmed 9:323–325, 2011; Urology 39:376–379, 1992; AD 125:417–422, 1989*

Leiomyosarcomas *Urol Clin NA 19:139–142, 1992; JAAD 20:290–292, 1989*

Leukemia–acute myelogenous leukemia *JAAD 21:410–413, 1989*

Lipoma *Arch Ital Urol Androl 89:243–244, 2017;* accessory scrotum and lipoma *Int J Health Sci (Qassim) 12:85–86, 2018; Ped Derm 29:522–524, 2012*

Liposarcoma *Urol Clin NA 19:139–142, 1992*

Lymphocytoma/lymphoma – testicular lymphoma–personal observation; primary cutaneous CD30+ lymphoma *J Dermatol 30:230–235, 2003;* primary cutaneous CD 8+ anaplastic large cell lymphoma *Eur J Dermatol 21:609–610, 2011*

Malignant mesothelioma–thick scrotum *Am J Dermatopathol 38:222–225, 2016; J Cut Pathol 10:213–216, 1983*

Melanocytic nevus

Melanoma *Urol Clinics NA 19:131–142, 1992*

Metastatic carcinoma–transitional cell carcinoma metastatic to scrotum demonstrating cobblestoned papules *AD 143:1067–1072, 2007;* rectal carcinoma; colon carcinoma *Dermatol Online J Jan 15, 2016;* prostate adenocarcinoma *J Cytol 32:121–123, 2015*

Multinucleate cell angiohistiocytoma–red to brown nodules *JAAD 30:417–422, 1994*

Neuroblastoma, metastatic – scrotal mass *J Pediatr Urol 7:495–497, 2011*

Perineurioma *Urology 60:515, 2002*

Sebaceous trichofolliculoma *Dermatologica 181:68–70, 1990*

Sebocystomas

Seborrheic keratosis

Calcifying Sertoli cell tumor in Peutz-Jegher's syndrome *Ped Derm 11:335–337, 1994*

Squamous cell carcinoma, including mule spinner's disease; squamous cell carcinoma in cotton textile workers *Am J Dermatopathol 37:5514, 2015; AD 121:370–372, 1985*

Superficial angiomyxoma – pink polypoid scrotal mass; may be associated with Carney complex *Ped Derm 28:200–201, 2011*

Sweat gland carcinosarcoma, primary *J Cutan Pathol 31:678–682, 2004*

Syringocystadenoma papilliferum *AD Syphilol 71:361–372, 1955*

Trichofolliculomas *Dermatologica 181:68–70, 1990*

Verrucous carcinoma (giant condylomata of Buschke and Lowenstein) *JAAD 23:723–727, 1990; Z Hautkr 58:1325–1327, 1983*

PRIMARY CUTANEOUS DISEASES

Atopic dermatitis

Erythema of Jacquet *Cutis 82:72–74, 2008*

Granuloma gluteale infantum *J Dermatol 40:1038–1041, 2013*

Hernia

Lichen myxedematosus–personal observation

Lichen planus

Lichen simplex chronicus *BJD 144:915–916, 2001*

Malakoplakia – red nodule *JAMADerm 153:1315–1316, 2017*

SYNDROMES

Angiokeratoma corporis diffusum

Dyskeratosis benigna intraepithelialis mucosae et cutis hereditaria – conjunctivitis, umbilicated keratotic nodules of scrotum, buttocks, trunk; palmoplantar verruca-like lesions, leukoplakia of buccal mucosa, hypertrophic gingivitis, tooth loss *J Cutan Pathol 5:105–115, 1978*

Gardner's syndrome

H syndrome (low height, heart, hallus valgus, hormonal, hypogonadism, hematologic) – autosomal recessive; sclerodermoid changes of middle and lower body with overlying hyperpigmentation sparing the knees and buttocks; starts on feet and legs and progresses upward; hypertrichosis, short stature, facial telangiectasia, ichthyosiform changes, gynecomastia, varicose veins, skeletal deformities (camptodactyly of 5th fingers), scrotal masses with massively edematous scrotum obscuring the penis, hypogonadism, micropenis, azospermia, sensorineural hearing loss, dilated scleral vessels, exophthalmos, cardiac anomalies, hepatosplenomegaly, mental retardation; mutation in nucleoside transporter Hent3 *JAAD 70:80–88, 2014; BJD 162:1132–1134, 2010; Ped Derm 27:65–68, 2010; JAAD 59:79–85, 2008*

Lipoid proteinosis *JAAD 39:149–171, 1998*

Neurofibromatosis

Steatocystoma multiplex

TOXINS

Chloracne – cysts *Clin Exp Dermatol 6:243–257, 1981*

TRAUMA

Posttraumatic spindle cell nodules *Arch Pathol Lab Med 118:709–711, 1994*

Scar

VASCULAR

Aggressive angiomyxoma–polypoid mass *JAAD 38:143–175, 1998*

Angiokeratoma corporis diffusum without metabolic abnormalities *AD 142:615–618, 2006*

Angiokeratoma of Fordyce

Angioma – unilateral with varicocoele *Scand J Urol 50:58–59, 2016*

Hemangioma *Urology 8:502–505, 1976*

Henoch-Schonlein purpura

Lymphangioma scroti – cobblestoned, furrowed scrotum; differentiate from hydrocele, hematocele, inguinal hernia, varicocele, spermatocele, dermoid cyst *Ped Derm 24:654–656, 2007*

Lymphatic malformation, microcystic of scrotum *JAMADerm 153:103–105, 2017*

PELVIS syndrome (may be part of urorectal septum malformation sequence) – macular telangiectatic patch; larger perineal hemangiomas, external genitalia malformations, including bifid scrotum, lipomyelomeningocele, vesicorenal abnormalities, imperforate anus, and skin tags *AD 142:884–888, 2006*

Pyogenic granuloma *Cutis 62:282, 1998*

Varix – varicoid tumor of scrotum, boys *J Urol 165:593–594, 2001*

Verrucous localized lymphedema of penis, scrotum, vulva, pubis, *JAAD 71:320–326, 2014*

SCROTAL ULCERATIONS

AUTOIMMUNE DISEASES AND DISEASES OF IMMUNE DYSFUNCTION

Allergic contact dermatitis

Juvenile dermatomyositis *BMJ Case Rep Jan 23, 2018; J Clin Rheumatol 26:e7–8, 2020*

Bullous pemphoid

Cicatricial pemphigiod–anti-laminin gamma 1 and anti-laminin 332 mucous membrane pemphigoid – lip erosions, nasal erosions, conjunctival erosions, scrotal ulcers *BJD 171:1257–1259, 2014*

Linear IgA disease

Pemphigus vulgaris

DRUG-INDUCED

All-trans retinoic acid – induction chemotherapy in acute promyelocytic leukemia *JAMADerm 153:1181–1182, 2017; JAAD 43:316–317, 2000; Clin Lab Haematol 22:171–174, 2000;* for acute promyelocytic leukemia *Cutis 91:246–247, 2013; Oman Medical J 28:207–209, 2013*

Capecitabine *Clin Colorectal Cancer 6:382–385, 2007*

Coumarin necrosis *JAAD 55:S50–53, 2006*

Linear IgA disease, drug-induced

Non-selective antiangiogenic multikinase inhibitors – sorafenib, sunitinib, pazopanib – hyperkeratotic hand foot skin reactions with knuckle papules, inflammatory reactions, alopecia, kinking of hair, depigmentation of hair; chloracne-like eruptions, erythema multiforme, toxic epidermal necrolysis, drug hypersensitivity, red scrotum with erosions, yellow skin, eruptive nevi, pyoderma gangrenosum-like lesions *JAAD 72:203–218, 2015*

EXOGENOUS AGENTS

Mustard gas exposure

INFECTIONS AND INFESTATIONS

Actinomycosis *J Urol 121:256, 1979*

AIDS–oral and scrotal ulcers of HIV–major aphthae

Amebiasis *J Cut Pathol 34:620–628, 2007; BJ Plast Surg 31:48, 1978; AD 24:1, 1931*

Anthrax *Ann Trop Ped 3:47, 1983*

Arthropod bite *JAAD 55:S50–53, 2006*

Bacillary angiomatosis

Brucella canis JAMA 598:172, 1978

Buruli ulcer *Prog Urol 15:736–738, 2005*

Candida–red bag

Cellulitis–personal observation

Chancroid *JAAD 55:S50–53, 2006*

Chikungunya fever – punctate or deep undermined ulcers *Indian J DV Leprol 74:383–384, 2008*

Chronic epidymo-orchitis and scrotal ulcers *BMJ Case Rep March 8, 2011*

Corynebacterium diphtheria – black necrotic ulcers of penis and scrotum *Indian J DV Leprol 74:187, 2008; Cutis 79:371–377, 2007*

renal transplant *J Cut Med Surg 20:567–569, 2016*

Corynebacterium urealyticum–necrotic scrotal ulcer *J Clin Inf Dis 22:851–852, 1996*

Cytomegalovirus

Ecthyma

Ecthyma gangrenosum *JAAD 55:S50–53, 2006*

Fournier's fulminating synergistic scrotal gangrene *Clin Inf Dis 40:990–996, 2005; JAAD 6:289–299, 1982; J R Soc Med 75:916–917, 1982; Am J Surg 129:591–596, 1975;* black necrotic scrotum and perineum *NEJM 376:1158*

Granuloma inguinale *AD 111:1464–1465, 1975*

Herpes simplex virus infection *JAAD 55:S50–53, 2006;* giant scrotal ulcer in immune reconstitution syndrome *JAAD 65:456–457, 2011;* multi-drug resistant *J Infect 80:232–254, 2020;* IRIS *JAAD 65:456–457, 2011*

Herpes zoster

Histoplasmosis

Human bite

Leishmaniasis *AD 130:1313, 1315–1316, 1994;* denudation of penis and scrotum in AIDS; punched out ulcers of penis and scrotum *BJD 160:311–318, 2009*

Meleney's synergistic gangrene

Mycobacterium haemophilum AD 138:229–230, 2002

Mycobacterium tuberculosis J Coll Phys Surg Pak 15:439–440, 2005; hematogenous disseminated tuberculosis – annular verrucous plaques of buttocks, scrotal ulcers, hyperkeratotic plaques of

sole *BMJ Case Rep Dec 19, 2018; Clin Inf Dis 49:1402–1404,1450–1451, 2009*

Onchocerciasis–calcified nodules

Pseudomonas sepsis–gangrenous scrotal ulcer in infants (noma neonatorum) *Lancet 2:289–291, 1978*

Rickettsial diseases

Salmonella (typhoid fever) *Trop Med Health 43:69–73, 2015*

Schistosomiasis – phagedenic ulceration

Serratia marcescens Int J Dermatol 56:e160–162, 2017; Eur J Dermatol 27:309–310, 2017

Snake bite *Br J Urol 47:334, 1975*

Spider bite

Staphylococcus aureus, methicillin-resistant *Int J STD AIDS 30:1229–1231, 2019; J Infects 1:e241–243, 2005*

Syphilis–primary, secondary, or tertiary (gumma)

INFILTRATIVE DISEASES

Langerhans cell histiocytosis in the adult – scrotal ulcer; solitary pink papule; red papules of trunk; ulceronecrotic plaque of scalp; perianal plaque; perianal dermatitis *BJD 167:1287–1294, 2012*

INFLAMMATORY DISEASES

Aphthae of HIV disease–personal observation

Crohn's disease *Scand J Urol Nephrol 38:436–437, 2004; Gut 11:18, 1970*

Fistulae
  Fecal *J Indian Med Assoc 73:192, 1979*
  Urethral *Urology 9:310, 1977*

Hidradenitis suppurativa *Ann Ital Chir 81:465–470, 2010; Med Gen Med 7:19, 2005*

Malakoplakia *JAAD 34:325–332, 1996*

Pyoderma gangrenosum *BJD 138:337–340, 1998; JAAD 34:1046–1060, 1996; AD 131:609–614, 1995; J Urol 144:984–986, 1990; Actas Urol Esp 9:263–266, 1985; J Urol 127:547, 1982;* Trisomy 8-myelodysplastic syndrome – scrotal ulcers, tongue ulcers *BJD 174:239–241, 2016*

Stevens-Johnson syndrome with Evans syndrome *J Clin Med Aug 22, 2018;* with trisomy MDS *BJD 174:239–241, 2016;* with Crohn's disease *Singapore Med J 50:e397–400, 2009*

Superficial granulomatous pyoderma *Acta DV 80:311–312, 2000*

METABOLIC

Acrodermatitis enteropathica

Calciphylaxia *Saudi J Kidney Dis Transpl 19:82–86, 2008*

Riboflavin deficiency (oculogenital syndrome)

NEOPLASTIC DISEASES

Basal cell carcinoma *JAMA 312:288–289, 2014; JAAD 26:574–578, 1992; J Urol 127:145, 1982*

Eccrine porocarcinoma *Can J Urol 12:2722, 2723, 2005*

Kaposi's sarcoma *Urology 9:686, 1977*

Leiomyoma *Urologe 38:370–371, 1999*

Leukemia cutis–acute myelogenous leukemia *Cutis 95:E18–20, 2015; JAAD 21:410–413, 1989;* acute promyelocytic leukemia *Mod Pathol 18:1569–1576, 2005*

Lymphoma – NK cell lymphoma *Am J Dermatopathol 20:582–585, 1998*

Malignant melanoma *Urology 71:1053–1054, 2008*

Metastatic carcinomas, including metastatic male breast carcinoma *JAAD 38:995–996, 1998*

Mesothelioma *Am J Dermatopathol 38:222–225, 2016*

Extramammary Paget's disease *Urol Oncol 28:28–33, 2010; Photodiagnosis Photodyn Ther 2:309–311, 2005*

Primary cutaneous mucinous carcinoma *Urol Ann 12:83–86, 2020*

Squamous cell carcinoma *J Urol 130:423, 1983; J Urol 108:760, 1972*

PARANEOPLASTIC DISEASES

Glucagonoma syndrome (necrolytic migratory erythema)–red scrotum *AD 121:389–404, 1985*

PRIMARY CUTANEOUS DISEASES

Erythema of Jacquet

Hailey-Hailey disease (benign familial pemphigus)

Hidradenitis suppurativa *J Urol 118:686, 1977*

Lichen planus, ulcerative *Cutis 79:37–40, 2007*

Lichen simplex chronicus

Pustular ulcerative dermatosis of the scalp with ulcerative scrotal lesions *J Dermatol 25:657–661, 1998*

PSYCHOCUTANEOUS DISEASES

Factitial dermatitis

Neurotic exoriations *Genital Skin Disorders, Fischer and Margesson, CV Mosby, 1998, p. 92*

SYNDROMES

Behcet's disease *JAAD 79:987–1006, 2018; BJD 159:555–560, 2008; BJD 157:901–906, 2007; JAAD 51:S83–87, 2004; JAAD 41:540–545, 1999; JAAD 40:1–18, 1999; NEJM 341:1284–1290, 1999; JAAD 36:689–696, 1997*

MAGIC syndrome – combination of relapsing polychondritis and Behcet's syndrome *AD 126:940–944, 1990*

Reactive arthritis

TRAUMA

Coma bullae

Giant inguinoscrotal ulcer *J Surg Case Rep Oct 1, 2010*

Human bite

Excoriations

Paraquat burn *J Tenn Med Assoc 72:109, 1979*

Mechanical trauma – zipper, etc *JAAD 55:S50–53, 2006*

Pressure ulcerations

Radiation necrosis

Voluminous unilateral hydrocele *Pan Afr Med J Aug 7, 2018*

VASCULAR DISEASES

Cholesterol emboli *BJD 150:1230–1232, 2004; SMJ 75:677, 1982*

Juvenile gangrenous vasculitis of the scrotum – necrotic ulcers of the scrotum *J Eur Acad DV 33:e459–461, 2019; JAAD 55:S50–53, 2006;*

Hemangioma *J Urol 160:182–183, 1998*

Henoch-Schonlein *JAAD 55:S50–53, 2006*

Small vessel vasculitis *JAAD 55:S50–53, 2006*

Weeping scrotum–cutaneous chylous reflux *AD 115:464–466, 1979*

SERPIGINOUS LESIONS

AUTOIMMUNE DISEASES AND DISEASES OF IMMUNE DYSFUNCTION

Allergic contact dermatitis – to temporary tattoo; to cashew apple *Cutis 92:174–176, 2013*

Bullous pemphigoid–IgA anti-p200 pemphigoid (p200 is laminin gamma 1) – blisters with serpiginous urticarial and annular plaques *AD 147:1306–1310, 2011;* mimicking erythema annulare centrifugum *Acta DV Croat 25:255–256, 2017*

Dermatitis herpetiformis *AD 126:527–532, 1990*

Epidermolysis bullosa acquisita

Fogo selvagem

Graft vs. host disease–serpiginous plaques–columnar epidermal necrosis in transfusion-associated chronic GVH *AD 136:743–746, 2000*

IgA pemphigus (intraepidermal IgA pustulosis)–vesiculopustules *JAAD 43:923–926, 2000*

Linear IgA disease–annular psoriasiform, serpiginous red plaques of palms *JAAD 51:S112–117, 2004*

Lupus erythematosus–neonatal lupus erythematosus *JAAD 29:848–852, 1993;* discoid lupus erythematosus; subacute cutaneous lupus erythematosus (erythema gyratum repens-like) *Ann DV 128:244–246, 2001; Dermatologica 173:146–149, 1986; SCLE AD 148:190–193, 2012;* SCLE in children – annular and polycyclic *Ped Derm 20:31–34, 2003;* lupus profundus – serpentine hypertrophy of scalp with deep ulcers *AD 147:1443–1448, 2011*

Morphea – "Addisonian keloid" *Case Rep Dermatol Med 2015:635481*

Pemphigus foliaceus of children – arcuate, circinate, polycyclic lesions *Ped Derm 36:236–241, 2019; JAAD 46:419–422, 2002; Ped Derm 3:459–463, 1986*

Pemphigus herpetiformis – concentric targetoid lesions; herpetiform lesions; serpiginous blisters *Ped Derm 30:760–762, 2013*

Pemphigus vegetans – serpiginous mucosal ulcers *Niger J Clin Pract 21:1238–1241, 2018*

Scleroderma–supravenous serpiginous hyperpigmentation *JAAD 11:265–268, 1984*

Serum sickness *NEJM 311:1407–1413, 1984*

Urticaria

CONGENITAL LESIONS

Median raphe cyst of the scrotum and perineum *JAAD 55:S114–115, 2006*

Neonatal skin markings

DRUG-INDUCED

Intra-articular corticosteroid injection – serpiginous hypopigmentation *Dermatol Online J April 15, 2017*

Docataxel recall after docataxel extravasation – annular serpiginous patch *AD 146:1190–1191, 2010*

Drug rash, serpiginous

5-fluorouracil serpentine hyperpigmentation *JAAD 71:203–214, 2014; JAAD 29:325–330, 1993; JAAD 25:905–908, 1991*

Lenalidomide – polycyclic pigmented purpuric eruption *JAAD 65:654–656, 2011*

Serpentine supravenous hyperpigmentation – 5-fluorouracil, vinorelbine, fotemustine, docataxel *NEJM 363:e8, 2010*

EXOGENOUS AGENTS

Coral dermatitis *JAMADerm 155:107, 2019; JAAD 52:534–535, 2005*

Cutaneous pili migrans (embedded hair) (migrating hair of plantar surface) (pili cuniculati) (creeping hair) – resembling cutaneous larva migrans *Ped Derm 27:628–630, 2010; Int J Derm 48:947–950, 2009; Clin Exp Dermatol 34:256–257, 2009; Dermatology 213:179–181, 2006; Ped Derm 21:612–613, 2004; BJD 144:219, 2001; BJD 93:349–351, 1975; AD 83:663, 1961; AD 76:254, 1957*

Pili migrans – linear and serpiginous red line of sole *Ped Derm 35:251–252, 2018*

Shiitake mushroom dermatitis

Tattoos

INFECTIONS AND INFESTATIONS

Amebiasis–serpiginous ulcer

Campylobacter – red, annular, and serpiginous plaques of lower leg in HIV+ patient *AD 142:1240–1241, 2006*

Chronic mucocutaneous candidiasis; candidiasis in cutaneous T-cell lymphoma *Ann DV 133:566–570, 2006*

Coccidioidomycosis

Coelenterate sting–recurrent eruptions following coelenterate envenomation *JAAD 17:86–92, 1987*

Cutaneous larva migrans–*Ancylostoma brasiliensis, A. caninum, Bunostomum phlebotomum, Uncinaria stenocephala, Gnathostoma spinigerum, Dirofilaria species, Strongyloides procyonis, S. stercoralis L. caninum, L.ceylonicum Cutis 95:126–128, 2015; JAMA 312:1458–1459, 2014; BJD 170:166–169, 2014; JAAD 70:961–963, 2014; Clin Inf Dis 53:167,205–206, 2011; AD 146:210–212, 2010; Cutis 82:239–240, 2008; Clin Inf Dis 31:493–498, 2000; Ped Derm 15:367–369, 1998; South Med J 89:609–611, 1996; Hautarzt 31:450–451, 1980*

Cytomegalovirus infections – ulcers of vulva and buttocks; serpiginous, morbilliform eruptions, petechiae, vesiculobullous lesions, hyperpigmented nodules, livedoid papules *JAMADerm 154:1217–1218, 2019; Dermatol Ther 23:533–540, 2010; Transpl Infect Dis 10:209–213, 2008; BJD 155:977–982, 2006; Dermatology 200:189–195, 2000*

Demodicidosis in childhood ALL–facial rash *J Pediatr 127:751–754, 1995*

Dracunculosis

Erysipelas

Fascioliasis *(Fasciola hepatica, F. gigantica)* – liver fluke; urticaria, jaundice, diarrhea, serpiginous tracts, subcutaneous nodules *JAAD 73:929–944, 2015; BJD 145:487–489, 2001;* vesicular end of serpiginous tract *Am J Trop Med Hyg 72:508–509, 2005*

Gnathostomiasis – cutaneous larva migrans *BJD 145:487–489, 2001*

Gongylonema pulchrum – nematode; migrating intraoral serpiginous tract of buccal mucosa, lower lip *Clin Inf Dis 32:1378–1380, 2001*

Granuloma inguinale – papule or nodule breaks down to form ulcer with overhanging edge; deep extension may occur; or serpiginous extension with vegetative hyperplasia; pubis, genitalia, perineum; extragenital lesions of nose and lips, or extremities *JAAD 54:559–578, 2006; JAAD 32:153–154, 1995; JAAD 11:433–437, 1984*

Herpes simplex – congenital herpes simplex – shawl-like giant erosion covering upper back; giant polycyclic erosive patches *JAAD 60:312–315, 2009*

Herpes zoster of S1 dermatome – long linear and serpiginous erythematous plaque of upper and lower leg *NEJM 370:2031, 2014*

HIV – persistent serpentine supravenous hyperpigmentation *Skin Med 11:93–94, 2013*

Jellyfish envenomation–serpiginous red plaque of wrist *JAMAADerm 156:348–350, 2020; Vet Hum Toxicol 43:203–205, 2001*

Larva currens *(Strongyloides) Clin Inf Dis 66:1636–1638, 2018; Dermatol Clin 7:275–290, 1989; AD 124:1826–1830, 1988*

Leprosy – lepromatous leprosy, reactional state *JAAD 68:879–881, 2013;* borderline leprosy – annular serpiginous plaques *JAMADerm 154:1076–1077, 2018;* Lucio's phenomenon – serpiginous polycyclic necrotic ulcers *J Clin and Aesthet Dermatol 12:35–38, 2019*

Loiasis – adult worm seen migrating through trunk, scalp, fingers, eyelids, tongue, penis, and conjunctivae *AD 108:835–836, 1973*

Lyme disease–personal observation of serpiginous lymphangitis and erythema chronicum migrans

Mycobacterium tuberculosis – scrofuloderma *JAAD 54:559–578, 2006;* tuberculosis verrucosa cutis; verrucous plaque of hand knees, ankles, buttocks; serpiginous outline with finger-like projections *Clin Exp Dermatol 13:211–220, 1988;* lupus vulgaris; starts as red-brown plaque, enlarges with serpiginous margin or as discoid plaques; apple-jelly nodules; vegetative linear serpiginous lesion of neck; plaque form – psoriasiform, irregular scarring, serpiginous margins *Ped Derm 36:955–957, 2019; Int J Dermatol 26:578–581, 1987; Acta Tuberc Scand 39(Suppl 49):1–137, 1960*

Myiasis causing creeping eruption (migratory myiasis); linear and serpiginous patches; *Gasterophilus intestinalis, Hypoderma spp. JAAD 75:19–30, 2016; JAAD 58:907–926, 2008*

North American blastomycosis – disseminated blastomycosis *Am Rev Resp Dis 120:911–938, 1979; Medicine 47:169–200, 1968*

Octopus tentacles – curvilinear lesions due to suction purpura *JAAD 61:733–750, 2009*

Oral hairy leukoplakia *Oral Dis 22 Suppl 1:120–127, 2016*

Paragonomiasis *BJD 145:487–489, 2001*

Portuguese man-of-war stings (*Physalis physalis*) – long curvilinear plaques *JAAD 61:733–750, 2009; J Emerg Med 10:71–77, 1992*

Pyomotes ventricosus dermatitis – mite of wood-boring beetle *Am J Trop Med Hyg 100:1041–1042, 2019*

Rheumatic fever – erythema marginatum–polycyclic pattern *Eur J Ped 162:655–657, 2003; JAAD 8:724–728, 1983; Ann Int Med 11:2223–2272, 1937–1938*

Scabies – serpiginous burrow; periaxillary, periareolar, abdomen, periumbilical, buttocks, thighs; scabies incognito – subcorneal pustules, ruptured, serpiginous *Rurkye Parazitol Derm 39:244–247, 2015*

Smallpox vaccination – with lymphangitis *Clin Inf Dis 37:241–250, 2003;* progressive vaccinia (vaccinia necrosum) *Clin Inf Dis 37:251–271, 2003*

Sparganosis (larvae of tapeworm) – serpiginous plaque *JAMADerm 152:831–832, 2016; BJD 145:487–489, 2001*

Streptococcal ulcers of the legs – serpiginous margins *AD 104:271–280, 1971*

Strongyloidiasis, hyperinfection – migratory, linear, serpiginous purpuric papules and plaques; aseptic meningitis *Clin Inf Dis 59:559,601–602, 2014; JAAD 70:113–1134, 2014;* anasarca, renal failure, serpiginous abdominal purpura *Clin Inf Dis 59:559, 601–602, 2014*

Syphilis – secondary- giant serpiginous lesion *An Bras Dermatol 93:590–591, 2018;,* late nodular, noduloulcerative lesions; tertiary *JAAD 24:832–835, 1991; AD 123:1707–1712, 1987;* lues tuber-ulcero-serpiginosa *Przegl Dermatol 53:419–423, 1966;* secondary syphilis mimicking tinea imbricate (atypical annular morphology) *Clin Inf Dis 51:929–930,980–982, 2010; JAAD 61:165–167, 2009;* painful shallow oral ulcers; may be serpiginous or as snail track ulcers *NEJM 362:740–748, 2010; Clinics (Sao Paulo) 61:161–166, 2006;* tertiary – tubero-ulcero-serpiginous syphilid *Dtsch Arztenl Int 115:750, 2018*

Tinea corporis treated with topical corticosteroids; generalized dermatophytosis; dermatophyte immune restoration inflammatory syndrome (IRIS) *Clin Inf Dis 40:113, 182–183, 2005*

Tinea faciei – treated with topical fluorinated corticosteroids

Tinea imbricata *Cutis 83:186–191, 2009*

Tinea versicolor

Trypanosomiasis

Wart

Yaws – serpiginous ulcers *Clin Dermatol 18:687–700, 2000*

INFILTRATIVE DISEASES

Amyloidosis, primary systemic *JAAD 15:379–382, 1986;* presenting as dilated veins *Am J Med 109:174–175, 2000;* lichen amyloidosis–personal observation

Diffuse cutaneous reticulohistiocytosis *AD 118:173–176, 1982*

Intralymphatic histiocytosis – linear and serpiginous (possibly paraneoplastic, associated with Merkel cell tumor, breast cancer, lung adenocarcinoma) *JAMADerm 155:960–961, 2019; Histopathol 24:265–268, 1994*

INFLAMMATORY DISORDERS

Eosinophilic fasciitis *Open Access Maced J Med Sci 7:2964–2968, 2019*

Erythema multiforme–personal observation

Hidradenitis suppurativa

Interstitial granulomatous dermatitis (interstitial granulomatous dermatitis with plaques, linear rheumatoid nodule, railway track dermatitis, linear granuloma annulare, palisaded neutrophilic granulomatous dermatitis) – tender red, linear, curvilinear, serpiginous plaques with arthritis; annular plaques, papules, linear erythematous cords (rope sign), urticarial lesions *JAMA Derm 149:609–614, 2013; JAAD 61:711–714, 2009; JAAD 47:319–320, 2002; JAAD 47:251–257, 2002; JAAD 46:892–899, 2002; JAAD 46:892–899, 2002; JAAD 45:286–291, 2001; JAAD 34:957–961, 1996; Dermatopathol Prac Concept 1:3–6, 1995*

Kawasaki's disease – polycyclic figurate erythema *Ped Derm 30:491–492, 2013*

Peristomal pyoderma gangrenosum – peristomal ulcer with serpiginous border *Digestion 85:295–301, 2012; J Crohn's Colitis Sep4, 2012; Int J Dermatol 29:129–133, 1990*

Pyostomatitis vegetans – oral serpiginous lesions; red swollen gingiva with serpiginous white tracking; association with ulcerative colitis and Crohn's disease *An Bras Dermatol 86:S137–140, 2011; Med Oral Patol Oral Cir Bucal 14:E114–117, 2009; Clin Exp Dermatol 29:1–7, 2004; JAAD 46:107–110, 2002*

Sarcoidosis *North Clin Istanb 1:114–116, 2014*

Sinus histiocytosis with massive lymphadenopathy (Rosai-Dorfman disease)

METABOLIC DISEASES

Cryoglobulinemia – scaly serpinous eythema with pustules and purpura of feet – pustular cryoglobulinemic vasculitis *AD 147:235–240, 2011*

Diabetes mellitus – migratory ichthyosiform dermatosis with type 2 diabetes mellitus and insulin resistance; polycyclic ichthyosiform rash *AD 135:1237–1242, 1999*

Fabry's disease–personal observation

Hereditary angioedema – prodromal serpiginous rash *BJD 161:1153–1158, 2009*

Hereditary LDH M-subunit deficiency–acroerythema *JAAD 27:262–263, 1992; JAAD 24:339–342, 1991*

Kwashiorkor–personal observation

Liver disease, chronic – telangiectasias

Necrobiosis lipoidica diabeticorum *Int J Derm 33:605–617, 1994; JAAD 18:530–537, 1988*

Necrolytic migratory erythema – recurrent seborrheic, serpiginous, annular papulosquamous eruptions; glucagonoma, chronic liver disease, inflammatory bowel disease, heroin abuse, pancreatitis, malabsorption syndromes *Int J Dermatol 49:24–29, 2010*

Pregnancy – lymphangiectasias–personal observation

Scurvy – coiled (corkscrew) hairs *AD 145:195–200, 2009; NEJM 357:392–400, 2007; AD 142:658, 2006; JAAD 41:895–906, 1999; JAAD 29:447–461, 1993; NEJM 314:892–902, 1986*

Uremia – serpiginous arterial calcification *Neurology 89:1530–1531, 2017*

Xanthomas–Type II hypercholesterolemia

Zinc deficiency – serpiginous crusted lesions of trunk *Ped Derm 35:255–256, 2018*

NEOPLASTIC DISEASES

Atrial myxoma, serpiginous lesions of distal finger pads *Cutis 62:275–280, 1998; Arthr Rheum 23:240–243, 1980*

Basal cell carcinoma–personal observation

Congenital smooth muscle hamartoma with livedo appearance – resembles cutis marmorata telangiectatica congenita with fibrotic appearance *Ped Derm 37:204–206, 2020*

Cutaneous horn

Disseminated superficial actinic porokeratosis *An Bras Dermatol 89:988–991, 2014*

Epidermal nevi – S-shaped in lines of Blaschko

Ganglion cyst of foot *JAAD 47:S266–267, 2002*

Inflammatory linear verrucous epidermal nevus–personal observation

Kaposi's sarcoma–personal observation

Keloid

Giant keratoacanthoma–serpiginous polycyclic border

Lymphoma–cutaneous T-cell lymphoma *JAAD Case Rep 1:82–84, 2015;*anaplastic large cell lymphoma *Cutis 60:211–214, 1997;* CD30+ anaplastic large cell lymphoma *BJD 157:1291–1293, 2007;* neoplastic angioendotheliosis *Nippon Hifuka Gakkai Zasshi 99:566–567, 1989;* Woringer-Kolopp disease *JAAD 55:276–284, 2006;* Hodgkin's disease *World J Clin Cases 7:2513–2518, 2019*

Metastatic cancer

Nevus marginatus – red plaque with surrounding hyperpigmented serpiginous verrucous margin; *HRAS* mutation *BJD 168:892–894, 2013*

Porokeratosis – of Mibelli *Cutis 72:391–393, 2003;* treated with topical corticosteroid *AD 136:1568–1569, 2000;* linear porokeratosis *Cutis 81:479–483, 2008;* porokeratosis ptychotropica – Blaschko-esque, serpiginous, annular, hyperpigmented verrucous plaques of intertriginoua areas and buttocks *Ped Derm 37:248–250, 2020; JAMA Derm 149:1099–1100, 2013; BJD 132:150–151, 1995*

Seborrheic keratoses, serpiginous *Indian J DV Leprol 78:775–776, 2012*

Woolly hair nevus–isolated woolly hair nevus, associated with epidermal nevus, keratosis pilaris atrophicans facei *XVI Congressus Internat Dermatol. Tokyo, 1982*; associated with Noonan's syndrome *BJD 100:409–416, 1979;* associated with cardiofaciocutaneous syndrome *JAAD 28:815–829, 1993*

PARANEOPLASTIC DISEASES

Erythema gyratum repens–seen with malignancy, benign breast hypertrophy, pulmonary tuberculosis, CREST syndrome, bullous pemphigoid, ichthyosis, palmoplantar hyperkeratosis, and pityriasis rubra pilaris *JAMADerm 156:912–2020; JAAD 54:745–762, 2006; JAAD 37:811–815, 1997; NEJM 380:e3, 2019; Int J Dermatol 58:408–415, 2019; JAAD 26:757–762, 1992; Am J Med Sci 2001;321 (5):302–305.doi.10.1097/00000441–200105000–00002; JAAD 26:757–762, 1992; J Eur Acad DV 28:112–115, 2012;* carcinoma of the breast *Arch Derm Syphilol 1952;66 (4);494–505. doi:10:1001/archderm 1952.01530290070010;*

Glucagonoma syndrome (necrolytic migratory erythema) – annular and serpiginous periorificial dermatitis with crusted papules, red tongue, brittle nails *Am J Dermatopathol 41:e29–32, 2019; JAMADerm 155:1180, 2019; Int J Dermatol 57:642–645, 2018; AD 148:385–390, 2012; Clin Exp Dermatol 36:161–164, 2012; J Eur Acad Dermatol 18:591–595, 2004; JAAD 21:1–30, 1989; AD 45:1069–1080, 1942*

Lymphoma – serpiginous, reticulated plaques due to cutaneous granulomas associated with systemic lymphoma *JAAD 51:600–605, 2004*

Necrobiotic xanthogranuloma with paraproteinemia

Paraneoplastic neutrophilic figurate erythema *BJD 156:396–398, 2007*

Acute varicocele – due to renal cancer; serpiginous varicose vein of scrotum *NEJM 374:2075, 2016*

PHOTODERMATOSES

Actinic granuloma

Annular elastolytic granuloma *Dermatol Online J April 16, 2015; BJD 160:1126–1128, 2009; JAAD 26:359–363, 1992*

Cutis rhomboidalis nuchae

Phytophotodermatitis from a plant (*Cneoridium dumosum*) *Cutis 54:400–402, 1994;* lime juice–personal observation

PRIMARY CUTANEOUS DISEASES

Acquired progressive kinking of hair *AD 125:252–255, 1989; AD 121:1031–1037, 1985*

Annular epidermolytic ichthyosis *JAAD 27:348–355, 1992*

Asteatotic dermatitis–personal observation

Atrophoderma vermiculatum – keratosis pilaris atrophicans; worm-eaten, reticular, or honeycomb atrophy *Cutis 83:83–86, 2009*

Blaschkitis–personal observation

Darier's disease – serpiginous plaques *JAAD 58:S116–118, 2008*

Elastosis perforans serpiginosa *JAAD 51:1–21, 2004; Hautarzt 43:640–644, 1992; AD 97:381–393, 1968;* folliculitis *J Derm 20:329–340, 1993*

Eosinophilic pustular folliculitis of Ofuji – circinate and serpiginous plaques with overlying papules and pustules in seborrheic areas; pustules are follicular *J Dermatol 16:388–391, 1989; Acta DV 50:195–203, 1970*

Epidermolysis bullosa pruriginosa – dominant dystrophic or recessive dystrophic; mild acral blistering at birth or early childhood; violaceous papular and nodular lesions in linear array on shins, forearms, trunk; lichenified hypertrophic and verrucous plaques in adults *BJD 146:267–274, 2002; BJD 130:617–625, 1994*

Epidermolysis bullosa simplex – migratory circinate erythema *Ped Derm 37:358–361, 2020*

Epidermolytic hyperkeratosis–personal observation

Erythema annulare centrifugum *Acta DV Croat 26:262–263, 2018*

Erythema cracquele (asteatotic dermatitis) *Cutis 83:75–76, 2009;*

Erythema dyschromicum perstans

Erythema elevatum diutinum – gyrate, serpiginous, annular lesions *BJD 67:121–145, 1955*

Erythema papulosa semicircularis recidivans – serpiginous annular eruption *JAMADerm 154:1340–1341, 2018; Eur J Dermtol 26:306–307, 2016; Dermatitis 23:44–47, 2012*

Erythrokeratoderma hiemalis (erythrokeratolysis hiemalis (Oudtshoorn disease)) – palmoplantar erythema, cyclical and centrifugal peeling of affected sites, targetoid lesions of the hands and feet; annular serpiginous lesions of lower legs, knees, thighs, upper arms, shoulders – seen in South African whites; precipitated by cold weather or fever *BJD 98:491–495, 1978*

Erythrokeratoderma variabilis *BJD 152:1143–1148, 2005; Ped Derm 19:510–512, 2002; AD 124:1271–1276, 1988;* with erythema gyratum repens-like lesions *Ped Derm 19:285–292, 2002*

Erythrokeratolysis–peeling skin syndrome

Geographic tongue

Granuloma annulare–personal observation

Harlequin fetus *Ped Derm 26:575–578, 2009*

Keratosis lichenoides chronica–in children *JAAD 56:S1–5, 2007*

Lichen planus–personal observation

Linear and whorled nevoid hypermelanosis

Mid-dermal elastolysis–personal observation

Necrolytic acral erythema – serpiginous, verrucous plaques of dorsal aspects of hands, legs; associated with hepatitis C infection *JAAD 50:S121–124, 2004*

Onychogryphosis *Cutis 68:233–235, 2001*

Parakeratosis variegate

Phylloid hypermelanosis – serpiginous hyperpigmentation with macrocephaly, frontal bossing, hypertelorism, internal strabismus, ear anomalies *Ped Derm 31504–506, 2014*

Pityriasis rubra pilaris–*JAAD 69:e32–e33, 2013;* familial pityriasis rubra pilaris with CARD14 mutation *BJD 179:969–972, 2018*

Progressive patterned scalp hypotrichosis – curly hair, thinning of parietal and vertex scalp, onycholysis, cleft lip and palate *JID Symp Proc 8:121–125, 2003*

Progressive symmetric erythrokeratoderma *JAAD 34:858–859, 1996*

Psoriasis, including erythema gyratum repens-like psoriasis *Int J Derm 39:695–697, 2000;* erythema gyratum repens in patient with psoriasis treated with acetretin *J Drugs Dermatol 3:314–316, 2003;* palatal psoriasis *J Can Dent Assoc 66:80–82, 2000;* pustular psoriasis–personal observation

Resolving pityriasis rubra pilaris resembling erythema gyratum repens *AD 129:917–918, 1993*

Ridgeback anomaly of scalp hair *AD 125:98–102, 1989*

Sebopsoriasis–personal observation

Seborrheic dermatitis

Spongiotic dermatitis–personal observation

Striae

Subcorneal pustular dermatosis of Sneddon-Wilkinson – pustules which expand to annular and serpiginous lesions with scaly edge; heal with hyperpigmentation *Ped Derm 20:57–59, 2003; BJD 145:852–854, 2001; J Dermatol 27:669–672, 2000; Cutis 61:203–208, 1998; JAAD 19:854–858, 1988; BJD 68:385–394, 1956*

Terra firme

Urticaria–personal observation

Urticaria multiforme – annular, serpiginous, urticarial lesions; edema of hands, feet, face *NEJM 375:470, 2016*

Vitiligo – serpiginous papulosquamous variant of inflammatory vitiligo *Dermatology 200:270–274, 2000;* overlying varicose veins

SYNDROMES

Acantholytic ectodermal dysplasia (similar to McGrath syndrome) – curly hair, palmoplantar keratoderma, skin fragility, hyperkeratotic fissured plaques with perioral involvement, red fissured lips, nail dystrophy *BJD 160:868–874, 2009*

Ankyloblepharon-nail dysplasia syndrome – curly hair *Birth Defects Original Article Ser 7:100–102, 1971*

Antiphospholipid antibody syndrome – unmasked by sclerotherapy with extensive thrombosis of treated superficial veins *BJD 146:527–528, 2002*

Ataxia telangiectasia

Carney complex – non-blanching annular and serpiginous macules of digital pads *JAAD 46:161–183, 2002*

Cardiofaciocutaneous syndrome

Carvajal syndrome

Carvajal-like syndrome–blisters, woolly hair, palmoplantar kertoderma, cardiac abnormalities; heterozygotes of *DSP* (desmoplakin) *BJD 166:894–896, 2012; Clin Genet 80:50–58, 2011; J Cutan Pathol 36:553–559, 2009*

CHAND syndrome – curly hair, ankyloblepharon, and nail dysplasia; ataxia *JAAD 59:1–22, 2008*

Costello syndrome – sparse curly hair, short stature, coarse facies, lax skin of hands and feet, nasal and perioral papillomata; risk of development of rhabdomyosarcoma, neuroblastoma, transitional cell carcinoma; HRAS mutations *JAAD 59:1–22, 2008; JAAD 32:904–907, 1995*

Down's syndrome – elastosis perforans serpiginoss Ehlers-Danlos syndrome type IV (vascular type) – elastosis perforans serpiginosa *JAMADerm 153:595–596, 2017*

Epidermal nevus syndrome *Dermatol Online J Sept 15, 2010*

Hereditary angioedema – prodrome of non-pruritic serpiginous eruption (erythema marginatum-like); other prodromes include tingling fatigue, asthenia, and discomfort *NEJM 382:1136–1148, 2020; Ped Derm 30:94–96, 2013*; triad of circumscribed edema of the skin, laryngeal edema, and abdominal pain *BJD 161:1153–1158, 2009; Sybert's Genetic Skin Disorders; Hosp TID No.40.1 rk 4:741–747, 1886; Monatsschr Prakt Dermatol 1:129–131, 1882*

Hypomelanosis of Ito

Incontinentia pigmenti

Keratosis-ichthyosis-deafness (KID) syndrome – reticulated severe diffuse hyperkeratosis of palms and soles, well marginated, serpiginous erythematous verrucous plaques, perioral furrows, leukoplakia, sensory deafness, photophobia with vascularizing keratitis, blindness *AD 117:285–289, 1981*

Lipoatrophic diabetes – curly hair *JAAD 59:1–22, 2008*

Macrocephaly-CMTC (cutis marmorata telangiectatica congenita syndrome) – macrocephalic neonatal hypotonia and developmental delay; distended linear and serpiginous abdominal wall veins, patchy reticulated vascular stain without atrophy; telangiectasias of face and ears; midline facial nevus flammeus, hydrocephalus, skin and joint hypermobility, polydactyly, 2–3 toe syndactyly, frontal bossing, hemihypertrophy with segmental overgrowth *JAAD 58:697–702, 2008; Ped Derm 24:555–556, 2007; JAAD 56:541–564, 2007* (Note: Beckwith-Wiedemann syndrome demonstrates dysmorphic ears, macroglossia, body asymmetry, midfacial vascular stains, visceromegaly with omphalocele, neonatal hypoglycemia, BUT NO MACROCEPHALY)

Netherton's syndrome – serpiginous papulosquamous ichthyosiform eruption, ichthyosis linearis circumflexa *JAMADerm 156:350–351, 2020; JAMADerm 152:435–442, 2016; AD 146:57–62, 2010; BJD 159:744–746, 2008; Ped Derm 25:253–254, 2008; AD 136:875–880, 2000; Ped Derm 13:183–199, 1996*

Noonan's syndrome – autosomal dominant; curly hair or woolly hair; dysmorphic facies, ear, eye, and cardiovascular anomalies, nevi, short stature, keratosis pilaris atrophicans, webbed neck; gain of function mutation in PTPN11 (encodes SHP-2 tyrosine phosphatase) *JAAD 59:1–22, 2008*

Pseudoglucagonoma syndrome – periorificial erythema, crusted migratory plaques, hair loss, brittle nails, poor weight gain, onycholysis; associated with cirrhosis, celiac disease inflammatory bowel disease, small cell lung cancers *Am J Med 126:387–389, 2013; Int J Derm 49:24–29, 2010*

Pseudoglucagonoma syndrome with alcoholic liver disease *AD 138:405–410, 2002;* with chronic liver disease, chronic pancreatitis, traumatic necrotizing pancreatitis, celiac disease, jejunal adenocarcinoma *AD 115:1429–1432, 1979*

Pseudoxanthoma elasticum–elastosis perforans serpiginosa with PXE; cutis laxa-like marked wrinkling with serpiginous streak *J Dermatol 36:288–292, 2009*

Reactive arthritis syndrome *JAAD 59:113–121, 2008*

Treacher-Collins syndrome with reactive perforating collagenosis *JAAD 36:982–983, 1997*

Tricho-odonto osseous syndrome – autosomal dominant; diffuse curly hair at birth, enamel hypoplasia, widely spaced teeth, otosclerosis, dolichocephaly, frontal bossing; mutation in *DLX3* (homeobox gene) *JAAD 59:1–22, 2008; Am J Med Genet 72:197–204, 1997*

Tumor necrosis factor (TNF) receptor 1-associated periodic fever syndromes (TRAPS) (same as familial hibernian fever, autosomal dominant periodic fever with amyloidosis, and benign autosomal dominant familial periodic fever) – Still's disease-like eruption with erythematous patches, tender red plaques, fever, annular, generalized serpiginous, polycyclic, reticulated, and migratory patches and plaques (migrating from proximal to distal), urticaria-like lesions, centrifugal migratory red patch overlying myalgia, red cheeks, morbilliform exanthems; lesions resolving with ecchymoses, conjunctivitis, periorbital edema, myalgia, arthralgia, abdominal pain, headache; Irish and Scottish predominance; mutation in tumor necrosis factor receptor superfamily 1A (*TNFRSF1A* gene)–gene encoding 55kDa TNF receptor *BJD 161:968–970, 2009; Medicine 81:349–368, 2002; Netherlands Journal of Medicine 59:118–125, 2001; AD 136:1487–1494, 2000; Mayo Clin Proc 62:1095–1100, 1987*

Uncombable hair syndrome (spun glass hair syndrome)

Wells' syndrome – blaschkolinear purpura *J Drugs Dermatol 16:1036–1038, 2017*

Winchester syndrome – annular and serpiginous thickenings of skin; arthropathy, gargoyle-like face, gingival hypertrophy, macroglossia, osteolysis (multilayered symmetric restrictive banding), generalized hypertrichosis, very short stature, thickening and stiffness of skin with annular and serpiginous thickenings of skin, multiple subcutaneous nodules *JAAD 50:S53–56, 2004*

Woolly hair, alopecia, premature loss of teeth, nail dystrophy, reticulate acral hyperkeratosis, facial abnormalities *BJD 145:157–161, 2001*

TRAUMA

Babinski sign, cutaneous

Cauliflower ears

Heel sticks – scarring

Lightning injury

Radiation dermatitis

Radiation-induced pemphigus foliaceus of the breast *JAAD 54:S251–252, 2006*

Surgical grounding plate burn–personal observation

VASCULAR

Angioma serpiginosum – red or purple punctae within background of erythema; serpiginous pattern *Ital J Ped 27:53, 2019; JAAD 37:887–920, 1997; AD 92:613–620, 1965*

Arteriovenous fistulae – congenital or acquired; red pulsating nodules with overlying telangiectasia and distal serpiginous varicosities of an extremity or trunk

Atrophie blanche (livedoid vasculopathy) *Stat Pearls Nov 4, 2019; JAAD 69:1033–1042, 2013*

Blue rubber bleb nevus *AD 129:1505–1510, 1993*

Capillary malformation in segmental distribution – central atrophy; serpiginous; geographic *JAAD 83:213–214, 2020*

Caput medusae – portal obstruction; hepatic vein thrombosis *QJM 112:231, 2019; Ann Int Med 62:133–161, 1965*

Diffuse dermal angiomatosis – serpiginous red plaque *AD 148:1411–1416, 2012*

Emboli – from cardiac myxomas; violaceous annular and serpiginous lesions *BJD 147:379–382, 2002*

Klippel-Trenaunay syndrome–personal observation

Lipodermatosclerosis with ankle flare – serpiginous vascular accentuation along the lower ankle and lateral foot

Lymphedema of abdomen in pregnancy *JAAD 12:930–932, 1985*

Lymphangiectasias

Lymphoangioendothelioma, benign serpiginous mass *J Cut Pathol 42:217–221, 2015*

Mondor's disease – periphlebitis of the chest wall *NEJM 352:1024, 2005; Ga Ox, Ong Yi Xue Ke Za Zhi 8:231–235, 1992*

Net-like superficial vascular malformation (lymphatic malformation); deep red, purple, or red-brown *BJD 175:191–193, 2016*

Nevus anemicus–personal observation

Non-venereal sclerosing lymphangitis of the penis *JAAD 49:916–918, 2003; Urology 127:987–988, 1982; BJD 104:607–695, 1981; Derm Z 78:24–27, 1938; Munchn Med Wschr 70:1167–1168, 1923*

Parkes-Weber syndrome – hypertrophy with pulasatile dilated veins and arteries, palpable thrill, giant arteriovenous malformation *NEJM 371:2114, 2014*

Pressure-induced vasodilatation from jeans mimicking Lichtenberg figures (lightning strike) *Ped Derm 31:522–523, 2014*

Subclavian vein occlusion–personal observation

Sunburst varicosities and telangiectasia *J Derm Surg Oncol 15:184–190, 1989*

Superficial thrombophlebitis

Superior vena cava syndrome – garland sign *Int J Med 103:707, 2010*

Telangiectasia

Temporal arteritis (giant cell arteritis)–personal observation of serpiginous palpable temporal artery

Urticarial vasculitis, including urticarial vasculitis associated with mixed cryoglobulins, hepatitis B or C infection, IgA multiple myeloma, infectious mononucleosis, monoclonal IgM gammopathy (Schnitzler's syndrome), fluoxetine ingestion, metastatic testicular teratoma, serum sickness, Sjogren's syndrome, systemic lupus erythematous *JAAD 38:899–905, 1998; Medicine 74:24–41, 1995; JAAD 26:441–448, 1992*

Varicosities *NEJM 355:488–498, 2006; Br Med J 300:763–764, 1990*

Vasculitis – leukocytoclastic vasculitis presenting as gyrate erythema *JAAD 47:S254–256, 2002*

Venous stasis

Verrucous hemangioma *J Cutan Pathol 38:740–746, 2011; Ped Derm 17:213–217, 2000*

Volkmann ischemic contracture – cutaneous ulcer with white necrosis of forearm in newborn; serpiginous border; muscle necrosis and nerve palsy due to increased intracompartmental pressure from amniotic band, oligohydramnios, or abnormal fetal position; begins as large bulla *Ped Derm 37:207–208, 2020*

    Differential diagnosis includes:
        Aplasia cutis congenita
        Protein C or S deficiency with disseminated intravascular coagulation
        Neonatal ecthyma gangrenosum from bacterial infection
        Aspergillosis
        Varicella zoster virus infection

SHORT STATURE

AUTOIMMUNE DISEASES AND DISORDERS OF IMMUNE DYSFUNCTION

Adenine deaminase deficiency – autosomal recessive; disproportionate short stature; short limb skeletal dysplasia type 1 (bowed femurs) *Am J Med Genet 66:378–398, 1996*

Chronic granulomatous disease – short stature, low weight *Ped Derm 21:646–651, 2004*

Hyper IgE syndrome – papular, pustular, excoriated dermatitis of scalp, buttocks, neck, axillae, groin; furunculosis; growth failure *Clin Exp Dermatol 11:403–408, 1986; Medicine 62:195–208, 1983*

Periodic fever, immunodeficiency, and thrombocytopenia – severe oral ulcers leading to scarring and microstomy; fever, poor growth, infections, thrombocytopenia *Ped Derm 33:602–614, 2016*

SCID with microcephaly, growth retardation, and sensitivity to radiation syndrome *BJD 178:335–349, 2018*

STAT5b deficiency – dwarfism, facial dysmorphism, high pitched voice *BJD 178:335–349, 2018*

CONGENITAL DISORDERS

Hydrocephalus *J Pediatr Endocrinol Metab 9:181–187, 1996*

Intrauterine growth restriction *NEJM 368:1220–1228, 2013*

DRUGS

Corticosteroid therapy *NEJM 368:1220–1228, 2013*

Stimulants therapy *NEJM 368:1220–1228, 2013*

Coumarin embryopathy *Atlas of Clinical Syndromes A Visual Aid to Diagnosis, 1992, pp.224–225*

Cri du chat syndrome *Atlas of Clinical Syndromes A Visual Aid to Diagnosis, 1992, pp.92–93*

Fetal hydantoin syndrome – short stature, hypertrichosis, hypoplastic distal phalanges *JAAD 46:161–183, 2002*

EXOGENOUS AGENTS

Stimulants therapy *NEJM 368:1220–1228, 2013*

INFILTRATIVE DISORDERS

Langerhans cell histiocytosis – growth hormone deficiency due to hypothalamic involvement *NEJM 292:332–333, 1975*

METABOLIC DISORDERS

Acrodermatitis enteropathica or acquired zinc deficiency – stunted growth in infant with vesiculobullous dermatitis of hands, feet, periorificial areas *Ped Derm 19:426–431, 2002; AD 116:562–564, 1980; Acta DV (Stockh) 17:513–546, 1936*

Celiac disease *JAMA 311:1787–1796, 2014; NEJM 368:1220–1228, 2013*

Chronic diseases (diabetes mellitus, renal, cardiac, pulmonary, hematologic) and increased caloric requirements (hyperthyroidism, diencephalic syndrome, neuroectodermal tumors) *JAMA 311:1787–1796, 2014;* mild chronic disease *NEJM 368:1220–1228, 2013*

Congenital dyserythropoietic anemia type I – small or absent nails; partial absence or shortening of fingers and toes, mesoaxial polydactyly, syndactyly of hands and feet; short stature, verterbral abnormalities and Madelung deformity; mutation in *CDAN1 Clin Exp Dermatol 515–517, 2020*

Congenital erythropoietic porphyria *Ped Derm 20:498–501, 2003*

Constitutional delay of growth and puberty – most common cause of delayed puberty *JAMA 311:1787–1796, 2014; NEJM 366:443–453, 2012*

Cushing's syndrome *NEJM 368:1220–1228, 2013;* glucocorticoid excess *JAMA 311:1787–1796, 2014*

Diabetes mellitus *JAMA 311:1787–1796, 2014*

DNA ligase I deficiency – short stature, photosensitivity *Am J Med Genet 66:378–398, 1996*

Failure to thrive *NEJM 368:1220–1228, 2013*

Familial hypophosphatemic rickets *Atlas of Clinical Syndromes A Visual Aid to Diagnosis, 1992, pp.254–255*

Fanconi's anemia – autosomal recessive; short stature; dyschromatosis with café au lait macules, guttate hypopigmentation, intertriginous hyperpigmentation, endocrine abnormalities with hypothyroidism, decreased growth hormone, diabetes mellitus, café au lait macules, diffuse hyperpigmented macules, guttate hypopigmented macules, intertriginous hyperpigmentation, skeletal anomalies (thumb hypoplasia, absent thumbs, radii, carpal bones), oral/genital erythroplasia and leukoplakia with development of squamous cell carcinoma, hepatic tumors, microphthalmia, ectopic or horseshoe kidney, broad nose, epicanthal folds, micrognathia, bone marrow failure, acute myelogenous leukemia, solid organ malignancies (brain tumors, Wilms' tumor) *Ped Derm 36:725–727, 2019; NEJM 370:2229–2236, 2014; BJD 164:245–256, 2011; JAAD 54:1056–1059, 2006*

Fucosidosis – red papules, purpura, short stature *Ped Derm 24:442–443, 2007*

Glycogen storage disease type I *Atlas of Clinical Syndromes A Visual Aid to Diagnosis, 1992, pp.110–111*

Growth hormone deficiency *JAMA 311:1787–1796, 2014; NEJM 368:1220–1228, 2013*

Hereditary Vitamin D-resistant rickets – autosomal recessive; normal hair at birth; alopecia, growth failure, developmental delay *Ped Derm 31:519–520, 2014*

Hunter's syndrome – decreased sulfoiduronate sulfatase *JAAD 48:161–179, 2003; Ped Derm 15:370–373, 1998*

Hurler's syndrome *JAAD 48:161–179, 2003; Syndromes of the Head and Neck p. 100, 1990*

Hurler-Schei syndrome *Syndromes of the Head and Neck p. 105, 1990*

Hypogonadism *NEJM 368:1220–1228, 2013*

Hypopituitarism – hypopituitary dwarf; hairless

Hypothyroidism *JAMA 311:1787–1796, 2014; NEJM 368:1220–1228, 2013*

Inflammatory bowel disease *JAMA 311:1787–1796, 2014; NEJM 368:1220–1228, 2013*

Iron deficiency in infants and children – retarded growth

Malabsorption (celiac disease, inflammatory bowel disease) *JAMA 311:1787–1796, 2014*

Nutritional deficiency *JAMA 311:1787–1796, 2014*

Mucolipidosis *Atlas of Clinical Syndromes A Visual Aid to Diagnosis, 1992, pp.134–135*

Phosphoglucomutase 1 deficiency – autosomal recessive; disorder of glycosylation with impaired glycoprotein production; liver dysfunction, bifid uvula, malignant hyperthermia, hypogonadotropic hypogonadism, growth retardation, hypoglycemia, myopathy, dilated cardiomyopathy, cardiac arrest *NEJM 370:533–542, 2014*

Pituitary dwarfism

Porphyria–congenital erythropoietic porphyria *Semin Liver Dis 2:154–63, 1982*

Progressive osseous heteroplasia

Prolidase deficiency – autosomal recessive; peptidase D mutation (PEPD); increased urinary imidopeptides; leg ulcers, anogenital ulcers, short stature (mild), telangiectasias, recurrent infections (sinusitis, otitis); mental retardation; splenomegaly with enlarged abdomen, atrophic scarring, dermatitis, hyperkeratosis of elbows and knees, low hairline, poliosis, canities, lymphedema, photosensitivity, hypertelorism, saddle nose deformity, frontal bossing, dull expression, mild ptosis, micrognathia, mandibular protrusion, exophthalmos, joint laxity, deafness, osteoporosis, high arched palate *JAAD 62:1031, 1034, 2010*

Sanfilippo syndrome (mucopolysaccharidosis type III) *JAAD 48:161–179, 2003;*

Atlas of Clinical Syndromes A Visual Aid to Diagnosis, 1992, pp.124–125

Starvation *JAMA 311:1787–1796, 2014*

Trichothiodystrophy – with *ERCC2* mutation (excision repair) – matted twisted hair with ichthyosis; collodion baby, neutropenia and hypogammaglobulinemia, poor growth *Ped Derm 36:668–671, 2019*

Variegate porphyria–homozygous variegate porphyria – erosions, photosensitivity, short stature *BJD 144:866–869, 2001*

Weight loss or more pronounced decline in weight gain than in linear growth *JAMA 311:1787–1796, 2014*

Zinc deficiency, endemic *Am J Clin Nutr 30:833–834, 1977; Arch Int Med 111:407–428, 1963*

PARANEOPLASTIC DISORDERS

Neutrophilic panniculitis of myelodysplasia – red nodules of legs and soles; *MYSM1* deficiency; short stature *Ped Derm 36:258–259, 2019*

PRIMARY CUTANEOUS DISEASES

Atopic dermatitis

Cutis laxa *J Med Genet 24:556–561, 1987*

Cutis laxa type II – autosomal recessive; facial dysmorphism with all the changes of wrinkly skin syndrome; pre and postnatal growth retardation, delayed motor development, delayed closure of large fontanelle, congenital hip dislocation, bone dysplasias, parallel strips of redundant skin of back *Ped Derm 23:225–230, 2006; Ped Derm 21:167–170, 2004*

Darier's disease

Epidermolysis bullosa, recessive dystrophic *Ped Derm 19:436–438, 2002*

Ichthyosis – rarely severe in infants due to failure to thrive *Ichthyosis Focus 23:1,4, 2004*

PSYCHOCUTANEOUS DISORDERS

Anorexia nervosa *JAMA 311:1787–1796, 2014*

SYNDROMES

Aagenaes syndrome (hereditary cholestasis with lymphedema) – autosomal recessive; lymphedema of legs due to congenital lymphatic hypoplasia; pruritus, growth retardation

Aarskog syndrome (facio-digito-genital syndrome) – X-linked recessive – anteverted nostrils, long philtrum, broad nasal bridge; short broad hands with syndactyly, scrotal shawl (scrotal fold which surrounds the base of the penis); skeletal defects; learning disabilities *Am J Med Genet 46:501–509, 1993; Am J Ophthalmol 109:450–456, 1990; Am J Med Genet 15:39–46, 1983; Hum Genet 42:129–135, 1978; J Pediatr 77:856–861, 1970*

Abruzzo-Erickson syndrome (cleft palate, eye coloboma, short stature, hypospadias) *J Med Genet 14:76–80, 1977*

Achondrogenesis *Atlas of Clinical Syndromes A Visual Aid to Diagnosis, 1992, pp.212–213*

Achondroplasia *Syndromes of the Head and Neck p. 171–175, 1990*

Acraniofacial dysostosis *Am J Med Genet 29:95–106, 1988*

Acrodystosis *Atlas of Clinical Syndromes A Visual Aid to Diagnosis, 1992, pp.190–191*

Acrogeria (Gottron's syndrome) – micrognathia, atrophy of tip of nose, atrophic skin of distal extremities with telangiectasia, easy bruising, mottled pigmentation or poikiloderma of extremities, dystrophic nails *BJD 103:213–223, 1980*

Acromesomelic dysplasia *Birth Defects 10:137–146, 1974*

Acroosteolysis (Hajdu-Cheney syndrome) *J Periodontol 55:224–229, 1984*

Adams-Oliver syndrome – autosomal dominant; terminal transverse limb anomalies, aplasia cutis congenita, cutis marmorata telangiectatica congenita, severe growth retardation, aplasia cutis congenita of knee, short palpebral fissures, dilated scalp veins, simple pinnae, skin tags on toes, hemangioma, undescended testes, supernumerary nipples, hypoplastic optic nerve, congenital heart defects *Ped Derm 24:651–653, 2007*

Aganglionic megacolon and cleft lip/palate *J Craniofac Genet Dev Biol 1:185–189, 1981*

Alagille syndrome – xanthomas of palmar creases, extensor fingers, nape of neck; growth retardation, delayed puberty *Ped Derm 22:11–14, 2005*

Albright's hereditary osteodystrophy (pseudohypoparathyroidism) – atrophic pink patches of neck with striations containing white papules (subcutaneous ossification); white papules of trunk and ear;

dry, rough keratotic puffy skin; short stature, obesity, frontal bossing, depressed nasal bridge; brachydactyly with dimples over 4th and 5th metacarpal bones; mutation in *GNAS1* gene *JAMA Derm 149:975–976, 2013; Ped Derm 28:135–137, 2011; BJD 162:690–694, 2010; Ergeb Inn Med Kinderheilkd 42:191–221, 1979; Endocrinology 30:922–932, 1942*

Angelman syndrome – short stature, unusual facies, severe mental retardation, spasticity, seizures; paternal uniparental isodisomy *Ped Derm 22: 482–487, 2005*

Ataxia telangiectasia – non-infectious cutaneous granulomas present as papules or nodules, red plaques with atrophy or ulceration; telangiectasias of bulbar conjunctivae, tip of nose, ears, antecubital and popliteal fossae, dorsal hands and feet; atrophy with mottled hypo- and hyperpigmentation, dermatomal CALMs, photosensitivity, canities, acanthosis nigricans, dermatitis; humoral and cellular immunodeficiency, lymphoreticular malignancy, growth retardation; *ATM* gene (phosphotidylinisitol-3'kinase) *JAAD 56:541–564, 2007; AD 134:1145–1150, 1998; JAAD 10:431–438, 1984; Ann Int Med 99:367–379, 1983*

Autosomal recessive blepharophimosis, ptosis, V-esotropia, syndactyly, and short stature *Clin Genet 41:57–61, 1992*

Ballard-Gerold syndrome – poikiloderma, craniosynostosis, radial ray defects, patellar and palatal abnormalities, dislocated joints, diarrhea, short stature, slender nose, normal intellect *RECQL4* mutations *JAAD 75:855–870, 2016; Soc Ped Dermatol Annual Meeting, 2006*

Barber-Say syndrome – autosomal dominant, X-linked *JAAD 48:161–179, 2003*

Bardet-Biedl syndrome *Atlas of Clinical Syndromes A Visual Aid to Diagnosis, 1992, pp.288–289*

Begeer syndrome – cataracts, deafness, short stature, ataxia, polyneuropathy *Clin Dysmorphol 4:283–288, 1995*

Berlin syndrome – no vellus hairs; mottled pigmentation and leukoderma, flat saddle nose, thick lips, fine wrinkling around the eyes and mouth (similar to Christ-Siemens ectodermal dysplasia); stunted growth, bird-like legs, mental retardation *Dermatologica 123:227–243, 1961*

Bloom's syndrome (congenital telangiectatic erythema and stunted growth) – autosomal recessive; blisters of nose and cheeks; slender face, prominent nose; facial telangiectatic erythema with involvement of eyelids, ear, hand and forearms; bulbar conjunctival telangiectasias; stunted growth; CALMs, clinodactyly, syndactyly, congenital heart disease, annular pancreas, high-pitched voice, testicular atrophy; no neurologic deficits *JAAD 75:855–870, 2016; Ped Derm 22:147–150, 2005; Curr Prob Derm 14:41–70, 2002; Ped Derm 14:120–124, 1997; JAAD 17:479–488, 1987; AD 114:755–760, 1978; Clin Genet 12:85–96, 1977; Am J Hum Genet 21:196–227, 1969; Am J Dis Child 116:409–413, 1968; AD 94:687–694, 1966; Am J Dis Child 88:754–758, 1954*

Bone dysplasia *NEJM 368:1220–1228, 2013*

Borrone dermatocardioskeletal syndrome – autosomal recessive or X-linked; gingival hypertrophy, coarse facies, late eruption of teeth, loss of teeth, thick skin, acne conglobata, osteolysis, large joint flexion contractures, short stature, brachydactyly, camptodactyly, mitral valve prolapse, congestive heart failure *Ped Derm 18:534–536, 2001*

Brachman-de Lange syndrome *Atlas of Clinical Syndromes A Visual Aid to Diagnosis, 1992, pp.182–183*

Braegger syndrome – proportionate short stature, IUGR, ischiadic hypoplasia, renal dysfunction, craniofacial anomalies, postaxial polydactyly, hypospadias, microcephaly, mental retardation *Am J Med Genet 66:378–398, 1996*

Buschke-Ollendorf syndrome – with or without precocious puberty; mutation in *LEMD3* (LEM domain-containing protein 3 gene) *BJD 174:723–729, 2016; Ped Derm 11:31–34, 1994; AD 106:208–214, 1972*

Camptomelic dysplasia *Atlas of Clinical Syndromes A Visual Aid to Diagnosis, 1992, pp.232–233*

Cardio-facio-cutaneous syndrome – autosomal dominant, xerosis/ichthyosis, eczematous dermatitis, alopecia, growth failure, hyperkeratotic papules, ulerythema ophryogenes (decreased or absent eyebrows), seborrheic dermatitis, CALMs, nevi, hemangiomas, keratosis pilaris, patchy or widespread ichthyosiform eruption, sparse curly scalp hair and sparse eyebrows and lashes, congenital lymphedema of the hands, redundant skin of the hands, short stature, abnormal facies with macrocephaly, broad forehead, bitemporal narrowing, hypoplasia of supraorbital ridges, short nose with depressed nasal bridge, high arched palate, low set posteriorly rotated ears with prominent helices, cardiac defects; gain of function sporadic missense mutations in *BRAF, KRAS, MEK1,* or *MEK2, MAP2K1/MAP2K2 BJD 163:881–884, 2010; Ped Derm 27:274–278, 2010; Ped Derm 17:231–234, 2000; JAAD 28:815–819, 1993; AD 129:46–47, 1993; JAAD 22:920–922, 1990;* port wine stain *Clin Genet 42:206–209, 1992; Eur J Pediatr 150:486–488, 1991; JAAD 22:920–922, 1990*

Cartilage-hair hypoplasia (metaphyseal chondrodysplasia of McKusick) (disproportionate short stature; short limb skeletal dysplasia) – autosomal recessive; short limb dwarfism, mild leg bowing with short limbs, short sparse, lightly colored hair; soft doughy skin, small dystrophic fingernails; some with total baldness, immune defects; mutation in mitochondrial RNA processing; endoribonuclease; 9p13 *JAAD 54:S8–10, 2006; Am J Med Genet 66:378–398, 1996; Eur J Pediatr 155:286–290, 1996; Eur J Pediatr 142:211–217, 1993; Am J Med Genet 41:371–380, 1991; Bull Johns Hopkins Hosp 116:285–326, 1965*

Catel-Schwartz-Jampel syndrome *Atlas of Clinical Syndromes A Visual Aid to Diagnosis, 1992, pp.508–509*

Chanarin-Dorfman disease – neutral lipid storage disease; ABHD5 mutation; a necessary cofactor for adipose triglyceride lipase-mediated lipolysis; hyperkeratosis of the knees; hepatomegaly, ataxia, neurosensory hearing loss, cataracts, nystagmus, short stature, leukocytes with lipid vacuoles *BJD 158:1378–1380, 2008*

CHARGE syndrome – short stature, coloboma of the eye, heart anomalies, choanal atresia, somatic and mental retardation, genitourinary abnormalities, ear anomalies, primary lymphedema *Ped Derm 20:247–248, 2003*

CHILD syndrome – X-linked dominant; linear hyperkeratosis with brownish scaling of fingers and toes *AD 142:348–351, 2006;* linear hyperkeratotic plaques of feet (unilateral inflammatory ichthyosiform nevus) with spontaneous involution; strawberry-like papillomatous lesions of toes; macrodactyly; ptychotropism, shortening and absence of limbs, short stature; ipsilateral involvement of bones, lung, kidney, heart, brain; epiphyseal stippling (chondrodysplasia punctata); short stature, scoliosis, clefting of hand or foot, hexadactyly; lateralization and mutations in *NSDHL* gene which encodes 3-beta hydroxysteroid dehydrogenase *JAAD 63:1–22, 2010; BJD 161:714–715, 2009*

Chondrodysplasia punctata, rhizomelic type – autosomal recessive *Atlas of Clinical Syndromes A Visual Aid to Diagnosis, 1992, pp.220221*

CHOPS syndrome – coarse facies, heart defects, obesity, pulmonary involvement, short stature, long eyelashes, synophrys *Am J Med Genet 179:1126–1138, 2019*

Chronic infantile neurological cutaneous articular syndrome (CINCA) (Neonatal onset multisystem inflammatory disorder

(NOMID)) – urticarial rash at birth, arthropathy, uveitis, mental retardation, short stature *AD 136:431–433, 2000; Eur J Ped 156:624–626, 1997; Scand J Rheumatol Suppl 66:57–68, 1987; J Pediatr 99:79–83, 1981*

Conradi-Hunermann syndrome – X-linked dominant ichthyosis; mutation in gene encoding 8- 7 sterol isomerase; collodion baby or generalized ichthyosiform erythroderma; Blaschko erythroderma and scaling; palmoplantar keratoderma; follicular atrophoderma and cicatricial alopecia in adults; short stature; asymmetric shortening of limbs; chondrodysplasia punctata, cataracts *Eur J Dermatol 10:425–428, 2000; Hum Genet 53:65–73, 1979*

Cleft lip-palate, posterior keratoconus, short stature, mental retardation, genitourinary anomalies *J Med Genet 19:332–336, 1982*

Cleft lip-palate and pituitary dysfunction *Syndromes of the Head and Neck p. 781, 1990*

Cleft palate, macular coloboma, short stature, skeletal abnormalities *Br J Ophthalmol 53:346–349, 1969*

Cleft palate, microcephaly, large ears, short stature (Say syndrome) *Humangenetik 26:267–269, 1975*

Cleft palate and sensorineural hearing loss *Helv Paediatr Acta 38:267–280, 1983*

Cleidocranial dysplasia *Syndromes of the Head and Neck p. 249–253, 1990*

Cockayne syndrome – xerosis with rough, dry skin, anhidrosis, erythema of hands, hypogonadism; autosomal recessive; short stature, facial erythema in butterfly distribution leading to mottled pigmentation and atrophic scars, premature aged appearance with loss of subcutaneous fat and sunken eyes, canities, mental deficiency, photosensitivity, disproportionately large hands, feet, and ears, ocular defects including retinal degeneration, demyelination *JAMA Derm 149:1414–1418, 2013; Ped Derm 20:538–540, 2003; Am J Hum Genet 50:677–689, 1992; J Med Genet 18:288–293, 1981;* birdheaded dwarfism

Cohen syndrome *Atlas of Clinical Syndromes A Visual Aid to Diagnosis, 1992, pp.290–291*

Coffin-Lowry syndrome – X-linked inheritance; straight coarse hair, prominent forehead, prominent supraorbital ridges, hypertelorism, large nose with broad base, thick lips with mouth held open, large hands, tapering fingers, severe mental retardation; loose skin easily stretched, cutis marmorata, dependent acrocyanosis, varicose veins *Clin Genet 34:230–245, 1988; Am J Dis Child 112:205–213, 1966*

Congenital cataracts, sensorineural deafness, hypogonadism, hypertrichosis, gingival hyperplasia, short stature *Clin Dysmorphol 4:283–288, 1995*

Congenital disorders of glycosylation (CDG-IIc) (Rambam-Hasharon syndrome) – GDP-L-fucose AKA leukocyte adhesion deficiency type 2 (LAD 2); localized cellulitis, neurologic abnormalities, distinctive facies, short stature *Ped Derm 22:457–460, 2005*

Congenital ichythyosis, hypogonadism, small stature, facial dysmorphism, scoliosis, and myogenic dystrophy *Ann Genet 42:45–50, 1999*

Congenital ichthyosis, retinitis pigmentosa, hypergonadotropic hypogonadism, small stature, mental retardation, cranial dysmorphism, abnormal electroencephalogram *Ophthalmic Genet 19:69–79, 1998*

Constitutional delay of growth and puberty ("late bloomer") *JAMA 311:1787–1796, 2014; NEJM 368:1220–1228, 2013*

Conradi-Hunermann syndrome–X-linked dominant ichthyosis (Happle's syndrome) – chondrodysplasia punctata, ichthyosis, cataract syndrome; collodion baby or ichthyosiform erythroderma; linear and whorled hyperkeratosis with Blaschko pattern of erythroderma and scaling; plantar hyperkeratosis; resolves with time to reveal swirls of fine scale, linear hyperpigmentation, follicular atrophoderma of arms and legs, cicatricial alopecia; skeletal defects with short stature severe autosomal rhizomelic type; X-linked recessive variant; mutation in emopamil binding protein (EBP) *JAAD 63:607–641, 2010; BJD 160:1335–1337, 2009;* chondrodysplasia punctata, X-linked recessive–with ichthyosis *Ped Derm 18:442–444, 2001;* rhizomelic form *Syndromes of the Head and Neck p. 190–191, 1990*

Cornelia de Lange (Brachmann-de Lange) syndrome – generalized hypertrichosis, confluent eyebrows, low hairline, hairy forehead and ears, hair whorls of trunk, single palmar crease, cutis marmorata, psychomotor and growth retardation with short stature, specific facies, hypertrichosis of forehead, face, back, shoulders, and extremities, bushy arched eyebrows with synophrys; long delicate eyelashes, skin around eyes and nose with bluish tinge, small nose with depressed root, prominent philtrum, thin upper lip with crescent shaped mouth, widely spaced, sparse teeth, hypertrichosis of forehead, posterior neck, and arms, low set ears, arched palate, antimongoloid palpebrae; congenital eyelashes *Ped Derm 24:421–423, 2007; JAAD 37:295–297, 1997; Am J Med Genet 47:959–964, 1993*

Corneodermatoosseous syndrome – autosomal dominant; premature birth; diffuse PPK; photophobia, corneal dystrophy, distal onycholysis, brachydactyly, short stature, medullary narrowing of digits, dental decay *Curr Prob Derm 14:71–116, 2002; Am J Med Genet 18:67–77, 1984*

Costello syndrome – failure to thrive; linear deep palmar creases; warty papules around nose and mouth, legs, perianal skin; coarse facial features, hypotonia, loose skin of neck, hands, and feet; acanthosis nigricans; low set protuberant ears, thick palmoplantar surfaces, gingival hyperplasia, hypoplastic nails, moderately short stature, craniofacial abnormalities, hyperextensible fingers, tight Achilles tendon, curly or fine sparse curly hair, perianal and vulvar papules, diffuse hyperpigmentation, generalized hypertrichosis, multiple nevi; rhabdomyosarcoma, neuroblastoma, transitional cell carcinoma of the bladder *BJD 164:245–256, 2011; Ped Derm 20:447–450, 2003; Am J Med Genet 82:187–193, 1999; JAAD 32:904–907, 1995; Am J Med Genet 47:176–183, 1993; Am J Med Genet 41:346–349, 1991; Aust Paediat J 13:114–118, 1977*

Cross-McKusick-Breen syndrome (oculocerebral syndrome with hypopigmentation) – autosomal recessive; albino-like hypopigmentation, silver-gray hair, gingival fibromatosis, microphthalmos, opaque cornea, nystagmus, spasticity, athetosis, mental retardation; post-natal growth retardation *Ped Derm 18:534–536, 2001; J Pediatr 70:398–406, 1967*

DeBarsy syndrome – autosomal recessive progeroid syndrome; cutis laxa with psychomotor retardation, cloudy corneas, mental retardation, athetoid movements, synophrys, pinched nose, thin skin, sparse hair, large malformed ears, thin lips; growth retardation *Eur J Pediatr 144:348–354, 1985*

Depigmented hypertrichosis with dilated follicular pores, short stature, scoliosis, short broad feet, dysmorphic facies, supernumery nipple, and mental retardation (cerebral-ocular malformations) *BJD 142:1204–1207, 2000*

DeSanctis-Cacchione syndrome – dwarfism, gonadal hypoplasia, mental deficiency, microcephaly, xeroderma pigmentosum

Diastrophic dysplasia – cystic ear during hemorrhagic phase; calcifies *J Bone Jt Surg 50A:113–118, 1968*

Disproportionate short stature; trunk is longer in comparison with limbs: *JAMA 311:1787–1796, 2014*
    Skeletal dysplasias

SHOX gene mutations
Spinal radiation

Distal aphalangia, syndactyly, extra metatarsal, short stature, microcephaly, borderline intelligence – autosomal dominant *Am J Med Genet 55:213–216, 1995*

Donahue syndrome (leprechaunism) – congenital insulin resistance; dwarfism; elfin-like face, large eyes, thick lips, low set ears, less subcutaneous fat, excessive folding of skin *Pediatr 83:18, 1994; AD 117: 531–535, 1981*

Down's syndrome – short stature, cutis marmorata, acrocyanosis, low-set, small ears *JAAD 46:161–183, 2002; Syndromes of the Head and Neck p. 35, 1990*

Dubowitz syndrome – autosomal recessive, microcephaly, sloping forehead, telecanthus, erythema and scaling of face and extremities in infancy, ichthyosiform eruption, sparse blond scalp and arched eyebrow hair, dysplastic low set ear pinnae, high pitched hoarse voice, delayed eruption of teeth, growth retardation, craniofacial abnormalities; syndactyly, cryptorchidism, hypospadius, developmental delay, transitory short stature, hyperactive behavior, blepharophimosis, ptosis of the eyelids, epicanthal folds, broad nose, palate anomalies, micrognathia, and severe atopic dermatitis *Ped Derm 22:480–481, 2005; Am J Med Genet 63:277–289, 1996; Clin Exp Dermatol 19:425–427, 1994; Am J Med Genet 47:959–964, 1993; Eur J Pediatr 144:574–578, 1986; Am J Med Genet 4:345–347, 1979; J Med Genet 2:12–17, 1965*

Dwarfism-alopecia-pseudoanodontia- cutis laxa; autosomal recessive; generalized atrichia, unerupted teeth, hyperconvex nails, cutis laxa with fragile skin, dwarfism, deafness, eye anomalies *Cien Cult 34(Suppl): 705, 1982*

Dwarfism, bilateral club feet, premature aging, progressive panhypogammaglobulinemia *J Rheumatol 21:961–963, 1994*

Dyggve-Melchior-Clausen syndrome – short trunk dwarfism and mental retardation *Clin Genet 14:24–30, 1978*

Dyschondrosteosis *Atlas of Clinical Syndromes A Visual Aid to Diagnosis, 1992, pp.202–203*

Dyschromatosis universalis hereditaria – mottled hyperpigmentation, small stature, high tone deafness *Ped Derm 24:566–570, 2007; Semin Cut Med Surg 16:72–80, 1997; Clin Exp Derm 2:45, 1977*

Dyskeratosis congenita *JAAD 77:1194–1196, 2017; J Blood Med 5:157–167, 2014; Br J Haematol 145:164–172, 2009; Semin Cut Med Surg 16:72–80, 1997*

Dysosteosclerosis – oligodontia *Birth Defects 11:349–351, 1975*

Ectodermal dysplasia/skin fragility syndrome – autosomal recessive (Carvajal-Huerta syndrome); skin peeling; generalized erythema and peeling at birth; very short stature, superficial skin fragility with crusts of face, knees, alopecia of scalp and eyebrows, perioral hyperkeratosis with fissuring and cheilitis, thick dystrophic cracking finger- and toenail dystrophy, keratotic plaques on limbs, diffuse or focal striate palmoplantar keratoderma with painful fissuring; *PKP1* gene (encoding plakophilin 1) or *DSP* (encoding desmoplakin); follicular hyperkeratosis of knees; woolly hair; perianal erythema and erosions; cardiomyopathy associated with mutation in desmoplakin not with plakophilin *BJD 160: 692–697, 2009; JAAD 55:157–161, 2006; Acta DV 85:394–399, 2005; JID 122:1321–1324, 2004; Curr Prob Derm 14:71–116, 2002; Hum Molec Genet 9:2761–2766, 2000; Hum Molec Genet 8:143–148, 1999*

Ectodermal dysplasia with sparse hair, short stature, hypoplastic thumbs, single upper incisor, and abnormal skin pigmentation *Am J Clin Genet 29:209–216, 1988*

Ehlers-Danlos syndrome type VII (arthrochalasis multiplex congenita) *J Med Genet 24:698–701, 1987; J Bone Jt Surg 40:663, 1958;* type IV

Ellis-van Creveld syndrome (chondroplastic dwarf with defective teeth and nails, and polydactyly) (chondroectodermal dysplasia) – autosomal recessive; very short stature; chondrodysplasia, ectodermal dysplasia with ulnar polydactyly, cone- and peg-shaped teeth or hypodontia, enamel hypoplasia, fused incisors, molars with extra cusps, dental fissures and pits, neonatal teeth, malocclusion; short upper lip bound down by multiple labiogingival frenulae; gingival hypertrophy, nail dystrophy, hair may be normal or sparse and brittle; cardiac defects; ichthyosis, palmoplantar keratoderma; asymmetric distal limb shortening; short distal phalanges with small dystrophic fingernails; congenital heart disease; hypospadias, cryptorchidism; mutations in EVC and EVC2 *Cutis 83;303–305, 2009; Ped Derm 18:485–489, 2001; J Med Genet 17:349–356, 1980; Arch Dis Child 15:65–84, 1940*

Familial dysautonomia (Riley-Day syndrome) (hereditary sensory and autonomic neuropathy type III) – delayed growth *AD 89:190–195, 1964*

Familial eosinophilic cellulitis, short stature, dysmorphic habitus, and mental retardation–bullae, vesicles, and red plaques *JAAD 38:919–928, 1998*

Familial partial lipodystrophy, mandibuloacral dysplasia variety – autosomal recessive; short stature, high pitched voice, mandibular and clavicular hypoplasia, dental anomalies, acro-osteolysis, stiff joints, cutaneous atrophy, alopecia, nail dysplasia *Am J Med 108:143–152, 2000*

Familial short stature *JAMA 311:1787–1796, 2014; NEJM 368:1220–1228, 2013*

Femoral hypoplasia-unusual facies syndrome *J Pediatr 86:107–111, 1975*

Fibrochondrogenesis *Atlas of Clinical Syndromes A Visual Aid to Diagnosis, 1992, pp.242–243*

Filippi syndrome – characteristic facies, polydactyly, syndactyly, microcephaly, growth retardation, and mental retardation *Am J Med Genet 87:128–133, 1999; Genet Couns 4:147–151, 1993*

Fleisher syndrome – X-linked, proportionate short stature, hypogammaglobulinemia, isolated growth hormone deficiency *Am J Med Genet 66:378–398, 1996*

Frydman syndrome – autosomal recessive; prognathism, syndactyly, short stature, blepharophimosis, weakness of extraocular and frontal muscles, synophrys *Clin Genet 41:57–61, 1992*

GAPO syndrome–growth retardation, alopecia, pseudoanodontia, and progressive optic atrophy; midface hypoplasia; frontal bossing, wide anterior fontanelle, saddle nose, protruding thick lips, low set ears, anti-Mongoloid slant, diffuse scalp hypotrichosis, prominent scalp veins, sparse eyebrows and eyelashes, absent teeth, slightly redundant skin, impacted teeth *Ped Derm 27:156–161, 2010; Ped Derm 19:226, 2002; J Craniofac Genet Dev Biol 19:189–200, 1999; Birth Defects 24:205–207, 1988; Am J Med Genet 19:209–216, 1984; Syndr Ident 8:14–16, 1982; Odont Tilster 55:484–493, 1947*

Geleophysic dysplasia *Am J Med Genet 19:483–486, 1984*

GEMSS syndrome (glaucoma, lens ectopia, microspherophakia (small, spherical lens)–autosomal dominant; glaucoma, lens ectopia, microspherophakia, stiff joints, shortness, gingival hypertrophy, flexion contractures of joints, osteolytic defects, stunted growth, stocky pseudoathletic build, cutaneous sclerosis of upper back and extremities *AD 131:1170–1174, 1995; Am J Med Genet 44:48–51, 1992*

Geroderma osteodysplastica (Bamatter syndrome) (osteodysplastic geroderma) – autosomal recessive; short stature, cutis laxa-like changes with drooping eyelids and jowls (sad characteristic facies), osteoporosis and skeletal abnormalities; lax wrinkled, atrophic skin and hyperextensible joints, osteoporosis, growth retardation *Ped Derm 25:66–71, 2008; Ped Derm 23:467–472, 2006; Ped Derm 16:113–117, 1999; Am J Med Genet 3:389–395, 1979; Hum Genet 40:311–324, 1978; J Genet Hum 17:137–178, 1969; Ann Paediatr 176:126–127, 1950*

Gingival fibromatosis, hypertrichosis, cherubism, mental and somatic retardation, and epilepsy (Ramon syndrome) *Am J Med Genet 25:433–442, 1986*

Goltz's syndrome (focal dermal hypoplasia) *Atlas of Clinical Syndromes A Visual Aid to Diagnosis, 1992, pp.334–335*

Gorlin-Chaudhry-Moss syndrome – short and stocky with craniosynostosis, midface hypoplasia, hypertrichosis of the scalp, arms, legs, and back, anomalies of the eyes, digits, teeth, and heart, and genitalia hypoplasia *Am J Med Genet 44:518–522, 1992*

H syndrome – autosomal recessive; coarse facies, orbital swelling, proptosis, facial telangiectasias; flexion contractures of fingers and toes, sclerodermoid changes of middle and lower body with overlying hyperpigmentation sparing the knees and buttocks; hypertrichosis, short stature, gynecomastia, camptodactyly of 5th fingers, scrotal masses with massively edematous scrotum obscuring the penis, hypogonadism, azospermia, sensorineural hearing loss, cardiac anomalies, hepatosplenomegaly; Arabic Palestinian population; gluteal lipoatrophy; hyperpigmentation, sensorineural hearing loss, diabetes mellitus, lymphadenopathy, heart anomalies, micropenis, hallus valgus, hyperpigmentation induration and hypertrichosis of inner thighs and shins (sclerodermoid), chronic diarrhea, anemia, dilated lateral scleral vessels, episcleritis, exophthalmos, eyelid swelling, varicose veins, chronic rhinitis, renal abnormalities, bone lesions (osteoporosis), arthritis, arthralgia; scrotal masses with massively edematous scrotum obscuring the penis, hypogonadism, azospermia, hallux valgus, hyperglycemia, hepatosplenomegaly; mutation in nucleoside transporter Hent3 (*SLC29A3*) *JAAD 70;80–88, 2014; BJD 162:1132–1134, 2010; Ped Derm 27:65–68, 2010; JAAD 59:79–85, 2008;* faci *BJD 162:1132–1134, 2010; Ped Derm 27:65–68, 2010; JAAD 59:79–85, 2008*

> Differential diagnostic considerations include:
>   Winchester syndrome – arthropathy, coarse facies, no hearing loss
>   POEMS syndrome–paraproteinemia

Hajdu-Cheney syndrome (acroosteolysis) – dissolution of the terminal phalanges, abnormally shaped skull, premature loss of teeth, short stature; thick scalp and eyebrow hair with synophrys; hypertrichosis and hyperelastic skin *Int J Oral Surg 14:113–125, 1985; J Periodontol 55:224–229, 1984; Am J Med 65:627–636, 1978; J Pediatr 88:243–249, 1976*

Hallermann-Streiff syndrome – partial anodontia, short stature, atrophy and telangiectasia of central face, parrot-like appearance, microphthalmia, cataracts, high-arched palate, small mouth, sutural alopecia pinched beak nose, extraordinary retrognathia, parrot-like appearance, frontal and/or occipital bossing, atrophy of skin especially of nose, proportionate dwarfism, microphthalmos, cataracts, sparse eyebrows and eyelashes *Clin Exp Dermatol 29:477–479, 2004; JAAD 50:644, 2004; Birth Defects 18:595–619, 1982*

Hennekam syndrome – autosomal recessive; intestinal lymphangiectasia, lymphedema of legs and genitalia, gigantic scrotum and penis, multilobulated lymphatic ectasias, small mouth, narrow palate, gingival hypertrophy, tooth anomalies, thick lips, agenesis of ear, pre-auricular pits, wide flat nasal bridge, frontal upsweep, platybasia, hypertelorism, pterygia colli, hirsutism, bilateral single palmar crease, mild mental retardation, facial anomalies, growth retardation, pulmonary, cardiac, hypogammaglobulinemia *JAAD*

56:353–370, 2007; Ped Derm 23:239–242, 2006; Am J Med Genet 34:593–600, 1989

Hoyeraal-Hreidarsson syndrome – reticulate

hyperpigmentation (resembles dyskeratosis congenita), growth retardation, microcephaly, mental retardation, cerebellar malformation, progressive bone marrow failure, and mucocutaneous lesions *J Pediatr 136:390–393, 2000*

Hunter's syndrome – reticulated 2–10mm skin colored papules over scapulae, chest, neck, arms; X-linked recessive; MPS type II; iduronate-2 sulfatase deficiency; lysosomal accumulation of heparin sulfate and dermatan sulfate; short stature, full lips, coarse facies, macroglossia, clear corneas (unlike Hurler's syndrome), progressive neurodegeneration, communicating hydrocephalus, valvular and ischemic heart disease, lower respiratory tract infections, adenotonsillar hypertrophy, otitis media, obstructive sleep apnea, diarrhea, hepatosplenomegaly, skeletal deformities (dysostosis multiplex), widely spaced teeth, dolichocephaly, deafness, retinal degeneration, inguinal and umbilical hernias *Ped Derm 21:679–681, 2004;* macrocephaly

Hurler's syndrome (mucopolysaccharidosis type I-H)– disorder of glycosaminoglycans accumulation; autosomal recessive; coarse facies, macroglossia, short stature, macrocephaly, hepatosplenomegaly, hernias, corneal clouding, vision and hearing loss; cardiac anomalies; respiratory infections; alpha-I-iduronate deficiency *Ped Derm 33:594–601, 2016*

Hurst syndrome – short stature, hypertonia, unusual facies, mental retardation, hemolytic anemia, delayed puberty *Am J Med Genet 29:107–115, 1988; Am J Med Genet 28:965–970, 1987*

Hutchinson-Gilford syndrome (progeria)–loss of subcutaneous tissue, hyper- and hypomelanosis, alopecia, mid-facial cyanosis around mouth and nasolabial folds, decreased sweating, sclerodermoid changes, cobblestoning of soft pebbly nodules *Am J Med Genet 82:242–248, 1999*

Hypertelorism-microtia-clefting syndrome (Bixler syndrome) *J Med Genet 387—388, 1982*

Hypertrichosis cubiti (hairy elbow) *JAAD 48:161–179, 2003; Clin Exp Dermatol 24:497–498, 1999; Clin Exp Dermatol 19:86–87, 1994; J Med Genet 26:382–385, 1989;* with facial asymmetry *Am J Med Genet 53:56–58, 1994*

Hypochondrodysplasia – acanthosis nigracans, short stature, frontal bossing, high forehead, prognathism, thick lips, large broad hands *Ped Derm 27:664–666, 2010; J Bone Jt Surg 51A:728–736, 1969*

Hypohidrotic ectodermal dysplasia

Hypoplastic anemia with triphalangeal thumbs *Atlas of Clinical Syndromes A Visual Aid to Diagnosis, 1992, pp.436–437*

Ichthyosis follicularis with atrichia and photophobia (IFAP) *Am J Med Genet 85:365–368, 1999; Med Genet 44:233–236, 1992*

Immuno-osseous dysplasia – short-limbed dwarfism, immunodeficiency, hypotonia, sparse scalp hair, bullae, facial dyschromatosis (mottled hyper- and hypopigmentation) *Ped Derm 23:373–377, 2006*

Incontinentia pigmenti *JAAD 47:169–187, 2002*

Infantile systemic hyalinosis – autosomal recessive; synophrys, thickened skin, perianal nodules, dusky red plaques of buttocks, gingival hypertrophy, joint contractures, juxta-articular nodules (knuckle pads), osteopenia, growth failure, diarrhea, frequent infections, facial red papules; mutation in CMG2 (capillary morphogenesis protein 2) *JAAD 58:303–307, 2008; JAAD 50:S61–64, 2004*

Keratitis-ichthyosis-deafness (KID) syndrome – postnatal growth deficiency in 50% of the cases *AD 115:467–471, 1979; AD 113:1701–1704, 1977*

Johanson-Blizzard syndrome–aplasia cutis congenita of the scalp, sparse hair, deafness, absence of permanent tooth buds, hypoplastic ala nasi, dwarfism, microcephaly, mental retardation, hypotonia, pancreatic insufficiency with malabsorption, hypothyroidism, genital and rectal anomalies *Clin Genet 14:247–250, 1978; J Pediatr 79:982–987, 1971*

Juvenile hyaline fibromatosis (infantile systemic hyalinosis) – nodular perianal lesions, ears, lips, gingival hypertrophy, hyperpigmentation, flexion contractures of joints, osteolytic defects, stunted growth *JAAD 55:1036–143, 2006; Dermatology 190:148–151, 1995; Ped Derm 11:52–60, 1994*

Kabuki makeup syndrome (Niikawa-Kuroki syndrome) – short stature, congenital heart defects, distinct expressionless face (frontal bossing, long palpebral fissures, eversion of the lower eyelids, sparse arched lateral eyebrows, epicanthus, telecanthus, prominent eyelashes, short flat nose with anteversion of the tip, short philtrum, large mouth with thick lips, high arched palate, cleft palate, dental malocclusion, micrognathia, large protuberant low set ears with thick helix), lowcut hairline, vitiligo, cutis laxa, hyperextensible joints, syndactyly of toes 2–3, brachydactyly, clinodactyly, fetal finger pads with abnormal dermatoglyphics, short great toes, blue sclerae, lower lip pits, cryptorchidism, mental retardation with microcephaly; preauricular dimple/fistula mutation in *MLL2 Ped Derm 30:253–255, 2013; Ped Derm 24:309–312, 2007; JAAD S247–251, 2005; Am J Med Genet 132A:260–262, 2005; Am J Med Genet 94:170–173, 2000; Am J Med Genet 31:565–589, 1988; J Pediatr 105:849–850, 1984; J Pediatr 99:565–569, 570–573, 1981*

Kearns-Sayre syndrome *Atlas of Clinical Syndromes A Visual Aid to Diagnosis, 1992, pp.500–501*

Kenny syndrome (tubular stenosis) *Clin Pediatr 28:175–179, 1989*

Kniest dysplasia (metatropic dysplasia) *Am J Med Genet 6:171–178, 1980*

Langer-Giedion syndrome *Atlas of Clinical Syndromes A Visual Aid to Diagnosis, 1992, pp.408–409*

Larsen syndrome *Atlas of Clinical Syndromes A Visual Aid to Diagnosis, 1992, pp.404–405*

Lenz microphthalmia syndrome *Z Kenderheilkd 77:384–390, 1955*

LEOPARD (Moynahan's) syndrome – autosomal dominant; CALMs, granular cell myoblastomas, steatocystoma multiplex, small penis, hyperelastic skin, low set ears, short webbed neck, short stature, syndactyly *Ped Derm 20:173–175, 2003; JAAD 46:161–183, 2002; JAAD 40:877–890, 1999; J Dermatol 25:341–343, 1998; Am J Med 60:447–456, 1976; AD 107:259–261, 1973; Am J Dis Child 117:652–662, 1969*

Leprechaunism – Donohue's syndrome – decreased subcutaneous tissue and muscle mass, characteristic facies, severe intrauterine growth retardation, broad nose, low set ears, hypertrichosis of forehead and cheeks, loose folded skin at flexures, gyrate folds of skin of hands and feet; breasts, penis, clitoris hypertrophic *Ped Derm 19:267–270, 2002; Endocrinologie 26:205–209, 1988*

Leri-Weill dyschondrosteosis – mesomelic short stature syndrome with Madelung's deformity; SHOX haploinsufficiency like Turner's syndrome *JAAD 50:767–776, 2004*

Lesch-Nyhan syndrome *Arch Int Med 130:186–192, 1972*

Leschke's syndrome – growth retardation, mental retardation, diabetes mellitus, genital hypoplasia, hypothyroidism *Bolognia, p.859, 2003*

Lymphedema-distichiasis syndrome – periorbital edema, vertebral abnormalities, spinal arachnoid cysts, congenital heart disease, thoracic duct abnormalities, hemangiomas, cleft palate, microphthalmia, strabismus, ptosis, short stature, webbed neck *Ped Derm 19:139–141, 2002*

Macrocephaly with cutis marmorata, hemangioma, and syndactyly syndrome – macrocephaly, hypotonia, hemihypertrophy, hemangioma, cutis marmorata telangiectatica congenita, internal arteriovenous malformations, syndactyly, joint laxity, hyperelastic skin, thickened subcutaneous tissue, developmental delay, short stature, hydrocephalus *Ped Derm 16:235–237, 1999*

Maffucci's syndrome (enchondromatosis) – enchondromas and multiple venous malformations; spindle cell hemangioendothelioma; oral and intra-abdominal venous and lymphatic anomalies; short stature, shortened long bones with pathologic fractures; enchondromas undergo sarcomatous change in 30–40%; breast, ovarian, pancreatic, parathyroid, pituitary tumors *JAAD 56:541–564, 2007; Ped Derm 17:270–276, 2000; Ped Derm 12:55–58, 1995;*

Malformation-retardation syndrome due to incomplete triploidy *Atlas of Clinical Syndromes A Visual Aid to Diagnosis, 1992, pp.150–151*

Marden- Walker syndrome – autosomal recessive; mental retardation, failure to thrive, microcephaly, immobility of facial muscles, blepharophimosis, congenital joint contractures, arachnodactyly, kyphoscoliosis, and transverse palmar creases *J Child Neurol 16:150–153, 2001*

Marinesco-Sjogren syndrome – – sparse, fine, short, fair, brittle hair, short stature, congenital cataracts, cerebellar ataxia; mental retardation, microcephaly, hypogonadism, ataxia, hypotonia *Clin Dysmorphol 4:283–288, 1995; J Ped 65:431–437, 1964*

Maroteaux-Lamy syndrome (pycnodysostosis) *Atlas of Clinical Syndromes A Visual Aid to Diagnosis, 1992, pp.126–127; Birth Defects 10:78–98, 1974*

Martsolf syndrome – cataracts, facial dysmorphism, microcephaly, short stature, hypogonadism *Am J Med Genet 1:291–299, 1978*

Mastocytosis of the skin, short stature, conductive hearing loss, and microtia *Clin Genet 37:64–68, 1990*

MC/MR syndrome with multiple circumferential skin creases – multiple congenital anomalies including high forehead, elongated face, bitemporal sparseness of hair, broad eyebrows, blepharophimosis, bilateral microphthalmia and microcornea, epicanthic folds, telecanthus, broad nasal bridge, puffy cheeks, microstomia, cleft palate, enamel hypoplasia, micrognathia, microtia with stenotic ear canals, posteriorly angulated ears, short stature, hypotonia, pectus excavatum, inguinal and umbilical hernias, scoliosis, hypoplastic scrotum, long fingers, overlapping toes, severe psychomotor retardation, resembles Michelin tire baby syndrome *Am J Med Genet 62:23–25, 1996*

Menkes' syndrome *Atlas of Clinical Syndromes A Visual Aid to Diagnosis, 1992, pp.108–109*

Mesomelic dysplasia type Langer *Atlas of Clinical Syndromes A Visual Aid to Diagnosis, 1992, pp.204–205*

Metaphyseal chondrodysplasia Schmid type *Atlas of Clinical Syndromes A Visual Aid to Diagnosis, 1992, pp.262–263*

Metaphyseal dysplasia Wiedemann-Spranger type *Atlas of Clinical Syndromes A Visual Aid to Diagnosis, 1992, pp.266*

Metatropic dysplasia *Atlas of Clinical Syndromes A Visual Aid to Diagnosis, 1992, pp.240–241*

Microcephalic osteodysplastic primordial dwarfism type II – autosomal recessive; craniofacial dysmorphism with slanting palpebral fissures, prominent nose, small mouth, micrognathia; fine sparse hair and thin eyebrows; café au lait macules; xerosis; mottling; dark pigmentation of neck and trunk; depigmentation; small pointed widely spaced teeth; low set ears missing lobule; widened metaphyses and relative shortening of distal limbs; cerebrovascular anomalies *Ped Derm 25:401–402, 2008*

Microcephaly-growth deficiency-retardation syndrome *Atlas of Clinical Syndromes A Visual Aid to Diagnosis, 1992, pp.172–173*

Microcephaly-lymphedema syndrome autosomal dominant; with short stature *Am J Med Genet 280:506–509, 1998*

Microphthalmia with linear skin defects (MIDAS syndrome) (MLS syndrome, Xp deletion syndrome, Xp 22.3 microdeletion syndrome) – Xp22.3 deletion – X-linked dominant; linear jagged skin defects of scalp, face, neck, and occasionally upper trunk, Blaschko-esque depressed patches of face, pre-auricular ear pit, severe short stature, congenital heart defects, agenesis of the corpus callosum, ambiguous genitalia, nail dystrophy *Ped Derm 25:548–552, 2008; Ped Derm 20:153–157, 2003*

Mietens syndrome *Atlas of Clinical Syndromes A Visual Aid to Diagnosis, 1992, pp.180–181*

Monosuperocentroincisivodontic dwarfism *Clin Genet 32:370–373, 1987*

Moore-Federman syndrome–short stature, stiffness of joints, characteristic facies *J Med Gen 26:320–325, 1989*

Morquio syndrome (mucopolysaccharidosis type IV) – autosomal recessive; short neck, skeletal abnormalities, corneal clouding, cardiac valvulopathies, odontoid hypoplasia, hypermobile joints *Ped Derm 33:594–601, 2016; Syndromes of the Head and Neck p. 100, 1990*

Mucopolysaccharidosis type IX – autosomal recessive; hyaluronidase 1 deficiency; soft tissue masses, short stature, coarse facies, hypertrichosis, synophrys; accumulation of hyaluronic acid *Ped Derm 33:594–601, 2016*

Mulibrey nanism – autosomal recessive; proportionate short stature, prenatal growth deficiency, muscle weakness, abnormal sella turcica, hepatomegaly, ocular fundi lesions *Am J Med Genet 66:378–398, 1996; Act Ophthalmol 52:162–171, 1974*

Multiple cartilaginous exostoses *Atlas of Clinical Syndromes A Visual Aid to Diagnosis, 1992, pp.406–407*

Multiple pterygium syndrome *Am J Dis Child 142:794–798, 1988; Eur J Pediatr 147:550–552, 1988; J Med Genet 24:733–749, 1987*

Myhre syndrome – low birth weight, short stature, muscular build, limited joint mobility, cardiac defects, deafness, skeletal abnormalities, facial dysmorphism, thick skin, keratosis pilaris, coarse facies

Naegeli-Franceschetti-Jadassohn syndrome variant – reticulate pigmentary dermatosis with hypohidrosis and short stature *Int J Dermatol 34:30–31, 1995*

Nager acrofacial dysostosis *Atlas of Clinical Syndromes A Visual Aid to Diagnosis, 1992, pp.50–51*

Netherton's syndrome – short stature, erythroderma, short sparse hair *Ped Derm 31:90–94, 2014*

Neu-Laxova syndrome – variable presentation; mild scaling to harlequin ichthyosis appearance; ichthyosiform scaling, increased subcutaneous fat and atrophic musculature, generalized edema and mildly edematous feet and hands, absent nails; microcephaly, intrauterine growth retardation, limb contractures, low set ears, sloping forehead, short neck; small genitalia, rudimentary eyelids, polyhydramnios, growth retardation, microcephaly, ichthyosis, thick hyperkeratotic skin; eyelid and lip closures, syndactyly, cleft lip and palate, micrognathia; autosomal recessive: uniformly fatal *Ped Derm 20:25–27,78–80, 2003; Curr Prob Derm 14:71–116, 2002; Am J Med Genet 43:602–605, 1992; Clin Dysmorphol 6:323–328, 1997; Am J Med Genet 35:55–59, 1990*

Neurofibromatosis

Nicolaides-Baraitser syndrome – congenital hypotrichosis, unusual facies (inverted triangular shaped face, low frontal hairline, mild facial hirsutism, deep set eyes, pointed nasal tip, thin nasal bridge, high arched palate, thick lower lip), interphalangeal swelling, short

metacarpals ("drumstick fingers"), growth and mental retardation *JAAD 59:92–98, 2008*

Niemann-Pick disease *Atlas of Clinical Syndromes A Visual Aid to Diagnosis, 1992, pp.112–113*

Nievergelt syndrome *Atlas of Clinical Syndromes A Visual Aid to Diagnosis, 1992, pp.206–207*

Nijmegen breakage syndrome – autosomal recessive; microcephaly, mental retardation, prenatal onset short stature, bird-like facies, café-au-lait macules; pink to red-brown firm papules and plaques with sclerosis and atrophy, clinodactyly, syndactyly, vitiligo, growth retardation, chromosomal instability, and combined immunodeficiency *Ped Derm 27:285–289, 2010;Am J Med Genet 66:378–398, 1996*

Noonan's syndrome – malformed ears, nevi, keloids, transient lymphedema, ulerythema ophyrogenes, keratosis follicularis spinulosa decalvans, joint hyperextensibility, hypertelorism, broad short webbed neck, down slanting of palpebral fissures, keratosis pilaris atrophicans, short stature or normal height, lymphedema of feet and legs, orbital edema, leukokeratosis of lips and gingiva, low posterior hairline, hypertrichosis of cheeks or shoulders, ulerythema oophyrogenes, chest deformity (pectus carinatum and pectus excavatum), cubitus valgus, radioulnar synostosis, clinobrachydactyly, congenital heart disease; *PTPN* 11 gene on chromosome 12; gain of function of non-receptor protein tyrosine phosphate SHP-2 or KRAS gene *NEJM 370:2229–2236, 2014; Ped Derm 24:417–418, 2007; JAAD 46:161–183, 2002; Cutis 67:315–316, 2001; Arch Dis Child 84:440–443, 2001; JAAD 40:877–890, 1999; J Med Genet 24:9–13, 1987; J Pediatr 63:468–470, 1963*

Oculocerebral hypopigmentation syndrome of Preus – very short with thin build, ptosis, high arched palate, dental malocclusion, prominent central upper incisors, hair and skin hypopigmented, deafness, severe mental retardation *Ped Derm 24:313–315, 2007*

Oculocutaneous albinism, dysmorphic features, short stature *Ophthalmic Paediatr Genet 11:209–213, 1990*

Oculo-palato-cerebral dwarfism *Clin Genet 27:414–419, 1985*

Odonto-trichomelic syndrome – autosomal recessive; severe hypotrichosis, few small conical teeth, hypoplastic or absent areolae, cleft lip, tetramelic dysplasia, short stature *Hum Hered 22:91–95, 1972*

Oligosymptomatic hypothyroidism *Atlas of Clinical Syndromes A Visual Aid to Diagnosis, 1992, pp.184–185*

Oliver-McFarlane syndrome–trichomegaly with mental retardation, dwarfism, and pigmentary degeneration of the retina *BJD 174:741–752, 2016; JAAD 37:295–297, 1997; Can J Ophthalmol 28:191–193, 1993*

Olmsted syndrome–periorificial keratotic plaques; congenital diffuse sharply marginated transgredient keratoderma of palms and soles, onychodystrophy, constriction of digits, diffuse alopecia, thin nails, chronic paronychia, leukokeratosis of oral mucosa, linear keratotic streaks, follicular keratosis, constriction of digits (ainhum), anhidrosis, small stature; differential diagnostic considerations include Clouston hidrotic ectodermal dysplasia, pachyonychia congenita, acrodermatitis enteropathica, Vohwinkel's keratoderma, mal de Meleda, and other palmoplantar keratodermas *Ped Derm 20:323–326, 2003; AD 132:797–800, 1996; JAAD 10:600–610, 1984*

Omenn syndrome – disproportionate short stature, short limb skeletal dysplasia type 1; alopecia, eosinophilia, ichthyosiform skin lesions, reticuloendotheliosis, erythroderma *Am J Med Genet 66:378–398, 1996*

Oral-facial-digital syndrome type 1 (Papillon-Leage-Psaume syndrome) – X-linked dominant; congenital facial milia which resolve with pitted scars; milia of face, scalp, pinnae, and dorsal hands;

short stature, hypotrichosis with dry and brittle hair, short upper lip, hypoplastic ala nasi and lower jaw, pseudoclefting of upper lip, hooked pug nose, hypertrophied labial frenulae, bifid or multilobed tongue with small white tumors within clefts, ankyloglossia, multiple soft hamartomas of oral cavity, clefting of hard and soft palate, teeth widely spaced with dental caries, trident hand or brachydactyly, syndactyly, clinodactyly, ulnar deviation of index finger, or polydactyly; hair dry and brittle, alopecic, numerous milia of face, ears, backs of hands, mental retardation with multiple central nervous system abnormalities, frontal bossing, hypertelorism, telecanthus, broad depressed nasal bridge; polycystic renal disease; combination of polycystic renal disease, milia, and hypotrichosis is highly suggestive of OFD 1 *Ped Derm 27:669–670, 2010; JAAD 59:1050–1063, 2008; Ped Derm 25:474–476, 2008; Ped Derm 9:52–56, 1992; Am J Med Genet 86:269–273, 1999; JAAD 31:157–190, 1994; Ped Derm 9:52–56, 1992; Pediatrics 29:985–995, 1962; Rev Stomatol 55:209–227, 1954*

Oral-facial-digital syndrome with acromelic short stature *Clin Dysmorphol 8:185–188, 1999;* type VI *Am J Med Genet 35:360–369, 1990*

Osteodysplastic geroderma (Walt Disney dwarfism) – short stature, cutis laxa-like changes with drooping eyelids and jowls, osteoporosis and skeletal abnormalities *Am J Med Genet 3:389–395, 1979*

Osteogenesis imperfect *Atlas of Clinical Syndromes A Visual Aid to Diagnosis, 1992, pp.366–369*

Osteoglophonic dysplasia *Eur J Pediatr 147:547–549, 1988*

Oto-palatal-digital syndrome – short stature, distinctive facies, cleft palate, hearing loss, short thumbs and big toes *Am J Dis Child 113:214–221, 1967*

Phosphoglucomutase 1 deficiency – autosomal recessive; disorder of glycosylation with impaired glycoprotein production; liver dysfunction, bifid uvula, malignant hyperthermia, hypogonadotropic hypogonadism, growth retardation, hypoglycemia, myopathy, dilated cardiomyopathy, cardiac arrest *NEJM 370:533–542, 2014*

Poikiloderma with neutropenia – autosomal recessive; Navajo Indians; erythematous rash of limbs, trunk, and face beginning in infancy; evolves into poikiloderma; recurrent infections; palmoplantar keratoderma; pachyonychia of great toenails, photosensitivity; growth retardation; dental caries; atrophic scars; mutation in *C16orf57 BJD 163:866–869, 2010; Am J Med Genet A 146A:2762–2769, 2008; Am J Hum Genet 86:72–76, 1991*

Prader-Willi syndrome – obesity, hypogonadism, cryptorchidism, mental retardation, hypotonia, disproportionately small hands *Dermatol Clin 10:609–622, 1992*

Premature aging syndrome (Mulvihill-Smith syndrome)–Mulvihill-Smith syndrome – autosomal dominant; short stature, microcephaly, unusual birdlike facies (broad forehead, small face, micrognathia) (progeroid with lack of facial subcutaneous tissue), multiple pigmented congenital melanocytic nevi, freckles, blue nevi, hypodontia, immunodeficiency with chronic infections, high pitched voice, xerosis, telangiectasias, thin skin, fine silky hair, premature aging, hypodontia, high-pitched voice, mental retardation, sensorineural hearing loss, hepatomegaly low birth weight, short stature, conjunctivitis, delayed puberty *Am J Med Genet 66:378–398, 1996; J Med Genet 31:707–711, 1994; Am J Med Genet 45:597–600, 1993*

Primordial microcephalic and osteodysplastic dwarfism *Atlas of Clinical Syndromes A Visual Aid to Diagnosis, 1992, pp.170–171*

Proportionate short stature: trunk is length expected in comparison with limbs: *JAMA 311:1787–1796, 2014*
    Intrinsic inherent limitations on bone growth
        Small for gestational age/intrauterine growth retardation
        Genetic or chromosomal abnormalities

Pyknodystosis *Atlas of Clinical Syndromes A Visual Aid to Diagnosis, 1992, pp.200–201*

Panhypopituitary dwarfism – short stature, excess subcutaneous fat, high pitched voice, soft, wrinkled skin, child-like facies *Birth Defects 12:15–29, 1976*

Pansclerotic morphea *Ped Derm 19:151–154, 2002*

Poikiloderma with neutropenia – autosomal recessive; Navajo Indians; erythematous rash of limbs, trunk, and face beginning in infancy; evolves into poikiloderma; recurrent infections; palmoplantar keratoderma; pachyonychia of great toenails, photosensitivity; growth retardation; dental caries; atrophic scars; cryptorchidism; hepatosplenomegaly; mutation in *USB1* gene; mutation in *C16orf57 BJD 168:665–666, 2013; Ped Derm 29:463–472, 2012; BJD 163:866–869, 2010; Am J Med Genet A 146A:2762–2769, 2008; Am J Hum Genet 86:72–76, 1991; Am J Hum Genet 49:A661, 1991*

Polydysplastic epidermolysis bullosa

Prader-Willi syndrome – albinoid skin; almond-shaped eyes, narrow bifrontal diameter, thin upper lip, short stature, central obesity, small hands and feet, mental retardation, hypogonadism, hypotonia at birth, excoriations, trichotillomania *Cutis 90;129–131, 2012; Growth Genet Hormones 2:1–5, 1986; Schweiz Med Wschr 86:1260–1261, 1956*

Premature aging syndrome with osteosarcoma, cataracts, diabetes mellitus, osteoporosis, erythroid macrocytosis, severe growth and developmental deficiency *Am J Med Genet 69:169–170, 1997*

Proteus syndrome *Atlas of Clinical Syndromes A Visual Aid to Diagnosis, 1992, pp.352–355*

Pseudoachondroplasia *Atlas of Clinical Syndromes A Visual Aid to Diagnosis, 1992, pp.268–269*

Pseudodiastrophic dysplasia *Atlas of Clinical Syndromes A Visual Aid to Diagnosis, 1992, pp.238–239*

Pseudohypoparathyroidism type Ia (Albright's hereditary osteodystrophy) – subcutaneous nodule (osteoma cutis); short stature, round face, obesity, subcutaneous ossifications, bilateral brachydactyly, mental retardation, hypothyroidism, saddle nose deformity *Ped Derm 36:355–359, 2019; Ped Derm 33:675–676, 2016*

Pseudohypothyroidism *Atlas of Clinical Syndromes A Visual Aid to Diagnosis, 1992, pp.188–189*

Pseudoxanthoma elasticum with osteoectasia – dwarfism, radiographic changes, increased alkaline phosphatase *Clin Exp Dermatol 7:605–609, 1982*

PYCR1-related cutis laxa – hair loss, prominent scalp veins, triangular shaped face, microcephaly, short stature, hypermobility of joints, thin atrophic skin, wrinkled skin, muscle weakness, finger contractures *Dtsch Arztebl Intl 16:489–496, 2019*

Rabson-Mendenhall syndrome – autosomal recessive; insulin-resistant diabetes mellitus, growth retardation, fissured tongue, unusual facies (prominent jaw), dental precocity, hypertrichosis, acanthosis nigricans, onychauxis, and premature sexual development, pineal hyperplasia *Ped Derm 19:267–270, 2002*

Ramon syndrome- cherubism, gingival fibromatosis, epilepsy, mental deficiency, hypertrichosis, and stunted growth *Am J Med Genet 25:433–441, 1986*

RAPADILINO syndrome – same as Ballard-Gerold syndrome, but without poikiloderma; radial ray defects, limb malformations, diarrhea in infancy, short stature; osteosarcoma *RECQL4* mutations *JAAD 75:855–870, 2016; AD 141:617–620, 2005*

Rapp-Hodgkin hypohidrotic ectodermal dysplasia–autosomal dominant; alopecia of wide area of scalp in frontal to crown area, short eyebrows and eyelashes, coarse wiry sparse hypopigmented scalp hair, sparse body hair, scalp dermatitis, ankyloblepharon, syndactyly, nipple anomalies, cleft lip and/or palate; nails narrow and dystrophic, small stature, hypospadius, conical teeth and anodontia or hypodontia; distinctive facies, short stature *JAAD 53:729–735, 2005; Ped Derm 7:126–131, 1990; J Med Genet 15:269–272, 1968*

Restrictive dermopathy (stiff skin syndrome) – severe intrauterine growth retardation; micrognathia, fixed facial expression, low set ears, pinched nose, O-shaped mouth, flexion contractures, rigid, translucent, inelastic skin *AD 138:831–836, 2002*

Reticulate hyperpigmentation with alopecia, nail changes, and growth retardation with or without blisters *Schweiz Med Wochenschr 100:228–233, 1970; Monatsschr Kinderheilkd 78:773–781, 1939*

Rhizomelic dwarfism – autosomal recessive; chondrodysplasia punctata with mild ichthyosis *Ped Derm 18:442–444, 2001*

Ricketts–personal observation

Ring chromosome 7, 11 – CALMs microcephaly, mental retardation *Am J Med Genet 30:911–916, 1988;* 12, and 15 syndromes *JAAD 40:877–890, 1999*

Ring chromosome 17 – multiple café au lait macules, short stature *Ped Derm 22:270–275, 2005*

Ritscher-Schinzel syndrome – autosomal recessive; Dandy Walker-like malformation, atrioventricular canal defect, short stature *Am J Med Genet 66:378–398, 1996*

Robert's syndrome (hypomelia-hypotrichosis-facial hemangioma syndrome) – autosomal recessive; mid-facial port wine stain extending from forehead to nose and philtrum, cleft lip +/- cleft palate, sparse silver-blond hair, limb reduction malformation, characteristic facies, malformed ears with hypoplastic lobules, marked growth retardation *Clin Genet 31:170–177, 1987; Clin Genet 5:1–16, 1974*

Robinow syndrome – overfolded helix *Eur J Pediatr 151:586–589, 1992; Am J Med Genet 35:64–68, 1990*

Rombo syndrome – autosomal dominant; acral erythema, cyanotic redness of hands and lips, follicular atrophy (atrophoderma vermiculata), milia-like papules and cysts of the face and trunk, telangiectasias, red face, red ears with telangiectasia, thin eyebrows, sparse beard hair, basal cell carcinomas, trichoepitheliomas, short stature with short trunk *Ped Derm 23:149–151, 2006; BJD 144:1215–1218, 2001; JAAD 39:853–857, 1998; Acta DV 61:497–503, 1981*

Rothmund-Thomson syndrome – poikiloderma, photosensitivity (early erythema, edema, blistering of face); sparse hair, sparse eyebrows, small stature, palmoplantar keratoderma, skeletal anomalies, cataractsosteosarcoma in 30% *JAAD 75:855–870, 2016; JAAD 67:1113–1127, 2012; Curr Prob Derm 14:41–70, 2002; BJD 139:1113–1115, 1998; Ped Derm 6:325–328, 1989; Ped Derm 6:321–324, 1989; JAAD 17:332–338, 1987;* mutations in DNA helicase gene *RECQL4 Nat Genet 22:82–84, 1999; Ped Derm 18:210–212, 2001; Am J Med Genet 22:102:11–17, 2001; Ped Derm 18:210212, 2001; Ped Derm 16:59–61, 1999; Dermatol Clin 13:143–150, 1995; JAAD 27:75–762, 1992; BJD 122:821–829, 1990; Ped Derm 6:325–328, 1989; Ped Derm 6:321–324, 1989; JAAD 17:332–328, 1987; JAAD 17:332–338, 1987; Arch Ophthalmol (German) 4:159, 1887*

Rubella embryopathy *Atlas of Clinical Syndromes A Visual Aid to Diagnosis, 1992, pp.528–529*

Rubinstein-Taybi syndrome – very short stature; mental deficiency, small head, broad terminal phalanges of thumbs and great toes, beaked nose, malformed low-set ears, capillary nevus of forehead, hypertrichosis of back and thick eyebrows, long eyelashes (trichomegaly) keratosis pilaris or ulerythema ophryogenes; arciform large keloids, cardiac defects; hemangiomas, nevus flammeus, café au lait macules, pilomatrixomas, hirsutism, keloids, scars; mutations or deletions of chromosome 16p13.3; human cAMP response element binding protein *Cutis 93:83–87, 2014; JAAD 56:541–564, 2007; Ped Derm 21:44–47, 2004; JAAD 46:161–183, 2002;JAAD 46:159, 2002; Ped Derm 19:177–179, 2002; Cutis 57:346–348, 1996; Am J Dis Child 105:588–608, 1963*

Russell-Silver syndrome – intrauterine and post-natal growth retardation; large head, short stature, premature sexual development, CALMs, clinodactyly, syndactyly of toes, triangular facies, childhood hyperhidrosis, limb asymmetry, café au lait macules, blue sclerae, achromia, 5th finger clinodactyly, genital dysmorphia *Ped Derm 30:150–151, 2013;JAAD 40:877–890, 1999; J Med Genet 36:837–842, 1999; Clin Genet 29:151–156, 1986; Am J Dis Child 13:447–451, 1977*

SADDAN syndrome – autosomal dominant; short stature, severe tibial bowing, severe achondroplasia with profound developmental delay and acanthosis nigricans *BJD 147:1096–1011, 2002; Am J Med Genet 85:53–65, 1999*

Saldino-Noonan syndrome *Atlas of Clinical Syndromes A Visual Aid to Diagnosis, 1992, pp.218–219*

San Filippo syndrome (A-D) – autosomal recessive; accumulation of glycosaminoglycans; decreased hearing, skeletal deformities *Ped Derm 33:594–601, 2016*

Satoyoshi syndrome – alopecia areata with progressive painful intermittent muscle spasms, diarrhea or unusual malabsorption, endocrinopathy with amenorrhea (hypothalamic dysfunction), very short stature, flexion contractures, skeletal abnormalities *Ped Derm 18:406–410, 2001; AD 135:91–92, 1999*

Say-Barber syndrome – short stature, microcephaly, large ears, flexion contractures, decreased subcutaneous fat; dermatitis in infancy with transient hypogammaglobulinemia *Am J Med Genet 86:165–167, 1999; Am J Med Genet 45:358–360, 1993*

Schimke immune-osseous dysplasia – disproportionate short stature, spondyloepiphyseal dysplasia, progressive nephropathy, episodic lymphopenia, pigmentary skin changes *Am J Med Genet 66:378–398, 1996*

Schwachman-Diamond syndrome – autosomal recessive; dry face with perioral dermatitis, palmoplantar hyperkeratosis; periodontal disease and caries; abscesses, short stature, delayed puberty, skeletal changes, pancreatic exocrine deficiency with malabsorption, pancytopenias, cyclic neutropenia, failure to thrive, hepatomegaly, pneumonia, otitis media, metaphyseal dysplasia, osteomyelitis *Ped Derm 28:568–569, 2011; J Pediatr 135:81–88, 1999; Am J Med genet 66:378–398, 1996; J Pediatr 65:645–663, 1964*

Schwartz-Jampel syndrome (chondrodystrophic myotonia) *Am J Med Genet 66:378–398, 1996; J Neurol Neurosurg Psychiat 41:161–169, 1978*

Seckel's syndrome – autosomal recessive; abnormal teeth, short stature, hypopigmented papules and macules, small deformed ears lacking lobules, syndactyly, clinodactyly; hair sparse and prematurely gray, growth retardation, beak-like nose, large eyes, skeletal defects *Ped Derm 24:53–56, 2007; Am J Med Genet 12:7–21, 1982*

SHORT syndrome – short stature, joint hyperextensibility, ocular depression (deep-set eyes), Rieger anomaly, teething delay; lipoatrophy of face *Clin Dysmorphol 8:219–221, 1999; Birth Am J Med Genet 61:178–181, 1996; J Med Genet 26:473–475, 1989; Defects 11:46–48, 1975*

Short limb skeletal dysplasia type 3 (disproportionate short stature) – metaphyseal dysplasia, exocrine pancreatic insufficiency, cyclic neutropenia *Am J Med Genet 66:378–398, 1996*

Short stature, alopecia, and macular degeneration

Short stature, characteristic facies, mental retardation, skeletal anomalies, and macrodontia *Clin Genet 26:69–72, 1984*

Short stature and delayed dental eruption *Oral Surg 41:235-243, 1976*

Short stature and macrocephaly, mental retardation *Am J Med Genet 21:697–705, 1985*

Short stature, mental retardation, facial dysmorphism, short webbed neck, skin changes, congenital heart disease–xerosis, dermatitis, low set ears, umbilical hernia *Clin Dysmorphol 5:321–327, 1996*

Short stature, mental retardation, ocular abnormalities *Helv Paediat Acta 27:463–469, 1972*

Short stature, oligodontia *Syndromes of the Head and Neck p. 873, 1990*

Short stature and osteopetrosis *Radiology 164:23–224, 1987*

Short stature, premature aging, pigmented nevi *J Med Genet 25:53–56, 1988*

Short stature, sensorineural hearing loss, low nasal bridge, cleft palate *Am J Med Genet 21:317–324, 1985*

Short stature and short thin dilacerated dental roots *Oral Surg 54:553–559, 1982*

Short stature and solitary maxillary central incisor *J Pediatr 91:924–928, 1977*

SHOX mutations–disproportionate short stature; trunk is longer or shorter than expected in comparison with limbs *JAMA 311:1787–1796, 2014*

Sjogren-Larsson syndrome *Ped Derm 20:180–182, 2003; Atlas of Clinical Syndromes A Visual Aid to Diagnosis, 1992, pp.468–469*

Skeletal dysplasias – disproportionate short stature; trunk is longer or shorter than expected in comparison with limbs *JAMA 311:1787–1796, 2014*

Smith-Fineman-Myers syndrome (unusual facies, short stature, and mental deficiency) *Am J Med Genet 22:301–304, 1985*

Smith-Lemli-Opitz syndrome *Atlas of Clinical Syndromes A Visual Aid to Diagnosis, 1992, pp.494–495*

Spondyloepiphyseal dysplasia congenita *Atlas of Clinical Syndromes A Visual Aid to Diagnosis, 1992, pp.246–247*

Spondyloepiphyseal dysplasia tarda *Atlas of Clinical Syndromes A Visual Aid to Diagnosis, 1992, pp.248–249*

Stanescu osteosclerosis syndrome – short stature, brachycephaly, hypoplastic midface, ocular proptosis, micrognathia, brachydactyly, dense cortices of long bones *J Genet Hum 29:129–139, 1981*

Stickler syndrome (hereditary arthro-ophthalmopathy) – autosomal dominant; flat midface, cleft palate, myopia with retinal detachment, cataracts, hearing loss, arthropathy *J Med Genet 36:353, 359, 1999; Birth Defects 11:77–103, 1975*

Stiff skin syndrome (congenital fascial dystrophy) *JAAD 75:163–168, 2016*

STING-associated vasculopathy with onset in infancy (SAVI) (type 1 interferonopathy) – red plaques of face and hands; chilblain-like lesions; atrophic plaques of hands, telangiectasias of cheeks, nose, chin, lips, acral violaceous plaques and acral cyanosis (livedo reticularis of feet, cheeks, and knees), distal ulcerative lesions with infarcts (necrosis of cheeks and ears), gangrene of fingers or toes with ainhum, nasal septal perforation, nail dystrophy ; small for gestational age; paratracheal adenopathy, abnormal pulmonary function tests; interstitial lung disease with fibrosis with ground glass and reticulate opacities; gain of function mutation in *TMEM173* (stimulator of interferon genes); mimics granulomatosis with

polyangiitis *JAMADerm 151:872–877, 2015; NEJM 371:507–518, 2014*

Tay syndrome – autosomal recessive, growth retardation, triangular face, cirrhosis, trident hands, premature canities, vitiligo

Thanatophoric dysplasia – autosomal dominant; micromelic dwarfism; defect in FGFR3 *BJD 147:1096–1011, 2002*

3-M syndrome *Birth Defects 11:39–47, 1975*

Tonoki syndrome – short stature, brachydactyly, nail dysplasia, mental retardation *Am J Med Genet 80:403–405, 1998*

Toriello syndrome – autosomal recessive; proportionate short stature, prenatal growth deficiency, delayed skeletal maturation, cataracts, enamel hypoplasia, neutropenia, microcephaly, mental retardation *Am J Med Genet 66:378–398, 1996*

Tricho-oculo-dermo-vertebral syndrome (Alves syndrome) – dry, sparse, brittle hair, dystrophic nails, plantar keratoderma, short stature, cataracts *Am J Med Genet 46:313–315, 1993*

Trichorhinophalangeal syndrome type I – autosomal dominant; slow growing short blond hair, receding frontotemporal hairline with high bossed forehead; thin nails, koilonychias, leukonychia, facial pallor, pear-shaped nose with bulbous nose tip, wide long philtrum, thin upper lip, triangular face, receding chin, tubercle of normal skin below the lower lip, protruding ears, distension and deviation with fusiform swelling of the PIP joints; hip malformation, brachydactyly, prognathism, fine brittle slow growing sparse hair, lateral eyebrows sparse and brittle,, dense medially, bone deformities (hands short and stubby), joint hyperextensibility, cone-shaped epiphyses of bones of hand, lateral deviation of interphalangeal joints, flat feet, hip malformations, high arched palate, supernumerary teeth, dental malocclusion, mild short stature; hypotonia, hoarse deep voice, recurrent respiratory infections, hypoglycemia, diabetes mellitus, hypothyroidism, decreased growth hormone, renal and cardiac defects, mutation in zinc finger nuclear transcription factor (*TRPS1* gene) *Cutis 89:56,73–74, 2012; Ped Derm 26:171–175, 2009; Ped Derm 25:557–558, 2008; BJD 157:1021–1024, 2007; AD 137:1429–1434, 2001; JAAD 31:331–336, 1994; Hum Genet 74:188–189, 1986; Helv Paediatr Acta 21:475–482, 1966*

Trichorhinophalangeal syndrome type II (Langer-Giedion syndrome) – microcephaly with mental retardation, deep set eyes, exotropia, long nose with bulbous tip, broad nasal bridge, thick ala nasi, high palate, crowded teeth, micrognathia, long neck, short metacarpals, thin nails, small feet with brachydactyly, vaginal stenosis, short stature, thin sparse hair, long face, prominent ears, madarosis, cartilaginous exostoses, foot deformities, joint laxity; EXT gene *BJD 171:1581–1583, 2014; BJD 157:1021–1024, 2007; Genetic Skin Disorders, Second Edition, 2010,pp.225–228; Atlas of Clinical Syndromes A Visual Aid to Diagnosis, 1992, pp.408–409420–421*

Trichorhinophalangeal syndrome type III (Sugio-Kajii syndrome) – autosomal dominant; like type I (alopecia (receding frontotemporal hairline), facial dysmorphism, high bossed forehead, bone deformities, severe brachydactyly, facial pallor, protruding low set ears, bulbous distal nose, elongated philtrum, thin upper lip, prognathism, micrognathia, dental malocclusion, high arched palate, supernumerary teeth, koilonychias, leukonychia, flat feet) with severe growth retardation; shortening of all phalanges; severe short stature; shortening of metacarpals and phalanges; facial dysmorphism with dental malocclusion *Ped Derm 26:171–175, 2009; BJD 159:476–478, 2008; Ped Derm 25:557–558, 2008; BJD 157:1021–1024, 2007*

Trichothiodystrophy syndromes–BIDS, IBIDS, PIBIDS – autosomal recessive; collodion baby, congenital erythroderma, poikiloderma, sparse or absent eyelashes and eyebrows, sulfur deficient short brittle hair with tiger tail banding on polarized microscopy, trichomegaly, brittle soft nails with koilonychia, premature aging, very short stature, microcephaly, sexual immaturity, ichthyosis, photosensitivity, hypohidrosis, high arched palate, dysmyelination of white matter, bird-like facies, abnormal teeth with dental caries; trichothiodystrophy with ichthyosis, urologic malformations, hypercalciuria and mental and physical retardation; recurrent infections with neutropenia; ocular abnormalities, osteopenia; socially engaging personality; mutation in one of 3 DNA repair genes (XPB, XPA, TTDA, or TTDN1 *Ped Derm 32:865–866, 2015; JAAD 63:323–328, 2010; Curr Prob Derm 14:71–116, 2002; JAAD 52:224–232, 2005; JAAD 44:891–920, 2001; Ped Derm 14:441–445, 1997; Am J Med Genet 35:566–573, 1990; JAAD 16:940–947, 1987; Eur J Pediatr 141:147–152, 1984;* trichothiodystrophy with ichthyosis, urologic malformations, hypercalciuria and mental and physical retardation; trichothiodystrophy, mental retardation, short stature, ataxia, and gonadal dysfunction *Am J Med Genet 35:566–573, 1990*

Turner's syndrome (XO in 80%) – peripheral edema at birth which resolves by age 2; redundant neck skin in newborn; small stature, broad shield-shaped cest with widely spaced nipples, arms show wide carrying angle, webbed neck, low posterior hairline, low misshapen ears, high arched palate, cutis laxa of neck and buttocks, short fourth and fifth metacarpals and metatarsals, hypoplastic nails, keloid formation, increased numbers of nevi; skeletal, cardiovascular, ocular abnormalities; increased pituitary gonadotropins with low estrogen levels *JAMA 311:1787–1796, 2014; NEJM 368:1220–1228, 2013; JAAD 46:161–183, 2002; JAAD 40:877–890, 1999; NEJM 335:1749–1754, 1996*

Trisomy 9 – short stature, bulbous nose, marked palmar folds, low set ears, long philtrum, thin lips, low palpebral folds, cryptorchidism, mental retardation *Ped Derm 26:482–484, 2009*

Trisomy 13 (Patau syndrome)–phylloid hypomelanosis – associated with trisomy 13 mosaicism; mental retardation, short stature, scoliosis, facial dysmorphism, asymmetric leg lengths *Ped Derm 14:278–280, 1997*

Tuomaala-Haapanen syndrome (brachymetapody, anodontia, hypotrichosis, albinoid trait) *Acta Ophthalmol 46:365–371, 1968*

Vertebral and eye anomalies, cutis aplasia, and short stature (VECS) *Am J Med Genet 77:225–227, 1998*

Watson's syndrome – café au lait macules, axillary and perianal freckling, pulmonic stenosis, low intelligence, short stature *JAAD 46:161–183, 2002; JAAD 40:877–890, 1999*

Werner's syndrome *Leuk Lymphoma 21:509–513, 1996; Medicine 45:177–221, 1966*

Westerhof syndrome–autosomal dominant, hyper- and hypopigmented macules on trunk and extremities, short stature, small sella turcica, cervical ribs *AD 114:931–936, 1978*

Whistling face syndrome (Freeman-Sheldon syndrome) *Atlas of Clinical Syndromes A Visual Aid to Diagnosis, 1992, pp.46–47*

Wiedemann-Rautenstrauch syndrome (neonatal progeroid syndrome) – autosomal recessive; aged facies at birth, frontal and biparietal bossing, scalp with sparse hair and prominent veins, retarded psychomotor development; death by age five *Eur J Pediatr 136:245–248, 1981*

Wiedemann-Steiner syndrome – hypertrichosis, prominent forehead, low hairline, small ears, hypertelorism, bushy eyebrows, localized thickened cutaneous plaques; dwarfism, peripheral corneal opacities, coarse facial features

Williams' syndrome – skin with soft texture, abnormal smoothness, easy mobility from underlying subcutaneous tissue, growth retardation, elfin-like facies, mental retardation, hoarse voice, supravalvular aortic stenosis; deletion of elastin gene *BJD 156:1052–1055, 2007*

Winchester syndrome (hereditary contractures with sclerodermatoid changes of skin) – scleredema-like skin changes, widespread nodules, joint contractures, gingival hyperplasia, hypertrichosis, dwarfism, arthritis of small joints (RA-like), osteolysis, corneal opacities *JAAD 55:1036–143, 2006; JAAD 50:S53–56, 2004; Am J Med Genet 26:123–131, 1987; J Pediatr 84:701–709, 1974; Pediatrics 47:360–369, 1971*

Wolf-Hirschhorn syndrome – 4p deletion; posterior midline scalp defects, cutaneous T-cell lymphoma, growth retardation *Ped Derm 22:270–275, 2005*

Wrinkly skin syndrome–autosomal recessive *Clin Genet 38:307–313, 1990;* same as cutis laxa with growth and developmental delay; increased palmoplantar creases, prominent venous pattern over chest, mental retardation, microcephaly, hypotonia (joint laxity), musculoskeletal (decreased muscle mass, hip dislocation, winging of scapulae, vertebral deformities), short stature, craniofacial abnormalities, and connective tissue abnormalities *Ped Derm 25:66–71, 2008; Ped Derm 23:225–230, 2006; Am J Med Genet 101:213–220, 2001; Ped Derm 6:113–117, 1999; Am J Med Genet 85:194, 1999; Clin Genet 4:186–192, 1973*

Xeroderma pigmentosum – short stature, conjunctivitis, photophobia, pyogenic granulomas in toddlers *BJD 168:1109–1113, 2013*

X-linked agammaglobulinemia with growth hormone deficiency and delayed growth and puberty *Acta Paediatr 83:99–102, 1994*

X-aneuploidy variants *Syndromes of the Head and Neck, p.58, 1990*

X-linked recessive ichthyosis with mild mental retardation, chondrodysplasia punctata and short stature *Clin Genet 34:31–37, 1988*

49,XXXXX syndrome *Syndromes of the Head and Neck, p.63, 1990*

49,XXXXY syndrome *Syndromes of the Head and Neck, p.59, 1990*

TOXINS

Fetal alcohol syndrome – short stature, angiomas, hypertrichosis *JAAD 46:161–183, 2002; Atlas of Clinical Syndromes A Visual Aid to Diagnosis, 1992, pp.480–483*

TRAUMA

Spinal radiation–disproportionate short stature; trunk is longer or shorter than expected in comparison with limbs *JAMA 311:1787–1796, 2014; NEJM 368:1220–1228, 2013*

VASCULAR DISORDERS

PHACES syndrome – hypopituitarism with growth hormone deficiency *Sem Cut Med Surg 35:108–116, 2016*

SICKLE CELL DISEASE, CUTANEOUS MANIFESTATIONS

Am J Hematol 618–625, 2009

SICKLE CELL DACTYLITIS (HAND-FOOT SYNDROME)

Acute pain
Swelling of hands and/or feet
Within first 4 years of life
May be first sign of sickle cell anemia
Occurs in 40% of all patients with sickle cell anemia
Bone infarction, necrosis

HEMATOLOGIC ULCERS

Painful, round, punched out, raised margins, deep base, necrotic slough with bacterial colonizations with *Staphylococcus aureus* and *Pseudomonas*
From a few mm to circumferential distal lower extremities
Lateral malleoli more frequent than medial malleoli
Less common over tibia, foot, Achilles tendon
Less subcutaneous fat, thin skin, decreased blood flow
Very slow to heal

PSEUDOXANTHOMA ELASTICUM

Rare *Ped Derm 36:e64–65, 2019; JAAD 56:170–171, 2007*
Seen in sickle cell anemia and beta thalassemia *J Med Imaging Radiat Oncol 60:74–82, 2016; Blood 99:30–35, 2007;* pseudoxanthoma elasticum-like syndrome *Rev Med Interne 29:15–18, 2008*

HYDROXYUREA ULCERS

Lateral malleolus
Hyperpigmentation
Nail discoloration

OTHER

"Boggy skull" – soft head syndrome; pain, spontaneous subgaleal hematoma; ultrasound of head for diagnosis *Clin Case Rep 7:2220–2224, 2019; J Neurol Surg Rep 76:e97–99, 2015; Am J Hematol 89:225–227, 2014*

Eccrine chromhidrosis *Ped Derm 34:e273–274, 2017*

Erythema ab igne *Ped Hem Oncol 35:225–230, 2018*

Fat embolism – painful erythematous plaques *Am J Hematol 89:233, 2014*

Livedoid vasculopathy with sickle cell trait *Int Wound J 9:344–347, 2012*

Purpura *Am J Dermatopathol 1:384–386, 1999*

Retiform purpura – exceptionally rare *Am J Dermatopathol 21:384–386, 1999*

SINUS TRACTS

AUTOIMMUNE DISEASES AND DISORDERS OF IMMUNE REGULATION

Chronic granulomatous disease–scrofula *JAAD 36:899–907, 1997*
Dermatomyositis – panniculitis with ulceration and sinuses
Leukocyte adhesion deficiency *JAAD 31:316–319, 1994*

Rheumatoid arthritis – fistulous rheumatism; tracking of nodules to skin *JAAD 53:191–209, 2005*

CONGENITAL LESIONS

Accessory auricles with congenital fistulae

Branchial cleft sinus and fistulae – pit in lower third of the neck along anterior border of sternocleidomastoid muscle; skin tag at opening *Arch Otolaryngol Head Neck Surg 123:438–441, 1997; Clin Otolaryngol 3:77–92, 1978;* Melnick-Fraser syndrome–preauricular pits, hearing loss, and renal anomalies

Bronchogenic cyst (overlying the suprasternal notch or manubrium sterni, scapular) – may drain mucoid fluid; may be either sinus tract or subcutaneous nodule *AD 142:1221–1226, 2006; JAAD 46:S16–18, 2002; AD 136:925–930, 2000; Ped Derm 16:285–287, 1999; Ped Derm 15:277–281, 1998; Ped Derm 12:304–306, 1995; Am J Dermatopathol 13:509–517, 1991; Ann DV 115:855–858, 1988; J Cutan Pathol 12:404–409, 1985; Am J Roentgenol Radium Ther Nucl Med 70:771–785, 1953; J Thoracic Cardiovasc Surg 14:217–220, 1945;* skin-colored nodule of chin *BJD 143:1353–1355, 2000;* papilloma *JAAD 11:367–371, 1984*

Cloacal sinuses – between anus and adjoining skin; urethra, perineum

Congenital dermal sinus – over lower spine; hair may protrude from opening *Pediatr Neurosurg 84:428–434, 2019; Pediatr Neurosurg 26:275, 1997; AD 112:1724–1728, 1976*

Congenital lip sinus

Congenital pilonidal sinus *Pediatrics 35:795–797, 1965*

Congenital sinus or cyst of genitoperineal raphe (mucous cysts of the penile skin) *Cutis 34:495–496, 1984; AD 115:1084–1086, 1979*

Dermoid cyst and sinus – pit *Ped Derm 33:e244–248, 2016; Ped Derm 32:161–170, 2015; Neurosurg Clin N Am 6:359–366, 1995; AD 107:237–239, 1973*

Dorsal dermal sinus – dimple in suboccipital or lumbosacral regions *AD 112:1724–1728, 1976; J Pediatr 87:744–750, 1975*

Ectopic or christomatous salivary gland (heterotopic salivary gland tissue) – skin colored nodule along lower surface of the sternocleidomastoid muscle *JAAD 58:251–256, 2008*

Fourth branchial sinus causing recurrent cervical abscess *Aust N Z J Surg 67:119–122, 1997*

Fistula in ano *Dis Colon Rectum 41:1147–1152, 1998*

Omphalomesenteric duct–patent peripheral portion of omphalomesenteric duct; red nodule with a fistula with fecal discharge or intestinal prolapse *Am J Surg 88:829–834, 1954*

Preauricular cyst and sinuses (pre-auricular fistula) *Ped Derm 37:40–51, 2020; J La State Med Soc 151:447–450, 1999; Plast Reconstr Surg 102:1405–1408, 1998*

Presternal sinus tracts, congenital – in and around midline *BJD 159:763–765, 2008;* peristernal dermal sinus connecting to pectoralis major – swelling, suppuration, and pain *Ped Derm 37:40–51, 2020*

Sinus sternoclavicularis – congenital cervical sinus; pit overlying anterior border of sternocleidomastoid muscle *Ped Derm 32:240–243, 2015*

Spinal dysraphism, occult–overlying protrusion, dimple, sinus, lipoma, faun tail nevus, dermoid cyst, hemangioma, port wine stain *Ped Derm 112:641–647, 2003; AD 114:573–577, 1978; AD 112:1724–1728, 1976*

Sternal clefts – associated with fistulae, ulceration or scarring, supra-umbilical midline raphe, and facial hemangiomas

Thyroglossal duct cyst and/or sinus–midline cervical cleft with sinus tract *Am J Neuroradiol 20:579–582, 1999; JAAD 26:885–902, 1992; J Pediatr Surg 19:437–439, 1984*

DEGENERATIVE DISORDERS

Neurotrophic ulcers including those associated with neuropathies – on metatarsal heads and heels with surrounding (hemorrhagic) callosities

DRUG REACTIONS

Alendronate – osteonecrosis of mandible; halitosis, hypesthesia of lower lip, submental sinus; necrosis of mandible underlying gingiva *NEJM 367:551, 2012*

EXOGENOUS AGENTS

Barber's hair sinus *Derm Surg 29:288–290, 2003; AD 112:523–524, 1976*

BCG vaccination with scrofuloderma *Ped Derm 22:179–180, 2005*

Foreign body

Hair sinus of the breast *Clin Exp Dermatol 7:445–447, 1982;*

hair sinuses of the feet; umbilical hair sinus

Paraffinoma – grease gun injury; nodule, plaque, sinus of hand *BJD 115:379–381, 1986*

Silicone, injected – draining sinuses *AD 141:13–15, 2005; Derm Surg 27:198–200, 2001*

INFECTIONS AND INFESTATIONS

Actinomycetoma – *Nocardia, Actinomadura, Streptomyces*

Actinomycosis (*A. israelii*)–cervicofacial – nodule of cheek or submaxillary area; board-like induration; multiple sinuses with puckered scarring; sulfur granules discharged *Cutis 60:191–193, 1997; Infect Dis Clin North Am 2:203–220, 1988; Arch Int Med 135:1562–1568, 1975;* perianal *Dis Colon Rectum 37:378–380, 1994;* thoracic actinomycosis with multiple sinuses *Ped Derm 30:504–505, 2013; Am J Clin Pathol 75:113–116, 1981;* abdominal *Hum Pathol 4:319–330, 1973;* primary cutaneous – subcutaneous nodules with draining sinuses *Hum Pathol 4:319–330, 1973;* actinomycetoma – forehead sinus tracts; *Nocardia brasiliensis, N. asteroides BJD 143:192–194, 2000; Nocardia brasiliensis;* pustules, scarring, sinus tracts, multilobulated nodules, grains *JAAD 62:239–246, 2010*

African blastomycosis

Alveolar echinococcosis *JAAD 34:873–877, 1996*

Amebiasis – perianal abscesses and fistulae *Proc R Soc Med 66:677–678, 1973; Entamoeba histolytica* in neonate

Botryomycosis – granulomatous reaction to bacteria with granule formation; single or multiple abscesses of skin and subcutaneous tissue break down to yield multiple sinus tracts; small papule; extremities, perianal sinus tracts, face *Cutis 80:45–47, 2007; JAAD 24:393–396, 1991; Int J Dermatol 22:455–459, 1983; AD 115:609–610, 1979*

Calymmatobacterium granulomatis (Donovanosis) *J Clin Inf Dis 25:24–32, 1997*

Carbuncle *Stat Pearls Feb 28, 2020*

Coccidioidomycosis *Ann NY* Acad *Sci 1111:411–421, 2007; JAAD 55:929–942, 2006; JAAD 26:79–85, 1992; South Med J 77:1464–1465, 1984*

Cryptococcosis *JAAD 32:844–50, 1995*

Dental sinus *Cutis 85:36–38, 2010; Cutis 70:264–267, 2002; J Am Dent Assoc 130:832–836, 1999; JAAD 14:94–100, 1986; JAAD 8:486–492, 1983; AD 114:1158–1161, 1978;* in edentulous patients with retained tooth fragments *J Craniofac Surg 11:254–257, 2000;* dual sinus tracts *Oral Surg Oral Med Oral Pathol 52:653–656, 1981;* periapical dental abscess *Cutis 43:22–24, 1989;* due to bisphosphonate-induced osteonecrosis of mandible *JAAD 62:672–676, 2010*

Eumycetoma – *Madurella, Fusarium, Acremonium, Pseudallescheria boydii, Exophiala, Curvularia; Phaeoacremonium sphinctrophorum* – white grains *JAMADerm 152: 1063–1065, 2016*

Giant condyloma of Buschke and Lowenstein *AD 136:707–710, 2000*

Glanders (*Burkholderia mallei*)

Granuloma inguinale (donovanosis) ("serpiginous ulcer") – *Calymmatobacterium granulomatis* – starts as skin colored subcutaneous nodule which breaks down into vulvar ulcer, vegetative perianal plaques with fistula formation, mutilation, and elephantine changes *JAAD 54:559–578, 2006*

Histoplasmosis with fistulae *AD 132:341–346, 1996*

Implant-associated infections *Chiurg 87:813–821, 2016*

Leprosy – histoid leprosy – scrotal sinuses *Indian J Lepr 76:231–232, 2004*

Linear bacterial dissection *Cutis 51:43–44, 1993*

Lymphogranuloma venereum – Jersild syndrome – perirectal abscesses, fistulae, sclerosis *JAAD 54:559–578, 2006;* inguinal adenitis with abscess formation and draining chronic sinus tracts; rectal syndrome in women with pelvic adenopathy, periproctitis with rectal stricture and fistulae; esthiomene – scarring and fistulae of the buttocks and thighs with elephantiasic lymphedema of the vulva; lymphatics may develop abscesses which drain and form ulcers *Int J Dermatol 15:26–33, 1976*

Malacoplakia *AD 134:244–245, 1998; Am J Dermatopathol 20:185–188, 1998; JAAD 34:325–332, 1996; JAAD 30:834–836, 1994*

Mamillary fistula (periareolar abscess) *Br J Surg 73:367–368, 1986*

Melioidosis *AD 135:311–322, 1999*

Milker's sinuses – fragments of cow hair; 2nd or 3rd finger web tender nodules and discharging sinuses

Mycetoma – tumefaction, multiple sinuses, fistulae, and granules; eumycetoma; *Acremonium falciforme, Madurella mycetomatis, Madurella grisea, Pseudallescheria boydii (North America), Exophiala jeanselmei, Leptosphaeria senegalensis, Leptosphaeria tompkinsii;* actinomycetoma – *Actinomadura, Actinomyces israelii, A. bovis, Nocardia asteroides, Nocardia brasiliensis, Actinomyces madurae (Actinomadura sp.), Streptomyces somaliensis The Dermatologist January 2014,pp.35–37; AD 147:609–614, 2011; JAAD 53:931–951, 2005; JAAD 32:311–315, 1995; Cutis 49:107–110, 1992; Australas J Dermatol 31:33–36, 1990; JAAD 6:107–111, 1982;* due to *Microsporum canis Mycopathologica 81:41–48, 1983; Scytalidium dimidiatum (formerly Hendersonula toruloidea) BJD 148:174–176, 2003*

Mycobacterium abscessus AD 142:1287–1292, 2006; Am J Respir Crit Care Med 156(pt. 2):S1–S25, 1997; J Clin Inf Dis 24:1147–1153, 1997; Clin Inf Dis 19:263–273, 1994; Rev Infect Dis 5:657–679, 1983

Mycobacterium avium complex JAAD 26:1108–1110, 1990; foot ulcer with sinus tracts Am Rev Resp Dis 106:469–471, 1972; ulcerated plaques with sinus tracts AD 126:1108–1110, 1990

Mycobacterium avium-intracellulare – cervicofacial lymphadenitis in children with fistulae Ped Derm 21:24–29, 2004

Mycobacterium chelonae AD 142:1287–1292, 2006; Am J Respir Crit Care Med 156 (pt. 2):S1–S25, 1997; J Clin Inf Dis 24:1147–1153, 1997; Clin Inf Dis 19:263–273, 1994; J Inf Dis 166:405–412, 1992; Rev Infect Dis 5:657–679, 1983

Mycobacterium fortuitum AD 142:1287–1292, 2006; Dermatol Surg 26:588–590, 2000; Am J Respir Crit Care Med 156(pt. 2):S1–S25, 1997; J Clin Inf Dis 24:1147–1153, 1997; Clin Inf Dis 19:263–273, 1994; Rev Infect Dis 5:657–679, 1983

Mycobacterium malmoense–cervicofacial lymphadenitis in children with fistulae Ped Derm 21:24–29, 2004

Mycobacterium szulgai – diffuse cellulitis, nodules, and sinuses Am Rev Respir Dis 115:695–698, 1977

Mycobacterium tuberculosis – scrofuloderma – infected lymph node, bone, joint, lacrimal gland with overlying red-blue nodule which breaks down, ulcerates, forms fistulae, scarring with adherent fibrous masses which may be fluctuant and draining JAAD 54:559–578, 2006; JAAD 52:S65–68, 2005; Ped Derm 20:309–312, 2003; Ped Derm 18:328–331, 2001; BJD 134:350–352, 1996; Thorax 16:77–81, 1967; tuberculous mastitis – nodular tuberculous mastitis (solitary or multiple palpable masses); sinus tract, ulcer Int J Inf Dis 87:135–142, 2019Nocardia brasiliensis – actinomycetomas of trunk, extremities, feet– N. brasiliensis, N. otitidiscaviarum, N. asteroides BJD 156:308–311, 2007; mycetoma or multiple subcutaneous draining nodules mimicking foreign body granuloma Cutis 60:191–193, 1997; JAAD 13:125–133, 1985; J Inf Dis 134:286–289, 1976; mediastinal infection with draining sternal sinus tracts West J Med 167:47–49, 1997; Nocardia asteroides–mycetoma BJD 144:639–641, 2001; N. otodiscavarium – multiple abscesses with draining sinus tracts AD 143:1086–1087, 2007; N. otodiscavarium actinomycetoma AD 142:101–106, 2006

North American blastomycosis (*Blastomyces dermatitidis*) JAAD 21:1285–1293, 1989; Oral Surg Oral Med Oral Pathol 54:12–14, 1982

Osteomyelitis *Radiology 173:355–359, 1989*

Paecilomycosis

Paracoccidioidomycosis *JAAD 31:S91–S102, 1994*

Pasteurella multocida (P. haemolytica, pneumotropica, and ureae) – cellulitis with ulceration with hemorrhagic purulent discharge with sinus tracts JAAD 33:1019–1029, 1995; Medicine 63:133–144, 1984

Pseudomycetoma, *Actinomyces*–personal observation

Schistosomal granuloma–perianal hypertrophic plaques; perianal fissuring; paragenital granulomas due to S. haematobium. May have communicating sinuses and fistulae Br J Vener Dis 55:446–449, 1979

Sporotrichosis – fistulae *Derm Clinics 17:151–185, 1999*

Subcutaneous phaeohyphomycosis *Am J Trop Med Hyg 29:901–911, 1980*

Syphilis–tabes dorsalis – callus with sinus tract of weight bearing regions of sole Arch Neurol 42:606–613, 1985

Tinea capitis (*T. verrucosum, T. mentagrophtes*) – kerion AD 114:371–372, 1978

Tinea corporis, invasive (*T.violaceum*) BJD 101:177–183, 1979

Trichosporon dermatis – ulcerated verrucous plaque with draining sinus tracts JAAD 65:434–436, 2011

INFILTRATIVE DISORDERS

Langerhans cell histiocytosis – draining sinuses over involved lymph nodes Curr Prob Derm VI Jan/Feb 1994; Clin Exp Derm 11:183–187, 1986; JAAD 13:481–496, 1985

INFLAMMATORY DISORDERS

Acquired lacrimal sac fistula due to dacryocysitis – ulcers around medial canthus BJD 168:1348–1350, 2013

Crohn's disease–enterocutaneous fistula NEJM 347:417–429, 2002; Gut 45:874–878, 1999; fistulae and sinus tracts BJD 80:1–8, 1968; penile sinus tracts /fistulae Cutis 72:432–437, 2003

Dissecting cellulitis of the scalp (perifolliculitis capitis abscedens et suffodiens) JAAD 62:534–536, 2010; BJD 159:506–507, 2008; Cutis 67:37–40, 2001; Minn Med 34:319–325, 1951; AD 23:503–518, 1931

Diverticulitis of sigmoid colon Int Surg 97:285–287, 2012; Hip Int 18:58–60, 2008; Dig Dis Sci 38:1985–1988, 1993

Esophago-pleuro-cutaneous fistula Jpn J Surg 14:139–142, 1984

Granulomatous mastitis – abscess, sinus tract, or subcutaneous nodule of breast The Breast Journal 14:588–590, 2008

Hidradenitis suppurativa BJD 175:882–891, 2016; JAMA Derm 149:1192–1194, 2013; BJD 165:415–418, 2011; BJD 161:831–839, 2009; JAAD 60:539–561, 2009; Ped Derm 24:465–473, 2007; AD 142:1110–1112, 2006; Derm Surg 26:638–643, 2000; BJD 141:231–239, 1999; retroauricular sinus anal fistulae Dis Colon Rectum 62:1278–1280, 2019; Dis Colon Rectum 33:731–734, 1990

 Diseases associated with hidradenitis suppurativa: JAAD 60:539–561, 2009; Dermatol Online J 19:18558, 2013

  Acanthosis nigricans
  Acne conglobata
  Acne vulgaris Br Med J 292:245–248, 1986; Surg Gynecol Obstet 95:455–464, 1952
  Bazex-Dupre-Christol syndrome
  Crohn's disease Inflammatory Bowel Dis 7:33–326, 2001; Int J Colorect Dis 8:117–119, 1993; BJD 126:523, 1992
  Dissecting cellulitis of the scalp
  Dowling-Degos disease Clin Exp Dermatol 31:454–456, 2006; Clin Exp Dermaol 29:622–624, 2004; Hautarzt 52:642–645, 2001; Australas J Dermatol 38:209–211, 1997; Clin Exp Dermatol 21:305–306, 1996; Ann DV 120:120:705–708, 1993; JAAD 24:888–892, 1991; Cutis 45:446–450, 1990
  Down's syndrome Dermatol Online J 19:18558, 2013
  Fox-Fordyce disease JID 31:127–135, 1958
  Interstitial keratitis AD 95:473–475, 1967
  Keratitis-ichthyosis-deafness syndrome Eur J Dermatol 15:347–352, 2005; JAAD 51:377–382, 2004
  Obesity Acta DV 85:225–232, 2005; J Eur Acad Dermatol Venereol 17:276–279, 2003
  Pachyonychia congenita JID Symp Proc 10:3–17, 2005; BJD 123:663–666, 1990; JAAD 19:705–711, 1988
  PAPA (pyogenic arthritis, pyoderma gangrenosum, acne) syndrome Mayo Clin roc 72:611–615, 1997
  PAPASH (pyogenic arthritis, pyoderma gangrenosum, acne, suppurative hidradenitis) JAAD Case Rep 3:70–73, 2017

PASH (pyoderma gangrenosum, acne, suppurative hidradenitis) *JAAD Case Rep 3:70–73, 2017*
Pilonidal cysts and sinuses *BJD 175:1103–1104, 2016*
Pyoderma gangrenosum
Reflex sympathetic dystrophy *Arch Phys Med Rehabil 82:412–414, 2001*
SAPPHO (synovitis, acne, pustulosis, periostitis, hyperostosis, osteitis) syndrome *J Clin Rheumatol 8:13–22, 2002*
Scrotal elephantiasis
Smith-Magenis syndrome *Cureus 11:e4970, 2019*
Smoking *Acta DV 85:225–232, 2005; J Cut Med Surg 8:415–423, 2004; J Eur Acad Dermatol Venereol 17:276–279, 2003; Dermatology 198:261–264, 1999*

Peristomal fistulae and ulcers *Ann Surg 197:179–182, 1982*

Peristomal hidradenitis suppurativa *J Wound Ostomy Continence Nurs 23:171–173, 1996*

Pseudofolliculitis barbae

Pyoderma fistulans sinifica (fox den disease) *Clin Inf Dis 21:162–170, 1995*

Pyodermia chronica glutealis *J Dermatol 25:242–245, 1998*

METABOLIC DISORDERS

Calcinosis cutis *Medicine 97:e12517, 2018;* in juvenile dermatomyositis *J Ped Orthoped 35:e43–46, 2015; Laryngoscope 118:75–77, 2008; Postgrad Med J 79:424–425, 2003*

Pancreatic cutaneous fistulas *Am J Surg 155:36–42, 1988*

NEOPLASTIC DISORDERS

Adenocarcinoma occurring in a chronic sinus tract *Cancer 47:2093–2097, 1981;* adenocarcinoma of the colon

Connective tissue nevus with sinus tract *Ped Derm 32:e298–299, 2015*

Nevus comedonicus *AD 116:1048–1050, 1980*

Pilonidal cyst and sinus *Surg Clin North Am 74:1309–1315, 1994;* pilonidal sinus *BJD 175:1103–1104, 2016*

Sacro-coccygeal chordoma – mimicking pilonidal sinus *J R Coll Surg Edinb 45:254–255, 2000*

Squamous cell carcinoma *Am J Orthop 28:253–256, 1999;* anal squamous cell carcinoma in situ–multiple fistulae *J Clin Inf Dis 21:603–607, 1995; Am J Gastroenterol 86:1829–1832, 1991;* penis (carcinoma cuniculatum) *Am J Surg Pathol 31:71–75, 2007*

Suppurative keloidosis *JAAD 15:1090–1092, 1986*

Verrucous carcinoma (epithelioma cuniculatum) *AD 136:547–548, 550–551, 2000; Cancer 49:2395–2403, 1982*

PRIMARY CUTANEOUS DISEASES

Acne conglobata *Ped Derm 17:123–125, 2000;* familial–plaque with sinus tracts *JAAD 14:207–214, 1986*

Acne keloidalis nuchae *JAAD 39:661, 1998*

Acne rosacea *Hautarzt 46:417–420, 1995*

Heterotopic cervical salivary glands *J Laryngol Otol 91:35–40, 1977*

Pyoderma faciale *AD 128:1611–1617, 1992*

SYNDROMES

Branchio-oculo-facial syndrome *Am J Ophthalmol 139:362–364, 2005*

Branchio-oto-renal syndrome–pre-auricular sinus tract or cyst, abnormal pinna, branchial cleft fistulae and/or cyst; autosomal dominant, chromosome 8q *Genomics 14:841–844, 1992; Clin Genet 9:23–34, 1976*

Mosaic partial trisomy 13 – pre-auricular fistulae, phylloid hypomelanosis, mental retardation, agenesis of the corpus callosum, conductive hearing loss, coloboma, skeletal defects, syndactyly, clinodactyly, dental malposition, oligodontia *AD 145:576–578, 2009*

SAPPHO syndrome

Trichothiodystrophy – pre-auricular pits *Ped Derm 32:865–866, 2015*

TRAUMA

Pressure ulcer *Am Fam Physician 78:1186–1194, 2008; Clin Geriatr Med 13:455–481, 1997*

VASCULAR DISEASES

Capillary malformations, branchial clefts, lip pseudoclefts, and unusual facies; anomalous retroverted ears, microphthalmia, cleft lip/palate *JAAD 56:541–564, 2007; J Laryngol Otol 71:597–603, 1957*

SPIKY SKIN

Chronic renal failure

Crohn's disease

Demodicidosis, spiculate *Ped Derm 35:244–245, 2018; BJD 138:901–903, 1998*

HIV follicular syndrome–pityriasis rubra pilaris, acne conglobate, and follicular spicules *BJD 179:774–775, 2018*

Keratosis pilaris

Lichen planopilaris

Lichen scrofulosorum

Lichen spinulosus

Lymphoma

Minute digitate hyperkeratosis (music box spicules)

Multiple myeloma – keratotic spicules – precipitates of monoclonal dysproteins identical to serum proteins *JAAD 32:834–839, 1995*

Phrynoderma – Vitamin A deficiency

Pityriasis rubra pilaris

Scurvy

Trichodysplasia spinulosa – polyoma virus *JAMADerm 154:1342–1343, 2018*

SPINAL DYSRAPHISM (CUTANEOUS STIGMATA)

AD 140:1109–1115, 2004; JAAD 31:892–896, 1994; AD 118:643–648, 1982

DEPRESSED LESIONS

Aplasia cutis congenita (denuded skin)
Dermal sinus
Deviated superior gluteal crease

Dimple (dermal pit) – large, greater than 2.5 cm from anal verge
Dimple – small; less than 2.5 cm from anal verge; low index of suspicion
Scar
Sinus tract (with or without dermoid cyst)

DERMAL LESIONS

Congenital scar
Connective tissue nevus
Hamartoma, unclassifiable
Hypertrophic skin
Neurofibroma

DYSCHROMIC LESIONS

Hyperpigmentation – low index of suspicion
Hypopigmentation or depigmentation

HAIRY LESIONS

Hypertrichosis (faun tail nevus)

NEOPLASMS (BENIGN OR MALIGNANT)

Ependymoma
Epidermal nevus *AD 118:643–648, 1982*
Hamartoma, unclassified
Lipoma, sacral
Melanocytic nevi – low index of suspicion
Neurofibroma
Teratoma – low index of suspicion

POLYPOID LESIONS

Acrochordon
Pseudotail
True tail (human tail)

SUBCUTANEOUS NODULES

Dermoid cyst or sinus
Lipoma
Neural tissue–includes ependymoma, lipomeningocele, lipomyelomeningocele, occult meningocele, neurofibroma

VASCULAR LESIONS

Port wine stain – low index of suspicion
Hemangioma
Lipoma with overlying port wine stain *AD 140:1109–1115, 2004*
Lumbar twin nevus – combined telangiectasia and nevus anemicus *Ped Derm 21:664–666, 2004*
Telangiectasia – low index of suspicion

TYPES OF SPINAL DYSRAPHISM

Dermal sinus tract
Diastemetamyelia

Filum terminale with tethered conus
Hydrosyringomyelia
Lipomyelomeningocele
Myelomeningocele
Neurofibroma

SPLINTER HEMORRHAGES

JAAD 50:289–292, 2004
Anti-phospholipid antibody syndrome
Arthritis
Behcet's disease
Blood dyscrasia
Buerger's disease
Cancer chemotherapy
Cirrhosis
Collagen vascular disease
Cryoglobulinemia
Cutaneous T-cell lymphoma
Darier's disease
Dermatitis
Diabetes mellitus
Emboli, arterial
Exfoliative dermatitis
Fungal endocarditis
Hemochromatosis
Hemodialysis
High altitude
Hypertension
Hypoparathyroidism
Idiopathic
Indwelling brachial artery cannula
Internal malignancy
Langerhans cell histiocytosis
Lupus erythematosus, subacute cutaneous LE
Mitral stenosis
Occupational trauma
Onychomycosis
Osler-Weber-Rendu syndrome
Peptic ulcer disease
Peritoneal dialysis
Psoriasis
Pterygium
Pulmonary disease
Radial artery puncture
Raynaud's disease
Renal disease
Sarcoidosis
Scurvy
Sepsis
Subacute bacterial endocarditis
Sweet's syndrome
Tetracycline
Thyrotoxicosis
Trauma
Trichinosis
Vasculitis

SPOROTRICHOID LESIONS

AD 131:1329–1334, 1995

EXOGENOUS AGENTS

Mercury granuloma *JAAD 43:81–90, 2000*

INFECTIONS AND INFESTATIONS

Acanthamebiasis *AD 147:857–862, 2011*

Alternaria infectoria – sporotrichoid ulcerated purpuric plaques *BJD 145:484–486, 2001*

Anthrax (*Bacillus anthracis*)

Aspergillus fumigatus Ped Derm 26:592–596, 2009

Bed bug bites *NEJM 359:1047, 2008*

Cat scratch fever

Chromomycosis *Cutis 85:73–76, 2010*

Coccidioidomycosis *JAAD 55:929–942, 2006*

Cowpox *BJD 122:705–708, 1990*

Cryptoccocus neoformans BJD 120:683–687, 1989; Cryptococcus diffluens

Ecthyma *Cutis 54:279–286, 1994*

Exophiala polymorpha Am Fam Physician 63:326–332, 2001; J Dermatol 40:638–640, 2013

Fonsecaea pedrosoi Am Fam Physician 63:326–332, 2001

Fusarium solani Med Mycol 48:103–109, 2010

Insect bites–personal observation

Histoplasmosis

Insect bites

Kaposi's sarcoma *JAAD 29:488, 1993*

Leishmaniasis – along lymphatics *Clin Dermatol 38:140–151, 2020; Dermatol Clin 33:579–593, 2015; JAAD 60:897–925, 2009; JAAD 51:S125–128, 2004; BJD 147:1022–1023, 2002; JAAD 36:847–849, 1997; South Med J 90:325–327, 1997;* American leishmaniasis (*L. brasiliensis*) and *L. major JAAD 73:897–908, 2015; BJD 153:203–205, 2005; Trans R Soc Trop Med Hyg 88:552–554, 1994; JAAD 17:759–764, 1987; L. tropica; L. panamensis Clin Inf Dis 61:1314,1342–1343, 2015; JAAD 73:897–908, 2015*

Leprosy, tuberculoid *JAAD 53:931–951, 2005;* sporotrichoid nerve abscesses *Indian J Lepr 86:103–113, 2014*

Lymphogranuloma venereum *Cutis 54:279–286, 1994*

Melioidosis (*Burkholderia pseudomallei*) *Am Fam Physician 63:326–332, 2001; Cutis 54:279–286, 1994*

Mycetoma *JAAD 49:S170–173, 2003*

Mycobacterium avium-intracellulare JAAD 47:S249–250, 2002; AD 129:1343–1344, 1993; AD 124:1545–1549, 1988

Mycobacterium bovis JAAD 43:535–537, 2000

Mycobacterium chelonei (abscessus) BJD 151:1101, 2004; J Cutan Med Surg 5:28–32, 2001; BJD 143:1345, 2000; Clin Inf Dis 18:999–1001, 1994; Clin Exp Dermatol 14:309–312, 1989; Ann DV 112:319–324, 1985

Mycobacterium fortuitum Dermatol Therapy 17:491–498, 2004

Mycobacterium kansasii JAAD 41:854–856, 1999; JAAD 36:497–499, 1997

Mycobacterium marinum Cutis 100:331–336, 2017; NEJM 373:1761, 2015; JAAD 65:1060–1062, 2011; Dermatol Therapy 21:154–161, 2008; JAAD 57:413–420, 2007; Cutis 79:33–36, 2007; Clin Inf Dis 31:439–443, 2000; Clin Exp Dermatol 23:214–221, 1998; facial *J Pediatr 130:324–326, 1997; AD 122:698–703, 1986; Nature 168:826, 1951*

Mycobacterium scrofulaceum AD 138:689–694, 2002

Mycobacterium szigai Clin Exp Derm 29:377–379, 2004

Mycobacterium tuberculosis–tuberculous gumma *Clin Dermatol 38:152–159, 2020;* extremities more than trunk *Scand J Infect Dis 32:37–40, 2000; Int J Dermatol 26:600–601, 1987; JAAD 6:101–106, 1982; Semin Hosp Paris 43:868–888, 1967;* primary tuberculosis; tuberculosis verrucosa cutis *Ped Derm 18:393–395, 2001;* lupus vulgaris *Int J Derm 40:336–339, 2001;* sporotrichoid pattern *Int J Derm 40:336–339, 2001;* scrofuloderma or lupus vulgaris *Ped Derm 30:7–16, 2013*

Mycobacterium xenopi Cutis 67:81–82, 2001

Nocardiosis, lymphocutaneous *Cutis 89:75–77, 2012; Cutis 85:73–76, 2010; J Inf Dis 134:286–289, 1976; Nocardia brasiliensis JAMADerm 151:895–896, 2015; Cutis 78:249–251, 2006; Cutis 76:33–35, 2005; N. asteroides BJD 144:639–641, 2001; AD 124:659–660, 1988; N. caviae JAAD 29:639–641, 1993; N. transvalensis JAAD 28:336–340, 1993; N. otitidiscaviarium Hand Surg 7:285–287, 2002;* primary cutaneous *AD 146:81–86, 2010;* sporotrichoid ulcers *Clin Dermatol 38:152–159, 2020*

North American blastomycosis

Paecilomyces lilacinus JAAD 39:401–409, 1998

Paracoccidiodomycosis *Cutis 85:73–76, 2010*

Phaeohyphomycosis – *Alternaria infectoria BJD 145:484–486, 2001*

Pseudoallescheria boydii AD 138:271–272, 2002

Pseudomonas pseudomallei

Rat bite fever

Scedosporiosis (*Scedosporium apiospermum* (asexual form of *Pseudallescheria boydii*)) – hyalohyphomycosis – fungal thrombophlebitis *JAMA Derm 150:83–84, 2014; BJD 133:805–809, 1995; Rev Inst Med Trop Sao Paulo 39:227–230, 1997;* sporotrichoid nodules of foot and leg *Australas J Dermatol 56:e39–42, 2015*

Sporotrichosis *Dermatol Clin 33:595–607, 2015; JAAD 53:931–951, 2005; Cutis 54:279–286, 1994; Dermatologica 172:203–213, 1986; brasiliensis, schenckii*

Staphylococcus aureus – nodular lymphangitis *Ped Derm 34:103–104, 2017; AD 146:1435–1437, 2010; Clin Inf Dis 21:433–434, 1995; Dermatologica 178:278–80, 1989*

Streptococcus pyogenes Am Fam Physician 63:326–332, 2001

Syphilis–extragenital chancre *JAAD 53:931–951, 2005*

Trichosporon beigelii

Tularemia – *Francisella tularensis*; skin, eye, respiratory, gastrointestinal portals of entry; ulceroglandular, oculoglandular, glandular types; toxemic stage heralds generalized morbilliform eruption, erythema multiforme-like rash, crops of red nodules on extremities *Medicine 54:252–269, 1985*

Yersinia pseudotuberculosis J Coll Physicians Surg Pak 17:120–121, 2017

INFILTRATIVE DISORDERS

Langerhans cell histiocytosis (adult onset) *J Drugs Dermatol 5:174–177, 2006*

METABOLIC DISORDERS

Calcium gluconate, intravenous – sporotrichoid metastatic calcification *BJD 166:892–894, 2012*

NEOPLASTIC DISORDERS

Epithelioid sarcoma *Am Fam Physician 63:326–332, 2001;* ankle ulcer, sporotrichoid nodules, and inguinal lymphadenopathy *Acta Med Iran 48:72–74, 2010; Eur J Dermatol 13:599–602, 2003*

Keratoacanthomas *Cureus 10:e3196, 2018; JAAD 74:1220–1223, 2016*

Lipomas

Lymphatic tumors

Lymphoma – primary cutaneous diffuse large cell B-cell lymphoma, leg type – red-violaceous sporotrichoid nodules of leg *JAAD Case Rep 6:815–818, 2020; AD 148:1199–1204, 2012;* primary peripheral T-cell lymphoma *J Cut Med Surg 21:568–571, 2017*

Metastases – melanoma *Indian J DV Leprol 29:823–825, 2015*

Methotrexate-related lymphoproliferative disorder – linear perilymphatic nodules of leg; linear bands; ulcerated and non-ulcerated red nodules *JAAD 61:126–129, 2009*

Spindle cell hemangioendotheliomas *Cutis 62:23–26, 1998*

Squamous cell carcinoma *Dermatol Online J 19:18174, 2013; Am J Dermatopathol 32:395–397, 2010; Cutis 64:261–264, 1999*

PRIMARY CUTANEOUS DISEASES

Sweet's syndrome *Cutis 71:469–472, 2003*

VASCULAR DISORDERS

Arteriosclerotic peripheral vascular disease–personal observation

SPOTTY PIGMENTATION OF THE FACE

Acro-dermato-ungual-lacrimal-tooth syndrome (ADULT syndrome) – ectrodactyly or syndactyly, freckling and dry skin, dysplastic nails, lacrimal duct atresia, primary hypodontia, conical teeth, and early loss of permanent teeth; small ears hooked nose, sparse hair, hypohidrosis, hypoplastic breasts and nipples, urinary tract anomalies mutation in *TP63* gene (encodes transcription factor p63); p63 mutations also responsible for EEC, AEC, limb mammary, and Rapp-Hodgkin syndromes *Ped Derm 27:643–645, 2010; Ped Derm 22:415–419, 2005; Hum Mol Genet 11:799–804, 2002; Am J Med Genet 45:642–648, 1993*

Carney complex *Rev Endocr Metab Disord 17:367–371, 2016*

Centrofacial lentiginosis – personal observation

Centrofacial neurodysraphic lentiginosis *BJD 94:39–43, 1976*

Cronkhite-Canada syndrome

Lentiginosis of African-Americans

LEOPARD syndrome *Orphanet J Rare Dis May 27 2008*

Noonan's syndrome *Orphanet J Rare Dis Jan 14, 2007*

Patterned lentiginosis *AD 125:1231–1235, 1989*

Peutz-Jegher's syndrome *J Med Genet 34:1007–1011, 1997*

Seborrheic keratoses, macular

Solar lentigines

Turner's syndrome

STRIAE DISTENSAE (STRETCH MARKS)

DRUGS

Bevacizumab and corticosteroids – ulcerations within striae *AD 148:385–390, 2012; J Neurooncol 101:155–159, 2011; AD 147:1227–1228, 2011*

Medroxyprogesterone (Depo-Provera) *Br J Fam Plann 26:104–105, 2000*

Prolonged therapy with ACTH or adrenocorticosteroids

Protease inhibitors – intra-abdominal fat ("crix belly") ("protease paunch"); indinavir *JAAD 41:467–469, 1991*

Topical corticosteroid therapy, either superpotent or under occlusion *Med Clin (Barc) 148:e25, 2017; JAAD 54:1–15, 2006*

EXOGENOUS AGENTS

Augmentation mammoplasty *Aesthet Plast Surg 36:894–890, 2012*

METABOLIC DISORDERS

Adolescent/pubertal striae from rapid growth *Acta Biomed 91:176–181, 2020*

Angiokeratoma corporis diffusum–personal observation

Cushing's syndrome/disease *Semin Dermatol 3:287–294, 1984;* bilateral macronodular adrenal hyperplasia *NEJM 369:2115–2125, 2013; NEJM 369:2105–2114, 2013;* diabetic ketoacidosis due to ultrapotent topical corticosteroids–personal observation

Eating disorders *Am J Clin Derm 6:165–173, 2005*

Liver disease, chronic – lower abdomen, thighs, buttocks

Obesity *JAAD 81:1037–1057, 2019*

Pregnancy (striae gravidarum)

PRIMARY CUTANEOUS DISEASES

Mid-dermal elastolysis *Int J Derm 28:426, 1989*

Linear focal elastosis – mimicking striae distensae *BJD 178:e278, 2018*

Pruritic urticarial papules and plaques of pregnancy (PUPPP); post-partum PUPPP *Cutis 95:344–347, 2015*

Rapid weight gain or loss

PSYCHOCUTANEOUS DISORDERS

Anorexia nervosa *Dermatoendocrinol 1:268–270, 2009*

SYNDROMES

Marfan's syndrome – progressive striae *JAAD 64:290–295, 2011; Int J Dermatol 28:291–299, 1989*

TRAUMA

Athletes, weight lifters

STROKE SYNDROMES, CUTANEOUS MANIFESTATIONS

VASCULAR DISORDERS

Large vessel atherosclerosis

Small vessel disease

Arterial disease
  Cerebral artery dissection
  Cerebrotendinous xanthomatosis
  Fat embolism syndrome – persistent somnolence, fever, tachycardia, respiratory symptoms, petechial eruption *NEJM 375:370–378, 2016; Circulation 123:1947–1952, 2011*
  Genetic or inherited arteriopathy
    Adenosine deaminase 2 (ADA2) mutation – mutation in *CECR1*; intermittent fevers, early onset lacunar strokes, livedoid eruption, hepatosplenomegaly, systemic vasculopathy; early onset polyarteritis nodosa *Ann Rheum Dis 76:1648–1656, 2017; JAAD 75:449–453, 2016; NEJM 370:911–920, 2014*
    Cerebral autosomal dominant arteriopathy with subcortical infarcts and leukoencephalopathy (CADASIL)
    3' repair exonuclease 1 (TREX1) mutation disorders
    Dolichoectasia
    Ehlers-Danlos disease type IV *J Neurol Sci 318:168–170, 2012*
    Fabry's disease *Continuum (Minneap Minn) 20:399–411, 2014*
    Fibromuscular dysplasia
    Hyperhomocysteinemia
    Mitochondrial encephalomyopathy with lactic acidosis and stroke-like episodes (MELAS syndrome) *Brain Dev 41:465–469, 2019*
    Neurofibromatosis type 1
    Susac's syndrome
  Illicit drug use
    Cocaine
    Amphetamines
    3,4-methylenedioxymethamphetamine ("ecstasy")
  Infectious arteriopathy
    Bacterial meningitis
    Coronovirus-2 (Covid 19)
    Fungal meningitis
    -
      Mucormycosis *E Cancer Medical Science Dec 19, 2013*
    Herpes zoster – vasculitis of cerebral arteries, confusion, seizures, stroke *NEJM 369;255–263, 2013*
    HIV disease
    Lyme disease *Cerebrovasc Dis 26:455–61, 2008; JAAD 49:363–392, 2003*
    Syphilis
    Tuberculosis
    Varicella
  Inflammatory arteriopathy
    Behcet's disease
    Cerebral amyloid angiopathy
    Eosinophilic granulomatosis with polyangiitis *Stroke Cerebrovasc Dis 26 e47–49, 2017; Acta Neurol Taiwan 21:169–175, 2012*
    Degos' disease
    Giant cell arteritis (temporal arteritis)
    Microscopic polyangiitis *J Neurol Sci 277:174–175, 2009*
    Primary angiitis of the central nervous system
    Polyarteritis nodosa
    Sneddon's syndrome – livedo racemosa *BMJ Case Rep Nov 21, 2019*
    Takayasu's arteritis
  Migraine-induced stroke
  Moyamoya disease
  Premature atherosclerosis or lipohyalinosis
  Radiation-induced arteriopathy
  Reversible cerebral vasoconstriction syndrome
  Sickle cell disease
  Transient cerebral arteriopathy of childhood

CARDIAC DISEASE

Arrhythmia (atrial fibrillation; sick sinus syndrome)
Cardiac surgery or catheterization
Cardiac tumors (atrial myxoma or papillary fibroelastoma)
Congenital heart disease
Dilated cardiomyopathy
Infectious and nonbacterial thrombotic endocarditis
NAME syndrome *J Assoc Physicians India 60:50–52, 2012*
Patent foramen ovale
Recent myocardial infarction
Rheumatic valvular heart disease

HEMATOLOGIC CAUSES

Heparin-induced thrombocytopenia (HIT syndrome)
Hypercoagulable state
  Anti-thrombin-3 mutation
  Factor V Leiden mutation
  Protein C deficiency
  Protein S deficiency
  Prothrombin G20210A
Acquired hypercoagulable state
  Anabolic steroids
  Antiphospholipid antibody syndrome
  Cancer
  Erythropoietin
  Nephrotic syndrome
  Oral contraceptive
  Pregnancy
Primary hematologic disorders
  Essential thrombocythemia
  Hypereosinophilic syndrome *J Stroke Cerebrovasc Dis 23:1709–1712, 2014; Acta Clin Croat 51:65–69, 2012*
  Leukemia
  Lymphoma
  Multiple myeloma
  Paroxysmal nocturnal hemoglobinuria
  Polycythemia vera
  Thrombotic thrombocytopenic purpura

SYNDROMES

Arterial tortuosity syndrome – fragmented elastic fibers and increase collagen deposition on skin biopsy *Genet Med 20:1236–1245, 2018*

Carney complex *Eur J Pediatr 168:1401–1404, 2009*

Deficiency of adenosine deaminase – ADA 1 – autosomal recessive; severe combined immunodeficiency; ADA 2 – loss of function mutation in cat eye syndrome chromosome candidate 1 gene (*CECR1*); painless leg nodules with intermittent livedo reticularis, Raynaud's phenomenon, cutaneous ulcers, morbilliform rashes,

Raynaud's phenomenon, digital gangrene, oral aphthae; vasculitis of small and medium arteries with necrosis, fever, early recurrent ischemic and hemorrhagic strokes, peripheral and cranial neuropathy, and gastrointestinal involvement (diarrhea); hepatosplenomegaly, systemic vasculopathy, stenosis of abdominal arteries *Ped Derm 37:199–201, 2020; NEJM 380:1582–1584, 2019; Ped Derm 33:602–614, 2016; NEJM 370:911–920, 2014; NEJM 370:921–931, 2014*

Ehlers-Danlos syndrome *Iran J Neurol 13:190–208, 2014*

Hereditary hemorrhagic telangiectasia (Osler-Weber-Rendu disease) – pulmonary arteriovenous fistulae with thrombotic or septic emboli *NEJM 381:2552, 2019; Handb Clin Neurol 135:185–197, 2015; Am J Med 82:989–997, 1987*

Kosaki overgrowth syndrome *Clin Genet April 14, 2020*

Leriche syndrome *Intern Med 57:1953–1954, 2018*

POEMS syndrome *Intern Med 58:3573–3575, 2019; BMJ Case Rep July 12, 2019*

Rabson-Mendenhall syndrome *Int J Dermatol 52:182–185, 2013*

Sturge-Weber syndrome *Pediatr Neurol 96:30–36, 2019*

SWOLLEN CALF

AUTOIMMUNE DISEASES AND DISORDERS OF IMMUNE DYSREGULATION

Deep morphea

DEGENERATIVE DISORDERS

Baker's cyst – "pseudothrombophlebitis syndrome" *Kaohsiung J Med Sci 20:600–603, 2004;* ruptured Baker's cyst *Singapore Med 37:175–180, 1996*

Ganglion cyst

Lumbosacral stenosis – compensatory work hypertrophy of non-denervated fibers *Spine 18:E406–409, 2002*

Radiculopathy – S1 radiculopathy *Lancet 365:1662, 2005; Arch Neurol 45:660–664, 1988;* focal myositis *J Neurol Sci 170:64–68, 1999*

INFECTIONS AND INFESTATIONS

Cellulitis – following knee replacement surgery *BMJ Case Rep Nov 21, 2019; SMJ 108:439–444, 2015*

Dengue fever – calf hematoma *BMJ Case Rep Jan 21, 2018*

Lyme disease – personal observation

Necrotizing fasciitis – *Serratia Age Aging 42:266–268, 2013*

Pyomyositis *Am J Orthoped 32:148–150, 2003*

Tuberculosis of muscle *BMJ Case Rep Nov 23, 2016; Phlebologie 45:185–189, 1992*

INFLAMMATORY DISORDERS

Eosinophilic fasciitis *Clin Med (London)20:105–106, 2010*

Fasciitis

Neurogenic muscle (pseudo)-hypertrophy – compensatory hypertrophy *Ned Tijdschr Geneeskd 147:2183–2186, 2003*

Panniculitis – atypical neutrophilic panniculitis in BCR-ABL negative chronic myelogenous leukemia *BMJ Case Rep Oct 8, 2019*

Polymyositis *J R Soc Med 96:236–237, 2003*

Rhabdomyolysis – mimics deep vein thrombosis *Postgrad Med J 63:653–655, 1987*

Ruptured popliteal cyst *Lancet 365:1662, 2005*

METABOLIC DISORDERS

Antiphospholipid antibody syndrome – hematoma within muscle *J Clin Rheumatol 8:346–349, 2002*

Diabetic myonecrosis *Ann Med Surg (London)35:141–145, 2018*

Scurvy *Skeletal Radiol 48:977–884, 2019*

NEOPLASTIC DISORDERS

Lipoma, intramuscular *Sarcoma 2:53–56, 1998*

Lymphoma – B-cell lymphoma *Oncol Lett 10:2156–2160, 2015*

Neural tumors

Sarcoma – leiomyosarcoma *BMJ Case Rep Oct 19, 2016;* myxoid chondrosarcoma *Zentrolbl Chir 135:83–86, 2010*

PRIMARY CUTANEOUS DISEASES

Lipedema – disproportionate obesity of legs in symmetric distribution *J Dtsch Dermatol Ges 11:225–233, 2013; Ann Rehabil Med 35:922–927, 2011*

TRAUMA

Achilles tendon rupture *China J Traumatol 19:290–294, 2016; Aust Fam Physician 29:35–40, 2000*

Compartment syndrome – trauma, fractures, surgery, vascular injuries, infection, myositis, insect bites *Medicine 97:e11613, 2018*

Dak-Bum devotees – tender swollen calf muscles and myoglobinuria *J Fam Med Prim Care 5:453–456, 2016*

Popliteus rupture – *Injury 25:200–201, 1994*

Tear of medial head of gastrocnemius or plantaris muscles

Trauma – hematoma *Lancet 365:1662, 2005*

VASCULAR DISORDERS

Aneurysm – pseudoaneurysm of anterior tibial artery *Am J Emerg Med 27:129.e3–4, 2009; Postgrad Med J 63:649–652, 1987*

Deep vein thrombosis *Zhonghua Liu Xing Bing Xue Za Zhi 29:716–719, 2008;* secondary to aortic aneurysm *Medicine 98:e16645, 2019*

Hemangioma

Popliteal artery pseudoaneurysm *J Surg Case Rep Nov 1, 2014*

Popliteal venous aneurysm *J Surg Case Rep Feb 15, 2020*

Polyarteritis nodosa *J Med Care Reports 15:450, 2011*

Vascular hamartoma *Proc R Soc Med 53:879, 1960*

Venous congestion – muscle edema *Rinsho Shinkeigaku 40:717–621, 2000*

Bilateral venous malformations – painless swollen calf muscles *World J Orthoped 8:602–605, 2017*

SYNDACTYLY

CLASSIFICATION

Eur J Hum Genet 20:817–824, 2012

DRUGS

Collagenase-induced syndactyly *J Hand Surg Eur Vol 41:665–666, 2016*

METABOLIC DISORDERS

Congenital dyserythropoietic anemia type I – small or absent nails; partial absence or shortening of fingers and toes, mesoaxial polydactyly, syndactyly of hands and feet; short stature, verterbral abnormalities and Madelung deformity; mutation in *CDAN1 Clin Exp Dermatol 515–517, 2020*

PRIMARY CUTANEOUS DISEASES

Epidermolysis bullosa – junctional EB, Herlitz type, recessive dystrophic EB, severe generalized, recessive dystrophic EB, generalized other *JAAD 58:931–950, 2008;* cicatricial junctional EB – scarring, alopecia, syndactyly, contractures *JAAD 12:836–844, 1985;* recessive dystrophic EB *Epidermolysis Bullosa: Basic and Clinical Aspects. New York: Springer, 1992: 135–151*

Hereditary acrokeratotic poikiloderma *AD 103:409–422, 1971*

Hidrotic ectodermal dysplasia *AD 113:472–476, 1977*

Lichen planus, ulcerative – webbing of toes *J R Soc Med 79:363–365, 1986*

Mal de Meleda – autosomal dominant, autosomal recessive transgrediens with acral erythema in glove-like distribution; syndactyly *Dermatology 203:7–13, 2001; AD 136:1247–1252, 2000; J Dermatol 27:664–668, 2000; Dermatologica 171:30–37, 1985*

Rapp-Hodgkin hypohidrotic ectodermal dysplasia–autosomal dominant; alopecia of wide area of scalp in frontal to crown area, short eyebrows and eyelashes, coarse wiry sparse hypopigmented scalp hair, sparse body hair, scalp dermatitis, ankyloblepharon, syndactyly, nipple anomalies, cleft lip and/or palate; nails narrow and dystrophic, small stature, hypospadius, conical teeth and anodontia or hypodontia; distinctive facies, short stature *JAAD 53:729–735, 2005; Ped Derm 7:126–131, 1990; J Med Genet 15:269–272, 1968*

Transient bullous dermolysis of the newborn with pseudosyndactyly – mutation in COL 7A1; subtype of dystrophic epidermolysis bullosa *BJD 157:179–182, 2007; AD 121:1429–1438, 1985*

SYNDROMES

Aarskog syndrome (facio-digito-genital syndrome) – X-linked recessive – anteverted nostrils, long philtrum, broad nasal bridge; short broad hands with syndactyly, scrotal shawl (scrotal fold which surrounds the base of the penis); skeletal defects; learning disabilities *J Pediatr 77:856–861, 1970*

Acrocallosal syndrome (Greig cephalopolysyndactyly syndrome) (Greig's polysyndactyly-cranial dysmorphism syndrome) – abnormal upper lids, frontonasal dysostosis, callosal agenesis, cleft lip/palate, redundant skin of neck, grooved chin, bifid thumbs, polydactyly, syndactyly *Am J Med Genet 43:938–941, 1992; Am J Med Genet 32:311–317, 1989; Clin Genet 24:257–265, 1983*

Acrodental dysostosis (polydactyly, conical teeth, nail dystrophy, short limbs) *Birth Defects 15:253–263, 1979*

Acrodermatitis continua of Hallopeau *BJD 152:1083–1084, 2005*

Acro-dermato-ungual-lacrimal-tooth syndrome (ADULT syndrome) – ectrodactyly or syndactyly, freckling and dry skin, dysplastic nails, superficial blisters and desquamation of hands and feet; lacrimal duct atresia, primary hypodontia, conical teeth, and early loss of permanent teeth; small ears hooked nose, sparse thin blond hair, frontal alopecia, hypohidrosis, lacrimal duct atresia, hypoplastic breasts and nipples, urinary tract anomalies; mutation in *TP63* gene (encodes transcription factor p63); p63 mutations also responsible for EEC, AEC, limb mammary, and Rapp-Hodgkin syndromes *BJD 172:276–278, 2015; Ped Derm 27:643–645, 2010; Hum Mol Genet 11:799–804, 2002; Am J Med Genet 45:642–648, 1993*

Acro-fronto-facio-nasal dysostosis *Am J Med Genet 20:631–638, 1985*

Acro-renal complex

Adams-Oliver syndrome

Albright's hereditary osteodystrophy

Amnion rupture malformation sequence (amniotic band syndrome)– congenital ring constrictions and intrauterine amputations; secondary syndactyly, polydactyly; distal lymphedema *JAAD 32:528–529, 1995; Am J Med Genet 42:470–479, 1992; Cutis 44:64–66, 1989*

AEC syndrome (Hay-Wells syndrome)–ankyloblepharon, ectodermal dysplasia, cleft lip/palate syndrome – blepharitis, eyelid papillomas, periorbital wrinkling; microcephaly, widespread congenital scalp erosions; alopecic ulcerated plaques of scalp, trunk, groin; alopecia of scalp and eyebrows; congenital erythroderma; depigmented patches; syndactyly; bony abnormalities; widely spaced nipples; TP63 mutation *Ped Derm 26:617–618, 2009; AD 141:1591–1594, 2005; AD 141:1567–1573, 2005; AD 134:1121–1124, 1998; Ped Derm 14:149–150, 1997;* generalized fissured erosions of trunk *BJD 149:395–399, 2003; TP63* mutations seen in AEC syndrome, EEC syndrome, Rapp-Hodgkin syndrome, limb-mammary syndrome, split-hand split-foot malformation type 4, acro-dermato-ungual-lacrimal-tooth syndrome *AD 141:1567–1573, 2005*

Apert's syndrome (acrocephalosyndactyly) – craniosynostosis, mid-facial malformations, symmetrical syndactyly; severe acne vulgaris; mutation of fibroblast growth factor receptor-2 *Ped Derm 24:186–188, 2007; Ped Derm 22:561–565, 2005; AD 102:381–385, 1970; Ann Hum Genet 24:151–164, 1960; Bull Soc Med Hop (Paris) 23:1310–1330, 1906*

Anderson-Tawil syndrome *Arq Neuropsiquiatr 72:899, 2014*

Aplasia cutis congenita Type II–scalp ACC with associated limb anomalies; hypoplastic or absent distal phalanges, syndactyly, club foot, others *Ped Derm 19:326–329, 2002*

Autosomal dominant syndactyly – *GJA1* mutation *Clin Chim Acta 459:73–78, 2016*

Autosomal dominant syndrome – camptodactyly, clinodactyly, syndactyly, and bifid toes *Am J Med Genet A 152A:2312–2317, 2010*

Auralcephalosyndactyly *J Med Genet 25:491–493, 1988*

Autosomal recessive blepharophimosis, ptosis, V-esotropia, syndactyly, and short stature *Clin Genet 41:57–61, 1992*

Autosomal recessive ectodermal dysplasia with corkscrew hairs, pili torti, syndactyly, keratosis pilaris, onychodysplasia, dental abnormalities, conjunctival erythema, palmoplantar keratoderma, cleft lip or palate, and mental retardation *JAAD 27:917–921, 1992*

Bannayan-Riley-Ruvalcaba-Zonana syndrome (PTEN phosphatase and tensin homolog hamartoma) – dolichocephaly, frontal bossing, macrocephaly, ocular hypertelorism, long philtrum, thin upper lip, broad mouth, relative micrognathia, lipomas, penile or vulvar lentigines, facial verruca-like or acanthosis nigricans-like papules, multiple acrochordons, angiokeratomas, transverse palmar crease, accessory nipple, syndactyly, brachydactyly, vascular malformations, arteriovenous malformations, lymphangiokeratoma, goiter, hamartomatous intestinal polyposis *JAAD 53:639–643, 2005*

Bilateral macrodystrophia lipomatosa *Hand Surg 18:267–272, 2013; J Plast Surg Hand Surg 45:303–306, 2011*

Bowen-Armstrong syndrome–ectodermal dysplasia, syndactyly, mental retardation, autosomal recessive *Clin Genet 9:35–42, 1976*

Buschke-Ollendorff syndrome *Ped Derm 29:6610662, 2012*

C syndrome (Opitz trigonocephaly syndrome) *Birth Defects 5:161–166, 1969*

Carpenter's syndrome *Turk Kardiyol Dern Ars 45:454–457, 2017; Klin Pediatr 189:120, 1977*

Cenani-Lenz syndactyly syndrome *Am J Med Genet A 179:266–279, 2019*

CHARGE syndrome – syndactyly, short stature, coloboma of the eye, heart anomalies, choanal atresia, somatic and mental retardation, genitourinary abnormalities, ear anomalies, primary lymphedema *Ped Derm 20:247–248, 2003; J Med Genet 26:202–203, 1989*

Cleft lip/palate-ectodermal dysplasia

Cleft lip-palate, mental and growth retardation, sensorineural hearing loss, and postaxial polydactyly *Syndromes of the Head and Neck, p. 772, 1990*

Cleft lip-palate, preaxial and postaxial polydactyly of hands and feet, congenital heart defect, and genitourinary anomalies *Syndromes of the Head and Neck, p. 751, 1990*

Cleft lip and palate, pili torti, malformed ears, partial syndactyly of fingers and toes, mental retardation *J Med Genet 24:291–293, 1987*

Cleft palate, absent tibiae, preaxial polydactyly of the feet, and congenital heart defect *Am J Dis Child 129:714–716, 1975*

Cleft palate, dysmorphic facies, digital defects *Syndrome Ident 5:14–18, 1977*

Cleft palate, microcephaly, short stature – large ears

Cleft uvula, preaxial and postaxial polysyndactyly, somatic and motor retardation *Eur J Pediatr 130:47–51, 1979*

Congenital cutis marmorata telangiectatica *Arch Argent Pod 114:e111–113, 2016*

Congenital erosive and vesicular dermatosis with reticulate supple scarring – widespread erosions, low set ears, syndactyly *Ped Derm 24:384–386, 2007; Ped Derm 22:55–59, 2005; JAAD 45:946–948,2001; Ped Derm 15:214–218, 1998; Dermatol 194:278–280, 1997; JAAD 32:873–877, 1995; AD 126:544–546, 1990; JAAD 17:369–376, 1987; AD 121:361–367, 1985*

Congenital onychodysplasia of the index fingers (COIF) (Iso Kikuchi syndrome) *J Hand Surg 15A:793–797, 1990*

Cornelia de Lange syndrome *Am J Med Genet 25:163–165, 1986*

Craniofrontonasal syndrome *Birth Defects 15:85–89, 1979*

Curry-Jones syndrome – linear hypo- or hyperpigmented lesions, palmoplantar pitting, streaks of atrophy, hypertrichosis, trichoblastomas and nevus sebaceous, polydactyly or preaxial polysyndactyly, dysmorphic facies, macrocephaly, microcephaly, dental anomalies, craniosynostosis, anal stenosis, myofibromas and smooth muscle hamartomas, medulloblastomas, cerebral malformations (agenesis of corpus callosum), developmental delay, cataracts, microphthalmia, coloboma, glaucoma, cryptorchidism; mutation in *SMOc.1234C>T BJD 182:212–217, 2020; Clin Dysmorphol 4:116–129, 1995*

del (3p) syndrome *J Med Genet 21:307–310, 1984*

Disorganization syndrome – filiform worm-like projections, syndactyly, popliteal pterygium, polydactyly, cleft lip/palate; ear abnormalities *Ped Derm 24:90–92, 2007; J Med Genet 26:417–420, 1989*

Distal aphalangia, syndactyly, extra metatarsal, short stature, microcephaly, borderline intelligence – autosomal dominant *Am J Med Genet 55:213–216, 1995*

Dubowitz syndrome

Duplication of the eyebrows, stretchable skin and syndactyly

Ectodermal dysplasia-syndactyly syndrome 1 – mutation in *PVRL4 Int J Dermatol 57:223–226, 2018; Ann Hum Genet 82:232–238, 2018*

Ectrodactyly-ectodermal dysplasia-clefting syndrome – alopecia of scalp, eyebrows, and eyelashes, xerosis, atopic dermatitis, nail dystrophy, hypodontia with peg shaped teeth, reduced sweat glands and salivary glands, syndactyly and split hand, mammary gland and nipple hypoplasia, conductive or sensorineural hearing loss, urogenital anomalies, lacrimal duct abnormalities; *TP63* mutations *BJD 162:201–207, 2010; Ped Derm 20:113–118, 2003; BJD 146:216–220, 2002; Dermatologica 169:80–85, 1984Ped Derm 20:113–118, 2003*

EEM syndrome *Arq Bras Oftalmol 81:440–442, 2018; J Med Genet 20:52–57, 1983*

Ellis-van Creveld syndrome *J Med Genet 17:349–356, 1980*

Epidermal (sebaceus) nevus syndrome

Familial milia and absent dermatoglyphics – digital flexion contractures, webbed toes, palmoplantar hypohidrosis, painful fissured calluses, acral blistering, simian crease *JAAD 59:1050–1063, 2008*

Familial syndactyly *Eur J Hum Genet 20:817–824, 2012*

FG syndrome (unusual facies, mental retardation, congenital hypotonia, imperforate anus) *Am J Med Genet 19:383–386, 1984*

Fibrolipomatous hamartoma of the nerve – macrodactyly and syndactyly *JAAD 70:736–742, 2014*

Filippi syndrome – short stature, microcephaly, characteristic face, polydactyly, syndactyly, mental retardation; *CKAPZL* mutation *Clin Genet 93:1109–1110, 2018; Am J Med Genet 87:128–133, 1999; Genet Couns 4:147–151, 1993*

Finlay-Marks syndrome (scalp-ear-nipple syndrome) – nipple or breast hypoplasia or aplasia, aplasia cutis congenita of scalp, abnormal ears and teeth, nail dystrophy, syndactyly, reduced apocrine secretion

Fontaine syndrome (ectrodacytyly of the feet and cleft palate) *J Genet Hum 22:289–307, 1974*

Fraser syndrome (cryptophthalmos-syndactyly syndrome) *Atlas of Clinical Syndromes A Visual Aid to Diagnosis, 1992, pp.74–75*

Frontonasal malformation *Clin Genet 10:214–217, 1976*

Frydman syndrome – autosomal recessive; prognathism, syndactyly, short stature, blepharophimosis, weakness of extraocular and frontal muscles, synophrys *Clin Genet 41:57–61, 1992*

Fused digits with micronychia

Generalized anhidrosis, diffuse reticular hyperpigmentation, syndactyly *J Dermatol 46:e154–155, 2019*

Goltz's syndrome (focal dermal hypoplasia) – syndactyly, hypoplasia or aplasia of digits, ectrodactyly, clawhand or foot (gampsodactyly), polydactyly, oligodactyly, asymmetric linear and reticulated streaks of atrophy and telangiectasia; yellow-red nodules; raspberry-like papillomas of lips, perineum, acrally, at perineum, buccal mucosa; linear alopecia, xerosis; scalp and pubic hair sparse and brittle; short stature; asymmetric face; syndactyly, polydactyly; ocular, dental, and skeletal abnormalities with osteopathia striata of long bones; iris colobomas *Ped Derm 31:220–224, 2014; AD 143:109–114, 2007; Cutis 53:309–312, 1994; J Dermatol 21:122–124, 1994; JAAD 25:879–881, 1991; AD 86:708–717, 1962;* male mosaic Goltz's syndrome; blaschko-linear white atrophic depigmented lines, hyperpigmented linear streaks, linear alopecia, syndactyly, hydronephrosis *Ped Derm 28:550–554, 2011*

Happle-Tinschert syndrome – segmental basaloid follicular hamartomas, basal cell carcinomas, linear hypo- or hyperpigmented lesions, linear atrophoderma, palmoplantar pitting, atrophoderma, ipsilateral hypertrichosis, hypotrichosis; polydactyly, syndactyly, rudimentary ribs, limb length disparities, dysmorphic facies, macrocephaly, jaw ameloblastomas, dental anomalies, imperforate anus, colon adenocarcinoma; medulloblastoma cerebral manifestation, developmental delay, optic glioma or meningioma, cataracts, microphthalmia, coloboma; mutation in *SMOc.1234>T BJD 182:212–217, 2020; BJD 169:1342–1345, 2013; Ped Derm 28:555–560, 2011; JAAD 65:e17–19, 2011; Dermatology 218:221–225, 2009; Acta DV 88:382–387, 2008*

Hemihyperplasia-Multiple Lipomatosis syndrome – extensive congenital vascular stain, compressible blue nodule, multiple subcutaneous nodules, hemihypertrophy, syndactyly, thickened but not cerebriform soles, dermatomyofibroma *Soc Ped Derm Annual Meeting, July 2005; Am J Med Genet 130A-111–122, 2004; Am J Med Genet 79:311–318, 1998*

Holoprosencephaly syndrome

Holt-Oram syndrome (Hand-heart syndrome type I)

Hydrolethalus syndrome *Am J Med Genet 27:935–942, 1987*

Hypohidrosis and diabetes insipidus (Fleck syndrome) – hypohidrosis, hypotrichosis, diabetes insipidus, syndactyly, coloboma, disturbed hematopoiesis *Dermatol Wochenschr 132:994–1007, 1955*

Hypomelanosis of Ito/pigmentary mosaicism

Kabuki makeup syndrome – short stature, congenital heart defects, distinct expressionless face (frontal bossing, long palpebral fissures, eversion of the lower eyelids, sparse arched lateral eyebrows, epicanthus, telecanthus, prominent eyelashes, short flat nose with anteversion of the tip, short philtrum, large mouth with thick lips, high arched palate, cleft palate, dental malocclusion, micrognathia, large protuberant low set ears with thick helix), lowcut hairline, vitiligo, cutis laxa, hyperextensible joints, syndactyly of toes 2–3, brachydactyly, clinodactyly, fetal finger pads with abnormal dermatoglyphics, short great toes, blue sclerae, lower lip pits, cryptorchidism, mental retardation with microcephaly; preauricular dimple/fistula *Ped Derm 24:309–312, 2007; JAAD S247–251, 2005; Am J Med Genet 132A:260–262, 2005; Am J Med Genet 94:170–173, 2000; Am J Med Genet 31:565–589, 1988; J Pediatr 105:849–850, 1984; J Pediatr 99:565–569, 570–573, 1981*

Kallman syndrome *J Coll Physicians Surg Pak 29:5101–5102, 2019*

Kaufman-McKusick syndrome – hydrometrocolpos, postaxial polydactyly, congenital heart defect *Eur J Pediatr 136:297–305, 1981*

Kindler's syndrome – webbing due to congenital blistering; pseudosyndactyly resembles that of dystrophic epidermolysis bullosa *JAMA 306:767–768, 2011; BJD 160:1119–1122, 2009; BJD 160:233–242, 2009; Ped Derm 23:586–588, 2006; AD 142:1619–1624, 2006; AD 142:620–624, 2006; AD 140:939–944, 2004; AD 1487–1490, 1996; BJD 66:104–111, 1954*

Klippel-Trenaunay syndrome – port wine stain with lymphatic malformation and lymphedema *JAAD 65:893–906, 2011; JAAD 61:621–628, 2009*

Koraxitrachitic syndrome – self-healing collodion baby; heals with mottled reticulated atrophy; alopecia, absent eyelashes and eyebrows, conjunctival pannus, hypertelorism, prominent nasal root, large mouth, micrognathia, brachydactyly, syndactyly of interdigital spaces *Am J Med Genet 86:454–458, 1999*

LADD syndrome Mol Vis 23:179–184, 2017; Eur J Pediatr 146:536–537, 1987

Lenz-Majewski syndrome *Radiology 149:129–131, 1983*

LEOPARD (Moynahan's) syndrome – CALMs, granular cell myoblastomas, steatocystoma multiplex, small penis, hyperelastic skin, low set ears, short webbed neck, short stature, syndactyly *JAAD 46:161–183, 2002; JAAD 40:877–890, 1999; Am J Med 60:447–456, 1976*

Macrocephaly-CMTC (cutis marmorata telangiectatica congenita syndrome) – renamed "macrocephaly-capillary malformation syndrome"–macrocephalic neonatal hypotonia and developmental delay; frontal bossing, segmental overgrowth, syndactyly, asymmetry, distended linear and serpiginous abdominal wall veins, patchy reticulated vascular stain without atrophy; telangiectasias of face and ears; midline reticulated facial nevus flammeus (capillary malformation) (vascular stains), hydrocephalus, skin and joint hypermobility, hyperelastic skin, thickened subcutaneous tissue, polydactyly, 2–3 toe syndactyly, post-axial polydactyly, hydrocephalus, frontal bossing, hemihypertrophy with segmental overgrowth; neonatal hypotonia, developmental delay *Ped Derm 29:384–386, 2012; Ped Derm 26:342–346, 2009; AD 145:287–293, 2009; JAAD 58:697–702, 2008; Ped Derm 24:555–556, 2007; JAAD 56:541–564, 2007; Ped Derm 16:235–237, 1999; Genet Couns 9:245–253, 1998; Am J Med Genet 70:67–73, 1997; Clin Dysmorphol 6:291–302, 1997;*

(Note: Beckwith-Wiedemann syndrome demonstrates dysmorphic ears, macroglossia, body asymmetry, midfacial vascular stains, visceromegaly with omphalocele, neonatal hypoglycemia, BUT NO MACROCEPHALY)

Meckel syndrome – microcephaly, microphthalmia, congenital heart defects, postaxial polydactyly, polycystic kidneys, cleft lip/palate *J Med Genet 8:285–290, 1971*

MEND – X-linked recessive; hypomorphic mutation of emopamil-binding protein; diffuse mild ichthyosis; telecanthus, prominent nasal bridge, low set ears, micrognathia, cleft palate large anterior fontanelle, polydactyly, 2–3 syndactyly, kyphosis, Dandy-Walker malformation, cerebellar hypoplasia, corpus callosal hypoplasia, hydrocephalus, hypotonia, developmental delay, seizures; bilateral cataracts, glaucoma, hypertelorism; cardiac valvular and septal defects, hypoplastic aortic arch; renal malformation, cryptorchidism, hypospadias *BJD 166:1309–1313, 2012*

Menkes' kinky hair syndrome – X-linked recessive; polydactyly, syndactyly, fine hypopigmented wiry hair, doughy skin, bone and connective tissue disturbances, progressive neurologic deterioration; intracranial hemorrhages *Cutis 90:183–185, 2012*

Nail-patella syndrome (Fong's syndrome, hereditary onychoosteodysplasia, Turner-Kieser syndrome) – autosomal dominant; webbing between digits and/or within popliteal fossa, cloverleaf iris (Lester iris); LMX1B mutation (dorsal/ventral patterning) *Ped Derm*

27:95–97, 2010; Dermatology 213:153–155, 2006; JAAD 49:1086–1087, 2003

Nasal alar colobomas, mirror hands and feet, and talipes *J Bone Jt Surg 52:367–370, 1970*

Neu-Laxova syndrome – variable presentation; mild scaling to harlequin ichthyosis appearance; ichythosiform scaling, increased subcutaneous fat and atrophic musculature, generalized edema and mildly edematous feet and hands, absent nails; microcephaly, intrauterine growth retardation, limb contractures, low set ears, sloping forehead, short neck; small genitalia, eyelid and lip closures, syndactyly, cleft lip and palate, micrognathia; autosomal recessive; uniformly fatal *Ped Derm 20:25–27,78–80, 2003; Curr Prob Derm 14:71–116, 2002; Clin Dysmorphol 6:323–328, 1997; Am J Med Genet 35:55–59, 1990; Am J Med Genet 13:445–452, 1982*

Nevoid basal cell carcinoma syndrome (Gorlin's syndrome) – autosomal dominant; macrocephaly, frontal bossing, hypertelorism, cleft lip or palate, papules of the face, neck, and trunk, facial milia, lamellar calcification of the falx cerebri and tentorium cerebelli, cerebral cysts, calcifications of the brain, palmoplantar pits, mandibular keratocysts, skeletal anomalies, including enlarged mandibular coronoid, bifid ribs, kyphosis, spina bifida, polydactyly of the hands or feet, syndactyly; basal cell carcinomas; multiple eye anomalies – congenital cataract, microphthalmia, coloboma of the iris, choroid, and optic nerve; strabismus, nystagmus, keratin-filled cysts of the palpebral conjunctivae; also medulloblastomas, ovarian tumors (fibromas), mesenteric cysts, cardiac fibromas, fetal rhabdomyomas, astrocytomas, meningiomas, craniopharyngiomas, fibrosarcomas, ameloblastomas; renal anomalies; hypogonadotropic hypogonadism, *BJD 165:30–34, 2011; AD 146:17–19, 2010; JAAD 53:S256–259, 2005; JAAD 39:853–857, 1998; Dermatol Clin 13:113–125, 1995; JAAD 11:98–104, 1984; NEJM 262:908–912, 1960;* linear unilateral nevoid basal cell nevus syndrome *JAAD 50:489–494, 2004*

Nevus comedonicus syndrome – with ipsilateral polysyndactyly and bilateral oligodontia *Ped Derm 27:377–379, 2010*

Nijmegen breakage syndrome – autosomal recessive; microcephaly, growth retardation, chromosomal instability, and combined immunodeficiency; pink to red-brown firm papules and plaques with sclerosis and atrophy, clinodactyly, syndactyly, vitiligo, café au lait macules *Ped Derm 27:285–289, 2010*

Oculo-dento-osseous (oculo-dento-digital) dysplasia – sparse scalp hair, eyebrows and eyelashes sparse or absent, small closely set sunken eyes, small mouth, enamel hypoplasia producing yellow teeth, syndactyly, camptodactyly, iris anomalies, hypertelorism *Cytogenet Genome Res 154:181–186, 2018; J Pediatr 63:69–75, 1963*

Opitz trigonocephaly syndrome (Smith-Lemli-Opitz syndrome)–syndactyly of 2nd and 3rd toes *BJD 138:885–888, 1998;*

Am J Dis Child 129:1348, 1975

Oral-facial-digital syndrome type I (Papillon-Leage syndrome) – X-linked dominant; short upper lip, hypoplastic ala nasi, hooked pug nose, hypertrophied labial frenulum, bifid or multilobed tongue with small tumors within clefts, clefting of hard and soft palate, teeth widely spaced, trident hand or brachydactyly, syndactyly, or polydactyly; hair dry and brittle, alopecic, numerous milia of face, ears, backs of hands, mental retardation *Ped Derm 9:52–56, 1992*

Oro-acral syndrome–microglossia to aglossia, cleft palate

Oto-palato-digital syndrome *J Craniofac Surg 28:1068–1070, 2017*

Pallister-Hall syndrome *Am J Med Genet 7:75–83, 1980*

Pfeiffer syndrome – syndactyly, craniosynostosis, broad great toes, pre-auricular tag, gingival hypertrophy *Z Kinderheilkd 90:301–320, 1964*

Pili torti, defective teeth, webbed fingers *JAAD 46:301–303, 2002*

Poland's chest wall deformity–breast and pectoralis muscle hypoplasia; absence of axillary hair, ipsilateral syndactyly, dermatoglyphic abnormalities *Hand (NX)11:389–395, 2016; Am J Clin Dermatol 16:295–301, 2015; Clin Exp Dermatol 25:308–311, 2000; Plast Reconstr Surg 99:429–436, 1997*

Polydactyly and syndactyly

Popliteal pterygium syndrome – autosomal dominant; bilateral popliteal pterygia, intercrural pterygium, hypoplastic digits, valgus or varus foot deformities, syndactyly, cryptorchidism, inguinal hernia, cleft scrotum, lower lip pits, mucous membrane bands, eyelid adhesions *J Med Genet 36:888–892, 1999; Int J Pediatr Otorhinolaryngol 15:17–22, 1988*

Postaxial acrofacial dysostosis *J Pediatr 95:970–975, 1979*

Postaxial polydactyly-dental-vertebral syndrome *J Pediatr 90:230–235, 1977*

Proteus syndrome *Cutis 83:255–261, 2009*

Rabenhorst syndrome–syndactyly of 2nd and 3rd toes

Reticulolinear aplasia cutis congenita of the face and neck – Xp deletion syndrome, MIDAS (microphthalmia, dermal aplasia, sclerocornea), MLS (microphthalmia and linear skin defects), and Gazali-Temple syndrome (syndactyly); lethal in males; residual facial scarring in females, short stature, organ malformations *BJD 138:1046–1052, 1998*

Riga-Fede disease *J Clin Pediatr Dent 43:356–359, 2019*

Robert's syndrome (pseudothalidomide syndrome)

Rosselli-Gulinetti syndrome – autosomal recessive, hypohidrosis, fine, dry, sparse scalp hair, dystrophic nails and teeth, cleft lip and palate, syndactyly, defects of external genitalia *J Plast Surg 14:190–204, 1961*

Rothmund-Thomson – syndactyly, absent thumbs *JAAD 75:855–870, 2016*

Russell-Silver syndrome – large head, short stature, premature sexual development, CALMs, clinodactyly, syndactyly of toes, triangular face *JAAD 40:877–890, 1999; J Med Genet 36:837–842, 1999*

Saethre-Chotzen syndrome – partial syndactyly of second and third fingers, craniosynostosis, low-set frontal hairline, facial asymmetry, ptosis, brachydactyly, other skeletal anomalies *Acta Anaesthesiol Belg 65:179–182, 2104; Dtsch Z Nerverneilkd 117:533–555, 1931*

Sataki syndrome *J Pediatr 79:104–109, 1971*

Say-Poznanski syndrome *Pediatr Radiol 17:93–96, 1987*

Scalp-ear-nipple syndrome – autosomal dominant; aplasia cutis congenita of the scalp, irregularly shaped pinna, hypoplastic nipple, widely spaced teeth, partial syndactyly *Am J Med Genet 50:247–250, 1994*

Sclerosteosis *Bone 116:321–322, 2018; Ped Radiol 45:1239–1243, 2015; Ann Int Med 84:393–397, 1976*

Seckel's syndrome – abnormal teeth, short stature, hypopigmented papules and macules, small deformed ears lacking lobles, syndactyly, clinodactyly *Ped Derm 24:53–56, 2007*

Short rib-polydactyly syndrome *Am J Roentgenol 114:257–263, 1972*

Smith-Lemli-Opitz syndrome – autosomal recessive; occasional immunodeficiency; hypospadias, cryptorchidism, hypospadias, partial syndactyly of 2nd and 3rd toes, polydactyly, dysmorphic facies with anteverted nostrils, cleft palate, congenital heart disease, severe photosensitivity, 7-dehydrocholesterol reductase deficiency (defect in cholesterol metabolism) *BJD 153:774–779, 2005; NEJM 351;2319–2326, 2004; JAAD 41:121–123, 1999; BJD 141:406–414, 1999; Am J Med Genet 66:378–398, 1996; Clin Pediatr 16:665–668, 1977; J Pediatr 64:210–217, 1964*

STAR syndrome plus *Am J Med Genet A 173:3226–3230, 2017*

Symphalangism-brachydactyly syndrome with conductive hearing impairment

Syndactyly, congenital

Timothy syndrome-like condition with syndactyly without QT prolongation *Am J Med Genet A 176:1657–1661, 2018; Clin Res Cardiol 100:1123–1127, 2011*

Townes-Brocks syndrome *J Pediatr 81:321–326, 1972*

Triploidy syndrome *Syndromes of the Head and Neck, p.64, 1990*

Trisomy 13 (Patau) syndrome *J Genet Hum 23:83–109, 1975*

Trisomy 21 *Eur J Med Genet 58:674–680, 2015*

Turner's syndrome *J Ped 45:85, 2019*

Type VI syndactyly – with skeletal dysplasia; a new syndrome? *Clin Dysmorphol 28:30–34, 2019*

Varadi syndrome (polydactyly, cleft lip/palate, lingual lump, cerebellar anomalies *J Med Genet 17:119–122, 1980*

Waardenburg syndrome, type 3 *Genet Mol Res Dec 2, 2016*

Zlotogora-Ogur syndrome–ectodermal dysplasia, syndactyly, mental retardation, autosomal recessive *J Med Genet 24:291–293, 1987*

TRAUMA

Burns *BJD 152:1083–1084, 2005*

Physical trauma *BJD 152:1083–1084, 2005*

VASCULAR DISORDERS

Macrocephaly-capillary malformation syndrome – body asymmetry, 2–3 toe syndactyly, hypotonia, developmental delay, midfacial vascular stains, joint laxity, loose skin *Ped Derm 33:570–584, 2016; Ped Derm 24:555–556, 2007*

SYNDACTYLY WITH CRANIODYSOSTOSIS

AD 128:1378–1386, 1992

Apert's syndrome

Cranioectodermal dysplasia

Craniosynostosis syndromes

SYNOPHRYS

Aging

Drug-induced – diazoxide

Familial

Bohring-Opitz syndrome – facial nevus flammeus, unexplained bradycardia, obstructive apnea, pulmonary infections *Am J Med Genet 182:201–204, 2020*

Broad thumb hallux syndrome–synophrys *JAAD 37:295–297, 1997*

Centrofacial lentiginosis – synophrys, high arched palate, sacral hypertrichosis, spina bifida, scoliosis *BJD 94:39–43, 1976*

Cerebrofaciothoracic dysplasia *Am J Med Genet 179:43–49, 2019*

CHOPS syndrome – coarse facies, heart defects, obesity, pulmonary involvement, short stature, long eyelashes, synophrys *Am J Med Genet 179:1126–1138, 2019*

Cornelia de Lange syndrome – specific facies, hypertrichosis of forehead, face, back, shoulders, and extremities, synophrys; long delicate eyelashes, cutis marmorata, skin around eyes and nose with bluish tinge, red nose *Ped Derm 19:42–45, 2002; JAAD 37:295–297, 1997; J Pediatr Ophthalmol Strabismus 27:94–102, 1990*

Cretinism – coarse facial features, lethargy, macroglossia, cold dry skin, livedo, umbilical hernia, poor muscle tone, coarse scalp hair, synophrys, no pubic or axillary hair at puberty

Del (3p) syndrome *Am J Med Genet 32:269–273, 1990*

Distichiasis-lymphedema syndrome *BJD 142:148–152, 2000*

3q duplication syndrome *Birth Defects 14:191–217, 1978*

Elsahy-Waters syndrome *Am J Med Genet 173:3143–3152, 2017*

Familial trichomegaly – increased length of forearm hair, synophrys, nonsyndromic oculocutaneous albinism; mutation in *FGF5* gene *BJD 174:741–752, 2016; Am J Med Genet A 136A:398, 2005; Arch Ophthalmol 115:1602–1603, 1997*

Fetal trimethadione syndrome *Teratology 3:349–362, 1970*

Frydman syndrome – autosomal recessive; prognathism, syndactyly, short stature, blepharophimosis, weakness of extraocular and frontal muscles, synophrys *Clin Genet 41:57–61, 1992*

Hajdu-Cheney syndrome (osteolysis)–broad eyebrows with synophrys *J Periodontol 55:224–229, 1984*

Hypertrichosis lanuginosa

Infantile systemic hyalinosis – autosomal recessive; synophrys, thickened skin, perianal nodules, dusky red plaques of buttocks, gingival hypertrophy, joint contractures, juxta-articular nodules (knuckle pads), osteopenia, growth failure, diarrhea, frequent infections, facial red papules *JAAD 50:S61–64, 2004*

KBG syndrome – autosomal dominant; macrodontia, characteristic facial features with triangular face, bushy eyebrows, bulbous nose, synophrys *Orphanet Rare Dis Dec 19, 2017*

Kwashiorkor

Mucopolysaccharidoses types I, II, III, IV, VI–thick eyebrows with synophrys *JAAD 37:295–297, 1997*

Pachyonychia congenita

Pigmented hairy epidermal nevus syndrome – unilateral brown hyperpigmented plaques with hypertrichosis; generalized checkerboard pattern, ipsilateral hypoplasia of the breast, skeletal abnormalities *JAAD 50:957–961, 2004*

Porphyrias – congenital erythropoietic porphyria, porphyria cutanea tarda

Waardenburg's syndrome – synophrys; widow's peak; sensorineural hearing loss, pigmentation abnormalities of hair and skin; hypoplastic blue eyes or heterochromia irides *JAAD 37–295–297, 1997*

TAILS

Apert syndrome *Oan Med J 29:e0580, 2014; Orphanet J Rare Dis 1:19, 2006*

Caudal appendage, short terminal phalanges, deafness, cryptorchidism, and mental retardation *Clin Dysmorphol 3:340–346, 1994*

Congenital isolated perineal lipoma – presenting as human pseudotail *Am Surg Treat Res 90:53–55, 2016*

Ectopic renal tissue – pedunculated sacral mass *Ped Derm 36:542–543, 2019*

FGFR1 mutation *Childs Nerv Syst 28:1221–1226, 2012*

Goltz's syndrome *AD 145:218–219, 2009*

Tail–like malformation (cervical braid) *Br J Plast Surg 43:369–370, 1990*

Human tail – with underlying spinal dysraphism

Persistent vestigial tail

Pseudotail with spinal dysraphism; tethered cord, spina bifida occulta

Sacrococcygeal eversion – in Goldenhaar syndrome, Turner's syndrome *Childs Nerv Syst 33:69–89, 2017*

True human tail – benign vestigial caudal cutaneous structure *Asian J Neurosurg 14:1–4, 2019; Sultan Qaboos Univ Med J 17:e109–111, 2017*

TALL STATURE SYNDROMES

Beckwith–Wiedemann syndrome

Congenital generalized lipodystrophy *Atlas of Clinical Syndromes A Visual Aid to Diagnosis, 1992, pp.280–281*

Contractural arachnodactyly *Atlas of Clinical Syndromes A Visual Aid to Diagnosis, 1992, pp.144–145*

Exomphalos–macroglossia–gigantism syndrome *Atlas of Clinical Syndromes A Visual Aid to Diagnosis, 1992, pp.136–137*

Fragile X syndrome *Am J Med Genet C Semin Med Genet 137C:32–37, 2005*

Homocystinuria *Atlas of Clinical Syndromes A Visual Aid to Diagnosis, 1992, pp.146–147*

Klinefelter's syndrome

Marfan's syndrome *Human Mut 37:524–531, 2016*

Normal variant tall stature/familial tall stature; constitutional advance of growth *Curr Pediatric Rev 15:10–21, 2019*

Proteus syndrome *Atlas of Clinical Syndromes A Visual Aid to Diagnosis, 1992, pp.352–355*

Simpson–Folabi–Behmel syndrome *Mol Genet Metab 72:279–286, 2001*

Soto syndrome *Atlas of Clinical Syndromes A Visual Aid to Diagnosis, 1992, pp.138–139*

Susceptibility to autism 18

Tatton–Brown Rahman syndrome *Wellcome Open Res 3:46, 2018*

Triple X syndrome

Weaver syndrome *Atlas of Clinical Syndromes A Visual Aid to Diagnosis, 1992, pp.140–141*

XYY syndrome *Atlas of Clinical Syndromes A Visual Aid to Diagnosis, 1992, pp.148–149*

TARGET LESIONS

AUTOIMMUNE DISEASES AND DISEASES OF IMMUNE DYSFUNCTION

Allergic contact dermatitis – to rubber gloves *Contact Dermatitis 45:311–312, 2001;* cardiac monitor electrodes; benzalkonium chloride *Contact Dermatitis Feb 28, 2020*

Alopecia areata – perinevoid alopecia *BJD 179:969–970, 2019*

Autoimmune estrogen dermatitis – erythema multiforme–like *JAAD 49:130–132, 2003*

Autoimmune progesterone dermatitis – bullous erythema multiforme; *J Dermatol 47:178–180, 2020; J R Soc Med 78:407–408, 1985; Cutis 33:490–491, 1984*

Bullous pemphigoid *J Dermatol Sci 78:5–10, 2015; Clin Exp Dermatol 24:263–265, 1999; AD 133:775–780, 1997;* pemphigoid en cocarde *JAAD 20:1125, 1989*

Common variable immunodeficiency with functional T–cell defect – granulomatous dermatitis – targetoid facial plaques *AD 142:783–784, 2006*

Dermatitis herpetiformis – targetoid lesions of palms *Clin Exp Dermatol 30:294–307, 2005*

Epidermolysis bullosa acquisita *AD 133:1122–1126, 1997*

Graft vs. host disease, chronic – targetoid lesions of palmar creases *JAAD 59:S127–128, 2008*

Herpes (pemphigoid) gestationis – erythema multiforme–like lesions *BJD 172:120–129, 2015; BJD 170:760–762, 2013; JAAD 55:823–828, 2006; JAAD 40:847–849, 1999;* concentric bullae *JAMADerm 150:445–446, 2014*

Linear IgA bullous dermatosis – rosette lesions *Ped Derm 26:28–33, 2009; AD 139:1121–1124, 2003; Ped Derm 13:509–512, 1996; Cutis 45:37–42, 1990; Int J Dermatol 26:513–517, 1987;* targetoid, urticarial, herpetiform lesions, confluent bullae *BJD 177:212–222, 2017;* targetoid bullae *BJD 169:210–211, 2013; Ped Derm 27:178–181, 2010;* mimicking Stevens–Johnson syndrome *BJD 178:786–789, 2018*

Lupus erythematosus – neonatal lupus erythematosus; bullous dermatosis of SLE (annular bullae) – face, neck, upper trunk, oral bullae *JAAD 27:389–394, 1992; Ann Int Med 97:165–170, 1982; Arthritis Rheum 21:58–61, 1978;* discoid LE resembling erythema multiforme (targetoid lesions) *Dermatologica 122:6–10, 1961;* subacute cutaneous LE *Acta DV 80:308–309, 2000; JAAD 35:147–169, 801–803, 1996;* lupus with erythema multiforme–like lesions (Rowell's syndrome) *BJD 142:343–346, 2000; Eur J Dermatol 10:459–462, 2000; Clin Exp Dermatol 24:74–77, 1999;* systemic lupus erythematosus – lesions of palate, buccal mucosa, gums; red or purpuric areas with red halos break down to form shallow ulcers *BJD 135:355–362, 1996; BJD 121:727–741, 1989*

Morphea

Pemphigus – IgG/IgA pemphigus – herpetiform, targetoid lesions *BJD 147:1012–1017, 2002*

Pemphigus herpetiformis – concentric targetoid lesions; herpetiform bullous lesions; serpiginous blisters *JAAD 70:780–787, 2014; Ped Derm 30:760–762, 2013*

Pemphigus vegetans – personal observation

Pemphigus vulgaris – personal observation; peristomal pemphigus vulgaris – personal observation

Rheumatoid vasculitis – personal observation

Serum sickness–like reaction *Clinics Dermatology 37:148–158, 2019*

Sjogren's syndrome – erythema multiforme

Urticaria – foods, drugs, hymenoptera stings, plasma expanders, blood products, anesthetic agents

DRUG

Acute generalized exanthematous pustulosis with erythema multiforme–like lesions *NEJM 375:471–475, 2016; Eur J Dermatol 12:475–478, 2002*

Drug reactions surrounding seborrheic keratoses

Clindamycin–induced acute generalized exanthematous pustulosis *AD 142:1080–1081, 2006*

Dermal hypersensitivity reaction – personal observation

Drug–induced linear IgA disease – amiodarone, captopril, cefamandole, cyclosporine, diclofenac, euglucon, furosemide, interleukin, lithium, phenytoin, somatostatin, sulfa, vigabatrin, piroxicam, vancomycin *JAAD 45:691–696, 2001; Cutis 44:393–396, 1989*

Drug reaction with eosinophilia and systemic symptoms (DRESS) – morbilliform eruption, cheilitis (crusted hemorrhagic lips), diffuse desquamation, areolar erosion, periorbital dermatitis, vesicles, bullae, targetoid plaques, purpura, pustules, exfoliative erythroderma, urticarial papular–confluent; facial edema, lymphadenopathy *BJD 168:391–401, 2013; Ped Derm 28:741–743, 2011; JAAD 68:693–705, 2013; AD 146:1373–1379, 2010; Ped Derm 26:536–546, 2009*

Erlotinib – painful annular pustular eruption; targetoid lesions *Cutis 88:281–283, 2012*

Fixed drug reactions; *AD 120:520–524, 1984;* clopidogrel *JAMADerm 152:1169–1170, 2016;* generalized fixed drug eruption *Clinics in Dermatology 37:148–158, 2019*

Interferon – erythema gyratum repens due to pegylated interferon *AD 148:1213–1214, 2012*

Non–selective antiangiogenic multikinase inhibitors – sorafenib, sunitinib, pazopanib – hyperkeratotic hand foot skin reactions with knuckle papules, inflammatory reactions, alopecia, kinking of hair, depigmentation of hair; chloracne–like eruptions, erythema multiforme, toxic epidermal necrolysis, drug hypersensitivity, red scrotum with erosions, yellow skin, eruptive nevi, pyoderma gangrenosum–like lesions *JAAD 72:203–218, 2015*

Propranolol – annular telangiectatic perivascular angiomatosis – red to violaceous hyperpigmented annular plaques with central clearing and radial telangiectasia *BJD 169:1369–1371, 2013*

Ranitidine drug rash

Sorafenib – targetoid plaques mimicking erythema multiforme *Postgrad Med J 94:535–536, 2018; JAMADerm 152:227–228, 2016*

Syringosquamous metaplasia associated with chemotherapy *Soc Ped Derm Annual Meeting, July 2005*

Trimethoprim – bullous fixed drug eruption; bulla of leg with surrounding erythema *AD 143:535–540, 2007*

Urticarial drug reactions *Clin Inf Dis 58:1140–1148, 2014*

Ustekinumab – leukocytoclastic vasculitis – purpuric necrotic targetoid bullae *J Drugs Dermatol 15:358–361, 2016*

Vincristine/vinblastine/vinorelbine – erythema multiforme–like lesions *JAAD 71:203–214, 2014*

Vitamin K reaction *Contact Dermatitis 77:343–345, 2017*

Vasculitis, drug–induced; systemic disease *Clinics in Dermatology 37:148–158, 2019; J Med Case Rep 7:34, 2013; BJD 135:972–975, 1996;* anti–tuberculous medications *J Eur Acad DV 21:135–136, 2007*

EXOGENOUS AGENTS

Acute iododerma, radiocontrast material – personal observation

Bath powder *BJD 148:171–172, 2003*

Rhus lacquer – ingestion resulting in erythema multiforme, exfoliative erythroderma, morbilliform exanthema *BJD 142:937–942, 2000*

INFECTIONS AND INFESTATIONS

Acremonium – target–like lesions with central necrosis

African trypanosomiasis *AD 131:1178–1182, 1995*

Anthrax – central eschar with surrounding vesicles *J Clin Inf Dis 19:1009–1014, 1994*

Brown recluse spider bite – *Loxosceles rufescens;* eschar, necrosis, targetoid: 6 eyes *JAMADerm 156:203, 2020*

Burkholderia pseudomallei (melioidosis) – disseminated; ecthyma–like lesions *Clin Inf Dis 40:988–989, 1053–1054, 2005*

Candida tropicalis – candidal sepsis; disseminated candidiasis; targetoid lesions with central necrosis *J Hosp Infect 50:316–319, 2002; Mycoses 40:17–20, 1997; AD 115:234–235, 1979*

Coccidioidomycosis – erythema multiforme as hypersensivity reaction in acute coccidioidomycosis *JAAD 55:929, 942, 2006; JAAD 46:743–747, 2002;* acute pulmonary coccidioidomycosis *AD 142:744–746, 2006;* targetoid lesions of exanthem *JAAD 55:929, 942, 2006*

Cowpox – tongue ulcer, targetoid and umbilicated indurated papules, vesicles, pustules with central necrosis; exposure to pet rat *Clin Inf Dis 68:1063–1064, 2019*

Coxsackie virus – erythema multiforme–like exanthem

Coxsackie virus A6(atypical hand, foot, and mouth disease) – red papulovesicles of fingers, palmar erythema, red papules of ears, red papules of antecubital fossa, perioral papulovesicles, vesicles of posterior pharynx; crusted papules of scalp, ears, and face; purpuric targetoid painful vesicular lesions of hands and feet, arthritis, fissured scrotum *Int J Dermatol 59:487–489, 2020; JAMA Derm 149:1419–1421, 2013; JAAD 69:736–741, 2013;* erythema multiforme–like lesions *JAAD Case Rep 3:49–52, 2017*

Cryptococcal panniculitis – erythema with central hyperpigmentation *Cutis 74:165–170, 2004*

Ecthyma gangrenosum

Erysipeloid (*Erysipelothrix insidiosa (rhusiopathiae)*) in neonate – erythema multiforme–like eruption *J Clin Inf Dis 24:511, 1997*

Fusarium – sepsis *Ped Derm 9:62–65, 1992; Fusarium solani* – target–like lesions with central necrosis *Eur J Clin Microbiol Infect Dis 13:152–161, 1994; F. falciforme BJD 157:407–409, 2007*

Gonococcemia – hemorrhagic pustules with halo of erythema; *AD 107:403–406, 1973*

Hepatitis B – erythema multiforme

Herpes simplex virus – personal observation

Herpes zoster with surrounding urticarial – personal observation

Histoplasmosis, disseminated – erythema multiforme–like lesions *J Cutan Pathol 29:215–225, 2002*

Insect bites – bed bug bites *JAMA Derm 149:751–756, 2013*

Leprosy – targetoid erythematous plaques *NEJM 364:1657, 2011; Eur J Dermatol 11:65–67, 2001;* targetoid red–brown plaques *Cutis 92:187–189, 2013;* erythema nodosum leprosum – targetoid red nodules with central necrosis *AD 144:821–822, 2008;* erythema multiforme–like erythema nodosum leprosum *Int J Mycobacteriol 8:29034, 2019*

Lyme disease (*Borrelia burgdorferi*) – erythema (chronicum) migrans *NEJM 370:1724–1731, 2014; JAAD 64:619–636, 2011; JAAD 49:363–392, 2003*

  Differential diagnosis: *NEJM 370:1724–1731, 2014*
    Cellulitis
    Erythema multiforme
    Granuloma annulare
    Hypersensitivity to insect bite
    Insect bite
    Nummular dermatitis
    Spider bite
    Tinea
    Urticaria
    Wells' syndrome
  Coinfections with Lyme disease *NEJM 370:1724–1731, 2014*
    Anaplasma phagocytoplilum
    Babesia microti
    Borrelia miyamotoi
    Deer tick virus (Powassan virus)
    Ehrlichia species

Meningococcemia

Milker's nodule (pseudocowpox, bovine papular stomatitis virus) – starts as flat red papule on fingers or face, progresses to red–blue tender nodule, which crusts; zone of erythema; may resemble pyogenic granulomas; vesiculopustules of dorsal hand *JAMADerm 156:93, 2020; JAAD 44:1–14, 2001; AD 111:1307–1311, 1975*

Molluscum contagiosum – molluscum dermatitis *Acta DV 82:217–218, 2002;* molluscum contagiosum surrounded by erythema annulare centrifugum *JAMADerm 151:1385–1386, 2015*

Mucormycosis – necrotic eschar with surrounding erythema *JAAD 61:172–174, 2009;* bulls eye infarct *JAAD 82:783–796, 2020; Mucor, Rhizopus oryzi, Rhizomucor, Lichtheimia, Saksenaea, Cunninhghamella, Apophysomyces JAAD 80:869–880, 2019; Rhizopus arrhizus;* bull's eye infarct *JAAD 51:996–1001, 2004; JAMA 2254:737–738, 1973;* annular bulla with central necrosis *Ped Derm 24:257–262, 2007*

Mycobacterium avium–intracellulare JAAD 39:493–495, 1998

Mycoplasma–induced rash with mucositis (MIRM) – atypical target lesions *Clinics in Dermatol 37:148–158, 2019; JAAD 79:110–117, 2018*

New Jersey novel polyoma virus – personal observation

Orf – Parapoxvirus (genus); family Poxviridae *Cutis 71:288–290, 2003; JAAD 44:1–14, 2001;* palmar bulla *JAMA 308:126–128, 2012;* generalized severe blistering eruptions (bullous orf) *JAAD 58:49–55, 2008*

Zoonotic orthopoxvirus – teats of cows as source; targetoid bullae of hands and fingers healing with eschars; edema of hands; fever; axillary lymphadenopathy *NEJM 372:223–230, 2015*

Parvovirus B19 infection – erythema multiforme–like *J Clin Inf Dis 21:1424–1430, 1995*

Novel poxvirus – equine exposure; targetoid pox–like bullae *Clin Inf Dis 60:195–202, 2015*

Psittacosis – erythema multiforme *Br Med J 2:1469–1470, 1965*

Rhizopus arjyzii – violaceous targetoid plaque of thigh *Ped Derm 24:560–561, 2007; JAAD 51:996–1001, 2004; Mycoses 45(Suppl 1):27–30, 2002*

Rickettsial pox – targetoid papule of foot *JAMADerm 150:203–204, 2014*

Sealpox (parapoxvirus) – gray concentric nodule with superimposed bulla on dorsum of hand *BJD 152:791–793, 2005*

Southern tick–associated rash infection (erythema migrans–like illness) – *Borrelia lonestari;* targetoid erythema migrans lesions without evidence of Borrelia infection; reported from Georgia, Kentucky, Maryland, Missouri, North Carolina, and South Carolina *JAAD 72:371–372, 2015; Clin Inf Dis 40:429, 475–476, 2005; J Clin Microbiol 42:1163–1169, 2004; JAAD 49:363–392, 2003; Emerg Inf Dis 7:471–473, 2001; AD 135:1317–1326, 1999; AD 134:955–960, 1998; Arch Int Med 157:2635–2641, 1997; J Inf Dis 172:470–480, 1995*

Spider bites – black widow spider (*Latrodectus mactans*) – punctum with erythema and edema *AD 123:41–43, 1987;* brown recluse spider (*Loxosceles reclusa*)– erythema, edema, central bulla; targetoid lesion with central blue/purple, ischemic halo, outer rim of erythema; at 3–4 days central necrosis, eschar, ulcer, scar *South Med J 69:887–891, 1976*

Streptococcus pyogenes – ecthyma gangrenosum–like lesion (erythematous plaque with central black necrosis) in disseminated streptococcal disease *JAMA 311:957–958, 2014*

Syphilis – congenital – targetoid erythema multiforme–like lesions *JAAD 55:S11–15, 2006; BJD 149:658–660, 2003;* secondary – corymbose lesions; erythema multiforme–like lesions *Int J STD AIDS 30:304–309, 2019; Dermatol Online J 19:20403, 2013; BJD 149:658–660, 2003*

Tick bite

Tick typhus (Boutonneuse fever, Kenya tick typhus, African and Indian tick typhus) (ixodid ticks) – small ulcer at site of tick bite (tache noire) – black necrotic center with red halo; pink morbilliform eruption of forearms, then generalizes, involving face, palms, and soles; may be hemorrhagic; recovery uneventful *JAAD 2:359–373, 1980*

Tinea corporis, cruris, faciei, bullous tinea *Cutis 6:661–668, 1970; Trichophyton tonsurans* – concentric bullae *AD 145:497, 2009*

Tinea imbricata

Toxic shock syndrome – targetoid spotty rashes *Clinics in Dermatol 37:148–158, 2019; Acta DV 82:449–452, 2002*

Trichosporon beigelii sepsis – personal observation

Trypanosomiasis – African; edema of face, hands, feet with transient red macular, morbilliform, targetoid, petechial or urticarial dermatitis (trypanids); circinate, annular of trunk *JAAD 60:897–925, 2009; AD 131:1178, 1995*

Tularemia – erythema multiforme *JAAD 49:363–392, 2003*

Tungiasis – white papule of toe tip with central brown dot *BJD 158:635–636, 2008*

Vaccinia – contact vaccinia – targetoid plaque *AD 146:667–672, 2010*

Varicella–zoster infection – varicella or herpes zoster; atypical recurrent varicella with vesiculopapular lesions with central necrosis *JAAD 48:448–452, 2003*

Verruca vulgaris – rosettes after cryotherapy

Yaws – primary red papule, ulcerates, crusted; satellite papules; become round ulcers, papillomatous or vegetative friable nodules which bleed easily (raspberry–like) (framboesia); heals with large atrophic scar with white center with dark halo

INFILTRATIVE DISEASES

Amyloid – purpuric halos surrounding cherry angiomas *Cutis 48:141–143, 1991; BJD 112:209–211, 1985*

Digital myxoid cyst

INFLAMMATORY DISORDERS

Erythema multiforme *JAMA 311:1152–1153, 2014; JAMA 312:426–427, 2014; Medicine 68:133–140, 1989; JAAD 8:763–765, 1983;* marginal ring of vesicles (herpes iris of Bateman) *Medicine 68:133–140, 1989; JAAD 8:763–765, 1983;* id reaction, erythema multiforme–like *J Eur Acad Dermatol Venereol 17:699–701, 2003;* associated with oral herpes simplex *JAMA 311:1152–1153, 2014*

Interstitial granulomatous dermatitis *BJD 152:814–816, 2005*

Kawasaki's disease *Ped Inf Dis 61:1272–1274, 2019*

Kikuchi's disease (histiocytic necrotizing lymphadenitis) – erythema multiforme lesions *Ped Derm 18:403–405, 2002*

Neutrophilic eccrine hidradenitis *Cutis 75:93–97, 2005*

Ofuji's disease (eosinophilic pustular folliculitis) *Cutis 58:135–138, 1996*

Pyoderma gangrenosum; bullous pyoderma gangrenosum *JAAD 51:996–1001, 2004* Sarcoid – erythema multiforme–like lesions *Cutis 33:461–463, 1984*

Relapsing idiopathic nodular panniculitis *BJD 152:582–583, 2005*

Sarcoidosis *Cutis 33:461–463, 1984*

Stevens–Johnson syndrome (erythema multiforme major) *BJD 174:1194–1227, 2016*

Toxic epidermal necrolysis *Australas J Dermatol 43:35–38, 2002*

Urticaria–like neutrophilic dermatosis – annular urticarial plaques without scale – IgA gammopathy *BJD 170:1189–1191, 2014; Medicine (Balt)88:23–31, 2009*

Urticaria multiforme – large polycyclic and annular wheals with dusky centers, acral and facial angioedema *Proc Baylor Univ Med Ctr 32:427–428, 2019; Ped Derm 28:436–438, 2011;* fever, arcuate, annular, polycyclic lesions; ecchymotic center or central pallor; edema of hands and feet; aged 4 months to 4 years *Cutis 89:260:262–264, 2012; Pediatrics 119:e1177–1183, 2007*

METABOLIC DISORDERS

Porphyria cutanes tarda *J Nepal Health Res Counc 17:119–121, 2019*

Pruritic urticarial papules and plaques of pregnancy – targetoid lesions *JAAD 39:933–939, 1998; JAAD 10:473–480, 1984; Clin Exp Dermatol 7:65–73, 1982; JAAD 5:401–405, 1981; JAMA 241:1696–1699, 1979*

NEOPLASTIC DISORDERS

Angioplasmocellular hyperplasia – red nodule with red rim, ulcerated nodule, vascular nodule of face, scalp, neck, trunk, and leg *JAAD 64:542–547, 2011*

Atypical nevus

Blue nevi – target blue nevi *AD 119:919–920, 1983*

Cytophagic histiocytic panniculitis – manifestation of hemophago-cytic syndrome; red tender nodules; T–cell lymphoma, B–cell lymphoma, histiocytic lymphoma, sinus histiocytosis with massive lymphadenopathy (Rosai–Dorfman disease) *JAAD 4:181–194, 1981; Arch Int Med 140:1460–1463, 1980*

Halo lesions (lesions with halos) *AD 92:14–35, 1965*
   Basal cell carcinoma
   Blue nevus
   Cafe au lait macules *Ped Derm 15:70–71, 1998*
   Congenital melanocytic nevus *NEJM 370:262, 2014; Ped Derm 19:73–75, 2002; J Derm Surg Oncol 16:377–380, 1990*
   Histiocytoma
   Nevocellular (melanocytic) nevus *JAAD 67:582–586, 2012*
   Primary melanoma
   Metastatic melanoma
   Neurofibroma *AD 112:987–990, 1976*
   Seborrheic keratosis
   Involuting flat wart

HTLV–1 leukemia, lymphoma *Int J Dermatol 47:390–392, 2008*

Kaposi's sarcoma

Leukemia cutis – acute myelogenous leukemia

Lymphoma – cutaneous T–cell lymphoma *Cutis 97:12,31–32, 2016;* CTCL mimicking erythema multiforme *JAAD 47:914–918, 2002;* nasal T–cell lymphoma *Pathology 21:164–168, 1989;* primary cutaneous epidermotropic aggressive CD8+ T–cell lymphoma – red plaques with central necrosis (targetoid); ulcerated nodule *J Cut Pathol 44:867–873, 2017; JAAD 67:748–759, 2012*

Lymphomatoid papulosis

Melanocytic nevus – signature nevi *JAAD 60:508–514, 2009;* cockarde nevus *Ped Derm 5:250–253, 1988;* eclipse nevus – tan center with stellate brown rim *BJD 145:1023–1026, 2001;* halo nevus (Sutton's nevus; leukoderma acquisitum centrifugum) *AD 92:14–35, 1965;* Myerson's nevus – melanocytic nevus with surrounding dermatitis *AD 103:510–512, 1971;* due to interferon–alpha and ribavirin *BJD 152:193–194, 2005;* atypical nevus *JAAD 34:357–361, 1996;* halo nevi around congenital nevi *Ped Derm 26:755–756, 2009;* congenital melanocytic nevus *NEJM 370:262, 2014;* halo nevi in vitiligo *BJD 172:1052–1057, 2015*

Melanoma – primary, metastatic *Semin Oncol 2:5–118, 1975;* eruptive pigmentation around nevi and seborrheic keratoses in stage III melanoma – hyperpigmented halo or "nottus" phenomenon *BJD 168:1140–1141, 2013*

Metastases – lung cancer, plurivisceral carcinoma *BJD 148:361, 2003*

Nevocentric lesions *JAAD 33:842–843, 1995*
   Eclipse nevus *AD 145:1334–1336, 2009*
      Erythema multiforme
      Halo dermatitis
      Halo nevus *JAAD 29:267–268, 1993*
      Nummular dermatitis (Meyerson's nevus – halo dermatitis) *BJD 118:125–129, 1988*
      Pityriasis rosea
      Psoriasis
      Targetoid halo nevus

Nevus – cockade nevus of scalp *BJD 165:137–143, 2011*

Spitz nevus *Am J Dermatopathol 17:484–486, 1995; JAAD 27:901–913, 1992*

Sutton's nevus *Ped Derm 30:281–293, 2013*

PARANEOPLASTIC DISORDERS

Glucagonoma syndrome – alpha cell tumor in the tail of the pancreas; 50% of cases have metastasized by the time of diagno-sis; skin rash, angular stomatitis, cheilosis, beefy red glossitis, blepharitis, conjunctivitis, alopecia, crumbling nails; rarely, associated with MEN I or IIA syndromes *AD 133:909, 912, 1997; JAAD 12:1032–1039, 1985; Ann Int Med 91:213–215, 1979*

Paraneoplastic pemphigus – targetoid erythema multiforme–like lesions *Clinics in Dermatol 37:148–158, 2019; BJD 145:127–131, 2001; Cutis 61:94–96, 1998; NEJM 323:1729–1735, 1990*

PHOTODERMATOSES

Hydroa vacciniforme

Polymorphic light eruption *Adv Exp Med Biol 996:61–70, 2017; Photodermatol Photoimmunol Photomed 26:101–103, 2010*

PRIMARY CUTANEOUS DISEASES

Acquired perforating collagenosis *AD 143:1201–1206, 2007*

Adrenergic urticaria – wheals surrounded by white halos (due to vasoconstriction) *BJD 158:629–631, 2008*; urticarial papules with pale halo (as opposed to cholinergic urticaria – urticarial papules with red halos) *JAAD 70:763–766, 2014*

Alopecia areata – targetoid hair regrowth *AD 134:1042, 1998*

Annular lichenoid dermatitis of youth *JAAD 49:1029–1036, 2003*

Epidermolysis bullosa simplex – Dowling–Meara type *AD 122:190–198, 1986*

Epidermolysis bullosa, dominant dystrophic – personal observation

Eruptive pseudoangiomatosis *AD 140:757–758, 2004*

Erythema annulare centrifugum

Erythrokeratoderma en cocardes *Ped Derm 19:285–292, 2002*

Erythrokeratolysis hiemalis – keratolytic winter erythema (Oudsthoorn disease) – palmoplantar erythema, cyclical and centrifugal peeling of affected sites, targetoid lesions of the hands and feet – seen in South African whites; precipitated by cold weather or fever *Ped Derm 19:285–292, 2002; BJD 98:491–495, 1978*

Febrile ulceronecrotic Mucha–Habermann disease *JAAD 49:1142–1148, 2003*

Granuloma annulare – giant inflammatory targetoid plaques *AD 128:979, 982, 1992; AD 105:928, 1972*

Nummular dermatitis may surround: *JAAD 33:842–843, 1995*
    Basal cell carcinoma
    Dermatofibromas
    Insect bites
    Keloids
    Lentigines
    Nevus – Meyerson's nevus
    Squamous cell carcinoma
    Seborrheic keratosis
    Stucco keratosis

Pityriasis rosea *Indian J Dermatol Online J 9:414–417, 2018; Indian J Dermatol Online 7:212–215, 2016; JAAD 15:159–167, 1986*; pityriasis rosea with erythema multiforme–like lesions *JAAD 17:135–136, 1987*

Psoriasis – Woronoff rings *BJD 148:170, 2003*; pustular psoriasis – personal observation

Relapsing annular erythema (neutrophilic figurate erythema of infancy) – facial, polycyclic borders; may be bullous, purpuric, or targetoid *Ped Derm 37:209–210, 2020*; recurrent annular erythema with purpura – leukocytoclastic vasculitis *BJD 135:972–975, 1996; Ann DV 192:457, 2002*

Toxic erythema of newborn

Urticaria *Ped 119:e1177–1183 2007*

Vitiligo – halo nevi in vitiligo *BJD 172:1052–1057, 2015*

PSYCHOCUTANEOUS DISORDERS

Factitial dermatitis

SYNDROMES

Behcet's disease *Yonsei Med J 38:380–389, 1997*

Erythrokeratoderma variabilis *Clinics in Dermatol 23:23–32, 2005*

Kawasaki's disease – erythema multiforme–like *JAAD 69:501–510, 2013; Cutis 72:354–356, 2003; JAAD 39:383–398, 1998; Jpn J Allergol 16:178–222, 1967*

Marshall's syndrome *AD 131:1175–1177, 1995*

Rowell's syndrome – lupus erythematosus and erythema multiforme–like syndrome – butterfly rash, facial dermatitis, exanthem, papules, annular, atypical targetoid lesions, vesicles, bullae, necrosis, ulceration, oral ulcers, and perniotic lesions *JAMADerm 153:461–462, 2017; BJD 142:343–346, 2000; Clin Exp Dermatol 24:74–77, 1999; JAAD 21:374–377, 1989: AD 88:176–180, 1963*

Sweet's syndrome *Ped Derm 29:38–44, 2012; Ped Derm 25:509–519, 2008; AD 141:881–884, 2005*; in chronic granulomatous disease *Ped Derm 11:237–240, 1994*; red annular targetoid plaques *AD 148:969–970, 2012*; chronic recurrent Sweet's syndrome of myelodysplasia – pustules, plaques, and papules *AD 142:1170–1176, 2006*; bullous Sweet's syndrome *Cutis 82:395,405–406, 2008*; Sweet's syndrome in infancy with acquired cutis laxa *Ped Derm 26:358–360, 2009*

Turner's syndrome – halo nevi *JAAD 51:354–358, 2004*

Vogt–Koyanagi–Harada syndrome – halo nevi; occurs primarily in Asians, blacks, and darkly pigmented Caucasians; Stage 1 – aseptic meningitis; Stage 2 – uveitis (iritis, iridocyclitis) and dysacusis (tinnitus, hearing loss); Stage 3 – depigmentation of skin (60% of patients), depigmentation of hair (poliosis – eyelashes, eyebrows, scalp, and body hair – 90% of patients), alopecia areata *Ann DV 127:282–284, 2000; AD 88:146–149, 1980*

Wells' syndrome *AD 142:1157–1161, 2006*

TRAUMA

Frostnip – targetoid papules *Ped Derm 32:869–870, 2015*

Radiation therapy *Australas Radiol 40:334–337, 1996*

Ricocheted action safety bullet marks *Am J Forensic Med Pathol 18:15–20, 1997*

Post-treatment with liquid nitrogen

VASCULAR DISORDERS

Acute hemorrhagic edema of infancy (Finkelstein's disease) (Seidlmayer's purpura) *JAMA 309:2159–2160, 2013; JAAD 59:684–695, 2008; Ped Int 45:697–700, 2003; Cutis 68:127–129, 2001; J Dermatol 28:279–281, 2001; Cutis 61:283–284, 1998; AD 130:1055–1060, 1994*

Angiokeratoma with pink halo *JAAD 76:S16–18, 2017*

Angiolymphoid hyperplasia with eosinophilia *Ped Derm 15: 91–96, 1998*

Arteriovenous malformation – personal observation

Bossed hemangioma with telangiectasia and peripheral pallor *AD 134:1145–1150, 1998*

Capillary malformation surrounding the nipple – with white halo around nipple (Bork–Baykal phenomenon) *Ped Derm 36:558–560, 2019*

Capillary malformation–AVM syndrome – autosomal dominant; port wine stain with multifocal <1–3cm round or oval pink macules of face, trunk, or extremities; 50% with blanched halo (white halo surrounding red patches); arteriovenous malformations of brain, spine, skin, bone, muscle; inactivating mutations of *RASA1* or *EPHB4 JAMADerm 155:733, 2019; Ped Derm 33:570–584, 2016; AD 148:1334–1335, 2012; Ped Derm 30:409–415, 2013;* red patch of eyelid with white halo *Ped Derm 37:64–68, 2020*

Cherry angioma *BJD 112:209–211, 1985*

Allergic granulomatous vasculitis – erythema multiforme–like exanthems *Autoimmun Rev 14:341–348, 2015; Dermatopathol 37:214–221, 2015; JAAD 37:199–203, 1997; JID 17:349–359, 1951; Am J Pathol 25:817, 1949*

Congenital plaque-type glomuvenous malformations – glomulin gene on 1p21; loss of function mutation; atrophic at birth; livedoid plaques, blue plaques, vascular nodules, red patches, cerebriform, targetoid *AD 142:892–896, 2006*

Degos' disease (malignant atrophic papulosis) – flat, white papules with erythematous telangiectatic halos *NEJM 370:2327–2337, 2014; JAAD 68:138–143 2013; BJD 100:21–36, 1979; Ann DV 79:410–417, 1954*

Eruptive pseudoangiomatosis – pink papules with pale, anemic halos *JAAD 76:S12–15, 2017; BJD 143:435–438, 2000*

Glomus tumors – congenital plaquelike glomuvenous malformations – targetoid blue blaschko–esque plaques *Cutis 84:16–18, 2009*

Granulomatosis with polyangiitis – personal observation

Hemangioma of pregnancy *JAAD 32:282–284, 1995*

Hemangioma, traumatized

Henoch–Schonlein purpura mimicking erythema multiforme – personal observation

Hereditary benign telangiectasia – punctuate telangiectasias with anemic halos *AD 146:98–99, 2010*

Hobnail hemangioma – violaceous central papule with thin pale ring and ecchymotic periphery *JAAD 81:1257–1270, 2019*

Leukocytoclastic vasculitis; Henoch–Schonlein purpura; urticarial vasculitis *AD 134:231–236, 1998;* erythema multiforme–like lesions

Non–involuting congenital hemangioma – blue plaque with central telangiectasia and peripheral rim of pallor *Ped Derm 36:835–853, 2019;* round to ovoid pink to purple papule or plaque with central or peripheral pallor, coarse telangiectasias *JAAD 50: 875–882, 2004*

Pustular vasculitis – annular pustular plaques with central necrosis

Rapidly involuting congenital hemangioma – red mass of elbow with white halo *Ped Derm 37:40–1, 2020*

Superficial lymphatic malformation (formerly targetoid hemosiderotic hemangioma/hobnail hemangioma) – purpuric plaque *AD 138:117–122, 2002;* brown to violaceous papule or nodule with ecchymotic halo; violaceous papule with ecchymotic or brown ring *JAAD 66:112–115, 2012; int J Dermatol 47:991–992, 2008; AD 142:1351–1356, 2006; Cutis 72:51–52, 2003; AD 138:117–122, 2002; AD 136:1571–1572, 2000; J Cutan Pathol 26:279–286, 1999; JAAD 41:215–224, 1999; JAAD 32:282–284, 1995; J Cutan Pathol 17:233–235, 1990; JAAD 19:550–558, 1988*

Urticarial vasculitis – personal observation

TATTOO, PALPABLE/LESIONS IN A TATTOO

AUTOIMMUNE DISEASES AND DISEASES OF IMMUNE DYSFUNCTION

Allergic contact dermatitis to paraphenylenediamine in temporary henna tattoo *Am J Contact Dermat 12:186–187, 2001; Australas J Dermatol 41:168–171, 2000; AD 136:1061–1062, 2000;* radiotherapy tattoos *Australas Radiol 43:558–561, 1999;* p–tertiary butyl phenol formaldehyde resin in temporary tattoo *Dermatitis 25:37–38, 2014*

Cadmium reaction – red *Cutis 23:71–72, 1979;* mercury–cadmium photoallergic reaction in red pigment *Ann Int Med 67:984–989, 1967;* yellow *South Med J 55:792–795, 1962*

Carbon – black *JAAD 35:477–479, 1996;* track marks of IVDA

Chrome salts (chromic oxide) – green pigment Contact Dermatitis *21:276–278, 1989; AD 82:237–243, 1960; Acta DV (Stockh) 39:23–29, 1959*

Cinnabar allergy (mercury) – red pigment *BJD 124:576–580, 1991;* organic pigments in red tattoos *Acta DV 71:70–73, 1991; Br J Plast Surg 30:84–85, 1977; Acta DV 48:103–105, 1968; US Armed Forces Med J 11:261–280, 1960;* due to thimerosol as preservative *Ann Int Med 88:428, 1978*

Cobalt chloride – light blue *Acta DV (Stockh) 41:259–263, 1961;* blue–black *JAAD 55:s71–73, 2006*

Lupus erythematosus, discoid *Lupus 28:241–243, 2019; AD 98:667–669, 1968*

Manganese reaction – purple *Contact Dermatitis 16:198–202, 1987; Cutis 23:71–72, 1979*

Nickel – blue–black *JAAD 55:s71–73, 2006*

Purple tattoo pigment – granulomatous reaction *Contact Dermatitis 16:198–202, 1987*

Red azo dye – delayed allergic reaction *Hautarzt 48:666–670, 1997*

EXOGENOUS AGENTS

Aluminum granuloma in a tattoo *JAAD 20:903–908, 1989*

Amalgam tattoo – personal observation

Black gun powder

Drug abuse – soot tattooing NY State J Med 68:3129–3134, 1968

Earrings – iron tattoo *JAAD 24:788–789, 1991*

Fireworks explosion – personal observation

Foreign body granulomas after ochre tattoos

Monsel's solution (ferric chloride) *JAAD 17:819–825, 1987*

INFECTIONS AND INFESTATIONS

AIDS – tattoo reaction to black pigment (carbon) – after immune restoration in AIDS *AD 137:669–670, 2001*

Aspergillus fumigatus – painful, purpuric necrotic papules and pustules in tattoo *BJD 170:1373–1375, 2014*

Cellulitis *JAAD 48:S73–74, 2003*

Erysipelas *JAAD 48:S73–74, 2003*

Herpes simplex *Med J Aust 187:598, 2007*

Influenza vaccine *Ann Int Med 88:428, 1978*

Leishmaniasis in HIV disease *Clin Inf Dis 45:220–221,267–268, 2007; JAAD 41:847–850, 1999*

Leprosy – inoculation leprosy; upgrading borderline tuberculoid leprosy *Int J Dermatol 26:332–333, 1987; Indian J Lepro 57:887–888, 1985*

Molluscum contagiosum *Br Med J 285:607, 1982*

Mycobacterium abscessus JAAD 48:S73–74, 2003

Mycobacteria chelonae – swelling and itching of red area *JAMA 314:2071–2072, 2015; JAAD 62:501–506, 2010;* palpable tattoo *JAAD 64:998–999, 2011;* in gray wash ink of tattoo *JAMADerm 152:205–206, 2016*

Mycobacterium tuberculosis – inoculation tuberculosis *AD 121:648–650, 1985*

Staphylococcal infection *Am J Emerg Med 30:2055–2063, 2012; MMWR 55:677–679, 2012*

Streptococcal infection – personal observation

Syphilis – in a tattoo, spares mercury – personal observation; secondary syphilis *Eur J Dermatol 20:544–545, 2010*

Tinea – *Trichophyton tonsurans Cutis 73:232, 2004; Cutis 28:541–542, 1981*

Vaccinia *JAAD 48:S73–74, 2003*

Verruca vulgaris *Int J Dermatol 53:882–884, 2014; Int J Dermatol 33:796–797, 1994;* in areas of black dye *AD 130L1453–1454, 1994*

Zygomycosis *Australas J Dermatol 27:107–111, 1986*

INFLAMMATORY DISEASES

Pseudolymphomatous reactions *JAAD 6:485–488, 1982*

Pyoderma gangrenosum *CMAJ 186:935, 2014; J Dermatol Treat 19:58–60, 2008*

Sarcoidosis – papules within a tattoo *NEJM 382:744, 2020; JAMA 313:1747–1748, 2015; Cutis 75:44–48, 2005; J Cutan Laser Ther 2:41–43, 2000; Cutis 59:113–115, 1997; Clin Exp Dermatol 22:254–255, 1997; BJD 130:658–662, 1994; Cutis 36:423–424, 1985;* confined to red tattoos *Clin Exp Dermatol 17:446–448, 1992;* in green tattoo *Wien Klin Wochenschr 99:14–18, 1987; Clin Exp Dermatol 1:395–399, 1976;* papules within tattoo; patients with hepatitis C treated with interferon and ribavirin *AD 145:321–326, 2009; Clin Exper Derm 131:387–389, 2006; Clin Exp Dermatol 1:395–399, 1976*

METABOLIC DISEASES

Osteoma cutis *Cureus 26:e4323, 2019*

Winged angel lung tattoos of cystic fibrosis *NEJM 372:351–362, 2015*

NEOPLASTIC DISEASES

Basal cell carcinoma *Dermatology 208:181–182, 2004; Cutis 39:125–126, 1987; Br J Plast Surg 36:258–259, 1983; Br J Plast Surg 29:288–290, 1976*

Dermatofibroma *J Cutan Pathol 35:696–698, 2008*

Dermatofibrosarcoma protuberans *J Drugs Dermatol 10:837–842, 2011; Sarcoma 9:37–41, 2005*

Hypertrophic scar *J Spec Oper Med 16:96–100, 2016*

Keloid

Keratoacanthoma *J Cutan Pathol 35:62–64, 2008; J Cutan Pathol 35:504–507, 2008; J Drugs Dermatol 6:931–932, 2007;* eruptive keratoacanthomas *AD 143:1457–1458, 2007*

Leiomyosarcoma *J Plast Reconstr Aesthet Surg 62:e79–80, 2009*

Lymphoma – primary non–Hodgkin's lymphoma *Plast Reconstr Surg 62:125–127, 1978;* CD30+ lymphoproliferative disorder – lesions in red tattoo *BJD 171:668–670, 2014*

Lymphocytoma cutis *JAAD 38:877–905, 1998*

Melanocytic nevus

Melanoma *Cutis 92:227–230, 2013; JAMA Derm 149:1087–1089, 2013; J Cut Med Surg 13:321–325, 2009; Dermatology 217:219–221, 2008; J Dtsh Dermatol Ges 5:1120–1121, 2007; Melanoma Res 16:375–376, 2006; Dermatology 206:345–346, 2003; Br J Plast Surg 52:598, 1999; Cutis 59:111–112, 1997; Int J Dermatol 32:297–298, 1993; Surg Oncol 25:100–101, 1984; Br J Radiol 53:913–914, 1980; Br J Plast Surg 27:303–304, 1974; Int J Dermatol 11:16–20, 1972; AD 99:596–598, 1969; Arch Dermatol Syphilol 37:301–306, 1938*

Milia *J Drugs Dermatol 16:621–624, 2017; Cutis 87:195–196, 2011*

Seborrheic keratosis – erupting in a tattoo *Ann DV 125:261–263, 1998*

Squamous cell carcinoma *Clin Exp Dermatol 42:601–606, 2017; JAAD 60:1073–1074, 2009; JAAD 56:1072–1073, 2007; JAAD 48:S73–74, 2003; Minn Med 49:799–801, 1966*

PHOTODERMATOSES

Photoallergy to cadmium sulfide

PRIMARY CUTANEOUS DISEASE

Lichen planus *Dermatology 233:100–109, 2017;* lichenoid reaction to red pigment *J Cosmet Dermatol Sept 10, 2019*

Perforating granuloma annulare *Indian Dermatol Online J 6:296–298, 2015; BJD 138:360–361, 1998*

Pseudoepitheliomatous hyperplasia in tattoo – verrucous plaques in white section of tattoo *JAMADerm 153:463–464, 2017; Am J Clin Dermatol 9:337–340, 2008; Am J Dermatopathol 25:338–340, 2003*

Psoriasis *J Drugs in Dermatol 10:1199–1200, 2011;* ostraceous psoriasis *J Drugs Dermatol 18:825–826, 2019*

Reactive perforating collagenosis *JAAD 48:S73–74, 2003*

Urticaria *JAAD 48:S73–74, 2003*

TRAUMA

Concentration camp tattoos

Cuban political tattoo – personal observation

Decorative tattoos – personal observation

Intravenous drug abuse – track marks, sooting tattoos *JAAD 69:135–142, 2013*

Loss of pigmentation

Mende – personal observation

Pachuco mark *JAAD 18:1066–1073, 1988*

Silversmith – traumatic silver tattoos

TEETH

NATAL TEETH

INFECTIONS AND INFESTATIONS

Pyelitis during pregnancy

Syphilis, congenital

METABOLIC DISORDERS

Adrenogenital syndrome

Febrile systemic illness

Hypovitaminosis

PRIMARY CUTANEOUS DISEASES

Idiopathic or familial

SYNDROMES

Chondroectodermal dysplasia (Ellis–van Creveld syndrome) *J Dent Child 47:28–31, 1980*

Craniofacial dysostosis

Cyclopia *Syndromes of the Head and Neck, p. 583, 1990*

Dyskeratosis congenita – taurodontism; short tooth roots *JAAD 77:1194–1196, 2017*

Ectodermal dysplasia

Ellis–van Creveld syndrome (chondroectodermal dysplasia) – neonatal teeth, partial anodontia, small early or late erupting teeth; malpositioned teeth *Atlas of Clinical Syndromes A Visual Aid to Diagnosis, 1992, pp.244–245*

Epidermolysis bullosa simplex

Gardner's syndrome – unerupted supernumerary teeth *JAAD 45:940–942, 2001*

Hallermann–Streiff (oculomandibular syndrome with hypotrichosis)

Natal teeth with patent ductus arteriosus and intestinal pseudo–obstruction *Clin Genet 9:479–482, 1976*

Pachyonychia congenita, Jadassohn Lewandowsky; type II – natal teeth, bushy eyebrows, follicular keratoses, angular cheilitis, unruly hair, thick nails, palmoplantar keratoderma with hyperhidrosis, hoarseness, cysts oral leukokeratosis; mutations in *KRT6A, KRT6B, KRT6C, KRT16, KRT17 BJD 171:343–355, 2014; JAAD 67:680–686, 2012; AD 147:1077–1080, 2011; BJD 159:500–501, 2008;* multiple epidermoid cysts of volar upper extremities; keratin 17 mutation *BJD 159:730–732, 2008*

Pallister–Hall syndrome (hypothalamic hamarblastoma) *Am J Med Genet 7:75–83, 1980*

Pfeiffer syndrome

Pierre–Robin syndrome

Restrictive dermopathy *Ped Derm 20:25–27, 2003*

Rubinstein–Taybi syndrome

Short rib–polydactyly syndrome, type II (Majewski) *Am J Med Genet 14:115–123m 1983*

Sotos syndrome

Steatocystoma multiplex *J Craniofac Genet Dev Biol 7:311–317, 1987*

Walker-Warburg syndrome

Wiedemann-Rautenstrauch (neonatal progeroid syndrome) – generalized lipoatrophy, macrocephaly, premature aging, wide open sutures, hypoplasia of facial bones, low set ears, beak-shaped nose, neonatal teeth, slender limbs, large hands and feet with long fingers, large penis *J Med Genet 34:433–437, 1997*

Witkop tooth and nail syndrome *Ped Derm 13:63–64, 1996*

TOXINS

Polychlorinated biphenyls – natal teeth, pigment anomalies

PREMATURE LOSS OF TEETH

AUTOIMMUNE DISORDERS

Scleroderma – missing teeth with xerostoma *JAAD 77:795–806, 2017*

INFECTIONS AND INFESTATIONS

AIDS

Caries

Paracoccidioidomycosis – granulomatous ulcerative gingivitis with loss of teeth *JAAD 53:931–951, 2005; Cutis 40:214–216, 1987*

Periodontal disease – destructive; rapidly progressive

INFILTRATIVE DISORDERS

Eosinophilic granuloma

Langerhans cell histiocytosis *JAAD 78:1035–1044, 2018; Med Oral Patol Oral Cir Bucal 14:E222–228, 2009; Curr Prob Derm 14:41–70, 2002*

INFLAMMATORY DISORDERS

Juvenile periodontitis

METABOLIC DISORDERS

Cyclic neutropenia *Ped Derm 18:426–432, 2001; Am J Med 61:849–861, 1976*

Hereditary Vitamin D–resistant rickets *JDR Clin Trans Res 3:28–34, 2018*

Hypophosphatasia

Hypoplasminogenemia – autosomal recessive; red eyes, oral ulcers, gingival edema; ligneous conjunctivitis with red eyes, ligneous periodontitis, blindness, tooth loss; decreased wound healing *JAMADerm 150:1227–12228, 2014*

Immune defects

Neutropenia

Scurvy *NEJM 379:282–289, 2018*

NEOPLASTIC DISORDERS

Tumors

PRIMARY CUTANEOUS DISEASES

Epidermolysis bullosa, recessive dystrophic severe generalized, dominant dystrophic (pretibial) and recessive dystrophic (pretibial), junctional EB, Herlitz type, non–Herlitz type generalized, non–Herlitz type, localized, junctional EB inverse, laryngo–onycho–cutaneous syndrome, – dental caries; enamel hypoplasia *JAAD 58:931–950, 2008; Ped Derm 19:436–438, 2002;* dystrophic epidermolysis bullosa inversa – flexural bullae, oral ulcers, dental caries, milia *Ped Derm 20:243–248, 2003*

SYNDROMES

Acro–dermato–ungual–lacrimal–tooth syndrome (ADULT syndrome) – ectrodactyly or syndactyly, freckling and dry skin, dysplastic nails, superficial blisters and desquamation of hands and feet; lacrimal duct atresia, primary hypodontia, conical teeth, and early loss of permanent teeth; small ears hooked nose, sparse thin blond hair, frontal alopecia, hypohidrosis, lacrimal duct atresia, hypoplastic breasts and nipples, urinary tract anomalies; mutation in *TP63* gene (encodes transcription factor p63); p63 mutations also responsible for EEC, AEC, limb mammary, and Rapp–Hodgkin syndromes *BJD 172:276–278, 2015; Ped Derm 27:643–645, 2010; Hum Mol Genet 11:799–804, 2002; Am J Med Genet 45:642–648, 1993*

Carvajal syndrome, variant *Int J Ped Dent 22:390–396, 2012*

Cockayne syndrome – caries

Coffin–Lowry syndrome *Int J Ped Dent 22:154–156, 2011*

Congenital analgia *Syndromes of the Head and Neck, p.598, 1990*

Congenital atrichia, palmoplantar keratoderma, mental retardation, early loss of teeth *JAAD 30:893–898, 1994*

Down's syndrome – periodontal disease; dental abnormalities

Ehlers–Danlos syndrome – EDS type IV – lobeless ears; periodontitis *JAAD 55:S41–45, 2006;* type VIII – autosomal dominant; skin fragility, abnormal scarring, severe early periodontitis with loss of adult dentition by end of third decade; cigarette paper scars of shin; marfanoid habitus (tall, long limbs, arachnodactyly); triangular face, prominent eyes, thin nose, prematurely aged appearance, thin skin with prominent veins, no joint hypermobility, easy bruising, blue sclerae *Am J Hum Genet 99:1005–1014, 2016; JAAD 55:S41–45, 2006; BJD 128:458–463, 1993*

Familial mandibuloacral dysplasia (craniomandibular dermatodysostosis) – onset at age 3–5 years; atrophy of skin over hands and feet with club-shaped terminal phalanges and acro–osteolysis, mandibular dysplasia, delayed cranial suture closure, short stature, dysplastic clavicles, prominent eyes and sharp nose, alopecia, sharp nose, loss of lower teeth, multiple Wormian bones, acro–osteolysis *Ped Derm 22:75–78, 2005; BJD 105:719–723, 1981; Birth Defects x:99–105, 1974*

Familial PDGFRA–mutation syndrome *Hum Pathol 76:52–57, 2018*

GAPO syndrome *Genet Couns 24:133–139, 2013*

Gingival fibromatosis–hypertrichosis syndrome – gingival fibromatosis which covers teeth, delays eruption of teeth, premature loss *Atlas of Clinical Syndromes A Visual Aid to Diagnosis, 1992, pp.310–311*

Haim–Munk syndrome (same as Papillon–Lefevre syndrome plus acro–osteolysis, acrachnodactyly, and pes planus) – congenital palmoplantar keratoderma, progressive periodontal destruction, recurrent skin infections (bacterial), arachnodactyly, claw–like deformity of terminal phalanges, onychogryphosis; also with cathepsin C mutation *JAAD 66:339–341, 2012; BJD 152:353–356, 2005; BJD 147:575–581, 2002; J Med Genet 37:88–94, 2000; Eur J Hum Genet 5:156–160, 1997; BJD 77:42–54, 1965*

Hajdu–Cheney syndrome

Hereditary sensory autoimmune neuropathy type VIII *J Med Case Rep 11:233 Aug 15, 2017*

Incontinentia pigmenti – delayed dentition, conical teeth, hypodontia *JAAD 81:1142–1149, 2019*

Juvenile hyaline fibromatosis (infantile systemic hyalinosis) *Ped Derm 23:458–464, 2006*

Kindler's syndrome – early onset periodontal disease with poor dentition; acral bullae in infancy; progressive poikiloderma with photosensitivity; nail dystrophy, webbing of digits, esophageal and urethral stenosis, ectropion, gingival fragility, aged hands with fine wrinkling and scarring, hyperkeratosis of hands and palms and soles, dyspigmentation, diffuse telangiectasias, hypshort arm chromosome 20; Kind 1; actin cytoskeleton–extracellular matrix interactions (membrane-associated structural and signaling protein *Gene Reviews March 3, 2016; AD 142:1619–1624, 2006; AD 142:620–624, 2006; BJD 66:104–111, 1954*

Olmsted syndrome *Odontology 103:241–245, 2015*

Papillon–Lefevre syndrome – autosomal recessive; diffuse transgradiens palmoplantar keratoderma; red scaly palms and soles; punctate hyperkeratosis of palms and soles; ichthyosis; hypotrichosis, nail fragility, periodontal disease with shedding of primary and permanent dentition; recurrent cutaneous and systemic pyodermas; psoriasiform plaques of elbows and knees; generalized psoriasiform dermatitis; hyperhidrosis, calcification of dura mater eyelid cysts; mutations and polymorphisms in cathepsin C gene defect on chromosome 11q14.1–14.3 encoding a cysteine–lysosomal protease (dipeptidyl protease I) *Mol Genet Genomic Med 2:217–228, 2014; Ped Derm 30:749–750, 2013; Eur J Ped 170:689–691, 2011; Cutis 79:55–56, 2007; JAAD 52:551–553, 2005; Australas J Dermatol 46:199–201, 2005; JAAD 49:S240–243, 2003; JAAD 48:345–351, 2003; Curr Prob Derm 14:71–116, 2002; JAAD 46:S8–10, 2002; JID 116:339–343, 2001; J Med Genet 36:881–887, 1999; JID 116:339–343, 2001; J Med Genet 36:881–887, 1999; J Periodontol 66:413–420, 1995; Ped Derm 11:354–357, 1994;* chromosome 11q14 *Eur J Hum Genet 5:156–160, 1997;* variant with arachnodactyly and acro–osteolysis *BJD 115:243–248, 1986; BJD 77:42–54, 1965;* late onset Papillon–Lefevre syndrome *JAAD 49:S240–243, 2003; J Periodontol 64:379–386, 1993*

Schwachman–Diamond syndrome – periodontal disease and caries; abscesses, short stature, delayed puberty, skeletal changes, pancreatic exocrine deficiency, pancytopenias, cyclic neutropenia, failure to thrive, hepatomegaly, pneumonia, otitis media, metaphyseal dysplasia, osteomyelitis *Ped Derm 28:568–569, 2011; Am J Med genet 66:378–398, 1996*

Sclerodactyly, non–epidermolytic palmoplantar keratoderma, multiple cutaneous squamous cell carcinomas, periodontal disease with loss of teeth, hypogenitalism with hypospadius, altered sex hormone levels, hypertriglyceridemia, 46XX *JAAD 53:S234–239, 2005*

Woolly hair, alopecia, premature loss of teeth, nail dystrophy, reticulate acral hyperkeratosis, facial abnormalities *BJD 145:157–161, 2001*

TOXINS

Acrodynia

TRAUMA

Physical trauma

VASCULAR DISORDERS

Erythromelalgia *Ped Dent 34:422–426, 2012*

HYPODONTIA

METABOLIC DISORDERS

Hurler's syndrome – widely spaced teeth with hypertrophic gums *Atlas of Clinical Syndromes A Visual Aid to Diagnosis, 1992, pp.118–119*

PRIMARY CUTANEOUS DISEASES

Anhidrotic ectodermal dysplasia – defective dentition *J Med Genet 38:579–585, 2001; Am J Med Genet 53:153–162, 1994*

Dyskeratosis congenita – hypodontia, edentulous, extensive caries; hypocalcification, thin enamel, increased mobility of widely separated, crowded, malformed teeth *J Oral Pathol Med 21:280–284, 1992; Oral Surg Oral Med Oral Pathol 37:736–744, 1974*

Epidermolysis bullosa, dystrophic – dental delay *JAAD 77:809–830, 2017*

Papillon–Lefevre syndrome – palmoplantar keratoderma and rapid periodontal destruction with loss of deciduous and permanent teeth *JAAD 60: 289–298, 2009; Quintessence Int 26:795–803, 1995; AD 124:533–539, 1988; Hum Genet 51:1–35, 1979*

Rapp–Hodgkin syndrome *J Med Genet 5:269–272, 1968*

Hypohidrotic ectodermal dysplasia – personal observation

Hypomelanosis of Ito – talon cusps *Clin Genet 21:65–68, 1982*; single maxillary central incisor *Clin Genet 31:370–373, 1987*; enamel defects, hypodontia, irregularly spaced teeth *JAAD 60:289–298, 2009*

SYNDROMES

Acro–dermato–ungual–lacrimal–tooth syndrome (ADULT syndrome) – ectrodactyly or syndactyly, freckling and dry skin, dysplastic nails, lacrimal duct atresia, primary hypodontia, conical teeth, and early loss of permanent teeth; small ears hooked nose, sparse hair, hypohidrosis, hypoplastic breasts and nipples, urinary tract anomalies; mutation in *TP63* gene (encodes transcription factor p63); p63 mutations also responsible for EEC, AEC, limb mammary, and Rapp–Hodgkin syndromes *Ped Derm 27:643–645, 2010; Hum Mol Genet 11:799–804, 2002; Am J Med Genet 45:642–648, 1993*

Ambras syndrome – hypertrichosis universalis congenital; fine silky light colored hair primarily of face, ears, shoulders, nose; associated minor facial dysmorphism, supernumerary nipples, dental anomalies *Clin Genet 44:121–128, 1993*

Ankyloblepharon–ectrodactyly–cleft lip/palate (AEC) syndrome – autosomal dominant; hypodontia, sparse hair, alopecia, nail dystrophy; mutation in p63 *BJD 166:134–144, 2012; AD 141:1591–1594, 2005*

Autosomal dominant hypodontia with nail dysgenesis *Oral Surg 39:409–423, 1975*

Autosomal recessive ectodermal dysplasia – alopecia, hypodontia *BJD 179:758–760, 2018;*

Birth Defects 24:205–207, 1988

Book syndrome *Am J Hum Genet 2:240–263, 1950*

Borrone dermatocardioskeletal syndrome – autosomal recessive or X–linked; gingival hypertrophy, coarse facies, late eruption of teeth, loss of teeth, thick skin, acne conglobata, osteolysis, large joint flexion contractures, short stature, brachydactyly, camptodactyly, mitral valve prolapse, congestive heart failure *Ped Derm 18:534–536, 2001*

Cherubism *Atlas of Clinical Syndromes A Visual Aid to Diagnosis, 1992, pp.106–107*

Cleft palate, stapes fixation, and oligodontia *Birth Defects 7:87–88, 1971*

Coffin–Lowry syndrome *J Pediatr 86:724–731, 1975*

Congenital hypertrichosis lanuginosa and dental anomalies *Clin Genet 10:303–306, 1976*

Cornelia de Lange (Brachmann–de Lange) syndrome – generalized hypertrichosis, confluent eyebrows, low hairline, hairy forehead and ears, hair whorls of trunk, single palmar crease, cutis marmorata, psychomotor and growth retardation with short stature, specific facies, hypertrichosis of forehead, face, back, shoulders, and extremities, bushy arched eyebrows with synophrys; long delicate eyelashes, skin around eyes and nose with bluish tinge, small nose with depressed root, prominent philtrum, thin upper lip with crescent-shaped mouth, widely spaced, sparse teeth, hypertrichosis of forehead, posterior neck, and arms, low set ears, arched palate, antimongoloid palpebrae; congenital eyelashes *Ped Derm 24:421–423, 2007; JAAD 48:161–179, 2003; JAAD 37:295–297, 1997; Am J Med Genet 47:959–964, 1993*

Cranioectodermal dysplasia – shortened arms, fingers, toes, fine sparse hair *Ped Derm 18:332–335, 2001; J Pediatr 90:55–61, 1977; Birth Defects XI:372–379, 1975*

Craniofacial dysostosis – hypoplastic teeth *JAAD 48:161–179, 2003*

Curry–Hall syndrome – small conical teeth, short limbs, polydactyly, nail dysplasia *Am J Med Genet 17:579–583, 1984*

Digitocutaneous dysplasia – X–linked dominant; digital fibromas, atrophic plaques with appearance of hyperpigmentation, metacarpal and metatarsal disorganization with resultant brachydactyly and clinodactyly, dysmorphic features including frontal bossing, broad nasal root, telecanthus and epicanthal folds, conical teeth, dental fissures, hypodontia, accessory gingival frenula, enamel hypoplasia *JAAD 56:S6–9, 2007*

Dysosteosclerosis – oligodontia *Birth Defects 11:349–351, 1975*

Ectrodactyly–ectodermal dysplasia–clefting syndrome – alopecia of scalp, eyebrows, and eyelashes, xerosis, atopic dermatitis, nail dystrophy, hypodontia with peg-shaped teeth, reduced sweat glands and salivary glands, syndactyly, mammary gland and nipple hypoplasia, conductive or sensorineural hearing loss, urogenital anomalies, lacrimal duct abnormalities; *TP63* mutations *BJD 162:201–207, 2010; Ped Derm 20:113–118, 2003; BJD 146:216–220, 2002; Dermatologica 169:80–85, 1984*

Ehlers–Danlos syndrome type VIII – periodontitis, loss of permanent teeth by second or third decade

Ellis–van Creveld syndrome (chondroplastic dwarf with defective teeth and nails, and polydactyly)(chondroectodermal dysplasia) – autosomal recessive; very short stature; chondrodysplasia, ectodermal dysplasia with ulnar polydactyly, cone– and peg–shaped teeth or hypodontia, enamel hypoplasia, fused incisors, molars with extra cusps, dental fissures and pits, neonatal teeth, malocculusion; short upper lip bound down by multiple labiogingival frenulae; gingival hypertrophy, nail dystrophy, hair may be normal or sparse and brittle; cardiac defects; ichthyosis, palmoplantar keratoderma; asymmetric distal limb shortening; short distal phalanges with small dystrophic fingernails; congenital heart disease; hypospadias, cryptorchidism; mutations in EVC and EVC2 *Cutis 83;303–305, 2009; Ped Derm 18:485–489, 2001; J Med Genet 17:349–356, 1980; Arch Dis Child 15:65–84, 1940*

FG syndrome (unusual facies, mental retardation, congenital hypotonia, imperforate anus) *Am J Med Genet 19:383–386, 1984*

Frontometaphyseal dysplasia – oligodontia *Radiol Clin N Am 10:225–243, 1972*

GAPO syndrome – growth retardation, alopecia, pseudoanodontia, and progressive optic atrophy; midface hypoplasia; frontal bossing, wide anterior fontanelle, saddle nose, protruding thick lips, low set ears, anti–Mongoloid slant, diffuse scalp hypotrichosis, prominent scalp veins, sparse eyebrows and eyelashes, absent teeth, slightly redundant skin, impacted teeth *Ped Derm 27156–161, 2010; Ped Derm 19:226, 2002; J Craniofac Genet Dev Biol 19:189–200, 1999; Birth Defects 24:205–207, 1988; Am J Med Genet 19:209–216, 1984; Syndr Ident 8:14–16, 1982; Odont Tilster 55:484–493, 1947*

Gardner's syndrome – unerupted teeth, supernumerary teeth, dentigerous cysts, odontomas, absent teeth

Goltz's syndrome (focal dermal hypoplasia) – hypodontia, enamel hypoplasia, dysplastic microdontia *JAAD 77:809–830, 2017;* asymmetric linear and reticulated streaks of atrophy and telangiectasia; yellow–red nodules; raspberry–like papillomas of lips, perineum, acrally, at perineum, buccal mucosa; xerosis; hypopigmented atrophic macules, Blaschko–esque hyperpigmentation, yellow nodulaes of hand, oligodontia, wide–spaced teeth, cleft hand, syndactyly, mammary hypoplasia, scalp and pubic hair sparse and brittle; short stature; asymmetric face; syndactyly, polydactyly; ocular, dental, and skeletal abnormalities with osteopathia striata of long bones; thin or atrophic nails *AD 148:85–88, 2012; AD 143:109–114, 2007; JAAD 25:879–881, 1991; AD 86:708–717, 1962;* aplasia cutis congenita *AD 145:218–219, 2009;* male mosaic Goltz's syndrome; blaschko–linear white atrophic depigmented lines, hyperpigmented linear streaks, linear alopecia, syndactyly, hydronephrosis *Ped Derm 28:550–554, 2011;* unilateral focal dermal hypoplasia, unilateral – PORCN gene mutation; PORCN encodes O–acyltransferase involved in palmitolylation and secretion of Wnt signaling proteins important in embryonic tissue development, fibroblast proliferation and osteogenesis *AD 148:85–88, 2012; AD 145:218–219, 2009*

Hair–nail–skin–teeth dysplasias (dermo–odonto–dysplasia, pilo–dento–ungular dysplasia, odonto–onycho–dermal dysplasia, odonto–onychial dysplasia, tricho–dermo–sysplasia with dental alterations) *Am J Med Genet 14:335–346, 1983*

Hallermann–Streiff syndrome – partial anodontia, short stature, atrophy and telangiectasia of central face, parrot–like appearance, microphthalmia, cataracts, high–arched palate, small mouth, sutural alopecia *JAAD 50:644, 2004*

Hay–Wells syndrome (AEC syndrome) *BJD 94:277–289, 1976*

Hemimaxillofacial dysplasia (segmental odontomaxillary dysplasia) (HATS – hemimaxillary enlargement, asymmetry of face, skin findings)– facial asymmetry, hypertrichosis of the face, unilateral maxillary enlargement, partial anodontia, delayed eruption of teeth, gingival thickening of affected segment, Becker's nevus, hairy nevus (hypertrichosis), lip hypopigmentation, depression of cheek, erythema, hypoplastic teeth *Ped Derm 21:448–451, 2004; JAAD 48:161–179, 2003; Oral Surg Oral Med Oral Pathol 64:445–448, 1987*

Hypodontia, sensorineural hearing loss and dizziness *Arch Otolaryngol 104:292–293, 1978*

Hypodontia, taurodontism, sparse hair *Birth Defects 11:39–50, 1975; Oral Surg 33:841–845, 1972*

Hypoglossia–hypodactylia *Syndromes of the Head and Neck, p. 666–670, 1990*

Hypohidrotic ectodermal dysplasia *Helv Paediatr Acta 11:604–639, 1956*

Hypomelanosis of Ito – anodontia, dental dysplasia

Kindler's syndrome – severe periodontitis with premature loss of teeth *AD 140:939–944, 2004*

Incontinentia pigmenti – pegged, conical teeth, accessory cusps; partial anodontia; delayed dentition; no enamel hypoplasia *JAAD 60:289–298, 2009; JAAD 47:169–187, 2002; J Pediatr 576:78–85, 1960*

Jakac–Wolf syndrome – palmoplantar keratoderma with squamous cell carcinoma, gingival dental anomalies, hyperhidrosis *JAAD 53:S234–239, 2005*

Johanson–Blizzard syndrome – hypodontia, microcephaly, hypoplastic alae nasi, hearing loss, pancreatic dysfunction, mental retardation *Birth Defects 24:205–207, 1988*

Kabuki syndrome – vitiligo, developmental delay, short stature, congenital heart defects, skeletal defects, cleft palate, dental abnormalities, cryptorchidism, lip pits, prominent fingertip pads, autoimmune disorders, blue sclerae, prominent eyelashes, thinning of central eyebrows, protuberant ears *Amer J Med Genet 132A:260–262, 2005*

KID syndrome – dental abnormalities *Ped Derm 19:232–236, 2002*

Kindler's syndrome – gingivitis leading to loss of teeth *BJD 160:233–242, 2009*

LADD syndrome *Eur J Pediatr 146:536–537, 1987*

Laryngo–onycho–cutaneous syndrome – autosomal recessive type of junctional epidermolysis bullosa; skin ulceration with prominent granulation tissue, early hoarseness and laryngeal stenosis; scarred nares; chronic erosion of corners of mouth (giant perleche); paronychia with periungual inflammation and erosions; onycholysis with subungual granulation tissue and loss of nails with granulation tissue of nail bed, conjunctival inflammation with polypoid granulation tissue, and dental enamel hypoplasia and hypodontia; only in Punjabi families; mutation in laminin alpha–3(*LAMA3A*) *BJD 169:1353–1356, 2013; Ped Derm 23:75–77, 2006; Biomedica 2:15–25, 1986*

Lelis syndrome – acanthosis nigricans with hypohidrosis, hypotrichosis, hypodontia, furrowed tongue, nail dystrophy, palmoplantar keratoderma *Genetic Skin Disorders, Second Edition, 2010, pp.94–97*

Microcephaly, short stature, characteristic facies – oligodontia *Syndromes of the Head and Neck, p. 871–872, 1990; Syndromes of the Head and Neck, 3rd Edition, p. 871–872*

Monosuperocentroincisivodontic dwarfism *J Pediatr 91:924–928, 1977*

Mosaic partial trisomy 13 – phylloid hypomelanosis, mental retardation, agenesis of the corpus callosum, conductive hearing loss, coloboma, skeletal defects, syndactyly, clinodactyly, dental malposition, oligodontia, pre–auricular fistulae *AD 145:576–578, 2009*

Multiple mucosal neuroma syndrome (MEN IIB) – dental diastema (gap) *JAAD 77:809–830, 2017*

Mulvihill–Smith syndrome (premature aging, multiple nevi, mental retardation) – oligodontia *J Med Genet 31:707–711, 1994; J Med Genet 25:53–56, 1988*

Neonatal ichthyosis–sclerosing cholangitis syndrome – autosomal recessive; lamellar ichthyosis, scalp hypotrichosis, scarring alopecia, sclerosing cholangitis; congenital paucity of bile ducts; oligodontia, hypodontia, dysplastic enamel; mutation in *CLDN1*(claudin–1; a tight junction component) *BJD 170:976–978, 2014; JAAD 63:607–641, 2010; BJD 163:205–207, 2010; Hum Mutat 27:408–410, 2006; Clin in Dermatol 23:47–55, 2005; Gastroenterol 127:1386–1390, 2004; JID 119:70–76, 2002*

Nevus comedonicus syndrome – with ipsilateral polysyndactyly and bilateral oligodontia *Ped Derm 27:377–379, 2010*

Nevus sebaceous syndrome (Schimmelpenning–Feuerstein–Mims syndrome) – anodontia, dysodontia *JAAD 52:S62–64, 2005; Ped Derm 13:22–24, 1996; Int J Oral Maxillofac Surg 12:437–443, 1983*

Odonto–onycho–dermal dyplasia – oligodontia with small widely spaced conical peg–shaped teeth, hypodontia, absence of secondary teeth; palmoplantar keratoderma, hyperhidrosis, dystrophic nails, erythematous telangiectatic, reticulated atrophic malar and ala nasal patches with vermiculate scarring *JAAD 57:732–733, 2007; Am J Med Genet 14:335–346, 1983*

Oligodontia, keratitis, skin ulceration and arthroosteolysis *Am J Med Genet 15:205–210, 1983*

Otodental dysplasia *Clin Genet 8:136–144, 1975*

Peutz–Jeghers syndrome *JAAD 77:809–830, 2017*

Pili torti, defective teeth, webbed fingers *JAAD 46:301–303, 2002*

Pili torti, enamel hypoplasia syndrome – keratosis pilaris, dry fair hair, enamel hypoplasia, widely spaced abnormal teeth *BJD 145:157–161, 2001*

Primary osteoma cutis – generalized osteomas; unilateral anodontia, hemihypertrophy, linear basal cell nevus

Pseudoacromegaly – autosomal recessive; skin ulcers, arthro–osteolysis, keratitis, oligodontia *Am J Med Genet 15:205–210, 1983*

Reticulolinear aplasia cutis congenita of the face and neck – Xp deletion syndrome, MIDAS (microphthalmia, dermal aplasia, sclerocornea), MLS (microphthalmia and linear skin defects), and Gazali–Temple syndrome; lethal in males; residual facial scarring in females, short stature, organ malformations *BJD 138:1046–1052, 1998*

Rieger syndrome – hypodontia and primary mesodermal dysgenesis of the iris *Trans Am Ophthalmol Soc 81:736–784, 1983*

Riga–Fede syndrome *Austral Dermatol J 42:225–227, 1997*

Rutherfurd syndrome – autosomal dominant; gum hypertrophy, failure of tooth eruption, corneal opacities, mental retardation, aggressive behavior *Ped Derm 18:534–536, 2001*

Schopf–Schulz–Passarge syndrome (hypotrichosis, palmoplantar hyperkeratosis, apocrine hidrocystomas of eyelid margins, nail dystrophy) – oligodontia; red palms and soles with focal dryness; maceration with hyperhidrosis; finger and toenail dystrophy; mutation in *WNT10A BJD 171:1211–1214, 2014; Ped Derm 30:491–492, 2013; JAAD 65:1066–1069, 2011; AD 140:231–236, 2004; Acta DV 88:607–612, 2008; JAAD 10:922–925, 1984*

Singleton–Merten syndrome – autosomal dominant; muscle weakness, failure to thrive, glaucoma, abnormal dentition, aortic calcification, acro–osteolysis, psoriasis; chilblains of helices of ears with edema, erythema, ulcers *BJD 173:1369–1370, 2015; BMJ Case Reports Sept 5, 2014; Am J Med GenetcsA 161A:360–370, 2013; IF1H1 gain of function mutation Am J Hum Genet 96:275–262, 2015*

Steatocystoma multiplex, partial congenital absence of secondary dentition, persistence of primary dentition; mutation in keratin 17 gene *BJD 161:1396–1398, 2009*

Trichodental syndrome – fine short hair, madurosis *BJD 116:259–263, 1987*

Trichodento–osseous syndrome – curly hair, sclerotic cortical bone, thin dental enamel, unerupted teeth *Oral Surg 77:487–493, 1994*

Tuomaala–Haapanen syndrome (brachymetapody, anodontia, hypotrichosis, albinoid trait) *Acta Ophthalmol 46:365–371, 1968*

Uncombable hair syndrome – enamel hypoplasia, oligodontia *Cutis 79:291–292, 2007*

Van der Woude syndrome – autosomal dominant; hypodontia, lip pits, cleft lip and/or palate; mutation in interferon regulatory factor 6(*IRF6*) *Ped Derm 29:768–770, 2012*

Waardenburg syndrome – caries

Witkop tooth–nail syndrome – autosomal dominant; hypodontia with nail dysgenesis; teeth widely spaced; narrow crowns; hypoplastic spoon-shaped nails, slow growing, prone to fracture; normal facies; mutation in *MSX1 Ped Derm 28:281–285, 2011; J Clin Pediatr Dent 28:107–112, 2004; Oral Surg 37:576–582, 1974*

X–linked anhidrotic ectodermal dysplasia – hypodontia with peg–shaped or pointed teeth *Oral Dis 7:163–170, 2001; Birth Defects 24:205–207, 1988*

OTHER DENTAL ANOMALIES

AUTOIMMUNE DISEASES AND DISORDERS OF IMMUNE DYSREGULATION

Autoimmune polyendocrinopathy–candidiasis–ectodermal dystrophy syndrome (APECED) – enamel hypoplasia; sparse scalp, facial, and body hair, chronic mucocutaneous candidiasis, adrenal insufficiency, hypoparathyroidism, nail dystrophy, keratoconjunctivitis, vitiligo; mutation in autoimmune regulator gene (AIRE) *Ped Derm 24:529–533, 2007*

Dermatitis herpetiformis – dental abnormalities including horizontal grooves, large enamel pits, defects in enamel color *JAAD 64:1017–1024, 2011*

Gain of function *STAT1* mutations – chronic mucocutaneous candidiasis; onychodystrophy, generalized dermatophytosis; disseminated coccidioidomycosis, histoplasmosis, sinopulmonary infections, herpes simplex infections; endocrine, dental gastrointestinal disease; diabetes mellitus, hypothyroidism, autoimmune hepatitis, cerebral aneurysms, oral and esophageal squamous cell carcinomas; increased levels of interferon results in decreased IL–17A and IL–22 *JAAD 73:255–264, 2015*

GATA2 deficiency (MONOMAC) – personal observation

Hyper IgE syndrome – retained primary teeth leading to double rows of teeth; lack of eruption of secondary teeth, delayed resorption of roots of primary teeth *JAAD 60:289–298, 2009; JAAD 54:855–865, 2006;* Job's syndrome (hyperimmunoglobulin E syndrome) – autosomal dominant; dermatitis, abscesses, retention of primary teeth with double rows of teeth; deep–set eyes, broad nasal bridge, wide fleshy nasal tip, prognathism, ocular hypertelorism; bone abnormalities, cyst–forming pneumonia, elevated IgE levels; *STAT3* mutations *NEJM 357:1608–1619;Clin Inf Dis 34:1213–1214,1267–1268, 2002; JAAD S268–269, 2002; Pediatr 141:572–575, 2002; Curr Prob in Derm 10:41–92, 1998*

Leukocyte adhesion deficiency types I–III – delay in separation of umbilical stump and omphalitis; mucositis; periodontitis; delayed wound healing *JAAD 72:1066–1073, 2015*

DRUGS

Doxycycline–induced brown staining of permanent teeth *AD 142:1081–1082, 2006*

Minocycline – gray teeth

Tetracycline (tetracycline teeth) – gray pigmentation

Thalidomide embryopathy – dental anomalies *Atlas of Clinical Syndromes A Visual Aid to Diagnosis, 1992, pp.370–371*

EXOGENOUS AGENTS

Cocaine abuse – dental caries *JAAD 59:483–487, 2008; Int Dent J 55:365–369, 2005*

Methamphetamine abuse – dental caries *JAAD 69:135–142, 2013*

Tea – brown stained teeth

INFECTIONS

Actinomycosis – carous teeth; dental abscess

Pseudoerythrodontia – red fluorescence of the teeth from poor dental hygiene with resultant dental plaque, tartar, and calculus; *Provotella intermedia, Actinomyces naeslundi, A. israelii, Lactobacillus fermentans, L. rhamnosus and L. casei* – red fluorescence; *Streptococcus oralis, S. salivarius, S. mutans, Fusobacterium nucleatum, and S. sobrinus* – green fluorescence *BJD 159:979–981, 2008*

Syphilis, congenital – Hutchinson's incisors – centrally notched, widely spaced, peg–shaped upper central incisors; present at age 6 *Tr Path Soc London 9:449–455, 1858;* mulberry molars *Br J Vener Dis 47:5–56, 1971*

INFILTRATIVE DISORDERS

Langerhans cell histiocytosis – destructive periodontitis which may simulate necrotizing gingivitis; "floating teeth"; gingival recession; may lead to severe alveolar bone loss *J Periodontol 60:57–66, 1989;* premature eruption of teeth

INFLAMMATORY DISORDERS

Desquamative gingivitis with loss of teeth *JAAD 78:839–848, 2018*
    Allergic contact dermatitis
    Behcet's disease
    Cicatricial pemphigoid
    Epidermolysis bullosa acquisita
    Erythema multiforme
    Graft vs host disease
    Irritant contact dermatitis
    Lichen planus
    Paraneoplastic pemphigus

    Pemphigus vulgaris

METABOLIC DISORDERS

Celiac disease – enamel defects with white color change *JAMA 315:81–82, 2016*

Congenital erythropoietic porphyria (Gunther's disease) – erythrodontia (purple teeth), fluorescent teeth, gingival recession; bullous photosensitivity, photomutilation, fixed flexion deformities, resorption of fingertips, blepharitis, ectropion, meibomian cysts, conjunctivitis, loss of eyebrows, dental caries, overcrowding of teeth, facial hypertrichosis, scarring alopecia due to recurrent blistering, dyschromatosis; neonatal jaundice, hemolytic anemia, splenomegaly due to pancytopenia *JAMA Derm 149:969–970, 2013; BJD 166:697–699, 2012; BJD 167:988–900, 2012; Ped Derm 30:484–489, 2013; Am J Med 45:624–627, 1968*

Congenital renal disease – dystrophic teeth – personal observation

Hepatoerythropoietic porphyria – extreme photosensitivity, skin fragility in sun–exposed areas, hypertrichosis, erythrodontia, pink urine, sclerodermoid changes *AD 146:529–533, 2010*

Hunter's syndrome – widely spaced teeth; reticulated 2–10mm skin-colored papules over scapulae, chest, neck, arms; X–linked recessive; MPS type II; iduronate–2 sulfatase deficiency; lysosomal accumulation of heparin sulfate and dermatan sulfate; short stature, full lips, coarse facies, macroglossia, clear corneas (unlike Hurler's syndrome), progressive neurodegeneration, communicating hydrocephalus, valvular and ischemic heart disease, lower respiratory tract infections, adenotonsillar hypertrophy, otitis media, obstructive sleep apnea, diarrhea, hepatosplenomegaly, skeletal deformities (dysostosis multiplex), dolichocephaly, deafness, retinal degeneration, inguinal and umbilical hernias *Ped Derm 21:679–681, 2004*

Morquio's syndrome – blue–grey teeth due to enamel hypoplasia *Atlas of Clinical Syndromes A Visual Aid to Diagnosis, 1992, pp.124–125*

NEOPLASTIC DISORDERS

Porokeratotic eccrine ostial and dermal duct nevus, generalized – blaschko–distributed verrucous plaques; non–scarring alopecia, hypohidrosis, teeth in disarray, deafness *JAAD 59:S43–45, 2008*

PRIMARY CUTANEOUS DISEASES

Alpha6–beta4 epidermolysis bullosa – onychogryphosis; yellow–brown discoloration of teeth with enamel defects *BJD 169:115–124, 2013*

Anhidrotic ectodermal dysplasia *Atlas of Clinical Syndromes A Visual Aid to Diagnosis, 1992, pp.456–457*

Epidermolysis bullosa – dental caries in both junctional EB and recessive dystrophic *JAAD 60:289–298, 2009; Pediatr Dent 16:427–432, 1994;* junctional epidermolysis bullosa – abnormal teeth with papular prurigo–like lesions *BJD 169:195–198, 2013;* junctional epidermolysis bullosa of late onset (formerly junctional epidermolysis bullosa progressive) – loss of dermatoglyphs, waxy hyperkeratosis of dorsal hand, atrophic skin of lower leg, transverse ridging and enamel pits of teeth, nail atrophy, amelogenesis imperfect, hyperhidrosis, blisters on elbows, knees, and oral cavity *BJD 164:1280–1284, 2011*

Epidermolysis bullosa, junctional – *COL17A1* mutations (GABEB); enamel hypoplasia; ulcers, crusts, and atrophy; anonychia; pitted enamel of teeth; hyperkeratotic lesions of legs *BJD 170:1056–1064, 2014; BJD 160:1094–1097, 2009; BJD 156:861–870, 2007; Arch Oral Biol 38:943–955, 1993*

Epidermolysis bullosa, junctional, Herlitz type – pitted teeth; laminin V mutation

Epidermolysis bullosa simplex – enamel hypoplasia *Ped Derm 167–168, 2006*

Happle–Tinschert syndrome – segmental basaloid follicular hamartomas, basal cell carcinomas, linear hypo– or hyperpigmented lesions, linear atrophoderma, palmoplantar pitting, atrophoderma, ipsilateral hypertrichosis, hypotrichosis; polydactyly, syndactyly, rudimentary ribs, limb length disparities, dysmorphic facies, macrocephaly, jaw ameloblastomas, dental anomalies, imperforate anus, colon adenocarcinoma; medulloblastoma cerebral manifestation, developmental delay, optic glioma or meningioma, cataracts, microphthalmia, coloboma; mutation in *SMOc.1234>T BJD 182:212–217, 2020; BJD 169:1342–1345, 2013; Ped Derm 28:555–560, 2011; JAAD 65:e17–19, 2011; Dermatology 218:221–225, 2009; Acta DV 88:382–387, 2008*

Hidrotic ectodermal dysplasia – "tiger teeth"

Incontinentia pigmenti achromians – personal observation

Junctional epidermolysis bullosa of late onset (skin fragility in childhood) – speckled hyperpigmentation of elbows; hemorrhagic bullae, teeth and nail abnormalities, oral blisters, disappearance of dermatoglyphs, palmoplantar keratoderma, small vesicles, atrophy of skin of hands *BJD 169:714–716, 2013*

Marie–Unna hereditary hypotrichosis – autosomal dominant; sparse curly hair; begins at puberty; at vertex; affects eyebrows, eyelashes, body and pubic hair; 50% with widely spaced incisors; 8p21 *Ped Derm 28:202–204, 2011; BJD 160:194–196, 2009; Ped Derm 19:250–252, 2002; Derm Wschr 82:1167–1178, 1925*

Rapp–Hodgkin hypohidrotic ectodermal dysplasia – autosomal dominant; alopecia of wide area of scalp in frontal to crown area, short eyebrows and eyelashes, coarse wiry sparse hypopigmented scalp hair, sparse body hair, scalp dermatitis, ankyloblepharon, syndactyly, nipple anomalies, cleft lip and/or palate; nails narrow and dystrophic, small stature, hypospadius, conical teeth and anodontia or hypodontia; distinctive facies, short stature *JAAD 53:729–735, 2005; Ped Derm 7:126–131, 1990; J Med Genet 15:269–272, 1968*

X–linked hypohidrotic ectodermal dysplasia, mosaicism – V–shaped hypopigmented linear lesions, patchy hypotrichosis, abnormal teeth *Ped Derm 24:551–554, 2007*

SYNDROMES

Acro–dermato–ungual–lacrimal–tooth syndrome (ADULT syndrome) – ectrodactyly or syndactyly, freckling and dry skin, dysplastic nails, lacrimal duct atresia, primary hypodontia, conical teeth, and early loss of permanent teeth; small ears hooked nose, sparse hair, hypohidrosis, hypoplastic breasts and nipples, urinary tract anomalies mutation in *TP63* gene (encodes transcription factor p63); p63 mutations also responsible for EEC, AEC, limb mammary, and Rapp–Hodgkin syndromes *Ped Derm 27:643–645, 2010; Ped Derm 22:415–419, 2005; Hum Mol Genet 11:799–804, 2002; Am J Med Genet 45:642–648, 1993*

Albright's hereditary osteodystrophy (pseudohypoparathyroidism) – defective teeth; poor dentition *JAMA Derm 149:975–976, 2013; Ergeb Inn Med Kinderheilkd 42:191–221, 1979*

Anhidrotic ectodermal dysplasia with immunodeficiency – conical teeth, sparse hair, hypohidrosis; mutation in NEMO with I–KB gain of function *JAAD 58:316–320, 2008*

Apert's syndrome (acrocephalosyndactyly) – delayed dental development and malocclusion *Ped Derm 24:186–188, 2007*

Carney complex – personal observation

Cleidocranial dysplasia – delayed dentition; supernumerary teeth *Atlas of Clinical Syndromes A Visual Aid to Diagnosis, 1992, pp.32–3*

Cockayne syndrome – dental caries, xerosis with rough, dry skin, anhidrosis, erythema of hands, hypogonadism; autosomal recessive; short stature, facial erythema in butterfly distribution leading to mottled pigmentation and atrophic scars, premature aged appearance with loss of subcutaneous fat and sunken eyes, canities, mental deficiency, photosensitivity, cyanotic livedo reticularis, disproportionately large hands, feet, and ears, sensorineural hearing loss, ocular defects including retinal degeneration, demyelination *JAAD 75:873–882, 2016; JAMA Derm 149:1414–1418, 2013; Ped Derm 20:538–540, 2003; Am J Hum Genet 50:677–689, 1992; J Med Genet 18:288–293, 1981;* birdheaded dwarfism

COG6 syndrome – hypohidrosis and intellectual disability; abnormal teeth, acquired microcephaly *J Med Genet 50:431–436, 2013*

Crouzon syndrome – narrowly spaced teeth *Atlas of Clinical Syndromes A Visual Aid to Diagnosis, 1992, pp.12–13*

Curly hair–ankyloblepharon–nail dysplasia syndrome – abnormal dentition (form of hypophidrotic ectodermal dysplasia) *Birth Defects Orig Art Ser 7:100–102, 1971*

Curry–Jones syndrome – linear hypo– or hyperpigmented lesions, palmoplantar pitting, streaks of atrophy, hypertrichosis, trichoblastomas and nevus sebaceous, polydactyly or preaxial polysyndactyly, dysmorphic facies, macrocephaly, microcephaly, dental anomalies, craniosynostosis, anal stenosis, myofibromas and smooth muscle hamartomas, medulloblastomas, cerebral malformations (agenesis of corpus callosum), developmental delay, cataracts, microphthalmia, coloboma, glaucoma, cryptorchidism; mutation in *SMOc.1234C>T BJD 182:212–217, 2020; Clin Dysmorphol 4:116–129, 1995*

Dentinogenesis imperfecta – personal observation

Ectodermal dysplasia and clefting – alopecia, tooth abnormalities, reticulated hyperpigmentation *Ped Derm 28:707–710, 2011*

Ectrodactyly–ectodermal dysplasia–clefting syndrome (EEC syndrome) – small carious teeth with hypoplastic enamel; missing teeth *Atlas of Clinical Syndromes A Visual Aid to Diagnosis, 1992, pp.386–387*

Ectodermal dysplasia with hair anomalies and syndactyly – atypical order of eruption of teeth *Atlas of Clinical Syndromes A Visual Aid to Diagnosis, 1992, pp.458–459*

Elejalde syndrome (neuroectodermal (neurocutaneous)–melanolysosomal disease) – silvery hair, central nervous system dysfunction; hypotonic facies, plagiocephaly, micrognathia, crowded teeth, narrow high palate, pectus excavatum, cryptorchidism *JAAD 38:295–300, 1998*

Erythrokeratoderma–cardiomyopathy syndrome – recurrent infections, wiry or absent hair, dental enamel defects, nail dystrophy, sudden onset congestive heart failure; early death; dominant mutation in desmoplakin *Cases of the Year, Pre–AAD Pediatric Dermatology Meeting*

Familial partial lipodystrophy, mandibuloacral dysplasia variety – autosomal recessive; short stature, high pitched voice, mandibular and clavicular hypoplasia, dental anomalies, acro–osteolysis, stiff joints, cutaneous atrophy, alopecia, nail dysplasia *Am J Med 108:143–152, 2000*

Finlay–Marks syndrome (scalp–ear–nipple syndrome) – nipple or breast hypoplasia or aplasia, aplasia cutis congenita of scalp, abnormal ears and teeth, nail dystrophy, syndactyly, reduced apocrine secretion

Frontonasal dysplasia – widely spaced *Atlas of Clinical Syndromes A Visual Aid to Diagnosis, 1992, pp.40–41*

Gardner's syndrome – supernumerary teeth, multiple non–erupted teeth, follicular odontomas, dentigerous cysts, impacted teeth, absent teeth, and caries; desmoid tumors (subcutaneous nodule/tumor); epidermoid cysts *JAAD 68:189–209, 2013; JAAD 60:289–298, 2009; Oral Disease 13:360–365, 2007; Br J Oral Maxillfoac Surg 24:410–416, 1986; Br J Surg 69:718–721, 1982*

Goldenhaar syndrome – dental anomalies *Atlas of Clinical Syndromes A Visual Aid to Diagnosis, 1992, pp.52–53*

Goltz's syndrome – vertically grooved teeth *AD 145:218–219, 2009*

Happle–Tinschert syndrome – segmental basaloid follicular hamartomas; ipsilateral hypertrichosis; hypo– and hyperpigmentation; linear atrophoderma; osseous, dental, and/or cerebral defects; mutation in *SMO BJD 175:1108, 2016; BJD 169:1342–1345, 2013; Ped Derm 28:555–560, 2011; JAAD 65:e17–19, 2011; Dermatology 218:221–225, 2009; Acta DV 88:382–387, 2008*

Hennekam syndrome – autosomal recessive; intestinal lymphangiectasia, lymphedema of legs and genitalia, gigantic scrotum and penis, multilobulated lymphatic ectasias, small mouth, narrow palate, gingival hypertrophy, tooth anomalies, thick lips, agenesis of ear, pre–auricular pits, wide flat nasal bridge, frontal upsweep, platybasia, hypertelorism, pterygia colli, bilateral single palmar crease, hirsutism, mild mental retardation, facial anomalies, growth retardation, pulmonary, cardiac, hypogammaglobulinemia *Ped Derm 23:239–242, 2006*

Ichthyosis follicularis with atrichia and photophobia (IFAP) – enamel dysplasia; collodion membrane and erythema at birth; ichthyosis, spiny (keratotic) follicular papules (generalized follicular keratoses), non–scarring alopecia, keratotic papules of elbows, knees, fingers, extensor surfaces, xerosis; punctate keratitis, photophobia; nail dystrophy, psychomotor delay, short stature; beefy red tongue and gingiva, angular stomatitis, atopy, lamellar scales, psoriasiform plaques, palmoplantar erythema *Curr Prob Derm 14:71–116, 2002; JAAD 46:S156–158, 2002; BJD 142:157–162, 2000; Am J Med Genet 85:365–368, 1999; Ped Derm 12:195, 1995; AD 125:103–106, 1989; Dermatologica 177:341–347, 1988*

Incontinentia pigmenti – anomalous crowns with extra cusps; supernumerary teeth *JAAD 47:169–187, 2002*

Jackli syndrome – generalized reticulated hyperpigmentation with alopecia, microdontia, and childhood cataracts

Kindler's syndrome (hereditary bullous acrokeratotic poikiloderma of Weary–Kindler) – poor dentition and premature loss of teeth due to periodontitis, gingivitis; teeth enamel defects; bullous disease in infancy, photosensitivity, poikiloderma, atrophic skin of dorsal hands, pseudoainhum; mutation in FERMT1 gene BJD 159:1192–1196, 2008; BJD 158:1375–1377, 2008; Ped Derm 23:586–588, 2006; AD 142:1619–1624, 2006; AD 142:620–624, 2006; AD 140:939–944, 2004; Int J Dermatol 36:529–533, 1997; AD 1487–1490, 1996; BJD 66:104–111, 1954

Keratosis–ichthyosis–deafness (KID) syndrome – abnormal teeth *Ped Derm 19:513–516, 2002*

Laryngo–onycho–cutaneous syndrome (Shabbir syndrome) – autosomal recessive; symblepharon, crusted erosions of elbows, anonychia, mucosal nodule of hard palate; hoarse cry, chronic granulation tissue, tooth enamel hypoplasia; laminin alpha 3A mutation (LAMA 3A) with N–terminal deletion of LAMA 3A *Ped Derm 24:306–308, 2007; Cornea 20:753–756, 2001; Arch Dis Child 70:319–326, 1994; JAAD 29:906–909, 1993; Clin Dysmorphol 1:3–14, 1992; Eye 5:717–722, 1991; Biomedica 2:15–25, 1986*

Lipodystrophy associated with mandibuloacral dysplasia – bird–like facies, acro–osteolysis, mottled cutaneous pigmentation, dental abnormalities, skin atrophy, alopecia *J Clin Endocrinol Metab 87:776–785, 2002*

Macrocephaly–alopecia–cutis laxa–scoliosis syndrome (MACS) – droopy eyelids, everted lips, gingival hypertrophy, dental anomalies, alopecia, high pitched voice; mutation in *RIN2 JAAD 66:842–851, 2012*

Melnick–Needlas syndrome – malalignment of teeth *Atlas of Clinical Syndromes A Visual Aid to Diagnosis, 1992, pp.30–31*

Microcephalic osteodysplastic primordial dwarfism type II – autosomal recessive; craniofacial dysmorphism with slanting palpebral fissures, prominent nose, small mouth, micrognathia; fine sparse hair and thin eyebrows; café au lait macules; xerosis; mottling; dark pigmentation of neck and trunk; depigmentation (nevus depigmentosus); small pointed widely spaced teeth; low set ears missing lobule; widened metaphyses and relative shortening of distal limbs; cerebrovascular anomalies *Ped Derm 25:401–402, 2008*

Naegeli–Franceschetti–Jadassohn syndrome – autosomal dominant; abnormally shaped teeth, polydontia, yellow spotted enamel, caries, early total loss; reticulate gray to brown pigmentation of neck, upper trunk and flexures, punctate or diffuse palmoplantar keratoderma, hypohidrosis with heat intolerance, onycholysis, subungual hyperkeratosis *BJD 177:945–959, 2017;*

JAAD 60: 289–298, 2009; Ped Derm 22:122–126, 2005; Semin Cutan Med Surg 16:72–80, 1997; JAAD 28:942–950, 1993

Nevoid basal cell carcinoma syndrome – odontogenic cysts *JAAD 60: 289–298, 2009; Swed Dent J13:131–139, 1989*

Nevus sebaceous syndrome (Schimmelpfenning syndrome) – variable anomalies *Atlas of Clinical Syndromes A Visual Aid to Diagnosis, 1992, pp.314–315*

Oculocerebral hypopigmentation syndrome of Preus – very short with thin build, ptosis, high arched palate, dental malocclusion, prominent central upper incisors, hair and skin hypopigmented, deafness, severe mental retardation *Ped Derm 24:313–315, 2007*

Oculodentodigital dysplasia – autosomal dominant; bilateral microphthalmos, nasal malformations, syndactyly, hypotrichosis, curly hair, nail dystrophy, enamel hypoplasia *Clinics in Dermatol 23:23–32, 2005; ASDC J Dent Child 53:131–134, 1986*

Odonto–onycho–dermal dysplasia – telangiectatic atrophic patches of face, sparse hair, conical teeth, oligodontia, hyperkeratosis of palms and soles, smooth tongue, dystrophic nails; WNT10A mutation *JAAD 65:1066–1069, 2011; Am J Med Genet 14:335–346, 1983*

Oral–facial–digital syndrome type 1 (Papillon–Leage–Psaume syndrome) – X–linked dominant; congenital facial milia which resolve with pitted scars; milia of face, scalp, pinnae, and dorsal hands; short stature, hypotrichosis with dry and brittle hair, short upper lip, hypoplastic ala nasi and lower jaw, pseudoclefting of upper lip, hooked pug nose, hypertrophied labial frenulae, bifid or multilobed tongue with small white tumors within clefts, ankyloglossia, multiple soft hamartomas of oral cavity, clefting of hard and soft palate, teeth widely spaced with dental caries, trident hand or brachydactyly, syndactyly, clinodactyly, ulnar deviation of index finger, or polydactyly; hair dry and brittle, alopecic, numerous milia of face, ears, backs of hands, mental retardation with multiple central nervous system abnormalities, frontal bossing, hypertelorism, telecanthus, broad depressed nasal bridge; polycystic renal disease; combination of polycystic renal disease, milia, and hypotrichosis is highly suggestive of OFD 1 *Ped Derm 27:669–670, 2010; JAAD 59:1050–1063, 2008; Ped Derm 25:474–476, 2008; Ped Derm 9:52–56, 1992; Am J Med Genet 86:269–273, 1999; JAAD 31:157–190, 1994; Ped Derm 9:52–56, 1992; Pediatrics 29:985–995, 1962; Rev Stomatol 55:209–227, 1954*

Osteogenesis imperfecta – gray–brown teeth *Am J Med Genet 31:1470–1481, 2014; Eur J Med Genet 51:383–408, 2008;* yellow teeth *JAAD 46:161–183, 2002*

Prader–Willi syndrome – hypoplasia of enamel, severe early caries *Atlas of Clinical Syndromes A Visual Aid to Diagnosis, 1992, pp.286–287*

Rabson–Mendenhall syndrome – insulin–resistant diabetes mellitus, unusual facies, dental precocity, fissured tongue, hypertrichosis, acanthosis nigricans, and premature sexual development *Ped Derm 19:267–270, 2002*

Rothmund–Thomson syndrome – dental dysplasia

Seckel's syndrome – abnormal teeth, short stature, hypopigmented papules and macules, small deformed ears lacking lobules, syndactyly, clinodactyly *Ped Derm 24:53–56, 2007*

Segmental odontomaxillary dysplasia (HATS – hemimaxillary enlargement, asymmetry of the face, tooth abnormalities, and skin findings) – localized facial hypertrichosis, commissural lip cleft, hyperlinear palms, abnormal teeth, missing teeth, abnormal spacing *Ped Derm 25:491–492, 2008*

Sensorineural hearing loss, periorificial erythrokeratoderma, dental enamel defects, excess granulation tissue *JID 121:1221–1223, 2003*

SHORT syndrome – short stature, hyperextensible joints, ocular depression, Reiger (ocular and dental) anomaly, teething delay, loss of subcutaneous fat of face, upper extremities, chest

Sjogren–Larsson syndrome – autosomal recessive; enamel dysplasia or hypoplasis; serrated teeth; caries, periodontitis, malocclusion *JAAD 60:289–298, 2009; Swed Dent 7:141–151, 1983*

Tetrasomy 13q – facies with long forehead, thick eyebrows, hypertelorism, broad nasal bridge, malposition of teeth, prominent central incisors with diastema, bilateral clinodactyly of fifth fingers *Ped Derm 32:263–266, 2015*

Tooth and nail syndromes *Ped Derm 28:281–285, 2011*
    Curry–Hall syndrome – polydactyly
    DOOR syndrome (deafness and onychoosteodystrophy with retardation)
    Fried syndrome – autosomal recessive; thin sparse hair and eyebrows; everted lower lip
    Witkop tooth and nail syndrome

Treacher–Collins–Franceschetti syndrome (mandibulofacial dysostosis) – autosomal dominant; prominent nose, sunken cheeks, stretching of skin to side of neck, recessed chin, large down–turned mouth, widespaced eyes with antimongoloid slants, lateral coloboma, absent eyelashes of lower lids, hairline extended to cheeks, small and crumpled pinnae; hypoplastic or deformed teeth in older children *Ped Derm 23:511–513, 2006*

Tricho–odonto osseous syndrome – autosomal dominant; diffuse curly hair at birth, enamel hypoplasia, widely spaced teeth, otosclerosis, dolichocephaly, frontal bossing; mutation in *DLX3* (homeobox gene) *JAAD 59:1–22, 2008; Am J Med Genet 72:197–204, 1997; Hum Molec Genet 7:563–569, 1998; J Med Genet 35:825–828, 1998; Pediatrics 37:498–502, 1966*

Trichorhinophalangeal syndrome type I – autosomal dominant; slow growing hair, receding frontotemporal hairline with high bossed forhead; thin nails, koilonychias, leukonychia, facial pallor, pear–shaped nose with bulbous nose tip, wide long philtrum, thin upper lip, triangular face, receding chin, tubercle of normal skin below the lower lip,protruding ears, distension and deviation with fusiform swelling of the PIP joints; hip malformation, brachydactyly, prognathism, fine brittle slow growing sparse hair, lateral eyebrows sparse and brittle, dense medially, bone deformities (hands short and stubby), cone–shaped epiphyses of bones of hand, lateral deviation of interphalangeal joints, flat feet, hip malformations, high arched palate, supernumerary teeth, dental malocclusion, mild short stature; hypotonia, deep voice, recurrent respiratory infections, hypoglycemia, diabetes mellitus, hypothyroidism, decreased growth hormone, renal and cardiac defects, mutation in zinc finger nuclear transcription factor (TRPS1 gene) *Cutis 89:56, 73, 74, 2012; Ped Derm 26:171–175, 2009; Ped Derm 25:557–558, 2008; BJD 157:1021–1024, 2007; AD 137:1429–1434, 2001; JAAD 31:331–336, 1994; Hum Genet 74:188–189, 1986; Helv Paediatr Acta 21:475–482, 1966*

Trichorhinophalangeal syndrome type II (Langer–Giedion syndrome) – microcephaly with mental retardation, deep set eyes, exotropia, long nose with bulbous tip, broad nasal bridge, thick ala nasi, high palate, crowded teeth, micrognathia, long neck, short metacarpals, thin nails, small feet with brachydactyly, vaginal stenosis, short stature, thin sparse hair, long face, prominent ears, madarosis, cartilaginous exostoses, foot deformities, joint laxity; *EXT gene BJD 171:1581–1583, 2014; BJD 157:1021–1024, 2007; Genetic Skin Disorders, Second Edition, 2010, pp.225–228; Atlas of Clinical Syndromes A Visual Aid to Diagnosis, 1992, pp.408–409420–421*

Trichorhinophalangeal syndrome type III (Sugio–Kajii syndrome) – facial dysmorphism with dental malocclusion *BJD 159:476–478, 2008*

Tuberous sclerosis – enamel pits *JAAD 49:163–166, 2003*

Turner's syndrome – malpositioned teeth *Atlas of Clinical Syndromes A Visual Aid to Diagnosis, 1992, pp.192–193*

Uncombable hair syndrome – enamel hypoplasia, oligodontia *Cutis 79:291–292, 2007*

Williams's syndrome – malpositioned teeth with abnormal enamel *Atlas of Clinical Syndromes A Visual Aid to Diagnosis, 1992, pp.484–485*

VASCULAR DISORDERS

Infantile hemangioma of upper lip – enamel hypoplasia *Ped Derm 36:899–901, 2019*

Port wine stain with gingival hypertrophy and dental abnormalities *Ped Derm 33:570–584, 2016; J Craniofac Surg 20:1629–1630, 2009*

Facial port wine stains (capillary malformation) – widened interdental spaces; abnormal bite *JAAD 67:687–693, 2012*

PHACES syndrome – dental root abnormalities *Ped Derm 36:505–508, 2019;* tooth enamel hypoplasia with intraoral hemangiomas *Ped Derm 31:455–458, 2014;* dental anomalies in adults *Ped Derm 36:618–622, 2019;* absence or severe malformation roots of permanent first molars, bilateral, and not restricted to segments affected by the cutaneous hemangioma *Ped Derm 36:505–508, 2019*

DENTAL PITS

JAAD 56:786–790, 2007

Amelogenesis imperfecta – *LAMB3* mutations *J Dent Res 92:899–904, 2013*

Junctional epidermolysis bullosa – dental pits due to enamel hypoplasia *JAAD 60:289–298, 2009; Pediatr Dent 16:427–432, 1994*

Pseudohypoparathyroidism *BMC Oral Health 2019 Dec 31. doi:101186/s12903–019–0978–z*

Tuberous sclerosis – pits due to reduction in amount of enamel matrix formed during amelogenesis *Ped Derm 32:563–570, 2015; JAAD 60:289–298, 2009; J Med Genet 34:637–639, 1997; Clin Genet 32:216–221, 1987*

Vitamin D–dependent rickets *OSOMOPORE 95:705–709, 2003; Shoni Shikagaka Zasshi 28:503–509, 1990*

SUPERNUMERARY TEETH

Am J Med Genet Part A 170A2611–2616, 2016

Cleidocranial dysplasia

Familial adenomatous polyposis syndrome

Nance–Moran syndrome

Oculofaciocardiodental syndrome

OpitzBBB/G syndrome

Robinow syndrome – autosomal dominant

Rubinstein–Taybi syndrome

Trichorhinophalangeal syndrome type 1

TELANGIECTASIAS

CONGENITAL AND/OR GENETIC SYNDROMES WITH TELANGIECTASIAS

Acrogeria (Gottron's syndrome) – micrognathia, atrophy of tip of nose, atrophic skin of distal extremities with telangiectasia, easy bruising, mottled pigmentation or poikiloderma of extremities, dystrophic nails *BJD 103:213–223, 1980*

Adams–Oliver syndrome – with widespread cutis marmorata telangiectasia congenita *Ped Derm 24:651–653, 2007*

Amyoplasia congenita disruptive sequence – mid–facial macular telangiectatic nevi *Am J Med Genet 15:571–590, 1983*

Angiokeratoma corporis diffusum (Fabry's disease (alpha galactosidase A) – X–linked recessive; especially of face *BJD 157:331–337, 2007; NEJM 276:1163–1167, 1967;* fucosidosis (alpha–l–fucosidase) *AD 107:754–757, 1973;* Kanzaki's disease (alpha–N–acetylgalactosidase) – telangiectasias on lips, intraorally *AD 129:460–465, 1993;* aspartylglycosaminuria (aspartylglycosaminidase) *Paediatr Acta 36:179–189, 1991;* adult–onset GM1 gangliosidosis (beta galactosidase) *Clin Genet 17:21–26, 1980;* galactosialidosis (combined beta–galactosidase and sialidase) *AD 120:1344–1346, 1984;* no enzyme deficiency – telangiectasias or small angiokeratomas *AD 123:1125–1127, 1987; JAAD 12:885–886, 1985*

Angioma serpiginosum *JAAD 42:384–385, 2000*

Arteriovenous fistulae – congenital; red pulsating nodules with overlying telangiectasia – extremities, head, neck, trunk

Ataxia telangiectasia (Louis–Bar syndrome) – telangiectasias of bulbar conjunctivae, tip of nose, ears, antecubital and popliteal fossae, dorsal hands and feet; atrophy with mottled hypo– and hyperpigmentation, dermatomal CALMs, photosensitivity, canities, acanthosis nigricans, dermatitis; cutaneous granulomas present as papules or nodules, red plaques with atrophy or ulceration *JAAD 68:932–936, 2013; Ped Derm 28:494–501, 2011 Neurology 73:430–437, 2009; JAAD 10:431–438, 1984; Ann Int Med 99:367–379, 1983*

Benign familial telangiectasias (hereditary benign telangiectasia) – idiopathic, skin and lips *An Bras Dermatol 92:162–163, 2017*

Bloom's syndrome (congenital telangiectatic erythema and stunted growth) – autosomal recessive; slender face, prominent nose; facial telangiectatic erythema with involvement of eyelids, ear, hand, and forearms; bulbar conjunctival telangiectasias; stunted growth; CALMs, clinodactyly, syndactyly, congenital heart disease, annular pancreas, high–pitched voice, testicular atrophy; no neurologic deficits *Ped Derm 27:174–177, 2010; Ped Derm 22:147–150, 2005; Am J Hum Genet 21:196–227, 1969; AD 94:687–694, 1966; Am J Dis Child 88:754–758, 1954*

Circumareolar telangiectasia, congenital *AD 126:1656, 1990*

Coats' disease – cutaneous telangiectasia or unilateral macular telangiectatic nevus with retinal telangiectasia *AD 108:413–415, 1973*

Cockayne's syndrome – autosomal recessive; short stature, facial erythema in butterfly distribution leading to mottled pigmentation and atrophic scars, premature aged appearance with loss of subcutaneous fat and sunken eyes, canities, mental deficiency, photosensitivity, disproportionately large hands, feet, and ears, ocular defects, demyelination *J Med Genet 18:288–293, 1981*

Congenital disorders of glycosylation (CDG–Ie) – eyelid telangiectasia, hemangiomas, inverted nipples, microcephaly; neurologic abnormalities; dolichol–phosphate–mannose synthase *Ped Derm 22:457–460, 2005*

Congenital hemangioma of eccrine sweat glands *Ped Derm 10:341–343, 1993*

Cutis marmorata telangiectatica congenita – reticulated capillary malformation with telangiectasias; ulceration over elbows and knees; atrophy, limb hypo– or hyperplasia; telangiectasias may be

prominent at birth *JAAD 56:541–564, 2007; BJD 137:119–122, 1997; JAAD 20:1098–1104, 1989; AD 118:895–899, 1982*

Diffuse neonatal hemangiomatosis

Dyskeratosis congenita *JAAD 6:1034–1039, 1982*

Essential progressive telangiectasia (progressive symmetric telangiectasis) *JAAD 64:217–219, 2018;* Symmetric ascending telangiectasia over extensive areas of skin with no systemic manifestations

Fabry's disease – linear perioral telangiectasia *AD 126:1544–1545, 1990;* telangiectasias of axillae and upper chest *BJD 157:331–337, 2007; JAAD 46:161–183, 2002;* telangiectasias of the neck *J Dermatol 33:652–654, 2006*

Fanconi's anemia

Fucosidosis *J Pediatr 84:727–780, 1974;* with angiokeratoma corporis diffusum on telangiectatic background *Genital Skin Disorders, Fischer and Margesson, CV Mosby, 1998, p. 198*

Generalized essential telangiectasia – familial or acquired *Cutis 75:223–224, 2005; JAAD 37:321–325, 1997; JAMA 185:909–913, 1963; JAMADerm 150:1103–1104, 2014*

Gingival and labial telangiectasia *Syndromes of the Head and Neck, p.119, 1990*

Goltz's syndrome – palmar telangiectasias *AD 114:1078–1079, 1978*

H syndrome – autosomal recessive; hyperpigmented hypertrichotic plaques; hepatosplenomegaly; heart anomalies including atrial septal defect, ventricular septal defect, mitral valve prolapse, cardiomegaly, varicose veins; dilated scleral vessels, facial telangiectasias, exophthalmos, gynecomastia, scrotal masses, flexion contractures of toes and PIP joints; sensorineural hearing loss; hypogonadism; short stature; mutation in *SLC29A3* gene (equilibrative nucleoside transporter) *Ped Derm 33:602–614, 2016*

Hallermann–Streiff syndrome *Quintessence Int 42:331–338, 2011*

Hemochromatosis – spider telangiectasias *AD 113:161–165, 1977; Medicine 34:381–430, 1955*

Hereditary acrolabial telangiectasia – blue lips, blue nails, blue nipples, telangiectasia of the chest, elbows, knees, feet, dorsa of hands, varicosities of the legs, migraine headaches *AD 115:474–478, 1979*

Hereditary benign telangiectasia – autosomal dominant; patterns of telangiectasia include plaquelike, radiating, arborizing, reticulated, mottled, spiderlike, and punctuate; lips, neck, trunk, arms, hands, and knees; photodistributed *Ped Derm 33:570–584, 2016; JAAD 57:814–818, 2007; Ped Derm 6:194–197, 1989; Trans St.Johns Hosp Dermatol Soc 57:148–156, 1971;* punctuate telangiectasias with anemic halos *JAMA Derm 149:633–634, 2013; AD 146:98–99, 2010*

Hereditary hemorrhagic telangiectasia (Osler–Weber–Rendu disease) *NEJM 381:2552, 2019; Am J Med 82:989–997, 1987;* gingival, oral telangiectasia *Oral Surg 66:440–444, 1988*

Homocystinuria

I–cell disease (mucolipidosis II) – puffy eyelids; small orbits, prominent eyes, fullness of lower cheeks; small telangiectasias; fish–mouth appearance, short neck; gingival hypertrophy *Clin Genet 23:155–159, 1983; Am J Med Genet 9:239–253, 1981; Birth Defects 5:174–185, 1969*

Incontinentia pigmenti – linear and macular telangiectasias *Dermatol Wochenschr 153:489–496, 1967*

Klinefelter variants – macular telangiectatic vascular nevi *J Urol 119:103–106, 1978*

Klippel–Trenaunay–Weber syndrome *Syndromes of the Head and Neck, p.380, 1990*

Lethal multiple pterygium syndrome – mid–facial macular telangiectatic nevi *Am J Med Genet 12:377–409, 1982*

Linear telangiectatic erythema and mild atrophoderma *Cutis 39:69–70, 1987*

Maffucci's syndrome

Morquio's syndrome

Multiple endocrine neoplasia syndrome (MEN I) – telangiectasias on face and lips *AD 133:853–857, 1997*

Neonatal lupus erythematosus – facial telangiectasias *Lupus 21:552–555, 2012*

Nevus flammeus

Non–involuting congenital hemangioma (NICH) – warm high–flow lesion with coarse telangiectasias over surface; less commonly ulcerated *Plast Reconstr Surg 107:1647–1654, 2001*

Odonto–onycho–dermal dysplasia – telangiectatic atrophic patches of face, sparse hair, conical teeth, hyperkeratosis of palms and soles, dystrophic nails *Am J Med Genet 14:335–346, 1983*

Pre–auricular skin defects *AD 133:1551–1554, 1997*

Prolidase deficiency – autosomal recessive; skin spongy and fragile with annular pitting and scarring; leg ulcers; photosensitivity, telangiectasia, purpura, premature graying, lymphedema *Ped Derm 13:58–60, 1996; JAAD 29:819–821, 1993; AD 127:124–125, 1991; AD 123:493–497, 1987*

Rapidly involuting congenital hemangioma (RICH) – palpable tumor with pale rim, coarse overlying telangiectasia with central depression or ulcer *Ped Dev Pathol 6:495–510, 2003; Ped Derm 19:5–11, 2002*

Rombo syndrome – acral erythema, cyanotic redness, follicular atrophy (atrophoderma vermiculata), milia–like papules, telangiectasias, red ears with telangiectasia, thin eyebrows, sparse beard hair, basal cell carcinomas, short stature *BJD 144:1215–1218, 2001*

Rothmund–Thomson syndrome (poikiloderma congenitale) – autosomal recessive *Am J Med Genet 22:102:11–17, 2001; Ped Derm 18:210212, 2001; Ped Derm 16:59–61, 1999; Dermatol Clin 13:143–150, 1995; JAAD 27:75–762, 1992*

Schinzel–Giedion syndrome – autosomal recessive; ectodermal dysplasia; midface retraction, hirsutism, telangiectasias of nose and cheeks, skeletal anomalies, mental retardation *Hum Genet 62:382, 1982; Am J Med Genet 1:361–375, 1978*

Short arm 4 deletion syndrome – macular telangiectatic vascular nevi *Am J Dis Child 122:421–425, 1971*

STING–associated vasculopathy with onset in infancy (SAVI)(type 1 interferonopathy) – red plaques of face and hands; chilblain–like lesions; atrophic plaques of hands, telangiectasias of cheeks, nose, chin, lips, acral violaceous plaques and acral cyanosis (livedo reticularis of feet, cheeks, and knees), distal ulcerative lesions with infarcts (necrosis of cheeks and ears), gangrene of fingers or toes with ainhum, nasal septal perforation, nail dystrophy; small for gestational age; paratracheal adenopathy, abnormal pulmonary function tests; interstitial lung disease with fibrosis with ground glass and reticulate opacities; gain of function mutation in *TMEM173*(stimulator of interferon genes); mimics granulomatosis

with polyangiitis *JAMADerm 151:872–877, 2015; NEJM 371:507–518, 2014*

Sturge–Weber syndrome

Telangiectasias, spondyloepiphyseal dysplasia, hypothyroidism, neovascularization, and tractional retinal detachments

Ped Derm 6:178–184, 1989

Trichothiodystrophy syndromes – BIDS, IBIDS, PIBIDS – telangiectasias, sparse or absent eyelashes and eyebrows, brittle hair, premature aging, sexual immaturity, ichthyosis, dysmyelination, bird–like facies, dental caries; trichothiodystrophy with ichthyosis, urologic malformations, hypercalciuria and mental and physical retardation *JAAD 44:891–920, 2001; Ped Derm 14:441–445, 1997;*

Unilateral nevoid telangiectasia *Dermatol Online J 17:2, 2011*

Vascular malformations, congenital

Vascular nevi

Von Hippel–Lindau disease – macular telangiectatic nevi, facial or occipitocervical; retinal angiomatosis, cerebellar or medullary or spinal hemangioblastoma, renal cell carcinoma. pheochromocytoma, café au lait macules *Arch Intern Med 136:769–777, 1976*

Warsaw breakage syndrome – livedo reticularis with telangiectasias of the legs *Eur J Med Genet 58:235–237, 2015*

Werner's syndrome

Wyburn–Mason (Bonnet–Duchaume–Blanc) syndrome – unilateral salmon patch with punctate telangiectasias or port wine stain; unilateral retinal arteriovenous malformation, ipsilateral aneurysmal arteriovenous malformation of the brain *Am J Ophthalmol 75:224–291, 1973*

Xeroderma pigmentosum – acute sunburn, persistent erythema, freckling – initially discrete, then fuse to irregular patches of hyperpigmentation, dryness on sun–exposed areas; with time telangiectasias and small angiomas, atrophic white macules develop; vesiculobullous lesions, superficial ulcers lead to scarring, ectropion; multiple malignancies; photophobia, conjunctivitis, ectropion, symblepharon, neurologic abnormalities *Adv Genet 43:71–102, 2001; Hum Mutat 14:9–22, 1999; Mol Med Today 5:86–94, 1999; Derm Surg 23:447–455, 1997; Dermatol Clin 13:169–209, 1995; Recent Results Cancer Res 128:275–297, 1993; AD 123:241–250, 1987; Ann Int Med 80:221–248, 1974; XP variant AD 128:1233–1237, 1992*

XXYY syndrome – macular telangiectatic vascular nevi *AD 94:695–698, 1966*

ACQUIRED DISORDERS WITH TELANGIECTASIAS

AUTOIMMUNE DISEASES AND DISEASES OF IMMUNE DYSFUNCTION

Chronic graft vs host disease *JAAD 38:369–392, 1998*

Dermatomyositis – dermatomyositis with anti–transcriptional intermediary factor–1gamma antibodies – hypopigmented and telangiectatic patches (red and white patches); palmar hyperkeratotic papules; psoriasiform plaques *JAAD 72:449–455, 2015*

Lupus erythematosus – systemic lupus – reticulated telangiectatic erythema of thenar and hypothenar eminences, finger pulps, toes, lateral feet, and heels; bluish red with small white scars; systemic, discoid, neonatal LE – facial telangiectasia *Ped Derm 10:177–178, 1993;* discoid lupus – facial, periungual and fingertip telangiectasias; tumid lupus (lupus erythematosus telangiectoides) – reticulate telangiectasias of face, neck, ears, hands, breasts, heels, sides of feet; punctate atrophy *JAAD 41:250–253, 1999;* subacute cutaneous lupus erythematosus – annular and polycyclic lesions resolve with hypopigmentation and telangiectasias *Dermatology 200:6–10, 2000; Med Clin North Am 73:1073–1090, 1989; JAAD 19:1957–1062, 1988;* palmar telangiectasias *Cutis 89:84–88, 2012*

Mixed connective tissue disease *Am J Dermatopathol 19:206–213, 1997*

Morphea – mimicking port wine stain *Ped Derm 31:591–594, 2014; JAAD 64:779–782, 2011*

Rheumatoid arthritis – periungual telangiectasias; spider telangiectasias

Scleroderma (CREST) – telangiectatic mats of face, palms, back of hands, soles, upper trunk, lips, tongue, mouth *Microvasc Res 111:20–24, 2017;* gingival telangiectasia CREST syndrome; palmar telangiectasias *Chest 130(Suppl):290S, 2006; Arch Int Med 140:1121, 1980;* sclerodermatomyositis – palmar telangiectasias *Indian J Dermatol Venereol Leprol 74:148–150, 2008*

Sjogren's syndrome with dorsal root ganglionitis *NEJM 364:1856–1865, 2011*

DEGENERATIVE DISORDERS

Reflex sympathetic dystrophy (complex regional pain syndrome) *AD 127;1541–1544, 1991*

DEVELOPMENTAL DISORDERS

Chiari I malformation – palmar telangiectasias *Pediatr Neurol 29:250–252, 2003*

DRUGS

Amlodipine – photo–induced telangiectasia *BJD 142:1255–1256, 2000; BJD 136:974–975, 1997; J Allergy Clin Immunol 97:852–855, 1996*

Antibody drug conjugate therapies – diffuse telangiectatic rash *JAMADerm 156:601–602, 2020*

Bleomycin – scaly linear erythema of dorsa of hands with atrophy and telangiectasia (dermatomyositis–like) *JAAD 48:439–441, 2003*

BCNU–treated cutaneous T–cell lymphoma *JAAD 46:325–357, 2002*

Calcium channel blockers – facial and truncal telangiectasia; felodipine, nifedipine, amlodipine, diltiazem – photodistributed telangiectasias *JAAD 74:247–270, 2016; JAAD 45:323–324, 2001; BJD 136:974–975, 1997*

Carmustine

Cefotoxime – photodistributed telangiectasia *BJD 143:674–675, 2000*

Cetuximab (epidermal growth factor receptor inhibitor) – rosacea–like telangiectasias *JAAD 58:545–570, 2008*

Corticosteroids – systemic, topical *JAAD 54:1–15, 2006; AD 126:1013–1014, 1990;* oral, inhaled, topical–induced acne rosacea – papules, pustules, atrophy, telangiectasia *Clin Exp Dermatol 18:148–150, 1993; AD Forsch 247:29–52, 1973;* palmar telangiectasias *Cutis 89:84–88, 2012*

Epidermal growth factor receptor inhibitors – telangiectasias of face, chest, back, and limbs, acneiform eruptions, xerosis, paronychia, hyperpigmentation, trichomegaly *JAAD 72:203–218, 2015; JAAD 56:302–316, 2007*

Erlotinib – rosacea–like telangiectasias *JAAD 58:545–570, 2008*

Estrogen therapy

Felodipine–induced photodistributed facial telangiectasia *JAAD 45:323–324, 2001;* after mastectomy and radiation *BJD 162:210–211, 2010*

Gefitinib – rosacea–like telangiectasias *JAAD 58:545–570, 2008*

Hydroxyurea *JAAD 36:178–182, 1997*

Interferon alpha *JAAD 37:118–120, 1997*

Interferon alpha

Loncastuximab tesirine – blanching reticulated telangiectatic patches of upper and lower extremities *JAMADerm 156:601–603, 2020*

Nifedipine – photodistributed facial telangiectasia *BJD 129:630–633, 1993; Lancet 339:365–366, 1992*

Propranolol – annular telangiectatic perivascular angiomatosis – red to violaceous hyperpigmented annular plaques with central clearing and radial telangiectasia *BJD 169:1369–1371, 2013*

Rovalpituzumab teserine – blanching reticulated telangiectatic patches of upper and lower extremities *JAMADerm 156:601–603, 2020*

Venlaxifine – photodistributed eruptive telangiectasias of face, forearms, dorsal hands *BJD 157:822–824, 2007*

Voriconazole – in immunosuppressed patients; chronic phototoxicity with aggressive squamous cell carcinomas; sunburn–like erythema, multiple lentigines, multiple actinic keratoses, cheilitis, exfoliative dermatitis, pseudo–porphyria cutanea tarda, telangiectasias *JAAD 62:31–37, 2010*

EXOGENOUS AGENTS

Chronic alcoholism

Aluminum plant workers – mat–like telangiectasias of upper back *NEJM 303:1278–1281, 1980*

Reticular telangiectatic erythema associated with implantable cardioverter defibrillator, pacemakers, knee prostheses, spinal cord stimulators, infusion pumps *Dermatitis 25:98–99, 2014; Mayo Clinic Proc 88:117–119, 2013; Contact Dermatitis 64:280–288, 2011; Cutis 78:329–331, 2006; AD 137:1239–1241, 2001;* overlying intrathecal pump *Soc Ped Derm Annual Meeting, July 2005; AD 141:106–107, 2005;* overlying a pacemaker *Hautarzt 32:651–654, 1981*

INFECTIONS

AIDS – chest wall *Ann Int Med 105:679–682, 1986;* periungual *Int J Dermatol 34:199–200, 1995;* neck, arms, shoulders

Cutaneous Borreliosis – acrodermatitis chronica atrophicans, cutis laxa–like changes, red patches, erythema migrans, erythema and edema of foot, poikilodermatous changes, red macules and telangiectasias *JAAD 72:683–689, 2015*

Echovirus 23,32 – telangiectatic macular lesions *Pediatrics 44:498–502, 1969*

Hepatitis C infection – unilateral nevoid telangiectasia *JAAD 36:819–822, 1997*

Leprosy – Lucio's phenomenon – widespread telangiectasias

Lyme disease – poikiloderma; acrodermatitis chronica atrophicans *Lancet Infect Dis 11:800, 2011*

Toxoplasmosis, congenital – telangiectatic macules *JAAD 60:897–925, 2009*

INFILTRATIVE DISEASES

Amyloidosis – poikiloderma–like cutaneous amyloidosis *Eur J Dermatol 18:289–291, 2008; Dermatologica 155:301–309, 1977*

Telangiectasia macularis eruptiva perstans (mastocytosis) *Eur J Dermatol 29:174–178, 2019; AD 147:932–940, 2011; AD 124:429–434, 1988; JAAD 7:709–722, 1982;* unilateral of the breast *Cutis 90:26–28, 2012*

Urticaria pigmentosa – palmar telangiectasias *Proc R Soc Med 27:144, 1933;* recurrent flushing – personal observation

INFLAMMATORY DISEASES

Sarcoidosis – angiolupoid sarcoid – orange–red, reddish–brown nodules with marked telangiectasia lupus pernio; red pretibial plaques with atrophic scars, telangiectasias, venous prominence *JAMADerm 154:955–956, 2018;*

METABOLIC DISEASES

Carcinoid syndrome – flushing, patchy cyanosis, hyperpigmentation, telangiectasia, pellagrous dermatitis, salivation, lacrimation, abdominal cramping, wheezing, diarrhea *Cureus 12:e7186, 2020; AD 77:86–90, 1958*

Acute congestive heart failure with telangiectasias of chest – personal observation

Cushing's disease *Semin Dermatol 3:287–294, 1984*

Cystinosis – skin atrophy and telangiectasia mimicking premature aging; normal skin; subcutaneous plaques *JAAD 62:AB26, 2010; JAAD 68:e111–116, 2013*

Fucosidosis – palmar telangiectasias *J Inherit Metab Dis 31:S313–S316, 2008*

Graves' disease – palmar telangiectasias *Cutis 89:84–88, 2012; Hormonal Res 69:189–192, 2008*

Hyperviscosity syndrome – spider telangiectasias *AD 128:860, 1992*

Hyperthyroidism, thyrotoxicosis – spider telangiectasias

Hypothyroidism – punctate telangiectasias of arms and fingertips

Liver disease, chronic – spider telangiectasias

Necrobiosis lipoidica diabeticorum *Int J Derm 33:605–617, 1994; JAAD 18:530–537, 1988*

Panhypopituitarism – personal observation

Polycythemia vera

Pregnancy – spider telangiectasias *J Drugs Dermatol 14:512–513, 2015; JAAD 6:977–998, 1982*

Primary biliary cirrhosis – gingival telangiectasia

Prolidase deficiency – autosomal recessive; peptidase D mutation (PEPD); increased urinary imidopeptides; leg ulcers, anogenital ulcers, short stature (mild), telangiectasias, recurrent infections (sinusitis, otitis); mental retardation; splenomegaly with enlarged abdomen, atrophic scarring, dermatitis, hyperkeratosis of elbows and knees, low hairline, poliosis, canities, lymphedema, photosensitivity, hypertelorism, saddle nose deformity, frontal bossing, dull expression, mild ptosis, micrognathia, mandibular protrusion, exophthalmos, joint laxity, deafness, osteoporosis, high arched palate *JAAD 62:1031, 1034, 2010*

Tyrosinemia type 1 with cirrhosis – personal observation

NEOPLASTIC DISEASES

Actinic keratosis

Atrial myxoma *BJD 147:379–382, 2002; Cutis 62:275–280, 1998; JAAD 32:881–883, 1995; JAAD 21:1080–1084, 1989;*

Basal cell carcinoma – palmar telangiectasias *AD 143:813–814, 2007*

Carcinoid, metastatic – unilateral nevoid telangiectasia *BJD 124:86–88, 1991;* foregut (stomach, lung, pancreas) – bright red geographic flush, sustained, with burning, lacrimation, wheezing, sweating; hindgut (ileal) – patchy, violaceous, intermixed with pallor, short duration; edema, telangiectasia, cyanotic nose and face, rosacea *Acta DV (Stockh) 41:264–276, 1961*

Carcinoma telangiectoides; *JAAD Case Rep 6:263–265, 2020; Cancer 19:162–168, 1966;* telangiectatic metastatic breast carcinoma of face and scalp mimicking cutaneous angiosarcoma *JAAD 48:635–636, 2003;* adenocarcinoma of the lung *JAAD 64:798–799, 2011*

Glomangioma, telangiectatic *BJD 139:902–905, 1998*

Kaposi's sarcoma – telangiectatic nodules *JAAD 59:179–206, 2008; G Ital DV 12:643–646, 1987; AD 118:1020–1021, 1982*

Leukemia – B–cell chronic lymphocytic leukemia – violaceous telangiectatic circumferential patches of legs *JAAD 60:772–780, 2009;* natural killer cell CD 56– large granular lymphocytic leukemia – leg ulcer associated with thigh telangiectasia *JAAD 62:496–501, 2010*

Lymphoma – angiotropic B–cell lymphoma *JAAD S260–262, 2002;* intravascular B–cell lymphoma (malignant angioendotheliomatosis) – red plaques with telangiectasias *Cutis 72:137–140, 2003; Ann DV 129:320324, 2002;* intravascular B–cell lymphoma – painful gray–brown, red, blue–livid patches, plaques, nodules, with telangiectasia and underlying induration; 40% of patients with intravascular lymphoma present with cutaneous lesions *Cutis 82:267–272, 2008; BJD 157:16–25, 2007; AD 128:255, 1992; Clin Exp Dermatol 45:269–271, 2020;* primary cutaneous follicle center lymphoma – extensive scalp telangiectasis *Br J Hematol 158:297, 2012;* poikilodermatous cutaneous T–cell lymphoma *Int J Dermatol 46:950–951, 2007*

Malignant angioendotheliomatosis (intravascular lymphomatosis) – purpuric papules, plaques, and nodules with overlying telangiectasias *AD 128:255, 258, 2003; JAAD 18:407–412, 1988*

(angiotropic B–cell lymphoma) – red to purple nodules and plaques on trunk and extremities with prominent overlying telangiectasias *AD 128:255–260, 1992*

Malignant myopericytoma *AD 141:1311–1316, 2005*

Medallion–like dermal dendrocyte hamartoma – yellow–brown, blue–brown annular or oval depression of back of neonate; wrinkled surface, telangiectasias; thin hair on surface *AD 142:921–926, 2006*

Metastases – cervical carcinoma; erythema, edema, and telangiectasia of entire central face *JAAD 56:S26–28, 2007;* intra–arterial metastatic telangiectatic breast cancer – – violaceous swelling with telangiectasia and necrosis *JAMADerm 155:615–616, 2019;* adenocarcinoma of the lung – telangiectatic metastases *JAAD 64:798–799, 2011;* prostate *BJD 156:598–600, 2007*

Mucinous carcinoma – telangiectatic nodule *JAAD 49:941–943, 2003*

Plasmacytosis, systemic *JAAD 38:629–631, 1998*

Stewart–Treves angiosarcoma – reddish–blue macules and/or nodules which become polypoid; pachydermatous changes, blue nodules, telangiectasias, palpable subcutaneous mass, ulcer *JAAD 67:1342–1348, 2012*

PARANEOPLASTIC DISORDERS

Telangiectasia of face and hands – paraneoplastic finding associated with bronchogenic carcinoma *Dermatolog Clin 26:45–57, 2008; BJD (Suppl 68):17, 2004; Dermatologica 165:620–623, 1982*

PHOTODERMATOSES

Dermatoheliosis – face, ears

Poikiloderma of Civatte *Dermatology 214:177–182, 2007; Eur Acad DV 20:1248–1251, 2006; Clin Exp Dermatol 24:385–387, 1999*

PRIMARY CUTANEOUS DISORDERS

Acne rosacea

Acquired bilateral telangiectatic macules *JAMADerm 150:974–977, 2014*

Coats' disease

Costal fringe telangiectasias *AD 127:1201–1202, 1991*

Degos' disease *JAAD 68:211,e1–33, 2013*

Keratosis lichenoides chronica (Nekam's disease) – reticulated keratotic papules, linear arrays, atrophy, comedo–like lesions, prominent telangiectasia *AD 144:405–410, 2008*

Lichen planus–induced poikiloderma *Indian J Dermatol 46:178–179, 2001*

Lichen sclerosus et atrophicus – of glabrous skin; of glans penis *JAAD 38:831–833, 1998*

Linear atrophoderma of Moulin *Dermatology 207:310–315, 2003*

Mid–dermal elastolysis *JAAD 51:165–185, 2004*

Parapsoriasis, poikilodermatous *Indian J Dermatol 54:S32–36, 2009*

Poikiloderma vasculare atrophicans

Progressive ascending telangiectasias *J Drugs Dermatol 16:280–282, 2017* Rosacea

SYNDROMES

Acrogeria (Gottron's syndrome)

Apert's syndrome – autosomal dominant; *FGFR–2* mutation; craniosynostosis with midfacial malformation; cone-shaped calvarium, proptosis, hypertelorism, short nose with bulbous tip; high arched palate; lips bow–shaped, unable to form a seal; telangiectasias of face and bulbar conjunctiva, often in butterfly distribution; mottled hyperpigmentation, hypopigmentation and poikiloderma; seborrheic dermatitis, atopic dermatitis, and xerosis common *Am J Med Genet 44:82–89, 1992;* severe pustular acne at puberty *Ped Derm 20:443–446, 2003*

Ataxia telangiectasia – non–infectious cutaneous granulomas present as papules or nodules, red plaques with atrophy or ulceration; telangiectasias of bulbar conjunctivae, tip of nose, ears, antecubital and popliteal fossae, dorsal hands and feet; atrophy with mottled hypo– and hyperpigmentation, dermatomal CALMs, photosensitivity, canities, acanthosis nigricans, dermatitis; humoral and cellular immunodeficiency, lymphoreticular malignancy, growth retardation; *ATM* gene (phosphatidylinisitol–3'kinase) *JAAD 56:541–564, 2007; AD 134:1145–1150, 1998; JAAD 10:431–438, 1984*

Bloom's syndrome – autosomal recessive; erythema with hyperpigmentation, telangiectasias, crusting and atrophy in photodistribution; hypogonadism, poor development of genitalia, cheilitis of upper and lower lips; clinodactyly, syndactyly; decreased IgM or IgA and IgG; recurrent respiratory and gastrointestinal infections; DNA repair defect with chromosomal breakage with increased sister chromatid exchanges (triradial and quadriradial chromosomes); recQ helicase mutation *JAAD 75:855–870, 2016; Ped Derm 27:174–177, 2010; Am J Dis Child 88:754–758, 1954*

Cockayne's syndrome – with associated xeroderma pigmentosum *Orphanet J Rare Dis 12:65, 2017*

Familial multiple discoid fibromas (Birt–Hogg–Dube look–alike) – red papules of cheeks, around nose, helices and posterior ears, skin-colored papules with overlying telangiectasias; white papules of face and ears *BJD 169:177–180, 2013; JAAD 66:259–263, 2012*

H syndrome – autosomal recessive; facial telangiectasias; sclerodermoid changes of middle and lower body with overlying hyperpigmentation sparing the knees and buttocks; hypertrichosis, short stature, facial telangiectasia, gynecomastia, camptodactyly of 5th fingers, scrotal masses with massively edematous scrotum obscuring the penis, hypogonadism, azospermia, sensorineural hearing loss, cardiac anomalies, hepatosplenomegaly; Arabic Palestinian population; gluteal lipoatrophy; hyperpigmentation, hearing loss, diabetes mellitus, lymphadenopathy, hypertrichosis, heart anomalies, micropenis, hallus valgus, hyperpigmentation induration and hypertrichosis of inner thighs and shins (sclerodermoid), chronic diarrhea, anemia, dilated lateral scleral vessels, episcleritis, exophthalmos, eyelid swelling, varicose veins, chronic rhinitis, renal abnormalities, bone lesions, arthritis, arthralgia; mutation in *SLC29A3 JAAD 70;80–88, 2014;JAAD 59:79–85, 2008*

Haber's syndrome – autosomal dominant; photo–aggravated rosacea–like rash of face; papules, pustules, scarring and telangiectasias; reticulate pigmented macules and keratotic plaques on trunk and extremities *Australas J Dermatol 38:82–84, 1997; AD 117:321, 1981; BJD 77:1–8, 1965*

Hypotrichosis–lymphedema–telangiectasis syndrome (chronic edema, monoclonal dysglobulinemia and profuse telangiectasia) – vascular nevi on palms and soles; autosomal recessive *Clin in Dermatol 23:47–55, 2005; Eur J Dermatol 11:515–517, 2001; Ann DV 124:717–720, 1997;* palmar telangiectasias *Am J Hum Genet 72:1470–1478, 2003; Eur J Dermatol 11:515–517, 2001*

Hypotrichosis–Lymphedema–Telangiectasia–Renal failure syndrome – diffuse reticulated capillary malformation, hypertensive emergency with transient ischemic attack, dilatation or aortic root, pleural effusions, acute kidney injury, thin facies with telangiectasias of cheeks, livedo reticularis of trunk and extremities; mutation in *SOX18* gene *Cases of the Year, Pre–AAD Pediatric Dermatology Meeting, 2016*

Infantile myofibromatosis – skin-colored multilobulated tumor with overlying telangiectasias *Ped Derm 27:29–33, 2010*

Keratosis follicularis spinulosa decalvans – facial telangiectasia *JAAD 53:1–37, 2005*

Kindler's syndrome – acral bullae in infancy; progressive poikiloderma with photosensitivity; nail dystrophy, webbing of digits, esophageal and urethral stenosis, ectropion, poor dentition, gingival fragility, aged hands with fine wrinkling and scarring, hyperkeratosis of hands and palms and soles, dyspigmentation, diffuse telangiectasias, hypshort arm chromosome 20; Kind 1; actin cytoskeleton–extracellular matrix interactions (membrane-associated structural and signaling protein) *Ped Derm 37:337–341, 2020; AD 142:620–624, 2006*

Macrocephaly–CMTC (cutis marmorata telangiectatica congenita syndrome) – macrocephalic neonatal hypotonia and developmental delay; patchy reticulated vascular stain without atrophy; telangiectasias of face and ears; midline facial nevus flammeus, hydrocephalus, skin and joint hypermobility, polydactyly, 2–3 toe syndactyly, frontal bossing, hemihypertrophy with segmental overgrowth, neonatal hypotonia, developmental delay *JAAD 58:697–702, 2008; Ped Derm 24:555–556, 2007; JAAD 56:541–564, 2007* (Note: Beckwith–Wiedemann syndrome demonstrates dysmorphic ears, macroglossia, body asymmetry, midfacial vascular stains, visceromegaly with omphalocele, neonatal hypoglycemia, BUT NO MACROCEPHALY)

Multiple endocrine neoplasia syndrome type I

Nijmegen breakage syndrome – autosomal recessive; chromosome instability syndrome; mutations in *NBS–1* gene which encodes bibirin (DNA damage repair); microcephaly, receding mandible, prominent midface, prenatal onset short stature, growth retardation, bird–like facies with epicanthal folds, large ears, sparse hair, clinodactyly/syndactyly; freckling of face, café au lait macules, vitiligo, photosensitivity of the eyelids, telangiectasias; pigmented deposits of fundus; IgG, IgA deficiencies, agammaglobulinemia, decreased CD3 and CD4 T cells with recurrent respiratory and urinary tract infections *Ped Derm 26:106–108, 2009; DNA Repair 3:1207–1217, 2004; Arch Dis Child 82:400–406, 2000; Am J Med Genet 66:378–398, 1996*

Phakomatosis pigmentokeratotica – coexistence of an organoid nevus (nevus sebaceous/epidermal nevus) and a contralateral segmental lentiginous or papular speckled lentiginous nevus; telangiectasias within the speckled lentiginous nevus *Ped Derm 25:76–80, 2008; Dermatology 194: 77–79, 1997;* speckled lentigines of soles *JAAD 55:S16–20, 2006*

Phakomatosis spilorosea (form of phakomatosis pigmentovascularis) – nevus spilus with a telangiectatic nevus *AD 141:385–388, 2005*

Phakomatosis cesiomarmorata – Mongolian spot and cutis marmorata telangiectatica congenita *AD 141:385–388, 2005*

POEMS syndrome – mat–like telangiectasias, hypertensive crisis, calciphylaxis *JAMADerm 130:667–668, 2014*

Proteus syndrome – telangiectatic nevi

Pseudoxanthoma elasticum

Rothmund–Thomsen syndrome

Reticular erythematous mucinosis syndrome – with telangiectasias, essential thrombocytosis, and lung cancer *Dur J Dermatol 15:179–181, 2005*

TEMPI syndrome – telangiectasias, elevated erythropoietin level and erythrocytosis, monoclonal gammopathy, perinephric fluid collections, and intrapulmonary shunting *NEJM 367:778–780, 2012; NEJM 366:1843–1845, 2012; NEJM 365:475–477, 2011*

Xeroderma pigmentosum

TOXINS

Aluminum foundry workers

Mustard gas *Int J Dermatol 30:684–686, 1991*

Vinyl chloride exposure – telangiectasias of face; thick skin of hands, face, and trunk *AD 106:219–223, 1972*

TRAUMA

Actinic damage

Multiple cardiac catheterizations – personal observation

Cardioversion (defibrillation) – hypopigmented, atrophic, telangiectatic, crusted erythematous plaque of back with rim of hyperpigmentation; delayed onset of years *AD 145:1411–1414, 2009*

Computer palms *JAAD 42:1073–1075, 2000*

Hematoma – following hip replacement *SKINMed 16:199–200, 2018*

Multiple mammograms – personal observation

Post–surgical sternal erythema – red patch with telangiectasia *JAAD 53:893–896, 2005*

Physical trauma

Post–surgical scars

Radiodermatitis – acute or chronic radiodermatitis *BJD 160:1237–1241, 2009;* gingival telangiectasia *JAAD 54:28–46, 2006;* fluoroscopy–induced radiation injury – red telangiectatic patch with ulceration of upper back or axilla *AD 143:637–640, 2007;* post–radiation vascular proliferations of breast (atypical vascular lesions of the breast) – erythema; erythema with underlying induration or ulceration, telangiectasias, papules, plaques, nodules, *JAAD 57:126–133, 2007*

VASCULAR DISORDERS

Abortive hemangiomas – telangiectasias with or without peripheral papules *Ped Derm 26:664–665, 2009*

Angiomas

Angiokeratoma – facial telangiectatic papule *Pan Afr Med J June 9, 2018;* in normal healthy individuals *Int J Dermatol 58:713–721, 2019*

Angioma serpiginosum – red or purple punctae within background of erythema; serpiginous pattern *Dermatology (Basel)213:256–258, 2006; JAAD 37:887–920, 1997; AD 92:613–620, 1965*

Arborizing telangiectasia – thighs and calves with restless legs *J Neurol Neurosurg Psychiatry 49:820–823, 1986*

Arteriovenous fistulae – acquired; red pulsating nodules with overlying telangiectasia – extremities, head, neck, trunk

Arteriovenous malformation – personal observation

Atrophie blanche (livedo with ulceration) – ivory white plaque of sclerosis with stippled telangiectasias and surrounding hyperpigmentation; venous insufficiency, thalassemia minor *Acta DV (Stockh)50:125–128, 1970;* cryoglobulinemia, systemic lupus erythematosus, *JAAD 8:792–798, 1983; AD 119:963–969, 1983*

Bilateral nevoid telangiectasia *BJD 172:1651–1653, 2015*

Capillary malformation–arteriovenous malformation syndrome – telangiectasias of chest; central punctate red spots; nevus anemicus surrounded by pale halo; absence of vellus hairs over the AVM *BJD 172:450–454, 2015*

Congenital circumareolar telangiectasia

Cutaneous collagenous vasculopathy (progressive ascending telangiectasia) – widespread telangiectasias, indistinguishable from generalized essential telangiectasia; telangiectatic patches of trunk and extremities; paresthesias and Raynaud's phenomenon; networks of telangiectasias of feet and lower legs *JAMADerm 150:451–452, 2014; JAMA Derm 149:97–102, 2013; Ped Derm 28:598–599, 2011; JAAD 63:882–885, 2010; Am J Clin Dermatol 11:63–66, 2010; Actas Dermosifiliogr 101:444–447, 2010; J Cutan Pathol 35:967–970, 2008; J Cutan Pathol 27:40–48, 2000*

Congenital hemangioma of eccrine sweat glands

Degos' disease (malignant atrophic papulosis) – porcelain white scar surrounded by rim of erythema and telangiectasia *JAAD 37:480–484, 1997; AD 122:90–91,93–94, 1986; BJD 100:21–36, 1979; Ann DV 79:410–417, 1954*

Familial cerebral cavernous malformation *Neurology 71:861–862, 2008*

Gingival and labial telangiectasia

Hemangiomas, proliferative – telangiectatic macules present at birth or in early infancy *JAAD 48:477–493, 2003; Cutis 66:325–328, 2000;* involuted hemangiomas – atrophy, telangiectasia, redundant skin *JAAD 48:477–493, 2003;* abortive or minimal growth infantile hemangiomas – reticulated red patch with telangiectasias *JAAD 58:685–690, 2008*

Hereditary hemorrhagic telangiectasia – arteriovenous malformation; pulmonary arteriovenous malformations; juvenile polyposis syndrome; mutation in *ENG* (endoglin) (a cell surface component of transforming growth factor beta complex) or *ALK1* gene (product is activin receptor–like tyrosine kinase1) (*ALK1* is endothelin cell receptor for TGF beta superfamily of ligands); both encode membrane glycoprotein on vascular endothelial cells as surface receptor for TGFRbeta superfamily which mediates vascular remodeling effects on extracellular matrix production; mutations in *SMAD4* and *BMPR1A* in juvenile polyposis syndrome; *NEJM 376:972–980, 2017; Cutis 89:69–72, 2012; JAAD 68:189–209, 2013; JAAD 56:541–564, 2007; BJD 145:641–645, 2001;* telangiectatic mats *Cutis 85:9,13–14, 2010;* palmar telangiectasias *Cutis 89:84–88, 2012*

Infantile hemangiomas with minimal or arrested growth – bruise–like appearance; telangiectatic patch; red plaques; more often on lower body *AD 146:971–976, 2010*

Kaposiform hemangioendothelioma – tender telangiectatic plaque or multiple telangiectatic papules *JAAD 38:799–802, 1998*

Nevus flammeus; acquired (Fegeler syndrome) *Vasa 29:225–228, 2000*

Non–involuting congenital hemangioma – round to ovoid pink to purple papule or plaque with central or peripheral pallor, coarse telangiectasias; red, white, and blue patch with central telangiectasia and peripheral pallor *Ped Derm 36:835–853, 2019; JAAD 70:899–903, 2014; JAAD 50: 875–882, 2004*

PELVIS syndrome (may be part of urorectal septum malformation sequence) – macular telangiectatic patch; larger perineal hemangiomas, external genitalia malformations, lipomyelomeningocele, vesicorenal abnormalities, imperforate anus, and skin tags *AD 142:884–888, 2006*

PHACES syndrome – facial telangiectasias of zosteriform distribution of V1 and V2 *Ped Derm 26:381–398, 2009; Pediatrics 124:1447–1456, 2009*

Purpura annularis telangiectoides (Majocchi's pigmented purpuric eruption)*; Dermatologica 140:45–53, 1970;* palmar telangiectasias *AD Syphilol 28:384–388, 1933*

Rapidly involuting congenital hemangioma – large violaceous gray–blue nodule of scalp with overlying telangiectasia *BJD 158:1363–1370, 2008; Soc Ped Derm Annual Meeting, 2005*

RASA1 mutations (capillary malformation–arteriovenous malformation syndrome) – arteriovenous malformations with multiple telangiectasias *Human Mutation 34:1632–1641, 2013; Eur J Med Genetics 55:191–195, 2012*

Raynaud's disease – face and mucous membranes

Sunburst varicosities and telangiectasia (arborizing telangiectasia) – thighs and calves *J Derm Surg Oncol 15:184–190, 1989*

Telangiectatic leg veins *BJD 169:365–373, 2013*

Tufted angioma – personal observation

Unilateral nevoid telangiectasia *BJD 172:1651–1653, 2015; AD 146:1167–1172, 2010; Dermatolology 209:215–217, 2004; JAAD 37:523–549, 1997; JAAD 8:468–477, 1983; Monatsschr Prakt Dermat 28:451, 1899;* palmar telangiectasias *AD 114:446–447, 1978*

Varicose veins *Med Clin NA 93:1333–1346, 2009*

Vascular malformations

Vein of Galen malformation – eyelid edema, telangiectatic patches of forehead and cheek, prominent superficial veins of forehead *JAMA Derm 149:249–251, 2013*

PALMAR TELANGICTASIAS

Cirrhosis *Clin Gastroenterol 4:439–460, 1975*

Computer palms

Fucosidosis *J Inherit Metab Dis 31:S313–316, 2008*

Graves' disease *Cutis 89:84–88, 2012*

Hereditary hemorrhagic telangiectasia

Pregnancy *Am J Clin Dermatol 7:65–69, 2006*

Prolonged smoking *Dermatology 233:390–395, 2017*

Purpura annularis telangiectoides

Unilateral nevoid telangiectasia

Urticaria pigmentosa

TESTICULAR ENLARGEMENT

INFECTIONS AND INFESTATIONS

Acute epididymitis *NEJM 378:1233–1240, 2018*
  Chlamydia trachomatis
  Neisseria gonorrhoeae
  Urinary pathogens of older men
Orchitis *NEJM 378:1233–1240, 2018*
  Mumps
  MMR vaccine
Tuberculosis *NEJM 378:1233–1240, 2018; Rev Port Pneumol 15:1193–1197, 2009*

INFLAMMATORY DISORDERS

Granulomatous orchitis *Human Pathol 45:844, 2014*

Hydrocele *NEJM 378:1233–1240, 2018*

Sarcoidosis *NEJM 378:1233–1240, 2018*

NEOPLASTIC DISORDERS

Germ cell tumors
  Seminoma
  Embryonal carcinoma
  Teratoma
  Yolk sac tumor
  Choriocarcinoma
Leydig cell tumors

Sertoli cell tumors

Mesothelioma

Sarcoma

Adenocarcinoma of the collecting system of the testis

Kaposi's sarcoma

Metastatic cancer – mucinous adenocarcinomas of colon *BMJ Case Reports Feb 25, 2013*

Testicular lymphoma, primary; diffuse large cell B–cell lymphoma

Burkitt's lymphoma

Pseudolymphoma

Plasmacytoma *Actas Urol Esp 32:1039–1042, 2008*

Rhabdomyosarcoma

Seminoma (germ cell tumoe) *NEJM 378:1233–1240, 2018*

Stromal tumors (Leydig cell, granulosa cell, and Sertoli cell tumors) *NEJM 378:1233–1240, 2018*

Teratoma *Urology 74:783–784, 2009*

SYNDROMES

McCune–Albright syndrome *J Ped Endocrin Metab 23:513–515, 2010*

TRAUMA

Testicular torsion *NEJM 378:1233–1240, 2018*

Inguinoscrotal hernia *NEJM 378:1233–1240, 2018*

VASCULAR LESIONS

Polyarteritis nodosa – testicular pain *NEJM 378:2518–2529, 2018*

Varicocele *NEJM 378:1233–1240, 2018*

Vasculitis – rheumatoid vasculitis *Rev Bras Rheum 53:365–367, 2013*

THUMBS

ANOMALIES OF THE THUMBS

TRIPHALANGEAL (FINGER–LIKE) THUMBS

Acrofacial dysostosis Genee–Wiedemann type *Atlas of Clinical Syndromes A Visual Aid to Diagnosis, 1992, pp.418–419*

Acro–renal complex *Atlas of Clinical Syndromes A Visual Aid to Diagnosis, 1992, pp.442–443*

Fanconi's anemia *Atlas of Clinical Syndromes A Visual Aid to Diagnosis, 1992, pp.440–441*

Holt–Oram syndrome (hand–heart syndrome) *Atlas of Clinical Syndromes A Visual Aid to Diagnosis, 1992, pp.438–439*

Hypoplastic anemia with triphalangeal thumbs syndrome (Aase–Smith syndrome) *Atlas of Clinical Syndromes A Visual Aid to Diagnosis, 1992, pp.436–437*

Nager acrofacial dysostosis *Atlas of Clinical Syndromes A Visual Aid to Diagnosis, 1992, pp.50–51*

Thalidomide embryopathy *Atlas of Clinical Syndromes A Visual Aid to Diagnosis, 1992, pp.370–371*

Tibial aplasia with polydactyly and triphalangeal thumbs – autosomal dominant *Atlas of Clinical Syndromes A Visual Aid to Diagnosis, 1992, pp.394–395*

HYPO– OR APLASIA OF THE THUMBS

Brachmann–de Lange syndrome *Atlas of Clinical Syndromes A Visual Aid to Diagnosis, 1992, pp.182–183*

Diastrophic dysplasia *Atlas of Clinical Syndromes A Visual Aid to Diagnosis, 1992, pp.236–237*

Fanconi's anemia *Atlas of Clinical Syndromes A Visual Aid to Diagnosis, 1992, pp.440–441*

Fibrodysplasia ossificans *Atlas of Clinical Syndromes A Visual Aid to Diagnosis, 1992, pp.444–445*

Holt–Oram syndrome (hand–heart syndrome) *Atlas of Clinical Syndromes A Visual Aid to Diagnosis, 1992, pp.438–439*

LADD syndrome *Atlas of Clinical Syndromes A Visual Aid to Diagnosis, 1992, pp.378–379*

Nager acrofacial dysostosis *Atlas of Clinical Syndromes A Visual Aid to Diagnosis, 1992, pp.50–51*

Oro–palatal–digital syndrome *Atlas of Clinical Syndromes A Visual Aid to Diagnosis, 1992, pp.26–27*

Thalidomide embryopathy *Atlas of Clinical Syndromes A Visual Aid to Diagnosis, 1992, pp.370–371*

Trichorhinophalangeal syndrome type I *Atlas of Clinical Syndromes A Visual Aid to Diagnosis, 1992, pp.420–421*

THYROID DISEASE, CUTANEOUS MANIFESTATIONS

HYPERTHYROIDISM

Alopecia

Exophthalmos

Facial flushing *JAAD 26:885–902, 1992*

Goiter

Hyperhidrosis

Hyperpigmentation

Metastatic nonseminomatous germ–cell tumor – hCG–mediated hyperthyroidism *NEJM 373:2358–2369, 2015*

Onycholysis (Plummer's nails)

Palmar erythema (Graves' disease) *Cutis 89:84–88, 2012;JAAD 26:885–902, 1992*

Pemphigus vulgaris – association with autoimmune thyroid disease, rheumatoid arthritis, type 1 diabetes mellitus *BJD 172:729–738, 2015*

Periorbital edema – hyperthyroidism, Graves' disease (endocrine exophthalmos) *Semin Neurol 20:43–54, 2000; Semin Ophthalmol 14:52–61, 1999;* hyperthyroidism – unilateral eyelid edema *JAAD 48:617–619, 2003;* Grave's disease – periorbital edema *NEJM 341:265–273, 1999*

Pretibial myxedema – cobblestoned yellow papules

Pruritus – hyperthyroidism, including thyrotoxicosis *JAAD 45:892–896, 2001; J Allergy Clin Immunol 48:73–81, 1971; South Med J 62:1127–1130, 1969*

Red feet

Thyroid acropachy *JAAD 26:885–902, 1992*

Thyrotoxicosis – splinter hemorrhages *JAAD 50:289–292, 2004*

Urticaria *JAMA 254:2253–2254, 1985; J Allergy Clin Immunol 48:73–81, 1971;* Graves' disease *JAAD 48:641–659, 2003*

Velvet skin

HYPOTHYROIDISM

Alopecia

Cretinism – multilobulated tongue; macroglossia

Cystinosis – white facial papules; renal failure, ocular, pancreatic, hepatic, muscular, dental, gonadal, and neurologic involvement, hypothyroidism *JAMADerm 152:108–109, 2016*

Delayed puberty

DRESS syndrome – hypothyroidism, liver failure, renal failure *JAAD 82:573–574, 2020*

Edema

Erythema multiforme/Stevens–Johnson syndrome – long term sequelae

Facial edema

Fanconi's anemia – autosomal recessive; endocrine abnormalities with hypothyroidism, decreased growth hormone, diabetes mellitus, café au lait macules, diffuse hyperpigmented macules, guttate hypopigmented macules, intertriginous hyperpigmentation, skeletal anomalies (thumb hypoplasia, absent thumbs, radii, carpal bones), oral/genital erythroplasia with development of squamous cell carcinoma, hepatic tumors, microphthalmia, ectopic or horseshoe kidney, broad nose, epicanthal folds, micrognathia, bone marrow failure, acute myelogenous leukemia, solid organ malignancies (brain tumors, Wilms' tumor) *BJD 164:245–256, 2011; JAAD 54:1056–1059, 2006*

Follicular papules *Ped Derm 22:447–449, 2005*

Frontal fibrosing alopecia – personal observation

Johanson–Blizzard syndrome – autosomal recessive; growth retardation, microcephaly, ACC of scalp, sparse hair, hypoplastic ala nasi, CALMs, hypoplastic nipples and areolae, hypothyroidism, sensorineural deafness *Clin Genet 14:247–250, 1978*

Keratoderma of myxedema *Aust Fam Physician 28:1217–1222, 1999; BJD 139:741–742, 1998; Clin Exp Derm 13:339–41, 1988; Acta DV 66:354–357, 1986*

Leschke's syndrome – growth retardation, mental retardation, diabetes mellitus, genital hypoplasia, hypothyroidism

Myxedema – yellow skin and yellow papules; ivory yellow skin color *JAAD 57:1051–1058, 2007; JAAD 26:885–902, 1992;* carotenemia prominent on palms and soles and nasolabial folds *JAAD 48:641–659, 2003;* congenital hypothyroidism

Myotonic dystrophy (Steinert syndrome) type 1 – autosomal dominant; muscular hypotonia, distal weakness of muscles, frontal alopecia, cataract, sensorineural hearing loss, dysarthria, dysphagia, diabetes mellitus, hypothyroidism, cardiac arrhythmias *Dtsch Arztebl Int 116:489–496, 2019; J Med Genet 19:341–348, 1982*

Oral ulcers *Oral Surg Oral Med Oral Pathol 46:216–219, 1978*

Pallor

Periorbital edema – hypothyroidism (myxedema) – puffy edema of eyelids *JAAD 26:885–902, 1992*

PHACES syndrome – hypothyroidism due to cutaneous and hepatic hemangiomas producing type III iodothyronine deiodinase deficiency and empty sella *Sem Cut Med Surg 35:108–116, 2016*

POEMS syndrome (Crowe–Fukasi syndrome, Takatsuki syndrome) (PEP syndrome – plasma cell dyscrasia, endocrinopathy, polyneuropathy) – plethora, angiomas (cherry, globular, glomeruloid) presenting as red nodules of face, trunk, and extremities, diffuse hyperpigmentation, hypertrichosis, scleroderma–like changes, either generalized or localized (legs), hyperhidrosis, clubbing, leukonychia, papilledema, pleural effusion, peripheral edema, ascites, pulmonary hypertension, weight loss, fatigue, diarrhea, thrombocytosis, polycythemia, fever, renal disease, artralgias; osteosclerotic myeloma (IgG or IgA lambda) bone lesions, progressive symmetric sensorimotor peripheral polyneuropathy, hypothyroidism, and hypogonadism; peripheral edema, thrombocytosis, cutaneous angiomas, blue dermal papules associated with

Castleman's disease (benign reactive angioendotheliomatosis), maculopapular brown–violaceous lesions, purple nodules; papilledema *JAAD 58:671–675, 2008; JAAD 55:149–152, 2006; JAAD 44:324–329, 2001, JAAD 40:808–812, 1999; AD 124:695–698, 1988, Cutis 61:329–334, 1998; JAAD 21:1061–1068, 1989; JAAD 12:961–964, 1985; Nippon Shinson 26:2444–2456, 1968*

Pruritus – hypothyroidism *JAAD 45:892–896, 2001; The Clinical Management of Itching; Parthenon; p. 26, 2000*

Pseudohypoparathyroidism type Ia (Albright's hereditary osteodystrophy) – subcutaneous nodule (osteoma cutis); short stature, round face, obesity, subcutaneous ossifications, bilateral brachydactyly, mental retardation, hypothyroidism, saddle nose deformity *Ped Derm 33:675–676, 2016; Atlas of Clinical Syndromes A Visual Aid to Diagnosis, 1992, pp188–189*

Purpura and ecchymoses *JAAD 26:885–902, 1992*

Telangiectasias, spondyloepiphyseal dysplasia, hypothyroidism, neovascularization, and tractional retinal detachments *Ped Derm 6:178–184, 1989*

Trichomegaly *Ped Derm 26:188–193, 2009*

Urticaria

Xanthoderma

Xerosis

MISCELLANEOUS DISORDERS

AUTOIMMUNE DISEASES AND DISORDERS OF IMMUNE DYSREGULATION

Gain of function *STAT1* mutations – chronic mucocutaneous candidiasis; onychodystrophy, generalized dermatophytosis; disseminated coccidioidomycosis, histoplasmosis, sinopulmonary infections, herpes simplex infections; endocrine, dental, gastrointestinal disease; diabetes mellitus, hypothyroidism, autoimmune hepatitis, cerebral aneurysms, oral and esophageal squamous cell carcinomas; increased levels of interferon results in decreased IL–17A and IL–22 *JAAD 73:255–264, 2015*

Sjogren's syndrome – increased risk of autoimmune thyroid disease *A Clinician's Pearls and Myths in Rheumatology pp.107–130; ed John Stone; Springer 2009*

DEVELOPMENTAL ANOMALIES

Ectopic thyroid gland *NEJM 363:1351, 2010*

Pyramidal lobe of thyroid gland – congenital nodule

Thyroglossal duct cyst and/or sinus – midline cervical cleft with sinus tract *Am J Neuroradiol 20:579–582, 1999; JAAD 26:885–902, 1992; J Pediatr Surg 19:437–439, 1984*

PRIMARY CUTANEOUS DISEASES

Hypopigmentation – white lunulae; hyper– or hypothyroidism – vitiligo

Vitiligo *JAAD 76:871–878, 2017*

SYNDROMES

APECED (autoimmune polyendocrinopathy, candidiasis, ectodermal dystrophy) syndrome (autoimmune polyendocrine syndrome type 1) – autosomal recessive; mutation in AIRE gene (autoimmune regulator gene); chronic mucocutaneous candidiasis, hypoparathyroidism, Addison's disease, diabetes mellitus type 1, thyroid autoimmune disease, gonadal failure, hepatitis, vitiligo, alopecia areata, pernicious anemia, intestinal malabsorption, keratinopathy, dystrophy of dental enamel and nails *JAAD 62:864–868, 2010;*

Bannayan–Riley–Ruvalcaba–Zonana syndrome (PTEN phosphatase and tensin homolog hamartoma) – dolicocephaly, frontal bossing, macrocephaly, ocular hypertelorism, long philtrum, thin upper lip, broad mouth, relative micrognathia, lipomas, penile or vulvar lentigines, facial verruca–like or acanthosis nigricans–like papules, multiple acrochordons, angiokeratomas, transverse palmar crease, accessory nipple, syndactyly, brachydactyly, vascular malformations, arteriovenous malformations, lymphangiokeratoma, goiter, hamartomatous intestinal polyposis *JAAD 53:639–643, 2005*

Carney complex – thyroid neoplasms *Ped Derm 36:160–162, 2019*

Cowden's syndrome (multiple hamartoma syndrome) – punctate palmar papules with central depressions; autosomal dominant with variable penetrance; facial trichilemmomas with cobblestone appearance around eyes and mouth; acrokeratosis verruciformis; punctate palmoplantar keratoderma; multiple angiomas and lipomas; café au lait macules; mucous membrane papillomas; craniomegaly; fibrocystic breast disease with associated breast cancer; goiter with thyroid carcinoma; other adenocarcinomas and melanoma *JAAD 68:189–209, 2013; JAAD 17:342–346, 1987; JAAD 11:1127–1141, 1984*

Hermansky–Pudlak syndrome type 2 – oculocutaneous albinism, hemorrhage, ceroid–like material deposited in several organs; granulomatous colitis, pulmonary fibrosis, renal failure, cardiomyopathy, hypothyroidism *Ped Derm 34:638–646, 2017; SKINMed 12:313–315, 2014*

IPEX syndrome – immune dysregulation (neonatal autoimmune enteropathy, food allergies), polyendocrinopathy (diabetes mellitus, thyroiditis), enteropathy (neonatal diarrhea), X–linked, rash (atopic dermatitis–like with exfoliative erythroderma and periorificial dermatitis; psoriasiform dermatitis, pemphigoid nodularis, painful fissured cheilitis, edema of lips and perioral area, urticaria secondary to foods); penile rash; thyroid dysfunction, diabetes mellitus, hepatitis, nephritis, onychodystrophy, alopecia universalis; mutations in *FOXP3*(forkhead box protein 3) gene – master control gene of T regulatory cells (Tregs); hyper IgE, eosinophilia *NEJM 378:1132–1141, 2018; JAAD 73:355–364, 2015; BJD 160:645–651, 2009; ichthyosiform eruptions Blood 109:383–385, 2007; BJD 152:409–417, 2005; NEJM 344:1758–1762, 2001; alopecia areata AD 140:466–472, 2004*

Multifocal idiopathic fibrosclerosis (hyper IgG4 syndrome) – sclerodermoid red plaque of breast; fibrosis of thyroid, mediastinum, retroperitoneum, orbits, pancreas, gallbladder *AD 148:1335–1336, 2012*

Wiedemann–Rautenstrauch (neonatal progeroid syndrome) – autosomal recessive; present at birth, generalized lipoatrophy, macrocephaly, sparse hair, premature aging, wide open sutures, aged and triangular face with hypoplasia of facial bones, persistent fontanelles, prominent scalp veins, growth retardation, low set ears, beak shaped nose, neonatal teeth, slender limbs, large hands and feet with long fingers, joint contractures, large penis, pseudohydrocephalus, psychomotor retardation; osteosarcoma, thyroid carcinoma, melanoma; mutation in helicase *BJD 164:245–256, 2011; Ped Derm 22:75–78, 2005; J Med Genet 34:433–437, 1997; Am J Med Genet 35:91–94, 1990; Eur J Pediatr 130:65–70, 1979; Eur J Pediatr 124:101–111, 1977*

VASCULAR DISORDERS

Hepatic hemangiomas associated with multiple cutaneous infantile hemangiomas – hypothyroidism *Seminars Cut Med Surg 35:108–116, 2016*

TONGUE, ENLARGED (MACROGLOSSIA)

Pediatrics 129:e431–437, 2012

TRUE MACROGLOSSIA

Primary muscular hypertrophy of the tongue (when histologic findings correlate with clinical evidence of an enlarged tongue) *Ped Derm 20:361–363, 2003; Plastic and Reconstructive Surgery 78:715–723, 1986; Laryngoscope 86:291–296, 1976; Arch Otolaryngol 93:378–383, 1971*

CONGENITAL ANOMALIES

Congenital macroglossia – autosomal dominant *Genet Couns 5:151–154, 1994*

Dermoid cyst, including sublingual dermoid *Br J Oral Maxillofac Surg 37:58–60, 1999; Oral Surg Oral Med Oral Pathol 50:217–218, 1980*

Fibrous hamartoma *Int J Pediatr Otorhinolaryngol 33:171–178, 1995*

Gland hyperplasia

Hemihyperplasia (congenital hemihypertrophy) *Am J Dis Child 120:372–373, 1970*

Idioathic muscle hypertrophy *Pediatrics 129:e431–437, 2012*

Lingual tonsil *Int J Pediatr Otorhinolaryngol 53:63–66, 2000; Am J Forensic Med Pathol 14:158–161, 1993*

Lingual thyroid *NEJM 358:1712, 2008; Thyroid 10:511–514, 2000*

Sublingual dermoid cyst

Thyroglossal duct cyst *J Pediatr Surg 31:1574–1576, 1996*

METABOLIC DISORDERS

Endocrine disorders

Fucosidosis type II

Ganglioside storage disease type 1

Glycogen storage disease

GM1 gangliosidosis type I – X–linked – gingival hypertrophy, macroglossia, coarse facies, micrognathia, loose skin, inguinal hernia, delayed growth, hepatosplenomegaly, neonatal hypotonia, delayed motor development *Ped Derm 18:534–536, 2001; Syndromes of the Head and Neck, p.118, 1990*

Hereditary gelsolin amyloidosis (AGel amyloidosis) – cutis laxa, corneal lattice dystrophy, cranial and peripheral polyneuropathy *BJD 152:250–257, 2005*

Hunter's syndrome (decreased sulfoiduronate sulfatase) – macroglossia; reticulated 2–10mm skin-colored papules over scapulae, chest, neck, arms; X–linked recessive; MPS type II; iduronate–2 sulfatase deficiency; lysosomal accumulation of heparin sulfate and dermatan sulfate; short stature, full lips, coarse facies, clear corneas (unlike Hurler's syndrome), progressive neurodegeneration, communicating hydrocephalus, valvular and ischemic heart disease, lower respiratory tract infections, adenotonsillar hypertrophy, otitis media, obstructive sleep apnea, diarrhea, hepatosplenomegaly, skeletal deformities (dysostosis multiplex), widely spaced teeth, dolichocephaly, deafness, retinal degeneration, inguinal and umbilical hernias *Ped Derm 21:679–681, 2004; Ped Derm 15:370–373, 1998; Syndromes of the Head and Neck, p. 101, 1990*

Hurler's syndrome *Acta Anaesthesiol Sin 37:93–96, 1999*

Hypothyroidism *Ped Neurol 94:82–83, 2019*

Mannosidosis – autosomal recessive; gingival hypertrophy, macroglossia, coarse features, prognathism, thick eyebrows, low anterior hairline, deafness, lens opacities, hepatosplenomegaly, recurrent respiratory tract infections, muscular hypotonia, mental retardation *Ped Derm 18:534–536, 2001*

Mucopolysaccharidoses (Hurler's, Hurler–Schei, Sanfilippo, Morquio, Maroteaux–Lamy, Sly syndromes) *Syndromes of the Head and Neck, p.113, 1990*

Pompe disease *Br J Oral Maxillofac Surg 57:831–838, 2019*

Sanfilippo type IIIb mucopolysaccharidosis *Bull Group Int Rech Sci Stomatol Odontol 35:5–12, 1992*

Transient neonatal diabetes mellitus *Pediatrics 129:e431–437, 2012; Clin Genet 78:580–584, 2010; J Perinatol 16:288–291, 1996*

NEOPLASTIC DISORDERS

Granular cell tumor

Lingual cyst – recurrent swelling in adult *J Oral Maxillofac Surg 59:908–912, 2001*

Malignant oncocytoma – base of tongue *J Otorhinolaryngol Relat Spec 62:104–108, 2000*

Neurofibroma *JAAD 81:43–56, 2019*

Palisaded encapsulated neuroma *JAAD 81:43–56, 2019*

Schwannoma *JAAD 81:43–56, 2019*

SYNDROMES

AKT1 somatic mosaicism – hemihypertrophy, hemimacroglossia, epidermal nevus, café au lait macules *BJD 175:612–614, 2016*

Angelman syndrome ("happy puppet syndrome") *Acta Paediatr Scand 73:398–402, 1984*

Beckwith–Wiedemann syndrome (Exomphalos–Macroglossia–Gigantism)(EMG) syndrome – autosomal dominant; zosteriform rash at birth, exomphalos, macroglossia (rhabdomyomas), hemihypertrophy of muscle fibers, visceromegaly, facial salmon patch of forehead, upper eyelids, nose, and upper lip and gigantism; linear earlobe grooves, circular depressions of helices; increased risk of Wilms' tumor, adrenal carcinoma, hepatoblastoma, and rhabdomyosarcoma *JAAD 37:523–549, 1997; Clin Genet 46:168–174, 1994; Am J Dis Child 122:515–519, 1971*

Canavan disease *Int J Pediatr Otorhinolaryngol 66:303–307, 2002*

Congenital macroglossal angiodysplasia (lymphanioendotheliomatosis) *Arch Pathol Lab Med 124:1349–1351, 2000*

Cornelia de Lange syndrome *Arch Kinderheikd 172:75–80, 1965*

Costello syndrome *JAAD 32:904–907, 1995*

Cretinism (congenital hypothyroidism) – coarse facial features, lethargy, macroglossia, cold dry skin, livedo, umbilical hernia, poor muscle tone, coarse scalp hair, synophrys, no pubic or axillary hair at puberty

Down's syndrome (trisomy 21) – fissured tongue, macroglossia *Adv Clin Exp Med 28:1587–1592, 2019; Ped Derm 24:317–320, 2007; J Laryngol Otol 104:494–496, 1990*

Ehlers–Danlos syndrome

Ellis–van Creveld syndrome – hypertrophied frenulum *J Am Dent Assoc 77:1090–1095, 1968*

Exomphalos–macroglossia–gigantism syndrome (EMG) *Int Ped 82:814–820, 1973*

Goldenhaar syndrome (oculo–auriculo–vertebral syndrome) – macroglossia, preauricular tags, abnormal pinnae, facial asymmetry, macrostomia, epibulbar dermoids, facial weakness, central nervous system, renal, and skeletal anomalies

Hereditary angioedema – of retropharyngeal space in an adult *Am J Otolaryngol 20:136–138, 1999*

Hunter's polydystrophy *Int J Pediatr Otorhinolaryngol 44:273–278, 1998; Laryngoscope 97:280–285, 1987*

Lipoid proteinosis *Pediatrics 129:e431–437, 2012*

Melkersson–Rosenthal syndrome *Pediatrics 129:e431–437, 2012*

Multiple endocrine neoplasia syndrome – type 2b *Int J Oral Maxillofac Surg 21:110–114, 1992*

Neurofibromatosis – usually unilateral macroglossia *J Laryngol Otol 101:743–745, 1987; Oral Surg Oral Med Oral Pathol 58:493–498, 1984; J Dent Child 47: 255–260, 1980*

Opitz trigonocephaly syndrome (C syndrome) – multiple frenula *Birth Defects 5:161–166, 1969*

Oral–facial–digital syndrome *Otolaryngol Pol 65:423–427, 2011*

Phakomatosis pigmentokeratotica – plaque of tongue; coexistence of large nevus sebaceous, epidermal nevus, and speckled lentiginous nevus; multilobulated pink nodules representing connective tissue nevus; seizures, hyperhidrosis, peripheral neuropathy; high incidence of vitamin D–resistant rickets *Ped Derm 28:715–719, 2011; JAAD 63:1–22, 2010; Ped Derm 25:76–80, 2008; Arch Surg 43:341–375, 1941*

Plummer–Vinson syndrome – lymphangiomatous macroglossia with upper airway obstruction and sleep apnea *Oto Head Neck Surg 2001, April p. 477–478*

Robinow syndrome (fetal face syndrome)

Simpson–Golabi–Behmel syndrome type I *Medicine 98:e17616, 2019*

Triploidy syndrome

Trisomy 4p syndrome

Complete trisomy 22 – primitive low–set ears, bilateral preauricular pit, broad nasal bridge, antimongoloid palpebral fissures, macroglossia, enlarged sublingual glands, cleft palate, micrognathia, clinodactyly of fifth fingers, hypoplastic fingernails, hypoplastic genitalia, short lower limbs, bilateral sandal gap, deep plantar furrows *Pediatrics 108:E32, 2001*

TRAUMA

Traumatic neuroma *JAAD 81:43–56, 2019*

VASCULAR DISORDERS

Angioma

Diffuse angiomatosis *Arch Otolaryng 93:83–89, 1971*

Hemangiolymphangiomas

Hemangiomas *Head Neck Surg 9:299–304, 1987*

Klippel–Trenaunay–Weber syndrome – hemihypertrophy *Oral Surg Oral Med Oral Pathol 63:208–215, 1987; Ann DV 114:665–669, 1987; Rev Stomatol Chir Maxillofac 87:320–326, 1986*

Lymphangiomas *J Indian Assoc Ped Surg 25:49–51, 2020; Oto Head Neck Surg 2001, April p. 477–478*

Lymphatic malformation *J Pediatr Surg 31:1648–1650, 1996*

Vascular malformations – venous and lymphatic malformations *Int J Oral Maxillofac Surg Jan 20, 2020*

ACQUIRED MACROGLOSSIA

AUTOIMMUNE DISEASES AND DISEASES OF IMMUNE DYSFUNCTION

Allergic contact dermatitis – tongue swelling *Contact Dermatitis 60:114–115, 2009*

Angioedema *Oral Dis 3:39–42, 1997; Dermatol Clin 3:85–95, 1985*

Contact urticaria – peanut butter *Contact Dermatitis 9:66–68, 1983*

GATA 2 deficiency *BJD 178:781–785, 2018*

Pemphigus vegetans *AD 121:1328–1329, 1985*

Pemphigus vulgaris *AD 121:1328, 1985*

Scleroderma *Rheumatologia 6:301–306, 1968*

DRUGS

ACE–inhibitor-induced angioedema *NEJM 355:295, 2006; J Forensic Sci 46:1239–1243, 2001;* lisinopril

Fidoxamicin (macrolide antibiotic) – facial, tongue, and throat swelling *Clin Inf Dis 58:537–538, 2014*

Mirtazapine *Med Clin Barcelona 115:78, 2000*

EXOGENOUS AGENTS

Chewing on house plant (dieffenbachia) leaves containing calcium oxalate *Oral Surg Oral Med Oral Pathol 78:631–633, 1994*

INFECTIONS AND INFESTATIONS

Abscess *Br Dent J 24:376–382, 1986*

Actinomycosis *Head Neck Pathol 13:327–330, 2019*

Amebic dysentery

Bacterial glossitis

Candidiasis – chronic mucocutaneous candidiasis *Med Cutan Ibero Lat Am 12:33–40, 1984; Ann Rev Med 32:491–497, 1981*

Cellulitis/erysipelas *Br Med J 300:24, 1990*

Diphtheria *Anesthesiology 50:132–145, 1979*

Histoplasmosis *Rev Med Chil 138:586–589, 2010*

Infection – chronic inflammation of "scrotal" tongue

Leishmaniasis – post kala–azar dermal leishmaniasis – in India, hypopigmented macules; nodules develop after years; tongue, palate, genitalia *E Afr Med J 63:365–371, 1986*

Leprosy – multilobulated tongue *Int J Leprosy 64:325–330, 1992*

Mycobacterium tuberculosis – tuberculosis *Cutis 60:201–202, 1997;* orofacial granulomatosis due to tuberculosis; enlarged tongue; vegetative plaques of nose and nasolabial folds *Ped Derm 26:108–109, 2009*

Syphilis – secondary *Oral Surg Oral Med Oral Pathol 45:540–542, 1978;* tertiary (gumma) (interstitial glossitis)

Wasp/bee stings of the tongue *Oto Head Neck Surg 122:778, 2000*

INFILTRATIVE DISEASES

Amyloidosis – primary systemic – myeloma, plasmacytomas *Postgrad Med J 64:696–698, 1988; Oral Surg 63:586–591, 1987; Clin Exp Dermatol 4:517–536, 1979;* dialysis–related amyloidosis – nodular macroglossia with combined light chain and beta–2 microglobulin deposition *Eur J Dermatol 13:393–395, 2003; J Nephrol 14:128–131, 2001; Kidney Int 52:832–838, 1997;* monoclonal light chains *NEJM 378:2321, 2018;* localized amyloidosis *Mol Clin Oncol 12:258–262, 2020*

Juvenile xanthogranuloma, giant *Am J Otolaryngol 20:241–244, 1999*

INFLAMMATORY DISEASES

Crohn's disease – cobblestoning, pyostomatitis vegetans

Ludwig's angina – "double tongue" *NEJM 381:163, 2019; BMJ Case Rep June 29, 2018*

Median rhomboid glossitis – tongue nodule *AD 135:593–598, 1999*

Sarcoidosis *Clin Exp Dermatol 17:47–48, 1992*

METABOLIC DISEASES

Acromegaly *Pituitary 19:448,–457, 2016; JAAD 42:511–513, 2000*

Adult onset acid maltase deficiency *Medicine 74:131, 1995*

Gigantism

Hypothyroidism, myxedema *Virchows Archives A Pathol Anat Histol 373:353–360, 1977*

Pellagra – swollen red tongue with erosions and furrows *BJD 164:1188–1200, 2011*

Uremia – uremic stomatitis *Clinics (Sao Paolo) 60:259–262, 2005;* mimicking oral hairy leukoplakia *OSOMOPOR Endod 83:350–353, 1997*

Vitamin B12 deficiency (pernicious anemia, sprue) – enlarged red tongue *AD 122:896–899, 1986*

NEOPLASTIC DISEASES

Alveolar rhabdomyosarcoma – neonatal lesion with massive macroglossia *Soc Ped Derm Annual Meeting, July 2005*

Ectomesenchymal chondromyxoid tumor of the anterior tongue *JAAD 59:S23–24, 2008; Oral Surg Oral Med Oral Pathol Oral Radiol Endod 82:417–422, 1996; Am J Surg Pathol 19:519–530, 1995*

Embryonal rhabdomyosarcoma *Ped Derm 22:218–221, 2005*

Epidermoid carcinoma

Fibroma

Granular cell myoblastoma *JAAD 81:43–56, 2019*

Kaposi's sarcoma *Case Rep Infec Dis 2015;851462*

Keratoacanthomas, eruptive *JAAD 29:299–304, 1993*

Leiomyoma

Leukemias – leukemic macrocheilitis *JAAD 14:353–358, 1986*

Lingual thyroid

Lipoma – facial infiltrating lipomatosis *Plast Reconstr Surg 108:1544, 1554, 2001;* symmetric lipomatosis of the tongue *J Cranio Maxillo Facial Surg 21:298–301, 1993;* atypical lipoma of tongue *J Laryngol Otol 115:859–861, 2001*

Lymphomas *Human Pathol 14:375–377, 1983*

Metastasis – rectal carcinoma *J Laryngol Otol 103:322–323, 1989*

Nerve sheath myxoma (neurothekoma) of the tongue *Oral Surg Oral Med Oral Pathol Oral Radiol Endod 90:74–77, 2000*

Neurilemmoma (schwannoma) – nodule

Neurinoma (sublingual) *Neuroradiology 20:87–90, 1980*

Neurofibromas

Oral florid papillomatosis (verrucous carcinoma) *NEJM 372:2049, 2015*

Osteoma (osseous choristoma) *Br J Oral Surg 25:79–82, 1987*

Plasmacytoma *Mund Kiefer Gesichtschir 3:46–49, 1999*

Pleomorphic adenoma *J Laryngol Otol 114:793–795, 2000*

Rhabdomyoma *Br J Oral Surg 23:284–291, 1985; Oral Surg 48:525–531, 1979*

Squamous cell carcinoma with lymphedema due to obstruction of lymphatics

Waldenstrom's macroglobulinemia *Rinsho Ketsueki 33:1708–1713, 1992*

PARANEOPLASTIC DISEASES

Generalized malignant acanthosis nigricans *AD 115:201–202, 1979*

PRIMARY CUTANEOUS DISEASES

Acanthosis nigricans *Oral Surg 56:372–374, 1983;*

Lichen nitidus – tongue papules *Ped Derm 36:189–192, 2019*

Madelung's disease (benign symmetrical lipomatosis) *JAAD 42:511–513, 2000; J Craniomaxillfacial Surg 21:298–301, 1993*

Malacoplakia *J Otolaryngol 14:179–182, 1985*

Partial lipodystrophy, complement abnormalities, vasculitis – macroglossia, polyarthralgia, mononeuritis, hypertrophy of subcutaneous tissue *Ann DV 114:1083–1091, 1987*

Pseudomacroglossia – tongue sits in abnormal position; tongue displaced
    Enlarged tonsils or adenoids
    Habitual posturing of tongue
    Hypotonia of tongue
    Low palate and decreased oral cavity volume (glossoptosis)
    Neoplasms displacing tongue
    Severe mandibular deficiency (retrognathism)

Scleredema of Buschke *Hautarzt 49:48–54, 1998; JAAD 11:128–134, 1984*

Scleromyxedema – personal observation

SYNDROMES

Blue rubber bleb nevus syndrome – sublingual angiomas *Arch Neurol 38:784–785, 1981*

Beckwith–Wiedemann syndrome – gigantism, omphalocele, macroglossia; hypoglycemia, tumors (Wilms', rhabdomyosarcoma, hepatoblastoma, adrenal tumors), centrofacial capillary malformations *JAAD 56:541–564, 2007*

Facial edema with eosinophilia

Hereditary angioedema – autosomal dominant; prodrome of erythema marginatum (annular urticarial eruption); facial, lip, eyelid, tongue, and hand edema *JAAD 65:843–850, 2011; Monatsh Prakt Derm 1:129–131, 1882; Edinb Med J 22:513–526, 1876*

Kabuki makeup syndrome – short stature, congenital heart defects, distinct expressionless face (frontal bossing, long palpebral fissures, eversion of the lower eyelids, sparse arched lateral eyebrows, epicanthus, telecanthus, prominent eyelashes, short flat nose with anteversion of the tip, short philtrum, large mouth with thick lips, high arched palate, cleft palate, dental malocclusion, micrognathia, large protuberant low set ears with thick helix), lowcut hairline, vitiligo, cutis laxa, hyperextensible joints, syndactyly of toes 2–3, brachydactyly, clinodactyly, fetal finger pads with abnormal dermatoglyphics, short great toes, blue sclerae, lower lip pits, cryptorchidism, mental retardation with microcephaly; preauricular dimple/fistula *Ped Derm 24:309–312, 2007; JAAD S247–251, 2005; Am J Med Genet 132A:260–262, 2005; Am J Med Genet 94:170–173, 2000; Am J Med Genet 31:565–589, 1988; J Pediatr 105:849–850, 1984; J Pediatr 99:565–569, 570–573, 1981*

Lipoid proteinosis – thickened tongue with thick sublingual frenulum; mutation in extracellular matrix protein-1(ECM1) *AD 147:857–862, 2011; Ped Derm 26:91–92, 2009; BJD 151:413–423, 2004; JID 120:345–350, 2003; Hum Molec Genet 11:833–840, 2002; Int J Derm 39:203–204, 2000; JAAD 39:149–171, 1998; Cutis 56:220–224, 1995; JAAD 27:293–297, 1992; Virchows Arch (Pathol Anat) 273:285–319, 1929*

Melkersson–Rosenthal syndrome

Multicentric reticulohistiocytosis *JAAD 20:530–532, 1989*

Neurofibromatosis

Partial lipodystrophy, complement abnormalities, vasculitis – macroglossia, polyarthralgia, mononeuritis, hypertrophy of subcutaneous tissue *Ann DV 114:1083–1091, 1987*

Primary lateral sclerosis (motor neuron disease) *Int J Neurosci 129:1189–1191, 2019*

Rabson–Mendenhall syndrome – autosomal recessive; insulin-resistant diabetes, acanthosis nigricans, coarse and senile appearance, precocious puberty *J Indian Soc Pedod Prev Dent 30:279–282, 2012*

Simpson–Golabi–Behmel syndrome (bulldog syndrome – X–linked recessive; macroglossia, protruding jaw and tongue, widened nasal bridge, upturned nasal tip, hands/feet short, broad dysplastic nails, supernumerary nipples, hypotonia

Winchester syndrome – annular and serpiginous thickenings of skin; arthropathy, gargoyle–like face, gingival hypertrophy, macroglossia, osteolysis (multilayered symmetric restrictive banding), generalized hypertrichosis, very short stature, thickening and stiffness of skin with annular and serpiginous thickenings of skin, multiple subcutaneous nodules *JAAD 50:S53–56, 2004*

TOXINS

Lead toxicity

TRAUMA

After posterior fossa and craniofacial surgery in children *Int J Oral Maxillofac Surg 47:428–436, 2018*

Direct trauma

Intubation injury

Physical trauma

Radiation therapy

Self–induced traumatic macroglossia *Case Rep Otolaryngol May 12, 2019*

VASCULAR DISORDERS

Giant cell arteritis *J Rheumatol 15:1026–1028, 1988*

Hemangioma

Lymphangioma (including cystic hygroma) *Otolaryngol Head Neck Surg 90:283, 1982*

Lymphatic malformation *Ped Derm 30:383–385, 2013; BJD 148:1279–1282, 2003*

Lymphatic obstruction

Port wine stain *JAMADerm 150:1336–1340, 2014*

Pyogenic granuloma *Br J Oral Surg 24:376–382, 1986*

Superior vena cava obstruction (SVC syndrome) *Cutis 79:362, 367–368, 2007; Am Rev Respir Dis 141:1114–1118, 1990; Q J Med 162:151–168, 1972*

Venous malformation

RELATIVE MACROGLOSSIA

(when histologic findings do not provide a pathologic explanation for an apparently enlarged tongue)

CONGENITAL

Angelman syndrome *Brain Dev 16:249–252, 1994*

Down's syndrome *Ped Derm 24:317–320, 2007; Plast Reconstr Surg 78:715–723, 1986*

Congenital hypothyroidism (cretinism)

ACQUIRED

Congenital macroglossia, idiopathic

Edentulous patients

Ludwig's angina (cellulitis/erysipelas) *Ear Nose Throat Journal 80:217–218;222–223, 2001*

Myxedema

Syphilis, tertiary – interstitial glossitis

Following operative correction of mandibular prognathism

PSEUDOMACROGLOSSIA (TONGUE SITS IN ABNORMAL POSITION, TONGUE DISPLACED)

Habitual posturing of tongue

Enlarged tonsils or adenoids

Low palate and decreased oral cavity volume (glossoptosis)

Severe mandibular deficiency (retrognathism)

Neoplasms displacing the tongue

Hypotonia of the tongue

TONGUE, HYPERPIGMENTATION

Ped Derm 9:123–125, 1992

AUTOIMMUNE DISEASES

Lupus erythematosus, systemic *Lupus 24:111–112, 2015*

DRUGS

Adriamycin *Cancer Treat Rep 60:1402–1404, 1976*

Amitryptiline – black tongue (not hairy) *AD 143:813, 2007; J Contemp Dent Pract 4:10–31, 2003*

Antimalarials – plaquenil

AZT (azidothymidine) therapy *Am J Med 86:469–470, 1989*

Benztropine – black tongue (not hairy) *AD 143:813, 2007; J Contemp Dent Pract 4:10–31, 2003*

Cancer chemotherapy *South Med J 72:1615–1616, 1979;* cisplatin, ifosfamide, temozolomide, and vincristine *J Drugs Dermatol 12:223–226, 2013*

Capecitabine *Indian J Pharmacol 42:326–328, 2010; Am J Clin Dermatol 10:261–263, 2009*

Cephalosporins – black tongue (not hairy) *AD 143:813, 2007; J Contemp Dent Pract 4:10–31, 2003*

Clarithromycin – black tongue (not hairy) *AD 143:813, 2007; J Contemp Dent Pract 4:10–31, 2003*

Clofazimine – in lepromatous leprosy; red to purple black

Clonazepam – black tongue (not hairy) *AD 143:813, 2007; J Contemp Dent Pract 4:10–31, 2003*

Corticosteroids – black tongue (not hairy) *AD 143:813, 2007; J Contemp Dent Pract 4:10–31, 2003*

Doxorubicin *Dermatol Online J 14:18, 2008; South Med J 72:1615–1616, 1979*

Fixed drug eruption *Ped Derm 12:51–52, 1995*

Fluoxetine – black tongue (not hairy) *AD 143:813, 2007; J Contemp Dent Pract 4:10–31, 2003*

Griseofulvin – black tongue (not hairy) *AD 143:813, 2007; J Contemp Dent Pract 4:10–31, 2003*

Hydroxyurea *Cureus 11:e6311, 2019; Ped Derm 21:124–127, 2004*

Imipramine – black tongue (not hairy) *AD 143:813, 2007; J Contemp Dent Pract 4:10–31, 2003*

Inhaled heroin smoke – black tongue (not hairy) *AD 143:813, 2007*

Interferon, pegylated and ribavirin therapy *JAAD 62:164–165, 2010; Gut 57:1697, 1727, 2008; J Eur Acad Dermatol Venereol 22:1389–1391, 2008; Am J Gastroenterol 102:1334–1335, 2007; Am J Gastroenterol 101:197–198, 2006; Indian J Gastroenterol 25:324, 2006; BJD 149:390–394, 2003*

Lansoprazole – black tongue *AD 137:968–969, 2001*

Methyldopa – black tongue *AD 137:968–969, 2001; AD 136:427–428, 2000*

Minocycline *AD 136:427–428, 2000; Arch Fam Med 9:687–688, 2000;* black tongue *AD 137:968–969, 2001; BJD 134:943–944, 1996; AD 131:620, 1995; AD 121:417–418, 1985*

Nortriptylene – black tongue (not hairy) *AD 143:813, 2007; J Contemp Dent Pract 4:10–31, 2003*

Penicillins – black tongue (not hairy) *AD 143:813, 2007; J Contemp Dent Pract 4:10–31, 2003*

Streptomycin – black tongue (not hairy) *AD 143:813, 2007; J Contemp Dent Pract 4:10–31, 2003*

Sulfonamides – black tongue (not hairy) *AD 143:813, 2007; J Contemp Dent Pract 4:10–31, 2003*

Tegafur *J Dermatol 137:937–938, 2010; Acta DV 77:80–81, 1997*

Tetracycline – black tongue (not hairy) *AD 143:813, 2007; J Contemp Dent Pract 4:10–31, 2003*

Tricyclic antidepressants *AD 136:427–428, 2000*

EXOGENOUS AGENTS

Amalgam tattoo *AD 136:427–428, 2000*

Betel quid chewing *Cutis 71:307–311, 2003*

Bismuth subsalicylate tablets (Pepto–Bismol) – black tongue (pseudo–black hairy tongue) *Cutis 105:288, 293, 2020; J Drugs Dermatol 8:1132–1135, 2009; AD 137:968–969, 2001*; black dots after oral ingestion of Pepto–Bismol *JAAD 37:489–490, 1997*

Crack cocaine smoking – black tongue *AD 143:813, 2007; J Contemp Dent Pract 4:10–31, 2003; AD 137:968–969, 2001*

Silver – silver dental amalgam *Quintessence Int 26:553–557, 1995*

Tobacco – black tongue *AD 143:813, 2007; J Contemp Dent Pract 4:10–31, 2003; AD 137:968–969, 2001*

Vegetable dyes – black tongue (not hairy) *AD 143:813, 2007; J Contemp Dent Pract 4:10–31, 2003; AD 137:968–969, 2001*

INFECTIONS AND INFESTATIONS

AIDS (HIV disease)*; Oral Surg Oral Med Oral Pathol 67:301–307, 1989*

Candidiasis

Golden tongue syndrome – *Ramichlordium schulzeri AD 121:892–894, 1985*

Relapsing fever – mustard tongue

METABOLIC DISORDERS

Addison's disease *Clin Exp Dermatol 36:429–430, 2011; Cutis 76:97–99, 2005*

Hemochromatosis

Vitamin B12 deficiency *Cutis 71:127–130, 2003*

NEOPLASTIC DISORDERS

Angioleiomyoma of the tongue – blue lesion *Clin in Derm 37:468–486, 2019*

Melanocytic nevi *AD 139:767–770, 2003; Cancer 25:812–823, 1970*

Melanoma *AD 139:767–770, 2003; Cancer 25:812–823, 1970*

Melanotic macules of the tongue *AD 139:767–770, 2003; JAAD 44:1048–1049, 2001; Ped Derm 9:123–125, 1992*

PARANEOPLASTIC DISORDERS

Occult malignancy *J Otolaryngol 7:389–394, 1978*

PRIMARY CUTANEOUS DISEASES

Acanthosis nigricans *AD 115:201–202, 1979*

Brown or black hairy tongue *AD 77:97–103, 1958*

Congenital lingual melanotic macules *AD 139:767–770, 2003*

Fungiform papillae, pigmented *JAAD 76:540–542, 2017; Ped Derm 27:398–399, 2010; AD 140:1275, 2004; AD 135:593–598, 1999; Cutis 58:410–412, 1996*

Green hairy tongue

Lichen sclerosus et atrophicus

Papillae, prominent pigmented *AD 95:394–396, 1967*

Physiologic melanin pigmentation *Malays Fam Physician 12:28–29, 2017; Ped Derm 9:123–125, 1992*

Racial variant – tip of tongue with isolated groups of pigmented filiform papillae *Cutis 69:215–217, 2002*

SYNDROMES

Albright's syndrome

Blue rubber bleb nevus syndrome – blue lesions

Carney complex (LAMB, NAME syndrome) *JAAD 10:72–82, 1984*

Dermatopathia pigmentosa reticularis – autosomal dominant; reticulate pigmentation of trunk, neck, and proximal extremities, alopecia, nail changes (mild onychodystrophy), palmoplantar hyperkeratosis, loss of dermatoglyphics, hyperpigmented tongue, hypo– or hyperhidrosis, non–scarring blisters of dorsal hands and feet, dark areolae, thin eyebrows, *Ped Derm 24:566–570, 2007; J Dermatol 24:266–269, 1997; JAAD 26:298–301, 1992; AD 126:935–939, 1990; Dermatol Wochenschr 138:1337, 1958*

Dyskeratosis congenita *AD 133:97–98, 101, 1997*

Laugier–Hunziker syndrome *AD 143:631–633, 2007; JAAD 49:S143–145, 2003; J Eur Acad DV 12:171–173, 1999*

Neurofibromatosis Type I

Peutz–Jegher's syndrome *Ann Plast Surg 36:394–397, 1996*

TOXINS

Lead

Mercury

TONGUE, MULTILOBULATED

AUTOIMMUNE DISEASES AND DISEASES OF IMMUNE DYSFUNCTION

Pemphigus vulgaris – personal observation

Pemphigus vegetans (cerebriform tongue) *Indian Dermatol Online J 11:87–90, 2019; BJD 104:587–591, 1981*

INFECTIONS AND INFESTATIONS

Abscess

Bartonella henselae–related pseudoangiomatous papillomatosis of the tongue accompanying graft vs. host disease; yellow–pink pseudomembranous pedunculated vegetations of the tongue *BJD 157:174–178, 2007*

Botryomycosis *Oral Surg 24:503–509, 1967*

Candida – chronic multifocal oral candidiasis (hyperplastic candidiasis, nodular candidosis) – personal observation

Herpes simplex in acute myelogenous leukemia *JAAD 20:1125–1127, 1989*; herpetic geometric glossitis – personal observation

Histoplasmosis in AIDS *J Dermatol Case Rep 30:25–26, 2013; Cutis 55:104–106, 1995*

Hydatid cyst (*Taenia echinococcus*)

Leishmaniasis – post kala–azar dermal leishmaniasis – tongue nodules *E Afr Med J 63:365–371, 1986*

Leprosy *Int J Dermatol 32:27–29, 2013*

Paracoccidioidomycosis *Dermatol Clin 26:257–269, 2008*

Syphilis – secondary syphilis *JAAD 54:S59–60, 2006;* gumma; interstitial glossitis *Scand J Inf Dis 38:822–825, 2006*

Tuberculosis – multilobulated tongue with ulcers *Clin Inf Dis 52:1231, 1276–1277, 2011*

Yaws – gumma

INFILTRATIVE DISEASES

Amyloidosis – primary systemic – nodules of tongue *JAAD 77:809–830, 2017; AD 126:235–240, 1990; Postgrad Med J 64:696–698, 1988; Clin Exp Dermatol 4:517–536, 1979*

Lipoid proteinosis

Plasma cell orificial mucositis *AD 122:1321–1324, 1986*

INFLAMMATORY DISEASE

Pyostomatitis vegetans

Sarcoid – nodules of central tongue *AD 147:989–991, 2011; Clin Exp Dermatol 17:47–48, 1992*

METABOLIC

Acromegaly

Hypothyroidism (cretinism)

Mucopolysaccaridosis

Pernicious anemia

NEOPLASTIC

Ectomesenchymal chondromyxoid tumor of the anterior tongue *Oral Surg Oral Med Oral Pathol Oral Radiol Endod 82:417–422, 1996; J Oral Pathol Med 25:456–458, 1996*

Chloroma *Ann Hematol 96:883–884, 2017*

Chondromyxoid tumor *Oral Oncol 39:83–86, 2003*

Christoma, lingual

Epidermal nevus *Australas J Dermatol 59:128–130, 2018*

Granular cell tumor (schwannoma)

Kaposi's sarcoma *Int J Dermatol 52:666–672, 2013; Int J Med Sci 8:709–710, 2011*

Keratoacanthomas, eruptive *JAAD 29:299–304, 1993*

Leukemia *JAAD 14:353–358, 1986*

Lymphoma, including cutaneous T–cell lymphoma *JAAD 22:569–577, 1990*

Nevus sebaceous *J Int Oral Health 5:139–142, 2013*

Oral verruciform xanthoma *Med Oral Patol Oral Cir Cuca l23:e429–455, 2018*

Rhabdomyomatous mesenchymal hamartoma – polypoid masses of tongue *Ped Derm 32:256–262, 2015*

Neurilemmoma *Am J Neurol Res 26:421–423, 2005*

Schwannoma *Indian J Dent Res 21:457–459, 2010*

Squamous cell carcinoma *JAAD 12:515–521, 1985*

Verrucous carcinoma

PRIMARY CUTANEOUS DISEASE

Acanthosis nigricans *Syndromes of the Head and Neck, p.355, 1990*

Angiolymphoid hyperplasia *JAAD 11:333–339, 1984*

Crenated tongue

Darier's disease

Fissured tongue *Indian J Dent Res 22:843–846, 2011*

Hypertrophy of circumvallate, foliate, or fungiform papillae

TRAUMA

Tension, scalloped tongue *JAAD 15:1289, 1986*

SYNDROMES

Blue rubber bleb nevus syndrome

Cowden's syndrome – scrotal tongue *JAAD 11:1127–1141, 1984*

Down's syndrome – scrotal tongue

Epidermal nevus syndrome

Focal epithelial hyperplasia (Heck's disease) – HPV 13,14,32,55; Eskimos and South Americans *Ped Derm 26:465–468, 2009; BJD 96:375–380, 1977*

Gardner's syndrome – multiple fibrous tumors

Goltz's syndrome

LAMB syndrome – myxoma *JAAD 10:72–82, 1984*

Maffucci's syndrome – multiple hemangiomas *BJD 99(Suppl 16):31–33, 1978; J Bone Jt Surg 55A:1465–1479, 1973*

Melkersson–Rosenthal syndrome – scrotal tongue; orofacial edema; edema of cheeks, forehead, eyelids, scalp *Oral Surg Oral Med Oral Pathol 75:220–224, 1993; Oral Surg Oral Med Oral Pathol 74:610–619, 1992; JAAD 21:1263–1270, 1989*

Multicentric reticulohistiocytosis *JAAD 20:530–532,535–536, 1989; Oral Surg Oral Med Oral Pathol 65:721–725, 1988*

Multiple mucosal neuroma syndrome (MEN IIB)(Gorlin's syndrome) – skin-colored papules and nodules of lips, tongue, oral mucosa *JAAD 77:809–830, 2017; NEJM 373:756, 2015; AD 139:1647–1652, 2003; JAAD 36:296–300, 1997; Oral Surg 51:516–523, 1981; J Pediatr 86:77–83, 1975; Am J Med 31:163–166, 1961*

Neurofibromatosis *Syndromes of the Head and Neck, p.395, 1990*

Nevus sebaceous syndrome (Schimmelpenning–Feuerstein–Mims syndrome) – papillomas of tongue, gingival hyperplasia, thickened mucosa, anodontia, dysodontia *JAAD 52:S62–64, 2005; Ped Derm 13:22–24, 1996; Int J Oral Maxillofac Surg 12:437–443, 1983*

Oral–facial–digital syndrome type 1(Papillon–Leage–Psaume syndrome) – X–linked dominant; congenital facial milia which resolve with pitted scars; milia of face, scalp, pinnae, and dorsal hands; short stature, hypotrichosis with dry and brittle hair, short upper lip, hypoplastic ala nasi and lower jaw, pseudoclefting of upper lip, hooked pug nose, hypertrophied labial frenulae, bifid or multilobed tongue with small white tumors within clefts, ankyloglossia, multiple soft hamartomas of oral cavity, clefting of hard and soft palate, teeth widely spaced, trident hand or brachydactyly, syndactyly, clinodactyly, ulnar deviation of index finger, or polydactyly; hair dry and brittle, alopecic, numerous milia of face, ears, backs of hands, mental retardation with multiple central nervous system abnormalities, frontal bossing, hypertelorism, telecanthus, broad depressed nasal bridge; polycystic renal disease; combination of polycystic renal disease, milia, and hypotrichosis is highly suggestive of OFD 1 *Ped Derm 27:669–670, 2010; JAAD 59:1050–1063, 2008; Ped Derm 25:474–476, 2008; Ped Derm 9:52–56, 1992; Am J Med Genet 86:269–273, 1999; JAAD 31:157–190, 1994; Ped Derm 9:52–56, 1992; Pediatrics 29:985–995, 1962; Rev Stomatol 55:209–227, 1954*

Oral–facial–digital syndrome type II – autosomal recessive; lobulated, bifid tongue; poly–, syn–, and brachydactyly, cleft palate, broad bifid nasal tip *Genetic Skin Disorders, Second Edition, 2010, pp.264–268; Clin Genet 2:261–266, 1971*

Oral–facial–digital syndrome type III – lobulated hamartomatous tongue, mental retardation, eye abnormalities, dental abnormalities, bifid uvula, skeletal anomalies *Clin Genet 2:248–254, 1971*

Pachyonychia congenita – scrotal tongue

Sjogren's syndrome – scrotal tongue

Werdnig–Hoffmann spinal muscular atrophy

VASCULAR DISORDERS

Arteriovenous malformation – personal observation

Cystic hygroma (macrocystic and microcystic lymphatic malformation) – personal observation

Lymphangioma, lingual cystic *Indian J DV Leprol 76:593, 2010*

Venous malformation *JAAD 56:353–370, 2007*

TONGUE NECROSIS (LINGUAL NECROSIS)

AUTOIMMUNE DISEASES

Lupus erythematosus with anti–phospholipid antibodies *J Clin Rheumatol 21:319, 2015; Am J Ob Gyn 208:e3–4, 2013*

DRUGS

Epirubicin and cyclophosphamide for invasive ductal carcinoma *Mund Kopfer Gesichtschir 7:175–179, 2003*

Ergotamine tartrate–induced vasospasm *J Internal Med 232:541–544, 1992; Eur J Dermatol 9:652–653, 1999; JAMA 225:514–515, 1973*

Intra–arterial chemotherapy – 5 fluorouracil and cisplatin to facial artery for buccal squamous cell carcinoma

Intra-arterial vasopressin therapy

EXOGENOUS AGENTS

Hyaluronic acid chin augmentation *Aesthetic Plast Surg 42:553–559, 2018*

INFECTIONS AND INFESTATIONS

Bite of a fer–de–lance (snake)

Mucormycosis *J Mycol Med 28:519–522, 2018; Br J Oral Maxillofac Surg 50:e96–98, 2012*

Septic shock *BMC Surg 16:48, July 19, 2016*

INFILTRATIVE DISORDERS

Primary systemic amyloid deposition in familial transthyretin amyloidosis *Hum Pathol 42:734–737, 2011*

METABOLIC DISORDERS

Disseminated intravascular coagulation *Int J Oral Maxillofac Surg 37:777–779, 2008*

Essential thrombocytosis (platelet 700Km JAK2V617F mutation)

NEOPLASTIC DISORDERS

Kaposi's sarcoma *Case Rep Infect Dis 2015; 851462*

TRAUMA

Endotracheal tube malpositioning/compression *Asian J Neurosurg 7:214–216, 2012; Laryngoscope 120 Suppl 4:S159, 2010;* prolonged oral intubation *J Surg Case Rep Nov 20, 2019*

Previous radiation of the head and neck *OSOMOPOR 123:e238–232, 2017*

Self–application of rubber band

VASCULAR DISORDERS

Cardiogenic shock with ischemic necrosis of the tongue *J Oral Maxillofacial Surg 60:322–323, 2002*

Carotid artery stenosis with embolic event *J Vasc Surg 54:837–839, 2011*

Carotid artery thrombosis after radiotherapy *Acta Otorinolaringol Esp 58:331–332, 2007*

Cholesterol emboli *Br J Oral Maxillofac Surg 56:340–342, 2018*

Disseminated intravascular coagulation *Int J Oral Maxillofac Surg 37:777–779, 2008*

Giant cell (temporal) arteritis – most common cause of tongue necrosis *Clin Med Insights Case Rep June 20, 2019; NEJM 378:2517, 2018; Rheumatol Int 32:799–800, 2012; Clin Rheumatol 28:S47–49, 2009*

Granulomatosis with polyangiitis

Lingual artery stenosis, bilateral – complication of chemoradiotherapy *Eur Ann Otorhinolaryngol Head Neck Dis 134:269–271, 2017*

Necrotizing vasculitis *J Otolaryngol Head Neck Surg 41:E38–40, 2012*

Polyarteritis nodosa *Br J Oral Maxillofac Surg 53:883–885, 2015; Acta Ped 84:1333–1336, 1993*

TONGUE NODULES, SOLITARY

Cutis 75:277, 2005

Angiosarcoma

Granular cell schwannoma

Intramuscular hemangioma

Lipomas

Liposarcomas

Malignant endovascular papillary angioendothelioma (Dabska tumor)

Rhabdomyomas

Thyroglossal duct cysts

TONGUE, RED

AUTOIMMUNE DISEASES AND DISEASES OF IMMUNE DYSFUNCTION

Allergic contact dermatitis – toothpaste *Contact Derm 33:100–103, 1995*

Dermatomyositis

Graft vs. host reaction *Am J Clin Dermatol 19:33–50, 2018; OSOMOP 66:130–138, 1988*

Scleroderma

Sjogren's syndrome – red, smooth, dry tongue

DRUG–INDUCED

Acute generalized exanthematous pustulosis – red tongue with pustules *NEJM 372:161, 2015*

Antibiotics

Anticholinergics

Chemotherapy

Drug rash

Hydroxyurea *Clin Exp Derm 26:141–148, 2001*

Interleukin–2 *JAMA 258:1624–1629, 1987*

Taxotere mucositis – personal observation

EXOGENOUS AGENTS

Mouthwash

Reverse smoking

INFECTIONS AND INFESTATIONS

Candidiasis – acute atrophic oral candidiasis *Am J Med 30:28–33, 1984; Candida* in psoriasis *JAAD 68:986–991, 2013*

Ebola virus hemorrhagic fever (Filovirus) – dark red discoloration of soft palate, pharyngitis, oral ulcers, glossitis, gingivitis; morbilliform exanthem which becomes purpuric with desquamation of palms and soles; high fever, body aches, myalgia, arthralgias, prostration, abdominal pain, watery diarrhea; disseminated intravascular coagulation *Int J Dermatol 51:1037–1043, 2012; JAMA 287:2391–2002; Int J Dermatol 51:1037–1043, 2012; JAAD 65:1213–1218, 2011; MMWR 44, No.19, 382, 1995*

Herpes simplex – herpetic geometric glossitis *South Med J 89:1231–1235, 1995*

HIV infection – acute retroviral syndrome – glossitis

Recurrent toxin–mediated perineal erythema – associated with pharyngitis due to *Staphylococcus aureus* or *Streptococcus pyogenes AD 144:2390243, 2008; AD 132:57060, 1996*

Scarlet fever – white or red strawberry tongue *JAAD 39:383–398, 1998*

Syphilis – secondary, tertiary (syphilitic atrophic glossitis) – red, smooth tongue with loss of papillae; plaques en prairie fauchee *Infect Dis Cases Dec 29, 2018; Case Rep Emerg Med 2016:1607583*

Toxic shock syndrome, either staphylococcal or streptococcal *JAAD 39:383–398, 1998*

INFILTRATIVE DISEASES

Amyloidosis, primary systemic – red nodule *AD 126:235–240, 1990*

INFLAMMATORY DISEASES

Acrodermatitis continua of Hallopeau *JAAD Case Rep 3:215–218, 2017*

Crohn's disease – glossitis

Eruptive lingual papillitis – tongue papules composed of fungiform papillae of tip and side of tongue *BJD 150:299–303, 2004*

Erythema multiforme major (Stevens–Johnson syndrome)

Foliate papillitis

Impetigo herpetiformis

Median rhomboid glossitis (central papillary atrophy) – possibly related to candidiasis *BJD 93:399–405, 1975*

METABOLIC DISEASES

Acrodermatitis enteropathica *Cutis 81:314, 324–326, 2008*

Celiac disease

Deficiency states
  Folic acid deficiency – glossitis *JAAD 12:914–917, 1985*
  Iron deficiency anemia *QJM 34:145, 1965;* Plummer Vinson syndrome
  Kwashiorkor *Cutis 51:445–446, 1993*
  Plummer–Vinson syndrome *AD 105:720, 1972*
  Protein deficiency – kwashiorkor *Cutis 67:321–327, 2001 ; Cutis 51:445–446, 1993*
  Sprue
  Tryptophan
  Vitamin B complex deficiencies
  Vitamin B1 deficiency (thiamine) – beriberi; edema, burning red tongue, vesicles of oral mucosa
  Vitamin B6 *Ped Derm 16:95–102, 1999; Clinics in Derm 17:457–461, 1999*
  Vitamin B12 deficiency (pernicious anemia, sprue) – enlarged red tongue *Cutis 71:127–130, 2003; AD 122:896–899, 1986;* linear erosions of lateral or dorsal tongue; linear erosions of hard and soft palate *JAAD 60:498–500, 2009;* Hunter's glossitis (Moeller's glossitis) – beefy red tongue with atrophy of lingual papillae *Ped Derm 35:796–799, 2018; JAAD 60:498–500, 2009*
  Niacin (Vitamin B3) (pellagra) – glossitis and glossodynia
  Nicotinic acid
  Pantothenic acid
  Pyridoxine
  Riboflavin (Vitamin B2) – smooth magenta glossitis *Ped Derm 16:95–102, 1999; JAAD 21:1–30, 1989*
  Thiamine

Zinc deficiency

Fucosidosis – autosomal recessive; angiokeratoma corporis diffusum with tongue lesions *J R Soc Med 87:707, 1994*

Liver disease

Malabsorption

Thalassemia trait – atrophic glossitis *J Formos Med Assoc 112:761–765, 2013*

Uremic glossitis

NEOPLASTIC DISORDERS

Erythroplasia, oral – underside of tongue, floor of mouth, soft palate *J Oral Pathol 12:11–29, 1983*

Kaposi's sarcoma *Case Rep Infect Dis 2015;851462*

Polycythemia vera *Postgrad Med J 70:768–769, 1994;* familial polycythemia vera – beefy red tongue *Hematol Rep 4:e02, 2012*

PARANEOPLASTIC DISORDERS

Glucagonoma syndrome – necrolytic migratory erythema; cheilitis and painful glossitis *JAMADerm 155:1180, 2019; JAAD 65:458–459, 2011; Int J Dermatol 49:24–29, 2010; JAAD 54:745–762, 2006; J Eur Acad Dermatol 18:591–595, 2004; JAAD 12:1032–1039, 1985*

Hypertrichosis lanuginosa acquisita (malignant down) – 41 cases; lung, colon carcinomas most common; also breast, gall bladder, uterus, urinary bladder; if accompanied by acanthosis nigricans; the malignancy is always an adenocarcinoma; hypertrophy of tongue papillae and glossitis often present; usually metastatic disease present at the time of diagnosis of hypertrichosis lanuginosa *JAMADerm 155:1180, 2019; Int J Dermatol 49:24–29, 2010; BJD 157:1087–1092, 2007; JAAD 56:S45–47, 2007; JAAD 54:745–762, 2006; J Surg Oncol 68:199–203, 1998; AD 122:805–808, 1986; AD 106:84, 1972; Med Times Gazette 2:507, 1865*

PRIMARY CUTANEOUS DISEASES

Geographic tongue (migratory glossitis)
   Atopic dermatitis *BJD 101:159–162, 1979*
   Diabetes mellitus *Oral Surg Oral Med Oral Pathol 63:68–70, 1987*
   Down's syndrome *Clin Genet 50:317–320, 1996*
   Fetal hydantoin syndrome *Ped Derm 6:130–133, 1989*
   Hereditary *Am J Hum Genet 24:124–133, 1972*
   Lichen planus *J Oral Med 29:58–59, 1974*
   Lithium carbonate *J Am Acad Child Adolesc Psychiatry 38:1069–1070, 1999; Int J Derm 31:368–369, 1992*
   Oral contraceptives *Br Dent J 171:94–96, 1991*
   Pustular bacterid of Andrews *Med Cutan Ibero Lat Am 3:453–458, 1975*
   Pustular psoriasis *AD 107:240–244, 1973*
   Reactive arthritis syndrome *AD 107:240–244, 1973*
Lichen planus, including atrophic and erosive lichen planus –
Plasma cell glossitis

SYNDROMES

Brook's disease

Dyskeratosis congenita

Hartnup's disease – red and inflamed tongue

Hereditary hemorrhagic telangiectasia – red papules of tongue with hemiparesis *NEJM 381:2552, 2019; JAMA 312:741–742, 2014; Cutis 80:109:121–122, 2007*

Hereditary mucoepithelial dysplasia *Ped Derm 11:133–138, 1994*

Ichthyosis follicularis with atrichia and photophobia (IFAP) – beefy red tongue; collodion membrane and erythema at birth; ichthyosis, spiny (keratotic) follicular papules (generalized follicular keratoses), non–scarring alopecia, keratotic papules of elbows, knees, fingers, extensor surfaces, xerosis; punctate keratitis, photophobia; nail dystrophy, psychomotor delay, short stature; enamel dysplasia, red gingiva, angular stomatitis, atopy, lamellar scales, psoriasiform plaques, palmoplantar erythema *Curr Prob Derm 14:71–116, 2002; JAAD 46:S156–158, 2002; BJD 142:157–162, 2000; Am J Med Genet 85:365–368, 1999; Ped Derm 12:195, 1995; AD 125:103–106, 1989; Dermatologica 177:341–347, 1988*

IgG4 disease (Mikulicz's syndrome) – personal observation

Kawasaki's disease – strawberry tongue; macular, morbilliform, urticarial, scarlatiniform, erythema multiforme–like pustular, erythema marginatum–like exanthems; non–suppurative conjunctivitis; cheilitis; edematous hands with lamellar desquamation; myocarditis and coronary artery thrombosis and aneurysms; arthralgia, arthritis *NEJM 373:467, 2015; JAAD 69:501–510, 2013; JAAD 39:383–398, 1998; Jpn J Allergol 16:178–222, 1967*

Progressive symmetric erythrokeratoderma

Recalcitrant erythematous desquamating (RED) syndrome – diffuse macular erythema, ocular and mucosal erythema, strawberry tongue, delayed desquamation in the setting of AIDS *JAAD 39:383–398, 1998*

Reactive arthritis syndrome *Semin Arthritis Rheum 3:253–286, 1974*

Riley–Day syndrome – strawberry tongue

TOXINS

Thallium – anagen effluvium *JAAD 50:258–261, 2004;* nausea, vomiting, stomatitis, painful glossitis, diarrhea; severe dysesthesias and paresthesias in distal extremities, facial rashes of cheeks and perioral region, acneiform eruptions of face, hyperkeratosis of palms and soles, hair loss, Mees' lines *AD 143:93–98, 2007*

Vitamin A intoxication

TRAUMA

Mouth breathing

VASCULAR DISEASES

Hemangioma *Clin Nucl Med 11:113–114, 1986*

Klippel–Trenaunay–Weber syndrome Temporal arteritis – glossitis; red tongue with blisters, desquamation, or necrosis *BJD 76:299–308, 1964*

Vascular malformation

TONGUE, SCROTAL (PLICATED TONGUE, FISSURED TONGUE)

AUTOIMMUNE DISORDERS

Pemphigus vegetans – cerebriform tongue *Indian Dermatol Online J 11:87–90, 2020*

CONGENITAL DISORDERS

Pure 15q deletion *Genet Counsel 27:1–8, 2016*

DRUGS

Tacrolimus, systemic

INFECTIONS AND INFESTATIONS

Herpes simplex – herpetic geometric glossitis (linear tongue fissures in HIV, other immunosuppressed patients); mimics scrotal tongue *JAAD 61:139–142, 2009; Am J Clin Oncol 20:567–568, 1997; South Med J 88:1231–1235, 1995; NEJM 329:1859–1860, 1993*

Tertiary syphilis

Trichinellosis – fissured ulcerated tongue *Clin Inf Dis 55:981–1022–1023, 2012*

METABOLIC DISORDERS

Acromegaly *Cutis 98:175–178, 2016*

Pernicious anemia *Clinics Dermatol 34:458–469, 2016*

NEOPLASTIC DISORDERS

Multiple myeloma – fissured tongue in 10% *Hematol Transfus Cell Ther May 15, 2019*

PARANEOPLASTIC DISORDERS

Hypertrichosis lanuginosa acquisita (malignant down) – 41 cases; lung, colon carcinomas most common; also breast, gall bladder, uterus, urinary bladder; if accompanied by acanthosis nigricans; the malignancy is always an adenocarcinoma; hypertrophy of tongue papillae and glossitis often present; usually metastatic disease present at the time of diagnosis of hypertrichosis lanuginosa *BJD 157:1087–1092, 2007; JAAD 56:S45–47, 2007; J Surg Oncol 68:199–203, 1998; AD 122:805–808, 1986; AD 106:84, 1972; Med Times Gazette 2:507, 1865*

Malignant acanthosis nigricans – verrucous papules at corners of mouth *Cutis 89:14–16, 2012*

PRIMARY CUTANEOUS DISEASES

Folliculitis spinulosa decalvans *Cutis 98:175–178, 2016*

Normal variant – 5% general population *Proc Finn Dent Soc 81:104–110, 1985;* age related *Swiss Dent J 126:886–897, 2016*

Psoriasis *JAAD 78:413–414, 2018;* pustular psoriasis *AD 129:1346, 1993; BJD 91:419–424, 1974*

SYNDROMES

Bazex–Dupre–Christol syndrome – congenital hypotrichosis, follicular atrophoderma, basal cell nevi and basal cell carcinomas, facial milia, hypohidrosis, pinched nose with hypoplastic alae, atopy with comedones, keratosis pilaris, joint hypermobility, scrotal tongue, hyperpigmentation of the forehead *BJD 153:682–684, 2005; Dermatol Surg 26:152–154, 2000; Hautarzt 44:385–391, 1993*

Coffin–Lowry syndrome *J Clin Diagn Res 7:1264–1265, 2019*

Cowden's syndrome *Int J Dermatol 51:1494–1499, 2012; JAAD 11:1127–1141, 1984*

Down's syndrome *Cutis 98:175–178, 2016; Ped Derm 24:317–320, 2007*

Goldenhaar syndrome *J Coll Physicians Surg Pak 29:1108–1110, 2019*

ECC syndrome *J Clin Diagn Res 7:1264–1265, 2019*

Fraser's syndrome *J Clin Diagn Res 7:1264–1265, 2019*

Hereditary mucoepithelial dysplasia (dyskeratosis)(Gap junction disease, Witkop disease) – autosomal dominant; fissured tongue; non–scarring alopecia; dry rough skin; red eyes, non–scarring alopecia, follicular keratosis (keratosis pilaris), erythema of oral (hard palate, gingival, tongue) and nasal mucous membranes, cervix, vagina, and urethra; perineal and perigenital psoriasiform dermatitis (perineal erythema); hyperpigmented hyperkeratotic lesions of flexures (neck, antecubital and popliteal fossae); esophageal stenosis; keratitis (visual impairment) increased risk of infections, fibrocystic lung disease *Ped Derm 29:311–315, 2012; BJD 153:310–318, 2005; Ped Derm 11:133–138, 1994; Am J Med Genet 39:338–341, 1991; JAAD 21:351–357, 1989; Am J Hum Genet 31:414–427, 1979; Oral Surg Oral Med Oral Pathol 46:645–657, 1978*

HOPP syndrome – hypotrichosis, striate, reticulated pitted palmo-plantar keratoderma, acro–osteolysis, psoriasiform plaques, lingua plicata, onychogryphosis, ventricular arrhythmias, periodontitis *BJD 150:1032–1033, 2004; BJD 147:575–581, 2002*

Hyper IgE syndrome *J Clin Diagn Res 10:2004–2005, 2016; Indian J Dermatol 60:324, 2015*

Maroteaux–Lamy syndrome *J Clin Diagn Res 7:1264–1265, 2019*

Melkersson–Rosenthal syndrome – scrotal tongue; orofacial edema; edema of cheeks, forehead, eyelids, scalp *Cutis 98:175–178, 2016; Oral Surg Oral Med Oral Pathol 75:220–224, 1993; Oral Surg Oral Med Oral Pathol 74:610–619, 1992; JAAD 21:1263–1270, 1989*

Moebius syndrome *Int J Ped Dent 12:446–449, 2002*

Mohr syndrome (OFD type II) *J Clin Diagn Res 7:1264–1265, 2019*

Oral–facial–digital (OFD) syndrome type 1 *J Clin Diagn Res 7:1264–1265, 2019*

Pachyonychia congenita *Eur J Dermatol 22:476–480, 2012*

Pierre–Robin syndrome *J Clin Diagn Res 7:1264–1265, 2019*

Rabson–Mendenhall syndrome – fissured tongue *Ped Derm 19:267–270, 2002*

Rapp–Hodgkin syndrome *J Indian Soc Pedod Prev Dent 34:192–195, 2016*

Sjogren's syndrome *Cutis 98:175–178, 2016*

Stuve–Wiedemann syndrome – clefted tongue and multiple eruptive vellus hair cysts *Ped Derm 37:381–382, 2020*

TONGUE, ULCERS

AUTOIMMUNE DISEASES AND DISEASES OF IMMUNE DYSFUNCTION

Allergic contact dermatitis – Balsam of Peru in diet cola; painful tongue ulcerations *Ear Nose Throat J 86:232–233, 2007*

Bullous pemphigoid – anti–p200 bullous pemphigoid *JAMADerm 152:897–904, 2016*

Cicatricial pemphigoid (mucous membrane pemphigoid) – desquamative gingivitis *BJD 174:436–438, 2016; NEJM 369:265–274, 2013; AD 138:370–379, 2002; JAAD 43:571–591, 2000; J Periodontol 71:1620–1629, 2000*

Dermatomyositis *Ryumachi 39:836–840, 1999;* anti–MDA5 dermatomyositis *JAAD 78:776–785, 2018*

Epidermolysis bullosa acquisita – personal observation

Good syndrome – adult acquired primary immunodeficiency in context of past or current thymoma; tongue ulcers; sinopulmonary infections; lichen planus, oral lichen planus of tongue, gingivitis *BJD 172:774–777, 2015; Am J Med Genet 66:378–398, 1996*

Graft vs. host disease *Aust NZ J Med 16:239–240, 1986*

Lichenoid reactions with antibodies to desmoplakins I and II – ulcers of hard palate and tongue *JAAD 48:433–438, 2003*

Linear IgA disease

Lupus erythematosus – systemic lupus with antiphospholipid antibodies – tongue necrosis *J Rheumatol 15:1281–1283, 1988;* DLE, bullous LE – personal observation

Pemphigus vegetans *Int J Dermatol 52:350–351, 2013*

Pemphigus vulgaris *J Dermatol Case 8:55–57, 2014; Indian J DV Leprol 67:267, 2001; JAAD 38:860–861, 1998*

CONGENITAL

Congential agranulocytosis (Kostman) *Dent Update 43:194–195, 2016*

Congenital vesicular and erosive dermatosis with supple and reticulated scarring – tongue erosions *JAAD 69:909–915, 2013; AD 121:361–367, 1985*

DRUGS

Alendronate *J Oral Pathol Med 29:514–518, 2000*

Aspirin *J Am Dent Assoc 91:130, 1975*

Bisphosphonate – heart-shaped tongue ulcer *J Dent Sci 13:182–183, 2018*

Captopril *AD 118:959, 1982*

Carbamazepine *An Otorhinolaringol Ibero Am 25:167–l71, 1998*

Chemotherapy mucositis – personal observation

Docataxel mucositis – personal observation

Ergotamine tartrate – tongue necrosis *Schweiz Med Wochenschr 19:1152–1156, 2000;* in temporal arteritis *AD 130:261–262, 1994*

Gold *Parodontol Stomalol (Nuova) 23:23–25, 1984*

Inhalers for respiratory disease *Br Dent J 182:350–352, 1997*

Iododerma – due to computed tomography scans; large ulcers on underside of tongue; red papules and plaques *J Drugs in Dermatol 12:574–576, 2013*

Intraarterial chemotherapy – 5–fluorouracil and cisplatin; tongue necrosis *Otolaryngology 121:655–657, 1999*

Methotrexate

Nicorandil *BJD 151:939–940, 2004; Oral Surg Oral Med Oral Pathol Oral Radiol Endod 91:189–193, 2001*

Opioids, sublingual injection *Med Org 19:212–215, 2004*

Pembrolizumab–induced mucous membrane pemphigoid – tongue ulcers, oral ulcers *BJD 179:993–994, 2018*

Retinoic acid syndrome *Int J Dermatol 53:912–916, 2014*

Stomatitis medicamentosa

Taxotere mucositis – personal observation

EXOGENOUS AGENTS

Ecstasy *J Craniofac Surg 30:e189–191, 2019*

Eugenol

INFECTIONS AND INFESTATIONS

Actinomycosis – *Actinomyces naeslundii Clin Inf Dis 64:370,384–385, 2017;* Actinomycosis *Otolaryngol Pol 53:103–104, 2001*

AIDS – giant aphthous ulcers

Aspergillosis *Mycoses 37:209–215, 1994*

Candida *NEJM 362:740–748, 2010*

Chancriform pyoderma *BJD 133:326–327, 1995*

Coccidioidomycosis

Cowpox – tongue ulcer, targetoid and umbilicated indurated papules, vesicles, pustules with central necrosis; exposure to pet rat *Clin Inf Dis 68:1063–1064, 2019*

Cryptococcosis *J Oral Maxillofac Surg 50:759–760, 1992*

Cytomegalovirus *AD 145:931–936, 2009; Otolaryngol Head Neck Surg 110:463–464, 1994;* CMV and HSV coinfected oral ulcers in HIV–positive patients *Oral Surg Oral Med Oral Pathol Oral Radiol Endod 81:55–62, 1996*

Epstein–Barr virus *Human Pathol 59:147–151, 2017*

Exanthem subitum – human herpesvirus 6 – uvulo–palatoglossal junctional ulcers *J Clin Virol 17:83–90, 2000; Med J Malaysia 54:32–36, 1999;*

Geotrichosis (Geotrichium candidum) *Oral Surg 73:726–728, 1992*

Gonococcemia *Br J Ven Dis 45:228–231, 1969*

Hand, foot, and mouth disease *Oral Surg Oral Med Oral Pathol 41:333, 1976*

Herpes simplex *NEJM 362:740–748, 2010; Cutis 83:181, 185–186, 2009; NEJM 329:1859–1860, 1993;* in acute myelogenous leukemia *JAAD 20:1125–1127, 1989;* herpetic geometric glossitis; in AIDS *Clin Dermatol 38:160–175, 2020*

Herpes zoster – Ramsay–Hunt syndrome *Clin Inf Dis 51:77–78,111–113, 2010;* herpes zoster mandibularis *NEJM 375:369, 2016*

Histoplasmosis *Clin Dermatol 38:152–159, 2020; JAAD 56:871–873, 2007; J Laryngol Otol 107:58–61, 1993; Oral Surg Oral Med Oral Pathol 70:631–636, 1990; Singapore Med J 31:286–288, 1990; Br J Oral Surg 16:234–240, 1979*

HIV disease – major aphthae *Oral Surg Oral Med Oral Pathol 71:68, 1991*

Leishmaniasis *Transpl Infect Dis 13:397–406, 2011*

Lymphogranuloma venereum *Sex Transm Infect 95:169–170, 2019*

Mycobacterium tuberculosis – primary lingual TB *NEJM 362:740–748, 2010; J Laryngol Otol 112:86–87, 1998;* tuberculosis cutis orificialis (acute tuberculous ulcer) – tongue ulcer *JAMA 235:2418, 1976;* tongue ulcer as first clinical sign of asymptomatic pulmonary TB *Gen Dent 48:458–461, 2000; J Infect 39:163–164, 1999; Cutis 60:201–202, 1997; Clin Inf Dis 19:200–202, 1994; BMC Oral Health 19:67, 2019;* mimicking squamous cell carcinoma *Indian J Tuberc 65:84–86, 2018*

Necrotizing bacterial infection

Non–tuberculous mycobacteria *NEJM 362:740–748, 2010*

Paracoccidioidomycosis *Mycopatholgia 177:325–329, 2014; J Clin Inf Dis 23:1026–1032, 1996*

Parvovirus B19 *Ann DV 123:735–738, 1996;* bullous papular–purpuric gloves and socks syndrome with aphthae of tongue *JAAD 60:691–695, 2009*

Pyoderma gangrenosum *Br J Oral Maxillofac surg 23:247–250, 1985*

Streptococcal gingivostomatitis

Syphilis – primary – chancre *NEJM 362:740–748, 2010; Rev Stomatol Chir Maxillofac 85:391–398, 1984;* secondary, tertiary *JAAD 49:749–751, 2003;* sublingual ulcer *NEJM 362:740–748, 2010;*

Otolaryngol Head Neck Surg 119:399–402, 1998; tertiary *Actas Dermatosifiliogr 69:145–148, 1978*

Trichinellosis – fissured ulcerated tongue *Clin Inf Dis 55:981–1022–1023, 2012*

Varicella – personal observation

Yaws

Zygomycosis *Lancet 336:282–284, 1991*

INFILTRATIVE DISEASES

Amyloidosis *OSOMOPOR Endod 108:e46–50, 2009*

Langerhans cell histiocytosis

INFLAMMATORY DISORDERS

Cancrum oris *JAAD 64:1200–1202, 2011*

Crohn's disease *NEJM 362:740–748, 2010*

Eosinophilic ulcer of the lip, tongue, or buccal mucosa *AD 137:815–820, 2001; Clin Exp Dermatol 22:154–156, 1997; Cutis 57:349–351, 1996; JAAD 33:734–740, 1995; Cutis 43:357–359, 1989*

Erythema multiforme, including Stevens–Johnson syndrome *NEJM 362:740–748, 2010*

Lethal midline granuloma

Lymphocytoma *J Contemp Dent Pract 15:111–119, 2005*

Malacoplakia *Palaminerva Med 44:159–161, 2002*

Periadenitis mucosae necrotica recurrens (Sutton's disease) *AD 133:1161–1166, 1997*

Malignant pyoderma – papulopustules, skin ulcers, violaceous nodules with central necrosis, tongue, pharyngeal, and nasal ulcers *AD 146:102–104, 2010; AD 98:561–576, 1968* Pyoderma gangrenosum *Br J Oral Maxillofac Surg 23:247–250, 1985*

Pyostomatitis vegetans – in ulcerative colitis *J Oral Maxillofac Pathol 22:199–203, 2018*

Sarcoid *NEJM 362:740–748, 2010*

Toxic epidermal necrolysis

METABOLIC DISEASES

Calciphylaxis – tongue necrosis *J Oral Maxillofac Surg 55:193–196, 1997*

Glycogen storage disease *Eur J Ped Dent 7:192–198, 2006*

Neutropenia or agranulocytosis *J Periodontol 58:51–55, 1987*

Pellagra – swollen red tongue with erosions and furrows *BJD 164:1188–1200, 2011*

NEOPLASTIC DISEASES

Atypical histiocytic granuloma – may be same as eosinophilic ulcer of the oral mucosa *BMJ Case Rep June 3, 2013; J Oral Maxillofac Surg 48:630–633, 1990*

Benign lymphoid hyperplasia – painless ulcer *J Contemp Dent Pract 15:111–119, 2005*

Foramen magnum meningioma – oral ulcers *Oral Surg Oral Med Oral Pathol Oral Radiol Endod 90:609–611, 2000*

Granular cell tumor

Keratoacanthoma – multiple eruptive keratoacanthomas of Grzybowski

Leiomyosarcoma *AME Case Rep April 18, 2018*

Leukemia cutis – HTLV–1 leukemia/lymphoma – ulcers of lips, hard palate, tongue *AD 146:804–805, 2010;* acute myelogenous leukemia – personal observation

Lymphoma – systemic lymphoma *NEJM 362:740–748, 2010;* CD8+ cutaneous T–cell lymphoma *Am J Dermatopathol 17:287–291, 1995;* cutaneous T–cell lymphoma *Oral Surg Oral Med Oral Pathol 57:267, 1984;* natural killer T–cell lymphoma *Ann Otol Rhinolaryngol 114:55–57, 2005*

Lymphomatoid papulosis *Dermatology 210:53–57, 2005; Oral Surg Oral Med Oral Pathol Oral Radiol Endod 90:195–204, 2000*

Meningioma – of foramen magnum *OSOMOPORE 90:609–611, 2000*

Metastases – small cell carcinoma; tongue necrosis *Otolaryngology 1995:782–784*

Minor salivary gland tumor *NEJM 362:740–748, 2010*

Monoclonal plasmacytic ulcerative stomatitis *Oral Surg Oral Med Oral Pathol 75:483–487, 1993*

Mucoepidermoid carcinoma

Squamous cell carcinoma *Gen Dent 67:e6–8, 2019; NEJM 362:740–748, 2010; JAAD 12:515, 1988*

PARANEOPLASTIC DISEASES

Paraneoplastic pemphigus *BJD 176:824–826, 2017; BJD 160:468–470, 2009; AD 141:1285–1293, 2005*

PRIMARY CUTANEOUS DISEASES

Aphthosis *NEJM 362:740–748, 2010; Dent Update 19:353, 1992*

Hailey–Hailey disease

Hydroa vacciniforme *Ped Derm 21:555–557, 2004*

Lichen planus *NEJM 362:740–748, 2010; JAAD 46:35–41, 2002; J Oral Maxillofac Surg 50:116–118, 1992*

Median rhomboid glossitis *BJD 93:399, 1975*

Necrotizing sialometaplasia

Pityriasis rosea *AD 121:14491451, 1985*

Submucous fibrosis of tongue *Indian J DV Leprol 75:56–59, 2009*

PSYCHOCUTANEOUS DISORDERS

Factitial *JAAD 17:339–341, 1987*

SYNDROMES

Behcet's disease *Bratisl Lek Listy 106:386–389, 2005*

Congenital insensitivity to pain – ulcers of fingers, lips, tongue, excoriations of face *BJD 179:1135–1140,2018*

Dyskeratosis congenita – X–linked *Ann Stomatol (Roma) 4(suppl 2)5–6, 2013*

Hypereosinophilic syndrome *AD 132:535–541, 1996; Ann Int Med 121:648, 1994*

Hyper IgM syndrome (hypogammaglobulinemia with hyper IgM)– X–linked with mutation in CD40 ligand gene; low IgA and IgG; sarcoid–like granulomas; multiple papulonodules of face, buttocks, arms *Ped Derm 21:39–43, 2004; Ped Derm 18:48–50, 2001*

Lesch–Nyan syndrome *J Clin Ped Dent 38:247–249, 2014*

Lipoid proteinosis *JAMADerm 155:977–979, 2019; JAAD 39:149–171, 1998*

MAGIC syndrome *AJM 79:65–71, 1985*

Obstructive sleep apnea syndrome *Br J Oral Maxillofac Surg 30:263–267, 1992*

Pyoderma gangrenosum–Trisomy 8–myelodysplastic syndrome – scrotal ulcers, tongue ulcers *BJD 174:239–241, 2016*

Reactive arthritis syndrome*; Semin Arthritis Rheum 3:253–286, 1974*

Sweet's syndrome *BMJ Casse Rep March 15, 2017*

Xeroderma pigmentosum – squamous cell carcinoma *JAAD 12:515–521, 1985*

TRAUMA

Chemical burn – ferrous sulfate tablets *Dent Update 33:632–633, 2006;* peppermint oil burn *Otolaryngol Head Neck Surg 133:801–802, 2005;* sodium hydroxide drain cleaner *Vet Hum Toxicol 46:319–321, 2009*

Congenital insensitivity to pain (analgesia congenita) *Int J Paediatr Dent 6:117–122, 1996*

Decubital lingual ulcers in myoclonus *ASDC J Dent Child 65:474–477, 438, 1998*

Electrical burn *Int J Pediatr Otorhinolaryngol 77:1325–1328, 2013*

Embolization of cavernous hemangioma – tongue necrosis

Epilepsy

Intubation – pressure necrosis *Anesthetis 24:136–137, 1975*

Mechanical *NEJM 362:740–748, 2010*

Neonatal sublingual traumatic ulceration (Riga–Fede disease) – natal or neonatal teeth with tongue ulceration; ulcer on underside of tongue due to rubbing on tooth *Ped Derm 26:640–641, 2009; Turk J Pediatr 41:113–116, 1999; Aust Dent J 42:225–227, 1997;* large ulcer *JAAD 77:445–447, 2002*

Paraquat poisoning *BMJ Case Rep Oct 21, 2014*

Phenol burn

Radiation glossitis

Self–application of rubber band *Br J Surg 62:956, 1975*

Surgery Thermal

Tongue biting

Traumatic eosinophilic ulcer of the tongue

Traumatic ulcerative granuloma with stromal eosinophilia *World J Surg Oncol 17:184, 2019;* self-healing CD30+T clonal proliferation of tongue *BMC Oral Health 19:186, 2019*

VASCULAR DISORDERS

Arteriosclerosis – tongue necrosis *Oral Surg Oral Med Oral Pathol 89:316–318, 2000*

Granulomatosis with polyangiitis *NEJM 362:740–748, 2010; Br J Clin Pract 46:268–269, 1992*

Necrotizing vasculitis in HIV *Schweiz Monatsschr Zahnmed 105:54–62, 1995*

Polyarteritis nodosa – tongue necrosis *Acta Pediatr 84:1333–1336, 1995*

Temporal arteritis (giant cell arteritis) – tongue necrosis *NEJM 378:2517, 2018; BJD 151:721–722, 2004; Oral Surg 74:582–586, 1992; Acta Med Scand 220:379–380, 1986; JAAD 6:1081–1088, 1982; BJD 76:299–308, 1964;* headache, loss of vision, tender temporal artery, muscle or joint pain, malaise, weight loss, loss of appetite, jaw claudication, tongue necrosis, absent temporal pulses; scalp necrosis *JAAD 61:701–706, 2009; AD 143:1079–1080, 2007; Clin Rheumatol 26:1169, 2007; Arthritis Rheum 42:1296, 1999; BJD 120:843–846, 1989; Q J Med 15:47–75, 1946;* gangrene of leg

TRICHOMEGALY

AUTOIMMUNE DISEASES AND DISORDERS OF IMMUNE DYSREGULATION

Allergic diseases – children *Ped Derm 21:534–537, 2004*

Alopecia areata *Ped Derm 26:188–193, 2009*

Dermatomyositis *BJD 174:741–752, 2016; Ped Derm 29:234–235, 2012; Dermatology 205:305, 2002*

Lupus erythematosus, systemic *Int J Trichology 9:79–81, 2017; BJD 174:741–752, 2016; Ped Derm 29:234–235, 2012; Clin Rheumatol 19:245–246, 2000*

DEGENERATIVE DISORDERS

Cataract and spherocytosis *Am J Ophthalmol 73:333–335, 1972;*Vitreochorioretinal degeneration *Ann Ophthalmol 8:811–815, 1976*

DRUGS

Bimatoprost *BJD 174:741–752, 2016; JAAD 51:S77–78, 2004*

Cetuximab (epidermal growth factor receptor inhibitor) – facial, eyelash, eyebrow hypertrichosis *JAAD 80:1179–1196, 2019; BJD 174:741–752, 2016; Supportive Care Cancer 21:1167–1174, 2013; BJD 161:515–521, 2009; JAAD 58:545–570, 2008; AD 142:1656–1657, 2006; Ann Oncol 16:1711–1712, 2005; Clin Oncol 17:492–493, 2005; BJD 151:1111–1112, 2004*

Cyclosporin A *BJD 174:741–752, 2016; JAAD 70:821–838, 2014; Nephrol Dial Transplant 11:1159–1161, 1996; Am J Ophthalmol 109:293–294, 1990*

Drug–induced – benoxaprofen, corticosteroids, cyclosporine *Ann Ophthalmol 24:465–469, 1992; Nephrol Dial Transplant 11:1159–1161, 1996;* diazoxide, interferon alpha *Lancet 359, 1107, March, 2002; J Interferon Cytokine Res 20:633–634, 2000; Eye 13:241–246, 1999;* latanaprost *Cutis 67:109–110, 2001; Clin and Exp Ophthalmol 29:272–273, 2001;* cetuximab *AD 142:248, 2006;* minoxidil, penicillamine, phenytoin, psoralen, streptomycin; zidovudine *AD 142:248, 2006;* acetazolamide, cetuximab, geftinib, panitumumab, tacrolimus *Ped Derm 26:188–193, 2009; Indian J Dermatol 60:378–380, 2015*

Dovitinib (selective pan–FGF–R inhibitor) – onycholysis, trichomegaly, straightening of scalp hair, hyperkeratosis of heels, xerostomia *JAMADerm 153:723–725, 2017*

Drug–induced – benoxaprofen, corticosteroids, cyclosporine *Ann Ophthalmol 24:465–469, 1992; Nephrol Dial Transplant 11:1159–1161, 1996;* diazoxide, interferon alpha *Lancet 359, 1107, March, 2002; J Interferon Cytokine Res 20:633–634, 2000; Eye 13:241–246, 1999;* latanaprost *Cutis 67:109–110, 2001; Clin and Exp Ophthalmol 29:272–273, 2001;* minoxidil, penicillamine, phenytoin, psoralen, streptomycin, zidovudine; cetuximab and erlotinib (epidermal growth factor receptor inhibitor) – excessive curling and growth of eyebrows and eyelashes *JAAD 56:317–326, 2007; JAAD 55:657–670, 2006; JAAD 55:429–437, 2006; Acta Oncol 42:345–346, 2003*

Epidermal growth factor receptor inhibitors – cetuximab and panitumumab; erlotinib and gefitinib; lapatinib; canertinib; vandetinib *JAAD 72:203–218, 2015*

Erlotinib ((epidermal growth factor receptor inhibitor) – trichomegaly and increased length of eyebrows *BJD 174:741–752, 2016; Oncol Lett 10:954–956, 2015; JAMAOphthalmol 132:1051, 2014; JAAD 70:821–838, 2014; JAAD 147:735–740, 2011; Clin in Dermatol 29:587–601, 2011; BJD 161:515–521, 2009; JAAD 58:545–570, 2008*Gefitinib (epidermal growth factor receptor inhibitor) *BJD 174:741–752, 2016; JAAD 58:545–570, 2008; BJD 151:1111–1112, 2004; Acta Oncol 42:345–346, 2003*

Interferon – interferon A *BJD 174:741–752, 2016; NEJM 311:1259, 1984;* interferon alpha 2b *Lancet 359:1107, 2002*

Latanoprost *BJD 174:741–752, 2016; JAAD 53:362–363, 2005*

Lucitanib (selective pan–FGF–R inhibitor) – onycholysis, trichomegaly, straightening of scalp hair, hyperkeratosis of heels, xerostomia *JAMADerm 153:723–725, 2017*

Panitumumab *BJD 174:741–752, 2016*

Prostaglandin analog – iris heterochromia and unilateral trichomegaly *JAMA 313:1967–1968, 2015*

Tacrolimus *AD142:248, 2006*

Topiramate *BJD 174:741–752, 2016; JAAD 53:362–363, 2005*

Zidovudine *BJD 174:741–752, 2016; NEJM 324:1896, 1991*

INFECTIONS AND INFESTATIONS

AIDS *AIDS 17:1695–1696, 2003; J Eur Acad Dermatol Venereol 11:89–91, 1998; Arch Ophthalmol 115:557–558, 1997; JAAD 28:513, 1993; AD 123:1599–1601, 1987*

HIV/AIDS and alopecia areata *BJD 174:741–752, 2016; Ped Derm 29:234–235, 2012; HIV AIDS 17:1695–1696, 2003; Dermatology 193:52–53, 1996*

Leishmaniasis – Kala–azar (Pitaluga's sign)

INFLAMMATORY DISORDERS

Uveitis *BJD 174:741–752, 2016; Ped Derm 26:188–193, 2009*

Vernal keratoconjunctivitis *BJD 174:741–752, 2016; Ped Derm 26:188–193, 2009*

METABOLIC DISORDERS

Cataract and spherocytosis *Am J Ophthalmol 73:333–335, 1972*

Hypothyroidism *Ped Derm 26:188–193, 2009*

Liver disease, chronic

Malnutrition *BJD 174:741–752, 2016; AD 142:248, 2006*

Phenylketonuria

Porphyria cutanea tarda *Ped Derm 26:188–193, 2009*

Pregnancy

Pretibial myxedema coma

NEOPLASTIC DISORDERS

Metastatic adenocarcinoma *Clin Exp Dermatol 20:237–239, 1995*

PARANEOPLASTIC DISORDERS

Malignancies *AD 142:248, 2006*

Metastatic adenocarcinoma *BJD 174:741–752, 2016; Clin Exp Dermatol 20:237–239, 1995*

PRIMARY CUTANEOUS DISEASES

Alopecia areata *Ped Derm 29:234–235, 2012; Ped Derm 26:188–193, 2009*

Atopic dermatitis – associated with hypotrichosis *BJD 174:741–752, 2016; J Eur Acad Dermatol Venereol 18:374–375, 2004*

Familial trichomegaly – increased length of forearm hair, synophrys, nonsyndromic oculocutaneous albinism; mutation in *FGF5* gene *BJD 174:741–752, 2016; Am J Med Genet A 136A:398, 2005; Arch Ophthalmol 115:1602–1603, 1997*

Hypertrichosis lanuginosa, congenital *J Genet Humaine 17:10–13, 1969*

Phylloid hypermelanosis – floral–like hypomelanosis, skeletal, cerebral, ocular defects, dental abnormalities *BJD 174:741–752, 2016; AD 145:576–578, 2009*

PSYCHOCUTANEOUS DISORDERS

Anorexia nervosa *Ped Derm 26:188–193, 2009*

SYNDROMES

Aghei–Dasthgeib syndrome – generalized hypertrichosis, bilateral nipple retraction, unilateral left–sided accessory nipple *BJD 174:741–752, 2016; Dermatol Online J 12: 19, 2006*

AIDS *AIDS 17:1695–1696, 2003; J Eur Acad Dermatol Venereol 11:89–91, 1998; Arch Ophthalmol 115:557–558, 1997; JAAD 28:513, 1993; AD 123:1599–1601, 1987*

Coffin–Siris syndrome – autosomal recessive; hypertrichosis of eyelashes, eyebrows, and lumbosacral areas *JAAD 48:161–179, 2003*

Cone–rod congenital amaurosis associated with congenital hypertrichosis and trichomegaly *BJD 174:741–752, 2016; J Med Genet 26:504–510, 1989*

Congenital polycoria – family history of congenital cataracts *BJD 174:741–752, 2016; J AApoS 17:619–620, 2013*

Cornelia de Lange syndrome (Brachmann de Lange) – trichomegaly, synophrys, low hairline, low birth weight, mental deficiency, abnormal speech development, malformed upper limbs; oral–dental abnormalities; mutations of genes related to chromosome function (*NIPBL, SMC1A, SMC3, HDAC8*) *BJD 174:741–752, 2016; Am J Med Genet 47:940–946, 1993; J Pediatr Ophthalmol Strabismus 27:94–102, 1990; Syndromes of the Head and Neck; Gorlin; 1990;p.300–304*

Costello syndrome – long eyelashes; warty papules around nose and mouth, legs, perianal skin; loose skin of neck, hands, and feet, thick, redundant palmoplantar surfaces, hypoplastic nails, short stature, craniofacial abnormalities; linear papillomatous papules of upper lip *BJD 168:903–904, 2013; Am J Med Genet 117:42–48, 2003; Eur J Eur Acad DV 34:601–607, 2020; J Dermatol 11:453–457, 2001; Am J Med Genet 82:187–193, 1999; JAAD 32:904–907, 1995; Am J Med Genet 47:176–183, 1993; Aust Paediat J 13:114–118, 1977*

Cutis laxa (dermatochalasis connata) – autosomal dominant; mild disease of late onset *Ped Derm 21:167–170, 2004;* bloodhound appearance of premature aging *Ped Derm 19:412–414, 2002; JAAD 29:846–848, 1993; Clin Genet 39:321–329, 1991; Ped Derm 2:282–288, 1985*

Goldstein–Hutt syndrome – trichomegaly, cataracts, hereditary spherocytosis *BJD 174:741–752, 2016; Ped Derm 26:188–193, 2009; Am J Ophthalmol 73:333–335, 1972*

H syndrome – autosomal recessive; hyperpigmented indurated plaques of legs with hypertrichosis, periorbital hyperpigmentation, diabetes mellitus, proptosis, sensorineural hearing loss, hemorrhage, hypogonadotropic hypogonadism, hallus valgus, flexion contractures; loss of function mutation of *SLC29A3*(same mutation as in cutaneous Rosai–Dorfman syndrome); gene encodes human equilibrative nuclear transporter3 (hENT3) protein which transports hydrophilic nucleoside, nucleobases, and nucleoside analog drugs across cell membranes and interacts with insulin signaling pathway *Ped Derm 32:731–732, 2015*

Hermansky–Pudlak syndrome – oculocutaneous albinism, trichomegaly, bleeding diathesis, lysosomal dysfunction; pulmonary fibrosis *BJD 174:741–752, 2016; Hematologie 34:301–309, 2014; AD 135:774–780, 1999*

Kabuki syndrome – vitiligo, developmental delay, short stature, congenital heart defects, skeletal defects, cleft palate, dental abnormalities, cryptorchidism, lip pits, prominent fingertip pads, autoimmune disorders, blue sclerae, prominent eyelashes, thinning of central eyebrows, protuberant ears *Amer J Med Genet 132A:260–262, 2005;*

J Pediatr 105:849–850, 1984

Oliver–McFarlane syndrome – autosomal recessive; trichomegaly, pigmentary degeneration of retina (retinitis pigmentosa), mental and growth retardation, peripheral neuropathy, progressive ataxia, retinitis pigmentosa, anterior pituitary deficiencies, primary amenorrhea, hypogonadism, short stature; mutation in *PBPLA6* gene encoding neuropathy target esterase; *BJD 174:741–752, 2016; Ped Derm 29:234–235, 2012; Br J Ophthalmol 87:119–120, 2003; Can J Ophthalmol 28:191–193, 1993; Genet Couns 2:115–118, 1991; Am J Med Genet 34:199–201, 1989; Am J Ophthalmol 101:490–491, 1986; Am J Dis Child 121:344–345, 1971; Arch Ophthalmol 74:169–171, 1965*

POEMS syndrome *Ped Derm 26:188–193, 2009*

Smith Magenis syndrome – distinctive facial and skeletal features; self–injurious behaviors *Ped Derm 32:337–341, 2015*

Trichothiodystrophy syndromes – BIDS, IBIDS, PIBIDS – autosomal recessive; collodion baby, congenital erythroderma, sparse or absent eyelashes and eyebrows, sulfur deficient short brittle hair with tiger tail banding on polarized microscopy, trichomegaly, brittle soft nails with koilonychia, premature aging, very short stature, microcephaly, sexual immaturity, ichthyosis, photosensitivity, hypohidrosis, high arched palate, dysmyelination of white matter, bird–like facies, abnormal teeth with dental caries; trichothiodystrophy with ichthyosis, urologic malformations, hypercalciuria and mental and physical retardation; recurrent infections with neutropenia; ocular abnormalities, osteopenia; socially engaging personality; mutation in one of 3 DNA repair genes (*XPB, XPA, TTDA, or TTDN1*) *JAAD 63:323–328, 2010; Curr Prob Derm 14:71–116, 2002; JAAD 44:891–920, 2001; Ped Derm 14:441–445, 1997*

TOXINS

Acrodynia *Ped Derm 26:188–193, 2009*

VASCULAR DISORDERS

Tetralogy of Fallot – short stature, generalized hypertrichosis lanuginose, brain atrophy and epilepsy *BJD 174:741–752, 2016; Clin Dysmorphol 13:247–250, 2004*

TROPICAL FEVER AND RASH

AUTOIMMUNE DISEASES

Systemic lupus erythematosus

DRUGS

DRESS – fever, skin rash, hepatitis, eosinophilia *Indian J Critical Care Med 21:29–231, 2017*

Drug eruptions

INFECTIONS AND INFESTATIONS

African trypanosomiasis (*Trypanosoma brucei rhodesiense*) – Tsetse fly, rural eastern and southeastern Africa, Tanzania, Uganda, Malawi, Zambia; cattle reservoir; chancre at fly bite site; more acute illness within days or weeks of bite, intermittent fever, headaches, rigors, muscle and joint pain and transient facial edema; 6–8 weeks later see erythematous urticarial or annular rashes

African trypanosomiasis (*Trypanosoma brucei gambiense*) – Democratic Republic of Congo, Angola, Sudan, Chad, Central African Republic; tsetse fly; more prolonged incubation period of weeks to months; enlarged cervical lymph nodes (Winterbottom's sign)

African tick bite fever (*Rickettsia africae*) – hemorrhagic pustule, purpuric papules; transmitted by *Amblyomma* ticks) – hemorrhagic pustule, purpuric papules; high fever, arthralgia, myalgia, fatigue, rash in 2–3 days, with eschar, maculopapules, vesicles, and pustules *JAAD 48:S18–19, 2003*

Alphavirus/flavivirus/bunyavirus

American trypanosomiasis – Chagas disease (*Trypanosoma cruzi*); triatome bugs (kissing bugs); Mexico, Central and South America; Romana's sign

Arenaviruses (hemorrhagic fevers) – Lassa fever (rats and mice) (West Africa), Junin virus (Argentine pampas), Machupo virus (Bolivian savannas), Guanarito virus (Venezuela), Sabia virus (Southeast Brazil), Whitewater virus (California, New Mexico), Tacaribe virus complex (mice) – swelling of face and neck, oral hemorrhagic bullae, red eyes *JAAD 49:979–1000, 2003*

Argentinian hemorrhagic fever

Arthropod bite reaction

Boutonneuse fever – *Rickettsia conorii*; diffuse morbilliform eruption; petechiae; palms and soles involved *JAAD 49:363–392, 2003*; Marseilles fever, South African tick fever, Kenya tick typhus, Israel tick typhus, and Indian tick typhus

Brazilian purpuric fever – *Haemophilus influenzae* biogroup aegyptius strains *J Infect Dis 171:209–212, 1995; Pediatr Infect Dis J 8:239–241, 1989*

Brucellosis – zoonosis; morbilliform, scarlatiniform, disseminated papulonodular, bullous, hemorrhagic eruptions *Cutis 63:25–27, 1999; AD 117:40–42, 1981;* erythema nodosum; widespread morbilliform eruption and fever *Am J Dermatopathol 31:687–690, 2009*

Bunyavirus hemorrhagic fever (Crimean Congo hemorrhagic fever, Rift Valley fever, Hantavirus) – ticks (*Hyalomma genus*) petechial eruption orally and on upper trunk *JAAD 49:979–1000, 2003*

Chikungunya fever – morbilliform exanthem of trunk and limbs

Congo Crimean hemorrhagic fever (Bunyavirus) – purpura

Cutaneous larva migrans – beach or sandy soil in Brazil, Jamaica, Malaysia, Thailand; dog or cat hookworm; linear serpiginous tracks (3mm wide, 15–20mm long), extends daily for 2–8 weeks; pruritic; self–limited

Cysticercosis – painless subcutaneous nodules

Dengue fever (Flavivirus) – classic dengue fever; morbilliform or scarlatiniform eruption on day 3–4, then becomes petechial; joint and bone pain with severe backache *JAAD 46:430–433, 2002; Dermatol Clinics 17:29–40, 1999; Inf Dis Clin NA 8:107, 1994; Bull Soc Pathol Exot 86:7–11, 1993;* exanthem with islands of sparing ("white islands in a sea of red") *Clin Inf Dis 36:1004–1005,1074–1075, 2003;* clinical differential diagnosis includes typhoid fever, leptospirosis, meningococcal disease, streptococcal disease, staph, rickettsial disease, malaria, arbovirus (chikungunya, o'nyong nyong fevers), Kawasaki's disease

Ebola viral hemorrhagic fever – morbilliform rash *MMWR 44:468–469, 1995*

Epidemic typhus (*Rickettsia prowazeki*)(body louse) – pink macules on sides of trunk, spreads centrifugally; flushed face with injected conjunctivae; then rash becomes deeper red, then purpuric; gangrene of finger, toes, genitalia, nose *JAAD 2:359–373, 1980;* transient red rash of trunk and face *Clin Inf Dis 32:979–982, 2001;* Brill–Zinsser disease – recrudescence of epidemic typhus

Filoviruses – Marburg and Ebola virus; transient morbilliform rashes, purpura, red eyes *JAAD 49:979–1000, 2003*

Gnathostomiasis – painless subcutaneous nodules

Guanarito – Venezuela

Hantavirus – infected rodent waste; flulike prodrome; nausea, vomiting, shock, extensive ecchymoses; oliguria, pulmonary edema, coagulopathy *AD 140:656, 2004*

Hemorrhagic fevers

HTLV–1 infection – infective dermatitis of scalp, eyelid margins, perinasal skin, retro–auricular areas, axillae, groin; generalized papular dermatitis Lancet 336:1345–1347, 1990; BJD 79:229–236, 1967; BJD 78:93–100, 1966

Infectious mononucleosis

Izumi fever – name in Japan for Far East scarlet fever–like eruption due to *Yersinia pseudotuberculosis;* red rash of face, elbows, and knees followed by desquamation; red strawberry tongue; conjunctival injection; toxic shock syndrome; mesenteric lymphadenitis and arthritis *Intern Med 57:437–440, 2018*

Kaposi's varicelliform eruption

Kenya tick typhus – *R. conorii*

Kyasanur Forest disease (Flavivirus)

Lassa fever (arenavirus) – morbilliform or petechial rash with conjunctivitis *J Infect Dis 155:445–455, 1985*

Leishmaniasis – tropical and subtropical Africa, Central and South America, Mediterranean region; sandfly bite (*Lutzomyia* of New World; *Phlebotomus* of Old World) on exposed skin of face or extremities; cutaneous painless skin ulcers with raised indurated margins and granulation tissue or eschar; heal with scars; Oriental sore, tropical sore Chiclero ulcer, Aleppo boil, Desert boil, Delhi boil; disseminated leishmaniasis *JAAD 50:461–465, 2004;* postkala–azar dermal leishmaniasis – papules of cheeks, chin, ears, extensor forearms, buttocks, lower legs; in India, hypopigmented macules; nodules develop after years; tongue, palate, genitalia *JAAD 34:257–272, 1996; E Afr Med J 63:365–371, 1986*

Leprosy – including erythema nodosum leprosum *AD 111:1575–1580, 1975*

Leptospirosis – recreational water sports and floods; infected animals; fever with hepatic syndrome (Weil's disease); non-catarrhal conjunctival injection; muscle tenderness; morbilliform *J Clin Inf Dis 21:1–8, 1995;* truncal red morbilliform, urticarial, pretibial, purpuric desquamative exanthem pretibial fever or canicola fever – blotchy erythema of legs

Loiasis – Western and Central Africa; filarial migrating under conjunctiva of eye; localized angioedema from migration of parasites; soft tissue swelling of hands, wrists, forearms lasting hours to days (Calabar swelling) *Int Marit Health 66:173–180, 2015*

Malaria

Marburg virus (filovirus) – maculopapular–vesicular *S Afr Med J 60:751–753, 1981*

Marseilles fever – *Rickettsia conorii*

Mayaro – arbovirus; Brazil and Trinidad

Measles

Mediterranean spotted fever – *Rickettsia conorii*; petechiae *JAAD 49:363–392, 2003*

Melioidosis

Meningococcemia

Monkeypox – exanthem indistinguishable from smallpox (papulovesiculopustular); Central Africa *J Infect Dis 156:293–298, 1987*; pronounced cervical, submandibular, and sublingual lymphadenopathy; lower mortality and lower person to person spread than smallpox

Murine typhus – *Rickettsia typhi* and ELB agent; flea bite fever headache, myalgia; blanching macular or morbilliform rash *MMWR 52:1224–1226, 2003; J Clin Inf Dis 21:991, 1995*

Mycobacterium tuberculosis – lichen scrofulosorum *Ped Derm 17:373–376, 2000; AD 124:1421–1426, 1988; Clin Exp Dermatol 1:391–394, 1976*

Myiasis – furuncular or wound myiasis; botfly (*Dermatobia hominis*)) or Tumbu fly (*Cordylobia anthropophaga*) larvae most common; pustular lesions resembling staphylococcal boils; pruritus and moving sensation with lancinating pain *Travel Med Inf Dis 7:125–146, 2009*

North Asian tick–borne typhus – *Rickettsia siberica*; Eastern Russia and China; resembles Rocky Mountain spotted fever; 50% develop unusual rope–like lymphangitis between inoculation eschar and draining lymph node

Omsk hemorrhagic fever (Flavivirus) *AD 140:656, 2004*

Onchocerciasis – intensely pruritic acute papular evanescent onchodermatitis – non–specific papular rash *BJD 121:187–198, 1989*

ONN – arbovirus; morbilliform eruption, fever, arthritis

Parvovirus B19

Picornavirus *Skin and Allergy News 30:38,1999*

Q fever – *Coxiella burnetii*; red macules, morbilliform, papular, urticarial, and purpuric eruptions *JAAD 49:363–392, 2003; Pediatr Inf Dis J 19:358, 2000*

Queensland tick typhus – *Rickettsia australis*

Rat bite fever– *Streptocbacillus moniliformis;* fever, headache, severe migratory arthralgias and myalgias; 2–4 days after fever see non–pruritic morbilliform or petechial eruptions of palms, soles, and extremities; asymmetric polyarthritis or septic arthritis; knees most common

Roseola

Rubella

Scarlet fever

Schistosomiasis – *S. hematobium* – Africa, Middle East; *S mansoni* – Africa; *S japonica* – Indonesia, Philippines; schistosomal dermatitis (cercarial dermatitis) – identical to swimmer's itch *Dermatol Clin 7:291–300, 1989*; S. japonicum – Katayama fever – fever, chills, abdominal pain, diarrhea, hepatosplenomegaly, lymphadenopathy, urticarial angioedema, and eosinophilia; purpura, arthralgia, systemic symptoms *Dermatol Clin 7:291–300, 1989*

Scrub typhus (*Orienta (Rickettsia) tsutsugamuchi*)(mites) – headache and conjunctivitis; eschar with black crust; generalized macular or morbilliform rash; 33% with lung involvement; pathognomonic hearing loss in 30% *Clin Inf Dis 18:624, 1994; JAAD 2:359–373, 1980*

Sepsis

Sindbis – arbovirus; fever, rash, arthritis; Europe, Asia, Africa, Australia

Smallpox – morbilliform exanthem as initial cutaneous manifestation *Cutis 71:319–321, 2003*

South American Arenaviruses (Junin, Machupo, Sabia, Guanarito)

Strongyloidiasis – larva currens; mostly perianal and buttock; rapid migration of 2–10 cm/hour; urticarial rash of buttock and trunk lasting 1–2 days, recurring regularly; acute fever, eosinophilia; disseminated erythematous macules *Travel Med Inf Dis 14:5350536, 2016*; hyperinfection strongyloides in immunocompromised host with periumbilical parasitic purpura

Syphilis

Tacaribe viruses – Argentinian, Bolivian, and Venezuelan hemorrhagic fevers – erythema of face, neck, and thorax with petechiae *Lancet 338:1033–1036, 1991; JAMA 273:194–196, 1994*

Talaromyces marneffei – HIV–associated disease of Southeast Asia; bamboo rats; fever weight loss anemia, hepatosplenomegaly; generalized papular or molluscum–like lesions of face, neck, upper trunk; pharyngeal and palatal lesions; pulmonary lesions *Lancet 344:110–113, 1994; Mycoses 34:245–249, 1991*

Togavirus – morbilliform, maculopapular–petechial (Sindbis) *BJD 135:320–323, 1996; BJD 80:67–74, 1968;* chikungunya *Trans R Soc Trop Med Hyg 49:28–32, 1955;* and O'Nyong–Nyong fever *Trans R Soc Med Hyg 55:361–373, 1961;* bunyavirus fevers) with joint pains; Ross River virus – morbilliform eruption and polyarthritis in Australia and Fiji *Med J Aust 159:159–162, 1993;* Barmah Forest virus – similar to Ross River virus *Med J Aust 152:463–466, 1990*

Tick typhus (Boutonneuse fever, Kenya tick typhus, African and Indian tick typhus)(ixodid ticks) – small ulcer at site of tick bite (tache noire) – black necrotic center with red halo; pink morbilliform eruption of forearms, then generalizes, involving face, palms, and soles; may be hemorrhagic; recovery uneventful *JAAD 2:359–373, 1980*

Trench fever – *Bartonella quintana*; human body louse; poor sanitation and personal hygiene; homeless; bout of fever lasting 4–5 days; truncal morbilliform eruption *Bull WHO 35:155–164, 1996;* associated with bacillary angiomatosis with subcutaneous and osseous lesions

Trypanosomiasis – African; edema of face, hands, feet with transient red macular, morbilliform, petechial or urticarial dermatitis; circinate, annular of trunk *AD 131:1178, 1995;* American – cutaneous inoculation (inoculation chagoma); edema with exanthems

Tunga penetrans – Chigoe (jigger) flea; Caribbean, South America, sub–Saharan Africa; under or near the toenails, interdigital, papule, vesicle or pustule 6–8mm with central black dot; gravid female increases in size to 1 cm creating a pruritic or painful nodule; secondary infection with sepsis, necrotic ulcer, osteomyelitis, or tetanus

Typhoid and paratyphoid fevers – rose spots, transient non–pruritic macules of upper abdomen

Typhus – epidemic (*Rickettsia prowazekii*) – human body louse; fever headache, red macules of trunk on day 5 and rapid spread to extremities; conjunctival injection

Typhus, murine (*Rickettsia typhus*); rat reservoir; flea vectors; fever, headache, myalgia, morbilliform rash of trunk or extremities, may be petechial

Varicella

Viral hemorrhagic fevers – including Argentine hemorrhagic fever, Bolivian hemorrhagic fever, Lassa fever, Venezuelan hemorrhagic fever, Kyasanur Forest disease, Omsk hemorrhagic fever, yellow fever and

Viral insect borne and hemorrhagic fevers *Dermatol Clinics 17:29–40, 1999*

Togavirus

    Sindbis fever – birds and *Culex* mosquitoes; Pogosta disease in Northern Europe; arthritis, pruritic rash, fever, muscle aches, headache

    Chikungunya fever – *Aedes* mosquito; Sub–Saharan Africa, Southeast Asia, Indian subcontinent; saddle back fever curve, polyarticular arthritis of small joints, myalgias, flush of face and neck becomes morbilliform, maybe pruritic; clinically indistinguishable from Mayaro, O'nyong nyong fever, Ross River, Sindbis, parvovirus, hepatitis B prodrome, juvenile rheumatoid arthritis, Dengue fever, and rubella *Clin Microbiol Infec* 24:240–245, 2018

    Mayaro virus – *Hemagogus Aedes* mosquitoes, Caribbean, Brazil; fever, morbilliform rash, marked arthralgia *Microbes Infec* 18:724–734, 2016

    O'nyong nyong fever

    Ross river fever – epidemic fever, rash, arthralgia, myalgia; Northern Australia

    Barmah forest fever – mosquitoes; Australia; fever, arthralgias, morbilliform, vesicular, or purpuric rash of trunk, limbs, and face *Clin Derm* 25:212–220, 2007

    Zika virus – *Aedes* mosquito; Florida, Caribbean; conjunctival hyperemia, headache, arthritis and/or arthralgia; pruritic morbilliform rash; distinctive painful periarticular edema of joints; microcephaly and other fetal CNS malformations *Clin Exp Derm* 44:4–12,13–19, 2019

Flavivirus

    Dengue fever – exanthema with islands of sparing (white islands in a sea of red) *Clin Inf Dis* 36:1004–1005,1074–1075, 2003; morbilliform or scarlatiniform rash on day 3–4 becomes petechial; joint and bone pain with severe backache (breakbone fever) *JAAD* 46:43–433, 2002

    West Nile fever – *Culex salinarius* mosquito bites; black birds, crows, blue jays; punctate (1–2mm) red macular, papular or morbilliform eruption of neck, trunk, arms, or legs in 20–50%of patients; flushed face, conjunctival injection and roseolar rash in some; encephalitis in elderly or immunocompromised *JAAD* 51:820–823, 2004; *JAAD* 49:979–1000, 2003; *Ann Int Med* 137:173–179, 2002; *Lancet* 358:261–264, 2001

    Kunjin fever

Arena virus

    Lassa fever – rats and mice; West Africa; morbilliform or petechial rash with conjunctivitis *J Inf Dis* 155:445–455, 1985; retro–orbital pain, myalgias, severe body pains, conjunctivitis, pharyngitis with tonsillar patches, generalized petechial eruption and facial edema

    Junin fever – Argentine pampas

    Machupo fever – Bolivian savannas

    Sabia – Brazil

Filovirus

    Marburg fever– Angola, Democratic Republic of Congo; fever, myalgias, headache, conjunctival injection, morbilliform rash prominent on trunk day 5; bleeding of skin and mucosa *JAAD* 49:979–1000, 2003; *Afr Med J* 60:751–753, 1981

    Ebola fever – Zaire, Sudan, Ivory Coast; morbilliform rash on day 5; fever, myalgias, headache, conjunctival injection; hemorrhage of skin and oral mucosa *MMWR* 44:468–469, 1995;

Bunyavirus

    Bwamba fever

    Rift valley fever – sub–Saharan Africa; *Aedes mcintoshi* mosquito bite; undifferentiated febrile disease; 10% macular and perimacular retinitis and vasculitis, permanent blindness

    Crimea/Congo fever – *Hyalomma* tick bite; severe hemorrhagic fever, shock, DIC, frequent extensive bleeding

    Hanta virus (hemorrhagic fever with renal syndrome (Hanta virus); striped field mouse, yellow–necked mouse, rats, bank vole; flu–like syndrome, thrombocytopenia, extensive ecchymoses, acute renal insufficiency (interstitial nephritis), shock, erythematous blanchable flush of trunk and face *AD* 140:656–, 2004

West Nile virus – *Culex salinarius*; punctate (1–2mm) red macular, papular, or morbilliform eruption of neck, trunk, arms, or legs in 20% of patients *JAAD* 51:820–823, 2004; *JAAD* 49:979–1000, 2003; *Ann Int Med* 137:173–179, 2002; *Ann DV* 128:656–658, 2001; *Lancet* 358:261–264, 2001

Yersinia pestis (bubonic plague, Black Death) – rat flea or squirrel flea – macular red, petechial or purpuric eruption *West Med J* 142:641–646, 1985

INFLAMMATORY DISORDERS

Stevens–Johnson syndrome

Toxic epidermal necrolysis

VASCULAR DISORDERS

Stroke

TUMORS, GIANT

AUTOIMMUNE DISORDERS OR DISORDERS OF IMMUNE DYSREGULATION

Chronic granulomatous disease – massive lymphadenopathy *NEJM* 367:753, 2012

CONGENITAL LESIONS

Congenital cellular blue nevus *Ped Derm* 29:651–655, 2012

Congenital cranial fasciitis – giant skin-colored nodule *Ped Derm* 24:263–266, 2007

Congenital granular cell tumor – giant intraoral tumor *Ped Derm* 33:663–664, 2016

Dermoid cyst *J Pediatr Orthop* 6:486–488, 1986

Ectopic thyroid gland *NEJM* 363:1351, 2010

Encephalocele

Fibrous hamartoma of infancy – occurs within first year of life (23% congenital); male:female ratio of 2.4:1; painless shoulder girdle or neck; solitary with rapid growth; 3–5cm *JAAD* 64:579–586, 2011; *Pediatr Dev Pathol* 2:236–243, 1999; *AD* 125:88–91, 1989

    Differentiate from:

        Infantile myofibromatosis – 50% congenital; occur within first 2 years of life; male>female; neck>extremities>viscera; solitary; affects skin, bone, soft tissues; generalized myofibromatosis with visceral involvement *Curr Prob Dermatol* 14:41–70, 2002;

giant necrotic ulcerated tumor *Ped Derm* 27:29–33, 2010

        Infantile fibrosarcoma – in first year of life; male>female; deep tissues of extremities; large solitary red painless dome-shaped 10–15cm tumor; vascular and ulcerated appearance; metastases uncommon *JAAD 64:579–586, 2011; JAAD 50:523–525, 2004;* congenital infantile fibrosarcoma – giant red tumor of lip *Ped Derm 31:88–89, 2014*

Hemangiopericytoma *Medicine 98:e17888, 2019; Ped Derm 10:267–270, 1993*

Herpes zoster – postherpetic pseudohernia (segmental paresis of abdominal musculature); large reducible protrusion of flank *JAMA 310:639–640, 2013*

Lipomyelomeningocele *Ped Derm 26:688–695, 2009*

Meningocele – in NF–1 *Hippokratia 21:63, 2017*

Myelomeningocele *Ped Derm 26:688–695, 2009*

DEGENERATIVE DISORDERS

Inguinal hernia (ventral hernia) – giant hanging protuberance *NEJM 368:171, 2013; NEJM 350:601, 2006;* umbilical hernia

Subcutaneous fat necrosis – giant lumbosacral tumor *BJD 171:183–185, 2014*

Transsternal gastric hernia *NEJM 370:1440, 2014*

INFECTIONS AND INFESTATIONS

Bacillary angiomatosis – giant tumor with ulceration in HIV disease *JAMADerm 150:1015–1016, 2014*

Condyloma acuminatum *Transpl Inf Dis 20:e129891, 2018; Ped Derm 26:488–489, 2009; Cutis 24:203–206,209, 1979*

Cryptococcosis and Kaposi's sarcoma, coexistent – giant purple tumor of lower face in HIV disease; satellite papules *Clin Inf Dis 58:540,596–597, 2014*

Echinococcosis – dog tapeworm; hydatid cyst

Giant condyloma of Buschke and Lowenstein – cerebriform, multilobulated giant tumor *Dermatol Ther 32:e12867, 2019; BJD 166:247–251, 2012;* giant disfiguring, exophytic cauliflower–like tumor *JAAD 66:867–880, 2012*

Granuloma inguinale (donovanosis)("serpiginous ulcer") – *Calymmatobacterium granulomatis* – starts as skin-colored subcutaneous nodule which breaks down into vulvar ulcer, vegetative perianal plaques with fistula formation, mutilation, and elephantine changes *JAAD 54:559–578, 2006*

Leprosy – giant histoid tumor *Int J Lepr Other Mycobact Dis 60:274–276, 1992*

Leishmaniasis – chronic cutaneous tumid leishmaniasis *Clin Dermatol 38:140–151, 2020*

Lobomycosis (Lobo's disease)(keloidal blastomycosis) *JAAD 53:931–951, 2005; Cutis 46:227–234, 1990; Int J Derm 17:572–574, 1978*

Lymphogranuloma venereum – *Chlamydia trachomatis;* elephantiasis of vulva, penis, scrotum (esthiomene) *JAAD 54:559–578, 2006; J Inf Dis 160:662–668, 1989*

Molluscum contagiosum with cyst formation *Clin Inf Dis 52:1029–1030,1077–1078, 2011; Acta DV 76:247–248, 1996; Am J Dermatopathol 17:414–416, 1995; Int J Dermatol 33:266–267, 1994; JAAD 19:912–914, 1988;* giant molluscum contagiosum *AD 147:652–654, 2011*

Mucor irregularis – multilobulated red nodule covering orbital skin *BJD 180:213–214, 2019*

Mycetoma

Mycobacterium tuberculosis – Pott's disease – giant subcutaneous multilobulated mass of lower back *Cutis 85:85–89, 2010*

North American blastomycosis (*Blastomyces dermatitidis*) – tumid mass of shoulder *Clin Inf Dis 70:973–975, 2020*

Orf *BJD 179:e132, 2018; JAAD 58::S39–40, 2008*

Phaeohyphomycosis – disseminated cutaneous phaeohyphomycosis – giant verrucous nodules *Ped Derm 28:30–31, 2011*

Pseudohernia – flaccid paralysis of abdominal musculature; diabetic radiculoneuropathy, poliomyelitis, ventral nerve root damage from intradural tumor excision, Lyme disease, syringomyelia, prolapsed intravertebral disk; must be differentiated from true abdominal hernia *JAMA 310:639–640, 2013; Hernia 10:364–366, 2006*

Rhinosporidiosis – vascular nodules of nose, extending to pharynx or lips *Mycopathologica 73:79–82, 1981*

Schistosoma mansoni – anal fissure with multilobulated giant anal polyp *AD 144:950–952, 2008*

Subcutaneous phaeohyphomycosis – personal observation

Tinea barbae (kerion) *AD 142:1059–1064, 2006*

Tropical pyomyositis – *Staphylococcus aureus JAAD 54:559–578, 2006*

Verrucae vulgaris *Cutis 80:145–148, 2007*

INFILTRATIVE DISORDERS

Amyloidosis – primary systemic amyloid with large tumefactions; beta–2 microglobulin amyloidosis associated with hemodialysis – giant linear tumors of back *JAMADerm 151:564–565, 2015*

Juvenile hyaline fibromatosis (infantile systemic hyalinosis) – limb contractures, sclerodermoid changes; gigantic lip fibromas, giant fibrous nodules of scalp and ears; giant nodules of frontal scalp and face; periarticular nodules of knees; gingival hypertrophy, bone deformities; mutation in gene encoding capillary morphogenesis protein 2(*ANTRX2(CMG2)*) *Ped Derm 23:458–464, 2006; JAAD 55:1036–143, 2006; Ped Derm 11:52–60, 1994; Pediatrics 87:228–234, 1991*

Juvenile xanthogranuloma – yellow–brown nodule *JAAD 76:S76–78, 2017; Ped Derm 26:709–712, 2009; AD 140:231–236, 2004; Ann DV 122:678–681, 1995; Ped Derm 11:227–230, 1994; AD 124:1723–1724, 1988; Arch Pathol Lab Med 110:911–915, 1986;* exophytic and endophytic *Ped Derm 7:185–188, 1990;* congenital giant xanthogranuloma *Ped Derm 21:121–123, 2004*

Langerhans cell histiocytosis *AD 127:1237–1238, 1991; AD 126:1617–1620, 1990*

Progressive nodular histiocytosis *JAAD 57:1031–1045, 2007*

Regressing atypical histiocytosis *AD 126:1609–1616, 1990*

Verruciform xanthoma – of gluteal crease *Ped Derm 21:432–439, 2004*

INFLAMMATORY DISORDERS

Pseudomalignant granuloma *JAAD 3:292–298, 1980*

Sarcoid – giant nodular form *JAAD 66:699–716, 2012;* tumoral sarcoidosis *Ann DV 122:783–785, 1995;* giant parotomegaly *Cutis 68:199–200, 2001*

Sinus histiocytosis with massive lymphadenopathy (Rosai–Dorfman disease) *JAAD 50:159–161, 2004*

METABOLIC DISORDERS

Diabetic lipohypertrophy – giant skin-colored tumid mass *BJD 171:1402–1406, 2014*

Gout – tophus *Cardiovasc Interv Ther July 10, 2019*

Pretibial myxedema of shoulders *AD 122:85–88, 1986*

NEOPLASTIC DISORDERS

Acrochordon Acta DV Croat 27:127–128, 2019

Acrospiroma (benign acrospiroma) *Cutis 83:12,21, 2009*

Adenoid cystic carcinoma, primary of skin *Cutis 87:237–239, 2011; Cancer 43:1463–1473, 1979*

Adenoma of the anogenital mammary–like glands – pedunculated; lobulated, tan–brown or gray–pink or white papules or nodules of vulva or perianal area; may ulcerate *JAAD 57:896–898, 2007; Breast J 9:113–116, 2003; J Reprod Med 47:949–951, 2002; Eur J Gynaecol Oncol 23:21–24, 2002; Gynecol Oncol 73:155–159, 1999*

Aggressive angiomyxoma – greater than 5 cm subcutaneous nodule *Am J Surg Pathol 7:463–475, 1983*

Aggressive digital papillary adenocarcinoma – exophytic friable tumor *JAAD 60:331–339, 2009*

Alveolar soft part sarcoma – tumor of muscle or fascial planes *Clin Exp Dermatol 10:523–539, 1985*

Angiokeratoma of Fordyce, multiple giant *An Bras Dermatol 90(suppl 1)150–152, 2015*

Angiolipoma *Ann R Coll Surg Eng 101:e91–93, 2019*

Angiomyxoma *Cutis 21:673–674, 1978*

Angiosarcoma *BJD 77:e27, 2017; Cutis 83:91–94, 2009; AD 142:1059–1064, 2006; BJD 149:1273–1275, 2003*

Apocrine cystadenoma *J Oral Maxillofac Surg 59:463–467, 2001*

Apocrine gland carcinoma *BJD 371–373, 2004; Am J Med 115:677–679, 2003*

Apocrine hidrocystoma *J Surg Oncol 27:146–151, 1984; AD 104:515–521, 1971*

Atypical palmar fibromatosis – with giant fibrous nodule *J Hand Surg Am 29:159, 2004; J Hand Surg Am 28:525–527, 2003*

Basal cell carcinoma *JAAD 71:1005–1008, 2014; J Drugs in Dermatol 13:601–606, 2014; Cutis 92:247–249, 2013; Cutis 80:60–66, 2007; JAAD 54:S50–52, 2006; JAAD 52:149–151, 2005; Cutis 67:73–76, 2001; Plast Reconstr Surg 106:653–656, 2000; Ann Plast Surg 41:444–447, 1998; J Dermatol 24:317–321, 1997; Int J Dermatol 35:222–223, 1996; Cutis 58:289–292, 1996; Neuroradiology 38:575–577, 1996; JAAD 30:856–859, 1994; BJD 127:164–167, 1992; J Derm Surg Oncol 12:459–464, 1986; AD 113:316–319, 1977;* with cerebral invasion *Eur J Surg Oncol 27:510–511, 2001;* polypoid *Cutis 58:289–292, 1996;* linear *Int J Dermatol 33:284, 1994;* fatal giant basal cell carcinoma *J Derm Surg Oncol 13:556–557, 1987; AD 113:316–319, 1977;* "horrifying basal cell carcinomas" *J Surg Oncol 5:431–463, 1973;* giant ulcer of scalp *JAMA Derm 149:639–641, 2013*

Benign adenoma – personal observation

Blastic plasmacytoid dendritic cell neoplasm – solitary or multiple nodules, plaques or bruise–like infiltrates; may involve lung, eyes, CNS *BJD 169:579–586, 2013; Arch Path Lab Med 134:1628–1638, 2010; Arch Path Lab Med 132:326–348, 2008*

Blue nevus *J Eur Acad DV 13:144–146, 1999; JAAD 28:653–654, 1993;* cellular blue nevus *J Surg Oncol 74:278–281, 2000; Br J Plast Surg 51:410–411, 1998;* giant alopecic nodule (cellular blue nevus) *BJD 126:375–377, 1992*

Primary breast carcinoma – personal observation

CD 30+ lymphoproliferative disorders – red tumors, red plaques with or without necrosis, giant tumor *JAAD 72:508–515, 2015*

Cephalohematoma

Chondroid syringoma *Clin Ther 165:207–209, 2014; J Cutan Med Surg 3:115–117, 1998*

Clear cell acanthoma (exophytic) *BJD 143:1114–1115, 2000; JAAD 21:313–315, 1989; JAAD 17:513–514, 1987*

Cutaneous horns *J Drugs Dermatol 18:697–698, 2019; Ann Plast Surg 43:674, 1999; Ann Plast Surg 39:654–655, 1997; Cutis 77–78, 1982; JAMA 210:2285, 1969*

Cylindroma *NEJM 351:2530, 2004*

Dendritic fibromyxolipoma – skin-colored pedunculated giant tumor *AD 144:795–800, 2008*

Dermal dendrocytoma of the face *AD 126:689–690, 1990*

Dermatofibroma *J Cut Pathol 45:774–776, 2018; BJD 143:655–657, 2000; Cutis 58:282–285, 1996; JAAD 30:714–718, 1994;* combined dermatofibroma *BJD 143:655–657, 2000;* xanthomatous dermatofibroma *Dermatology 190:67–71, 1995;* hemosiderotic dermatofibroma *Am J Dermatopathol 37:778–782, 2015;* aneurysmal benign fibrous histiocytoma presenting as giant acrochordon *Indian Dermatol Online J 6:436–438, 2005*Dermatomyofibroma – up to 8cm; oval nodule or firm plaque of shoulders, axillae, upper arms, neck, or abdomen *Clin Exp Dermatol 21:307–309, 1996*

Dermatofibrosarcoma protuberans *Dermatol Ther 21:428–432, 2008; JAAD 53:76–83, 2005;* giant vulvar DFSP *J Buon 24:1289–1295, 2019;* giant scalp DFSP *Ophthal Plast Reconstr Surg 35:e36–39, 2019*

Desmoid tumors – in Gardner's syndrome; subcutaneous mass in subumbilical paramedian region; arise in thoracotomy scar *AME Case Rep Nov 17, 2017; Thoracic Cardiovasc Surg 40:300–302, 1992*

Eccrine acrospiroma *JAAD 23:663–668, 1990*

Eccrine hidrocystoma of eyelid *Indian J DV Leprol 83:267, 2017*

Eccrine poroma *Cutis 88:227–229, 2011; AMA Arch Derm 74:511–521, 1956*

Eccrine spiradenoma *Diagn Inter Imaging 98:89–91, 2017; Int J Dermatol 37:221–223, 1998; Ann DV 104:485–487, 1977;* malignant eccrine spiradenoma of scalp *Derm Surg 25:45–48, 1999;* vascular eccrine spiradenoma *J Dermatol 40:853–854, 2013*

Embryonal rhabdomyosarcoma *Ped Derm 22:218–221, 2005*

Enchondroma of the forefinger *Hautarzt 36:168–169, 1985*

Epidermoid cyst – multiloculated epidermoid cyst – often of plantar surface *JAAD 58:S120–122, 2008; Dermatol Surg 31:1323–1324, 2005; BJD 151:943–945, 2004; Dermatol Surg 28:639–640, 2002; BJD 144:217–218, 2001;* of the skull *Plast Reconstr Surg 97:1246–1248, 1996*

Epithelioid sarcoma – fungating giant mass *AD 145:589–594, 2009*

Extramammary Paget's disease of the genital areas *Dermatology 202:249–251, 2001*

Fibrokeratoma – acquired digital fibrokeratoma *JAAD 48:S67–68, 2003;* acquired fibrokeratoma of the nail bed *Dermatology 190:169–171, 1995*

Folliculosebaceous cystic hamartoma – scrotal cobblestoned plaque; pedunculated, dome–shaped and umbilicated papules *BJD 157:833–835, 2007*

Giant cell fibroblastoma (variant of dermatofibrosarcoma protuberans)

Giant cell tumor of soft tissue *J Orth Case Rep 9:70–73, 2019*

Giant pore and hair–shaft acanthoma *Hautarzt 34:209–216, 1983*

Glomus tumor, subungual *Dermatol Online J Oct 15, 2016*

Hibernoma – giant multilobulated tumor of neck *NEJM 367:1636, 2012*

Hidradenocarcinoma *Pathol Int 48:818–823, 1998*

Histiocytic lymphoma (reticulum cell sarcoma) – gigantic tumor *G Ital Dermatol Venereol 115:143–145, 1980*

Infantile digital fibrokeratoma – giant tumor of 2nd toe *Cutis 105:16, 20, 2020*

Intramuscular hydatid cyst – giant skin-colored subcutaneous tumor (25x15cm) *Clin Inf Dis 61:1707, 1759–1760, 2015*

Hypertrophic scar – plantar giant nodule *BJD 145:1005–1007, 2001*

Kaposi's sarcoma *BJD 145:847–849, 2001; Cutis 68:50–52, 2001;* AIDS–related giant KS *Medicine 97:e12530, 2018*

Keloid – personal observation; keloid following BCG vaccination Ped Derm 20:460, 2003

Keratoacanthoma *Dermatology 200:317–319, 2000; Otolaryngol Head Neck Surg 93:112–116, 1985; Ann Plast Surg 3:172–176, 1979;* in epidermolysis bullosa, recessive dystrophic *Ped Derm 19:436–438, 2002;* keratoacanthoma centrifugum marginatum *BJD 163:633–637, 2010; JAAD 54:S218–219, 2006; Cutis 73:257–262, 2004; JAAD 48:282–285, 2003; JAAD 30:1–19, 1994; AD 111:1024–1026, 1975; Hautarzt 13:348–352, 1962*

Leiomyosarcoma *Am J Case Rep 17:35–38, 2016*

Leukemia – HTLV–1(acute T–cell leukemia) *JAAD 49:979–1000, 2003*

Lipoblastoma *Ped Derm 23:514–515, 2006*

Lipomas *J of Ultrasound June 2012, 124–126; Pan African Medical J 2011; JAAD 28:266–268, 1993; Zentralbl Chir 91:1608–1611, 1966;* diffuse lipomatosis *AD 122:1298–1302, 1986; World J Plast Surg 7:368–371, 2018*

Liposarcoma – diffuse nodular infiltration of leg or buttock, retroperitoneum, inguinal, paratesticular *JAAD 38:815–819, 1998;* swollen neck *NEJM 363:864, 2010;* giant subcutaneous nodule *JAAD 64:1202–1203, 2011*

Lymphoma – cutaneous T–cell lymphoma *JAAD 70:205–220, 2014; JAAD 122:135–136, 1986;* Woringer–Kolopp disease *AD 128:526–529, 1992;* granulomatous slack skin *BJD 142:353–357, 2000;* T–cell lymphoma presenting as giant ulcer *Clin Exp Dermatol 17:379–381, 1992;* HTLV–1 lymphoma *BJD 144:1244–1248, 2001;* cutaneous type adult T–cell leukemia/lymphoma – multilobulated purple giant tumor *JAAD 57:S115–117, 2007;* CD30+ T–cell lymphoma *JAAD 48:S28–30, 2003; BJD 146:1091–1095, 2002;* large cell B–cell lymphoma of the leg *JAAD 49:223–228, 2003;* B–cell lymphoblastic lymphoma *Ped Derm 21:525–533, 2004;* primary cutaneous follicle center B–cell lymphoma *BJD 157:1205–1211, 2007;* pyogenic lymphoma – primary cutaneous neutrophil–rich CD30+ anaplastic large–cell lymphoma *BJD 148:580–586, 2003;* primary cutaneous epidermotropic CD8+ T–cell lymphoma – giant hand; mixture of patches, plaques, papulonodules with central ulceration, necrosis, and hemorrhage *JAAD 62:300–307, 2010;* extranodal NK/T–cell lymphoma, nasal type – multilobulated giant tumor of leg *JAMADerm 150:1109–1110, 2014;* epidermotropic CTCL *BJD 172:819–821, 2015;* Epstein–Barr virus-associated plasmablastic lymphoma (HIV–defining lesion) – ulcerated fungating giant perianal tumor *BJD 174:398–401, 2016;* diffuse large cell B–cell non–Hodgkin's lymphoma *Medicine 96:e6270, 2017*

Malignant clear cell hidradenoma – giant axillary metastasis *Ann Plast Surg 45:102, 2000*

Malignant eccrine spiradenoma of the scalp *Derm Surg 25:45–48, 1999*

Malignant peripheral nerve sheath tumors (neurofibrosarcoma) *BJD 153:79–82, 2005; AD 137:908–913, 2001*

Malignant proliferating trichilemmal tumor *BJD 148:180–182, 2003*

Malignant sacrococcygeal teratoma *Am Surg 57:425–430, 1991*

Melanocytic nevi – congenital – cobblestoned, cerebriform, localized hypertrichosis, hyperpigmented discrete annular plaque *JAAD 68:441–451, 2013; JAAD 54:778–782, 2006; Clin Exp Dermatol 25:7–11, 2000; J Pediatr 120:906–911, 1992;* giant congenital melanocytic nevus sparing nipple *Ped Derm 32:514–517, 2015;* congenital neuroid melanocytic nevus *AD 116:318–320, 1980;* giant cerebriform intradermal nevus *Ped Derm 25:43–46, 2008; Ann Plast Surg 19:84–88, 1987;* giant congenital melanocytic nevi with proliferative nodules *AD 140:83–88, 2004;* atypical proliferative nodules in congenital melanocytic nevi of scalp *BJD 165:1138–1142, 2011;* congenital dermal melanocytic nevus *JAAD 49:732–735, 2003; AD 134:245–246, 1998; AD 127:1702–1704, 1991;* congenital lentiginous dermal nevus *Ann Plast Surg 43:546–550, 1999;* desmoplastic giant congenital nevus *JAAD 56:S10–14, 2007*

Melanoma *Curr Prob Derm 14:41–70, 2002; Eur J Surg Oncol 26:189–190, 2000;* metastatic melanoma *J Dermatol 21:442–446, 1994; Ann Plast Surg 27:583–585, 1991;* melanoma arising in a giant cerebriform nevus *AD 96:536–539, 1967;* amelanotic melanoma *AD 145:1198–1199, 2009; AD 138:1245–1250, 2002;* primary scrotal melanoma *AD 145:1071–1072, 2009;* primary melanoma – giant vascular tumor *JAMADerm 150:574–575, 2014;* metastatic melanoma – sessile giant inframammary mass *NEJM 372:2073–2074, 2015*

Merkel cell carcinoma – scalp tumor *Cutis 103:261,280–282, 2019; J Cut Med Surg 17:351–355, 2013; Derm Surg 27:493–494, 2001; JAAD 24:827–831, 1991; Surv Ophthalmol 35:171–187, 1990; Cancer 57:178–182, 1986; AD 123:653–658, 1987;* exophytic Merkel cell carcinoma *Cutis 44:295–299, 1989*

Metastases – breast cancer – personal observation

Microcystic adnexal carcinoma *Derm Surg 27:678–680, 2001*

Mixed tumor of the face *J Dermatol 23:369–371, 1996*

Monophasic synovial sarcoma – giant subcutaneous tumor; *SYT–SSXI* or *SYT–SSX2* translocation *Cutis 93:13–16, 2014*

Mucinous carcinoma of skin *JAAD 36:323–326, 1997;* scalp *Clin Exp Dermatol 18:375–377, 1993*

Mucocutaneous papillomatoses, giant *AD 99:499–502, 1969*

Myofibroma – giant tumor of scalp with surface telangiectasias *Ped Derm 27:525–526, 2010*

Neurofibrosarcoma

Nevus comedonicus *Przegl Dermatol 75:305–307, 1988(Polish)*

Nevus lipomatosis superficialis *Actas Dermosifiliogr 110:e1, 2019; JAAD 67:E168–170, 2012; J Dermatol 27:16–19, 2000; J Dermatol 15:543–545, 1988; J Derm Surg Oncol 9:279–281, 1983*

Nevus sebaceous *Ped Derm 25:355–358, 2008; Ann Chir Infant 11:243–253, 1970;* exophytic nevus sebaceous *Pediatr Neurosurg 44:144–147, 2008; Ped Derm 25:366–358, 2008; Ped Derm 8:84–86, 1991;* papillomatous pedunculated nevus sebaceous *BJD 176:204–208, 2017*

Nevus spilus *Acta DV 75:327, 1995; AD 125:1284–1285, 1989*

Osteoma – platelike cutaneous osteoma *JAAD 16:481–484, 1987*

Pigment synthesizing melanocytic neoplasm with protein kinase C alpha (*PRKCA*) fusion – ATPase calcium transporting plasma membrane4(ATp2B4)–protein kinase C–alpha (PRKCA) fusion transcript *JAMADerm 152:318–322, 2016*

Pilar cyst *Plast Reconstr Surg 92:1207–1208, 1993*

Piloleiomyoma *Ann Dermatol 23(suppl 2) S144–146, 2011*

Pilomatrix carcinoma – multiple of head and neck *Otolaryngol Head Neck Surg 109:543–547, 1993; JAAD 23:985–988, 1990*

Pilomatrixoma *Ped Derm 25:449–451, 2008; JAAD 58:535–536, 2008; BJD 155:208–210, 2006; Australas J Dermatol 42:120–123, 2001; Arch Otolaryngol Head Neck Surg 114:1042–1045, 1998; Arch Otolaryngol 102:753–755, 1976; Arch Surg 111:86–87, 1976;* multiple giant pilomatrixomas *J Dermatol 27:276–279, 2000;* pedunculated giant pilomatrixoma *Ann Plast Surg 41:337–338, 1998;* proliferating pilomatrixoma *Australas J Dermatol 58:e91–93, 2017*

Plexiform fibrohistiocytic tumor of the soft tissues and bone *Cesk Patol 36:106–110, 2000; Ann Plast Surg 38:306–307, 1997; Am J Surg Pathol 21:235–241, 1997*

Pleomorphic fibroma *Clin Exp Dermatol 45:97–99, 2020*

Plexiform schwannoma – mimics giant hemangioma *BJD 157:838–839, 2007*

Porocarcinoma *BJD 152:1051–1055, 2005*

Porokeratosis *Dermatol Surg 44:580–581, 2018; BJD 141:936–938, 1999; Dermatology 189:78–80, 1994*

Post–transplant lymphoproliferative disorder *JAAD 52:S123–124, 2005*

Proliferating trichilemmal tumor of the scalp *J Dermatol 27:687–688, 2000; Ann Plast Surg 43:574–575, 1999; Mund Kiefer Gesechtschir 2:216–219, 1998;* with malignant transformation *Ann Plast Surg 41:314–316, 1998*

Rhabdomyosarcoma – large solitary tumor of the head and neck; differential diagnosis includes infantile hemangioma, lymphatic malformation, myofibroma, lipoblastoma, teratoma, fibrosarcoma *Acta Oncol 35:494–495, 1996; Hautkr 53:887–892, 1978;* congenital – giant skin-colored tumor *Ped Derm 32:143–144, 2015; Ped Derm 28:299–301, 2011; Ped Derm 20:335–338, 2003*

Sacrococcygeal teratoma – personal observation

Schwannoma *Eur J Dermatol 9:493–495, 1999*

Sebaceoma *Am J Dermatopathol 24:294–304, 2002; J Dermatol 21:367–369, 1994*

Sebaceous adenoma *Cancer 33:82–102, 1974; Arch Derm Syphilol 57:102–111, 1948*

Sebaceous gland carcinoma *BJD 149:441–442, 2003; AD 137:1367–1372, 2001; Nippon Ganka Gakkai Zasshi 104:740–745, 2000;* cystic sebaceous carcinoma – multilobulated nodule of nose *J Drugs Dermatol 6:540–543, 2007; Indian J Surg Oncol 4:366–367, 2013*

Seborrheic keratosis *G Ital DV 152:383–386, 2017; Plast Reconstr Surg 99:1466–1467, 1997; J Dermatol 12:341–343, 1985*

Squamous cell carcinoma *AD 143:889–892, 2007; JAAD 55:S81–85, 2006; JAAD 54:740–741, 2006; Derm Surg 28:268–273, 2002; JAAD 23:1174–1175, 1990; JAAD 10:372–378, 1984;* of lip *Ped Derm 26:59–61, 2009;* of face and scalp – giant verrucous plaque *BJD 176:498–502, 2017;* vulvar *Genital Skin Disorders, Fischer and Margesson, CV Mosby, 1998, p. 215;* in epidermolysis bullosa, recessive dystrophic *Ped Derm 19:436–438, 2002;* of foot periungual *Cutis 78:173–174, 2006;* of face *JAAD 55:S81–85, 2006;* of hand *JAAD 55:S81–85, 2006;* HPV 26–associated squamous cell carcinoma of nail beds *BJD 157:788–794, 2007;* in xeroderma pigmentosum *BJD 152:545–551, 2005*

Syringocystadenoma papilliferum in a giant comedone *Tokai J Exp Clin Med 11:47–50, 1986;* giant multilobulated linear tumor *Ped Derm 26:758–759, 2009*

Syringoma of the vulva *BJD 141:374–375, 1999*

Trichoblastic carcinoma – giant red beefy tumor *Arch Craniofac Surg 19:275–78, 2018; BJD 173:1059–1062, 2015*

Trichoblastoma – scalp *Am J Dermatopathol 15:497–502, 1993*

Trichoepithelioma *South Asian J Cancer 4:41–44, 2015; Dermatology Online J 5:1, 1999; Am J Dermatopathol 14:155–160, 1992;* perianal *BJD 118:563–566, 1988; BJD 115:91–99, 1986; AD 120:797–798, 1984*

Undifferentiated sarcoma – giant pendulous cystic lesion of cheek *Soc Ped Derm Annual Meeting, July 2005*

Verrucous carcinoma – Buschke–Lowenstein tumor – giant, multilobulated, disfiguring, exophytic cauliflower–like tumor *JAAD 66:867–880, 2012; AD 145:950–952, 2009; Acta DV 79:253–254, 1999; Dermatol Monatsschr 175:247–250, 1989; Z Hautkr 58:1325–1327, 1983;* epithelioma cuniculatum – of the foot *NEJM 352:488, 2005;* of the hand *Ir J Med Sci 163:379–380, 1994;* oral florid papillomatosis *Cutis 21:207–211, 1978;* of the lip *BJD 151:727–729, 2004;* arising in a burn scar *Cutis 79:133–135, 2007;* giant tumor of ankle in epidermolysis bullosa simplex *BJD 167:929–936, 2012*

Woringer–Kolopp disease (pagetoid reticulosis) *JAAD 59:706–712, 2008; Ann Dermatol Syph 10:945–958, 1939*

PRIMARY CUTANEOUS DISEASES

Café au lait macule *Acta DV 79:496, 1999*

Giant comedone *BJD 133:662–663, 1995*

Lipedema *JAAD 50:969–972, 2004*

Malakoplakia – perianal nodules, vulvar nodules, skin-colored nodules, ulcerations, abscesses, red papules, masses *Arch Pathol Lab Med 132:113–117, 2008*

SYNDROMES

Benign symmetric lipomatosis (Madelung's disease, Launois–Bensuade syndrome) *J Oral Maxillofac Surg 65:1365–1369, 2007; Aesthetic Plastic Surg 28:108–112, 2004*

Birt–Hogg–Dube syndrome – giant disfiguring lipomas *JAAD 50:810–812, 2004*

Blue rubber bleb nevus syndrome (Bean syndrome) – giant subcutaneous vascular malformations; blue lesions of skin and mucous membranes *JAAD 50:S101–106, 2004; Cutis 62:97–98, 1998; Trans Pathol Soc 11:267, 1860*

Brooke–Spiegler syndrome – giant eccrine spiradenomas *Int J Surg Case Rep 51:277–281, 2018*

CHILD syndrome – verruciform xanthoma giant red plaque of lateral foot; cobblestoned, verrucous giant tumor; enlarged foot; exophytic mass; X–linked dominant; mutation in *NSDHL* (NAD(P)–dependent steroid dehydrogenase-like gene) *Cutis 88:269–272, 2012; Ped Derm 27:551–553, 2010*

CLOVES syndrome (congenital lipomatous overgrowth with vascular, epidermal, and skeletal abnormalities – mutation in *PIK3CA JAAD 68:885–896, 2013; Am J Hum Genet 90:1108–1115, 2012*

Congenital self–healing reticulohistiocytosis *Ped Derm 6:28–32, 1989*

Fibrodysplasia ossificans progressiva – heterotopic bone formation within soft tissues; multiple neonatal scalp nodules associated with malformation of the great toes (hallux valgus); hypoplastic great toes; development of tumors is cranial to caudal, dorsal to ventral and proximal to distal; ossification after infections or trauma; scalp nodules large, firm, and immobile; mutation in *ACVR1* gene *JAAD 64:97–101, 2011*

Flood syndrome – sudden rush of ascitic fluid with spontaneous rupture of umbilical hernia in longstanding ascites and end-stage liver disease *JAAD Case Reports 2015:1:5–6*

Gardner's syndrome – osteomas, desmoid tumors, epidermoid cysts, neurofibromas, lipomas *Contemp Clin Dent 5:252–255, 2014*

Goltz's syndrome (focal dermal hypoplasia) with giant papillomas *BJD 133:997–999, 1995;* giant cell tumor of bone (large subcutaneous nodule); protruding ears, mid–facial hypoplasia, pointed chin, lower limb hypoplasia, blaschko–esque atrophy, red and hypopigmented blaschko streaks, painful exophytic granulation tissue *BJD 160:1103–1109, 2009*

Juvenile hyaline fibromatosis

Maffucci's syndrome (enchondromatosis) – enchondromas and multiple venous malformations; spindle cell hemangioendothelioma; oral and intra–abdominal venous and lymphatic anomalies; short stature, shortened long bones with pathologic fractures; enchondromas undergo sarcomatous change in 30–40%; breast, ovarian, pancreatic, parathyroid, pituitary tumors *JAAD 56:541–564, 2007; Ped Derm 17:270–276, 2000; Ped Derm 12:55–58, 1995*

Neurofibromatosis – neurofibroma pendulans *Zentralbl Chir 110:1193–1195, 1985;* rugose and plexiform neurofibromas; *NEJM 382:1430–1442, 2020; JAAD 52:191–195, 2005; Ann Plast Surg 45:442–445, 2000;* elephantiasis neurofibromatosa – diffuse neurofibromatosis of nerve trunks with overgrowth of skin and subcutaneous tissues yielding a wrinkled and pendulous appearance *J Plast Reconstr Aesthet Surg 65:176–177, 2012*

Olmsted syndrome – plantar squamous cell carcinoma *BJD 145:685–686, 2001*

Proteus syndrome – port wine stains, subcutaneous hemangiomas and lymphangiomas, lymphangioma circumscriptum, hemihypertrophy of the face, limbs, trunk; macrodactyly, cerebriform hypertrophy of palmar and/or plantar surfaces, macrocephaly; verrucous epidermal nevi, sebaceous nevi with hyper– or hypopigmentation *Am J Med Genet 27:99–117, 1987;* vascular nevi, soft subcutaneous masses; lipodystrophy, café au lait macules, linear and whorled macular pigmentation somatic mosaic mutation of *AKT1 NEJM 365:611–619, 2011; Pediatrics 76:984–989, 1985; Am J Med Genet 27:87–97, 1987; Eur J Pediatr 140:5–12, 1983; Arch Fr Pediatr 47:441–444, 1990(French)*

Rubinstein–Taybi syndrome – multiple large keloids (red tumors) *BJD 171:615–621, 2014; Cutis 57:346–348, 1996;* broad thumb *Ped Derm 11:21–25, 1994;* mental deficiency, small head, broad thumbs and great toes, beaked nose, malformed low–set ears, capillary nevus of forehead, hypertrichosis of back and eyebrows, cardiac defects; mutation in *CREBBP* and *EP300 BJD 171:615–621, 2014; Am J Dis Child 105:588–608, 1963*

SCALP syndrome – sebaceous nevus syndrome, central nervous system malformations, aplasia cutis congenital, limbal dermoid, pigmented nevus (giant congenital melanocytic nevus) with neurocutaneous melanosis *JAAD 58:884–888, 2008*

Tuberous sclerosis – giant angiofibromas *JAAD 67:1319–1326, 2012; J Dermatol 24:132–134, 1997; AD 114:1843–1844, 1978*

TOXINS

Arsenic – squamous cell carcinoma of lateral hand or trunk; arsenic toxicity due to contaminated ground water consumption; especially in Bangladesh and West Bengal, India; also in India, Argentina, China, Chile, Thailand, and Mexico *SkinMed 11:211–216, 2013*

TRAUMA

Hematoma – personal observation

Rectus femoris tear – subcutaneous thigh mass *JAMADerm 153:945–946, 2017*

VASCULAR DISORDERS

Agminated eruptive pyogenic granuloma–like lesions over congenital vascular stains (capillary malformations) *Ped Derm 29:186–190, 2012*

Arteriovenous malformation *AD 143:1043–1045, 2007*

Congenital hemangioma – *GNA11* mutation *JAMADerm 152:1015–1020, 2016*

Cystic hygroma (macrocystic lymphatic malformation) – personal observation

Glomus tumor *J Cutan Pathol 24:384–389, 1997; JAAD 14:1083–1084, 1986; BJD 90:229–231, 1974; JAMA 214:1562, 1970; plaque type; patch-like JAAD 40:826–828, 1999*

Hemangiomas, giant – zosteriform infantile hemangioma of face *Ped Derm 30:151–154, 2013;* life–threatening *AD 133:1567–1571, 1997;* arising in port wine stain *JAAD 31:675–676, 1994;* multiple giant hemangiomas with heart failure *Jpn Heart J 33:493–497, 1992;* with diffuse neonatal hemangiomatosis *J Dermatol 18:286–290, 1991; Clin Pediatr (Phila) 23:498–502, 1984;* of scalp *S Afr Med J 55:47–49, 1979;* non–involuting capillary hemangioma (NICH) – large purple tumor *Semin Cut Med Surg 35:124–127, 2016; Ped Derm 29:182–185, 2012;* partially involuting congenital hemangioma *JAAD 70:75–79, 2014*

Hemangiopericytoma, congenital *Medicine 98:e17888, 2019;* Infantile hemangioma of face *AD 147:1049–1056, 2011*

Kassabach-Merritt syndrome *Arch Dis Child 65:790–791, 1990;* swollen face and neck with deep red infiltrated tumor; Kaposiform hemangioendothelioma *Ped Derm 31:595–598, 2014*

Lymphatic malformation – giant tumor of cheek *JAAD 70:1050–1057, 2014;*

lymphangiomatosis – fluctuant swellings *Am J Surg Pathol 16:764–771, 1992*

Klippel–Trenaunay syndrome – microcystic lymphatic malformation *JAMADerm 152:1058–1059, 2016*

Lymphatic malformation, microcystic of vulva *J Ob Gyn Res 44:978–982, 2018*

Massive localized lymphedema in the morbidly obese – giant pendulous masses of the medial thighs *Lymphology 39:181–184, 2006; Obes Surg 16:1126–1130, 2006; Obes Surg 16:88–93, 2006; Plast Surg Reconstr Surg 106:1663–1664, 2000; Human Pathol 31:1162–1168, 2000; Am J Surg Pathol 22:1277–1283, 1998*

PHACES syndrome giant multilobulated hemangioma with hemihypertrophy of face

Pyogenic granuloma; multiple congenital pyogenic granulomas – multifocal nodules of thigh, giant *J Eur Acad DV 31:e512–513, 2017; J Craniofac Surg 27:e433–435, 2016; Society Pediatric Dermatology Annual Meeting, July, 2015*

Rapidly involuting congenital hemangioma *Sem Cut Med Surg 35:124–127, 2016; JAMADerm 151:422–425, 2015; BJD 158:1363–1370, 2008*

Retiform hemangioendothelioma – exophytic masses of scalp, arms, legs, and penis *JAAD 38:143–175, 1998*

Tufted angioma *J Dermatol 38:942–944, 2011; AD 145:847–848, 2009*

Venous malformation – of scalp *Zentralbl Neurochir 59:274–277, 1998;* of trunk *JAAD 56:353–370, 2007*

ULCERS, LEG

JAAD 25:965–987, 1991

AUTOIMMUNE DISEASES AND DISEASES OF IMMUNE DYSFUNCTION

Allergic contact dermatitis *BJD 148:388–401, 2003*

Anti-centromere antibodies – ulcers and gangrene of the extremities *Br J Rheumatol 36:889–893, 1997*

Antineutrophil cytoplasmic antibody syndrome – purpuric vasculitis, orogenital ulceration, fingertip necrosis, pyoderma gangrenosum-like ulcers *BJD 134:924–928, 1996*

Antiphospholipid antibody syndrome *Clin Exp Rheum 9:63–66, 1991*

Bare lymphocyte syndrome – ulcers of the legs and feet; severe reduction in cell surface expression of HLA molecules (HLA class I, type I BLS; HLA class II, type II BLS); TAP1 and TAP2 mutations (transporter-associated antigen-processing heterodimers) (transportation of cytoplasmic peptides into the endoplasmic reticulum) *AD 146:96–98, 2010; Lancet 354(9190):1598–1603, 1999; Science 265:237–241, 1994*

Bullous pemphigoid

Dermatomyositis

Graft-versus-host reaction, chronic *AD 134:602–612, 1998;* calcinosis cutis in GVHD – umbilicated nodules, leg ulcers, rippled appearance *JAMADerm 156:814–817, 2020*

Immune complex disease

Immunodeficiency disease with *RAG* mutations and granulomas – ulcers of the face and extremities *NEJM 358:2030–2038, 2008*

Leukocyte adhesion deficiency type 1 (beta 2 integrin deficiency) (congenital deficiency of leucocyte adherence glycoproteins (CD11a (LFA-1), CD11b, CD11c, CD18) – autosomal recessive; delayed separation of umbilical stump; necrotic cutaneous abscesses, cellulitis, skin ulcerations (pyoderma gangrenosum leg ulcers healing with flaccid scarring), abnormal wound healing; psoriasiform dermatitis, ulcerative stomatitis; gingivitis, stomatitis, recurrent skin and systemic infections (tonsillitis, periodontitis, septicemia, ulcerative stomatitis, pharyngitis, otitis media, pneumonia, sinusitis, peritonitis) *Ped Derm 28:156–161, 2011; Ped Derm 27:500–503, 2010; Nat Rev Immunol 7:678–689, 2007; BJD 139:1064–1067, 1998; JAAD 31:316–319, 1994; J Pediatr 119:343–354, 1991; BJD 123:395–401, 1990; Bone Marrow Transplant 24:1261–1263, 1990; Ann Rev Med 38: 175–194, 1987; J Infect Dis 152:668–689, 1985*

Lupus erythematosus, systemic – malleolar, foot ulcers in areas of livedo or vasculitis *J Rheumatol 6:204–209, 1979;* SLE with calcinosis and ulcer – personal observation; discoid *BJD 148:388–401, 2003*

Morphea, including pansclerotic morphea of childhood *JAAD 53:S115–119, 2005; Ped Derm 16:245–247, 1999*

Mixed connective tissue disease *Acta DV 61:225–231, 1981*

Pemphigus vulgaris *Clin Exp Dermatol 25:224–226, 2000*

Polymyalgia rheumatica *BJD 148:388–401, 2003*

Pyrin-associated autoinflammatory neutrophilic disease (PAAND) – autosomal dominant; facial pustules, pyoderma gangrenosum lesions; mutation in *MEFV Ped Derm 33:602–614, 2016*

Rheumatoid arthritis *BJD 152:1062–1064, 2005; J Rheumatol 10:507–509, 1983; AD 92:489–494, 1965*
    Arteritis
    Dystrophic calcification *J Med Inves 64:308–310, 2017*

Felty's syndrome *JAAD 53:191–209, 2005; BJD 148:388–401, 2003; Sem Arthr Rheum 21:129–142, 1991*
    Gravitational ulcers
    Lymphedema due to immobility with ulceration
    Associated with mononeuritis multiplex
    Pyoderma gangrenosum
    Pressure ulcers
    Rheumatoid vasculitis – ulcers of the lateral malleolus or pretibial area *JAAD 53:191–209, 2005*
    Vasculitis, necrotizing *BJD 147:905–913, 2002; Med J Aust 153:585–587, 1990*
    Rheumatoid nodules, ulcerated at pressure sites
    Traumatic ulcers

Scleroderma – painful ulcers over bony prominences *Acta DV 98:677–682, 2018; AD 84:359–374, 1961*

Sjogren's syndrome – vasculitis *A Clinician's Pearls and Myths in Rheumatology pp.107–130; ed John Stone; Springer 2009*

Still's disease

CONGENITAL LESIONS

Aplasia cutis congenita with epidermolysis bullosa

DEGENERATIVE

Neuropathic ulcer (trophic ulcer)
    Charcot-Marie-Tooth syndrome with neurotrophic foot ulcer
    Decubitus
    Diabetes
        Hereditary sensory neuropathy *Clin Exp Derm 1:91–92, 1976*
    Leprosy
    Neuropathy
    Paraplegias
    Syringomyelia – trophic ulcer
    Tabes dorsalis
    Trigeminal trophic syndrome *J Dermatol 18:613–615, 1991*

DRUG-INDUCED

Corticosteroid-induced leg ulcers – systemic, intralesional, topical *AD 92:52–53, 1965*

Coumarin necrosis *AD 122:1408, 1412, 1986*

Ergot

Granulocyte colony-stimulating factor *BJD 148:388–401, 2003*

Halogenoderma *BJD 148:388–401, 2003*

Heparin necrosis

Hydroxyurea – ulcers of the lower legs and feet *AD 143:1310–1313, 2007;* often over lateral malleoli; atrophic, scaling, poikilodermatous patches with erosions on the backs of the hands, sides of the feet *J Korean Med Sci 21:177–179, 2006; JAAD 45:321–322, 2001; AD 137:467–470, 2001; Leuk Lymphoma 35:109–118, 1999; AD 135:818–820, 1999; JAAD 39:372–374, 1998; JAAD 36:178–182, 1997; Cutis 52:217–219, 1993;* dermatomyositis-like rash *Clin Exp Dermatol 25:256–257, 2000*

Levophed ischemic necrosis

Methotrexate *BJD 148:388–401, 2003*

Methimazole – antithyroid drug-induced ANCA+ vasculitis; round ulcers of the legs *JAMADerm 153:223–224, 2017; J Clin Endocrinol Metab 94:2806–2811, 2009*

Nicorandil *BJD 156:394–396, 2007*

Pentazocine abuse *Int J Dermatol 55:e49–51, 2016*

Vasculitis, drug-induced – furosemide, captopril

EXOGENOUS AGENTS

Calcium gluconate extravasation – calcinosis cutis *Ped Derm 26:311–315, 2009*

Contact dermatitis, irritant

Marijuana – cannabis arteritis – peripheral necrosis over the legs *JAAD 69:135–142, 2013*

Silicone injection

Tibial cement extrusion *J Arthroplasty 13:826–829, 1998*

INFECTIONS AND INFESTATIONS

Acanthamebiasis in AIDS *AD 131:1291–1296, 1995*

Actinomycosis

Aeromonas hydrophila

Alternariosis *Clin Inf Dis 32:1178–1187, 2001*

Amebiasis

Animal bites

Anthrax *BJD 148:388–401, 2003*

Arcanobacterium haemolyticum J Clin Inf Dis 18:835–836, 1994

Aspergillosis, primary cutaneous *JAAD 31:344–347, 1994;* resembling pyoderma gangrenosum *JAAD 29:656–658, 1993;* leg ulcer in chronic GVHD *JAAD 66:535–550, 2012*

Bacillary angiomatosis *AD 131:963–964, 1995*

Bacillus cereus JAAD 47:324–325, 2002

Bacterial endocarditis *BJD 148:388–401, 2003*

BCG vaccination *BJD 148:388–401, 2003*

Bipolaris spicifera AD 125:1383–1386, 1989

Botryomycosis

Brucellosis

Candida albicans – granulomatous panniculitis *JAAD 28:315–317, 1993; J Cut Pathol 16:183–193, 1989*

Cat scratch disease

Chromomycosis – feet, legs, arms, face, and neck *AD 113:1027–1032, 1997; BJD 96:454–458, 1977; AD 104:476–485, 1971*

Clostridial gas gangrene – acute ulcer *BJD 148:388–401, 2003*

Coccidioidomycosis *BJD 148:388–401, 2003*

Corynebacterium pyogenes Int J Dermatol 21:407–409, 1987; epidemic leg ulcers of children in Thailand *Southeast Asian J Trop Med Public Health 13:568–574, 1982*

Corynebacterium ulcerans – medial and lateral lower leg ulcers mimicking cutaneous diphtheria with gray membrane and sweet smell *Clin Inf Dis 33:1598–600, 2001*

Cryptococcosis *JAAD 5:32–36, 1981*

Cytomegalovirus JAMADerm 151:661–662, 2015

Desert sore (Veldt sore) – acute leg ulcer

Diphtheria (*Corynebacterium diphtheriae*) – after international travel *MMWR 68:281–284, 2019;* in drug users *Clin Inf Dis 18:94–96, 1994;* cutaneous diphtheria *BJD 148:388–401, 2003;* mimicking pyoderma gangrenosum *JAMADerm 154:227–228, 2018*

Dracunculosis – bulla which ruptures leaving an ulcer *J Clin Inf Dis 25:749, 1997*

Ecthyma *Clin Inf Dis 48:1213–1219, 2009*

Ecthyma gangrenosum – *Pseudomonas, Escherichia coli, Aeromonas hydrophila BJD 148:388–401, 2003*

Epstein-Barr virus (infectious mononucleosis) – cold urticaria with cold agglutinins and leg ulcers *Acta DV 61:451–452, 1981*

Erysipelas *BJD 148:388–401, 2003*

Erythema induratum *JAMADerm 154:355–356, 2018; Dermatology 231:195–200, 2015; Am J Dermatopathol 31:263–267, 2009; JAAD 49:1029–1036, 2008*

Filariasis – secondary lymphedema

Furuncle

Fusarium, localized *JAAD 47:659–666, 2002*

Glanders

Helicobacter bilis – leg ulcer in X-linked agammaglobulinemia *AD 146:523–526, 2010*

Helicobacter cinaedi – pyoderma gangrenosum-like ulcers in hypogammaglobulinemia *J Dermatol 44:e334–335, 2017*

Herpes simplex, chronic in AIDS *BJD 148:388–401, 2003*

Histoplasmosis *BJD 148:388–401, 2003*

Hyalohyphomycosis – *Acremonium* species *BJD 150:789–790, 2004*

Insect bites *BJD 148:388–401, 2003*

Klebsiella pneumonia – grossly swollen cellulitic thigh with focal ulcerations, crepitus, fever, impaired state of consciousness *Clin Inf Dis 56:1457,1505–1506, 2013*

Lacazia loboi (lobomycosis) – leg ulcer *Clin Inf Dis 59:264,314–315, 2014*

Leishmaniasis – tumoral cutaneous leishmaniasis *Clin Dermatol 38:140–151, 2020;* impetigo- and ecthyma-like lesions of the legs (Bauru ulcers) *Ped Derm 34:721–723, 2017; JAAD 73:897–908, 2015; JAAD 60:897–925, 2009; BJD 151:1165–1171, 2004; Trans R Soc Trop Med Hyg 81:606, 1987; Cutis 38:198–199, 1986; L. brasiliensis JAAD 73:897–908, 2015;* multiple ulcers of the legs and feet in AIDS *BJD 160:311–318, 2009; L. tropica* with viscerotropic lesions *AD 145:1023–1026, 2009*

Leprosy – lepromatous leprosy with ulcerated nodules of the legs and feet; Lucio's phenomenon *JAAD 71:795–803, 2014; JAAD 48:958–961, 2003; AD 135:983–988, 1999*

Lyme borreliosis (*Borrelia burgdorferi*) – acrodermatitis chronica atrophicans – red to blue nodules or plaques; sclerosis of lower legs with ulceration *BJD 121:263–269, 1989; Int J Derm 18:595–601, 1979*

Meleney's synergistic gangrene

Melioidosis – pretibial ulcerative vegetative plaque *Cutis 72:310–312, 2003*

Meningococcemia *BJD 148:388–401, 2003*

Mosquito bite hypersensitivity syndrome in EBV-associated natural killer cell leukemia/lymphoma – clear or hemorrhagic bullae with necrosis, ulceration, and scar formation *JAAD 45:569–578, 2001*

Mucormycosis resembling pyoderma gangrenosum *JAAD 29:462–465, 1993*

Mycetoma *BJD 148:388–401, 2003*

Mycobacterium abscessus Ped Derm 32:488–494, 2015; BJD 152:727–734, 2005

Mycobacterium avium complex – traumatic inoculation leg ulcers, ulcerated nodules, panniculitis, folliculitis, or papules *BJD 130:785–790, 1994; JAAD 19:492–495, 1988*

Mycobacterium chelonae AD 129:1189–1194, 1993; Am Rev Resp Dis 119:107–159, 1979

Mycobacterium fortuitum JAAD 57:413–420, 2007

Mycobacterium haemophilum – ulcerated plaque *Ann Int Med* 120:118–125, 1994

Mycobacterium intracellulare

Mycobacterium kansasii

Mycobacterium marinum

Mycobacterium scrofulaceum

Mycobacterium szulgai

Mycobacterium tuberculosis – scrofuloderma, lupus vulgaris, erythema induratum *JAAD 14:738–742, 1986;* tuberculous chancre *Clin Dermatol 8(3/4):49–65, 1990;* papulonecrotic tuberculid *BJD 148:388–401, 2003;* mimicking systemic vasculitis *Trop Doct 47:158–164, 2017*

Mycobacterium ulcerans (Buruli ulcer) (Bairnsdale, Kakerifu, Kasongo, Searls' ulcer) – lower leg ulcer with undermined margins; differential diagnosis includes tropical phagedenic ulcer or necrotizing fasciitis *Clin Inf Dis 62:342–350, 2016; JAMADerm 151:1137–1139, 2015; Dermatol Clinics 29:1–8, 2011; JAAD 54:559–578, 2006; NEJM 348:1065–1066, 2003; Trans R Soc Trop Med Hyg 94:277–279, 2000; Med Trop(Mars) 57:83–90, 1997(French); Clin Inf Dis 21:1186–1192, 1995; Med Trop(Mars) 55:363–373, 1995; Aust J Dermatol 26:67–73, 1985; Pathology 17:594–600, 1985;* leg ulcers with osteomyelitis *Clin Inf Dis 59:1256–1264, 2014*

Necrotizing fasciitis *BJD 148:388–401, 2003*

Nocardia Clin Dermatol 38:152–159, 2020; granulomatous panniculitis *Case Rep Dermatol 9:117–129, 2017*

North American blastomycosis – ulcers of the leg and foot

Osteomyelitis *J Derm Surg Oncol 10:384–388, 1984;* chronic ulcer of the heel with underlying osteomyelitis – personal observation

Pasteurella multocida (also P. haemolytica, pneumotropica, and *ureae)* – cellulitis with ulceration with hemorrhagic purulent discharge with sinus tracts *Medicine 63:133–144, 1984*

Phagedenic ulcer *BJD 148:388–401, 2003*

Phaeohyphomycosis – *Curvularia pallescens JAAD 32:375–378, 1995*

Pinta

Prototothecosis *AD 136:1263–1268, 2000*

Pseudomonas aeruginosa

Pyoderma *BJD 148:388–401, 2003*

Pyomyositis

Pythium insidiosum (pythiosis) (alga) (aquatic oocyte) – necrotizing hemorrhagic plaque; ascending gangrene of the legs; Thailand; painful subcutaneous nodules, eyelid swelling and periorbital cellulitis, facial swelling, ulcer of the arm or leg, pustules evolving into ulcers *BJD 175:394–397, 2016; J Infect Dis 159:274–280, 1989*

Rat bite fever

Rhizopus azygosporus BJD 153:428–430, 2005

Scorpion stings

Septic emboli

Serratia marcescens – sepsis *JAAD 58:S55–56, 2008; JAAD 49:S193–194, 2003*

Shewanella alga Clin Inf Dis 22:1036–1039, 1996

Snakebites

Spider bites

Sporotrichosis *BJD 148:388–401, 2003*

Streptococcal ulcers of the legs – serpiginous margins with granular base *AD 104:271–280, 1971*

Syphilis – secondary (malignant lues), tertiary (gumma) tabes dorsalis – trophic ulcer; tertiary syphilis with chronic leg ulcers *Clin Dermatol 8(3/4):157–165, 1990*

Tinea corporis, pedis, Majocchi's granuloma

Tropical phagedenic ulcers – mixed infection; mixed infection with *Fusobacterium ulcerans, anaerobic cocci, Bacteroides* species, *Borrelia vincentii, Bacillus fusiformis, Treponema vincentii,* and other organisms; papule or bulla which breaks down to form very painful rapidly growing ulcer with undermined border *JAAD 54:559–578, 2006; BJD 148:388–401, 2003; Int J Dermatol 27:49–53, 1988; Trans R Soc Trop Med Hyg 82:185–189, 1988; BJD 116:31–37, 1987;* tropical ulcers – anaerobic (35%) and coliform (60%) organisms;

Trypanosoma brucei rhodesiense J Clin Inf Dis 23:847–848, 1996

Tularemia *Clin Inf Dis 20:174–175, 1995; Cutis 54:279–286, 1994*

Vibrio extorquens

Vibrio vulnificus JAAD 46:S144–145, 2002

Yaws – mother yaw; leg ulcer in a 15-year-old boy *NEJM 372:693–695, 2015;* gumma *Clin Dermatol 8:157–165, 1990*

Zygomycosis *JAAD 30:904–908, 1994*

INFILTRATIVE DISEASES

Familial amyloid polyneuropathy due to mutation in transthyretin – ulcers of the knees *BJD 164:1398–1400, 2011*

Langerhans cell histiocytosis *BJD 148:388–401, 2003*

INFLAMMATORY DISEASES

Chronic recurrent multifocal osteomyelitis (CRMO) – seen with varied neutrophilic dermatoses including SAPHO syndrome, pyoderma gangrenosum, acne fulminans, pustular psoriasis, Sweet's syndrome *JAAD 70:767–772, 2014; Ped Derm 26:497–505, 2009*

Crohn's disease, metastatic – granulomatous ulcer *JAAD 41:476–479, 1999; JAAD 28:115–117, 1993*

Erythema multiforme *BJD 148:388–401, 2003*

Fibrosis from longstanding edema – ischemic ulcers

Hidradenitis suppurativa – personal observation

Pancreatic panniculitis (fat necrosis) *BJD 178:388–401, 2003*

Panniculitis, including Weber-Christian disease, lupus profundus, alpha-1 antitrypsin deficiency *AD 123:1655–1661, 1987;*

Pyoderma gangrenosum *BJD 175:882–891, 2016; BJD 165:1244–1250, 2011; JAAD 61:730–732, 2009; Ped Derm 25:509–519, 2008; Dermatology 195:50–51, 1997; J Derm Surg Oncol 20:833–836, 1994; JAAD 18:559–568, 1988;* pyoderma gangrenosum with C7 deficiency *JAAD 27:356–359, 1992; AD 22:655–680, 1930;* bullous pyoderma gangrenosum; associations with solid tumors – gastric, renal, oral, parotid, hypopharynx, breast, colon *JAAD 64:1208–1211, 2011;* giant ulcer with Achilles tendon rupture *BJD 172:522–526, 2015*

Sarcoid – ulcerative sarcoid – tender, "punched-out," and often bilateral *JAMA Derm 149:1040–1049, 2013; JAAD 66:699–716, 2012; JAAD 53:917, 2005; AD 133:215–219, 1997; AD 123:1531–1534, 1987; AD 118:9331–933, 1982*

Superficial granulomatous pyoderma (pyoderma gangrenosum vegetans) *Ped Derm 27:496–499, 2010; BJD 153:684–686, 2005;*

BJD 146:141–143, 2002; J Eur Acad Dermatol Venereol 16:159–161, 2002; J Eur Acad Dermatol Venereol 16:97, 2002; Hautarzt 45:635–638, 1994; BJD 129:718–722, 1993; Mayo Clin Proc 64:37–43, 1989; J Dermatol 16:127–132, 1989; JAAD 18:511–521, 1988

METABOLIC

Acrodermatitis enteropathica – foot ulcers – personal observation

Antiphospholipid deficiency *BJD 148:388–401, 2003*

Antithrombin III deficiency *JAAD 65:880–881, 2011; BJD 148:388–401, 2003*

C3 deficiency *BJD 148:388–401, 2003*

Calcinosis – ulcerative calcinosis cutis *J Drugs in Dermatol 10:1042–1044, 2011;* calcinosis cutis; calcinosis of muscles or subcutaneous tissue – overlying ulceration; dystrophic calcifications in end-stage renal disease – personal observation

Calciphylaxis (vascular calcification cutaneous necrosis syndrome) (cutaneous calcinosis in end-stage renal disease) – necrotic cutaneous ulcers, livedo racemosa, hemorrhagic patches, indurated plaques, hemorrhagic bullae *JAMA Derm 149:163–167, 2013; JAAD 56:569–579, 2007; AD 143:152–154, 2007; AD 142:900–906, 2006; AD 140:1045–1048, 2004; BJD 143:1087–1090, 2000; JAAD 40:979–987, 1999; JAAD 33:53–58, 1995; JAAD 33:954–962, 1995*

Cold agglutinins *BJD 148:388–401, 2003*

Cryofibrinogenemia *Am J Med 116:332–337, 2004*

Cryoglobulinemia – type I *JAMADerm 150:426–428, 2014; NEJM 347:1412–1418, 2002; JAAD 45:S202–206, 2001;* mixed – bilateral in 87% of patients *JAAD 82:799–816, 2020; AD 139:391–393, 2003;* hemorrhagic crusted leg ulcer *Cutis 70:319–323, 2002*

Defective organization of the extracellular matrix of fibronectin *BJD 142:166–170, 2000*

Defective fibrinolysis *BJD 148:388–401, 2003*

Diabetes mellitus *Diabet Med 16:889–909, 1999; Diabetes 40:1305–1313, 1991;* necrobiosis lipoidica diabeticorum, ulcerative; neuropathic and large vessel and microvascular foot ulcers (mal perforans)

Factor V Leiden deficiency *BJD 148:388–401, 2003;* Factor V Leiden mutation and cryofibrinogenemia *JAAD 51:S122–124, 2004;* heterozygous factor V Leiden deficiency *BJD 143:1302–1305, 2000*

Factor XIII deficiency *BJD 148:388–401, 2003*

Gamma heavy-chain disease

Gaucher's disease

Gout – subcutaneous tophus *BJD 148:388–401, 2003; AD 134:499–504, 1998;Am J Pathol 32:871–895, 1956*

Hematologic disease
  Dysproteinemias – cryoglobulinemia *JAAD 45:S202–206, 2001;* cold agglutinins, macroglobulinemia, cryofibrinogenemia, myeloma, polyclonal dysproteinemia *BJD 148:388–401, 2003*
  Red blood cell disorders – sickle cell disease *Plast Surg Nurs 38:99–100, 2018;* hereditary spherocytosis *Ped Derm 20:427–428, 2003; Clin Exp Dermatol 16:28–30, 1991;* in atypical locations (backs of the feet) *Dermatologica 181:56–59, 1990;* thalassemia, polycythemia vera, G-6PD deficiency,
hereditary elliptocytosis, hereditary nonspherocytic hemolytic anemia *BJD 148:388–401, 2003*
  White blood cell disease – leukemia, granulocytopenia *BJD 148:388–401, 2003*

Platelet disorders – essential thrombocythemia *Hautarzt 35:259–262, 1984; Br J Surg 60(5):377–380, 1973;* thrombotic thrombocytopenic purpura *BJD 148:388–401, 2003*

Edema due to cardiac or renal failure

Extramedullary hematopoiesis *JAAD 4:592–596, 1981*

Homocysteinemia *Ned Tijdschr Geneeskd 142:2706–2707, 1998(Dutch)*

Hyperparathyroidism *BJD 83:263–268, 1970*

Hyperviscosity – paraproteinemia, leukemia *BJD 148:388–401, 2003*

Iron deficiency anemia with pruritus – personal observation

Malnutrition

Myxedema *BJD 148:388–401, 2003;* pretibial myxedema masquerading as venous ulcer *Wounds 29:77–79, 2017*

Necrobiosis lipoidica diabeticorum *Dermatol Clinics 33:343–360, 2015; Cutis 95:252, 265–266, 2015; JAAD 69:783–791, 2013; JAMA Derm 149:879–881, 2013; Ped Derm 27:178–181, 2010; AD 145:437–439, 2009; AD 142:20–22, 2006; JAAD 17:351–354, 1987*

Oxalosis (primary oxalosis) – autosomal recessive; livedo reticularis, acrocyanosis, peripheral gangrene, ulcerations, sclerodermoid changes (woody induration of extremities), eschar of the hand (calcium oxalate); acral and/or facial papules or nodules; end-stage renal disease; primary hyperoxalosis – deficiency of alanine-glyoxylate aminotransferase; primary hyperoxalosis – deficiency of D-glycerate dehydrogenase/glyoxylate reductase *AD 147:1277–1282, 2011; JAAD 49:725–728, 2003; AD 136:1272–1274, 2000*

Primary hyperoxaluria – livedo reticularis *AD 147:1302–1305, 2011; Clin Exper Dermatol 16:367–370, 1991;* peripheral (digital) ischemia *Hemodial Int 13:266–270, 2009; AD 136:1272–1274, 2000;* ulcers *AD 131:821–823, 1995*
  Primary hyperoxaluria type I – decreased peroxisomal, liver-specific alanine-glyoxylate aminotransferase *BJD 169:227–230, 2013*
  Primary hyperoxaluria type II – glyoxylate/hydroxypyruvate reductase; *GRHPR* gene mutation *BJD 169:227–230, 2013*
  Primary hyperoxaluria type III – decreased 4-hydroxy-2-oxoglutarate aldolase *BJD 169:227–230, 2013*

Paget's disease of the bone – leg ulcer overlying focus of Paget's disease *AD 141:1050, 2005*

Paraproteinemia

Paroxysmal nocturnal hemoglobinuria – petechiae, ecchymoses, hemorrhagic bullae; ulcers; red plaques which become hemorrhagic bullae with necrosis; lesions occur on the legs, abdomen, chest, nose, and ears; fever; deficiency of enzymes – decay-accelerating factor (DAF) and membrane inhibitor of reactive lysis (MIRL) *AD 148:660–662, 2012; AD 138:831–836, 2002; AD 122:1325–1330, 1986; AD 114:560–563, 1978*

Porphyria cutanea tarda *BJD 148:388–401, 2003*

Prolidase deficiency – autosomal recessive; peptidase D mutation (PEPD); increased urinary imidopeptides; leg ulcers, anogenital ulcers, short stature (mild), telangiectasias, recurrent infections (sinusitis, otitis); mental retardation; splenomegaly with enlarged abdomen, atrophic scarring, spongy fragile skin with annular pitting and scarring; dermatitis, xerosis, hyperkeratosis of the elbows and knees, lymphedema, purpura, low hairline, poliosis, canities, lymphedema, photosensitivity, hypertelorism, saddle nose deformity, frontal bossing, dull expression, mild ptosis, micrognathia, mandibular protrusion, exophthalmos, joint laxity, deafness, osteoporosis, high-arched palate *JAAD 62:1031, 1034, 2010; BJD 144:635–636,*

2001; Ped Derm 13:58–60, 1996; JAAD 29:819–821, 1993; AD 127:124–125, 1991; AD 123:493–497, 1987

Protein C or S deficiency *BJD 148:388–401, 2003*

Scurvy – hemorrhagic leg ulcers *Ann DV 127:510–512, 2000; JAAD 41:895–906, 1999*

Sickle cell disease – chronic leg ulcers *Clin Sci(Lond) 98:667–672, 2000; J Trop Med Hyg 85:205–208, 1982*

Spherocytosis, hereditary – thrombotic vasculitis *South Med J 104:150–152, 2011; Ped Derm 20:427–428, 2003;* pyoderma gangrenosum *Indian J Low Extrem Wounds 15:92–95, 2016*

Subcutaneous calcification (postphlebitic subcutaneous calcification) – chronic venous insufficiency; nonhealing ulcers; fibrosis *Radiology 74:279–281, 1960*

Subcutaneous fat necrosis

TAP1 mutation *BJD 148:388–401, 2003*

NEOPLASTIC

Angiosarcoma *Cutis 102:E8–11, 2018*

Atrial myxoma – leg ulcers, acral red papules with claudication *JAAD 32:881–883, 1995;* tender red fingertip papule *JAAD 21:1080–1084, 1989*

Basal cell carcinoma *AD 148:704–708, 2012; JAAD 25:47–49, 1991;* complicating venous stasis ulcers *J Derm Surg Oncol 19:150–152, 1993;* mimicking venous stasis ulcer *Adv Skin Wound Care 31:130–134, 2018*

Eccrine syringofibroadenoma – in a burn scar *BJD 143:591–594, 2000*

Epithelioid sarcoma *BJD 118:843–844, 1988*

Epithelioma cuniculatum (verrucous carcinoma) *Ann Pathol 4:223–229, 1984*

Kaposi's sarcoma – gangrene and ulcerations of the legs *JAMA Derm 149:1319–1322, 2013*

Leiomyosarcoma *AD 148:704–708, 2012*

Leukemia – hairy cell leukemia, chronic myelogenous leukemia *South Med J 60:567–572, 1967;* natural killer cell CD5 – large granular lymphocytic leukemia – leg ulcer associated with thigh telangiectasia *JAAD 62:496–501, 2010*

Lymphoma – cutaneous T-cell lymphoma *AD 145:677–682, 2009; Cutis 28:43–44, 1981;* gamma/delta T-cell lymphoma *JAAD 56:643–647, 2007;* gamma/delta T-cell lymphoma with hemophagocytic syndrome *Am J Dermatopathol 16:426–433, 1994;* angiocentric T-cell lymphoma *AD 132:1105–1110, 1996;* lymphomatoid granulomatosis *AD 117:196–202, 1981;* Hodgkin's disease *BJD 148:388–401, 2003; Br J Derm 80:555–560, 1968;* subcutaneous panniculitis-like T-cell lymphoma *BJD 148:516–525, 2003; JAAD 39:721–736, 1998;* primary cutaneous diffuse large B-cell lymphoma, leg type; Bcl-2 expression *JAAD 69:343–354, 2013; AD 143:1144–1150, 2007;* cutaneous large B-cell lymphoma *BJD 146:144–147, 2002;* CD30+ anaplastic large cell T-cell lymphoma *JAAD 57:S103–105, 2007; AD 143:255–260, 2007; BJD 149:542–553, 2003;* CD56+ lymphoma *BJD 147:1017–1020, 2000;* extranodal NK/T-cell lymphoma *BJD 160:333–337, 2009;* syringotropic cutaneous T-cell lymphoma – red plaques, leg ulcers, comedo-like lesions, palmoplantar hyperkeratosis *JAAD 71:926–934, 2014*

Lymphomatoid granulomatosis – Epstein-Barr-related angiocentric T-cell-rich B-cell lymphoproliferative disorder; papules and dermal nodules with or without ulceration, folliculitis-like lesions, maculopapules, indurated plaques, ulcers *BJD 157:426–429, 2007; JAAD 54:657–663, 2006*

Lymphoproliferative disorder of granular lymphocytes – ulcerated plaque *JAAD 30:339–344, 1994*

Marjolin's ulcer – squamous cell carcinoma arising in a chronic ulcer; may present as induration and persistence of ulceration, elevated border at edge of ulcer, breakdown of burn scar with indurated base, nodule formation within burn scar *AD 148:704–708, 2012; Cutis 56:168–170, 1995; Dictionnaire de Medicine. In:Adelon N(ed.)Paris:Bechet, 1828:31–50;* complicating venous stasis ulcers *South Med J 58:779–781, 1965;* bilateral Marjolin's ulcers *Clin Inf Dis 61:1147,1199–1200, 2015*

Melanoma *AD 148:704–708, 2012; BJD 148:388–401, 2003;* mimicking toe gangrene in diabetic *Eur J Endovasc Surg 56:18, 2018*

Metastases *BJD 148:388–401, 2003*

Myelofibrosis – extramedullary hematopoiesis in myelofibrosis *JAAD 4:592–596, 1981*

Neoplastic obstruction with lymphedema

Osteoclastoma (giant cell tumor of bone)

Osteosarcoma – extraskeletal *J Coll Physicians Surg Pak 21:429–430*

Polycythemia vera – thrombotic vasculitis

Porocarcinoma *BJD 152:1051–1055, 2005*

Porokeratosis – congenital linear porokeratosis *Ped Derm 12:318–322, 1995*

Posttransplantation lymphoproliferative disorder *JAAD 54:657–663, 2006*

Rhabdomyosarcoma *BJD 148:388–401, 2003*

Soft tissue sarcoma *BJD 148:388–401, 2003*

Waldenstrom's macroglobulinemia *AD 134:1127–1131, 1998;*

PARANEOPLASTIC DISEASES

Leukocytoclastic vasculitis – associated with T-large granular lymphocytic leukemia *BJD 157:631–633, 2007*

Necrobiotic xanthogranuloma with paraproteinemia *AD 145:279–284, 2009; AD 133:97–102, 1997; JAAD 29:466–469, 1993; Medicine(Baltimore) 65:376–388, 1986; BJD 113:339–343, 1985; JAAD 3:257–270, 1980*

Pyoderma gangrenosum, bullous – associated with acute myelogenous leukemia *Leuk Lymph 47:147–150, 2006*

Sweet's syndrome, bullous – associated with myelodysplasias

Vasculitis – paraneoplastic vasculitis *J Rheumatol 18:721–727, 1991;* leukocytoclastic vasculitis; thrombotic vasculitis associated with plasma cell dyscrasias

PRIMARY CUTANEOUS DISEASES

Acute parapsoriasis (Mucha-Habermann disease)

Epidermolysis bullosa including pretibial epidermolysis bullosa *JAAD 22:346–350, 1990*

Erosive pustular dermatosis (chronic atrophic erosive dermatosis of the scalp and extremities) *JAAD 57:421–427, 2007*

Erythema elevatum diutinum *BJD 148:388–401, 2003*

Fibrosis

Lichen planus – bullous *BJD 148:388–401, 2003;* erosive lichen planus of the soles

Lipedema *BJD 148:388–401, 2003*

Malakoplakia – ulcerated papule *JAAD 30:834–836, 1994*

Nummular dermatitis

Psoriasis

Reactive perforating collagenosis

Verrucous hyperplasia of the amputation stump – personal observation

PSYCHOCUTANEOUS DISEASE

Factitial dermatitis

SYNDROMES

Antiphospholipid antibody syndrome *BJD 157:389–392, 2007; NEJM 347:1412–1418, 2002; Semin Arthritis Rheum 31:127–132, 2001; JAAD 36:149–168, 1997; JAAD 36:970–982, 1997; BJD 120:419–429, 1989;* anticardiolipin syndrome

Behcet's syndrome – pyoderma gangrenosum-like lesion *J Dermatol 31:806–810, 2004; Arch Int Med 145:1913–1915, 1985*

Congenital indifference to pain

Defective expression of HLA class I and CD1a molecules with Marfanoid habitus *JAAD 35:814–818, 1996*

Ehlers-Danlos syndrome

Felty's syndrome – arthritis, leucopenia, splenomegaly, rheumatoid arthritis *JAAD 53:191–209, 2005*

Hereditary sensory neuropathy (ulceromutilating type 2) – primary *Wounds 30:E25–28, 2018*

Kawasaki's disease *BJD 148:388–401, 2003*

Klinefelter syndrome – leg ulcers with stasis ulcers, hyperpigmentation, or atrophie blanche *J Eur Acad EV 17:62–64, 2003; AD 131:230, 1995*

Marfan's syndrome with venous stasis leg ulcer – personal observation

Neurofibromatosis – vasculopathy *JAAD 51:656–659, 2004*

Pachydermoperiostosis (Touraine-Solente-Gole syndrome) *Clin Rheumatol 14:705–707, 1995*

PAPA (pyogenic arthritis with pyoderma gangrenosum) syndrome – pyoderma gangrenosum, cystic acne, acne fulminans, non-axial destructive aseptic arthritis; sterile abscesses at injection sites; attacks last 5 days; mutation in CD2-binding protein 1 *Ped Derm 22:262–265, 2005; Proc Natl Acad Sci USA 100:13501–13506, 2003; Mayo Clin Proc 72:611–615, 1997*

Pyogenic sterile arthritis, pyoderma gangrenosum, and acne – autosomal dominant; mutation in proline-serine-threonine phosphatase-interacting protein 1 (CD2-binding protein 1) *JAAD 70:767–773, 2014*

Reactive arthritis syndrome – keratoderma blenorrhagicum

SAPHO syndrome

Sneddon's syndrome – noninflammatory thrombotic vasculopathy; cerebrovascular disease and livedo racemosa *Clin Exp Dermatol 33:377–379, 2008; BJD 148:388–401, 2003*

Werner's syndrome – senile appearance, short stature, premature gray hair, birdlike face, sclerodermoid skin changes, leg ulcers, cataracts, osteoporosis, hypogonadism, diabetes, ischemic heart disease *An Bras Dermatol 92:271–272, 2017; AD 133:1293–1295, 1997; Acta DV 50:237–239, 1970*

TRAUMA

Amputation stump friction blisters with ulceration

Burns

Charcot foot *Am Family Physician 97:594–599, 2018*

Chemical injury – corrosive agents, sclerotherapy *BJD 148:388–401, 2003*

Cold injury – perniosis (erythrocyanosis frigida); frostbite *BJD 148:388–401, 2003*

Coma bullae with ulcers *Dermatology 203:233–237, 2001*

Decubitus – heels and ankles *BJD 148:388–401, 2003*

Drug abuse – intravenous (IVDA); skin popping; delayed cutaneous ulcers at sites of prior drug abuse *BJD 150:1–10, 2004; JAAD 29:1052–1054, 1993*

Hematoma *BJD 148:388–401, 2003*

Nerve injury, traumatic – surgical injury to lateral femoral cutaneous nerve with bulla and subsequent ulceration of lateral lower leg *Dermatol Wochenschri 136:971–973, 1957;*

Obesity – chronic venous insufficiency with ulcers *JAAD 81:1037–1057, 2019*

Physical trauma – ulcers of shins and ankles

Pressure – decubitus ulcer *BJD 148:388–401, 2003*

Radiation – ischemic ulcers

Reflex sympathetic dystrophy – bulla and leg ulceration *JAAD 44:1050, 2001; JAAD 28:29–32, 1993*

Scar tissue – ischemic ulceration

Sclerotherapy – extravasation of sclerosant

Trench foot *BJD 148:388–401, 200*

VASCULAR

Acroangiodermatitis of Mali (Stewart-Bluefarb syndrome) (pseudo-Kaposi's sarcoma) – ulceration of the lower leg signifies chronic venous insufficiency or *paralysis Int Wound J 12:169–172, 2015; BJD 148:388–401, 2003; BJD 148:388–401, 2003*

Acro-osteopathia ulceromutilans (Bureau-Barriere syndrome) *BJD 148:388–401, 2003*

Angiosarcoma, including Stewart-Treves syndrome *Cutis 102:E8–11, 2018; J Dermatol Case Rep 3:8–10, 2009*

Anterior tibial syndrome

Arterial thrombosis *BJD 148:388–401, 2003*

Arteriovenous fistulae and venous malformation (arteriovenous malformation) *BJD 148:388–401, 2003*

Atherosclerosis – punched-out ischemic ulcers over pretibial areas or toes *BJD 148:388–401, 2003;* peripheral vascular disease with foot ulcerations

Atrophie blanche (livedo with ulceration) – ivory white plaque of sclerosis with telangiectasias and surrounding hyperpigmentation; venous insufficiency, thalassemia minor *Acta DV(Stockh)50:125–128, 1970;* cryoglobulinemia, systemic lupus erythematosus, scleroderma *JAAD 8:792–798, 1983; AD 119:963–969, 1983;* mimicking pyoderma gangrenosum *Dermatology Reports May 14, 2018;* livedo vasculitis with summer ulcerations (livedoid vasculopathy) – ulcers of the ankles and legs *BJD 168:898–899, 2013; Ann Rheum Dis 67:1055–1056, 2008; BJD 148:388–401, 2003; BJD 149:647–652, 2003; NEJM 347:1412–1418, 2002; Int J Dermatol 40:153–157, 2001; AD 96:489–499, 1967; Circulation 13:196–216, 1956*

Buerger's disease (thromboangiitis obliterans) *BJD 148:388–401, 2003; AD 134:1019–1024, 1998; Cutis 51:180–182, 1993; Am J Med Sci 136:566–580, 1908*

Cholesterol emboli – foot ulcers *BJD 146:1107–1108, 2002; Semin Arth Rheum 18(4):240–246, 1989*

Congenital absence of veins

Congenital hypoplasia of venous valves *BJD 148:388–401, 2003*

Diffuse dermal angiomatosis with arteriosclerotic peripheral vascular disease *AD 138:456–458, 2002*

Disseminated intravascular coagulation *BJD 148:388–401, 2003*

Eosinophilic granulomatosis with polyangiitis *BJD 148:388–401, 2003*

Erythrocyanosis

Erythromelalgia *BJD 143:868–872, 2000;* associated with thrombocythemia – may affect one finger or toe; ischemic necrosis *JAAD 22:107–111, 1990;* primary (idiopathic) – lower legs, no ischemia *JAAD 21:1128–1130, 1989;* secondary to peripheral vascular disease *JAAD 43:841–847, 2000; AD 136:330–336, 2000;* all types exacerbated by warmth; may be associated with systemic lupus erythematosus, dermatomyositis, neuropathy, hypertension and vasculitis, calcium antagonists *BJD 143:868–872, 2000*

Fat embolism *BJD 148:388–401, 2003*

Fibromuscular dysplasia *BJD 148:388–401, 2003*

Granulomatosis with polyangiitis *Cutis 99:E12–15, 2017; BJD 151:927–928, 2004; NEJM 347:1412–1418, 2002; JAAD 28:710–718, 1993*

Hemangioma *BJD 148:388–401, 2003*

Hemangiosarcoma in leg ulcer *AD 124:1080–1082, 1988*

Henoch-Schonlein purpura *BJD 148:388–401, 2003*

Hypertensive ulcer (Martorell's ulcer) – very painful ulcer of the lower lateral leg (above lateral malleolus) with livedo at edges *BJD 148:388–401, 2003; Phlebology 3:139–142, 1988; Mayo Clin 21:337–346, 1946; J Cardiovasc Surg(Torino) 19:599–600, 1978*

Klippel-Trenaunay-Weber syndrome *NEJM 347:1412–1418, 2002*

Lipodermatosclerosis *Burns Trauma June 15, 2018*

Lymphangiosarcoma *BJD 148:388–401, 2003*

Lymphedema *BJD 148:388–401, 2003*

Malignant angioendothelioma

Malignant atrophic papulosis (Degos disease) *Eur J Pediatr 149:457–458, 1990*

May-Thurner syndrome *Int Wound 14:578–582, 2017*

Mixed arterial and venous ulceration

Nodular vasculitis (erythema induratum of Bazin) *JAAD 36:99–101, 1997*

Peripheral vascular disease – personal observation

Polyarteritis nodosa *BJD 159:615–620, 2008; NEJM 347:1412–1418, 2002; Ann Int Med 89:66–676, 1978;* PAN associated with hepatitis B infection; cutaneous PAN (microscopic polyarteritis nodosa) – livedo reticularis with surrounding erythema; acrocyanosis, leg ulcers, papules, petechiae, palpable purpura, ecchymoses, fever arthralgias *JAAD 57:840–848, 2007; BJD 136:706–713, 1997; AD 128:1223–1228, 1992*

Purpura fulminans *BJD 148:388–401, 2003*

Scars

Small vessel occlusive arterial disease *NEJM 347:1412–1418, 2002*

Superficial thrombophlebitis

Takayasu's arteritis (giant cell arteritis) *JAAD 17:998–1005, 1987*

Temporal arteritis *BJD 76:299–308, 1964*

Thrombophlebitis, ulcerated *BJD 148:388–401, 2003*

Vasculitis (small, medium, and large vessel) *AD 120:484–489, 1984*

Venous gangrene – foot ulcers

Venous stasis ulceration (chronic venous insufficiency) – medial lower leg and medial malleolus *NEJM 355:488–498, 2006; NEJM 347:1412–1418, 2002; AD 133:1231–1234, 1997; Semin Dermatol 12:66–71, 1993;* with subcutaneous calcification *J Derm Surg Oncol 16:450–452, 1990;* venous stasis due to compression or obstruction of veins (pelvic tumors, lymphadenopathy, or pelvic vein thrombosis); dependency syndrome (immobility, arthritis, paralysis, orthopedic malformations); post-thrombotic venous ulcer

ULCERS, LEG, IN A YOUNG PATIENT

JAAD 29:802–803, 807, 1993

AUTOIMMUNE DISEASES AND DISORDERS OF IMMUNE REGULATION

Anti-centromere antibodies – ulcers and gangrene of the extremities *Br J Rheumatol 36:889–893, 1997*

Antineutrophil cytoplasmic antibody syndrome – purpuric vasculitis, orogenital ulceration, fingertip necrosis, pyoderma gangrenosum-like ulcers *BJD 134:924–928, 1996*

Defective expression of HLA class I and CD 1a molecules with Marfanoid habitus *JAAD 35:814–818, 1996*

Graft-versus-host reaction, chronic *AD 134:602–612, 1998*

Lupus erythematosus, systemic *Ital J Pod 36:72, 2010*

Morphea – pansclerotic morphea *JAAD 53:S115–119, 2005; Ped Derm 16:245–247, 1999*

Rheumatoid vasculitis *BJD 147:905–913, 2002*

Scleroderma *J Pediatr 159:698, 2011*

Still's disease

CONGENITAL DISORDERS

Aplasia cutis congenita with epidermolysis bullosa

Congenital insensitivity to pain (HSANV)

Familial dysautonomia (HSAN type IV)

Hereditary sensory neuropathy of ulceromutilating type (type 2) (HSAN)

Subcutaneous fat necrosis of the newborn *Dermatology 197:261–263, 1998*

DEGENERATIVE DISORDERS

Neuropathy

DRUG-INDUCED

Calcium gluconate extravasation

Hydroxyurea *JAAD 49:339–341, 2003*

EXOGENOUS AGENTS

Silicone injection

INFECTIONS AND INFESTATIONS

Acanthamoeba J Clin Inf Dis 20:1207–1216, 1995; JAAD 42:351–354, 2000

Anthrax

Bacillary angiomatosis in HIV disease *AD 131:963, 1995*

Bacillus cereus JAAD 47:324–325, 2002

Cat scratch disease

Bordetella trematum BMC Inf Dis 19:485, 2019

Corynebacterium diphtheriae in drug users *Clin Inf Dis 18:94–96, 1994*

Cryptococcosis – mimicking pyoderma gangrenosum *JAAD 5:32–36, 1981*

Diphtheria

Dracunculosis *Clin Inf Dis 25:749–750, 1997*

Ecthyma

Ecthyma gangrenosum – *Pseudomonas, Escherichia coli, Aeromonas hydrophila*

Epstein-Barr virus (infectious mononucleosis) – cold urticaria with cold agglutinins and leg ulcers *Acta DV 61:451–452, 1981*

Herpes simplex in atopic dermatitis; in AIDS

Histoplasmosis

Leishmaniasis *Trans R Soc Trop Med Hyg 81:606, 1987; Cutis 38:198–199, 1986*

Melioidosis – pretibial ulcerative vegetative plaque *Cutis 72:310–312, 2003*

Mosquito bite hypersensitivity syndrome in EBV-associated natural killer cell leukemia/lymphoma – clear or hemorrhagic bullae with necrosis, ulceration, and scar formation *JAAD 45:569–578, 2001*

Mycetoma of the foot

Mycobacterium avium complex – traumatic inoculation leg ulcers, ulcerated nodules, panniculitis, folliculitis, or papules *BJD 130:785–790, 1994; JAAD 19:492–495, 1988*

Mycobacterium tuberculosis – scrofuloderma, lupus vulgaris *JAAD 14:738–742, 1986;* tuberculous chancre *Clin Dermatol 8(3/4):49–65, 1990;* foot ulcer *Indian Ped 43:255–257, 2006*

Mycobacterium ulcerans (Buruli ulcer) – leg ulcer with undermined margins *JAAD 54:559–578, 2006; NEJM 348:1065–1066, 2003; Med Trop(Mars) 57:83–90, 1997(French); Clin Inf Dis 21:1186–1192, 1995; Med Trop(Mars) 55:363–373, 1995; Aust J Dermatol 26:67–73, 1985; Pathology 17:594–600, 1985*

Mycobacteria, nontuberculous, including *M. chelonae Am Rev Resp Dis 119:107–159, 1979; M. marinum, M. kansasii*

Necrotizing fasciitis

Nocardia

North American blastomycosis – primary infection *Ped Derm 20:128–130, 2003*

Pasteurella multocida (also *P. haemolytica, pneumotropica,* and *ureae*) – cellulitis with ulceration with hemorrhagic purulent discharge with sinus tracts *Medicine 63:133–144, 1984*

Rat bite fever

Scorpion stings

Septic emboli

Shewanella algae Infez Med 27:179–192, 2019

Snakebites

Spider bites

Syphilis – secondary (malignant lues)

Tropical phagedenic ulcers – mixed infection; mixed infection with *Fusobacterium ulcerans,* anaerobic cocci, *Bacteroides* species, and other organisms; papule or bulla which breaks down to form ulcer with undermined border *Int J Dermatol 27:49–53, 1988; BJD 116:31–37, 1987; Trans R Soc Trop Med Hyg 82:185–189, 1988*

Tularemia *Clin Inf Dis 20:174–175, 1995; Cutis 54:279–286, 1994*

Yaws (*Treponema pertenue*)

INFLAMMATORY DISORDERS

Pyoderma gangrenosum *Dermatology 195:50–51, 1997; J Derm Surg Oncol 20:833–836, 1994; JAAD 18:559–568, 1988;* pyoderma gangrenosum with C7 deficiency *JAAD 27:356–359, 1992; AD 22:655–680, 1930*

METABOLIC DISEASES

Antithrombin III deficiency

Calciphylaxis

Metastatic Crohn's disease – granulomatous ulcer *JAAD 41:476–479, 1999*

Cryofibrinogenemia

Cryoglobulinemia

Diabetes mellitus – juvenile, longstanding, poor control

Essential thrombocythemia *JAAD 24:59–63, 1991*

Factor XII deficiency – livedo with ulceration *BJD 143:897–899, 2000*

Gaucher's disease

Hemoglobinopathy (sickle cell anemia) *Int Wound 16:897–902, 2019*

Hereditary spherocytosis *Ped Derm 20:427–428, 2003*

Homocystinuria *JAAD 40:279–281, 1999; Ned Tijdschr Geneeskd 142:2706–2707, 1998(Dutch)*

Porphyrin retention

Prolidase deficiency – autosomal recessive; recurrent infection; skin spongy and fragile with annular pitting and scarring; recalcitrant leg ulcers; photosensitivity, telangiectasia, purpura, premature graying, lymphedema *BJD 147:1227–1236, 2002; Ped Derm 13:58–60, 1996; AD 127:124–125, 1991; AD 123:493–497, 1987*

Protein C deficiency – including IV catheter-induced thrombosis in protein S deficiency *JAAD 23:975–989, 1990*

Protein S deficiency

Red blood cell disorders – sickle cell disease, hereditary spherocytosis, thalassemia, polycythemia vera,

hereditary elliptocytosis, hereditary nonspherocytic hemolytic anemia

Sickle cell ulcer *Hematol Oncol Clin North Amer 10:1333–1344, 1996*

Thalassemia

NEOPLASTIC DISEASES

Kaposi's sarcoma

Lymphoma – subcutaneous panniculitis-like T-cell lymphoma *BJD 148:516–525, 2003*

Melanoma

Posttransplantation lymphoproliferative disorder *JAAD 54:657–663, 2006*

PRIMARY CUTANEOUS DISEASES

Epidermolysis bullosa, including pretibial epidermolysis bullosa *JAAD 22:346–350, 1990*

Lichen planus, erosive, ulcerative

PSYCHOCUTANEOUS DISEASES

Factitial dermatitis

SYNDROMES

Antiphospholipid antibody syndrome *NEJM 347:1412–1418, 2002; Semin Arthritis Rheum 31:127–132, 2001; JAAD 36:149–168, 1997; JAAD 36:970–982, 1997; BJD 120:419–429, 1989*

Behcet's syndrome *Arch Int Med 145:1913–1915, 1985*

Felty's syndrome – leg ulcers, granulocytopenia, rheumatoid arthritis, skin nodules, pigmentation, splenomegaly *BJD 148:388–401, 2003; Semin Arthr Rheum 21(3):129–142, 1991*

Klinefelter's syndrome – venous and arterial ulcers; leg ulcers with hyperpigmentation or atrophie blanche *AD 133:1051–1052, 1997; AD 131:230, 1995; Cutis 38:110–111, 1986*

Lesch-Nyhan syndrome

Neurofibromatosis – vasculopathy *JAAD 51:656–659, 2004*

PAM1 (PSTPIP1-associated myeloid-related proteinemia) – autoin-flammatory syndrome – acne vulgaris, pyoderma gangrenosum, thrombocytopenia, anemia, sterile osteomyelitis, sterile arthritis *BJD 179:982–983, 2018*

PAPA (pyogenic arthritis with pyoderma gangrenosum) syndrome – pyoderma gangrenosum, cystic acne, acne fulminans, non-axial destructive aseptic arthritis; sterile abscesses at injection sites; attacks last 5 days; mutation in CD2-binding protein 1 *Ped Derm 22:262–265, 2005; Proc Natl Acad Sci USA 100:13501–13506, 2003; Mayo Clin Proc 72:611–615, 1997*

PASH syndrome (pyoderma gangrenosum, acne, and hidradenitis suppurativa) *JAAD 66:409–415, 2012*

Phakomatosis pigmentovascularis IIb – with hypoplasia of the inferior vena cava and iliac and femoral veins with stasis leg ulcers *JAAD 49:S167–169, 2003*

Reflex sympathetic dystrophy – bulla and leg ulceration *JAAD 44:1050, 2001; JAAD 28:29–32, 1993*

Sneddon's syndrome – livedo racemosa with leg ulcers *JAMADerm 152:726–727, 2016*

Werner's syndrome *AD 133:1293–1295, 1997*

TRAUMA

Burn *J Burn Care Rehab 25:129–133, 2004*

Chemical injury

Chilblains

Immersion foot due to ice, cold water, and fans – acral cyanosis, mottled coloration, marked edema of the feet, maceration, bullae, erosions, painful ulcers, pain *JAAD 69:169–171, 2013*

Intravenous drug abuse (IVDA) *BJD 150:1–10, 2004;* shooter's patch – ulceration of the anterior thigh *Cutis 88:61, 65–66, 2011*

VASCULAR DISORDERS

Atrophie blanche (livedoid vasculitis) (livedoid vasculopathy) (atrophie blanche en plaque; atrophie blanche with summer ulceration) – painful purpuric papules and plaques; leg and ankle ulcers; stellate atrophic white scars; livedo reticularis *JAAD 69:1033–1042, 2013; Cutis 90:302–306, 2012; AD 148:385–390, 2012; JAAD 58:512–515, 2008*

Congenital agenesis of the inferior vena cava *Vascular 24:106–108, 2016*

Cutaneous polyarteritis nodosa – angioedema; livedo reticularis, lower leg ulcers *JAMADerm 150:880–884, 2014;* ankle ulcer with livedo reticularis *Ped Derm 36:932–935, 2019*

Erythromelalgia *BJD 143:868–872, 2000;* associated with thrombo-cythemia – may affect one finger or toe; ischemic necrosis *JAAD 22:107–111, 1990;* primary (idiopathic) – lower legs, no ischemia *JAAD 21:1128–1130, 1989;* secondary to peripheral vascular disease *JAAD 43:841–847, 2000; AD 136:330–336, 2000;* all types exacerbated by warmth; may be associated with systemic lupus erythematosus, dermatomyositis, neuropathy, hypertension and vasculitis, calcium antagonists *BJD 143:868–872, 2000*

Granulomatosis with polyangiitis *Dermatol Clin 33:509–630, 2015*

Marijuana – cannabis arteritis – peripheral necrosis over the legs *JAAD 69:135–142, 2013*

Martorell hypertensive ulcer (hypertensive ischemic leg ulcer) – vio-laceous black necrotic ulcer *AD 146:961–968, 2010; JID 9:285–298, 1947; Proc Staff Meet Mayo Clin 21:337–346, 1946; Policlinico Barcelona 1(1):6–9, 1945*

Methylenetetrahydrofolate reductase (MTHFR) polymorphisms – thrombophilia and vasculopathy; leg nodules and leg ulcers; treated with folic acid, vitamins B6 and B12 *JAMADerm 150:780–781, 2014; AD 147:450–453, 2011; Int J Dermatol 46:431–434, 2007; AD 142:75–78, 2006; J Endocrinol Metab 91:2021–2026, 2006;* livedo vasculopathy and MTHFR polymorphisms *BJD 155:850–852, 2006*

Polyarteritis nodosa *Ann Int Med 89:66–676, 1978;* cutaneous polyarteritis nodosa (livedo with nodules) – arthritis; arthralgias; painful or asymptomatic red or skin-colored multiple nodules with livedo reticularis of the feet, legs, forearms face, scalp, shoulders, trunk; leg ulcers, atrophie blanche-like lesions; reticulate hyperpig-mentation *JAAD 63:602–606, 2010; JAAD 57:840–848, 2007; BJD 146:694–699, 2002;* anti-phosphatidylserine-prothrombin complex *JAAD 63:602–606, 2010; BJD 136:706–713, 1997; AD 128:1223–1228, 1992;* microscopic polyarteritis nodosa – arthralgias, leg ulcers, fever, palpable purpura, petechiae, ecchymoses, acral bullae, plantar red plaque *JAAD 57:840–848, 2007;* in children *Ann Rheum Dis 54:134–136, 1995;* familial polyarteritis nodosa of Georgian Jewish, German, and Turkish ancestry – oral aphthae, livedo reticularis, leg ulcers, Raynaud's phenomenon, digital necrosis, nodules, purpura, erythema nodosum; systemic manifes-tations include fever, myalgias, arthralgias, gastrointestinal symptoms, renal disease, central and peripheral neurologic manifestations; mutation in adenosine deaminase 2(*CECR1*) *NEJM 370:921–931, 2014*

Post-thrombotic syndrome *Acta Hematologica 115:207–213, 2016*

Reactive glomeruloid angioendotheliomatosis – livedo reticularis with hemorrhagic ulcers of distal extremities *JAAD 77:1145–1158, 2017*

Stewart-Bluefarb syndrome – arteriovenous malformation of the leg with multiple fistulae and port-wine stain-like purplish lesions (Mali's acroangiodermatitis/pseudo-Kaposi's sarcoma) – brown macules, purple nodules and plaques, edema, varicose veins, hypertrichosis, cutaneous ulcers, enlarged limb *Int Wound J 12:169–172, 2015; JAAD 65:893–906, 2011*

Vasculitis

Venous gangrene

Venous stasis ulcers *BJD 165:541–545, 2011*

ULCERS

AUTOIMMUNE DISEASES AND DISEASES OF IMMUNE DYSFUNCTION

Allergic contact dermatitis – contact vulvitis *NEJM 347:1412–1418, 2002;* peristomal ulcers *AD 142:1372–1373, 2006*

Anti-centromere antibodies – ulcers and gangrene of the extremities *Br J Rheumatol 36:889–893, 1997*

Antineutrophil cytoplasmic antibody syndrome – purpuric vasculitis, orogenital ulceration, fingertip necrosis, pyoderma gangrenosum-like ulcers *BJD 134:924–928, 1996*

Bare lymphocyte syndrome – ulcers of the legs and feet; severe reduction in cell surface expression of HLA molecules (HLA class I, type I BLS; HLA class II, type II BLS); TAP1 and TAP2 mutations (transporter-associated antigen-processing heterodimers) (transportation of cytoplasmic peptides into the endoplasmic reticulum) *AD 146:96–98, 2010; Lancet 354(9190):1598–1603, 1999; Science 265:237–241, 1994*

Bowel-associated dermatitis arthritis syndrome (BADAS)

Brunsting-Perry cicatricial pemphigoid – scalp erosions, bullae, oral bullae and ulcers, scarring alopecia *BJD 170:743–745, 2014*

Brunsting-Perry IgG epidermolysis bullosa acquisita – scalp ulcers *BJD 165:92–98, 2011*

Common variable immunodeficiency (Gottron-like papules) – granulomas presenting as acral red papules and plaques with central scaling, scarring, atrophy, ulceration *Cutis 52:221–222, 1993*

Chronic granulomatous disease – necrotic ulcers; bacterial abscesses, perianal abscesses *JAAD 36:899–907, 1997; AD 130:105–110, 1994; NEJM 317:687–694, 1987; AD 103:351–357, 1971*

Deficiency of adenosine deaminase – ADA 1 – autosomal recessive; severe combined immunodeficiency; ADA 2 – loss of function mutation in cat eye syndrome chromosome candidate 1 gene (*CECR1*); painless leg nodules with intermittent livedo reticularis, Raynaud's phenomenon, cutaneous ulcers, morbilliform rashes, Raynaud's phenomenon, digital gangrene, oral aphthae; vasculitis of small and medium arteries with necrosis, fever, early recurrent ischemic and hemorrhagic strokes, peripheral and cranial neuropathy, and gastrointestinal involvement (diarrhea); hepatosplenomegaly, systemic vasculopathy, stenosis of abdominal arteries *Ped Derm 37:199–201, 2020; NEJM 380:1582–1584, 2019; Ped Derm 33:602–614, 2016; NEJM 370:911–920, 2014; NEJM 370:921–931, 2014*

Dermatitis herpetiformis

Dermatomyositis *Cutis 62:89–93, 1998; AD 126:633–637, 1990;* livedo reticularis and multiple ulcers *J Eur Acad DV 11:48–50, 1998;* calcinosis cutis with ulcers due to extrusion of calcium *Rook p. 2560, 1998, Sixth Edition;* ulcers of the knuckles; punched-out ulcers of the arms, chest, and back; tender hyperkeratotic palmar papules in palmar creases of the fingers with central white coloration; dermatomyositis with MDA-5 (CADM-40) (melanoma differentiation-associated gene 5) MDA 5 – RNA-specific helicase; all with interstitial lung disease; ulcers of nail folds, Gottron's

papules, and elbows; these patients demonstrate oral ulcers, hair loss, hand edema, arthritis/arthralgia, diffuse hair loss, punched-out ulcers of the shoulder or metacarpophalangeal joints, digital necrosis, erythema of the elbows and knees (Gottron's sign), and tender gingiva *JAAD 78:776–785, 2018; JAAD 65:25–34, 2011*

Epidermolysis bullosa acquisita – Brunsting-Perry IgG; epidermolysis bullosa acquisita – scalp ulcers *BJD 165:92–98, 2011*

Familial chilblain lupus – autosomal dominant; violaceous erythema and scaling of the toes; ulcers, arthralgias and arthritis; mutation in *SAMHD1* and *TREX 1 JAMADerm 155:342–346, 2019; Ped Derm 33:602–614, 2016*

Familial pyoderma gangrenosum with common variable immunodeficiency – vegetative cheilitis; cutaneous ulcers *BJD 169:944–946, 2013*

Graft-versus-host disease, chronic – sclerodermoid GVHD with ulcerations *JAAD 66:515–532, 2012;* deep ulcers of the buttocks and legs *AD 138:924–934, 2002; Arch Neurol 39:188–190, 1982*

Immunodeficiency disease with *RAG* mutations and granulomas – ulcers of the face and extremities *NEJM 358:2030–2038, 2008*

Leukocyte adhesion deficiency (beta 2 integrin deficiency) (congenital deficiency of leucocyte adherence glycoproteins (CD11a(LFA-1), CD11b, CD11c, CD18)) – autosomal recessive; delayed separation of umbilical stump; deep nonhealing sacral wound; recurrent skin and systemic infections; abnormal wound healing *Ped Derm 27:500–503, 2010; Nat Rev Immunol 7:678–689, 2007; BJD 139:1064–1067, 1998; NEJM 376:1158, 2017;* necrotic cutaneous abscesses, cellulitis, skin ulcerations (pyoderma gangrenosum leg ulcers healing with flaccid scarring), psoriasiform dermatitis, ulcerative stomatitis; gingivitis, stomatitis, tonsillitis, periodontitis, septicemia, ulcerative stomatitis, pharyngitis, otitis media, pneumonia, sinusitis, peritonitis; delayed separation of umbilical stump and omphalitis *BJD 178:335–349, 2018; JAAD 72:1066–1073, 2015; Ped Derm 28:156–161, 2011; BJD 139:1064–1067, 1998; JAAD 31:316–319, 1994; J Pediatr 119:343–354, 1991; BJD 123:395–401, 1990; Bone Marrow Transplant 24:1261–1263, 1990; Ann Rev Med 38: 175–194, 1987; J Infect Dis 152:668–689, 1985*

Lupus erythematosus, systemic – malleolar, foot ulcers in areas of livedo or vasculitis *J Rheumatol 6:204–209, 1979;* generalized discoid lupus erythematosus; vasculitis – punched-out ulcers *JAAD 48:311–340, 2003; Lupus 235–242, 1997;* chronic pyoderma gangrenosum in hydralazine-induced LE *NEJM 347:1412–1418, 2002; JAAD 10:379–384, 1984;* DLE; palmar ulcer in SLE *AD 135:845–850, 1999;* lupus profundus *Lupus 10:514–516, 2001;* lupus profundus – serpentine hypertrophy of the scalp with deep ulcers *AD 147:1443–1448, 2011*

Marasmus – severe protein and caloric deprivation; skin ulcers due to wrinkled, loose, dry skin; extensive loss of subcutaneous fat *JAAD 21:1–30, 1989*

Pansclerotic morphea *Ped Derm 26:59–61, 2009*

Pemphigus vulgaris – bilateral foot ulcers *Clin Exp Dermatol 25:224–226, 2000*

Perforating neutrophilic and granulomatous dermatitis of the newborn – cutaneous eruption of immunodeficiency; papules, plaques, vesicles, crusts, ulcers; prominent involvement of the palms and soles; sparing of the trunk *Ped Derm 24:211–215, 2007*

PLAID (*PLCG2*-associated antibody deficiency and immune dysregulation) – ulcerated plaques; evaporative cold urticaria; neonatal ulcers in cold-sensitive areas; granulomatous lesions sparing flexures; blotchy pruritic red rash, spontaneous ulceration of nasal tip with eschar of the nose; erosion of nasal cartilage, neonatal small papules and erosions of the fingers and toes; brown granulomatous plaques with telangiectasia and skin atrophy of the cheeks, forehead, ears, chin; atopy; recurrent sinopulmonary infections *JAMADerm 151:627–634, 2015*

Pyrin-associated autoinflammatory neutrophilic disease (PAAND) – autosomal dominant; facial pustules, pyoderma gangrenosum lesions; mutation in *MEFV Ped Derm 33:602–614, 2016*

Rheumatoid arthritis – rheumatoid vasculitis *Rheum Dis Clin North Am 16:445–461, 1990; JAAD 18:140–141, 1988; Semin Arthritis Rheum 14:280–286, 1985;* ulcers *JAAD 48:311–340, 2003;* ulceration of sacrum; ulcerated rheumatoid nodule *Br Med J iv:92–93, 1975;* neutrophilic dermatitis *Cutis 60:203–205, 1997;*

SAVI – STING (stimulator of interferon genes)-associated vasculopathy with onset in infancy syndrome – autosomal dominant; gain-of-function mutation in transmembrane protein 173(STING) leading to chronic activation of type I interferon pathway; facial erythema and telangiectasia, progressive digital necrosis, swelling of the fingers, amputation of several digits, violaceous and telangiectatic malar plaques, nasal septal destruction, chronic leg myalgias, atrophic skin over the knees – red-purpuric plaques over cold-sensitive areas (acral areas) (cheeks, nasal tip, ears), reticulate erythema of the arms and legs; painful ulcers, eschars violaceous scaling plaques of the fingers, toes, nose, ears, cheeks; red ears which ulcerate with necrosis; nail loss, nail dystrophy, nasal septal perforation, severe interstitial lung disease *JAAD 74:186–189, 2016; Ped Derm 33:602–614, 2016*

Overlaps with:
   Familial chilblain lupus (interferonopathy)
   Aicardi-Goutieres syndrome

Scleroderma, systemic *J Rheumatol 25:1540–1543, 1998; Semin Cutan Med Surg 17:48–54, 1998;* ulcers over knuckles; ulcers overlying calcinosis cutis

CONGENITAL LESIONS

Aplasia cutis congenita
   Type 1 – ACC without associated anomalies *JAAD 13:429–433, 1985; AD 108:252–253, 1973;* extensive scalp ulcer *Ped Derm 27:540–542, 2010; AD 141:554–556, 2005;* aplasia cutis congenita in surviving co-twins *Ped Derm 18:511–515, 2001*
   Type 2 – ACC with distal limb reduction abnormalities (Adams-Oliver syndrome) – autosomal dominant; persistent cutis marmorata; aplasia cutis congenita of arm and radial dysplasia *Ped Derm 31:356–359, 2014;* congenital heart disease in 8%; differentiate from ACC with split-hand deformities *Birth Defects 18:123–128, 1982;* differentiate from ACC with postaxial polydactyly *Hum Genet 71:86–88, 1985; J Med Genet 24:493–496, 1987*
   Type 3 – ACC of the scalp with epidermal nevi *Clin Res 33:130, 1985;* including bullous ACC *J Med Genet 30:962–963, 1993*
   Type 4 – ACC overlying developmental malformations – hair collar sign; surface is translucent or membranous *AD 125:1253–1256, 1989;* may overlie defects of the vertebrae and spinal cord *J Pediatr 96:687–689, 1980*
   Type 5 – ACC associated with fetus papyraceus – delivery of dead twin or triplet (death during the second trimester) *Ped Derm 32:138–140, 2015; AD 141:554–556, 2005;* cutaneous ulcers, linear atrophic scars, atrophic scars of the scalp, dystrophic nails *Ped Derm 32:858–861, 2015;* ACC on the trunk and extremities with linear or stellate configuration; *Ped Derm 31:261–263, 2014; JAAD 25:1983–1985, 1991;* fibrous constriction bands of extremities *Aust Paediatr J 18:294–296, 1982*
   Type 6 – Bart's syndrome – congenital localized absence of the skin; ACC as presentation of junctional and dystrophic epider-

molysis bullosa; ulcerations of the feet and lower legs *AD 128:1087–1090, 1992; AD 93:296–303, 1966*
   Type 7 – ACC caused by teratogens – methimazole or carbimazole *Ped Derm 3:327–330, 1986; Can Med Assoc 130:1264, 1984*
   Type 8 – ACC as sign of intrauterine infection – herpes simplex *JAAD 15:1148–1155, 1986;* varicella-zoster – linear ulcers or scars; zosteriform *NEJM 314:1542–1546, 1986*
   Type 9 – ACC as feature of malformation syndromes
      Trisomy 13 – ACC of the scalp with holoprosencephaly, eye anomalies, cleft lip and/or palate, polydactyly, port-wine stain of forehead *Am J Dis Child 112:502–517, 1966*
      Deletion of short arm of chromosome 4 (4p- syndrome) – ACC of the scalp with hypertelorism, beaked or broad nose, microcephaly, low-set ears, preauricular tags or pits, mental retardation *Am J Dis Child 122:421–425, 1971*
      Oculocerebrocutaneous syndrome (Delleman-Oorthuys syndrome) – ACC of the scalp, neck, lumbosacral area; orbital cysts, microphthalmia, skull defects, porencephaly, agenesis of corpus callosum, skin tags around the eyes and nose *Am J Med Genet 40:290–293, 1991*
      Johanson-Blizzard syndrome – autosomal recessive; growth retardation, microcephaly, ACC of the scalp, sparse hair, hypoplastic alae nasi, CALMs, hypoplastic nipples and areolae, hypothyroidism, sensorineural deafness *Clin Genet 14:247–250, 1978*
   Focal dermal hypoplasia
   Facial focal dermal dysplasias
      Autosomal dominant focal facial dermal dysplasia without other facial anomalies – oval symmetrical scarred areas on the temples, cheeks, rim of fine lanugo hairs *BJD 84:410–416, 1971*
      Autosomal recessive focal facial dermal dysplasia without other facial anomalies *JAAD 27:575–58, 1992*
      Focal facial dermal dysplasia with other facial anomalies (Setleis syndrome) – leonine aged facies with absent eyelashes, eyebrows, puckered periorbital skin, scar-like defects of the temples *AD 110:615–618, 1974*
   Amniotic band syndrome
   Congenital erosive and vesicular dermatosis with reticulate supple scarring
   Lumpy scalp, odd ears, and rudimentary nipples *BJD 99:423–430, 1978*
   ACC with nipple and breast hypoplasia, nail dysplasia, delayed dentition *Am J Med Genet 14:381–384, 1983*
   ACC with tricho-odonto-onychodermal ectodermal dysplasia *BJD 105:371–382, 1981*
   ACC with EEC *Minerva Pediatr 34:627–632, 1982* and AEC syndromes *Ped Derm 10:334–340, 1993*
   ACC with intestinal lymphangiectasia *Am J Dis Child 139:509–513, 1985*
   ACC with 46 XY gonadal dysgenesis, cleft lip and palate, ear deformity, and preauricular pits *J Pediatr 97:586–590, 1980*
   Delleman syndrome (oculocerebrocutaneous syndrome) *J Med Genet 25:773–778, 1988*

Congenital absence of the skin *JAAD 2:203–206, 1980*

Congenital erosive and vesicular dermatosis with reticulated scarring – most infants premature; extensive symmetrical erosions with scattered vesicles; vesicles of the trunk and extremities, erosions, ulcers, erythroderma, collodion baby, ectropion, reticulated soft scarring, scarring patchy alopecia, absent eyebrows, hypohidrosis with compensatory hyperhidrosis *Ped Derm 29:756–758, 2012; JAAD 45:946–948, 2001; Ped Derm 15:214–218, 1998; JAAD 32:873–877, 1995; AD 121:361–367, 1985;* most infants premature; extensive symmetrical erosions with scattered vesicles; scarring with hypohidrosis, patchy alopecia, hypoplastic nails *Ped*

Derm 30:387–388, 2013; Ped Derm 26:735–738, 2009; JAAD 58:S104–106, 2008; Ped Derm 24:384–386, 2007; Ped Derm 22:55–59, 2005; Clin Exp Derm 30:146–148, 2004; Dermatol 194:278–280, 1997; JAAD 32:873–877, 1995; AD 126:544–546, 1990; JAAD 17:369–376, 1987
   Differential diagnosis:
   Aplasia cutis congenita
   Amniotic adhesions
   Cutaneous trauma
   Epidermolysis bullosa
   Focal dermal hypoplasia
   Intrauterine infection
   Intrauterine or perinatal trauma

Congenital ulcer of the buttock with pits of the knees *Ped Derm 31:726–728, 2014*

Cutis marmorata telangiectatica congenita

Epidermal necrosis, intrauterine *JAAD 38:712–715, 1998*

Erosive pustular dermatosis – scalp ulcer following aplasia cutis congenita *Ped Derm 34:695–696, 2017*

Halo scalp ring – pressure necrosis with neonatal scalp ulcer *JAMADerm 154:473–474, 2018*

Noma neonatorum – deep ulcers with bone loss, mutilation of the nose, lips, intraorally, anus, genitalia; *Pseudomonas*, malnutrition, immunodeficiency

Porokeratosis – congenital linear porokeratosis *Ped Derm 12:318–322, 1995*

Occult spinal dysraphism – aplasia cutis congenita-like lesion *J Pediatr 96:687–689, 1980*

DEGENERATIVE DISEASES

Cervical trophic syndrome – variant of trigeminal trophic syndrome *JAAD 63:724–725, 2010*

Channelopathy-associated insensitivity to pain – self-mutilating behavior and recurrent ulcerations; recurrent ulcerations of the lips and hands; sensory neuropathy due to loss of function mutation of *SCN9A* gene (encodes voltage-gated channels); decreased nociception and decreased sweating vs. neurotropic tyrosine kinase receptor 1 (*NTRK1*) – mental delay (congenital insensitivity to pain with anhidrosis (CIPA) or hereditary sensory autonomic neuropathy (HSAN) *BJD 171:1268–1270, 2014*

Digital mucous cyst

Hypesthesia following encephalitis

Neuropathic ulcer of the scalp – C2 radiculo-neuropathy after atlantoaxial fixation *JAMADerm 155:981–982, 2019*

Neurotrophic ulcers (mal perforans) (Charcot foot); including those associated with neuropathies – on metatarsal heads and heels with underlying sinus tract to joint or subfascial abscess

Peripheral neuropathy – painless acral cutaneous ulcers with deformity

Reflex sympathetic dystrophy *JAAD 35:843–845, 1996; AD 127:1541–1544, 1991*

Syringomyelia – painless ulcer

Trophic ulcers
   Acrodystrophic neuropathy of Bureau and Barriere
   Alcoholism
   Amantadine-induced peripheral neuropathy
   Autonomic trophic disorder of the cerebral hemispheres
   Beta thalassemia major and intermedia
   Carpal tunnel syndrome
   Cauda equina syndrome
   Charcot-Marie-Tooth syndrome, type 2A
   Chronic obliterating arteriopathies
   Compression syndrome
   Congenital acro-osteolysis
   Congenital dyserythropoietic anemia type II
   Cutaneous-mucous trophic disorder
   Diabetes mellitus
   Distal hyperirrigation syndrome
   Familial amyloid polyneuropathy type I
   Giaccai syndrome
   Gilbert's syndrome
   Hereditary sensory and autonomic neuropathies (HSAN), four types *Int J Dermatol 23:664–668, 1984*
   Hereditary spastic paraplegia with sensory neuropathy
   Klinefelter's syndrome
   Klippel-Trenaunay syndrome
   Leprosy
   Lipomeningocele
   Multiple sclerosis
   Multiple symmetric lipomatosus
   Neuroacropathy
   Peripheral arterial occlusive disease (Fontaine stage III, IV)
   Peripheral neuropathy
   Poliomyelitis
   Post-external fixation in quadriplegia
   Post-femoropopliteal shunt
   Post-keratoplasty
   Post-retroperitoneoscopic lumbar sympathectomy
   Post-spinal anesthesia
   Post-surgery of trigeminal nerve
   Post-varicose vein surgery
   Reflex sympathetic dystrophy
   Rheumatoid arthritis
   Spina bifida
   Split cord malformation with meningomyelocele (complex spina bifida)
   Syringomyelia
   Tabes dorsalis
   Trigeminal trophic syndrome (Wallenberg's syndrome)
   Ulcerative-mutilating acropathy – inherited (Thavenard's syndrome) or acquired (Bureau-Barriere syndrome)
   Venous insufficiency
   Werner's syndrome with torpid trophic ulcera cruris

Trigeminal trophic syndrome with scalp ulcers *Cutis 92:291–296, 2013*

DRUG-INDUCED

BCG – lupus vulgaris at site of BCG vaccine; ulcer of arm *Ped Derm 30:147:–148, 2013*

Bevacizumab and corticosteroids – ulcerations within striae *AD 148:385–390, 2012; J Neurooncol 101:155–159, 2011; AD 147:1227–1228, 2011*

Bromoderma *JAAD 58:682–684, 2008; NEJM 347:1412–1418, 2002*

Corticosteroids, topical; Lotrisone atrophy of the breast with ulceration and extrusion of fat *JAAD 54:1–15, 2006*

Coumarin necrosis – eschar and ulceration *JAAD 47:766–769, 2002*

Epidermal growth factor receptor inhibitors – cetuximab and panitumumab; erlotinib and gefitinib; lapatinib; canertinib; vandetanib – pyoderma gangrenosum-like lesions *JAAD 72:203–218, 2015*

Etretinate – ulcerated atrophic striae *Cutis 65:327–328, 2000*

Heparin necrosis – eschar and ulceration *JAAD 47:766–769, 2002*

Hydralazine-induced SLE (pyoderma gangrenosum-like ulcers) *JAAD 10:379–384, 1984;* acute vasculitis after urography with iopamidol *BJD 129:82–85, 1993*

Hydroxyurea – ulcers of the lower legs and feet; atrophic, scaling, poikilodermatous patches with erosions on the backs of the hands, sides of the feet *NEJM 347:1412–1418, 2002; JAAD 45:321–322, 2001; AD 135:818–820, 1999; Leuk Lymphoma 35:109–118, 1999*

Ibuprofen vasculitis

Interferon alpha – necrotic ulcerations at injection site *JAAD 46:611–616, 2002; J Eur Acad DV 13:141–143, 1999; JAAD 35:788–789, 1996;* interferon beta-1b injection sites *JAAD 37:553–558, 1997; JAAD 37:488–489, 1997; JAAD 34:365–367, 1996*

Iododerma *JAAD 36:1014–1016, 1997*

Meperidine – ulcer and fibrosis of the forearm *JAMADerm 151:331–332, 2015*

Methimazole, carbimazole – congenital skin defects (aplasia cutis congenita) *Ped Derm 28:743–745, 2011; Ann Int Med 106:60–61, 1987*

Methotrexate – ulcers in psoriatic plaques or normal skin *JAAD 11:59–65, 1984*

Mycophenolate mofetil – personal observation

Nicorandil – multiple cutaneous ulcerations *BJD 169:956–57, 2013*

Nivolumab – ulcer of the scalp; scalp necrosis; giant cell arteritis (temporal arteritis) due to nivolumab *JAMADerm 155:1086–1087, 2019*

Pentazocine *AD 132:1365–1370, 1996; JAAD 2:47–55, 1980*

Propranolol – treatment of PHACES syndrome *Ped Derm 30:71–89, 2013*

Radiation recall – capecitabine, doxorubicin, taxanes, gemcitabine; erythema and desquamation; edema; vesicles and papules; ulceration and skin necrosis *The Oncologist 15:1227–1237, 2010*

Sirolimus/acitretin *Clin Exp Dermatol 44:62–65, 2019*

Sunitinib – pyoderma gangrenosum *BJD 159:242–243, 2008*

Vascular endothelial growth factor receptor (VEGFR)inhibitors – bevacizumab, ranibizumab – mucocutaneous hemorrhage, disturbed wound healing *JAAD 72:203–218, 2015*

Vasculitis, drug-induced

EXOGENOUS AGENTS

Anabolic steroids – acne fulminans with necrotic ulcers *AD 148:1210–1212, 2012*

Caustics

Chemical burns
    Acids and alkalis
    Cement (lime) (calcium hydroxide) *Br Med J i:1250, 1978*
    Chromic acid
    Hydrofluoric acid
    Lime dust – necrosis with ulcers *Contact Dermatitis 1:59, 1981*
    Phosphorus
    Phenol

Chrome ulcers of the skin and nasal mucosae – tanners, electroplaters

Irritant contact dermatitis – peristomal ulcers *AD 142:1372–1373, 2006*

Levamisole-contaminated cocaine – ulcers *Clin Inf Dis 61:1840–1849, 2015;* pyoderma gangrenosum *JAAD 74:892–898, 2016*

Percutaneous long line – extravascular location; neck ulcer in infant *AD 147:512–514, 2011*

Sodium silicate – ulcerative contact dermatitis due to primary irritant contact dermatitis with contact urticaria *AD 118:518–520, 1982*

Suture granulomas – peristomal ulcers *AD 142:1372–1373, 2006*

INFECTIONS AND INFESTATIONS

Abscess – bacterial, fungal, parasitic; bone abscess

Actinomycosis

Aeromonas hydrophila

African histoplasmosis (*Histoplasma duboisii*) (*Histoplasma capsulatum* var. *duboisii*) – exclusively in Central and West Africa and Madagascar *Clin Inf Dis 48:441, 493–494, 2009; BJD 82:435–444, 1970*

African trypanosomiasis *AD 131:1178, 1995*

AIDS – acute HIV infection; genital ulcers *AD 134:1279–1284, 1998*

Alternaria alternata (phaeohyphomycosis) *Cutis 56:145–150, 1995; Clin Exp Dermatol 18:156–158, 1993;* cellulitis with ulceration *JAAD 52:653–659, 2005;* multiple ulcers *BJD 145:484–486, 2001*

Amebiasis (*Entamoeba histolytica*) – nasal destruction; malodorous ulcer with gray-white necrotic base; penile and perianal ulcers *Cutis 90:310–314, 2012; NEJM 347:1412–1418, 2002;* foot ulcer, perianal ulcer

Acanthamoeba Cutis 73:241–248, 2004; JAAD 42:351–354, 2000; J Clin Inf Dis 20:1207–1216, 1995; amebic ulcers (*Entamoeba histolytica*) – ulcers of vulva and perineum; often accompanied by diarrhea; serpiginous ulcer *JAAD 60:897–925, 2009; AD 144:1369–1372, 2008; Ped Derm 23:231–234, 2006; Ped Derm 10:352–355, 1993; Pediatrics 71:595–598, 1983; Arch Dis Child 55:234–236, 1980; Mod Probl Paediatr 17:259–261, 1975; Am J Proctol 17:58–63, 1966; Entamoeba histolytica* in neonate *Textbook of Neonatal Dermatology, p.234, 2001*

Animal bite

Anthrax – *Bacillus anthracis*; malignant pustule; face, neck, hands, arms; starts as papule then evolves into bulla on red base; then hemorrhagic and necrotic crust with edema and erythema with small satellite vesicles; edema of the surrounding skin; black eschar then painless ulcer; ulceroglandular disease *JAAD 65:1213–1218, 2011; JAAD 47:766–769, 2002; Am J Dermatopathol 19:79–82, 1997; J Clin Inf Dis 19:1009–1014, 1994; Br J Opthalmol 76:753–754, 1992; J Trop Med Hyg 89:43–45, 1986; Bol Med Hosp Infant Mex 38:355–361, 1981*

Arcanobacterium haemolyticum – trophic ulcer *Clin Inf Dis 18:835–836, 1994*

Aspergillosis – necrotic ulcers *JAAD 80:869–880, 2019; NEJM 347:1412–1418, 2002;* giant ulcer of abdominal wall *Cutis 81:127–130, 2008;* ulcers with satellite abscesses *Ped Derm 19:439–444, 2002;* eschar and ulceration *JAAD 47:766–769, 2002; Ped Inf Dis 12:673–682, 1993; Aspergillus flavus*, primary cutaneous – necrotic ulcer *AD 141:1035–1040, 2005;* primary cutaneous in neonate *Ped Derm 8:253–255, 1991; Clin Exp Dermatol 15:446–450, 1990*

Bacillus cereus – cutaneous infection begins with vesicle and/or pustule and becomes cellulitis; then a nonhealing ulcer with a black eschar *Cutis 79:371–377, 2007; Lancet Mar 18;1(8638):601–603, 1989*

Basidiobolomycosis *Ped Derm 8:325–328, 1991*

BCG vaccination site in Kawasaki's disease – ulcerated plaque *JAAD 37:303–304, 1997;* disseminated BCG in X-linked severe combined immunodeficiency *Ped Derm 23:560–563, 2006*

Bilophila wadsworthia – cellulitis *J Clin Inf Dis(Suppl 2):S88–93, 1997*

Botryomycosis *Cutis 80:45–47, 2007; JAAD 24:393–396, 1991*

Boutonneuse spotted fever – *Rickettsia conorii;* black eschar (tache noir) *JAAD 49:363–392, 2003*

Brown recluse spider bite *NEJM 347:1412–1418, 2002*

Brucellosis (*Brucella melitensis*) *Med Clin(Barc)100:417–419, 1993*

Calymmatobacterium granulomatis (Donovanosis) – buttock ulcer *J Clin Inf Dis 25:24–32, 1997*

Candida albicans Clin Exp Dermatol 14:295–297, 1989; granuloma-tous panniculitis with multiple leg ulcers *JAAD 28:315–317, 1993;* peristomal ulcers *AD 142:1372–1373, 2006*

Carbuncle – personal observation

Cat scratch disease – ulceroglandular disease *JAAD 47:766–769, 2002*

Chagas disease

Chancriform pyoderma (*Staphylococcus aureus*) – ulcer with indurated base; eyelid, near the mouth, genital *AD 87:736–739, 1963*

Chancroid – resembling granuloma inguinale; ulceroglandular disease *JAAD 47:766–769, 2002;* phagedenic chancroid

Chikungunya fever – vasculitic ulcers *Ped Derm 35:408–409, 2018; Indian J DV 76:671–676, 2010*

Chromobacterium violaceum JAAD 54:S224–228, 2006

Chromomycosis – feet, legs, arms, face, and neck *AD 133:1027–1032, 1997; BJD 96:454–458, 1977; AD 104:476–485, 1971*

Citrobacter freundii – ecthyma, ulcers, red plaque with central ulceration and caseation *AD 143:124–125, 2007*

Clostridium welchii

Clostridial gas gangrene – acute ulcer

Coccidioidomycosis *JAAD 46:743–747, 2002;* primary cutaneous coccidioidomycosis *JAAD 49:944–949, 2003*

Colletotrichum gloeosporioides (plant pathogen) – necrotic ulcers *JAMADerm 1511383–1384, 2015*

Corals (true corals) (Anthozoa) – erythema, bullae, ulcers *JAAD 61:733–750, 2009*

Corynebacterium diphtheria – superficial round ulcer with overhang-ing edge; gray adherent membrane; later edge thickens and becomes raised and rolled; umbilicus, postauricular, groin, finger or toe web; heals with scarring; crusts around the nose and mouth with faucial diphtheria *Schweiz Rundsch Med Prax 87:1188–1190, 1998; Postgrad Med J 72:619–620, 1996; Am J Epidemiol 102:179–184, 1975;* painful vesicle evolving into pustule then anesthetic shallow punched-out ulcer with gray-black membrane *Cutis 79:371–377, 2007;* heel ulcerations, bullae; fatal heart block *Ped Cardiol 21:282–283, 2000; J Med Assoc Thai 56:670–674, 1973*

Corynebacterium jeikeium – ulcers, subcutaneous nodules *Scand J Infect Dis 27:581–584, 1995; JAAD 16:444–447, 1987*

Corynebacterium pseudodiphtheriticum – hand ulcer *Clin Infect Dis 29:938–939, 1999*

Corynebacterium pyogenes – epidemic leg ulcers in Thailand *Int J Dermatol 21:407–409, 1987*

Corynebacterium ulcerans – ulcer mimicking diphtheria with gray membrane and sweet smell *Clin Inf Dis 33:1598–1600, 2001*

Cowpox (*Orthopoxvirus* infection) – papule progresses to vesicle to hemorrhagic vesicle to umbilicated pustule, then eschar with ulcer *JAAD 44:1–14, 2001; BJD 133:598–607, 1994*

Cryptococcosis – punched-out ulcers with rolled edge *NEJM 347:1412–1418, 2002; AD 124:429–434, 1988; AD 112:1734–1740, 1976; BJD 74:43–49, 1962; AD 77:210–215, 1958;* verrucous ulcer *Cutis 51:377–380, 1993;* herpetiform ulcers *JAAD 10:387–390, 1984;* mimicking pyoderma gangrenosum *JAAD 5:32–36, 1981*

Curvularia lunata – sternal wound infection with chest ulcer *J Clin Inf Dis 19:735–740, 1994; Arch Int Med 139:940–941, 1979*

Cytomegalovirus – usually small ulcers of the perineum, buttocks, proximal thighs; sharply marginated, crusted, or purulent ulcers *JAAD Case Rep 6:57–59, 2020; Dermatology 200:189–195, 2000; JAAD 38:349–351, 1998; J Rheumatol 20:155–157, 1993; AD 127:396–398, 1991;* ulcers of the back – reactivation of CMV due to corticosteroid therapy *JAAD 68:721–728, 2013;* punched-out ulcers in pemphigus *JAAD 71:284–292, 2014;* necrotic ulcers of the scalp *Ped Derm 31:729–731, 2014;* generalized pustules and punched-out ulcers *JAMADerm 151:1380–1381, 2015*

Dematiacious fungal infections in organ transplant recipients – all lesions on the extremities
Alternaria
Bipolaris hawaiiensis
Exophiala jeanselmi, E. spinifera, E. pisciphera, E. castellani
Exserohilum rostratum
Fonsecaea pedrosoi
Phialophora parasitica

Deep fungal infections – peristomal ulcers *AD 142:1372–1373, 2006*

Dracunculosis – small papule or vesicle which ruptures; ulcer forms from which worm can be removed *Dermatol Clinic 7:323–330, 1989*

Ecthyma – streptococcal or staphylococcal *Clin Inf Dis 48:1213–1219, 2009;* ulcer with thick hard crust; eschar and ulceration *JAAD 47:766–769, 2002*

Ecthyma gangrenosum – *Pseudomonas aeruginosa, Candida, Aspergillus, Escherichia coli, Aeromonas hydrophila*

Chronic active *Epstein-Barr virus* – vulvitis, hemorrhagic cheilitis, necrotic ulcers, periorbital erythema and edema, maxillary sinusitis, hepatosplenomegaly *BJD 173:1266–1270, 2015*

Filariasis – elephantiasis of the dorsum of the foot with ulceration

Fire coral (*Millepora* spp.) – scuba divers; dermatitis, bullae, hemorrhagic bullae, necrosis, ulceration, urticaria; late lichenoid and granulomatous reactions *JAAD 61:733–750, 2009*

Fusarium solani Rev Soc Bras Med Trop 30:323–328, 1997(Spanish); J Med Vet Mycol 28:209–213, 1990; Sabouradis 17:219–223, 1979

Glanders – *Pseudomonas mallei* – cellulitis which ulcerates with purulent foul-smelling discharge, regional lymphatics become abscesses; nasal and palatal necrosis and destruction; metastatic papules, pustules, bullae over the joints and face, then ulcerate; deep abscesses with sinus tracts occur; polyarthritis, meningitis, pneumonia; eschar and ulceration; ulceroglandular (nodule progressing to ulcer) *JAAD 54:559–578, 2006; JAAD 47:766–769, 2002*

Gram-negative web space infection

Granuloma inguinale – papule or nodule breaks down to form ulcer with overhanging edge; deep extension may occur; or serpiginous extension with vegetative hyperplasia; pubis, genitalia, perineum; extragenital lesions of the nose and lips, or extremities *JAAD 11:433–437, 1984*

Herpes simplex *NEJM 347:1412–1418, 2002; AD 132:1157–1158, 1996; JAMA 241:592–594, 1979;* extensive ulcers of the buttocks *AD 143:1340–1342, 2007;* kidney-shaped (reniform) ulcer of the hand (HSV2) *Cutis 89:78–80, 2012;* neonatal HSV – widespread erosions *J Pediatr 101:958–960, 1982;* congenital absence of the skin *J Pediatr 101:958–960, 1982;* ulceroglandular disease *JAAD 47:766–769, 2002;* eczema herpeticum – personal observation

Herpes zoster – chronic ulcerating acyclovir-resistant *varicella-zoster Scand J Infect Dis 27:623–625, 1995*

Histoplasmosis *AD 132:341–346, 1996; JAAD 29:311–313, 1993; Medicine 60:361–373, 1990; Cutis 43:535–538, 1989;* punched-out ulcers *Arch Derm Syphilol 56:715–739, 1947*

Impetigo

Insect bites – eschar and ulceration *JAAD 47:766–769, 2002;* necrosis and ulceration due to hypersensitivity to mosquito bites in patients with *Epstein-Barr virus* infection *JAAD 72:1–19, 2015*

Kerion

Leishmaniasis – impetigo- and ecthyma-like lesions of the legs (Bauru ulcers) *Dermatol Clin 33:579–593, 2015; JAAD 60:897–925, 2009; JAAD 51:S125–128, 2004; Clin Inf Dis 33:815,897–898, 2001; Clin Inf Dis 32:1304–1312, 2001; Trans R Soc Trop Med Hyg 81:606, 1987; Cutis 38:198–199, 1986;* mucocutaneous leishmaniasis *J Emerg Med 20:353–356, 2001; AD 134:193–198, 1998; J Clin Inf Dis 22:1–13, 1996;* kala-azar – Leishmania donovani – pedal edema; primary ulcer; hyperpigmented skin of the face, hands, feet, abdomen *JAAD 60:897–925, 2009;* leishmaniasis recidivans (lupoid leishmaniasis) – crusted ulcer *Clin Inf Dis 33:1076–1079, 2001;* eschar and ulceration *JAAD 47:766–769, 2002;* ulcerated papules, nodules, and plaques *Cutis 77:25–28, 2006;* large ulcer of the hand – New World leishmaniasis *Cutis 95:208,229–230, 2015*

Leprosy (*Mycobacterium leprae*) – lepromatous leprosy *Int J Dermatol 29:156–157, 1990;* plantar ulcers due to involvement of common peroneal and posterior tibial nerve leading to foot drop *Indian J Lepr 71:437–450, 1999;* neurotrophic ulcers; Lucio's phenomenon – generalized ulcers *AD 135:983–988, 1999;* Lucio's phenomenon – polycyclic necrotic ulcers *Cutis 105:35–38, 2019;* relapsing erythema necroticans *SKINmed 12:103–104, 2014;* eschar and ulceration *JAAD 47:766–769, 2002;* painless ulcers *JAAD 48:958–961, 2003;* immune reconstitution inflammatory syndrome (IRIS) in HIV disease – ulcerated plaque *AD 140:997–1000, 2004;* tender ulcerations of the buttocks and legs *AD 116:201–204, 1980;*

Leprosy – Lucio's phenomenon – serpiginous polycyclic necrotic ulcers *J Clin Aesthet Dermatol 12:35–38, 2019*

Lobomycosis (lacaziosis) (*Lacazia loboi*) – chronic ulcer of the arm *Clin Inf Dis 59:264,314–315, 2014; Brasil Med 44:1227, 1930*

Lymphogranuloma venereum – ulceroglandular disease; inguinal ulcer *JAAD 54:559–578, 2006; J Inf Dis 160:662–668, 1989; JAAD 47:766–769, 2002*

Meleney's synergistic gangrene

Melioidosis – *Burkholderia pseudomallei;* septic arthritis, abscesses, ulcers *Ped Derm 29:692, 2012; Clin Inf Dis 31:981–986, 2000;* ulceroglandular disease *JAAD 47:766–769, 2002;* ulcerative vegetative plaque *Cutis 72:310–312, 2003;* pneumonia and cutaneous ulcers *MMWR 64:1–9, July 3, 2015*

Meningococcemia – necrotic purpura with ulcerations *Pediatrics 60:104–106, 1977*

Milker's nodule – eschar and ulceration *JAAD 47:766–769, 2002*

Mosquito bite hypersensitivity syndrome in EBV-associated natural killer cell leukemia/lymphoma – clear or hemorrhagic bullae with necrosis, ulceration, and scar formation *JAAD 45:569–578, 2001*

Mucormycosis *Clin Exp Dermatol 28:157–159, 2003; Clin Inf Dis 19:67–76, 1994; JAAD 21:1232–1234, 1989;* eschar and ulceration

JAAD 47:766–769, 2002; ulcer of arm *Acta Chir Belg 105:551–553, 2005*

Mycetoma

Mycobacterium abscessus JAAD 57:413–420, 2007; AD 142:1287–1292, 2006; Am J Respir Crit Care Med 156(pt 2):S1–S25, 1997; Clin Inf Dis 19:263–273, 1994; Rev Infect Dis 5:657–679, 1983

Mycobacterium avium-intracellulare BJD 142:789–793, 2000; BJD 136:260–263, 1997; Clin Inf Dis 19:263–273, 1994; JAAD 19:492–495, 1988; ecthyma-like ulcer *AD 126:1108–1110, 1990; Mycobacterium avium complex* – foot ulcer with sinus tracts *Am Rev Resp Dis 106:469–471, 1972;* ulcers *Clin Exp Dermatol 8:323–327, 1983*

Mycobacterium chelonae BJD 171:79–89, 2014; AD 142:1287–1292, 2006; Am J Respir Crit Care Med 156(pt 2):S1–S25, 1997; Clin Inf Dis 19:263–273, 1994; AD 129:1190–1191, 1193, 1993; Rev Infect Dis 5:657–679, 1983; postsurgical wound infection *J Infect Dis 143:533–542, 1981*

Mycobacterium fortuitum JAAD 57:413–420, 2007; AD 142:1287–1292, 2006; Am J Respir Crit Care Med 156(pt 2):S1–S25, 1997; Clin Inf Dis 19:263–273, 1994; Rev Infect Dis 5:657–679, 1983; postsurgical wound infection *J Infect Dis 143:533–542, 1981*

Mycobacterium haemophilum – necrotic ulcer *Clin Inf Dis 33-330–337, 2001; Clin Inf Dis 19:263–273, 1994; J Infection 23:303–306, 1991;* inguinal ulcer *AD 138:229–230, 2002*

Mycobacterium kansasii JAAD 36:497–499, 1997; Clin Inf Dis 19:263–273, 1994; swollen fingers with ulcers *JAAD 45:620–624, 2001*

Mycobacterium marinum – ecthyma-like ulcers *Clin Inf Dis 19:263–273, 1994;* ulcers mimicking *M. ulcerans Med J Austral ii:434–437, 1973*

Mycobacterium scrofulaceum Clin Inf Dis 20:549–556, 1995; Clin Inf Dis 19:263–273, 1994

Mycobacterium tuberculosis NEJM 347:1412–1418, 2002; Ned Tidjschr Geneeskd 145:1523–1524, 2001; tuberculous ulcer *JAAD 19:1067–1072, 1988;* chancre, primary inoculation – begins as red-brown papulonodular lesion with well-demarcated ulcer with red, blue, or undermined borders *Am J Clin Dermatol 3:319–328, 2002;* scrofuloderma (ulceroglandular disease) – ulcers of lateral chest wall *Clin Dermatol 38:152–159, 2020; Ped Derm 30:7–16, 2013; JAAD 54:559–578, 2006; Ped Derm 22:440–443, 2005; JAAD 47:766–769, 2002; Ped Derm 18:328–331, 2001;BJD 134:350–352, 1996;* miliary tuberculosis; large crops of vesicles, vesicles become necrotic to form ulcers *Practitioner 222:390–393, 1979; Am J Med 56:459–505, 1974; AD 99:64–69, 1969;* tuberculous gumma *Cutis 66:277–279, 2000;* malakoplakia of tuberculous origin – scalp ulcer *JAAD 18:577–579, 1988;* erythema induratum; papulonecrotic tuberculid *Ped Derm 15:450–455, 1998; Ped Derm 7:191–195, 1990;* ulcer of the nose *Ann DV 110:731–732, 1983;* phagedenic tuberculous ulcers *Int J Dermatol 9:283–289, 1970;* lupus vulgaris; starts as red-brown plaque; ulcerative and mutilating forms, vegetating forms – ulcerate, areas of necrosis, invasion of mucous membranes with destruction of cartilage (lupus vorax; head, neck, around nose, extremities, trunk *Int J Dermatol 26:578–581, 1987; Acta Tuberc Scand 39(Suppl 49):1–137, 1960;* eschar and ulceration *JAAD 47:766–769, 2002;* tuberculous mastitis; nodular tuberculous mastitis (solitary or multiple palpable masses); sinus tract, ulcer *Int J Inf Dis 87:135–142, 2019*

Mycobacterium ulcerans (Buruli ulcer) (Bairnsdale, Kakerifu, Kasongo, Searls' ulcer) – leg ulcer with undermined margins; differential diagnosis includes tropical phagedenic ulcer or necrotizing fasciitis *Clin Inf Dis 62:342–350, 2016; Dermatol Clinics 29:1–8,*

2011; JAAD 54:559–578, 2006; NEJM 348:1065–1066, 2003; Trans R Soc Trop Med Hyg 94:277–279, 2000; Lancet 354:1013, 1018, 1999; Med Trop(Mars) 57:83–90, 1997(French); Clin Inf Dis 21:1186–1192, 1995; Med Trop(Mars) 55:363–373, 1995; Aust J Dermatol 26:67–73, 1985; Pathology 17:594–600, 1985

Mycoplasma-induced rash and mucositis (MIRM) – oral ulcers, lip ulcers, penile ulcers JAMA 322, 2019

Myiasis, erosive AD 117:59–60, 1981

Necrotizing fasciitis – necrotic ulcer Ped Derm 29:264–269, 2012

Nocardiosis AD 130:243–248, 1994; Nocardia brasiliensis J Inf Dis 134:286–289, 1976; N. brasiliensis – ulcerated plaque, eschar, cellulitis, sporotrichoid pattern JAMADerm 151:895–896, 2015

Nontuberculous mycobacteria – peristomal ulcers AD 142:1372–1373, 2006

North American blastomycosis Ped Derm 30:749–750, 2013; Clin Inf Dis 22(suppl 2) S102–111, 1996; ulceration of the lip Rook p. 3135, 1998, Sixth Edition; primary inoculation blastomycosis – chancriform ulcer AD 104:408–411, 1971

Orf – eschar and ulceration JAAD 47:766–769, 2002

Osteomyelitis – leg ulcer overlying osteomyelitis

Paracoccidioidomycosis – near mouth, anus, or genitalia JAAD 53:931–951, 2005; J Clin Inf Dis 23:1026–1032, 1996; ulceration of the lip; ulcer of the hand Clin Dermatol 38:152–159, 2020

Pasteurella multocida (P. haemolytica, pneumotropica, and ureae) – cellulitis with ulceration with hemorrhagic purulent discharge with sinus tracts Medicine 63:133–144, 1984

Talaromyces (Penicillium) marneffei NEJM 347:1412–1418, 2002; Clin Inf Dis 18:246–247, 1994

Perirectal abscess

Phaeohyphomycosis – inoculation phaeohyphomycosis AD 137:815–820, 2001

Plague – eschar and ulceration; ulceroglandular JAAD 47:766–769, 2002; pustule or ulcer at site of flea bite; bubonic plague – fever, chills, headache, exhaustion, painful lymphadenitis which becomes necrotic and drains JAAD 65:1213–1218, 2011

Portuguese man o' war stings

Prevotella species J Clin Inf Dis(Suppl 2):S88–93, 1997

Prototothecosis JAAD 32:758–764, 1995; AD 125:1249–1252, 1989; red plaque with pustules and ulcers BJD 146:688–693, 2002; red plaque with focal ulcers covering the entire arm Clin Inf Dis 56:271, 307, 2013

Pseudomonas – interdigital web space infection; periumbilical pustules with necrotic ulcers; extensive necrosis in neutropenic patients JAAD 11:781–786, 1984; AD 97:312–318, 1968; Pseudomonas sepsis – bullae which rupture to yield necrotic ulcers (ecthyma gangrenosum) – eschar and ulceration JAAD 47:766–769, 2002; Ped Derm 4:18–20, 1987; Medicine 64:115–133, 1985

Pyoderma

Pythiosis (Pythium insidiosum) (alga) – cellulitis, infarcts, ulcers JAAD 52:1062–1068, 2005

Rat bite fever – eschar and ulceration JAAD 47:766–769, 2002

Rickettsial pox – eschar and ulceration JAAD 47:766–769, 2002

Scedosporium apiospermum – ulcer of the hand JAAD 39:498–500, 1998

Schistosomiasis Derm Clinics 17:151–185, 1999

Scopulariopsis brevicaulis

Scorpion stings

Scrub typhus – punched-out ulcer with adherent crust, then morbilliform eruption Clin Inf Dis 18:624, 1994; JAAD 2:359–373, 1980; eschar and ulceration JAAD 47:766–769, 2002

Sea anemones – erythema, bullae, ulcers JAAD 61:733–750, 2009

Serratia marcescens JAAD 49(Suppl):S193–194, 2003; JAAD 25:565, 1991

Snakebites

Sparganosis – Spirometra proliferum Derm Clinics 17:151–185, 1999

Spiders – necrotic arachnidism – brown recluse spider, wolf spider, sac spider, jumping spider, fishing spider, hobo spider, green lynx spider JAAD 44:561–573, 2001; Int Surg 46:24–28, 1966; eschar and ulceration JAAD 47:766–769, 2002

Sporotrichosis – finger ulcer Cutis 69:371–374, 2002; mimicking pyoderma gangrenosum NEJM 347:1412–1418, 2002; Derm Clinics 17:151–185, 1999; AD 122:691–694, 1986; three ulcers Cutis 78:337–340, 2006

Stonefish sting

Staphylococcal adenitis – ulceroglandular disease JAAD 47:766–769, 2002

Staphylococcus aureus – peristomal ulcers AD 142:1372–1373, 2006

Streptococcal adenitis – ulceroglandular disease JAAD 47:766–769, 2002

Streptococcus pneumoniae Clin Inf Dis 21:697–698, 1995; necrotizing fasciitis Acta Chir Belg 98:102–106, 1998; JAAD 20:774–781, 1989; Surgery 92:765–770, 1982; Group B streptococcal disease – foot ulcers, decubitus ulcers Clin Inf Dis 33:556–561, 2001

Subcutaneous phaeohyphomycosis – Exophiala jeanselmei; finger ulcer BJD 150:597–598, 2004; inoculation AD 137:815–820, 2001

Syphilis – primary (chancre), secondary (noduloulcerative syphilis, lues maligna) AD 113:1027–1028, 1030–1031, 1997; BJD 136:946–948, 1997; Cutis 45:119–122, 1990; Jarisch-Herxheimer reaction – reactivation of primary chancre Acta DV 76:91–92, 1996; tertiary – gumma – breast ulcerations NEJM 373:2069, 2015; tabes dorsalis – painless neurotrophic ulcer of weight-bearing regions of the sole Arch Neurol 42:606–613, 1985; syphilitic aortic aneurysm eroding through the sternum Dur M Cardiothorac Surg 10:922–924, 1996

Tick bites – especially soft ticks JAAD 49:363–392, 2003

Tick typhus (Boutonneuse fever, Kenya tick typhus, African and Indian tick typhus) (ixodid ticks) – small ulcer at site of tick bite (tache noire) – black necrotic center with red halo; pink morbilliform eruption of the forearms, then generalizes, involving the face, palms, and soles; may be hemorrhagic; recovery uneventful JAAD 2:359–373, 1980; eschar and ulceration JAAD 47:766–769, 2002

Trichophyton rubrum in AIDS JAAD 34:1090–1091, 1996

Trichosporosis, neonatal – cellulitis evolving into necrotic ulcer

Tropical phagedenic ulcer – due to Klebsiella Ped Derm 30:367–369, 2013; Corynebacterium pyogenes – fusiform bacilli; eschar and ulceration JAAD 47:766–769, 2002; also Proteus, Streptococcus, Vincent's spirochetes

Tularemia – Francisella tularensis – ulceroglandular tularemia – starts as papule, then pustule, then ulcer, then lymph node; fever, chills, headache, body aches, coryza, sore throat; punched-out painful ulcer with raised ragged edges and necrotic base with regional lymphadenopathy, lymphadenitis, or nodular lymphangitis (ulceroglandular disease) NEJM 374:573–581, 2016;

MMWR 62:963–966, 2013; JAAD 65:1213–1218, 2011; JAAD 47:766–769, 2002; Clin Inf Dis 33:573–576, 2001; Cutis 63:49–51, 1999; eschar and ulceration; scalp ulcer with lymphadenopathy *AD 140:1531–1536, 2004;* linear axillary ulcer with surrounding erythema with lymphocytic meningitis *Clin Inf Dis 48:1266–1267,1327–1328, 2009*

Typhoid fever *J Trop Med Hyg 97:298–299, 1994*

Ulcers with regional adenopathy – anthrax, ecthyma, *Pasteurella multocida* infection, sporotrichosis, cat scratch disease, plague, glanders, lymphogranuloma venereum, tularemia *JAAD 49:363–392, 2003*

Varicella – congenital varicella syndrome – linear and unilateral ulceration and scarring; congenital absence of the skin; maternal varicella in the last trimester *J Infect Dis 7:77–78, 1983*

Vibrio extorquens JAAD 9:262–8, 1983

Vibrio haemolyticum

Vibrio vulnificus sepsis *JAAD 24:397–403, 1991; J Infect Dis 149:558–564, 1984*

Wound infection

Yaws *Clin Dermatol 8:157–165, 1990*

Yersinia enterocolitica J Clin Inf Dis 21:223–224, 1995

Zygomycosis *NEJM 347:1412–1418, 2002;* neonatal – cellulitis evolving into necrotic ulcer

INFILTRATIVE DISEASES

Amyloidosis – familial amyloid polyneuropathy – atrophic scars and poorly healed ulcers *BJD 152:250–257, 2005*

Interstitial cryoglobulinosis – non-palpable petechial purpura, necrotic ulcers, hemorrhagic bullae; renal failure *JAAD 77:1145–1158, 2017*

Eosinophilic granuloma

Langerhans cell histiocytosis *NEJM 347:1412–1418, 2002;* axillary, vulvar ulcers *AD 137:1241–1246, 2001;* extensive paravertebral skin ulcers *BJD 145:137–140, 2001*

Mucinosis, primary cutaneous

Xanthogranuloma – scalp ulcer in adult-onset xanthogranuloma *AD 148:968–969, 2012*

INFLAMMATORY DISEASES

Chronic recurrent multifocal osteomyelitis (CRMO) – seen with varied neutrophilic dermatoses including SAPHO syndrome, pyoderma gangrenosum, acne fulminans, pustular psoriasis, Sweet's syndrome *Ped Derm 26:497–505, 2009*

Crohn's disease – local extension, fissures, metastatic Crohn's disease – postauricular ulcer *NEJM 347:1412–1418, 2002; JAAD 36:986–988, 1996; AD 129:1607–1612, 1993; AD 126:645–648, 1990; JAAD 10:33–38, 1984;* peristomal ulcers *AD 142:1372–1373, 2006*

Cytophagic histiocytic panniculitis *J Eur Acad DV 10:267–268, 1998; AD 121:910–913, 1985*

Dermatitis gangrenosum infantum – multiple necrotic ulcers complicating varicella, seborrheic dermatitis, etc. *BJD 75:206–211, 1963*

Edematous scarring vasculitic panniculitis – hydroa vacciniforme-like lesions with vesicles, deep ulcers, varicelliform scars *JAAD 32:37–44, 1995*

Frontal sinus fistula tract – ulcerated eyelid *AD 148:1411–1416, 2012*

Hidradenitis suppurativa *BJD 175:882–891, 2016; JAAD 60:539–561, 2009*

Diseases associated with hidradenitis suppurativa: *JAAD 60:539–561, 2009*

Acanthosis nigricans

Acne conglobata

Acne vulgaris *Br Med J 292:245–248, 1986; Surg Gynecol Obstet 95:455–464, 1952*

Bazex-Dupre-Christol syndrome

Crohn's disease *Inflammatory Bowel Dis 7:33–326, 2001; Int J Colorect Dis 8:117–119, 1993; BJD 126:523, 1992*

Dissecting cellulitis of the scalp

Dowling-Degos disease *Clin Exp Dermatol 31:454–456, 2006; Clin Exp Dermatol 29:622–624, 2004; Hautarzt 52:642–645, 2001; Australas J Dermatol 38:209–211, 1997; Clin Exp Dermatol 21:305–306, 1996; Ann DV 120:120:705–708, 1993; JAAD 24:888–892, 1991; Cutis 45:446–450, 1990*

Fox-Fordyce disease *JID 31:127–135, 1958*

Interstitial keratitis *AD 95:473–475, 1967*

Keratitis-ichthyosis-deafness syndrome *Eur J Dermatol 15:347–352, 2005; JAAD 51:377–382, 2004*

Obesity *Acta DV 85:225–232, 2005; J Eur Acad Dermatol Venereol 17:276–279, 2003*

Pachyonychia congenita *JID Symp Proc 10:3–17, 2005; BJD 123:663–666, 1990; JAAD 19:705–711, 1988*

PAPA (pyogenic arthritis, pyoderma gangrenosum, acne) syndrome *Mayo Clin roc 72:611–615, 1997*

Pilonidal cysts and sinuses

Pyoderma gangrenosum *AD 146:1265–1270, 2010*

Reflex sympathetic dystrophy *Arch Phys Med Rehabil 82:412–414, 2001*

SAPHO (synovitis, acne, pustulosis, hyperostosis, osteitis) syndrome *J Clin Rheumatol 8:13–22, 2002*

Scrotal elephantiasis

Smoking *Acta DV 85:225–232, 2005; J Cut Med Surg 8:415–423, 2004; J Eur Acad Dermatol Venereol 17:276–279, 2003; Dermatology 198:261–264, 1999*

Inflammatory bowel disease – fissures

Kikuchi's histiocytic necrotizing lymphadenitis *JAAD 36:342–346, 1997*

Malakoplakia *JAAD 34:325–332, 1996*

Neutrophilic dermatosis of the dorsal hands (variant of Sweet's syndrome) *AD 142:57–63, 2006*

Panniculitis

Pyoderma gangrenosum *JAAD 79:1009–1022, 2018; JAAD 62:646–654, 2010; NEJM 347:1412–1418, 2002; Dermatology 195:50–51, 1997; J Derm Surg Oncol 20:833–836, 1994; JAAD 18:559–568, 1988; Arch Dermatol Syph 22:655–680, 1930;* pyoderma gangrenosum with C7 deficiency *BJD 178:335–349, 2018; JAAD 27:356–359, 1992;* scalp ulcers and destruction of the calvarium *BJD 5:32–36, 1995;* peristomal pyoderma gangrenosum *BJD 143:1248–1260, 2000;* associations with Crohn's disease, ulcerative colitis, arthritis, HIV infection, sarcoid, hereditary hypogammaglobulinemia *JAAD 53:273–283, 2005;* breast ulcers *BJD 157:1279–1281, 2007; JAAD 55:317–320, 2006;* ulcer extending to retrosternal space *JAAD 56:696–699, 2007;* peristomal pyoderma gangrenosum – peristomal ulcer with serpiginous border *Digestion 85:295–301, 2012; J Crohn's Colitis Sep4, 2012; J Drugs in Dermatol 10:1059–1061, 2011Int J Dermatol 29:129–133, 1990;* peristomal ulcers *BJD 157:618–619, 2007; AD 142:1372–1373, 2006;* leg ulcers *BJD 165:1244–1250, 2011;* atypical pyoderma gangrenosum – ulcer of the hand *Clin in Dermatol 29:622–632, 2011*

Pyoderma sinifica pustulans (fox den disease)

Pyoderma vegetans – crusted hyperplastic plaques, mimic blastomycosis; ulceration mimicking pyoderma gangrenosum; crusted red plaques with pustules *JAAD 20:691–693, 1989; J Derm Surg Onc 12:271–273, 1986*

Sarcoidosis – ulcerative sarcoidosis *Dermatology 202:367–370, 2001; J Eur Acad Dermatol Venereol 12:78–79, 1999; AD 133:215–219, 1997; J Derm Surg Oncol 15:679–683, 1989; AD 123:1531–1534, 1987; Dermatologica 174:135–139, 1987;* ulcerative sarcoid of the scalp with alopecia *JAMADerm 155:238, 2019*

Superficial granulomatous pyoderma

Toxic epidermal necrolysis *BJD 68:355–361, 1956*

Ulcerative colitis – peristomal ulcers *AD 142:1372–1373, 2006*

METABOLIC DISEASES

Acrodermatitis enteropathica

Calcinosis cutis – ulcerative calcinosis cutis *J Drugs in Dermatol 10:1042–1044, 2011;* exogenous calcinosis cutis – ulcerated plaque *Ped Derm 15:27–30, 1998;* calcium gluconate extravasation – calcinosis cutis with ulcer of the arm *Ped Derm 26:311–315, 2009*

Calciphylaxis (vascular calcification cutaneous necrosis syndrome) (cutaneous calcinosis in end-stage renal disease) – necrotic cutaneous ulcers, livedo racemosa, hemorrhagic patches, indurated plaques, hemorrhagic bullae *NEJM 378:1704–1714, 2018; JAAD 56:569–579, 2007; Ped Derm 23:266–272, 2006; J Dermatol 28:272–275, 2001; Am J Clin Pathol 113:280–287, 2000; JAAD 40:979–987, 1999; JAAD 33:53–58, 1995; JAAD 33:954–962, 1995; AD 131:63–8, 1995*

Chronic renal failure – prolonged wound healing

Crohn's disease, metastatic – ulcerated plaques in perigenital, inframammary, intertriginous distribution *JAMADerm 154:609–610, 2018*

Diabetes mellitus – small vessel disease, neurotrophic ulcers (mal perforans) – painless circular punched-out ulcer in middle of a callus; necrobiosis lipoidica diabeticorum *Int J Dermatol 28:195–197, 1989;* arteriosclerotic ulcers – ulcers at the side or back of the ankle, along the heel

Gaucher's disease

Gigantomastia of pregnancy – ulceration of breast *Br J Surg 74:585–586, 1987*

Gout

Hematologic diseases
  Dysproteinemia
    Cryopathies
    Cold agglutinins
    Cryofibrinogenemia *JAAD 48:311–340, 2003; Am J Med 116:332–337, 2004; JAAD 28:71–74, 1993; Lancet 338(8763):347–348, 1991*
    Cryoglobulinemia *JAAD 25:21–27, 1991;* mixed cryoglobulinemia with *hepatitis C virus Am J Med 96:124–132, 1994;* cryoglobulinemia type I or mixed cryoglobulinemia *JAAD 48:311–340, 2003; NEJM 347:1412–1418, 2002;* cryoglobulin-associated ulcers in Waldenstrom's macroglobulinemia *JAAD 45:S202–206, 2001*
    Macroglobulinemia
  Red cell disease
    Sickle cell anemia
    Thalassemia
    Spherocytosis
    Polycythemia vera
  White blood cell disease
    Leukemia
  Platelet disorders – essential thrombocythemia *JAAD 24:59–63, 1991*

Hemolytic anemia, congenital

Hyperparathyroidism and calcinosis *Arch Pathol Lab Med 114:484–484, 1990*

Iron deficiency – generalized pruritus – personal observation

Marasmus – severe protein and caloric deprivation; skin ulcers due to wrinkled, loose, dry skin; extensive loss of subcutaneous fat *JAAD 21:1–30, 1989*

Methylenetetrahydrofolate reductase deficiency – pyoderma gangrenosum-like lesions *AD 147:450–453, 2011*

Necrobiosis lipoidica diabeticorum *NEJM 347:1412–1418, 2002; Int J Derm 33:605–617, 1994; JAAD 18:530–537, 1988; JAAD 17:351–354, 1987;* foot ulcers *BJD 143:668–669, 2000*

Osteoma cutis – ulcerating yellow-white plaques *BJD 146:1075–1080, 2002*

Paroxysmal nocturnal hemoglobinuria – petechiae, ecchymoses, hemorrhagic bullae; ulcers; red plaques which become hemorrhagic bullae with necrosis; lesions occur on the legs, abdomen, chest, nose, and ears; fever; deficiency of enzymes – decay-accelerating factor (DAF) and membrane inhibitor of reactive lysis (MIRL) *AD 148:660–662, 2012; AD 138:831–836, 2002; AD 122:1325–1330, 1986; AD 114:560–563, 1978;* livedo racemosa, painful ecchymoses, purpura, hemorrhagic bullae, ulcers; mutation *PIGA* gene which encodes glycosylphosphatidylinositol-anchored proteins (decrease in GPI proteins in cell membranes); complement-induced intravascular hemolysis; increased thrombosis *BJD 171:908–910, 2014*

Porphyria – porphyria cutanea tarda; congenital erythropoietic porphyria (Gunther's disease) *Semin Liver Dis 2:154–63, 1982;* congenital erythropoietic porphyria – blisters, scarring, hyperpigmentation, mutilating ulcers, hypertrichosis, erythrodontia, corneal scarring, keratoconjunctivitis, cataracts *JAAD 67:1093–1110, 2012*

Prolidase deficiency – autosomal recessive; peptidase D mutation (PEPD); increased urinary imidopeptides; leg ulcers, anogenital ulcers, short stature (mild), telangiectasias, recurrent infections (sinusitis, otitis); mental retardation; splenomegaly with enlarged abdomen, atrophic scarring, spongy fragile skin with annular pitting and scarring; dermatitis, xerosis, hyperkeratosis of the elbows and knees, lymphedema, purpura, low hairline, poliosis, canities, lymphedema, photosensitivity, hypertelorism, saddle nose deformity, frontal bossing, dull expression, mild ptosis, micrognathia, mandibular protrusion, exophthalmos, joint laxity, deafness, osteoporosis, high-arched palate *JAAD 62:1031, 1034, 2010; BJD 144:635–636, 2001; Ped Derm 13:58–60, 1996; JAAD 29:819–821, 1993; AD 127:124–125, 1991; BJD 121:405–409, 1989; Hautarzt 39:247–249, 1988; AD 123:493–497, 1987*

NEOPLASTIC DISEASES

Atrial myxoma *Cutis 62:275–280, 1998; JAAD 32:881–883, 1995; JAAD 21:1080–1084, 1989*

Basal cell carcinoma, including basal cell arising in venous ulcers *JAAD 71:1005–1008, 2014; J Derm Surg Oncol 19:150–152, 1993;* giant ulcer – basal cell carcinoma with bony metastases *Cutis 80:60–66, 2007;* giant ulcer of the scalp *JAMA Derm 149:639–641, 2013;* metastatic basal cell carcinoma *JAAD 59:S1–3, 2008;* basal cell carcinoma with squamous cell carcinoma within – scalp ulcer

JAMADerm 150:970–973, 2014; giant ulcer *JAAD 75:113–125, 2016*

Basaloid squamous cell carcinoma of the skin – ulcerated plaque of inguinal crease; necrotic linear ulcer of inguinal crease *JAAD 64:144–151, 2011*

Basosquamous carcinoma – giant scalp ulcer *BJD 175:1382–1386, 2016*

Bowen's disease

Chordoma – sacral ulcers *JAAD 52:S105–108, 2005*

Cutaneous blastic plasmacytoid dendritic cell neoplasm – ulceronecrotic lesions of the scalp; red nodules of the back *BJD 172:298–300, 2015*

Elastofibroma dorsi *JAAD 21:1142–1144, 1989*

Epithelioid sarcoma – ulcer of dorsal hand *AD 145:589–594, 2009*

Extramedullary hematopoiesis in chronic idiopathic myelofibrosis – ulcerated red plaque *JAAD 55:S28–31, 2006*

Fibrosarcoma/spindle cell sarcoma – extensive local destruction

Hemophagocytic syndrome *AD 128:193–200, 1992*

Keratoacanthoma

Leukemia – large granular lymphocytic leukemia – pyoderma gangrenosum-like ulcer *NEJM 347:1412–1418, 2002; JAAD 27:868–871, 1992; JAAD 27:553–559, 1992*

Lymphoma *JAAD 27:553–559, 1992; JAAD 11:121–128, 1984;* angiocentric T-cell lymphoma *NEJM 347:1412–1418, 2002; AD 132:1105–1110, 1996;* cutaneous T-cell lymphoma *JAAD 31:819–822, 1994;* pyoderma gangrenosum-like ulcers as manifestation of CTCL *J Eur Acad DV 16:401–404, 2002; Hautarzt 53:114–117, 2002;* anaplastic large cell T-cell lymphoma *NEJM 347:1412–1418, 2002;* mycosis fungoides bullosa *NEJM 347:1412–1418, 2002;* lymphomatoid granulomatosis *AD 127:1693–1698, 1991;* HTLV-1 adult T-cell lymphoma/leukemia *JAAD 46:S137–141, 2002;* cytotoxic T-cell lymphoma – psoriasiform dermatitis with widespread ulcerations *AD 145:801–808, 2009;* primary cutaneous B-cell lymphoma – pyoderma gangrenosum-like lesion *BJD 151:250–252, 2004;* Hodgkin's disease – scalp ulcer *Cutis 39:247–248, 1987;* extranodal nasal type natural killer T-cell lymphoma *AD 142:1658–1659, 2006; JAAD 54:S192–197, 2006;* primary B-cell lymphoma – necrotic ulcer of the lower back *JAAD 55:S24–27, 2006;* primary cutaneous anaplastic large cell lymphoma *AD 143:255–260, 2007; Epstein-Barr virus-associated hydroa vacciniforme-like cutaneous lymphoma;* variant of extranodal NK/T-cell lymphoma, nasal type/ CD8+ cytotoxic T cells – recurrent papulovesicles, necrosis, ulceration, facial edema, atrophic scars, lip ulcers, edema of the hands, subcutaneous nodules; systemic manifestations; occurs on both sun-exposed and non-sun-exposed skin *JAAD 81:23–41, 2019; JAAD 69:112–119, 2013; Ped Derm 27:463–469, 2010; AD 142:587–595, 2006; BJD 151:372–380, 2004; JAAD 38:574–579, 1998;* hydroa vacciniforme-like cutaneous T-cell lymphoma, *Epstein-Barr virus-related* with hemophagocytic lymphohistiocytosis – gangrenous ulceredema, blisters, vesicles, ulcers, scarring, facial scars, swollen nose, lips, and periorbital edema, crusts with central hemorrhagic necrosis, facial dermatitis, photodermatitis, facial edema, facial papules and plaques, crusting of ears, fever *JAAAD 72:21–34, 2015; J Dermatol 41:29–39, 2014; JAAD 69:112–119, 2013;* angioimmunoblastic lymphoma with granulomatous vasculitis *JAAD 14:492–501, 1986*

Lymphomatoid granulomatosis – ulcers, dermal nodules, maculopapules, plaques *JAAD 54:657–663, 2006*

Lymphomatoid papulosis – personal observation

Malignant fibrous histiocytoma *JAAD 47:463–464, 2002; AD 121:529–531, 1985*

Melanocytic nevus, congenital – giant ulcer *JAAD 49:752–754, 2003*

Melanoma, including melanoma in Marjolin's ulcer *JAAD 32:1058–9, 1995;* acral melanoma – plantar ulcer *JAAD 76:S34–36, 2017*

Metastases – peristomal red plaque with ulcers – metastatic adenocarcinoma of the rectum *AD 142:1372–1373, 2006; ;* prostate cancer *Dermatology Online J 11:24, 2005;* carcinoma of the breast; carcinoma en cuirasse – personal observation

Mucinous eccrine carcinoma

Mucoepidermoid carcinoma – index finger *BJD 149:1091–1092, 2003*

Multiple myeloma – hyperkeratotic filiform follicular spicules and ulcers *JAAD 49:736–740, 2003*

Myelodysplastic syndrome *JAAD 33:187–191, 1995*

Plasmacytoma – extramedullary plasmacytoma *Transplantation 68:901–904, 1999*

Porocarcinoma *BJD 152:1051–1055, 2005*

Porokeratosis *Dermatology 196:256–259, 1998*

Posttransplant *Epstein-Barr virus-*associated lymphoproliferative disorder – ulcerated plaques *JAAD 51:778–780, 2004*

Proliferating pilar cyst

Pseudo-cutaneous T-cell lymphoma in HIV disease *AD 131:1281–1288, 1995*

Squamous cell carcinoma *Derm Surg 28:268–273, 2002;* Marjolin's ulcer – squamous cell carcinoma arising in a chronic ulcer; may present as induration and persistence of ulceration, elevated border at edge of ulcer, breakdown of burn scar with indurated base, nodule formation within burn scar *Dictionnaire de Medicine. In:Adelon N(ed.)Paris:Bechet, 1828:31–50;* scalp ulcer *AD 147:1338–1339, 2011;* scalp ulcer – squamous cell carcinoma with perineural invasion *BJD 168:899–901, 2013*

Stewart-Treves angiosarcoma – reddish-blue macules and/or nodules which become polypoid; pachydermatous changes, blue nodules, telangiectasias, palpable subcutaneous mass, ulcer *JAAD 67:1342–1348, 2012*

Transient myeloproliferative disorder associated with mosaicism for trisomy 21 – vesiculopustular rash *NEJM 348:2557–2566, 2003;* in trisomy 21 or normal patients; periorbital vesiculopustules, red papules, crusted papules, and ulcers; with periorbital edema *Ped Derm 21:551–554, 2004*

Trichoepitheliomas

Verrucous carcinoma (epithelioma cuniculatum) – ulcerated verrucous plaque of the sole *JAAD 54:S233–235, 2006*

Waldenstrom's macroglobulinemia *AD 134:1127–1131, 1998;*

PARANEOPLASTIC

Bullous pyoderma gangrenosum *Int J Dermatol 40:327–329, 2001*

Glucagonoma syndrome – necrolytic migratory erythema

Necrobiotic xanthogranuloma with paraproteinemia *AD 133:97–102, 1997; JAAD 29:466–469, 1993; Medicine(Baltimore) 65:376–388, 1986; BJD 113:339–343, 1985; JAAD 3:257–270, 1980*

Paraneoplastic vasculitis – ulcers of the buttocks *J Rheumatol 18:721–727, 1991; Medicine(Baltimore) 67:220–230, 1988*

PRIMARY CUTANEOUS DISEASES

Acne fulminans *JAAD 52:S118–120, 2005; AD 124:414–417, 1988*

Atopic dermatitis

Epidermolysis bullosa, multiple types

Erosive pustular dermatosis (chronic atrophic erosive dermatosis of the scalp and extremities) *JAAD 57:421–427, 2007*

Erythema of Jacquet – erosive diaper dermatitis; shallow, round ulcers with raised edges

Febrile ulceronecrotic Mucha-Habermann disease (acute parapsoriasis) – painful hemorrhagic ulcers *JAAD 55:557–572, 2006; JAAD 54:1113–1114, 2006; Ped Derm 22:360–365, 2005; BJD 152:794–799, 2005; JAAD 49:1142–1148, 2003; BJD 147:1249–1253, 2002; Ped Derm 8:51–57, 1991; AD 100:200–206, 1969; Ann DV 93:481–496, 1966*

Lichen planus *AD 93:692–701, 1966;* ulcerative lichen planus of the soles *Acta DV 81:378–379, 2001; AD 127:405–410, 1991; Acta DV 66:366–367, 1986; AD 93:692–671, 1966*

Lichen sclerosus et atrophicus *BJD 144:387–392, 2001*

Lichen simplex chronicus

Malakoplakia – perianal nodules, vulvar nodules, skin-colored nodules, ulcerations, abscesses, red papules, masses *Arch Pathol Lab Med 132:113–117, 2008*

Reactive perforating collagenosis

PSYCHOCUTANEOUS DISEASE

Delusions of parasitosis – Delusions of parasitosis – white atrophic scars with erosions and ulcers *NEJM 371:2115–2123, 2014;* crusted ulcers of the hands *AD 142:352–355, 2006*

Factitial dermatitis *JAAD 76:779–791, 2017; Cutis 84:247–251, 2009; Ped Derm 21:205–211, 2004; NEJM 347:1412–1418, 2002; Klin Wochenschr 64:149–164, 1986; JAAD 11:1065–1069, 1984;* factitial panniculitis – ulcers of the thigh and buttocks *JAAD 2:47–55, 1980;* peristomal ulcers *AD 142:1372–1373, 2006;* scalp ulcer *BJD 168:889–891, 2013*

Neurotic excoriations *Cutis 85:149–152, 2010*

Self-mutilation

SYNDROMES

Acro-osteolysis associated with spinal dysraphism – blister, ulcers of the foot, hyperhidrosis of the affected limb *Ped Derm 18:97–101, 2001*

Adams-Oliver syndrome – congenital scalp ACC and amniotic bands with reduction of terminal phalanges of the fingers and toes (terminal transverse limb defects); bony abnormalities of cranium; congenital cardiac abnormalities *BJD 157:836–837, 2007; Am J Med Genet 136A:269–274, 2005; Ped Derm 15:48–50, 1998; Plast Reconstr Surg 100:1491–1496, 1997; Clin Genet 47:80–84, 1995; Int J Dermatol 32:52–53, 1993; Eur J Pediatr 126:289–295, 1977; JAAD 56:541–564, 2007; J Hered 36:3–7, 1945*

AEC syndrome (Hay-Wells syndrome) – ankyloblepharon, ectodermal dysplasia, cleft lip/palate syndrome – blepharitis, eyelid papillomas, periorbital wrinkling; microcephaly, widespread congenital scalp erosions; alopecic ulcerated plaques of the scalp, trunk, groin; alopecia of the scalp and eyebrows; congenital erythroderma; depigmented patches; syndactyly; bony abnormalities; widely spaced nipples; *TP63 mutation Ped Derm 26:617–618, 2009; AD 141:1591–1594, 2005; AD 141:1567–1573, 2005; AD 134:1121–1124, 1998; Ped Derm 14:149–150, 1997;* generalized fissured erosions of the trunk *BJD 149:395–399, 2003; TP63* mutations seen in AEC syndrome, EEC syndrome, Rapp-Hodgkin syndrome, limb-mammary syndrome, split-hand split-foot malformation type 4, acro-dermato-ungual-lacrimal-tooth syndrome *AD 141:1567–1573, 2005*

Antiphospholipid antibody syndrome *NEJM 347:1412–1418, 2002; Semin Arthritis Rheum 31:127–132, 2001; JAAD 36:149–168, 1997; JAAD 36:970–982, 1997; Semin Thromb Hemost 20:71–78, 1994; JAAD 15:211–219, 1986;* eschar and ulceration *JAAD 47:766–769, 2002;* IgA antiphospholipid antibodies *J Rheumatol 25:1730–1736, 1998;* ulcer resembling pyoderma gangrenosum *J La State Med Soc 147:357–361, 1995;* lupus anticoagulant – pyoderma gangrenosum-like *Dermatology 189:182–184, 1994*

Ataxia telangiectasia – ulcerated plaque of cutaneous granuloma of ataxia telangiectasia *AD 134:1145–1150, 1998*

Atypical progeroid syndrome – autosomal recessive; diffuse mottled hyperpigmentation, foot ulcers, facial dysmorphism, recurrent infections, intellectual disability; prolidase deficiency; peptidase D deficiency *Ped Derm 36:926–928, 2019*

Behcet's syndrome – extragenital ulcers *JAAD 36:689–696, 1997*

Branchiooculofacial syndrome – autosomal dominant; congenital bilateral cervical ulcerations (bilateral ectopic thymus glands); congenital ulcerated neck mass (ectopic thymus), flattened nasal tip, pseudo-cleft lip, posterior rotated ears, preauricular pit, cleft lip, microphthalmia, coloboma, nasolacrimal duct stenosis or atresia, dolichocephaly; mutation in *TFAP2A* (retinoic acid responsive gene) *Ped Derm 29:759–761, 2012; Mol Vis 16:813–818, 2010; Arch Otolaryngol Head Neck Surg 128:714–717, 2002*

Carpal tunnel syndrome *Dermatology 201:165–167, 2000*

Charcot-Marie-Tooth syndrome – neurotrophic ulcer

Chediak-Higashi syndrome

Congenital fibromuscular dysplasia – aneurysm in skin *BJD 163:1362–1364, 2010; JAAD 27:883–885, 1992*

Didymosis aplasticosebacea – nevus sebaceus with aplasia cutis congenita *JAAD 58:884–888, 2008; Ped Derm 24 514–516, 2007; Dermatology 202:246–248, 2001*

Ectodermal dysplasias

Ectodermal dysplasia-skin fragility syndrome – autosomal recessive; plakophilin gene mutation (PKP1) – generalized erythema and peeling at birth; widespread skin fragility, alopecia of the scalp and eyebrows, focal palmoplantar keratoderma with painful fissures, hypohidrosis; skin peeling; perioral fissuring and cheilitis; perianal erythema and erosions, follicular hyperkeratosis *JAAD 55:157–161, 2006; Acta DV 85:394–399, 2005; JID 122:1321–1324, 2004*

Ehlers-Danlos syndrome

Familial dysautonomia(Riley-Day syndrome)

Flynn-Aird syndrome – skin atrophy, ulceration, alopecia, and dental caries *J Neurol Sci 2:161–182, 1965*

Goltz syndrome

Hereditary sensory and autonomic neuropathy type IV (congenital insensitivity to pain) – ulcers with self-mutilation *Ped Derm 19:333–335, 2002;* congenital insensitivity to pain *Cutis 51:373–374, 1993;* congenital sensory neuropathy with anhidrosis (self-mutilation) *AD 124:564–566, 1988*

Hereditary sensory radicular neuropathy – plantar ulcers *Int J Dermatol 23:664–668, 1984*

Hermansky-Pudlak syndrome – mucocutaneous granulomatous disease in Hermansky-Pudlak syndrome; butterfly red plaques of the face; linear ulcers of the groin and vulva; pink plaques of the thighs; swollen vulva; indurated nodules of the vulva; axillary ulcers, red face *JAMADerm 150:1083–1087, 2014*

Histiophagocytic syndrome *AD 128:193–200, 1992*

Hyper IgM syndrome – diaper area ulcers *Ped Derm 18:48–50, 2001*

Hypereosinophilic syndrome, idiopathic *Blood 83:2759–2779, 1994;*

digital ulcers *Semin Dermatol 14:122–128, 1995*

Johanson-Blizzard syndrome – aplasia cutis congenita of the scalp, sparse hair, deafness, absence of permanent tooth buds, hypoplastic alae nasi, dwarfism, microcephaly, mental retardation, hypotonia, pancreatic insufficiency with malabsorption, hypothyroidism, genital and rectal anomalies *Clin Genet 14:247–250, 1978; J Pediatr 79:982–987, 1971*

Kawasaki's disease – crusting and ulceration of prior BCG vaccination site *JAAD 69:501–510, 2013*

Laryngo-onycho-cutaneous syndrome – autosomal recessive type of junctional epidermolysis bullosa; skin ulceration with prominent granulation tissue, early hoarseness and laryngeal stenosis; scarred nares; chronic erosion of the corners of the mouth (giant perleche); paronychia with periungual inflammation and erosions; onycholysis with subungual granulation tissue and loss of nails with granulation tissue of nail bed, conjunctival inflammation with polypoid granulation tissue, and dental enamel hypoplasia and hypodontia; only in Punjabi families; mutation in laminin alpha-3 (*LAMA3A*) *BJD 169:1353–1356, 2013; Ped Derm 23:75–77, 2006; Biomedica 2:15–25, 1986*

Lesch-Nyhan syndrome – X-linked recessive; hypoxanthineguanine phosphoribosyltransferase deficiency; self-mutilation; biting of lower lip *AD 94:194–195, 1966*

Lumpy scalp syndrome – autosomal dominant; scalp ulcers at birth heal as irregular scalp nodules; deformed pinnae, rudimentary nipples *Clin Exp Dermatol 15:240, 1989*

Marfan-like phenotype – deep skin ulcers *JAAD 35:814–818, 1996*

Neurofibromatosis type I – vasculopathy with acral necrosis, livedoid painful ulcerations *BJD 172:253–256, 2015; Pediatrics 100:395–397, 1997*

Neutrophilic dermatosis (pustular vasculitis of the dorsal hands) (variant of Sweet's syndrome) – ulcers *AD 138:361–365, 2002; JAAD 32:1192–1198, 1995*

Oligodontia, keratitis, skin ulceration, and arthroosteolysis *Am J Med Genet 15:205–210, 1983*

PAPA (pyogenic arthritis with pyoderma gangrenosum) syndrome – autosomal dominant; pyoderma gangrenosum, cystic acne, acne fulminans, non-axial destructive aseptic arthritis; sterile abscesses at injection sites; attacks last 5 days; mutation in CD2-binding protein 1 *JAAD 68:834–853, 2013; Ped Derm 22:262–265, 2005; Proc Natl Acad Sci USA 100:13501–13506, 2003; Mayo Clin Proc 72:611–615, 1997*

PAPA-like syndrome (autoinflammatory syndrome) – autosomal recessive; acneiform lesions; skin ulcers; mutation in proline-serine-threonine phosphatase-interacting protein 1 *JAMA Derm 149:209–215, 2013*

PASH syndrome – pyoderma gangrenosum, acne, hidradenitis suppurativa; *PSTPIP3* mutation *BJD 176:1588–1598, 2017; BJD 175:194–198, 2016*

Partial trisomy 2p – scalp defect

Patau's syndrome (non-mosaic trisomy 13) – parieto-occipital scalp defects, cleft lip/palate, abnormal helices, low-set ears, loose skin of the posterior neck, simian crease of the hand, hyperconvex narrow nails, polydactyly, microcephaly, microphthalmia, severe central nervous system anomalies, congenital heart defects, holoprosencephaly; death in the first year *Am J Med Genet 143A:1739–1748, 2007; Ped Derm 22:270–275, 2005*

POEMS syndrome *JAAD 37:887–920, 1997*

Prader-Willi syndrome – self-induced ulcers *Ann DV 124:390–392, 1997*

Pseudoacromegaly – autosomal recessive; skin ulcers, arthroosteolysis, keratitis, oligodontia *Am J Med Genet 15:205–210, 1983*

Reflex sympathetic dystrophy *JAAD 44:1050, 2001*

Rowell's syndrome – lupus erythematosus and erythema multiforme-like syndrome – papules, annular targetoid lesions, vesicles, bullae, necrosis, ulceration, oral ulcers; perniotic lesions *JAAD 21:374–377, 1989*

SAPHO syndrome

SCALP syndrome – aplasia cutis congenita, pigmented nevus, nevus sebaceus; limbal dermoid, CNS malformations *JAAD 63:1–22, 2010*

Scalp-ear-nipple syndrome – autosomal dominant; aplasia cutis congenita of the scalp, irregularly shaped pinna, hypoplastic nipple, widely spaced teeth, partial syndactyly *Am J Med Genet 50:247–250, 1994*

Sneddon syndrome – cutaneous thrombosis, cerebrovascular thrombosis, and lupus anticoagulant *Int J Dermatol 29:45–49, 1990*

Trigeminal trophic syndrome (Wallenberg's syndrome) *JAAD 6:52–57, 1982*

Werner's syndrome *AD 133:1293–1295, 1997; Acta DV 50:237–239, 1970*

Xeroderma pigmentosum – acute sunburn, persistent erythema, freckling – initially discrete, then fuse to irregular patches of hyperpigmentation, dryness on sun-exposed areas; with time telangiectasias and small angiomas, atopic white macules develop; vesiculobullous lesions, superficial ulcers lead to scarring, ectropion; multiple malignancies; photophobia, conjunctivitis, ectropion, symblepharon, neurologic abnormalities *Adv Genet 43:71–102, 2001; Hum Mutat 14:9–22, 1999; Mol Med Today 5:86–94, 1999; Derm Surg 23:447–455, 1997; Dermatol Clin 13:169–209, 1995; Recent Results Cancer Res 128:275–297, 1993; AD 123:241–250, 1987; Ann Int Med 80:221–248, 1974; XP variant AD 128:1233–1237, 1992*

TOXINS

Caustic substances *NEJM 382:1739–1748, 2020*
- Alkalis
  - Ammonium hydroxide
  - Sodium hydroxide or potassium hydroxide
  - Sodium hypochlorite
- Acids
  - Acetic acid
  - Hydrochloric acid
  - Oxalic acid
  - Phosphoric acid
  - Selenous acid
  - Sulfuric acid
- Miscellaneous caustics
  - Cationic detergents – benzalkonium chloride
  - Hydrofluoric acid
  - Hydrogen peroxide
  - Phenol
  - Zinc chloride

TRAUMA

Burns – actinic, thermal; electrical burns from enuresis blanket; galvanic burn

Chilblains – in elderly with peripheral arterial disease; with ulcers on the fingers, toes, nose, and ears in patients with monocytic leukemia *AD 121:1048, 1052, 1985*

Decubitus ulcers – overlying sacrum, greater trochanter, ischial tuberosity, calcaneal tuberosity, lateral malleolus, point of the shoulder

Elder abuse *JAAD 68:533–542, 2013*

Galvanic burn – battery and coins in pants pocket

Gunshot wound – round ulcer of entry wound; stellate ulcer of exit wound *JAAD 64:811–824, 2011*

Ice pack dermatosis – red plaque, retiform purpura with purpuric papules and ulcers *JAMA Derm 149:1314–1318, 2013*

Intravenous drug abuse *BJD 150:1–10, 2004; NEJM 347:1412–1418, 2002;* ulcers of the hands (skin popping) *AD 145:375–377, 2009*

Laser burns

Neurotic excoriations – personal observation

Octopus bite – *Vibrio alginolyticus Ann DV 135:225–227, 2008*

Physical injury

Perinatal scalp monitor – scalp ulcer *AD 135:697–703, 1999*

Prenatal amniography with accidental injection of contrast material *AD 135:697–703, 1999*

Pressure *Clin Inf Dis 35:1390–1396, 2002; Adv Wound Care 9:35–38, 1996; Prev Med 22:433–450, 1993;* pressure necrosis of the scalp due to cardiac surgery

Radiation injury *JAAD 49:417–423, 2003; JAAD 42:453–458, 2000; JAAD 30:719–723, 1994;* radiation therapy *Head Neck Surg 6:836–841, 1984;* fluoroscopy-induced radiation injury – red telangiectatic patch with ulceration of the upper back or axilla *AD 143:637–640, 2007;* postradiation vascular proliferations of breast (atypical vascular lesions of the breast) – erythema; erythema with underlying induration or ulceration, telangiectasias, papules, plaques, nodules, *JAAD 57:126–133, 2007*

Spinal cord injury – decubitus ulcers *AD 83:379–385, 1961*

VASCULAR

Acroangiodermatitis – ulceration of the hand signifies arteriovenous shunt

Arteriosclerosis – ischemic ulcers at pressure sites; linear fissure of the heel; arteriosclerosis obliterans in patients with chronic renal failure *JAAD 57:322–326, 2007; AD 138:1296–1298, 2002*

Arteriovenous fistula steal syndrome – personal observation

C2 deficiency vasculitis *Am J Gastroenterol 78:1–5, 1983*

Cholesterol emboli – ulcers of the toes, feet, and leg *JAAD 55:786–793, 2006; BJD 146:511–517, 2002; Medicine 74:350–358, 1995; AD 122:1194–1198, 1986; Angiology 38:769–784, 1987*

Eosinophilia with granulomatosis and polyangiitis *JAAD 47:209–216, 2002; JAAD 37:199–203, 1997*

Cutis marmorata telangiectatica congenita – reticulated capillary malformation with telangiectasias; ulcerated over elbows and knees; atrophy; limb hypoplasia *JAAD 56:541–564, 2007*

Diffuse dermal angiomatosis – breast ulcer *AD 142:348–351, 2006; JAAD 45:462–465, 2001;* reticulated ulcerations of the breasts *AD 144:693–694, 2008*

Disseminated intravascular coagulation

Erythromelalgia – all types exacerbated by warmth; associated with thrombocythemia; may affect one finger or toe; ischemic necrosis *JAAD 22:107–111, 1990;* primary (idiopathic) – lower legs, no ischemia *JAAD 21:1128–1130, 1989;* secondary to peripheral vascular disease *JAAD 43:841–847, 2000; AD 136:330–336, 2000*

Granulation tissue – personal observation

Granulomatosis with polyangiitis – necrotic ulcers *JAAD 48:311–340, 2003; NEJM 347:1412–1418, 2002; JAAD 31:605–612, 1994; AD 130:861–867, 1994; Ann Int Med 116:488–498, 1992; JAAD 10:341–346, 1984;* ulcer of arm *Ped Derm 16:277–280, 1999;* ulcer of posterior neck *JAMADerm 152:1375–1376, 2016;* malignant pyoderma – head and neck variant of pyoderma gangrenosum (cephalic variant of granulomatosis with polyangiitis) *Eur J Dermatol 11:595–596, 2001; AD 122:295–302, 1986; JAAD 13:1021–1025, 1985*

Granulomatous vasculitis, cutaneous – necrosis with ulcers *JAAD 58:S93–95, 2008*

Hemangiomas – ulceration more commonly in hemangiomas of the head and neck, lip, perioral area, perineal area, segmental *Ped Derm 22:383–406, 2005*

Hemangiosarcoma

Hypertensive ulcer

Klippel-Trenaunay-Weber syndrome *NEJM 347:1412–1418, 2002*

Livedo reticularis

Livedoid vasculopathy (atrophie blanche en plaque; atrophie blanche with summer ulceration) – painful purpuric papules and plaques; leg and ankle ulcers; atrophic white scars; livedo reticularis *JAAD 69:1033–1042, 2013; NEJM 347:1412–1418, 2002*

Malignant hemangioendothelioma *J Dermatol 22:253–261, 1995*

Polyarteritis nodosa *NEJM 347:1412–1418, 2002; JAAD 31:561–566, 1994;* punched-out ulcers *JAAD 48:311–340, 2003;* in children *Ann Rheum Dis 54:134–136, 1995;* microscopic polyangiitis (polyarteritis nodosa) – livedo reticularis with surrounding erythema; acrocyanosis, ulcers, papules *JAAD 57:840–848, 2007*

Purpura fulminans, neonatal – purpura or cellulitis-like areas evolving into necrotic bullae or ulcers

Pustular vasculitis of the hands *JAAD 32:192–198, 1995*

Raynaud's disease or phenomenon *Lancet 342(8863):80–83, 1993*

Reactive angioendotheliomatosis – red-purple purpuric patches and plaques with necrotic ulcers; includes acroangiomatosis, diffuse dermal angiomatosis, intravascular histiocytosis, glomeruloid angioendotheliomatosis, angioperictomatosis (angiomatosis with luminal cryoprotein deposition), reactive angiomatosis-like reactive angioendotheliomatosis; associated with subacute bacterial endocarditis, hepatitis, cholesterol emboli, cryoglobulinemia, arteriovenous shunt, antiphospholipid antibody syndrome, chronic lymphocytic leukemia, monoclonal gammopathy, chronic renal failure, rheumatoid arthritis, severe peripheral vascular disease, arteriovenous fistulae *JAAD 49:887–896, 2003; BJD 147:137–140, 2002*

Reticular infantile hemangioma – refractory punctate and scattered ulcerations of the buttocks, and/or perineum, involve the legs of females, enlarged foot and limb; associated with ventral-caudal anomalies such as omphalocele, femoral artery hypoplasia, imperforate anus, solitary or duplicate kidney, tethered cord; congestive heart failure *Ped Derm 24:356–362, 2007*

Sclerosing lymphangitis of the penis (non-venereal sclerosing lymphangitis of the penis)

Sinus pericranii *JAAD 46:934–941, 2002*

Small vessel occlusive arterial disease *NEJM 347:1412–1418, 2002*

Subcutaneous calcification (postphlebitic subcutaneous calcification) – chronic venous insufficiency; nonhealing ulcers; fibrosis *Radiology 74:279–281, 1960*

Takayasu's arteritis – cutaneous necrotizing vasculitis *NEJM 347:1412–1418, 2002; Dermatology 200:139–143, 2000*

Temporal arteritis – ulcer of the scalp; scalp necrosis; giant cell arteritis due to nivolumab *JAMADerm 155:1086–1087, 2019;* large scalp ulcer

Thromboangiitis obliterans (Buerger's disease) *Am J Med Sci 136:567–580, 1908*

Vasculitis – small *AD 120:484–489, 1984;* medium (polyarteritis nodosa) *JAAD 31:561–566, 1994;* and large vessel (temporal arteritis) – scalp ulcer *BJD 120:843–846, 1989; AD 126:1225–1230, 1990;* leukocytoclastic vasculitis *AD 134:309–315, 1998;* idiopathic hypersensitivity vasculitis *Int J Dermatol 34:786–789, 1995;* leukocytoclastic vasculitis with secondary infection *NEJM 347:1412–1418, 2002*

Venous gangrene

Venous stasis ulcers *NEJM 347:1412–1418, 2002*

Volkmann's ischemic contracture (neonatal compartment syndrome) – of the forearm – asymmetric, well-demarcated, stellate ulcers of the arms with neuromuscular defects; in newborn; serpiginous border; muscle necrosis and nerve palsy due to increased intracompartmental pressure from amniotic band, oligohydramnios, or abnormal fetal position; begins as large bulla

Differential diagnosis includes:
    Aplasia cutis congenita
    Epidermolysis bullosa
    Necrotizing fasciitis
    Subcutaneous fat necrosis
    Protein C or S deficiency with disseminated intravascular coagulation
    Neonatal ecthyma gangrenosum from bacterial infection
    Aspergillosis
    Varicella-zoster virus infection *Ped Derm 37:207–208, 2020; JAMADerm 150:978–980, 2014; Ped Derm 25:352–354, 2008*

UMBILICAL LESIONS

JAAD 72:1066–1073, 2015

AUTOIMMUNE DISEASES AND DISEASES OF IMMUNE DYSFUNCTION

Allergic contact dermatitis – medications *JAAD 72:1066–1073, 2015;* nickel allergic contact dermatitis with periumbilical dermatitis in children *Ped Derm 19:106–109, 2002*

Autoantibodies to BP 230 and laminin gamma 1 – bullae of the lips, periumbilical bullae, giant bullae of the palms *BJD 175:619–621, 2016*

Bullous pemphigoid

Cicatricial pemphigoid

Leukocyte adhesion deficiency types IIII – delay in separation of umbilical stump and omphalitis; mucositis; periodontitis; delayed wound healing *JAAD 72:1066–1073, 2015*

Linear IgA disease *JAAD 72:1066–1073, 2015*

Morphea

Pemphigoid (herpes) gestationis – periumbilical papules, bullae, and vesicles *JAAD 72:1066–1073, 2015; JAAD 70:957–959, 2014; JAAD 40:847–849, 1999; JAAD 17:539–556, 1987; Clin Exp Dermatol 7:65–73, 1982*

Pemphigoid vegetans *AD 115:446–448, 1979*

Pemphigus foliaceus *Cutis 63:271–274, 1999; Dermatologica 180:102–105, 1990*

Pemphigus vulgaris

CONGENITAL LESIONS

AD 90:160, 1964

Abdominal wall defects – extrophy of the bladder (associated with bladder cancer); gastroschisis (extrusion of abdominal contents); omphalocele – partial absence of abdominal wall with externalization of abdominal contents; Beckwith-Wiedemann syndrome *JAAD 72:1066–1073, 2015*

Associated anomalies of GU/GI tract

Associated fistulas

Choristia, periumbilical – intestinal mucosal cells; crusted, red periumbilical plaques *Ann DV 105:601–606, 1978*

Congenital band

Embryologic rests *AD 123:105–110, 1987*

Umbilical hernia – seen in Ehlers-Danlos syndrome; Beckwith-Wiedemann syndrome; mucopolysaccharidosis, cutis laxa, congenital hypothyroidism *JAAD 72:1066–1073, 2015;*

omphalocele *Postgrad Med 57:635–639, 1981;* herniation of umbilical cord

Omphalomesenteric duct (connects yolk sac to midgut) remnants – cutaneous remnants of the omphalomesenteric duct – completely patent duct – red nodule (raspberry tumor) with a fistula with fecal discharge or intestinal prolapse; melena, anemia, abdominal pain, intussusception, intestinal obstruction *JAAD 72:1066–1073, 2015; Am J Surg 88:829–834, 1954;* patent peripheral portion – red, polypoid nodule (ectopic gastrointestinal mucosa) (umbilical polyp); discharges mucus; resemble prolapsed urachal mucosa and talc granuloma; fistulae, cysts *Ped Derm 4:341–343, 1987; AD 90:463–470, 1964;* remnants of the most external aspect of omphalomesenteric duct leads to polyps, cysts, sinus tracts *JAAD 81:1072–1073, 2019; JAAD 72:1066–1073, 2015*

Urachal malformations – urachus connects the bladder to the umbilicus – umbilical sinus with recurrent periumbilical dermatitis or cellulitis; patent urachus – drainage of urine, painful mass under the umbilicus *JAAD 72:1066–1073, 2015;* patent urachal duct *AD 90:160–165, 1964*

Patent vitellointestinal duct (persistent urachal fistula, vitelline fistula) (yolk sac remnant) – vascular nodule of the umbilicus of infancy; communicates from ileum to the umbilicus, discharge of fecal contents at the umbilicus *AD 145:1447–1452, 2009*

Persistent vascular anomalies

Persistent vitelline duct and polyp, vitelline cyst – fecal or mucoid umbilical discharge; caused by failed obliteration of the middle portion of omphalomesenteric duct *Dermatologica 150:111–115, 1975*

Prolapsed urachal mucosa

Prune belly syndrome – hypoplastic abdominal musculature, cryptorchidism, urinary tract abnormalities *JAAD 72:1066–1073, 2015*

Supernumerary nipple – on each side of the umbilicus *JAAD 72:1066–1073, 2015*

Umbilical granuloma or granulation tissue – most common umbilical mass; due to delayed or irregular separation of cord stump

Urachal and vascular abnormalities (ectopic transitional epithelium of the bladder) –urachal remnants with cyst, sinus, or fistula *Cutis 62:83–84, 1998;* complete patency of the urachus – urine emanating from the umbilicus; nodule *Ped Clin N Am 6:1085–1116, 1959;* urachal cyst (partial patency of the urachus) – tender midline swellings between the umbilicus and symphysis pubis *Br J Urol 28:253–256, 1956;* urachal sinus; urachal sinus presenting as periumbilical psoriasiform dermatitis *BJD 157:419–420, 2007*

Vitelline sinus – opens at the umbilicus; caused by failed obliteration of distal omphalomesenteric duct; may have umbilical discharge of mucus *JAAD 81:1072–1073, 2019*

DEGENERATIVE DISORDERS

Acquired umbilical hernia *JAAD 72:1066–1073, 2015*

Extropy of the bladder

EXOGENOUS AGENTS

Foreign body granuloma *AD 139:1497–1502, 2003;* secondary infection

Irritant dermatitis

Talc granuloma – older individuals *BJD 83:151–156, 1970*

Umbilical ring

INFECTIONS

Candidiasis – candidal intertrigo; Candidal sepsis

Cellulitis

Chigger mite bites

Clostridial cellulitis *AD 113:683–684, 1977*

Condylomata acuminata *JAAD 72:1066–1073, 2015; Int J Dermatol 27:150–156, 1988*

Cysticercosis *J Trop Med Hyg 88:25–29, 1985*

Diphtheria – superficial round ulcer with overhanging edge; gray adherent membrane; later edge thickens and becomes raised and rolled; umbilicus, postauricular, groin, finger or toe web; heals with scarring; crusts around the nose and mouth with faucial diphtheria *Schweiz Rundsch Med Prax 87:1188–1190, 1998; Postgrad Med J 72:619–620, 1996; Am J Epidemiol 102:179–184, 1975*

Erythrasma *Cutis 31:541–542, 1983*

Herpes simplex

Herpes zoster

Impetigo

Lyme disease *CJEM 18:158–160, 2016*

Molluscum contagiosum

Mycobacterium tuberculosis – granuloma

Necrotizing fasciitis – periumbilical erythema *JAAD 72:1066–1073, 2015; JAAD 53:527–528, 2005; Critical Care Med 29:1071–1073, 2001*

Omphalitis – neonatal omphalitis and cellulitis; coagulase-negative staphylococcus *JAAD 72:1066–1073, 2015; Arch Derm 113:683, 1977*

Pediculosis pubis

Peritonitis – umbilical erythema *JAAD 72:1066–1073, 2015; J Clin Gastroenterol 11:192–200, 1989*

Pseudomonas

Rubella, congenital – hyperpigmentation of the forehead, cheeks, umbilical area *J Pediatr 71:311–331, 1967*

Salmonella typhi/paratyphi – rose spots *BMJ 4:397–398, 1974*

Scabies – periumbilical papules

Schistosomiasis – ectopic cutaneous granuloma – periumbilical papules skin-colored papule, 2–3 mm; group to form mamillated plaques; nodules develop with overlying dark pigmentation, scale, and ulceration; periumbilical *Dermatol Clin 7:291–300, 1989; BJD 114:597–602, 1986; Ann DV 107:759–767, 1980; Br J Vener Dis 55:446–449, 1979*

Staphylococcus aureus

Staphylococcal scalded skin syndrome

Strongyloidiasis – periumbilical parasitic purpura or thumbprint sign *JAAD 72:1066–1073, 2015; JAAD 256:1170–1171, 1986*

Syphilis – condyloma lata *BJ Vener Dis 53:391–393, 1977*

Tinea corporis *JAAD 72:1066–1073, 2015*

Typhoid fever (*Salmonella typhi, S. paratyphi*) – rose spots *JAAD 72:1066–1073, 2015; Br Med J 1:98–100, 1973; AD 105:252–253, 1972*

Umbilical papilloma – if congenital presumed maternal fetal transmission of HPV *Cureus 11:E5309, 2019*

Urachal abscess *J Clin Ultrasound 19:203–208, 1991*

Verruca vulgaris *Genitourin Med 70:49–50, 1994*

INFILTRATIVE DISORDERS

Primary systemic amyloidosis, myeloma – periumbilical purpura, ecchymoses *JAAD 72:1066–1073, 2015*

INFLAMMATORY DISEASES

Crohn's disease – metastatic *Clin Exp Dermatol 21:318–319, 1996;* pyoderma gangrenosum; umbilical fistulae *JAAD 72:1066–1073, 2015*

Cullen's sign – periumbilical purpura; acute pancreatitis, ruptured ectopic pregnancy, perforated duodenal ulcer *JAAD 72:1066–1073, 2015; Br Med J i:154, 1971*

Deep umbilicus – purulent umbilical drainage *JAAD 44:687–688, 2001*

Endometriomas (32% of all umbilical tumors, most common); cutaneous endometrioma *J Derm Surg 20:693–695, 1994; South Med J 70:147–152, 1977; AD 112:1435–1436, 1976; JAMA 191:167, 1965*

Erythema multiforme

Funisitis – inflammation of the umbilical cord or stump; increased secretions and/or foul odor

Pilonidal sinus of the umbilicus (hair sinus) – pain, tenderness, and discharge in hirsute men *Cutis 62:83–84, 1998; J Fam Pract 29:205–209, 1989*

Hidradenitis suppurativa *Gastro 157:1480–1482, 2019*

Omphalitis – periumbilical erythema *JAAD 53:527–528, 2005; Scand J Gastroenterol 39:1021–1024, 2004*

Pilonidal sinus with granuloma

METABOLIC DISEASES

Amyloidosis, primary systemic – periumbilical purpura, petechiae, ecchymosis *JAAD 72:1066–1073, 2015*

Angiokeratoma corporis diffusum (Fabry's disease (alpha-galactosidase A) – X-linked recessive; periumbilical rosette *NEJM 276:1163–1167, 1967;* fucosidosis (alpha-l-fucosidase) *AD 107:754–757, 1973;* Kanzaki disease (alpha-N-acetylgalactosidase) *AD 129:460–465, 1993*; aspartylglycosaminuria (aspartylglycosaminidase) *Paediatr Acta 36:179–189, 1991;* umbilical hernia *Clin Genet 23:427–435, 1983*

adult-onset GM1 gangliosidosis (beta-galactosidase) *Clin Genet 17:21–26, 1980;* galactosialidosis (combined beta-galactosidase and sialidase) *AD 120:1344–1346, 1984;* no enzyme deficiency) – telangiectasias or small angiokeratomas; periumbilical red papules *JAAD 72:1066–1073, 2015*

Ascites with umbilical hernia – personal observation

Calcified nodule *Int J Surg Pathol 26:417–422, 2018*

Cirrhosis – ulceration of umbilical vein; umbilical hemorrhage *Postgrad Med 57:461–462, 1981*

Colonic mucosa implantation – umbilical nodule *BJD 90:108, 1974*

Cow's milk protein intolerance – umbilical erythema *JAAD 72:1066–1073, 2015; J Pediatr Gastroenterol Nutr 42:531–534, 2006*

Cretinism – coarse facial features, lethargy, macroglossia, cold dry skin, livedo, umbilical hernia, poor muscle tone, coarse scalp hair, synophrys, no pubic or axillary hair at puberty *JAAD 72:1066–1073, 2015*

Mannosidosis – umbilical hernia *Johns Hopkins Med J 151:113–117, 1982*

Mucopolysaccharidoses (Hunter's, Hurler-Scheie, Sanfilippo, Morquio, Maroteux-Lemy, Sly syndromes) – congenital umbilical and inguinal hernias *Hol J Ped 44(supp1 2)133;2018; JAAD 72:1066–1073, 2015*

Pruritic urticarial papules and plaques of pregnancy (PUPPP)

Ruptured ectopic pregnancy – periumbilical hemorrhage and pigmentation *JAAD 72:1066–1073, 2015; Can Med Assoc J 85:1003–1004, 1961*

Stein-Leventhal syndrome (polycystic ovarian disease)

NEOPLASTIC DISEASES

Acrochordon *JAAD 72:1066–1073, 2015; Dermatologica 174:180–183, 1987*

Adenocarcinoma of urachal elements *JAAD 72:1066–1073, 2015*

Basal cell carcinoma *JAAD 72:1066–1073, 2015; Cutis 71:123–126, 2003*

Bowen's disease – plaque *JAAD 72:1066–1073, 2015; Cutis 42:321–322, 1988*

Carcinoid tumor *AD 114:570–572, 1978*

Clear cell papulosis *JAAD 72:1066–1073, 2015*

Dermatofibroma *JAAD 72:1066–1073, 2015; Int J Dermatol 27:150–156, 1988*

Desmoid tumor – subcutaneous mass in subumbilical paramedian region *JAAD 72:1066–1073, 2015; Int J Dermatol 27:150–156, 1988*

Endosalpingosis – ectopic fallopian tube epithelium; umbilical nodule *BJD 151:924–925, 2004;* postoperative endosalpingosis *AD 116:909–912, 1980*

Epidermal inclusion cyst *JAAD 72:1066–1073, 2015; Int J Dermatol 27:150–156, 1988*

Epidermal nevus *JAAD 72:1066–1073, 2015; Int J Dermatol 27:150–156, 1988*

Extramammary Paget's disease *JAAD 72:1066–1073, 2015; Dermatol Online J 17:13, 2011*

Fibroepithelial papilloma

Fibrous umbilical polyp – fasciitis-like proliferation; early childhood; male predominance *Am J Surg Pathol 25:1438–1442, 2001*

Granular cell tumor *JAAD 72:1066–1073, 2015; Int J Dermatol 27:150–156, 1988*

Keloid *JAAD 72:1066–1073, 2015; AD 139:1497–1502, 2003; Int J Dermatol 27:150–156, 1988*

Langerhans cell tumor, malignant – periumbilical red nodule *JAAD 49:527–529, 2003*

Leiomyosarcoma

Lipoma *JAAD 72:1066–1073, 2015; Int J Dermatol 27:150–156, 1988*

Lymphoma – cutaneous T-cell lymphoma; Sister Mary Joseph nodule *JAAD 72:1066–1073, 2015; Ann DV 127:732–734, 2000;* granulomatous slack skin syndrome (CTCL); retroperitoneal large B-cell lymphoma – periumbilical erythema *JAAD 53:527–528, 2005*

Melanocytic nevus *JAAD 72:1066–1073, 2015; Int J Dermatol 27:150–156, 1988;* atypical nevus

Melanoma *JAAD 72:1066–1073, 2015; AD 139:1497–1502, 2003*

Metastases – Sister Mary Joseph nodule *JAAD 72:1066–1073, 2015*; stomach *AD 111:1478–1479, 1975;* renal cell carcinoma *J Comput Assist Tomogr 22:756–757, 1998;* ovarian *JAAD 10:610–615, 1984;* pancreas *Cutis 31:555–558, 1983;* uterus *Br J Clin Pract 46:69–70, 1992;* leiomyosarcoma *AD 120:402–403, 1984;* peritoneal mesothelioma *Am J Dermatopathol 13:300–303, 1991*

Milia

Neurofibroma *JAAD 72:1066–1073, 2015; Int J Dermatol 27:150–156, 1988*

Omphalith (umbolith, umbilicolith, omphalokeratolith) – inspissated umbilical bolus *Dermatol Online J Sept 15, 2019; JAAD 72:1066–1073, 2015; Cutis 40:144–146, 1987; AD 103:221, 1971*

Omphaloma *AD 123:105–110, 1987*

Paget's disease *BJD 128:448–450, 1993*

Polyp of the umbilicus – mucosal remnants of vitelline duct includes ectopic mucosa, gastric or pancreatic (rarely colonic) in origin *JAAD 72:1066–1073, 2015; Int J Dermatol 27:150–156, 1988; Ped Derm 4:341–343, 1987; J Pediatr Surg 14:741–744, 1979*

Porokeratosis – linear porokeratosis

Primary umbilical adenocarcinoma *Arch Pathol 99:95–99, 1975*

Seborrheic keratosis *JAAD 72:1066–1073, 2015; AD 139:1497–1502, 2003; Int J Dermatol 27:150–156, 1988*

Serous cystadenoma *Int J Surg Pathol 26:417–422, 2018*

Squamous cell carcinoma *JAAD 72:1066–1073, 2015; AD 139:1497–1502, 2003; J Surg Oncol 47:67–69, 1991*

Syringoma *J Dermatol 58:326, 2013*

Teratoma *JAAD 72:1066–1073, 2015; Int J Dermatol 27:150–156, 1988*

PHOTODERMATOSES

Disseminated superficial actinic porokeratosis

PRIMARY CUTANEOUS DISEASES

Acanthosis nigricans *Cut Ocul Toxicol 32:173–175, 2013*

Atopic dermatitis

Cholesteatoma – umbilical nodule

Cutis laxa – congenital umbilical hernia *JAAD 72:1066–1073, 2015; Ped Derm 18:365–366, 2001*

Endometriosis (villar nodule) – umbilical multilobulated red nodule *AD 148:1331–1332, 2012; JAAD 72:1066–1073, 2015; Int J Dermatol 27:150–156, 1988*

Epidermolysis bullosa – absent navel syndrome *BJD 98:584, 1978*

Epidermolytic hyperkeratosis

Erythema annulare centrifugum

Fox-Fordyce disease *Dermatol Online J 18:28, 2012*

Hailey-Hailey disease *Am J Clin Dermatol Oct 9, 2019*

Ichthyosis bullosa of Siemens

Intertrigo

Lichen nitidus – personal observation

Lichen planus – *Case Rep Dermatol Med 2015:840193*

Lichen sclerosus et atrophicus

Mid-dermal elastolysis *Int J Women's Dermatol 1:126–130, 2015*

Periumbilical (perforating) pseudoxanthoma elasticum *JAMADerm 155:1418–1419, 2019; JAAD 39:338–344, 1998; JAAD 26:642–644, 1992; South Med J 84:788–789, 1991; AD 115:300–303, 1979*

Post-partum pseudoxanthoma elasticum-like dermatosis

Progressive symmetric erythrokeratoderma – personal observation

Prurigo nodularis – personal observation

Psoriasis *JAAD 72:1066–1073, 2015*

Pseudomyxoma peritonei – blue translucent umbilical lesion *AD 96:462–463, 1967*

Seborrheic dermatitis (intertrigo) *JAAD 72:1066–1073, 2015*

Supraumbilical mid-abdominal raphe *Ped Derm 10:71–76, 1998*

Umbilical granuloma (granulation tissue) – red umbilical papule *JAAD 72:1066–1073, 2015*

Vitiligo

PSYCHOCUTANEOUS DISEASES

Factitial dermatitis

SYNDROMES

Aarskog syndrome – prominent umbilicus with protruding buttonlike central area surrounded by deep ovoid depression *J Pediatr 86:885–891, 1975*

Beare-Stevenson syndrome – cutis gyrata (furrowed skin), acanthosis nigricans, hypertelorism, swollen lips, swollen fingers, prominent eyes, ear anomalies, and umbilical hernia *Ped Derm 20:358–360, 2003*

Beckwith-Wiedemann syndrome – congenital hernia *JAAD 72:1066–1073, 2015;* omphalocele or other umbilical anomalies; gigantism, macroglossia; hypoglycemia, tumors (Wilms', rhabdomyosarcoma, hepatoblastoma, adrenal tumors), centrofacial capillary malformations *JAAD 72:1066–1073, 2015; JAAD 56:541–564, 2007; Syndromes of the Head and Neck, 1990:323–328*

Blue rubber bleb nevus syndrome – personal observation

Carpenter syndrome (acrocephalosyndactyly) – omphalocele *Am J Med Genet 28:311–324, 1987*

Coffin-Siris syndrome – webbed neck, bifid scrotum, umbilical and inguinal hernias *JAAD 46:161–183, 2002*

Congenital total lipodystrophy (Lawrence-Seip syndrome lipoatrophic diabetes; Berardinelli syndrome, Seip syndrome) – umbilical hernia; extreme muscularity and generalized loss of body fat from birth, acanthosis nigricans, acromegalic features, hyperinsulinemia (fasting and postprandial), early-onset diabetes mellitus or glucose intolerance, hypertriglyceridemia/low HDL-C level, hirsutism, clitoromegaly *J Clin Endocrinol Metab 85:1776–1782, 2000; AD 91:326–334, 1965*

Cornelia de Lange (Brachmann-de Lange) syndrome – hypoplastic nipples and umbilicus, umbilical hernia *Syndromes of the Head and Neck, p.303, 1990;* generalized hypertrichosis, confluent eyebrows, low hairline, hairy forehead and ears, hair whorls of the trunk, single palmar crease, cutis marmorata, psychomotor and growth retardation with short stature, specific facies, hypertrichosis of the forehead, face, back, shoulders, and extremities, bushy arched eyebrows with synophrys; long delicate eyelashes, skin around the eyes and nose with bluish tinge, small nose with depressed root, prominent philtrum, thin upper lip with crescent-shaped mouth, widely spaced, sparse teeth, hypertrichosis of the forehead, posterior neck, and arms, low-set ears, arched palate, antimongoloid palpebrae; congenital eyelashes; xerosis, especially over the hands and feet, nevi, facial cyanosis, lymphedema *Ped Derm 24:421–423, 2007; JAAD 56:541–564, 2007; JAAD 48:161–179, 2003; JAAD 37:295–297, 1997; Am J Med Genet 47:959–964, 1993*

DeBarsey syndrome – umbilical hernia *Ped Derm 18:365–366, 2001*

Dup(3q) syndrome – omphalocele *Birth Defects 14:191–217, 1978*

Dyskeratosis congenita

Ehlers-Danlos syndrome type IX – congenital umbilical hernia *JAAD 72:1066–1073, 2015; Ped Derm 18:365–366, 2001*

Elejalde syndrome (acrocephalopolydactylous dysplasia) – omphalocele *Birth Defects 13:53–67, 1977*

Goltz syndrome – umbilical hernia

Fabry's disease – periumbilical red papules *JAAD 72:1066–1073, 2015*

Hunter's syndrome – umbilical and inguinal hernias; reticulated 2–10 mm skin-colored papules over scapulae, chest, neck, arms; X-linked recessive; MPS type II; iduronate-2 sulfatase deficiency; lysosomal accumulation of heparin sulfate and dermatan sulfate; short stature, full lips, coarse facies, macroglossia, clear corneas (unlike Hurler's syndrome), progressive neurodegeneration, communicating hydrocephalus, valvular and ischemic heart disease, lower respiratory tract infections, adenotonsillar hypertrophy, otitis media, obstructive sleep apnea, diarrhea, hepatosplenomegaly, skeletal deformities (dysostosis multiplex), widely spaced teeth, dolichocephaly, deafness, retinal degeneration *Ped Derm 37:369–370, 2020; Ped Derm 21:679–681, 2004*

I-cell disease (mucolipidosis II) – umbilical hernia *Helv Paediatr Acta 35:85–95, 1980*

Idaho syndrome – umbilical hernia; premature fusion of the sagittal suture, micrognathia, anomalous pulmonary venous return, anterior dislocation of the tibiae, contractures of PIP joints *J Neurosurg 47:886–898, 1977*

Lethal omphalocele and cleft palate *Hum Genet 64:99, 1983*

Marshall-Smith syndrome – omphalocele *Syndromes of the Head and Neck, p. 340–342, 1990*

MC/MR syndrome with multiple circumferential skin creases – multiple congenital anomalies including high forehead, elongated face, bitemporal sparseness of hair, broad eyebrows, blepharophimosis, bilateral microphthalmia and microcornea, epicanthic folds, telecanthus, broad nasal bridge, puffy cheeks, microstomia, cleft palate, enamel hypoplasia, micrognathia, microtia with stenotic ear canals, posteriorly angulated ears, short stature, hypotonia, pectus excavatum, inguinal and umbilical hernias, scoliosis, hypoplastic scrotum, long fingers, overlapping toes, severe psychomotor retardation, resembles Michelin tire baby syndrome *Am J Med Genet 62:23–25, 1996*

Menkes syndrome – umbilical hernia; puffy face with pudgy cheeks (cutis laxa-like), horizontal eyebrows, cupid's bow of the upper lip, short blond hair with pili torti; prolonged hypothermia, pectus excavatum, umbilical and inguinal hernias; loose skin with wrinkling *Ped Derm 14:347–350, 1997;* silvery hair, generalized hypopigmentation, lax skin of the brows, neck, and thighs *Ped Derm 15:137–139, 1998;* bone fractures with Wormian bones, cervical bone abnormalities, rib fractures, spurring of long bone metaphyses mimicking child abuse *Society Pediatric Dermatology Annual Meeting, July, 2015; Pediatr Int 41:423–429, 1999; Atlas of Clinical Syndromes A Visual Aid to Diagnosis, 1992, pp.108–109;* Menke gene variant – umbilical hernia *Ped Derm 18:365–366, 2001*

Occipital horn syndrome – umbilical hernia *Ped Derm 18:365–366, 2001*

Olmsted syndrome – periumbilical fissured keratotic plaques

Pseudoxanthoma elasticum *JAAD 72:1066–1073, 2015*

Rieger syndrome (hypodontia and primary mesodermal dysgenesis of the iris) – failure of periumbilical skin to involute; redundant umbilical skin; exomphalos *Br J Ophthalmol 67:529–534, 1983*

Short stature, mental retardation, facial dysmorphism, short webbed neck, skin changes, congenital heart disease – xerosis, dermatitis, low-set ears, umbilical hernia *Clin Dysmorphol 5:321–327, 1996*

Simpson-Golabi-Behmel syndrome – pre- and post-natal overgrowth, large cystic kidneys, limb abnormalities, wide mouth, cleft palate, midline facial clefts, umbilical hernia, supernumerary nipples *Clin Genet 51:375–378, 1997*

Sjogren-Larsson syndrome – verrucous hyperkeratosis of flexures, neck, and periumbilical folds; mental retardation, spastic diplegia, short stature, kyphoscoliosis, retinal changes, yellow pigmentation, intertrigo – deficiency of fatty aldehyde dehydrogenase *Ped Derm 22:569–571, 2005; Chem Biol Interact 130–132:297–307, 2001; Am J Hum Genet 65:1547–1560, 1999; JAAD 35:678–684, 1996*

Stein-Leventhal syndrome – hypertrichosis of the umbilicus

Trisomy 13 syndrome (Patau syndrome) – omphalocele *J Genet Hum 23:83–109, 1975;* umbilical hernia; total body milia; polydactyly, congenital cystic adenomatoid malformation, pulmonary hypertension, apnea, atrial septal defect, epilepsy, dislocated hip joint, ocular hypertelorism, microphthalmia, retinal hypoplasia, irideremia, small ears, deafness, broad flat nose, cleft palate, micrognathia, mental retardation *Ped Derm 27:657–658, 2010*

TRAUMA

Hernia *AD 139:1497–1502, 2003;* incarcerated hernias – umbilical nodules

Ileoumbilical fistula – after surgery for Crohn's disease *Dig Dis Sci 24:316–318, 1979*

Neonatal umbilical hemorrhage from slipped ligatures

VASCULAR DISORDERS

Angiokeratoma

Caput medusa – portal hypertension *JAAD 72:1066–1073, 2015*

Cullen's sign

Gangrenous bowel – umbilical erythema *JAAD 72:1066–1073, 2015; J Clin Gastroenterol 11:192–200, 1989*

Granulation tissue, exuberant

Hemangioma *Arch Gyn Ob 283 suppl1:15–17, 2011;* umbilical cord hemangiomas *Medicine 95:e5196, 2016*

Henoch-Schonlein purpura – periumbilical purpura prior to gastrointestinal involvement *Am J Clin Dermatol 10:127–130, 2009*

Lymphangiomas – benign lymphangiomatous papules (BLAP) in periumbilical region; sign of intra-abdominal tumor with lymphatic compression *JAAD 56:S41–44, 2007;* BLAP often seen postradiation therapy or postsurgically *JAAD 52:912–913, 2005; Am J Surg Pathol 26:328–337, 2002; Histopathology 35:319–327, 1999*

Pyogenic granuloma *JAAD 72:1066–1073, 2015; Int J Dermatol 27:150–156, 1988; Ped Derm 4:341–343, 1987*

Umbilical hemorrhage due to ulceration of the umbilical vein

Vasculitis

UMBILICAL NODULES

AD 128:1265–1270, 1992

CONGENITAL ANOMALIES

Embryologic rests *AD 123:105–110, 1987*

Mesodiverticular band *JAAD 81:1120–1126, 2019*

Omphalomesenteric duct remnants (vitelline duct remnant) – umbilical mucosal polyp (cherry red nodule), congenital red umbilical nodule; may vary from simple mucosal protrusion to moderate or complete prolapse of the duct and herniation of the ileum to complete prolapse of the duct and prolapse of the ileum; combined omphalomesenteric and urachal remnants; differential diagnosis includes pyogenic granuloma (umbilical granuloma), sarcomas congenital hemangiomas, patent urachus (passage of urine through the umbilicus), ligated umbilical hernia; ileoumbilical fistula (patent omphalomesenteric duct) *JAAD 81:1120–1126, 2019; Ped Derm 29:363–364, 2012; Ped Derm 28:404–407, 2011; Cutis 76:224,233–235, 2005; AD 126:1639–1644, 1990;* other omphalomesenteric duct remnants (deep cyst, Meckel's diverticulum or sinuses with ectopic gastrointestinal tissue) *JAAD 81:1120–1126, 2019; Cutis 62:83–84, 1998;* remnant may persist as open umbilical enteric fistula or patent vitellointestinal duct connecting the lumen of the small intestine to the umbilicus *Ped Derm 24:65–68, 2007; Cutis 76:233–235, 2005*

Patent urachal duct *AD 123:105–110, 1987;* urachal cyst – congenital red umbilical papule *Ped Derm 28:404–407, 2011*

Patent vitellointestinal duct (persistent urachal fistula) – vascular nodule of the umbilicus of infancy *JAMADerm 153:597–598, 2017; AD 145:1447–1452, 2009*; differential diagnosis includes:

    Umbilical cyst *JAAD 81:1120–1126, 2019*

    Umbilical granuloma – vascular nodule *Ped Derm 36:561–563, 2019; Ped Derm 36:393–394, 2019;* congenital *Ped Derm 28:404–407, 2011*

    Umbilical skin sinus *JAAD 81:1120–1126, 2019*

    Patent urachus fistula

    Osteomyelitis of the osteum

    Ectopic gastric mucosa

    Meckel's diverticulum

Persistent vitelline duct and polyp *AD 123:105–110, 1987*

Supraumbilical mid-abdominal raphe *Ped Derm 10:71–76, 1998*

Umbilical hernia *JAAD 81:1120–1126, 2019*

Urachal and vascular abnormalities (patent urachus) (ectopic transitional epithelium of the bladder) – urachal remnants with cyst, sinus, or fistula *JAAD 81:1120–1126, 2019; Cutis 62:83–84, 1998*

Yolk sac remnant – umbilico-ileal fistula

DEGENERATIVE DISORDERS

Extropy of the bladder

Hernia – incarcerated hernia *AD 139:1497–1502, 2003*

EXOGENOUS AGENTS

Foreign body granuloma *AD 139:1497–1502, 2003*

Talc granuloma – older individuals *BJD 83:151–156, 1970*

Umbilical hair granuloma and/or sinus

INFECTIONS AND INFESTATIONS

Abscess of the umbilicus

Condyloma acuminata

Mycobacterium tuberculosis – granuloma; of the urachal sinus *BMC Inf Dis Feb 5, 2016*

Schistosomiasis – ectopic cutaneous granuloma – skin-colored papule, 2–3 mm; group to form mamillated plaques; nodules develop with overlying dark pigmentation, scale, and ulceration; periumbilical *Dermatol Clin 7:291–300, 1989; BJD 114:597–602, 1986*

Tanapox infection *NEJM 350:361–366, 2004*

INFLAMMATORY DISORDERS

Hidradenitis suppurativa

Omphalitis

METABOLIC DISEASES

Colonic mucosa implantation *BJD 90:108, 1974*

Endometriomas (32% of all umbilical tumors, most common); cutaneous endometrioma – blue-red nodule *AD 147:1317–1322, 2011; AD 112:1435–1436, 1976; JAMA 191:167, 1965;* primary

umbilical endometriosis – solitary vascular appearing umbilical nodule *JAMADerm 156:339–340, 2020*

Differential diagnosis includes:

    Keloid

    Urachal duct cyst

    Omphalomesenteric duct remnant

    Metastatic adenocarcinoma

    Abdominal hernia

    Nodular melanoma

Endosalpingosis – ectopic fallopian tube epithelium; umbilical nodule *BJD 151:924–925, 2004;* postoperative endosalpingosis *AD 116:909–912, 1980*

NEOPLASTIC DISORDERS

Adenocarcinoma of the umbilicus *JAAD 81:1120–1126, 2019*

Basal cell carcinoma *AD 139:1497–1502, 2003*

Bowen's disease – plaque *Cutis 42:321–322, 1988*

Carcinoid tumor *AD 114:570–572, 1978; Mt Sinai J Med 44:257, 1977*

Dermatofibroma

Desmoid tumor *Cutis 81:124–126, 2008*

Epidermal inclusion cyst *JAAD 81:1120–1126, 2019; Cutis 81:124–126, 2008*

Fibroepithelial papilloma *JAAD 81:1120–1126, 2019*

Fibrous umbilical polyp – fasciitis-like proliferation; early childhood; male predominance *Am J Surg Pathol 25:1438–1442, 2001*

Granular cell tumor

Keloid *AD 139:1497–1502, 2003*

Leiomyosarcoma

Lipoma

Melanocytic nevus

Melanoma *AD 139:1497–1502, 2003*

Malignant Langerhans cell tumor – periumbilical red nodule *JAAD 49:527–529, 2003*

Malignant tumors (8.4% of all tumors) *SA Med Jnl Sept 1980, p, 457; Cancer 18:907, 1965*

53% Adenocarcinoma

23% Sarcomas

18% Melanomas

3% Squamous cell carcinoma

3% Basal cell carcinoma

Mesothelioma, primary – skin-colored nodule *JAAD 55:S101–102, 2006;* metastatic peritoneal malignant mesothelioma *Cutis 81:124–126, 2008*

Metaplastic synovial cyst – blue-gray periumbilical nodule near surgical scar *AD 142:775–780, 2006*

Metastases – Sister Mary Joseph nodule *BJ Surg 76:728–729, 1989;* stomach – crusted nodule *Cutis 98:253–256, 2016; AD 111:1478–1479, 1975;* multilobulated nodule of the umbilicus; metastatic gastric adenocarcinoma *Cutis 85:90–92, 2010;* renal cell carcinoma *J Comput Assist Tomogr 22:756–757, 1998;* ovarian *NEJM 380:1061, 2019; JAAD 10:610–615, 1984;* pancreas *Cutis 31:555–558, 1983;* uterus *Br J Clin Pract 46:69–70, 1992;* leiomyosarcoma *AD 120:402–403, 1984;* peritoneal mesothelioma *Am J Dermatopathol 13:300–303, 1991; BJ Surg 76:728–729, 1989; JAAD 10:610–615, 1984;* acute promyelocytic leukemia *AD 140:1161–1166, 2004;* colon *Cutis 80:469–472, 2007; J Chron Dis 19:1113–1117, 1966;* endometrial, pulmonary, cervical *Cutis 85:90–92, 2010;* serous papillary carcinoma *JAMADerm 155:956, 2019*

Neurofibroma

Nevus, intradermal, ulcerated *An Bras Dermatol 93:905–906, 2018*

Omphaloma *AD 123:105–110, 1987*

Periumbilical choristia

Sarcoma, congenital *Cutis 76:233–23235, 2005;*

Seborrheic keratosis *AD 139:1497–1502, 2003*

Squamous cell carcinoma *AD 139:1497–1502, 2003*

Umbilical mucosal polyp – vascular umbilical polyp *JAMADerm 153:597–598, 2017; Cutis 81:124–126, 2008; Ped Derm 4:341–343, 1987*

Verrucous carcinoma *AD 141:779–784, 2005*

PRIMARY CUTANEOUS DISEASES

Cholesteatoma

Cutis laxa – umbilical hernia *Ped Derm 18:365–366, 2001*

Omphalith (omphalokeratolith) – the inspissated umbilical bolus *AD 103:221, 1971; Cutis 40:144–146*

Periumbilical perforating pseudoxanthoma elasticum *JAAD 39:338–344, 1998; AD 132:223–228, 1996; JAAD 26:642–644, 1992; AD 115:300–303, 1979*

Pilonidal granulomata

Pilonidal sinus of the umbilicus *Cutis 62:83–84, 1998*

Umbilical granuloma – vascular nodule *Ped Derm 36:393–394, 2019*

Umbilical hernia, ligated *Cutis 76:233–23235, 2005;*

Umbilicolith

SYNDROMES

DeBarsey syndrome – umbilical hernia *Ped Derm 18:365–366, 2001*

Ehlers-Danlos syndrome type IX – umbilical hernia *Ped Derm 18:365–366, 2001*

Menke gene variant – umbilical hernia *Ped Derm 18:365–366, 2001*

Mucopolysaccharidoses

Occipital horn syndrome – umbilical hernia *Ped Derm 18:365–366, 2001*

TRAUMA

Rectus hematoma

VASCULAR DISORDERS

Hemangioma *Cutis 76:233–23235, 2005;*

Microcystic lymphatic malformation *Dermatopathol 26:105–110, 2019*

Pyogenic granuloma *Cutis 76:233–23235, 2005; Ped Derm 4:341–343, 1987*

Umbilical cord hemangioma *JAAD 81:1120–1126, 2019*

UMBILICATED LESIONS

AUTOIMMUNE DISEASES AND DISEASES OF IMMUNE DYSFUNCTION

Bowel-associated dermatitis arthritis syndrome – umbilicated pustules *BJD 142:373–374, 2000*

Bullous pemphigoid – acquired perforating disease in bullous pemphigoid *BJD 180:231–232, 2019*

Graft-versus-host disease – calcinosis cutis in GVHD – umbilicated nodules, leg ulcers, rippled appearance *JAMADerm 156:814–817, 2020*

Linear IgA disease – umbilicated bullae of the face *Ped Derm 29:111–112, 2012*

Lupus erythematosus – discoid lupus erythematosus – umbilicated papular eruption of the back with acneiform hypertrophic follicular scars *BJD 87:642–649, 1972;* neonatal lupus erythematosus – personal observation

Palisaded neutrophilic and granulomatous dermatitis of collagen vascular diseases (rheumatoid arthritis); cutaneous extravascular necrotizing granuloma; Churg-Strauss granuloma, rheumatoid papule, rheumatoid neutrophilic dermatosis *Cutis 78:133–136, 2006; JAAD 47:251–257, 2002; JAAD 34:753–759, 1996; AD 130:1278–1283, 1994*

CONGENITAL LESIONS

Dermoid cyst and sinus – central dimple *JAAD 46:934–941, 2002*

DRUG-INDUCED

BRAF inhibitors – keratoacanthomas *Cancer 121:60–68, 2015; BJD 170:475–477, 2014*

Cyclosporine – sebaceous hyperplasias *JAAD 35:696–699, 1996*

Dabrafenib – keratoacanthomas; plantar calluses, seborrheic keratosis, acneiform eruptions, epidermoid cysts, alopecia, verruca vulgaris *BJD 167:1153–1160, 2012*

Fresolimumab (transforming growth factor beta antibody) *Cancer Immunol Immunother 64:437–446, 2016*

Leflunomide – eruptive keratoacanthomas *JAMADerm 152:105–106, 2016*

Lenalidomide-induced perforating folliculitis – hyperkeratotic umbilicated nodules *BJD 173:618–620, 2015*

Pembrolizumab – eruptive keratoacanthomas *JAMADerm 15 3:694, 2017*

Transepidermal elimination of collagen after steroid injections *AD 120:539–540, 1984*

Vismodegib – keratoacanthomas *JAMADerm 149:242–243, 2013*

Vemurafenib – multiple eruptive keratoacanthomas *BJD 167:987–994, 2012; AD 148:363–366, 2012*

EXOGENOUS AGENTS

Caustic drilling fluid in petrochemical industry (acquired perforating disease in oil field workers) – papules with central umbilication due to perforation of calcium *JAAD 14:605–611, 1986*

Calcium-containing EEG paste – papules with central umbilication due to perforation of calcium *Neurology 15:477–480, 1965*

Foreign body granulomas from lava lamp – umbilicated keratotic papules *Ped Derm 31:623–624, 2014*

Hydrocarbon(tar) keratosis – flat-topped papules of the face and hands; keratoacanthoma-like lesions on the scrotum *JAAD 35:223–242, 1996*

Acute iododerma – radiocontrast material – personal observation

Suture material, transepidermal elimination *AD 120:539–540, 1984*

INFECTIONS AND INFESTATIONS

Acanthamoeba – disseminated infection; umbilicated pustules – *Transpl Inf Dis 12:529–537, 2018*

African histoplasmosis (*Histoplasma duboisii*) – umbilicated papules *J Mycol Med Oct 16, 2019; BJD 82:435–444, 1970*

AIDS – cutaneous mucinosis of AIDS – personal observation

Alternaria alternata – molluscum contagiosum-like lesions *AD 121:901, 1985*

Aspergillosis – primary cutaneous *AD 128:1229–1232, 1992;* perforating aspergillosis *AD 128:1229–1232, 1992; JAAD 15:1305–1307, 1986;* molluscum contagiosum-like lesions *JAAD 80:869–880, 2019*

BCG vaccination, disseminated – umbilicated facial papules *Ped Derm 18:205–209, 2001; Ped Derm 14:365–368, 1997; Ped Derm 13:451–454, 1996*

Botryomycosis *Cutis 80:45–47, 2007*

Candida albicans sepsis – umbilicated red papule with white center *JAMADerm 155:846–847, 2019;* transepidermal extrusion of *Candida albicans*

Candida parapsilosis – personal observation

Cladosporium carrioni – molluscum contagiosum-like lesions

Coccidioidomycosis – crateriform nasal nodule *AD 146:789–794, 2010*

Cowpox (*Orthopoxvirus* infection) – umbilicated pustule; hemorrhagic pustule; tongue ulcer, targetoid and umbilicated indurated papules, vesicles, pustules with central necrosis; exposure to pet rat *Clin Inf Dis 68:1063–1064, 2019; JAAD 54(suppl 2)) 51–54, 2006; JAAD 44:1–14, 2001*

Cryptococcosis – umbilicated papules with central necrosis *NEJM 370:1741, 2014; AD 142:921–926, 2006; AD 142:25–27, 2006;* molluscum contagiosum-like lesions *AD 132:545–548, 1996; JAAD 26:122–124, 1992; JAAD 13:845–852, 1985; AD 121:901–902, 1985;* keratoacanthoma-like

Cytomegalovirus infection – perinatal CMV *JAAD 54:536–539, 2006*

Dermatophytosis – *Trichophyton rubrum BJD 178:e328, 2018*

Draining sinus tract

Fire ant stings (*Solenopsis invicta*) – clusters of vesicles evolve into umbilicated pustules on red swollen base; crusting, heal with scars; urticaria *Ann Allergy Asthma Immunol 77:87–95, 1996; Allergy 50:535–544, 1995*

Fusarium sepsis

Herpes simplex infection, including eczema herpeticum (Kaposi's varicelliform eruption) *Cutis 75:33–36, 2005*

Herpes zoster *NEJM 369;255–263, 2013;* purpuric, umbilicated, necrotic bullae of the leg *AD 147:235–240, 2011*

Histoplasmosis with transepidermal elimination – molluscum contagiosum-like lesions *Am I TropMed Hyg 46:141–145, 1992; JAAD 13:842–844, 1985;* umbilicated facial papules *Cutis 91:291–294, 2013*

Insect bites

Leishmaniasis – umbilicated ulcerated nodule of the leg *JAAD 73:897–908, 2015*

Leprosy – histoid leprosy *Ped Derm 30:e261–262, 2013; BJD 160:305–310, 2009; Int J Lepr Other Mycobact Dis 65:101–102, 1997; Int J Dermatol 34:295–296, 1995; J Indian Med Assoc 90:106, 1992;* lepromatous leprosy *Indian J Leprol 77:155–161, 2005*

Milker's nodule

Molluscum contagiosum
  With primary immunodeficiency disorders *BJD 178:335–349, 2018*
    CD40 ligand (CD154) deficiency (X-chromosomal hyper IGM syndrome(HIGM1)
    DOCK8 deficiency
    Wiskott-Aldrich syndrome

Monkeypox – exanthem indistinguishable from smallpox – papulovesiculopustular; vesicles, umbilicated pustules, crusts *CDC Health Advisory, June 7,2003; JAAD 44:1–14, 2001; J Infect Dis 156:293–298, 1987*

Mycetoma – eumycetoma *AD 141:793–794, 2005*

Mycobacterium chelonae J Dermatol 30:485–491, 2003

Mycobacterium tuberculosis – congenital tuberculosis – red papule with central necrosis *AD 117:460–464, 1981;* molluscum contagiosum-like lesions; miliary tuberculosis *JAAD 50:S110–113, 2004; Clin Inf Dis 23:706–710, 1996;* papulonecrotic tuberculid *Indian J Dermatol Venereol Leprol 50:267–268, 1984;* miliary; inoculation tuberculosis of chest wall – umbilicated ulcerated crateriform nodule of chest wall *Ped Derm 33:349–350, 2016*

Orf – reddish-blue papule becomes hemorrhagic umbilicated pustule or bulla surrounded by gray-white or violaceous rim which is surrounded by a rim of erythema *Clin Inf Dis 56:1613, 1675–1676, 2013;AD 126:356–358, 1990;* large lesions may resemble pyogenic granulomas or lymphoma; rarely widespread papulovesicular or bullous lesions occur *Int J Dermatol 19:340–341, 1980*

Paecilomyces lilacinus – resemble molluscum contagiosum *JAAD 39:401–409, 1998*

Paracoccidioides brasiliensis Clin in Dermatol 38:52–62, 2020

Syphilis, secondary – multiple umbilicated papules of the penis *Int J STD AIDS 30:707–709, 2019*

Talaromyces (Penicillium) marneffei – molluscum contagiosum-like lesions *JAAD 54:730–732, 2006; JAAD 53:931–951, 2005; NEJM 344:1763, 2001; JAAD 37:450–472, 1997; Clin Inf Dis 18:246–247, 1994; JAAD 31:843–846, 1994*

Perforating folliculitis

Plague (*Yersinia pestis*) – umbilicated vesicles and pustules *J Infect Dis 129:S78–84, 1974*

Pneumocystis carinii – molluscum contagiosum-like lesions *AD 127:1699–1701, 1991*

Scabies-associated acquired perforating dermatosis *JAAD 51:665–667, 2004*

Smallpox

Smallpox – macular and papular exanthem of the face and extremities develop vesicles, pustules, and umbilicated crusts; hemorrhagic smallpox more severe *JAAD 65:1213–1218, 2011;* vaccination site *Clin Inf Dis 37:241–250, 2003;* generalized vaccinia – umbilicated vesicopustules *Clin Inf Dis 37:251–271, 2003*

Sporotrichosis – molluscum contagiosum-like lesions *West Afr J Med 11:216–220, 1992*

Staphylococcal sepsis (MRSA) – diffuse umbilicated vesicles *JAMA Derm 149:641–642, 2013*

Syphilis – extragenital chancre (KA-like) *JAAD 13:582–584, 1985;* multiple umbilicated papules of the penis *Int J STD AIDS 30:707–709, 2019*

Tanapox – umbilicated papule *NEJM 350:361–366, 2004; JAAD 44:1–14, 2001*

Trombiculosis – fowl mite bites

Tungiasis – *Tunga penetrans JAAD 20:941–944, 1989;* hemorrhagic crusted umbilicated papule of the heel *JAMA Derm 149:1235–1236, 2013*

Vaccinia – umbilicated vesicle (Jennerian vesicle) *JAAD 44:1–14, 2001;* sycosis vaccinatum – folliculocentric pustules of bearded region *JAMADerm 151:799–800, 2015*

Varicella *Asian Prac J Allergy Immunol 21:63–68, 2003*

Warts (HPV) *Open Forum Inf Dis Nov 12, 2018*

INFILTRATIVE LESIONS

Acral papular persistent mucinosis – personal observation

Generalized eruptive histiocytosis *Am J Dermatopathol March, 2015; An Bras Dermatol 88:105–108, 2013; JAAD 50:116–120, 2004; Am J Dermatopathol 18:490–504, 1996; AD 88:586–596, 1963*

Langerhans cell histiocytosis – masquerading as molluscum contagiosum *Ped Blood Cancer 65:e27047, 2018; JAAD 45:S233–234, 2001; JAAD 13:481–496, 1985;* umbilicated blisters and pustules *Hematol Oncol Clin North Amer 12:269–286, 1998;* congenital self-healing reticulohistiocytosis (Hashimoto-Pritzker disease) *AD 147:345–350, 2011*

INFLAMMATORY

Necrotizing infundibular crystalline folliculitis – red umbilicated follicular papules with waxy keratotic plugs of the face, neck, and back *JAMA Derm 149:1233–1234, 2013; BJD 145:165–168, 2001; BJD 143:310–314, 1999*

Pyoderma gangrenosum-like lesions, polyarthritis, and lung cysts with ANCA to azurocidin – umbilicated necrotic lesions *Clin Exp Immunol 103:397–402, 1996;* pustular pyoderma gangrenosum – personal observation

Sarcoid *JAAD 44:725–743, 2001*

METABOLIC

Calcinosis cutis – transepidermal elimination of dystrophic or metastatic calcinosis cutis *AD 134:97–102, 1998;* subepidermal calcified nodule *JAAD 49:900–901, 2003;* neonatal osteoma cutis; mutation in *GNAS* (pseudohypoparathyroidism) *Ped Derm 36:732–734, 2019*

Chronic renal disease – acquired perforating dermatosis of chronic renal disease *Int J Derm 32:874–876, 1993; Int J Dermatol 31:117–118, 1992; AD 125:1074–1078, 1989*

Hemophagocytic lymphohistiocytosis *Ped Derm 23:358, 2006*

Phrynoderma – hyperkeratotic, umbilicated follicular papules *JAAD 41:322–324, 1999*

Xanthomas, eruptive *AD 137:85–90, 2001*

NEOPLASTIC

Acantholytic acanthoma *AD 131:211–216, 1995*

Agminated syringocystadenoma papilliferum *Dermatol Online J Aug 15, 2013*

Basal cell carcinoma

Dermatofibroma, mimicking keratoacanthoma *JAAD 76:s57–59, 2017*

Desmoplastic trichoepithelioma

Eccrine poroma *BJD 146:523, 2002*

Epstein-Barr virus-associated lymphoproliferative lesions *BJD 151:372–380, 2004*

Eruptive vellus hair cysts *AD 131:341–346, 1995*

Fibrofolliculomas *JAAD 17:493–496, 1987*

Follicular tumors *JAAD 15:1123–1127, 1986*

Folliculosebaceous cystic hamartoma – skin-colored papule or nodule of central face or scalp; pedunculated or dome-shaped and umbilicated *BJD 157:833–835, 2007; Clin Exp Dermatol 31:68–79, 2006; AD 139:803–808, 2003; JAAD 34:77–81, 1996; Am J Dermatopathol 13:213–220, 1991; J Cutan Pathol 7:394–403, 1980*

Giant sebaceous hyperplasia *AD 122:1101–1102, 1986*

Hidradenoma papilliferum *JAAD 41:115–118, 1999*

Histiocytoma; generalized eruptive histiocytoma *BJD 144:435–437, 2001*

Keratoacanthoma *JAAD 74:1220–1233, 2016; AD 120:736–740, 1984;* eruptive keratoacanthomas of Grzybowski *AD 112:835–836, 1976;* due to blunt trauma *JAAD 48:S35–38, 2003;* sharp trauma *Derm Surg 50:753–758, 2004; Int J Derm 21:349, 1982;* thermal burn *Cutis 47:410–412, 1991;* in a donor graft site *Br J Plast Surg 50:560–561, 1997;* at site of scratch *JAAD 48:S35–38, 2003;* vaccination site *J Derm Surg Onc 9:381–382, 1983; BJD 90:689–690, 1974;* laser therapy *Derm Surg 25:666–668, 1999*

Leiomyosarcoma *Sem Cut Med Surg 21:159–165, 2002; JAAD 38:137–142, 1998; J D Surg Oncol 9:283–287, 1983*

Leukemia – molluscum-like papules of HTLV-1 associated ATLL *JAMA Derm 149:1101–1102, 2013; Indian J Dermtol 57:219–221, 2012; Acta DV 90:287–290, 2010;* acute myelomonocytic leukemia – personal observation; acute myelogenous leukemia *Indian J DV Leprol 78:752–754, 2012*

Lichen planus-like keratosis

Lymphoma – CD 30+ anaplastic large cell lymphoma *Cutis 98:253–256, 2016; JAAD 49:1049–1058, 2003;* HTLV-1 granulomatous T-cell lymphoma – umbilicated red-orange papulonodules *JAAD 44:525–529, 2001;* folliculotropic CTCL – umbilicated follicular papules *AD 146:607–613, 2010*

Lymphomatoid papulosis

Melanoma – amelanotic desmoplastic neurotropic melanoma – umbilicated papule of the nose *AD 139:1209–1214, 2003*

Metastases – salivary gland adenocarcinoma – keratoacanthoma-like lesions – personal observation; cutaneous metastases *AD 143:613–620, 2007;* adenocarcinoma of the lung; squamous cell carcinoma

Nevus comedonicus – personal observation

Nevus lipomatosus superficialis *BJD 153:209–210, 2005*

Palisaded encapsulated neuroma (red papule) *AD 130:369–374, 1994*

Pilar cyst

Pilar sheath acanthoma – umbilicated skin-colored papule with central keratinous plug of mustache area *AD 114:1495–1497, 1978*

Porokeratotic eccrine ostial and dermal duct nevus – resemble nevus comedonicus; linear keratotic papules with central plugged pit; may be verrucous; filiform; anhidrotic or hyperhidrotic; most common on the palms and soles *AD 138:1309–1314, 2002; JAAD 43:364–367, 2000; JAAD 24:300–301, 1991; Cutis 46:495–497, 1990*

Rhabdomyomatous mesenchymal hamartoma (striated muscle hamartoma) (congenital) – associated with Delleman syndrome – multiple skin tag-like lesions of infancy *Ped Derm 15:274–276, 1998*

Sebaceous adenoma

Sebaceous hyperplasia *BJD 118:397–402, 1988; Berlin:Verlag A Hirschfeld:1874*

Spitz nevus *AD 134:1627–1632, 1998*

Squamous cell carcinoma – personal observation

Syringocystadenoma papilliferum – umbilicated volcanic nodule of the trunk (shoulders, axillae, genitalia) *JAMADerm 153:725–727, 2017; AD 71:361–372, 1955;* linear syringocystadenoma papilliferum *AD 121:1197–1202, 1985; AD 112:835–836, 1976*

Syringoma

Trichoblastoma – umbilicated scalp nodule with central follicular plug *BJD 144:1090–1092, 2001*

Trichofolliculoma – tuft of white hair issuing from central pore

Verrucous acanthoma

Verrucous perforating collagenoma *Dermatologica 152:65–66, 1976*

Waldenstrom's IgM storage papules (macroglobulinosis) – skin-colored translucent papules on extensor extremities, buttocks, trunk; may be hemorrhagic, crusted, or umbilicated *JAAD 45:S202–206, 2001; AD 128:377–380, 1992*

Warty dyskeratoma

PARANEOPLASTIC DISEASES

Eruptive xanthogranulomas and hematologic malignancies *JAAD 59:488–493, 2008*

PHOTODERMATOSES

Hydroa vacciniforme – red macules progress to tender papules, hemorrhagic vesicles or bullae of the face and hands, umbilication and crusting; varioliform (pock-like) scars; keratoconjunctivitis and uveitis, blistering of the lips *JAAD 67:1093, 1110, 2012; Ped Derm 18:71–73, 2001; JAAD 42:208–213, 2000; Dermatology 189:428–429, 1994; JAAD 25:892–895, 1991; JAAD 25:401–403, 1991; BJD 118:101–108, 1988; AD 118:588–591, 1982;* familial *BJD 140:124–126, 1999; AD 114:1193–1196, 1978; AD 103:223–224, 1971;* late onset *BJD 144:874–877, 2001*

PRIMARY CUTANEOUS DISEASES

Acne necrotica miliaris (necrotizing lymphocytic folliculitis) *Aust J Dermatol e53–58, 2019*

Acne necrotica varioliformis *AD 132:1365–1370, 1996; JAAD 16:1007–1014, 1987*

Acrokeratoelastoidosis of Costa – umbilicated hyperkeratotic papules of the palms and soles *AD 140:479–484, 2004; Ped Derm 19:320–322, 2002; JAAD 22:468–476, 1990; Acta DV 60:149–153, 1980; Dermatologica 107:164–168, 1953*

Darier's disease – umbilicated white papules on oral mucosa *Clin Dermatol 19:193–205, 1994; JAAD 27:40–50, 1992*

Degenerative collagenous plaques of the hands – linear crateriform papules; may coalesce to form a band *JAAD 47:448–451, 2002; AD 82:362–366, 1960*

Degos disease – personal observation

Elastosis perforans serpiginosa *J Dermatol 20:329–340, 1993; Hautarzt 43:640–644, 1992; JAAD 10:561–581, 1984; AD 97:381–393, 1968*

    Acrogeria

    Down's syndrome

    Ehlers-Danlos syndrome type IV

    Osteogenesis imperfect

    Pseudoxanthoma elasticum

    Rothmund-Thomson syndrome

    Scleroderma *Dermatol Online J May 15, 2011*

Epidermolysis bullosa pruriginosa – dominant dystrophic or recessive dystrophic; mild acral blistering at birth or early childhood; violaceous papular and nodular lesions in linear array on shins, forearms, trunk; red, crusted, and lichenified papules; lichenified hypertrophic and verrucous plaques in adults *BJD 159:464–469, 2008; BJD 146:267–274, 2002; BJD 130:617–625, 1994*

Erythema of Jacquet – erosive diaper dermatitis with umbilicated papules *Pediatr Clin North Am 47:909–919, 2000; Ped Derm 15:46–47, 1998; Ped Derm 8:160–161, 1991*

Focal acral hyperkeratosis (acrokeratoelastoidosis without elastorrhexis) – autosomal dominant; crateriform papules of the sides of the hands and feet *JAAD 47:448–451, 2002; AD 120:263–264, 1984; BJD 109:97–103, 1983*

Fox-Fordyce disease *JAAD 48:453–455, 2003*

Granuloma annulare – in HIV disease *JAAD:S184–186, 2003;* perforating granuloma annulare *JAAD 75:457–465, 2016;* umbilicated papular granuloma annulare *Ped Derm 33:89–90, 2016; Ped Derm 23:72–74, 2006; AD 140:877–882, 2004; Int J Dermatol 36:207–209, 1997; AD 128:1375–1378, 1992;* perforating granuloma annulare *Int J Dermatol 36:340–348, 1997; AD 103:65–67, 1971*

Kyrle's disease (hyperkeratosis follicularis et parafollicularis in cutem penetrans) *Int J Dermatol 36:340–348, 1997; J Derm 20:329–340, 1993; JAAD 16:117–123, 1987; AD 103:65–67, 1971*

Lichen planus *Dermatol Online J Jan 15, 2013*

Lichen sclerosus et atrophicus – personal observation

Necrotizing infundibular crystalline folliculitis *BJD 145:165–168, 2001*

Papular elastorrhexis *Dermatology 205:198–200, 2002; Clin Exp Dermatol 27:454–457, 2002; JAAD 19:409–414, 1988; AD 123:433–434, 1987*

Perforating folliculitis *JAAD 40:300–302, 1999; Am J Dermatopathol 20:147–154, 1998; AD 97:394–399, 1968*

Peristomal pseudoverrucous papules – umbilicated papules *Ped Derm 36:713–715, 2019*

Periumbilical pseudoxanthoma elasticum *AD 132:223–228, 1996*

Pityriasis rosea, vesicular

Prurigo nodularis – personal observation

Reactive perforating collagenosis – early childhood, precipitated by trauma; skin-colored umbilicated papules; heal with hypopigmentation or scar *BJD 140:521–524, 1999; Int J Dermatol 36:340–348, 1997; AD 121:1554–1555, 1557–1558, 1985; AD 103:65–67, 1971;* familial RPC – umbilicated facial papules *Ped Derm 30:762–764, 2013*

SYNDROMES

Birt-Hogg-Dube syndrome – fibrofolliculomas – skin-colored papule with central keratinous plug *AD 135:1195–1202, 1999*

Dyskeratosis benigna intraepithelialis mucosae et cutis hereditaria – conjunctivitis, umbilicated keratotic nodules of the scrotum, buttocks, trunk; palmoplantar verruca-like lesions, leukoplakia of buccal mucosa, hypertrophic gingivitis, tooth loss *J Cutan Pathol 5:105–115, 1978*

Muir-Torre syndrome – autosomal dominant; sebaceous adenomas, sebaceous carcinomas, keratoacanthomas *JAAD 74:558–566, 2016; JAMADerm 151:1365–1366, 2015; Cutis 75:149–155, 2005; Curr Prob Derm 14:41–70, 2002; BJD 136:913–917, 1997; JAAD 33:90–104, 1995; JAAD 10:803–817, 1984; AD 98:549–551, 1968; Br J Surg 54:191–195, 1967*

Sweet's syndrome

VASCULAR

Eosinophilic granulomatosis with polyangiitis – umbilicated nodules of the elbows *BJD 150:598–600, 2004;* umbilicated nodules with central necrosis of the elbows and knees *BJD 127:199–204, 1992*

Degos disease – umbilicated papules *Aust J Dermatol 49:86–90, 2008; Ann DV 79:410–417, 1954*

Hemophagocytic lymphohistiocytosis – hemophagocytosis of erythrocytes, leukocytes, thrombocytes in the bone marrow, spleen, liver, or lymph nodes *Ped Derm 23:35–38, 2006*

Infantile hemangioma with central necrosis of the face *AD 147:1049–1056, 2011*

Granulomatosis with polyangiitis *JAAD 31:605–612, 1994;* palisaded neutrophilic and granulomatous dermatitis – tender umbilicated papules *Cutis 70:37–38, 2002*

Lymphomatoid granulomatosis – destruction of midline nasal structures; necrotic plaque of the nose; crateriform nodule of cheek *JAMADerm 155:113–114, 2019*

UNILATERAL FOOT EDEMA

Pedal muscle abscess without trauma *Clin Pediatr 56:975–978, 2017*

Amputee

Arthropod bite, envenomation, sting

Factitial dermatitis

Filariasis *Natl Med J India 15:192–2002*

Freiberg's infarction

Giant cell arteritis *Clin Rheumatol 18:82–84, 1999*

Ileocecal arteriovenous fistula *Ann Vasc Surg 5):298ei–298.e5, 2018*

Lymphoma – primary cutaneous gamma-delta T-cell lymphoma *Int J Clin Exp Pathol 7:5337–5352, 2014*

Melkersson-Rosenthal syndrome *Dermatol Online J 14:7, 2008*

Plantar fasciitis *Am J Roentgenol 173:699–701, 1999*

Plantar neuroma

Reflex sympathetic dystrophy

RS3PE (remitting seronegative symmetrical synovitis with pitting edema) *J Rheumatol 212:372, 1974*

Synovial sarcoma *Clin Orthop 364:220–226, 1999*

Tenosynovitis

Venous thrombosis – swelling and pain of the calf; edema of the ankle *BMJ 320:1453–1456, 2000*

URTICARIA AND URTICARIA-LIKE LESIONS

Cutis 79:41–49, 2007

AUTOIMMUNE DISORDERS AND DISEASES OF IMMUNE DYSFUNCTION

Allergic contact dermatitis – contact urticaria – foods, food additives, drugs, animal saliva or dander, pollen, caterpillars, rubber gloves, algae, lichens *JAAD 62:541–555, 2010;* contact urticaria to curcumin (spice) *Dermatitis 17:196–197, 2006;;* contact urticaria to lip plumper *JAAD 60:861–863, 2009;* contact urticarial to formaldehyde *Dermatitis 27:232, 2016; Contact Dermatitis 8: 333–334, 1982;* nickel – generalized urticaria after transfusions *Lancet ii:741–742, 1960;* chronic urticaria due to surgical metal skin clips *NEJM 329:1583–1584, 1993;* implanted alloys *Br Med J 4:36, 1967;* apple – perioral urticarial dermatitis *JAAD 53:736–737, 2005;* generalized urticarial following diphencyprone to treat warts *J Drugs Dermatol 6:529–530, 2007;*plants – fruits, vegetables, wheat bran, potato, eggs, beef, chicken, fish, pears, peanut butter, kiwi, apple, plum, pear birch pollen, alcohol, nickel, NCR paper, formalin, teak, fur, silk, horse saliva, rubber, ammonium persulfate, cinnamaldehyde, benzoic acid, guinea pig saliva and fur, streptomycin, vinylpyridine, balsam of Peru, pig gut, cow and pig blood; nettles; plant irritant contact dermatitis – urticarial dermatitis; buttercup, spurge, manzanillo tree, milfoil, mayweed; DEET-containing insect repellant *Contact Dermatitis 35:186–187, 1996;* chlorinated pool water *Contact Dermatitis 3:279, 1977;* rubber *JAAD 25:831–839, 1991;* spices, cornstarch *J Derm Surg Oncol 13:224, 1987;* globe artichoke *J Allergy Clin Immunol 97:710–711, 1996;* litchi fruit *Contact Dermatitis 33:67, 1995;* kiwi fruit *Contact Dermatitis 22:244. 1990;* watermelon *Contact Dermatitis 28:185–186, 1993;* shiitake mushrooms *JAAD 24:64–66, 1991;* rice *BJD 132:836–837, 1995;* buckwheat flour *Ann Allergy 63:149–152, 1989;* mold on salami casing *Contact Dermatitis 32:120–121, 1995;* nickel *Contact Dermatitis 17:187, 1987;* beef *Contact Dermatitis 27:188–189, 1992;* cow's milk *Allergy 42:151–153, 1987;* pork, fish *Contact Dermatitis 17:182, 1987;* dog saliva *Contact Dermatitis 26:133, 1992;* tobacco *Contact Dermatitis 16:225–226, 1987;* locusts *BJD 118:707–708, 1988;* mouse hair *Contact Dermatitis 28:200, 1993;* Red Sea coral – contact dermatitis *Int J Derm 30:271–273, 1991*

Alpha-gal syndrome – urticarial; IgE-mediated allergy to mammalian meat *JAMADerm 155:115–116, 2019*

Anaphylactoid reactions – aspirin, radiocontrast media, alcohol, foods

Autoimmune estrogen dermatitis *JAAD 32:25–31, 1995*

Autoimmune progesterone dermatitis – premenstrual urticaria *AD 145:341–342, 2009; BJD 133:792–794, 1995; Semin Dermatol 8:26–29, 1989; BJD 121(suppl 34):64, 1989*

Autoinflammatory syndrome with lymphedema (AISLE) – fever and urticarial, progressive edema of the scrotum and legs; mutation in *MyoD* family inhibitor domain-containing protein *Ped Derm 33:602–614, 2016*

Bruton's agammaglobulinemia

Bullous disease with IgA vs. collagen VII and IgG vs laminin 332 – urticarial plaques and bullae and oral erosions *BJD 167:938–941, 2012*

Bullous pemphigoid, urticarial phase *JAAD 81:355:363, 2019; BJD 165:1133–1137, 2011; JAAD 62:541–555, 2010; JAAD 29:293–299, 1993;* early signs of bullous pemphigoid (bullous pemphigoid without blisters); urticarial lesions, dermatitis, excoriations *JAMA Derm 149:950–953, 2013; BJD 167:1111–1117, 2012;* IgA anti-p200 pemphigoid (p200 is laminin gamma 1) – blisters with serpiginous urticarial and annular plaques; erosions *JAMADerm 153:1185–1186, 2017; JAAD 71:185–191, 2014; AD 147:1306–1310, 2011;* urticaria and bullae in 3-month-old infant *BJD 169:191–192, 2013;* bullous pemphigoid in infancy – urticarial and bullae *BJD 66:1140–1142, 2012*

Postvaccination bullous pemphigoid in infancy – bullae and urticarial papules *Ped Derm 30:741–744, 2013*

C1 esterase deficiency

C3 deficiency

Common variable immunodeficiency – chronic urticaria *JAAD 59:S40–41, 2008*

Complement deficiencies *Ped Derm 28:494–501, 2011*

Dermatitis herpetiformis – chronic urticaria *Ped Derm 21:564–567, 2004;* urticaria-like lesions *JAAD 62:541–555, 2010*

Dermatomyositis *J R Soc Med 77:137–138, 1984;* urticarial plaques with neutrophilic infiltrate *AD 144:1486–1490, 2008*

Epidermolysis bullosa acquisita – urticaria-like lesions *BJD 171:1022–1030, 2014; BJD 169:100–105, 2013; JAAD 62:541–555, 2010* IPEX syndrome – immune dysregulation (neonatal autoimmune enteropathy, food allergies), polyendocrinopathy (diabetes mellitus, thyroiditis), enteropathy (neonatal diarrhea), X-linked, rash (atopic dermatitis-like with exfoliative erythroderma and periorificial dermatitis; psoriasiform dermatitis, pemphigoid nodularis, painful fissured cheilitis, edema of the lips and perioral area, urticaria secondary to foods); penile rash; thyroid dysfunction, diabetes mellitus, hepatitis, nephritis, onychodystrophy, alopecia universalis; mutations in *FOXP3* (forkhead box protein 3) gene – master control gene of T regulatory cells (Tregs); hyper IgE, eosinophilia *JAAD 73:355–364, 2015; BJD 160:645–651, 2009;* ichthyosiform eruptions *Blood 109:383–385, 2007; BJD 152:409–417, 2005; NEJM 344:1758–1762, 2001;* alopecia areata *AD 140:466–472, 2004*

Gain-of-function mutation of NLRC4 (inflammasome) – fever, periodic urticarial rash, conjunctivitis, arthralgias, painful red nodules of the foot or leg, enterocolitis, splenomegaly, macrophage activation syndrome; increased IL-18 *BJD 176:244–248, 2017; Nat Genet 46:1135–1139, 2014; Nat Genet 46:1140–1146, 2014; J Exp Med 211:2385–2396, 2014*

Juvenile rheumatoid arthritis – personal observation

Linear IgA disease – targetoid, urticarial, herpetiform lesions, confluent bullae *BJD 177:212–222, 2017;* urticaria-like lesions *JAAD 62:541–555, 2010*

Lupus erythematosus, systemic – urticaria-like lesions *JID 75:495–499, 1980; BJD 99:455–457, 1978; AD 114:879–883, 1978;* urticaria *BJD 135:355–362, 1996;* hypocomplementemic vasculitis with urticarial lesions *J Rheumatol 14:854–855, 1987;* lupus vasculitis *JAAD 48:311–340, 2003;* urticarial vasculitis progressing to SLE *AD 124:1088–1090, 1988*

Mixed connective tissue disease *J Dermatol 11:195–197, 1984*

Pemphigoid gestationis (herpes gestationis) – urticaria-like lesions *JAAD 62:541–555, 2010; BJD 157:388–389, 2007; JAAD 55:823–828, 2006; JAAD 40:847–849, 1999; JAAD 17:539–536, 1987; Clin Exp Dermatol 7:65–73, 1982;* associated with anhydramnios *JAMADerm 154:484–486, 2018*

Pemphigus herpetiformis – red plaque with vesicles, circinate desquamation, erosions, urticarial lesions *Ped Derm 34:342–346, 2017; JAAD 62:611–620, 2010*

PLAID (*PLCG2*-associated antibody deficiency and immune dysregulation) – evaporative cold urticaria; neonatal ulcers in cold-sensitive areas; granulomatous lesions sparing flexures; blotchy pruritic red rash, spontaneous ulceration of nasal tip with eschar of the nose; erosion of nasal cartilage, neonatal small papules and erosions of the fingers and toes; brown granulomatous plaques with telangiectasia and skin atrophy of the cheeks, forehead, ears, chin; atopy; recurrent sinopulmonary infections *Ped Derm 37:147–149, 2020; JAMADerm 151:627–634, 2015*

Rheumatoid arthritis – Still's disease-like lesions *Q J Med 49:377–387, 1956;* palisaded neutrophilic granulomatous dermatitis of rheumatoid arthritis (rheumatoid neutrophilic dermatosis, interstitial granulomatous dermatitis with plaques, railway track dermatitis, linear granuloma annulare) – urticarial plaques on the backs of the hands and arms, back of the neck, trunk, over joints *JAAD 48:311–340, 2003; JAAD 47:251–257, 2002; AD 133:757–760, 1997; AD 125:1105–1108, 1989*

Serum sickness *Dermatol Clin 3:107–117, 1985; NEJM 311:1407–1413, 1984;* purple urticaria *Ped Derm 36:274–282, 2019*

Sjogren's syndrome – annular urticarial-like erythema, localized cutaneous nodular amyloidosis (brown nodule), leukocytoclastic vasculitis, photosensitivity *JAAD 79:736–745, 2018;* annular erythema *JAAD 48:311–340, 2003; JAAD 20:596–601, 1989;* urticarial vasculitis *Dermatol in Gen Med, 7th Edition, 2008,pp.1579*

Still's disease (systemic-onset juvenile idiopathic arthritis) – salmon pink urticaria-like lesions *Medicine 96:d6318, 2017; JAAD 50:813–814, 2004;* adult-onset Still's disease – urticaria and angioedema *J Eur Acad Dermatol Venereol 19:360–363, 2005;–* episodic fevers, polyarticular arthritis of both large and small joints; typical rash – evanescent salmon pink urticarial rash with fever on the trunk, proximal extremities, pressure areas, face; atypical rash persistent eruption, periorbital edema, dermatomyositis-like rash; heliotrope *AD 148:947–952, 2012;* severe periorbital edema *Rheumatol Int 32:2233–2237, 2012; Ped Derm 21:580–588, 2004; Sem Hop 59:1848–1851, 1983*

Urticaria – acute; idiopathic, foods (eggs, cheese, fruit, fish, milk, nuts, seafood), food additives (dyes, tartrazine), drugs, hymenoptera stings, plasma expanders, blood products, anesthetic agents *JAAD 79:599–614, 2018; Cutis 79:41–49, 2007;* peanut allergy – urticaria, angioedema, anaphylaxis *JAAD 66:136–143, 2012;* chronic – subclinical foci of infection, parasites

    Adrenergic urticaria

    Aquagenic urticaria

    Cholinergic urticaria

    Cold urticaria

    Contact urticaria – stinging nettles, jellyfish, cinnamon aldehyde, sorbic acid, latex, food handlers

    Delayed pressure urticaria

    Dermatographism *Clin Exp Dermatol 14:25–28, 1989;* delayed dermatographism *Ann Allergy 21:248–255, 1963*

    Familial cold autoinflammatory syndrome

    Gleich syndrome

    Heat urticaria

    NOMID syndrome

Phospholipase Cg2-associated antibody deficiency (temperature-dependent intracellular signaling) – infections, granulomatous, autoimmunity, cold-induced urticarial

Schnitzler's syndrome – increased serum IgM with angioedema

Solar urticaria

Vibratory angioedema

Urticaria, fever, and eosinophilia – personal observation

Urticaria with preceding vomiting *Semin Dermatol 6:286–291, 1987*

Urticaria, asthma, anaphylaxis *Semin Dermatol 6:286–291, 1987*

CONGENITAL LESIONS

Neonatal dermatographism *Ped Derm 25:130–131, 2008*

DRUG-INDUCED

ACE inhibitors – lisinopril *AD 133:972–975, 1997*

Anti-PD-1 therapy (atezolizumab, nivolumab, pembrolizumab, durvalumab) – bullous dermatoses (bullous pemphigoid, IgA dermatosis) – hemorrhagic bullae urticarial plaques, oral ulcers *JAAD 79:1081–1088, 2018*

Azathioprine hypersensitivity syndrome – fever, chills, erythema nodosum, Sweet's syndrome, leukocytoclastic vasculitis, pustular drug eruption, urticarial, purpuric eruption, leukocytosis, nausea, vomiting, diarrhea *JAAD 65:184–191, 2011*

Cisplatin, carboplatin, oxaliplatin – urticaria *JAAD 71:203–214, 2014*

Cyclophosphamide *JAAD 71:203–214, 2014*

Doxorubicin – focal pegylated liposomal doxorubicin – urticarial *JAMADerm 153:475–476, 2017*

Doxycycline – solar urticaria *J Drugs Dermatol 14:1358–1359, 2015*

Drug reaction with eosinophilia and systemic symptoms (DRESS) – morbilliform eruption, cheilitis (crusted hemorrhagic lips), diffuse desquamation, areolar erosion, periorbital dermatitis, vesicles, bullae, targetoid plaques, purpura, pustules, exfoliative erythroderma, urticarial papular-confluent; facial edema, lymphadenopathy *BJD 168:391–401, 2013; Ped Derm 28:741–743, 2011; JAAD 68:693–705, 2013; AD 146:1373–1379, 2010*

Foscarnet – urticarial rash with or without exanthem – eosinophilic pustular folliculitis due to foscarnet *JAAD 44:546–547, 2001*

Corticosteroids, inhaled (budesonide) *Clin Exp Allergy 23:232–233, 1993*

Interleukin-2 *JAAD 28:66–70, 1993*

Iododerma *JAAD 36:1014–1016, 1997*

MEK inhibitors (selumetinib, cobimetinib, trametinib) – urticarial plaques; pityriasis rosea-like hypersensitivity reactions *JAMADerm 151:78–81, 2015*

Prostaglandin E1 – neonatal urticaria *Ped Derm 17:58–61, 2000*

Radiocontrast dye

Urticarial drug reactions *Clin Inf Dis 58:1140–1148, 2014*

EXOGENOUS AGENTS

Alcohol urticarial syndrome – aldehyde dehydrogenase deficiency *Dermatitis 22:352–353, 2012*

Ammonium persulfate – hairdressers; contact urticaria

Animal dander

Aquagenic urticaria – familial or sporadic *Ped Derm 31:116–117 2014; AD 147:1461–1462, 2011; JAAD 47:611–613, 2002; JAAD 15:623–627, 1986; Dermatologica 158:468–470, 1979; JAMA 189:895–898, 1964*

Blood products

Chlorhexidine

Cocaine abuse – urticaria and urticarial vasculitis *Clin Exp Dermatol 45:630–632, 2020; Clin Inf Dis 61:1840–1849, 2015; JAAD 69:135–142, 2013; JAAD 59:483–487, 2008*

DEET (N,N-diethyl-meta-toluamide) – contact urticarial *Cutis 91:280–282, 2013*

Drug abuse – local urticaria from leakage of heroin or methadone

Ethanol *BJD 132:464–467, 1995*

Dermatographism – follicular, delayed *Ann Allergy 21:248–255, 1963;* cholinergic, cold-precipitated, exercise-induced, red, yellow, white; familial *Am J Med Genet 39:201–203, 1991*

Glove-related urticaria *BJD 174:1137–1140, 2016*

Hedgehog hives *AD 135:561–563, 1999*

Heroin *JAAD 69:135–142, 2013*

Heparin – anaphylaxis (without urticaria) *JAAD 61:325–332, 2009*

Histamine-releasing agents

Implants – metal orthopedic pins *Br Med J iv:36, 1967*; dental prostheses *Contact Dermatitis 21:204–205, 1989*; dental amalgams; *N Y State J Med 43:1648–1652, 1943*

Inhalants – grass pollens, molds, animal danders, house dust, tobacco smoke, foods

Intrauterine device – copper-containing *Int J Derm 15:594–595, 1976*

Kit and BCR-ABL inhibitors – imatinib, nilotinib, dasatinib – facial edema morbilliform eruptions, pigmentary changes, lichenoid reactions, psoriasis, pityriasis rosea, pustular eruptions, DRESS, Stevens-Johnson syndrome, urticarial, neutrophilic dermatoses, photosensitivity, pseudolymphoma, porphyria cutanea tarda, small vessel vasculitis, panniculitis, perforating folliculitis, erythroderma *JAAD 72:203–218, 2015*

Latex – urticaria *Am J Contact Dermatitis 4:4–21, 1993; Contact Dermatitis 17:270–275, 1987; BJD 101:597–598, 1979;* anaphylaxis *Allergy 42:46–50, 1987;* cross-reactivity to bananas, lychee nuts, chestnuts, avocado *Clin Exp Allergy 26:416–423, 1996*

Mold spores

Platinum – refiners; contact urticaria

Postcoital urticaria – penicillin allergy, seminal fluid allergy *JAMA 254:531, 1985;* seminal vulvitis – widespread urticaria *Am J Obstet Gynecol 126:442–444, 1976*

Rhus – ingestion of *Rhus* as folk medicine remedy *BJD 142:937–942, 2000*

Simvastatin – urticarial vasculitis *Dermatitis 21:223–224, 2010*

Zinc fumes *Am J Industr Med 12:331–337, 1987*

INFECTIONS AND INFESTATIONS

Acripito itch – papulourticarial rash (*Hylesia* moths) *JAAD 13:743–747, 1985*

Adenovirus

AIDS (HIV) – acute infection *AD 127:1383–1391, 1991;* in children *JAAD 18:1089–1102, 1988*

Amblyomma americanum – Lone star tick

Amebiasis

Ancylostomiasis – papular or papulovesicular rash; feet; generalized urticaria; late changes resemble kwashiorkor *Dermatol Clin 7:275–290, 1989*

Arcanobacterium haemolyticum – annular urticarial lesions *JAAD 48:298–299, 2003; J Clin Inf Dis 21:177–181, 1995*

Ascariasis *JAAD 73:929–944 2015; The Clinical Management of Itching; Parthenon; p. 53, 2000*

Campylobacter jejuni Lancet i:954, 1984

Candidiasis – chronic urticaria *BJD 84:227–237, 1971*

Cat scratch disease *JAAD 41:833–836, 1999; JAAD 31:535–536, 1994*

Caterpillar dermatitis – urticarial papules surmounted by vesicles, urticaria, eyelid edema, bruising in children; conjunctivitis; *Megalopyge* caterpillars – burning pain, spreading erythema, edema, lymphangitis *JAMA 175:1155–1158, 1961;* woolly bear caterpillar (*Euproctis edwardsii*), brown tail moth (*Euproctis chrysorrhoea*), tea tussock moth (*Euproctis pseudoconspersa*) – urticarial wheals *Australas J Dermatol 38:193–195, 1997;* Spanish pine processionary caterpillar (*Thaumetopoea pityo-campa*) – urticaria, angioedema, anaphylaxis *JAAD 62:1–10, 2010; Cutis 80:110–112, 2007;* saddleback caterpillar (*Limacodidae*) (*Acharia stimulea*) – urticaria or vesicles; painful sting *JAAD 62:1–10, 2010*

Chikungunya fever – generalized urticaria *JAAD 75:1–16, 2016*

Cholecystitis, chronic *AD 115:638, 1979*

Coccidioidomycosis – urticarial toxic erythema *Dermatol Clin 7:227–239, 1989;* acute pulmonary coccidioidomycosis – urticarial lesions of acute exanthem *JAAD 55:929, 942, 2006; AD 142:744–746, 2006*

Coelenterate envenomation, delayed reaction *JAAD 22:599–601, 1990*

Coxsackie A9 and B

Cutaneous larva migrans – urticarial migratory lesions – personal observation

Chronic infection – cystitis, cholecystitis, diverticulitis, sinusitis, dental abscess

Cytomegalovirus Dermatology 200:189–195, 2000

Dengue fever – hyperpigmentation of the nose (chik sign); transient flushing, purpuric lesions, scleral injection, morbilliform exanthem with circular islands of sparing, aphthous ulcers, lichenoid papules, flagellated pigmentation, urticarial lesions, erythema multiforme-like *Ped Derm 36:737–739, 2019; Indian Dermatol Online J 8:336–342, 2017; Indian J DV Leprol 76:671–676, 2010*

Dental abscess *The Clinical Management of Itching; Parthenon; p. 105, 2000*

Dirofilaria Cutis 72:269–272, 2003

Dracunculosis – *Dracunculus medinensis* – initially fever, pruritus, urticaria, edema; painful popular lesions, red papulonodular lesions become vesiculobullous; cellulitis lesions *JAAD 73:929–944, 2015; Int J Zoonoses 12:147–149, 1985*

Echinococcosis – dog tapeworm; cystic echinococcosis of the liver with acute generalized exanthematous pustulosis and urticaria, subcutaneous nodules *JAAD 73:929–944, 2015; BJD 148:1245–1249, 2003*

Enterobiasis (*Enterobius vermicularis*) (pin worm) – anal and perineal pruritus with localized urticaria; *AD 84:1026–1029, 1961*

Enterovirus infection – personal observation

Epstein-Barr virus (infectious mononucleosis) – presenting with acute urticaria *Ann Allergy 27:182–187, 1969;* cold urticaria with cold agglutinins and leg ulcers *Acta DV 61:451–452, 1981*

Escherichia coli sepsis – rose spots

Fascioliasis (*Fasciola hepatica, F. gigantica*) – liver fluke; urticarial, jaundice, diarrhea, serpiginous tracts, subcutaneous nodules *JAAD 73:929–944, 2015*

Filariasis – may present with acute urticaria *Dermatol Clin 7:313–321, 1989*

Fire ant stings (*Solenopsis invicta*) – clusters of vesicles evolve into umbilicated pustules on red swollen base; crusting, heal with scars; urticaria *Ann Allergy Asthma Immunol 77:87–95, 1996; Allergy 50:535–544, 1995*

Fire corals – urticarial lesions followed by vesiculobullous rash, chronic granulomatous, and lichenoid lesions *JAAD 61:733–750, 2009; Contact Dermatitis 29:285–286, 1993; Int J Dermatol 30:271–273, 1991*

Gianotti-Crosti syndrome (papular acrodermatitis of childhood) – urticaria-like lesions – personal observation

Giardiasis *Am J Dis Child 137:761–763, 1983*

Gnathostomiasis – including urticarial migratory lesions; intermittent migratory swellings and nodules; subcutaneous hemorrhages along tracks of migration; abdominal pain, nausea and vomiting, diarrhea; South East Asia *JAAD 73:929–944, 2015; JAAD 73:929–944, 2015; JAAD 11:738–740, 1984; AD 120:508–510, 1984*

Helicobacter pylori – chronic urticaria *JAAD 34:685–686, 1996*

Hepatitis B *JAAD 8:539–548, 1983*

Hepatitis C *Cutis 61:90–92, 1998; AD 131:1185–1193, 1995*

Herpes simplex – urticaria-like appearance

Herpes zoster – urticaria-like appearance – personal observation

Infectious mononucleosis (*Epstein-Barr virus*) – urticarial exanthem; urticaria and cold urticaria

Influenza

Insect bites – *JAAD 62:541–555, 2010;* bee and wasp stings *NEJM 133:523–527, 1994;* yellow jacket sting; urticaria-like lesions *The Clinical Management of Itching; Parthenon; p. 60, 2000;* tropical rat mite (O. baconi) *Cutis 42:414–416, 1988*

Jellyfish sting – acquired cold urticaria *Contact Dermatitis 29:273, 1993*

Katayama fever (acute schistosomiasis) – red papular exanthem, fever, cough, urticarial eruption, fatigue, pulmonary nodules *NEJM 374:469, 2016*

Larva currens – personal observation

Lepidopterism – moths, butterflies, caterpillars *JAAD 62:1–28, 2010*

Loiasis – migratory angioedema (Calabar swellings) *Clin Inf Dis 17:691–694, 1993*

Lyme disease – secondary urticarial lesions of Lyme disease *NEJM 370:1724–1731, 2014;* generalized urticaria, urticarial vasculitis *JAAD 22:1114–1116, 1990*

Malaria – *Plasmodium vivax Postgrad Med J 65:266–267, 1989*

Melioidosis (*Burkholderia pseudomallei*), pulmonary *SE Asian J Trop Med Public Health 44:862–865, 2013; AD 99:80–81, 1969*

Meningococcemia – urticaria-like lesions *Clin Exp Rheumatol 20:553–554, 2002; Pediatrics 60:104–106, 1977*

Moon jellyfish stings (*Aurelia aurita*) – urticarial-like eruption *JAMADerm 151:454–456, 2015*

Nematodes – *Anisakis simplex, Ascaris* spp., *Dirofilaria, Enterobius vermicularis* (pinworm) *AD 84:1026, 1961 Gnathostoma* spp., *Loa loa, Mansonella streptocerca, Necator americanus, Onchocerca volvulus, Strongyloides stercoralis, Toxocara* spp., *Trichinella* spp., *Wuchereria bancrofti Allergy Asthma Proc 39:86–95, 2018*

Octopus bite – blue-ringed octopus *J Emerg Med 10:71–77, 1992*

Onchocerciasis, acute – urticaria-like papules *AD 133:381–386, 1997;* acute urticaria in Zaire

Parvovirus B19 infection *Clin Exp Dermatol 31:473–474, 2006*

Portuguese man o' war stings (*Physalis physalis*) *JAAD 61:733–750, 2009; The Clinical Management of Itching; Parthenon; p. 65, 2000; J Emerg Med 10:71–77, 1992*

Pseudomonas – swimming pool or hot tub folliculitis; macules, papules, pustules, urticarial lesions *JAMA 239:2362–2364, 1978; JAMA 235:2205–2206, 1976*

Q fever – *Coxiella burnetii;* urticarial lesions *JAAD 49:363–392, 2003*

Rat bite fever

Rheumatic fever – urticarial eruption; erythema marginatum *Ped Derm 16:288–291, 1999*

Rose spots – typhoid fever, *Escherichia coli* sepsis

Scabies *Cutis 33:277–279, 1984*

Scarlet fever – urticaria-like lesions

Schistosomiasis (*S. japonicum*) – Katayama fever – purpura, arthralgia, systemic symptoms; fever, diarrhea, edema, urticarial eruption, headache, arthralgias, abdominal pain, hypereosinophilia occurring 4–6 weeks after infection *JAAD 73:929–944, 2015; Dermatol Clin 7:291–300, 1989*

Seabather's eruption – *Cnidaria* larvae (*Linuche unguiculata* (thimble jellyfish)); *Edwardsiella lineata* (sea anemone)

Sparganosis – linear migratory erythema with or without pustules; subcutaneous sparganosis (infective larvae of pseudophyllidean tapeworm of genus *Spirometra*) – urticaria-like lesions *BJD 170:741–743, 2014*

Streptococcal pharyngitis; Group B

Strongyloides stercoralis – urticarial lesions, including array of zebra stripes *Cutis 81:409–412, 2008; Br Med J ii:572–574, 1979;* larva currens (linear urticaria) *JAAD 73:929–944 2015; AD 124:1826–1830, 1988; BJD 80:108–110, 1968*

Tarantula hairs *Am J Trop Med Hyg 22:130–133, 1973*

Tooth abscess

Toxocariasis (urticarial migratory lesions) (*T. canis, T. cati, T. leonensis*) visceral larva migrans *JAAD 75:19–30, 2016; JAAD 59:1031–1042, 2008; Dermatologica 144:129–143, 1972*

Toxoplasmosis – chronic urticaria *BJD 162:80–82,2010*

Trichinosis – periorbital edema, conjunctivitis; transient urticarial and morbilliform eruption, splinter hemorrhages *JAAD 73:929–944, 2015; Can J Public Health 88:52–56, 1997; Postgrad Med 97:137–139, 143–144, 1995; South Med J 81:1056–1058, 1988*

Trypanosomiasis, African; edema of the face, hands, feet with transient red macular, morbilliform, petechial or urticarial dermatitis; circinate, annular of the trunk

Tularemia *Clin Exp Dermatol 43:770–774, 2018*

Unilateral laterothoracic exanthem – personal observation

Viral infection

INFILTRATIVE DISORDERS

Intralymphatic histiocytosis – red patch overlying swollen knee; livedo reticularis, papules, nodules, urticaria, unilateral eyelid edema *AD 146:1037–1042, 2010*

Langerhans cell histiocytosis, urticating Langerhans cell histiocytosis (Hashimoto-Pritzker disease) *Ped Derm 18:41–44, 2001; JAAD 14:867–873, 1986*

Lichen myxedematosus (4th variant) (scleromyxedema) – urticaria-like lesions *JAAD 38:289–294, 1998; Int J Derm 26:91–95, 1987;* papular mucinosis *AD Syphilol 199:71–91, 1954*

Juvenile xanthogranuloma – Darier's sign *J Dermatol 10:283–285, 1983*

Mastocytosis – urticaria pigmentosa *JAAD 62:541–555, 2010; The Clinical Management of Itching; Parthenon; p. 107, 2000;* Darier's sign *Acta DV(Stockh) 42:433–439, 1962;* mastocytosis, systemic – Darier's sign; diffuse cutaneous mastocytosis – urticarial wheals *AD 146:557–562, 2010*

Scleromyxedema – urticarial papules *JAAD 38:289–294, 1998*

Urticaria-like follicular mucinosis *JAAD 62:541–555, 2010*

Xanthomas – diffuse normolipemic plane xanthomas – urticaria-like lesions *JAAD 35:829–832, 1996*

INFLAMMATORY DISEASES

CAPS (cryopyrin-associated periodic syndromes) – familial cold autoinflammatory syndrome, Muckle-Wells syndrome, neonatal-onset multisystem inflammatory disorder (NOMID) – non-pruritic urticarial-like papules, confluent geographic plaques; conjunctivitis, episcleritis, uveitis; sensorineural hearing loss, chronic meningitis; secondary amyloidosis; IL-1beta increased; mutations in *NLRP3* gene (*CIAS1*) (cold-induced autoinflammatory syndrome 1) or *NALP3* (nacht domain-, leucine-rich repeat-, and PYD-containing protein) *JAAD 68:834–853, 2013; Ped Derm 31:228–231, 2014*

Eosinophilic myositis/perimyositis *JAAD 37:385–391, 1997;* eosinophilic cellulitis-like lesions associated with eosinophilic myositis – urticaria-like lesions *AD 133:203–206, 1997*

Eosinophilic pustular folliculitis *Dermatology Times p.39, Aug 1997*

Erythema multiforme – urticaria-like lesions *The Clinical Management of Itching; Parthenon; p. 107, 2000*

Inflammatory bowel disease

Interstitial granulomatous dermatitis *JAAD 62:541–555, 2010*

Kikuchi's disease (histiocytic necrotizing lymphadenitis) – red papules of the face, back, arms; red plaques; erythema and acneiform lesions of the face; morbilliform, urticarial, and rubella-like exanthems; red or ulcerated pharynx; cervical adenopathy; associations with SLE, lymphoma, tuberculous adenitis, viral lymphadenitis, infectious mononucleosis, and drug eruptions *AD 142:641–646, 2006; BJD 146:167–168, 2002; BJD 144:885–889, 2001; Ped Derm 18:403–405, 2001; Am J Surg Pathol 14:872–876, 1990*

Neutrophilic eccrine hidradenitis – urticarial papules resembling insect bites *JAAD 52:963–966, 2005; JAAD 35:819–822, 1996*

Pruritic linear urticarial rash, fever, and systemic inflammatory disease of adolescents – urticaria, linear lesions, periorbital edema and erythema, and arthralgia *Ped Derm 21:580–588, 2004*

Relapsing polychondritis – papular and annular fixed urticarial eruption; associated with myelodysplasia *JAAD 65:1161–1166, 2011*

Urticaria multiforme – large polycyclic and annular wheals with dusky centers, acral and facial angioedema *Ped Derm 28:436–438, 2011;* fever, arcuate, annular, polycyclic lesions; ecchymotic center or central pallor; edema of the hands and feet; aged 4 months to 4 years *NEJM 375:470, 2016; Cutis 89:260:262–264, 2012; Pediatrics 119:e1177–1183, 2007*

Whipple's disease – urticarial lesions, macular and reticulated erythema; Addisonian hyperpigmentation; *Tropheryma whipplei JAAD 60:277–288, 2009*

METABOLIC DISEASES

Adrenergic urticaria – urticarial papules with pale halo (as opposed to cholinergic urticarial – urticarial papules with red halos) *JAAD 70:763–766, 2014; Acta DV 70:82–84, 1990; Lancet 2:1031–1033, 1985*

Celiac disease *Int J Dermatol 378:15–19, 1998*

Cholinergic dermatographism – red line with punctate wheals *BJD 115:371–177, 1986*

Cholinergic erythema *BJD 109:343–348, 1983*

Cholinergic urticaria *AD 123:462–467, 1987;* cholinergic urticarial with anaphylaxis *Cutis 95:241–243, 2015*

Cryoglobulinemia – urticaria *JAAD 48:311–340, 2003;* cold urticaria *JAAD 13:636–644, 1985*

Cystic fibrosis-associated episodic arthritis – pink macules, urticarial papules, arthritis, purpura of the legs, erythema nodosum, cutaneous vasculitis *JAMADerm 155:375–376, 2019; Respir Med 88:567–570, 1994; Am J Dis Child 143:1030–1032, 1989; Ann Rheum Dis 47:218–223, 1988; Arch Dis Child 59:377–379, 1984*

Diabetes – adverse drug reaction or relapse of underlying autoimmune urticaria *Indian J Med Res 149:423–425, 2019*

Hyperparathyroidism *Ann Allergy Asthma Immunol 117:724–725, 2016; Lancet 1:1476, 1984*

Hyperthyroidism *JAMA 254:2253–2254, 1985; J Allergy Clin Immunol 48:73–81, 1971;* Graves' disease *JAAD 48:641–659, 2003*

Hypothyroidism *Allergy 72:1440–1460, 2017*

Menstrual urticaria and anaphylaxis *Allergy 42:477–479, 1987*

Paroxysmal cold hemoglobinuria – cold urticaria *NEJM 297:538–542, 1977*

Porphyria – porphyria cutanea tarda presenting as solar urticaria *BJD 141:590–591, 1999;* erythropoietic protoporphyria – urticaria-like plaques; solar urticaria *Eur J Pediatr 159:719–725, 2000; J Inherit Metab Dis 20:258–269, 1997; BJD 131:751–766, 1994; Curr Probl Dermatol 20:123–134, 1991; Am J Med 60:8–22, 1976*

Pregnancy

Pruritic urticarial papules and plaques of pregnancy *JAAD 10:473–480, 1984; Clin Exp Dermatol 7:65–73, 1982; JAMA 241:1696–1699, 1979*

Renal disease *The Clinical Management of Itching; Parthenon; p. 37, 2000; Semin Dermatol 14:297–301, 1995*

NEOPLASTIC DISORDERS

Angioimmunoblastic lymphadenopathy (T-cell lymphoma) *Dermatol Online J July 15, 2019; JAAD 46:325–357, 2002*

Essential thrombocythemia *JAAD 24:59–63, 1991*

Ganglioneuroblastoma – urticaria to water, light, and cold *Clin Exp Dermatol 14:25–28, 1989*

Leukemia cutis – acute basophilic leukemia *Ann DV 114:169–173, 1987;* urticaria-like lesions *AD 121:1497–1502, 1990;* acute lymphoblastic leukemia with eosinophilia *JAAD 51:S79–83, 2004; Ped Derm 20:502–505, 2003;* acute lymphocytic leukemia in children *AD 126:1497–1502, 1990;* juvenile chronic myelogenous leukemia with figurate lesions *JAAD 9:423–427, 1983;* eosinophilic leukemia; chronic lymphocytic leukemia – urticaria in 3%

Dermatologica 96:350–356, 1948; acute lymphoblastic leukemia with Darier's sign *JAAD 34:375–378, 1996;* acute myeloblastic leukemia with Philadelphia chromosome – painful urticaria *Clin Lab Haematol 8:161–162, 1986*

Lymphoma, including Hodgkin's disease; non-Hodgkin's B-cell lymphoma *JAAD 62:557–570, 2010;* intravascular lymphoma – painful gray-brown, red, blue-livid patches, urticarial plaques, nodules, with telangiectasia and underlying induration; 40% of patients with intravascular lymphoma present with cutaneous lesions *Cutis 82:267–272, 2008; BJD 157:16–25, 2007;* angioimmunoblastic T-cell lymphoma (angioimmunoblastic lymphadenopathy with dysproteinemia) – morbilliform eruption; arthralgias, purpura, petechiae, urticaria, nodules *JAAD 65:855–862, 2011; NEJM 361:900–911, 2009; BJD 144:878–884, 2001; JAAD 36:290–295, 1997; JAAD 1:227–32, 1979*

Lymphomatoid granulomatosis – *Epstein-Barr-*related angiocentric T-cell-rich B-cell lymphoproliferative disorder; presents as urticarial dermatitis; papules and dermal nodules with or without ulceration, folliculitis-like lesions, maculopapules, indurated plaques, ulcers *BJD 157:426–429, 2007; JAAD 54:657–663, 2006*

Polycythemia vera *JAAD 62:557–570, 2010*

Smooth muscle hamartoma, congenital – myokymia (smooth muscle fasciculations) (pseudo-Darier's sign) *Ped Derm 24:678–681, 2007*

Waldenstrom's macroglobulinemia *JAAD 45:S202–206, 2001; AD 134:1127–1131, 1998; Dermatologica 181:41–43, 1990;* cryoglobulin-associated cold urticaria *JAAD 45:S202–206, 2001*

PARANEOPLASTIC DISEASES

Carcinoid syndrome *AD 144:691–692, 2008*

Internal malignancy (urticaria and myelodysplasia) – chronic lymphocytic leukemia, hairy cell leukemia, lymphoma, solid tumor *Cutis 61:147–148, 1998;* carcinoma of lung *Cutis 69:49–50, 2002*

Paraneoplastic vasculitis – leukocytoclastic vasculitis with urticarial lesions *J Rheumatol 18:721–727, 1991; Medicine 67:220–230, 1988*

PHOTODERMATITIS

Fixed solar urticaria *JAAD 60:695–697, 2009; Photodermatol Photoimmunol Photomed 17:39–41, 2001; JAAD 29:161–165, 1993; Arch Dermatol Res 281:545–546, 1990*

Solar urticaria *JAAD 65:336–340, 2011; JAAD 59:909–920, 2008; AD 144:765–769, 2008; Am J Contact Dermat 11:89–94, 2000; BJD 142:32–38, 2000; Int J Dermatol 38:411–418, 1999; AD 134:71–74, 1998; JAAD 21:237–240, 1989; AD 124:80–83, 1988;* in an infant *BJD 136:105–107, 1997*

PRIMARY CUTANEOUS DISEASES

Alopecia mucinosa (follicular mucinosis) – urticaria-like *Dermatologica 170:133–135, 1985; Ann DV 107:491–495, 1980*

Anetoderma of Jadassohn – initial stages may be urticarial *AD 120:1032–1039, 1984*

Chronic urticaria *JAAD 46:645–657, 2002;* idiopathic

Cutis laxa, acquired – after urticaria and angioedema *AD 103:661–669, 1971;* acquired cutis laxa *Ped Derm 2:282–288, 1985;* palmar urticaria in acral localized acquired cutis laxa *JAAD 21:33–40, 1989*

Delayed pressure urticaria, bullous form – urticarial and bullae *BJD 166:1151–1152, 2012*

Episodic angioedema with eosinophilia – swollen feet *BJD 159:738–740, 2008; NEJM 310:1621–1626, 2008*

Erythema annulare centrifugum – urticaria-like lesions

Erythrokeratoderma variabilis – urticaria-like lesions

Exercise-induced urticaria and/or anaphylaxis *JAAD 55:290–301, 2006; Sports Med 15:365–373, 1993; J Allergy Clin Immunol 68:432–437, 1981*

Familial annular erythema – annular urticarial plaques *Ped Derm 28: 56–58, 2011; BJD 78:60–68, 1966*
   vs. Erythema gyratum repens – desquamation and vesiculation
   vs. Annular erythema of infancy – arcuate and polycyclic plaques with central scale *Cutis 44:139–140, 1989*

Ichthyosis congenita type IV – erythrodermic infant with follicular hyperkeratosis and positive Darier's sign mimicking diffuse cutaneous mastocytosis *BJD 136:377–379, 1997*

Mid-dermal elastolysis – preceding urticaria *JAAD 51:165–185, 2004*

Non-episodic angioedema with eosinophilia – erythema, livedo reticularis, edema of the legs, urticaria *Cutis 93:33–37, 2014*

Pityriasis rosea – urticarial PR *JAMA 82:178–183, 1924*

Prurigo pigmentosa – red papules with vesiculation and crusting arranged in reticulated pattern or reticulate plaques in young women; heals with reticulated hyperpigmentation; urticarial red pruritic papules, papulovesicles, vesicles, and plaques with reticulated hyperpigmentation *JAMADerm 153:353–354, 2017; JAMADerm 151:796–797, 2015; J Eur Acad Dermatol Venereol 26:1149–1153, 2012; Ped Derm 24:277–279, 2007; JAAD 55:131–136, 2006; Am J Dermatopathol 25:117–129, 2003; Cutis 63:99–102, 1999; JAAD 34:509–11, 1996; AD 130:507–12, 1994; BJD 120:705–708, 1989; AD 125:1551–1554, 1989; JAAD 12:165–169, 1985; Jpn J Dermatol 81:78–91, 1971*

Urticarial dermatitis *JAAD 62:541–555, 2010*

PSYCHOCUTANEOUS DISORDERS

Factitial dermatitis – fixed urticaria *JAAD 1:391–407, 1979*

Psychological factors – stress *Cutis 43:340, 1989*

SYNDROMES

AHA syndrome (arthritis or arthralgia, hives, angioedema) *Rheumatol Int 7:277–279, 1987*

BASCULE – Bier anemic spots, cyanosis, with urticarial-like eruption *BJD 175:218–220, 2016*

Blau syndrome *JAAD 62:557–570, 2010*

CANDLE syndrome (chronic atypical neutrophilic dermatosis with lipodystrophy and elevated temperature) – annular erythematous edematous plaques of the face (periorbital erythema) and trunk which become purpuric and result in residual annular hyperpigmentation; urticarial papules; limitation of range of motion with plaques over interphalangeal joints; periorbital edema with violaceous swollen eyelids, edema of the lips (thick lips), lipoatrophy of the cheeks, nose, and arms, chondritis with progressive ear and saddle nose deformities, hypertrichosis of the lateral forehead, gynecomastia, wide-spaced nipples, nodular episcleritis and conjunctivitis, epididymitis, myositis, aseptic meningitis; short stature, anemia, abnormal liver functions, splenomegaly, protuberant abdomen; pleuritic chest pain; lymphadenopathy; arthralgia/oral ulcers *BJD 170:215–217, 2014; JAAD 68:834–853, 2013; Ped Derm 28:538–541, 2011; JAAD 62:487–495, 2010*

Chediak-Higashi syndrome

CINCA syndrome (chronic infantile neurologic cutaneous articular syndrome) NOMID – (neonatal-onset multisystem inflammatory disease) – sporadic; generalized evanescent urticarial macules and papules (also includes CINCA (chronic infantile neurological cutaneous and articular syndrome) – urticarial lesions at birth, chronic meningitis, arthralgias of the knees and ankles with deforming arthropathy with epiphyseal bone formation, deafness, hepatosplenomegaly, uveitis, vitreitis, papilledema, corneal stromal keratopathy; frontal bossing; angelic facies, mental retardation; sensorineural hearing loss, fever and rash more severe in the evening; mutation in NALP3 (CIAS 1) which encodes cryopyrin *AD 142:1591–1597, 2006; NEJM 355:581–592, 2006; JAAD 54:319–321, 2006; Ped Derm 22:222–226, 2005; AD 141:248–263, 2005; Arthritis Rheum 52:1283–1286, 2005; Eur J Pediatr 156:624–626, 1997;* chronic urticaria *AD 136:431–433, 2000; J Pediatr 99:79–83, 1981*

Chronic recurrent multifocal osteomyelitis and Majeed syndrome *JAAD 62:557–570, 2010*

Familial cold autoinflammatory syndrome (cold urticaria) – non-pruritic urticarial rash precipitated by cold; conjunctivitis, arthralgias of the knees and ankles and arthritis; fever and rash more severe in the evening; mutation in gene encoding NALP3 (cryopyrin); CIAS1 *BJD 178:335–349, 2018; Ped Derm 24:85–89, 2007; AD 142:1591–1597, 2006; JAAD 54:319–321, 2006; BJD 150:1029–1031, 2004; JAMA 114:1067–1068, 1940;* CAPS (cryopyrin-associated periodic syndromes) – familial cold autoinflammatory syndrome, Muckle-Wells syndrome, neonatal-onset multisystem inflammatory disorder (NOMID) – non-pruritic urticarial-like papules, confluent geographic plaques; conjunctivitis, episcleritis, uveitis; sensorineural hearing loss, chronic meningitis; secondary amyloidosis; IL-1beta increased; mutations in *NLRP3* gene (*CIAS1*) (cold-induced autoinflammatory syndrome 1) or *NALP3* (nacht domain-, leucine-rich repeat-, and PYD-containing protein) *JAAD 68:834–853, 2013*

Familial cold urticaria – autosomal dominant *Cutis 97:59–62, 2016; AD 129:343–346, 1993; J Allergy Clin Immunol 85:965–981, 1990; Semin Dermatol 6:292–301, 1987*

Systemic atypical

Cold-dependent dermatographism
   Cold erythema

Cold-induced cholinergic urticaria *J Allergy Clin Immunol 68:438–441, 1981*

Delayed cold urticaria *Proc Royal Soc Med 58:622–631, 1965*
   Immediate cold-contact urticaria *JAAD 13:636–644, 1985;* Localized cold-reflex urticaria *J Allergy Clin Immunol 85:52–54, 1990;* localized cold urticaria of the face – red facial plaques *Ped Derm 27:266–269, 2010; BJD 132:666–667, 1995; J Allergy Clin Immunol 88:682, 1991; J Allergy Clin Immunol 86:272–273, 1990*

Leukocytoclastic vasculitis

Infections – mononucleosis, syphilis

Cold agglutinins

Cold hemolysins

Cold fibrinogens
Cryoglobulins

Acquired cold urticaria – painful erythema *JAMA 180:639–642, 1962*

Familial Mediterranean fever – autosomal recessive; urticaria-like lesions *AD 134:929–931, 1998*

Gleich's syndrome (episodic angioedema with eosinophilia) – angioedema, urticaria, fever, periodic weight gain, eosinophilia, increased IgM *AD 141:633–638, 2005; JAAD 20:21–27, 1989; NEJM 310:1621–1626, 1984*

Hereditary angioneurotic edema – transitory prodromal non-pruritic urticarial eruption *JAAD 53:373–388, 2005*

Hypereosinophilic syndrome, idiopathic; red macules, red papules, plaques, and nodules, urticaria, angioedema *AD 142:1215–1218, 2006; Allergy 59:673–689, 2004; Am J Hematol 80:148–157, 2005; AD 132:535–541, 1996; Medicine 54:1–27, 1975;BJD 144:639, 2001; AD 132:583–585, 1996; Blood 83:2759–2779, 1994; AD 114:531–535, 1978;* urticaria and/or angioedema *Med Clin(Barc)106:304–306, 1996; AD 132:535–541, 1996; Sem Derm 14:122–128, 1995*

Hyper IgD syndrome – recurrent urticarial; transient and fixed pink plaques and nodules of the face and extremities; cephalic pustulosis; mevalonate kinase deficiency; periodic fever, red macules or papules, urticaria, annular erythema, red nodules, arthralgias, abdominal pain, lymphadenopathy; combinations of fever, arthritis, and rash, annular erythema, and pustules; mevalonate kinase gene *Ped Derm 35:482–485, 2018; AD 136:1487–1494, 2000; Ann DV 123:314–321, 1996; AD 130:59–65, 1994*

Hyper IgE syndrome (Job's syndrome) (Buckley's syndrome) – contact urticaria; dermatitis of the scalp, axillae, and groin; recurrent bacterial infections of the skin with cold abscesses, infections of nasal sinuses and respiratory tract *Curr Prob in Derm 10:41–92, 1998; Medicine 62:195–208, 1983*

Ichthyosis prematurity syndrome ("self-healing congenital verruciform hyperkeratosis") – autosomal recessive; red and white dermatographism; erythrodermic infant with caseous vernix-like desquamation; evolves into generalized xerosis and mild flexural hyperkeratosis and of lower back; cutaneous cobblestoning; keratosis pilaris-like changes; fine desquamation of the ankles; focal erythema, diffuse alopecia, fine scaling of the scalp, in utero polyhydramnios with premature birth, thick caseous desquamating skin (thick vernix caseosa-like covering) (hyperkeratotic scalp) neonatal asphyxia; later in childhood, dry skin with follicular keratosis; mutation in fatty acid transporter protein 4 (FATP4) *JAAD 66:606–616, 2012; JAAD 63:607–641, 2010; JAAD 59:S71–74, 2008*

IgG4-related disease – cutaneous plasmacytosis (papulonodules); pseudolymphoma; angiolymphoid hyperplasia with eosinophilia; Mikulicz's disease; psoriasiform dermatitis; morbilliform eruption; hypergammaglobulinemic purpura; urticarial vasculitis; ischemic digits; Raynaud's disease and digital gangrene *BJD 171:929,959– 967, 2014*

IPEX syndrome – X-linked; immune dysregulation, polyendocrinopathy (diabetes mellitus, thyroiditis), autoimmune enteropathy; mutation of *FOXP3* gene encodes DNA-binding protein that suppresses transcription of multiple genes involved in cytokine production and T-cell proliferation (Tregs); atopic-like or nummular dermatitis, urticaria, scaly psoriasiform plaques of the trunk and extremities, penile rash, alopecia universalis, trachyonychia, bullae; pemphigoid nodularis (bullae and prurigo nodularis) *BJD 160:645– 651, 2009; JAAD 55:143–148, 2006; AD 140:466–472, 2004; J Pediatr 100:731–737, 1982*

Kawasaki's disease – macular, morbilliform, urticarial, scarlatiniform, erythema multiforme-like, pustular, erythema marginatum-like exanthems *Ped Derm 36:274–282, 2019; JAAD 69:501–510, 2013; JAAD 39:383–398, 1998*

Loeffler's syndrome (acute larval migration, *Ascaris* hookworm, *Strongyloides*) *NEJM 380:2052–2060, 2019*

Muckle-Wells syndrome – autosomal dominant; macular erythema (evanescent red macules), urticaria (cold air urticaria), deafness, extremity pain, arthralgias of the knees and ankles with arthritis; nephropathy, AA amyloidosis with neuropathy; fever and rash more severe in the evening; mutation in gene encoding NALP3 (cryopyrin) *BJD 178:335–349, 2018; SkinMed 11:80–83, 2013; AD 142:1591– 1597, 2006; BJD 151:99–104, 2004; Arthritis Rheum 50:607, 2004; Nature Genet 29:301, 2001; JAAD 39:290–291, 1998; QJMed 31:235–248, 1962;* CAPS (cryopyrin-associated periodic syndromes) – familial cold autoinflammatory syndrome, Muckle-Wells syndrome, neonatal-onset multisystem inflammatory disorder (NOMID) – non-pruritic urticarial-like papules, confluent geographic plaques; conjunctivitis, episcleritis, uveitis; sensorineural hearing loss, chronic meningitis; secondary amyloidosis; IL-1beta increased; mutations in *NLRP3* gene (*CIAS1*) (cold-induced autoinflammatory syndrome 1) or *NALP3* (nacht domain-, leucine-rich repeat-, and PYD-containing protein) *JAAD 68:834–853, 2013*

Neutrophilic urticarial dermatosis – urticaria with systemic inflammation, urticaria, night sweats, fever, polyarticular arthritis; increased IL-1; treated with anakinra polymorphonuclear leukocytes, joint inflammation; increased white blood cell count, increased C-reactive protein *JAMADerm 149:1244–1245, 2013; Medicine(Baltimore)88:23–31, 2009;*

JAAD 62:557–570, 2010; Acta DV(Stockh)68:129–133, 1988

NOD 2 mutations (nucleotide-binding oligomerization domain 2 – dermatitis, weight loss with gastrointestinal symptoms, episodic self–limiting fever, polyarthritis, polyarthralgia, red plaques of the face and forehead, urticarial plaques of the legs, patchy erythema of chest, pink macules of the arms and back *JAAD 68:624–631, 2013*

NOMID – neonatal-onset multisystem inflammatory disease – neonatal urticarial in 2/3 patients; generalized evanescent urticarial macules and papules; cerebral atrophy, aseptic meningitis, high-frequency hearing loss; arthropathy with osseous overgrowth; gain-of-function mutation in *NLRP3 AD 144:392–402, 2008; Ped Derm 22:222–226, 2005;* CAPS (cryopyrin-associated periodic syndromes) – familial cold autoinflammatory syndrome, Muckle-Wells syndrome, neonatal-onset multisystem inflammatory disorder (NOMID) – non-pruritic urticarial-like papules, confluent geographic plaques; conjunctivitis, episcleritis, uveitis; sensorineural hearing loss, chronic meningitis; secondary amyloidosis; IL-1beta increased; mutations in *NLRP3* gene (*CIAS1*) (cold-induced autoinflammatory syndrome 1) or *NALP3* (nacht domain-, leucine-rich repeat-, and PYD-containing protein) *JAAD 68:834–853, 2013*

PAPA (pyogenic arthritis, pyoderma gangrenosum-acne) syndrome *JAAD 62:557–570, 2010*

Periodic diseases with cyclic edema/periodic edema – may include hereditary angioedema, familial Mediterranean fever, capillary leak syndrome and autoimmune progesterone urticaria *Int J Dermatol 18:824–827, 1979*

Polyarteritis nodosa – systemic polyarteritis nodosa and microscopic polyarteritis – urticarial vasculitis *BJD 159:615–620, 2008*

Relapsing polychondritis *Clin Exp Rheumatol 20:89–91, 2002*

Schnitzler's syndrome – non-pruritic chronic urticaria with neutrophilic infiltrate on skin biopsy, intermittent fever, and IgM monoclonal gammopathy (macroglobulinemia); IgM kappa or IgM lambda, occasionally IgG kappa or lambda; high ESR, leukocytosis, arthralgia, arthritis, with disabling bone pain (osteosclerotic) of distal femur and proximal tibia, palpable lymphadenopathy, hepatosplenomegaly; marginal zone B-cell lymphoma *Rheumatology 58(suppl 6) vi31–43, 2019; Curr Rheum Rep 19:46, 2017; JAAD 68:834–853, 2013; JAAD 67:1289–1295, 2012; AD 147:1097–1102, 2011; Medicine(Balt)88:23–31, 2009; JAAD 61:1070–1075, 2009; Int J Dermatol 48:1190–1194, 2009; JAAD 57:361–364, 2007; AD 143:1046–1050, 2007; JAAD 56:S120–122, 2007; Semin Arthritis*

Rheum 37:137–148, 2007; J Eur Acad Dermatol Venereol 16:267–270, 2007; Medicine(Baltimore) 80:37–44, 2001; BJD 142:954–959, 2000; JAAD 30:316–318, 1994; AD 130:1193–1198, 1994; JAAD 20:855–857, 1989; JAAD 20:206–211, 1989; BJD Angers28(Abstract 46), 1922

> Differential diagnosis of Schnitzler's syndrome includes:
> > Acquired C1 inhibitor deficiency
> > Hyper IgD syndrome
> > Hypocomplementemic urticarial vasculitis
> > Still's disease

Sweet's syndrome *Ann Allergy Asthma Immunol 100:181–188, 2008*

Systemic capillary leak syndrome (Clarkson syndrome) *Ann Allergy Asthma Immunol 118:631–632, 2017*

Tumor necrosis factor (TNF) receptor 1-associated periodic fever syndromes (TRAPS) (same as familial hibernian fever, autosomal dominant periodic fever with amyloidosis, and benign autosomal dominant familial periodic fever) – Still's disease-like eruption with erythematous patches, tender red plaques, fever, annular, generalized serpiginous, polycyclic, reticulated, and migratory patches and plaques (migrating from proximal to distal), urticaria-like lesions, centrifugal migratory red patch overlying myalgia, red cheeks, morbilliform exanthems; lesions resolving with ecchymoses, conjunctivitis, periorbital edema, myalgia, arthralgia, abdominal pain, headache; Irish and Scottish predominance; mutation in tumor necrosis factor receptor superfamily 1A (*TNFRSF1A* gene) – gene encoding 55kDa TNF receptor *BJD 178:335–349, 2018; BJD 161:968–970, 2009; Medicine 81:349–368, 2002; Netherlands Journal of Medicine 59:118–125, 2001; AD 136:1487–1494, 2000; Mayo Clin Proc 62:1095–1100, 1987*

Wells' syndrome (eosinophilic cellulitis) – red plaques resembling urticaria or cellulitis *AD 142:1157–1161, 2006; JAAD 18:105–114, 1988; JAAD 14:32–38, 1986; Trans S.Johns Hosp Dermatol Soc 51:46–56, 1971*

TOXINS

Eosinophilia myalgia syndrome (l-tryptophan related) – morphea, urticaria, papular lesions; arthralgia *BJD 127:138–146, 1992; Int J Dermatol 31:223–228, 1992; Mayo Clin Proc 66:457–463, 1991; Ann Int Med 112:758–762, 1990*

Mustard gas exposure *AD 128:775–780, 1992; JAAD 32:765–766, 1995, JAAD 39:187–190, 1998*

Scombroid fish poisoning – urticaria-like lesions *Br Med J 281:71–72, 1980*

Toxic oil syndrome *JAAD 18:313–324, 1988*

TRAUMA

Acquired cold-contact urticaria – painful erythema *JAMA 180:639–642, 1962*

Chemical burn – inducing bullous pemphigoid *JAAD 38:337–340, 1998*

Heat urticaria – urticarial, angioedema, weakness, wheezing, headache, flushing, nausea and vomiting, diarrhea, tachycardia, syncope *BJD 175:473–476, 2016; Management of Itching; Parthenon; p. 103, 2000;* immediate heat urticaria *JAMA 83:3–8, 1924;* localized heat urticaria *BJD 147:994–997, 2002; BJD 90:289–292, 1974;* familial localized heat urticaria *Acta DV 51:279–283, 1971*

Pressure urticaria, including delayed pressure urticaria *JAAD 29:954–958, 1993*

Radiation dermatitis – urticaria *JAAD 54:28–46, 2006*

Red dermatographism – repeated rubbing produces punctate wheals *BJD 104:285–288, 1981*

Vibratory angioedema – familial or acquired *J Allergy Clin Immunol 50:175–182, 1972; BJD 120:93–99, 1989; Am J Med Genet 9:307–315, 1981*

Vibration urticaria *The Clinical Management of Itching; Parthenon; p. 104, 2000*

VASCULAR

Acute hemorrhagic edema of infancy – purpura in cockade pattern of the face, cheeks, eyelids, and ears; may form reticulate pattern; edema of the penis and scrotum *JAAD 23:347–350, 1990;* necrotic lesions of the ears, urticarial lesions; oral petechiae *JAAD 23:347–350, 1990; Ann Pediatr 22:599–606, 1975;* edema of limbs and face *Cutis 68:127–129, 2001*

Allergic granulomatous vasculitis with eosinophilia *JAAD 47:209–216, 2002; J Dermatol 22:46–51, 1995; JID 17:349–359, 1951*

Cutaneous necrotizing eosinophilic vasculitis – urticaria, angioedema *AD 130:1159–1166, 1994*

Degos disease – urticaria-like lesions *Ann DV 79:410–417, 1954*

Granulomatosis with polyangiitis

Henoch-Schonlein purpura – 30% of patients with urticarial lesions admixed with purpura *BJD 82:211–215, 1970*

Hypocomplementemic urticarial vasculitis *Int J Dermatol 57:1363–1364, 2018*

Leukocytoclastic vasculitis – urticaria-like lesions *Sem Arthr Rheum 46:367–371, 2016*

Polyarteritis nodosa *Ann Int Med 89:66–676, 1978*

Recurrent cutaneous eosinophilic vasculitis – urticarial plaques *BJD 149:901–902, 2003*

Urticarial vasculitis, including urticarial vasculitis associated with hypocomplementemia, mixed cryoglobulins, hepatitis B or C infection, IgA multiple myeloma, infectious mononucleosis, monoclonal IgM gammopathy (Schnitzler's syndrome), fluoxetine ingestion, cimetidine, diltiazem, cold, and solar urticaria, metastatic testicular teratoma, serum sickness, Sjogren's syndrome, systemic lupus erythematous *BJD 160:470–472, 2009; BJD 157:392–393, 2007; Clin Rev Allergy Immunol 23:201–216, 2002; JAAD 38:899–905, 1998; Medicine 74:24–41, 1995; JAAD 26:441–448, 1992;* hypocomplementemic vasculitis in childhood *Ped Derm 26:445–447, 2009;* monoclonal gammopathy of uncertain significance *JAAD 62:557–570, 2010*

UVEITIS, CUTANEOUS MANIFESTATIONS

AUTOIMMUNE DISEASES

Autoimmune uveitis associated with vitiligo, alopecia areata

Adult-onset Still's disease *BMC Ophthalmol 16:196, 2016*

Systemic lupus erythematosus

DRUGS

DRESS syndrome – carbamazepine *J Ophthalmol Vis Res 14:382–388, 2019*

Ipilimumab – uveitis, iridocyclitis *JAAD 71:217–227, 2014*

INFECTIONS AND INFESTATIONS

Actinomycosis – keratitis, conjunctivitis, anterior uveitis *Eye and Skin Disease, pp. 567–570, Lippincott, 1996*

Bartonella henselae Case Rep Ped 2013:726826

Cat scratch disease *Int Ophthalmol 30:553–558, 2010*

Chikungunya fever *Inf Dis Clin NA 33:1003–1025, 2019; Oculo Immunol Inflamm 26:677–679, 2018*

Herpes simplex virus – follicular conjunctivitis, episcleritis, keratitis, dendritic ulcer, anterior uveitis, central retinal vein occlusion, eczema herpeticum, periocular zosteriform eruption *NEJM 370:159–166, 2014; J Virol 75:5069, 5075, 2001; Medicine 78:395–409, 1999; Arch Ophthalmol 107:1155–1159, 1989; Nephron 50:368–370, 1988; Am J Med Sci 277:39–47, 1979*

Herpes zoster *Ped Int 61:1216–1220, 2019*

Infectious mononucleosis (*Epstein-Barr virus*) – conjunctivitis, keratitis, uveitis, choroiditis, retinitis, papillitis *Clin Inf Dis 31:184–188, 2000*

Leishmaniasis – Leishmania major uveitis *Clin Inf Dis 34:1279–1280, 2002;* post kala-azar dermal leishmaniasis – conjunctivitis *BJD 157:1032–1036, 2007*

Leprosy – lepromatous leprosy with infiltration of corneal nerves leading to anesthesia, infection, blindness *Chin Med J(Engl) 116:682–684, 2003;* erythema nodosum leprosum with uveitis, edema, and hyperemia *AD 138:1607–1612, 2002*

Leptospirosis *Travel Med Infect Dis 14:143–147, 2016*

Lyme disease *J Fr Ophthalmol 35:17–22, 2012*

Rickettsia conorii skin rash, fever, erythromelalgia, cholestatic hepatitis, and uveitis *Ticks Tick Borne Dis 7:338–341, 2016*

Syphilis, secondary *Oculo Immunol Inflamm 26:171–177, 2018; Ann Dermatol 21:399–401, 2009*

Varicella *BMJ Case Rep Sept 17, 2010*

Zika virus Oculo Immunol Inflamm 26:654–659, 2018

INFILTRATIVE DISORDERS

Cutaneous sinus histiocytosis (Rosai-Dorfman disease) – chronic uveitis *Oculo Immunol Inflamm 14:305–307, 2006; Practical Dermatology August 2014;pp.56,60; Ped Derm 17:377–380, 2000*

Juvenile xanthogranuloma – hemorrhage into anterior chamber, uveitis, iritis; anterior uveitis and glaucoma *Ped Derm 26:232–234, 2009*

INFLAMMATORY DISORDERS

Ankylosing spondylitis – associated findings include psoriasis, anterior uveitis, inflammatory bowel disease, lung abnormalities, heart conduction defects, aortic insufficiency, renal abnormalities, osteoporosis, vertebral fractures *Euro J Intern Med 2011:1–7; Int J Rheumatol 2011:1–10*

Crohn's disease – uveitis, conjunctivitis *Arch Int Med 148:297–302, 1988*

Familial histiocytic dermoarthritis – uveitis, arthritis

Juvenile idiopathic arthritis *Am J Ophthalmol 148:696–703, 2009*

Juvenile rheumatoid arthritis *Korean J Ped 53:921–930, 2010*

Rosai-Dorfman disease – clustered erythematous papules of the thigh; associated with uveitis *Practical Dermatol August 2014, pp.56,60*

Sarcoid – conjunctivitis, iridocyclitis, uveitis

NEOPLASTIC DISORDERS

Lymphoma – cutaneous T-cell lymphoma – keratitis, uveitis *Arch Ophthalmol 99:272–274, 1981;* peripheral T-cell lymphoma – tubulointerstitial nephritis, uveitis *BMC Nephrol 19:3–12, 2018*

PARANEOPLASTIC DISORDERS

Necrobiotic xanthogranuloma with paraproteinemia –conjunctivitis, keratitis, uveitis, iritis *AD 128:94–100, 1992*

PRIMARY CUTANEOUS DISEASES

Hydroa vacciniforme *BMJ Case Rep Apr 13, 2011*

Psoriasis *JAMADerm 151:1200–1205, 2015*

SYNDROMES

Behcet's disease *Joint Bone Spine 73:567–569, 2006*

Blau or Jabs syndrome (familial juvenile systemic granulomatosis) – autosomal dominant; translucent skin-colored papules (noncaseating granulomas) of the trunk and extremities; may resolve with pitted scars with follicular atrophoderma; with uveitis, synovitis, arthritis; polyarteritis, multiple synovial cysts; red papular rash in early childhood; camptodactyly (flexion contractures of PIP joints) mutations in NOD2 (nucleotide-binding oligomerization domain 2) (caspase recruitment domain family, member 15; *CARD* 15) *AD 143:386–391, 2007; Clin Exp Dermatol 21:445–448, 1996*

CAPS (cryopyrin-associated periodic syndromes) – familial cold autoinflammatory syndrome, Muckle-Wells syndrome, neonatal-onset multisystem inflammatory disorder (NOMID) – non-pruritic urticarial-like papules, confluent geographic plaques; conjunctivitis, episcleritis, uveitis; sensorineural hearing loss, chronic meningitis; secondary amyloidosis; IL-1beta increased; mutations in *NLRP3* gene (*CIAS1*) (cold-induced autoinflammatory syndrome 1) or *NALP3* (nacht domain-, leucine-rich repeat-, and PYD-containing protein) *JAAD 68:834–853, 2013*

Granulomatous synovitis, uveitis, and cranial neuropathies – JABS syndrome *J Pediatr 117:403–408, 1990*

Incontinentia pigmenti – iritis, uveitis *JAAD 47:169–187, 2002; Curr Prob in Derm VII:143–198, 1995; AD 112:535–542, 1976*

Kawasaki's disease *Am J Ophthalmol 129:101–192, 2000*

NOMID – (neonatal-onset multisystem inflammatory disease) – sporadic; generalized evanescent urticarial macules and papules (also includes CINCA (chronic infantile neurological cutaneous and articular syndrome) – urticarial lesions, chronic meningitis, arthralgias of the knees and ankles with deforming arthropathy with epiphyseal bone formation, deafness, hepatosplenomegaly, uveitis, vitreitis, papilledema, corneal stromal keratopathy; mental retardation; fever and rash more severe in the evening; mutation in NALP3 (CIAS 1) which encodes cryopyrin *AD 142:1591–1597, 2006; NEJM 355:581–592, 2006; JAAD 54:319–321, 2006; Ped Derm 22:222–*

226, 2005; AD 141:248–263, 2005; Arthritis Rheum 52:1283–1286, 2005

Reactive arthritis syndrome – conjunctivitis, uveitis, keratitis – sterile mucopurulent discharge *Ophthalmology 93:350–356, 1986; Ann Rheum Dis 38(Suppl.):8–11, 1979*

Sweet's syndrome *Neuroopthalmology 41:202–206, 2017*

Vogt-Koyanagi-Harada syndrome – granulomatous panuveitis *Eye and Skin Disease, pp.303–309, Lippincott, 1996*

TRAUMA

Cobalt – light blue; uveitis *Lancet ii:27–28, 1969*

VASCULAR DISORDERS

Granulomatosis with polyangiitis – keratoconjunctivitis, granulomatous scleritis or uveitis *NEJM 352:392, 2005; JAAD 49:335–337, 2003; Mayo Clin Proc 60:227–232, 1985;* scleritis

Henoch-Schonlein purpura *Rheumatol Int 30:1377–1379, 2010*

Urticarial vasculitis – conjunctivitis, uveitis, episcleritis with urticarial vasculitis *JAAD 49:S283–285, 2003; JAAD 38:899–905, 1998; JAAD 26:441–448, 1992; Arthr Rheum 32: 1119–1127, 1989;* hypocomplementemic vasculitis – iritis, uveitis, episcleritis *JAAD 48:311–340, 2003*

UVULA, ENLARGED

AUTOIMMUNE DISEASES AND DISEASES OF IMMUNE DYSFUNCTION

Angioedema (Quincke's disease) *NEJM 349:867, 2003; Auris Nasus Larynx 27:261–264, 2000*

DiGeorge syndrome – bifid uvula

Hypogammaglobulinemia *Ann Allergy Asthma Immunol 93:417–424, 2004*

CONGENITAL ANOMALIES

Bifid uvula – normal variant

DRUGS

Angiotensin-converting enzyme inhibitors

EXOGENOUS AGENTS

Smoking cannabis *Int Emerg Nurs 16:207–216, 2008; Emerg Med 14:106–108, 2002*

Smoking cocaine *Int Emerg Nurs 16:207–216, 2008; Emerg Med 14:106–108, 2002*

Ecballium elaterium – wild or squirting cucumber

INFECTIONS AND INFESTATIONS

Candida

Diphtheria *Scand J Inf Dis 28:37–40, 1996*

Epiglottitis with uvulitis *Auris Nasus Larynx 27:261–264, 2000*

Hemophilus influenzae uvulitis

Histoplasmosis

Infectious mononucleosis

Infectious uvulitis *Auris Nasus Larynx 27:261–264, 2000*

Leishmaniasis

Leprosy

Mycobacterium tuberculosis J Oral Pathol Med 35:123–125, 2006; lupus vulgaris

North American blastomycosis

Paracoccidioidomycosis *JAAD 53:931–951, 2005*

Roseola infantum – red papules on uvula and soft palate – Nagayama's spots *Pediatrics 93:104–108, 1994*

Group A streptococcal uvulitis

Syphilis

Warts – intraoral warts

INFILTRATIVE DISEASES

Amyloidosis

Langerhans cell histiocytosis

INFLAMMATORY DISEASES

Crohn's disease

Sarcoid *J Laryngol Otrol 118:385–387, 2004*

NEOPLASTIC DISEASE

Kaposi's sarcoma – personal observation

Leukemic infiltrates – acute myelomonocytic leukemia (AMML)

Lymphoma – cutaneous T-cell lymphoma – personal observation; NK/T-cell lymphoma nasal type *Am J Otolaryngol 36:80–83, 2015*

Melanoma *Hautarzt 56:156–159, 2005*

Papilloma *Auris Nasus Larynx 27:261–264, 2000*

Salivary gland carcinoma

Squamous cell carcinoma *Otolaryngol Head Neck Surg 146:81–87, 2012; Auris Nasus Larynx 27:261–264, 2000*

PRIMARY CUTANEOUS DISEASES

Simple elongation of the uvula *Auris Nasus Larynx 27:261–264, 2000*

SYNDROMES

Beare-Stevenson cutis gyrata syndrome – bifid uvula *Ped Derm 20:358–360, 2003*

Cowden's disease

Hereditary angioneurotic edema *JAAD 45:968–969, 2001*

Lipoid proteinosis (Urbach-Wiethe disease) *Int J Derm 39:203–204, 2000; JAAD 27:293–297, 1992*

Loeys-Dietz syndrome – joint hypermobility, thin skin with prominent veins, Marfanoid body habitus, triangular delicate face, hypertelorism, bifid uvula or cleft palate, arterial dissection and rupture, prominent eyes, blue sclerae, aortic aneurysms, generalized arterial tortuosity; type I and II TGF-beta receptor *JAAD 55:S41–45, 2006; Nature Genet 37:275–281, 2005*

Multiple endocrine neoplasia syndrome type II

MMMM syndrome – enlarged uvula *Turk J Pediatr 44:274–277, 2002*

Neurofibromatosis

Phosphoglucomutase 1 deficiency – autosomal recessive; disorder of glycosylation with impaired glycoprotein production; liver dysfunction, bifid uvula, malignant hyperthermia, hypogonadotropic hypogonadism, growth retardation, hypoglycemia, myopathy, dilated cardiomyopathy, cardiac arrest *NEJM 370:533–542, 2014*

Pierre-Robin syndrome – personal observation

Stickler syndrome – bifid uvula

Teebi hypertelorism syndrome – enlarged uvula *Am J Med Genetics 117:A181–183, 2003*

Werner's syndrome

TRAUMA

Self-inflicted (to induce vomiting)

Solid object in the mouth

Surgical trauma (adenoidectomy, tonsillectomy) – intubation, suction

VASCULAR

Hemangioma

Lymphangioma

Sturge-Webver syndrome

VALVULAR HEART DISEASE, CUTANEOUS MANIFESTATIONS

AUTOIMMUNE DISEASES

Antiphospholipid antibody syndrome – vegetations and/or thickening valve leaflets; valvular abnormalities – mitral>tricuspid

Dermatomyositis *J Cardiovasc Med(Hagerstown)11:906–911, 2010*

Lupus erythematosus, systemic – Libman-Sacks endocarditis, pericarditis, conduction defects, valvular damage, aortic insufficiency and mitral regurgitation>stenosis, heart failure *Am J Med Case Rep 6:180–183, 2018*

Scleroderma *Cleve Clin J Med 86:685–695, 2019*

Relapsing polychondritis – aortic regurgitation or aneurysm

INFECTIONS AND INFESTATIONS

Acute or subacute bacterial endocarditis – Osler's nodes, splinter hemorrhages, conjunctival petechiae

Rheumatic fever – erythema marginatum, subcutaneous nodules; pancarditis acutely, mitral and/or aortic valve disease late *NEJM 375:2480, 2016; JAAD 8:724–728, 1983*

Syphilis – aortic valvular insufficiency, aortic aneurysm, aortic root dilatation, coronary ostial stenosis

METABOLIC DISEASES

Fabry's disease – hypertrophic cardiomyopathy, valvular abnormalities, conduction defects, hypertension, progressive atherosclerotic disease of the coronary and cerebral arteries

Biophys Rev 10:1107–1119, 2018

Ochronosis (alkaptonuria) – aortic stenosis, arthropathy, blue-black pigmentation of the skin and sclerae, ochronotic bladder stones *Heart Lung Circ 22:870–872, 2013*

Porphyria – congenital erythropoietic porphyria with ventricular septal defect *Ped Derm 35:833–835, 2018; Heart Lung Cir 22:870–872, 2013*

NEOPLASTIC DISORDERS

Marantic endocarditis

Metastatic melanoma – pulmonary stenosis, tricuspid stenosis *J Card Surg 28:124–128, 2013*

Neuroendocrine tumor, metastatic – tricuspid regurgitation; abdominal pain, facial flushing, intermittent diarrhea *NEJM 371:260, 2014*

PRIMARY CUTANEOUS DISEASES

Cutis laxa – aortic dilatation and rupture, pulmonic stenosis with right heart failure *Circulation 124:100–102, 2011*

Pectus excavatum – mitral valve prolapse, aortic root enlargement *J Laparoendosc Adv Surg Tech A 22:508–513, 2012*

Psoriasis – increased risk of aortic stenosis *Eur Heart J 36:2177–2183, 2015*

SYNDROMES

Behcet's disease – aortic valve disease *Interact Cardiovasc Thoracic Surg 24:342–347, 2017;* aortic regurgitation *Anatol J Cardiol 16:529–533, 2016; J Card Surg 27:39–44, 2012; Ann Thoracic Surg 68:2136–2140, 1999*

Blue rubber bleb nevus syndrome *Indian Ped 53:525–527, 2016*

Borrone dermatocardioskeletal syndrome – autosomal recessive or X-linked; gingival hypertrophy, coarse facies, late eruption of teeth, loss of teeth, thick skin, acne conglobata, osteolysis, large joint flexion contractures, short stature, brachydactyly, camptodactyly, mitral valve prolapse, congestive heart failure *Eur J Hum Genet 22:741–747, 2014; Ped Derm 18:534–536, 2001*

Carcinoid syndrome – tricuspid valve regurgitation *Cardiol Rev 20:164–176, 2012; J Cardiovasc Ultrasound 19:45–49, 2011; Acta Ceidid 65:261–264, 2010*

Cardiofaciocutaneous syndrome – ulerythema ophryogenes, generalized keratosis pilaris, palmoplantar hyperkeratosis, melanocytic nevi, lack of CALM, pulmonic stenosis, hypertrophic cardiomyopathy, atrial septal defect, patent ductus arteriosus, developmental delay, short stature, failure to thrive

Costello syndrome – lax skin of hands and feet, papillomas, deep palmoplantar creases, sparse curly hair, pulmonic stenosis, hypertrophic cardiomyopathy, arrhythmia, supraventricular tachycardia, atrial tachycardia, chaotic atrial rhythm, ectopic atrial tachycardia; hypotonia, short stature, developmental delay, failure to thrive *JAAD 68:156–166, 2013*

Down's syndrome – bicuspid aortic valve, atrioventricular and ventricular septal defects

Ehlers-Danlos syndrome – joint hypermobility and laxity; hyperextensible skin; tenascin-X deficiency *BJD 163:1340–1345, 2010;* type VI – blue sclerae, scleral fragility, joint hypermobility, skin hyperextensibility, easy bruising, atrophic scarring, marfanoid habitus, scoliosis, neonatal hypotonia, arterial dissection; *Eur Heart J Case Rep June 1, 2019; Cutis 82:242–248, 2008;* mitral valve prolapse *Am J Med Genet A 176:1838–1844, 2018*

Familial hypercholesterolemia and supravalvular aortic stenosis *Ann Thorac Surg 105:e171–174, 2018; Ped Cardiol 27:282–285, 2006*

H syndrome – atrial septal defect, ventricular septal defect, mitral valve prolapse *JAAD 59:79–85, 2008*

Hereditary sclerosing poikiloderma – familial calcific aortic and mitral stenosis *Cardiovascular Pathol 25:195–199, 2016*

Kawasaki's disease – ruptured chordae tendineae *Cardiol Young 29:30–35, 2019; Ped Derm 35:743–747, 2018*

LEOPARD syndrome – lentigines, EKG abnormalities, ocular hypertelorism, pulmonic stenosis, abnormalities of genitalia, growth retardation, deafness; *PTPN11* mutation *Dermatol Online J Oct 16, 2015*

Marfan's syndrome – dilatation and dissection of ascending aorta, aortic regurgitation, mitral valve prolapse and regurgitation *Hum Mut 37:524–531, 2016*

Moynahan's syndrome – lentigines, congenital mitral stenosis, dwarfism, mental retardation, genital hypoplasia

Mucopolysaccharidosis I, Hurler's – thickening and stiffness of valve leaflets, mitral>aortic regurgitation

Neurofibromatosis type I – hypertension, pulmonic stenosis, aortic valve stenosis or coarctation, pulmonary valve dysplasia, mitral valve anomalies, septal defects

Noonan syndrome – cutis verticis gyrata, congenital lymphedema, pulmonary stenosis, hypertrophic cardiomyopathy, atrial septal defect, ventricular septal defect, tetralogy of Fallot

Osteogenesis imperfecta type 1 – mitral valve prolapse *Am J Med Genet A 164A:386–391, 2014*

Pseudoxanthoma elasticum – mitral valve prolapse, restrictive cardiomyopathy *NEJM 307:228–231, 1982; Chest 78:113–115, 1980*

Reactive arthritis syndrome – erosions with marginal erythema; circinate erosions *JAAD 59:113–121, 2008; NEJM 309:1606–1615, 1983; Semin Arthritis Rheum 3:253–286, 1974*

    Keratoderma blenorrhagicum; soles, pretibial areas, dorsal toes, feet, fingers, hands, nails, scalp; may be associated with HIV disease *Ann Int Med 106:19–26, 1987; Semin Arthritis Rheum 3:253–286, 1974;* following gastroenteritis due to *Salmonella enteritidis, Shigella, Yersinia, Campylobacter* species, and *Clostridium difficile* or following non-gonococcal arthritis *Clin Inf Dis 33:1010–1014, 2001*

    Aortic insufficiency

    Cardiac conduction abnormalities

    Seronegative non-suppurative arthritis – polyarticular knees, ankles, metatarsophalangeal, sacroiliac joints; relative sparing of hands and wrists; occasionally monoarticular; enthesitis

Singleton-Merten syndrome – autosomal dominant; muscle weakness, failure to thrive, glaucoma, abnormal dentition, aortic calcification, acro-osteolysis, psoriasis; chilblains of helices of ears with edema, erythema, ulcers *BJD 173:1369–1370, 2015; BMJ Case Reports Sept 5, 2014; Am J Med GenetcsA 161A:360–370, 2013; IF1H1 gain of function mutation Am J Hum Genet 96:275–262, 2015*

Sneddon's syndrome – aortic valve stenosis, mitral valve stenosis *Clin Res Cardiol 104:453–455, 2015*

Stickler's syndrome – mitral valve prolapse; distinctive facies – prominent eyes, small nose with scooped out facial appearance and receding chin, ocular problems, hearing loss, joint and skeletal problems

Turner's syndrome – bicuspid aortic valve, left-sided heart obstructive disease from hypoplastic left-sided heart syndrome to minimal aortic stenosis or coarctation of the aorta

Watson syndrome – autosomal dominant; intertriginous (axillary and perianal) freckling, CALMs, short stature, intellectual deficit, pulmonary valve stenosis *Clin in Dermatol 23:56–67, 2005; JAAD 46:161–183, 2002; JAAD 40:877–890, 1999; Curr Prob in Derm VII:143–198, 1995*

Werner's syndrome (pangeria) – mitral regurgitation, aortic stenosis, frequent valvular calcification *Cardiovasc Pathol 9:53–54, 2000; Ann Thoracic Surg 57:1319–1320, 1994*

Williams-Beuren syndrome – soft skin, premature graying of hair, "elfin" facial appearance, low nasal bridge, developmental delay, supravalvular aortic stenosis *Am J Med Genet A 170:1832–1842, 2016; Am J Med Genet A 164A2217–2225, 2014*

VASCULAR DISORDERS

Granulomatosis with polyangiitis – aortic valve insufficiency *Echocardiography 35:1456–1463, 2018; Cardiovasc Pathol 23:1363–1365, 2014; Rheum Int 33:1055–1058, 2013; Am J Kidney Dis 24:205–208, 1994*

Microscopic polyangiitis – aortic valve insufficiency *Rheumatol Int 33:1055–1058, 2013*

Mitral stenosis – malar flush

PHACES syndrome – coarctation of aorta; aortic arch anomalies, ventricular septal defect, double aortic arch, atrial septal defect, patent foramen ovale, tricuspid atresia, pulmonary stenosis *Ped Cardiol 29:793–799, 2008; J Ped 139:117–123, 2001*

Takayasu's arteritis – most with aortic regurgitation; mild mitral and tricuspid regurgitation; valve stenosis rare *Am J Med Sci 356:357–364, 2018; Vasa 22:347–351, 1993*

VASCULITIS, GRANULOMATOUS

Eosinophilic granulomatosis with polyangiitis – small vessel

Giant cell arteritis (large vessel granulomatous vasculitis)

Polyarteritis nodosa

Takayasu's disease (arteritis) – large vessel

Granulomatosis with polyangiitis – small vessel *JAAD 26:579–584, 1992*

VASCULITIS, LEUKOCYTOCLASTIC

AUTOIMMUNE DISEASES AND DISORDERS OF IMMUNE DYSREGULATION

RHEUMATIC DISEASES

ANA negative disease; urticarial vasculitis with systemic lupus erythematosus *JAAD 38:899–905, 1998*

ANCA positive disease

DADA2 (deficiency of adenosine deaminase 2) – autosomal recessive; recurrent fevers, early onset stroke, livedo racemosa, polyarteritis nodosa, hepatosplenomegaly; mutation in *CECR1 JAAD 75:449–453, 2016;* vasculopathy associated with mutations in ADA2 – syndrome of livedoid rash, intermittent fevers, early onset lacunar strokes and other neurovascular manifestations, hepatosplenomegaly, and systemic vasculopathy; loss of function mutations in *CECR1 NEJM 370:911–920, 2014*

Dermatomyositis

Hypersensitivity vasculitis (Zeek's; small vessel)

Mixed connective tissue disease

Relapsing polychondritis

Rheumatoid arthritis

Schnitzler's syndrome

Serum sickness

Sjogren's syndrome

Systemic lupus erythematosus

Urticarial vasculitis

DRUGS

Curr Rheumatol Rep 17:71, 2015

Additives

Allopurinol

Aminosalicylic acid

Amiodarone

Amphetamine

Ampicillin

Aspirin

BCG vaccination

Captopril

Carbamazepine

Cimetidine

Ciprofloxacin *Cureus 8:e900, 2016*

Coumadin

Didanosine

Enalapril

Erlotinib *Exp Ther Med 17:1128, 1131, 2019*

Erythromycin

Ethacrynic acid

Fluoroquinolone antibiotics

Fluoxetine ingestion – urticarial vasculitis *JAAD 38:899–905, 1998*

Furosemide

GM-CSF injection sites *AD 126:1243–1244, 1990*

Griseofulvin

Granulocyte colony-stimulating factor *JAAD 31:213–215, 1994*

Guanethidine

Hydralazine

Hydroxyurea *JAAD 36:178–182, 1997*

Iodides

Levamisole

Maprotiline

Mefloquine

Methotrexate

Nicotine patch

Non-steroidal anti-inflammatory drugs

Penicillin

Phenacetin

Phenothiazines

Phenylbutazone

Phenytoin

Piperazine

Procainamide

Propylthiouracil *J Burn Care Res 38:e678–685, 2017*

Quinidine

Radiocontrast media *JAAD 10:25–29, 1984*

Staphylococcal protein A column immunoadsorption therapy *AD 131:707, 1995*

Streptomycin

Sulfonamides

Sulfonylureas

Tetracyclines

Thiazides *Lancet ii:982–983, 1965*

Trazodone

Trimethadione

Vaccination

Vancomycin

Vitamin B6

Zidovudine

EXOGENOUS AGENTS

Amphetamine abuse

Cocaine – levamisole-induced vasculitis/vasculopathy

Drug additives – tartrazine, sodium benzoate, 4-hydroxybenzoic acid *JAAD 30:854, 1994*

INFECTIONS AND INFESTATIONS

Acute respiratory infection

Cystic fibrosis *J Ped 95:197, 1979*

Cytomegalovirus *Clin Exp Rheumatol 32(Suppl 82):573–575, 2014; Medicine 73:246–255, 1994*

Dental abscess *Acta DV(Stockh) 32:274–277, 1952*

Echovirus

Epstein-Barr virus

Escherichia coli

Gonococcemia *JAAD 29:276–278, 1993*

Hepatitis B-associated polyarteritis nodosa

Hepatitis C – cryoglobulinemia – thrombotic and/or leukocytoclastic vasculitis *AD 131:1119–1123, 1995*

Herpes simplex virus, disseminated *Am J Dermatopathol 6:561–565, 1984; Arch Pathol Lab Med 106:64–67, 1982*

HIV – chronic leukocytoclastic vasculitis in HIV in children *JAAD 22:1223–1231, 1990*

Leprosy – erythema nodosum leprosum *Int J Dermatol 35:389–392, 1996*; Lucio's phenomenon – granulomatous and necrotizing panvasculitis *Am J Dermatopathol 30:555–560, 2008*

Mycoplasma pneumoniae

Mycobacterium tuberculosis

Post-streptococcal glomerulonephritis *Medicine 49:433–463, 1970*

Rheumatic fever

Rickettsia – Rocky Mountain spotted fever

Staphylococcus aureus

Subacute bacterial endocarditis – *Streptococcus viridans*

Syphilis

Varicella zoster *Lancet Neurology 8:731–740, 2009*

INFLAMMATORY DISORDERS

Sarcoid

Inflammatory bowel disease – ulcerative colitis, Crohn's disease

METABOLIC DISORDERS

Paraproteinemia

Cryoglobulinemia, essential

Hyper IgD *AD 126:1621–1624, 1990*

Macroglobulinemia; urticarial vasculitis with monoclonal IgM gammopathy (Schnitzler's syndrome) *JAAD 38:899–905, 1998*

Mixed cryoglobulinemia; urticarial vasculitis with mixed cryoglobuli-nemia *JAAD 38:899–905, 1998*

    Causes of mixed cryoglobulinemia

        Infections – hepatitis B, syphilis, borreliosis, subacute bacterial endocarditis, leprosy, kala-azar

        Autoimmune diseases – lupus erythematosus, rheumatoid arthritis, Sjogren's syndrome, vasculitis

        Lymphoproliferative diseases – multiple myeloma, lymphoma

        Liver disease

Respiratory

    Cystic fibrosis *Ped Derm 4:108–111, 1987*

    Serous otitis media

NEOPLASTIC DISORDERS

Castleman's disease *JAAD 26:105–109, 1992*

Multiple myeloma *AD 127:69–74, 1991*

Waldenstrom's macroglobulinemia *AD 134:1127–1131, 1998*

PARANEOPLASTIC DISORDERS

Hairy cell leukemia

Henoch-Schonlein purpura

Malignancy – lymphoreticular malignancies metastatic testicular teratoma with urticarial vasculitis *JAAD 38:899–905, 1998*; metastatic hypopharyngeal carcinoma mimicking vasculitis *Cutis 49:187–188, 1992*; myeloma *AD 127:69–74, 1991*

Paraneoplastic – T-cell lymphoma *JAAD 19:973–978, 1988*; ovarian, leukemias, lung, prostate, colon, renal, breast, squamous cell carcinoma *JAAD 40:287–289, 1999*; myeloma

PRIMARY CUTANEOUS DISEASES

Erythema elevatum diutinum – HIV associated *JAAD Case Rep 5:1093–1096, 2019*

Granuloma faciale

SYNDROMES

Behcet's disease – necrotizing vasculitis *JAAD 41:540–545, 1999; JAAD 40:1–18, 1999; NEJM 341:1284–1290, 1999; JAAD 36:689–696, 1997*

Bowel-associated dermatitis-arthritis syndrome

Cogan's syndrome

Hypereosinophilic syndrome

Kawasaki's disease

POEMS syndrome (Takatsuki syndrome, Crow-Fukase syndrome) – osteosclerotic bone lesions, peripheral polyneuropathy, hypothyroid-ism, and hypogonadism *Cutis 61:329–334, 1998; JAAD 40:808–812, 1999; JAAD 21:1061–1068, 1989*

TOXINS

Arsenic

VASCULAR DISORDERS

Chronic necrotizing venulitis

Cutaneous polyarteritis nodosa

Eosinophilic granulomatosis with polyangiitis *JAAD 37:199–203, 1997*

Exercise-induced vasculitis *Am J Clin Dermatol 17:635–642, 2016*

Granulomatosis with polyangiitis *JAAD 26:579–584, 1992*

Henoch-Schonlein purpura

Lymphocytic thrombophilic arteritis

Microscopic polyangiitis (arteritis nodosum)

Polyarteritis nodosa

VASCULITIS, THROMBOTIC

AUTOIMMUNE DISEASES AND DISORDERS OF IMMUNE DYSREGULATION

Adenosine deaminase 2 (ADA2) mutation – mutation in *CECR1*; compromised endothelial integrity, endothelial cell activation, and inflammation; intermittent fevers, early onset lacunar strokes, livedoid eruption, hepatosplenomegaly, systemic vasculopathy *NEJM 370:911–920, 2014*

Antiphospholipid antibody syndrome with or without associated collagen vascular disease

Lupus anticoagulant; Sneddon's syndrome *JAAD 19:117, 1988*

DRUGS

Coumarin necrosis

Renal transplant patient treated with cyclosporine

Heparin necrosis *AD 132:341–346, 1996*

INFECTIONS AND INFESTATIONS

Hepatitis C – cryoglobulinemia – thrombotic and/or leukocytoclastic vasculitis *AD 131:1119–1123, 1995*

Septic vasculitis

    Bacterial

        Gonorrhea

        Meningococcus

        Pseudomonas – ecthyma gangrenosum

        Staphylococcal and streptococcal subacute bacterial endocarditis

    Fungal

        Aspergillosis

        Mucormycosis

    Viral

        Varicella zoster virus

    Rickettsia

        Rocky Mountain spotted fever

METABOLIC DISORDERS

Cold agglutinin disease *JAAD 19:356, 1987*

Cryofibrinogenemia *JAAD 24: 342, 1991*

Cryoglobulinemia

Paroxysmal nocturnal hemoglobinuria

Protein C deficiency

Protein S deficiency

Thrombocythemia *JAAD 24:59, 1991*

PRIMARY CUTANEOUS DISEASES

Sneddon-Wilkinson disease

SYNDROMES

Behcet's disease *JAAD 21:576, 1989*

Hemolytic uremic syndrome

VASCULAR DISORDERS

Degos disease – malignant atrophic papulosis

Disseminated intravascular coagulation, including purpura fulminans, symmetric peripheral gangrene

Embolic lesion – SBE, ABE, Libman-Sacks, atrial myxomas, cholesterol emboli, coral reef aorta, intimal angiosarcoma of the aorta, hydrophilic polymer (stents, grafts, catheters)

Ischemic ulcers of hematologic origin

   Hereditary spherocytosis

      Hemolytic anemia

      Sickle cell disease (SS)

   Polycythemia vera

Livedoid vasculitis (atrophie blanche en plaque)

Thrombotic thrombocytopenic purpura

Waldenstrom's hyperglobulinemic purpura

VASCULITIS, TYPES

AD 130:899–906, 1994
  Direct infections of vessels
    Bacterial vasculitis (neisserial)
    Fungal (mucor)
    Mycobacterial (tuberculosis)
    Rickettsial vasculitis (Rocky Mountain spotted fever)
    Spirochetal
    Viral
  Immunologic injury
  ANCA-associated or ANCA-mediated
    Churg-Strauss disease
    Some drug-induced (thiouracil)
    Microscopic polyarteritis nodosa
    Wegener's granulomatosis
  Cell-mediated
  Direct antibody attack – mediated
    Goodpasture's syndrome (anti-BM ABs)
    Kawasaki's disease
  Immune complex
    Behcet's disease
    Cryoglobulins
    Some drug-induced vasculitis (sulfonamides)
    Erythema elevatum diutinum
    Henoch-Schonlein purpura
    Infection-induced immune complex vasculitis
      Bacterial (*Streptococcus*)

      Viral (hepatitis B and C)
    Lupus erythematosus
    Paraneoplastic vasculitis
    Rheumatoid arthritis – nodules, pyoderma gangrenosum-like, digital gangrene, ulcers, petechiae, purpura, mononeuritis multiplex
    Serum sickness vasculitis
      Heterologous proteins
      Whole serum
  Unknown
    Allograft acute cellular vascular rejection
    Pyoderma gangrenosum-like, nodules, erythema nodosum-like,
    Raynaud's phenomenon
    Erythema nodosum
    Giant cell arteritis
    Polyarteritis nodosa
    Takayasu's arteritis

POLYMORPHONUCLEAR

Allergic vasculitis

Erythema elevatum diutinum – localized; HIV-associated

Henoch-Schonlein purpura

HIV-associated

Sweet's syndrome

Zeek's hypersensitivity vasculitis

Collagen vascular disease

Erythema nodosum (early)

Bowel-associated dermatitis-arthritis syndrome

Behcet's syndrome

Urticarial vasculitis

LYMPHOCYTIC

Drug reaction

Erythema multiforme

Erythema nodosum

Pityriasis lichenoides et varioliformis acuta

Dysproteinemia – macroglobulinemia

Degos' disease – idiopathic, HIV-associated *JAAD 38:852–856, 1998*

Lupus erythematosus – lymphocytic large vessel vasculitis

Macroglobulinemia

Malignant atrophic papulosis

Perniosis

GRANULOMATOUS VASCULITIS

SYSTEMIC

Eosinophilic granulomatosis with polyangiitis

Granulomatosis with polyangiitis

Infections – Hansen's disease, tuberculosis, syphilis, HIV-associated

Lymphomatoid granulomatosis (angiocentric T-cell lymphoma)

Polyarteritis nodosa – including HIV-associated

FOCAL

Lethal midline granuloma

Eosinophilic and necrotizing focal granuloma

Cogan's syndrome

Granuloma faciale

Nodular vasculitis

LARGE VESSEL VASCULITIS

POLYMORPHONUCLEAR

Polyarteritis nodosa

Superficial migratory thrombophlebitis

Lymphangitis

LYMPHOCYTIC

Peripheral vascular disease

Lupus erythematosus

GRANULOMATOUS

Giant cell arteritis

Erythema induratum

Takayasu's arteritis

VEGETATING LESIONS

AUTOIMMUNE DISEASES AND DISEASES OF IMMUNE DYSFUNCTION

Bullous pemphigoid *AD 117:56–57, 1981*

Chronic granulomatous disease *Minerva Ped 30:899–905, 1978*

Cicatricial pemphigoid *Arch Derm Res 279 Suppl:S30–37, 1987*

Familial pyoderma gangrenosum with common variable immunodeficiency – vegetative cheilitis; cutaneous ulcers *BJD 169:944–946, 2013*

Fogo selvagem (endemic pemphigus) – vegetative plaques *JID 107:68–75, 1996; JAAD 32:949–956, 1995*

Pemphigoid vegetans – vegetating plaque *JAAD 64:206–208, 2011; JAAD 30:649–650, 1994; JAAD 29:293–299, 1993; AD 115:446–448, 1979*; concurrent pemphigus vegetans and pemphigoid vegetans – vegetative plaques of groin *BJD 170:1192–1194, 2014*

Pemphigus foliaceus *Dermatologica 180:102–105, 1990*

Pemphigus vegetans *Int J Derm 23:135–141, 1984*; drug-induced (captopril) *JAAD 27:281–284, 1992*; pemphigus vegetans, Neumann type – giant cobblestoning with vegetative intertriginous plaques and blisters; oral bullae *AD 145:715–720, 2009*; giant vegetative plaque of the vulva; IgG anti-desmocollin-3 antibodies *JAMA Derm 149:1209–1213, 2013*; concurrent pemphigus vegetans and pemphigoid vegetans – vegetative plaques of groin *BJD 170:1192–1194, 2014*

Pemphigus vegetans variant of intraepidermal neutrophilic IgA dermatosis *JAAD 38:635–638, 1998*

Pemphigus vulgaris *BJD 161:313–319, 2009; BJD 146:684–687, 2002; BJD 109:459–463, 1983*

CONGENITAL LESIONS

Ectopic respiratory mucosa *JAAD 43:939–942, 2000*

DRUG-INDUCED

Amiodarone-induced iododerma *Ann DV 124:260–263, 1997*

Bromoderma – single or multiple papillomatous nodules or plaques studded with pustules on face or extremities *Ped Derm 18:336–338, 2001; AD 115:1334–1335, 1979*; ingestion of soft drink (Ruby Red Squirt) *NEJM 348:1932–1934, 2003*; vegetating bromoderma; pustular red plaque with pustules at margins to distinguish it from pyoderma gangrenosum *JAAD 58:682–684, 2008*

Iododerma, vegetating *JAMA Derm 149:1231–1232, 2013; Dermatology 198:295–297, 1999; JAAD 36:1014–1016, 1997; Ped Derm 13;51–53, 1996; JAAD 22:418–422, 1990; AD 123:387–388, 1987*; iododerma in chronic renal failure *Dermatology 198:295–297, 1999; Dermatologica 171:463–468, 1985*; intravenous contrast material in setting of chronic renal failure *BJD 170:1377–1379, 2014*

Lithium – halogenoderma-like lesion *AD 136:126–127, 2000*

INFECTIONS AND INFESTATIONS

Actinomycosis *JAAD 48:456–460, 2003*; actinomycotic mycetoma *J Eur Acad Dermatol Venereol 29:1873–1883, 2015JAAD 17:443–438, 1987*; perianal vegetating lesions *Ann DV 109:789–790, 1982*; actinomycetoma (*Gordonia terrae*) *J Clin Microbiol 45:1076–1077, 2007*

Alternariosis *BJD 145:484–486, 2001; BJD 143:910–912, 2000; Ann DV 109:841–846, 1982; Ann DV 108:653–662,1981; Alternaria tenuissima* – ulcerated vegetative nodule *BJD 142:840–841, 2000*

Amebic granulomas – vegetating plaque of genitalia, perineum, and anus *JAAD 48:456–460, 2003; Entamoeba histolytica* in neonate *Derm Clinics 17:151–185, 1999*

Aspergillosis *BJD 85(suppl 17):95–97, 1971*

Bartonellosis *Am J Trop Med Hyg 50:143–144, 1994*

BCG granuloma *Clin Infect Dis 29:1569–1570, 1999*

Bejel

Blastomyces dermatitidis

Blastomycosis-like pyoderma *Dermatol Clin 33:509–630, 2015; AD 142:1643–1648, 2006; JAAD 48:456–460, 2003; AD 115:170–173, 1979*; pseudomonas *JAAD 23:750–752, 1990*; *Staphylococcus aureus*; beta hemolytic *Streptococcus, Proteus mirabilis, Escherichia coli*

Botryomycosis

Calymmatobacterium granulomatis (Donovanosis) *J Clin Inf Dis 25:24–32, 1997*

Candida parapsilosis – superficial candidiasis; verrucous vegetative nodules of dorsal hands *JAMA Derm 149:1431–1432, 2013*

Candidal granuloma, chronic mucocutaneous candidiasis *Rev Inst Med Trop Sao Paolo 28:364–367, 1986; Ann Rev Med 32:491–497, 1981*; candida in KID syndrome – vegetative plaques of feet *Ped Derm 34:201–203, 2017*

Chancroid *Acta DV 64:452–5, 1984*

Chromomycosis – verrucous plaques, cauliflower-like masses, nodules, large vegetations; feet, legs, arms, face, and neck; common causative organisms include *Phialophora verrucosa, Fonsecaea pedrosoi, F. compactum, Wangiella dermatitidis,* and

Cladophialophora (Cladosporium) carrionii, Rhinocladiella aquaspersa, R. cerphilum, Exophiala spinifera, Cladophialophora boppii, and *Aureobasidium pullulans*; large pigmented round thick-walled bodies with septation in two planes (muriform cells) *JAAD 53:931–951, 2005; AD 141:1457–1462, 2005; BJD 152:560–564, 2005; JAAD 48:456–460, 2003; AD 133:1027–1032, 1997; BJD 96:454–458, 1977; AD 104:476–485, 1971*

Coccidioidomycosis – vegetative facial plaques *Cutis 85:25–27, 2010; JAAD 48:456–460, 2003*

Condyloma acuminata

Cryptococcosis *J Inf Dis 56:117,159–160, 2013; J Dermatol 23:209–213, 1996;* vegetative plaque of cheek *JAAD 63:177–179, 2010*

Cytomegalovirus infection – vegetative ulcer of the face *BJD 170:223–224, 2014*

Dermatophyte infection – deep dermatophytosis in inherited autosomal recessive CARD9 deficiency; vegetative plaques, verrucous plaques, and nodules; perianal vegetative plaques *NEJM 1704–1714, 2013;* tinea capitis; kerion; *T. rubrum* – exophytic nodules *Cutis 67:457–462, 2001*

Dissecting cellulitis

Ecthyma

Filariasis

Fusospirochetal or mixed infection, penile – uncircumcised

Granuloma inguinale – papule or nodule breaks down to form ulcer with overhanging edge; deep extension may occur; or serpiginous extension with vegetative hyperplasia; pubis, genitalia, perineum; extragenital lesions of the nose and lips or extremities *JAAD 54:559–578, 2006; JAAD 32:153–154, 1995; JAAD 11:433–437, 1984*

Herpes simplex – perianal vegetative tumid mass *JAMADerm 156:453–454, 2020;* in HIV *JAAD 37:860–863, 1997;* perianal in HIV disease *Pathology 33:532–535, 2001;* chronic herpes simplex – vegetative nodule *JAMA Derm 149:881–883, 2013*

Herpes zoster *Klin Med(Mosk) 43:42–44, 1965*

Histoplasmosis in AIDS *JAAD 23:422–428, 1990*

Klebsiella pneumoniae Am J Med 118:925–927, 2005

Leishmaniasis – chicleros ulcer *JAAD 73:897–908, 2015; J Drugs in Dermatol 13:210–215, 2014;* framboesoid leishmaniasis *JAAD 48:456–460, 2003; Leishmania mexicana* – weeping vegetative plaque of the face *Dermatol Clin 33:579–593, 2015;* of lips *JAAD 81:1013–1015, 2019;* espundia (mucocutaneous leishmaniasis) – facial edema, erythema, verrucous plaques, dermatitis, edema of lips; *Am J Trop Med Hyg 59:49–52, 1998;* vegetating tumor of the hard palate *Oral Dis 8:59–61, 2002; L. braziliensis BJD 173:571–573, 2015;* leishmania recidivans – central atrophy with vegetative border *Clin Dermatol 38:140–151, 2020*

Leprosy

Lymphogranuloma venereum

Melioidosis (*Burkholderia pseudomallei*) *Cutis 72:310–312, 2003*

Molluscum contagiosum in AIDS *JAAD 35:266–267, 1996*

Mycetoma

Mycobacterium haemophilum

Mycobacterium tuberculosis – vegetative lupus vulgaris (lupus vorax); vegetative linear serpiginous lesion of the neck *Ped Derm 36:955–957, 2019; JAAD 48:456–460, 2003; Ped Derm 16:264–269, 1999;* starts as red-brown plaque; vegetating forms – ulcerate, areas of necrosis, invasion of mucous membranes with destruction of cartilage (lupus vorax); tumorlike forms – deeply infiltrative; soft

smooth nodules or red-yellow hypertrophic plaque; head, neck, around nose, extremities, trunk *Int J Dermatol 26:578–581, 1987; Acta Tuberc Scand 39(Suppl 49):1–137, 1960;* orofacial granulomatosis due to tuberculosis; enlarged tongue; vegetative plaques of the nose and nasolabial folds *Ped Derm 26:108–109, 2009;* orificial tuberculosis – perioral crusted vegetative plaque *Am J Clin Dermatol 3:319–328, 2002;* scrofulous gumma *Ped Derm 30:7–16, 2013;* lupus vulgaris, tuberculosis verrucosa cutis

Mycobacteriosis, non-tuberculous *JAAD 48:456–460, 2003*

Nocardiosis – vegetative plaque *JAAD 41:338–340, 1999*

North American blastomycosis – beefy red vegetative plaques *Clin Inf Dis 55:1390–1391, 1426–1428, 2012; AD 143:1323–1328, 2007; Dermatol Int 6:44–48, 1967 (Spanish)*

Paracoccidioidomycosis – vegetative lesions of lip and nose *AD 145:1325–1330, 2009; Dermatol Clin 26:257–269, 2008*

Phaeoacremonium phaeohyphomycosis *JAAD 66:333–335, 2012*

Phaeohyphomycosis *JAAD 61:977–985, 2009; JAAD 23:363–367, 1990; JAAD 18:1023–1030, 1988;* linear vegetative plaques of the legs; *Coniothyrium Cutis 73:127–130, 2004; Alternaria Revista Iberoamericana de Micologia 27:44–46, 2012*

Prototothecosis *JAAD 48:456–460, 2003*

Rhinosporidiosis *Clinics in Dermatol 32:47–65, 2014*

Schistosomal granulomas

Scopulariopsis brevicaulis – vegetative ulcerative nodule of the forearm *Clin Inf Dis 30:820–823, 2000*

Serratia marcescens Cutis 66:461–463, 2000

Sporotrichosis – vegetative plaque of the penis *AD 139:1647–1652, 2003*

Syphilis – condylomata lata; nodular secondary syphilis *AD 113:1027–1032, 1997;* granulomatous secondary syphilis; framboesiform secondary syphilides; tertiary lues (gumma) *AD 134:365–370, 1998*

Tinea capitis

Warts, including condylomata acuminata; toe web warts; HPV–7 *BJD 162:579–586, 2010*

Yaws – primary red papule, ulcerates, crusted; satellite papules; become round ulcers, papillomatous or vegetative friable nodules which bleed easily (raspberry-like) (framboesia)

INFILTRATIVE LESIONS

Plasma cell balanitis (Zoon's balanitis) *J Urol 153:424–426, 1995; Genitourin Med 71:32–34, 1995; BJD 105:195–199, 1981*

Rosai-Dorfman disease (sinus histiocytosis with massive lymphadenopathy) – vegetative plaque resembling hidradenitis suppurativa *Soc Ped Derm Annual Meeting, July, 2006*

Verruciform xanthoma – of the penis *Urology 23:600–603, 1984*

INFLAMMATORY DISORDERS

Crohn's disease, cutaneous perianal vegetative linear plaque *Ped Derm 23:49–52,2006; JAAD 48:456–460, 2003;* annular vegetative perianal plaque *JAAD 63:165–166, 2010*

Pyoderma gangrenosum *Hautarzt 50:217–220, 1999*

Pyoderma vegetans – crusted hyperplastic plaques, mimic blastomycosis; ulceration mimicking pyoderma gangrenosum; crusted red plaques with pustules, often in intertriginous areas; vegetative nodules of the face, elbows, arm *JAMADerm 155:243–*

244, 2019; JAAD 75:578–584, 2016; Case Reports Dermatol 3:80–84, 2011; Cutis 84:201–204, 2009; JAAD 50:785–788, 2004; BJD 144:1224–1227, 2001; J Cut Med Surg 5:223–237, 2001; JAAD 20:691–693, 1989; J Derm Surg Onc 12:271–273, 1986; pyoderma vegetans (pseudoepithelioma of Azua; hyperinflammatory proliferative pyoderma; blastomycosis-like pyoderma) – ulcerated vegetative plaques and rhinophymatous changes of the nose *JAMADerm 150: 773–774, 2014; Arch Dermatol Syphilol 43:289–306, 1898*

Pyostomatitis vegetans – pustular lips and nose; erosive plaques of lips with yellow crusts; association with ulcerative colitis and Crohn's disease *JAMADerm 156:335, 2020; Int J Dermatol 56:1457–1459, 2017; JAAD 75:578–584, 2016*; vegetative plaques of the legs; *An Bras Dermatol 86:S137–140, 2011; Med Oral Patol Oral Cir Bucal 14:E114–117, 2009; Ann DV 135:753–756, 2008; Dermatology 217:146–148, 2008; Clin Exp Dermatol 29:1–7, 2004; Acta DV 81:134–136, 2001; JAAD 31:336–341, 1994*

Sarcoid *JAAD 48:456–460, 2003*

Superficial vegetative granulomatous pyoderma (pyoderma gangrenosum vegetans) *Ped Derm 27:496–499, 2010; BJD 153:684–686, 2005; BJD 146:141–143, 2002; J Eur Acad Dermatol Venereol 16:159–161, 2002; J Eur Acad Dermatol Venereol 16:97, 2002; Hautarzt 45:635–638, 1994; BJD 129:718–722, 1993; Mayo Clin Proc 64:37–43, 1989; J Dermatol 16:127–132, 1989; JAAD 18:511–521, 1988*

NEOPLASTIC DISEASES

Bowen's disease – penile

Buschke-Lowenstein tumor (giant condylomata acuminate) *JAMA Derm 149:1068–1070, 2013*

Kaposi's sarcoma

Keratoacanthoma *JAAD 74:1220–1233, 2016*

Leukemia – acute promyelocytic leukemia *Dermatologica 151:184–190, 1975*

Lymphoma – vegetating cutaneous T-cell lymphoma *Hautarzt 29-219–221, 1978*; malignant pyoderma (angiocentric lymphoma) *JAAD 48:456–460, 2003*; pyogenic lymphoma – primary cutaneous neutrophil-rich CD30+ anaplastic large cell lymphoma *BJD 148:580–586, 2003*

Malignant blue nevus – scalp *Int J Derm 37:126–127, 1998*

Melanoma, including acral lentiginous melanoma; metastatic melanoma

Metastatic carcinoma

Squamous cell carcinoma – complicating venous stasis ulcers *South Med J 58:779–781, 1965*; vegetative lesions of the penis *J Urol 104:291–297, 1970*

Verrucous carcinoma – epithelioma cuniculatum *AD 136:547–548, 550–551, 2000*; giant condyloma of Buschke-Lowenstein, oral florid papillomatosis *JAAD 32:1–21, 1995; JAAD 14:947–950, 1986; Int J Derm 18:608–622, 1979*; sacrum *BJD 143:459–460, 2000*; leg amputation stump *Dermatologica 182:193–195, 1991*

PRIMARY CUTANEOUS DISEASES

Acrodermatitis continua of Hallopeau

Darier's disease (keratosis follicularis) – malodorous vegetative plaques in flexures *Am J Clin Dermatol 4:97–105, 2003; AD 128:399, 1992*

Erythema elevatum diutinum

Hailey-Hailey disease – vegetative multilobulated malodorous friable plaques of the cheek *JAMA 319:1499–1500, 2018; JAAD 65:223–224, 2011*

Lichen simplex chronicus

Nummular dermatitis

Pustulosis vegetans *AD 120:1355–1359, 1984*

Subcorneal pustular dermatosis *Z Haut Geschlechtskr 45:1–10, 1970; Dermatol Int 7:132–133, 1968*

PSYCHOCUTANEOUS DISEASES

Factitial dermatitis

SYNDROMES

Epidermodysplasia verruciformis – giant cobblestoning *BJD 155:218–220, 2006*

Sweet's syndrome – vegetative neutrophilic dermatosis of the dorsal hands – personal observation

TRAUMA

Verruciform xanthoma – red-orange plaque; multilobulated, vegetative, cobblestoned; perigenital; seen in KID and CHILD syndromes and recessive dystrophic epidermolysis bullosa; usually at site of friction or frequent trauma *Ped Derm 37:176–179, 2020*

VASCULAR

Granulomatosis with polyangiitis *JAAD 48:456–460, 2003*

Lymphostasis verrucosa cutis

VERRUCOUS LESIONS OF THE LEGS

AUTOIMMUNE DISEASES AND DISEASES OF IMMUNE DYSFUNCTION

Fogo selvagem (endemic pemphigus) – verrucous prurigo nodularis-like lesions *JID 107:68–75, 1996; JAAD 32:949–956, 1995*

Lichen planus pemphigoides

Lupus erythematosus – hypertrophic DLE

Pemphigus vulgaris

DRUG-INDUCED

Lichen planus-like drug eruption

INFECTIONS AND INFESTATIONS

Blastomycosis-like pyoderma

Chromomycosis – feet, legs, arms, face, and neck *AD 133:1027–1032, 1997; BJD 96:454–458, 1977; AD 104:476–485, 1971*; squamous cell carcinoma arising in chromomycosis *Clin Inf Dis 60:1500–1504, 2015*

Cryptococcosis

Leishmaniasis – diffuse cutaneous leishmaniasis – multiple red verrucous nodules of the knees; multilobulated skin colored nodules of the ears *BJD 156:1328–1335, 2007*; leishmaniasis recidivans (lupoid leishmaniasis) – brown-red or brown-yellow papules close to scar of previously healed lesion; resemble lupus vulgaris; may ulcerate or form concentric rings; keloidal form, verrucous form of the legs, extensive psoriasiform dermatitis

Leprosy *An Bras Dermatol 89:481–484, 2014*

Mycetoma

Mycobacterium marinum AD 134:365–370, 1998; JAAD 24:208–215, 1991

Mycobacterium tuberculosis – lupus vulgaris, tuberculosis verrucosa cutis *Dermatol Therapy 21:154–161, 2008*

North American blastomycosis – disseminated blastomycosis *Am Rev Resp Dis 120:911–938, 1979; Medicine 47:169–200, 1968*

Paracoccidioidomycosis

Phaeohyphomycosis – *Alternaria JAAD 59:905–907, 2008*

Sporotrichosis

Trichophyton rubrum, invasive

Trichosporon dermatis – ulcerated verrucous plaque with draining sinus tracts above ankle *JAAD 65:434–436, 2011*

Warts – giant disseminated verrucosis (HPV2) (giant verrucous claw hands and feet) associated with idiopathic CD4 lymphopenia *AD 146:69–73, 2010*; verrucae vulgaris of amputation stump

INFILTRATIVE DISEASES

Amyloidosis – lichen amyloidosis

Lichen myxedematosus

Pretibial myxedema

Sarcoidosis *AD 133:882–888, 1997; AD 102:665–669, 1970*; mimicking hypertrophic lichen planus *Int J Derm 28:539–541, 1989*

NEOPLASTIC DISEASES

Epidermal nevus, linear; inflammatory linear verrucous epidermal nevus (ILVEN) *Cutis 102:111–114, 2018*

Hyperkeratotic lichen planus-like reactions combined with infundibulocystic hyperplasia *AD 140:1262–1267, 2004*

Kaposi's sarcoma

Keratoacanthoma – classical; keratoacanthoma centrifugum marginatum *JAAD 30:1–19, 1994; AD 111:1024–1026, 1975*

Lymphoma – cutaneous T-cell lymphoma *JAAD 60:359–375, 2009*; primary cutaneous diffuse large cell B-cell lymphoma, leg type – verrucous plaques *Clin Exp Dermatol 35:e87–89, 2010*

Melanoma – verrucous melanoma

Porocarcinoma *BJD 152:1051–1055, 2005*

Porokeratosis, linear *Ped Derm 21:682–683, 2004*

Porokeratosis of Mibelli *J Dermatol 37:475–479, 2010*

Squamous cell carcinoma

Verrucous carcinoma – of feet and legs *JAAD 56:S2–32, 2007*; of leg *JAAD 57:516–519, 2007*

Woringer-Kolopp disease (pagetoid reticulosis) *JAAD 59:706–712, 2008; Ann Dermatol Syph 10:945–958, 1939*

PRIMARY CUTANEOUS DISEASES

Acanthosis nigricans, generalized

Darier's disease (keratosis follicularis) *Clin Dermatol 19:193–205, 1994; JAAD 27:40–50, 1992*

Epidermolysis bullosa pruriginosa – mild acral blistering at birth or early childhood; violaceous papular and nodular lesions in linear array on shins, forearms, trunk; lichenified hypertrophic and verrucous plaques in adults *BJD 130:617–625, 1994*

Erythema elevatum diutinum

Hypertrophic lichen planus *Cutis 6:e3555, 2018*; *AD 139:933–938, 2003*

Lichenoid pigmented purpuric eruption

Lichen simplex chronicus

Necrolytic acral erythema – serpiginous, verrucous plaques of dorsal aspects of the hands and legs; associated with hepatitis C infection *JAAD 50:S121–124, 2004*

Psoriasis, elephantine

SYNDROMES

Incontinentia pigmenti *JAAD 47:169–187, 2002; Dermatol 191(2):161–163, 1995*

Netherton's syndrome – verrucous hyperplasia of the lower legs *BJD 131:615–621, 1994*

Reactive arthritis syndrome – keratoderma blenorrhagicum; pretibial areas *Semin Arthritis Rheum 3:253–286, 1974*

TRAUMA

Verrucous hyperplasia of the amputation stump *AD 74:448–449, 1956*

VASCULAR

Lymphostasis verrucosa cutis (chronic lymphedema) (elephantiasis nostras verrucosa) – brawny edema with overlying hyperkeratosis; congenital lymphedema, lymphangitis, cellulitis, filariasis, malaria, schistosomiasis, morphea, radiation, scleredema, surgical trauma, venous stasis *NEJM 370:2520, 2014; BJD 163:1358–1360, 2010*

Stasis dermatitis

Vasculitis

Verrucous hemangioma – verrucous plaque of the leg *JAMADerm 152:1269–1270, 2016*

VERRUCOUS LESIONS, PERIUNGUAL

AD 130:204–209, 1994

AUTOIMMUNE DISEASES AND DISORDERS OF IMMUNE DYSREGULATION

Pemphigus vegetans *Eur J Dermatol 29: 209–210, 2019; Clin Exp Dermatol 41:316–317, 2016*

Pemphigus vulgaris *Dermatology Online J 9:14, 2003*

INFECTIONS AND INFESTATIONS

Chromomycosis *JAAD 53:931–951, 2005*

Herpes vegetans (HSV in HIV disease) – personal observation

Mycobacterium marinum AD 134:365–370, 1998; JAAD 24:208–215, 1991

Mycobacterium tuberculosis – tuberculosis verrucosa cutis *Dermatol Clin 33:541–562, 2015*

Onychomycosis

Verrucae vulgaris
   Warts associated with immunodeficiency disorders *BJD 178:335–349, 2018; J Allergy Clin Immunol 130:1030–1048, 2012*
      Common variable immunodeficiency – epidermodysplasia verruciformis-like lesions in common variable immunodeficiency *Clin Inf Dis 51:195–196,248–249, 2010*
      DOCK8 deficiency – autosomal recessive hyper IgE syndrome
      Epidermodysplasia verruciformis
      GATA2 deficiency
      ICF syndrome
      Idiopathic CD4 lymphopenia
      LAD-1 (CD18 deficiency)
      Mammalian sterile 20-like 1 deficiency
      NEMO
      Netherton's syndrome – *SPINK5* mutation
      Severe combined immunodeficiency
      STK4 deficiency *J Clin Immunol 36:117–122, 2016*
      TWEAK syndrome *Proc Nat Acad Sci 110:5127–5132, 2013*
      WHIM syndrome
      WILD syndrome
      X-linked hyper IgM syndrome

NEOPLASTIC DISORDERS

Amelanotic melanoma

Bowen's disease *J Eur Acad DV 30:1503–1506, 2016*

Epidermal nevus *AD 97:273–285, 1968*

Keratoacanthoma

Squamous cell carcinoma – associated with human papillomavirus 16,18,34 *JAAD 64:1147–1153, 2011; AD 127:1813–1818, 1991; AD 125:666–669, 1989*

Subungual exostosis

Verrucous carcinoma (epithelioma cuniculatum) *Dermatology 186:217–221, 1993*

PRIMARY CUTANEOUS DISEASES

Epidermodysplasia verruciformis *BJD 121:463–469, 1989; Arch Dermatol Res 278:153–160, 1985*; in common variable immunodeficiency *Clin Inf Dis 51:195–196, 248–249, 2010*

SYNDROMES

Ataxia telangiectasia

Lipoid proteinosis

Reactive arthritis syndrome – keratoderma blenorrhagicum *Semin Arthritis Rheum 3:253–286, 1974*

Wiskott-Aldrich syndrome

VASCULAR DISORDERS

Lymphostasis verrucosa cutis (chronic lymphedema, multiple causes) – brawny edema with overlying hyperkeratosis

Pyogenic granuloma

VERRUCOUS PLAQUES

AUTOIMMUNE DISEASES AND DISEASES OF IMMUNE DYSFUNCTION

Chronic mucocutaneous candidiasis – crusted plaques, cicatricial alopecia, leukoplakia, dystrophic nails *Ped Derm 34:609–611, 2017*

GATA2 deficiency (includes MonoMAC syndrome, DCML, Emberger syndrome (lymphedema and myelodysplasia) (familial acute leukemia and myelodysplasia) – monocytopenia, B-cell and natural killer cell lymphopenia, myeloid leukemias, multiple soft tissue infections, disseminated mycobacterial infection, human papilloma virus infection (multiple warts), fungal infection; GATA2 transcription factor in early hematopoietic differentiation and lymphatic and vascular development with primary lower leg lymphedema; sensorineural deafness, primary alveolar proteinosis; panniculitis; erythema nodosum-like lesions; skin tumors including squamous cell carcinomas Sweet's syndrome with myelodysplastic syndrome; GATA2 – zinc finger transcription factor that regulates vascular and lymphatic development and hematopoietic maturation *BJD 178:593–594, 2018; JAAD 73:367–381, 2015; JAAD 71:577–580, 2014; BJD 170:1182–1186, 2014; JAAD 71:577–580, 2014; Blood 118:2653–2655, 2011; Hematologica 96:1081–1083, 2011*; dendritic cell, monocyte, B lymphocyte, and NK lymphocyte deficiency (DCML); Emberger syndrome – primary lymphedema with myelodysplasia – susceptibility to acute myelogenous leukemia; congenital neutropenia; histoplasmosis, cryptococcosis, *Mycobacterium avium*, aspergillosis; pulmonary alveolar proteinosis

Graft vs. host disease – columnar epidermal necrosis in transfusion-associated chronic GVH *AD 136:743–746, 2000*

Interleukin 7 (IL-7) deficiency, inherited – CD4 lymphopenia with generalized warts (HPV-3) *JAAD 72:1082–1084, 2015*

Lichen planus pemphigoides

Lupus erythematosus hypertrophicus – hypertrophic discoid lupus erythematosus *JAAD 9:82–90, 1983; Cutis 28:290–300, 1981*; lupus profundus; LE hypertrophicus et profundus – verrucous brown-black plaque *BJD 96:75–78, 1977*

Pemphigoid nodularis *BJD 142:143–147, 2000*

Pemphigoid vegetans – vegetating plaque *JAAD 30:649–650, 1994; AD 115:446–448, 1979*

Pemphigus erythematosus

Pemphigus foliaceus – widespread verrucous plaques *Clin Exp Dermatol 45:584–585, 2020*

Pemphigus vegetans – 1–2% of all cases of pemphigus; Neumann type – bullae with small peripheral pustules evolve into vegetative plaques; denuded areas develop after plaques slough; Hallopeau type – pustules, not bullae, are the primary lesions; verrucous plaques then develop; no denuded areas; cerebriform tongue; spontaneous resolution not uncommon *JAMA 314:2296–2297, 2015; Dermatol Clinics 11:429–452, 1993*

Scleroderma – axillary verrucous pigmentation resembling acanthosis nigricans *Br Med J ii:1642–1645, 1966*

CONGENITAL

Subepidermal calcified nodule in children – verrucous papule *Ped Derm 12:307–310, 1995*

DEGENERATIVE

Collagenous and elastotic marginal plaques of the hands – thick plaques on radial aspects of second fingers and ulnar aspects of thumbs *AD 147:499–504, 2011*

Diabetic neuropathy *BJD 133:1011–1012, 1995*

DRUG-INDUCED

Bleomycin *JAAD 33:851–852, 1995*

Dabrafenib – keratoacanthomas; plantar calluses, seborrheic keratosis, acneiform eruptions, epidermoid cysts, alopecia, verruca vulgaris *BJD 167:1153–1160, 2012*

Halogenoderma – iodides – nasal congestion, conjunctivitis, and a range of systemic symptoms or bromides with weakness, restlessness, headache, ataxia, and personality changes; both produce vegetative nodules or plaques often studded with pustules; in iododerma, the verrucous plaques are often closer to the eye, and in bromoderma, they are below the eye

EXOGENOUS AGENTS

Exogenous calcium from EEG paste *Ped Derm 15:27–30, 1998; Neurology 15:477–480, 1965*

Podoconiosis – silica microparticles in sole; non-filarial lymphedema *JAAD 59:324–331, 2008*

Tattoo – verrucous plaques in white part of tattoo; invasive pseudoepitheliomatous hyperplasia *JAMADerm 153:463–464, 2017; Am J Dermatopathol 25:338–340, 2003*

INFECTIONS AND/OR INFESTATIONS

Acremonium mucorum – mycetoma *JAAD 55:1095–1100, 2006;* verrucous plaque of dorsal hand *Cutis 88:293–295, 2012*

Actinomycosis – cervicofacial, thoracic, abdominal, primary cutaneous, and pelvic

AIDS – neutrophilic dermatosis of AIDS *JAAD 31:1045–1047, 1994*

Alternariosis *BJD 145:484–486, 2001; Clin Inf Dis 32:1178–1187, 2001; Alternaria alternata AD 141:1171–1173, 2005; A. tenuissima* – ulcerated verrucous nodule *BJD 142:840–841, 2000*

Bartonellosis – verruga peruana; bacillary angiomatosis

Bipolaris – verrucous plaque of nasal conchae *J Med Vet Mycol 24:461–465, 1986*

Blastomycosis-like pyoderma (pyoderma vegetans) – crusted or verrucous plaques which may weep, ulcerate, or clear centrally, often involve the flexures, and do not respond to antibiotics alone despite the regular presence of *Staph aureus* or Group A streptococci *Ann Dermatol 23:365–368, 2011; Int J Dermatol 49:1336–1338, 2010; Cutis 84:201–204, 2009; Acta DV 89:186–188, 2009; AD 142:1643–1648, 2006; JAAD 48:456–460, 2003; JAAD 20:691–693, 1989; AD 115:170–173, 1979*

Botryomycosis – usually on the limbs, reported on the trunk, face, and perianal area; causative organisms include *Actinobacillus actinomycetemcomitans, Staphylococcus aureus, Escherichia coli, Proteus spp., Actinobacillus lignieresii*, alpha hemolytic *Streptococcus, Propionibacterium acnes, Serratia marcescens, Peptostreptococcus, Moraxella nonliquefaciens, Neisseria* spp. *Cutis 80:45–47, 2007; Cutis 79:293–296, 2007; JAMA 123:339–341, 1943; JAAD 24:393–396, 1991;* due to *Moraxella nonliquefaciens Cutis 43:140–142, 1989*

Candida parapsilosis – superficial candidiasis; verrucous vegetative nodules of dorsal hands *JAMA Derm 149:1431–1432, 2013*

Candidal granuloma – chronic mucocutaneous candidiasis *JAAD 21:1309–1310, 1989; Ann Rev Med 32:491–497, 1981*

Chromomycosis – verrucous plaques, cauliflower-like masses, nodules, large vegetations; feet, legs, arms, face, and neck; common causative organisms include *Fonsecaea pedrosoi, F. compactum, Phialophora verrucosa, Cladophialophora (Cladosporium) carrionii, Rhinocladiella aquaspersa, Wangiella dermatitidis*, and *R. cerphilum, Exophiala spinifera, Exophiala jeanselmei, Cladophialophora boppii* and *Aureobasidium pullulans*; large pigmented round thick-walled bodies with septation in two planes (muriform cells) *Cutis 102:223, 230–231, 2018; Cutis 101:442,447–448, 2018; Clin Inf Dis 58:1734–1737, 2014; AD 145:195–200, 2009; JAAD 53:931–951, 2005; AD 141:1457–1462, 2005; BJD 152:560–564, 2005; AD 133:1027–1032, 1997; BJD 96:454–458, 1977; AD 104:476–485, 1971; Chaetomium funicola BJD 157:1025–1029, 2007;* psoriasiform plaque due to *Fonsecaea pedrosoi Clin Inf Dis 58:1734–1737, 2014; Cladophialophora bantiana* – renal transplant patient *SkinMed 13:251–254, 2015*

Coccidioidomycosis *JAAD 46:743–747, 2002; AD 134:365–370, 1998;* verrucous facial plaques *JAAD 55:929–942, 2006; Philadelphia Med J5:1471–1472, 1900; An Circ Med Argent 15:585–597, 1892*

Condyloma acuminata *JAAD 66:867–880, 2012*

Cryptococcosis *Clin Inf Dis 56:117, 159–160, 2013; JAAD 32:844–850, 1995; AD 112:1734–1740, 1976; BJD 74:43–49, 1962;* coexistent cryptococcosis and Kaposi's sarcoma in AIDS *Cutis 41:159–162, 1988*

Cytomegalovirus – verrucous plaques occur in patients with AIDS; retinitis and colitis in HIV patients *Dermatology 200:189–195, 2000; JAAD 38:349–351, 1998; JAAD 27:943–950, 1992; AD 125:1243–1246, 1989*

Dermatophyte infection – deep dermatophytosis in inherited autosomal recessive CARD9 deficiency; vegetative plaques, verrucous plaques, and nodules; perianal vegetative plaques *NEJM 1704–1714, 2013*

Ecthyma (RPC-like)

Emmonsia pasteuriana – dimorphic fungus; disseminated infection in South Africa; lichenoid diffuse papulosquamous eruption; crusted verrucous facial nodules and plaques *JAMADerm 151:1263–1264, 2015; NEJM 369:1416–1424, 2013*

Epidermodysplasia verruciformis *BJD 121:463–469, 1989; Arch Dermatol Res 278:153–160, 1985*

Erythrasma – disciform erythrasma

Filariasis

Fusarium solani – granulomatous hyalohyphomycosis due to *Fusarium solani AD 127:1735–1737, 1991*

Granuloma inguinale (*Calymmatobacterium granulomatis*) – pleomorphic non-motile gram negative bacillus; 3–6% have extragenital lesions on the nose, lips, or extremities

Herpes simplex virus – perianal and genital verrucous papules and plaques *JAAD 57:737–763, 2007;* acyclovir-resistant *JAAD 17:875–880, 1987;* herpes simplex and tinea nodule in AIDS *JAAD 16:1151–1154, 1987;* hyperkeratotic plaques of chronic HSV may also be culture positive for other organisms including *Mycobacterium avium-intracellulare* and *Candida*

Herpes zoster – chronic disseminated lesions in AIDS

Histoplasmosis – fever, cough, and skin lesions in the HIV positive patient *Int J Derm 30:104–108, 1991; JAAD 23:422–428, 1990*

Kerion *Ped Derm 21:444–447, 2004*

Leishmaniasis – paronychial verrucous plaque *Ped Derm 33:93–94, 2016*; verrucous plaque of arm *Ped Derm 23:78–80, 2006*; verrucous form of legs; *BJD 151:1165–1171, 2004; JAAD 51:S125–128, 2004; JAAD 48:893–896, 2003; JAAD 27:227–231, 1992*; of face *JAAD 56:612–616, 2007*; verrucous plaques *JAAD 60:897–925, 2009*; leishmaniasis recidivans (lupoid leishmaniasis) – brown-red or brown-yellow papules close to scar of previously healed lesion; resemble lupus vulgaris; may ulcerate or form concentric rings; keloidal form, extensive psoriasiform dermatitis *Cutis 77:25–28, 2006*; espundia (mucocutaneous leishmaniasis) – facial edema, erythema, verrucous plaques, dermatitis, edema of lips *Am J Trop Med Hyg 59:49–52, 1998*; post-kala-azar dermal leishmaniasis *BJD 143:136–143, 2000*; diffuse cutaneous leishmaniasis; *L. aethiopica, L. mexicana* – large hypopigmented areas, xanthomatous appearance, verrucous plaques, leonine facies *JAAD 73:897–908, 2015*; chronic cutaneous tumid leishmaniasis *Clin Dermatol 38:140–151, 2020*

Leprosy *BJD 131:747–748, 1994; Ind J Lepr 64:183–187, 1992*

Lobomycosis (lacaziosis) (*Lacazia loboi*) *Mycoses 55:298–309, 2012; JAAD 53:931–951, 2005; Int J Derm. 32:324–332, 1993*

Malassezia pachydermatis – verrucous plaque of the face *AD 142:1181–1184, 2006*

Molluscum contagiosum in AIDS *JAAD 27:943–950, 1992*

Mycetoma
    Fungi
        Cladophialophora bantiana JAAD 52:S114–117, 2005
        Exophiala jeanselmei
        Madurella mycetomatis
        M. grisea (New World)
        Leptosphaeria senegalensis
        Pyrenochaeta romeroi
        Curvularia lunata
        Pseudallescheria boydii
        Neotestudina rosatii
        Acremonium spp.
        Fusarium spp.
        Dermatophytes
    Aerobic actinomycetes
        Actinomadura madurae
        A. pelletieri
        Streptomyces somaliensis (Sudan and Middle East)
        Nocardia brasiliensis
        N. asteroides (Central America and Mexico)
        N. otitidiscaviarum

Mycobacterium avium complex Cutis 89:175–179, 2012

Mycobacterium marinum-like organism – on island of Satowan, Micronesia *Dermatol Clinics 29:9–13, 2011*

Mycobacterium tuberculosis – tuberculosis verrucosa cutis *Ped Derm 33:264–274, 2016; Dermatol Clin 33:541–562, 2015;*

J Drugs in Dermatol 12:117–118, 2013; SKINmed 10:28–33, 2012; Cutis 87:30–33, 2011; Dermatol Therapy 21:154–161, 2008; Am J Clin Dermatol 3:319–328, 2002; hand (prosector's wart), knees, ankles, buttocks; serpiginous outline with fingerlike projections; central involution and scarring; purplish, red, brown; occasional psoriasiform plaque or keloidal, crusting, and exudation; infiltrated papillomatous excrescences; deep papillomatous and sclerotic forms *AD 142:1221–1226, 2006; Ped Derm 18:393–395, 2001; Clin Exp Dermatol 13:211–220, 1988*; lupus vulgaris *Ped Derm 30:7–16, 2013; Dermatol Clin 26:285–294, 2008; Dermatol Therapy 21:154–161, 2008; Ped Derm 16:264–269, 1999*; hematogenous disseminated tuberculosis – annular verrucous plaques of buttocks, scrotal ulcers, hyperkeratotic plaques of sole *Clin Inf Dis 49:1402–1404, 1450–1451, 2009*; lupus vulgaris *Dermatol Clin 33:541–562, 2015*

Non-tuberculous mycobacterial infection, including *M. marinum Dermatol Therapy 21:154–161, 2008; Cutis 79:33–36, 2007; JAAD 24:208–215, 1991; AD 134:365–370, 1998; M. kansasii JAAD 40:359–363, 1999; JAAD 16:1122–1128, 1987; JAAD 36:497–499, 1997*

Nocardiosis, lymphocutaneous – crusted verrucous plaques with sporotrichoid nodules, abscesses, and pustules *Cutis 85:73–76, 2010*

North American blastomycosis – Mississippi valley; central Kentucky is endemic area; wood debris or soil close to rivers; primary cutaneous, pulmonary, and disseminated forms *Clin Inf Dis 70:973–975, 2020; Cutis 102:363–366, 2018; Practical Dermatology October 2015;pp.33–35; The Dermatologist pp.38–42, May 2013; Clin Inf Dis 55:1390–1391, 1426–1428, 2012*; verrucous nodules of toes *AD 143:653–658, 2007;AD 136:547, 550, 2000; Cutis 58:402–404, 1996; J Cutan Gen Dis 12:496–499, 1894*; ulcerated verrucous plaque *Ped Derm 30:23–28, 2013; NEJM 373:955–961, 2015*; primary cutaneous blastomycosis *Ped Derm 35:671–672, 2018*

Orf – papillomatous stage

Paracoccidioidomycosis (South American blastomycosis) (*Paracoccidioides brasiliensis*) *JAAD 53:931–951, 2005*; near mouth, anus, or genitalia *J Clin Inf Dis 23:1026–1032, 1996*; exophytic verrucous nodules of feet *BJD 158:624–626, 2008*; verrucous multinodular plaque of nose *Clin Dermatol 38:152–159, 2020*

Phaeohyphomycosis – subcutaneous phaeohyphomycosis refers to cyst-like or encapsulated subcutaneous nodular abscesses *JAAD 13:877–881, 1985*; verrucous nodule *JAAD 33:309–311, 1995; Derm Clinics 17:151–185, 1999; Alternaria alternata AD 137:815–820, 2001; JAAD 59:905–907, 2008*; subcutaneous phaeohyphomycosis – *Exophiala jeanselmei, Wangiella, Cladosporium, Bipolaris, Alternaria AD 138:973–978, 2002*; inoculation phaeohyphomycosis of finger and foot; multiple subcutaneous nodules (*Exophiala*) *JAAD 61:977–985, 2009*; disseminated cutaneous phaeohyphomycosis – giant verrucous nodules *Ped Derm 28:30–31, 2011*

Pinta

Prototheocosis *JAAD 31:920–924, 1994; BJD 146:688–693, 2002; Int J Derm 25:54–55, 1986*

Pyoderma

Scabies – crusted scabies – first described in 1848 by Danielssen and Boeck in Norway; seen in patients after renal transplants, with systemic vasculitis, Down's syndrome, collagen vascular disease, corticosteroids (systemic or topical), on immunosuppressive therapy, lymphoreticular malignancy, tabes dorsalis, syringomyelia, Parkinsonism, cerebrovascular disease, diabetes and malnutrition, vitamin A deficiency, Kaposi's sarcoma, and AIDS *BJD 158:1247–1255, 2008; Clin Exp Dermatol 17(5):339–341, 1992;Cutis 43:325–329, 1989*

Schistosomal granuloma, seen especially around the vulva and anus *JAAD 73:929–944, 2015; Derm Clinics 17:151–185, 1999*

Serratia marcescens Cutis 66:461–463, 2000

Sporotrichosis *JAAD 52:451–459, 2005*; fixed cutaneous sporotrichosis *JAAD 53:931–951, 2005; Derm Clinics 17:151–185, 1999; JAAD 25:928–932, 1991, AD 122:413–417, 1986 Ped Derm 3:311–314, 1986*

Syphilis – condyloma lata in toe webs *Cutis 57:38–40, 1996*; nodular secondary syphilis *AD 113:1027–1032, 1997*; annular verrucous perianal dermatitis in secondary syphilis *BJD 152:1343–1345, 2005*; malignant secondary syphilis; tertiary lues (gumma) nodules (arcuate and circinate, psoriasiform, granuloma annulare-like, serpiginous noduloulcerative), gummas (which result in punched out ulcers), gummatous infiltration of the tongue, perforation of the hard palate, destruction of the uvula

Tinea corporis, including invasive *Trichophyton rubrum* infection

Trichosporon dermatis – ulcerated verrucous plaque with draining sinus tracts above ankle *JAAD 65:434–436, 2011*

Tungiasis – verrucous plaque *BJD 144:118–124, 2001*

Tyzzer's disease (*Bacillus piliformis*) – papules *JAAD 34:343–348, 1996*

Varicella – chronic varicella zoster in AIDS *Clin Exp Derm 24:346–353, 1999; JAAD 28:306–308, 1993; JAAD 27:943–950, 1992*

Verrucae vulgaris *BJD 178:527–534, 2018; JAAD 55:907–908, 2006; JAAD 55:533–535, 2006; AD 140:13–14, 2004; JAAD 43:340–343, 2000; Cutis 63:91–94, 1999; JAAD 36:850–852, 1997*; large verrucae in selective IgM deficiency, immunoglobulin deficiency with hyper IgM; condyloma acuminate; giant disseminated verrucosis (HPV2) (giant verrucous claw hands and feet, annular plaques of trunk) associated with idiopathic CD4 lymphopenia *AD 146:69–73, 2010*; in AIDS *Clin Dermatol 38:160–175, 2020*

SYNDROMES WITH EXTENSIVE WARTS

AD 144:366–372, 2008

Clouston syndrome – alopecia, hyperpigmentation, sparse facial and body hair, dystrophic nails, keratoderma, mental retardation
Common variable immunodeficiency *JAAD 66:292–311, 2012*
GATA2 deficiency
Klinefelter syndrome – infertile, small testes, sparse facial and body hair, delayed motor function, gynecomastia
Mulvihill-Smith syndrome – low birth weight, growth delays, premature aged facial appearance, multiple pigmented nevi, hearing impairment, mental retardation
Netherton's syndrome
WHIM syndrome – warts, hypogammaglobulinema, infections, myelokathexis *AD 144:366–372, 2008*
WILD syndrome – disseminated warts, diminished cell-mediated immunity, primary lymphedema, anogenital dysplasia; perianal hypertrophic plaque *AD 144:366–372, 2008*
Wiskott-Aldrich syndrome
X-linked hyper-IgM immunodeficiency syndrome – oral ulcers, pneumonia, yaws (mother yaw) – *Treponema pallidum* subsp. *pertenue*; 10–13 micron long by .15 micron wide; replicate in 30 hours; non-venereal; transmitted by skin contact; primarily in children; primary lesions on feet, legs, and buttocks; Africa, Asia, South and Central America, and Pacific Islands *JAAD 29:519–535, 1993; Cutis 38:303–305, 1986*

INFILTRATIVE

Amyloidosis – lichen amyloidosis

Osteoma cutis – congenital plate-like osteoma cutis *Ped Derm 10:182–186, 1993; AD 69:613–615, 1954*

Verrucous (verruciform) xanthoma – normolipemic; most commonly on mucosal surfaces, especially the oral mucosa; also nose, axilla, neck, and scalp; may be multifocal or associated with lymphedema; seen in CHILD syndrome and with ILVEN; may be a non-X histiocytosis; scrotum, penis, vulva, anogenital area, sacrum, digits, periorificial, and on lymphedematous extremity *Cutis 91:198–202, 2013; Ped Derm 29:113–114, 2012; AD 147:1087–1092, 2011; Int J Derm 46:955–959, 2007; AD 138:689–694, 2002; JAAD 27:1021–1023, 1992; Am J Surg Pathol 22:479–487, 1998; Histopathology 9:245–252, 1985; J Cut Pathol 20:84–86, 1993; AD 118:686–691,*

1982; of glans penis *Genital Skin Disorders, Fischer and Margesson, CV Mosby, 1998, p. 80; Cutis 51:369–372, 1993;* of the scrotum *BJD 150:161–163, 2004;* of scalp *AD 143:1067–1072, 2007;* in recessive dystrophic epidermolysis bullosa *Ped Derm 26:747–748,2009*

Xanthoma disseminatum (Montgomery's syndrome) – red-yellow-brown papules and nodules of flexural surfaces, trunk, face, proximal extremities, and oral mucosa; become confluent into xanthomatous plaques; verrucous plaques *JAAD 56:302–316, 2007; NEJM 338:1138–1143, 1998; JAAD 23:341–346, 1990; AD Syphilol 37:373–402, 1938*

INFLAMMATORY

Mucinous syringometaplasia (papules) – mimics plantar wart or verruca vulgaris; metaplastic mucin containing cells lining glandular structures *JAAD 11:503–508, 1984*

Pseudoverrucous peristomal dermatitis (urostomy) – skin surrounding urostomy site may be normal or may show erythematous-erosive lesions or pseudoverrucous lesions *JAAD 19:623–628, 1988*

Pyoderma gangrenosum

Pyoderma vegetans – vegetating tissue reaction with localized bacterial infection in immune-compromised patient; associated with ulcerative colitis, defective cellular immunity, cutaneous T-cell lymphoma, large cell lymphoma, alcoholism; *Staph aureus* or beta hemolytic Strep common *J Cut Med Surg 5:223–227, 2001; JAAD 20:691–693, 1989*

Rosai-Dorfman disease (sinus histiocytosis with massive lymphadenopathy) – verrucous plaques with satellite lesions *JAAD 51:931–939, 2004; Semin Diagn Pathol 7:19–73, 1990*

Sarcoidosis *Dermatol Clin 33:509–630, 2015; JAAD 66:699–716, 2012; AD 133:882–888, 1997; AD 102:665–669, 1970;* mimicking hypertrophic lichen planus *Int J Derm 28:539–541, 1989*

Superficial granulomatous (vegetating) pyoderma *AD 136:1263–1268, 2000; JAAD 18:11–21, 1988*

Toxic epidermal necrolysis – healing with verrucous hyperplasia *BJD 149:1082–1083, 2003*

METABOLIC

Calcinosis cutis – overlying verrucous changes *Ann Acad Med Singapore 33:107–109, 2004*

Necrolytic acral erythema – cutaneous marker for hepatitis C; serpiginous, psoriasiform hyperpigmented, hyperkeratotic verrucous plaques of acral palmar, plantar, dorsal surfaces of hands and feet; darker, more velvety and verrucous than psoriasis *JAAD 53:247–251, 2005; AD 141:85–87, 2005; Int J Derm 44:916–921, 2005; JAAD 50:s121–124, 2004, Int J Derm 35:252–256, 1996*

Thyroid acropachy

Pretibial myxedema *JAAD 46:723–726, 2002*

NEOPLASTIC

Acrosyringeal epidermolytic papulosis neviformis *Dermatologica 171:122–125, 1985*

Actinic keratosis

Adnexal tumors

Anal intraepithelial neoplasia – verrucous perianal hyperpigmented patches, white and/or red plaques *JAAD 52:603–608, 2005*

Anogenital carcinoma *BJD 143:1217–1223, 2000*

Basal cell carcinoma

Bowen's disease – of the foot *AD 123:1517–1520, 1987;* of both feet *BJD 151:227–228, 2004*

Clear cell acanthoma

Collagenome perforans verruciforme – may occur in scars; transepidermal elimination disorder; other transepidermal elimination disorders include calcinosis cutis, chondrodermatitis nodularis chronica helicis, reactive perforating collagenosis, elastosis perforans serpiginosa, granuloma annulare, perforating folliculitis, blastomycosis, chromomycosis, botryomycosis, tuberculosis, histoplasmosis *Ped Derm 36:739–740, 2019; AD 122:1044–1046, 1986; Ann DV 90:29–36, 1963*

Connective tissue nevus – mimicking epidermal nevus *JAAD 16:264–266, 1987;* purplish verrucous plantar plaque *BJD 146:164–165, 2002*

Dermatofibroma

Eccrine angiomatous hamartoma *BJD 141:167–169, 1999; Dermatologica 143:100–104, 1971*

Eccrine dermal duct tumor

Eccrine poroma

Eccrine porocarcinoma (porocarcinoma) *BJD 152:1051–1055, 2005;*

JAAD 49:S252–254, 2003; JAAD 27:306–311, 1992

Eccrine syringofibroadenoma (acrosyringeal hamartoma) – tapioca pudding-like or mosaic surface; multiple lesions associated with hidrotic ectodermal dysplasia; ESFA associated with other tumors – papillary syringocystadenoma, clear cell acanthoma, verrucous eccrine poroma *JAAD 41:650–651, 1999; JAAD 36:569–576, 1997; AD 126:945–949, 1990;* reactive peristomal eccrine syringofibroadenoma – cerebriform verrucous plaque *JAAD 58:691–696, 2008*

Epidermal nevus *Ped Derm 16:211–213, 1999; JAAD 41:824–826, 1999;* epidermal nevus syndrome *J Clin Diagn Res 9:WD01–WD02, 2015; Ped Clin North Amer 57:1177–1198, 2010; Seminar Cutan Med surg 26:221–230, 2007; Ophthalmol Plast Reconstr Surg 10:262–266, 1994*

Epidermoid cyst

Erythroplasia of Queyrat *JAAD 37:1–24, 1997*

Fibroepithelioma of Pinkus *AD 134:861–866, 1998*

Granular cell tumor (nodule) *Cutis 69:343–346, 2002; Cutis 62:147–148, 1998; Cutis 43:548–550, 1989*

Hidroacanthoma simplex – extremities *J Cutan Pathol 21:274–279, 1994*

Infundibulocystic hyperplasia – hyperkeratotic lichen planus-like reactions combined with infundibulocystic hyperplasia *AD 140:1262–1267, 2004*

ILVEN – inflammatory linear verrucous epidermal nevus *J Dermatol 26:599–602, 1999; AD 133:567–568, 1997*

Intraepidermal pilar epithelioma *JAAD 18:123–132, 1988; Cutis 37:339–341, 1986*

Kaposi's sarcoma – verrucous nodules and plaques; hyperkeratotic Kaposi's sarcoma in AIDS with massive lymphedema *BJD 142:501–505, 2000; JAAD 38:143–175, 1998*

Keratoacanthoma – giant type, multiple keratoacanthomas; keratoacanthoma centrifugum marginatum *Cutis 73:257–262, 2004; JAAD 48:282–285, 2003; JAAD 30:1–19, 1994; AD 111:1024–1026, 1975; Hautarzt 13:348–352, 1962*

Large cell acanthomas *JAAD 8:840–845, 1983*

Lymphoma – cutaneous T-cell lymphoma *JAAD 60:359–375, 2009;* cutaneous T-cell lymphoma – verrucous plaque of the nose with red facial plaques *NEJM 372:2437, 2015;AD 140:441–447, 2004; J Eur Acad Derm Venereol 18:218–220, 2004; JAAD 46:325–357, 2002; Am J Dermatopathol 21:518–524, 1999; Clin Exp Derm 21:205–208, 1996; AD 124:655–657, 1988; AD 113:57–60, 1977;* Ki+1(CD 30) anaplastic lymphoma *AD 136:1559–1564, 2000;* anaplastic large cell lymphoma *Ped Derm 29:498–503, 2012;* CD8+ cytotoxic cutaneous T-cell lymphoma *NEJM 357:2496–2505, 2007;* primary cutaneous diffuse large cell B-cell lymphoma, leg type – verrucous plaques *Clin Exp Dermatol 35:e87–89, 2010;* Woringer-Kolopp disease (pagetoid reticulosis) – verrucous psoriasiform plaque of the leg *JAMADerm 156:585–586, 2020; Ann Dermatol Syphilol 67:945–958, 1939*

Malignant fibrous histiocytoma in DLE *AD 124:114–116, 1988*

Melanocytic nevus *Eyelid and Conjunctival Tumors, Shields JA and Shields CL, Lippincott Williams and Wilkins, 1999, p.80;* congenital melanocytic *Hum Pathol 4:395–418, 1973;* inflammatory nevi evolving into halo nevi in children *BJD 152:357–360, 2005*

Melanoma (verrucous melanoma) *Histopathology 23:453–458, 1993; JAAD 24:505–506, 1991; AD 124:1534–1537, 1988;* acral lentiginous melanoma *JAAD 48:183–188, 2003*

Metastatic carcinoma – personal observation

Mucinous nevus *BJD 148:1064–1066, 2003*

Neurocristic hamartoma – verrucous blue plaque *JAAD 49:924–929, 2003*

Nevoid hyperkeratosis of the nipple *JAAD 46:414–418, 2002*

Nevus lipomatosus superficialis *Ped Derm 20:313–314, 2003; AD Syphilol 130:327, 1921*

Nevus marginatus – red plaque with surrounding hyperpigmented serpiginous verrucous margin; *HRAS* mutation *BJD 168:892–894, 2013*

Nevus sebaceus *Curr Prob in Derm 8:137–188, 1996*

Nevus tricholemmocysticus – multiple pilar cysts; filiform hyperkeratoses of the face and arm, comedo-like plugs, osteomalacia, bone lesions; verrucous papules, yellow plaques, cysts; Blaschko distribution *Ped Derm 28:286–289, 2011; JAAD 57(Suppl):S72–77, 2007*

Pagetoid reticulosis *JAAD 59:706–712, 2008; AD 125:402–406, 1989; Ann Dermatol Syph 10:945–958, 1939*

  Two variants – (1) Localized – Woringer-Kolopp disease. (2) Generalized – Ketron-Goodman disease; intraepidermal large atypical cells expressing CD 30 (Ki-1) antigen; small lymphocytes in dermis

Papillomatosis cutis carcinoides *Cutis 62:77–80, 1998*

Plasmacytoma – extramedullary plasmacytoma *JAAD 34:146–148, 1996*

Porokeratosis of Mibelli – hyperkeratotic variant *Cutis 72:391–393, 2003; Arch Derm Res 279 Suppl:S38–47, 1987;* linear porokeratosis *Ped Derm 21:682–683, 2004;* perianal inflammatory verrucous porokeratosis (porokeratosis ptychotropica) – hyperpigmented verrucous plaques of intertriginous areas *JAMADerm 155:845, 2019; Australasian J Derm 58:e149–150, 2017; JAMA Derm 149:1099–1100, 2013; AD 146:911–916, 2010; BJD 140:553–555, 1999; BJD 132:150–151, 1995*

Porokeratotic eccrine ostial and dermal duct nevus (filiform wartlike lesions) – Blaschko red plaque with hyperkeratosis *Ped Derm 26:473–474, 2009; JAAD 43:364–367, 2000; JAAD 24:300–301, 1991; Cutis 46:495–497, 1990; AD 122:892–895, 1986;* generalized porokeratotic eccrine ostial and dermal duct nevus – Blaschko-distributed verrucous plaques; non-scarring alopecia, hypohidrosis, teeth in disarray, deafness *JAAD 59:S43–45, 2008*

Poroma – acral verrucous papule of fingertip *AD 144:1051–1056, 2008*

Seboacanthoma – verrucous sessile papules *AD 84:642–644, 1961*

Seborrheic keratosis – giant lesion mimicking verrucous carcinoma *J Dermatol 12:341–343, 1985*

Seborrheic keratosis – malignancies arising in seborrheic keratoses include adenocarcinoma, squamous cell carcinoma in situ (Bowen's disease), squamous cell carcinoma, basal cell carcinoma, keratoacanthomas, and malignant melanoma *AD 127:1738–1739, 1991*

Squamous cell carcinoma – giant verrucous plaque of the face and scalp *BJD 176:498–502, 2017; Derm Surg 22:243–254, 1996;* associated with human papillomavirus 16, 18 *AD 127:1813–1818, 1991; AD 125:666–669, 1989;* vulvar squamous cell carcinoma – papular and polypoid lesions; verrucous white cobblestoned plaque *JAAD 66:867–880, 2012;* of nail bed *JAAD 69:253–261, 2013*

Superficial acral fibromyxoma – verrucous changes of papules of fingers, toes, palms and soles *BJD 159:1315–1321, 2008*

Syringocystadenocarcinoma papilliferum *AD 138:1091–1096, 2002;* cauliflower-like verrucous plaque *JAAD 45:755–759, 2001;*

verrucous linear plaque *AD 71:361–372, 1955;* linear multilobulated verrucous plaque *Ped Derm 28:61–62, 2011;* verrucous papules of upper lip *Sultan Qaboos Univ Med J 14:e575–577, 2014*

Trichoadenoma of the forehead – linear yellow verrucous L-shaped plaque *JAAD 57:905–906, 2007;* solitary verrucous trichoadenoma, resembling seborrheic keratosis *J Cutan Pathol 16:145–148, 1989*

Vascular and myxoid fibromas of the fingers (papules)

Verrucous carcinoma – epithelioma cuniculatum *NEJM 352:488, 2005; AD 136:547–548, 550–551, 2000;* ulcerated verrucous plaque of the sole *JAAD 54:S233–235, 2006;* giant condyloma of Buschke-Lowenstein – penis *AD 145:950–952, 2009;* groin or perianal *Cutis 96:82,89–90, 2015; Cutis 24:203–206,209, 1979;* oral florid papillomatosis *NEJM 372:2049, 2015; JAAD 32:1–21, 1995; JAAD 14:947–950, 1986; Int J Derm 18:608–622, 1979;* sacrum *BJD 143:459–460, 2000;* of leg *JAAD 57:516–519, 2007;* of leg amputation stump *Dermatologica 182:193–195, 1991;* of feet and legs *JAAD 56:S2–32, 2007;* of the scalp *JAAD 56:506–507, 2007;* arising in a burn scar *Cutis 79:133–135, 2007;* of lip *BJD 157:813–815, 2007*

Verrucous cyst *Eur J Dermatol 8:186–188, 1998*

Verrucous perforating collagenoma – red verrucous plaque *Ped Derm 36:739–740, 2019; Ann DV 90:29–36, 1963*

PARANEOPLASTIC DISEASES

Acanthosis nigricans, malignant – verrucous papules at corners of mouth *Cutis 89:14–16, 2012; BJD 153:667–668, 2005*

Bazex syndrome

Florid cutaneous papillomatosis – generalized; multiple 0.5–1 cm verrucous papules distributed over the hands, wrists, ankles, and lower legs *JAAD 57:907–908, 2007;* palmar *Rook p.1555, 1998 Sixth Edition*

Keratoacanthoma visceral carcinoma syndrome – cancers of the genitourinary tract *AD 139:1363–1368, 2003; AD 120:123–124, 1984*

Necrobiotic xanthogranuloma with paraproteinemia – periorbital site most common, but multiple lesions always present; ulceration common; central clearing and atrophy; IgG-kappa most common,

then IgG-lambda; mucous membrane, lung, myocardial lesions, and associated lymphoreticular malignancy

AD 128:94–100, 1992

Paraneoplastic pemphigus *JAAD 39:876–871, 1998*

PRIMARY CUTANEOUS DISEASE

Acanthosis nigricans

Acral mucinous syringometaplasia – associated with verrucous hyperplasia *Arch Pathol Lab Med 110:248–249, 1986*

Adolescent onset ichthyosiform erythroderma – verrucous rippling *BJD 144:1063–1066, 2001*

Atopic dermatitis

Confluent and reticulated papillomatosis *J Dermatol 31:682–686, 2004*

Darier's disease (keratosis follicularis) *Clin Dermatol 19:193–205, 1994; JAAD 27:40–50, 1992;* of foot *Caputo, 2000, p.124*

Dermatitis – personal observation

Epidermolysis bullosa pruriginosa – mild acral blistering at birth or early childhood; violaceous papular and nodular lesions in linear array on shins, forearms, trunk; lichenified hypertrophic and verrucous plaques in adults *BJD 130:617–625, 1994*

Epidermolytic hyperkeratosis – overlying bony prominences, scalp, nipples

Erythema elevatum diutinum *JAAD 50:652–653, 2004;* of knuckles *BJD 164:675–677, 2011*

Granular parakeratosis (axillary (or submammary) granular hyperkeratosis) (axillary granular parakeratosis) *Cutis 80:55–56, 2007; AD 137:1241–1246, 2001; JAAD 40:813–814, 1999; JAAD 39:495–496, 1998; JAAD 33:373–375, 1995; JAAD 37:789–790, 1997; JAAD 24:541–544, 1991*

Perforating granuloma annulare – personal observation

Hailey-Hailey disease – genital papules *JAAD 26:951–955, 1992*

Hyperkeratosis of the nipple (hyperkeratosis areolae mammae) *JAAD 41:274–276, 1999; AD 113:1691–1692, 1977*

Ichthyosis hystrix, Curth-Macklin type – hyperkeratotic lesions of elbows, knees in parallel grooves (zebra stripe pattern); verrucous plaques; exophytic spiky hyperkeratosis; palmoplantar keratoderma; *KRT1* mutation *BJD 168:456–458 2013AD 147:999–1001, 2011; AD 141:779–784, 2005; Am J Hum Genet 6:371–382, 1954*

Kyrle's disease – chronic scattered generalized papules with hyperkeratotic cone shaped plugs; chronic genetically determined disorder *JAAD 16:117–123, 1987*

Keratosis lichenoides chronica *JAAD 49:511–513, 2003; BJD 144:422–424, 2001; AD 129:914–915, 1993; AD 105:739–743, 1972*

Lichen myxedematosus

Lichen planus – hypertrophic lichen planus *The Dermatologist June 2019, p. 47–49; AD 139:933–938, 2003*

Lichen sclerosus et atrophicus *JAAD 38:831–833, 1998*

Lichen simplex chronicus, including giant lichenification of Pautrier – genitocrural lichenification with solid tumorous plaques with verrucous cribriform surface *AD Syphilol 39:1012–1020, 1939*

Lichen striatus

Malignant pyoderma – rare potentially lethal disease characterized by necrotizing pyodermatous ulcers predominantly involving the face, neck, and upper trunk with a predilection for the preauricular areas; malignant pyoderma is distinct from pyoderma gangrenosum with an unrelenting destructive progression if untreated, a different clinical distribution, an earlier age of onset, a lack of deeply undermined necrotic borders, and the lack of association with any underlying diseases *Int J Derm 26:42, 1987*

Palmoplantar keratodermas

Perianal pseudoverrucous papules and nodules in children – perianal hypertrophic plaques *Cutis 67:335–338, 2001; AD 128:240–242, 1992*

Periumbilical pseudoxanthoma elasticum – verrucous plaque *JAAD 39:338–344, 1998; South Med J 84:788–789, 1991*

Prurigo nodularis

Pseudoepitheliomatous keratotic and micaceous balanitis *Cutis 35:77–79, 1985; Bull Soc Fr Dermatolog Syphiligr 68:164–167, 1961*

Psoriasis, elephantine, rupioid *Am J Dermatopathol 27:204–207, 2005*

Seborrheic dermatitis – personal observation

Progressive symmetric erythrokeratoderma

Urostomy site – pseudoverrucous peristomal lesions – warty papules at mucocutaneous junction *JAAD 19:623–632, 1988*

Terra firme (dermatosis neglecta) *AD 135:728–729, 1999*; verrucous plaque of distal shaft of penis *Ped Derm 33:455–456, 2016*

PSYCHOCUTANEOUS DISEASES

Factitial cheilitis – cobblestoned lips *Ped Derm 16:12–15, 1999*

SYNDROMES

CHILD syndrome – verruciform xanthoma giant red plaque of lateral foot; cobblestoned, verrucous giant tumor; enlarged foot; exophytic mass; X-linked dominant; mutation in *NSDHL* (NAD(P)-dependent steroid dehydrogenase-like gene) *Cutis 88:269–272, 2012; Ped Derm 27:551–553, 2010; Ped Derm 15:360–366, 1998*; verruciform xanthoma – Blaschko red cobblestoned verrucous hypertrophic plaque of the vulva with linear extension onto leg *Ped Derm 32:135–137, 2015*

Cobb's syndrome (cutaneomeningospinal angiomatosis) – segmental port wine stain and vascular malformation of the spinal cord *AD 113:1587–1590, 1977; NEJM 281:1440–1444, 1969; Ann Surg 62:641–649, 1915*; port wine stain may be keratotic *Dermatologica 163:417–425, 1981*; angiokeratoma-like lesions *Cutis 71:283–287, 2003*; with verrucous hemangioma *Dermatologica 163:417–425, 1981*

Ectodermal dysplasias

Focal epithelial hyperplasia – verrucous papules of lips, tongue, hard palate, buccal mucosa *Ped Derm 26:465–468, 2009*

Gall-Galli syndrome – Dowling-Degos disease with acantholysis – hyperkeratotic follicular papules *JAAD 45:760–763, 2001*

Garcia-Hafner-Happle syndrome – fibroblast growth factor receptor 3 epidermal nevus syndrome *BJD 166:202–204, 2012*

Goltz's syndrome (focal dermal hypoplasia) (papule) –

X-linked dominant, possible autosomal dominant; terminal deletion of the short arm of the X chromosome; cutaneous, musculoskeletal (80%), ocular (80%), and oral abnormalities; hypoplastic and atrophic skin changes, linear and reticulated hypo- and hyperpigmentation, lipomatous lesions, periorificial and mucous membrane papillomas and telangiectasias; xerosis, photosensitivity, nail changes, alopecia, sparse brittle hair; musculoskeletal involvement

includes syndactyly, hypoplastic or absent digits, asymmetry of the body, scoliosis, hand and foot bony anomalies; ocular changes include colobomas, microphthalmia, strabismus, nystagmus, lens subluxation; oral anomalies include enamel defects, dysplastic teeth, irregular spacing, agenesis of teeth, oral papillomas, microdontia, high-arched palate *JAAD 28:839–843, 1993*

Haber's syndrome – rosacea-like acneiform eruption, verrucous papules (seborrheic keratosis-like) of flexures, palmoplantar keratoderma, perioral pitted scars *BJD 160:215–217, 2009*

Hyper IgE syndrome (Buckley's syndrome)

Incontinentia pigmenti – X-linked dominant. Xp28 or Xp11.21 locations; progressive persistent verrucous plaques; skin lesions present in 50% at birth and in 90% by 2 weeks of life; dental abnormalities in 2/3 of patients, ocular in 25–35%, and CNS defects in 1/3 *JAAD 47:169–187, 2002; AD 124:29–30, 1988*; verrucous subungual lesions *Dermatol 191(2):161–163, 1995; AD 122: 1431–1434, 1986*; linear warty lesions of palms in late incontinentia pigmenti *BJD 143:1102–1103, 2000*

Keratitis-ichthyosis-deafness (KID) syndrome – autosomal recessive; verrucous plaques of the elbows, knees, face, helices, scalp, groin, skin over joints, dorsal feet; dotted waxy, fine granular, stippled, or reticulated surface pattern of severe diffuse hyperkeratosis of the palms and soles (palmoplantar keratoderma), ichthyosis with well marginated, serpiginous erythematous verrucous plaques, hyperkeratotic elbows and knees, perioral furrows, leukoplakia, follicular occlusion triad, scalp cysts, nodules (trichilemmal tumors, squamous cell carcinoma), bilateral sensorineural deafness, photophobia with vascularizing keratitis, blindness, hypotrichosis of the scalp, eyebrows, and eyelashes, dystrophic nails, chronic mucocutaneous candidiasis, otitis externa, abscesses, blepharitis; connexin 26 or connexin 30 mutation *JAAD 69:127–134, 2013; Ped Derm 27:651–652, 2010; Ped Derm 23:81–83, 2006; JAAD 51:377–382, 2004; BJD 148:649–653, 2003; Cutis 72:229–230, 2003; Ped Derm 19:285–292, 2002; Ped Derm 15:219–221, 1998; Ped Derm 13:105–113, 1996; JAAD 19:1124–1126, 1988; AD 123:777–782, 1987; AD 117:285–289, 1981; J Cutaneous Dis 33:255–260, 1915*

Klippel-Trenaunay-Weber – angiokeratomas; epidermal nevi *BJD 123:539, 1990*

Lipoid proteinosis (Urbach-Wiethe disease) – autosomal recessive; yellow verrucous plaques and nodules on extensor surfaces and sides of fingers; asymptomatic visceral involvement of multiple organs; extracellular hyaline-like material in dermis; PAS positive and diastase resistant; probably represents glycoproteins and/or proteoglycan complexes *JAMADerm 155:977–979, 2019; BJD 151:413–423, 2004; JID 120:345–350, 2003; BJD 148:180–182, 2003; Hum Molec Genet 11:833–840, 2002; JAAD 39:149–171, 1998; Ped Derm 14:22–25, 1997; JAAD 21:599–601, 605, 1989*

Mal de Meleda – keratotic (verrucous) plaques of the elbows *AD 136:1247–1252, 2000*

McCune-Albright syndrome – epidermal nevi *Eur J Pediatr 154:102–104, 1995*

Netherton's syndrome – flexural verrucous hypertrophy

Olmsted syndrome (nose and lips) – congenital palmoplantar and periorificial keratoderma which improves in adolescence; linear keratoses in flexures; keratosis pilaris-like lesions; leukokeratosis of the tongue; alopecia, onychodystrophy, anhidrosis of the palms and soles; missing premolar; hyperlaxity of the joints *Ped Derm 21:603–605, 2004; Ped Derm 20:323–326, 2003; BJD 136:935–938, 1997; AD 132:797–800, 1996; AD 131:738–739, 1995; JAAD 10:600–610, 1984*

Pachyonychia congenita *Ped Derm 14:491–493, 1997*

Phakomatosis pigmentokeratotica – coexistence of an organoid nevus (epidermal nevus/nevus sebaceus) and a contralateral segmental lentiginous or papular speckled lentiginous nevus (nevus spilus) *SkinMed 11:125–128, 2013; Dermatology 194: 77–79, 1997*

Phakomatosis pigmentovascularis – port wine stain, oculocutaneous (dermal and scleral) melanosis, CNS manifestations; type I – port wine stain and linear epidermal nevus; type II – port wine stain and dermal melanocytosis; type III – port wine stain and nevus spilus; type IV – port wine stain, dermal melanocytosis, and nevus spilus *J Dermatol 26:834–836, 1999; AD 121:651–653, 1985*

Proteus syndrome – epidermal nevi, port wine stains, subcutaneous hemangiomas and lymphangiomas, lymphangioma circumscriptum, hemihypertrophy of the face, limbs, trunk; macrodactyly, cerebriform hypertrophy of palmar and/or plantar surfaces, macrocephaly *JAAD 52:834–838, 2005; AD 140:947–953, 2004; AD 137:219–224, 2001*, sebaceous nevi with hyper- or hypopigmentation *Am J Med Genet 27:99–117, 1987;* vascular nevi, soft subcutaneous masses; lipodystrophy, café au lait macules, linear and whorled macular pigmentation *Arch Fr Pediatr 47:441–444, 1990(French); Am J Med Genet 27:87–97, 1987; Pediatrics 76:984–989, 1985; Eur J Pediatr 140:5–12, 198;*

Reactive arthritis syndrome – keratoderma blenorrhagicum; soles, pretibial areas, dorsal toes, feet, fingers, hands, nails, scalp *Semin Arthritis Rheum 3:253–286, 1974*

Rothmund-Thomson syndrome (poikiloderma congenitale) – autosomal recessive; photodistributed poikiloderma with juvenile cataracts, short stature, absent or shortened digits, partial or total alopecia, defects of nails and teeth, hypogonadism, triangular face, verrucous hyperkeratoses of the hands, feet, knees, and elbows *Ped Derm 8:58–60, 1991; JAAD 17:332–338, 1987*

Sjogren-Larsson syndrome – verrucous hyperkeratosis of flexures, neck, and periumbilical folds; mental retardation, spastic diplegia, short stature, kyphoscoliosis, retinal changes, yellow pigmentation, intertrigo – deficiency of fatty aldehyde dehydrogenase *Chem Biol Interact 130–132:297–307, 2001; Am J Hum Genet 65:1547–1560, 1999; JAAD 35:678–684, 1996*

WILD syndrome – disseminated warts, diminished cell-mediated immunity, primary lymphedema, anogenital dysplasia; perianal hypertrophic plaque *AD 144:366–372, 2008*

TOXIC

Arsenical keratosis

Foreign body granuloma

TRAUMA

Verrucous hyperplasia of the amputation stump *AD 74:448–449, 1956*

VASCULAR

Angiokeratomas

Angiokeratoma corporis diffusum with normal enzyme activities *AD 140:353–358, 2004*

Angiosarcoma *Histopathology 32:556–561, 1998*

Arteriovenous malformation – personal observation

Chylous reflux – from dilated chylous vesicles (lymphatics); yellow/cream-colored verrucous plaques

Elephantiasis nostras verrucosa *Cutis 62:77–80, 1998; Int J Derm 20:177–187, 1981*

Fibroangioma – digital verrucous fibroangioma – verrucous papule *Acta DV 72:303–304, 1992*

Glomus tumor, plaque type *BJD 127:411–416, 1992; J Dermatol 17:423–428, 1990*

Hemangioma – cutaneous keratotic hemangioma *AD 132:703–708, 1996;* verrucous hemangioma – verrucous plaque of the leg *JAMADerm 152:1269–1270, 2016;* verrucous plaque of the heel *Cutis 99:158,169, 2017;* keratotic blue plaque *BJD 171:466–473, 2014; AD 132:703–708, 1996; Int J Surg Pathol 2:171–176, 1995; J Derm Surg Oncol 13:1089–1092, 1987; Ped Derm 2:191–193, 1985; AD 96:247–253, 1967;* linear *JAAD 42:516–518, 2000*

Lymphatic malformations

Lymphangioma circumscriptum (localized microcystic lymphatic malformations) *JAAD 56:353–370, 2007; Ped Derm 16:423–429, 1999;* blue-black *BJD 83:519–527, 1970;* perianal verrucous plaque *Pediatrics 98:461–463, 1996;* acquired lymphangioma (lymphangiectasia) – due to scarring processes such as recurrent infections, radiotherapy, scrofuloderma, scleroderma, keloids, tumors, tuberculosis, repeated trauma *BJD 132:1014–1016, 1996*

Lymphedema, congenital (Milroy's disease), lymphedema praecox, lymphedema tarda *BJD 163:1358–1360, 2010*

Lymphostasis verrucosa cutis (chronic lymphedema, multiple causes) – brawny edema with overlying hyperkeratosis *NEJM 370:2520, 2014; BJD 163:1358–1360, 2010*

Pseudo-Kaposi's sarcoma due to arteriovenous fistula (Stewart-Bluefarb syndrome) – ulcerated purple plaque *Ped Derm 18:325–327, 2001; AD 121:1038–1040, 1985*

Pyogenic granuloma

Stasis dermatitis

Vasculitis

Verrucous localized lymphedema of the penis, scrotum, vulva, pubis, *JAAD 71:320–326, 2014*

Verrucous lymphovascular malformation – verrucous plaque of toes *Cutis 81:390–396, 2008*

Verrucous venous malformation *JAAD 80:556–558, 2019*

VULVA, HYPERTROPHIC, AND/OR EDEMATOUS LESIONS

AUTOIMMUNE DISEASES AND DISEASES OF IMMUNE DYSFUNCTION

Allergic contact dermatitis *Genital Skin Disorders, Fischer and Margesson, CV Mosby, 1998, p. 224;* unilateral vulvar edema *Ped Derm 22:554–557, 2005*

Angioedema *Genital Skin Disorders, Fischer and Margesson, CV Mosby, 1998, p. 224*

Lupus erythematosus – hypertrophic discoid lupus erythematosus

Pemphigus vegetans – giant vegetative plaque of the vulva; IgG anti-desmocollin-3 antibodies *JAMA Derm 149:1209–1213, 2013*

CONGENITAL LESIONS

Congenital labial hypertrophy *Genital Skin Disorders, Fischer and Margesson, CV Mosby, 1998, p. 111*

DRUG REACTIONS

Fixed drug eruption *Genital Skin Disorders, Fischer and Margesson, CV Mosby, 1998, p. 163*

EXOGENOUS AGENTS

Benzocaine – erosive papulonodular vulvar dermatitis *JAAD 55:S74–80, 2006*

INFECTIONS AND INFESTATIONS

Abscess – Bartholin's duct; vulvar edema *Genital Skin Disorders, Fischer and Margesson, CV Mosby, 1998, p. 224*

Actinomycosis – vulvar edema *Genital Skin Disorders, Fischer and Margesson, CV Mosby, 1998, p. 224*

Amebiasis – vegetating plaque of the genitalia, perineum, and anus *Derm Clinics 17:151–185, 1999;* vulvar edema *Genital Skin Disorders, Fischer and Margesson, CV Mosby, 1998, p. 224*

Bejel – condylomata

Candidiasis – vulvar edema *Genital Skin Disorders, Fischer and Margesson, CV Mosby, 1998, p. 224;* unilateral vulvar edema *Ped Derm 22:554–557, 2005*

Cellulitis (streptococcal) – chronic edema *Genital Skin Disorders, Fischer and Margesson, CV Mosby, 1998, p. 222–224*

Chronic infection – lymphedema *Genital Skin Disorders, Fischer and Margesson, CV Mosby, 1998, p. 222–223*

Condylomata acuminata *Genital Skin Disorders, Fischer and Margesson, CV Mosby, 1998, p. 128–130;* condylomata acuminate and molluscum contagiosum *SKINmed 12:310–311, 2014*

Entamoeba histolytica – multilobulated vulvar nodule (late cutaneous) *JAMADerm 156:96–97, 2020*

Enterobiasis – unilateral vulvar edema *Ped Derm 22:554–557, 2005*

Filariasis – vulvar edema *Genital Skin Disorders, Fischer and Margesson, CV Mosby, 1998, p. 224*

Granuloma inguinale (*Klebsiella granulomatis*) – multilobulated vulvar nodule *JAMADerm 156:96–97, 2020;* vulvar edema *Genital Skin Disorders, Fischer and Margesson, CV Mosby, 1998, p. 224; PNG Med J 25:283–285, 1982*

Herpes simplex virus – perianal and genital verrucous papules and plaques *JAAD 57:737–763, 2007;* rapidly growing giant genital mass *BJD 149:216–217, 2003*

Leishmaniasis

Lymphogranuloma venereum – esthiomene – scarring and fistulae of the buttocks and thighs with elephantiasic lymphedema of the vulva *JAAD 54:559–578, 2006; Int J Dermatol 15:26–33, 1976*

Mycobacterium tuberculosis – multilobulated vulvar nodule *JAMADerm 156:96–97, 2020; J Ob Gyn India 64(suppl 1)85–87, 2014; Ob Gyn 51:215–225, 1978*

Necrotizing fasciitis – unilateral vulvar edema *Ped Derm 22:554–557, 2005*

North American blastomycosis – vulvar edema *Genital Skin Disorders, Fischer and Margesson, CV Mosby, 1998, p. 224*

Rhinosporidiosis – vascular nodules; may resemble condylomata *Arch Otolaryngol 102:308–312, 1976*

Schistosoma haematobium – multilobulated vulvar nodule (late cutaneous bilharziasis) *JAMADerm 156:96–97, 2020;* verrucous lesion *AD 138:1245–1250, 2002; Eur J Obstet Gynecol Reprod Biol 79:213–216, 1998;* vulvar edema *Genital Skin Disorders, Fischer and Margesson, CV Mosby, 1998, p. 224;* unilateral vulvar edema *Ped Derm 22:554–557, 2005*

Syphilis – congenital syphilis – verrucous papules *Ped Derm 23:43–48, 2006;* secondary (condyloma lata); tertiary

Warts – personal observation

Yaws – secondary (daughter yaws, pianomas, framboesiomas) – small papules which ulcerate, become crusted; resemble raspberries; periorificial (around the mouth, nose, penis, anus, vulva); extend peripherally (circinate yaws) *JAAD 29:519–535, 1993*

INFILTRATIVE DISEASES

Amyloidosis

Erdheim-Chester disease (multisystem non-Langerhans cell histiocytosis) – infiltration of the vulva and clitoris *Cut Opin Rheumatol 24:53–59, 2012;* CD68+ and factor XIIIa+; negative for CD1a and S100; xanthoma and xanthelasma-like lesions (red-brown-yellow papules and plaques) (resemble xanthoma disseminatum); flat wartlike papules of the face; lesions occur in folds; the skin becomes slack with atrophy of folds and the face; also lesions of the eyelids, axillae, groin, neck; bony lesions; involvement of the heart (congestive heart failure), lungs (pulmonary fibrosis), central nervous system, gastrointestinal tract, endocrine; death; diabetes insipidus and exophthalmos *JAAD 57:1031–1045, 2007; AD 143:952–953, 2007; Hautarzt 52:510–517, 2001; Medicine (Baltimore) 75:157–169, 1996; Virchow Arch Pathol Anat 279:541–542, 1930*

Juvenile xanthogranuloma *Ped Derm 25:97–98, 2008*

Langerhans cell histiocytosis *JAAD 78:1035–1044, 2018*

Mastocytosis – unilateral vulvar edema *Ped Derm 22:554–557, 2005*

Verruciform xanthoma *Am J Clin Path 71:224–228, 1979*

Vulvitis circumscripta plasmacellularis – vegetating tumor *JAAD 19:947–950, 1988*

Xanthoma disseminatum *JAAD 25:433–436, 1991*

INFLAMMATORY DISEASES

Chronic edema of the vulva (granulomatous vulvitis) – unilateral vulvar edema *Ped Derm 22:554–557, 2005*

Crohn's disease (vulvitis granulomatosa) – vulvar erythema and swelling; bilateral or unilateral *Ped Derm 26:604–609, 2009; Ped Derm 23:49–52, 2006;* unilateral vulvar edema *Ped Derm 22:554–557, 2005; JAAD 36:697–704, 1997; Int J Gynecol Pathol 14:352–359, 1995; Gut 11:18–26, 1970*

Hidradenitis suppurativa *J Reprod Med 36:113–117, 1991;* unilateral vulvar edema *Ped Derm 22:554–557, 2005;* giant vulva with cobblestoning – severe lymphedema with lymphangiectasias *JAAD 64:1223–1224, 2011*

Pyostomatitis vegetans *BJD 149:181–184, 2003*

METABOLIC DISEASES

Calcinosis cutis – vaginal nodules due to urinary incontinence *BJD 150:169–171, 2004*

Masculinization

Ovarian hyperstimulation syndrome – unilateral vulvar edema *Ped Derm 22:554–557, 2005*

Pregnancy – vulvar edema due to lymphatic obstruction *Genital Skin Disorders, Fischer and Margesson, CV Mosby, 1998, p. 224*; unilateral vulvar edema *Ped Derm 22:554–557, 2005*

Pseudo-masculinization *Plast Reconstr Surg 68:787–788, 1981*

Virilizing tumors

NEOPLASTIC

Acrochordon *Genital Skin Disorders, Fischer and Margesson, CV Mosby, 1998, p. 197*

Aggressive angiomyxoma – enlarged labia majora *JAAD 58:S40–41, 2008*

Androgen-producing tumors – clitoromegaly *Genital Skin Disorders, Fischer and Margesson, CV Mosby, 1998, p. 111*

Angiomyofibroblastoma – vulvar labial enlargement *BJD 157:189–191, 2007*

Basal cell carcinoma – red and white vulvar plaque mimicking extramammary Paget's disease *AD 142:385–390, 2006*

Bowen's disease *Ann DV 109:811–812, 1982; Cancer 14:318–329, 1961*

Bowenoid papulosis *JAAD 29:644–646, 1993*

Caruncle – vascular papillary growth of urinary meatus *JAAD 57:371–392, 2007*

Epidermal inclusion cyst – due to genital mutilation *Genital Skin Disorders, Fischer and Margesson, CV Mosby, 1998, p. 118*; clitoral hypertrophy

Epidermal nevus *Ped Derm 17:1–6, 2000*

Erythroplasia of Queyrat

Extramammary Paget's disease – hypertrophic vulva with red plaque *JAAD 65:192–194, 2011; Obstet Gynecol 39:735–744, 1972*

Giant cell fibroblastoma (congenital) – vulvar hypertrophy *Ped Derm 18:255–257, 2001*

Granular cell tumor – cobblestoning of the vulva *Ped Derm 10:153–5, 1993*

Inflammatory linear verrucous epidermal nevus (ILVEN) *Ped Derm 17:1–6, 2000*

Leiomyomas – clitoral hypertrophy *J Iowa Med Soc 63:535–538, 1973*

Lipoblastoma – enlarged labia majora *Ped Derm 23:152–156, 2006*

Lipoma *Genital Skin Disorders, Fischer and Margesson, CV Mosby, 1998, p. 204*

Lymphoma, including cutaneous T-cell lymphoma

Malignant granular cell schwannoma

Melanocytic nevus – giant congenital melanocytic nevus (bulky perineal nevocytoma) *JAAD 53:S139–142, 2005*

Melanoma

Metastases – metastatic mucinous carcinoma – painful red indurated plaques and nodules *JAMADerm 155:1073–1074, 2019*; lymphangiectasis secondary to intralymphatic metastases

Nevus sebaceus

Pelvic tumor with lymphatic obstruction *Genital Skin Disorders, Fischer and Margesson, CV Mosby, 1998, p. 224*

Sarcoma botryoides (embryonal rhabdomyosarcoma) – "bunch of grapes" protruding from vagina *JAAD 57:371–392, 2007*

Sebaceous gland hypertrophy of the labia minora *Genital Skin Disorders, Fischer and Margesson, CV Mosby, 1998, p. 104*

Seborrheic keratosis

Squamous cell carcinoma – squamous cell carcinoma in ILVEN *Cutis 89:273–275, 2012*; metastatic epidermotropic squamous cell carcinoma of the vagina *JAAD 11:353–356, 1984*; squamous cell carcinoma in situ *Derm Surg 21:890–894, 1995*

Syringomas – hypertrophic, cobblestoned labia majora *JAAD 74:1234–1240, 2016; Ped Derm 23:369–372, 2006*

Tumors, various types – unilateral vulvar edema *Ped Derm 22:554–557, 2005*

Verrucous carcinoma – giant condylomata of Buschke and Lowenstein; verrucous plaque of the vulva and perianal area *Cutis 96:82,89–90, 2015; Cutis 21:207–211, 1978*

Vulvar intraepithelial neoplasia – hyperkeratotic verrucous papillomatous plaques *BJD 176:227–230, 2017*

PRIMARY CUTANEOUS DISEASES

Acantholytic dermatosis of the vulvocrural area – vulvar papules, cobblestoning of the vulva and thighs *Cutis 67:217–219, 2001*

Acanthosis nigricans *JAAD 31:1–19, 1994*

Benign hypertrophy of the labia minora *Eur J Obstet Gynecol Reprod Biol 8:61–64, 1978*

Childhood asymmetric labium majus enlargement mimicking a neoplasm *Am J Surg Pathol 29:1007–1016, 2005*

Darier's disease *Ped Derm 10:146–148, 1993*

Elephantiasis

Genitoperineal papular acantholytic dyskeratosis – hypertrophic cobblestoned vulva; perianal hypertrophic dermatitis; mutation in ATP2C1 *BJD 166:210–212, 2012*

Hailey-Hailey disease – verrucous plaque *AD 135:203–208, 1999*

Infantile gluteal granuloma

Lichen planus – hypertrophic lichen planus

Lichen sclerosus et atrophicus – lichen sclerosus of the vulva and vagina – cobblestoned vagina, white atrophic plaques *JAAD 82:1287–1298, 2020; JAMA Derm 149:1199–1202, 2013*

Lichen simplex chronicus *J Reprod Med 36:309–311, 1991*

Lipodystrophia centrifugalis abdominalis – vulvar atrophy *Ped Derm 21:538–541, 2004; AD 104:291–298, 1971*

Papular acantholytic dyskeratosis of the vulva *AD 148:755–760, 2012; Ped Derm 22:237–239, 2005; Am J Dermatopathol 6:557–560, 1984*; papular acantholytic dyskeratosis of the penis *J Dermatol 36:427–429, 2009; Am J Dermatopathol 8:365–366, 1986*

Pityriasis rosea

Psoriasis *Genital Skin Disorders, Fischer and Margesson, CV Mosby, 1998, p. 168*

Pyoderma vegetans *AD 116:1169–1171, 1980*

Ureterocoele *JAAD 57:371–392, 2007*

Urethral prolapse *JAAD 57:371–392, 2007*

Vulvar vestibular papillomatosis – filiform projections of inner labial mucosa and vaginal introitus; angiofibromas; vestibular papillae; papules *Cutis 90:300–301, 2012; AD 126:1594–1598, 1990*

SYNDROMES

CHILD syndrome *AD 142:348–351, 2006;* verruciform xanthoma – Blaschko red hypertrophic plaque of the vulva with linear extension onto leg *Ped Derm 32:135–137, 2015*

Lawrence-Seip syndrome (congenital generalized lipodystrophy) – lipoatrophic diabetes – clitoromegaly *AD 91:326–334, 1965*

Netherton's syndrome – intertriginous and perigenital dermatitis, edema, papillomatosis resembling cellulitis; vulvar edema and hypertrophy *BJD 131:615–621, 1994*

Neurofibromatosis – hypertrophy of the clitoral hood *Eur J Gyn Oncol 24:447–451, 2003; Urology 37:337–339, 1991*

Steatocystoma multiplex

TRAUMA

Physical trauma – vulvar edema *Genital Skin Disorders, Fischer and Margesson, CV Mosby, 1998, p. 224*

Thermal burn – child abuse; vulvar edema *Genital Skin Disorders, Fischer and Margesson, CV Mosby, 1998, p. 116*

Radiation therapy – lymphatic obstruction *Genital Skin Disorders, Fischer and Margesson, CV Mosby, 1998, p. 224*

Sexual abuse – unilateral vulvar edema *Ped Derm 22:554–557, 2005*

Surgical trauma – vulvar hematoma, vulvar fissure *Genital Skin Disorders, Fischer and Margesson, CV Mosby, 1998, p. 122*

Unilateral vulvar hypertrophy in competitive female cyclists *B J Sports Med 36:463–464, 2002*

Vulvar hematoma *Genital Skin Disorders, Fischer and Margesson, CV Mosby, 1998, p. 116*

VASCULAR

Hemangiomas *Genital Skin Disorders, Fischer and Margesson, CV Mosby, 1998, p. 200*

Lymphedema *Arch Pathol Lab Med 124:1697–1699, 2000;* congenital *Genital Skin Disorders, Fischer and Margesson, CV Mosby, 1998, p. 224*

Lymphangiectasia (acquired lymphangioma) – hypertrophic vesicular lesions of the vulva; due to scarring processes such as hysterectomy and radiation; recurrent infections, radiotherapy, scrofuloderma (tuberculous adenitis), tumors, genital Crohn's disease *AD 148:755–760, 2012; BJD 132:1014–1016, 1996*

Lymphangioma circumscriptum *JAAD 55:S106–107, 2006; Genital Skin Disorders, Fischer and Margesson, CV Mosby, 1998, p. 205–206;* acquired vulvar lymphangioma mimicking genital warts *J Cutan Pathol 26:150–154, 1999*

PELVIS syndrome (may be part of urorectal septum malformation sequence) – macular telangiectatic patch; larger perineal hemangiomas, external genitalia malformations, including hypertrophied labia, or undifferentiated asymmetric genitalia, lipomyelomeningocele, vesicorenal abnormalities, imperforate anus, and skin tags *AD 142:884–888, 2006*

Varicosity *Genital Skin Disorders, Fischer and Margesson, CV Mosby, 1998, p. 229*

Vascular malformations – unilateral vulvar edema *Ped Derm 22:554–557, 2005*

Verrucous localized lymphedema of the vulva *JAAD 71:320–326, 2014*

VULVAR EDEMA

Cutis 86:148–152, 2010

AUTOIMMUNE DISEASES AND DISORDERS OF IMMUNE DYSREGULATION

Angioedema *JAAD 25:155–161, 1991*

Contact dermatitis *Contact Dermatitis 7:226–227, 2018*

Urticaria

DRUGS

Methotrexate *Medicine 98:e16895, 2019*

DEGENERATIVE DISORDERS

Inguinal hernia *Taiwan J Ob Gyn 55:446–447, 2016*

INFECTIONS AND INFESTATIONS

Bartholin cyst abscess

Recurrent vulvovaginal candidiasis

Chancroid

Condylomata acuminata

Chronic active Epstein-Barr virus – vulvitis, hemorrhagic cheilitis, necrotic ulcers, periorbital erythema and edema, maxillary sinusitis, hepatosplenomegaly *BJD 173:1266–1270, 2015*

Erysipelas

Filariasis – *Wuchereria bancrofti, Brugia malayi, B. timori* – mosquito vector; lymphadenopathy of the groin, scrotal edema, vulvar edema, breast edema, edema of the legs

vs. Podoconiosis – non-infectious tropical lymphedema, lymphedema below the knee; offensive odor due to edema, hyperkeratosis, and fissures

Furuncle

Granuloma inguinale

Herpes simplex infection

Herpes zoster

Lipschutz ulcers (ulcus vulvae acuta) – due to Epstein-Barr virus; vulvar edema and ulcers *Cutis 91:273–276, 2013*

Lymphogranuloma venereum

Mycobacterium tuberculosis – vulvar lymphangiectasia due to gastrointestinal tuberculosis *Ped Derm 37:215–216, 2020*

Necrotizing fasciitis

Paragonimiasis (*Paragonimus westermani*) – edematous plaque of the vulva *JAAD Case Reports 1:239–240, 2015*

Syphilis

Trichomoniasis *Clin Obstet Gynecol 24:407–438, 1981*

INFILTRATIVE DISORDERS

Intralymphatic histiocytosis – swelling of the labia majora *JAAD 70:927–933, 2014*

Langerhans cell histiocytosis *Turk J Ped 58:675–678, 2016*

Mastocytosis *Ann DV 14:685–689, 2015*

INFLAMMATORY DISORDERS

Crohn's disease – edematous vulva with or without erythema *JAAD 82:1287–1298, 2020; Ped Derm 35:566–574, 2018; Ped Derm 33:553–554, 2016; JAMADerm 150:769–770, 2014; Genitourin Med 65:335–337, 1989*

Hidradenitis suppurativa *Urology 44:606–608, 1994;* severe lymphedema with lymphangiectasias; giant vulva with cobblestoning *JAAD 64:1223–1224, 2011*

Pyoderma gangrenosum – vulvar edema *BJD 157:1235–1239, 2007*

Sarcoidosis

METABOLIC DISORDERS

Anemia

Antepartum labial edema *Case Reports Ob Gyn 2018:7651254*

Ascites

Congestive heart failure

Eclampsia/pre-eclampsia *Niger J Med 20:380–382, 2011*

Hypoalbuminemia

Hypertension

Malnutrition

Multiple gestations

Nephrotic syndrome

Preterm ovarian hyperstimulation *Am J Case Rep 20:238–241, 2019; NEJM 372:2336, 2015*

Pre-eclampsia

Renal failure

NEOPLASTIC DISORDERS

Adenoma of round ligament

Angiomatoid fibrous histiocytoma *Mod Pathol 24:1560–1570, 2011*

Pelvic obstruction due to tumor, radiation or surgery; lipoma, cyst squamous cell carcinoma in long-standing hidradenitis suppurativa *Int J Dermatol 52:808–812, 2013*

Labial or vulvar neoplasm

Nuck hydrocele

Syringomas *JAAD 74:1234–1240, 2016*

PRIMARY CUTANEOUS DISEASES

Aphthae with edema *JAAD 82:1287–1298, 2020*

Atopic dermatitis

Ectopic breast tissue

SYNDROMES

Ehlers-Danlos hyperextensibility type *J Sex Med 10:2347–2350, 2013*

Hereditary angioedema

Hermansky-Pudlak syndrome – mucocutaneous granulomatous disease in Hermansky-Pudlak syndrome; butterfly red plaques of face; linear ulcers of the groin and vulva; pink plaques of the thighs; swollen vulva; indurated nodules of the vulva; axillary ulcers, red face *JAMADerm 150:1083–1087, 2014*

Mirror syndrome – triad of fetal hydrops, maternal edema, and placentomegaly with sudden and massive vulvar edema *J Matern Fetal Neonatal Med 26:313–315, 2013*

Retractile mesenteritis (IgG4 disease) – edema of abdominal wall, lower extremities, genitalia

TRAUMA

Birthing chair

Hematoma

Obstructed labor/prolonged delivery

Pancreas-kidney transplant with bladder drainage *J Low Genit Tract Dis 23:82–83, 2019*

Physical trauma – cycling *J Low Genit Tract Dis 18:e84–89, 2014*

Postparacentesis syndrome (Conn syndrome)

Tourniquet syndrome

VASCULAR DISORDERS

Capillary leak syndrome

Lymphatic malformation – multilobulated nodule with edematous vulva *Cutis 93:297–300, 2014*

Localized lymphedema of the vulva *Indian J Gyn Pathol 30:306–313, 2011*

Verrucous localized lymphedema of the penis, scrotum, vulva, pubis – vulvar edema; polypoid, verrucous, cobblestoned lesions *JAAD 71:320–326, 2014*

VULVAR ERYTHEMA WITH OR WITHOUT PRURITUS

AUTOIMMUNE DISEASES AND DISEASES OF IMMUNE DYSFUNCTION

Allergic contact dermatitis – anesthetics (benzocaine) *JAAD 68:351–352, 2013;* antibiotics (neomycin), antihistamine creams, nail polish, vaginal perfumes, douches, preservatives or active ingredients in topical creams and ointments (parabens, imidazolidinyl urea), moisturizers (lanolin), poison ivy, rubber (gloves, condoms, diaphragms), contraceptives, clothing dyes, fragrances in laundry products *BJD 126:52–56, 1992;* pigmented purpuric clothing dermatitis to disperse dyes *Contact Dermatitis 43:360, 2000*

Bullous pemphigoid *BJD 145:994–997, 2001*

Cicatricial pemphigoid *Ped Derm 21:51–53, 2004*

Food allergy – vaginal itching *Ann Allergy 72:546, 1994*

Graft vs. host disease, chronic – oral and vaginal lichen planus-like lesions *JAAD 66:515–532, 2012*

Lichenoid reactions with antibodies to desmoplakins I and II – *JAAD 48:433–438, 2003*

Lupus erythematosus – discoid lupus erythematosus *Genital Skin Disorders, Fischer and Margesson, CV Mosby, 1998, p. 172; BJD 121:727–741, 1989;* systemic lupus erythematosus *BJD 121:727–741, 1989*

Pemphigus foliaceus *JAAD 67:409–416, 2012; BJD 158:478–482, 2008; Obstet Gynecol 106:1005–1012, 2005*

Pemphigus vulgaris *JAAD 67:409–416, 2012; BJD 158:478–482, 2008; Obstet Gynecol 106:1005–1012, 2005;*

Seasonal allergic disease – vulvar itching *J Allergy Clin Immunol 95Z:780–782, 1995*

DRUG

Capecitabine (Xeloda) *JAAD 45:790–791, 2001*

Corticosteroids – topical corticosteroid withdrawal *Genital Skin Disorders, Fischer and Margesson, CV Mosby, 1998, p. 232*

Enalapril – vaginal itching *Ann Int Med 112:217–222, 1990*

Fixed drug eruption *Genital Skin Disorders, Fischer and Margesson, CV Mosby, 1998, p. 163*

Toxic epidermal necrolysis *Genital Skin Disorders, Fischer and Margesson, CV Mosby, 1998, p. 184*

EXOGENOUS AGENTS

Benzocaine – erosive papulonodular dermatitis (granuloma gluteale infantum, pseudoverrucous papules, Jacquet's erosive diaper dermatitis *JAAD 55:S74–80, 2006*

Irritant contact dermatitis – bubble baths in children, soap, detergents, fabric softener, feminine hygiene products, chemicals, deodorant sprays, friction, thermal damage (hot water bottles), trauma *JAAD 82:1287–1298, 2020; Contact Dermatitis 5:375–377, 1979*

INFECTIONS OR INFESTATIONS

Bacterial cellulitis/erysipelas *Genital Skin Disorders, Fischer and Margesson, CV Mosby, 1998, p. 140*
  Streptococcus pyogenes (group A beta hemolytic)
  Haemophilus influenzae
  Streptococcus pneumoniae
  Staphylococcus aureus
  Neisseria meningitidis
  Shigella
  Yersinia

Candidiasis *Ob Gyn Clin NA 44:353–370, 2017; Clin Obstet Gynecol 24:407–438, 1981*

Candidiasis (mucocutaneous candida infection) *BJD 178:335–349, 2018;*
  APECED syndrome
  Cardiac defects, vertebral anomalies – vulvovaginal candidiasis
  Chronic mucocutaneous candidiasis

Dectin-1 deficiency – vulvovaginal candidiasis
  DiGeorge syndrome – vulvovaginal candidiasis
  DOCK8 syndrome
  IL12/23 – vulvovaginal candidiasis
  Job's syndrome
  Mammalian sterile 20-like 1 deficiency – vulvovaginal candidiasis
  Severe combined immunodeficiency (SCID) – vulvovaginal candidiasis
  T-lymphocyte defects (CD4 lymphopenia, IL2 deficiency, IL2R mutations) – vulvovaginal candidiasis
  TYK2 deficiency – vulvovaginal candidiasis

Enterobiasis (Enterobius vermicularis) (threadworm) – vulvar dermatitis *Br J Vener Dis 49:314–315, 1973*

Erythrasma

Folliculitis *Genital Skin Disorders, Fischer and Margesson, CV Mosby, 1998, p. 141*

Gardnerella vaginalis – non-specific vaginitis (*Gardnerella* and *Mobiluncus*) *J Clin Microbiol 28:28:2033–2039, 1990; Clin Obstet Gynecol 24:439–460, 1981*

Gonorrhea

Haemophilus vulvovaginitis Ped Derm 17:1–6, 2000

Herpes simplex *Genital Skin Disorders, Fischer and Margesson, CV Mosby, 1998, p. 131–132*

Herpes zoster *Genital Skin Disorders, Fischer and Margesson, CV Mosby, 1998, p. 134*

Pediculosis *The Clinical Management of Itching; Parthenon; p. 123, 2000*

Pinworm

Scabies *The Clinical Management of Itching; Parthenon; p. 120, 2000*

Scarlet fever

Shigella vulvovaginitis Adolesc Pediatr Gynecol 7:86–89, 1994

Streptococcal vulvovaginitis/cellulitis *Ped Derm 17:1–6, 2000; South Med J 75:446–447, 1982*

Tinea cruris *AD 118:446, 1982*

Trichomoniasis *Clin Obstet Gynecol 24:407–438, 1981*

Vaginitis – bacterial vaginosis; *Haemophilus vaginalis, Gardnerella vaginalis,* anaerobic bacteria *The Clinical Management of Itching; Parthenon; p. 123, 2000*

INFILTRATIVE DISEASES

Langerhans cell histiocytosis – vulvar erythema with erosions and papules *Ped Derm 34:484–485, 2017*

Zoon's (plasma cell) vulvitis – red vulva *JAAD 82:1287–1298, 2020; AD 141:789–790, 2005;* red plaque *JAAD 19:947–950, 1988; Dermatologica 111:157, 1955*

INFLAMMATORY DISEASES

Crohn's disease – vulvar erythema and edema *JAAD 82:1287–1298, 2020; JAMADerm 150:769–770, 2014*

Desquamative inflammatory vaginitis – marked erythema of the labia minora *Cutis 85:39–46, 2010; Cutis 81:75–78, 2008*

Hidradenitis suppurativa *JAMA Derm 149:1192–1194, 2013*

Pseudolymphoma *Eur J Obstet Gynecol Reprod Biol 47:167–168, 1992*

Pyostomatitis vegetans *BJD 149:181–184, 2003*

Salivary vulvitis *Obstet Gynecol 37:238–240, 1971*

Seminal vulvitis – familial, allergic, vulvar edema, erythema, pruritus *Am J Obstet Gynecol 126:442–444, 1976*

Stevens-Johnson syndrome *Ped Derm 19:52–55, 2002*

Ulcus vulvae acutum (Lipschutz ulcer) – necrotic, painful vulvar ulcer with fever and lymphadenopathy; often associated with acute Epstein-Barr virus infection with positive serology to capsid antigens (IgM and IgG) *Ped Derm 25:364–367, 2008; Cutis 65:387–389, 2000; BJD 135:663–665, 1996; Acta DV (Stockh) 45:221–222,*

1965; Arch Dermatol Syph (Berlin) 114:363–395, 1913; Obstet Gynecol 38:440–443, 1971

Vulvar vestibulitis *Genital Skin Disorders, Fischer and Margesson, CV Mosby, 1998, p. 173; J Reprod Med 36:413–415, 1991*

METABOLIC DISEASES

Acrodermatitis enteropathica *Genital Skin Disorders, Fischer and Margesson, CV Mosby, 1998, p. 228*

Fucosidosis – with angiokeratoma corporis diffusum on telangiectatic background *Genital Skin Disorders, Fischer and Margesson, CV Mosby, 1998, p. 198*

Kwashiorkor (protein and caloric deprivation) – vulvitis and vulvovaginitis *Cutis 67:321–327, 2001; JAAD 21:1–30, 1989*

Pellagra – vulvar erythema (vulvitis) *BJD 164:1188–1200, 2011*

Vitamins B1 and B2 deficiency *JAAD 15:1263–1274, 1986*

Zinc deficiency

NEOPLASTIC DISEASES

Basal cell carcinoma – red plaque *AD 143:426–427, 2007;* anogenital pruritus *Am J Obstet Gynecol 121:173–174, 1975*

Bowen's disease

Cloacogenic carcinoma – anogenital pruritus *JAAD 23:1005–1008, 1990*

Extramammary Paget's disease *Genital Skin Disorders, Fischer and Margesson, CV Mosby, 1998, p. 217; Cancer 46:590–594, 1980; Am J Clin Pathol 27:559–566, 1957;* anogenital pruritus *Br J Surg 75:1089–1092, 1988*

Squamous cell carcinoma in situ – squamous cell carcinoma in lichen sclerosus – red plaque *JAMADerm 155:844, 2019;* anogenital pruritus *The Clinical Management of Itching; Parthenon; p. 125, 2000*

Syringoma *Obstet Gynecol 55:515–518, 1980*

Vulvar intraepithelial neoplasia – anogenital pruritus *The Clinical Management of Itching; Parthenon; p. 125, 2000*

PRIMARY CUTANEOUS DISEASES

Atopic dermatitis *Ped Derm 17:1–6, 2000*

Granulomatous periorificial dermatitis – extrafacial and generalized periorificial dermatitis *AD 138:1354–1358, 2002*

Hailey-Hailey disease *Genital Skin Disorders, Fischer and Margesson, CV Mosby, 1998, p. 178*

Intertrigo

Lichen planus *Sem Cut Med Surg 34:182–186, 2015; AD 125:1677–1680, 1989;* erosive lichen planus *JAAD 82:1287–1298, 2020; BJD 147:625–627, 2002;* vulvovaginal gingival syndrome *JAAD 55:98–113, 2006*

Lichen sclerosus et atrophicus – wrinkled lesions, atrophic vulva with shrinkage *Cutis 67:249–250, 2001 Trans St John's Hosp Dermatol Soc 57:9–30, 1971;* vulvar purpura *Ped Derm 31:95–98, 2014*

Lichen simplex chronicus *Genital Skin Disorders, Fischer and Margesson, CV Mosby, 1998, p. 157*

Lipschutz ulcer (ulcus vulvae acutum) – vulvar erythema and edema accompanying aphthous ulcers of the vulva *Ped Derm 25:113–115, 2008*

Psoriasis *JAAD 82:1287–1298, 2020; Ped Derm 17:1–6, 2000;* napkin psoriasis *Contact Dermatitis 26:248–252, 1992; BJD 773:445–447, 1961*

Seborrheic dermatitis

PSYCHOCUTANEOUS DISEASES

Psychogenic vulvar itching – pruritus, erythema, burning *BJD 104:611–619, 1981*

SYNDROMES

Behcet's disease – personal observation

CHILD syndrome *AD 142:348–351, 2006*

Hereditary mucoepithelial dysplasia (dyskeratosis) – red eyes, non-scarring alopecia, keratosis pilaris, erythema of oral (palate, gingiva) and nasal mucous membranes, cervix, vagina, and urethra; perineal and perigenital psoriasiform dermatitis; increased risk of infections, fibrocystic lung disease *BJD 153:310–318, 2005; Ped Derm 11:133–138, 1994; JAAD 21:351–357, 1989; Am J Hum Genet 31:414–427, 1979; Oral Surg Oral Med Oral Pathol 46:645–657, 1978*

Papular-purpuric "gloves and socks" syndrome *JAAD 41:793–796, 1999*

Reactive arthritis syndrome – circinate vulvitis *Dan Med Bull32:272–273, 1985*

Red vulva syndrome – due to chronic topical corticosteroid use *JAMADerm 154:731–733, 2018*

Wells' syndrome *JAAD 48:S60–61, 2003*

TRAUMA

Burns – thermal, chemical

Child abuse

Dermatographism *JAAD 31:1040–1041, 1994*

Enuresis

Radiation dermatitis *Genital Skin Disorders, Fischer and Margesson, CV Mosby, 1998, p. 123*

Trauma, physical

VASCULAR LESIONS

Hemangiomas *Genital Skin Disorders, Fischer and Margesson, CV Mosby, 1998, p. 200*

Klippel-Trenaunay-Weber syndrome *Genital Skin Disorders, Fischer and Margesson, CV Mosby, 1998, p. 201*

VULVAR PAPULES AND NODULES

AUTOIMMUNE DISEASES AND DISEASES OF IMMUNE DYSFUNCTION

Allergic contact dermatitis – poison ivy – personal observation

Angioedema

Pemphigus vulgaris/vegetans

Rheumatoid nodule *J Clin Pathol 49:85–87, 1996*

Urticaria

CONGENITAL LESIONS

Dermoid cyst

Lipomas *AD 118:447, 1982;* congenital vulvar lipoma with accessory labioscrotal fold – labial enlargement with subcutaneous nodule *Ped Derm 28:424–428, 2011*

Supernumerary breasts *Br Med J ii:1234–1236, 1962*

Supernumerary nipples *Obstet Gynecol 52:225–228, 1978; Cancer 38:2570–2574, 1976*

DRUGS

Corticosteroid-induced fat necrosis

Fixed drug eruption

EXOGENOUS AGENTS

Contact dermatitis – allergic or irritant

Foreign body

Sclerosing lipogranuloma *Am J Obstet Gynecol 101:854–856, 1968*

INFECTIONS

Actinomycosis

Amebic dysentery in infants – granuloma *Pediatrics 71:595–598, 1983*

Bacillary angiomatosis *Clin Dermatol 38:160–175, 2020; Obstet Gynecol 88:709–711, 1996*

Bartholin's abscess – *Escherichia coli, Streptococcus faecalis, Staphylococcus, gonococcus, Chlamydia trachomatis Br J Vener 54:409–413, 1978*

Bejel (endemic syphilis) – condyloma-like lesions

Botryomycosis – *Staphylococcus aureus*; disseminated papules, pustules, and eschars *J Drugs in Dermatol 13:976–978, 2014*

Candida

Condyloma acuminata

Epstein-Barr virus (HHV4) – primary cutaneous Epstein-Barr virus-related lymphoproliferative disorders; ulcerated vulvar nodule *JAAD 58:74–80, 2008*

Furunculosis – *Staphylococcus aureus*

Granuloma inguinale (donovanosis) – initial nodule

Herpes simplex *AD 135:203–208, 1999;* recalcitrant pseudotumoral anogenital herpes simplex virus type 2 – ulcers and hypertrophic nodules *Clin Inf Dis 57:1648–1655, 2013*

Leishmaniasis *Lancet i:127–132, 1960;* post-kala azar dermal leishmaniasis – in India, hypopigmented macules; nodules develop after years; tongue, palate, genitalia *E Afr Med J 63:365–371, 1986*

Lymphogranuloma venereum – initial papule or papulovesicle

Malakoplakia – vulvar nodules, abscesses, red papules; *Escherichia coli, Pseudomonas* species, *Staphylococcus aureus*; soft plaques; indurated ulcer *Arch Pathol Lab Med 132:113–117, 2008; J Ind Med Assoc 72:254–255, 1979; Clin Exp Dermatol 2:131–135, 1977*

Molluscum contagiosum

Mycobacterium tuberculosis – periorificial; Bartholin's gland infection *Clin Obstet Gynecol 2:530–548, 1959;* lichen scrofulosorum *Ped Derm 24:573–575, 2007*

North American blastomycosis

Rhinosporidiosis – vascular nodules; may resemble condylomata *Arch Otolaryngol 102:308–312, 1976*

Scabies

Schistosoma haematobium – genital sandy patches or rubbery papules *NEJM 381:2493–2495, 2019;* resemble condyloma acuminata *Clin Exp Dermatol 8:189–194, 1983;* vulvar cobblestoned nodule *Am J Surg Pathol 8:787–790, 1984*

Syphilis – secondary; condyloma lata – white moist papules gummas

Yaws – secondary (daughter yaws, pianomas, framboesiomas) – small papules which ulcerate, become crusted; resemble raspberries; periorificial (around the mouth, nose, penis, anus, vulva); extend peripherally (circinate yaws) *JAAD 29:519–535, 1993*

INFILTRATIVE DISEASES

Amyloidosis – nodular cutaneous amyloidosis *JAAD 39:149–171, 1998; AD 121:518–521, 1985*

Langerhans cell histiocytosis – vulvar papules, vesicles, pustules, ulcers; vulvar red papules *Eur J Gyn Onc 30:691–694, 2009; Obstet Gynecol 67:46–49, 1986*

Mastocytosis – localized mastocytosis; vulvar papules *Ped Derm 31:111–113, 2014;* vulvar nodules *J Ped Adolesc Gyn 31:156–157, 2018*

Primary chylous reflux – vulvar vesicles *AD 146:683–684, 2010*

Vulvitis chronica circumscripta plasmacellularis (plasma cell vulvitis) (Zoon's vulvitis) *BJD 149:638–641, 2003; AD 126:1351–1356, 1990;* red plaque *JAAD 19:947–950, 1988*

Verruciform xanthoma – yellow-orange verrucous plaques *AD 147:1087–1092, 2011; Am J Clin Pathol 71:224–228, 1979*

Vulvitis granulomatosis

INFLAMMATORY DISEASES

Crohn's disease – granulomas *J Obstet Gynecol 80:376–378, 1973; BJD 80:1–8, 1968;* unilateral labial hypertrophy; erythema, edema, induration *Ped Derm 27:279–281, 2010; JAAD 36:986–988, 1996; JAAD 27:893–895, 1992; AD 126:1351–1356, 1990; Ped Derm 5:103–106, 1988*

Edema

Endometriosis (cutaneous deciduosis) – blue cutaneous nodule *duVivier p.686, 2003;* firm blue nodules of the vulva *JAAD 43:102–107, 2000; Obstet 40:28–34, 1972*

Erythema of Jacquet – eroded violaceous nodules of the vulva and pubic area *AD 149:475–480, 2013*

Granuloma gluteale infantum (erosive papulonodular dermatitis) (granuloma gluteale infantum, pseudoverrucous papules, Jacquet's erosive diaper dermatitis) *JAAD 55:S74–80, 2006; Ped Derm 23:43–48, 2006; Ped Derm 17:141–143, 2000; AD 125:1703–1707, 1989; Arch Emerg Med 5:113–115, 1988; Clin Exp Dermatol 6:23–29, 1981; Cutis 28:644–648, 1981; Australas J Dermatol 18:20–24, 1977; Hautarzt 22:383–388, 1971;* in adults *J Dermatol 18:671–675, 1991; AD 114:382–383, 1978;* benzocaine – Hidradenitis suppurativa *BJD 119:345–350, 1988*

Infantile pyramidal protrusion – vulvar pyramidal protrusion associated with lichen sclerosus *JAAD 56:S49–50, 2007*

Lymphocytoma cutis *Hautarzt 15:657–661, 1964*

Midline granuloma *Proc R Soc Med 57:289–297, 1964*

Neutrophilic eccrine hidradenitis – violaceous perivulvar nodules *JAMADerm 150:1003–1004, 2014*

Nodular fasciitis *Obstet Gynecol 69:513–516, 1987*

Pseudoepitheliomatous hyperplasia

Sarcoid *JAAD 44:725–743, 2001; JAAD 39:281–283, 1998*

INTERLABIAL MASSES IN GIRLS

Hydrocolpos

Paraurethral duct cyst (Skene's duct cyst)

Prolapsed ectopic ureterocele

Rhabdomyosarcoma of the vagina (botryoid sarcoma)

Urethral prolapse – polypoid edematous vascular-appearing violaceous mass at urethral opening *JAAD 57:377–391, 2007*

METABOLIC DISEASES

Calcinosis cutis, idiopathic *J Pediatr Adolesc Gynecol 12:157–160, 1999; Cutis 41:273–275, 1988;* metastatic calcinosis *BJD 157:622–624, 2007*

Congenital adrenal hyperplasia – clitoromegaly *Genital Skin Disorders, Fischer and Margesson, CV Mosby, 1998, p. 108*

Endometriosis (cutaneous deciduosis) – red papule or nodule *JAAD 43:102–107, 2000;* firm blue nodules *Obstet 40:28–34, 1972*

Verrucous xanthoma *Genitourin Med 65:252–254, 1989; Am J Clin Pathol 71:224–228, 1979*

NEOPLASTIC DISEASES

Adenocarcinoma – undifferentiated carcinoma *Am J Surg Pathol 15:990–1001, 1991*

Adenoma of the anogenital mammary-like glands – pedunculated; lobulated, tan-brown or gray-pink or white papules or nodules of the vulva or perianal area; may ulcerate *JAAD 57:896–898, 2007; Breast J 9:113–116, 2003; J Reprod Med 47:949–951, 2002; Eur J Gynecol Oncol 23:21–24, 2002; Gynecol Oncol 73:155–159, 1999*

Aggressive angiomyxoma *AD 146:911–916, 2010; Histopathology 40:505–509, 2002;* polypoid mass *JAAD 38:143–175, 1998*

Angiomyofibroblastoma – painful red nodule *Ped Derm 29:217–218, 2012; BJD 157:189–191, 2007; Histopathology 40:505–509, 2002; JAAD 38:143–175, 1998*

Apocrine cystadenoma *JAAD 31:498–499, 1994*

Apocrine hamartomas – benign pigmented apocrine hamartomas *Ped Derm 10:123–124, 1993*

Apocrine nevi *Ped Derm 10:123–124, 1993*

Bartholin's gland carcinoma (adenocarcinoma) *Obstet Gynecol 35:578–584, 1970*

Bartholin's gland cyst *Genital Skin Disorders, Fischer and Margesson, CV Mosby, 1998, p. 199*

Basal cell carcinoma *Genital Skin Disorders, Fischer and Margesson, CV Mosby, 1998, p. 211; Cancer 24:460–470, 1969;* multiple hereditary infundibulocystic basal cell carcinomas *AD 135:1227–1235, 1999*

Blue nevus *AD 139:1209–1214, 2003;* epithelioid blue nevus *BJD 145:496–501, 2001*

Bowenoid papulosis – verrucous, lichenoid, dry, brown, whitish papules or plaques *Cancer 57:823–836, 1986*

Ciliated cyst of the vulva *JAAD 32:514–515, 1995*

Cellular angiofibroma *Histopathology 40:505–509, 2002*

Dermatofibrosarcoma protuberans *Gynecol Oncol 30:149–152, 1988; Br J Obstet Gynecol 88:203–205, 1981*

Embryonal rhabdomyosarcoma *AD 138:689–694, 2002*

Endometriosis *JAAD 43:102–107, 2000*

Epidermal nevus

Epidermoid cyst *Genital Skin Disorders, Fischer and Margesson, CV Mosby, 1998, p. 203;* near clitoris; clitoromegaly *Eur J Obstet Gynecol Reprod Biol 87:163–165, 1999*

Epithelioid sarcoma *Acta Cytol 39:100–103, 1995; Cancer 52:1462–1469, 1983*

Extramammary Paget's disease – red plaque of the vulva *JAMADerm 153:689–693, 2017;* vulvar pigmented extramammary Paget's disease; hyperpigmented plaque *BJD 142:1190–1194, 2000*

Fibroadenomas (accessory mammary tissue)

Fibromas

Giant cell fibroblastoma (congenital) – vulvar hypertrophy *Ped Derm 18:255–257, 2001*

Granular cell tumor (nodule or cobblestoning) *AD 136:1165–1170, 2000; Ped Derm 10:123–124, 1993; Ped Derm 4:94–97, 1987*

Hidradenoma (vulvar hidradenoma) – blue nodule of interlabial sulcus of the vulva *JAAD 75:380–384, 2016*

Hidradenoma papilliferum – vulvar or perianal nodule *Genital Skin Disorders, Fischer and Margesson, CV Mosby, 1998, p. 204; J Derm Surg Onc 16:674–676, 1990; Acta Obstet Gynecol Scand 52:387–389, 1973*

Inflammatory linear verrucous epidermal nevus (ILVEN)

Kaposi's sarcoma *Ann Dermatol 27:336–337, 2015*

Keratoacanthoma *JAAD 74:1220–1233, 2016; APMIS 114:562–565, 2006; G Ital DV 124:285–287, 1989; Oral Surg Oral Med Oral Pathol 54:663–667, 1982; Gazz Int Med Chir 67:1032–1038, 1962*

Leukemia – myeloid sarcoma of acute myelogenous leukemia *BJD 174:234–236, 2016;* chronic lymphocytic leukemia *J Gyn Oncol 23:205–206, 2012*

Leiomyoma *J Reprod Med 10:75–76, 1973*

Leiomyosarcoma – blue-black; also red, brown, yellow, or hypopigmented *JAAD 46:477–490, 2002*

Lipoblastoma – multilobulated nodule *Ped Derm 23:152–156, 2006; Histopathology 40:505–509, 2002*

Lipoma *Ghana Med J 45:125–127, 2011*

Lymphomas – B-cell lymphoma *JAAD Case Rep 4:962–967, 2018; Cureus 10:e3713, 2018; Medicine 95:e3041, 2016*

Lymphomatoid papulosis – ulcerated vulvar nodule *JAAD 44:339–341, 2001*

Mammary-like glands of the vulva – cysts *Int J Gynecol Pathol 14:184–188, 1995*

Merkel cell carcinoma *Obstet Gynecol 63 (Suppl):61–63, 1984*

Melanocytic nevi *JAAD 71:1241–1249, 2014; J Cutan Pathol 14:87–91, 1987*

Melanoma – hyperpigmented papule of the vulva *JAAD 71:1241–1249, 2014;* polypoid pigmented nodule of the vulva *JAAD 71:366–375, 2014; Mayo Clin Proceed 72:362–366, 1997; JAAD 22:428–435, 1990*

Mesonephric cyst (Gartner's cyst)

Metastases – cervical carcinoma *Gynecol Oncol 48:349–354, 1993;* endometrial or cervical carcinoma *Genital Skin Disorders, Fischer and Margesson, CV Mosby, 1998, p. 219*

Microcystic adnexal carcinoma *Gynecol Oncol 82:571–574, 2001*

Mullerian cyst

Multinucleated atypia of the vulva – white flat-topped papules *Cutis 75:118–120, 2005*

Myelodysplasia – primary cutaneous lesion – personal observation

Myofibroma – skin-colored to hyperpigmented nodules of the hand, mouth, genitals, shoulders *JAAD 46:477–490, 2002*

Neuroblastoma – vulvar blue nodules *Ped Derm 26:473–474, 2009*

Neurofibromas

Nodular fasciitis

Papillary apocrine fibroadenoma *J Cutan Pathol 24:256–260, 1997*

Retention cysts

Rhabdomyomatous mesenchymal hamartoma – red vascular polypoid mass *Ped Derm 26:753–755, 2009*

Rhabdomyosarcoma – vascular plaque of the vulva *Ped Derm 34:352–355, 2017*

Sarcoma – epithelioid, leiomyosarcoma, rhabdomyosarcoma, myxoid, hemangiosarcoma, liposarcoma

Schwannoma (neuroma)

Sebaceous gland hyperplasia *Obstet Gynecol 68(Suppl 3):635–655, 1986*

Seborrheic keratoses

Skene's duct cyst – paraurethral duct cyst *Genital Skin Disorders, Fischer and Margesson, CV Mosby, 1998, p. 208–209*

Skin tags (fibroepithelial polyps)

Squamous cell carcinoma – red plaque *JAAD 81:1387–1396, 2019*; pedunculated red tumor of the labia majora *BJD 171:7709–785, 2014*; fungating mass of the vaginal wall *NEJM 370:2032–2041, 2014*; squamous cell carcinoma associated with lichen planus – multilobulated, ulcerated, red nodule and plaque *JAAD 71:698–707, 2014*; metastatic epidermotropic squamous cell carcinoma of the vagina *JAAD 11:353–356, 1984*

Sweat gland tumors

Syringomas *JAAD 76:S37–39, 2017; AD 135:203–208, 1999; Ped Derm 13:80–81, 1996; JAAD 19:575–577, 1988; AD 121:756–760, 1985; AD 103:494–496, 1971*; giant syringoma of the vulva *BJD 141:374–375, 1999*; brown papules, skin-colored papules, discrete white cystic papules, lichenoid papules *JAAD 48:735–739, 2003*; giant cobblestoned vulvar nodules *SKINmed 11:305–306, 2013*

Trichoepithelioma *J Reprod Med 33:317–319, 1988*

Tubular apocrine adenoma – hyperpigmented papule of the vulva *Ped Derm 27:200–201, 2010*

Urethral caruncle *Genital Skin Disorders, Fischer and Margesson, CV Mosby, 1998, p. 209*

Verrucous carcinoma *BJD 143:1217–1223, 2000*

Vestibular mucous cyst *Genital Skin Disorders, Fischer and Margesson, CV Mosby, 1998, p. 210*

White sponge nevus

NORMAL

Vestibular papillae of the vulva (angiofibromas) (papillomatosis labialis, hirsuties papillaris vulvae, hirsutoid papilloma of the vulva, pseudocondylomas, vestibular microwarts, vulvar squamous papillomatosis) – cloudy white papules *JAAD 60:353–355, 2009AD 126:1594–1598, 1991; Geburtshilfe Frauenheilkd 41:783–786, 1981*; vestibular papillomatosis – large numbers of vestibular papillae

PRIMARY CUTANEOUS DISEASES

Angiolymphoid hyperplasia with eosinophilia *Clin Exp Dermatol 15:65–67, 1990*

Breast tissue – aberrant breast tissue of the vulva; ectopic breast tissue

Darier's disease *Ped Derm 10:146–148, 1993*

Erythema of Jacquet *Ped Derm 23:43–48, 2006*

Fox-Fordyce disease – papules

Granuloma faciale *JAAD 53:1002–1009, 2005*

Hailey-Hailey disease (white topped papules) *AD 78:446–453, 1958*

Lichen sclerosus – white vulvar plaques *BJD 176:307–316, 2017*

Lichen simplex chronicus

Papular acantholytic dyskeratosis of the vulva *AD 148:755–760, 2012; Ped Derm 22:237–239, 2005; Am J Dermatopathol 6:557–560, 1984*; papular acantholytic dyskeratosis of the penis *J Dermatol 36:427–429, 2009; Am J Dermatopathol 8:365–366, 1986*; vulvar papules, cobblestoning of the vulva and thighs *Cutis 67:217–219, 2001; AD 129:1344–1345, 1993*

Ureterocoele *JAAD 57:371–392, 2007*

Urethral prolapse – polypoid, edematous, vascular-appearing, violaceous mass at urethral opening *JAAD 57:371–392, 2007*

Warty dyskeratoma – keratotic nodule

PSYCHOCUTANEOUS DISEASES

Factitial granuloma

SYNDROMES

Angiokeratoma corporis diffusum (Fabry's disease)

Bazex-Dupre-Christol syndrome – multiple vulvar trichoepitheliomas *BJD 153:682–684, 2005*

Carney complex – acromegaly, facial lentigines, cutaneous myxoma, blue nevus of the vulva; gain of function mutation of *PRKACB* (catalytic subunit alpha of cAMP-dependent protein kinase *NEJM 370:1065–1067, 2014*

Costello syndrome – perianal and vulvar papules; warty papules around the nose and mouth, legs, perianal skin; loose skin of the neck, hands, and feet; acanthosis nigricans; low set protuberant ears, thick palmoplantar surfaces with single palmar crease, gingival hyperplasia, hypoplastic nails, moderately short stature, craniofacial abnormalities, hyperextensible fingers, sparse curly hair, diffuse hyperpigmentation, generalized hypertrichosis, multiple nevi *Ped Derm 20:447–450, 2003; JAAD 32:904–907, 1995; Aust Paediat J 13:114–118, 1977*

Goltz's syndrome – vulvar papillomas *Am J Med Genet 172:Issue 1, 2016*

Hermansky-Pudlak syndrome – mucocutaneous granulomatous disease in Hermansky-Pudlak syndrome; butterfly red plaques of face; linear ulcers of the groin and vulva; pink plaques of the thighs; swollen vulva; indurated nodules of the vulva; axillary ulcers, red face *JAMADerm 150:1083–1087, 2014*

Melkersson-Rosenthal syndrome – granuloma *Dermatologica 182:128–131, 1991*

Multiple mucosal neuroma syndrome – *MCT of Vulva In Vivo 24:791–794, 2010*

Neurofibromatosis *BJD 127:540–541, 1992; AD 88:320–321, 1963*

Nevoid basal cell carcinoma syndrome (Gorlin syndrome) *Eur J Gyn Oncol 27:519–522, 2006; J Lower Genital Tract Dis 20:e40–41, 2016*

Reactive arthritis syndrome – red and white papules; circinate vulvovaginitis *AD 128:811–814, 1992; Hautarzt 39:748–739, 1988*

Steatocystoma multiplex

TRAUMA

Inguinal hernia – vulvar swelling *Taiwanese J Ob Gyn January 2015*

VASCULAR

Angiokeratoma of Fordyce *JAAD 12:561–563, 1985; BJD 83:409–411, 1970*

Cherry angioma

Angiomyofibroblastoma *JAAD 38:143–175, 1998*

Blue rubber bleb nevus (purple) *Acta Obstet Gyn Scand 72:310–331, 1993*

Hemangiomas – intact or ulcerated nodules

Lymphangiectasia *Int J Dermatol 55:e482–487, 2016; Indian J Sex Transm-AIDS 33:35–37, 2012; GU Medicine 65:335–337, 1989*

Lymphangioma or lymphangioma circumscriptum *Cutis 67:229–232, 2001; BJD 129:334–336, 1993;* secondary to radiation therapy *Cutis 67:239–240, 2001*

Lymphedema – primary or secondary

Pyogenic granuloma *Ped Derm 21:614–615, 2004*

Thrombophlebitis of the vulva

Varicosity *Int J Women's Health 9:463–475, 2017; Int J Dermatol 55:e482–487, 2016; Indian J Sex Transm-AIDS 33:35–37, 2012; GU Medicine 65:335–337, 1989*

VULVAR ULCERS

AUTOIMMUNE DISEASES AND DISEASES OF IMMUNE DYSFUNCTION

Allergic contact dermatitis – contact vulvitis *NEJM 347:1412–1418, 2002;* vulvar fissure *Genital Skin Disorders, Fischer and Margesson, CV Mosby, 1998, p. 120*

Bullous pemphigoid, including localized childhood vulvar pemphigoid *Ped Derm 36:349–351, 2019; JAAD 22:762–764, 1992; Ped Derm 2:302–307, 1985; AD 128:804–807, 1992;* desquamative vaginitis *Dermatologica 176:200–201, 1988;* anti-p200 and anti-alpha-3 chain of laminin 5 *JAAD 52:S90–92, 2005*

Cicatricial pemphigoid *Ped Derm 21:51–53, 2004; BJD 118:209–217, 1988; Oral Surg 54:656–662, 1982;* end stage scarring may result in introital shrinkage

Dermatitis herpetiformis – juvenile *Trans St John's Hosp Dermatol Soc 54:128–136, 1968*

Epidermolysis bullosa acquisita

Graft vs. host disease

Linear IgA disease (chronic bullous disease of childhood) – annular polycyclic bullae *Ped Derm 15:108–111, 1998*

Lupus erythematosus, systemic *J Drugs in Dermatol 13:1285–1286, 2014; BJD 121:727–741, 1989*

Mixed connective tissue disease – orogenital ulcers *Am J Med 52:148–159, 1972*

Pemphigus foliaceus – erythema and erosions *JAAD 67:409–416, 2012; BJD 158:478–482, 2008; Obstet Gynecol 106:1005–1012, 2005;*

Pemphigoid gestationis

Pemphigus vegetans – personal observation

Pemphigus vulgaris – erythema and erosions *JAAD 73:655–659, 2015; JAAD 67:409–416, 2012; BJD 158:478–482, 2008; Obstet Gynecol 106:1005–1012, 2005; Obstet Gynecol 33:264–266, 1969*

Rheumatoid nodule *J Clin Pathol 49:85–87, 1996*

Severe combined immunodeficiency in Athabascan American-Indian children *AD 135:927–931, 1999*

DRUG-INDUCED

All-trans retinoic acid induction chemotherapy in acute promyelocytic leukemia – fever, scrotal, vulvar, or perineal necrotic ulcers *JAMADerm 153:1181–1182, 2017*

Fixed drug eruption *J Drugs in Dermatol 13:1285–1286, 2014*

Foscarnet-induced ulcer *Cutis 99:14,38, 2017; JAAD 28:799, 1993*

Lithium carbonate *Cutis 48:65–66, 1991*

Nicorandil *BJD 156:394–396, 2007; BJD 155:494–496, 2006; Eur J Dermatol 7:132–133, 1997*

Non-steroidal anti-inflammatory drugs *J Oral Pathol Med 24:46–48, 1995*

EXOGENOUS AGENTS

Benzocaine – erosive papulonodular vulvar dermatitis *JAAD 55:S74–80, 2006*

Foreign bodies *JAAD 57:371–392, 2007*

Irritation – vulvar aphthosis *Ped Derm 26:514–518, 2009*

Quaternary ammonium solutions on a speculum

Tampon use – recurrent vulvar ulcers *JAMA 250:1430–1431, 1983*

INFECTIONS AND INFESTATIONS

Actinomycosis

African histoplasmosis (*Histoplasma capsulatum* var. *duboisii*) – exclusively in central and west Africa and Madagascar *Clin Inf Dis 48:441, 493–494, 2009*

Amebic abscesses – *Entamoeba histolytica Derm Clinics 17:151–185, 1999;* amebic dysentery *Int J Derm 2:259–261, 1963;* amebic ulcers (*Entamoeba histolytica*) – ulcers of the vulva and perineum; often accompanied by diarrhea; serpiginous ulcer *AD 144:1369–1372, 2008; Ped Derm 23:231–234, 2006; Ped Derm 10:352–355, 1993; Pediatrics 71:595–598, 1983; Arch Dis Child 55:234–236, 1980; Mod Probl Paediatr 17:259–261, 1975; Am J Proctol 17:58–63, 1966*

Anaerobic streptococcal infections

Brown recluse spider bite (*Loxosceles reclusa*) *Am J Obstet Gynecol 140:341–343, 1981*

Brucellosis

Candidiasis – vulvar fissure *Sex Transm Dis 12:193–197, 1985*

Chancriform pyoderma (pyogenic ulcer) (*Staphylococcus aureus*) – ulcer with indurated base; eyelid, near mouth, genital *AD 87:736–739, 1963*

Chancroid – ulcerated papule *Genital Skin Disorders, Fischer and Margesson, CV Mosby, 1998, p. 145;* phagedenic chancroid (deformity and mutilation) – round or oval ragged undermined ulcer with satellite ulcers *Int J STD AIDS 8:585–588, 1997; JAAD 19:330–337, 1988*

Cryptococcosis *JAAD 37:116–117, 1997; Genitourin Med 63:341–343, 1987*

Cytomegalovirus infections – ulcers of the vulva and buttocks; serpiginous, morbilliform eruptions, petechiae, vesiculobullous lesions, hyperpigmented nodules, livedoid papules *JAMADerm 154:1217–1218, 2019; Dermatol Ther 23:533–540, 2010; Transpl Infect Dis 10:209–213, 2008; BJD 155:977–982, 2006; Dermatology 200:189–195, 2000*

Diphtheria – gray pseudomembrane

Ecthyma gangrenosum *JAAD 11:781–787, 1984*

Epstein-Barr virus – acute infection (infectious mononucleosis) (Lipschutz ulcer) (ulcus vulvae acuta) – vulvar ulcer in young girl; accompanying tonsillitis and fever with flu-like symptoms *JAAD 72:1–19, 2015; Ped Derm 29:147–153, 2012; Dermatol Ther 23:533–540, 2010; AD 145:38–45, 2009; AD 144:547–552, 2008; Ped Derm 24:130–134, 2007; Act DV 86:439–442, 2006; JAAD 51:824–826, 2004; Dermatol Clin 20:283–289, 2002; Obstet Gynbecol 92:642–644, 1998; J Pediatr Adolesc Gynecol 11:185–187, 1998; Sex Transm Infect Dis 74:296–297, 1998; Genitourin Med 70:356–357, 1993; NEJM 311:966–968, 1984; Am J Obstet Gynecol 127:673–674, 1977*

Furunculosis

Fusospirochetal infection

Gangrenous ecthyma of infancy *Ann DV 108:451–455, 1981*

Gonorrhea with vaginal discharge – round or oval ulcers *Acta DV (Stockh) 43:496, 1963*

Granuloma inguinale (donovanosis) ("serpiginous ulcer") – *Calymmatobacterium granulomatis* – starts as skin-colored subcutaneous nodule which breaks down into vulvar ulcer, vegetative perianal plaques with fistula formation, mutilation, and elephantine changes *JAAD 54:559–578, 2006;* ulcer with rolled border *Genital Skin Disorders, Fischer and Margesson, CV Mosby, 1998, p. 146–148*

Hand foot and mouth disease

Herpes simplex – superficial erosions of the vulva *NEJM 375:666–674, 2016; BJD 172:278–280, 2015; JAAD 60:484–486, 2009; J Inf Dis 177:543–550, 1998; Pediatr Clin North Am 28:397–435, 1981; Am J Obstet Gynecol 135:553–554, 1979;* recalcitrant pseudotumoral anogenital herpes simplex virus type 2 – ulcers and hypertrophic nodules *Clin Inf Dis 57:1648–1655, 2013*

Herpes virus 7 *Acta DV 96:1002–1003, 2016*

Herpes zoster *Genital Skin Disorders, Fischer and Margesson, CV Mosby, 1998, p. 241*

Histoplasmosis *Ob Gyn 122(pt 2)449–452, 2013*

HIV infection, acute *Dermatol Ther 23:533–540, 2010; AD 134:1279–1284, 1998; J Acquir Immune Defic Syndr Hum Retrovirol 13:343–347, 1996*

Impetigo *Genital Skin Disorders, Fischer and Margesson, CV Mosby, 1998, p. 241*

Influenza A *Dermatol Ther 23:533–540, 2010*

Leprosy

Lyme disease *JAMADerm 150:1202–1204, 2014*

Lymphogranuloma venereum – fluctuant lymph nodes ulcerate; fistula formation

Malakoplakia – *Escherichia coli, Pseudomonas* species, *Staphylococcus aureus*; indurated ulcer *J Ind Med Assoc 72:254–255, 1979; Clin Exp Dermatol 2:131–135, 1977*

Morganella morganii G Hal DV 153:291–293, 2018

Mumps *Dermatol Ther 23:533–540, 2010*

Mycobacterium tuberculosis – primary tuberculous chancre *JAAD 26:342–344, 1992;* periorificial tuberculosis *Int J Ob Gyn 48:2234, 1995;* ulcers with ragged edges *Case Rep Ob Gyn 2014:815401*

Mycoplasma pneumoniae JAAD 56:S117–118, 2007

Myiasis *J Nepal Med Assoc 53:288–290, 2015*

Nonsexual acute genital ulcers *Dermatol Ther 23:533–540, 2010*
 Cytomegalovirus
 Epstein-Barr virus
 HIV disease
 Influenza A
 Mumps
 Mycoplasma
 Toxoplasmosis

Osteomyelitis *Genitourinary Med 69:460–461, 1993*

Paratyphoid fever *Eur J Dermatol 13:297–298, 2003*

Phagedenic ulcer

Pneumonia

Pseudomonas aeruginosa J Eur Acad DV 33:781–785, 2019

Pyoderma

Salmonella paratyphi (paratyphoid fever) *Eur J Dermatol 13:297–298, 2003*

Scabies *Genitourinary Med 67:322–326, 1991*

Schistosomiasis *Genital Skin Disorders, Fischer and Margesson, CV Mosby, 1998, p. 241*

Smallpox

Staphylococcus aureus – vulvar fissure; botryomycosis *J Low Genital Tract Dis 18:e80–83, 2014*

Streptococci, beta hemolytic – vaginitis; vulvar fissure *JAAD 57:371–392, 2007;* anaerobic streptococci

Syphilis – primary chancre *Genital Skin Disorders, Fischer and Margesson, CV Mosby, 1998, p. 143;* secondary; tertiary (gummas) *Genitourin Med 65:1–3, 1989*

Tinea cruris – vulvar fissure *Genital Skin Disorders, Fischer and Margesson, CV Mosby, 1998, p. 120*

Trichomonas vaginalis Int J Dermatol 53:e472–473, 2014

Toxoplasmosis *Dermatol Ther 23:533–540, 2010*

Typhoid fever – aphthous ulcer *Ned Tijdschr Geneekd 115:1080–1082, 1971*

Vaccinia *Clin Inf Dis 51:420–421,472–473, 2010*

Varicella *Genital Skin Disorders, Fischer and Margesson, CV Mosby, 1998, p. 241*

Yaws

INFILTRATIVE DISEASES

Amyloidosis *Am J Ob Gyn 180:1041–1044, 1999*

Langerhans cell histiocytosis *Ped Derm 34:484–485, 2017; JAMADerm 150:325–326, 2014; Pan Afr Med J Jul 6, 2014; AD 137:1241–1246, 2001; Cancer 85:2278–2290, 1999; J Dermatol 21:259–263, 1994; Ann Dermatol 2:128–131, 1990;* postmenopausal women *Int J Gyn Pathol 36:111–114, 2017*

Vulvitis circumscripta plasmacellularis (Zoon's plasma cell vulvitis); *BJD 149:638–641, 2003*

INFLAMMATORY DISEASES

Aphthosis

Crohn's disease *Sem Cut Med Surg 34:182–186, 2015;; AD 129:1607–1612, 1993; JAAD 36:986–988, 1996; AD 126:1351–1356, 1990;* mimicking herpes simplex infection *Int J STD AIDS 4:54–56, 1993;* knife-cut ulcer (linear) *JAAD 82:1287–1298, 2020*

Desquamative inflammatory vaginitis *Genitourin Med 66:275–279, 1990*

Erythema multiforme *Medicine 68:133–140, 1989; JAAD 8:763–765, 1983;* Stevens-Johnson syndrome

Erythema of Jacquet *Ped Derm 8:160–161, 1991*

Focal vulvitis

Hidradenitis suppurativa *Sem Cut Med Surg 34:182–186, 2015;*

Pilonidal sinuses *Am J Obstet Gynecol 101:854–856, 1968*

Pyoderma gangrenosum *Sem Cut Med Surg 34:182–186, 2015; BJD 157:1235–1239, 2007; JAAD 27:623–625, 1992; Int J Gynaecol Obstet 35:175–178, 1991*

Stevens-Johnson syndrome – adhesions of the labia *BJD 177:924–935, 2017*

Toxic epidermal necrolysis *Genital Skin Disorders, Fischer and Margesson, CV Mosby, 1998, p. 241*

Ulcus vulvae acutum (Lipschutz ulcer) – necrotic, painful vulvar ulcer with fever and lymphadenopathy; often associated with acute Epstein-Barr virus infection with positive serology to capsid antigens (IgM and IgG) *J Eur Acad DV Dec 19, 2019; Ped Derm 370–372, 2012; Ped Derm 25:113–115, 2008; Ped Derm 25:364–367, 2008; Cutis 65:387–389, 2000; BJD 135:663–665, 1996; Acta DV (Stockh) 45:221–222, 1965; Arch Dermatol Syph (Berlin)114:363–395, 1913; Obstet Gynecol 38:440–443, 1971;* inflammatory dermatoses – any inflammatory dermatosis may result in vulvar erosions and ulcers; Lipschutz ulcer (ulcus vulvae acutum) (genital ulcers in teenagers) – acute genital (vulvar) ulcer accompanying tonsillitis and fever with flu-like symptoms; Epstein-Barr virus in 1/3 of patients *Cutis 91:273–276, 2013; JAAD 63:44–51, 2010; AD 145:38–45, 2009; Ped Derm 25:113–115, 2008; Eur J Dermatol 13:297–298, 2003; J Pediatr 11:185, 1998; Obstet Gynecol 92:642, 1998; Sex Transm Infec 74:296–297, 1998; BJD 135:663–665, 1996; Genitourin Med 70:356, 1994; Acta DV 45:221–222, 1965; Archives of Dermatology Syphilol 20:363–396, 1912;* associated with upper respiratory infections, viral gastroenteritis, Epstein-Barr virus, cytomegalovirus, *Mycoplasma fermentans,* influenza A, streptococcal pharyngitis, mumps *JAMADerm 151:1388–1389, 2015; JAAD 68:885–896, 2013*

Vulvovaginitis, non-specific *JAAD 57:371–392, 2007*

METABOLIC DISEASES

Acrodermatitis enteropathica *Genital Skin Disorders, Fischer and Margesson, CV Mosby, 1998, p. 228*

Estrogen deficiency – atrophic vulvitis with vulvar fissure *Genital Skin Disorders, Fischer and Margesson, CV Mosby, 1998, p. 120*

Pellagra vaginitis

Uremia

NEOPLASTIC

Basal cell carcinoma *Sem Cut Med Surg 34:182–186, 2015*

Bowen's disease

Eccrine porocarcinoma *J Med Case Rep 10:319, 2016*

Extramammary Paget's disease *Sem Cut Med Surg 34:182–186, 2015; J Cutan Aesthet Surg 6:40–44, 2013*

Kaposi's sarcoma

Leukemia – myelomonocytic leukemia – presenting with vaginal ulcers *Dermatology 199:346–348, 1999;* myelocytic *South Med J 86:293–294, 1993*

Lymphoma *JAAD 51:824–826, 2004*

Melanoma *Oncology 10:1017–1024, 1996*

Metastases – metastases from anal squamous cell carcinoma *Cutis 91:125–126, 2013;* ulcerated nodule *Genital Skin Disorders, Fischer and Margesson, CV Mosby, 1998, p. 219;* infiltrating ductal carcinoma of the breast *J Egypt Natl Cancer Instit 27:243–246, 2015*

Myelodysplasia – primary cutaneous lesion – personal observation

Squamous cell carcinoma *Sem Cut Med Surg 34:182–186, 2015; Gynecol Oncol 134:314–318, 2014;* squamous cell carcinoma of the vagina with condylomata acuminata with high-grade squamous intraepithelial lesion of the cervix due to high risk papillomavirus infection *NEJM 370:2032–2041, 2014;* squamous cell carcinoma associated with lichen planus *JAAD 71:698–707, 2014*

Vulvar intraepithelial neoplasia *Genital Skin Disorders, Fischer and Margesson, CV Mosby, 1998, p. 212–213*

PARANEOPLASTIC DISORDERS

Necrobiotic xanthogranuloma with paraproteinemia *JAAD December 2014;e247–248*

Necrolytic migratory erythema (glucagonoma syndrome) *Genital Skin Disorders, Fischer and Margesson, CV Mosby, 1998, p. 241; Lancet ii:1–4, 1974*

Paraneoplastic pemphigus *Ped Derm 20:238–242, 2003*

PRIMARY CUTANEOUS DISEASES

Acute parapsoriasis (pityriasis lichenoides et varioliformis acuta) (Mucha-Habermann disease) *AD 123:1335–1339, 1987; AD 118:478, 1982*

Anovaginal fistula – vulvar ulceration *J Reprod Med 33:857–858, 1988*

Aphthosis (complex aphthosis) (nonsexually acquired genital ulceration) *Sem Cut Med Surg 34:187–191, 2015; JAAD 68:797–802, 2013*

Atopic dermatitis – excoriations *JAAD 57:371–392, 2007*

Epidermolysis bullosa – polydysplastic epidermolysis bullosa

Hailey-Hailey disease *Bull Soc Fr Dermatol Syphiligr 75:352–355, 1975*

Hailey-Hailey disease *Bull Soc Fr Dermatol Syphiligr 75:352–355, 1975*

Intertrigo – with fissuring *Genital Skin Disorders, Fischer and Margesson, CV Mosby, 1998, p. 164*

Keratosis lichenoides chronica *JAAD 49:511–513, 2003*

Lichen planus – erosive *JAAD 79:789–804, 2018; Sem Cut Med Surg 34:182–186, 2015; BJD 135:89–91, 1996; AD 130:1379–1382, 1994; AD 125:1677–1680, 1989; Int J Dermatol 28:381–384, 1989;* vulvovaginal gingival syndrome (lichen planus) *JAAD 55:98–113, 2006*

Lichen sclerosus et atrophicus – bullous or non-bullous; vulvar fissure *Genital Skin Disorders, Fischer and Margesson, CV Mosby, 1998, p. 120–121*

Lichen simplex chronicus *J Reprod Med 36:309–311, 1991;* vulvar fissure *Genital Skin Disorders, Fischer and Margesson, CV Mosby, 1998, p. 120*

Psoriasis – vulvar fissure *Genital Skin Disorders, Fischer and Margesson, CV Mosby, 1998, p. 120*

PSYCHOCUTANEOUS DISEASES

Factitial *Genital Skin Disorders, Fischer and Margesson, CV Mosby, 1998, p. 241; Obstet Gynecol 41:239–242, 1973*

Self-mutilation *Genital Skin Disorders, Fischer and Margesson, CV Mosby, 1998, p. 123–124*

SYNDROMES

AEC syndrome (Hay-Wells syndrome) – vaginal erosions, mild hypohidrosis *Ped Derm 16:103–107, 1999*

Behcet's disease *JAAD 79:987–1006, 2018; BJD 159:555–560, 2008; BJD 157:901–906, 2007; JAAD 51:S83–87, 2004; Ulster Med J 56:74–76, 1987;* giant vulvar ulcers *JAAD 62:162–164, 2010;* in children *Ped Derm 32:714–717, 2015*

Hemophagocytic syndrome *Ped Hem Oncol 20:421–425, 2003*

Hypereosinophilic syndrome *AD 132:535–541, 1996*

Kindler's syndrome – vaginal stenosis following blistering *BJD 160:233–242, 2009*

MAGIC syndrome *AD 126:940–944, 1990*

Periodic fever, aphthosis, pharyngotonsillitis, cervical adenopathy (PFAPA) – aphthous ulcers, vulvar ulcers *Ped Derm 28:290–294, 2011*

Reactive arthritis syndrome – erosions with marginal erythema; circinate erosions *JAAD 59:113–121, 2008; NEJM 309:1606–1615, 1983; Semin Arthritis Rheum 3:253–286, 1974; Dtsch Med Wochenschr 42:1535–1536, 1916*
  Urethritis
  Ulcerative vulvitis – red crusted plaques of the vulva and perineum *JAAD 48:613–616, 2003; Arch Int Med 145:822–824, 1985*

Sweet's syndrome *JAAD 51:824–826, 2004*

TRAUMA

Blunt/sharp injury *Genital Skin Disorders, Fischer and Margesson, CV Mosby, 1998, p. 241*

Chemical trauma *Genital Skin Disorders, Fischer and Margesson, CV Mosby, 1998, p. 241*

Child abuse – transaction of the posterior hymenal ring *JAAD 57:371–392, 2007*

Excoriations

Female genital mutilation

Lacerated hymen *Genital Skin Disorders, Fischer and Margesson, CV Mosby, 1998, p. 115*

Mechanical *Genital Skin Disorders, Fischer and Margesson, CV Mosby, 1998, p. 241*

Pressure ulcers *Wounds 29:e28–31, 2017; Sem Cut Med Surg 34:182–186, 2015*

Radiation necrosis *Am J Obstet Gynecol 164:1235–1238, 1991*

Sexual abuse *Genital Skin Disorders, Fischer and Margesson, CV Mosby, 1998, p. 125–127*

Sexual injury *Aust NZ J Obstet Gynecol 6:291–293, 1966*

VASCULAR LESIONS

Atherosclerotic peripheral vascular disease *Genital Skin Disorders, Fischer and Margesson, CV Mosby, 1998, p. 230*

Hemangioma, ulcerated *JAAD 57:371–392, 2007; Plast Reconstr Surg 87:861–866, 1991; Clin Pediatr 27:213–215, 1988*

VULVAR ULCERS IN YOUNG GIRLS

Ped Derm 29:147–153, 2012

Behcet's disease

Bullous pemphigoid

Child abuse

Cytomegalovirus infection

Epstein-Barr virus – acute infection (infectious mononucleosis) (Lipschutz ulcer) (ulcus vulvae acuta) – vulvar ulcer in young girl; accompanying tonsillitis and fever with flu-like symptoms

Fixed drug eruption

Idiopathic

Inflammatory bowel disease

Influenza

Lipschutz ulcer (ulcus vulvae acutum) *Ped Derm 29:370–372, 2012; Ped Derm 25:113–115, 2008*

MAGIC syndrome

Mumps

Mycoplasma pneumonia

Paratyphoid

Pemphigus vulgaris

Pyoderma gangrenosum

Salmonella

Stevens-Johnson syndrome

Trauma

WHITE FEET

AUTOIMMUNE DISEASES AND DISEASES OF IMMUNE DYSFUNCTION

Allergic contact dermatitis

Bullous pemphigoid

Dermatomyositis

Hypersensitivity vasculitis

Lupus erythematosus, systemic

Pemphigus

Rheumatoid arthritis

Scleroderma

Vitiligo

CONGENITAL ANOMALIES

Syringomyelia

DRUG-INDUCED

Intra-arterial injection of vasopressors

Vasoconstrictors – nicotine, ergot

EXOGENOUS

Overhydration – maceration

INFECTIONS AND INFESTATIONS

Pitted keratolysis

Tinea pedis

INFLAMMATORY DISEASES

Stevens-Johnson syndrome/toxic epidermal necrolysis *BJD 174:1194–1227, 2016*

METABOLIC DISEASES

Cold proteins

Cystic fibrosis – aquagenic wrinkling of the palms *Ped Derm 23:39–42, 2006; AD 141:621–624, 2005*

Hyperviscosity

Macroglobulinemia

PARANEOPLASTIC DISEASES

Tripe soles *J Clin Oncology 7:669–678, 1989*

PRIMARY CUTANEOUS DISEASES

Dyshidrosis

Palmoplantar keratoderma

Pustular psoriasis

Symmetrical lividity of the soles (hyperhidrosis) *BJD 37:123–125, 1925*

Weber-Cockayne epidermolysis bullosa with plantar blisters

TOXINS

Perchloroethylene-induced Raynaud's phenomenon

Vinyl chloride exposure

TRAUMA

Delayed deep pressure urticaria

Friction blisters

Tropical immersion foot

VASCULAR DISEASES

Arteriosclerosis – pallor

Raynaud's phenomenon *NEJM 368:1344, 2013*

Thromboangiitis obliterans

WHITE MACULES

AUTOIMMUNE DISEASES AND DISEASES OF IMMUNE DYSFUNCTION

Allergic contact dermatitis – azo dyes *Contact Dermatitis 38:189–193, 1998;* monobenzyl ether of hydroquinone; rubber allergic contact dermatitis with post-inflammatory depigmentation; rubber wristwatch band; biking suit

Acquired agammaglobulinemia – vitiligo

APECED (autoimmune polyendocrinopathy, candidiasis, ectodermal dystrophy) syndrome (autoimmune polyendocrine syndrome type 1) – autosomal recessive; mutation in AIRE gene (autoimmune regulator gene); chronic mucocutaneous candidiasis, hypoparathyroidism, Addison's disease, diabetes mellitus type 1, thyroid autoimmune disease, gonadal failure, hepatitis, vitiligo, alopecia areata, pernicious anemia, intestinal malabsorption, keratinopathy, dystrophy of dental enamel and nails *JAAD 73:255–264, 2015; Ped Derm 24:529–533, 2007; JAAD 62:864–868, 2010*

Bullous pemphigoid – white coating to oral lesions *ENT J 95:e1–5, 2016*

Dermatomyositis – with Degos disease-like lesions *JAAD 50:895–899, 2004;* avascular areas – personal observation

Graft vs. host disease – hypopigmented patches or total leukoderma *BJD 134:780–783, 1996;* acute GVHD – vitiligo of the central face *AD 147:1460–1461, 2011;* confetti-like depigmentation *JAAD 66:515–532, 2012;* vitiligo and alopecia areata in chronic graft vs. host disease *JAMADerm 151:23–332, 2015*

Lupus erythematosus – systemic lupus – reticulated telangiectatic erythema of thenar and hypothenar eminences, finger pulps, toes, lateral feet, and heels; bluish red with small white scars; striate leukonychia discoid lupus erythematosus; Degos disease-like lesions *BJD 95:649–652, 1976; Arch Int Med 134:321–323, 1974;* vitiligo-like patches after resolution of subacute cutaneous LE *JAAD 44:925–931, 2001; Dermatology 200:6–10, 2000; SCLE JAAD 33:828–830, 1995, Z. Hautkr 69:123–126, 1994;* discoid lupus erythematosus *NEJM 269:1155–1161, 1963;* neonatal lupus – vitiligo-like patches *Clin Exp Dermatol 19:409–411, 1994;* neonatal lupus – depigmented raccoon eyes *Ped Derm 47:647, 2002*

Morphea – guttate; linear morphea (en coup de sabre) – early bleaching of hair; pansclerotic morphea; morphea resembling vitiligo *JAAD 65:364–373, 2011*

Pemphigus vulgaris

Rheumatoid arthritis – Degos disease-like lesions *J Dermatol 24:488–490, 1997;* atrophie blanche-like lesions in rheumatoid vasculitis *BJD 147:905–913, 2002*

Scleroderma (progressive systemic sclerosis) – Raynaud's phenomenon *NEJM 369:1638, 2013;* Degos disease-like lesions *AD 100:575–581, 1969*

CONGENITAL LESIONS

Facial fusion defect (focal preauricular dermal dysplasia) (form of aplasia cutis congenital) – white atrophic patches of lateral cheeks *Ped Derm 25:344–348, 2008*

DEGENERATIVE DISEASES

Atrophic genitourinary syndrome of menopause – pale white firm vagina *JAAD 82:1287–1298, 2020*

Idiopathic guttate hypomelanosis *JAAD 23:681–684, 1990*

Morgagnian cataract (hypermature corticonuclear cataract) *NEJM 370:2326, 2014*

DRUGS

Afloqualone – photoleukomelanoderma *J Dermatol 21:430–433, 1994*

Anti-PD-1 therapy (nivolumab/pembrolizumab) – lichenoid eruptions, vitiligo, dermatitis *JAAD 76:863–870, 2017; JAAD 74:455–461, 2016;* pembrolizumab depigmentation *RJO 178:265–269, 2018*

Cabozantinib – VEGFR2 inhibitor; c-met; RET multitargets; tyrosine kinase inhibitor; hand foot skin reactions with bullae, hyperkeratosis, acral erythema; skin and hair depigmentation, splinter hemorrhages, xerosis, red scrotum *JAMADerm 151:170–177, 2015*

Chloroquine *Cutis 91:129–136, 2013; NEJM 360:160–169, 2009; JAAD 48:981–983, 2003;* phototoxicity leading to vitiligo *J R Army Med Corps 144:163–165, 1998;* loss of hair pigmentation

Corticosteroids – topical; following steroid injection; inhaled corticosteroids – hair depigmentation *J Drugs Dermatol 12:119–120, 2013*

CTLA-4 inhibitors – ipilimumab, tremelimumab – vitiligo, morbilliform eruption *JAAD 72:221–236, 2015*

Dasatinib (thiazole carboxamide derivative) – leukotrichia *JAMA Derm 149:636–638, 2013*

Diphencyprone *Dermatologica 177:146–148, 1988*

DRESS syndrome – resulting in vitiligo *BJD 175:642–644, 2016*

Epidermal growth factor receptor inhibitors – cetuximab and panitumumab; erlotinib and gefitinib; lapatinib; canertinib; vandetanib – poliosis *JAAD 72:203–218, 2015*

Fluphenazine *NEJM 360:160–169, 2009*

Flutamide – with residual vitiligo *Contact Dermatitis 38:68–70, 1998*

Guanonitrofuracin

Hydroquinone – hypopigmentation of skin and hair

Imatinib mesylate – vitiligo-like lesions *NEJM 360:160–169, 2009; Ped Derm 23:175–178, 2006;* extension of vitiligo *BJD 153:691–692, 2005;* generalized hypopigmentation *Cancer 98:2483–2487, 2003;* hypopigmentation of distal fingers *J Natl Med Assoc 95:722–724, 2003;* progression of vitiligo *BJD 153:691–692, 2005; Cancer 98:2483–2487, 2003; J Natl Mead Assoc 95:722–724, 2003; J Clin Oncol 20:869–870, 2002*

Imiquimod *Cutis 91:129–136, 2013; NEJM 360:160–169, 2009*

Interferon alpha – induction of vitiligo *Cutis 60:289–290, 1997*

Ipilimumab – vitiligo *JAAD 71:161–169, 2014*

IL-2 reaction *AD 130:890–893, 1995*

Melanoma vaccine-associated leukoderma – gp100/MART-1-transduced dendritic cell vaccine *AD 138:799–802, 2002*

Mercaptoamines

Mercurial ointments – periorbital depigmentation

Niacinamide *Cutis 91:129–136, 2013*

Non-selective antiangiogenic multikinase inhibitors – sorafenib, sunitinib, pazopanib – hyperkeratotic hand foot skin reactions with knuckle papules, inflammatory reactions, alopecia, kinking of hair, depigmentation of hair; chloracne-like eruptions, erythema multiforme, toxic epidermal necrolysis, drug hypersensitivity, red scrotum with erosions, yellow skin, eruptive nevi, pyoderma gangrenosum-like lesions *JAAD 72:203–218, 2015*

Phenobarbital – depigmentation of skin and hair *Ann DV 119:927–929, 1992*

Phenols

Phenylthiourea – hypopigmentation of the skin and hair

Physostigmine *Cutis 91:129–136, 2013; NEJM 360:160–169, 2009*

Prolixin *Cutis 91:129–136, 2013*

Serine protease inhibitors *Cutis 91:129–136, 2013*

Sulfhydryls *Cutis 91:129–136, 2013*

Sunitinib – facial depigmentation *JAAD 61:905–906, 2009*

Thiotepa eyedrops – periorbital depigmentation *Cutis 91:129–136, 2013; AD 115:973–974, 1979*

Tremelimumab – depigmented hair *JAAD 80:1179–1196, 2019*

Tretinoin *Cutis 91:129–136, 2013*

Triparanol – hypopigmented hair

Tyrosine kinase inhibitors

Valproic acid – hypopigmented hair

Vasoconstrictors – nicotine, ergot

Vasopressors – intra-arterial injections of vasopressors

EXOGENOUS AGENTS

Chemical leukoderma *NEJM 360:160–169, 2009*
  Aloesin *Cutis 91:129–136, 2013*
  Alstroemeria *Cutis 91:129–136, 2013*
  Amyl nitrite *Cutis 91:129–136, 2013*
  Arsenic *Cutis 91:129–136, 2013*
  Ascorbic acid *Cutis 91:129–136, 2013*
  Azelaic acid *Cutis 91:129–136, 2013*
  Azo dyes – eyeliner, lipliner, lipstick, "alta," fur dye, amulet string color *BJD 160:40–47, 2009*
  Benzyl alcohol
  Carbyne *Cutis 91:129–136, 2013*
  C2 ceramides *Cutis 91:129–136, 2013*
  Cerium oxide *Cutis 91:129–136, 2013*

Cinnamic aldehyde *Cutis 91:129–136, 2013*
Co-enzyme Q10-triggered vitiligo *BJD 169:1333–1336, 2013*
Corticosteroids *Cutis 91:129–136, 2013*
Diisopropyl fluorophosphates
4-S-cysteaminylphenol *Cutis 91:129–136, 2013*
4-S-cysteinylphenol *Cutis 91:129–136, 2013*
Diphencyprone *Cutis 91:129–136, 2013*
Ellagic acid *Cutis 91:129–136, 2013*
Hydroquinone *Cutis 91:129–136, 2013; BJD 105(Suppl.21):51–56, 1981*
4-hydroxyanisole *Cutis 91:129–136, 2013*
Kojic acid *Cutis 91:129–136, 2013*
Lectins *Cutis 91:129–136, 2013*
Lysophosphatidic acid *Cutis 91:129–136, 2013*
Mercurials
Methyl gentisate *Cutis 91:129–136, 2013*
Monobenzone *Cutis 91:129–136, 2013*
Monobenzyl ether of hydroquinone *BJD 105(Suppl.21):51–56, 1981;* rubber sandals *BJD 160:40–47, 2009*
Monobenzyl ether *Cutis 91:129–136, 2013*
Neoglycoproteins *Cutis 91:129–136, 2013*
Paraphenylenediamine – hair dye, black socks and shoes *BJD 160:40–47, 2009;* paraphenylenediamine in cosmetic strings – linear depigmentation *JAAD 61:909–910, 2009*
Para-tertiary butyl phenol *Cutis 91:129–136, 2013; BJD 105(Suppl.21):51–56, 1981; Dermatologica 135:54–59, 1967;* deodorant, spray perfume, detergent, cleansers, adhesive "bindi" *BJD 160:40–47, 2009*
Para-tertiary amyl phenol *Cutis 91:129–136, 2013; BJD 105(Suppl.21):51–56, 1981*
Para-tertiary butyl catechol *BJD 105(Suppl.21):51–56, 1981*
Phenols/catechols
Physostigmine
Rubber gloves *Dermatitis 25:155–162, 2014*
Sulfhydryls
Lymphocyte infusion – vitiligo *BJD 145:1015–1017, 2001*
Nickel *Cutis 91:129–136, 2013*
Synthetic opioid MT-45 – hair depigmentation, hair loss, Mees' lines *BJD 176:1021–1027, 2017*
Phospholipids D2 *Cutis 91:129–136, 2013*
PPD *Cutis 91:129–136, 2013*
Primula *Cutis 91:129–136, 2013*
PUVA therapy for cutaneous T-cell lymphoma – vitiligo-like leukoderma *BJD 145:1008–1014, 2001*
Resveratrol *Cutis 91:129–136, 2013*
Squaric acid dibutyl ester *Cutis 91:129–136, 2013*
Swim goggles – periorbital leukoderma (raccoon-like) *Contact Dermatitis 10:129–131, 1984*
Tazarotene *Cutis 91:129–136, 2013*
Vitamin E – white hair at injection sites of infants *Cutis 91:129–136, 2013; Dermatologica 145:56–59, 1972*

INFECTIONS AND INFESTATIONS

Dengue fever (*Flavivirus*) – exanthem with islands of sparing ("white islands in a sea of red") *Clin Inf Dis 36:1004–1005,1074–1075, 2003;* initially (first 24 hours) flushing of the face, neck, and chest; morbilliform or macular eruption with white islands of sparing and petechiae; acral and/or periorbital edema, petechial mucosae, headache, retro-orbital pain, arthralgia, myalgia, leucopenia; incubation period 3–14 days; *Aedes aegypti/A. albopictus JAAD*

58:308–316, 2008; JAAD 46:430–433, 2002; Dermatol Clinics 17:29–40, 1999; Inf Dis Clin NA 8:107, 1994; clinical differential diagnosis includes typhoid fever, leptospirosis, meningococcal disease, streptococcal disease, staph, rickettsial disease, malaria, arbovirus (chikungunya, o'nyong nyong fevers), Kawasaki's disease

Gram-negative toe web space infection – white maceration

Herpes zoster – post-inflammatory depigmentation *Int J Derm 25:624–628, 1986*

Leishmaniasis – post-kala azar dermal leishmaniasis; depigmented macules *JAAD 60:897–925, 2009*

Leprosy – indeterminate – hypopigmented macules of the face, arms, buttocks, or trunk; borderline tuberculoid, tuberculoid – ill-defined hypopigmented macules and patches with dry, hairless anesthetic surface with fine wrinkling *Indian J Opin 57:74–76, 208; Int J Lepr Other Mycobact Dis 67:388–391, 1999;* lepromatous leprosy; borderline lepromatous; white lunulae

Measles – Koplik's spots

Onchocerciasis – hypopigmented and depigmented atrophic macules of pretibial, inguinal areas, and bony prominences (leopard skin); dermatitis *JAAD 73:929–944, 2015; BJD 171:1078–1083, 2014; Cutis 65:293–297, 2000*

Oral hairy leukoplakia – Epstein-Barr + tongue lesion *Med Oral Pathol Oral Cir Buccal 24:e799–803, 2019*

Parvovirus B19 – Koplik's spots

Pinta – late secondary phase hypopigmented, depigmented hyperpigmented atrophic skin *JAAD 54:559–578, 2006; AD 135:685–688, 1999;* tertiary (late phase) – achromia over the elbows, knees, ankles, wrists back of hands

Pitted keratolysis

Syphilis – secondary; as macular syphilid fades get depigmented macules with hyperpigmented background (leukoderma syphiliticum) ("necklace of Venus") on back and sides of the neck (necklace of Venus) *JAAD 82:1–14, 2020*

Tinea pedis

Tinea versicolor *NEJM 360:160–169, 2009; Semin Dermatol 4:173–184, 1985*

Tungiasis – white papule of toe tip with central brown dot *BJD 158:635–636, 2008*

Verruca – involuting flat wart with halo

Yaws – primary red papule, ulcerates, crusted; satellite papules; become round ulcers, papillomatous or vegetative friable nodules which bleed easily (raspberry-like) (framboesia); heals with large atrophic scar with white center with dark halo

INFLAMMATORY DISEASES

Crohn's disease – Degos disease-like lesions *Acta DV (Stockh) 75:408–409, 1995*

Leukoderma following erythema multiforme *Ped Derm 18:120–122, 2001;* also following SLE, SCLE, CTCL, actinic dermatitis, Darier's disease

Post-inflammatory hypopigmentation of the skin and hair

Sarcoid *AD 123:1557–1562, 1987; Am J Med 35:67–89, 1963;* extensive depigmented scars of scalp *JAAD 59:S126–127, 2008;* white patches of vulva *JAMADerm 130:666–667, 2014*

Sympathetic ophthalmia – depigmentation of eyebrows and eyelashes

METABOLIC DISEASES

Acrodermatitis enteropathica – vitiligo-like acral depigmentation *Ped Derm 24:668–669, 2007*

Addison's disease – vitiligo-like patches; generalized bronze hyperpigmentation *Trans Ped 6:300–312, 2017*

Anemia – generalized pallor

Metastatic calcification – personal observation

Canities in infant *JAMADerm 150:1116–1117, 2014*
  Micronutrient deficiency
  Pernicious anemia
  Premature aging syndrome

Cold proteins – cryoglobulins, cryofibrinogens, cold agglutinins

Hyperviscosity

Hypopituitarism – diffuse loss of pigment

Kwashiorkor – hypochromotrichia and hypopigmentation of the skin *Cutis 67:321–327, 2001; Cutis 51:445–446, 1993*

Malabsorption – AIDS, inflammatory bowel disease, vitamin B12 deficiency; hypopigmented hair; white lunulae

Necrobiosis lipoidica diabeticorum – of the scalp with central depigmentation *Trans St John's Hosp Dermatol Soc 57:202–220, 1971*

Nephrogenic systemic fibrosis – personal observation

Panhypopituitarism – pale, yellow tinged skin

Pernicious anemia – vitiligo, canities

Phenylketonuria – phenylalanine hydroxylase deficiency; fair skin and hair; lichen sclerosus-like changes *JAAD 49:S190–192, 2003*

Congenital erythropoietic porphyria – photodistributed bullae, hypertrichosis of the face and neck, depigmented scars, milia, sclerosis of the hands; mutation of URO III synthase *Ped Derm 35:833–834, 2018;* or GATA1 *Eur J Haematol 94:491–497, 2015*

Prolidase deficiency – autosomal recessive; atrophie blanche lesions; skin spongy and fragile with annular pitting and scarring; leg ulcers; photosensitivity, telangiectasia, purpura, premature graying, lymphedema *Ped Derm 13:58–60, 1996; JAAD 29:819–821, 1993; AD 127:124–125, 1991; AD 123:493–497, 1987*

Renal disease – hypopigmented hair; generalized pallor

Schnyder's crystalline corneal dystrophy – deposition of cholesterol and phospholipids in corneal stroma; decreased day vision *NEJM 363, 275, 2010*

Thyroid disease – hyper- or hypothyroidism – vitiligo

Vitamin A deficiency – Bitot spots – triangular foamy white lesions at temporal paralimbal areas of both eyes

Vitamin B12 deficiency – hair depigmentation *JAAD 68:211–243, 2013;* hyperpigmentation of the palms and soles and intertriginous areas, oral mucosa; atrophic glossitis, vitiligo *Cut Oculo Tox 33:70–73, 2014*

Zinc deficiency – canities in infant *JAMADerm 150:1116–1117, 2014*

NEOPLASTIC DISEASES

Basal cell carcinoma – with depigmented halo

Blue nevus – with depigmented halo

Clear cell papulosis – white macules on the lower abdomen in infancy with later development of these lesions in the milk line *AD 143:358–360, 2007; BJD 138:678–683, 1998; Am J Surg Pathol 11:827–834, 1987*

Dermatofibroma – with depigmented halo

Eccrine syringomatous carcinoma – facial scar-like lesion *JAMADerm 151:1034–1036, 2015*

Extramammary Paget's disease – white patches of the vulva *BJD 151:1049–1053, 2004*

Histiocytosis, malignant – multiple erythematous plaques with depigmentation *Am J Dermatopathol 19:299–302, 1997*

Lymphoma – hypopigmented cutaneous T-cell lymphoma *NEJM 360:160–169, 2009; J Dermatol 27:543–546, 2000; AD 128:1265–1270, 1992;* depigmented macules of erythrodermic CTCL *JAAD 46:325–357, 2002;* in childhood *Ped Derm 14:449–452, 1997; AD 130:476–480, 1994; JAAD 17:563–570, 1987;* hydroa vacciniforme-like cutaneous T-cell lymphoma, Epstein-Barr virus-related – edema, blisters, vesicles, ulcers, white scars, facial scars, swollen nose, lips, and periorbital edema, crusts with central hemorrhagic necrosis, facial dermatitis, photodermatitis, facial edema, facial papules and plaques, crusting of ears, fever *JAAD 81:23–41, 2019; JAAD 69:112–119, 2013;*

Melanocytic nevus, congenital or acquired – halo nevus *JAAD 67:582–586, 2012; JAAD 60:508–514, 2009;* atypical nevi, non-pigmented *AD 113:992–994, 1997*
  Congenital melanocytic nevus with areas of depigmentation *Ped Derm 33:307–310, 2016*
  Halo nevus (Sutton's nevus; leukoderma acquisitum centrifugum) – depigmented skin and hair *Clin in Derm 37:561–579, 2019; AD 92:14–35, 1965*
  Halo nevus without nevus

Melanoma – melanoma-associated leukoderma *NEJM 360:160–169, 2009;* hypopigmented hair; regressed melanoma – white scar *JAAD 53:101–107, 2005;* primary cutaneous melanoma – vitiligo-like patch *Practical Dermatology pp.55–56, May, 2014;* melanoma response to pembrolizumab – onset of vitiligo *JAMADerm 152:45–51, 2016*

Neurofibroma – with halo

Nevus depigmentosus

Retinoblastoma – white pupil (leucocoria) *JAMA 311:1799–1800, 2014*
  Differential diagnosis of leucocoria in a child:
    Cataract
    Coats' disease
    Persistent fetal vasculature
    Retinal detachment
    Retinoblastoma
    Toxocariasis
    Uveitis

Seborrheic keratosis – with halo

Tumor of the follicular infundibulum

Waldenstrom's macroglobulinemia – pallor, IgM storage papules, livedo reticularis *Ann Dermatol 30:87–90, 2018;* exposed acral areas exposed to low temperatures *Clin Dermatol 37:610–617, 2019*

White sponge nevus

PARANEOPLASTIC DISORDERS

Carcinoid syndrome – white macules surrounded by erythema and telangiectasia *BJD 90:547–551, 1974*

Melanoma-associated leukoderma *JAAD 75:1198–1204, 2016*

Tripe palms

PHOTODERMATOSES

Annular elastolytic granuloma (actinic granuloma) – annular lesion with central wrinkling, atrophy, and white depigmentation *JAMADerm 152:1045–1046, 2016*

Chronic actinic dermatitis with vitiligo-like depigmentation *Clin Exp Dermatol 17:38–43, 1992*

Stellate pseudoscars *BJD 159:479–480, 2008; AD 105:551–554, 1972*

PRIMARY CUTANEOUS DISEASES

Adrenergic urticaria – wheals surrounded by white halos (due to vasoconstriction) *BJD 158:629–631, 2008*

Albinism – tyrosinase negative (type IA), yellow mutant (type IB), platinum, tyrosinase positive (type II), minimal pigment, brown, rufous; Hermansky-Pudlak syndrome – hypopigmented skin and hair *JAAD 19:217–255, 1988;* Elejalde syndrome, Cross-McKusick-Breen syndrome, Chediak-Higashi syndrome

Albinoidism *JAAD 19:217–255, 1988*

Alopecia areata – white overnight (Marie Antoinette syndrome) *AD 145:656, 2009*

Atopic dermatitis – white dermatographism; pallor around the mouth, nose, and ears; post-inflammatory depigmentation in dark-skinned patients secondary to rubbing and lichenification

Atrophoderma of Pasini and Pierini

Bier's spots *J Eur Acad DV 33:e78–79, 2019*

Darier's disease – perifollicular depigmented macules *BJD 827–830, 1989;* linear white streaks of nails *JAAD 27:40–50, 1992;* white lunulae

Dyshidrosis

Epidermolysis bullosa – Weber-Cockayne variant with plantar bullae

Fibroelastolytic papulosis of the neck *BJD 137:461–466, 1997*

Granuloma multiforme – upper trunk and arms; papules evolving into annular plaques with geographical, polycyclic borders; heal centrally with depigmented macules; Central Africa

Idiopathic guttate hypomelanosis *Clin in Derm 37:561–579, 2019*

Lichen planus, atrophic

Lichen sclerosus et atrophicus (balanitis xerotica obliterans (lichen sclerosus of the glans)) – non-bullous or bullous *JAAD 82:1287–1298, 2020; World J Urol 18:382–387, 2000; AD 123:1391–1396, 1987;* purpuric *Ped Derm 10:129–131, 1993;* guttate variant; of the scalp *BJD 103:197–200, 1980;* lichen sclerosus and morphea *AD 148:24–28, 2012;* vitiligoid lichen sclerosus *Ped Derm 35:198–201, 2018*

Lichen striatus *Clin in Derm 37:561–579, 2019*

Palmoplantar keratoderma – diffuse non-epidermolytic of Bothnian type with hyperhidrosis; *Corynebacterium* infections; mutation in AQP5 *BMC Dermatol Jul 3, 2015*

Perifollicular macular atrophy (perifollicular elastolysis) – gray-white finely wrinkled round areas of atrophy with central hair follicle *BJD 83:143–150, 1970*

Pili annulati – spangled hair *Cutis 91:254–257, 2013*

Pityriasis alba

Pityriasis lichenoides chronica *BJD 100:297–302, 1979*

Progressive macular hypomelanosis

Psoriasis – Woronoff ring; pustular psoriasis

Striae – depigmentation *Cutis 91:129–136, 2013*

Symmetrical lividity of the soles

Vitiligo – face, axillae, groin, areolae, genitalia, areas of trauma or friction *JAAD 80:1215–1231, 2019; JAAD 65:473–491, 2011; Ped Derm 28:209–210, 2011; BJD 164:759–764, 2011; BJD 160:861–863, 2009; NEJM 360:160–169, 2009; JAMA 293:730–735, 2005; JAAD 38:647–666, 1998;* segmental vitiligo *BJD 166:240–246, 2012; BJD 165:44–49, 2011; Ped Derm 27:624–625, 2010;* Blaschko-esque vitiligo *JAAD 65:965–971, 2011;* follicular vitiligo *JAAD 74:1178–1184, 2016*

   Differential diagnosis of vitiligo
     Alezzandrini syndrome
     Anti-PD-1 immunotherapy
     Halo nevi
     Kabuki syndrome
     Lichen sclerosus
     Melanoma-associated leukoderma
     MELAS syndrome
     Onchocerciasis
     Pinta
     Post-inflammatory depigmentation
     Post-steroid injections
     Regressed nevi
     Scleroderma
     Vogt-Koyanagi-Harada syndrome

PSYCHOCUTANEOUS DISEASES

Acarophobia

Delusions of parasitosis – white atrophic scars with erosions and ulcers *NEJM 371:2115–2123, 2014*

Factitial dermatitis

SYNDROMES

Acroleukopathy – hypopigmentation around nail folds and distal interphalangeal joints *AD 92:172–173, 1965*

Alezzandrini syndrome – unilateral degenerative tapetoretinal degeneration (retinitis), ipsilateral facial vitiligo, poliosis, with or without deafness *Arch Iranian Med 4, April, 2001; Ophthalmologica 147:409–419, 1964*

Angelman syndrome – hypopigmentation, mental retardation *Am J Med Genet 40:454, 1991*

AEC syndrome (Hay-Wells syndrome) – ankyloblepharon, ectodermal dysplasia, cleft lip/palate syndrome – blepharitis, eyelid papillomas, periorbital wrinkling; microcephaly, widespread congenital scalp erosions; alopecic ulcerated plaques of the scalp, trunk, groin; alopecia of the scalp and eyebrows; congenital erythroderma; depigmented patches; syndactyly; bony abnormalities; widely spaced nipples; *TP63* mutation *Ped Derm 26:617–618, 2009; AD 141:1591–1594, 2005; AD 141:1567–1573, 2005; AD 134:1121–1124, 1998; Ped Derm 14:149–150, 1997; BJD 94:287–289, 1976;* generalized fissured erosions of the trunk *BJD 149:395–399, 2003; TP63* mutations seen in AEC syndrome, EEC syndrome, Rapp-Hodgkin syndrome, limb-mammary syndrome, split-hand split-foot malformation type 4, acro-dermato-ungual-lacrimal-tooth syndrome *AD 141:1567–1573, 2005*

Antiphospholipid antibody syndrome – porcelain white scars (atrophie blanche-like) *JAAD 36:149–168, 1997; JAAD 36:970–982, 1997*

Apert syndrome – cutaneous and ocular hypopigmentation; craniosynostosis, midface malformation, syndactyly, severe acne and seborrhea

Ataxia telangiectasia – vitiligo and canities *JAAD 42:939–969, 2000*

Bloom's syndrome – hypopigmented macules *Ped Derm 14:120–124, 1997*

Chediak-Higashi syndrome – autosomal recessive; oculocutaneous hypopigmentation, pigment dilution, silvery hair, neurologic dysfunction, defective polymorphonuclear cell chemotaxis *Ped Derm 24:182–185, 2007; Ped Derm 21:479–482, 2004; Curr Probl Dermatol 18:93–100, 1989; Arch Int Med 119:381–386, 1987*

Congenital plasminogen deficiency – autosomal recessive; chronic mucosal pseudomembranous lesions with white membranes of gingivae and eyelids; blepharitis, gingival hyperplasia, leukoplakia, ligneous conjunctivitis; thick nodular eyelids *Ped Derm 448–451, 2009*

Conradi-Hunermann syndrome – hypochromic areas, linear hyperkeratotic bands with diffuse erythema and scale, follicular atrophoderma, scalp alopecia *Ped Derm 15:299–303, 1998; AD 127:539–542, 1991,*

Cross-McKusick-Breen syndrome (oculocerebral syndrome with hypopigmentation) – autosomal recessive; albino-like hypopigmentation, microphthalmos, opaque cornea, nystagmus, spasticity, mental retardation *J Pediatr 70:398–406, 1967*

Crouzon's syndrome – hypopigmentation in surgical scars; mutation in *FGFR2 Ped Derm 13:18–21, 1996*

Crouzon syndrome with acanthosis nigricans (CAN) – white hypopigmented scars; onset of acanthosis nigricans during childhood, dark melanocytic nevi, craniosynostosis, ocular proptosis, midface hypoplasia, choanal atresia, hypertelorism, anti-Mongoloid slant, posteriorly placed ears, hydrocephalus; mutation in *FGFR3 JAMA Derm 149:737–741, 2013; Ped Derm 27:43–47, 2010; Am J med Genet 84:74, 1999*

Darier's disease – leukoderma *Dermatology 188:157–159, 1994;* unilateral Darier's and guttate leukoderma *JAAD 48:955–957, 2003*

Deafness, vitiligo, and muscle wasting of the hands, feet, and legs *Arch Otolaryngol 93:194–197, 1971*

Depigmented bilateral Blaschko hypertrichosis with dilated follicular orifices and cerebral and ocular malformations *BJD 142:1204–1207, 2000*

Down's syndrome – hypopigmented hair; vitiligo

Dyskeratosis congenita

Eosinophilic fasciitis

Epidermal nevus syndrome – hypochromic nevi *Ped Derm 6:316–320, 1989*

Goltz's syndrome – male mosaic Goltz's syndrome; Blaschko-linear white atrophic depigmented lines, hyperpigmented linear streaks, linear alopecia, syndactyly, hydronephrosis *Ped Derm 28:550–554, 2011*

Griscelli syndrome – silvery hair, eyelashes, and eyebrows, pigment dilution (partial albinism), and cellular and humoral immunodeficiency, recurrent infections; mutations in *MYO5A, RAB27A, MLPH BJD 176:1086–1019, 2017; Ped Derm 21:479–482, 2004; JAAD 38:295–300, 1998; Am J Med 65:691–702, 1978*

Hermansky-Pudlak syndrome – white skin and hair *BJD 178:335–349, 2018; AD 135:774–780, 1999; Am J Hematol 26:305–311, 1987; Blood 14:162–169, 1959*

Hypomelanosis of Ito (incontinentia pigmenti achromians) – whorled depigmented patches in Blaschko pattern; associated musculoskel-etal, teeth, eye, and central nervous system abnormalities *NEJM 360:160–169, 2009; JAAD 19:217–255, 1988*

Incontinentia pigmenti – anhidrotic and achromians lesions *BJD 116:839–849, 1987*

Kabuki syndrome – vitiligo, developmental delay, short stature, congenital heart defects, skeletal defects, cleft palate, dental abnormalities, cryptorchidism, lip pits, prominent fingertip pads, autoimmune disorders, blue sclerae, prominent eyelashes, thinning of central eyebrows, protuberant ears *JAAD 65:473–491, 2011; Amer J Med Genet 132A:260–262, 2005*

LIG4 syndrome *BJD 178:335–349, 2018*

MAUIE syndrome – erythroderma with skip areas; micropinnae, alopecia, ichthyosis, and ectropion *JAAD 37:1000–1002, 1997*

MELAS syndrome (mitochondrial encephalomyopathy, lactic acidosis, stroke-like episodes); central nervous system abnormalities, neurosensory hearing loss, dermatomyositis, cardiomyopathy *JAAD 65:473–491, 2011*

Mukamel syndrome – autosomal recessive; premature graying in infancy, lentigines, depigmented macules, mental retardation, spastic paraparesis, microcephaly, scoliosis

Multiple endocrine neoplasia syndrome type I – hypopigmented macules *JAAD 42:939–969, 2000*

Multiple lentigines syndrome – hypopigmented macules *Ped Derm 13:100–104, 1996*

Neurofibromatosis type I – neurofibroma presenting as gray-white atrophic patch *Ped Derm 26:231–232, 2009; Cutis 57:100–102, 1996; BJD 112:435–441, 1985; AD 118:577–581, 1982;* nevus anemicus in neurofibromatosis type 1 *JAAD 69:768–775, 2013*

Nijmegen breakage syndrome – autosomal recessive; chromosome instability syndrome; mutations in *NBS-1* gene which encodes bibirin (DNA damage repair); microcephaly, receding mandible, prominent midface, prenatal onset short stature, growth retardation, bird-like facies with epicanthal folds, large ears, sparse hair, clinodactyly/syndactyly; freckling of face, café au lait macules, vitiligo, photosensitivity of the eyelids, telangiectasias; pigmented deposits of fundus; IgG, IgA deficiencies, agammaglobulinemia, decreased CD3 and CD4 T cells with recurrent respiratory and urinary tract infections *BJD 178:335–349, 2018; Ped Derm 27:285–289, 2010; Ped Derm 26:106–108, 2009; DNA Repair 3:1207–1217, 2004; Arch Dis Child 82:400–406, 2000; Am J Med Genet 66:378–398, 1996*

Oculocutaneous albinism *Dermatol Clin 6:217–228, 1988; JAAD 19:217, 1988;* OCA1A – white hair and hypopigmentation *BJD 166:896–898, 2012*

Oculocutaneous albinism, dysmorphic features, short stature *Ophthalmic Paediatr Genet 11:209–213, 1990*

P14/LAMTOR2 deficiency *BJD 178:335–349, 2018*

Patau syndrome (trisomy 13) – depigmented spots

Phakomatosis pigmentovascularis – nevus anemicus *Ped Derm 13:33–35, 1996*

Piebaldism – autosomal dominant; white forelock, white patches on the upper chest, abdomen, extremities with islands of hyperpigmentation within *BJD 168:910–912, 2013; BJD 161:468–469, 2009; NEJM 360:160–169, 2009; Cutis 80:411–414, 2007; JAAD 44:288–292, 2001;* mutations and deletions of *c-kit* (steel factor receptor) *Am J Hum Genet 56:58–66, 1995*

Piebaldism, multiple café au lait macules, and intertriginous freckling – *KIT* and *SPRED1* mutations *Ped Derm 30:379–382, 2013*

Prader-Willi syndrome – hypopigmentation, mental retardation *Am J Med Genet 40:454, 1991*

Pseudocleft of upper lip, cleft lip-palate, and hemangiomatous branchial cleft – canities *Plast Reconstr Surg 83:143–147, 1989*

Russell-Silver syndrome – achromia *JAAD 40:877–890, 1999; J Med Genet 36:837–842, 1999*

Symmetrical progressive leukopathy – Japan and Brazil; punctate leukoderma on shins, extensor arms, abdomen, interscapular areas *Ann Dermatol Syphiligr 78:452–454, 1951*

Tay syndrome – autosomal recessive; growth retardation, triangular face, cirrhosis, trident hands, premature canities, vitiligo

Tietze syndrome – autosomal dominant; absence of pigment, deaf-mutism, hypoplastic eyebrows *Am J Hum Genet 15:259–264, 1963*

Tuberous sclerosis – ash leaf macules, confetti hypopigmentation, white eyelashes, poliosis *NEJM 360:160–169, 2009; Int J Dermatol 37:911–917, 1998; BJD 135:1–5, 1996; JAAD 32:915–935, 1995; Ped Clin North Amer 38:991–1017, 1991; S Med J 75:227–228, 1982;* scalp poliosis, hypomelanotic macules, confetti hypopigmentation *Ped Derm 32:563–570, 2015*

Tuomaala-Haapanen syndrome (brachymetapody, anodontia, hypotrichosis, albinoid trait) *Acta Ophthalmol 46:365–371, 1968*

Unusual facies, vitiligo, canities, progressive spastic paraplegia *Am J Med Genet 9:351–357, 1981*

Vogt-Koyanagi-Harada syndrome – poliosis and vitiligo; occurs primarily in Asians, blacks, and darkly pigmented Caucasians; stage 1 – aseptic meningitis; stage 2 – uveitis (iritis, iridocyclitis) and dysacusis (tinnitus, hearing loss); stage 3 – depigmentation of skin (60% of patients), depigmentation of hair (poliosis – eyelashes, eyebrows, scalp, and body hair – 90% of patients), alopecia areata or diffuse hair loss; halo nevi *Ped Derm 34:612–613, 2017; Autoimmun Rev 13:550–555, 2014; Ped Derm 31:99–101, 2014; JAAD 69:625–633, 2013; J Drugs in Dermatol 11:1004–1005, 2012; Ped Derm 27:624–625, 2010; Ann DV 127:282–284, 2000; AD 88:146–149, 1980; Neurology 20:965–974, 1970*

von Willebrand disease with albinism

Waardenburg syndrome – type I – white forelock; dystopia canthorum, broad nasal root, synophrys, iris heterochromia, deafness, canities, piebaldism; hypoplasia of the nasal alae, terminal hair on tip of the nose; PAX 3 gene mutation; type II – sensorineural hearing loss, heterochromia iridis, absence of dystopia canthorum; MITF mutations; type III (Waardenburg-Klein syndrome) – features of type I, limb abnormalities; PAX 3 gene mutations; type IV (Waardenburg-Shah syndrome) – extensive depigmentation; Hirschsprung's disease; endothelin receptor B gene mutations *NEJM 360:160–169, 2009; Dermatol Clin 6:205–216, 1988*

Woolf syndrome – autosomal recessive; piebaldism with congenital nerve deafness *JAAD 48:466–468, 2003; Arch Otolaryngol 82:244–250, 1965*

Xeroderma pigmentosum – acute sunburn, persistent erythema, freckling – initially discrete, then fuse to irregular patches of hyperpigmentation, dryness on sun-exposed areas; with time telangiectasias and small angiomas, atrophic white macules develop; vesiculobullous lesions, superficial ulcers lead to scarring, ectropion; multiple malignancies; photophobia, conjunctivitis, symblepharon, neurologic abnormalities *Adv Genet 43:71–102, 2001; Hum Mutat 14:9–22, 1999; Mol Med Today 5:86–94, 1999; Derm Surg 23:447–455, 1997; Dermatol Clin 13:169–209, 1995; Recent Results Cancer Res 128:275–297, 1993; AD 123:241–250, 1987; Ann Int Med 80:221–248, 1974;* XP variant *AD 128:1233–1237, 1992*

X-linked dominant chondrodysplasia punctate (Happle syndrome) – white eyelashes, growth retardation, cataracts, temporary ichthyosiform erythroderma *Clin in Derm 37:561–579, 2019*

Ziprkowski-Margolis syndrome – X-linked recessive, deaf-mutism, heterochromia iridis, piebald-like hypomelanosis, hyperpigmented macules with geographic appearance *Cutis 80:411–414, 2007; JAAD 48:466–468, 2003*

TOXINS

Perchloroethylene-induced Raynaud's phenomenon

Thallium – anagen effluvium *JAAD 50:258–261, 2004;* nausea, vomiting, stomatitis, painful glossitis, diarrhea; severe dysesthesias and paresthesias in distal extremities, facial rashes of the cheeks and perioral region, acneiform eruptions of the face, hyperkeratosis of the palms and soles, hair loss, Mees' lines *AD 143:93–98, 2007*

Vinyl chloride exposure

TRAUMA

Burns – post-burn leukoderma *AD 147:1023–1026, 2011*

Cryotherapy

Delayed deep pressure urticaria

Eyebrow plucking *Cutis 91:129–136, 2013*

Friction blisters

Frostbite – waxy white appearance

Ice pack depigmentation – personal observation

Immersion foot due to ice, cold water, and fans – maceration, acral cyanosis, mottled coloration, marked edema of feet, bullae, erosions, painful ulcers, pain *JAAD 69:169–171, 2013*

Laser resurfacing – depigmentation *Cutis 91:129–136, 2013*

Paintball injury – annular white scars *Cutis 80:49–50, 2007*

Physical trauma – post-inflammatory depigmentation

Post-traumatic leukoderma *NEJM 360:160–169, 2009*

Radiation therapy – depigmentation *Cutis 91:129–136, 2013*

Scars

Scratching – depigmentation *Cutis 91:129–136, 2013*

Sun damage – pseudoscars

Tropical immersion foot

Ultraviolet light-induced leukoderma *Clin in Derm 37:561–579, 2019*

Vibration white finger (hand-arm vibration syndrome) *Clin in Derm 37:561–579, 2019; Int Arch Occup Environ Health 73:150–155, 2000*

VASCULAR DISORDERS

Arteriosclerosis – pallor

Bier spots – anemic macules or ivory white spots on erythrocyanotic background; exaggerated vasoconstrictive response in stasis associated hypoxia; or with mixed cryoglobulinemia *BJD 146:921–922, 2002; AD 136:674–675, 2000*

Buerger's disease – elevation of the leg – white leg and foot

Capillary malformation-arteriovenous malformation syndrome – telangiectasias of the chest; central punctate red spots; nevus anemicus surrounded by pale halo; absence of vellus hairs over the AVM *BJD 172:450–454, 2015*

Constitutive speckled vascular mottling *AD 136:674–675, 2000*

Degos disease – flat, white papules with erythematous telangiectatic halos *JAMADerm 153:1183–1184, 2017; NEJM 370:2327–2337, 2014;* malignant atrophic papulosis *AD 145:321–326, 2009; Int J Derm 39:361–362, 2000; Ann DV 79:410–417, 1954;* familial Degos disease *JAAD 50:895–899, 2004*

Eruptive pseudoangiomatosis – white halos *Eur J Dermatol 10:455–458, 2000*

Hemangioma, pre-proliferative phase – avascular patch; early white discoloration of infantile hemangiomas – a sign of impending ulceration *AD 146:1235–1239, 2010*

Livedoid vasculopathy – ulcers and stellate scars of ankles; (atrophie blanche en plaque; atrophie blanche with summer ulceration) – painful purpuric papules and plaques; atrophic white scars; livedo reticularis *JAAD 69:1033–1042, 2013; AD 148:385–390, 2012; AD 134:491–493, 1998; JAAD 8:792–798, 1983; AD 119:963–969, 1983;* with Degos disease-like lesions *JAAD 50:895–899, 2004*

Nevus anemicus *BJD 134:292–295, 1996*

Nevus oligemicus

Polyarteritis nodosa – atrophie blanche-like lesions *BJD 148:789–794, 2003; Rheum Dis Clin NA 27:677–728, 2001;* cutaneous (livedo with nodules) – arthritis; arthralgias; painful or asymptomatic red or skin-colored multiple nodules with livedo reticularis of the feet, legs, forearms, face, scalp, shoulders, trunk; leg ulcers, atrophie blanche-like lesions; reticulate hyperpigmentation *JAAD 73:1013–1020, 2015; JAAD 63:602–606, 2010; JAAD 57:840–848, 2007; BJD 146:694–699, 2002;* anti-phosphatidylserine-prothrombin complex *JAAD 63:602–606, 2010*

Pseudoleucoderma angiospaticum *Clin Dermatol 37:610–617, 2019*

Raynaud's phenomenon – vasoconstriction *NEJM 369:1638, 2013; JAAD 59:633–653, 2008;* Raynaud's phenomenon in breast feeding – white blanching of the nipple *JAMADerm 149:300–306, 2013*

Vasculitis

Venous ulcer scars – mimicking atrophie blanche – personal observation

Congenital Volkmann ischemic contracture (neonatal compartment syndrome) – upper extremity circumferential contracture from the wrist to elbow; necrosis, cyanosis, edema, eschar, bullae, purpura; irregular border with central white ischemic tissue with formation of bullae, edema, or spotted bluish color with necrosis, a reticulated eschar or whorled pattern with contracture of arm; differentiate from necrotizing fasciitis, congenital varicella, neonatal gangrene, aplasia cutis congenita, amniotic band syndrome, subcutaneous fat necrosis, epidermolysis bullosa *Ped Derm 37:207–208, 2020; BJD 150:357–363, 2004*

LINEAR HYPOPIGMENTATION

Epidermal nevus

Goltz's syndrome

Hypomelanosis of Ito

Incontinentia pigmenti, fourth stage

Intralesional corticosteroid injection

Lichen striatus

Linear keratosis follicularis and linear basaloid follicular hamartoma with guttate macules

Menkes kinky hair syndrome (female carrier)

Nevus comedonicus

Nevus depigmentosus

Pigmentary mosaicism

Segmental vitiligo

Segmental ash leaf macule

WHITE PAPULES, NODULES, AND PLAQUES

AUTOIMMUNE DISEASES AND DISEASES OF IMMUNE DYSFUNCTION

Dermatomyositis – Degos-like lesions *JAMADerm 156:218–220, 2020;* calcinosis cutis *JAMADerm 150:724–729, 2014;* white papules resembling malignant atrophic papulosis *JAAD 36:317–319, 1997;* tender hyperkeratotic palmar papules in palmar creases of the fingers with central white coloration; dermatomyositis with MDA-5 (CADM-40) (melanoma differentiation-associated gene 5) MDA 5 – RNA-specific helicase; all with interstitial lung disease; ulcers of nail folds, Gottron's papules, and elbows; these patients demonstrate oral ulcers, hair loss, hand edema, arthritis/arthralgia, diffuse hair loss, punched out ulcers of shoulder or metacarpophalangeal joints, digital necrosis, erythema of the elbows and knees (Gottron's sign), and tender gingiva *JAAD 65:25–34, 2011*

Graft vs. host disease, chronic – lichen sclerosus-like lesions *JAAD 66:515–532, 2012; JAAD 53:591–601, 2005; AD 138:924–934, 2002*

Lupus erythematosus – white papules resembling malignant atrophic papulosis (Degos disease) *JAAD 36:317–319, 1997; Dermatologica 175:45–46, 1987; BJD 95:649–652, 1976; Arch Int Med 134:321–323, 1974;* dystrophic calcification – personal observation; nodular episcleritis; discoid lupus erythematosus – calcinosis cutis of scalp *JAMA Derm 149:246–248, 2013*

Morphea – white plaque; guttate morphea generalized morphea; superficial morphea – personal observation; hyperpigmented white scaly Blaschko-esque plaques – morphea/lichen sclerosus overlap *AD 147:857–862, 2011*

Rheumatoid arthritis – white eyelid papules – personal observation; rheumatoid nodule

Scleroderma – white papules resembling malignant atrophic papulosis (Degos disease) *Cutis 75:101–104, 2005; JAAD 36:317–319, 1997; AD 100:575–581, 1969;* ivory subcutaneous nodules of the trunk and extremities *BJD 101:93–96, 1979;* calcinosis; CREST syndrome

CONGENITAL LESIONS

Calcinosis cutis of the ear, congenital *JAAD 49:117–119, 2003*

Cartilaginous rest of the neck, congenital *Cutis 58:293–294, 1996*

Ectopic meningothelial hamartoma – white linear plaque of occipital-posterior scalp; may be orange or yellow *Ped Derm 34:99–100, 2017; Ped Derm 31:208–211, 2014; Ped Derm 28:677–680, 2011; Am J Surg Pathol 14:1–11, 1980*

   Differential diagnosis:

      Angiosarcoma

      Membranous aplasia cutis congenita

      Atretic meningocele

      Epithelioid hemangioma

Giant cell fibroblastoma

Hypertrophic scar

Intravascular papillary endothelial hyperplasia

Spindle cell hemangioendothelioma

Epstein's pearls (Bohn's pearls (milia) of the neonate) – keratinous cysts (milia) of palatal, gingival, or alveolar mucosa in neonates *Int Dent J 27:261–262, 1988*

Milia – profuse familial congenital milia *Ped Derm 26:62–64, 2009*

Urethral retention cyst – white papule at urethral opening of males

DRUG-INDUCED

Intramuscular corticosteroid injections – personal observation

Lichen planus

Palifermin white tongue *NEJM 360:326, 2009*

Pegylated alpha-interferon injection sites – Degos disease (atrophic papulosis) *BJD 170:992–994, 2014*

EXOGENOUS AGENTS

Aquagenic wrinkling of the palms – white cobblestoned plaques *BJD 167:575–582, 2012; AD 147:609–614, 2011*

Contact dermatitis – personal observation

Foreign body granuloma

Silicone granuloma

INFECTIONS

Adiaspiromycosis – cutaneous adiaspiromycosis (*Chrysosporium* species) – hyperpigmented plaque with white-yellow papules, ulcerated nodules, hyperkeratotic nodules, crusted nodules, multilobulated nodules *JAAD S113–117, 2004*

Coxsackie A16 – Koplik's spots

Demodex folliculitis – white spiky papules in a 6-year-old child *Ped Derm 35:244–245, 2018*

Ebola virus hemorrhagic fever (filovirus) – gray exudate of the soft palate with white clear lesions (tapioca granules), dark red discoloration of the soft palate, pharyngitis, oral ulcers, glossitis, gingivitis; morbilliform exanthem which becomes purpuric with desquamation of the palms and soles; high fever, body aches, myalgia, arthralgias, prostration, abdominal pain, watery diarrhea; disseminated intravascular coagulation *Int J Dermatol 51:1037–1043, 2012; JAMA 287:2391–2002; Int J Dermatol 51:1037–1043, 2012; JAAD 65:1213–1218, 2011; MMWR 44, No.19, 382, 1995*

Echovirus 9 – Koplik's spots

Epidermodysplasia verruciformis

Fusarium and *Mucormycosis* – black plaques and white nodules *JAMADerm 150:1355–1356, 2014*

Maggots *Clin Inf Dis 35:1566–1571, 2002*

Measles – Koplik's spots *NEJM 372:2218–2223, 2015; NEJM 372:2217, 2015*

Molluscum contagiosum, including molluscum folliculitis *BJD 142:555–559, 2000*

Mycetoma – *Pseudallescheria boydii, Acremonium* sp. – white and yellow grains; *Actinomadura madurae, Nocardia asteroides* – white grains; *Nocardia brasiliensis* – white or orange grains; *Nocardiopsis dassonvillei* – white or yellow *JAAD 53:931–951, 2005; Cutis 60:191–193, 1997*

Mycobacterium tuberculosis – red eye with white conjunctival plaque *Clin Inf Dis 68:525–529, 2019*

Parvovirus B19 – Koplik's spots

Prototheocosis *Nippon Ishinkin Gakkai Zasshi 42:143–147, 2001*

Pitted keratolysis – personal observation

Syphilis – condyloma lata – white moist papules; interdigital and perianal papules *Clin Inf Dis 55:1106,1164–1166, 2012*

Tungiasis

INFILTRATIVE LESIONS

Amyloid – amyloid elastosis (primary systemic amyloid) – white cobblestoned plaque around urethral meatus *BJD 158:858–860, 2008*; white gingival papules *BJD 148:154–159, 2003*

Cutaneous mucinosis of infancy – days 1–6; firm grouped white to translucent papules of the arms, hands, and trunk; may be linear *AD 119:272–273, 1983; AD 116:198–200, 1980*

Focal mucinosis – solitary asymptomatic skin colored to white papule, nodule, or plaque anywhere on the body or oral mucosa *An Bras Dermatol 94:334–336, 2019*

Scleromyxedema *JAAD 33:37–43, 1995*

Self-healing juvenile cutaneous mucinosis – red nodules of the face, scalp, hand; macrodactyly (enlarged thumbs); periarticular painless papules and nodules, painful polyarthritis; linear ivory white papules, multiple subcutaneous nodules, indurated edema of periorbital and zygomatic areas *JAAD 55:1036–1043, 2006; AD 131:459–461, 1995; Ann DV 107:51–57, 1980; Lyon Med 230:470–474, 1973*

INFLAMMATORY LESIONS

Sarcoid *AD 123:1559, 1562, 1987*; white patches of the vulva *JAMADerm 130:666–667, 2014*

METABOLIC DISEASES

Calcinosis cutis – idiopathic solitary congenital calcified nodule of the ear *Ped Derm 34:195–196, 2017; Am J Dermatopathol 4:377–380, 1982;* perforating congenital calcinosis cutis – white papule of the helix *Ped Derm 23:185–186, 2006;* papular or nodular calcinosis cutis secondary to heel sticks *Ped Derm 18:138–140, 2001;* cutaneous calculus *BJD 75:1–11, 1963;* disseminated idiopathic calcinosis cutis – white nodules *Cutis 91:291–294, 2013;* uremic tumoral calcinosis *JAMA 309:181–182, 2013;* extravasation of calcium carbonate or gluconate solution; metastatic calcification – deposition of calcium in the media of blood vessels – extensive bone destruction, milk-alkali syndrome, primary or secondary hyperparathyroidism, primary hypoparathyroidism, pseudohypo-parathyroidism, chronic renal failure, sarcoid, vitamin D intoxication – umbilicated white papules of the wrist (pseudohypoparathyroidism); mutation in *GNAS Ped Derm 36:732–724, 2019; Ped Derm 23:235–238, 2006; JAAD 33:693–706, 1995; Cutis 32:463–465, 1983;* milia-like calcinosis cutis in Down's syndrome *J Dtsch Dermatol Ges 17:340–341, 2019; Ped Derm 19:271–273, 2002;* heel sticks *Cutis 32:65–66, 1983;* vaginal nodules due to urinary incontinence *BJD 150:169–171, 2004;* subepidermal calcified nodule (Winer's nodular calcinosis) – yellow-white papule *Ped Derm 28:191–192, 2011; Ped Derm 25:253–254, 2008; Arch Dermatol Syph 66:204–211, 1952;* dystrophic calcification *AD 144:585–587, 2008;* calcified elastin – personal observation; idiopathic calcinosis of the scrotum – personal observation

Calcium phosphate

Chylous reflux – white milky blisters *JAAD 55:1108–1109, 2006*

Cystinosis – white facial papules; renal failure, ocular, pancreatic, hepatic, muscular, dental, gonadal, and neurologic involvement, hypothyroidism *JAMADerm 152:108–109, 2016*

Cystic fibrosis – aquagenic wrinkling of the palms *BJD 179:494–495, 2018*

Gout – tophus – monosodium urate *AD 143:1201–1206, 2007; Cutis 64:233–236, 1999; AD 134:499–504, 1998;* white papule of helix *Cutis 92:190–192, 2013;* miliary gout – brown plaques and milky white fluid *JAMADerm 150:569–570, 2014*

Idiopathic calcinosis of the scrotum *NEJM 365:647, 2011; Br J Plast Surg 42:324–327, 1989; Eur Urol 13:130–131, 1987; Int J Derm 20:134–136,1981; AD 114:957, 1978;* dystrophic calcinosis of benign epithelial cyst *BJD*

Jaundice – personal observation

Kwashiorkor – personal observation

Miliaria – giant centrifugal miliaria profunda – white papule

Osteoma cutis – primary osteoma cutis including multiple military osteomas *BJD 164:544–552, 2011;* congenital plate-like osteoma cutis, multiple miliary facial osteomas, Albright's hereditary osteodystrophy, and fibrodysplasia ossificans progressiva *BJD 146:1075–1080, 2002; JAAD 38:906–910, 1998;* plate-like osteoma cutis *AD 143:109–114, 2007*

Oxalosis, primary – distal digital white papule *Am J Dermatopathol 40:456–458, 2018*

Progressive osseous heteroplasia – papules and nodules *J Bone Joint Surg Am 76:425–436, 1994*

Pseudogout – pseudotophi (calcium pyrophosphate)

Renal disease, chronic – nodular calcinosis

Uremic frost *Mayo Clin Proc 93:1535, 2018*

Zinc deficiency – personal observation

NEOPLASTIC DISEASES

Acrochordon

Anal intraepithelial neoplasia – perianal hyperpigmented patches, white and/or red plaques *JAAD 52:603–608, 2005*

Basal cell carcinoma, morpheaform; of nose *BJD 180:229–230, 2019*

Bowenoid papulosis – vulvar whitish papules or plaques *Cancer 57:823–836, 1986*

Clear cell papulosis – hypopigmented macules and slightly elevated 1–10 mm papules along milk line on lower abdomen and pubic area *AD 143:358–360, 2007; Ped Derm 22:268–269, 2005; Ped Derm 14:380–382, 1997; JAAD 33:230–233, 1995*

Connective tissue nevus *Ped Derm 22:153–157, 2005;* eruptive collagenoma *J Dermatol 29:79–85, 2002;* eruptive collagenomas in pregnancy *JAAD 53:S150–153, 2005;* familial cutaneous collagenomas *BJD 101:185–195, 1979;* connective tissue nevus with elastorrhexis – multiple 3mm papules *Ped Derm 31:2014; Ann Dermatol 23:S53–56, 2011*

Desmoplastic trichilemmoma – white papule of eyelid; lip papule *JAAD 76:S22–24, 2017*

Desmoplastic trichoepithelioma – single papule *Cancer 40:2979–2986, 1977;* multiple familial *JAAD 39:853–857, 1998*

Elastic nevus *Dermatology 198:307–309, 1999*

Epidermoid cyst

Eruptive vellus hair cysts – skin colored, red, white, blue, yellow eyelid papules *Ped Derm 19:26–27, 2002*

Fibroma – personal observation

Large cell acanthomas – white to red flat-topped papules *JAAD 53:335–337, 2005*

Leiomyoma

Leiomyosarcoma – blue-black; also red, brown, yellow or hypopigmented *JAAD 46:477–490, 2002*

Lymphoma – lymphomatoid granulomatosis *Am J Surg Pathol 25:1111–1120, 2001;* cutaneous T-cell lymphoma mimicking lichen sclerosus *BJD 157:411–413, 2007; Am J Dermatopathol 19:446–455, 1997;* syringotropic cutaneous T-cell lymphoma – atrophic white papules *AD 145:77–82, 2009*

Mantleoma – 2–4mm yellow or white papules *Cutis 28:429–432, 1981*

Marginal cysts of eyelids – occluded glands of Moll; painless white or yellow cyst of the lower eyelid close to lacrimal punctum

Melanocytic nevus – atypical nevi, non-pigmented *AD 113:992–994, 1997;* congenital nevus – red, white, and blue plaque on flank of newborn mimicking a vascular tumor *Ped Derm 30:749–750, 2013*

Melanoma – desmoplastic melanoma

Metastatic carcinoma

Milia, including multiple eruptive milia – face, earlobe *JAAD 37:353–356, 1997; Cutis 60:183–184, 1997; Clin Exp Dermatol 21:58–60, 1996;* after blistering (epidermolysis bullosa, EBA, bullous lupus erythematosus) or trauma (porphyria cutanea tarda, friction) of the nipple *Ped Derm 26:485–486, 2009;* milia en plaque *JAAD Case Rep 59:167–169, 2019*

Mucoepidermoid carcinoma *JAAD Case Report 75:739–741, 2019*

Neuroma (solitary neurofibroma) – palisaded encapsulated neuroma *AD 140:1003–1008, 2004;* white penile papules – traumatic neuromas *JAAD 54:S54–55, 2006*

Nevus sebaceus

Osteochondroma – white-yellow nodule *Derm Surg 27:591–593, 2001*

Palisaded encapsulated neuroma *JAAD 76:S84–85, 2017*

Perforating follicular hybrid cyst (pilomatrixoma and steatocystoma) of the inner eyelid (tarsus) *JAAD 48:S33–34, 2003*

Persistent actinic epidermolytic hyperkeratosis – hypopigmented papules *J Cutan Pathol 6:272–279, 1979*

Pilar cyst, calcified

Pilomatrixoma – papule with white inclusions – personal observation; *Eyelid and Conjunctival Tumors, Shields JA and Shields CL, Lippincott Williams and Wilkins, 1999, p.71*

Porokeratosis of Mibelli – white plaque *Cutis 79:22,53–54, 2007; JAAD 52:553–555, 2005; Gior Ital d Mal Ven 28:313–355, 1893*

Reactive fibrous papule of the fingers (giant-cell fibroma) – fingers and palms *Dermatologica 143:368–375, 1971*

Retention cyst from glands of Zeis

Retinoblastoma – white pupil *JAMA 311:1799–1800, 2014*

Sclerotic fibromas of the skin *JAAD 20:266–271, 1989*

Seborrheic keratosis, irritated; stucco keratosis

Squamous cell carcinoma – white plaque of penis *JAAD 66:867–880, 2012; JAAD 62:284–290, 2010;* vulvar squamous cell carcinoma – papular and polypoid lesions; verrucous white cobblestoned plaque *JAAD 66:867–880, 2012*

Syringomas, vulvar – discrete white cystic papules *JAAD 48:735–739, 2003*

Trichodiscoma – hypopigmented papules *AD 126:1093,1096, 1990*

Trichoepithelioma; Blaschko distribution – hypopigmented papules *Ped Derm 23:149–151, 2006;*

Tumors of the follicular epithelium, multiple eruptive – hypopigmented papules of the face and extremities *AD 135:463–468, 1999; JAAD 39:853–857, 1998*

Vulvar intraepithelial neoplasia – white vulvar plaques *JAAD 81:1–21, 2019*

White sponge nevus – white plaques of lips and/or buccal mucosa *Ped Derm 29:495–497, 2012*

PHOTODERMATOSES

Actinic lichen planus *AD 135:1543–1548, 1999*

Weathering nodules (elastotic nodules of the ear) – white papules of helices *Indian J Dermatol 6:433–436, 2016; AD 149:475–480, 2013; JAAD 50:100, 2004; BJD 135:550–554, 1996; Cutis 44:452–454, 1989*

PRIMARY CUTANEOUS DISEASES

Acne vulgaris – closed comedones (whiteheads); osteoma cutis

Anetoderma *BML Dermatol 4:9, 2004*

Aquagenic acrosyringeal keratoderma – personal observation

Balanitis xerotica obliterans – white papules of penis *JAMA Derm 149:23–24, 2013*

Darier's disease, hypopigmented – personal observation

Degos disease *JAAD 50:895–899, 2004*

Degos-like lesions – connective tissue disease; systemic lupus erythematosus, dermatomyositis, systemic sclerosis *Clin Cosmet Investig Dermatol Nov 7, 2019*

Digitate dermatosis – personal observation

Epidermolysis bullosa, dominant dystrophic; epidermolysis bullosa, albopapuloidea (Pasini) – ivory white papules *BJD 146:267–274, 2002*

Epidermolysis bullosa pruriginosa – reticulate scarring, dermatitis with lichenified plaques, violaceous linear scars, albopapuloid lesions of the trunk, prurigo nodularis-like lesions, milia, hyperkeratosis of nails *JAMA Derm 149:727–731, 2013; BJD 152:1332–1334, 2005*

Eruptive tooth

Fibroelastic papulosis – variants; PXE-like papillary dermal elastolysis; papillary dermal elastolysis; white fibrous papulosis of the neck *Am J Dermatopathol 41:46, 2019*

Focal epithelial hyperplasia (Heck's disease)

Follicular fibrosis – personal observation

Follicular keratosis of the chin – frictional dermatitis; yellow-white to skin colored papules *Ped Derm 24:412–414, 2007; JAAD 26:134–135, 1992; Int J Dermatol 24:320–321, 1985; J Cutan Pathol 10:376, 1983; J Dermatol 6:365–369, 1979*

Frictional dermatitis of children – pinhead-sized white papules or warty lesions of backs of the hands, elbows, and knees

Granuloma annulare

Lichen myxedematosus – personal observation

Lichen nitidus

Lichen planus – personal observation; perianal

Lichen sclerosus et atrophicus – vulvar white plaques *JAAD 82:1287–1298, 2020; BJD 176:307–316, 2017; JAMADerm 151:1061–1067, 2015; BJD 171:388–396, 2014; JAMADerm 150:621–627, 2014; Ped Derm 31:95–98, 2014; JAAD 71:84–91, 2014; BJD 168:1316–1324, 2013;* guttate variant; of the scalp *BJD 103:197–200, 1980;* generalized extragenital lichen sclerosus et atrophicus – white plaques; intertriginous distribution; bullae *AD 145:1303–1308, 2009;* lichen sclerosus of the vulva and vagina – cobblestoned vagina, white atrophic plaques *JAMA Derm 149:1199–1202, 2013;* penile lichen sclerosus *BJD 174:687–689, 2016*

Lichen striatus – personal observation

Nevus anelasticus *Ped Derm 22:153–157, 2005*

Papular acantholytic dyskeratosis of the vulva *AD 148:755–760, 2012; Ped Derm 22:237–239, 2005; Am J Dermatopathol 6:557–560, 1984;* papular acantholytic dyskeratosis of the penis *J Dermatol 36:427–429, 2009; Am J Dermatopathol 8:365–366, 1986*

Papular elastorrhexis – non-follicular white papules *Int J Dermatol 58:543–544, 2019; Ped Derm 22:153–157, 2005; Ped Derm 19:565–567, 2002; JAAD 19:409–414, 1988*

Pearly penile papules – angiofibromas *JAMA Derm 149:748–750, 2013*

Perifollicular elastolysis – gray or white follicular papules of neck, earlobes *JAAD 51:165–185, 2004*

Pseudoepitheliomatous keratotic and micaceous balanitis *Clin Exp Dermatol 42:424–426, 2017; Bull Soc Fr Dermatol Syphiligr 68:164–167, 1966*

Pseudoxanthoma elasticum-like papillary dermal elastolysis *AD 136:791–796, 2000; JAAD 26:648–650, 1992*

Psoriasis

Reactive perforating collagenosis

Trichodysplasia spinulosa (viral-associated trichodysplasia spinulosa) – acneiform; follicular crusted papules with keratotic spines; lesions of the face, neck with eyebrow alopecia; trichodysplasia spinulosa-associated polyomavirus *AD 148:863–864, 2012; AD 147:1215–1220, 2011;* perioral papules with white spicules – in nevoid basal cell carcinoma syndrome treated with vismodegib *JAMADerm 150:1016–1018, 2014*

White fibrous papulosis of the neck *JAAD 51:165–185, 2004; BJD 127:295–296, 1992; Clin Exp Derm 16:224–225, 1991; JAAD 20:1073–1077, 1989*

SYNDROMES

Albright's hereditary osteodystrophy (pseudohypoparathyroidism) – atrophic pink patches of the neck with striations containing white papules (subcutaneous ossification); white papules of the trunk and ear; dry, rough keratotic puffy skin; short stature, obesity, frontal bossing, depressed nasal bridge; brachydactyly with dimples over 4th and 5th metacarpal bones; mutation in *GNAS1* gene *BJD 162:690–694, 2010; Ergeb Inn Med Kinderheilkd 42:191–221, 1979; Endocrinology 30:922–932, 1942*

Birt-Hogg-Dube syndrome – trichofolliculomas, trichodiscomas *AD 147:499–504, 2011; AD 146:1316–1318, 2010; JAAD 48:111–114, 2003; AD 113:1674–1677, 1977;* collagenomas *JAAD 56:877–880, 2007; AD 135:1195–1202, 1999;* comedo-like white papules of back, pedunculated lip papules of mucosal surface, thyroid nodules or cysts; mutation in *FLCN* (folliculin) gene *BJD 162:527–537, 2010*

Buschke-Ollendorff syndrome – connective tissue nevi and osteopoikilosis; single or multiple yellow, white, or skin colored papules, nodules, plaques of extremities *JAAD 48:600–601, 2003; BJD 144:890–893, 2001*

Cowden's syndrome – collagenomas (sclerotic fibromas) *JAAD 56:877–880, 2007; J Cutan Pathol 19:346–351, 1992*

Dermochondrocorneal dystrophy – white nodules of feet

Down's syndrome – milia-like idiopathic calcinosis cutis *Cutis 91:291–294, 2013; BJD 134:143–146, 1996;* milia-like syringomas with calcification – white eyelid papules *BJD 157:612–614, 2007*

Familial keratosis alba (familial hypochromic seborrheic keratosis) *SKINMed 15:77–78, 2017*

Familial multiple discoid fibromas (Birt-Hogg-Dube look-alike) – white papules of the face and ears *JAAD 66:259–263, 2012*

Fibrodysplasia ossificans progressiva – osteoma cutis

Hunter's syndrome – white to skin-colored papules over the scapulae, shoulders, upper arms, chest, thighs, and nape of the neck; sometimes arranged in linear ridges and plaques or cobble-stoned *Ped Derm 7:150, 1991; AD 113:602–605, 1977*

Hurler's syndrome

Juvenile hyaline fibromatosis – pearly white papules of the face and neck; larger papules and nodules around the nose, behind ears, on fingertips; multiple subcutaneous nodules of the scalp, trunk, and extremities; papillomatous perianal papules; joint contractures, skeletal lesions, gingival hyperplasia, stunted growth

Lipoid proteinosis – yellow-white papules of the tongue, lips, pharynx *Int J Derm 39:203–204, 2000; JAAD 27:293–297, 1992*

Multiple endocrine neoplasia syndrome (MEN I) – multiple dome-shaped papules; collagenomas *JAAD 56:877–880, 2007; J Clin Endocrinol Metab 89:5328–5336, 2004; AD 133:853–857, 1997*

Nevoid basal cell carcinoma syndrome with type 2 mosaicism – Blaschko-esque atrophy, Blaschko-esque pits of the palms; linear papules of foot; white papules and plaques; segmental hyper- and hypopigmented patches *BJD 169:1342–1345, 2013*

Oral-facial-digital syndrome – white nodules of tongue

ROMBO syndrome – peripheral vasodilatation and cyanosis; vermiculate atrophoderma, milia, trichoepitheliomas *Ped Derm 23:149–151, 2006; BJD 144:1215–1218, 2001; Acta DV 61:497–503, 1981*

Tuberous sclerosis – connective tissue nevus *JAAD 56:877–880, 2007; AD 135:1195–1202, 1999;* white epidermal nevi at birth *Ped Derm 31:360–362, 2014; Ped Derm 10:16–18, 1993*

TRAUMA

Extruding tooth – white papule *Cutis 54:253–254, 1994*

Piezogenic pedal papules *AD 106:597–598, 1972*

Scar

VASCULAR DISEASES

Angiofibroma – personal observation

Cutaneous polyarteritis nodosa – atrophie blanche lesions, acrocyanosis, Raynaud's phenomenon, peripheral gangrene, red plaques and peripheral nodules, myalgias; macular lymphocytic arteritis – red or hyperpigmented reticulated patches of legs *JAAD 73:1013–1020, 2015*

Degos disease (malignant atrophic papulosis) – visual and neurologic impairment; pleuritis, pericarditis *JAMADerm 156:204, 2020; JAAD 75:1274–1277, 2016; JAMA Derm 150:96–97, 2014; JAAD 68:138–143 2013; Ped Derm 28:302–305, 2011; JAAD 37:480–484, 1997; AD 122:90–91,93–94, 1986; BJD 100:21–35, 1979; Ann DV 79:410–417, 1954; Arch Dermatol Syphilol 181:783–784, 1941*

Livedoid vasculopathy – ulcers and stellate scars of the ankles *AD 148:385–390, 2012*

Primary lymphedema with lymphorrhea – thick white drops *The Dermatologist pp.47–49 May 2013*

WOOLLY HAIR

JAAD 61:813–818, 2009

Acantholytic ectodermal dysplasia (similar to McGrath syndrome) – curly hair, palmoplantar keratoderma, skin fragility, hyperkeratotic fissured plaques with perioral involvement, red fissured lips, nail dystrophy *BJD 160:868–874, 2009*

Acquired progressive kinking of hair *AD 125:252–255, 1989; AD 121:1031–1037, 1985*

Ankyloblepharon-nail dysplasia syndrome – curly hair *Birth Defects Original Article Ser 7:100–102, 1971*

Autosomal recessive ectodermal dysplasia with corkscrew hairs, pili torti, syndactyly, keratosis pilaris, onychodysplasia, dental abnormalities, conjunctival erythema, palmoplantar keratoderma, cleft lip or palate, and mental retardation *JAAD 27:917–921, 1992*

Cardio-facio-cutaneous syndrome – autosomal dominant, xerosis/ ichthyosis, eczematous dermatitis, alopecia, growth failure, hyperkeratotic papules, ulerythema ophryogenes (decreased or absent eyebrows), seborrheic dermatitis, CALMs, nevi, hemangiomas, keratosis pilaris, patchy or widespread ichthyosiform eruption, sparse curly scalp hair and sparse eyebrows and lashes, congenital lymphedema of the hands, redundant skin of the hands, short stature, abnormal facies with macrocephaly, broad forehead, bitemporal narrowing, hypoplasia of supraorbital ridges, short nose with depressed nasal bridge, high arched palate, low set posteriorly rotated ears with prominent helices, cardiac defects; gain of function sporadic missense mutations in *BRAF, KRAS, MEK1,* or *MEK2, MAP2K1/MAP2K2 BJD 163:881–884, 2010; Ped Derm 27:274–278, 2010; Ped Derm 17:231–234, 2000; JAAD 28:815–819, 1993; AD 129:46–47, 1993; JAAD 22:920–922, 1990;* port wine stain *Clin Genet 42:206–209, 1992*

Carvajal syndrome

Carvajal-like syndrome – blisters, woolly hair, palmoplantar keratoderma, cardiac abnormalities; heterozygotes of *DSP* (desmoplakin) *BJD 166:894–896, 2012; Clin Genet 80:50–58, 2011; J Cutan Pathol 36:553–559, 2009*

CHAND syndrome – curly hair, ankyloblepharon, and nail dysplasia; ataxia *JAAD 59:1–22, 2008*

Costello syndrome – sparse curly hair, short stature, coarse facies, lax skin of the hands and feet, nasal and perioral papillomata; risk of development of rhabdomyosarcoma, neuroblastoma, transitional cell carcinoma; HRAS mutations *JAAD 59:1–22, 2008; JAAD 32:904–907, 1995*

Curly hair-ankyloblepharon-nail dysplasia syndrome – abnormal dentition (form of hypohidrotic ectodermal dysplasia) *Birth Defects Orig Art Ser 7:100–102, 1971*

Ectodermal dysplasia/skin fragility syndrome – autosomal recessive (Carvajal-Huerta syndrome); skin peeling; generalized erythema and peeling at birth; very short stature, superficial skin fragility with crusts of the face, knees, alopecia of the scalp and eyebrows, perioral hyperkeratosis with fissuring and cheilitis, thick dystrophic cracking finger- and toenail dystrophy, keratotic plaques on the limbs, diffuse or focal striate palmoplantar keratoderma with painful fissuring; *PKP1* gene (encoding plakophilin 1) or *DSP* (encoding desmoplakin); follicular hyperkeratosis of knees; woolly hair;

perianal erythema and erosions; cardiomyopathy associated with mutation in desmoplakin not with plakophilin *BJD 160: 692–697, 2009; JAAD 55:157–161, 2006; Acta DV 85:394–399, 2005; JID 122:1321–1324, 2004; Curr Prob Derm 14:71–116, 2002; Hum Molec Genet 9:2761–2766, 2000; Hum Molec Genet 8:143–148, 1999*

Epidermolysis bullosa simplex with ectodermal dysplasia and skin fragility – autosomal recessive; plakophilin 1 mutation; palmoplantar keratoderma, woolly hair and alopecia, anhidrosis until first year

Hypotrichosis simplex with woolly hair – autosomal recessive; mutation in lipase H *JAAD 61:813–818, 2009*

Keratoderma, woolly hair, follicular keratoses, blistering *Retinoids Today Tomorrow 37:15–19, 1994*

Marie-Unna hereditary hypotrichosis – autosomal dominant; sparse curly hair; begins at puberty; at vertex; starts affects eyebrows, eyelashes, body, and pubic hair; 50% with widely spaced incisors; 8p21 *Ped Derm 28:202–204, 2011; BJD 160:194–196, 2009; Ped Derm 19:250–252, 2002; Derm Wschr 82:1167–1178, 1925*

Menkes kinky hair syndrome – X-linked recessive; polydactyly, syndactyly, fine hypopigmented wiry hair, doughy skin, bone and connective tissue disturbances, progressive neurologic deterioration; intracranial hemorrhages *Cutis 90:183–185, 2012*

Naxos syndrome

Noonan's syndrome – autosomal dominant; curly hair or woolly hair; dysmorphic facies, ear, eye, and cardiovascular anomalies, nevi, short stature, keratosis pilaris atrophicans, webbed neck; gain of function mutation in PTPN11 (encodes SHP-2 tyrosine phosphatase) *JAAD 59:1–22, 2008*

Palmoplantar keratoderma with woolly hair *AD 130:522–524, 1994;* rolled and spiraled hairs *Acta DV 65:250–254, 1985;* PPK, woolly hair, endomyocardial fibrodysplasia *TIG 13:229, 1997*

Palmoplantar keratoderma with hypotrichosis, alopecia totalis, steel hair, curly hair, rolled hair, woolly hair, heliotrichosis, congenital atrichia, canities

Skin fragility-woolly hair syndrome – mutation in desmoplakin *BJD 166:894–896, 2012;* autosomal recessive; woolly hair, palmoplantar keratoderma, skin fragility; desmoplakin abnormality *JID 118:232–238, 2002*

Tricho-dento-osseous syndrome – autosomal dominant; diffuse curly hair at birth, enamel hypoplasia, widely spaced teeth, otosclerosis, dolichocephaly, frontal bossing; mutation in *DLX3* (homeobox gene) *JAAD 59:1–22, 2008; Am J Med Genet 72:197–204, 1997*

Woolly hair nevus, Blaschko-linear pigmentation, epidermal nevi; *HRAS* mutation *Ped Derm 36:368–371, 2019*

Woolly hair, alopecia, premature loss of teeth, nail dystrophy, reticulate acral hyperkeratosis, facial abnormalities *BJD 145:157–161, 2001*

Woolly hair hypotrichosis – keratosis pilaris; mutations in *LPAR6 (P2RY5)* or *LIPH* genes *BJD 165:425–431, 2011*

Woolly hair nevus – isolated woolly hair nevus, associated with epidermal nevus, keratosis pilaris atrophicans faciei *XVI Congressus Internat Dermatol. Tokyo, 1982;* associated with Noonan's syndrome *BJD 100:409–416, 1979;* associated with cardiofaciocutaneous syndrome *JAAD 28:815–829, 1993*

Woolly hair and skin fragility syndrome – blistering of the heels and lower legs, focal and diffuse palmoplantar keratoderma; mutation in desmoplakin *JAAD 59:1–22, 2008*

XANTHOMATOUS LESIONS

EXOGENOUS AGENTS

Titanium dioxide pigmentation – plane xanthoma-like lesion *AD 121:656–658, 1985*

INFECTIONS AND INFESTATIONS

Leishmaniasis – diffuse cutaneous leishmaniasis; *L. aethiopica, L. mexicana* – large hypopigmented areas, xanthomatous appearance, verrucous plaques, leonine facies *JAAD 73:897–908, 2015*

INFILTRATIVE DISORDERS

Amyloidosis – periorbital xanthoma-like lesions with multiple myeloma *Eur J Dermatol 29:566–567, 2019*

Erdheim-Chester disease *JAMADerm 155:483–484, 2019*

Langerhans cell histiocytosis – xanthoma-like cutaneous lesions in an adult *JAAD 34:688–689, 1996*

Xanthoma disseminatum *NEJM 338:1138–1143, 1998; Clin Investig 7:233–238, 1993; JAAD 23:341–346, 1990; AD Syphilol 37:373–402, 1938*

INFLAMMATORY DISORDERS

Rosai-Dorfman disease *Am J Dermatopathol 20:393–398, 1998*

METABOLIC DISORDERS

APO E11/E111 phenotype

Axillary perifollicular xanthomatosis *Aust J Dermatol 45:146–148, 2004*

Cerebrotendinous xanthomatosis

Eruptive xanthoma *Cutis 50:31–32, 1992*

Hereditary tendinous and tuberous xanthomas

High-density lipoprotein deficiency

Hyper-apoprotein B

Normocholesterolemic dysbetalipoproteinemia

Normocholesterolemic xanthomatosis *AD 122:1253–1257, 1986*

Beta sitosterolemia

Serum lipoprotein deficiency

NEOPLASTIC DISORDERS

Leukemia – chronic myelomonocytic leukemia *Clin Exp Dermatol 21:145–147, 1996; AD 121:1318–1320, 1985;* juvenile chronic myelogenous leukemia, neurofibromatosis type 1, and xanthomas *J Dermatol 26:33–35, 1999*

Lymphoma – B-cell lymphoma – xanthomatous infiltration of the neck *Eur J Derm 10:481–483, 2000;* papular xanthomatosis *JAAD 26:828–832, 1992;* dystrophic xanthoma in cutaneous T-cell lymphoma *AD 123:91–94, 1987;* xanthomatous CTCL *AD 128:1499–1502, 1992*

Metastases – histiocytoid breast carcinoma *Dermatology 205:63–66, 2002*

PARANEOPLASTIC DISORDERS

Necrobiotic xanthogranuloma with paraproteinemia *Orbit 23:65–76, 2004*

Normolipemic eruptive xanthomas

Normolipemic plane xanthomas – multiple myeloma; Castleman's syndrome *JAAD 39:439–442, 1998; JAAD 26:105–109, 1991;* relapsing polychondritis *Acta DV 74:221–223, 1994*

PRIMARY CUTANEOUS DISEASES

Epidermolysis bullosa, dystrophica – verruciform xanthoma

Normolipemic papular xanthomas – in erythrodermic atopic dermatitis *JAAD 32:326–333, 1995*

Normolipemic subcutaneous xanthomatosis

Normolipemic tendinous and tuberous xanthomas

Papular xanthomas

Verruciform xanthoma *JAAD 42:343–347, 2000; Am J Surg Pathol 22:479–487, 1998*

Xanthomas following erythroderma

SYNDROMES

Alagille syndrome – triangular facies, cardiovascular anomalies (peripheral pulmonary stenosis), butterfly-like vertebral arch defects, ocular abnormalities *Ped Derm 15:199–202, 1998*

CHILD syndrome – xanthomatous pattern *Dermatologica 180:263–266, 1990*

POEMS syndrome with xanthomatous cells *Am J Dermatopathol 21:567–570, 1999*

TRAUMA

Liposuction *BJD 180:E103, 2019*

VASCULAR DISORDERS

Granulomatosis with polyangiitis – yellow eyelid papules (florid xanthelasmata) *JAAD 37:839–842, 1997; Br J Ophthalmol 79:453–456, 1995; Eyelid and Conjunctival Tumors, Shields JA and Shields CL, Lippincott Williams and Wilkins, 1999, p.167*

XEROSIS, ASSOCIATIONS AND CAUSES

AUTOIMMUNE DISEASES AND DISEASES OF IMMUNE DYSFUNCTION

Graft vs. host disease – asteatotic graft vs. host disease *JAAD 66:515–532, 2012; Biol Blood Marrow Transplant 12:1101–1113, 2006; JAAD 53:591–601, 2005*

Job's syndrome (hyper IgE syndrome) – autosomal dominant or sporadic; atrophoderma vermiculatum; coarse facial features with broad nose, rough thickened skin with prominent follicular ostia; papular and papulopustular folliculitis-like eruptions; oral candidiasis; chronic paronychia; cold abscesses of the neck and trunk; otitis media common; mutation in *STAT3* (transcription 3 gene activator and signal transducer) *JAAD 65:1167–1172, 2011*

Lupus erythematosus

Sjogren's syndrome – anhidrosis *JAAD 16:233–235, 1987;* xerosis, annular urticarial-like erythema, localized cutaneous nodular amyloidosis (brown nodule), leukocytoclastic vasculitis, photosensitivity *JAAD 79:736–745, 2018;*

DEGENERATIVE DISEASES

Senescence *BJD 122 Suppl 35:97–103, 1990*

Sympathetic nerve dystrophy – anhidrosis with xerosis

DRUG-INDUCED

Afatinib (epidermal growth factor receptor-tyrosine kinase inhibitors) – xerosis, paronychia, acneiform eruptions, pruritus *JAMADerm 152:340–342, 2016*

Beta-blockers *The Clinical Management of Itching; Parthenon; p. 35, 2000*

Busulfan *The Clinical Management of Itching; Parthenon; p. 35, 2000*

Cabozantinib – VEGFR2 inhibitor; c-met; RET multitargets; tyrosine kinase inhibitor; hand-foot skin reactions with bullae, hyperkeratosis, acral erythema; skin and hair depigmentation, splinter hemorrhages, xerosis, red scrotum *JAMADerm 151:170–177, 2015*

Cetuximab (epidermal growth factor receptor inhibitor) *BJD 161:515–521, 2009; JAAD 58:545–570, 2008; JAAD 56:317–326, 2007; JAAD 55:657–670, 2006; JAAD 55:429–437, 2006; JAAD 53:291–302, 2005*

Cimetidine *AD 118:253–254, 1982*

Clofazimine

Clofibrate *The Clinical Management of Itching; Parthenon; p. 35, 2000*

Diazocholesterol

Epidermal growth factor receptor inhibitors – cetuximab and panitumumab; erlotinib and gefitinib; lapatinib; canertinib; vandetanib *JAAD 72:203–218, 2015; JAAD 56:460–465, 2007*

Erlotinib (epidermal growth factor receptor inhibitor) – xerosis, paronychia, acneiform eruptions, pruritus *JAMADerm 152:340–342, 2016; JAAD 69:463–472, 2013; Clin in Dermatol 29:587–601, 2011; BJD 161:515–521, 2009; JAAD 58:545–570, 2008; JAAD 56:317–326, 2007; JAAD 55:657–670, 2006; JAAD 55:429–437, 2006*

Fenretinide *Clin Can Res 9:2032–2039, 2003*

Flutamide

Gefitinib/erlotinib/cetuximab/panitumumab (epidermal growth factor receptor inhibitors) – papulopustular eruptions; xerosis, paronychia, acneiform eruptions, pruritus *JAMADerm 152:340–342, 2016; JAAD 71:217–227, 2014; JAAD 58:545–570, 2008; JAAD 56:317–326, 2007; AD 142:939, 2006*

Hydroxyurea *AD 135:818–820, 1999; AD 111:183–187, 1975*

Indinavir (protease inhibitor) – retinoid-like side effects *JAAD 63:549–561, 2010; JAAD 46:284–293, 2002*

Interferon alpha *Semin Oncol 14:1–12, 1987*

Itraconazole – photodermatitis and retinoid-like dermatitis *J Eur Acad Dermatol Venereol 14:501–503, 2000*

Lithium carbonate *AD 111:1073–1074, 1975*

MEK inhibitors – C1-1040, selumetinib, trametinib – morbilliform eruptions, papulopustular eruptions, xerosis, paronychia *JAAD 72:221–236, 2015*

Nafoxidine *The Clinical Management of Itching; Parthenon; p. 35, 2000*

Niacin *The Clinical Management of Itching; Parthenon; p. 35, 2000*

Pemetrexed (Alimta) – anti-folate agent; asteatotic dermatitis *BJD 166:1359–1360, 2012*

PUVA *J Formosa Med Assoc 98:335–340, 1999*

Retinoid dermatitis – isotretinoin, etretinate, acitretin *Clin Pharm 2:12–19, 1983*

Sorafenib *JAAD 60:299–305, 2009*

Tamoxifen *The Clinical Management of Itching; Parthenon; p. 35, 2000*

Targeted anti-cancer therapies *JAAD 72:656–667, 2015*

Trametinib (MAP kinase inhibitor) (MEK inhibitor) – angular cheilitis, xerosis, bacterial folliculitis, acneiform eruptions, paronychia, thinning hair *Ped Derm 34:90–94, 2017*

Triparanol

Vandetanib (kinase and growth factor receptor inhibitor) – photosensitivity, xerosis, and blue-gray perifollicular macules; also blue-gray pigment within scars *JAAD 72:203–218, 2015; AD 48:1418–1420, 2012; AD 145:923–925, 2009*

Voriconazole – photodermatitis and retinoid-like dermatitis *Ped Derm 21:675–678, 2004; Pediatr Infect Dis J 21:240–248, 2002; Clin Exp Dermatol 26:648–653, 2001*

EXOGENOUS AGENTS

Chloracne *Clin Exp Dermatol 18:523–525, 1993*

Cryosurgery *Arch Ophthalmol 99:460–463, 1981*

Dry environment *BJD 149:240–247, 2003*

Irritant contact dermatitis – resembles xerosis

Kava dermopathy – xerosis with scaly yellow pigmentation *JAAD 53:S105–107, 2005; JAAD 31:89, 1994*

Methamphetamine *JAAD 69:135–142, 2013*

Water sports

Winter itch

INFECTIONS AND INFESTATIONS

AIDS *JAAD 22:1270–1277, 1990*

Amebiasis

Chikungunya fever *JAAD 75:1–16, 2016*

Generalized dermatophytosis – personal observation

HTLV-1-associated myelopathy/tropical spastic paraparesis *Clin Inf Dis 36:507–513, 2003;* HTLV-1 (acute T-cell leukemia) *JAAD 49:979–1000, 2003*

HTLV-II

Leishmaniasis – post-kala azar leishmaniasis *J Inf Dis 173:758, 1996*

Leprosy

Onchocerciasis – atrophic changes; earliest of the buttock, shoulders, and legs; fine wrinkling and xerotic skin (lizard skin) *AD 140:1161–1166, 2004; BJD 121:187–198, 1989*

Scabies, crusted

INFLAMMATORY DISEASES

Sarcoid – ichthyosis-like

METABOLIC DISEASES

Chronic renal failure *Nephrol Dial Transplant 10:2269–2273, 1995*

Cretinism – coarse facial features, lethargy, macroglossia, cold dry skin, livedo, umbilical hernia, poor muscle tone, coarse scalp hair, synophrys, no pubic or axillary hair at puberty

Diabetes mellitus *Skin Res Technol 8:250–254, 2002*

Essential fatty acid deficiency – severe xerosis with underlying erythema, hair loss with hypopigmentation, and weeping intertriginous rash *Ped Derm 16:95–102, 1999*

Hypoparathyroidism *JAAD 15:353–356, 1986*

Hemochromatosis – ichthyosis-like atrophic dry skin *AD 113:161–165, 1977; Medicine 34:381–430, 1955*

Hypopituitarism – Sheehan's syndrome – skin is yellow, dry

Hypothyroidism (myxedema) – pale, cold, scaly, wrinkled skin *JAAD 26:885–902, 1992;* erythema craquele *BJD 89:289–291, 1973*

Kwashiorkor – personal observation

Liver disease

Multiple nutritional deficiencies – erythema craquele-like appearance

Malabsorption syndromes

Marasmus – severe protein and caloric deprivation; wrinkled, loose, dry skin *JAAD 21:1–30, 1989*

Panhypopituitarism

Prolidase deficiency – autosomal recessive; peptidase D mutation (PEPD); increased urinary aminopeptidase; leg ulcers, anogenital ulcers, short stature (mild), telangiectasias, recurrent infections (sinusitis, otitis); mental retardation; splenomegaly with enlarged abdomen, atrophic scarring, spongy fragile skin with annular pitting and scarring; dermatitis, xerosis, hyperkeratosis of the elbows and knees, lymphedema, purpura, low hairline, poliosis, canities, lymphedema, photosensitivity, hypertelorism, saddle nose deformity, frontal bossing, dull expression, mild ptosis, micrognathia, mandibular protrusion, exophthalmos, joint laxity, deafness, osteoporosis, high-arched palate *JAAD 62:1031, 1034, 2010; BJD 144:635–636, 2001; Ped Derm 13:58–60, 1996; JAAD 29:819–821, 1993; AD 127:124–125, 1991; AD 123:493–497, 1987*

Selenium deficiency – xerosis, alopecia, leukotrichia, leukonychia; pancytopenia, muscle weakness, muscle pain, cardiac arrhythmia, unsteady gait, distal paresthesias *JAAD 80:1215–1231, 2019; Nutrition 23:782–787, 2007; Nutrition 12:40–43, 1996*

Vitamin A deficiency (phrynoderma) – follicular hyperkeratotic papules, xerosis with decreased fatty acids, patchy hyperpigmentation *Ped Derm 28:346–349, 2006; JAAD 41:322–324, 1999*

Vitamin A intoxication *J Pediatr Orthop 5:219–221, 1985; Exp Eye Res 7:388–393, 1968*

Zinc deficiency, acquired – dry skin *JAAD 69:616–624, 2013*

PARANEOPLASTIC DISORDERS

Generalized erythema craquele as a paraneoplastic phenomenon; lymphoma *BJD 97:323–326, 1977;* breast, cervix, lung, Kaposi's sarcoma, leiomyosarcoma, T-cell lymphoma; angioimmunoblastic lymphadenopathy *AD 115:370, 1979;* gastric carcinoma *BJD 109:277–278, 1983;* breast cancer *BJD 110:246, 1984*

Lymphoma *BJD 97:323–326, 1977;* adnexotropic T-cell lymphoma *JAAD 38:493–497, 1998*

PRIMARY CUTANEOUS DISEASES

Asteatotic dermatitis – in hypoesthetic skin *JAMADerm 150:1088–1090, 2014*

Atopic dermatitis *AD 127:1689–1692, 1991*

Erythema craquele *Cutis 83:75–76, 2009*

Hidrotic ectodermal dysplasia *JAAD 27:917–921, 1992*

Ichthyosis – epidermolytic hyperkeratosis, ichthyosis vulgaris, lamellar ichthyosis, non-bullous congenital ichthyosis, Refsum's syndrome, KID syndrome

Ichthyosis bullosa of Siemens – autosomal dominant; xerosis with desquamation on a background of hyperkeratosis; hyperkeratosis of the elbows, knees, dorsal hands, and ankles; palms and soles spared *Ped Derm 27:653–654, 2010; BJD 140:689–695, 1999; Arch Derm Res 282:1–5, 1990; Arch Derm Syph 175:590–608, 1937*

Idiopathic guttate hypomelanosis *BJD 103:635–642, 1980*

Monilethrix – alopecia, keratosis pilaris, xerosis; autosomal recessive – *Dsg4* mutation; autosomal dominant *KRT81, KRT83, KRT86 BJD 165:425–431, 2011*

Nummular dermatitis *Dermatology 199:135–139, 1999*

X-linked ichthyosis *JAAD 72:617–627, 2015*

PSYCHOCUTANEOUS DISEASES

Anorexia nervosa/bulimia nervosa *Am J Clin Dermatol 6:165–173, 2005; Dermatology 203:314–317, 2001; Int J Dermatol 39:348–353, 2000; Ped Derm 16:90–94, 1999; AD 123:1386, 1987*

SYNDROMES

Ablepharon macrostomia – absent eyelids, ectropion, abnormal ears, rudimentary nipples, dry redundant skin, macrostomia, ambiguous genitalia *Hum Genet 97:532–536, 1996*

Acro-dermato-ungual-lacrimal-tooth syndrome (ADULT syndrome) – ectrodactyly or syndactyly, freckling and dry skin, dysplastic nails, superficial blisters and desquamation of the hands and feet; lacrimal duct atresia, primary hypodontia, conical teeth, and early loss of permanent teeth; small ears hooked nose, sparse thin blond hair, frontal alopecia, hypohidrosis, lacrimal duct atresia, hypoplastic breasts and nipples, urinary tract anomalies; mutation in *TP63* gene (encodes transcription factor p63); p63 mutations also responsible for EEC, AEC, limb mammary, and Rapp-Hodgkin syndrome *BJD 172:276–278, 2015; Ped Derm 27:643–645, 2010; Hum Mol Genet 11:799–804, 2002; Am J Med Genet 45:642–648, 1993*

Albright's hereditary osteodystrophy – atrophic pink patches of the neck with striations containing white papules (subcutaneous ossification); white papules of the trunk and ear; dry, rough keratotic puffy skin; short stature, obesity, frontal bossing, depressed nasal bridge; brachydactyly with dimples over 4th and 5th metacarpal bones; mutation in *GNAS1* gene *BJD 162:690–694, 2010; Endocrinology 30:922–932, 1942*

Angiokeratoma corporis diffusum (Fabry's disease (alpha galactosidase A)) – X-linked recessive; skin dry or anhidrotic *JAAD 17:883–*

887, 1987; NEJM 276:1163–1167, 1967; anhidrosis *JAAD 37:523–549, 1997*

Anhidrotic ectodermal dysplasia (Christ-Siemens-Touraine syndrome) *J Dermatol 26:44–47, 1999;* X-linked recessive – premature aged appearance with soft, dry, finely wrinkled skin, especially around eyes; absent or reduced sweating, hypotrichosis, and total or partial anodontia *J Med Genet 28:181–185, 1991;* autosomal recessive *Ped Derm 7:242, 1990*

Apert syndrome – autosomal dominant; *FGFR-2* mutation; craniosynostosis with midfacial malformation; cone-shaped calvarium, proptosis, hypertelorism, short nose with bulbous tip; high arched palate; lips bow-shaped, unable to form a seal; telangiectasias of the face and bulbar conjunctiva, often in butterfly distribution; mottled hyperpigmentation, hypopigmentation, and poikiloderma; seborrheic dermatitis, atopic dermatitis, and xerosis common *Am J Med Genet 44:82–89, 1992;* severe pustular acne at puberty *Ped Derm 20:443–446, 2003*

Cardio-facio-cutaneous syndrome – xerosis/ichthyosis, eczematous dermatitis, alopecia, growth failure, hyperkeratotic papules, ulerythema ophryogenes, seborrheic dermatitis, CALMs, nevi, keratosis pilaris *Ped Derm 30:665–673, 2013; Ped Derm 17:231–234, 2000*

Cockayne syndrome *AD 133:1293–1295, 1997*

Congenital insensitivity to pain – autosomal recessive; anhidrosis with palmoplantar keratoderma; unilateral plantar ulcer; mutation in *NTRK1 Ped Derm 30:754–756, 2013*

Conradi-Hunermann syndrome (chondrodysplasia punctata – X-linked dominant) – linear and whorled hyperkeratosis, follicular atrophoderma of the forearms in Blaschko distribution; linear atrophic lesions with follicular plugging of the scalp; cicatricial alopecia of the scalp; patchy patterned alopecia, generalized xerosis; cataracts, chondrodysplasia punctata; asymmetric shortening of long bones epiphyseal stippling, short stature, short limbs, kyphoscoliosis, craniofacial abnormalities; short arms and legs; cataracts – X-linked; mutation in emopamil-binding protein (EBP) *Ped Derm 31:493–496, 2014; BJD 160:1335–1337, 2009; Curr Prob in Derm VII:143–198, 1995; AD 121:1064–1065, 1985;* ichthyotic and psoriasiform lesions (Blaschko hyperkeratotic scaling), nail defects, cicatricial alopecia, follicular pitted scars, skeletal anomalies *JAAD 33:356–360, 1995; Hum Genet 53:65–73, 1979;* neonatal transient scaly plaques of the limbs, trunk, and scalp; scaly rash disappears in months leaving hypo- or hyperpigmented streaks with follicular atrophoderma and patchy scarring alopecia; *CDPX2* – X-linked lethal in males; X-linked dominant (mosaic for emopamil-binding protein); X-linked recessive – male EBP disorder with neurologic defects *BJD 166:1309–1313, 2012*

Crouzon's syndrome

Down's syndrome *Dermatology 205:234–238, 2002*

Ectodermal dysplasia – ankyloblepharon, absent lower eyelashes, hypoplasia of the upper lids, coloboma, seborrheic dermatitis, cribriform scrotal atrophy, ectropion, lacrimal duct hypoplasia, malaligned great toenails, gastroesophageal reflux, ear infections, laryngeal cleft, dental anomalies, scalp hair coarse and curly, sparse eyebrows, xerosis, hypohidrosis, short nose absent philtrum, flat upper lip *BJD 152:365–367, 2005*

Ectrodactyly-ectodermal dysplasia-clefting syndrome – alopecia of the scalp, eyebrows, and eyelashes, xerosis, atopic dermatitis, nail dystrophy, hypodontia with peg-shaped teeth, reduced sweat glands and salivary glands, syndactyly, mammary gland and nipple hypoplasia, conductive or sensorineural hearing loss, urogenital anomalies, lacrimal duct abnormalities; *TP63* mutations *BJD 162:201–207, 2010*

Goltz's syndrome (focal dermal hypoplasia) – asymmetric linear and reticulated streaks of atrophy and telangiectasia; yellow-red nodules; raspberry-like papillomas of lips, perineum, acrally, at perineum, buccal mucosa; xerosis; scalp and pubic hair sparse and brittle; short stature; asymmetric face; syndactyly, polydactyly; ocular, dental, and skeletal abnormalities with osteopathia striata of long bones *Cutis 53:309–312, 1994; JAAD 25:879–881, 1991*

Haber's syndrome *AD 117:321–324, 1981*

Hallermann-Streiff syndrome

Hereditary mucoepithelial dysplasia (dyskeratosis) (Gap junction disease, Witkop disease) – dry rough skin; red eyes, non-scarring alopecia, keratosis pilaris, erythema of oral (hard palate, gingival, tongue) and nasal mucous membranes, cervix, vagina, and urethra; perineal and perigenital psoriasiform dermatitis; increased risk of infections, fibrocystic lung disease *BJD 153:310–318, 2005; Ped Derm 11:133–138, 1994; Am J Med Genet 39:338–341, 1991; JAAD 21:351–357, 1989; Am J Hum Genet 31:414–427, 1979; Oral Surg Oral Med Oral Pathol 46:645–657, 1978*

Hutchinson-Gilford syndrome – hypohidrosis

Hypohidrotic ectodermal dysplasias
  Hypohidrotic ED – X-linked
  Hypohidrotic ED – autosomal recessive
  Hypohidrotic ED with corkscrew hairs *JAAD 27:917–921, 1992*
  Rapp-Hodgkin ED
  Ectrodactyly-ectodermal dysplasia-cleft lip/palate (EEC) syndrome
  Rosselli-Gulienetti syndrome
  Alopecia-onychodysplasia-hypohidrosis-deafness
  Basan syndrome
  Greither type
  Xeroderma-talipes-enamel defect
  Ankyloblepharon-ectodermal dysplasia-cleft lip/palate (AEC) syndrome
  Anonychia with flexural pigmentation
  Tricho-onycho-dental dysplasia
  Hypohidrosis-diabetes insipidus syndrome
  Hypohidrosis with neurolabyrinthitis
  Hypoplastic enamel-onycholysis-hypohidrosis (Witkop-Brearley-Gentry syndrome) – marked facial hypohidrosis, dry skin with keratosis pilaris, scaling and crusting of the scalp, onycholysis and subungual hyperkeratosis, hypoplastic enamel of the teeth *Oral Surg 39:71–86, 1975*

Ectodermal dysplasia with cataracts and hearing defects

Ichthyosis follicularis with atrichia and photophobia (IFAP) – collodion membrane and erythema at birth; generalized follicular keratoses, non-scarring alopecia, keratotic papules of the elbows, knees, fingers, extensor surfaces, xerosis; punctate keratitis *BJD 142:157–162, 2000; Am J Med Genet 85:365–368, 1999; AD 125:103–106, 1989; Dermatologica 177:341–347, 1988*

Keratosis follicularis spinulosa decalvans – X-linked dominant and autosomal dominant; alopecia, xerosis, thickened nails, photophobia, spiny follicular papules (keratosis pilaris), scalp pustules, palmoplantar keratoderma *Ped Derm 22:170–174, 2005*

Ichthyosis prematurity syndrome("self-healing congenital verruciform hyperkeratosis") – autosomal recessive; erythrodermic infant with caseous vernix-like desquamation; evolves into generalized xerosis and mild flexural hyperkeratosis and of lower back; cutaneous cobblestoning; keratosis pilaris-like changes; fine desquamation of the ankles; focal erythema, diffuse alopecia, fine scaling of the scalp, red and white dermatographism; in utero polyhydramnios with premature birth, thick caseous desquamating skin (thick vernix caseosa-like covering) (hyperkeratotic scalp) neonatal asphyxia; later in childhood, dry skin with follicular keratosis; mutation in fatty acid transport protein 4 (FATP4) *JAAD 66:606–616, 2012; JAAD 63:607–641, 2010; JAAD 59:S71–74, 2008*

MELAS syndrome – mitochondrial encephalomyopathy with lactic acidosis – scaly itchy diffuse erythema with xerosis *JAAD 41:469–473, 1999*

Microcephalic osteodysplastic primordial dwarfism type II – autosomal recessive; craniofacial dysmorphism with slanting palpebral fissures, prominent nose, small mouth, micrognathia; fine sparse hair and thin eyebrows; café au lait macules; xerosis; mottling; dark pigmentation of the neck and trunk; depigmentation (nevus depigmentosus); small pointed widely spaced teeth; low set ears missing lobule; widened metaphyses and relative shortening of the distal limbs; cerebrovascular anomalies *Ped Derm 25:401–402, 2008*

Mucoepithelial dysplasia (gap junction disease) – dry rough skin

Naxos syndrome – personal observation

NERDS syndrome *Dermatology 191:133–138, 1995*

Peeling skin syndrome – red macules, erosions, desquamation, xerosis; mutation in corneodesmosin *JAMADerm 151:225–226, 2015*

Pseudohypoparathyroidism – dry, scaly, hyperkeratotic puffy skin; multiple subcutaneous osteomas, collagenoma *BJD 143:1122–1124, 2000*

Shwachman syndrome – neutropenia, malabsorption, failure to thrive; generalized xerosis, follicular hyperkeratosis, widespread dermatitis, palmoplantar hyperkeratosis *Ped Derm 9:57–61, 1992; Arch Dis Child 55:531–547, 1980; J Pediatr 65:645–663, 1964*

Scleroatrophic and keratotic dermatosis of the limbs (scleroatrophic syndrome of Huriez) – autosomal dominant; scleroatrophy of the hands, sclerodactyly, palmoplantar keratoderma, xerosis, hypoplastic nails *BJD 143:1091–1096, 2000; BJD 134:512–518, 1996; Bull Soc Fr Dermatol Syphiligr 70:24–28, 1963;* dry hands and feet; 50% of patients with hypohidrosis *Ped Derm 15:207–209, 1998*

Short stature, mental retardation, facial dysmorphism, short webbed neck, skin changes, congenital heart disease – xerosis, dermatitis, low set ears, umbilical hernia *Clin Dysmorphol 5:321–327, 1996*

Tricho-odonto-onychodysplasia syndrome – multiple melanocytic nevi, freckles, generalized hypotrichosis, parietal alopecia, brittle nails, xerosis, supernumerary nipples, palmoplantar hyperkeratosis, enamel hypoplasia, deficient frontoparietal bone *JAAD 29:373–388, 1993; Am J Med Genet 15:67–70, 1983*

Trichothiodystrophy – PIBIDS *Ped Derm 32:865–866, 2015*

Turner's syndrome *JAAD 36:1002–1004, 1996*

Xeroderma pigmentosum

TRAUMA

Excessive cleansing, washing, obsessive-compulsive disorder

Radiation dermatitis, chronic *JAAD 54:28–46, 2006*

Reflex sympathetic dystrophy (complex regional pain syndrome) *AD 127:1541–1544, 1991*

VASCULAR DISEASES

Arteriosclerosis – xerosis as part of distal trophic changes

Edema, acute of legs – xerosis with erythema craquele *BJD 145:355–357, 2001*

Raynaud's disease – xerosis of hands *SKINmed 12:80–82, 2014;*

Venous stasis

YELLOW NAILS

CONGENITAL DISORDERS

Hereditary yellow nails without a syndrome *SKINMed 19:73–74, 2019*

DRUG-INDUCED

Amphotericin B – yellow nails

Gold therapy – yellow nails *BJD 145:855–856, 2001*

Penicillamine – yellow nails

Tetracycline – yellow nails, lunulae *s JAAD 57:1051–1058, 2007*

EXOGENOUS AGENTS

Boots – personal observation

Carotenemia

Insecticides – yellow lunulae *JAAD 57:1051–1058, 2017*
  Dinitro-ortho-cresol
  Diquat and paraquat

Nail hardener

Nail polish

Nicotine – yellow nails

Tar – yellow nails

INFECTIONS AND INFESTATIONS

Candida albicans – yellow nails

Dermatophytoma – linear white or yellow nail band *JAAD 66:1014–1016, 2012; AD 147:1277–1282, 2011; BJD 138:189–190, 1998*

Onychomycosis – yellow nails

METABOLIC DISORDERS

Hyperbilirubinemia

NEOPLASTIC DISORDERS

Onychomatrixoma – onycholysis with linear yellow band *JAAD 70:395–397, 2014;* banded or diffuse thickening of nail with yellowish discoloration, splinter hemorrhages, and transverse overcurvature (thick yellow nail) *Cutis 96:121–124, 2015;* parallel white and yellow nail bands with thickening of the nail plate; multiple subungual perforations *JAAD 76:S19–21, 2017; Dermatol Clin 33:197–205, 2015*
  Differential diagnosis of onychomatricoma
    Acquired digital fibrokeratoma
    Aggressive angiomyxoma
    Angiokeratoma
    Basal cell carcinoma of nail unit
    Glomus tumor
    Juvenile xanthogranuloma of the proximal nail fold
    Langerhans cell histiocytosis
    Malignant proliferating onycholemmal cyst
    Melanocytic nevus
    Nail psoriasis
    Neurofibroma
    Onychodystrophy
    Onychogenic Bowen's disease
    Onychogryphosis
    Onycholemmal horn
    Onychomycosis
    Pachyonychia congenita
    Periungual and subungual warts
    Pyogenic granuloma
    Longitudinal melanonychia
    Nail bed fibrosarcoma
    Subungual exostosis
    Subungual keratoacanthoma
    Subungual melanoma
    Subungual metastasis
    Subungual osteochondroma
    Subungual porocarcinoma
    Subungual eccrine syringofibroadenoma
    Subungual squamous cell carcinoma
    Superficial acral fibromyxoma
    Yellow nail syndrome
  Onychopapilloma

PRIMARY CUTANEOUS DISEASES

Psoriasis – yellow oil droplets of the nail beds *JAAD 57:1051–1058, 2007;* pustular psoriasis

SYNDROMES

Yellow nail syndrome – yellow slow growing thick nails, lymphedema, respiratory symptoms *Ped Derm 27:675–676, 2010; JAAD 56:537–538, 2007; BJD 156:1230–1234, 2007; JAAD 22:608–611, 1990; BJD 76:153–157, 1964; Acta Paediatr 49:748–751, 1960; Arch Dis Child 35:192–196, 1960; Orphanet J Rare Dis 12:42, 2017; J Dtsch Dermatol Ges 12:131–137, 2014; Case Rep Dermatol 3:251–258, 2011; Ped Derm 27:533–534, 2010; Chest 134:375–381, 2008; JAAD 56:537–538, 2007; BJD 156:1230–1234, 2007; JAAD 28:792–794, 1993*

VASCULAR DISEASES

Lymphedema

YELLOW OR SKIN-COLORED PAPULES OF THE NECK

DRUG REACTIONS

Corticosteroid acne

Penicillamine *Dermatology 184:12–18, 1992*

EXOGENOUS AGENTS

Saltpetre-induced pseudoxanthoma elasticum *Acta DV 58:323–327, 1978*

INFECTIONS

Cryptococcosis in AIDS *BJD 121:665–667, 1989*

Histoplasmosis *Infect Dis Clin North Am 2:841, 1988*

Leishmaniasis – Old World leishmaniasis or leishmaniasis recidivans *BJD 74:127–131, 1962*

Molluscum contagiosum

Mycobacterium tuberculosis – lichen scrofulosorum *AD 124:1421, 1988;* lupus vulgaris *JAAD 6:101, 1982*

Scrub typhus (*Orientia (Rickettsia) tsutsugamushi*) (larval stage of trombiculid mites(chiggers)) – headache and conjunctivitis; eschar with black crust ("cigarette burn-like: eschar); generalized macular or morbilliform rash; jaundice and abdominal pain *Clin Inf Dis 60:1828,1864–1865, 2015; Clin Inf Dis 39:1329–1335, 2004; AD 139:1545–1552, 2003; JAAD 2:359–373, 1980;* eschar and ulceration *JAAD 47:766–769, 2002*

Syphilis – papular syphilid *JAMA 249:3069, 1983*

Verrucae planae

INFILTRATIVE DISORDERS

Amyloidosis *AD 121:498, 1985*

Amyloid elastosis

Benign cephalic histiocytosis *AD 122:1038, 1986*

Colloid milium *AD 105:684, 1972*

Langerhans cell histiocytosis

Scleromyxedema (papular mucinosis)

Papular xanthoma *JAAD 22:1052, 1992*

Plane xanthomas – normolipemic plane xanthomas *AD 114:425–431, 1978; BJD 93:407–415, 1975*

Xanthoma disseminatum (Montgomery's syndrome) *Ped Pul 39:84–87, 2005; AD Syphilol 208:373, 1938*

INFLAMMATORY DISEASES

Sarcoid, papular *AD 123:1557, 1987*

METABOLIC DISEASES

Hyperphosphatemia

Pseudoxanthoma elasticum-like lesions with hyperphosphatemia *Am J Med 83:1157–1162, 1987*

Osteitis deformans (Paget's disease of bone)

Osteoectasia

Pseudoxanthoma elasticum-like changes with osteoectasia *Clin Exp Derm 7:605–609, 1982*

Xanthoma papuloeruptivum *JAAD 13:1, 1985*

NEOPLASTIC DISEASES

Acrochordon

Actinic keratosis

Basal cell carcinoma

Clear cell hidradenoma (eccrine acrospiroma) *Cancer 23:641, 1969*

Connective tissue nevi *JAAD 3:441, 1980;* eruptive collagenoma *JID 76:284, 1981*

Dermatofibromas

Eccrine angiomatous hamartoma *Ped Derm 14:401–402, 1997*

Eccrine spiradenoma *JID 46:347, 1966*

Elastoma – juvenile elastoma

Juvenile xanthogranuloma *Br J Plast Surg 52:591–593, 1999; Cutis 11:499–501, 1973*

Leiomyomas

Melanoma – amelanotic melanoma

Merkel cell carcinoma

Metastases – from oral cavity, lung, breast *JAAD 33:161, 1995*

Milia *AD 120:300, 1984*

Mucoid milia

Neurofibromas

Nevus sebaceous *JAAD 18:429, 1988*

Sebaceous epithelioma *JAAD 34:47–50, 1996; AD 89:711, 1964*

Sebaceous adenoma

Squamous cell carcinoma

Syringomas, including eruptive syringomas *J Eur Acad Derm Vener 15:242–246, 2001; AD 121:756, 1985*

Trichoepitheliomas, multiple *AD 68:517, 1953*

PARANEOPLASTIC DISEASES

Necrobiotic xanthogranuloma *JAAD 3:257, 1980*

PRIMARY CUTANEOUS DISEASES

Benign symmetric lipomatosis (Madelung's disease) *South Med J 79:1023, 1986*

Closed comedones

Cutis laxa *Acta Paediatr Scand 67:775–780, 1978*

Elastosis perforans serpiginosa

Granuloma annulare, disseminated

Lichen nitidus

Lichen spinulosus

Pseudoxanthoma elasticum *BJD 161:635–639, 2009; JAAD 42:324–328, 2000; Dermatology 199:3–7, 1999; AD 124:1559, 1988*

Perforating pseudoxanthoma elasticum *AD 121:1321, 1985*

Pseudoxanthoma elasticum and acrosclerosis *Proc Roy Soc Med 70:567–570, 1977*

PXE-like papillary dermal elastolysis – side of the neck, axilla; postmenopausal and elderly women *JAAD 67:128–135, 2012*

SYNDROMES

Acrogeria with late onset focal dermal elastosis *Dermatology 192:264–268, 1996*

Birt-Hogg-Dube syndrome

Buschke-Ollendorff syndrome

Cowden's disease

Ehlers-Danlos syndrome

Hunter's syndrome – dermal nodules

Muir-Torre syndrome *JAAD 10:803, 1984*

Multicentric reticulohistiocytosis *Oral Surg Oral Med Oral Pathol 65:721–725, 1988*

Niemann-Pick disease *Ann Int Med 82:257, 1975*

Steatocystoma multiplex

VASCULAR DISORDERS

Lymphangioma circumscriptum

YELLOW PAPULES AND PLAQUES

AUTOIMMUNE DISEASES AND DISEASES OF IMMUNE DYSFUNCTION

CREST syndrome with cutaneous plate-like calcinosis

Lupus erythematosus – systemic lupus with nodular episcleritis

Morphea – personal observation

Relapsing polychondritis – normolipemic plane xanthomas in relapsing polychondritis *Acta DV 74:221–223, 1994*

Rheumatoid arthritis – rheumatoid neutrophilic dermatitis *AD 133:757–760, 1997*

Urticaria with jaundice – "yellow hives"

CONGENITAL LESIONS

Aplasia cutis congenita

Chin hamartoma – multipapillated yellow-pink papules of the chin with underlying infantile hemangioma; biopsy demonstrates sebaceous hamartoma of dermal fibroplasia with prominent vessels *Ped Derm 37:78–85, 2020*

Juvenile xanthogranuloma – yellow-brown nodule *Ped Derm 26:709–712, 2009*

Median raphe canal of the ventral penis – with or without median raphe cysts; yellow cystic papules *Ped Derm 27:667–669, 2010*

Median raphe cysts of the ventral penis – yellow cystic papules *Ped Derm 27:667–669, 2010;* differential diagnosis includes epidermoid or dermoid cysts, urethral diverticulosis, apocrine hidrocystoma

Median raphe cyst of the scrotum and perineum *JAAD 55:S114–115, 2006*

Rudimentary meningocele (primary cutaneous meningioma) – yellow plaque of the scalp *Ped Derm 15:388–389, 1998*

Sebaceous gland hyperplasia of the newborn

DEGENERATIVE DISORDERS

Morgagnian cataract – yellow opacity *NEJM 370:2326, 2014*

DRUGS

Calcium chloride extravasation – calcinosis cutis *AD 124:922–925, 1988*

Corticosteroid atrophy

Cyclosporine – sebaceous hyperplasias *JAAD 35:696–699, 1996; Dermatologica 172:24–30, 1986*

Indomethacin – eruptive xanthomas *AD 139:1045–1048, 2003; Acta DV 55:489–492, 1975*

Olanzapine – eruptive xanthomas *AD 139:1045–1048, 2003*

Penicillamine *JAAD 30:103–107, 1994;* pseudoxanthoma elasticum-like changes *Dermatology 184:12–18, 1992*

Ritonavir – hyperlipidemia with xanthomas *JAAD 52:S86–89, 2005*

EXOGENOUS AGENTS

Acquired pseudoxanthoma elasticum – farmers exposed to saltpeter (calcium-ammonium-nitrate salts); antecubital fossa; yellow macules and papules *JAAD 51:1–21, 2004; Acta DV 78:153–154, 1998; Acta DV 58:319–321, 1978*

Exogenous calcium – EEG or EMG paste *Ped Derm 15:27–30, 1998; AD 89:360–363, 1964*

Titanium dioxide-induced plane xanthoma-like lesions *AD 121:656–658, 1985*

INFECTIONS

Adiaspiromycosis – cutaneous adiaspiromycosis (*Chrysosporium* species) – hyperpigmented plaque with white-yellow papules, ulcerated nodules, hyperkeratotic nodules, crusted nodules, multilobulated nodules *JAAD S113–117, 2004*

Favus – scutulum of favus

Hepatitis B – urticaria with jaundice (yellow hives)

Leishmaniasis *JAAD 34:257–272, 1996*

Leprosy – histoid leprosy; xanthomatous lesions *BJD 160:305–310, 2009; Indian J Lepr 73:353–358, 2001;* lepromatous leprosy *Cutis 83:66,73–74, 2009*

Lyme borreliosis – acrodermatitis chronica atrophicans; small yellow papules or nodules *JAAD 49:363–392, 2003*

Mycetoma – *Pseudallescheria boydii, Acremonium* sp. – white and yellow grains; *Nocardiopsis dassonvillei* – white or yellow; *Streptomyces somaliensis* – yellow grains *JAAD 53:931–951, 2005; Cutis 60:191–193, 1997*

Mycobacterium tuberculosis – lupus vulgaris; starts as red-brown plaque, enlarges with serpiginous margin or as discoid plaques; apple-jelly nodules; tumorlike forms – deeply infiltrative; soft smooth nodules or red-yellow hypertrophic plaque; head, neck, around nose, extremities, trunk *Int J Dermatol 26:578–581, 1987; Acta Tuberc Scand 39(Suppl 49):1–137, 1960;* lichen scrofulosorum – yellow-brown papules

Scutular favus-like tinea cruris et pedis *JAAD 34:1086–1087, 1996*

Trichomycosis axillaris (*Corynebacterium tenuis*) – yellow concretions *JAMADerm 151:1023–1024, 2015; NEJM 369:1735, 2013*

Verrucae – yellow subungual papules *Ped Derm 35:521–522, 2018*

INFILTRATIVE DISEASES

Amyloid elastosis (primary systemic amyloid) – neck, axillae, flexor surfaces, trunk, and groin *AD 121:498–502, 1985;* primary cutaneous nodular amyloidosis – yellow nodules *Cutis 84:87–92, 2009*

Amyloidosis *NEJM 349:583–596, 2003; JAAD 18:19–25, 1988; AD 122:1425–1430, 1986; AD 121:498, 1985;* xanthoma-like lesions *BJ Clin Pract 27:271–273, 1973;* lichen amyloidosis; familial lichen amyloidosis; primary cutaneous amyloidosis of the penis – translucent yellow plaques of the penis *JAMADerm 151:910–911, 2015*

Benign cephalic histiocytosis – pink-yellow papules of the face *Ped Derm 31:547–550, 2014 JAAD 47:908–913, 2002; Ped Derm*

11:164–167, 1994; Am J Dermatopathol 15:315–319, 1993; AD 120:650–655, 1984; Bull Soc Fr Dermatol Syphiligr 78:232–233, 1971

Colloid milium *Clin Exp Dermatol 18:347–350, 1993; BJD 125:80–81, 1991; AD 105:684, 1972;* juvenile colloid milium – yellow facial plaques; eyelids, nose, gingiva, conjunctiva *JAAD 49:1185–1188, 2003; Clin Exp Dermatol 25:138–140, 2000*

Erdheim-Chester disease (non-Langerhans cell histiocytosis) (lipoid granulomatosis) – CD68+ and factor XIIIa+; negative for CD1a and S100; xanthoma and xanthelasma-like lesions (red-brown-yellow papules and plaques); flat wartlike papules of the face; lesions occur in folds; the skin becomes slack with atrophy of the folds and face; also lesions of the eyelids, axillae, groin, neck; bony lesions; diabetes insipidus, painless exophthalmos, retroperitoneal, renal, and pulmonary histiocytic infiltration *JAAD 74:513–520, 2016; JAAD 57:1031–1045, 2007; AD 143:952–953, 2007; Hautarzt 52:510–517, 2001; JAAD 37:839–842, 1997; Medicine (Baltimore) 75:157–169, 1996; Virchow Arch Pathol Anat 279:541–542, 1930*

Focal cutaneous mucinosis

Generalized eruptive histiocytosis *JAAD 50:116–120, 2004; JAAD 17:449–454, 1987; AD 88:586–596, 1963*

Langerhans cell histiocytosis – xanthoma-like lesions *JAAD 34:688–689, 1996;* yellow-red-brown papules *Curr Prob in Derm VI:1–24, 1994;* Hashimoto-Pritzker disease; congenital single yellow-red nodule with central ulceration *Ped Derm 26:121–126, 2009*

Mastocytosis – solitary mastocytoma *AD 84:806–815, 1961;* urticaria pigmentosa; xanthelasmoidea (infiltrative diffuse cutaneous mastocytosis) *BJD 144:355–358, 2001; AD 112:1270–1271, 1976;* bullous mastocytosis; cutaneous mastocytosis simulating tuberous xanthomas *Przegl Dermatol 77:40–46, 1990(Polish)*

Systemic non-Langerhans cell histiocytosis (juvenile xanthogranuloma) – progressing to hemophagocytic lymphohistiocytosis *J Pediatr Hematol Oncol 34:222–225, 2012; Pediatr Blood Cancer 47:103–106, 2006; J Pediatr Hematol Oncol 26:591–595, 2004*

Papular xanthoma *Ped Derm 15:65–67, 1998; Ped Derm 10:139–141, 1993; JAAD 22:1052, 1992; JAAD 22:1052–1056, 1990;* disseminated primary papular xanthoma *AD 143:667–669, 2007*

Progressive nodular histiocytosis – yellow-pink/yellow –brown papules *JAAD 57:1031–1045, 2007*

Verruciform xanthoma *JAAD 42:343–347, 2000; Am J Surg Pathol 22:479–487, 1998;* of scrotum – yellow cauliflower-like appearance *J Dermatol 16:397–401, 1989;* verruciform xanthoma of the toes in patient with Milroy's disease due to persistent leg edema *Ped Derm 20:44–47, 2003;* disseminated verruciform xanthoma *BJD 151:717–719, 2004;* of the vulva – yellow-orange verrucous plaques *AD 147:1087–1092, 2011*

Xanthogranuloma – juvenile xanthogranuloma *JAAD 56:54–55, 2007; Am J Pathol 30:625–626, 1954; BJD 124:85–89, 1912; BJD 17:222–223, 1905;* disseminated JXG *JAAD 58:S12–15, 2008; BJD 17:222, 1905;* generalized lichenoid juvenile xanthogranuloma – face, neck, scalp, upper trunk *BJD 126:66–70, 1992;* disseminated JXG *Ped Derm 26:475–476, 2009;* of the penis *JAAD 62:524, 2010; J Urol 150:456–457, 1993;* yellow papules of the penis *Ped Derm 34:603–604, 2017*

Xanthoma disseminatum (Montgomery's syndrome) – red-yellow-brown cobblestoned papules and nodules of the flexural surfaces (inguinal folds, axillae), trunk, face, proximal extremities, eyelids, and oral mucosa; become confluent into xanthomatous plaques; verrucous plaques *JAMADerm 153:813–814, 2017; JAMADerm 152:715–716, 2016; AD 147:459–464, 2011; JAAD 56:302–316,*

2007; Ped Derm 22:550–553, 2005; JAAD 55:185–187, 2006; NEJM 338:1138–1143, 1998; Clin Invest 7:233–238, 1993; JAAD 23:341–346, 1990; AD Syphilol 37:373–402, 1938; zosteriform juvenile xanthogranuloma *Ped Derm 31:615–617, 2014*

INFLAMMATORY DISEASES

Crohn's disease – metastatic – personal observation

Lipogranulomas – orbital lipogranulomas – yellow eyelid papules *JAAD 37:839–842, 1997*

Malacoplakia *JAAD 34:325–332, 1996*

Rosai-Dorfman disease (sinus histiocytosis with massive lymphadenopathy) – xanthoma-like lesions with grouped yellow-red papules and nodules of the head, neck, ears, trunk, arms, and legs; cervical lymphadenopathy; also axillary, inguinal, and mediastinal adenopathy; hypergammaglobulinemia; emperipolesis (histiocytes with intracellular inflammatory cells and debris) *JAAD 65:1069–1071, 2011; JAAD 56:302–316, 2007; BJD 148:1060–1061, 2003; Int J Derm 37:271–174, 1998; Am J Dermatopathol 17:384–388, 1995; Semin Diagn Pathol 7:19–73, 1990;Cancer 30:1174–1188, 1972; Arch Pathol 87:63–70, 1969;* red-brown plaque with yellow nodules *JAMADerm 150:177–181, 2014*

Sarcoidosis *AD 123:1557, 1987*

METABOLIC

Amyloidosis – hereditary apolipoprotein A1 amyloidosis – yellow papules *BJD 152:250–257, 2005*

Benign monoclonal gammopathies – normolipemic plane xanthomas *JAAD 49:119–122, 2003*

Biliary atresia, congenital – multiple xanthomas *Ped Derm 25:403–404, 2008*

Calcinosis cutis – secondary to subcutaneous calcium heparin injections *JAAD 50:210–214, 2004;* cutaneous calculus *BJD 75:1–11, 1963;* idiopathic calcinosis of the scrotum; calcinosis cutis following intravenous calcium infusion; subepidermal calcified nodule (Winer's nodular calcinosis) – yellow-white papule *Ped Derm 25:253–254, 2008; Arch Dermatol Syph 66:204–211, 1952;* tumoral calcinosis – progressively growing red-yellow lobulated masses *Ped Derm 27:299–300, 2010;* soft tumoral calcinosis – personal observation

Cerebrotendinous xanthomatosis – autosomal recessive; tendon (Achilles tendon) and tuberous xanthomas *Ped Derm 17:447–449, 2000*

Chylous ascites – xanthomas secondary to chylous ascites *JAAD 51:75–78, 2004*

Cryoglobulinemia – normolipemic plane xanthomas *JAAD 49:119–122, 2003*

Familial chylomicronemia – autosomal recessive; eruptive xanthomas; due to lipoprotein lipase or apolipoprotein II deficiency or inhibitors of lipoprotein lipase *Ped Derm 24:323–325, 2007*

Gout – tophus *Cutis 48:445–451, 1991; Ann Rheum Dis 29:461–468, 1970*

Hypercholesterolemia, familial – tuberous xanthomas *Ped Derm 17:447–449, 2000*

Marginal cysts of the eyelids – occluded glands of Moll; painless white or yellow cyst of lower eyelid close to lacrimal punctum

Myxedema; hypothyroidism

Necrobiosis lipoidica diabeticorum *JAMA 311:2328, 2014; Ped Derm 27:178–181, 2010; Int J Derm 33:605–617, 1994; JAAD 18:530–537, 1988;* yellow nodules *AD 143:546–548, 2007*

Osteitis deformans (Paget's disease of bone) *Ann Int Med 82:257, 1975*

Osteoma cutis, primary *Cutis 68:103–106, 2001*

Porphyria cutanea tarda with sclerodermoid lesions

Pretibial myxedema

Pseudogout – pseudotophi (calcium pyrophosphate)

Retention cyst from glands of Zeis

Tangier's disease – enlarged yellow tonsils (alpha-lipoprotein deficiency) – personal observation

Tendinous xanthomas
    Cerebrotendinous xanthomatosis – mutation in sterol 27-hydroxy-lase; increased serum cholestanol and urinary bile alcohols; normal serum cholesterol *JAAD 45:292–295, 2001*
    Phytosterolemia (beta sitosterolemia) *Ped Derm 17:447–449, 2000*
    Familial hypercholesterolemia
    Familial combined hyperlipidemia
    Familial type III hyperlipoproteinemia

Tuberous xanthoma
    Alagille syndrome
    Familial combined hyperlipidemia
    Familial hypercholesterolemia *Ped Derm 17:447–449, 2000*
    Familial type III hyperlipoproteinemia
    Cerebrotendinous xanthomatosis
    Phytosterolemia

Xanthelasmas
    Cerebrotendinous xanthomatosis *JAAD 45:292–295, 2001*
    Familial hypercholesterolemia (decrease LDL receptors)
    Phytosterolemia – excessive absorption of plant sterols; normal LDL *Clin Biochem Rev 25:49–68, 2004*
    Familial type III hyperlipoproteinemia (abnormal apoprotein E)
    Sitosterolemia – tuberous and tendon xanthomas *Ped Derm 17:447–449, 2000*

Xanthomas
    Diffuse plane xanthomas – apolipoprotein A-1 deficiency
    Familial hypercholesterolemia *Ped Derm 24:230–234, 2007*
    Niemann-Pick disease
    Plane xanthomas – normolipemic plane xanthomas *AD 114:425–431, 1978; BJD 93:407–415, 1975*

Xanthoma striatum palmare
    Familial type III hyperlipoproteinemia

Eruptive xanthomas – yellow-red papules *JAMA 313:83–84, 2015; Cutis 89:141–144, 2012; Cutis 50:31–32, 1992*
    Familial hypertriglyceridemias (type V)
    Familial lipoprotein lipase deficiency (apolipoprotein C II deficiency)
    Familial combined hyperlipidemia (increased plasma apo-beta-lipoprotein)
    Familial type III hyperlipoproteinemia
    HAART therapy – protease inhibitors *Ped Infect Dis 21:259–260, 2002; J Infect Dis 42:181–188, 2001; AIDS 12:1393–1394, 1998*

Xanthoma papuloeruptivum *AD 141:1595–1600, 2005; JAAD 13:1, 1985*

NEOPLASTIC

Atypical lymphoid infiltrate (hyperplasia) – xanthelasma-like periorbital plaque *JAAD 37:839–842, 1997*

Basal cell carcinoma, including morpheaform basal cell carcinoma of the eyelid – papule *Eyelid and Conjunctival Tumors, Shields JA and Shields CL, Lippincott Williams and Wilkins, 1999, p.25*

Basaloid follicular hamartoma – yellow plaque *AD 129:915–917, 1993*

Cellular neurothekeoma *Ped Derm 12:191–194, 1995*

Chalazion – yellow, skin-colored, or red papule or nodule *Ophthalmology 87:218–221, 1980; Eyelid and Conjunctival Tumors, Shields JA and Shields CL, Lippincott Williams and Wilkins, 1999, p.165*

Cholesterotic fibrous histiocytoma *AD 126:506–508, 1990*

Connective tissue nevus (collagenomas) including eruptive collagenomas *JID 76:284, 1981; BJD 72:217–220, 1960;* familial cutaneous collagenomas *Ped Derm 21:33–38, 2004;* connective tissue nevus with elastorrhexis or upper chest – skin-colored or hypopigmented or yellow papules, plaques, nodules in cobblestoned pattern *Ped Derm 32:518–521, 2015*

Dermatofibroma, myxoid – multiple eruptive myxoid dermatofibro-mas; 3–8 mm yellow-pink papules *BJD 157:382–385, 2007;* xanthomatous dermatofibroma

Dermatofibrosarcoma protuberans *JAAD 35:355–374, 1996*

Eccrine angiomatous hamartoma – vascular nodule; macule, red plaque, acral nodule of infants or neonates; painful, red, purple, blue, yellow, brown, skin colored *JAAD 47:429–435, 2002; JAAD 37:523–549, 1997; Ped Derm 13:139–142, 1996*

Elastoma – face, abdomen, trunk, buttock, thigh, scrotum *JAAD 51:1–21, 2004;* Dubreuilh elastoma – thick yellow plaque of the face, neck, or chest mistaken for basal cell carcinoma *JAAD 32:1016–1024, 1995*

Epidermal nevus

Epidermoid cyst

Eruptive vellus hair cysts – skin-colored, red, white, blue, yellow eyelid papules *Ped Derm 19:26–27, 2002;* yellow brown papules of the chest and arms *Cutis 84:295–298, 2009*

Fibroepithelioma of Pinkus

Folliculosebaceous cystic hamartoma – skin-colored or yellow papule or nodule of the central face or scalp; pedunculated or dome-shaped and umbilicated *BJD 157:833–835, 2007; Clin Exp Dermatol 31:68–79, 2006; AD 139:803–808, 2003; JAAD 34:77–81, 1996; Am J Dermatopathol 13:213–220, 1991; J Cutan Pathol 7:394–403, 1980*

Folliculosebaceous smooth muscle hamartoma – pink-yellow dome-shaped facial papule *JAAD 56:1021–1025, 2007*

Granular cell tumor – personal observation

Kaposi's sarcoma, anaplastic – yellow hyperkeratotic plantar nodules *BJD 164:209–211, 2011*

Leiomyomas

Leiomyosarcoma – blue-black; also red, brown, yellow, or hypopig-mented *JAAD 46:477–490, 2002*

Leukemia cutis – acute myelogenous leukemia in children, yellow-violaceous oval nodules *Ped Derm 36:658–663, 2019*

Lipoblastoma – yellow nodule of the eyelid *Am J Dermatopathol 12:408–411, 1990*

Lipoma, mobile encapsulated lipoma *AD 145:931–936, 2009*

Lymphoma – papular xanthomatosis *JAAD 26:828–832, 1992;* dystrophic xanthoma in cutaneous T-cell lymphoma (CTCL) *AD 123:91–94, 1987;* xanthomatous CTCL *AD 128:1499–1502, 1992;* B-cell lymphoma – xanthomatous infiltration of the neck *Eur J Derm 10:481–483, 2000*

Mantleoma – 2–4mm yellow or white papules *Cutis 28:429–432, 1981*

Microcystic adnexal carcinoma of lip *JAAD 29:840–845, 1993*

Metastases – oral cavity, lung, breast *JAAD 33:161, 1995;* histiocytoid breast carcinoma *Dermatology 205:63–66, 2002*

Microcystic adnexal carcinoma *Derm Surg 27:979–984, 2001; JAAD 29:840–845, 1993; AD 122:286–289, 1986*

Neurilemmoma (schwannoma) – yellowish nodules of the head and neck

Nevus lipomatosus superficialis – grouped skin-colored to yellow papules *Ped Derm 29:119–21, 2012; Cutis 72:237–238, 2003; Int J Dermatol 14:273–276, 1975*

Nevus sebaceous *JAAD 18:429, 1988; Arch Dermatol Syphilol 33:355–394, 1895*

Oncocytoma – benign tumor of oxyphil epithelial cells; bright red or yellow papule of the eyelid *Arch Ophthalmol 102:263–265, 1984*

Onychomatricoma – localized yellow thickening with transverse overcurvature *Dermatol Clin 33:197–205, 2015*

Osteochondroma – white-yellow nodule *Derm Surg 27:591–593, 2001*

Pilomatrixomas

Progressive nodular histiocytomas – yellow-brown papules; coalesce to form large disfiguring plaques *BJD 146:138–140, 2002; BJD 143:678–679, 2000; JAAD 29:278–280, 1993; JAAD 57:1031–1045, 2007; AD 114:1505–1508, 1978*

Reticulohistiocytoma – yellow papule *JAAD 46:801, 2002*

Sebaceous adenoma (sebaceoma) – yellow ulcerated papules *J Cutan Pathol 11:396–414, 1984;* intraoral *J Ral Surg 26:593–595, 1968*

Sebaceous carcinoma *Br J Ophthalmol 82:1049–1055, 1998; Br J Plast Surg 48:93–96, 1995; JAAD 25:685–690, 1991; J Derm Surg Oncol 11:260–264, 1985*

Sebaceous epithelioma *JAAD 34:47–50, 1996; AD 89:711, 1964*

Sebaceous hyperplasia of the face *JAAD 61:549–560, 2009; BJD 118:397–402, 1988; Berlin: Verlag A Hirschfeld: 1874;* of the vulva *Obstet Gynecol 68:63S–65S, 1986*

Seborrheic keratosis

Smooth muscle hamartoma

Spitz nevus

Syringomas, including eruptive syringomas *AD 121:756, 1985*

Trichoadenoma of the forehead – linear yellow verrucous L-shaped plaque *JAAD 57:905–906, 2007*

Trichoepithelioma – single or multiple *AD 68:517, 1953*

Xanthomatous giant cell tumor of the tendon sheath – yellow nodule of the fingertip *AD 145:931–936, 2009*

PARANEOPLASTIC DISORDERS

Eruptive xanthogranulomas and hematologic malignancies *JAAD 59:488–493, 2008; JAAD 50:976–978, 2004*

Generalized eruptive histiocytosis – associated with *FIPIL1-PDGFRA* + chronic eosinophilic leukemia *JAMADerm 151:766–769, 2015;* associated with acute myelogenous leukemia *JAAD 49:S233–236, 2003;* associated with chronic myelogenous leukemia *J Cutan Pathol 40:725–729, 2013; Actos Dermosifilogr 103:643–644, 2012*

Necrobiotic xanthogranuloma with paraproteinemia – yellow-red plaques *JAMADerm 156:696, 2020; J Eur Acad DV 31:221–235,* *2017; SkinMed 11:121–123, 2013;* prominent periorbital lesions; red eyes – scleritis, uveitis; IgG kappa most common *AD 147:1215–1220, 2011; AD 145:279–284, 2009; JAAD 56:302–316, 2007; Ann Hematol 86:303–306, 2007; Eyelid and Conjunctival Tumors, Shields JA and Shields CL, Lippincott Williams and Wilkins, 1999, p. 141; JAAD 29:466–469, 1993; AD 125:287–292, 1992; JAAD 3:257–270, 1983; JAAD 3:257–270, 1980;* yellow linear plaques within scars *Int J Derm 43:293–295, 2004* (burn scar)*; Orbit 27:191–194, 2008; Mayo Clin Proc 72:1028–1033, 1997; AD 128:94–100, 1992* (surgical scars)

Neurofibromatosis, juvenile xanthogranulomas, and juvenile myelomonocytic leukemia *Ped Derm 36:114–118, 2017*

Normolipemic plane xanthomas – multiple myeloma; Castleman's syndrome *JAAD 39:439–442, 1998; JAAD 26:105–109, 1991;* non-Hodgkin's lymphoma *JAAD 49:119–122, 2003;* paraproteinemia *JAAD 49:119–122, 2003*

PHOTODERMATOSES

Actinic granuloma

Dermatoheliosis (solar or actinic elastosis) (sun damage; basophilic alteration of collagen) *JAAD 51:1–21, 2004*

Dubreuilh's elastoma *JAAD 32:1016–1024, 1995*

Favre-Racouchot syndrome (nodular elastosis with cysts and comedones) *JAAD 51:1–21, 2004*

Keratoelastoidosis marginalis (degenerative collagenous plaques of the hands) *JAAD 51:1–21, 2004; AD 82:362–366, 1960*

Solar elastotic bands – forearms *JAAD 15:650–656, 1986*

PRIMARY CUTANEOUS DISEASE

Atopic dermatitis – normolipemic papular xanthomas in erythrodermic atopic dermatitis *JAAD 32:326–333, 1995*

Elastosis perforans serpiginosa with pseudoxanthoma elasticum-like changes in Moya-Moya disease (bilateral stenosis and occlusion of basa intracranial vessels and carotid arteries) *BJD 153:431–434, 2005*

Erythema elevatum diutinum *Medicine (Baltimore) 56:443–455, 1977; BJD 67:121–145, 1955*

Focal acral hyperkeratosis – yellow papules on lateral aspect of the palms *AD 132:1365, 1368, 1996*

Follicular keratosis of the chin – frictional dermatitis; yellow-white to skin-colored papules *Ped Derm 24:412–414, 2007; JAAD 26:134–135, 1992; Int J Dermatol 24:320–321, 1985; J Cutan Pathol 10:376, 1983; J Dermatol 6:365–369, 1979*

Fordyce spots (ectopic sebaceous glands) – yellow papules of buccal mucosa, lip, penile shaft *BJD 121:669–670, 1989;* areola of the nipple *J Dermatol 21:524–526, 1994*

Frontal fibrosing alopecia with yellow facial papules *JAAD 77:764–766, 2017*

Granuloma annulare – disseminated *JAAD 3:217–230, 1980;* perforating granuloma annulare *BJD 147:1026–1028, 2002*

Granuloma faciale *JAAD 53:1002–1009, 2005*

Hereditary papulotranslucent acrokeratoderma *Cutis 61:29–30, 1998*

Herniated lacrimal gland – personal observation

Idiopathic non-familial acro-osteolysis – yellow digital papules *Indian J Dermatol 57:486–488, 2012*

Late-onset focal dermal elastosis – yellow papules of the thighs and lower abdomen; peau d'orange appearance of the neck, thighs, groin, axillae, antecubital and popliteal fossae in older men *JAAD 51:1–21, 2004; BJD 133:303–305, 1995*

Lichen planus of the palms and soles

Linear focal elastosis – linear yellow bands of the lumbosacral area, lower legs, or face in older men *BJD 145:188–190, 2001; JAAD 36:301–303, 1997; AD 127:1365–1368, 1991*

Miescher's granuloma – personal observation

Orbital fat herniation (vs. dermolipoma) *JAMADerm 150:1115, 2014*

Papular elastorrhexis *AD 123:433–434, 1987*

Periumbilical perforating pseudoxanthoma elasticum – yellow macules and papules *JAAD 51:1–21, 2004; JAAD 26:642–644, 1992; AD 115:300–303, 1979*

Pingueculae

Punctate porokeratotic keratoderma (spiny keratoderma) – yellow keratotic palmar papules *AD 147:609–614, 2011; AD 124:1678–1682, 1988; JAAD 13:908–912, 1985; Dermatologica 147:206–213, 1973*

Waxy keratoses of childhood (disseminated hypopigmented keratoses) – generalized dome-shaped yellow or skin-colored keratotic papules *Ped Derm 18:415–416, 2001; Clin Exp Dermatol 19:173–176, 1994*

White fibrous papulosis – back or sides of the neck *JAAD 67:128–135, 2012; Cut Ocul Toxicol 30:69–71, 2011; Ann DV 119:925–926; JAAD 20:1073–1077, 1989*; Xanthoerythroderma perstans *JAAD 36:301–303, 1997; Cutis 60:41–42, 1997*

SYNDROMES

Adult onset asthma with periocular xanthogranuloma *Ophthalmol Plast Reconstr Surg 29:104–108, 2013; AD 147:1230–1231, 2011; Br J Ophthalmol 90:602–608, 2006*

Alagille syndrome – obstructive cholestatic liver disease (paucity of interlobular hepatic ducts) – tendinous, planar, and tuberous xanthomas; xanthomas of palmar creases, extensor fingers, the nape of the neck; growth retardation, delayed puberty; autosomal dominant; pruritus and failure to thrive; wispy hair, triangular face, broad forehead, deep-set eyes, mild hypertelorism, straight nose, small pointed chin, ventricular hypertrophy, pulmonary artery stenosis; supernumerary digital flexion creases of the middle phalanges *JAAD 58:S9–11, 2008; Ped Derm 22:11–14, 2005; Ped Derm 17:447–449, 2000*

Benign symmetric lipomatosis (Madelung's disease) *SMJ 79:1023, 1986*

Birt-Hogg-Dube syndrome – fibrofolliculomas – autosomal dominant; white or yellow facial and nose papules *AD 135:1195–1202, 1999; AD 133:1161–1166, 1997; JAAD 16:452–457, 1987*

Blau or Jabs syndrome (familial juvenile systemic granulomatosis) – autosomal dominant; onset under 4 years of age; generalized papular rash of infancy; translucent skin-colored papules (non-caseating granulomas) of the trunk and extremities or dense lichenoid yellow to red-brown papules with grainy surface with anterior or panuveitis, synovitis, symmetric polyarthritis; polyarteritis, multiple synovial cysts; red papular rash in early childhood; exanthema resolves with pitted scars; camptodactyly (flexion contractures of PIP joints); no involvement of the lung or hilar nodes; activating mutations in NOD2 (nucleotide-binding oligomerization domain 2) (caspase recruitment domain family, member 15; *CARD* 15) *Ped Derm 27:69–73, 2010; AD 143:386–391, 2007; Clin Exp Dermatol 21:445–448, 1996; J Pediatr 107:689–693, 1985*

Buschke-Ollendorff syndrome (dermatofibrosis lenticularis disseminata) – autosomal dominant; connective tissue nevi and osteopoikilosis; single or multiple yellow, white, or skin-colored papules, nodules, plaques of extremities; skin-colored to yellow papules; loss of function mutation in *LEMD3* (inner nuclear membrane protein that antagonizes transforming growth factor beta and bone morphogenetic protein signaling) *AD 146:63–68, 2010; Ped Derm 22:133–137, 2005; Nat Genet 36 (11):1213–1218, 2004; JAAD 49:1163–1166, 2003; JAAD 48:600–601, 2003; BJD 144:890–893, 2001; Derm Wochenschr 86:257–262, 1928;* juvenile elastoma; large yellowish nodules and plaques *Clin Exp Dermatol 7:109–113, 1982*

CHILD syndrome – congenital hemidysplasia, ichthyosis, limb defects, ichthyosiform erythroderma with verruciform xanthoma, linear eruptions, and hypopigmented bands; fingertip nodules (verruciform xanthomas) *JAAD 50:S31–33, 2004; Ped Derm 15:360–366, 1998;* xanthomatous pattern *Dermatologica 180:263–266, 1990*

Congenital self-healing reticulohistiocytosis *JAAD 11:447–454, 1984*

Cowden's syndrome

Ehlers-Danlos syndrome

Encephalocraniocutaneous lipomatosis (Haberland syndrome) – red soft plaque of the bulbar conjunctiva (limbal dermoids) (pterygium like lesion) lipomatous hamartomas of the scalp and eyelids; linear yellow papules of the forehead extending to the eyelids; alopecia and ocular christomas; scalp nodules, skin-colored nodules, facial and eyelid papules, lipomas, and fibrolipomas; ophthalmologic manifestations; seizures, mental retardation; mandibular or maxillary ossifying fibromas and odontomas; cranial asymmetry; developmental delay, mental retardation, seizures, spasms of contralateral limbs; unilateral porencephalic cysts with cortical atrophy *Ped Derm 35:825–826, 2018; Ped Derm 30:491–492, 2013; Ped Derm 23:27–30, 2006; Ped Derm 22:206–209, 2005; JAAD 47:S196–200, 2002; Am J Med Genet 191:261–266, 2000; JAAD 37:102–104, 1998; BJD 104:89–96, 1981; Arch Neurol 22:144–155, 1970*

Farber's disease (lipogranulomatosis) – xanthoma-like papules of the face and hands

Francois syndrome (idiopathic carpotarsal osteolysis) – xanthoma-like nodules of the hands, elbows, and face, gingival hyperplasia, osteochondrodystrophy, bilateral corneal dystrophy *JAAD 55:1036–143, 2006*

Goltz's syndrome (focal dermal hypoplasia) – asymmetric linear and reticulated streaks of atrophy and telangiectasia; yellow-red nodules; raspberry-like papillomas of lips, perineum, acrally, at perineum, buccal mucosa; xerosis; scalp and pubic hair sparse and brittle; short stature; asymmetric face; syndactyly, polydactyly; ocular, dental, and skeletal abnormalities with osteopathia striata of long bones *JAAD 25:879–881, 1991*

Hereditary progressive mucinous histiocytosis – yellow dome-shaped papules of the face, gingiva, hard palate *BJD 141:1101–1105, 1999*

Lipoid proteinosis – yellow-white papules of the tongue, lips, pharynx *Int J Derm 39:203–204, 2000;* xanthoma-like nodules of the elbows *Acta Paediatr 85:1003–1005, 1996; JAAD 27:293–297, 1992*

Muir-Torre syndrome – autosomal dominant; sebaceous adenomas, sebaceous carcinomas, keratoacanthomas; mutation of mismatch repair genes (*MLH1, MSH2, MSH6*) *JAAD 74:558–566, 2016; JAAD 68:189–209, 2013; JAAD 61:563–578, 2009; Cutis 75:149–155, 2005;* Curr Prob Derm 14:41–70, 2002; BJD 136:913–917, 1997; JAAD 33:90–104, 1995; JAAD 10:803–817, 1984; AD 98:549–551, 1968; Br J Surg 54:191–195, 1967*

Multicentric reticulohistiocytosis – yellow papules and plaques *Oral Surg Oral Med Oral Pathol 65:721–725, 1988*; *Pathology 17:601–608, 1985*; *JAAD 11:713–723, 1984*; *AD 97:543–547, 1968*

Multiple mucosal neuroma syndrome (MEN IIB) – yellow to skin-colored papules and nodules of the oral mucosa, tongue, eyelids, conjunctivae *JAAD 36:296–300, 1997*; *Oral Surg 51:516–523, 1981*; *J Pediatr 86:77–83, 1975*; *Am J Med 31:163–166, 1961*

Neurofibromatosis type I – juvenile xanthogranulomas (and possible juvenile myelomonocytic leukemia) *JAAD 61:1–14, 2009*

Nevus sebaceus syndrome (Schimmelpenning-Feuerstein-Mims syndrome) *JAAD 61:563–571, 2009*; *Fortschr Geb Rontgenstr Nuklearmed 87:716–720, 1957*

Niemann-Pick disease – autosomal recessive; sphingomyelinase deficiency; waxy induration with transient xanthomas overlying enlarged cervical lymph nodes *Medicine 37:1–95, 1958*

Oculocutaneous albinism

Phakomatosis pigmentokeratotica – coexistence of an organoid nevus (nevus sebaceus) and a papular speckled lentiginous nevus *Ped Derm 25:76–80, 2008*

Proteus syndrome – sebaceous nevi with hyper- or hypopigmentation *Am J Med Genet 27:99–117, 1987*; port wine stains, subcutaneous hemangiomas and lymphangiomas, lymphangioma circumscriptum, hemihypertrophy of the face, limbs, trunk; macrodactyly, cerebriform hypertrophy of palmar and/or plantar surfaces, macrocephaly; verrucous epidermal nevi, vascular nevi, soft subcutaneous masses; lipodystrophy, café au lait macules, linear and whorled macular pigmentation *Am J Med Genet 27:87–97, 1987*; *Pediatrics 76:984–989, 1985*; *Eur J Pediatr 140:5–12, 1983*

Pseudoxanthoma elasticum *BJD 161:635–639, 2009*; *JAAD 42:324–328, 2000*; *Dermatology 199:3–7, 1999*; *AD 124:1559, 1988*; PXE and acrosclerosis *Proc Roy Soc Med 70:567–570, 1977*

Pseudoxanthoma elasticum-like lesions
   Beta thalassemia *JAAD 44:33–39, 2001*
   Calcinosis – idiopathic, tumoral calcinosis, calciphylaxis *JAAD 44:33–39, 2001*
   Cutis laxa *JAAD 44:33–39, 2001*
   Focal dermal elastolysis *JAAD 27:113–115, 1992*
   Hyperphosphatemia *JAAD 44:33–39, 2001*; *Am J Med 83:1157–1162, 1987*
   Periumbilical perforating PXE *AD 132:224–225, 227–228, 1996*; *JAAD 19:384–388, 1988*; *AD 121:1321, 1985*
   PXE-like lesions in eosinophilia myalgia syndrome (l-tryptophan toxicity) *JAAD 24:657–658, 1991*; *Dermatologica 183:57–61, 1991*
   PXE-like papillary dermal elastolysis (upper dermal elastolysis) – yellow papules of the neck with coarse furrows or wrinkles postmenopausal and elderly women *JAAD 67:128–135, 2012*; *JAAD 51:165–185, 2004*; *AD 136:791–796, 2000*; *JAAD 26:648–650, 1992*
   PXE-like papillary mid-dermal elastolysis – yellowish-white papules resembling PXE on the neck and supraclavicular areas of elderly people (photoaging) *JAAD 47:S189–192, 2002*; *JAAD 28:938–942, 1993*; *JAAD 26:648–650, 1992*
   Saltpeter (calcium ammonium nitrate salts) ingestion *JAAD 51:1–21, 2004*; *JAAD 44:33–39, 2001*
   Elastosis perforans serpiginosa with PXE

Refsum's disease – melanocytic nevi may be yellow due to lipids

Rothmund-Thomson syndrome – calcinosis cutis *JAAD 33:693–706, 1995*

SCALP syndrome – aplasia cutis congenita, pigmented nevus, nevus sebaceus; limbal dermoid, CNS malformations *JAAD 63:1–22, 2010*

Steatocystoma multiplex – personal observation

Xanthogranulomas – syndrome of juvenile xanthogranuloma, neurofibromatosis type I, and juvenile chronic myelogenous leukemia *JAAD 36:355–367, 1997*; *Cutis 11:499–501, 1973*; in the adult *Clin Exp Dermatol 18:462–463, 1993*

TOXINS

Arsenical keratoses of palms *Cancer 312–339, 1968*

Toxic oil syndrome – rapeseed oil denatured with aniline; early see morbilliform exanthem then yellow or brown papules *JAAD 18:313–324, 1988*

TRAUMA

Piezogenic pedal papules *AD 106:597–598, 1972*

Verruciform xanthoma – red-orange plaque; multilobulated, vegetative, cobblestoned; perigenital; seen in KID and CHILD syndromes and recessive dystrophic epidermolysis bullosa; usually at site of friction or frequent trauma *Ped Derm 37:176–179, 2020*

VASCULAR DISEASES

Angioendotheliomatosis *JAAD 13:903–908, 1985*

Angiosarcoma – yellow plaques of the eyelids *JAAD 34:308–310, 1996*

Chylous lymphedema – xanthomas of the toes and feet *BJD 146:134–137, 2002*

Lymphangioma circumscriptum

Lymphedema – xanthomas associated with lymphedema *JAMA 211:1372–1374, 1970*

Granulomatosis with polyangiitis – yellow eyelid papules (florid xanthelasmata) *Eyelid and Conjunctival Tumors, Shields JA and Shields CL, Lippincott Williams and Wilkins, 1999, p.167*; *JAAD 37:839–842, 1997*; *Br J Ophthalmol 79:453–456, 1995*

Superficial hemosiderotic lymphovascular malformation (hobnail hemangioma) (targetoid hemosiderotic hemangioma) – red-brown papule; blue-purple papule; yellow/green blue/papule *Ped Derm 31:281–285, 2014*

YELLOW PLAQUE

AUTOIMMUNE DISEASES AND DISORDERS OF IMMUNE DYSFUNCTION

Diffuse plane xanthomas in common variable immunodeficiency *Ped Derm 28:65–66, 2011*

Pansclerotic morphea – yellow ulcerated plaque covering the entire scalp *AD 144:125–126, 2008*

CONGENITAL DISORDERS

Ectopic meningothelial hamartoma – white linear plaque of the occipital-posterior scalp; may be orange or yellow *Ped Derm 34:99–100, 2017*; *Ped Derm 31:208–211, 2014*; *Ped Derm 28:677–680, 2011*; *Am J Surg Pathol 14:1–11, 1980*
   Differential diagnosis:
      Angiosarcoma
      Membranous aplasia cutis congenita
      Atretic meningocele

Epithelioid hemangioma
Giant cell fibroblastoma
Hypertrophic scar
Intravascular papillary endothelial hyperplasia
Spindle cell hemangioendothelioma

Median raphe cyst of the scrotum and perineum *JAAD 55:S114–115, 2006*

Nasal dermoid cyst – congenital ill-defined yellow plaque *Ped Derm 23:556–559, 2006*

DRUG-INDUCED

Corticosteroid atrophy

Dabrafenib – hand-foot skin reaction – thick yellow hyperkeratotic plaques of the soles with erythematous borders *JAMADerm 151:102–103, 2015*

Penicillamine *JAAD 30:103–107, 1994*

EXOGENOUS AGENTS

Exogenous calcium – EEG or EMG paste *AD 89:360–363, 1964*

Saltpeter – acquired pseudoxanthoma elasticum – farmers exposed to saltpeter (calcium-ammonium-nitrate salts); antecubital fossa; yellow macules and papules *JAAD 51:1–21, 2004; Acta DV 78:153–154, 1998; Acta DV 58:319–321, 1978*

Titanium dioxide-induced plane xanthoma-like lesions *AD 121:656–658, 1985*

INFECTIONS AND INFESTATIONS

Dermatophytoma *J Drugs Dermatol 14:524–526, 2015*

Leishmaniasis – diffuse cutaneous leishmaniasis; *L. aethiopica, L. mexicana* – large hypopigmented areas, xanthomatous appearance, verrucous plaques, leonine facies *JAAD 73:897–908, 2015*

Malakoplakia – pink-yellow plaque of the intra-abdominal fold *JAAD 62:896–897, 2010*

Mycobacterium tuberculosis – lupus vulgaris; starts as red-brown plaque, enlarges with serpiginous margin or as discoid plaques; apple-jelly nodules; tumorlike forms – deeply infiltrative; soft smooth nodules or red-yellow hypertrophic plaque; head, neck, around nose, extremities, trunk *Int J Dermatol 26:578–581, 1987; Acta Tuberc Scand 39(Suppl 49):1–137, 1960*

INFILTRATIVE DISEASES

Amyloidosis – xanthoma-like lesions *BJ Clin Pract 27:271–273, 1973;* plane xanthoma-like dermatosis in primary systemic amyloidosis (amyloid elastosis) *BJD 148:154–159, 2003;* primary cutaneous nodular amyloidosis – yellow plaque *Cutis 84:87–92, 2009*

Colloid milium *Clin Exp Dermatol 18:347–350, 1993; BJD 125:80–81, 1991;* juvenile colloid milium – yellow facial plaques *JAAD 49:1185–1188, 2003*

Erdheim-Chester disease (non-Langerhans cell histiocytosis) – CD68+ and factor XIIIa+; negative for CD1a and S100; xanthoma and xanthelasma-like lesions; flat wartlike papules of the face; bony lesions; retroperitoneal fibrosis *JAMADerm 155:483–484, 2019; Rheumat Clin NA 39:299–311, 2013; AD 143:952–953, 2007; Hautarzt 52:510–517, 2001; Medicine (Baltimore) 75:157–169, 1996*

Mastocytosis – xanthelasmoidea *BJD 144:355–358, 2001; AD 112:1270–1271, 1976; Med Chir Trans 66:329–347, 1883;* xanthelasmoid mastocytosis – flexural yellow papules and plaques *Ped Derm 21:520, 2004*

Verruciform xanthoma of scrotum – yellow cauliflower-like appearance *J Dermatol 16:397–401, 1989;* disseminated verruciform xanthoma – hyperkeratotic yellow plaques; subungual pink papules *Cutis 93:307–310, 2014*

Xanthogranuloma – juvenile xanthogranuloma *JAAD 36:355–367, 1997;* juvenile xanthogranuloma en plaque *Ped Derm 24:670–671, 2007*

INFLAMMATORY DISEASES

Sarcoidosis – yellow-red plaque of the face and scalp *BJD 175:1111–1112, 2016;* necrobiosis lipoidica-like lesions *J Dermatol 25:653–656, 1998*

METABOLIC

Calcinosis cutis – yellow reticulated plaques *JAAD 49:1131–1136, 2003;* metastatic calcification of the forehead, cheek, mandibular area, and neck at sites of old sun damage *JAAD 64:296–301, 2011;* dystrophic calcinosis cutis – yellow ulcerated plaque of the foot of 8-week-old infant *Ped Derm 33:555–556, 2016*

Necrobiosis lipoidica diabeticorum *JAMA 311:2328–2329, 2014; Int J Derm 33:605–617, 1994; JAAD 18:530–537, 1988;* yellow ulcerated plaques *JAAD 69:783–791, 2013*

Osteoma cutis – ulcerating yellow-white plaques *BJD 146:1075–1080, 2002*

Plane xanthomas – normolipemic plane xanthomas *AD 114:425–431, 1978; BJD 93:407–415, 1975;* normolipemic plane xanthomas in AIDS *BJD 142:571–573, 2000; Am J Surg Pathol 21:54–549, 1997;* associated with type III dysbetalipoproteinemia

Pretibial myxedema

Thalassemia – pseudoxanthoma elasticum-like cutaneous changes of beta thalassemia and sickle cell disease *Blood 99:30–35, 2002*

Xanthelasma

NEOPLASTIC

Angiosarcoma – yellow plaques of the eyelids *Aust NZ J Opththalmol 23:69–72, 1995*

Atypical lymphoid infiltrate (hyperplasia) – xanthelasma-like periorbital plaque *JAAD 37:839–842, 1997*

Basaloid follicular hamartoma – yellow plaque *AD 129:915–917, 1993*

Connective tissue nevus

Epidermal nevus

Kaposi's sarcoma – yellow-green penile plaques *Cutis 88:14–16, 2011*

Lymphoma – CD30+ T-cell lymphoma – yellow plaque after radiotherapy *JAAD 48:S28–30, 2003*

Microcystic adnexal tumor – skin-colored to yellow plaque *AD 143:791–796, 2007; Sem Cut Med Surg 21:159–165, 2002; Derm Surg 27:979–984, 2001*

Nevus sebaceus – yellow-orange plaque *Ped Derm 26:236–237, 2009; BJD 82:99–117, 1970*

Nevus tricholemmocysticus – multiple pilar cysts; filiform hyperkeratoses of the face and arm, comedo-like plugs, osteomalacia, bone lesions; verrucous papules, yellow plaques, cysts; Blaschko distribution *Ped Derm 28:286–289, 2011; JAAD 57(Suppl):S72–77, 2007*

Onychomatricoma – thick yellow discoloration of the nail plate; longitudinal ridging *Ped Derm 24:46–48, 2007*

Orbital fat hernia *AD 150:1115, 2014*

Seborrheic keratosis

PARANEOPLASTIC DISEASES

Necrobiotic xanthogranuloma with paraproteinemia *AD 145:279–284, 2009; Medicine(Baltimore) 65:376–388, 1986; BJD 113:339–343, 1985; JAAD 3:257–270, 1980;* yellow plaques of the eyelids *JAMADerm 156:696, 2020; J Eur Acad DV 31:221–235, 2017*

PRIMARY CUTANEOUS DISEASES

Linear focal elastosis – yellow linear bands on lower back of elderly men *JAAD 20:633–636, 1989; JAAD 36:301–303, 1997*

Normolipemic papuloeruptive cutaneous xanthomatosis (red-yellow plaques of the face) *Ped Derm 26:360–362, 2009; J Dermatol 18:235–239, 1991; AD 122:1294–1297, 1986*

Periumbilical pseudoxanthoma elasticum *JAMADerm 155:1418–1419, 2019*

Pityriasis rubra pilaris – hyperkeratotic yellow palms and soles

SYNDROMES

Adult onset asthma with periocular xanthogranuloma *Ophthalmol Plast Reconstr Surg 29:104–108, 2013; AD 147:1230–1231, 2011; Br J Ophthalmol 90:602–608, 2006*

Didymosis aplasticosebacea – nevus sebaceus with aplasia cutis congenita *JAAD 58:884–888, 2008; Ped Derm 24 514–516, 2007; Dermatology 202:246–248, 2001*

Encephalocranial lipomatosis – lipomas with overlying alopecia, scalp nodules, skin-colored nodules, facial and eyelid papules and nodules; lipomas and fibrolipomas; organoid nevi (nevus sebaceus) *JAAD 47:S196–200, 2002*

Neutrophilic dermatosis (pustular vasculitis) of the dorsal hands – variant of Sweet's syndrome – ulcerated yellow plaque *AD 138:361–365, 2002*

Phakomatosis pigmentokeratotica – nevus sebaceus and popular nevus spilus *JAAD 63:1–22, 2010*

Proteus syndrome – port wine stains, subcutaneous hemangiomas and lymphangiomas, lymphangioma circumscriptum, hemihypertrophy of the face, limbs, trunk; macrodactyly, cerebriform hypertrophy of palmar and/or plantar surfaces, macrocephaly; verrucous epidermal nevi, sebaceous nevi with hyper- or hypopigmentation *Am J Med Genet 27:99–117, 1987;* vascular nevi, soft subcutaneous masses; lipodystrophy, café au lait macules, linear and whorled macular pigmentation *Am J Med Genet 27:87–97, 1987; Pediatrics 76:984–989, 1985; Eur J Pediatr 140:5–12, 1983*

Pseudoxanthoma elasticum – linear and reticulated yellow papules and plaques *JAAD 42:324–328, 2000; Dermatology 199:3–7, 1999; AD 124:1559, 1988*

SCALP syndrome – nevus sebaceous syndrome, central nervous system malformations, aplasia cutis congenita, limbal dermoid, pigmented nevus (giant congenital melanocytic nevus) with

neurocutaneous melanosis *Ped Derm 29:365–367, 2012; JAAD 58:884–888, 2008*

Schimmelpenning syndrome – nevus sebaceus with involvement of the brain (hemimegalencephaly), eyes (lipodermoid of the conjunctiva or coloboma), and bones *JAAD 63:1–22, 2010; Fortschr Rontgenstr 87:716–720, 1957*

VASCULAR DISORDERS

Acquired progressive lymphangioma – brown, red, violaceous, yellow, or apple-jelly plaque; plantar red plaques *JAAD 49:S250–251, 2003*

Chylous reflux – from dilated chylous vesicles (lymphatics); yellow/cream-colored verrucous plaques

YELLOW SKIN (XANTHODERMA)

JAAD 57:1051–1058, 2007; Cutis 412:100–102, 1988

AUTOIMMUNE DISEASES AND DISEASES OF IMMUNE DYSFUNCTION

Morphea

Rheumatoid arthritis

Urticaria with jaundice *Cutis 70:41–44, 2002*

DRUG-INDUCED

Atabrine (mepacrine) – greenish-yellow pigmentation of the face, hands, feet; then diffuse *Am J Med Sci 192:645–650, 1936*

Dapsone gel and topical benzoyl peroxide – yellow-orange pigmentation *AD 145:1027–1029, 2009*

Dipyridamole intoxication *Lakartidningen 100:4194–4195, 2003*

Quinacrine *Cutis 71:441–442, 448, 2003*

Sunitinib (multikinase inhibitor) – yellow coloration of the face *JAAD 71:217–227, 2014; JAAD 58:545–570, 2008*

Tetracycline – yellow lunulae *JAAD 57:1051–1058, 2007*

EXOGENOUS AGENTS

Acriflavine

Aniline dye – yellow stain *AD 121:1022–1027, 1985*

Anthralin – yellow hair

Boots – yellow nails – personal observation

Cigarette smoke – yellow hair; yellow forelock; yellow-brown fingers

Dihydroxyacetone *JAAD 50:706–713, 2004; Skin Res Technol 6:199–204, 2000*

Dinitrophenols *Cutis 71:441–442, 448, 2003*

Fluorescein by intravenous injection *Cutis 63:103–106, 1999*

Kava dermopathy – xerosis with scaly yellow pigmentation *JAAD 53:S105–107, 2005; JAAD 31:89, 1994*

Lycopene – tomatoes, rose hips, bittersweet berries; deep orange *JAAD 43:1–16, 2000; NEJM 262:263–269, 1960*

Man-Tan palms (dihydroxyacetone)

Methylenedianiline – used in manufacture of plastics; yellow skin, hair, and nails *AD 121:1022–1027, 1985*

Non-selective antiangiogenic multikinase inhibitors – sorafenib, sunitinib, pazopanib – hyperkeratotic hand-foot skin reactions with knuckle papules, inflammatory reactions, alopecia, kinking of hair, depigmentation of hair; chloracne-like eruptions, erythema multiforme, toxic epidermal necrolysis, drug hypersensitivity, red scrotum with erosions, yellow skin, eruptive nevi, pyoderma gangrenosum-like lesions *JAAD 72:203–218, 2015*

Phenol (carbolic acid) *JAAD 57:1051–1058, 2007*

Picric acid – yellow skin and hair; blue lips and fingernails *Cutis 71:441–442, 448, 2003; Pigment Cell Res 15:119–126, 2002;*

Resorcin – stains hair yellow

Saffron *Cutis 71:441–442, 448, 2003*

Santonin

Tetryl acid

Trinitrotoluene

INFECTIONS AND INFESTATIONS

Erysipelas – personal observation

Hepatitis B – urticaria with jaundice (yellow hives)

Millipedes – yellow-brown stain on contact

INFILTRATIVE DISEASES

Colloid milium

Mastocytosis, including urticaria pigmentosum; diffuse cutaneous mastocytosis (xanthelasmoidea) (pseudoxanthomatous mastocytosis) *BJD 65:296–297, 1963*

METABOLIC DISEASES

Carotenemia – food faddists, hyperlipidemia, diabetes, chronic renal disease, hypothyroidism; alfalfa, apples, apricots, asparagus, beans, beet greens, broccoli, Brussel sprouts, butter, cabbage, cantaloupes, carrots, cheese, collard greens, cucumbers, eggs, figs, kale, kiwi, lettuce, mangoes, milk, mustard, oranges, palm oil, papayas, parsley, peaches, pineapples, plums, seaweed, spinach, squash, sweet potatoes, tomatoes, yams, yellow corn *JAAD 57:1051–1058, 2007; Ped Derm 23:571–573, 2006; JAAD 43:1–16, 2000; JAMA 73:1743–1745, 1919;* beta carotene – yellow skin

Diabetes mellitus – carotenemia *JAAD 57:1051–1058, 2007; Cutis 71:441–442, 448, 2003*

Gaucher's disease type I – yellow-brown pigmentation

Hepatic dysfunction *JAAD 57:1051–1058, 2007*

Hyperbilirubinemia (jaundice) *JAAD 43:1–16, 2000*

Hyperlipidemia

Hypopituitarism – yellow tinge to the skin with pallor; Sheehan's syndrome – yellow, dry skin

Hypothyroidism; myxedema – ivory yellow skin color *JAAD 57:1051–1058, 2007; JAAD 26:885–902, 1992;* carotenemia prominent on the palms and soles and nasolabial folds *JAAD 48:641–659, 2003;* congenital hypothyroidism

Kwashiorkor – yellow brittle hair *JAMADerm 150:910–911, 2014;*

Lycopenia

Necrobiosis lipoidica diabeticorum

Nephrotic syndrome *JAAD 57:1051–1058, 2007*

Retroperitoneal bile leakage – after cholecystectomy; well-demarcated jaundice of the hips, extending to 3 cm below the clavicles (to the fascia of Scarpa) *Ann Int Med 142:389–390, 2005*

Riboflavinemia *NEJM 294:177–183, 1976*

Uremia

Vitamin A intoxication – yellow-orange skin *JAAD 4:675–682, 1982*

Vitamin B12 deficiency

NEOPLASTIC DISEASES

Nevus lipomatosis superficialis

Onychopapilloma

PARANEOPLASTIC DISEASES

Normolipemic plane xanthomas

Myeloma with xanthoderma – IgG lambda monoclonal anti-flavin IgG antibody *JAAD 57:1051–1058, 2007; Mol Immunol 27:385–394, 1990; NEJM 294:177–183, 1976*

PHOTODERMATOSES

Nodular elastoidosis – yellow furrowed skin with large folds

PRIMARY CUTANEOUS DISEASES

Aplasia cutis congenita

Collodion baby (lamellar desquamation of the newborn)

Epidermolysis bullosa, junctional – letalis (atrophicans generalisata gravis, Herlitz type) – extensive blistering and erosions at birth; yellow teeth

Harlequin fetus (ichthyosis congenital fetalis) – severe non-bullous ichthyosiform erythroderma or mild erythrodermic ichthyosis *JAAD 212:335–339, 1989; Ped Derm 6:216–221, 1989; Int J Derm 21:347–348, 1982*

Linear focal elastosis *AD 127:1365–1368, 1991*

Pityriasis rubra pilaris – yellow tinge to the skin; hyperkeratotic yellow palms and soles

Unna-Thost palmoplantar keratoderma – diffuse non-epidermolytic palmoplantar keratoderma – autosomal dominant; mutations in keratin 16 *Hum Mol Genet 4:1875–1881, 1995;* mutation in keratin 1 *JID 103:764–769, 1994*

Xanthoerythroderma perstans *Cutis 60:41–42, 1997*

PSYCHOCUTANEOUS DISORDERS

Anorexia nervosa – carotenemia *JAAD 57:1051–1058, 2007; Am J Clin Dermatol 6:165–173, 2005; JAMA 205:533–534, 1968*

SYNDROMES

Alagille syndrome

Albinism – oculocutaneous albinism

Eosinophilia myalgia syndrome

Lipoid proteinosis – autosomal recessive; early lesions with crusted erosions, small vesicles, linear cribriform scars; over time diffuse thickening and yellowing of the skin; loss of function mutation in extracellular matrix protein 1 (*ECM1*) gene *Ped Derm 26:91–92, 2009; Ped Derm 23:1–6, 2006; BJD 151:413–423, 2004; JID 120:345–350, 2003; BJD 148:180–182, 2003; Hum Molec Genet 11:833–840, 2002; Acta Paediatr 85:1003–1005, 1996; JAAD 27:293–297, 1992; Virchows Arch Pathol Anat 273:286–319, 1929*

Niemann-Pick disease

Oculocutaneous albinism – personal observation

Pseudoxanthoma elasticum – cutaneous and oral yellow patches and plaques

Rombo syndrome – yellow tone to the skin

Sjogren-Larsson syndrome – ichthyosis, mental retardation, spastic diplegia, short stature, kyphoscoliosis, retinal changes, yellow pigmentation, intertrigo *JAAD 35:678–684, 1996*

TRAUMA

Post-surgical bile leakage – demarcation of yellow skin to flanks and groin bilaterally due to retroperitoneal bile leakage after cholecystectomy *Ann Int Med 142:389–340, 2005*

VASCULAR DISEASES

Ecchymoses, resolving

ZEBRA STRIPES

AUTOIMMUNE DISEASES AND DISEASES OF IMMUNE DYSFUNCTION

Allergic contact dermatitis – cactus, biking pants, poison ivy

Bullous pemphigoid – erythema gyratum repens-like pemphigoid *BJD 96:343, 1977*

Dermatomyositis – centripetal flagellate erythema *Ped Derm 35:676–677, 2018; J Drugs in Dermatol 10:902–904, 2011; J Rheumatol 26:692–695, 1999; Clin Exp Dermatol 21:440–441, 1996;* Wong type dermatomyositis

Still's disease in the adult – brown coalescent scaly papules; persistent psoriasiform papular lesions; persistent plaques and linear pigmentation; flagellate erythema *JAMA Derm 149:1425–1426, 2013; AD 143:1461–1462, 2007; JAAD 52:1003–1008, 2005; J Eur Acad DV 19:360–363, 2005; Dermatology 188:241–242, 1994*

CONGENITAL DISORDERS

Dysmature or small-for-dates neonates vernix caseosa – "crazed" with long transverse splits on the trunk which peels

Horizontal neonatal linear hyperpigmentation of creases of the abdomen and knees (transient horizontal bands) *Ped Derm 26:768, 2009*

DRUG-INDUCED

Bleomycin – flagellate erythema, dermatitis, and/or hyperpigmentation *J Drugs Dermatol 13:983–984, 2014; JAAD 71:203–214, 2014; AD 143:1461–1462, 2007; Clin Exp Dermatol 16:216–217, 1991; AD 123:393–398, 1987; JAAD 13:464,1985*

Corticosteroid (topical)-induced striae

Docetaxel chemotherapy – flagellate erythema *Clin Exp Dermatol 33:276–277, 1999;* transverse nail bands *AD 133:1466–1467, 1997*

FGFR1 inhibitor – calcinosis cutis presenting as corrugated pink plaque *JAMADerm 155:122–123, 2019*

5-Fluorouracil serpentine hyperpigmentation *JAAD 25:905–908, 1991*

Furosemide – papuloerythroderma of Ofuji induced by furosemide *JAAD 58:S54–55, 2008*

Imatinib-induced exfoliative dermatitis – deck chair sign

Iopamidol (non-ionic contrast media)-induced laser recall dermatitis *JAMADerm 150:212–213, 2014*

EXOGENOUS AGENTS

African tribal scarring – personal observation

Aquagenic wrinkling of the palms *Ped Derm 21:180, 2004*

Argon laser depigmentation after treatment of poikiloderma of Civatte *AD 121:714, 1985*

Collier's stripes

Coral dermatitis; Red sea coral granulomatous reaction *BJD 145:849–851, 2001*

Explosion tattoo *JAAD 50:479–480, 2004*

Grass – wrestling in the grass – personal observation

Gravel tattoo

Rubber – elastic biking suit depigmentation

Shiitake mushroom (*Lentinula edodes*) – flagellate dermatitis due to ingestion of shiitake mushrooms (toxicoderma) (*Lentinula edodes*) (lentinan) *Cutis 104:335–336, 2019; Dermatitis 29:43–44, 2018; Cutis 91:287–290, 2014; J Drugs in Dermatol 13:87, 2014; The Dermatologist pp.47–49, March 2013; JAAD 65:453–455, 2011; AD 146:1301–1306, 2010; Dermatitis 21:290–291, 2010; Clin Exp Dermatol 34:e910–913, 2009; AD 144:1241–1242, 2008; Dermatology 197:255–257, 2008; AD 143:1461–1462, 2007; BJD 154:800–801, 2006; BJD 148:178–179, 2003; J Kyoto City Hospital 23:44–47, 2003; Australas J Dermatol 44:155–157, 2003; Korean J Dermatol 36:477–481, 1998; BJD 131:700–702, 1994; Contact Dermatitis 27:65–70, 1992; JAAD 24:64–66, 1991; Jpn J Clin Dermatol 31:65–68, 1977*

Tefillin dermatitis *JAAD 32:812–813, 1995*

INFECTIONS AND INFESTATIONS

Caterpillar envenomation – puss caterpillar (*Megalopyge opercularis*) envenomation yielding parallel purpuric linear patches *Cutis 32:114–119, 1990*

Chikungunya fever, congenital – flagellate pigmentation of the trunk and extremities *Ped Derm 33:209–212, 2016*

Coelenterate envenomation – acute jellyfish stings (cnidarian envenomation); recurrent eruptions following coelenterate envenomation *The Clinical Management of Itching; Parthenon Publishing, 2000; p. xiii; JAAD 17:86–92, 1987*

Dengue fever – hyperpigmentation of the nose (chik sign); transient flushing, purpuric lesions, scleral injection, morbilliform exanthem with circular islands of sparing, aphthous ulcers, lichenoid papules, flagellated pigmentation, urticarial lesions, erythema multiforme-like *Ped Derm 36:737–739, 2019; Indian Dermatol Online J 8:336–342, 2017; Indian J DV Leprol 76:671–676, 2010*

Herpes simplex infection

Jellyfish envenomation – personal observation

Larva currens – *Strongyloides stercoralis*; urticarial zebra stripes *Cutis 81:409–412, 2008*

Lepromatous leprosy – deck chair sign *Lepr Rev 84:252–254, 2013*

Lyme disease – recurrent erythema migrans *AD 129:709–716, 1993*

Oral hairy leukoplakia – AIDS-associated lesion; Epstein-Barr virus *JAAD 22:79–86, 1990;* also seen in immunosuppressed *BJD 124:483–486, 1991;* and immunocompetent patients *Oral Surg Oral Med Oral Pathol 74:332–333, 1992*

Syphilis – secondary syphilis mimicking oral hairy leukoplakia *JAAD 49:749–751, 2003*

INFILTRATIVE DISEASES

Amyloidosis, macular *AD 143:255–260, 2007; AD 133:381–386, 1997; BJD 84:199–209, 1971;* lichen amyloidosis

Localized lichen myxedematosus (papular mucinosis) in morbid obesity *BJD 148:165–168, 2003*

Mastocytosis – diffuse cutaneous mastocytosis (xanthelasmoidea) (pseudoxanthomatous mastocytosis) – exaggeration of the skin folds in axillae and inguinal creases *BJD 65:296–297, 1963*

Scleromyxedema – zebra stripe striations of the forehead *JAAD 44:273–281, 2001; JAAD 33:37–43, 1995;* Shar-Pei sign (scleromyxedema) *JAAD 69:66–72, 2013;* lichen myxedematosus

Self-healing juvenile cutaneous mucinosis *Ann DV 107:51–57, 1980; JAAD 11:327–332, 1984*

METABOLIC DISEASES

Acrodermatitis enteropathica or acquired zinc deficiency – linear bullae in palmar creases

Calcinosis cutis – iatrogenic metastatic calcinosis cutis *Ped Derm 20:225–228, 2003*

Iron deficiency anemia – flagellate hyperpigmentation – personal observation

Multiple nutritional deficiencies – personal observation

Pregnancy – pigmentary demarcation lines of pregnancy *Cutis 38:263–266, 1986*

Pruritic urticarial papules and plaques of pregnancy *JAAD 39:933–939, 1998; JAAD 10:473–480, 1984; Clin Exp Dermatol 7:65–73, 1982; JAMA 241:1696–1699, 1979*

Scurvy in AIDS – petechial zebra stripes *JAAD 13:845–852, 1985*

NEOPLASTIC DISEASES

Epidermal nevus, including epidermal nevus syndrome

Large plaque parapsoriasis – deck chair sign

Lymphoma – cutaneous T-cell lymphoma *JAAD 60:359–375, 2009;* small- to medium-sized pleomorphic T-cell lymphoma *JAAD 46:531–535, 2002;* Angioimmunoblastic T-cell lymphoma – deck chair sign

Metastases – carcinoma telangiectoides – personal observation

Seborrheic keratoses – eruptive linear seborrheic keratoses *JAAD 18:1316–1321, 1988*

Smooth muscle hamartoma – personal observation

Syringomas – peri-axillary *AD 140:1161–1166, 2004*

Waldenstrom's macroglobulinemia *JAAD 52:45–47, 2005*

PARANEOPLASTIC DISEASES

Erythema craquele – paraneoplastic – personal observation

Erythema gyratum repens *JAAD 12:911–913, 1985*

Malignant acanthosis nigricans – deck chair sign *Int J Dermatol 52:377–378, 2013*

Tripe palms *J Clin Oncol 7:669–678, 1989; JAAD 16:217–219, 1987*

PHOTODERMATITIS

Berloque dermatitis

Cutis rhomboidalis nuchae

Erythema of Jacquet – inflammatory diaper dermatitis *Cutis 82:72–74, 2008*

Phytophotodermatitis – linear and bullous lesions; meadow dermatitis (Umbelliferae)

Poikiloderma of Civatte

Striated beaded lines (dermatoheliosis) *JAAD 32:1016–1024, 1995*

PRIMARY CUTANEOUS DISEASES

Acanthosis nigricans *JAAD 21:461–469, 1989*

Adolescent onset ichthyosiform erythroderma *BJD 144:1063–1066, 2001*

Adolescent striae – personal observation

Axillary granular parakeratosis – personal observation

Confluent and reticulated papillomatosis

Congenital cutis laxa *Atlantic Dermatological Society Meeting May 1994*

Congenital ichthyosiform dermatosis with linear keratotic flexural papules and sclerosing palmoplantar keratoderma *AD 125:103–106, 1989*

Digitate dermatosis *Cutis 49:457–458, 1991*

Epidermolysis bullosa pruriginosa – reticulated linear hypopigmented plaques; bullae; scars; zebra stripe appearance; dyschromatosis *Ped Derm 32:549–550, 2015*

Epidermolytic ichthyosis (hyperkeratosis) *Cutis 47:277–280, 1991*

Erythema craquele (asteatotic dermatitis) – personal observation

Harlequin ichthyosis *JAAD 21:999–1006, 1989*

Ichthyosis – X-linked ichthyosis

Ichthyosis bullosa of Siemens – personal observation

Ichthyosis hystrix, Curth-Macklin type – hyperkeratotic lesions of the elbows, knees in parallel grooves (zebra stripe pattern); palmoplantar keratoderma; *KRT1* mutation *AD 147:999–1001, 2011; AD 141:779–784, 2005; Am J Hum Genet 6:371–382, 1954*

Juxta-clavicular beaded lines

Keratosis lichenoides chronica (Nekam's disease) – reticulated, flat-topped keratotic papules, linear arrays, atrophy, comedo-like lesions, prominent telangiectasia, conjunctival injection, seborrheic dermatitis-like eruption *AD 145:867–69, 2009; AD 144:405–410, 2008; JAAD 49:511–513, 2003; Dermatology 201:261–264, 2000; JAAD 38:306–309, 1998; JAAD 37:263–264, 1997; AD 131:609–614, 1995; AD 105:739–743, 1972; Arch Dermatol Syph (Berlin) 31:1–32, 1895;* in children *JAAD 56:S1–5, 2007*

Lichen planus pigmentosus inversus – linear gray-brown macules of intertriginous areas in folds of the chest, abdomen, and groin *AD 147:1097–1102, 2011*

Lichen sclerosus – personal observation

Lichen striatus *Int J Dermatol 25:584–585, 1986*

Linear focal elastosis *BJD 145:188–190, 2001; JAAD 30:874–877, 1994; AD 127:1365–1368, 1991; JAAD 20:633–636, 1989*

Linear and whorled nevoid hypermelanosis

Mid-dermal elastolysis

Notalgia paresthetica

Papuloerythroderma of Ofuji – deck chair sign *JAMADerm 155:979–980, 2019; Dermatology 220:311–320, 2010; Clin Exp Dermatol 25:293–295, 2000; Clin Exp Dermatol 23:79–83, 1998; JAAD 26:499–501, 1992;* in CTCL *J Dermatol 25:185–189, 1998; JAAD 20:927–931, 1989*

  Deck chair sign

    Angioimmunoblastic T-cell lymphoma

    Imatinib-induced exfoliative dermatitis

    Lepromatous leprosy *Lepr Rev 84:252–254, 2013*

    Malignant acanthosis nigricans *Int J Dermatol 52:377–378, 2013*

    Waldenstrom's macroglobulinemia *JAAD 52:45–47, 2005*

    Large plaque parapsoriasis

Parakeratosis variegata (retiform parapsoriasis) – personal observation

Pigmentary lines of the newborn *JAAD 28:893, 1993*

Pigmented purpuric eruption – personal observation

Pityriasis rubra pilaris

Poikiloderma vasculare atrophicans

Pseudoxanthoma elasticum

Psoriasis with tripe palms *Clin Exp Dermatol 5:181–189, 1980*

Raised limb bands *BJD 149:436–437, 2003; BJD 147:359–363, 2002*

Reticulated pigmented anomaly of the flexures (Dowling-Degos disease)

Striae distensae (striae atrophicans)

Striate palmoplantar keratoderma *Cutis 61:18–20, 1998*

Striped hyperpigmentation of the torso *Textbook of Neonatal Dermatology, p.379, 2001*

Transient infantile patterned hyperpigmentation *Ped Derm 29:372–373, 2012*

Terra firme – personal observation

PSYCHOCUTANEOUS DISEASES

Factitial dermatitis – linear bullae due to deodorant spray *Ped Derm 37:559–560, 2020*

Neurotic excoriations

SYNDROMES

Alagille syndrome – obstructive cholestatic liver disease (paucity of interlobular hepatic ducts) – supernumerary digital flexion creases of the middle phalanges; tendinous, planar, and tuberous xanthomas; xanthomas of palmar creases, extensor fingers, nape of the neck; growth retardation, delayed puberty; autosomal dominant; pruritus and failure to thrive; wispy hair, triangular face, broad forehead, deep-set eyes, mild hypertelorism, straight nose, small pointed chin, ventricular hypertrophy, pulmonary artery stenosis *JAAD 58:S9–11, 2008; Ped Derm 22:11–14, 2005; Ped Derm 17:447–449, 2000*

Basaloid follicular hamartoma syndrome – multiple skin-colored, red, and hyperpigmented papules of the face, neck chest, back, proximal extremities, and eyelids; syndrome includes milia-like cysts, comedones, sparse scalp hair, palmar pits, and parallel bands of papules of the neck (zebra stripes) *JAAD 43:189–206, 2000*

Beare-Stevenson cutis gyrata syndrome – localized redundant skin of the scalp, forehead, face, neck, palms, and soles, acanthosis nigricans, craniofacial anomalies, anogenital anomalies, skin tags, and large umbilical stump; bifid uvula *Genetic Skin Disorders, Second Edition, 2010, pp.477; Ped Derm 20:358–360, 2003; Am J Med Genet 44:82–89, 1992*

Behcet's syndrome – superior vena cava syndrome – superior and inferior vena cava obstruction; dilated and tortuous veins of the chest wall (garland sign), facial edema, thickening of the neck with neck vein distension, upper body edema and edema of the arms and legs, proptosis; superficial and deep thrombophlebitis *BJD 159:555–560, 2008*

Blau or Jabs syndrome (familial juvenile systemic granulomatosis) – autosomal dominant; translucent skin-colored papules (non-caseating granulomas) in linear arrays or as zebra stripes of the trunk and extremities with uveitis, synovitis, arthritis; polyarteritis, multiple synovial cysts; red papular rash in early childhood; camptodactyly (flexion contractures of PIP joints) mutations in NOD2 (nucleotide-binding oligomerization domain 2) (caspase recruitment domain family, member 15; CARD 15) *AD 143:386–391, 2007; Clin Exp Dermatol 21:445–448, 1996*

Buschke-Ollendorff syndrome – connective tissue nevi and osteopoikilosis; single or multiple yellow, white, or skin-colored papules, nodules, plaques of the extremities; skin-colored to yellow papules *JAAD 49:1163–1166, 2003*

Conradi-Hunermann syndrome *AD 130:325–333, 1994; JAAD 21:248–256, 1989*

Cutis laxa type II – autosomal recessive; parallel strips of redundant skin of back *Ped Derm 21:167–170, 2004*

Fibroblastic rheumatism – linear parallel cords of the neck *Cutis 100:354, 356–357, 2017*

Franceschetti-Jadassohn syndrome – personal observation

Gardner-Diamond syndrome (painful bruising syndrome) (auto-erythrocyte sensitization) – arms and legs *JAAD 27:829–832, 1992; Ann Med Interne (Paris) 125:323–332, 1974; Blood 10:675–690, 1955;* autosensitization to DNA *Ann Int Med 60:886–891, 1964;* zebra stripe and annular purpura *BJD 164:672–673, 2011*

Geroderma osteodysplastica (Bamatter syndrome) (osteodysplastic geroderma) – autosomal recessive; parallel hyperlinear plantar skin; short stature, cutis laxa-like changes with drooping eyelids and jowls (characteristic facies with hypoplastic midface), osteoporosis and skeletal abnormalities; lax wrinkled, atrophic skin, joint hyperextensibility, growth retardation *Ped Derm 23:467–472, 2006; Ped Derm 16:113–117, 1999; Am J Med Genet 3:389–395, 1979; Hum Genet 40:311–324, 1978; Ann Paediatr 174:126–127, 1950*

Goltz's syndrome – streaky telangiectatic atrophic patches

Hypotrichosis, striate, reticulated pitted palmoplantar keratoderma, acro-osteolysis, psoriasiform plaques, lingua plicata, ventricular arrhythmias, periodontitis *BJD 147:575–581, 2002*

Keratosis-ichthyosis-deafness (KID) syndrome – ichthyotic elbows *JAAD 19:1124–1126, 1988*

Multiple endocrine neoplasia syndrome type 2A (MEN 2A) (multiple mucosal neuroma syndrome) – macular or lichen amyloidosis occur in more than one third of patients with MEN 2A (Sipple's syndrome) *Clin Endocrinol 59:156–161, 2003;* linear cutaneous neuromas with striated pigment in Sipple's syndrome (MEN 2A) *J Cut Path 14:43, 1972*

Reticulated erythematous mucinosis (REM) syndrome

Sjogren-Larsson syndrome – personal observation

Trichothiodystrophy – curly wood and tiger tails of hair under polarized light *AD 139:1189–1192, 2003;* also may be seen with loose anagen syndrome, argininosuccinic aciduria, pseudopili annulati; rarely seen in normal infants

TOXINS

Eosinophilia myalgia syndrome – l-tryptophan

TRAUMA

Child abuse – burn from heating grill; zebra stripe sparing of the skin folds *JAAD 57:371–392, 2007; Ped Derm 23:311–320, 2006; AD 138:318–320, 2002*

Coin rubbing

Coma pressure necrosis – personal observation

Excoriations

Facial scarification and tattooing on Santa Catalina Island (Solomon Islands) *Cutis 60:201–202, 1997*

Frictional melanosis *Acta DV 111:1063–1071, 1984*

Forceps marks of the face

Lightning strike – Lichtenberg figures; frond-like (ferning pattern) transient non-blanching pink-red erythema beginning 20 minutes to 3 1/2 hours after the strike and lasting up to 48 hours *Cutis 80:141–143, 2007; Arch Neurol 61:977, 2005; Injury 34:367–371, 2003; Burns Incl Thermal Inj 13:141–146, 1987; Proc IEE 123:1163–1180, 1976; AD 111:1466–1468, 1975; Memoirs Med Soc London 2:493–507, 1794*

Nail habit tic deformity

Scars

Splash burn

VASCULAR

Hemosiderin staining

Lymphangitis

Lymphedema tarda

Sunburst varicosities and telangiectasia (arborizing telangiectasia) – thighs and calves *J Derm Surg Oncol 15:184–190, 1989*

Superior vena cava syndrome *AD 128:953–956, 1992*

ZOSTERIFORM LESIONS/SEGMENTAL DISORDERS

AUTOIMMUNE DISEASES AND DISEASES OF IMMUNE DYSFUNCTION

Graft vs. host disease, chronic – lichenoid GVHD occurring on lesions of resolved herpes zoster *BJD 173:1050–1053, 2015; AD 147:1121–1122, 2011; AD 138:924–934, 2002;* lichenoid *JAAD 38:369–392, 1998; AD 134:602–612, 1998; J Cutan Pathol 23:576–581, 1996;* linear lichenoid graft vs. host reaction *AD 130:1206–1207, 1994; South Med J 87:758–761, 1994;* zosteriform GVHD *JAAD 57:690–699, 2007; Int J Derm 42:562–564, 2003*

Lupus erythematosus – discoid lupus erythematosus

Morphea, linear; including en coup de sabre – facial, truncal, and extremity hemiatrophy at site of healed herpes zoster *JAAD 46:90–94, 2002*

Pemphigus vulgaris, unilateral – in radiation portal *JAAD 56:S82–85, 2007*

Rheumatoid nodules *Int J Derm 27:645–646, 1988*

Scleroderma *AD 144:1215–1217, 1978*

CONGENITAL LESIONS

Congenital dermatofibrosarcoma protuberans – zosteriform red plaques *Cutis 90:285–288, 2012*

Congenital segmental dermal melanocytosis *AD 128:521–525, 1992*

Congenital varicella syndrome – unilateral segmental scars, limb hypoplasia, low birth weight, mild mental retardation, cataract,

chorioretinitis; *Ped Derm 13:341–344, 1996; Lancet i:1547–1550, 1994; Helv Paed Acta 40:399–404, 1985*

Harlequin color change – blanchable erythema on dependent side; aberrant dilatation of peripheral vasculature due to incomplete development of the hypothalamus *NEJM 382:456, 2020; NEJM 369:373, 2013*

DEGENERATIVE DISEASES

Notalgia paresthetica – hyperpigmentation of centrolateral back; association with MEN2A *JAAD 74:215–228, 2016; Nervenarzt 133:188–196, 1934*

Degenerative joint disease – dermatomal pruritus *J Dermatol 14:512–513, 1987*

DRUG-INDUCED

Erlotinib – radiation recall *JAAD 61:1086, 2009*

5-bromodeoxyuridine – desquamative or erosive dermatitis from intra-arterial 5-bromodeoxyuridine and radiation *JAAD 21:1235–1240, 1989*

Methotrexate photorecall in old herpes zoster

EXOGENOUS AGENTS

Drinking black tea – dermatomal pruritus *BJD 143:1355–1356, 2000*

INFECTIONS AND INFESTATIONS

Aspergillus flavus JAAD 38:488–490, 1998

Bacillary angiomatosis

Candidal sepsis

Cellulitis – following treatment for breast cancer *NEJM 357:488, 2007*

Condyloma acuminata – at site of healed herpes simplex *Int J Derm 39:705–706, 2000*

Echovirus 6 – zoster-like eruption *AJDC 133:283–284, 1979*

Erysipelas

Herpes simplex – personal observation; with Bell's palsy; zosteriform herpes simplex *Singapore Med J 49:e59–60, 2008; Pediatr Infec Dis J 20:226–228, 2001; Arch Ophthalmol 112:1515–1516, 1994; Cutis 52:99–100, 1993; JAAD 23:928–930, 1990; Am J Med 81:775–778, 1986*

Herpes zoster *NEJM 369;255–263, 2013;* V1 herpes zoster – confluent hypertrophic crusting of the scalp, forehead, and eyelids *NEJM 369:255–263, 2013; NEJM 362:1128, 2010;* Ramsay-Hunt syndrome (herpes zoster of geniculate ganglion) *Cutis 91:181–184, 2013; Clin Inf Dis 51:77–78,111–113, 2010;* post-zoster hyperpigmentation; nodules *JAAD 32:908–911, 1995;* chronic ulcerating acyclovir-resistant varicella zoster *Scand J Infect Dis 27:623–625, 1995;* post-herpetic neuralgia; post-herpetic pruritus *BJD 172:1672–1673, 2015; Acta DV 76:45–47, 1996;* multisegmental herpes zoster *Cutis 89:36–37, 2012;* herpes zoster in a 4-year-old boy with intrauterine varicella zoster exposure *Cutis 91:127–128,140, 2013;* satellite lesions in herpes zoster *BJD 172:1530–1534, 2015*

Eruptions occurring after herpes zoster *JAAD 24:429–433, 1991*

Abscesses following herpes zoster – personal observation

Allergic contact dermatitis – poison ivy (unilateral); at site of healed herpes zoster *Int J Derm 34:341–348, 1995*

Comedones (acneiform eruption) *AD 133:1316–1317, 1997*
Discoid lupus erythematosus *Cutis 101:370–372, 2018*
Eosinophilic dermatosis – at site of healed herpes zoster *BJD 137:465–466, 1997*
Furunculosis *Int J Derm 34:341–348, 1995*
Graft vs. host disease, chronic *AD 138:924–934, 2002*
Granuloma annulare *JAAD 14:764–770, 1986; Cutis 34:177–179, 1984;* perforating granuloma annulare in herpes zoster scars *JAAD 75:467–479, 2016; JAAD 29:859–862, 1993*
Granulomas in herpes zoster scars *Clin Exp Dermatol 44:197–199, 2019; Dermatologica 179:45–46, 1989;* granulomas at site of herpes zoster *BJD 156:1369–1371, 2007;* post-herpetic granuloma annulare-like reaction (Wolf isotopic response) *AD 145:589–594, 2009;* granulomatous zosteriform eruption *SKINmed 10:50–51, 2012*
Granulomatous vasculitis *JAAD 33:268–269, 1994; JAAD 24:429–433, 1991*
Hypohidrosis – post-herpes zoster *JAAD 76:160–162, 2017*
Kaposi's sarcoma *JAAD 18:448–451, 1988*
Keloids- personal observation
Leishmaniasis *AD 133:1316–1317, 1997*
Lichen planus *AD 38:615–618, 1938*
Lichen simplex chronicus with syringomyelia *BJD 138:904–927, 1998*
Lymphoma in herpes zoster scars *JAAD 41:884–886, 1999; Hautarzt 41:455–457, 1990; JAAD 22:130–131, 1990;* lymphoplasmacytic lymphoma *JAAD 32:854–857, 1995;* Methotrexate photorecall
Morphea *JAAD 46:90–94, 2002*
Nodular solar degeneration – at site of healed herpes zoster *BJD 134:606, 1996*
Pseudolymphoma (lymphocytoma cutis) *JAAD 38:877–905, 1998; AD 130:661–663, 1994*
Psoriasis *BJD 62:314–316, 1950;* personal observation
Sarcoidal granuloma *AD 119:788–789, 1983*
Staphylococcus aureus – cellulitis *NEJM 369;255–263, 2013*
Streptococcus – cellulitis *NEJM 369;255–263, 2013*
Tinea faciei (*Trichophyton rubrum*) *Cutis 60:51–52, 1997*
Trigeminal autonomic cephalalgia – S/P herpes zoster *JAAD 69:625–633, 2013*
Tuberculoid granuloma

Insect bites – personal observation

Leishmaniasis *Clinics in Derm 14:425–431, 1996*

Leprosy – dermatomal hypopigmented macular lesions *Experientia 39:723–725, 1983*

Lymphangitis

Microsporum canis Mycoses 54:463–465, 2011

Molluscum contagiosum

Phaeohyphomycosis (*Exserohilum rostratum*) mimicking hemorrhagic herpes zoster *SKINmed 13:275–281, 2015; JAAD 25:852–854, 1991*

Rhizopus arrhizus JAAD 32:357–361, 1995

Schistosomiasis – ectopic cutaneous granuloma – skin-colored papule, 2–3mm; group to form mammillated plaques; nodules develop with overlying dark pigmentation, scale, and ulceration; zosteriform *Dermatol Clin 7:291–300, 1989; BJD 114:597–602, 1986*

Staphylococcus aureus SKINmed 13:275–281, 2015

Syphilis *Br Med J 1:685, 1968; BJD 64:97–103, 1952*

Tinea corporis

Tinea faciei (*Trichophyton rubrum*) in healing herpes zoster lesions *Cutis 60:51–52, 1997; Int J Derm 24:539, 1985*

Tinea versicolor

Unilateral laterothoracic exanthem of childhood – scarlatiniform or dermatitic *AD 138:1371–1376, 2002; JAAD 34:979–984, 1996; JAAD 29:799–800, 1993; JAAD 27:693–696, 1992*

Zygomycosis *JAAD 32:357–361, 1995*

INFILTRATIVE DISEASES

Juvenile xanthogranuloma *Ped Derm 31:615–617, 2014*

Lymphocytoma cutis – personal observation

Telangiectasia macularis eruptiva perstans – unilateral of face *AD 142:641–646, 2006; JAAD 16:250–252, 1987;* unilateral *Actas Dermatosifiliogr 92:358–361, 2001; Int J Derm 32:123–124, 1993; Ann DV 17:109–111, 1990*

INFLAMMATORY DISEASES

Annular elastolytic granuloma at site of previous herpes zoster (Wolf's isotopic response) *SKINmed 13:267–269, 2015*

Encephalitis – hyperesthesias – personal observation

Granulomatous nodules – after mastectomy for breast carcinoma *BJD 146:891–894, 2002*

Hair repigmentation of the scalp at site of herpes zoster *AD 146:569–570, 2010*

Pseudolymphoma – at site of healed herpes zoster *AD 117:377, 1981*

Sarcoid *Arch Derm Research 119:788–789, 1983*

Tuberculoid granulomas *JAAD 16:1261–1263, 1987*

Zosteriform pruritus – due to transverse myelitis *BJD 149:204–205, 2003*

METABOLIC DISEASES

Mixed cryoglobulinemia – palpable purpura at site of previous herpes zoster *J Derm 28:256–258, 2001*

Xanthomas *AD 37:864–869, 1957; Arch Int Med 59:793–822, 1937*

NEOPLASTIC DISEASES

Acantholytic dyskeratotic epidermal nevus *JAAD 39:301–304, 1998*

Achromic nevi *BJD 144:187–188, 2001; JAAD 39:330–333, 1998;* achromic nevus and agminated Spitz nevi simultaneously appearing *BJD 144:187–188, 2001*

Acrochordons – personal observation

Adnexal carcinoma *JAAD 32:854–857, 1995*

Agminated angiofibromas *Dermatology 195:176–178, 1997*

Agminated Spitz nevi *Ped Derm 22:546–549, 2005*

Angiofibromas – unilateral facial angiofibromas (possible form fruste for tuberous sclerosis) *Cutis 80:284–288, 2007; J Eur Acad DV 18:641–642, 2004; JAAD 43:127–129, 2000; Ann DV 125:325–327, 1998; Dermatology 195:176–178, 1997; Ann Derm Syphilol 4:563–571, 1903*

Basal cell carcinoma *JAAD 32:854–857, 1995; BJD 64:97–103, 1952;* multiple familial basal cell carcinomas, segmental *J Dermatol 27:434–439, 2000*

Basaloid follicular hamartoma – unilateral *BJD 146:1068–1070, 2002; J Eur Acad Dermatol Venereol 13:210–213, 1999*

Becker's nevus – dermatomal pigmentation

Blue nevi, acquired *JAAD 36:268–269, 1997*

Cervicothoracic syrinx and thoracic spinal cord tumor – dermatomal lichen simplex chronicus *Neurosurgery 30(3):418–421, 1992*

Connective tissue nevus *Ped Derm 24:557–558, 2007; Am J Dermatopathol 29:303–305, 2007; Int J Derm 9:720–722, 2003; Cutis 36:77–78, 1985; Arch Dermatol Syphilol 50:183–190,1944*

Dermal melanocytosis – in distribution of C3 *JAAD 60:1072–1073, 2009*

Desmoplastic hypopigmented hairless nevus – indurated papule *Ped Derm 29:336–340, 2012*

Eccrine nevus – segmental hypopigmented patch *Ped Derm 25:613–615, 2008*

Eccrine porocarcinoma *JAAD 32:854–857, 1995*

Eccrine poromas *AD 112:841–844, 1976*

Eccrine spiradenomas *Dermatol Online J Aug 2017; AD 138:973–978, 2002; Ped Derm 17:384–386, 2000; JAAD 2:259–261, 1980*

Epidermal nevus – epidermal nevus with verruciform xanthoma within *BJD 159:493–496, 2008*

Epithelioid sarcoma *Actas Dermosif 83:203–208, 1992*

Hair follicle hamartoma – unilateral *BJD 143:1103–1105, 2000*

Hemifacial mixed appendageal tumor *Ped Derm 3:405–409, 1986*

Kaposi's sarcoma *JAAD 32:854–857, 1995; Clin Exp Dermatol 26:402–404, 2001*

Keloids – following herpes zoster – personal observation

Keratoacanthomas – multiple self-healing keratoacanthomas of Ferguson-Smith – one reported unilateral case *AD 74:525–532, 1956*

Leiomyomas – nevoidal pilar leiomyomas *AD 144:1217–1222, 2008; J Dermatol 28:759–761, 2001; Eur J Dermatol 10:590–592, 2000; JAAD 38:272–273, 1998; Cutis 27:484–486, 1981;* bilateral zosteriform leiomyomas *Cutis 82:33–36, 2008;* unilateral red painful papules *JAMA Derm 149:865–866, 2013; NEJM 369:1344–1355, 2013*

Lentiginosis, segmental (unilateral lentiginosis, partial unilateral lentiginosis) *JAAD 44:387–390, 2001; JAAD 43:361–363, 2000; JAAD 29:693–695, 1993; Am J Dermatopathol 14:323–327, 1992;* with ocular involvement *JAAD 44:387–390, 2001*

Lentiginous nevus *BJD 98:693–698, 1978;* large segmental speckled lentiginous nevi *JAAD 64:1190–1193, 2011*

Leukemia cutis *BJD 143:773–779, 2000; JAAD 37:1022, 1997; JAAD 32:854–857, 1995; AD Syphilol 37:238–246, 1938;* chronic lymphocytic leukemia – cutaneous infiltrates in resolved herpes zoster *Cancer 76:26–31, 1995*

Linear rhabdomyomatous mesenchymal hamartoma – unilateral facial depressions, atrophy, and hyperpigmentation of chin *Ped Derm 36:716–717, 2019*

Lymphomatoid papulosis *BJD 141:1125–1128, 1999;* persistent agminated lymphomatoid papulosis *Ped Derm 26:762–764, 2009*

Lymphoma – cutaneous T-cell lymphoma *Eur J Dermatol 15:489–491, 2005; Dermatology 205:176–179, 2002; Ped Derm 21:558–560, 2004; JAAD 32:127–128, 1995; Int J Derm 30:432–434, 1991;* primary cutaneous B-cell lymphoma *JAAD 41:884–886, 1999;* B-cell lymphoma *J Dermatol 29:748–753, 2002; BJD 142:180–182, 2000;* erythrodermic cutaneous T-cell lymphoma with sparing of site of healed herpes zoster *JAAD 123–126, 2004;* Hodgkin's disease *BJD 151:722–724, 2004*

Melanocytic nevi – congenital melanocytic nevus *BJD 133:315–316, 1995;* congenital agminated segmental nevi *BJD 133:315–316,*

1995; melanocytic nevi, nevi, and lentigines *AD 124:926–929, 1988;* atypical nevi *J Dermatol 18:649–653, 1991;* atypical nevi (quadrant distribution of atypical mole syndrome) *AD 124:926–930, 1988*

Melanoma *Melanoma Res 13:635–639, 2003; BMJ 10:1025–1026, 2003; Cutis 62:143–146, 1998; JAAD 32:854–857, 1995*

Metastases – zosteriform metastases *Dermatol Surg 35:1355–1363, 2009; Tech Coloproctol 7:105–107, 2003; Clin Exp Dermatol 27:199–201, 2002; Acta DV 80:391–392, 2000; BJD 142:182–183, 2000; J Derm Surg Oncol 14:774–778, 1988; Int J Dermatol 18:142–145, 1979;* breast *JAAD 60:891–893, 2009; JAAD 43:733–751, 2000;* male breast carcinoma *JAAD 55:1101–1102, 2006; JEADV 19:593–596, 2005; BJD 135:502–503, 1996;* colon *BJD 142:182–183, 2000; Acta DV 79:90–91, 1999;* melanoma *Cutis 62:143–146, 1998;* squamous cell carcinoma *BJD 142:573–574, 2000;* lung, ovary, transitional cell carcinoma of the bladder, transitional cell carcinoma of the renal pelvis *JAAD 37:1008–1009, 1997; JAAD 31:284–286, 1994; BJD 45:418–423, 1933;* zosteriform erythema from metastatic transitional cell carcinoma *AD 122:1357–1358, 1986;* angiosarcoma *Int J Derm 23:404–407, 1984;* prostatic carcinoma metastases *AD 76:402–406, 1957; JAAD 32:854–857, 1995;* tonsillar adenocarcinoma *JAAD 32:854–857, 1995;* carcinoma telangiectoides; bronchogenic carcinoma *Acta DV 80:391–392, 2000;* rectal carcinoma *Tech Coloproctol 7:105–107, 2003;* cutaneous squamous cell carcinoma *Am J Dermatopathol 23:216–220, 2001; Clin Exp Dermatol 27:199, 2001; BJD 142:573–574, 2000; Clin Exp Dermatol 23:116–118, 1998; JAAD 37:1008–1009, 1997;* T-cell lymphoma *J Dermatol 34:68–73, 2007;* zosteriform lung cancer *Respirol Case Rep 18:e00515, 2019;* zosteriform cutaneous metastases – breast, colon *Clin Exp Dermatol 43:734–736, 2018*

Mucinous nevus (nevus mucinosis (mucinous connective tissue nevus)) *Ped Derm 25:288–289, 2008; BJD 148:1064–1066, 2003; JAAD 37:312–313, 1997; BJD 131:368–370, 1994;* congenital mucinous nevus *Ped Derm 20:229–231, 2003*

Neurilemmomas, agminated *JAAD 17:891–894, 1987*

Nevus comedonicus *JAAD 21:1085–1088, 1989*

Nevus depigmentosus *JAAD 55:423–428, 2006*

Nevus lipomatosus superficialis *AD 143:1583–1588, 2007; Cutis 72:237–238, 2003; AD 128:1395–1400, 1992*

Nevus of Ito (nevus fuscoceruleus acromiodeltoideus) *Tohoku J Exp Med 60:10–20, 1954*

Nevus of Ota (nevus fuscoceruleus ophthalmomaxillaris) *JAAD 47:S257–259, 2002; Clin Dermatol 7:11–27, 1989; AD 85:195–208, 1962; BJD 67:317–319, 1955*

Nevus spilus (speckled lentiginous nevus (zosteriform lentiginous nevus) *JAAD 27:106–108, 1992; AD 107:902–905, 1973;* dermatomal pigmentation *Ped Derm 21:516–517, 2004; Curr Prob in Derm VII:143–198, 1995; AD 107:902–905, 1973*

Pilomatrixoma *Wiad Lek 28:673–675, 1975(Polish)*

Plasmacytoma *Int J Derm 29:562–565, 1990*

Porokeratosis of Mibelli *JAAD 58:S49–50, 2008; Dermatologica 155:340–349, 1977*

Porokeratotic eccrine ostial and dermal duct nevus *BJD 138:684–688, 1998*

Segmentally arranged seborrheic keratosis with impending atypia (SASKIA) *BJD 172:1642–1645, 2015*

Smooth muscle hamartoma – personal observation

Spiradenomas *JAAD 2:59–61, 1980*

Spitz nevi, agminated *BJD 144:187–188, 2001*

Squamous cell carcinoma *Am J Dermatopathol 23:216–220, 2001; JAAD 32:854–7, 1995; J Derm Surg Oncol 10:718–720, 1984*

Syringocystadenoma papilliferum *Int J Derm 24:520–521, 1985*

Syringomas – unilateral *AD 117:308, 1981*

Trichoepithelioma *JAAD 13:927–930, 1986; AD 87:102–114, 1963*

PARANEOPLASTIC DISORDERS

Eruptive segmental neurofibromas – esophageal, lung, colon, gastric cancer *JAAD 60:880–881, 2009; Clin Exp Dermatol 32:43–44, 2007; Dermatology 209:342, 2004; J Dermatol 29:350–353, 2002*

Unilateral hyperhidrosis and hypothermia – manifestation of contralateral intrathoracic tumor *BJD 174:1147–1148, 2016;* apical pulmonary adenocarcinoma and contralateral hyperhidrosis *AD 117:659–661, 1981*

PHOTODERMATOSES

Favre-Racouchot syndrome – unilateral elastosis with cysts and comedones *Ann DV 121:721–723, 1994*

PRIMARY CUTANEOUS DISEASES

Acanthosis nigricans, nevoid – unilateral and localized *Int J Dermatol 30:452–453, 1991*

Acne in irradiated area *AD 125:1005, 1989*

Atrophoderma of Moulin (linear atrophoderma of Moulin) – unilateral acquired atrophic pigmented band-like lesions following Blaschko's lines *JAMADerm 156:583–584, 2020; Ann DV 119:729–736, 1992*

Atrophoderma of Pasini and Pierini *JAAD 30:441–446, 1994; Int J Derm 29:281–283, 1990*

Atrophoderma vermiculatum *JAAD 43:310–312, 2000;* folliculitis ulerythematosa reticulata (atrophoderma vermiculata) – unilateral *Ped Derm 15:285–286, 1998*

Darier's disease (keratosis follicularis) *BJD 173:587–589, 2015; Mt Sinai J Med 68:339–341, 2001;* segmental; mosaicism for *ATP2A2* mutations *JID 115:1144–1147, 2000*

Familial progressive hyperpigmentation

Granuloma annulare *JAAD 57:690–699, 2007; Ann DV 133:623–624, 2006; Int J Dermatol 31:672, 1992; JAAD 14:746–770, 1986;* in herpes zoster scars *Cutis 87:240–244, 2011*

Hailey-Hailey disease *Dermatology 210:182–183, 2005; JAAD 49:712–714, 2003; Eur J Dermatol 10:265–268, 2000*

Hyperkeratosis lenticularis perstans (Flegel's disease) *JAAD 39:655–657, 1998*

Hypermelanocytic guttate and macular segmental hypomelanosis *BJD 151:701–705, 2004*

Hyperhidrosis – idiopathic unilateral circumscribed hyperhidrosis *AD 137:1241–1246, 2001; Ped Derm 17:25–28, 2000;* following herpes zoster *JAAD 41:119–121, 1999*

Keratosis pilaris – unilateral generalized keratosis pilaris *Cutis 94:203–205, 2014*

Lichen aureus *Cutis 69:145–148, 2002; Hautarzt 49:135–138, 1998; Int J Derm 30:654–657, 1991*

Lichen planus *BJD 158:1145–1146, 2008; JAAD 57:690–699, 2007; J Dermatol 29:339–342, 2002; AD 142:836–837, 2000; Acta DV 77:491–492, 1997; Dermatology 192:375–377, 1996; AD 126:665–670, 1990; Cutis 4:1076–1078, 1968;* lichen planus pigmentosus *J Dermatol 24:193–197, 1997*

Lichen simplex chronicus with syringomyelia *Neurosurgery 30:418–421, 1992*

Lichen striatus *Int J Dermatol 25:584–585, 1986*

Lichen sclerosus – bilateral zosteriform *SKINmed 12:123–125, 2014*

Mosaic pigmentation – personal observation

Perioral dermatitis

Pigmentary mosaicism (Happle mosaic zosteriform pigmentation) – personal observation

Pityriasis lichenoides chronica – segmental distribution *JAAD 55:557–572, 2006*

Pityriasis rosea – unilateral *Int J Dermatol 22:312–313, 1983; JAMA 82:178–183, 1924; BJD 26:329, 1914*

Progressive cribriform and zosteriform hyperpigmentation *SKINmed 13:271–273, 2015; AD 114:98–99, 1978*

Progressive zosteriform macular pigmented lesions

Prurigo pigmentosa – reticulated crusted papules *Ped Derm 31:523–525, 2014*

Psoriasis – unilateral *Cutis 65:167–170, 2000; BJD 120:837–841, 1989; BJD 62:314–316, 195;* following herpes zoster – personal observation

Reactive perforating collagenosis, acquired *JAAD 36:778–779, 1997*

Seborrheic dermatitis – unilateral associated with trigeminal nerve disease *JAAD 55:356–357, 2006; AD 73110–115, 1956*

Segmental hyperpigmentation disorder *BJD 162:1337–1341, 2010; Acta DV 63:167–169, 1983*

Transient acantholytic dermatosis (Grover's disease) *JAAD 35:653–666, 1996; JAAD 29:797–798, 1993*

Unilateral hyperhidrosis of the trunk *Acta Med Scand 168:17–20, 1960*

Vitiligo – segmental vitiligo *BJD 168:56–64, 2013; BJD 166:240–246, 2012; BJD 165:44–49, 2011; BJD 164:1004–1009, 2011; Ped Derm 27:624–625, 2010; NEJM 360:160–169, 2009; JAAD 57:690–699, 2007; J Cutan Med Surg 10:104–107, 2006; BJD 118:223–228, 1988; JAAD 16:948–954, 1987;* Blaschko-esque vitiligo *JAAD 65:965–971, 2011*

Waxy keratoses of childhood – segmental *Ped Derm 18:415–416, 2001*

Zosteriform reticulate hyperpigmentation *BJD 121:280, 1989;* in children *BJD 117:503–17, 1987; AD 114:98–99, 1978;* unilateral dermatomal pigmentary dermatosis *Semin Cut Med Surg 16:72–80, 1997; JAAD 27:763–764, 1992*

SYNDROMES

Alezzandrini's syndrome – unilateral degenerative retinitis, ipsilateral facial vitiligo, poliosis, with or without deafness *Ophthalmologica 147:409–419, 1964*

Ataxia telangiectasia – telangiectasias of bulbar conjunctivae, tip of the nose, ears, antecubital and popliteal fossae, dorsal hands and feet; atrophy with mottled hypo- and hyperpigmentation, dermatomal CALMs, photosensitivity, canities, acanthosis nigricans, dermatitis; cutaneous granulomas present as papules or nodules, red plaques with atrophy or ulceration *JAAD 10:431–438, 1984*

Auriculotemporal syndrome (Frey syndrome) – zosteriform flush and sweating of the cheek *AD 133:1143–1145, 1997*

Basaloid follicular hamartoma syndrome, segmental – osseous, dental, and cerebral anomalies *Dermatology 218:221–225, 2009*

Beckwith-Wiedemann syndrome (Exomphalos-Macroglossia-Gigantism) (EMG) syndrome – autosomal dominant; zosteriform rash at birth, exomphalos, macroglossia, visceromegaly, facial nevus flammeus and gigantism; earlobe grooves, circular depressions of helices *JAAD 37:523–549, 1997; Am J Dis Child 122:515–519, 1971*

Buschke-Ollendorff syndrome – segmental connective tissue nevi and osteopoikilosis; single or multiple yellow, white, or skin-colored papules, nodules, plaques of the extremities; skin-colored to yellow papules *JAAD 49:1163–1166, 2003*

CHILD syndrome – unilateral *Am J Med Genet 90:328–335, 2000*

Coats' disease – cutaneous telangiectasia or unilateral macular telangiectatic nevus with retinal telangiectasia *AD 108:413–415, 1973*

Cobb's syndrome (cutaneomeningospinal angiomatosis) – segmental port wine stain and vascular malformation of the spinal cord *AD 113:1587–1590, 1977; NEJM 281:1440–1444, 1969; Ann Surg 62:641–649, 1915*; port wine stain may be keratotic *Dermatologica 163:417–425, 1981;* segmental angiokeratoma-like lesions *Cutis 71:283–287, 2003*

Cutaneous segmental heterotopic meningeal tissue with multifocal neural and mesenchymal hamartomas – skin-colored pedunculated papules of the forehead, eyelids, scalp, ala nasi; hypertrichotic heterotopic meningeal nodule *BJD 156:1047–1050, 2007*

Encephalocraniocutaneous lipomatosis – unilateral lesions *Ped Derm 10:164–168, 1993*

Fegeler syndrome – acquired port wine stain following trauma *Ped Derm 21:131–133, 2004*

Focal dermal hypoplasia, unilateral – PORCN gene mutation *AD 148:85–88, 2012; AD 128:1108–1111, 1992*

Happle-Tinschert syndrome – segmental basaloid follicular hamartomas; ipsilateral hypertrichosis; hypo- and hyperpigmentation; linear atrophoderma; osseous, dental, and/or cerebral defects *BJD 169:1342–1345, 2013; Ped Derm 28:555–560, 2011; JAAD 65:e17–19, 2011; Dermatology 218:221–225, 2009; Acta DV 88:382–387, 2008*

Harlequin syndrome – damage to sympathetic innervation of one side of the face; decreased sweating and flushing on one side of the face; compensatory increased sweating and flushing on normal side of the face *BJD 169:954–956, 2013*

Incontinentia pigmenti in boys *Ped Derm 23:523–527, 2006*

McCune-Albright syndrome

Melorheostosis – cutaneous lesions resemble linear morphea overlying bony lesions (endosteal bony densities resembling candle wax) *BJD 86:297–301, 1972*

Neurofibromatosis, segmental *NEJM 372:963, 2015; Cutis 87:45–50, 2011; Hum Genet 114:284–290, 2004; Am J Med Genet 30:121A:132–135, 2003; Dermatol 204:296–297, 2002; Neurology 56:1433–1443, 2001; JAAD 37:864–869, 1997; Ped Derm 10:43–45, 1993; JAAD 23:866–869, 1990; AD 113:837–838, 1977;* regional eruptive neurofibromas *J Dermatol 24:198–201, 1997;* blue-red pseudoatrophic plaques *Cutis 94:149–152, 2014*

Nevoid basal cell carcinoma syndrome; may be with comedones *JAAD 20:973–978, 1989; AD 100:187–190, 1969; BJD 74:20–23, 1962*

Nevoid basal cell carcinoma syndrome with type 2 mosaicism – Blaschko-esque atrophy, Blaschko-esque pits of the palms; linear papules of the foot; white papules and plaques; segmental hyper- and hypopigmented patches *BJD 169:1342–1345, 2013*

Partial unilateral lentiginosis – multiple lentigines and café au lait macules in segmental distribution

Phakomatosis pigmentokeratotica – coexistence of an organoid nevus (epidermal nevus) and a contralateral segmental lentiginous or papular speckled lentiginous nevus *Dermatology 194:77–79, 1997*

Romberg syndrome (facial hemiatrophy) – unilateral *Arch Neurol 39:44–46, 1982*

Ross' syndrome – unilateral tonic pupils, generalized areflexia, progressive segmental anhidrosis with compensatory band of hyperhidrosis *AD 142:264, 2006*

Speckled lentiginous nevus syndrome – speckled lentiginous nevus with ipsilateral sensory and motor neuropathy, hyperhidrosis, spinal muscle atrophy with fasciculations, dysesthesias, muscle weakness *Ped Derm 26:298–301, 2009; Eur J Dermatol 12:133–135, 2002;* ipsilateral shortening of the limb and vertebral malformations *Acta DV(Stockh)74:327–334, 1994*

Stiff skin syndrome – unilateral (segmental); mutation in fibrillin-1 *JAAD 75:163–168, 2016*

Sweet's syndrome – zosteriform red plaques in acute myelogenous leukemia *AD 142:235–240, 2006*

Tuberous sclerosis – unilateral agminated angiofibromas *J Coll Phys Surg Pak 14:628–630, 2004; JAAD 49:S164–166, 2003; Eur J Dermatol 12:262, 2002; Dermatology 195:176–178, 1997; BJD 134:727–730, 1996; Arch Dermatol Syphilol 14:483, 1926; Proc R Soc Med 18:55, 1925*

Wallenberg's syndrome (trigeminal trophic syndrome) *AD 144:984–986, 2008*

Bullous Wells' syndrome – segmental facial vesicles and bullae *JAMADerm 155:617–618, 2019*

Wiskott-Aldrich syndrome

Wyburn-Mason (Bonnet-Dechaume-Blanc) syndrome – unilateral salmon patch with punctate telangiectasias or port wine stain; unilateral retinal arteriovenous malformation, ipsilateral aneurysmal arteriovenous malformation of the brain *Am J Ophthalmol 75:224–291, 1973*

TRAUMA

Coma bullae – personal observation

Electrical skin injury *Amer J Forensic Med and Pathol 12:222–226, 1991*

Ionizing radiation-induced pemphigus *AD 126:1319–1323, 1990*

VASCULAR

Acral pseudolymphomatous angiokeratoma in children (APACHE) – unilateral multiple persistent papules on the hands and feet *JAAD 38:143–175, 1998*

Angiofibromas – unilateral facial angiofibromas *Ped Derm 23:303–305, 2006*

Angiokeratoma circumscriptum *AD 117:138–139, 1981*

Angiosarcoma *JAAD 32:854–857, 1995; Int J Derm 23:404–407, 1984*

Arteriovenous malformation

Cherry angiomas, unilateral- personal observation

Cutis marmorata telangiectatica congenita *JAAD 56:541–564, 2007; Ped Derm 8:329–331, 1991*

Glomangioma – segmental glomangiomas of the leg; hemi-facial *JAAD 45:239–245, 2001;* glomus tumors with linear trichilemmal cysts *Dermatology 200:75–77, 2000*

Glomerulovenous malformation *Ped Derm 25:381–382, 2008; BJD 154:450–452, 2006; AD 140:971–976, 2004*

Hemolymphangioma

Infantile hemangioma *BJD 169:1252–1256, 2013; Ped Derm 30:151–154, 2013; Ped Derm 28:658—662, 2011; JAAD 65:320–327, 2011; Ped Derm 28:108–114, 2011;* diffuse hemangioma *AD 139:869–875, 2003;* infantile hemangiomas with unusually prolonged growth phase – often are segmental *AD 144:1632–1637, 2008;* biker glove pattern of segmental infantile hemangioma – high risk of ulceration *JAAD 71:542–547, 2014;* segmental hemangiomas of infancy with visceral hemangiomatosis *AD 140:591–596, 2004;* segmental proliferating hemangioma

Infantile hemangioma of the beard region associated with subglottic hemangioma *Seminars Cut Med Surg 35:108–116, 2016*

Infantile hemangiomas of the extremities – zosteriform or segmental *JAAD 75:556–563, 2016*

Kaposiform hemangioendothelioma – gray-violaceous plaque with red papules *Ped Derm 24:570–571, 2007*

Klippel-Trenaunay-Weber syndrome

LUMBAR syndrome (PELVIS syndrome) – segmental cutaneous infantile hemangiomas of the lower body; myelopathy, cutaneous defects, urogenital abnormalities, bony deformities, anorectal abnormalities, arterial anomalies, renal anomalies *JAAD 68:885–896, 2013; Ped Derm 27:588, 2010; J Pediatr 157:795–801, 2010; AD 42:884–888, 2006; Dermatology 214:40–45, 2007*

Lymphangioma circumscriptum (benign lymphangiectasia) (microcystic lymphatic malformation) *Cutis 76:310–311, 2005; AD 124:263–268, 1988; AD 114:394–396, 1978*

Non-involuting congenital hemangioma – segmental blue plaque with central telangiectasia and peripheral rim of pallor *Ped Derm 36:835–853, 2019*

PHACES syndrome – posterior fossa malformations, cervicofacial hemangiomas, often segmental, arterial anomalies, cardiac defects, eye anomalies, and sternal clefting or supraumbilical raphe *Ped Derm 23:476–480, 2006;* segmental port wine stain in PHACES syndrome; segmental telangiectasias *BJD 173:242–246, 2015; Ped Derm 28:180–184, 2011; Ped Derm 26:381–398, 2009; Pediatrics 124:1447–1456, 2009; Neuroradiology 31:544–546, 1990;* ventral linear midline blanching with segmental infantile hemangioma *Ped Derm 32:180–187, 2015;* segmental hemangiomas of the arm and/or trunk without facial angiomas *Ped Derm 28:235–241, 2011*

Pigmented purpuric eruptions (lichen aureus-like) *AD 143:1599–1600, 2007; AD 141:1311–1316, 2005; Hautarzt 49:135–18, 1998; Int J Dermatol 30:654–655, 1991; Dermatologica 180:93–95, 1990; Hautarzt 40:373–375, 1989;* unilateral Schamberg's disease *J Dtsch Dermatol Ges 2:931–934, 2004; Ped Derm 19:517–519, 2002; BJD 144:190–191, 2001*

Port wine stain (nevus flammeus) *Eyelid and Conjunctival Tumors, Shields JA and Shields CL, Lippincott Williams and Wilkins, 1999, p.114*

Sturge-Weber syndrome (encephalofacial angiomatosis) – facial port wine stain with homolateral leptomeningeal angiomatosis *Ped Derm 29:32–37, 2012; Oral Surg Oral Med Oral Pathol 22:490–497, 1966*

Telangiectasia (unilateral dermatomal superficial telangiectasia) *J Dermatol 17:638–642, 1990*

Tufted angioma – personal observation

Unilateral nevoid telangiectasia *AD 146:1167–1172, 2010; Dermatology 209:215–217, 2004; JAAD 37:523–549, 1997; JAAD 8:468–477, 1983; Monatsschr Prakt Dermat 28:451, 1899*

Vascular malformations, dermatomal – isolated *BJD 143:888–891, 2000*

Vascular malformations – syndromes

    Cobb syndrome – nevus flammeus with underlying spinal cord defect *JAAD 37:523–549, 1997; Dermatologica 163:417–425, 1981*
    Klippel-Trenaunay-Weber syndrome *Cutis 60:127–132, 1997*

Venous malformation (cavernous hemangiomatosis) *Dermatologica 161:347–354, 1980;* zosteriform venous malformations *AD 144:861–867, 2008; AD 139:1409–1416, 2003; Dermatologica 161:347–354, 1980; AD 113:848–849, 1977*